PHARMACOTHERAPEUTICS

A Primary Care Clinical Guide

PHARMACOTHERAPEUTICS

A Primary Care Clinical Guide

Second Edition

Ellis Quinn Youngkin, PhD, RNC, ARNP
Professor and Associate Dean for Academic Programs
Christine E. Lynn College of Nursing
Women's Health Care Nurse Practitioner
University Student Health Services
Florida Atlantic University
Boca Raton, Florida

Kathleen J. Sawin, DNS, RN, FAAN
Professor and Joint Reseach Chair in the Nursing of Children
Children's Hospital of Wisconsin and College of Nursing
University of Wisconsin-Milwaukee
Milwaukee, Wisconsin

Jeanette F. Kissinger, EdD, RN, CS, CANP
Professor Emeritus, School of Nursing
Medical College of Virginia Campus
Virginia Commonwealth University
Certified Adult Nurse Practitioner
The Cross-Over Ministry, Inc.
Richmond, Virginia

Debra S. Israel, PharmD, BCPS
Medical Liaison
Roche Labs, Inc.
Austin, Texas

PEARSON
Prentice Hall

Upper Saddle River, New Jersey 07458

Library of Congress Cataloging-in-Publication Data

Pharmacotherapeutics : a primary care clinical guide / Ellis Quinn Youngkin . . .
[et al.].—2nd ed.
p. cm.
Includes bibliographical references and index.
ISBN 0-13-049762-2
1. Chemotherapy. 2. Pharmacology. 3. Primary care (Medicine)
[DNLM: 1. Drug Therapy—methods. 2. Pharmaceutical Preparations—administration & dosage. 3. Primary Health Care—methods. WB 330 P5352 2005] I. Youngkin, Ellis Quinn.
RM262.P466 2005
615.5'8—dc22

2004015064

Publisher: Julie Levin Alexander
Assistant to Publisher: Regina Bruno
Editor-in-Chief: Maura Connor
Executive Editor: Barbara Krawiec
Development Editor: Sheba Jalaluddin
Editorial Assistant: Jennifer Dwyer
Director of Production and Manufacturing: Bruce Johnson
Managing Production Editor: Patrick Walsh
Production Liaison: Mary C. Treacy
Production Editor: Jessica Balch, Pine Tree Composition
Manufacturing Manager: Ilene Sanford
Manufacturing Buyer: Pat Brown
Design Director: Cheryl Asherman
Senior Design Coordinator: Maria Guglielmo Walsh
Senior Marketing Manager: Nicole Benson
Marketing Coordinator: Janet Ryerson
Channel Marketing Manager: Rachele Strober
Composition: Pine Tree Composition, Inc.
Printer/Binder: Courier Westford
Cover Printer: Phoenix Color Corp.

Notice: This volume is intended to educate students and healthcare providers, not to be a guide for any individual therapy. The authors and the publisher of this volume have taken care to make certain that the doses of drugs and schedules of treatments are correct and compatible with the standards generally accepted at the time of publication. Nevertheless, as new information becomes available, changes in treatment and in the use of drugs, devices, and other therapies become necessary. The reader is advised to carefully consult the instruction and information material included in the package insert of each drug, device, or therapy agent, as well as appropriate, current references before administration. This advice is especially important when using, administering, or recommending new or infrequently used drugs/devices/agents. The authors and publisher advise that an individual with a particular problem consult a primary care provider or a specialist in the field of medicine or advanced practice nursing appropriate for that problem. Under no circumstances should the reader use this volume in lieu of or to substitute for the judgment of the treating provider. The authors and the publisher disclaim all responsibility for any liability, loss, injury, or damage incurred as a consequence, directly or indirectly, of the use and application of any of the contents of this volume.

Pearson Education LTD.
Pearson Education Singapore, Pte. Ltd
Pearson Education, Canada, Ltd
Pearson Education—Japan
Pearson Education Australia PTY, Limited
Pearson Education North Asia Ltd
Pearson Educación de Mexico, S.A. de C.V.
Pearson Education Malaysia, Pte. Ltd
Pearson Education, Upper Saddle River, New Jersey

PEARSON
Prentice Hall

10 9 8 7 6 5 4 3 2 1
ISBN 0-13-049762-2

DEDICATIONS

This book is dedicated to the following very important people who supported and loved us during the past months of preparation:

To my dear husband, Carroll Youngkin, who has willingly helped me with this second edition, patiently supported my efforts in writing, and still loves me. To my mother-in-law, Marian Youngkin, who has overcome so much these past years. And to my dear children, Dottie Youngkin Kouba and Glenn Youngkin, their spouses, Chris Kouba and Suzanne Youngkin; and our wonderful grandchildren: Valarie Quinn, Julianne Elizabeth, and Emily Rose Kouba; and Grant McDaniel, Anna Elizabeth, John Ellis, and Thomas Glenn Youngkin. **(EQY)**

To my children Marc Hedahl and Melissa Kirkendall, and their spouses Abby Hedahl and Jeremy Kirkendall, my granddaughter Annabelle Grace Kirkendall, and our many family members from California to Massachusetts and North Dakota to South Carolina who have always been there for me to multiply my joys and divide my challenges. And to the colleagues, students, and families that have influenced my teaching, research, and practice. You have indeed given me a gift. My work on this book brought much pleasure to my mother, Annabelle Roth Sawin, and I dedicate my efforts in it to her memory. **(KJS)**

Many thanks go to my loving family, colleagues, students, and friends who were part of the potter's wheel that shaped my life, but I dedicate my efforts in this book to my grandchildren, John, Elizabeth, Jeanette, and Lydia, whose unconditional love for "Nana K" is truly a gift from God. **(JFK)**

To my husband, Lonny Gorban, who has continued to give me his love and support through all of my endeavors. To my children, Matthew, Rachel, and Sarah, whose unconditional love, unbounded energy, wonderful curiosity, and sense of humor continue to amaze and inspire me. **(DSI)**

CONTENTS

Contributors

Jeanne Archer, PhD, APN
Clinical Associate Professor
College of Nursing
University of Arkansas for Medical Sciences
Little Rock, Arkansas

Catherine M. Berardelli, PhD, RN, CS, FNP
Assistant Professor, RN-Studies Coordinator
University of Maine, School of Nursing
Orono, Maine

Geneva Clark Briggs, PharmD, BCPS
Clinical Associate
MedOutcomes, Inc.
Richmond, Virginia

Laurie Ann Buchwald, MS, RNC, WHNP, CFNP
Women's Health Nurse Practitioner
Family Nurse Practitioner
Obstetrics and Gynecology of Radford
Radford, Virginia

Candace M. Burns, PhD, ARNP
Associate Professor
University of South Florida College of Nursing
Tampa, Florida

Thomas J. Comstock
Associate Professor
Department of Pharmacy
Medical College of Virginia
Virginia Commonwealth University
Richmond, Virginia

Michael A. Crouch, PharmD, BCPS
Assistant Professor of Pharmacy
School of Pharmacy
Virginia Commonwealth University–MCV Campus
Richmond, Virginia

Robert V. DiGregorio, PharmD
Associate Professor
Arnold & Marie Schwartz College of Pharmacy
Long Island University
New York, New York

Glen E. Farr, PharmD
Professor of Pharmacy
University of Tennessee
College of Pharmacy
Knoxville, Tennessee

Margaret A. Fitzgerald, MS, APRN, BC, NP-C, FAANP
President, Fitzgerald Health Education Associates, Inc.
FNP, Greater Lawrence (MA) Family Health Center
Visiting Professor, U Mass Worcester
Andover, Massachusetts

William R. Garnett, PharmD
Professor of Pharmacy and Neurology
Medical College of Virginia Campus
Virginia Commonwealth University
Richmond, Virginia

Denese C. Gomes, RN, MSN, PNP, FNP
Medical College of Virginia/VCU Health System
Richmond, Virginia

Katharine A. Gracely-Kilgore, RN, MSN, CS, CPNP
Pediatric Nurse Practitioner
Drs. Meyer, Day and Lovings
Richmond, Virginia

Debra K. Hearington, MS, RN, CS, PNP
Clinical Assistant Professor
Virginia Commonwealth University
Richmond, Virginia

Janet C. Horton, MS, RN, APRN-BC
Family Nurse Practitioner
Cold Harbor Family Medicine and Bon Secours Care-A-Van
Richmond, Virginia

Karen W. Jefferson RN, MSN, GNP-C
Instructor/Gerontological Nurse Practitioner
School of Nursing
Division of Family Nursing Care
University of Texas Health Science Center at San Antonio
San Antonio, Texas

Kathleen F. Jett, ARNP, GNP, CS, PhD
Assistant Professor
Christine E. Lynn College of Nursing
Florida Atlantic University
Boca Raton, Florida

Sharon Ann Jung, PharmD, BCPS
Geriatrics Clinical Pharmacy Specialist,
South Texas Veterans Health Care System,
Audie L. Murphy Division
Clinical Assistant Professor,
Division of Pharmacotherapy
College of Pharmacy
The University of Texas at Austin
San Antonio, Texas

Daniel J. Kent, RPh, CDE
Clinical Diabetes Specialist II
Group Health Cooperative
Seattle, Washington

B. J. Landis, PhD, APN
Director Nursing Education
AHEC-Fort Smith
Fort Smith, Arkansas

Pamela Brinker Lester, ARNP, MS
Instructor
Christine E. Lynn College of Nursing
Florida Atlantic University
Boca Raton, Florida
Family Nurse Practitioner, Western Communities Family Practice
Wellington, Florida

Ruth G. McCaffrey, ND, ARNP
Assistant Professor
Family and Gerontologic Nurse Practitioner
Christine E. Lynn College of Nursing
Florida Atlantic University
Boca Raton, Florida

Chuck C. Marsh, PharmD, BCPS
Clinical Science Manager
Global Clinical Sciences
Pharmacia
Fort Smith, Arkansas

Stephanie G. Metzger, MS, RN, CS, PNP
Clinical Assistant Professor
Virginia Commonwealth University School of Nursing
Richmond, Virginia

Michael Sean Monaghan, PharmD
Associate Professor
Department of Pharmacy Practice
School of Pharmacy and Allied Health Professions
Creighton University
Omaha, Nebraska

Linda O. Morphis, ND, WHNP
Clinical Associate Professor
College of Nursing
University of South Carolina
Columbia, South Carolina

David H. Nelson, PharmD
Assistant Professor
Orvis School of Nursing
University of Nevada
Reno, Nevada

C. Fay Parpart, RN-C, MS, ANP, AOCN
Director of Clinical Services
RW IIIB EIS (TIPS) Program
HIV/AIDS Center
Virginia Commonwealth University
Richmond, Virginia

Ginette A. Pepper, PhD, RN, FAAN
Colby Bamberger Presidential Endowed Chair
University of Utah College of Nursing
Salt Lake City, Utah

Martha J. Price, DNSc, NP
Associate Clinical Professor
School of Nursing
University of Washington
Seattle, Washington

Susan Rawlins, MS, RNC, WHNP
Faculty Associate, University of Texas Southwestern Medical School, Dallas
Instructor, Planned Parenthood Federation of America, OB-Gyn Nurse Practitioner Program
Education Consultant, National Association of Nurse Practitioners in Women's Health
Dallas, Texas

Karen D. Rich, PharmD
Pharmacotherapy Specialist Consultant
Heritage Information Systems, Inc.
Richmond, Virginia

Linda D. Scott, DNS, FNP-BC
Clinical Nurse Practitioner
Spectrum Healthcare Resources
Joel Clinic
Fort Bragg, North Carolina

Cynthia Jane Simonson, RN, MS, CS, AOCN
Massey Cancer Center
Division of Hematology/Oncology
Virginia Commonwealth University Health System
Richmond, Virginia

Joanne K. Singleton, PhD, RN, CS, FNP
Professor
Pace University
Lienhard School of Nursing
New York, New York

Maca Sharm Steadman, PharmD, BCPS, FASHP
Professor, Department of Family and Preventive Medicine
University of South Carolina School of Medicine
Columbia, South Carolina

Kathleen M. Tauer, MS, RN, CPNP
Department of Juvenile Justice, Adolescent Correctional Health
Richmond, Virginia

Sharon A. Thrush, MSN, ARNP
Adjunct Assistant Professor
Family Nurse Practitioner
Christine E. Lynn College of Nursing
Florida Atlantic University
Boca Raton, Florida

Adrianne Kathleen Tillmanns, PharmD
Oklahoma City, Oklahoma

Gene White, RPh, JD
Associate Professor Emeritus
School of Pharmacy
Medical College of Virginia Campus
Virginia Commonwealth University
Richmond, Virginia
Adjunct Faculty of Pharmacy
Shenandoah University
Winchester, Virginia

J. Claire Whiting, MS, RN, CFNP
Cross Over Health Care Clinic
Richmond, Virginia

Jill E. Winland-Brown, EdD, MSN, ARNP
Professor and Director, Treasure Coast Campus
Christine E. Lynn College of Nursing
Florida Atlantic University
Boca Raton, Florida

Victor Joe Yim, MD
Clinical Associate Professor
Pace University
Lienhard School of Nursing
Attending Physician
New York Eye & Ear Infirmary
New York, New York

CONTRIBUTORS TO FIRST EDITION

A special thank you and recognition go to those who contributed to the first edition of the book:

Mary L. Brubaker
Cardiovascular Disorders

Stephen G. Bryant
Mental Health Disorders

Douglas F. Covey
Dermatological Disorders

Jessie Drew-Cates
Neurologic Disorders

Mai Duong
Sexually Transmitted Diseases, Vaginitis, and Pelvic Inflammatory Disease

Aimee Gelhot
Musculoskeletal Disorders

Sandra Graves
Migrant and Homeless Populations

Robert A. Gross
Neurologic Disorders

Lauwana E. Hollis
Lower Respiratory Disorders

Angela B. Hoth
Musculoskeletal Disorders

Vivien E. James
Contraceptives

Thomas E. Johns
Upper Respiratory Disorders

Patricia J. Kelly
Gastrointestinal Disorders

Lori W. Lush
Individuals with Chronic Pain

Robert L. Martin
Menopause and Hormonal Replacement Therapy

Mary S. Peery
Immune System Disorders: HIV/AIDS, Mononucleosis and Allergic Responses

Judith B. Sellers
Cardiovascular Disorders

Candice Smith-Scott
Gastrointestinal Disorders

Constance R. Uphold
Upper Respiratory Disorders

Reviewers

Nancy Balkon, PhD, ANP
Clinical Associate Professor School of Nursing
SUNY Stony Brook
Stony Brook, New York

Karen Stuart Champion, RN, MS
Professor
Indian River Community College
Ft. Pierce, Florida

Christine Colella, MSN, RN, CS, C-ANP
Assistant Professor of Clinical Nursing
University of Cincinnati College of Nursing
Cincinnati, Ohio

Denise Coppa, PhD, RNP
Director Family Nurse Practitioner Program
University of Rhode Island
Kingston, Rhode Island

Kimberly Couch, PharmD
Professor
University of Delaware School of Nursing
Newark, Delaware

Linda Dumas, RN, PhD, ANP
Associate Professor of Nursing
University of Massachusetts Boston
Boston, Massachusetts

Laurel A. Eisenhauer, RN, PHD, FAAN
Professor of Nursing and Associate Dean
for Graduate Programs
Boston College School of Nursing
Chestnut Hill, Massachusetts

Marilyn E. Hess, Ph.D
Professor of Pharmacology
University of Pennsylvania Medical School
Philadelphia, Pennsylvania

Cindy Munro, RN, ANP, PhD
Associate Professor
Virginia Commonwealth University
Richmond, Virginia

Jacqueline S. Shrock, RN, BSN
Instructor
Wayne Adult School of Practical Nursing
Smithville, Ohio

PREFACE

Pharmacotherapeutics: A Primary Care Clinical Guide is the second edition of our vision to create a pharmacotherapeutics text in primary care that provides the information needed by the clinician to choose the correct drug or device for therapy and monitor the results for effectiveness and safety. Practitioners across the country have validated that this book, developed with an interdisciplinary team, is useful to primary care providers and is organized the way clinicians think.

Fulfilling this vision involved the extraordinary efforts of many very knowledgeable and established professionals in nursing, pharmacy, and medicine. Most of the chapters, especially those in Unit IV on specific conditions and disorders, were written by a team consisting of a nurse practitioner and a doctor of pharmacy. This collaboration provides contemporary and accurate management regimen options and logical monitoring information with factors such as patient-related variables (age, organ function, concomitant disease states, etc.) and drug-related variables (toxicity, monitoring parameters, interactions, costs, etc.) as considerations. It is our belief that the members of an interdisciplinary team all share the responsibility for the therapeutic outcomes of our patients.

The book is aimed at the practicing primary care clinician (physician, nurse practitioner, physican's assistant, pharmacist) or the graduate student who will be a practitioner in primary care. It is designed to be a clinical reference from which information may be easily retrieved, with enough depth for efficacy and safety. A major concern with a pharmacotherapy book is that new drugs or devices are constantly made available. We hope the reader will use the book for guidance for therapy, even as it "ages," and will be stimulated to keep abreast of the newest therapies, using additional research to discern if they are truly the safest, the best, and the most economical for the patient.

We attempt to maintain a focus on more common conditions that must be managed in primary care practice, and so the book delves into selected areas of tertiary care only where hospitalization is indicated as a condition worsens or complexity increases. Supporting data, found in the first three units of the book, aid the provider in implementing care from a more holistic viewpoint. We recognize that some approaches may vary from those with which the reader is familiar, but this diversity should serve to stimulate the clinician to compare regimens and anticipate outcomes while deciding on the therapy best suited for the particular patient in a specific situation.

The book is organized uniquely to guide decision making and action by the clinician in providing primary care. The five main units are:

Unit I. Principles of Pharmacotherapy. Principles of pharmacokinetics and pharmacodynamics as well as the impact of drugs on renal and hepatic dysfunction are presented in this section, in which we put particular focus on the importance of underlying concepts in basic pharmacology.

Unit II. General Issues. Issues presented in this section include patient safety, psychological, sociological, and cultural factors, legal considerations, pharmacotherapy resources for providers, adverse drug events and drug interactions, evaluation of over-the-counter therapies, herbal therapies, and immunizations.

Unit III. Special Issues and Patient Populations. This section provides insights for pharmacotherapy of children, the elderly, people with disabilities, migrant and homeless populations, individuals with chronic pain, and pregnant and lactating women. Contraception, menopause, and hormonal replacement therapy are also covered. More than ever, special populations require special care measures, and we want the practicing provider to have increased understanding in these areas.

Unit IV. Pharmacotherapy for Common Primary Care Disorders. Chapters in this unit address commonly encountered conditions and disorders across the age span in primary care. Diagnoses and conditions are categorized by systems. Although for each condition we assume the provider has reached an established, accurate diagnosis and is at the point of making an appropriate pharmacotherapeutic selection, definitions, epidemiologic and etiologic data, as well as history, physical examination, and diagnostic assessment findings are provided. A template is used for each condition for this section of the book to aid the reader in finding information consistently. By using this format, we intend to emphasize the necessity in primary care of looking at short-term management of conditions while still considering long-term goals in treating the patient. We focus on considerations such as when first line therapies would not be appropriate or when nonpharmacologic therapies should be tried first; in other words, we look holistically at the patient's care on a long timeline.

Unit V. Tables of Pharmacotherapeutic Agents. These comprehensive drug tables, from antibiotics to miscellaneous agents, are referenced throughout Unit IV. The tables provide information to guide the reader in the specific details about drugs that may be considered for therapy: drug and dosage forms, spectrum of activity and usual dosage range, administration issues and drug-drug, drug-food interactions, common adverse drug reactions and pharmacokinetics, contraindications, pregnancy category, and lactation issues. Also included are tables of fat- and water-soluble vitamins and major and trace minerals.

The reader is reminded that the scope of prescribing varies for advanced practice nurses and physician assistants from state to state, and that the individual provider is responsible for knowing the legal limits of the scope of practice for the state in which he or she is practicing. With the advent of telemedicine and distance learning, this reminder may apply to more than one state as clinicians cross state lines to practice. Additionally, providers must constantly stay abreast of new standards based on evolving knowledge for practice. Readers are urged to recognize that this book is as current as possible, considering that new drugs are being continuously approved and removed from the market. Thus it is up to each practitioner to keep apprised of the newest drug additions and deletions for safe practice.

As you read and use this book, we hope you find that it enhances your practice, and we urge you to send us ideas to improve future editions. We want this book to be a valuable resource to you in the ever-changing healthcare world in which we all live.

ACKNOWLEDGMENTS

We wish to extend heartfelt thanks to our excellent contributing authors for their fine chapters. With their individual and collective expertise and hard work, the book has evolved as an expression of true collaborative efforts. We extend sincere thanks to Barbara Krawiec and the editorial staff at Prentice Hall, Sheba Jalaluddin, Jennifer Dwyer, and Regina Bruno; and Jessica Balch and staff at Pine Tree Composition, Inc., for their help in the publication of this book. A special thank you to our co-author, Deb Israel, for her work in reviewing and polishing the tables into useful references. We want to direct a large measure of appreciation to the faculty, students, and preceptor colleagues we work with who make our professions possible and who give so generously to the development of our next generation of clinicians. Last, but certainly not least, deep appreciation goes to our families and friends who have encouraged us and withstood the pressures of deadlines in the years of preparation. We celebrate the unveiling of this second edition book—healthy, settled, safe, and certainly relieved. We wish you all health, safety, and love.

Ellis Quinn Youngkin
Kathleen J. Sawin
Jeanette F. Kissinger
Debra S. Israel

Foreword

Occasionally a book comes along that fits nicely with the way the clinician using diagnostic reasoning thinks though a problem and makes appropriate decisions for care management. *Pharmacotherapeutics: A Primary Care Clinical Guide,* Second Edition, is such a book. Editors Youngkin, Sawin, Kissinger, and Israel have used their combined understanding of primary care, advanced practice nursing, and pharmacotherapeutics to craft a needed supplement to clinical practice for primary care providers. A strength of this book is its overall holistic approach to primary care with priority given to nonpharmacologic management, followed by complete pharmacologic approaches to caring for patients. Many books of this type are organized by drug classification or by organ system, while in reality most clinicians diagnose first and then formulize their pharmacologic management based on a comprehensive database about the individual patient.

As well, this text is an excellent companion for health professions students who are engaged in clinical primary care courses and who are beginning to formulate their own individualized approach to diagnosis and management of patient problems. In my view, this format is exceptionally well suited to both students and practitioners because it matches the way they practice and think through a clinical situation. It allows primary care providers to view the basic disease process, assess the patient, and make pharmacologic and nonpharmacologic decisions based on outcomes management that includes appropriate selection from a group of drug choices based on efficacy, drug interactions, toxicity, and socioeconomic and cultural influences.

Most importantly, the interdisciplinary team of author contributors is uniquely well suited to address pharmacotherapeutics across the age span. A comprehensive view across life stages is important for clinicians who practice in primary care venues and offers the readers a single resource for all age groups. The early chapters lay the groundwork for pharmacotherapeutics and pharmacodynamics and play out important but practical pediatric, gerontologic, and cultural differences that are critical to high-quality patient management. The inclusion of nonpharmacologic alternatives allows the practitioner to incorporate a holistic approach while exploring the selection of drugs necessary to treat the problem.

Each chapter presents important information around a specific primary care concern. For example, the chapter on lower respiratory problems offers an excellent overview of adult and pediatric asthma including assessment parameters, diagnostic tests, classification of asthma severity, information about flow meters, and step-by-step asthma treatment based on national guidelines. National guidelines are becoming the norm to assure appropriate outcomes in primary care and are assuredly the way of the future. A powerful component of this book is the incorporation of national guidelines that support quality decision-making thoughout this process.

As well, the mental health disorders chapter presents a mix of therapy choices for anxiety, depression, substance and nicotine abuse, insomnia, and eating disorders that is often a missing component of pharmacotherapeutics texts. Unique to this book is the addition of specific chapters that focus on the practice realities of caring for the special and expanding populations such as migrant/homeless persons and people with disabilities who comprise the core of primary healthcare.

The tables of pharmacotherapeutic agents that encompass Unit V are of prime importance. These tables offer complete information about individual pharmacologic agents, including spectrum of activity and dosage range, administration, interactions, common adverse reactions, and contraindications including pregnancy and fetal concerns. The tables allow the reader to select the most appropriate drug for the individual patient and health problem after the assessment and diagnosis has been made.

The interdisciplinary, holistic approach offered in *Pharmacotherapeutics: A Primary Care Clinical Guide,* Second Edition is a welcome addition to any primary care clinician's bookshelf and is a book that will support the health professions student who is preparing for practice. From the point of view of faculty who are preparing graduate students, it provides an important adjunct to other clinical textbooks and is a valuable resource for students who are engaged in experiences within a clinical setting. Youngkin, Sawin, Kissinger, and Israel and the competent team of authors who shared in this collaborative venture are to be commended for their efforts in bringing this important resource to the many clinicians who serve primary care patients.

Charlene M. Hanson, EdD, FNP, CS, FAAN
Professor Emerita and Family Nurse Practitioner
Georgia Southern University
Statesboro, Georgia

I ❖ Principles of Pharmacotherapy

CHAPTER ❖ 1

INTRODUCTION TO PHARMACOTHERAPY

Ellis Quinn Youngkin ◆ Kathleen J. Sawin ◆ Jeanette F. Kissinger ◆ Debra S. Israel

This book now moves into its second edition as a resource to offer guidance for providers related to pharmacotherapeutic management of patients' conditions. Questions confronting the clinician include:

- Which pharmacotherapy would be best for this condition?
- What specific assessments need to be made relative to the patient?
- If the patient has these particular personal characteristics, would this medication be preferred over that one?
- What outcome should be expected if this medication is used, and how soon?
- What if the outcome is not as expected, and a change in pharmacotherapy is indicated? What should be used next?
- What concerns should be kept in mind when using a particular pharmacotherapy?
- What should the patient and family be told about using this drug?

These are but a few of the questions that arise in making pharmacotherapy decisions. Situations like the following raise such questions:

- Ms. E. brings Bryan, a 10-year-old Caucasian boy, to your office with complaints of a runny nose, itchy eyes, and constant postnasal drip. What is the safest, most effective treatment for Bryan?
- Mr. T., a 65-year-old African American man, has hypertension that is not responding to the calcium channel blocker you prescribed. What is the best course of medication change or addition?
- Ms. J., a 48-year-old Hispanic woman, has hot flashes that are keeping her awake at night. She is still having some periods, but they are somewhat irregular. She was diagnosed with essential hypertension two years ago. She was doing well on her medications but ran out three weeks ago. Her blood pressure is elevated significantly today. What pharmacotherapies are indicated?
- Ms. N., a 19-year-old Asian woman, presents with burning with urination, frequency, and hematuria. The urine test indicates significant infection. She is allergic to sulfa and nitrofurantoin. This is her third urinary tract infection (UTI) in eighteen months. What further information do you need to prescribe an effective medication? Does Ms. N. need any further diagnostic tests? A referral to a urologist?
- Mr. P., a 68-year-old Indian man with asthma, calls complaining of more difficulty breathing. He is using several inhalers—a steroid, a long-acting bronchodilator, and a short-acting bronchodilator—but states these are not working as well as they used to. Is Mr. P.'s use of the inhalers correct and timely? Is he taking any cultural treatments for his asthma?
- Ms. G., a 20-year-old Caucasian woman, is 8 weeks pregnant. She has been diagnosed with trichomonas vaginitis and complains of severe pruritis. What are the treatment options at this stage of pregnancy?

The questions raised by the aforementioned cases take on a heightened importance in light of the multitude of critical factors influencing health care today. "New" is the definitive adjective describing trends in pharmacotherapies: *new drugs and devices,* such as antivirals, oral contraceptives, and experimental drugs that may restore sight; *new guidelines* from the nation's leading authorities, such as the new STD guidelines from the CDC and the new guidelines for bipolar management; *new risks* with some drugs, such as SSRIs, Vioxx, and HT; *new clinical trials* with alternative as well as traditional therapies, such as St. John's wort and SSRIs; *new controversies* with therapies, such as hormone replacement therapy; *new uses* for old drugs, such as methotrexate for rheumatoid arthritis; *new data on side effects* related to increased or decreased therapy, such as topamax for migranes; *new forms of old drugs,* such as controlled-release and long-acting oral drugs; *new concerns* about drug resistance; *new ethical worries* about companies masking dangerous data on drugs; *new desired effects* with some drugs such as with aspirin and statins; *new information* about drugs taken off the market; *new support* that some new drugs may be riskier than old ones; *new costs* for prescription drugs driven by a few high-priced medications; and *new plans* to try to decrease costs for those with less means.

Literally thousands of drugs are available today to the clinician and the patient for wellness and illness care, either over-the-counter or by prescription, and what is "new" must be factored in with all other influences when considering any clinical pharmacotherapy question. If this thought is not daunting enough to the clinician, reflect on the myriad concerns and considerations surrounding safe and correct drug therapy. Attaining desired therapy outcomes depends on the interactions and influences of hundreds of variables. Everything possible must be taken into consideration from the route of administration and expected action of the drug to political, legal, economic, and ethical concerns, to interactions between the therapy and other drugs, foods, herbs, and legal and nonlegal substances, as well as environmental toxins. In addition, the patient's hereditary disease background and personal characteristics, such as age, sex, race, culture, beliefs, physical factors such as weight, illness status, family influences, and education and learning style must be factored in. Even the biologic rhythm of the person in relation to the specific drug is becoming an important variable.

Choosing the least expensive therapy may not be the best therapy for the patient or for the health care system (Sanchez, 1999). A balance of cost, clinical appropriateness based on evidence-based findings, and humanistic quality of life and health outcome is necessary. The clinician is required to determine these components logically, responsibly, and involve the patient, the payer, and society in determining a therapy. Health maintenance and promotion become the focus along with prevention in this age of increasing chronic diseases, longer lives of those with disabilities, and ever-increasing age spans. Achieving better quality of life with dignity must be an outcome of treatment.

With such an array of influences challenging the clinician with each drug therapy decision, the primary goal of a clinical guidebook is for it to be logically and efficiently useful in practice. Thus, this book is intended first to be a practical, easy-to-use resource for the clinician, and second to be a learning tool for advanced practice professional students. The major thrust of the book is to present information on pharmacotherapeutic management of commonly encountered conditions in primary care practice with an emphasis on monitoring therapy outcomes. Table 1–1 gives definitions for common terms frequently encountered in this text.

TABLE 1–1. Definitions of Terms

Pharmaceutic or pharmaceutical: relating to pharmacy or to pharmaceutics.
Pharmaceutics: the science of pharmaceutical systems—that is, preparations, dosage forms, and so on. A synonym is pharmacy.
Pharmacodynamics: the study of drug actions on the living organism.
Pharmacoeconomics: the analysis and determination of cost-benefit in choosing pharmacotherapy for the greatest health result for the resources invested (Sanchez, 1999, p.1).
Pharmacognosy: a branch of pharmacology concerned with the physical characteristics and botanical sources of crude drugs.
Pharmacokinetic: relating to the disposition of drugs in the body.
Pharmacokinetics: movements of drugs within biologic systems as affected by uptake, distribution, elimination, and biotransformation.
Pharmacologic or pharmacological: relating to pharmacology or to the composition, properties, and actions of drugs.
Pharmacology: the science concerned with drugs and their sources, appearance, chemistry, actions, and uses.
Pharmacotherapeutics: the study of drug therapy to treat illness associated with patient care.
Pharmacotherapy: the treatment of disease by means of drugs.

Sources: Adapted from Guttierrez, 1999; McDonough, 1994; Sanchez, 1999.

DETERMINING PHARMACOTHERAPY: PRINCIPLES OF PLANNING AND PROCESS

Ten essential considerations enter into the actual decision-making process for a specific therapy for a specific individual. These are (adapted from DiPiro & Wells, 1999; DiPiro et al., 1992; DiPiro et al., 1997; Mathews & Johnson, 2000; Melmon & Morrelli, 1978):

1. The diagnosis must be accurate and the application of a therapy for a patient must be justifiable based on the diagnosis and the pathophysiology.
2. The practitioner must understand the pathophysiology and the actions of the therapy selection on the processes, including the best route for safety and effectiveness.
3. Risks/benefits, hypersensitivity, toxicity, and teratogenicity must be weighed.
4. The use of the lowest effective dosage and time needed for a therapy for a given condition is essential. This implies the use of only one therapy if that therapy alone will accomplish the effect desired.
5. The implementation of measures to assist the patient with adherence to the therapy regimen is required, including appropriate oral and written information.
6. Convenience, cost, comfort, simplicity of use, acceptance, and response by the patient, based on culture, race, ethnicity, gender, beliefs, and values, must be considered.
7. The use of other therapeutic modalities that may enhance the effectiveness of the pharmacotherapy, such as nutrition, exercise, or cessation of alcohol use should be employed.
8. The application of pharmaceutics, pharmacoeconomics, pharmakinetics, pharmacodynamics, and pharmacotherapy must be consistent in choosing a therapy for the patient (see Table 1–1).
9. The recognition of any adverse effects, whether from the drug or from drug-drug/drug-substance/drug-food/or drug-environment interactions, and the appropriate cessation or change of the therapy must be timely.
10. The specific therapeutic outcome based on the relationship of the variables for an individual patient must be set and anticipated. This means knowing the patient-specific influences that will impact the outcome and knowing what diagnostic tests to order and what clinical manifestations to assess to properly monitor the patient.

SELECTING THE BEST PHARMACOTHERAPEUTIC REGIMEN FOR THE CONDITION

The assumption with this book is that the correct diagnosis has been made before the most appropriate drug can be selected. An inadequate or incorrect diagnosis can result in incorrect or no therapy. Risks and benefits of each drug considered for therapy must be weighed (DiPiro et al., 1997). Specific information about selected drugs in a class is presented in the drug tables in Unit V. Cross-references to these tables appear throughout the text. Drug tables are arranged alphabetically by classifications and alphabetically by generic drug names within the tables. The index of the book indicates where the classification table is found and where the drug is listed in Unit V. For convenience the index lists both generic and trade names.

When the final drug choice is made, the specific regimen is determined. This includes dose per each 24 hours, interval between doses, length of total therapy, route and method of administration, and form of drug to enhance adherence by the patient (DiPiro et al., 1997). Since this book focuses on outpatient, ambulatory care, it will be the patient's or caretaker's responsibility (once the provider has selected the drug regimen and the pharmacist has filled the prescription) to be sure the drug therapy is delivered on time and in a correct dose and manner. If an essential part of monitoring and evaluation requires knowledge by the patient and/or caretaker, the clinician must be sure this knowledge is correctly understood. Other measures for monitoring and evaluation will require gathering subjective information by history and performing diagnostic tests and/or physical examination measures for objective data. Definitive alternative plans must be made in case of adverse effects or unmet therapeutic goals. Quality care can be maintained only through monitoring of patient outcomes.

In conclusion, pharmacotherapy requires careful prerequisite planning in order to select and implement the appropriate therapy for a given condition with a specific individual who has numerous influencing variables. Improving or maintaining the quality of life for the patient is a guiding objective. In addition, effective pharmacotherapy requires meticulous monitoring and evaluation based on measurable, expected outcomes in order to provide continuing therapy, alter the therapy, or take other appropriate action for effective therapeutic management of the patient and the condition. This book offers a comprehensive consideration of pharmacotherapy management for selected populations and conditions in primary care.

REFERENCES

DiPiro, J. T., Talbert, R. L., Hayes, P. E., Yee, G. C., Matzke, G. R., & Posey, L. M. (Eds.). (1992). *Pharmacotherapy: A pathophysiologic approach* (2nd ed.). New York: Elsevier.

DiPiro, J. T., Talbert, R. L., Yee, G. C., Matzke, G. R., Wells, B. G., & Posey, L. M. (Eds.). (1997). *Pharmacotherapy: A pathophysiologic approach* (3rd ed.). Stamford, CT: Appleton & Lange.

DiPiro, J. T., & Wells, B. G. (1999). Guiding principles of pharmacotherapy. In J. DiPiro, R. Talbert, et al. (Eds.), *Pharmacotherapy: A pathophysiologic approach* (4th ed.). Stamford, CT: Appleton & Lange.

Guttierrez, K. (1999). *Pharmacotherapeutics: Clinical decision-making in nursing.* Philadelphia: W. B. Saunders Co.

Matthews, H. W., & Johnson, J. (2000). Racial, ethnic, and gender differences in response to drugs. In E. T. Herfindal & D. R. Gourley (Eds.), *Textbook of therapeutics: Drug and disease management.* Philadelphia. Lippincott Williams & Wilkins.

Melmon, K. L., & Morrelli, H. F. (Eds.). (1978). *Clinical pharmacology basic principles in therapeutics* (p. 3). New York: Macmillan.

McDonough, Jr., J. T. (Ed.). (1994). *Stedman's concise medical dictionary* (2nd ed.). Baltimore: Williams & Wilkins.

Sanchez, L. (1999). Pharmoceconomics: Principles. In J. DiPiro, R. Talbert, et al. (Eds.), *Pharmacotherapy: A pathophysiologic approach* (4th ed.). Stamford, CT: Appleton & Lange.

CHAPTER ❖ 2

PHARMACOKINETICS AND PHARMACODYNAMICS

Ginette A. Pepper

The study of the interaction of drugs and other chemicals with living systems is *pharmacology,* which is a broad field of knowledge with several subdivisions. *Pharmacokinetics* focuses on changes in the concentrations of drugs over time resulting from absorption, distribution, metabolism, and excretion. *Pharmacodynamics* is the science of the molecular interactions of drugs with receptors and the subsequent reactions that result in the clinically observed drug response. Some other subdivisions of pharmacology are *toxicology* (the effects and detection of and antidotes for poisons and overdoses of drugs), *pharmacogenetics* (the relationship of genetics to variations in drug response), *pharmaceutics* (the compounding and preparation of dosing units), and *chronopharmacology* (the relationship of biologic rhythms to variations in drug response). Pharmacology, a scientific field, is distinguished from *pharmacy,* which is a practice discipline, just as sociology is a scientific field and social work is a practice discipline. The safe and effective use of drugs in the prevention, diagnosis, and treatment of disease and modification of physiologic functions, such as reproduction, is the applied field of *pharmacotherapeutics.* Practice disciplines involved in pharmacotherapeutics include medicine, nursing, pharmacy, dentistry, veterinary medicine, podiatry, and all others involved in prescribing, dispensing, administering, and monitoring drug therapy and informing patients about their medications.

VARIABILITY IN DRUG RESPONSE

If all patients with a particular diagnosis were identical, pharmacotherapeutics would require little more than application of a universal protocol. Because factors such as age, gender, race, body build, organ function, diet, genetic inheritance, concurrent medications, and comorbidity can alter the pharmacokinetics and pharmacodynamics of drugs, the clinician optimally individualizes drug therapy based upon his or her understanding of how these variables affect drug response. The understanding of pharmacokinetic and pharmacodynamic variability can guide the prescriber in the selection of drug, dosage, form, route, frequency, and titration, as well as in patient education and monitoring of drug therapy. For example, recognizing that a patient with renal impairment taking digoxin would be at risk for accumulation of this renally excreted drug, the prescriber should monitor the patient more carefully and educate the patient to detect and report symptoms of toxicity. In some cases, the prescriber may need to reduce the dosage or extend the dosing interval of the drug, Figure 2–1 illustrates that the relationship between administration of a drug and the response to the drug is determined by three phases of drug action: pharmaceutics, pharmacokinetics, and pharmacodynamics. Anything that modifies one of the phases of drug action can affect drug response, as manifested by the intended

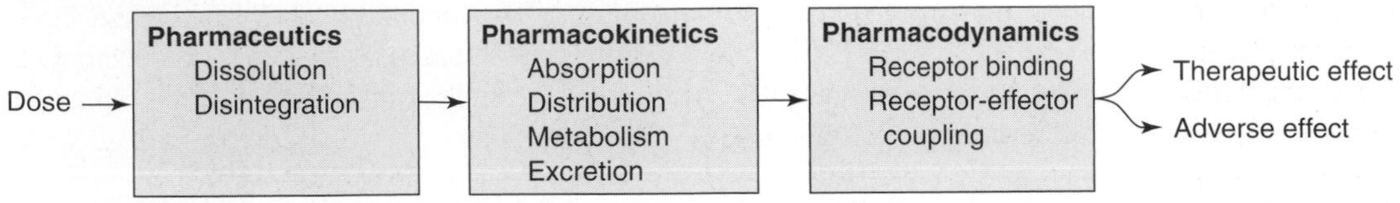

FIGURE 2–1. Phases of drug action. *Source: Modified from Pepper, G. A. & Wiener, M. B. (1985). Biophysical and psychosocial principles of drug action. In M. B. Wiener & G. A. Pepper (Eds.), Clinical pharmacology and therapeutics in nursing (2nd ed.). New York: McGraw-Hill, p. 56.*

therapeutic effects and unintended adverse effects. The purposes of this chapter are to define the processes of each phase of drug action, to describe what factors modify the processes, to identify how the processes are measured, and to discuss the clinical implications of alterations in the phases of drug action.

PLASMA PROFILE

Figure 2–2 illustrates the typical graphic representation of the plasma concentration of drugs over time after oral drug administration. This plasma profile reflects important clinical markers of the pharmaceutic and pharmacokinetic phases. During the absorptive phase of the curve, the *onset* of drug action occurs when the concentration of drug in the plasma (C_p) first exceeds the minimum effective concentration, and the peak of drug action occurs when the highest plasma concentration (sometimes referred to as the C_{max} or maximum concentration) is attained. The elimination phase of the curve is characterized by *termination* of the drug's effect when the plasma concentration falls below the minimum effective concentration. The *duration* of drug action is the time during which the plasma concentration exceeds the minimum effective concentration. *Toxicity* occurs when the plasma concentration exceeds the toxic level. The *therapeutic range* reflects the target serum concentrations for optimal drug response. This range is large in drugs with a wide margin of safety and small in drugs with a narrow margin of safety. An important parameter of the plasma profile commonly used in pharmaceutic and pharmacokinetic research studies is the *area under the curve* (AUC). Usually derived from computer calculations, the area under the curve is a measure of

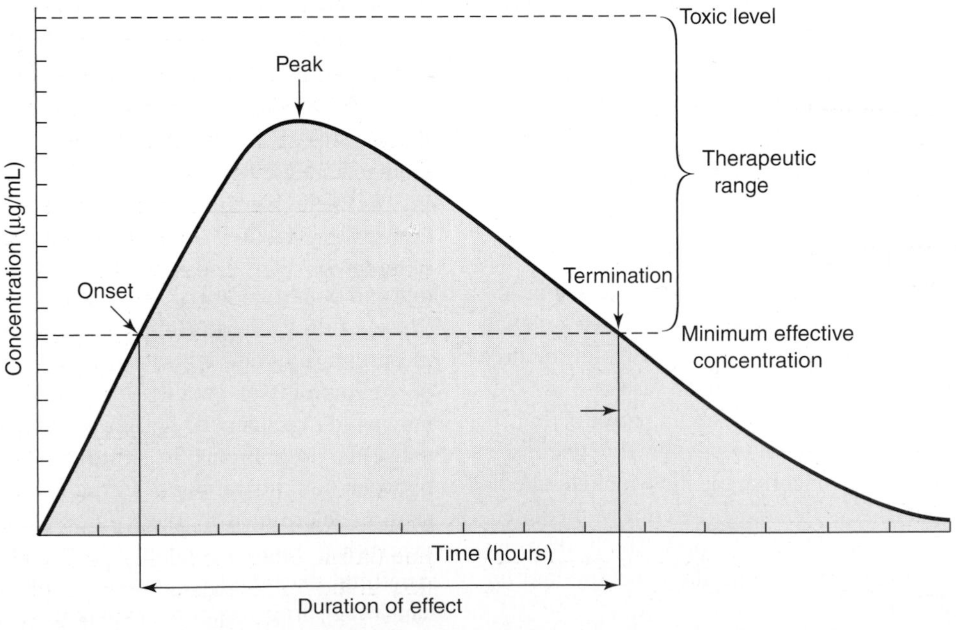

FIGURE 2–2. Plasma profile for a single dose. Shaded area represents area under the curve (AUC).

total exposure to the drug. Conceptualizing how unique variables alter the plasma profile can provide the clinician with guidance for individualizing pharmacotherapeutic decisions. For example, if taking a drug with food increases the rate of absorption, it can be anticipated that the peak concentration would be higher and the drug effect would be more intense for a shorter period of time.

PHARMACEUTIC PHASE

The pharmaceutic phase involves the liberation of the drug from the dosing unit. Because a drug must be in solution to be absorbed and safely distributed in the body, the pharmaceutic phase is called the *rate-limiting step* of drug action; that is, the onset of the drug's effect can occur no faster than the rate at which the drug is released into solution from the product. Liquid dosing forms, such as injectables and elixirs, are already in solution and are immediately available for absorption and transport. The pharmaceutic phase for solid oral preparations, such as tablets and capsules, requires a two-step process: (1) disintegration into smaller particles and (2) dissolution of the particles so molecules of the diluent and drug intermingle in the solution. This phase is comparable to dissolving sugar cubes in tea. The cube must first disintegrate into sugar granules, and then the granules dissolve in the tea. The amount of fluid and intensity of stirring will influence how readily the sugar dissolves. Similarly, the fluid ingested with a drug and the motility of the gut will promote drug dissolution. Diseases or drugs that reduce gut motility will slow the liberation of drugs from solid preparations. Although they appear to be liquid, suspensions are actually particles of the drug suspended in liquid, so drugs in suspension must dissolve before they are available for absorption.

IMMEDIATE-RELEASE PREPARATIONS

How a medication is compounded by the manufacturer determines the release characteristics of the drug product and onset of drug action, as illustrated in Figure 2–3. The preparation may be produced to speed the dissolution of the drug, frequently by formulation of the drug as a salt. For example, naproxen is available in tablet form as naproxen (Naprosyn) and as the salt, naproxen sodium (Aleve, Anaprox), which is more rapidly released from the tablet and has a faster onset. The dosage of naproxen sodium is 10% greater due to the weight of the sodium (200 mg of naproxen is equivalent to 220 mg of naproxen sodium). The naproxen oral suspension and naproxen suppositories share the slower-release characteristics and dose of the naproxen tablets. Figure 2–3*a* compares the plasma profiles of a hypothetical drug with its more rapidly released salt, revealing that the peak concentration is higher and the onset and time to peak effect are twice as rapid for the salt form. Some salts and compounds are formulated to prolong drug release. For example, imipramine hydrochloride tablets (Tofranil, others) release the drug rapidly and require three or four times daily dosing. Imipramine pamoate (Tofranil PM) capsules with slow-release properties are dosed once daily at bedtime, which improves compliance and restricts the sedative effects of this antidepressant to nighttime. The clinician must know the characteristics of various formulations well to avoid confusion and overdose. Solutions for injection or topical use may also be formulated as salts or compounds to ensure solubility, which is especially important for intravenous or ophthalmic administration in which crystals or particles in the solution can have serious consequences.

Liberation of a drug from a dosing unit may also be modified to minimize adverse effects. Nitrofurantoin capsules (Macrodantin) contain macrocrystals of the drug that slow dissolution and absorption, causing less gastrointestinal irritation than the microcrystals in nitrofurantoin tablets and suspensions. Nitrofurantoin is also available as a macrocrystal monohydrate extended-release capsule (Macrobid, others). This formulation has even slower release of the active ingredient, which allows it to be dosed twice daily compared to three to four times daily dosing required for the other formulations. Drugs such as bisacodyl (Dulcolax, others) are enteric-coated to prevent dissolution of the tablet in the acid environment of the stomach, reducing gastric irritation, nausea, and vomiting, but delaying drug onset (Figure 2–3*b*). However, decreased production of hydrochloric acid, which occurs with aging, some diseases, and drugs for peptic ulcer disease (histamine blockers, antacids, and proton pump inhibitors), can increase the pH of the stomach enough to promote premature dissolution of enteric-coated drugs in the stomach.

Some dosing systems that target delivery of the drug directly to the receptors in high concentrations provide minimal absorption and very low systemic drug concentrations. Topical decongestant sprays such as oxymetazoline (Afrin, others) are delivered directly to the site of action in the nasal mucosa and have few of the cardiac and central nervous system adverse effects of the oral decongestant pseudoephedrine (Sudafed, others). Similarly,

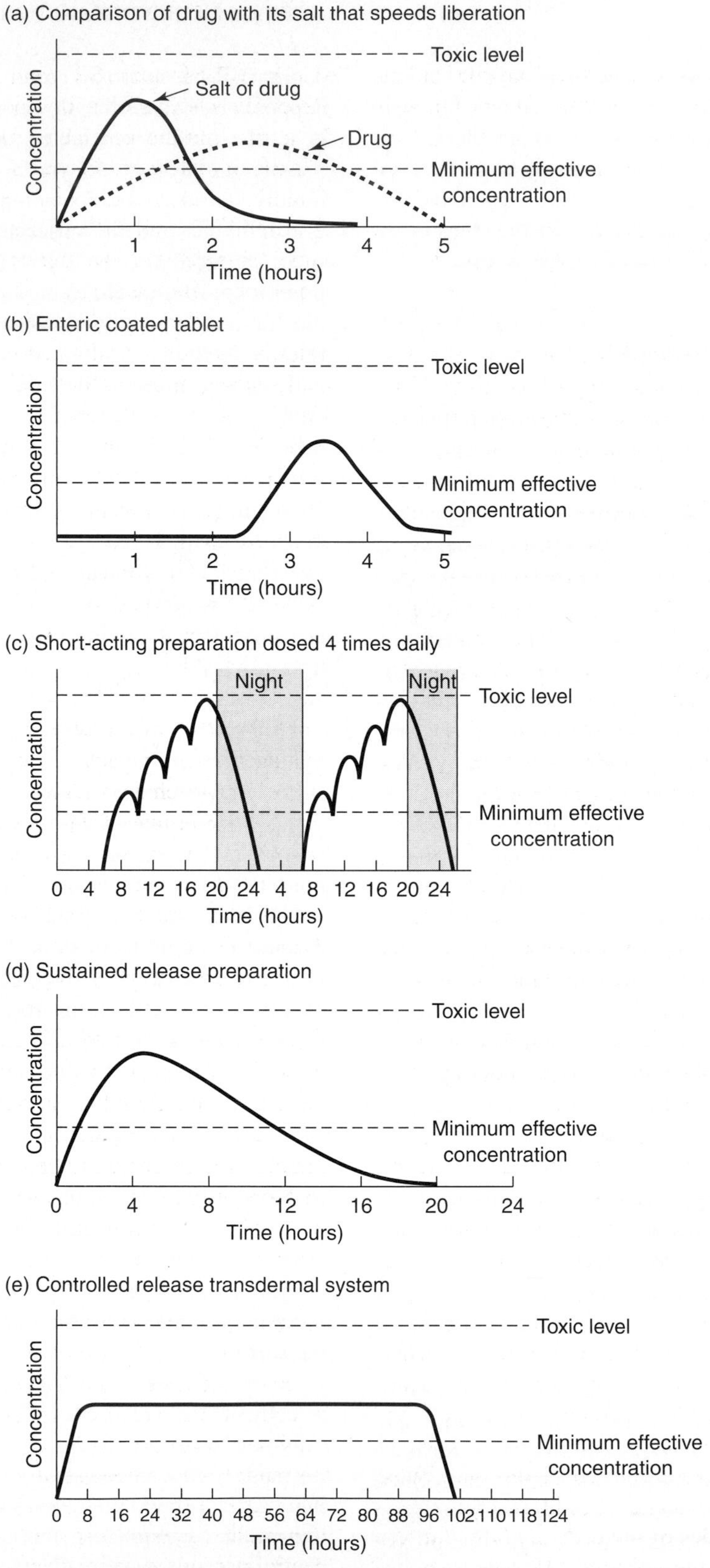

FIGURE 2–3. Plasma profiles for various pharmaceutic preparations.

metered dose inhalers for corticosteroids provide the advantages of steroid treatment of asthma without the serious metabolic effects of oral therapy.

PROLONGED-RELEASE PREPARATIONS

When immediate-release preparations are used, there are fluctuations in drug concentration over the span of a dosing interval, resulting in peaks in drug concentration that can approach toxic concentrations and trough plasma concentrations below the minimum effective concentration, especially during the night, when the drug is not administered (Figure 2–3*c*). Prolonged-release formulations decrease the required frequency of dosing, improving both convenience and compliance. Further, the decreased fluctuation in plasma concentrations can enhance therapeutic benefit. Immediate-release calcium channel blockers such as nifedipine (Adalat, Procardia) may be associated with increased incidence of coronary heart events compared to prolonged-release formulations (Adalat CC, Procardia XL), because the rapid absorption and sudden onset of hypotension can trigger reflex sympathetic stimulation. Additionally, plasma concentrations of the shorter-acting immediate-release calcium channel blockers are low in the early morning hours, providing no protection during the period of highest incidence of coronary events, and patients are more likely to omit doses of drugs requiring multiple daily doses. (Freher et al., 1999; Pepper, 1999; Trujillo & Nolan, 2001).

The first prolonged-release formulations consisted of capsules containing coated pellets of medication that dissolved at various rates depending on the amount of coating. The delayed dissolution of pellets prolongs the liberation of the drug and extends the duration of action (Figure 2–3*d*). In prolonged-release intramuscular injectables, the drug is combined with an oil- or water-insoluble substance, called *depot* injections. Examples of these products, which are injected at intervals of a week to months and gradually release the drug, are penicillin G benzathine (Bicillin L-A), medroxyprogesterone acetate suspension (Depo-Provera), and haloperidol decanoate (Haldol LA). Recently, the development of prolonged-release dosage forms has focused on drug-polymer systems using either a *matrix* or *reservoir* configuration. These polymers are synthetically produced chains of molecules. In matrix systems molecules of the drug are bound to the polymers and released as the polymer dissolves or is hydrated; examples are delayed-release verapamil tablets (Calan SR, Isoptin SR) and morphine (MS Contin). Reservoir systems contain a pool of the drug surrounded by a rate-limiting polymeric membrane that controls the release of the drug. Products using a reservoir system (Figure 2–3*e*) include oral extended-release tablets of nifedipine (Procardia XL), as well as transdermal fentanyl (Duragesic), nitroglycerin (Nitro-Dur, others), and clonidine (Catapres-TTS).

Many abbreviations, suffixes, and terms are used by manufacturers for prolonged-release dosage forms, such as sustained-release (SR), delayed-release, extended-release, controlled-release (CR, CD, CC), transdermal systems (TDS, TTS), and long-acting (LA, XL), so the nomenclature for these forms can be quite confusing. Because prolonged-release tablets and capsules contain two to four times as much medication as an immediate-release form of the drug, it is essential that both patients and clinicians distinguish these products.

BIOEQUIVALENCE

Although pharmaceutically equivalent drugs contain identical amounts of the active drug, the excipients or inactive ingredients, such as buffers, fillers, coloring, and flavoring, in a tablet may differ widely from one manufacturer to another. These ingredients and the manufacturing process can cause clinical variability in the rate and extent of liberation of a drug from the dosing unit and its subsequent absorption. During the 1970s, studies showed that the digoxin tablets made by different manufacturers—and even different lot numbers from the same manufacturer—had as much as twofold differences in the area under the curve. This much variability could have harmful effects, especially for a drug like digoxin that has a narrow therapeutic range. Federal legislation passed in the 1980s mandated that manufacturers demonstrate that generic drugs are bioequivalent to the innovator drug, which is generally the first brand of a drug to be marketed. Although most generic drugs on the market have proven bioequivalence to the innovator, some drug groups such as hormones, oral and transdermal extended-release products, and a few older drugs do not have bioequivalence among manufacturers. Most agents are legally required to demonstrate bioequivalence within the range of −20% to +25% of the innovator, since experts have judged that this difference in the plasma concentration of a drug will not cause clinically detectable differences. Some researchers and clinicians have argued that this much difference may be clinically significant for some populations and diseases, such as the very young, the very old, and patients who are very difficult to regulate on cardiac, psychiatric, or other drugs. Clinicians should also note that bioequivalence has not yet been established for most drugs among the same strengths of different dosage forms; that is, a 40-mg capsule may not yield the same plasma profile as a 40-mg tablet, although a federal requirement for research on comparability of bioavailability of dosage forms applies to investigational drugs. Food and Drug Administration (FDA) information on bioequivalence is available online as the *Electronic Orange Book* on the Web at http://www.fda.gov/cder/ob/default.htm

CLINICAL IMPLICATIONS OF PHARMACEUTICS

When taking oral medications, including liquids and suspensions, patients should ingest a full glass of water, which promotes the dissolution of drugs and their passage into the stomach. Generally, medications prescribed to be taken at bedtime should be taken at least 30 minutes before retiring, since an upright position aids the transport of medication into the stomach. Erosive esophagitis has resulted when drugs such as alendronate (Fosamax) or tetracycline were used without these precautions. Suspensions must be shaken before measurement to disperse the drug particles equally throughout the liquid, whereas solutions do not require agitation. Clinicians need to be mindful that patients with conditions that slow peristalsis, such as diabetic gastroparesis, or those taking anticholinergic drugs may have delayed or decreased drug absorption, especially for poorly soluble drugs such as digoxin (Lanoxin, others) or phenytoin (Dilantin, others). Similarly, it should be noted that enteric-coated medications might not afford protection against gastrointestinal irritation if the patient is taking antiulcer medications. Prescribers familiar with the range of dosage forms available and the plasma profile for each can provide alternatives that enhance the efficacy of drug therapy.

Patients must be well educated when a prolonged-release drug is substituted for immediate-release forms, as there have been numerous incidents of drug toxicity in patients taking prolonged-release preparations on a schedule appropriate for immediate-release form. The prohibition against crushing or chewing prolonged-release forms should also be emphasized. Some matrix forms are scored and may be divided without danger, but reservoir preparations must remain intact. Prescribers and patients should consult the pharmacist for proper use of dosage forms. Used transdermal patches must be disposed of in a location where pets or children cannot access the used product. Some reservoir systems such as the gastrointestinal system (GITS) used for nifedipine extended-release tablets (Procardia XL) may appear intact in the stool. Patients should be reassured that this is normal and that the drug has actually been released and absorbed.

Generally, it is recommended that immediate-release forms of a drug should be used to titrate the dosage of a drug, with the switch to an extended-release preparation being made after the optimal daily dosage has been identified, although some calcium channel blockers may be an exception (Pepper, 1999). If a patient's response to a medication suddenly changes, the clinician should inquire whether there has been a prescription refill, since the pharmacist may have substituted a generic equivalent. For some patients the legal variability in bioequivalence can manifest as changes in disease control. In these cases, and when the products are not bioequivalent, the prescriber can specify that the prescription be filled using a consistent manufacturer. This may be done by indicating the brand or manufacturer on the prescription and writing "DAW" (dispense as written) or "PBO" (prescribed brand only) or by communicating with the pharmacist orally or in writing of the need for consistent products. It is not essential that the drug be the innovator brand, which is often more expensive. Rather, it is important that the product used to titrate to optimal dosage is also used for maintenance therapy. Working together, the pharmacist and prescriber can ensure both quality and cost control.

BIOTRANSPORT

Drug molecules must cross biologic membranes to reach the sites of action and sites where they will undergo the pharmacokinetic processes. The transport of chemicals across biologic membranes is called *biotransport.* How readily a drug crosses membranes is determined by the characteristics of biologic membranes and the characteristics of the particular drug molecule. *Biologic membranes* are composed of layers of individual cells, and drugs must usually pass through the cells to cross the membranes. Surrounding each cell is the *cell membrane,* consisting of a double layer of phospholipids oriented so that the lipid portions of the molecule are surrounded by the phosphate-containing portion of the molecule. Figure 2–4 shows several types of proteins embedded in the lipid bilayer. Some proteins form channels through which ions

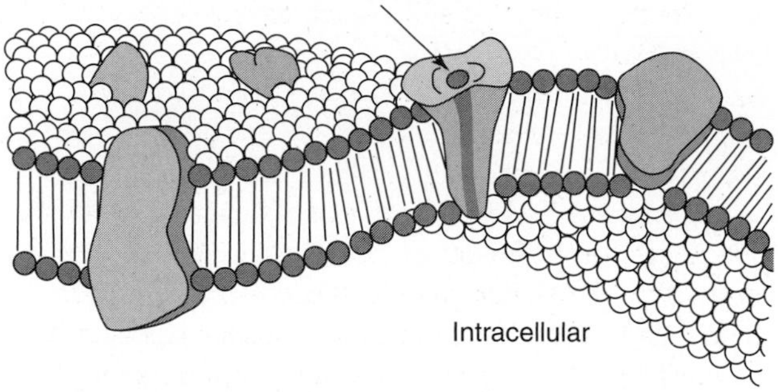
Extracellular
Ion channel
Intracellular

FIGURE 2–4. Structure of the cell membrane. The cell membrane is a double layer of phospholipid molecules with the highly polar phosphate heads of the molecules oriented outward and the nonpolar chains of fatty acids inside the membrane. Embedded in the membrane are proteins that include transport carriers, ion channels, and receptors.

can traverse the membrane rapidly. Other proteins are carriers, capable of binding to a chemical and transporting it across the membrane. Drug receptors are also located on proteins embedded in membranes. Unless it can pass through a channel or is one of the few chemicals transported by a carrier, a drug must dissolve in the lipid layer as it crosses the cell membrane.

Features of drugs that affect their ability to cross membranes are size, lipid solubility, polarity, and ionization. Small molecules cross membranes more readily than large molecules. In fact, molecules with molecular weights in excess of 1000 are usually too large to be used as drugs because they cannot cross biologic membranes to access sites of action. Drugs that are lipid-soluble (*lipophilic*) dissolve easily in the lipid layer of the cell membrane and cross biologic membranes readily. Drugs that are water-soluble (*hydrophilic*) do not dissolve easily in the lipid layer and cross membranes poorly, if at all. *Polarity* and *ionization* are characteristics that make drugs hydrophilic (see Figure 2–5). Polar molecules have an uneven distribution of charge, with the positive and negative charges congregating at different parts of the molecule. However, polar molecules do not have a net charge. Ions are molecules that have a net charge, either positive or negative, which is represented by the plus or minus sign in the chemical formula, such as the bicarbonate ion (HCO_3^-) or calcium ion (Ca^{2+}). In general, polar molecules and ions do not cross biologic membranes.

Many drugs are weak acids or weak bases. Acids and bases exist in ionized or nonionized states, depending upon the pH of the solution. Acids are molecules that can release a proton (H^+), becoming ionized with a net negative charge. Bases are molecules that can accept a proton, resulting in a positively charged ion. The ionized and nonionized forms of the acid (or base) are at equilibrium in a solution of a given pH, with some portion of total number of molecules in the ionized state and some portion in the nonionized state. Only drug molecules that are nonionized cross biologic membranes, but when the nonionized molecules cross the membrane, some of the remaining ionized drug molecules become nonionized to maintain the equilibrium. Acids in acid environments are predominantly in the nonionized form and cross biologic membranes rapidly. For example, acetylsalicylic acid (aspirin) is primarily nonionized in the acid environment of the stomach and is readily absorbed. Acids in alkaline environments are predominantly ionized, so the majority of the aspirin molecules in the small intestine cannot cross biologic membranes. However, even enteric-coated aspirin, which does not dissolve until it reaches the small intestine, is almost completely absorbed, because the small portion of aspirin that is nonionized is rapidly absorbed. Eventually, because of the shift of ionized aspirin to nonionized aspirin to maintain equilibrium, virtually all of the aspirin is absorbed. Conversely, bases in alkaline environments are predominantly nonionized; bases in acid environments are predominantly ionized. A base such as amphetamine in the stomach will be mainly in the ionized state and will have negligible absorption, but in the small intestine, it is absorbed rapidly.

Mechanisms of Biotransport

Figure 2–6 shows four major mechanisms by which chemicals cross biologic membranes: filtration, pinocytosis, carrier-mediated transport, and passive diffusion. Two types of drug interactions, competition for protein carriers and ion trapping, are related to these mechanisms.

Filtration. In filtration, the drug passes through channels or pores in the cell membrane or passes through the gaps between cells. Only very small molecules can cross by filtration through cell membranes, but if small enough, even polar molecules or ions such as potassium or lithium can cross by this mechanism. Filtration is also the mechanism by which drugs exit the vasculature, since the epithelial cells that form the walls of the capillaries have gaps between them and all but the largest molecules readily exit. However, in some parts of the body, such as the brain, the cells of the capillaries have very tight junctures

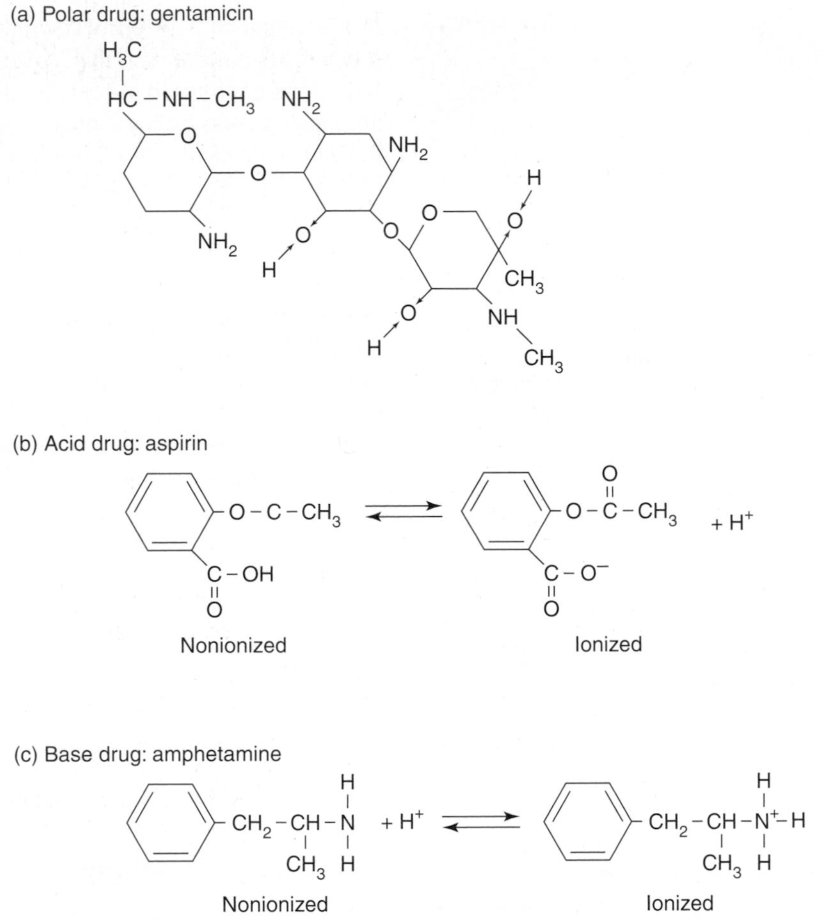
(a) Polar drug: gentamicin
(b) Acid drug: aspirin
Nonionized
Ionized
(c) Base drug: amphetamine
Nonionized
Ionized

FIGURE 2–5. Hydrophilic drug molecules. (a) Polar molecule. Oxygen atoms in the −OH groups of the structure of gentamicin attract electons (schematically represented by arrows), displacing the center of negative charge from the center of positive charge, resulting in a polar molecule. (b) Acid molecule. Aspirin is an acid that becomes ionized when it releases the protein (H^+), resulting in a net negative charge. (c) Base molecule. Amphetamine is a base that becomes polarized when it accepts a proton (H^+), resulting in a net positive charge.

with no gaps between cells, and drugs cannot exit these capillaries by filtration.

Pinocytosis. In pinocytosis the cell wall engulfs the molecule, and it is transferred across the membrane in a vacuole. It is thought that antibodies cross the placenta by pinocytosis, transferring immunity from mother to infant. Currently pinocytosis is not significant in biotransport of drugs, but ongoing research suggests that in the future it may be possible to chemically induce pinocytosis by cell membranes. This would allow large molecules like heparin to be taken orally or facilitate the entry of macromolecules such as the missing enzyme in phenylketonuria into cells.

Carrier-Mediated Transport. Drugs can be transported across biologic membranes by protein carrier molecules embedded in the cell membrane. Carrier-mediated transport has been proposed as the mechanism for transport of some drugs during absorption from the gastrointestinal tract, into the brain, and into cells. The elimination of drugs by active transport into the kidney tubule using pro-

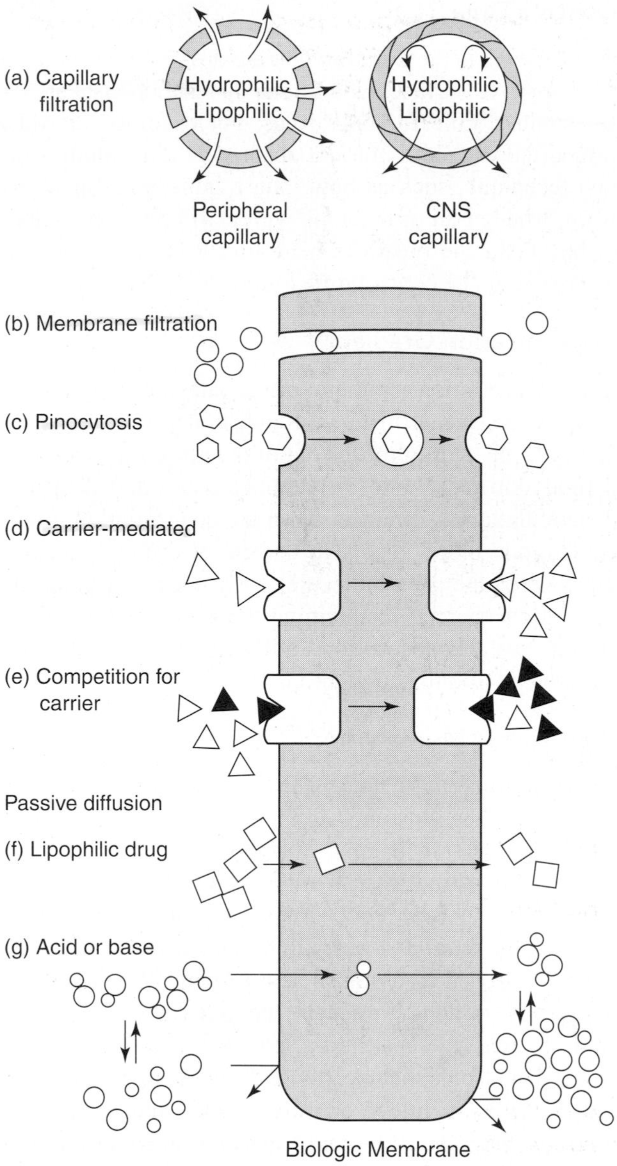

FIGURE 2–6. Mechanisms of biotransport. (a) Both lipophilic and hydrophilic drugs can filter out of peripheral capillaries, but drugs exiting central nervous system (CNS) capillaries must be lipophilic to pass through cells. (b) Small molecules can filter through channels in cell membranes. Larger and polar molecules can cross by (c) pinocytosis and (d) carrier-mediated transport, but (e) competition for the protein carrier can impair transport. (f) Lipophilic drugs diffuse through membranes readily, but (g) only nonionized forms of acids and bases can cross membranes.

tein carriers is called tubular secretion. When drugs are transported across membranes by protein carriers, it is possible that two drugs, or a drug and an endogenous chemical (i.e., one that naturally occurs in the body) will use the same carrier protein. The concurrent presence of both molecules may overwhelm the carrier mechanism and result in decreased transfer of one or both substances. For example, levodopa competes with amino acids for carrier transport during absorption in the gastrointestinal tract, so taking levodopa with protein foods can cause erratic absorption. Instructing the patient to take levodopa with low-protein meals may help to stabilize the response to therapy.

Passive Diffusion. In passive diffusion chemicals cross through the lipid bilayer of the cell membrane. Because passive diffusion is the major mechanism of drug biotransport, most drugs are relatively small molecules that are nonpolar and lipid-soluble, or are acids or bases that are nonionized at some physiologic pH. Polar or ionized drugs can be effective if administered parenterally. For example, the antibiotic gentamicin is a polar molecule (molecular weight 1500) that is administered intravenously for systemic infections because it is not absorbed orally unless there are lesions in the gastrointestinal tract.

Passive diffusion, as well as filtration, is driven by the concentration gradient, with drug molecules moving from areas of higher concentration to areas of lower concentration. If a biologic membrane intervenes between areas of different concentration of the drug, the drug moves "down" the gradient through the membrane until the concentration is equal on the two sides of the biologic membrane. When blood containing a drug passes through tissues with lower concentration than that in the plasma, drug molecules exit the blood vessels into the tissues. Thus, a drug does not usually accumulate in greater concentration on one side of a biologic membrane unless it is actively transported by a carrier-mediated mechanism. However, drugs that are acids or bases can accumulate unequally on either side of a membrane if there is a different pH on each side of the membrane. This phenomenon is called *ion trapping* or *pH partitioning.* For example, amphetamine molecules, which are nonionized in the alkaline pH of the plasma, become more ionized when they are filtered or diffused into the mammary gland, since human milk is slightly more acidic than plasma. The ionized drug becomes trapped in the milk because it cannot diffuse back across membranes. Thus, drugs that are bases can occur in higher concentration in the milk than in the maternal plasma.

PHARMACOKINETIC PHASE

The pharmacokinetic phase has been described as what the body does to the drug during its sojourn in the organism. The processes of pharmacokinetics are absorption, distribution, metabolism, and excretion. The concentration of a drug available at the site of action over time depends upon these four processes, so the duration of action and magnitude of the drug's effect are governed by pharmacokinetics. Any alteration in the fundamental chemical or physiologic mechanisms underlying a pharmacokinetic process due to age, gender, disease, drug interaction, or other source of variation can modify the time-concentration relationship of the plasma profile. When this occurs, patient response to the drug, either therapeutic or adverse, can be altered. Although the pharmacokinetic processes of absorption, distribution, metabolism, and excretion actually occur simultaneously, with changes in one process affecting other processes, they are best learned as discrete sequential events.

ABSORPTION

Absorption is defined as the passage of the drug from the site of administration into the systemic circulation. Drugs administered intravenously are delivered directly into the systemic circulation, bypass the absorptive process, and are totally and immediately absorbed. The rate and extent of absorption of drugs delivered by other routes of administration are influenced by four physical or physiologic mechanisms: (1) surface area, (2) contact time, (3) concentration gradient, and (4) presystemic metabolism.

Surface Area

The rate and completeness of absorption are proportional to the area of the absorptive surface. The reason that enteric-coated aspirin is well absorbed in the small intestine, where most of this acid drug is ionized, is that the small intestine has a large absorptive surface that rapidly absorbs the nonionized aspirin. Because the absorptive surface of the lungs is even larger, drugs delivered through the lungs, such a nicotine in cigarette smoke, achieve high peak levels very rapidly. Transdermal nicotine skin patches release the nicotine at a steady rate, which does not produce a plasma profile at all similar to that for the actual smoking of cigarettes. Other delivery systems for nicotine, such as nasal sprays, which more closely mimic the rapid peak in the plasma profile of smoking, may be more effective in promoting smoking cessation.

Contact Time

Contact time is the duration that the drug is contiguous to an absorptive surface. Conditions that alter peristalsis affect contact time for oral drugs. For example, diarrhea can curtail drug and nutrient absorption. The administration technique, such as how long a transdermal patch is worn, whether an ointment is wiped off after application, or how long the breath is held after a metered dose inhaler, affects the contact time of topical drugs.

Concentration Gradient

The concentration gradient drives the movement of a drug by passive diffusion through biologic membranes. For example, a drug moves out of the reservoir in a transdermal skin patch into the dermal tissues and then into the circulation as it moves down the concentration gradient. A good blood supply to the site of drug administration sweeps the drug molecules away once they enter the circulation, thereby maintaining the concentration gradient that sustains absorption until virtually all of the drug has crossed into the circulation.

Presystemic Metabolism

Before a drug enters the systemic circulation, there are a number of sites illustrated in Figure 2–7 where it may be metabolized to an inactive metabolite. Some drugs are destroyed by the acid in the stomach. Penicillin G is an example of an acid-labile drug—only 30 to 40% of an orally administered dose will be absorbed because the rest is destroyed by stomach acid. If penicillin G is taken with food, which stimulates the release of additional stomach acid, the absorption may be decreased to 20%. Drugs can also be metabolized by bacteria in the small intestine. Digoxin undergoes presystemic metabolism by intestinal bacteria, and toxicity can be triggered by antibiotic therapy that kills intestinal bacteria, because more of the digoxin is available for absorption. The venous circulation for most of the intestinal tract, excluding the mouth and lower one-third of the rectum, passes first through the portal circulation into the liver, where toxins and impurities ingested with food are eliminated, before the portal blood merges with the systemic circulation in the inferior vena cava. Drugs can be metabolized on this initial pass through the liver, a phenomenon known as *first-pass metabolism.* Drugs susceptible to the first-pass effect (listed in Table 2–1) will have marked differences between oral and parenteral dosages. For example, in the patient regularly receiving opioids 30 mg of morphine administered orally is required to achieve the pain relief given by 10

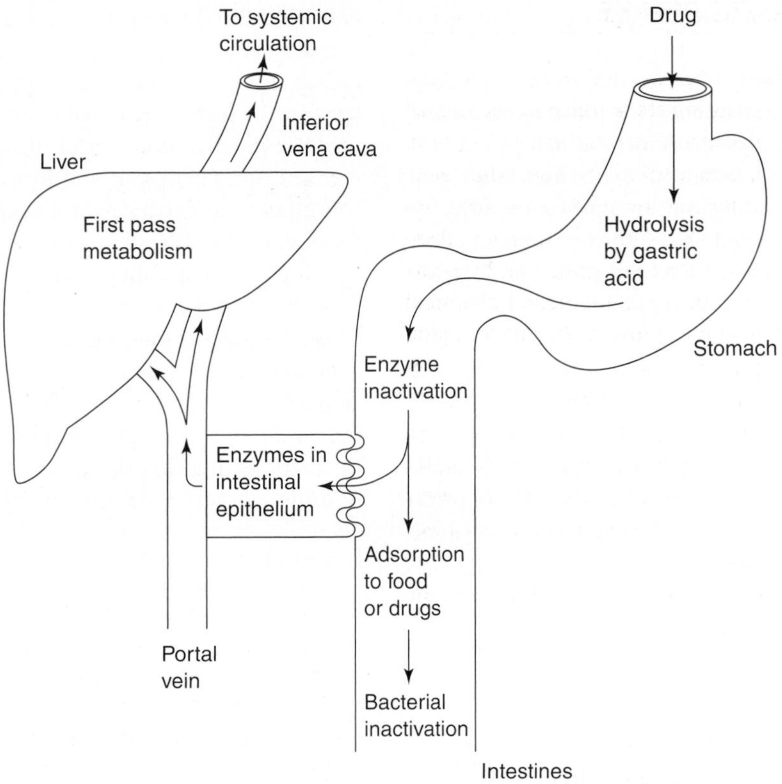

FIGURE 2–7. Presystemic metabolism. Drugs can be metabolized before absorption is complete by gastric acid, bacterial action in the intestine, and enzymes in the intestine or cell wall. The first pass effect involves metabolism because drugs absorbed into the portal circulation pass through the liver before entering the systemic circulation.

mg parenterally, since the majority of morphine is lost through first-pass metabolism. In addition, drugs that undergo first-pass metabolism often have variable dosage requirements among individuals because the genetic variability in drug-metabolizing enzymes causes variation in drug absorption from person to person.

TABLE 2–1. Examples of Drugs with Extensive First-Pass Metabolism

Drug	Oral Bioavailability, F
Diltiazem (Cardizem)	0.44
Imipramine (Tofranil)	0.40
Isosorbide dinitrate (Isordil)	0.22
Labetalol (Normodyme, Trandate)	0.18
Lidocaine (Xylocaine)	0.35
Meperidine (Demerol)	0.52
Metoprolol (Lopressor)	0.38
Morphine	0.24
Nifedipine (Procardia)	0.50
Nortriptyline (Aventyl, Pamelor)	0.51
Propranolol (Inderal)	0.26
Verapamil (Isoptin, Calan)	0.22

Factors That Alter Absorption

Any condition that alters surface area, contact time, concentration gradient, or presystemic metabolism can affect absorption. The route of administration is a major variable in absorption. Intramuscular injection yields a faster onset and shorter duration than subcutaneous injection because muscular anatomy is characterized by flat planes of muscle tissue that promote the spread of the injected drug across a larger absorptive surface area. Further, the greater blood flow to muscles than to subcutaneous tissue promotes the concentration gradient. Exercise can increase the absorption of a drug injected into a muscle or subcutaneous tissue of an extremity by increasing blood flow, just as hypoperfusive states resulting from shock or vascular and cardiac diseases can decrease absorption of injected drugs. Sublingual, lingual (metered dose spray), and buccal administration are advantageous for drugs that undergo first-pass metabolism. Nitroglycerin is used to treat acute anginal attacks by these routes, which not only bypass its extensive first-pass metabolism, but also promote the rapid absorption essential for immediate onset. Rectal administration also may bypass first-pass metabolism, but rectal absorption is erratic due to the small absorptive surface area and tendency for the drug to ascend into segments subject to first-pass metabolism.

Acute or chronic malabsorptive diseases alter oral drug absorption by affecting the amount or integrity of the absorptive surface and by altering contact time through changes in peristalsis. Liver disease can decrease first-pass metabolism so that a greater portion of the administered dosage reaches the systemic circulation. Topical or transdermal absorption is increased in the presence of a rash, sunburn, or irritation, since the blood flow to the absorptive surface is increased. The effects of pregnancy and age on drug absorption are complex. In addition, decreased first-pass metabolism in the elderly probably contributes to higher plasma concentrations of some drugs in this population (see Chapter 13). Clinically significant changes in absorption are also reported in neonates and young children (Chapter 12).

Absorption Drug Interactions

Mechanisms of drug interaction that alter absorptive processes include chelation, adsorption, alteration of peristalsis, alteration of hydrochloric acid production, alteration of intestinal flora, and competition for protein carriers. Coadministration of tetracycline or ciprofloxacin (Cipro) with food or medication that contains a divalent cation (Ca^{2+}, Mg^{2+}, Fe^{2+}) or trivalent cation (Fe^{3+}, Al^{3+}) results in the formation of an insoluble chelate that prevents the absorption of the antibiotic. The therapeutic benefit of cholestyramine (Questran), attapulgite (Kaopectate) or kaolin and pectin (Kaopectolin) is due to the ability of these agents to adsorb (attract and combine with) toxins and chemicals like cholesterol, preventing their absorption. These adsorbent agents also decrease the absorption of drugs such as digoxin and diuretics. Either increased or decreased gastrointestinal peristalsis affects drug absorption. The prokinetic agents metoclopramide (Reglan) and cisapride (Propulsid) speed intestinal transit and decrease the absorption of many drugs. Drugs with anticholinergic properties (e.g., tricyclic antidepressants, phenothiazines, antihistamines, antiparkinsonian agents, antispasmodics) slow peristalsis, which delays gastric emptying and prolongs intestinal transit time. Because little absorption occurs in the stomach, delayed gastric emptying delays drug onset. Once the drug passes into the intestine, contact time is increased by the slowed peristalsis, which enhances overall absorption. Changes in stomach pH alter the absorption of drugs such as the antifungal ketoconazole (Nizoral), which requires a low pH for absorption and may be poorly absorbed when antiulcer drugs that decrease stomach acidity are given concurrently. Since bacteria in the intestines metabolize digoxin and other drugs presystemically, broad-spectrum antibiotic therapy can increase drug absorption and lead to toxicity. Competition for the protein carrier for transport across absorptive surfaces is a rare drug interaction; the erratic absorption of levodopa in competition with amino acids is the most significant example. Chelation, adsorption, competition for protein carriers, and alteration of gastric acidity with antacids require the interacting drugs to be present in the stomach at the same time. Therefore, timing of drug administrations as far apart as possible will minimize these interactions, but this strategy is ineffective for other types of drug interactions involving absorption.

Bioavailability

The measure of liberation and absorption of drugs is bioavailability, which is computed by comparing the area under the curve of the plasma profile for oral administration (or another route) to the area under the curve for intravenous administration, which represents complete absorption. The abbreviation for bioavailability is F for fraction of the drug absorbed, but bioavailability is often reported as the percentage absorbed. Drugs with significant first-pass metabolism (like those listed in Table 2-1) have low bioavailability, because the drug is metabolized before it reaches the systemic circulation. Other drugs with low bioavailability are those with poor solubility, which retards dissolution, and drugs susceptible to other types of presystemic metabolism.

DISTRIBUTION

Distribution is defined as the transport of drugs to sites of action and elimination, as well as storage of the drug in the organs. Figure 2–8 represents how potential distribution space for a drug is conceptualized as containing a central compartment consisting of the plasma and a peripheral compartment consisting of the rest of the extracellular fluid and tissues. Drugs that distribute primarily to the central compartment circulate through the kidneys and liver frequently and thus are subject to elimination, whereas drugs stored in the peripheral compartment may persist for weeks. Physiologic mechanisms that determine the distribution characteristics of a drug are (1) blood flow, (2) special membrane barriers, (3) plasma protein binding, and (4) amount and characteristics of storage tissues.

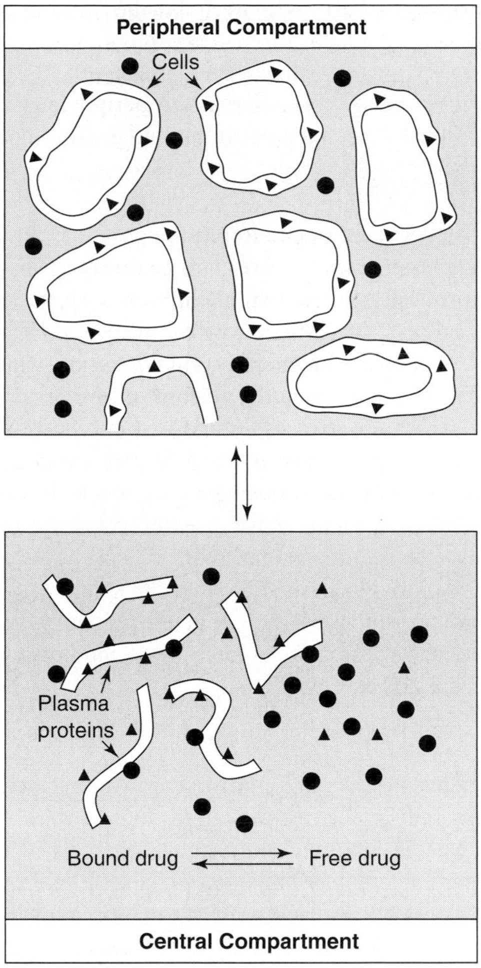

FIGURE 2–8. Conceptual distribution compartments. The distribution spaces for drugs are conceptualized as a central compartment (also called plasma compartment) and the peripheral compartment (also called tissue compartment). In the central compartment are a drug (▲) that is 80% plasma protein bound and a drug (●) that is 30% bound. In the peripheral compartment the lipophilic drug (▲) is sequestered in the lipid membranes, while the hydrophilic drug (●) distributes to extracellular fluid.

Blood Flow

Once drug molecules enter the systemic circulation, they are initially distributed to organs in proportion to blood flow to the organ. Since the brain receives 20% of cardiac output even though it is less than 5% of body mass, its potential exposure to drugs is considerable. When short-acting barbiturates are administered intravenously for the induction of anesthesia, the patient falls asleep rapidly because of the initial exposure from the intravenous bolus, but will awaken in a few minutes unless other anesthetics are administered. The half-life of these agents averages over 20 h, so it is not the elimination of the drug that causes the termination of effect. Rather, it is the *redistribution phenomenon* that occurs when the concentration of drug molecules distributed to the brain from the initial bolus is higher than that in the plasma, so the molecules move out of the brain and are redistributed to organs with lower blood flow. Blood flow is also critical during antibiotic therapy. If the site of the infection is well perfused, the antibiotic is more effective than if blood flow is restricted by peripheral vascular disease or some other condition.

Special Membrane Barriers

A number of membrane barriers have been identified that restrict the passage of chemicals, including the placental barrier, the blood-testicular barrier, and the blood-milk barrier. The blood-brain barrier is a function of the anatomy of capillaries in the brain that have tight junctures between the cells, rather than the gaps that characterize other capillaries. Glia, the connective tissues of the brain, also play a role in limiting access of chemicals to the brain. Drug molecules must pass through the cells to gain access to the central nervous system, and only lipophilic substances achieve significant concentrations in the brain. This can be a problem when there is an infection of brain tissue, because most antibiotics are hydrophilic. However, meningitis causes vasodilation of the capillaries and increases penetration of hydrophilic drugs. To circumvent the blood brain barrier, drugs can be administered directly into the cerebrospinal fluid or administered as precursors that can cross the blood-brain barrier. For example, precursor therapy is used in Parkinson's disease, which is associated with reduced concentrations of dopamine in certain areas of the brain. Dopamine is a polar molecule that cannot cross the blood-brain barrier and causes marked cardiovascular effects in the peripheral tissues. The precursor levodopa crosses the blood-brain barrier and is converted to dopamine by the enzyme dopa decarboxylase. Unfortunately, levodopa is also converted to dopamine by dopa decarboxylase in peripheral tissues, resulting in adverse cardiovascular effects. Combining levodopa and an inhibitor of dopa decarboxylase that does not cross the blood-brain barrier in the combined product, carbidopa-levodopa (Sinemet) results in a beneficial effect in the brain with decreased dosage requirements, because levodopa is converted to dopamine in the brain, but not in the peripheral tissues where dopa decarboxylase is inhibited.

Plasma Protein Binding

Figure 2–8 illustrates that many drugs are transported in plasma bound to proteins, which increases their water solubility and renders them pharmacologically inactive. That is, as long as the drug is bound to plasma protein, it is pharmacodynamically inert because it cannot exit the vascular space to get to receptors, and it is pharmacokinetically inert because it cannot be metabolized or excreted. The drug in the plasma exits in an equilibrium of bound and free drug. Highly bound drugs have greater than 90% of the drug in the plasma bound to plasma protein and less than 10% as the pharmacologically active free drug. Warfarin (Coumadin) is an example of a highly bound drug with 98% of the drug bound to plasma albumin. The 2% free warfarin molecules interact with receptors in the liver to alter production of clotting factors, but are also eliminated by metabolism. Then 2% of the remaining drug in the body is freed from the albumin to react with receptors and be metabolized. Thus, plasma protein binding can act as the body's physiologic sustained-release mechanism. If warfarin were not protein-bound, it would be too toxic to use clinically unless given by intravenous infusion. Plasma proteins that bind drugs include albumin, globulins, and lipoproteins (Table 2–2). Albumin binds acidic drugs at several different binding sites, whereas α_1-acid glycoprotein (AAG) binds bases. Drugs like warfarin that are highly bound concentrate in the plasma compartment, because the plasma protein binding sequesters the drug in the blood vessels. However, many drugs like fluoxetine (Prozac, others) are so lipophilic that they sequester in the peripheral compartment in spite of plasma protein binding greater than 90%.

Tissue Storage

Drug molecules not bound to plasma proteins can distribute to the peripheral compartment. Hydrophilic drugs distribute primarily to the extracellular water, intracellular water, and the muscles. Lipophilic drugs distribute to lipids in cell membranes and adipose tissue, which can store the drug and gradually release it over time. Drugs can also be stored by being bound to other peripheral tissues. For example, digoxin binds to protein in muscles. The amount of tissue influences how much drug can be stored. Obese patients have greater capacity to store lipophilic drugs, and patients with muscle wasting have decreased digoxin storage potential. This depot storage of drugs prolongs their duration of action, because the molecules are in the peripheral compartment and not subject to metabolism and excretion.

Factors That Alter Distribution

Age, gender, disease, and nutrition are variables that alter drug distribution by affecting blood flow, special barriers, plasma protein binding, and tissue storage. The distribution of cardiac output, competence of the blood-brain barrier, amount and capacity of plasma proteins to bind drugs, and body composition vary with developmental

TABLE 2–2. Extent and Primary Site of Binding to Plasma Proteins

Albumin	Percentage Bound	α_1-acid Glycoprotein	Percentage Bound	Lipoproteins	Percentage Bound
Amoxicillin	18	Bupavicaine	98	Amitriptyline (Elavil)	95
Aspirin	49	Disopyramide (Norpace)	*	Nortriptyline (Pamelor)	92
Chlorpropamide (Diabinese)	96	Imipramine (Tofranil)	90		
Diazepam (Valium)	99	Lidocaine	70		
Fluoxetine (Prozac)	98	Prazosin (Minipress)	95		
Glipizide (Glucotrol)	98†	Propranolol (Inderal)	87		
Ibuprofen (Motrin)	99	Quinidine	87		
Meperidine (Demerol)	58	Verapamil (Calan)	90		
Phenobarbital	51				
Phenytoin (Dilantin)	89				
Simvastatin (Zocor)	95				
Sulfamethoxazole (in Bactrim, Septra)	62				
Tetracycline	65				
Tolbutamide (Orinase)	96				
Valproic acid (Depakene, Depakote)	93				
Warfarin (Coumadin)	98				

*Binding varies by concentration.
†Nonionic binding; does not displace other albumin-bound drugs.

stage and pregnancy, resulting in age-related differences in drug distribution. Gender differences in drug distribution due to body composition commence at puberty and account for substantial variability in drug response. Women have less lean mass and greater fat mass than men. A woman taking an identical "dose" of ethanol as a man of the same weight would have a higher blood level of the drug because ethanol is distributed to lean mass, which constitutes a smaller percentage of the total weight of women. Diseases that cause fluid retention change the distribution of drugs by increasing total body water. Nephrotic syndrome depletes plasma albumin, and uremia impairs the binding of drugs because the waste products accumulated in plasma bind to albumin, decreasing binding sites available for drugs. Although it is known that α_1-acid glycoprotein is increased in inflammatory diseases and cancer, the effect of these changes on drug binding and clinical response has not been established. Malnutrition and obesity also affect body composition and the amount of plasma albumin available to bind drugs.

Distribution Drug Interactions

The number of binding sites on plasma protein is limited, so two drugs that bind to the same site on plasma protein compete for binding if they are present in the plasma simultaneously. Competition for plasma protein binding can also occur between a drug and an endogenous substance such as bilirubin, which is highly bound to albumin. Newborns receiving sulfonamides have developed kernicterus when bilirubin displaced from binding sites by the sulfonamides was deposited in the brain. The immediate effect of adding a highly protein bound drug to the regimen of a patient already taking another drug bound to the same site is a magnified effect of one or both drugs, because there is a greater free drug concentration available to interact with receptors. Figure 2–9 shows that over time the free drug is subject to increased elimination and the initial concentration of free drug will be restored, reducing the total drug (bound drug + free drug) concentration. Therefore, the clinical effects of competition for plasma protein binding are usually self-limiting and of short duration. However, if the interaction involves a highly plasma protein bound drug with a narrow therapeutic range or if the elimination of the free drug is impaired by organ disease or drug interaction, drug toxicity can develop. Further, this drug interaction must be considered in the interpretation of laboratory assays for plasma concentrations of drugs ("blood levels"). Since these assays measure the total drug in the plasma, the plasma concentration may appear subtherapeutic due to the accelerated excretion of free drug, even though the remaining free drug is sufficient to control the disease clinically. If the clinician fails to recognize the drug interaction and does not ascertain that the clinical response to the drug is appropriate, raising the dosage to achieve the "therapeutic range" could cause drug toxicity. When it is important to know the free drug concentration, the clinician can order "free" or "unbound" drug concentrations for some drugs. For example, in the patient with

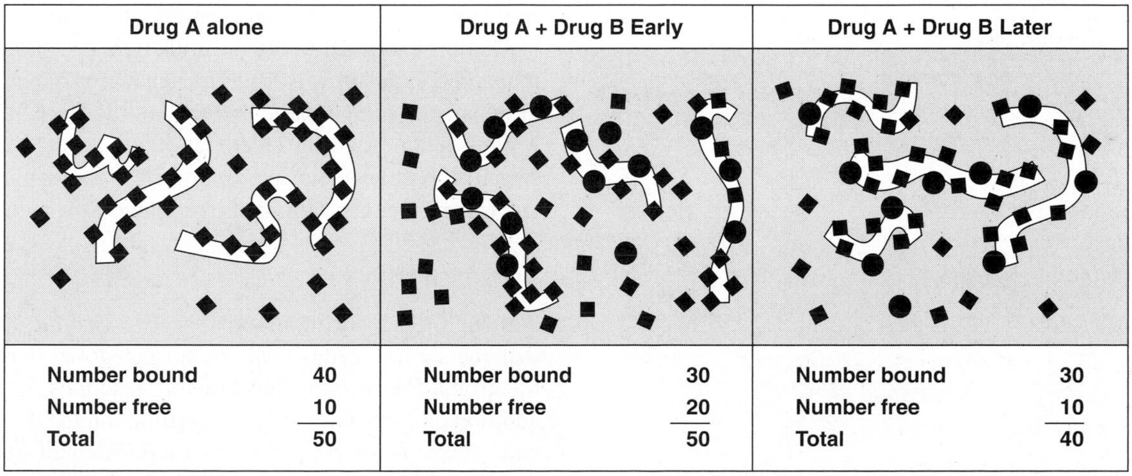

FIGURE 2–9. Competition for protein binding. When present alone, Drug A (◆) is 80% bound to plasma protein. Addition of Drug B (●), which is avidly bound to the same sites on plasma protein, causes competition and release of Drug A, doubling the concentration of its free fraction and increasing its clinical effect. Over time the increased free Drug A is eliminated and the free drug concentration returns to baseline. Although the total drug is less, only the pharmacologically inert bound drug is decreased.

uremia, hypoalbuminemia, or acute trauma, the therapeutic *free* phenytoin (Dilantin, others) concentration is 0.8 to 2 μg per mL, compared to the usual therapeutic *total* phenytoin concentration of 10 to 20 μg per mL.

Volume of Distribution

The distribution characteristics of a drug are quantified by the *apparent volume of distribution,* which is abbreviated V_D. The apparent volume of distribution is defined as the volume required to contain the dose if it was distributed equally at the concentration in the plasma. Of course, drugs are not distributed equally throughout the body at the concentration in the plasma. Some drugs are stored in the peripheral tissues, and only a fraction of the total drug is in the plasma. These drugs have a large V_D; for example, the V_D of fluoxetine (Prozac) is 2520 L in a 70-kg man, which is physically impossible since 2520 L of water weighs 2520 kg. Because fluoxetine is lipophilic and distributes to the peripheral compartment, leaving only a fraction of the dose in the plasma, the plasma concentration from a 40-mg dose averages approximately 30 ng/mL (1 nanogram = 1000 micrograms). If it is assumed that the dose is equally distributed at 30 ng/mL, it would *apparently* require 2520 L, or 36 L/kg, to contain the dose. Although the apparent volume of distribution is an abstraction rather than an actual volume, V_D can be used to characterize the distribution of a drug according to the values in Table 2–3. V_D is also useful in pharmacokinetic calculations and in computing loading doses (see Appendix 2–1, Calculating Loading Doses).

TABLE 2–3. Interpretation of Volume of Distribution

If V_d is approximately . . .			Examples	
L/kg	*L/70 kg*	*Drug Distributes to . . .*	*Drug*	*V_D, L/kg*
0.6	40	Total body water	Enalapril (Vasotec)	0.6
			Erythromycin	0.8
			Lithium	0.8
			Nifedipine (Procardia)	0.8
			Theophylline	0.5
0.2	15	Extracellular fluid	Amoxicillin	0.2
			Gentamicin	0.2
			Cephalexin (Keflex)	0.2
0.04	3	Plasma	Chlorpropamide (Diabinese)	0.04
			Warfarin	0.13
			Furosemide (Lasix)	0.05
>0.7	>46	Sequestered in peripheral tissues	Acetaminophen	1.0
			Diazepam (Valium)	1.1
			Digoxin	6.2
			Fluoxetine (Prozac)	36

METABOLISM

Metabolism and excretion are the two processes by which drugs are eliminated from the body. Metabolism, also called *biotransformation,* is the elimination of a drug through enzymatic alteration of the chemical structure of the drug molecule to form a metabolite. The drug is eliminated from the body by conversion to a new chemical entity that is more water soluble and more readily excreted from the body. The resulting metabolites may be active or inactive. Active metabolites retain the ability to interact with the target receptor and cause therapeutic and adverse effects of the parent drug. Some medicinals, called *prodrugs,* are not active in the form administered but are activated by metabolism in the intestinal wall or during the first pass through the liver. It is even possible for a metabolite to be more toxic than the parent drug. For example, one of the intermediary metabolites of acetaminophen (Tylenol) can cause liver necrosis if it is present in the high concentrations that occur in overdose or hepatic impairment. Although the major organ of metabolism is the liver, drugs undergo metabolism in many different organs. Physiologic mechanisms that determine the liver metabolism of drugs are (1) amount of liver blood flow and (2) enzyme activity.

Liver Blood Flow

Since the liver is the major organ of metabolism, liver blood flow is critical to drug elimination, because it determines the exposure of drugs to hepatic enzymes. Drugs designated as high hepatic extraction drugs (see Table 2–6 in the section on drug clearance below) are particularly sensitive to changes in liver blood flow and can accumulate to toxic concentrations if liver blood flow is impaired.

Enzyme Activity

Although there are numerous specific enzyme reactions that metabolize drugs, two broad categories have been identified. *Phase I,* or nonsynthetic, reactions involve the addition or unmasking of a polar group on the drug molecule. *Phase II,* or conjugation, reactions entail joining of the drug molecule to a polar molecule. Two common conjugation reactions are *glucuronidation,* bonding the drug to a glucose molecule, and *acetylation,* bonding the drug molecule to an acetate molecule. Although the terms suggest that a Phase I reaction always precedes a Phase II reaction, drugs can undergo only Phase II metabolism or only Phase I metabolism, or can undergo both processes in any order. Drugs often have multiple pathways for metabolism and several active or inactive metabolites.

An important group of enzyme systems for metabolizing drugs and endogenous lipophilic substances such as steroidal hormones is the *cytochrome P-450 enzymes,* which have also been called the *mixed-function oxidases* or the *microsomal enzymes.* Cytochrome, like hemoglobin, is a hemoprotein. Eleven isozyme families of cytochrome P-450 have been identified, designated by "CYP" to indicate human cytochrome P-450, followed by the Arabic number to designate the P-450 family, followed by a capital letter to designate the subfamily, followed by a second Arabic number to designate the particular gene encoding the isozyme (Table 2–4). The cytochrome P-450 enzymes catalyze primarily Phase I reactions. A notable characteristic of these enzyme systems is their responsiveness to environmental chemicals. Some chemicals increase the density and activity of cytochrome P-450 enzymes, a process called *induction.* Other chemicals can decrease the amount and activity of the cytochrome P-450 enzymes, which is referred to as enzyme *inhibition.* Induction and inhibition are the mechanism for important interactions of drugs with foods, environmental pollutants, and other drugs.

Factors That Alter Metabolism

Metabolism is the most individual of pharmacokinetic processes, varying among individuals and within the same individual over time. Genetic inheritance is the major source of individual difference in drug metabolism. For example, in some racial groups, 5 to 20% of the population may lack one of the isozymes of cytochrome P-450, utilizing different pathways to metabolize drugs usually processed by that isozyme (Otani & Aoshima, 2000). In the United States about half of the population are slow acetylators, more prone to develop certain adverse effects with drugs that are metabolized by acetylation, such as isoniazid (INH) and procainamide (Pronestyl). Relatively little of the genetic basis of drug metabolism has been adequately studied, so this important source of variation in drug response remains poorly understood.

Developmental and environmental factors also have profound effects on drug metabolism. The very young and the very old have less effective hepatic metabolism than young adults, but children actually have accelerated elimination of some drugs metabolized by cytochrome P-450. Since the constituents of cytochrome P-450 and other drug-metabolizing enzymes are iron, proteins, and vitamin cofactors, nutritional deficiency can impair drug metabolism. Thyroid function can speed or slow drug metabolism, and correction of hyperthyroid or hypothyroid states will alter dose requirements for many drugs. Diseases like cirrhosis and hepatitis decrease both the hepatic blood flow and enzyme activity, resulting in decreased drug elimination. Although patients with abnormal values on liver function tests often have impairment of drug metabolism, it is not possible to adjust dosages of metabolized drugs based upon laboratory tests of liver function. The clinician must rely on an assay of plasma concentration of the drug or evaluation of the clinical response to titrate dosages of hepatically eliminated drugs.

Metabolism Drug Interactions

A growing list of chemicals, including drugs, foods, and pollutants, have been identified that can induce or inhibit cytochrome P-450 enzyme systems, and recent research has identified the specific isozymes involved for some interactions. Table 2–4 lists the isozyme, the substrates metabolized by the isozyme, the drugs that induce the isozyme, and the drugs that inhibit the isozyme. When a cytochrome P-450 isozyme is induced by a drug or chemical, the rate of metabolism of any substrate of that isozyme is increased, which lowers the serum concentration and results in decreased drug effect. For example, a cigarette smoker metabolizes theophylline more rapidly and needs a higher dosage to attain the therapeutic effect. Conversely, when an isozyme is inhibited by a drug, any substrate of that isozyme will be metabolized more slowly, accumulating in the body with the potential to cause toxicity. At high serum concentrations astemizole (Hismanal) and cisapride (Propulsid), which are metabolized by CYP3A4, causing potentially lethal cardiovascular adverse effects and withdrawal of these drugs from the market. Patients taking these agents and inhibitors of CYP3A4 such as erythromycin and ketoconazole Nizoral developed lethal dysrhythmias. CYP3A4 is also located in intestinal mucosa where grapefruit juice may inhibit it during presystemic metabolism, increasing bioavailability and causing toxicity of diltiazem (Cardizem) and other CYP3A4 substrates (Flockhart & Tanus-Santos, 2002; Hansten & Horn, 2000; Pepper, 1997; Tatro, 2002). Drugs such as cimetidine (Tagamet) and albuterol (Proventil) alter hepatic blood flow and affect metabolism of high hepatic extraction drugs.

TABLE 2–4. Cytochrome P-450 Isozymes, Substrates, Inducers, and Inhibitors

Isozyme	Substrates	Inducers	Inhibitors
CYP1A2	Acetaminophen (Tylenol) Caffeine Clozapine (Clozaril) Imipramine (Tofranil) Tacrine (Cognex) Theophylline R-warfarin (Coumadin) Tamoxifen	Charbroiled foods Cigarette smoke Cruciferous vegetables Rifampin Omeprazole (Prilosec) Phenobarbital	Cimetidine (Tagamet) Ciprofloxacin (Cipro) Grapefruit juice (?) Enoxacin (Penetrex) Erythromycin Fluvoxamine (Luvox) Mexiletine (Mexitil) Norfloxacin (Noroxin) Tacrine (Cognex)
CYP2C9	Diclofenac (Voltaren) Ibuprofen (Motrin) S-warfarin (Coumadin) Cimetidine (Tagamet) Fluvastatin	Fluconazole (Diflucan) Fluoxetine (Prozac) Barbiturates Carbamazepine	Cimetidine (Tagamet) Disulfiram (Antabuse) Co-trimoxazole (Bactrim, Septra) Metronidazole (Flagyl) Isoniazid
CYP2C18-19	Diazepam (Valium) Imipramine (Tofranil) Naproxen (Anaprox) Omeprazole (Prilosec) Phenytoin (Dilantin) Propranolol (Inderal) Tolbutamide (Orinase)	Barbiturates	Felbamate (Felbatol) Fluoxetine (Prozac) Fluvoxamine (Luvox) Omeprazole (Prilosec) Tolbutamide (orinase)
CYP2D6	Amitriptyline (Elavil) Clomipramine (Anafranil) Codeine Desipramine (Norpramin) Dextromethorphan Fluoxetine (Prozac) Haloperidol (Haldol) Imipramine (Tofranil) Metoprolol (Lopressor) Nortriptyline (Aventyl) Paroxetine (Paxil) Pentazocine (Talwin) Propranolol (Inderal) Risperidone (Risperdal) Thioridazine (Mellaril) Type 1c antiarrhythmics (e.g., encainide, flecainide, propafenone) Venlafaxine (Effexor)		Amiodarone Fluoxetine (Prozac) Haloperidol (Haldol) Paroxetine (Paxil) Quinidine Ranitidine (Zantac) Thioridazine (Mellaril) Venlafaxine (Effexor) Cloroquine Cimetidine (Tagamet) Propoxyphene (Daron) Vinblastine
CYP3A4 (also in intestinal mucosa)	Alprazolam (Xanax) Atorvastatin (Lipitor) Carbamazepine (Tegretol) Cisapride (Propulsid) Corticosteroids Cyclosporine Diazepam (Valium) Diltiazem (Cardizem) Felodipine (Plendil) Lidocaine Lovastatin (Mevacor) Midazolam (Versed) Nifedipine (Procardia) Quinidine Simvastatin (Zocor) Testosterone Triazolam (Halcion) Verapamil (Isoptin, Calan)	Carbamazepine (Tegretol) Corticosteroids Phenobarbital Phenytoin (Dilantin) Rifampin Rifabutin	Cimetidine (Tagamet) Clarithromycin (Biaxin) Diltiazem (Cardizem) Erythromycin Fluconazole (Diflucan) Fluoxetine (Prozac) Miconazole (Monistat) Nefazodone (Serzone) Norfloxacin Paroxetine (Paxil) Quinidine Fluvoxamine (Luvox) Grapefruit juice Itraconazole (Sporanox) Ketoconazole (Nizoral) Sertraline (Zoloft) Protease inhibitors (e.g., indinavir, ritonavir)

Sources: Hansten & Horn, 2000; Pepper, 1997; Tatro, 2002.

EXCRETION

Excretion involves the removal of drugs, active metabolites, or inactive metabolites from the body. Although drugs and metabolites are excreted through the sweat, saliva, and other secretions, renal elimination through the urine is the most common route of excretion. Biliary excretion is another common route of elimination. For drugs eliminated unchanged (that is, unmetabolized) or as active metabolites, decreased excretion results in accumulation of the drug and toxicity. The four physiologic processes that determine excretion are (1) glomerular filtration, (2) tubular secretion, (3) passive reabsorption, and (4) enterohepatic recirculation. The first three mechanisms, which are illustrated in Figure 2–10, are relevant to renal excretion, while enterohepatic recirculation involves biliary excretion.

Glomerular Filtration

Molecules of drugs and metabolites in plasma that are not bound to plasma protein filter into the renal tubular filtrate at Bowman's capsule. Blood flow to the kidneys maintains filtration pressure, and decreased blood flow impairs drug excretion. Creatinine clearance is a valid laboratory indicator of glomerular filtration used to adjust dosages of renally excreted drugs. Molecules in the filtrate that are not reabsorbed will be excreted from the body in the urine.

Tubular Secretion

Located in the walls of the tubule are protein carriers that actively transport substances into the renal tubules, even against a concentration gradient. The tubules have two types of transport systems, one for acids and one for

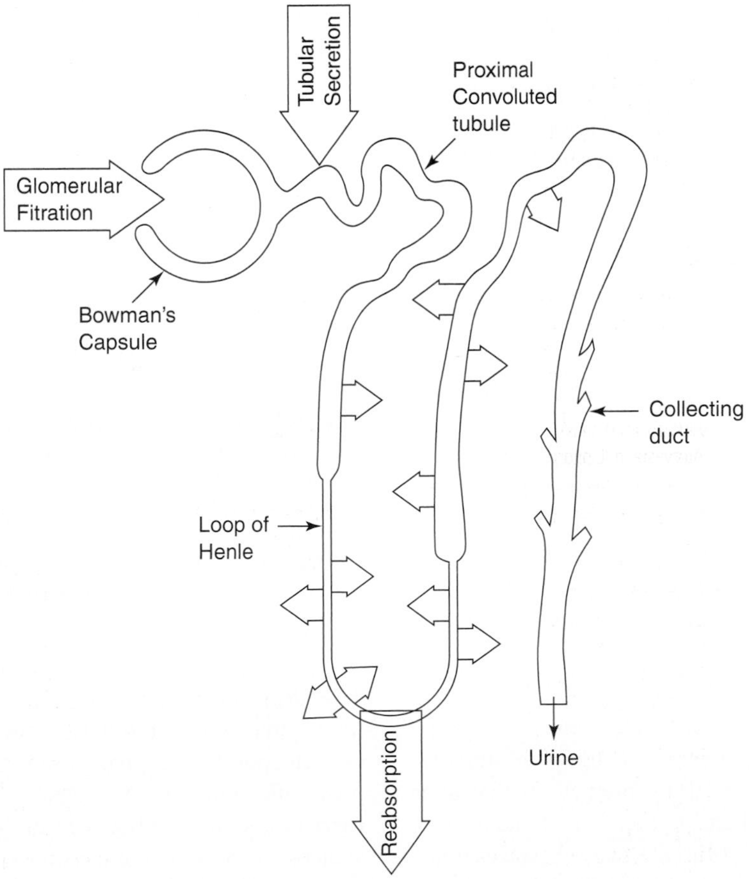

FIGURE 2–10. Processes of renal excretion. Drug molecules are excreted by glomerular filtration into the renal tubule and active tubular secretion by protein carriers in the proximal convoluted tubule. During passage through the nephron lipid soluble, nonionized drug molecules are reabsorbed, and remaining molecules are excreted in the urine.

bases. Penicillin is transported by the acid transport system from the plasma into the proximal convoluted tubule by a carrier-mediated process called tubular secretion. This mechanism accounts for the very short half-life of penicillin of one-half hour.

Passive Reabsorption

Drug molecules in the renal tubules can be reabsorbed by passive diffusion back into the body. Lipid-soluble, nonpolar, nonionized substances will be readily returned to the circulation. Because the pH of urine has wide variability, an acid or base may be nonionized and reabsorbed at one urine pH and ionized and eliminated at a different urine pH.

Enterohepatic Recirculation

After Phase II metabolism, conjugates excreted into the bile come into contact with intestinal bacteria that can hydrolyze the bond between the drug and the conjugate, which restores the drug to its pharmacologically active, lipid-soluble form, which is then reabsorbed. Figure 2–11 illustrates how this recycling of the drug extends its duration of action. For example, estrogens undergo enterohepatic recirculation, so that a small amount of hormone has prolonged effects.

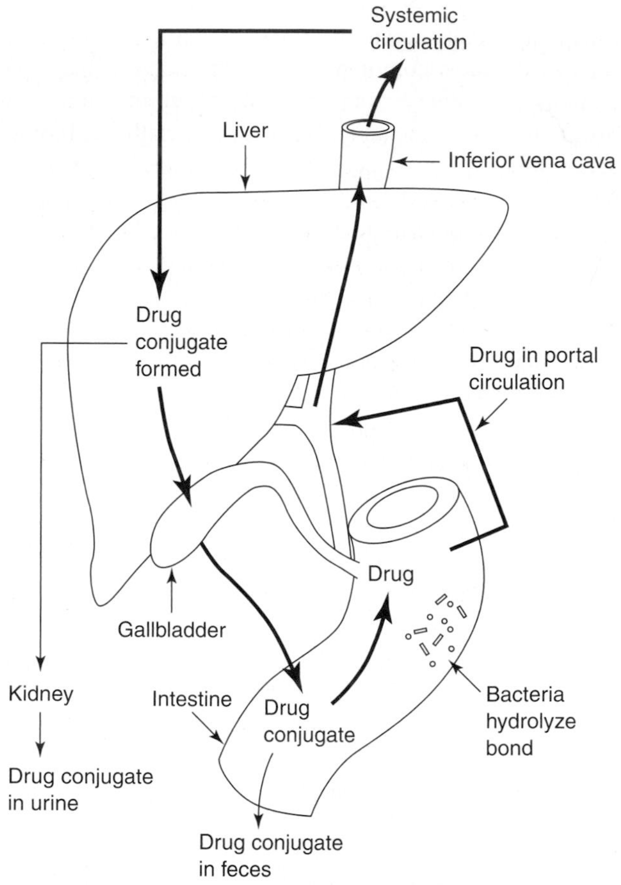

FIGURE 2–11. Enterohepatic recirculation. Drug molecules from the systemic circulation are conjugated in the liver and excreted via the bile into the intestines. Bacteria in the intestines enzymatically hydrolyze the bond of the drug conjugate, releasing drug in its lipid soluble form, which is reabsorbed through the portal system to the systemic circulation. During each cycle, some hydrophilic drug conjugate is excreted with the urine or feces.

Factors That Alter Excretion

The renal function of the very young (preterm infants and neonates) and the elderly is not as effective as other age groups, so dosages of drugs that are renally excreted unchanged or as active metabolites must be reduced for patients in these groups. Pregnancy can actually increase excretion secondary to the effects of increased blood volume on renal blood flow, so dosage increases of some drugs may be required to treat serious disorders during pregnancy (see Chapter 17). Renal disease and dehydration impair excretion of drugs. Drugs eliminated by biliary excretion can have impaired elimination in gallbladder disease.

Excretion Drug Interactions

Competition for protein carriers, ion trapping, and decreased renal blood flow are drug interactions that alter renal drug excretion. When probenecid (Benemid) is given concurrent with penicillin, the two substances compete for the protein carrier responsible for tubular secretion of penicillin in the nephron, prolonging the half-life of the penicillin and raising its peak serum concentration. This drug interaction has been used therapeutically; patients receiving tubularly secreted penicillins and cephalosporins are given probenecid (Benemid) to improve the antibiotic response. Competition for protein carriers also occurs between drugs and endogenous substances, such as the competition of uric acid with thiazide and loop diuretics for the same tubular secretion carrier. As a result, these diuretics raise serum uric acid and can trigger acute gout in genetically susceptible patients.

Acidic drugs are trapped in alkaline urine, and conversely alkaline drugs are trapped in acidic urine; both conditions promote excretion of the drugs. Treatment of poisoning often involves modification of urine pH so that the ionized drug is trapped in the urine and excreted. Overdose of the acid, phenobarbital, is managed with sodium bicarbonate infusion to alkalinize the urine. Amphetamine overdose is treated by acidification of the urine. Table 2–5 shows drugs that may have altered excretion due to ion trapping. For example, a patient on quinidine who uses megadose ascorbic acid therapy to treat a cold can develop recurrence of the arrhythmia because the basic drug will be ion-trapped in the acidic urine and excreted. Conversely, using sodium bicarbonate (baking soda) for gastric upset could trigger toxicity because the drug would be nonionized and reabsorbable in alkaline urine.

Decreased blood pressure reduces glomerular filtration, so antihypertensive drugs and other agents that decrease blood pressure impair elimination of drugs cleared by the kidneys. Nonsteroidal antiinflammatory agents also reduce renal blood flow and drug elimination by decreasing synthesis of prostaglandins. Prostaglandins are endogenous chemicals that dilate the renal artery and sustain renal blood flow, especially in conditions like congestive heart failure when compensatory mechanisms decrease renal blood flow.

Enterohepatic recirculation is interrupted when antibiotic therapy kills the bacteria that normally hydrolyze the bond in the drug conjugate, causing the plasma concentration of drugs that are normally recycled to decline. Women taking oral contraceptives are advised to use a backup contraception method for the remainder of the cycle after a course of broad-spectrum antibiotics. Similarly, women on hormone replacement therapy may experience return of hot flashes during antibiotic therapy.

TABLE 2–5. Drugs with Elimination Dependent on Urine pH

Elimination Increased by Acid Urine (Bases)	Elimination Increased by Alkaline Urine (Acids)
Amphetamines	Aspirin
Chloroquine (Aralen)	Acetazolamide (Diamox)
Ephedrine	Choline salicylate (Arthropan)
Mexiletine (Mexitil)	Choline magnesium trisalicylate (Trilisate)
Quinidine	Nitrofurantoin (Furadantin, Macrodantin)
Quinine	Phenobarbital
	Probenecid (Benemid)
	Salsalate (Disalcid)

Drug Clearance

The measure of drug elimination by all routes of metabolism and excretion is clearance, which is defined as the rate of removal of a drug in proportion to plasma concentration. Clearance (CL) is reported as the volume of plasma cleared of the drug per unit of time. The clearances of some common drugs are shown in Table 2–6. If the plasma concentration of a hypothetical drug is 2 μg/mL and it is eliminated at 2 mg/h, the clearance would be 1 L/h or about 17 mL/min. (This is because 1000 mL or 1 L of plasma would be needed to contain 2 mg at a concentration of 2 μg/mL.) Like volume of distribution, clearance is a useful abstraction, rather than a representation of absolute reality. That is, after 1 h there would not be 1 L of plasma somewhere in the patient's body with no drug and the remaining 2 L of plasma with 2 μg/mL of the drug. Rather, the overall plasma concentration would decline slightly, depending on how much drug stored in the peripheral compartment moved into the central compartment to replace the drug that was eliminated. The concept of clearance is useful in understanding the elimination characteristics of a drug and in pharmacokinetic calculations, particularly in the computation of maintenance dose (see Appendix 2–2, Calculating Maintenance Doses).

TABLE 2–6. Examples of Route and Rate of Clearance of Common Drugs

Drug Types	Clearance, L/h per kg*
High Hepatic Extraction Drugs	
Imipramine (Tofranil)	0.9
Labetalol (Normodyne, Trandate)	1.5
Lidocaine (Xylocaine)	0.549
Meperidine (Demerol)	1.02
Morphine	3.286
Propranolol	0.72
Verapamil (Isoptin, Calan)	0.9
Other Drugs Eliminated by Liver	
Acetaminophen	0.3
Carbamazepine (Tegretol)	0.076
Metronidazole (Flagyl)	0.077
Theophylline	0.041
Drugs with Primarily Renal Elimination as Unchanged Drug	
Ampicillin	0.23†
Ciprofloxacin (Cipro)	0.36†
Digoxin	0.111
Gentamicin	0.077
Vancomycin	0.084

*Assuming normal renal and hepatic function.
†High clearance due to tubular secretion.

HALF-LIFE

The elimination half-life of a drug is the amount of time required for half of the drug to be eliminated from the body. Figure 2–12 illustrates that elimination half-life is measured as the amount of time it takes for the plasma concentration to decline by 50%. Because the drug in the peripheral compartment and the drug in the plasma compartment are at equilibrium, changes in concentration of the drug in the plasma represent changes of the total amount in the body, regardless of whether the drug is primarily located in the blood or primarily sequestered in the peripheral tissues. Therefore, a drop in plasma concentration of 50% means that the amount of drug in the whole body has declined by 50%.

Half-life ($t_{1/2}$) is determined by the volume of distribution and clearance of a drug according to the following formula:

$$t_{\frac{1}{2}} = 0.7\left[\frac{V_D}{CL}\right]$$

Analysis of this formula reveals why it is important to consider both the volume of distribution and the clearance of a drug. Fluoxetine (Prozac) has a clearance of 0.58 L/h per kilogram, which ranks it with the high hepatic extraction drugs, yet its half-life averages 53 h because it has an extraordinary volume of distribution of 36 L/kg. Even though any fluoxetine that passed through the liver would be immediately metabolized, most of it is sequestered in peripheral tissues and is not subject to elimination. Although fluoxetine is over 90% bound to plasma proteins and drug interaction with other highly plasma protein bound drugs is theoretically possible, only a tiny fraction of the drug is in the plasma compartment, rendering clinically significant drug interaction unlikely.

The duration of drug action corresponds roughly with the half-life for many drugs, because the plasma concentration often falls below the minimum effective concentration after one half-life, but the effects of some drugs last well beyond one elimination half-life. Corticosteroids initiate a series of chemical reactions, but need to be present only for the initial reaction. Thus, the biologic

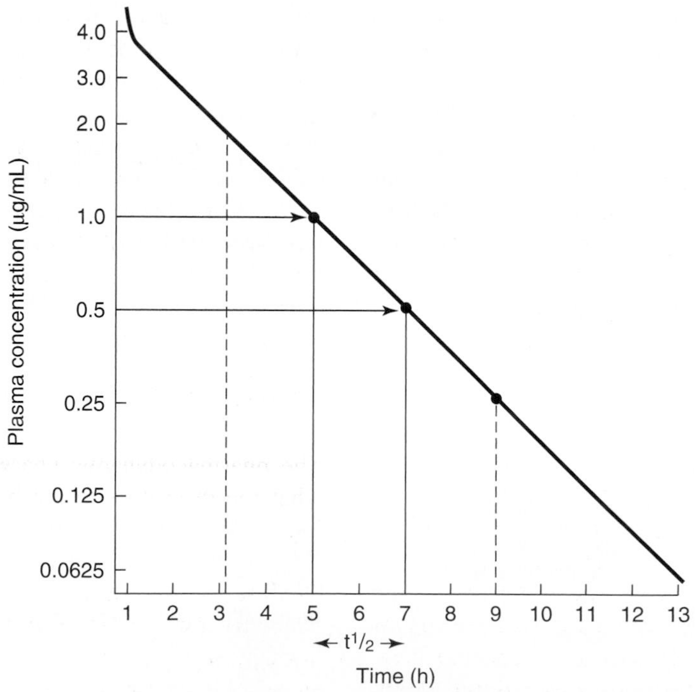

FIGURE 2–12. Elimination half-life. The plasma profile for intravenous administration plotted with concentration on a log scale demonstrates linear drug elimination with a constant fraction of the drug removed per period of time. For the hypothetical drug in this figure, the elimination half-life is 2 hours, the time required for the plasma concentration to decrease by half.

half-life of corticosteroids far exceeds the elimination half-life. For drugs like the angiotensin-converting enzyme inhibitors, the peak drug level is so much greater than the minimum effective concentration that the plasma concentration exceeds the minimum effective concentration even after several half-lives have passed. A drug is largely eliminated from the body in about four half-lives, because half of the remaining drug is removed during each subsequent half-life:

Number of Half-Lives	Percentage of Drug Eliminated
1	50.0
2	75.0
3	87.5
4	93.75

Dose-Dependent Kinetics

For most drugs a constant *proportion* of the drug is eliminated per unit of time, so that during each half-life 50% of the drug is eliminated. This is called *first-order kinetics,* which is how most drugs are eliminated. When there is not excess enzyme capacity for metabolism of a drug, the drug is removed at a constant *amount* per unit of time. This is called *dose-dependent* or *zero-order* kinetics. Common drugs with dose-dependent kinetics are aspirin, phenytoin (Dilantin), and ethanol. Aspirin has a half-life of 3 to 4 h and first-order kinetics at usual analgesic dosages (650 mg every 4 h). At antiarthritis dosages (4 g per day), the half-life of aspirin is 18 h and the drug is eliminated by dose-dependent kinetics. For drugs with dose-dependent kinetics, the clinician should titrate dosages in small increments, as well as monitor plasma concentration and clinical response frequently.

STEADY STATE

In Figure 2–2 the plasma profile represented is for a single oral dose. Most drugs are given on a repetitive basis, with the repeat dose administered before the previous dose has been eliminated. When a drug is repeatedly administered, a *steady state* occurs after approximately four half-lives. A steady state occurs when absorption and elimination are equal and the average plasma concentration reaches a plateau. Regardless of whether the total daily dosage is administered as a single dosage, four times daily, ten times daily, or as a constant intravenous infusion, a steady state is approximated after four half-lives. With less frequent dosage, the plasma concentration fluctuates widely around the average concentration—that is, the peaks are higher and the troughs are lower than with more frequent dosing.

CLINICAL IMPLICATIONS OF PHARMACOKINETICS

Rational pharmacotherapeutics requires thorough assessment and analysis of patient factors that may alter pharmacokinetics. Thinking in terms of how diseases and drugs alter the mechanisms of each of the pharmacokinetic processes, rather than trying to remember all the contraindications and precautions for each drug, is an effective outline for this analysis. One of the most important clinical implications of pharmacokinetics is the need for dosage reduction and meticulous patient monitoring when drug elimination is impaired. A drug excreted by the kidneys more than 30% unchanged or as an active metabolite will accumulate when there is renal impairment. For many drugs there are formulas and tables to guide the dosing of renally excreted drugs based upon creatinine clearance. Because there is no comparable laboratory test to guide dosage in hepatic impairment, it is prudent to start doses at one-fourth to one-third the usual starting dose and titrate slowly upward. Since dose adjustments should be made only after a steady state is approximated, the interval between increments during dose titration should be longer in both renal and hepatic impairment, which decrease clearance and cause prolonged half-life and extended time to a steady state. After the initial dosage is selected, plasma concentration is a useful measurement to use in dosage adjustment for drugs with a valid drug assay procedure (see Appendix 2–3, Adjusting Dosage Using Laboratory Drug Levels).

PHARMACODYNAMIC PHASE

The pharmacodynamic phase has been characterized as what the drug does to the body to elicit the pharmacologic effect. The processes of pharmacodynamics are *drug-receptor binding* and *receptor-effector coupling.* Binding is the interaction of the drug with receptors, whereas coupling is how the interaction, directly or through a series of chemical and physiologic steps, evokes the therapeutic and adverse effects of the drug. Whereas the pharmacokinetic processes determine the concentration of a drug at the receptor, the pharmacodynamic processes determine the relationship between the concentration at the receptor and the nature and degree of the response.

MECHANISMS OF ACTION

Drugs work by chemical, mechanical, general membrane, and receptor mechanisms. An example of a chemical mechanism is the acid-base interaction of antacids with gastric hydrochloric acid, or the inactivation of heparin (an acid) by protamine sulfate (a base). When bulk laxatives adsorb fluids and lipids in the gastrointestinal tract, the increased mass stimulates peristalsis through a mechanical action. General anesthetics do not interact with any specific receptor, but rather dissolve in the lipid layer of cell membranes in the central nervous system. This general membrane effect disrupts membrane function, resulting in loss of consciousness. However, most drugs elicit their pharmacologic responses through specific receptor interactions.

DRUG-RECEPTOR BINDING

Drug-receptor interactions involve the reversible joining of a drug (D) and a receptor (R) to form a drug-receptor complex (DR), represented by the following equation for receptor binding:

$$D + R \Leftrightarrow DR$$

Because the bonds between drugs and receptors are usually electrostatic (weak chemical bonds), the interaction is reversible. Otherwise, drug effects would not terminate until new receptors were synthesized to replace those complexed with the drug.

Dose-Response Relationships

Figure 2–13*a* illustrates the relationship between the dose of a drug and the response. As the dose is incremented, the response increases until all of the receptors are filled and the curve plateaus. Once the receptors are saturated, further dose increments do not increase the effect. Because pharmacokinetic factors affect the dose-response relationship, a more precise representation of pharmacodynamic processes is the concentration-response graph, which depicts the relationship between the concentration *at the receptor* and the response. Figure 2–13*b* demonstrates that plotting the concentration-response data on a log scale results in the more easily interpretable S-shaped curve.

Maximal efficacy (E_{max}), the response attained when the receptors are saturated, is one important parameter of the concentration-response curve used to compare drugs. Another useful measure is the concentration or dose which elicits half of the maximal response (EC_{50} or ED_{50}), which is the measure of drug *potency.* The meanings of *drug potency* and *drug efficacy* are often confused. Sales promotions often hype the potency of a product, which means only that each dose requires fewer milligrams than an equally effective dose of the comparison drug. For example, famotidine (Pepcid) is the most potent H_2 blocker, which means only that it takes 40 mg of famotidine to achieve the same effect as 300 mg of ranitidine (Zantac). It does not mean that famotidine is any more effective than ranitidine—that is, both drugs have the same E_{max}.

Ligands

Any chemical that interacts with a receptor is referred to as a ligand. Substances that interact with receptors can be either exogenous drugs or endogenous chemicals naturally occurring in the body such as a hormones, neurotransmitters, peptides, or prostaglandins. The term *ligand* encompasses both endogenous substances and drugs. Classical receptors are regulatory proteins that mediate the actions of endogenous ligands. When drugs interact with classical receptors, they may act either as agonists or as antagonists. *Agonists* bind to and activate the receptor, causing the change in function of the receptor that elicits the pharmacologic response. *Antagonists* also bind to the receptor, but do not alter their function. Rather, by occupying the receptor, antagonists prevent the endogenous ligand from binding to it, which is why antagonists are also called *blockers.* For example, terbutaline is an adrenergic agonist that interacts with $beta_2$ receptors on smooth muscle in the bronchi, eliciting bronchial dilation. This response is the same as occurs when the endogenous ligand norepinephrine interacts with these receptors. Propranolol is an antagonist that blocks $beta_2$ receptors, which prevents norepinephrine from binding to the $beta_2$ receptor and results in bronchial constriction due to the absence of adrenergic stimulation. Besides classical receptors, a frequent receptor site for drugs is on enzymes, large proteins that catalyze biochemical interactions. By binding to the enzyme a drug may change the shape of the enzyme or otherwise inhibit its interaction with the substrate. For example, clavulanic acid is an inhibitor of beta-lactamase, an enzyme produced by some penicillin-

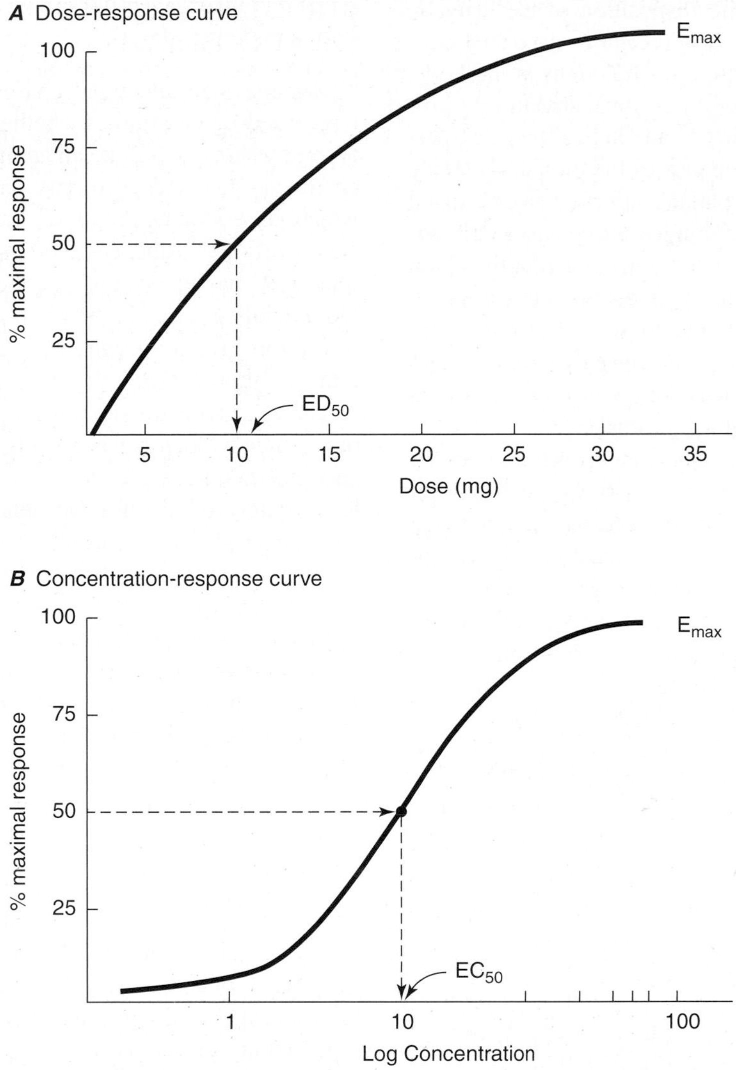

FIGURE 2–13. Dose-response and concentration-response relationships. Graph of dose-response relationship with dose on an arithmetic scale results in a hyperbolic curve. Graph of concentration response with concentration on a logarithmic scale results in the readily interpreted S-shaped curve. [E_{max} is maximal efficacy; ED_{50} is the dose that elicits 50% of the maximal response; EC_{50} is the concentration at the receptor that elicits 50% of the maximal response.]

resistant bacteria. When clavulanic acid and amoxicillin are combined (Augmentin), beta-lactamase–producing strains of *Haemophilus influenzae, Moraxella cattarhalis,* gonococci, and other organisms are susceptible to the amoxicillin. The clavulanic acid inhibits the inactivation of the amoxicillin by the beta-lactamase, permitting the amoxicillin to impair bacterial cell wall synthesis and kill the organism.

Receptors. Receptors are large protein molecules, such as lipoproteins, glycoproteins, or enzymes, which are often embedded in cell membranes with the ligand binding sites located on the outer surfaces of cells. It is important to distinguish receptor binding, which is pharmacodynamic and related to the drug effect, from other kinds of protein binding with drugs, such as plasma protein binding and binding to protein carriers, which are pharmacokinetic and involve the disposition of the drug by the body. Proteins are ideal drug receptors since they have many reactive sites and regulatory functions in the body. In addition, due to the three-dimensional structure of proteins, consisting of folds, sheets, and helical shapes, interaction of the ligand with one part of the protein molecule can cause a change in the spatial conformation of a distal section of the molecule, bringing it into contact with another chemical, which activates the next step in the chain of events that results in drug response. Ligands must be large enough molecules to bind to several reactive sites that make up the receptor, so drugs usually have a molecular weight between 100 and 1000, large enough to fit the receptor, but small enough for biotransport.

Most classical receptors are named for their endogenous ligand, although opioid receptors were labeled for drugs used centuries before the receptors were identified. The earliest receptors to be characterized were the receptors for acetylcholine, called cholinergic receptors, and the receptors for norepinephrine, called adrenergic receptors. More recently, receptors have been identified for serotonin, gamma-aminobutyric acid (GABA), histamine, dopamine, opioids, adenosine, glycine, insulin, and numerous other hormones, neurotransmitters, and peptides. Receptor subtypes have been identified for most receptors. It is thought that the subtypes represent slight variants in the structure of the receptor protein, but subtypes may also have different coupling mechanisms. Because the receptor subtypes often mediate different effects, it has been possible to develop drugs for specific subtypes to target particular therapeutic responses or to avoid adverse effects. For example, once it was known that the histamine receptor involved in allergic responses (H_1 receptor) was distinct from the histamine receptor that controlled gastric acid secretion (H_2 receptor), pharmacologists were able to synthesize cimetidine (Tagamet) and other drugs that selectively block the H_2 receptor. Such "designer drugs" are now a common source of new drug products. Many receptor subtypes have been identified by a numeric subscript like the histamine receptors H_1, H_2, and H_3. Some receptor subtypes received Greek letter names, like the alpha- and beta-adrenergic receptors and mu, kappa, epsilon, and delta opioid receptors. Subdivisions of receptor subtypes have also been given subscript numbers, as in $beta_1$- and $beta_2$-adrenergic receptors. Cholinergic receptors are unique in that the major subtypes were named muscarinic and nicotinic by early pharmacologists who discovered that they could be distinguished by their response to plant extracts from a mushroom and the tobacco plant, respectively.

STRUCTURE-ACTIVITY RELATIONSHIPS

The shape, size, electrical charge, and atomic composition of a drug determines whether it will bind to a receptor and whether it will be an agonist or an antagonist. The chemical structure also governs its receptor *affinity,* which is defined as propensity to bind to a receptor. Receptor affinity influences the concentration of a drug required at the receptor to elicit a desired response. The more avidly a drug binds to a receptor, the lower the concentration of drug required. This structure-activity relationship allows selectivity of drug molecules for specific receptors or receptor subtypes. For example, at low doses propranolol (Inderal) has affinity for both $beta_1$ and $beta_2$ subtypes of adrenergic receptors, but atenolol (Tenormin) has greatest affinity for the $beta_1$ subtype. Thus, at low doses only propanolol causes dyspnea. At higher doses, such as usual antihypertensive and antianginal dosages, selectivity is lost and both propranolol and atenolol cause dyspnea in susceptible patients. Thus, even when drugs are selective—that is, have low affinity for a receptor subtype—they will bind to the receptor when the concentration at the receptor is sufficiently high.

Dissociation Constant

The dissociation content for the drug-binding equation presented above is called the equilibrium dissociation constant (K_D). K_D is defined as the concentration of drug at which half of the receptors are occupied. K_D is the measure of affinity of a drug for the receptor and reflects the potency of a drug. A low K_D means that the drug has high affinity for the receptor.

Stereoselectivity

Many drugs exhibit chirality; that is, they have paired forms with the same atomic composition existing in mirror-image spatial orientation, called enantiomers. Like the right and left hands of a human, the enantiomers are nonsuperimposable pairs, as illustrated in Figure 2–14. In pure solution one of the enantiomers rotates polarized light to the right (dextrorotary), whereas a pure solution of the other enantiomer will rotate polarized light to the left (levorotary). From this optical property is derived the convention of naming the pairs as the *d*- and *l*-enantiomers, such as *d*-propoxyphene (the analgesic Darvon). Other nomenclature uses the S- and R- or D- and L- prefixes, which are based on the absolute configuration of the atoms in the molecule independent of rotation of

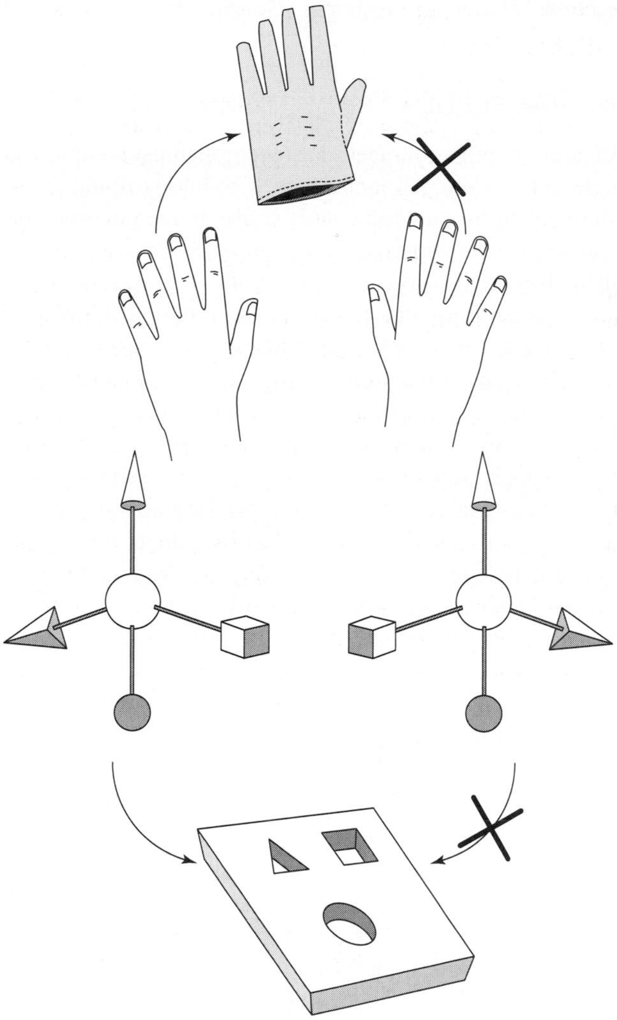

FIGURE 2–14. Stereoselectivity. The right and left human hands are nonsuperimposable mirror images and only the left hand fits well in the left glove. Chiral drugs are also nonsuperimposable mirror images with paired enantiomers. The enantiomer that fits the receptor best has more affinity and elicits the greatest response.

light, such as L-epinephrine. Because the shape of a ligand must be complementary to the receptor, two enantiomers might not fit the receptor equally well, just as a right and left hand do not fit equally well into the left glove. This is called stereoselectivity because one enantiomer has greater affinity for the receptor. Most of the activity of beta blockers is attributed to the *l*-isomers because they have greater affinity (lower K_D) for the receptors than the *d*-isomers. The alpha-beta blocker, labetalol (Normodyne, Trandate), is a chiral drug with an *l*-enantiomer that blocks beta receptors and a *d*-enantiomer that blocks the alpha receptors. For some enantiomers, such as the intravenous anesthetic ketamine, the bronchodilator albuterol, and methylphenidate (Ritalin), it has been hypothesized that one enantiomer causes the beneficial effect and the other enantiomer causes the adverse effects (Brocks & Jamali, 1995). Newly released pure enantiomers levalbuterol (Xopenex) and dexmethylphenidate (Focalin) were developed to exploit the chiral characteristics of albuterol and methylphenidate (Ritalin, others), respectively. The pharmacokinetics of enantiomers may differ, and enantiomer-specific drug interactions with warfarin (Coumadin) have been identified. Drug groups that include numerous agents with chiral properties are nonsteroidal antiinflammatory drugs, beta agonists, beta blockers, calcium channel blockers, warfarin, antiarrhythmics, psychotropics, and anesthetics. Over half of these chiral agents are currently marketed as the racemic mixture containing equal concentrations of the active enantiomer and the inactive (or actively toxic) enantiomer. For example, timolol and naproxen are supplied as the pure active enantiomers, while other beta-blockers and nonsteroidal antiinflammatory drugs are racemates. In the future, researchers, regulatory agencies, and manufacturers are expected to increase emphasis on evaluating the significance of chirality for each drug and modifying the products as necessary. Clinicians can anticipate several new pure enantiomers of established drugs to be released each year.

RECEPTOR-EFFECTOR COUPLING

Coupling encompasses all the chemical and physiologic processes between the drug-receptor binding and the observed clinical effect. As the couplings on a train hold the railroad cars together, receptor-effector coupling is the aspect of pharmacodynamics that links the drug-receptor interaction to the reactions leading to the drug effect, represented by the unidirectional arrows in the equation below:

$$D + R \Leftrightarrow DR \rightarrow \rightarrow \rightarrow \text{Effect}$$

For example, when a patient receives digoxin for congestive heart failure, the clinician may monitor the clinical response using weight and lung sounds. The pharmacologic effects of digoxin are initiated when the digoxin binds to its receptor site on an enzyme in the cardiac muscle cell membrane called Na^+, K^+-ATPase. This enzyme, also known as the sodium pump, normally pumps Na^+ out of the cell in exchange for K^+. The binding of the digoxin to the enzyme decreases its effectiveness, causing accumulation of Na^+ inside the cell that is removed by another pump in exchange for Ca^{2+}. This increases the intracellular concentration of Ca^{2+}. The interaction of the contractile proteins actin and myosin in muscles is inhibited by a protein called troponin C. During the cardiac cycle, Ca^{2+} is released intermittently and it interacts with troponin C to remove the inhibition of actin and myosin, resulting in the periodic muscle contraction of the myocardium. The increased Ca^{2+} inside the cell when digoxin inhibits the sodium pump increases myosin-actin interaction, which is manifested as increased force of myocardial contraction. This improves both pulmonary circulation, resulting in disappearance of rales, and systemic circulation, which decreases edema and triggers weight loss. All these steps represent coupling of digoxin's clinical effects to its drug-receptor interaction.

SIGNAL TRANSDUCTION

In recent years the first step in coupling, signaling, or signal transduction, has been the focus of intense research. Signal transduction involves the molecular mechanisms whereby the binding of drug and receptor, which usually occurs extracellularly, is translated into intracellular messages that control cell function. These mechanisms provide an explanation for the action of some drugs that do not act at receptors such as metformin (Glucophage), and they may provide targets for the development of new drug classes. Figure 2–15 schematically represents the four signaling mechanisms that have been characterized for classical receptor systems: intracellular receptors, transmembranous enzymes, gated channels, and G protein–second messenger systems (Bourne & von Zastrow, 2001).

INTRACELLULAR RECEPTORS

Ligands acting at intracellular receptors must be lipid soluble to cross the cell membrane. The highly lipid-soluble steroidal hormones (glucocorticoids, mineralocorticoids, and sex hormones) bind to receptors in the cytoplasm of the cell. The ligand-receptor complex migrates to the nucleus where it affects genetic transcription by binding to DNA sequences near the gene whose expression is stimulated. The onset of action of drugs working by this mechanism requires a lag period of 30 min to several hours for the synthesis of new proteins that produce the drug effects. This is why corticosteroid therapy is used to prevent rather than treat an asthmatic attack. Similarly, this mechanism is associated with long-lasting effects that persist until the new proteins stimulated by the drugs are metabolized. Other ligands known to work by directly affecting genetic transcription are thyroid hormone and vitamin D. Nitric oxide, an endogenous ligand with an intracellular enzyme, is probably involved in the pharmacodynamics of nitroglycerin and other nitrates.

Transmembranous Enzymes

These transmembranous enzymes consist of a ligand-binding component on the outside of the cell and an enzyme on the cytoplasmic side of the membrane. When the extracellular component binds to the ligand, the protein receptor undergoes conformational change that activates the intracellular enzyme to catalyze a biochemical reac-

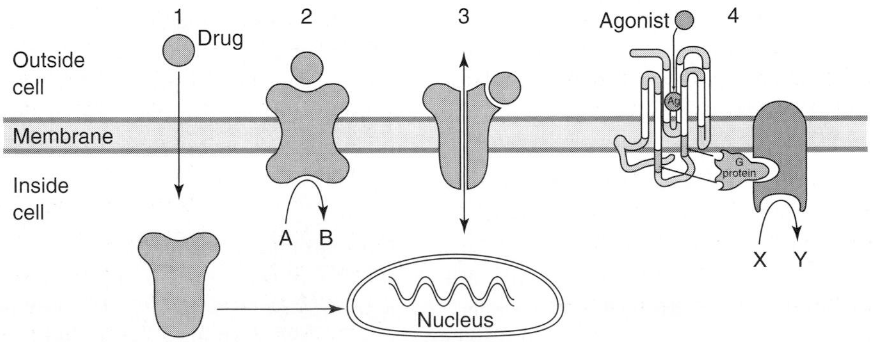

FIGURE 2–15. Signal transduction mechanisms. There are four known signal transduction mechanisms: (**1**) A lipid soluble ligand crosses the membrane and acts on an intracellular receptor, which may be an enzyme or regulator of gene transcription, (**2**) the ligand binds to the extracellular domain of a transmembranous protein, thereby activating an enzymatic activity of its cytoplasmic domain, (**3**) the ligand binds directly to and directly regulates the opening of an ion channel, and (**4**) the ligand binds to a cell surface receptor linked to an effector second messenger by a G protein.

tion. Insulin, growth factors, and atrial natriuretic factor are endogenous ligands with this signaling mechanism.

Gated Channels

Acetylcholine nicotinic receptors, receptors for GABA, and the receptors for the excitatory amino acids glycine, aspartate, and glutamate are proteins that function as gates on ion channels through cell membranes. Binding of ligands to the receptors causes a conformational change that closes or opens the channel. For example, the antianxiety effects of diazepam (Valium) are attributed to binding with a receptor near the GABA receptor, resulting in increased affinity of GABA for its receptor. GABA binding opens chloride channels, and the influx of chloride into the cell inhibits neuronal depolarization. This mechanism occurs within milliseconds, so gated channels are often the signaling mechanism in the nervous system where information must be processed rapidly.

G Proteins and Second Messengers

By binding to an extracellular receptor, a ligand can cause increased concentration of a chemical within the cell called the second messenger. The second messenger goes on to interact with intracellular constituents. Common second messengers are calcium ions, phosphoinositides, and cyclic adenosine 3′,5′-monophosphate (cyclic AMP, or cAMP). These receptor systems usually have three components, the extracellular surface receptor, the G protein located on the internal surface of the membrane, and the second messenger. Interaction of the ligand with the surface receptor, which is commonly of the serpentine type, causes a conformational change in the receptor protein, bringing it into contact with the G protein. This activates an effector element, usually an enzyme or an ion channel, causing an increase in the concentration of the second messenger. For example, the G protein may activate the enzyme adenyl cyclase that catalyzes the conversion of intracellular ATP to cAMP, which goes on to stimulate protein kinases that initiate many intracellular reactions. G proteins with second messengers are the signaling mechanisms for muscarinic receptors for acetylcholine and $alpha_1$ and beta receptors for norepinephrine, serotonin receptors, and many peptide receptors.

RESPONSE VARIABILITY

Some variability in response to drugs can be attributed to changes in the number and coupling efficacy of receptors. This may be due to hormonally induced changes in receptor number and sensitivity, such as occurs with beta-adrenergic receptors in thyrotoxicosis. In addition, drugs can induce receptor changes. Agonist therapy can cause *down-regulation* of the number of receptors, which manifests clinically as tolerance, increasing dose requirements to achieve the therapeutic response. The tolerance to $beta_2$-adrenergic agonist bronchodilators in asthma has been attributed to receptor down-regulation in which the receptors are taken into the cell by endocytosis and metabolized. Antagonist therapy can result in *up-regulation,* an increase in the number of receptors. Beta blockers must be tapered when they are discontinued, because abrupt withdrawal can cause rebound hypertension, angina, or even fatal myocardial infarction. The rebound is attributed to beta receptor up-regulation during therapy; with sudden discontinuation of the blocker, the increased number of receptors is suddenly accessible to endogenous norepinephrine.

TYPES OF ANTAGONISTS

Receptor antagonists are classified as *competitive antagonists* and *irreversible antagonists.* Competitive or surmountable antagonism exists when increased concentration of agonist will overcome the receptor blockade. Opioid receptor blockade by naloxone (Narcan) is reversed if more opioid agonist, such as morphine, is administered. This blockade is called *competitive* because the agonist and antagonist molecules compete to occupy the receptors, and the ligand with the greatest affinity (lowest K_D and greatest concentration at the receptor site) will dominate. Figure 2-16*a* shows that a competitive antagonist shifts the concentration-response curve to the right, requiring a greater dose of the agonist to get the maximal effect. *Irreversible antagonism* occurs if increased concentration of agonist does not overcome the blockade. Also called *noncompetitive antagonism,* it is thought to be due to binding of the antagonist by strong covalent chemical bonds or binding near the receptor, causing a conformational change in the receptor that prevents the agonist from binding to it. Figure 2-16*a* indicates that an irreversible antagonist decreases the maximal efficacy attainable from the agonist. An example of an irreversible antagonist is the alpha-adrenergic blocker phenoxybenzamine (Dibenzyline) used to treat pheochromocytoma, a hypertensive disease characterized by periodic release of large amounts of norepinephrine. If a competitive antagonist like prazosin (Minipress) is used in pheochromocytoma, it is displaced by norepinephrine when the hypertensive crisis occurs, but phenoxybenza-

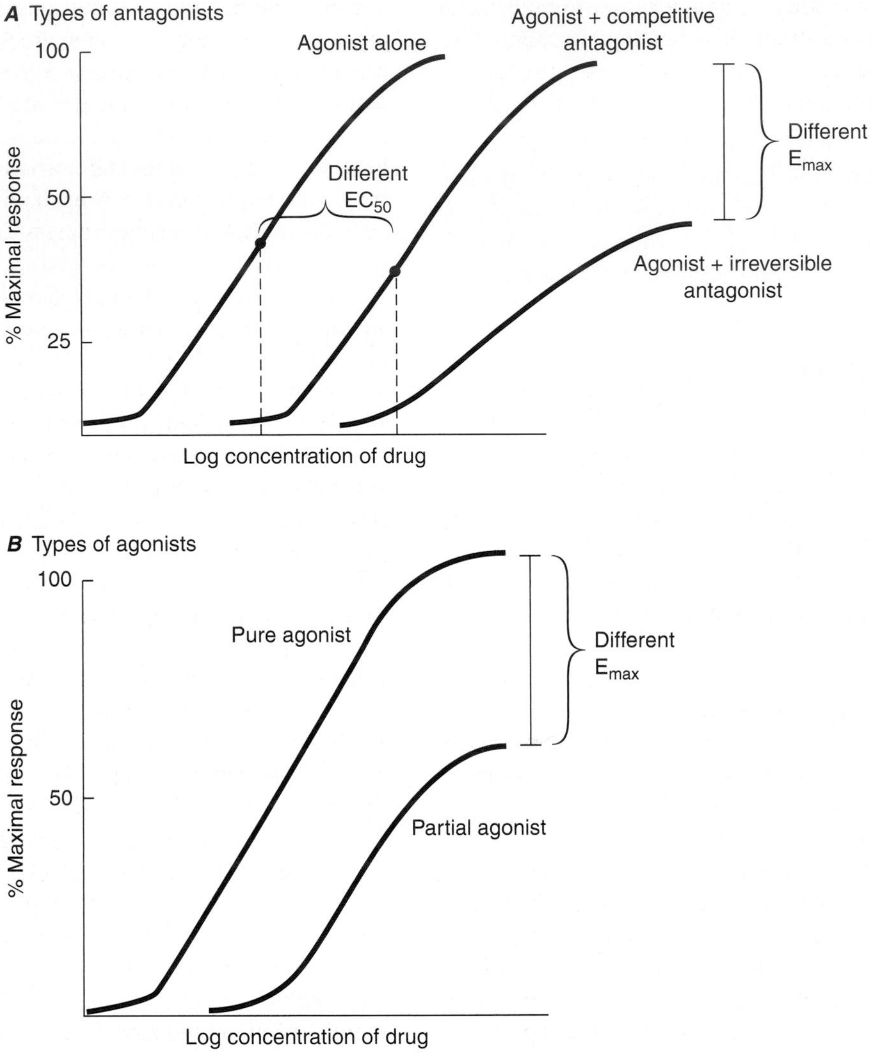

FIGURE 2–16. Concentration-response curves for various agonists and antagonist types. (a) There are two types of receptor antagonists. Competitive antagonists do not affect the maximal efficacy (E_{max}) of an agonist, but do increase the dosage required to elicit a response of a particular magnitude (EC_{50}). Irreversible antagonists decrease maximal efficacy and cannot be reversed regardless of the amount of agonist added. (b) Partial agonists do not elicit the magnitude of maximal effect (E_{max}) as do full agonists.

mine is not displaced regardless of how much norepinephrine is released.

The term *antagonism,* which has specific meaning related to receptor antagonists, is also used generally for neutralization of the effects of one drug by another, regardless of mechanism. Even drugs that interact pharmacokinetically, such as drugs that prevent absorption of other drugs, are sometimes called antagonists. In addition to pharmacokinetic antagonism and receptor antagonism, drugs can counteract the effects of others drugs through *chemical antagonism* and *functional antagonism.* An example of chemical antagonism is the acid-base reaction that causes the reversal of heparin effects by protamine sulfate. Functional or physiologic antagonism involves the counteracting of one drug by another through a different receptor system on a different physiologic pathway. For example, bradycardia caused by the beta-adrenergic receptor blocker propranolol (Inderal) can be reversed by administering the cholinergic receptor blocker atropine. Propranolol decreases the heart rate by blocking receptors in the sympathetic nervous system, whereas atropine antagonizes the inhibitory action of the parasympathetic nervous system by blocking receptors for the vagus nerve.

TYPES OF AGONISTS

Two types of agonists have been identified based on the maximum pharmacologic effect attained when all the receptors are occupied. Most drugs are *full agonists* that elicit the total capability of the receptor system when given in sufficient doses. As shown in Figure 2-16*b*, *partial agonists* do not elicit this maximal response, and have a lower E_{max} even when the receptors are fully occupied. In fact, in the presence of a full agonist, a partial agonist functions as a competitive antagonist, reversing the agonist effects. Buprenorphine (Buprenex) is a partial agonist at the mu opioid receptors and cannot provide, even at maximal doses, as much analgesia as the full mu agonist morphine. Some drugs are *agonist-antagonists,* operating as agonists at one receptor subtype and antagonists at another subtype. The opioid nalbuphine (Nubain) is an agonist at kappa receptors and an antagonist at mu receptors. Agonist-antagonists also can reverse the effects of full agonists. Administered to a patient who has a full mu receptor agonist present, such as morphine, nalbuphine reverses the analgesic effects of the mu receptor. If the patient is physically dependent on morphine, nalbuphine will elicit withdrawal symptoms.

PHARMACODYNAMIC DRUG INTERACTIONS

Many pharmacodynamic drug interactions involve antagonism by one of the mechanisms described above. Other important interactions are additive effects, in which the combination of two drugs increases the intensity of a drug response. This can occur through the same receptor system, such as the combination of prazosin (Minipress) for high blood pressure and thioridazine (Mellaril) for schizophrenia. Both block alpha receptors, so they have additive hypotensive effects. Additive effects also can occur through separate physiologic and pharmacologic pathways. Both prazosin (Minipress) and the diuretic hydrochlorothiazide decrease blood pressure, but through entirely different mechanisms. Although the prescriber purposely can use drugs for their additive therapeutic benefits, many additive effects result in an adverse response. In both of the previous examples, the additive effects could lead to hypotension, syncope, and falls.

ADVERSE DRUG EFFECTS

The nomenclature for adverse drug effects includes many overlapping and imprecise terms, such as iatrogenic disease, drug-induced disease, side effect, toxic effect, and idiosyncratic reaction. In 1986 Kellaway formulated the classification of adverse drug effects shown in Table 2–7 for use in helping patients to identify harmful and nuisance adverse effects. An important distinction in this classification is the differentiation of *unwanted pharmacologic effects,* which are predictable based upon the drug-receptor interactions, and pathologic reactions that are the unpredictable emergence of a disease condition unrelated to the activity of the drug at receptors, such as the development of anaphylaxis, cancer, or neutropenia. The first column of Table 2-7 lists Kellaway's five types of adverse drug effects (ADE). The second column describes the mechanism. For adverse drug effects that are receptor mediated, the mechanism depends on whether the adverse effect is elicited at the same receptor or same effector organ as the beneficial effect. Often the pathologic mechanism is hypersensitivity, an antigen-antibody allergic reaction mediated by the immune system.

CLINICAL IMPLICATIONS OF PHARMACODYNAMICS

The understanding of pharmacodynamic properties plays a major role in the selection of a drug to treat a disease or symptom. To ignore this consideration is prescribing by rote, putting patients at risk for inappropriate or harmful therapy. The pharmacodynamics of adverse drug effects also merits attention, since appropriate prevention, management, and patient education derives from a thorough understanding of the mechanisms of the adverse effects. Too often patient education about adverse effects is merely a list of potential effects, but unless patients are taught how to detect the effects and what to do if an

TABLE 2–7. Classification of Adverse Drug Effects

Category	Mechanism	Examples	
		Drug/Group	*Adverse Effect*
Excessive therapeutic effect	Same receptor/same effector	Metoclopramide (Reglan)	Diarrhea
		Anticoagulants	Bleeding
		Thrombolytics	Bleeding
		Antidiabetic agents	Hypoglycemia
		Antihypertensives	Hypotension
		Sedatives	Stupor/coma
Unwanted pharmacologic effect	Same receptor/different effector	Opioids	Constipation
		Haloperidol (Haldol)	Parkinsonism
		Trihexyphenidyl (Artane)	Dry mouth
		Terbutaline (Brethine)	Hyperglycemia
		Nitroglycerin	Headache
		Verapamil (Isoptin, Calan)	Constipation
	Different receptor/different effector	Propranolol (Inderal)	Dyspnea
		Chlorpheniramine (Chlor-Trimeton)	Drowsiness
		Haloperidol (Haldol)	Dry mouth
		Erythromycin	Diarrhea
		Penicillin	Seizures
		Thioridazine (Mellaril)	Hypotension
		ACE inhibitors	Nonproductive cough
Pathological reactions	Hypersensitivity	Captopril (Capoten)	Neutropenia
		Penicillin	Anaphylaxis
		Sulfonamides	Stevens-Johnson syndrome
	Teratogenesis	Lithium	Cardiovascular defects
		Warfarin (Coumadin)	Hypoplastic nasal bridge, chondrodysplasia
	Carcinogenesis	Chemotherapeutic agents	Various cancers
		Glucocorticoids	Various cancers
	Other, unknown	Acetaminophen (Tylenol)	Nephritis
		HMG CoA reductase inhibitors	Rhabdomyolysis
Superinfection	Inhibits normal flora	Tetracycline	Vaginal candidiasis
		Broad-spectrum antibiotics	Pseudomembranous colitis
Drug interaction	Pharmacokinetic	Erythromycin theophylline	Theophylline toxicity
	Pharmacodynamic	Opioid + Antihistamine	Somnolence

effect occurs, their ability to participate in self-care is limited. Not all adverse effects need to be reported to the clinician in a midnight call, but evaluation of many adverse effects should not be deferred until the next visit. Based upon the classification of adverse effects in Table 2–7, excessive therapeutic effects, pathological reactions, superinfection, and drug interaction require consultation with the prescriber or healthcare provider within hours to days of when they are first detected. Most unwanted pharmacologic effects are transient and can be managed by the patient, but if the effect is severe, bothersome, or continuous, it should be reported to a healthcare professional. Since these effects are predictable based upon the pharmacodynamics of the drug, the clinician can provide anticipatory counseling on how to avoid the effect and how to minimize its impact on comfort and functional status if it occurs.

Prevention and management of adverse effects will vary depending upon the type of adverse effect. The two most common types are excessive therapeutic effects and unwanted pharmacologic effects. Excessive therapeutic effects occur when the adverse and therapeutic responses are produced at the same receptor on the same effector, such as postural hypotension caused by the antihypertensive prazosin (Minipress). Pharmacologic options for prevention or management of excessive therapeutic effects are minimizing the dose, which could compromise the therapeutic response; choosing a drug from a different drug group; or prescribing multidrug therapy to minimize the dose of each agent, such as adding a diuretic to another antihypertensive. Replacing the drug with nonpharmacologic therapy could be considered, depending upon severity and sequelae of the condition. Using a drug to treat an adverse effect of another drug is usually contraindicated, but nonpharmacologic interventions such as teaching the patient with postural hypotension to change position slowly and keep well-hydrated may render the adverse effects tolerable.

There are two types of unwanted pharmacologic effects. The first occurs when the therapeutic and adverse effects involve the same receptor subtype on different effector organs, such as hyperglycemia from oral albuterol (Proventil) for asthma. Any of the options listed for managing an excessive therapeutic effect may be beneficial, but consideration should also be given to prescribing the medication via a route that maximizes the drug concentration at the site of the receptors for the therapeutic effect, such as administering albuterol by inhalation. The second mechanism of unwanted pharmacologic effects involves different receptors on different organs for the therapeutic and adverse effects, which can be avoided by prescribing a more selective drug in the same drug group. For example, if a nonselective beta blocker such as propranolol (Inderal) causes dyspnea, a cardioselective agent like atenolol (Tenormin) could be tried, or any of the strategies proposed above for other mechanisms of adverse effects could also be used.

CONCLUSION

Three phases of drug action—pharmaceutics, pharmacokinetics, and pharmacodynamics—mediate variability in drug response. By understanding the processes and mechanisms for each phase, the prescriber is able to select optimal drug therapy for each patient's unique response patterns. One of the greatest challenges of pharmacotherapeutics is keeping up with the rapid advances in the field of pharmacology; it has been proposed that the half-life of pharmacology knowledge is less than five years. Understanding of the underlying principles of pharmaceutics, pharmacokinetics, and pharmacodynamics also allows the clinician to adapt to this rapidly changing environment and to critically appraise the therapeutic significance of the new developments.

REFERENCES

Bourne, H. R., & von Zastrow, W. (2001). Drug receptors and pharmacodynamics. In B. G. Katzung (Ed.), *Basic and clinical pharmacology* (8th ed.). Norwalk, CT: Appleton & Lange.

Brocks, D. R., & Jamali, F. (1995). Stereochemical aspects of pharmacotherapy. *Pharmacotherapy, 15,* 551–564.

Flockhart, D. A., & Tanus-Santos, J. E. (2002). Implications of cytochrome P450 interactions when prescribing medication for hypertension. *Archives of Internal Medicine, 162* (4), 405–12,

Food and Drug Administration. (2002). *Electronic Orange Book of approved drug products with therapeutic equivalence evaluations.* http://www.fda.gov/cder/ob/default.htm.

Freher, M., Challapalli, S., Pinto, J. V., Schwartz, J., & Bonow, R. O., & Gheorgiade, M. (1999). Current status of calcium channel blockers in patients with cardiovascular disease. *Current Problems in Cardiology, 24* (5), 236–340.

Hansten, P. D. & Horn, J. R. (2000). *Hansten and Horn's drug interactions, analysis and management.* St. Louis, MO: Facts and Comparisons.

Kellaway, G. (1986). The patient. In W. H. W. Inman (Ed.), *Monitoring for drug safety* (2nd ed., pp. 637–649). Boston: MTP Press.

Otani, K., & Aoshima, T. (2000). Pharmacogenetics of classical and new antipsychotic drugs. *Therapeutic Drug Monitoring, 22* (1), 118–121.

Pepper, G. A. (1997). The perils of P450. *Clinical Letter for Nurse Practitioners, 1* (1), 7–8.

Pepper, G. A. (1999). Pharmacology of antihypertensive drugs. *JOGNN, 28,* 649–659

Tatro, D. S. (2002). *Drug interaction facts.* St. Louis, MD: Facts and Comparisons.

Trujillo, T. C., & Nolan, P. E. (2001). Ischemic heart disease: Anginal syndromes. In M. A. Koda-Kimble & L. L. Young (Eds.), *Applied therapeutics: The clinical use of drugs* (7th ed., pp. 15.17–15.18). Philadelphia: Lippincott Williams & Wilkins.

APPENDIX 2–1

CALCULATING LOADING DOSES

Because the danger of exceeding toxic levels is substantial, loading doses are reserved for urgent situations when it is critical to attain steady-state plasma concentrations immediately. Usually loading doses are given by intravenous bolus and followed by an intravenous infusion to maintain the desired plasma concentration, but a loading dose can be given orally as a single dose or divided into several doses given at intervals of several hours to allow the drug to distribute between doses. Digoxin is sometimes "loaded" in hospitalized patients using this divided oral dose method. Since the function of a loading dose is to fill up the distribution volume in a single dose, rather than over the four half-lives usually required to approximate the steady state, the key parameters required to compute the loading dose are volume of distribution (V_D) and the desired plasma concentration (C_p). If the drug is given orally, bioavailability (F) must also be considered. All three parameters can be found in standard references. The formula for computing loading dose is:

$$\text{Loading dose} = \frac{V_D \times C_p}{F}$$

Example: To compute the loading dose of theophylline for a 50-kg adolescent female, the clinician must first determine the target plasma concentration (C_p). The therapeutic range for theophylline is 10 to 20 μg/mL. Because it is prudent to begin in the lower end of the therapeutic range, the C_p selected is 10 μg/mL. The V_D reported in standard references must be adjusted for the weight of the patient. From Table 2–3 the V_D of theophylline is 0.5 L/kg or 25 L for this 50-kg patient. Since the bioavailability of theophylline is 0.96, it is virtually 1.0, which is used in the calculation. The loading dose of 250 mg was calculated as follows:

$$\begin{aligned}\text{Loading dose} &= \frac{25\text{L} \times [10\ \mu\text{g/mL}]}{1.0} \\ &= 25{,}000\ \text{mL} \times 10\ \mu\text{g/mL} \\ &= 250{,}000\ \mu\text{g} = 250\ \text{mg}\end{aligned}$$

APPENDIX 2–2

CALCULATING MAINTENANCE DOSES

The dose of a drug prescribed is generally based upon the usual dosage recommended by the manufacturer, modified by clinical considerations such as patient weight. For drugs with narrow therapeutic ranges that are followed by laboratory drug assays (blood levels), computation of maintenance dose individualizes the dosage for a desired plasma concentration. The goal of maintenance dosing is to replace the drug that is eliminated during each dosing interval, so that the target plasma concentration is sustained. Therefore, the critical parameters in calculating maintenance dose are the clearance (CL) and the desired therapeutic concentration (C_p). Since maintenance doses are usually given orally, bioavailability (F) and dosing interval (τ or tau) are considered. The formula for calculation of maintenance dose is:

$$\text{Maintenance dose} = \frac{C_L \times C_p}{F} \times \tau$$

Example: The clinician wants to compute the maintenance dose of theophylline required to sustain a plasma concentration of 12 μg/mL for a 50-kg adolescent using an immediate-release dosage form administered three times daily. The target C_p was historically determined from patient responses to various plasma concentrations of theophylline. CL may be computed from individualized pharmacokinetic studies or obtained from standard references. The dosing interval (τ) is 8 h, based upon the usual frequency of dosing with the preparation selected. Bioavailability *(F)* of 0.96 is used for illustration, although it is so close to 1.0 that it might be omitted from the calculation. The CL of 0.04 L/h per kg from Table 2–6 adjusted for the patient's weight is 2.0 L/h. The maintenance dose of 200 mg t.i.d. was computed as follows:

$$\begin{aligned}\text{Maintenance dose} &= \frac{2\text{L/h} \times 12\ \mu\text{g/mL}}{0.96} \times 8\text{h} \\ &= \frac{2000\ \text{mL/h} \times 12\ \mu\text{g/mL}}{0.96} \times 8\text{h} \\ &= \frac{24{,}000\ \mu\text{g/h}}{0.96} \times 8\text{h} \\ &= 200{,}000\ \mu\text{g/dose} \\ &= 200\ \text{mg t.i.d.}\end{aligned}$$

APPENDIX 2–3

ADJUSTING DOSAGE USING LABORATORY DRUG LEVELS

Even if a maintenance dose was calculated for a particular patient using values from standardized tables, the measured plasma concentration might not equal the target plasma concentration. Patients vary widely from the average values in standardized tables in actual absorption, liver function, and renal function. The dose (D_2) required to attain a desired plasma concentration for a particular patient can be computed from the current dose (D_1), the current plasma concentration (C_1), and the desired plasma concentration (C_2) using the following formula:

$$\frac{D_1}{D_2} = \frac{C_1}{C_2}$$

Example: The plasma concentration for a 14-year-old girl taking theophylline 200 mg t.i.d. is 10 μg/mL. She is experiencing dyspnea and wheezing and her past history indicates plasma theophylline concentrations of 14 μg/mL are required for disease control. The new dose of theophylline of 280 mg t.i.d. was computed as follows:

$$\frac{200\ \text{mg}}{D_2} = \frac{10\ \mu\text{g/mL}}{14\ \mu\text{g/mL}}$$
$$D_2 = 280\ \text{mg}$$

If the dose is raised to 280 mg and the target plasma concentration is not attained, the clinician should check to see that the blood samples for drug assay are collected at the proper time to ensure appropriate values.

CHAPTER ❖ 3

PHARMACOTHERAPEUTIC IMPACT OF RENAL OR HEPATIC DYSFUNCTION

Thomas J. Comstock

GENERAL CONSIDERATIONS

Dosage regimen design for patients with renal and/or hepatic impairment requires knowledge of the pharmacokinetic characteristics of a drug as well as the physiologic changes that occur as a result of the decreased organ function. Pharmacokinetic changes that accompany organ dysfunction usually are manifested as decreased elimination, such as decreased metabolism by the liver and decreased excretion by the kidneys, but also may be manifested as changes in absorption and distribution.

Overall drug elimination from the body can be considered as the sum of elimination by two primary pathways, such that the total rate of elimination from the body is equal to renal plus nonrenal elimination, where nonrenal elimination is predominantly hepatic metabolism.

As a general rule, when a drug is eliminated more than 30% by an organ system, then impairment of that organ system may necessitate changes in the dosage regimen in order to avoid excessive accumulation of the drug and subsequent toxicity. The degree of organ impairment and the fraction of the drug that normally is eliminated by that route determine the amount of change in a dosage regimen. Drugs with a narrow therapeutic range—for example, digoxin 1 to 2 μg/L or phenytoin 10 to 20 mg/L—will require more individualization of the regimen and closer monitoring compared to those with a wider therapeutic range, such as many analgesic compounds.

Although drug elimination is an important consideration, changes in absorption and distribution of drugs also may occur with organ dysfunction. This chapter will focus on the pharmacokinetic alterations that occur with drugs administered to patients with liver or kidney disease and the actions the clinician should take to optimize the dosage regimen in order to obtain the desired clinical outcome and avoid unnecessary toxicity.

ASSESSMENT OF ORGAN FUNCTION

Adjustment of dosage regimens is dependent on some knowledge of organ function. Whereas renal function can be estimated using several clinical tools, hepatic function is not easily quantified. Despite this limitation, an understanding of the processes involved in drug elimination by the liver is useful as a guide to clinical decision making.

HEPATIC FUNCTION

The levels of the hepatic enzymes aspartate aminotransferase (AST) and alanine aminotransferase (ALT), commonly referred to as "liver function tests," are not useful as quantitative measures of hepatic drug metabolism. These enzymes are increased under conditions of hepatic inflammation, such as acute hepatitis, but do not reflect drug elimination capability. Drug clearance by the liver is complex and related to hepatic blood flow, plasma protein binding of a drug, and intrinsic hepatic clearance. A drug is delivered to the liver via the portal vein (~1050 mL/min) and hepatic artery (~350 mL/min) and is present within the blood in equilibrium between the protein-bound and unbound states. The primary driving force for hepatic blood flow is cardiac output, which may be significantly reduced during heart failure. As a drug flows through the liver, the unbound drug is able to move into the hepatocyte, where it may undergo metabolism and/or biliary excretion. Formed metabolites then are able to reenter the systemic circulation or be excreted in the bile. The fraction of a drug that is removed, or cleared, as it passes through the liver is the hepatic extraction ratio (E), which has a range in value from 0 to 1. The pharmacokinetic parameter that best describes drug elimination is clearance. As discussed in Chapter 2, clearance is the volume of plasma that is cleared totally of a drug per unit time. For example, the clearance of theophylline in a nonsmoking adult is 40 mL/min. Clearance of a drug by an individual organ is the product of the flow through the organ and the extraction ratio of the drug. For drugs with a high extraction ratio, the hepatic clearance approaches hepatic blood flow, and any change in hepatic blood flow will have a proportionate effect on hepatic elimination of the drug.

Drugs eliminated by hepatic metabolism can be considered as high-, middle-, or low extraction drugs based on the fraction of the drug that is removed as blood flows through the liver. High extraction drugs are characterized by $E > 0.7$, middle as $0.3 < E < 0.7$, and low as $E < 0.3$. Whereas hepatic blood flow is the primary determinant for the removal of high extraction ratio drugs, elimination of low extraction ratio drugs is dependent on plasma protein binding and intrinsic clearance. Intrinsic clearance refers to the ability of the liver (hepatocytes) to eliminate the drug without the restrictions of blood flow or protein binding. Generally, this refers to the ability of the liver to metabolize the drug. Drugs in this category are susceptible to drug interactions from drugs such as cimetidine that compete for metabolizing enzymes or to induction of enzymes by drugs such as rifampin and phenobarbital, resulting in an increased elimination of other drugs and subtherapeutic plasma concentrations. Examples of high and low extraction drugs are included in Table 3–1.

TABLE 3–1. Examples of High and Low Hepatic Extraction Drugs

High Extraction	Low Extraction
Propranolol	Theophylline
Lidocaine	Warfarin
Verapamil	Phenytoin
Meperidine	Ibuprofen
Morphine	Procainamide
Nitroglycerin	Phenobarbital

Drug metabolizing enzymes of the liver are categorized broadly as being responsible for Phase I reactions (synthetic) or Phase II reactions (conjugation). Phase I reactions consist of oxidation, reduction, hydrolysis, and others, and may result in formation of an "active" metabolite, such as the demethylation of codeine to form morphine. A large group of enzymes responsible for many of the Phase I oxidative reactions is the cytochrome P-450 system (sometimes referred to as microsomal enzymes). This set of enzymes can be subdivided into approximately twenty different isozymes, such as CYP2D6 and CYP3A4. Each isozyme is responsible for a different metabolic pathway. The presence and quantity of these isozymes is genetically determined, which in part accounts for variability in pharmacokinetics among individuals. As a result of these oxidative pathways, metabolites then may be further metabolized to other species or eliminated in the urine. Metabolism of a drug by Phase II or conjugation reactions (such as glucuronidation, sulfation, or acetylation) results in larger, more polar compounds, which are subsequently eliminated either in the urine or through the biliary system into the gastrointestinal tract (GIT). Active metabolites also may result from this process as well, such as the formation of *N*-acetylprocainamide from the acetylation of procainamide. Elimination of some glucuronide conjugates into the GIT may undergo hydrolysis by β-glucuronidase with subsequent reabsorption of the parent compound, a process known as enterohepatic recycling (Rowland & Tozer, 1995).

The numerous metabolic pathways through which drug elimination occurs in the liver have precluded identification of a single test to quantitate hepatic metabolic function. Furthermore, hepatic blood flow and plasma protein binding are also determinants of hepatic drug clearance. Attempts have been made to use markers representative of the various drug elimination pathways through the liver, including antipyrine and aminopyrine for Phase I metabolism, lorazepam for Phase II metabolism, and indocyanine green (ICG) for hepatic blood flow. These markers have been shown to distinguish between patients with hepatic cirrhosis and normal subjects, but have not been proven effective for quantitation of hepatic function within these extremes. The tests are potential research tools but have limited use in the clinic.

More appropriate clinical tools to assess hepatic drug metabolism include a combination of the serum albumin and bilirubin concentrations as well as the prothrombin time. Individually, abnormal tests are not indicative of hepatic dysfunction, but when taken together may reflect severe hepatic disease such as cirrhosis. For example, several conditions may lead to hypoalbuminemia, including not only cirrhosis, but also malabsorption, malnutrition, and nephrotic syndrome. An albumin value of <2.5 g/dL is consistent with hepatic cirrhosis, since it reflects the decreased synthetic capacity of the liver. Likewise, a prolonged prothrombin time > 15 s in a patient not receiving warfarin may suggest severe hepatic disease, reflecting decreased synthesis of clotting factors and other synthetic activity within the liver. Elevation of the bilirubin concentration is suggestive of an inability to excrete bilirubin and thus hepatobiliary disease. Together, abnormalities in these markers point toward severe hepatic dysfunction and should be considered as a sign of decreased drug elimination by the liver. A scoring system for cirrhosis, which includes these tests as well as other clinical signs, has been used as a semi-quantitative assessment of hepatic function and is shown in Table 3–2 (Pugh, Murray-Lyon, Dawson, Pietroni, & Williams, 1973).

RENAL FUNCTION

Each kidney normally consists of approximately 1 million nephrons, the functional unit. Excretion of a drug through the nephron is achieved through the net combination of filtration, secretion, and reabsorption. Filtration is accomplished at the glomerulus and allows for the passive movement of protein-free plasma from the glomerulus into the proximal tubule. The concentration of solute in the early proximal tubule is similar to the unbound concentration in the plasma. Secretion occurs by an active transport process whereby drug is carried from the peritubular capillary circulation, across the tubular cell, and into the tubular lumen. Reabsorption of drug generally occurs as a passive process in the collecting tubule, moving from the tubule into the circulation. Factors such as urine flow and pH of the urine may influence tubular reabsorption. Increased urine flow will decrease reabsorption, and an increase in urine pH for weak acids (e.g., salicylate) or decreased pH for weak bases (e.g., amphetamine) will decrease reabsorption by trapping the ionized form of the drug in the lumen, resulting in increased urinary excretion.

Measurement of kidney function is based on the premise that filtration, secretion, and reabsorption all change in parallel when there is a loss of functional nephrons. This concept is known as *Bricker's intact nephron hypothesis,* which states that net kidney function is proportional to the number of functional nephrons. Based on this, measurement of the glomerular filtration rate (GFR) provides an assessment of overall function.

Approximately 20% of cardiac output perfuses the kidney, at 1200 mL/min. Renal plasma flow is therefore about 625 mL/min, after correcting the renal blood flow for hematocrit. The filtration fraction of plasma across the glomerulus is 20%, and the resultant glomerular filtration rate is about 125 mL/min in individuals with normal kidney function. Determination of the GFR can be accomplished by measuring the renal clearance of a solute that is freely filtered across the glomerulus, is not protein-bound, and does not undergo tubular secretion or reabsorption. The "gold standard" test for measurement of GFR is inulin clearance, but it has limited use in the clinical setting. A more common marker for GFR is creatinine, an endogenous product of muscle metabolism. Creatinine is also not bound to plasma proteins, is freely filtered across the glomerulus, and is not reabsorbed. Unlike inulin, approximately 10% of the elimination of creatinine by the kidneys is due to tubular secretion in subjects with normal kidney function. As renal function declines, the fraction of creatinine that is secreted increases to about 50%, so that the creatinine clearance overestimates GFR in patients with reduced kidney function. Despite this limitation, it is the most useful clinical marker for renal function and drug elimination by the kidneys (Comstock, 1997). Urea, or the blood urea nitrogen (BUN) concentration, has also been suggested as a marker of renal function. Although it also is freely

TABLE 3–2. Pugh's Criteria for the Assessment of Hepatic Cirrhosis

Criterion	1 point	2 points	3 points
Encephalopathy (grade)	None	1 or 2	3 or 4
Ascites	Absent	Slight	Moderate
Bilirubin (mg/dL)	1–2	2–3	>3
Albumin (g/dL)	>3.5	2.8–3.5	<2.8
Prothrombin time (s > control)	1–4	4–10	>10

Scoring system: 5–6 total points = mild dysfunction; 7–9 = moderate dysfunction; > 9 = severe dysfunction
Source: Pugh et al. (1973).

filtered at the glomerulus and is not protein-bound, it does undergo substantial reabsorption, particularly under conditions of decreased effective circulating volume, such as volume depletion, congestive heart failure, ascites, or nephrotic syndrome. Urea is an ineffective osmole and is able to freely cross cell membranes. It follows water, and the above conditions all result in increased water reabsorption from the proximal tubule. The subsequent decrease in urea excretion, and elevated BUN are not a reflection of kidney function or GFR. Creatinine does not undergo appreciable reabsorption, which accounts for the elevated BUN:creatinine ratio under these conditions.

Creatinine clearance can be determined by direct measurement of the creatinine excretion rate or estimated using population-based equations. Measurement of creatinine clearance requires collection of a timed urine sample, usually 24 h, although shorter collection times may be used (2 to 4 h) and are as accurate as 24-h collections. Ideally, a midpoint serum creatinine concentration is measured, although it is more convenient to collect the sample at the end of the timed interval, as long as the patient has stable kidney function. Calculation of the measured creatinine clearance is as follows:

$$CL_{cr}, \text{mL/min} = (V_{urine} \times C_{urine})/(C_{serum} \times \text{time})$$

where:

V_{urine} = total volume of the urine collection
C_{urine} = concentration of creatinine in the urine sample
C_{serum} = concentration of creatinine in the serum sample
time = duration of the urine collection

For example, a 55-year-old man (70 kg), who is instructed to collect his urine for 24 h, returns to the clinic with a container holding 1360 mL of urine. The concentration of creatinine in the urine is reported to be 92 mg/dL, and his plasma creatinine concentration is 1.4 mg/dL. His creatinine clearance is:

$$CL_{cr} = \frac{1360 \text{ mL} \times 92 \text{ mg/dL}}{1.4 \text{ mg/dL} \times 1440 \text{ min}} = 62 \text{ mL/min}$$

It often is inconvenient to perform a measured creatinine clearance, and inaccurate collections can lead to falsely low measures of kidney function (e.g., if all of the urine is not collected). Often it is more convenient to estimate kidney function. The Cockcroft–Gault estimation method for creatinine clearance was described initially in 1976 and has served as a useful tool to estimate kidney function in adult patients:

$$CL_{cr}\ (\text{male}), \text{mL/min} = \frac{(140 - \text{age})\text{IBW}}{72(S_{cr})}$$

$$CL_{cr}\ (\text{female}) = CL_{cr}\ (\text{male}) \times 0.85$$

where:

S_{cr} = serum creatine concentration (mg/dL)
IBW = ideal body weight, kg
IBW(male) = 50 kg + 2.3 kg for every 1 in > 5 ft in height
IBW(female) = 45.5 kg + 2.3 kg for every 1 in > 5 ft in height

This method provides the individualized creatinine clearance. A normalized clearance based on 72 kg is:

$$CL_{cr}\ (\text{male}), \text{mL/min/72 kg} = (140 - \text{age, years})/S_{cr}$$

$$CL_{cr}\ (\text{female}) = CL_{cr}(\text{male}) \times 0.85$$

For the previous example, the creatinine clearance is estimated as:

$$CL_{cr} = \frac{140 - 55}{1.4} = 61 \text{ mL/min/72 kg}$$

The measured and estimated creatinine clearances are not always similar, and consideration must be given to factors that will alter the plasma creatinine concentration, since it is the primary measured determinant of the estimated creatinine clearance.

Patients with very low body mass or those with spinal cord injuries are not good candidates for estimation of creatinine clearance since the creatinine production rate is very low and the creatinine clearance is falsely elevated. Furthermore, false elevations of the serum creatinine concentration may occur with exercise or some medications, such as cimetidine or trimethoprim, and may falsely lower the estimate of kidney function. The blood sample for measurement of creatinine should be not be obtained following the ingestion of a meat meal, as the creatinine in the meat will be absorbed and falsely elevate the patient's

TABLE 3–3. Common Factors Interfering with the Interpretation of Creatinine Clearance as a Measure of Kidney Function

Elevation of Serum Creatinine	Mechanism
Acetoacetate	Analytical interference
Ascorbic acid	Analytical interference
Cephalosporins	Analytical interference
5-Flucytosine	Analytical interference
Exercise	Increased production
Diet (meat ingestion)	Absorption
Drugs (cimetidine, trimethoprim, probenecid)	Decreased tubular secretion

creatinine concentration. Preferably, the sample should be obtained in the morning before a meal is ingested. These conditions and others are listed in Table 3–3.

Estimation of kidney function in pediatric patients can be accomplished after considering developmental changes in renal function following birth. Renal function rapidly approaches normal values, corrected for body size, within the first year of life and can be estimated according to Schwartz, Feld, and Langford (1984), as follows:

$$CL_{cr}\ \text{mL/min per } 1.73\ \text{m}^2 = (0.45 \times \text{height, cm})/S_{cr}$$

For patients in the range of 1 to 12 years, the following equation by Schwartz, Haycock, Edelman, and Spitzer (1976) should be used:

$$CL_{cr}\ \text{mL/min per } 1.73\ \text{m}^2 = (0.55 \times \text{height, cm})/S_{cr}$$

DOSING ISSUES

HEPATIC IMPAIRMENT

Whereas it is difficult to quantify hepatic metabolic function because of the vast array of factors influencing drug elimination and the multiple metabolic pathways, certain pharmacokinetic changes may be anticipated based on drug characteristics in patients with hepatic cirrhosis (Brouwer, Dukes, & Powell, 1992). The half-life ($t_{1/2}$) for elimination of a drug is determined by both the clearance (CL) of the drug from the body and its volume of distribution (V_D). A decreased clearance or an increased V_D results in a prolonged elimination half-life. The relationship between these parameters is $t_{1/2} = (0.693 \times V_D)/\text{CL}$. When the clearance of a drug is reduced in hepatic failure and the volume of distribution is increased, such as for a protein-bound, high extraction drug such as lidocaine, there will be pronounced effects on the elimination half-life and caution must be exercised in patients with severe hepatic disease.

Drug absorption following oral administration involves disintegration (for solid dosage forms), dissolution, and absorption. The absorption process involves passage of drug molecules through the wall of the GIT and into the portal circulation where they are then delivered to the liver before entry into the systemic circulation. Both the GIT and liver are capable of drug metabolism during the absorption process, and the bioavailability of the absorbed drug is dependent on the fraction that escapes metabolism. For a high E drug, bioavailability is very low, and a relatively large oral dose must be administered in order to achieve adequate plasma concentrations, such as for propranolol. Lidocaine administered orally results in subtherapeutic concentrations of lidocaine and toxic concentrations of an active metabolite, thus precluding the oral administration of lidocaine to achieve systemic effects. Hepatic cirrhosis results in a significant reduction in effective hepatic blood flow as well as metabolic activity, resulting in as much as a twofold increase in absorption of high E drugs, necessitating dose reduction.

Volume of distribution is determined by the physiologic compartments for drug distribution—that is, extracellular and intracellular spaces—and protein binding of the drug in both the plasma and tissue compartments. Significant changes in the physiologic volume of distribution are not likely to occur in patients with hepatic disease, unless the drug has a small volume of distribution, such as is the case for the aminoglycoside antibiotics, which are limited to the extracellular space. For these drugs, in the presence of severe ascites, the V_D may increase by as much as 50%. Most changes in the V_D of patients with hepatic disease, however, are attributed to hypoalbuminemia. Decreased plasma protein binding as a result of fewer available binding sites will lead to the increased unbound drug moving into the extravascular space, thus resulting in an increased V_D. These changes are only significant for highly protein bound drugs (>90%). The impact of V_D changes on the elimination parameters of a drug depend on whether it is characterized as a low or high E compound. The low E drug will show an increased V_D, and the net effect on elimination will depend on whether the drug is eliminated by Phase I or Phase II enzymes. Phase I–eliminated drugs will most likely show a reduced clearance, and therefore a significantly prolonged elimination half-life, when combined with the increased V_D. Phase II–eliminated drugs may show a minimal effect on half-life since the hepatic clearance may actually increase because more of the drug is available for metabolism, and Phase II processes tend to be spared from the effects of cirrhosis. Highly protein bound drugs that are also high E compounds will show an increased V_D and decreased hepatic clearance and therefore a significantly prolonged elimination half-life.

Altered hepatic clearance of drugs in patients with liver disease is dependent on the drug and its elimination characteristics. Low extraction drugs eliminated by Phase I processes will have a reduced hepatic clearance, whereas those eliminated by Phase II processes will retain near-normal clearance. High extraction drugs will show reduced clearance as a result of a decreased effective hepatic blood flow. These changes in elimination should be reflected in the dosage regimen for the patient.

RENAL IMPAIRMENT

The new dosage regimen in the patient with reduced kidney function must take into consideration the changes in absorption and distribution as well as the expected changes in excretion. Factors to consider include concomitant drug therapy, organ dysfunction, and secondary effects of the disease (Lam, Banerji, Hatfield, & Talbert, 1997; Matzke & Frye, 1997).

Absorption

Although not well studied, altered absorption of drugs may occur in the patient with renal dysfunction. For the patient with end-stage renal disease (ESRD), numerous medications are often prescribed in order to manage secondary complications. Among these are calcium products for binding dietary phosphorus, iron supplements for the treatment of anemia, and multivitamin preparations. Absorption of fluoroquinolone antibiotics is significantly impaired when coadministered with these products, and digoxin bioavailability may be reduced when administered with antacids. These interactions may also occur in patients with normal kidney function. Generally, these interactions can be avoided by separating the administration of interacting drugs by at least 1 h, and 2 h if following a meal.

Another consideration with regard to absorption is the potential effect of renal failure and uremia on the function of other organs. For example, hepatic drug metabolism of high hepatic extraction drugs has been shown to be impaired in renal failure. As a result, the absorption of high extraction drugs may be expected to increase when administered to patients with ESRD. This has been demonstrated for propranolol and propoxyphene, where the absorption was increased by severalfold. This effect has not been observed with all high extraction compounds; the calcium antagonists show similar bioavailability in patients with normal and impaired renal function. Additional therapeutic monitoring is warranted when high hepatic extraction drugs are administered to patients with ESRD.

Distribution

Two potential changes in distribution may occur in patients with renal impairment, including volume and protein binding. Increased body water content is not likely to have a significant effect on drug distribution, although those patients receiving a drug with distribution limited to the extracellular volume (e.g., aminoglycoside antibiotics) may show an increased volume of distribution for the drug.

A more important consideration is the change in protein binding that may occur in the patient with renal disease. These changes may be related to decreased albumin concentration and thus a reduced number of binding sites available for the drug molecule, competition from uremic toxins for the drug-binding site, or altered conformation of the albumin molecule that results in a decreased affinity for the drug. Each of these conditions may result in a decreased fraction of the drug that is bound to the albumin molecule and an increased amount of the drug available for distribution to the tissue and available for elimination (e.g., metabolism). These changes in protein binding are only of concern for drugs bound more than 90% to plasma albumin. Changes in binding for drugs bound less than 90% generally do not result in significant changes in the free concentration of the drug to warrant concern. The best example of changes in protein binding in patients with kidney disease is phenytoin (Dilantin). In subjects with normal kidney function and serum albumin concentration, phenytoin is bound 90% to albumin. The usual therapeutic plasma concentration range is 10 to 20 mg/L based on the total plasma concentration; therefore, the unbound or free therapeutic concentration range is 1 to 2 mg/L. Patients with ESRD have a reduced plasma protein binding of 80%. Considering the goal of therapy is to have the same unbound concentration (the fraction available to interact with the receptor), the therapeutic total concentration range is then 5 to 10 mg/L since the 20% unbound will provide the same unbound concentration range, 1 to 2 mg/L. In patients with renal function between normal and end-stage there is an intermediate reduction in protein binding, and the total therapeutic plasma concentration range should be adjusted accordingly. Despite the change in the therapeutic range for phenytoin, the impact of these binding changes on the phenytoin dosage regimen is negligible. Although there is an increase in the volume of distribution of phenytoin, there is a proportionate increase in its hepatic clearance since more drug is available to the hepatocyte for metabolism.

Changes in tissue binding also may affect the volume of distribution for a drug. For example, digoxin is distributed mostly to the tissue compartment and has an apparent distribution volume of approximately 500 L. In patients with renal impairment, digoxin is displaced from tissue, binding sites and redistributes to the plasma compartment, resulting in a lowered volume of distribution. In ESRD it may be reduced to approximately 200 L. The impact of this change for the clinician is to administer a lower loading dose in order to avoid potentially toxic concentrations. The reduced maintenance dose necessary in patients with renal impairment is mostly a result of decreased renal elimination of digoxin, not changes in distribution.

Elimination

The most important changes in dosage regimens for patients with renal impairment are due to decreased renal elimination of a drug excreted by the kidneys. As a general rule, if a drug is eliminated more than 30% by the kidneys, then dosage regimen adjustment will usually be necessary in the patient with reduced kidney function. Dosage regimen adjustment for these drugs is based on several assumptions: Drug excretion is proportional to kidney function; dose individualization is based on concentrations of the parent compound; and metabolites, which may accumulate with renal dysfunction, are not considered to be pharmacologically active. This is not always true; some compounds accumulate as active metabolites, such as normeperidine following meperidine (Demerol) administration, and *N*-acetylprocainamide following procainamide administration.

For drug elimination from the body, it is useful to consider renal and nonrenal processes. Generally, renal impairment will result in a proportionate decrease in the renal component of drug elimination. The greater the loss of kidney function, the more of an effect on overall drug elimination, resulting in prolongation of the elimination half-life. Figure 3–1 illustrates this general principle. The *y*-axis intercept is considered the fixed, or nonrenal, clearance and is independent of kidney function, whereas the line represents the renal clearance as a function of kidney function, generally assessed as creatinine clearance. This approach to modifying the dosage regiment for a drug in patients with renal impairment is often applied to drugs eliminated at least in part by the kidneys. Figure 3–2 illustrates the principle applied to the anticonvulsant gabapentin. Note the *y*-intercept is 0, indicating there is no nonrenal elimination of gabapentin, and all of the elimination is dependent on renal function. For gabapentin, dose adjustments are recommended at various degrees of kidney function, and guidelines are presented in the package insert. The process for dosage adjustment is (1) defining the goals of therapy, (2) assessment of kidney function, and (3) appropriate dose adjustment based on kidney function.

Consider the normal dosage regimen for a patient, expressed as a dose administered at a specified frequency, such as 200 mg every 12 h. At the steady state, this regimen will result in a plasma concentration within the therapeutic range. Unless there are pharmacodynamic changes or alterations in protein binding of the drug, the patient with renal disease should be expected to maintain the same therapeutic plasma concentration range. The new dosage regimen for the patient can be expressed using the patient-specific drug clearance obtained from its relationship to kidney function. Often the summary guidelines are available from the manufacturer of the drug product. Except for the circumstances described previously, the fraction of dose absorbed is usually unchanged in patients with renal failure.

Although this method for individualizing therapy in the patient with renal impairment is useful in determining a new dose rate for the patient, it does not specify whether the dose, dosing interval, or both variables should be changed. As a general guideline, the dosage should remain constant and the interval prolonged for antibiotics. This approach will maintain similar peak plasma concentrations, which may be necessary for antibacterial effect. It is also reasonable to prolong the interval when the normal dosage regimen is inconvenient, such as every 6 h. It would be beneficial to extend the dosing interval to every 12 or 24 h in order to improve the ease of the dosing schedule rather than reducing the dose.

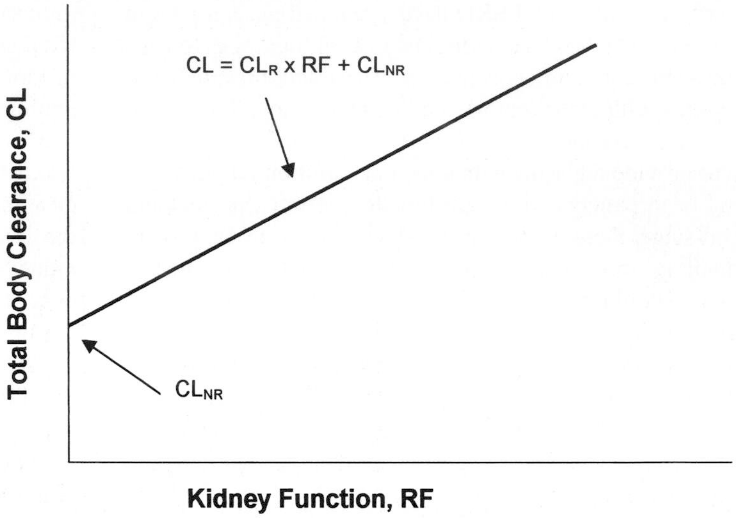

FIGURE 3–1. The linear relationship between total body drug clearance (CL) as a function of renal function (RF). The *y*-intercept denotes non-renal clearance, CL_{NR}, considered constant as renal function changes. The general form of the equation is $CL = (CL_R \times RF) + CL_{NR}$. Renal function (RF) is sometimes presented as creatinine clearance.

On occasion, it may be necessary to maintain the dose for nonantibiotics and adjust the interval. This method is appropriate when the dosing interval is already at a convenient frequency, such as once per day, or there is a narrow therapeutic range and there is a need to minimize the peak-to-trough fluctuation in plasma concentrations. Figure 3–3 illustrates the resulting plasma concentration-versus-time profile when the dose, dosing interval, or both variables are modified in the process of individualizing therapy.

This approach to dosage regimen adjustment in patients with renal disease includes several assumptions such as stable kidney function, a linear relationship between drug clearance and renal function as assessed using the creatinine clearance, normal hepatic function, normal cardiovascular function, normal protein binding and volume of distribution, no changes in bioavailability, similar therapeutic plasma concentration ranges compared to normal subjects, and no active metabolites. Each of these factors should be considered when drugs are administered to patients with impaired renal function.

Dialysis

Maintenance dialysis for patients with ESRD occurs primarily through either chronic hemodialysis (HD), three times weekly, or continuous ambulatory peritoneal dialy-

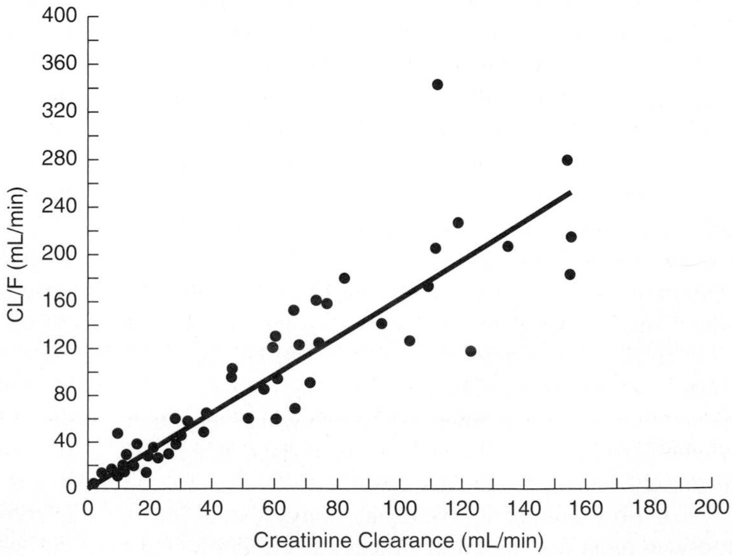

FIGURE 3–2. Relationship between gabapentin apparent oral clearance (CL/F) and creatinine clearance (CL_{CR}): $CL/F = (1.61 \times CL_{CR}) + 3.57$; Pearson correlation coefficient = 0.90 ($p < 0.05$). Bioavailability (F) of gabapentin is approximately 50% and independent of kidney function. *Source: Blum et al. (1994).*

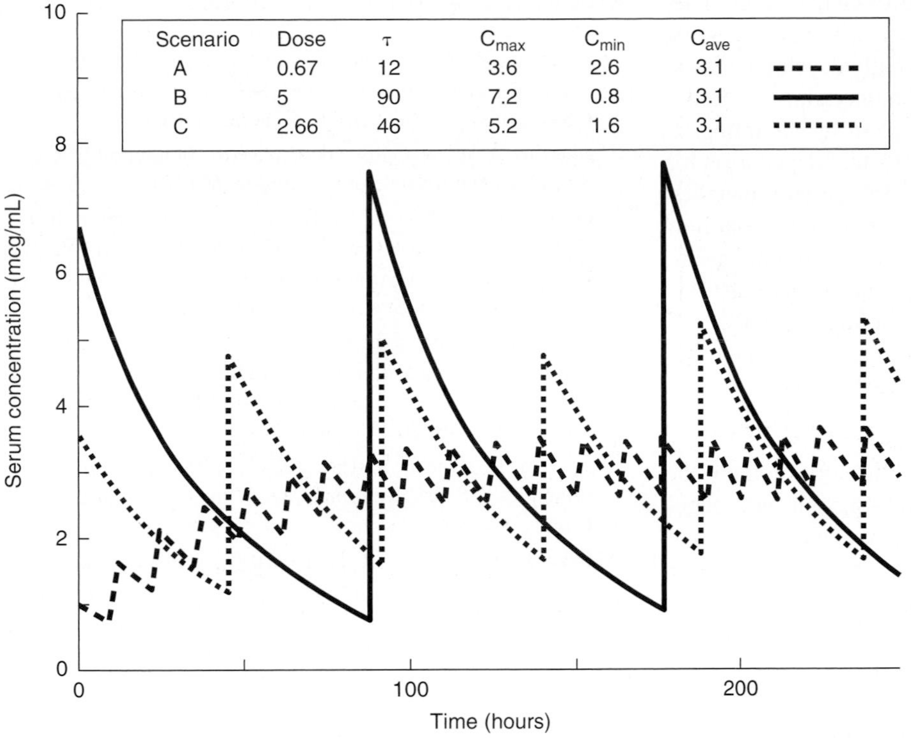

Scenario Dose τ Cmax Cmin Cave
A 0.67 12 3.6 2.6 3.1
B 5 90 7.2 0.8 3.1
C 2.66 46 5.2 1.6 3.1
Serum concentration (mcg/mL)
0
2
4
6
8
10
0
100
200
Time (hours)

FIGURE 3–3. Representation of the consequences of (**A**) altering the dose and maintaining the dosing interval; (**B**) changing the interval and maintaining the same dose; or (**C**) changing both the dose and interval. Note the peak-to-trough fluctuation with each scenario. *Source: Matzke & Frye (1997).*

sis (CAPD). During HD, the patient's blood is pumped through an artificial kidney that contains a semipermeable membrane across which the accumulated toxins in the blood diffuse into a dialysate solution on the opposing side. The rate of solute movement across the membrane depends on several variables, such as molecule size, plasma protein binding, membrane pore size, membrane thickness and surface area, and blood and dialysate flow rates. The amount of solute removed also depends on the length of the dialysis procedure, which is usually 3 to 4 h.

Drugs with a molecular weight of less than 500 and not bound to plasma proteins are removed from the plasma across conventional hemodialysis membranes (e.g., cellulose acetate and cuprophane), but the total amount removed depends on how readily the drug moves from the tissue compartment into the plasma. Drugs with a much higher molecular weight, such as vancomycin (~1500) and erythropoietin (~35,000) are not able to cross the membrane. Drugs bound to plasma proteins, such as albumin or α_1-acid glycoprotein, are functionally not able to cross the membrane due to the large size of the drug-protein complex (>65,000). The more a drug is bound to protein, the less likely it is that significant elimination will occur through dialysis. For example, phenytoin is bound 90% in patients with normal kidney function, and this is reduced to 80% in patients with ESRD. Although the free fraction is twice the normal value, most of the drug remains bound to albumin and is not removed by dialysis. Newer membranes, commonly known as *high-flux* membranes, which have a larger pore size (e.g., polysulfone, polyacrylonitrile, and polymethylmethacrylate), are able to permit the clearance of molecules up to 10,000 Da. For example, vancomycin supplementation must be administered to patients undergoing high-flux dialysis therapy, whereas conventional cellulose membranes often permitted a single dose of vancomycin to treat an infection because of its prolonged elimination half-life (DeSoi, Sahm, & Umans, 1992). These considerations are important when assessing the need for supplemental delivery of a drug following dialysis therapy. As a guideline, replacement dosing will be necessary when dialysis increases drug elimination by at least 30%.

Peritoneal dialysis is a slow, continuous dialysis, which usually consists of four exchanges of dialysate in the peritoneal cavity per day. Drug clearance is dependent on molecular size and protein binding, such that smaller and lesser-bound drugs have a higher clearance. Since the dialysate flow is very low with CAPD, the net removal of most drugs is insignificant relative to clearance by other routes, and dose adjustments are generally not necessary. Patients undergoing CAPD occasionally develop peritonitis and require intraperitoneal administration of antibiotics. Absorption of drugs administered by the intraperitoneal route may vary from 50 to 90% and depends on the residence time in the peritoneal cavity. Larger molecules, such as proteins, are not as efficiently absorbed, but they may be absorbed sufficiently to meet systemic needs, such as for insulin in patients with diabetes mellitus (Taylor, Abdel-Rahman, Zimmerman, & Johnson, 1996).

SUMMARY

Dosage regimen design must take into consideration the hepatic and renal functions of patients. Significant changes in the elimination profile of a drug may occur in the patient with altered organ function, and an alternative choice of drug may be appropriate. Choosing a drug eliminated by hepatic metabolism will minimize the risk of excessive accumulation in the patient with renal dysfunction. Furthermore, the clinician must adjust the regimen for changes in absorption and distribution that may accompany organ disease. Multiple organ dysfunction will require additional monitoring and care to ensure that the risk of toxicity is minimized while achieving therapeutic goals. For patients with end-stage renal disease, maintenance dialysis regimens may also influence dosage regimen design, depending on the type of dialysis performed. Recognition that dialysis methods may vary greatly and affect drug elimination will minimize the risk of adverse effects in that population.

REFERENCES

Blum, R. A., Comstock, T. J., Sica, D. A., Schultz, R.W., Keller, E., Reetze, P., Bockbader, H., Tuerck, D., Busch, J.A., Reece, P.A., & Sedman, A. J. (1994). Pharmacokinetics of gabapentin in subjects with various degrees of renal function. *Clinical Pharmacology and Therapeutics, 56,* 154–159.

Brouwer, K. L. R., Dukes, G. E., & Powell, J. R. (1992). Influence of liver function on drug disposition. In W. E. Evans, J. J. Schentag, & W. J. Jusko (Eds.), *Applied pharmacokinetics: Principles of therapeutic drug monitoring* (3rd ed.; pp. 6/1–6/59). Vancouver, WA: Applied Therapeutics.

Cockcroft, D. W., & Gault, M. H. (1976). Prediction of creatinine clearance from serum creatinine. *Nephron, 16,* 31–41.

Comstock, T. J. (1997). Quantification of renal function. In J. T. DiPiro, R. L. Talbert, G. C. Yee, G. R. Matzke, B. G. Wells, & L. M. Posey (Eds.), *Pharmacotherapy: A pathophysiologic approach* (3rd ed). Stamford, CT: Appleton & Lange.

DeSoi, C. A., Sahm, D. F., & Umans, J. G. (1992). Vancomycin elimination during high-flux hemodialysis: Kinetic model and comparison of four membranes. *American Journal of Kidney Diseases, 20,* 354–360.

Lam, Y. W. F., Banerji, S., Hatfield, C., & Talbert, R. L. (1997). Principles of drug administration in renal insufficiency. *Clinical Pharmacokinetics, 32,* 30–57.

Matzke, G. R., & Frye, R. F. (1997). Drug therapy individualization for patients with renal insufficiency. In J. T. DiPiro, R. L. Talbert, G. C. Yee, G. R. Matzke, B. G. Wells, & L. M. Posey (Eds.), *Pharmacotherapy: A pathophysiologic approach* (3rd ed). Stamford, CT: Appleton & Lange.

Pugh, R. N., Murray-Lyon, I. M., Dawson, J. L., Pietroni, M. C. & Williams, R. (1973). Transection of the oesophagus for bleeding oesophageal varices. *British Journal of Surgery, 60,* 646–649.

Rowland, M., & Tozer, T. N. (Eds.). (1995). *Clinical pharmacokinetics: Concepts and applications* (3rd ed). Baltimore: Williams & Wilkins.

Schwartz, G. J., Feld, L. G. & Langford, D. J. (1984). A simple estimate of glomerular filtration rate in full-term infants during the first year of life. *Journal of Pediatrics, 104,* 849–854.

Schwartz, G. J., Haycock, G. B., Edelman, C. M. Jr., & Spitzer, A. (1976). A simple estimate of glomerular filtration rate in children derived from body length and plasma creatinine. *Pediatrics, 58,* 259–263.

Taylor, C. A., III, Abdel-Rahman, E., Zimmerman, S. W., & Johnson, C. A. (1996). Clinical pharmacokinetics during continuous ambulatory peritoneal dialysis. *Clinical Pharmacokinetics, 31,* 293–308.

II ❖ General Issues

CHAPTER ❖ 4

SAFETY IN PHARMACOTHERAPY

Lea Ann Hansen

Every therapeutic process is more than picking a drug "recipe" from a book for a given diagnosis. After a pharmacotherapeutic regimen has been implemented, proper monitoring is critical to a successful outcome for the patient. This step may, in fact, be more difficult to carry out than the initial diagnosis and therapy selection since very little information is available in texts or in scientific papers about the best way to follow up. Knowing how, what, and who to monitor comes from experience—yet it is this ability that distinguishes the astute clinician from others. Patient responses to a specific therapy are generally unpredictable. Sometimes, we can predetermine if a patient is more or less likely to have a good outcome, but it is rarely an exact science.

Even in settings where followup programs have been studied, there are wide-ranging results. Virgo, Vernava, Longo, McKirgan, and Johnson (1995) describe in detail the literature on followup after potentially curative colorectal cancer treatment; the points raised in the article and accompanying editorial (Loprinzi, 1995) can be extrapolated to any disorder. Bottom line, they found that even though different strategies can vary in cost by as much as $800 million for a national cohort of patients, there are few data to support better outcomes for the more intensive programs.

When developing a monitoring plan for an individual patient, it is important to have a logical, comprehensive strategy to use even if it may seem cumbersome at first. Later, your experience will streamline the process. One such strategy, with examples, follows:

1. Outline all of the parameters that could be used to monitor efficacy. The decision to actually use any or all of these parameters will be a later step. How can you determine if the medication is working? The patient's symptoms (e.g., pain, shortness of breath) related to the disease state should lessen and possibly resolve. A physical finding (e.g., elevated blood pressure, edema), laboratory test (e.g., urinalysis, CBC), or radiological test (e.g., chest x-ray) used for diagnosis should normalize with proper therapy. If additional sequelae of the disease that were not present in the patient initially (e.g., suicidal thoughts in a depressed patient) represent worsening of the illness, how would you detect them? Familiarize yourself with the usual course of events in treating the condition.
2. Consider all the parameters that can be used to monitor side effects of treatment. Many drug references can provide you with an extensive list of possible side effects. How can they be detected? Ask your patients to report symptoms (e.g., call you if they have bleeding or bruising) or question them about specific possibilities at a later time. Consider an additional physical exam or laboratory test to detect frequently reported problems (e.g., transaminase levels for hepatic toxicity).

3. Decide which of these parameters you will actually monitor. Many facets of this decision relate primarily to the need to detect either poor efficacy or development of toxicity—that is, consequences of an undetected problem. Availability of testing and feasibility contribute to the decision. Not all references will provide adequate information to determine the relative importance of each issue. Be aware of situations that could cause mortality or severe morbidity. For example, for a patient on allopurinol, a seemingly simple rash can progress into Stevens–Johnson syndrome, a potentially fatal condition. Although such an occurrence is rare, evaluation for rash should be part of the monitoring plan. Also consider the frequency of occurrence for a certain problem: If a problem occurs in more than 1% of patients, it is likely to be encountered at some point in a busy practice. If it occurs in 10% of patients or more, specific procedures to handle the problem should be in place.
4. Decide how frequently each parameter will be monitored. Obviously, it is not feasible to monitor every parameter all the time, so the interval must coincide with how quickly a patient's status is likely to change (e.g., a few days for a minor bacterial infection compared to a few weeks to months for hyperlipidemia), feasibility (e.g., a reliable patient with a high level of interest in his or her health can be taught self-monitoring), and economics of the testing. Structured telephone followup is a useful tool that is probably not implemented as frequently as it could be. One study assessed the impact of doubling the time interval between face-to-face interactions and substituting three telephone calls for the omitted clinic visit. The group receiving the telephone calls had decreased total clinic visits, less need for medication, fewer hospital admissions, and fewer hospital days than did the group with routine followup. The subset of the population whose health was poor or fair, especially, used fewer healthcare resources when telephone interaction was used (Wasson et al., 1992).

The ability to change the overall outcome by detecting a problem should also be considered. For example, a patient on the most aggressive triple therapy for HIV has few additional options if it is ineffective. The most important focus for the monitoring plan is, therefore, to detect toxicity. Documentation of efficacy in this example can be somewhat less stringent, although the financial costs of monitoring may be justified if the cost of unrecognized ineffective therapy is high.

Documentation in the medical record should include the therapy plan with the specific drug(s) and doses, in addition to the monitoring plan described above. Mechanisms should be used to facilitate collection of that data. Patient self-reports should be logged. Laboratory values are frequently written on a flowsheet. Other types of data can be brought to the same level of prominence by documenting them in a similar manner: for example, pain ratings and bowel movement frequency in a patient on opioid analgesics, number of nitroglycerin tablets used for angina, or number of hours of sleep obtained by an insomniac.

COMPLIANCE WITH PHARMACOTHERAPEUTIC REGIMEN

The best drug therapy available will not help the patient if it is does not reach the site of action in the body. Incorrect use of medications is common in patients of all ages. Originally this behavior was described as *noncompliance.* This term has more recently been replaced by *nonadherence,* implying more patient involvement in determining the course of treatment. Since the majority of research uses the term noncompliance, it will be used here.

Noncompliance can lead to increased overall yearly expenditures (hospitalizations, lost wages, and decreased productivity) of over $100 billion per year (Levy, Zamacona, & Jusko, 2000). Noncompliers are also more likely to die, as in the beta blocker heart attack trial (2.6 times higher mortality in one year) (Coons et al., 1994). Most formal studies of compliance use an assessment of the proportion of a prescribed regimen used by the patient. Simple measures such as pill counts or patient diaries can be inaccurate and can potentially overestimate compliance rates. Studies frequently fail to consider inappropriately administered medication as a type of noncompliance.

Obviously, an informed patient is more likely to make correct decisions about treatment. Patient education issues are discussed in the next section. Besides knowledge deficit, other factors that can lead to suboptimal compliance include:

- Drug side effects
- Complexity of the regimen
- Adaptation to the lifestyle change
- Age greater than 75 years
- Female sex
- Living alone
- Lack of a support system

Socioeconomic status has not been consistently predictive (Coons et al., 1994). Previous experience leads patients to their own unique appraisal of the situation and the importance of the treatment, although belief in the importance of health does not always translate into compliant behavior (Wierenga & Hewitt, 1994). Previous success with behavioral change seems to be a strong predictor of future success with health habit changes (Rakowski, Wells, Lasater, & Carelton, 1991). Adapting the medication to the patient's lifestyle may be more effective than vice versa. Patients with serious illnesses, such as myocardial infarction, may be less compliant if they are highly prone to psychological distress (Rose, Conn, & Rodeman, 1994). Anxiety management may promote adherence as much as education.

Elderly patients may have impairments that hinder their ability to take medication, such as decreased vision, decreased physical functioning, or cognitive impairment. Atkin, Finnegan, Ogle, and Shenfield (1994) found that of 120 elderly patients admitted to a hospital who were well enough to give consent, 63% were unable to open at least one of seven types of medication containers. A screw-top bottle could be opened by 92.7% and a flip-top by 85.8%. A childproof container could only be opened by 43.4%. Even 7-day medication organizers, promoted to assist compliance, caused difficulty for 24%. Seventy-two percent could not break a scored tablet. Men were significantly less likely than women to have difficulties in opening containers.

TEACHING AND COUNSELING

Initially, a patient educational program should include an assessment of the patient's willingness to learn, any barriers to learning, and specific learning needs. A patient may understand the basic issues of treatment but develop a more negative attitude toward it if a situation arises that he or she feels incapable of handling (e.g., a missed dose of medication). Simple written medication leaflets in conjunction with oral counseling are preferred by patients, especially by middle-aged adults (Harvey & Plumridge, 1991). Clearly though, those education tools may not be enough for some patients. Cline et al. (1999) studied elderly patients with heart failure to determine the extent of non-compliance along with the ability of these patients to recall information given to them about their medication. Overall, 27% of patients were found to be noncompliant. Many of these patients were unable to state the correct name or prescribed dose of their medication even after receiving standardized verbal and written information regarding their medication. In addition, low-literacy patients may react to a complicated learning situation by withdrawing while indicating the material was understood even if it was not (Hussey, 1991).

Sophisticated training programs have been shown to increase knowledge and compliance. A program such as Medication Management Module for Schizophrenic Patients (Eckman, Liberman, Phipps, & Blair, 1990) consists of sessions held 3 h per week for 15 to 20 weeks. The program has specific educational objectives, goal setting, redundancy of information, multimedia instructional techniques, checking for assimilation of material presented, modeling, use of positive reinforcement and shaping techniques, role playing, coaching and active prompting of correct responses, homework assignments, and immediate positive or corrective feedback. This program increased the patients' ability to utilize certain medication-related skills from 40 to 50% and their compliance from 67 to 82%. Unfortunately, an assessment of healthcare resource utilization after completion of this extensive intervention was not reported.

Dividing educational material into understandable pieces is important, but it is very difficult in many healthcare systems to identify which person is responsible for education in every setting. It is important that each subsequent educator be aware of previous activity. Otherwise, useless repetition of basic information and omission of the more difficult material can result. Therefore, educational programs are incomplete unless content, patient comprehension, and ongoing needs are documented in the medical record.

MISUSE OF MEDICATIONS

When a medication is not used as prescribed or is used at a different dosage, it is being misused (Düsing, Lottermoser, & Mengden, 2001; Finch, 1993). Usually this is unintentional. Education or a strengthened support system may be needed. Instances of intentional misuse should not always be considered abuse—for example, lack of understanding may lead a person to use leftover antibiotics for a new symptom.

Over-the-counter medications or herbal therapies can also be misused, often without the knowledge of the healthcare provider. Patients may not consider that such medications might be dangerous and disregard the label directions. Fung, Weintraub, and Bowen (1995) reported a case of a 69-year-old woman who was admitted to the intensive care unit with symptoms resembling a stroke. Only after intubation and discussions of withdrawing medical therapy had taken place was it discovered that the patient's magnesium level was 6.65 mmol/L (normal, 0.80–1.20 mmol/L). After fluid diuresis, the patient recovered and admitted to taking two large bottles of magnesium-containing antacids per day for chronic GI complaints. A similar but milder presentation had resulted in a hospital admission just four months earlier.

It is estimated that approximately 5 to 7% of hospital admissions are due to adverse drug reactions (Green et al., 2000). Compounding this problem is the issue of inappropriate medication prescribing, which constitutes another type of medication misuse. A study by Lindley, Tully, Paramsothy, and Tallis (1992) found that, of the admissions due to adverse drug reactions, about half of these were due to inappropriate prescriptions. This included the use of contraindicated and unnecessary medications plus those that interacted with previous therapy. This supports the adage that "a drug that is not indicated is contraindicated." Lindley et al. also found that the drug-related admission rate was significantly higher for inappropriate drugs compared to appropriate drugs (5.1% vs. 1.1%). Willcox, Himmelstein, and Woolhandler (1994) found that 23.5% of a cohort of 6171 elderly patients were taking a medication that had been previously deemed inappropriate by a panel of geriatrics experts and of those, 20.4% were taking two or more. Spore et al. (1997) evaluated the prevalence of inappropriate prescriptions among residents, aged 65 and older, of board and care facilities. These authors found that between 20 and 25% of residents had at least one inappropriate prescription. Critical evaluation of all components of a medication profile should be a regular part of patient care. It can be difficult to obtain a complete medication history when multiple prescribers are involved.

ABUSE OF DRUGS

Abuse refers to drug use outside the normally accepted standard for that drug such that negative consequences occur. According to the National Institute on Drug Abuse, 4 million Americans 12 years or older had used a prescription medication for nonmedical reasons in 1999 (Vastag, 2001). Health professionals have a responsibility to detect substance abuse and intervene when it is suspected. However, this responsibility, coupled with fear that patients may be deceptive or that regulatory authorities may take action, can cause excessive vigilance. Prescribers must recognize the difference between addiction and physical dependence with its associated withdrawal symptoms. The latter can occur with appropriate therapy.

Waldrop and Mandry (1995) surveyed the perceptions of health professionals at an urban teaching hospital about opioid dependence among patients in pain. Staff physicians had the lowest percentage of perceived dependency (4% of all patients, 8% of sickle cell anemia patients). Resident physicians believed 9% of all patients and 17% of sickle cell patients were dependent. Nurses' ratings were 7% and 13% for the two groups. All these values are higher than any incidence of dependence documented in the literature: generally less than 1%. This example implies that unnecessary withholding of therapy for legitimate problems could occur, potentially a greater overall harm than allowing a few abusers to have access to medications.

Many categories of drugs have abuse potential. Agents acting on the central nervous system are most prominent, but others, such as anabolic steroids or thyroid medications, have been used outside of medical indications. An excellent review by Finch (1993), outlines characteristics of patients who are potent medication abusers, including:

- Previous substance abuse (assess this in every patient)
- Changes in functional status or personal relationships
- Early requests for refills (because a prescription was allegedly lost or stolen)
- Missed clinic appointments, with subsequent after-hours calls for prescription renewals
- Forgery of prescriptions
- Strong preference for a particular drug ("allergic" to others, "nothing" else works)
- Solicitation of prescriptions from multiple prescribers

Some healthcare systems have established multidisciplinary committees to identify and intervene when medication abuse is suspected (Britton, Lobeck, & Kelly, 1994). Actions that can be taken include limitations on quantity dispensed, requiring that the patient sign a receipt for a specific quantity of drug at each refill, restricting the prescription of the abused drug to one provider, or referral to a substance abuse treatment program.

REFERENCES

Atkin, R. A., Finnegan, T. P., Ogle, S. J., & Shenfield, G. M. (1994). Functional ability of patients to manage medication packaging: A survey of geriatric inpatients. *Age and Ageing, 23,* 113–116.

Britton, M. L., Lobeck, F. G., & Kelly, M. W. (1994). Multidisciplinary committee on the abuse of prescription medications. *American Journal of Hospital Pharmacy, 51,* 85–88.

Cline, C. M., Bjorck-Linne, A. K., Israelsson, B. Y., Willenheimer, R. B., & Erhardt, L. R. (1999). Non-compliance and knowledge of prescribed medication in elderly patients with heart failure. *European Journal of Heart Failure, 1,* 145–149.

Coons, S. T., Sheahan, S. L., Martin, S. S., Hendricks, J., Robbins, C. A., & Johnson, J. A. (1994). Predictors of medication noncompliance in a sample of older adults. *Clinical Therapeutics, 16,* 110–117.

Düsing, R., Lottermoser, K., & Mengden, T. (2001). Compliance with drug therapy—new answers to an old question. *Nephrology Dialysis Transplantation, 16,* 1317–1321.

Eckman, T. A., Liberman, R. P., Phipps, C. C., & Blair, K. E. (1990). Teaching medication management skills to schizophrenic patients. *Journal of Clinical Psychopharmacology, 10,* 33–38.

Finch, J. (1993). Prescription drug abuse. *Primary Care, 20,* 231–238.

Fung, M. C., Weintraub, M., & Bowen, D. L. (1995). Hypermagnesemia: Elderly over-the-counter drug users at risk. *Archives of Family Medicine, 4,* 718–723.

Green, C. F., Mottram, D. R., Rowe, P. H., Pirmohamed, M. (2000). Adverse drug reactions as a cause of admission to an acute medical assessment unit: A pilot study. *Journal of Clinical Pharmacy and Therapeutics, 25,* 355–361.

Harvey, J. L., & Plumridge, R. J. (1991). Comparative attitudes to verbal and written medication information among hospital outpatients. *Annals of Pharmacotherapy, 25,* 925–928.

Hussey, L. C. (1991). Overcoming the clinical barriers of low literacy and medication noncompliance among the elderly. *Journal of Gerontology Nursing, 17,* 27–29.

Levy, G., Zamacona, M. K., & Jusko, W. J. (2000). Developing compliance instructions for drug labeling. *Clinical Pharmacology and Therapeutics, 68,* 586–591.

Lindley, C. M., Tully, M. P., Paramsothy, V., & Tallis, R. C. (1992). Inappropriate medication is a major cause of adverse drug reactions in elderly patients. *Age and Ageing, 21,* 294–300.

Loprinzi, C. L. (1995). Follow-up testing for curatively treated cancer survivors: what to do? *Journal of the American Medical Association, 273,* 1877–1878.

Rakowski, W., Wells, B. L., Lasater, T. M., & Carelton, R. A. (1991). Correlates of expected success at health habit change and its role as a predictor in health behavior research. *American Journal of Preventive Medicine, 7,* 89–94.

Rose, S. K., Conn, V. S., & Rodeman, B. J. (1994). Anxiety and self-care following myocardial infarction. *Issues in Mental Health Nursing, 15,* 433–444.

Spore, D. L., Mor, V., Larrat, P., Hawes, C., & Hiris, J. (1997). Inappropriate drug prescriptions for elderly residents of board and care facilities. *American Journal of Public Health, 87,* 404–409.

Vastag, B. (2001). Mixed messages on prescription drug abuse. *Journal of the American Medical Association, 285,* 2183–2184.

Virgo, K. S., Vernava, A. M., Longo, W. E., McKirgan, L. W., & Johnson, F. E. (1995). Cost of patient follow-up after potentially curative colorectal cancer treatment. *Journal of the American Medical Association, 273,* 1837–1841.

Waldrop, R. D., & Mandry, C. (1995). Health professional perceptions of opioid dependence among patients with pain. *American Journal of Emergency Medicine, 13,* 529–531.

Wasson, J., Gaudette, C., Whaley, E., Sauvigne, A., Baribeau, P., & Welch, H. G. (1992). Telephone care as a substitute for routine clinic follow-up. *Journal of the American Medical Association, 267,* 1788–1793.

Wierenga, M. E., & Hewitt, J. B. (1994). Facilitating diabetes self-management. *The Diabetes Educator, 20,* 138–142.

Willcox, S. M., Himmelstein, D. U., & Woolhandler, S. (1994). Inappropriate drug prescribing for the community-dwelling elderly. *Journal of the American Medical Association, 272,* 292–296.

CHAPTER ❖ 5

PSYCHOLOGICAL, SOCIOLOGICAL, AND CULTURAL FACTORS

Jeanette F. Kissinger ◆ Kathleen J. Sawin

Two recent reports have documented the dramatic and pervasive disparities in health care and call for sweeping reform (AHRQ, 2004; IOM, 2003). The IOM report indicates that

- Racial and ethnic minorities tend to receive a lower quality of healthcare than non-minorities, even with access-related factors such as patient's insurance status and income, are controlled.
- Stereotyping, biases, and uncertainty on the part of the healthcare provider can contribute to unequal treatment.

The AHRQ (2004) report also found that

- Inequality in quality exists
- Disparities come at a personal and societal price
- Differential access may lead to disparities in quality
- Opportunities to provide preventive care are frequently missed by HCP

Further the AHRQ report indicates that data that explain why disparities exist is limited but improvement is clearly possible.

Exemplifying the challenges is a 36-year-old Hispanic male who presents at an ambulatory clinic complaining of "pain in my left hand." The hand is edematous, with erythematous induration extending 4 in. above the wrist. The client came to the clinic because the pain was interfering with driving his truck. Examination revealed two small healed abrasions on the dorsal side of the hand. When queried about the healed wounds, he stated that he had been punctured and cut on barbed wire the previous week and had been treated at this clinic. His past records at the clinic documented the treatment given at the time of the initial injury and showed that he was given a prescription for Augmentin. When asked if he had taken the Augmentin, he said he had not. When asked why, he stated, "I lost the prescription in my truck." He had been on a delivery to Chicago and had just returned from that run. He had not sought any other medical or over-the-counter (OTC) treatment for his hand and stated that the swelling and redness began 2 days prior. Told of the seriousness of the resulting cellulitis, he was given the appropriate treatment—all now at greater expense, monetarily and physically, to the patient as well as at a higher total cost of healthcare.

As healthcare providers, we must ask ourselves: Did he understand the health risk if he did not take the prescribed medication? Did he know that a phone call would have replaced the lost prescription, if it was lost? Did he understand he was at risk (susceptible) for complications? Was there a financial/insurance *or any other* reason for not following through and getting the prescription filled? Did he believe in preventive measures, or did he believe you can treat the problem when it occurs? Did his health orientation (seek help when it hurts or interferes with your occupation) or family tradition prevent him from taking the Augmentin?

When we prescribe a drug, we need to factor in the characteristics of the drug or drug schedule (see Chapter 4 in this book on safety), of the person we wish to take the medication, and of the provider/patient relationship associated with the likelihood of the drug actually being taken. If healthcare providers wish to achieve positive health outcomes from the therapies and medications they prescribe, they must consider all influences on the clients' medication-taking behavior and adherence (compliance) to the prescribed regime.

Rubel and Carro (1992) state that the major barrier to successful health outcomes from the treatment of tuberculosis (TB) today is the lack of adherence to the prescribed medications. Many studies have found that patients evaluate their prescribed medical regimes before deciding on a course of action, and these evaluations are based on their own beliefs, values, and knowledge (Bailey, 2000). Often, healthcare professionals and patients disagree on the definition of compliance. Subjects felt they were compliant if they were feeling well, heard their doctors' comments that they were doing fine, and in some instances were checking their own blood pressure or sugar levels. For some, treatment regimes were found to be more problematic than illness.

Healthcare professionals who assume that the prescribed drug regimen is the patient's only approach and treatment and that compliance is static need to examine their own beliefs. The literature uses both *adherence* and *compliance* synonymously. Many find that *compliance* conveys a negative connotation. *Adherence* implies a collaborative relationship in which the client and healthcare provider come to an agreement regarding the desired outcome and the treatment to achieve it. Indeed perhaps neither term is accurate and we should be focusing on teaching self-management which conveys working collaboratively with healthcare providers and learning the skills necessary to mange one's condition. This approach supports the belief structure of the patient and is likely to increase medication-taking behavior. In many cases, patient input in the decision is critical and avoiding that step may decrease the likelihood of an effective use of prescribed drugs. It is not the intent of the authors to discuss the entire range of factors that influence adherence, so this chapter focuses on beliefs, culture, religion, traditions, world views, and relevant psychosocial theories. It is important, however, as these patterns are explored, to remember to assess each individual and not assume he or she fits a "predetermined pattern."

DEMOGRAPHICS OF THE HEALTHCARE CONSUMER

AGE AND SEX

Dramatic changes are occurring in the age pyramid—and, thus, the "market profile" of healthcare consumers—due in part to the baby boom, the increasing growth of the 65+ age group now constituting 12.4% of the U.S. population (U.S. Census Bureau, 2001), and females outliving males by more than 7 years. Not only are women the major decision makers regarding consumption of healthcare, they use health services more frequently than men, particularly during childbearing and their senior years. As the population ages, the healthcare system will overwhelmingly be dominated by women. Why is this important? Their needs are different, most research has been done on men, and women constitute a large percentage of the workforce. All these facts contribute to the reality that the healthcare provider desiring positive health outcomes must approach prescribing therapies to women in a more collaborative manner. The increased aging of the population has necessitated further differentiations in what constitutes "old." The active 60s, the declining 70s, and the frail 80s not only have different health needs but also have different views of who should control their health behavior and how the health problem should be fixed (Bailey, 2000).

RACIAL AND ETHNIC DIVERSITY

When the census was taken in both 1990 and 2000, respondents were asked to indicate their ancestry. It was interpreted that the responses would indicate the ethnic group the person identified with and still had some strong attachment with regardless of how many generations they were removed from it. In the 2000 census a large percent of respondents reported double or triple ancestry, bringing into question the current categorization of race/ethnicity. Among the white population, English, German, and Irish were the most often cited ethnic groups. French and Italian came next, followed by Scottish, Polish, and Mexican at slightly lesser rates. The five states with the largest European ancestry groups are California, New York, Minnesota, Illinois, and Pennsylvania. The assimilation of the European immigrants is such that they share many of the "American" values and norms concerning healthcare and health behavior. However, diversity does exist in many health traditions and beliefs.

During the 1990s, immigrants, and the children born to recent immigrants, reached 20 million, nearly two-thirds of America's population growth during the past decade. Asians, Hispanics, and African Americans, although still minorities, are increasing faster than non-Hispanic whites, in part because birthrates among nonimmigrants are close to replacement levels (Dillin, 2001). Their influence on society is increasing commensurate with their numbers. By 2033 it is estimated that ethnic minorities will constitute 40% of the total U.S. population (Rexroth & Davidhizar, 2003). Three states—California, Texas, and Florida—will have a "minority majority."

African Americans constitute 12.3% of the U.S. population, a gain of 0.3% of the population during the 1990s. This segment of the population has a higher proportion of children and lower proportion of elderly than the total population.

Twelve and a half percent of the population is Hispanic, which increased from 9% in 1990. This ethnic group, as with the Asians, continues to grow much faster than the African American population because of the combined effects of immigration and fertility.

Considering all these trends, 24.9% of the U.S. population and nearly two-thirds of the nation's children in the year 2000 are racial or ethnic minorities. The immigrant pool will continue to diversify. The Immigration Act of 1990 had this as an intent and also ensures a continuous flow of immigrants into the United States. Unlike the typical European immigrant who shared many of the norms and values of middle America, these new immigrants have different attitudes towards the healthcare system and different patterns of health behavior and health traditions. Their intent is also different: They come to the United States to work and then retire in their original homeland. They tend to stay within their own ethnic group and often manage to neither need nor desire to learn English or interact outside their enclaves.

EDUCATION

Current trends point to a huge divergence of educational levels. If this trend continues, in the early part of the new century, patients will be either highly educated or close to functionally illiterate. This will have a great bearing on whether patients understand directions for their therapy. On the other hand, those who are well educated will demand to collaborate in the process of decision making regarding their treatment. Knowledge has been consistently shown to be necessary for informed patients but not sufficient to predict health behavior (Bradley, 1995; Conway, Pond, Hamnett, & Watson 1996; del Rosario, 2001; Montgomery, 1996). Intervention programs based on knowledge alone have not been successful in behavior change. However, behaviors, including medication use, have been changed with interventions that integrate knowledge with experiences, that change expectations, that encourage confidence in performing behaviors, and that enhance skills necessary for behavior change (assertiveness, communication skill, psychomotor skill) (Cowell, 2001; Philis-Tsimikas & Walker, 2001; van Balen & Gerrits, 2001). Clinicians cannot expect prescriptive behavior to change just because they have "taught" the patient new knowledge.

SELECTED CULTURAL FACTORS INFLUENCING MEDICATION-TAKING BEHAVIOR

Belief categories related to health/illness, culture, religion, traditions, and world view are not distinct. There is overlap among all these factors given the holism of people and the process of socialization. *Culture,* as defined by *The American Heritage Dictionary,* is "the aggregate of socially transmitted beliefs, traditions, behavior patterns, skills, and all other products of human work and convictions characteristic of a community or population" (Morris, 1993). All the factors listed above are included in the broad term *culture.* Ethnicity is not a synonym; it is subsumed under the umbrella term. Culture is used here to refer to specific socialization effects for the particular ethnic group addressed.

The groups discussed here are the white ethnic (German Americans, Irish Americans, Italian Americans, and Polish Americans) and the minority ethnic (Asian Americans, Hispanic Americans, African Americans, and Native Americans). The literature uses these classifications without differentiating status of citizenship. The authors can attempt here only to address those ethnic groups of the U.S. population that constitute the largest percentages.

WHITE ETHNIC GROUPS

- *German Americans: Beliefs:* Health is the ability to enjoy life and have energy to do things; illness is caused by stress, environmental changes, drafts, and germs, but also can be punishment or caused by an "evil eye." *Culture:* Strong family ties; everything in life has a purpose; the year is measured by the church calendar. *Religion/tradition:* Holy days are celebrated with festivities and take precedence over other commitments. *World view:* Emphasis is on the past and present, but also on plan for future. *Relevant Provider Tips:* Help this group see the connection between past and present activities and their illness. Include family in prescriptive, therapeutic plan.

- *Irish Americans: Beliefs:* Flesh is weak; ignore bodily complaints. *Culture:* Strong extended family ties; high alcohol use; problem expressing love and affection; male dominance. *Religion:* Strong faith in God, and the Catholic church's saints. *Tradition:* Celebrate saints' days with festivities and alcohol. *World view:* Past, present, and future oriented. *Relevant Provider Tips:* Explain expected change in symptoms by taking the medicine. Explain warning symptomology of worsening illness and/or adverse reaction to medication.
- *Polish Americans: Beliefs:* Health is when you are feeling OK; keep healthy by being pure; walk and exercise; be happy and put faith in God; illness is because of a poor diet and perhaps an "evil eye." *Culture:* Use folk medicine and faith healers. *Religion:* Strong faith in God and the Mother of God. *Traditions:* Wear scapulars for protection; celebrate saints' days and have special rituals, i.e., blessing of the throats, to protect health; honor relics of the saints; make novenas and pilgrimages. *World view:* Major focus on past and present. *Relevant Provider Tips:* Connect effects of folk medicine in illness and medication efficacy. Review diet that may influence both illness and medication.
- *Italian Americans: Beliefs:* Health is being able to take advantage of the present; illness is caused by drafts, contamination, suppression of emotions, stress, grief, fear, anxiety, "evil eye," and "curses." *Culture:* Male is the head of household, while female is the heart; rely on family to provide continuity in life and for coping; avoid talk of sex or menstrual cycle; expect immediate treatment for illness; report symptoms very dramatically; expect explanations of illness and treatment to be given in great detail. *Religion:* Strong faith in God; death is God's will and should not be discussed. *Tradition:* Most celebrations center around family; rituals to avoid "evil eye" and undo "curses." *World view:* Focus on present and future; internal locus of control—belief that they can effect the outcome of a situation by their actions. *Relevant Provider Tips:* Involve family in deciding the details of scheduling medications; explain expected symptom resolution.

Some general commonalties of the white ethnic group are: Time is money; the future is valued more than the present; small talk and personal space are valued.

MINORITY ETHNIC GROUPS

- *Asian Americans: Beliefs:* Illness is due to poor working conditions, poverty, crowding, imbalance of yin and yang; cannot treat a "hot" illness with a "hot" herb or "hot" medication; there are seven pulses that are used for diagnosis, using three fingers; 100 conditions can be diagnosed by the color and texture of the tongue; many diagnostic tests are not needed and need not be so painful; blood is the source of life and cannot be regenerated; immunizations and x-rays are acceptable. *Culture:* Value silence; avoid confrontation; self-expression should be repressed; loyalty of the young to the old; accept without questioning; family is multigenerational and is the chief social network; father is the main decision maker; male is valued more than female; the body is a gift; believe in prevention of illness; the health care system's task is to prevent illness; should not have to pay when one is ill; best to die with body intact. *Religion:* Evil is removed by purification; rituals are used to prevent illness and restore balance in yin and yang. *Tradition:* Use both Western and Oriental healing; use medicinal herbs and folk healers; fortune tellers can tell of the event that caused the illness; family takes care of the disabled. *World view:* Major focus is on the present; communication is largely nondirect; use strong self-control to avoid an incident that would bring shame. *Relevant Provider Tips:* Involve father or significant male in decisions regarding medications. Explore possible interactions between drugs and medicinal herbs being used. Explain health behaviors to prevent recurrence of illness.
- *Hispanic Americans: Beliefs:* Health is a gift from God as a reward for good behavior—it is the result of good luck; illness is an imbalance of hot/cold or wet/dry—a punishment; if the four body humors are disrupted, you will have a disease; malaise, fatigue, or a headache are caused by a "bad eye" (an unwanted condition resulting from the look/gaze of an individual thought to possess special powers). The

solution is to find the person who gave the bad eye and have him care for the ill person; illness is also caused by a "soul loss" (a depressed emotional state). *Culture:* "Envidia"—Belief that one's success may provoke the envy of friends, thus the potential of illness from a "bad eye"; father is the decision maker; traditional gender and family roles, but women are the primary healers; men are considered "macho"; strong effort to retain cultural identity. *Religion:* Demonstratively religious; have shrines in homes; wear medals and amulets and pray to prevent illness. *Tradition:* Use teas, herbs, spices, and folk healers; will not take a "hot" medication to treat a "hot" condition; make pilgrimages, visit shrines, offer medals, candles, and make promises to God to be cured from a severe illness; hold big celebrations for holidays, birthdays, and other family or religious occasions; parental assistance, physical and financial, continues to the children long after they have become adults. *World view:* Focus is on the present; time is relative—day, afternoon, or night—with a wider frame of reference; there is a lack of focus on clock time, i.e., being on time for appointments, taking medications, etc.; have an external locus of control (believe that their actions will not influence the outcome of situations); in communication, eye contact is important. *Relevant Provider Tips:* Involve significant female in scheduling of medications; being specific as to time of "day—afternoon, or night." Connect the medication time with a usual, routine activity. Caution is advised in prescribing beta blockers, calcium channel blockers (e.g., Plendil) or diuretics (e.g., Aldactone) that have the potential adverse effects of gynocomastia and/or impotence.

- *African Americans: Beliefs:* Health is a gift from God; trouble and pain are God's will; do not view illness as a burden; illness is a natural occurrence because of disharmony caused by demons, sin, and evil spirits; the cure is to get rid of the evil by voodoo, herbs, roots, and laxatives. *Culture:* Female is the dominant family force; grandmother is the major decision maker; elderly are held in high esteem; strong bonds in the extended family; nonrelatives often live in same household; the healthcare system is not considered for prevention. *Religion:* Reliance on the healing power of religion; social network; trust the advice of the preacher. *Traditions:* Use healers and folk medicine for most problems, i.e., prevent colds by taking cod liver oil, use sulfur and molasses as a spring tonic, wear copper or silver bracelets to protect (harm will occur if they are removed); use of alcohol (greatest health problem). *World view:* In communication, eye contact is important but is not synonymous with attention; have a closer personal space; present oriented, but those with a strong religious belief are future oriented as well; time is flexible; a person with status is expected to arrive late. *Relevant Provider Tips:* Consider recent/current use of folk medicine and herbs with the use of prescribed drugs. Involve dominant family female in drug selection and schedule. Focus on present symptoms.
- *Native Americans: Beliefs:* Health is equanimity with nature and the universe; disregard germ theory; illness has a mythical component associated with evil spirits; cure is to rid the body of the evil spirits; they are not to be blamed for their illness, since the cause is external. *Culture:* Treat body with regard; believe in self-control; witches have power to interact with the evil spirits and can bring illness and misery on those who chafe them; lineage is from mother; close relationship with nature; are true ecologists. *Religion:* Intertwined with their relationship with nature; give libation to the god of the earth, offer prayer sticks, and dance to the god of the wind, etc.; healer and medicine man are wise in the ways of the land and nature and have the ability to know supernatural effects. *Traditions:* Wear or carry amulets, etc., to guard against the power of witches; use herbs and rituals; follow advice of the medicine person; consult with singers and healers; are hesitant to use Western medicine because of conflicting perceptions of what the illness is, what the cause is, and how it should be treated; use of alcohol (greatest health problem). *World view:* Present time orientation; patterns of their social life are not bound by clock time, but by patterns in nature and need; the locus of control is both external (victim when ill) and internal (believe they have the power to control themselves); in communication, non-verbal cues are very important; it is proper to avoid eye contact when speaking and using a soft and low voice conveys respect; direct questions are considered an intrusion on privacy; the pointing of an object at another is considered an insult and a threat. *Relevant Provider Tips:* Consider current use of prescriptions from healers, medicine persons or singers. Since not focused on clock time, tie schedule of medication taking in with usual routine daily activities.

SELECTED PSYCHOSOCIAL FACTORS INFLUENCING MEDICATION-TAKING BEHAVIOR

Several of the most useful models or concepts worth considering when exploring medication use are discussed briefly below.

THE HEALTH BELIEF MODEL

The health belief model (HBM) was originated by social scientists in the 1950s who wondered why people did not use free chest screening for TB. The model has been revised and focused on a wide variety of health behaviors. The central concepts of the current version are susceptibility, seriousness, benefits, barriers, and cues to action. To act, individuals have to see themselves as susceptible to a condition, see the condition as serious, see benefits to the behavior undertaken to prevent or treat the condition, see few barriers to performing these behaviors, and be prompted to act by cues in the environment. A literature review indicates the majority of studies support barriers and susceptibility as the major predictors of health behavior (Hand & Bradley, 1996).

However, it is important to look at patterns. Barriers, such as time, transportation, schedules, financial cost, change in habits—real or perceived—are the most important variable to explore when patients are not able to follow the prescribed treatment or drug regime. For example, Marlenga (1995) found that even though dairy farmers knew they were susceptible to sun-mediated cancer and it was a serious problem, they did not use protective sunscreen because of barriers. In addition, Patel and Spaeth (1995) found barriers a significant predictor to eyedrop use for glaucoma. Similarly, barriers were cited as reasons for not using inhalers (Hand & Bradley, 1996).

Benefits, on the other hand, are useful to understand why people do follow through with prescribed behavior. This assessment was supported by a study of 251 low-income women that related intention to use folic acid with HBM constructs. Although seriousness, susceptibility, benefits, and barriers all had significant relationship to the medication behavior, benefits most consistently predicted intention to use folic acid (Kloeblen & Batish, 1999). In addition, patients took antipsychotic medication if they saw benefits of the medication and saw the condition as severe and themselves as susceptible (Budd, Hughes, & Smith, 1996). Bonin (1999) identified being female, being elderly, living with a partner, and perceived treatment benefits and obstacles as factors determining lithium compliance. Further, tools based on the HBM have been identified as valid and reliable to study TB-related medication behavior in Mexican migrant farm workers (Poss, 1999).

Providers need to explore the issues of threat and benefit/barrier ratio when discussing drugs with patients. Questions that assess barriers and susceptibility might be routinely assessed when the clinician gives a prescription. Asking, "Is there anything that will make it hard for you to get this prescription filled today?" could be a first-line screening question for all prescriptions. If the clinician feels the patient does not see himself or herself at risk, say, "I think you are at high risk for this to develop into a bigger problem and I want you to take this medicine for 7 days. What do you think about that?" In working with patients who have chronic illness, all four variables may need to be explored so that the clinician can determine which of the concepts is most important to the individual patient being seen. Interventions can then be targeted to individual patterns.

THE THEORY OF PLANNED BEHAVIOR

Two social scientists (Ajzen & Fishbein, 1980; Fishbein & Ajzen, 1975) advocated three constructs to explain why persons did or did not participate in health behavior. The three constructs of the theory of reasoned action are: (1) individuals' attitude toward the behavior; (2) their "subjective norm," or perception of what those important to them thought about the behavior; and (3) their intention to perform the behavior. For example, 41% of the use of gloves was accounted for by attitude and the importance of significant others and intention to use gloves (Jennings-Dozier, 1999; Levin, 1999). In addition, Kalichman et al. (2001) examined cognitive and behavioral factors associated with HIV treatment adherence in a study of 112 women. Results showed that women who missed at least one dose of their HIV medications in the previous week reported lower intentions to remain adherent and lower adherence self-efficacy (skills). Treatment-related information did not predict treatment adherence. In this model, behavioral intention is the only variable directly related to the behavior itself.

Overall evidence for the predictive utility of the model was found as long as attitude was measured specifically (Morrison, Gilmore, & Baker, 1995; Pender, 1996). That is, attitude toward a specific medication regime would need to be measured. Overall attitude toward taking medication would not be helpful in predicting hypertension medication use, or attitudes toward hypertension medications would not be helpful in predicting birth control medication use.

The theory of planned behavior is an extension of the theory of reasoned action (Ajzen, 1988, 1991). The dimension added was "perceived behavioral control," which is proposed to affect behavior directly and indirectly through intentions. Perceived behavioral control has been conceived as perceived ease or difficulty engaging in behavior and is viewed as a reflection of past experiences and anticipated impediments or obstacles (Ajzen, 1988). For example, intention to use, susceptibility, perception of personal control, and parent and peer attitudes predicted sunscreen use in 9- to 13-year-old Florida youth (Jennings-Dozier, 1999; Levin, 1999). The perceived control concept has been seen as somewhat similar to Bandura's self-efficacy (Ajzen, 1991). However, the conceptual definition of ease/difficulty of engaging in the behavior cannot be equated with the conceptual definition of self-efficacy and may in fact be closer to the conceptual definition of the benefit/barriers concept of the HBM. The support for this added variable is mixed (Pellino, 1997; Wambach, 1997).

In addition, several researchers have identified three variables that moderate the model's effectiveness: the measure of intention employed, the type of behavior, and the presence of a choice among alternatives. Modification to account for goal intentions, choice situations, and differences between intention and estimation measures has been proposed (Sheppard, Hartwick, & Warshaw, 1988).

SELF-EFFICACY

More recently, several theorists have tested the addition of the self-efficacy variable developed by Bandura (1986) to both the health-belief model and the theory of reasoned action. In social cognition theory, it is not only the specific value attitude toward the behavior (i.e., good idea vs. bad idea) that is thought to be predictive but the specific belief that the subject can perform the behavior change needed. An increasingly complex body of literature supports the effect of self-efficacy on the development of outcome behavior. The majority of this literature is in health promotion activities, such as smoking cessation and exercise behavior. The "lessons learned" indicate that self-efficacy is often a powerful predictor of behavior if measured specifically.

A growing number of studies have evaluated self-efficacy in medication-taking behavior. Their findings parallel the literature on health promotion behaviors (Scherer & Bruce, 2001). Measured specifically, self-efficacy predicted medication-taking behaviors for persons with epilepsy, diabetes, and AIDS. It is important to ask the client, "What do you think the likelihood is that you can take this medication three times a day [or however prescribed]?"

VALUE OF THE PROVIDER/ PATIENT RELATIONSHIP

The patient/provider relationship is another variable scientists are recently suggesting we add to these models of behavior. Several studies suggest that the provider has a powerful impact on health behavior (Elliot, 1994; Paskett, Carter, Chu, & White, 1990; Rosenberg, Burnhill, Waugh, Grimes, & Hillard, 1995; Somkin, 1993). The impact may be cumulative or inconsistent, but when studies addressing contraceptive use, mammogram use, or inhaler use are analyzed using multivariate techniques, provider relationship is a frequent predictor (Hand & Bradley, 1996; Rosenberg et al., 1995). Specifically, provider recommendation for a test (Champion, 1996; Van Essen, Kuyvenhoven, & de Melker, 1997) or a change in behavior (smoking) is frequently predictive even when other predictors are accounted for. The provider needs to realize the power of the relationship and use it: "Will you try this for me for 2 weeks to see if it is useful? You will need to take the medication every day for 2 weeks for us to evaluate its use. Do you think you can do that for me?" However, part of the relationship with the provider may be the attitude that all regimes are not appropriate for all patients and a willingness on the provider's part to explore options. The provider might say, "We have two choices: an injection or a 10-day course of antibiotics. Since you choose the 10-day course, can we count on you to complete that treatment? Is that something you can do for us?"

INTEGRATION OF MODELS PREDICTING MEDICATION-TAKING BEHAVIOR

Several studies have indicated that integrating variables from a variety of models increases precision. Results of Champion's work indicate that the predisposing variables of seriousness, benefits, health motivation, control, knowledge of breast cancer and mammography guidelines, socioeconomic status, age, physician recommendation for mammography, and prior breast symptoms were significantly related, to having had recent mammography

(Champion & Miller, 1996). Forty to fifty percent of medication usage was predicted by enhancing perceived control over adherence, emphasizing susceptibility, and addressing seriousness (Abraham, Clift, & Grabowski, 1999). In addition, the predictor variables suggested by Ajzen and Fishbein (1980), plus gender and the specific measure of condom use self-efficacy, were predictive of intentions to use condoms 3 months later (Jemmott & Jemmott, 1992; Morrison et al., 1995). The traditional theory of reasoned action worked well to predict condom use intentions and behavior. Support was also found for inclusion of gender and self-efficacy, but not behavior in the prediction of intention to use condoms, but not behavior (Morrison et al., 1995). Other studies have found that interventions provided by creditable providers, which address knowledge, attitude, and skills, can have a long-term impact on health behavior (J. B. Jemmott, L. S. Jemmott, & Fong, 1992; L. S. Jemmott & J. B. Jemmott, 1991). A recent study from the March of Dimes, conducted by the Gallup Poll (2002), found that fewer than 40% of women with childbearing potential were taking folic acid to prevent birth defects. A significant number indicted they would be more likely to take the supplement if it was recommended by their healthcare provider.

Pender (1996) has revised her model combining the predictive variables of other theories. The expectancy-value theory (the basis of the health belief model and the theory of reasoned action) and social cognitive theory (renamed from social learning theory, and the basis of self-efficacy) are articulated as the theoretical underpinnings of this model. The model also includes individual characteristics and experiences, such as previous experience with the behavior, since past behavior is repeatedly shown to be the best predictor of future behavior. For components of the model, see Figure 5–1. Pender reports that the model explains health-promoting lifestyles such as exercise, fitness, and cardiac rehabilitation program participation, as well as hearing protection programs. She recommends that researchers testing this revised model develop rigorous measures of behavior-specific variables if they do not already exist.

One particularly intriguing study suggests an important relationship to be tested in clinical practice. With a large sample in a experimental study, pretreatment perceptions of barriers were found to be predictive of short-term behavior change. After the treatment was initiated, self-efficacy was found to be predictive of long-term success. In getting patients to adopt an important drug regime, combating barriers may be critical for short-term prescriptions. However, once the treatment is initiated and the initial barriers are overcome, building self-efficacy for a program of long-term pharmacotherapy may be crucial. As the patient overcomes these barriers and builds new behaviors, continuing to reinforce the patient's confidence may prove to be a powerful force in increasing self-efficacy (Mudde, Kok, & Strecher, 1995). This may indeed be a part of the behavior of providers that patients have reacted to and report as a "positive relationship" with the provider. This finding also supports the need for the clinician to be familiar with the most recent theory impacting medication-taking behavior, discussed in the next section (Prochaska, Velicier, Rossi, & Goldstein, 1994).

THE TRANSTHEORETICAL MODEL OF BEHAVIOR CHANGE

Usually in chronic illness, when we begin, modify, or increase the medications prescribed, we are asking patients to make a fundamental change in their behavior for the long term. Thus, understanding not only factors associated with behavior but also stages of behavior change becomes very important. Currently, the dominant theory in the literature explaining the process is the *transtheoretical model of behavior change.* Prochaska et al. (1994) used their work with smoking cessation to identify the stages of change that a person goes through, whether the person is adopting a new behavior or quitting a health-threatening behavior. This model has five stages:

1. *Precontemplation:* A person is not thinking about adopting a particular behavior.
2. *Contemplation:* A person is seriously thinking about adopting a particular behavior.
3. *Planning or preparation:* A person who has tried to change a behavior is seriously thinking about engaging in the contemplated change (making small or sporadic changes).
4. *Action:* This phase covers the first period during which the person has made the behavior change consistently.
5. *Maintenance:* This period begins 6 months after action has started and continues indefinitely.

Each stage gives healthcare providers unique opportunities for influence. The movement between each stage is a balance of pros and cons discussed as variables in the previous theories. Minor changes in the balance of pros and cons are predicted as the force that moves a person from one stage to another. This work suggests different

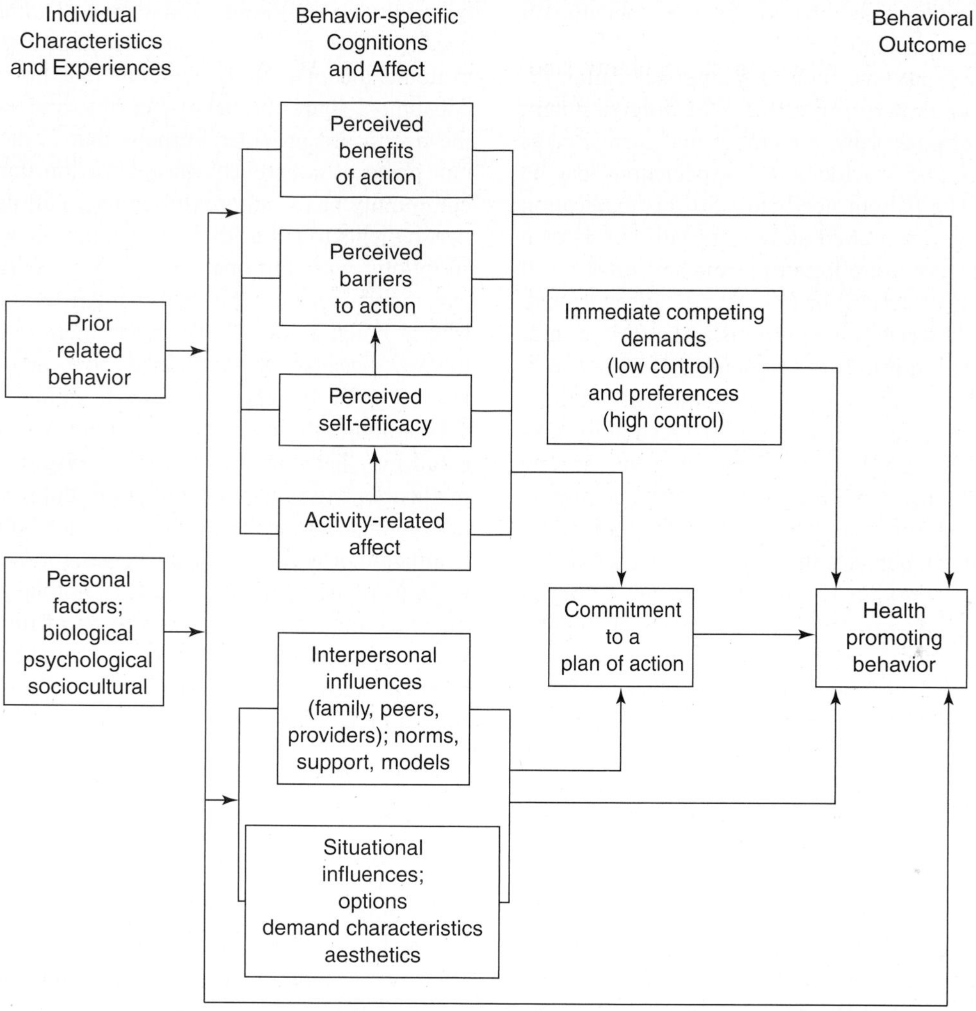

FIGURE 5–1. Pender Model.

interventions to use at various stages to maximize change. Consciousness raising and self-reevaluation are more important in the early stages and behavioral processes—such as reinforcement, counterconditioning, support from providers/significant others, and stimulus control—are more important for understanding and predicting transition from preparation to action and from action to maintenance. Thus, the provider using data such as lab results or a log of weekly blood pressure readings could raise a patient's consciousness that change is needed, and positive outcome data—such as hemoglobin A_{IC} (used to monitor long-term control of blood glucose level), serum levels, and decrease in bothersome symptoms—could reinforce changed medication-taking behavior. It is particularly important for the clinician to assess the patient's willingness to maintain the medication regime when immediate clinical results are not evident.

The transtheoretical model of behavior change is congruent with the findings of the previously cited study that identified barriers as the critical variable in initiating the behavior and self-efficacy as the critical variable in maintaining behavior change. Indeed, several authors have found that HBM constructs and self-efficacy differ by stages of behavior change (Champion & Huster, 1995; DeVries, Mudde, Dijkstra, & Willemsen, 1998). The health provider may need to combine several interventions to impact medication behavior change depending on the stage of behavior change.

In complex situations, such as taking medication for chronic illness or monitoring efficacy of drug treatment with measures of peak flow, remember that change takes time to establish. The provider's own expectations may be as follows: (1) The patient needs to start this medication or treatment program immediately (after all, I've known about this medication for a long time and am convinced it is the best course of action) or (2) relapses are avoidable. For the patient, however, changing his or her life to integrate this medication into it is a new idea, and one she or he might have to consider before adopting. In addition, relapses or inappropriate cessation of medication for limited or prolonged periods occur frequently. Marlatt and Gordon (1985) indicate that relapses are most common in times of negative emotional states (anger, frustration, depression, boredom), social situations (negative situations such as conflict with other significant persons), or physical craving (for food or substances). Persons attempting to establish long-term therapeutic use of prescriptive medications are at high risk for relapse. Relapse prevention might include maximizing intention with contracts, assessing barriers, *and* making a plan to deal with them, increasing skills necessary to perform the behavior, assessing social support and making a plan to optimize it if there is a deficit, or creating interventions that maximize a person's sense of confidence in the targeted behavior.

Simons studied interventions used by nurses that they believed to be effective in enhancing patient adherence to a prescribed regime. Thirty-eight nurses reviewed interventions and five interventions met the stringent criteria of the intervention content validity used. Nurses reported that behavior modification, coping enhancement, mutual goal setting, patient contracting, and self-modification were interventions appropriate to impact client behavior. The researchers identified multiple activities used in each of these intervention categories (Simons, 1992).

DISCUSSION

The review of the literature reveals in many instances where the patient sees the healthcare provider as a consultant who gives advice that can be acted upon, adapted, or ignored. The patient evaluates the regime based on the variables discussed in this chapter. In the past the healthcare provider assumed that his or her advice would automatically be followed. Today, the healthcare provider needs to explore all the variables that a patient uses to evaluate the plan. It is apparent that not all healthcare consumers share the beliefs, norms, and expectations of the healthcare provider. Perhaps that is the most important piece of adherence: the realization that the provider community has a culture (broad term) all its own. We expect patients to tell us their symptoms and to take our prescriptions with minimal questioning, follow them, and pay for the service. We expect them to value preventive care as much as we do. We expect them to complete their therapy because we explained how important it was. However, the beliefs, perceptions, values, and traditions vary among ethnic groups. A patient who is present oriented may hear the advice for exercise or take away the medications to prevent an infection, but never do them or take them because he or she does not believe that's the healthcare providers' task; or the patient may only be able to focus on here and now and does not value the future as much as the present. The perception of time by someone who is present oriented may not be ruled by the clock but by social activities or physical need. Telling this person or the parent to take or give the medication three times a day may not hold any meaning. Those who have an external locus of control may not follow through on the prescribed activities—warm soaks, stretching exercises, etc.—because they do not really believe that their actions will affect the outcome. They may need a significant other to remind and prod them to adhere.

Roles in the family are important, and their significance varies among ethnic groups. If the patient is not the major decision maker regarding health by virtue of his or her role in the family, the person who is (grandmother, father, nonrelative) needs to understand the regime and its importance to achieve adherence.

The literature has shown that respect is an important factor in adherence or self-management. We may think we are being respectful, but if we are talking in a medium voice and saying, "What did you say?" to a Native American, it is interpreted as disrespectful. If we avoid eye contact while taking notes or writing prescriptions in the presence of the patient, this may be considered disrespect by a majority of patients. If a negative comment is made regarding the use of folk medicine or a healer the patient has already consulted, the patient may disregard all that is prescribed. The external-locus-of-control belief that health is a matter of luck and mostly controlled by external forces in nature is the basis of folk medicine. Violating a person's personal space while doing a routine exam may be offensive to the patient and cause nonadherence to the prescriptive regime.

If a patient's concept of time is flexible and based on social life and need rather than a clock, giving him or her an appointment for 10:00 A.M. on Monday may hold no meaning except that it is in the morning. It may be more expeditious for this patient to be followed at a walk-in clinic (Inglehart, Basanez, & Moreno, 1998). The same applies to taking medications three or four times a day.

With cultural information in mind, the healthcare provider needs to assess specific attitudes regarding medication-taking behavior. Although each of the frameworks can be useful to the provider, the evidence suggests barriers, self-efficacy, and stages of behavior change have the most pragmatic value. The healthcare provider may gain further guidance through the emerging evidence that to affect medication-taking behavior, strategies need to be stage-specific.

IMPLICATIONS FOR PRACTICE

Based on the variation in the ethnic groups, individual belief patterns, and patient/provider relationships, how can healthcare providers optimize medication-taking behavior, enhancing the possibility of a positive health outcome? The following are some suggestions, by no means inclusive:

1. When patients present for care, ask them how you can help them; what is it they want to happen (goal).
2. When possible, relate their actions to the symptoms or the problem, i.e., moving furniture 2 days ago to musculoskeletal pain, or a high-sodium/high-fat breakfast at the local Shoney's buffet to ankle edema and elevated blood pressure.
3. Ask them what they think caused their symptoms.
4. Ask them if they have used any home remedies, broader than OTC treatment, or consulted anyone else for their problem. This will give you an idea of how strongly they follow the traditions of their ethnic group.
5. When there are several equally effective options for treatment, give the patient the choice, i.e., IM injection or 10 days of medication.
6. When the treatment is collaboratively decided upon, explain it thoroughly, using terms at the level of the patient's knowledge. The collaborative decision may be made with the family's major decision maker, if possible. If the patient has an external locus of control, it is important to know if he or she believes the treatment will take care of the problem. It is recognized that many patients will say, "You're the doc, what do you think?"
7. Ask if any family, ethnic, or religious belief would make them uneasy in following the prescribed therapy, i.e., no hot medications for hot illnesses; does not believe in prevention, so stops therapy when symptoms disappear; using certain appliances on the Sabbath (Baldonado, 1996).
8. Ask patients to tell you how they will fit the therapy into their lifestyle, i.e., children cannot take medicine at school; a diabetic works the night shift. Guide patients in problem solving, but let them come up with the solution. Let them own the problem and the solution.

When developing a long-term medication regime, all of the above, especially the barriers addressed in items 7 and 8, need to be considered, in addition to the following:

9. What possible reinforcement does this plan need to support long-term success?
10. What projected stress or changes would put the plan in jeopardy? What substitute strategies can be developed to support the plan?
11. If relapse is imminent, what plans are there for immediate access to healthcare personnel? Is the patient agreeable to a contract that specifies no modification of medication regime without contacting the provider?

The following considerations are applicable for both short- and long-term medication regimes:

12. Assess the patients' beliefs regarding seriousness, susceptibility, benefits, and barriers to the course of action. Design an explanation of the medication needed that is congruent with the your assessment of the patients' beliefs in these areas.
13. Get a commitment from the patients to follow through on the plan. Have them verbalize whether they think they will be able to carry out the plan. If it is a smoking cessation contract, have them sign the discharge slip, i.e., "I will decrease the cigarettes smoked by one each day this week." The literature shows that a commitment on the part of patients results in better adherence.
14. Consider including the following in your instructions: "If anything comes up that makes you consider changing this plan or stopping the medication, will

you contact me to discuss it before you change the plan if possible, but at least as soon as you can?"

The above suggestions are certainly not inclusive. Healthcare providers need to ask themselves this bottom-line question, "What do I need to know about these clients to help them effectively use pharmacological and other therapies to achieve the desired positive health outcomes?" The issues discussed in this chapter such as culture, norms, beliefs, theories, and patient/provider relationships provide a framework to make these decisions.

REFERENCES

Abraham, C., Clift, S., & Grabowski, P. (1999). Cognitive predictors of adherence to malaria prophylaxis regimens on return from a malarious region: A prospective study. *Social Science & Medicine, 48,* 1641–1654.

AHRQ (2004). *National Healthcare Disparities Report: Summary,* Agency for Healthcare Research and Quality: Rockville, MD. http://www.ahrq.gov/qual/nhdr03/nhdrsum03.htm

Ajzen, I. (1988). *Attitudes, personality and behavior.* Chicago: Dorsey Press.

Ajzen, I. (1991). The theory of planned behavior. *Organizational Behavior and Human Decision Processes, 50,* 179–211.

Ajzen, I., & Fishbein, M. (1980). *Understanding attitudes and predicting social behavior.* Englewood Cliffs, NJ: Prentice-Hall.

Amaro, H., & Zambrana, R. (2000). Criollo, Mestizo, Mulato, LatiNegro, Indigina, White or Black? The U.S. Hispanic/Latino population and multiple responses in the 2000 census. *American Journal of Public Health, 90* (11), 1724–1727.

Bailey, E.J. (2000). *Medical anthropology and African American health.* Westport, CT: Bergin & Garvey.

Baldonado, A. A. (1996). Transcending the barriers of cultural diversity in health care. *Journal of Cultural Diversity, 3* (1), 20–22.

Bandura, A. (1986). *Social foundations of thought and action: A social cognitive theory.* Englewood Cliffs, NJ: Prentice Hall.

Bonin J. (1999). Psychosocial determinants for lithium compliance in bipolar disorder. *Canadian Journal of Nursing Research, 31,* 25–40.

Bradley, C. (1995). Health beliefs and knowledge of patients and doctors in clinical practice and research. *Patient Education and Counseling, 26* (1–3), 99–106.

Budd, R. J., Hughes, I. C., & Smith, J. A. (1996). Health beliefs and compliance with antipsychotic medication. *British Journal of Clinical Psychology, 35* (Pt 3), 393–397.

Champion, V. L., & Huster, G. (1995). Effect of interventions on stage of mammography adoption. *Journal of Behavioral Medicine, 18* (2), 169–187.

Champion, V., & Miller, A. M. (1996). Recent mammography in women aged 35 and older: Predisposing variables. *Health Care of Women International, 17* (3), 233–245.

Conway, S. P., Pond, M. N., Hamnett, T., & Watson, A. (1996). Compliance with treatment in adult patients with cystic fibrosis. *Thorax, 51* (1), 29–33.

Cowell, C. (2001). Nutrition and women's health: Challenge for the 21st century. *Journal of the American Medical Women's Association, 56* (2), 73–74, 78.

del Rosario, V. M. (2001). A metaphor for HIV-positive Mexican and Puerto Rican women. *Western Journal of Nursing Research, 23* (5), 517–535.

DeVries, J., Mudde, A. N., Dijkstra, A., & Willemsen, M. C. (1998). Differential beliefs, perceived social influences and self-efficacy expectations among smokers in various motivational phases. *Preventive Medicine, 27* (5 part 1), 681–689.

Dillin, J. (2001 January 3). Behind population gains: Immigrant influx: Surprising growth rate in 2000 census reflects influx into Sun Belt from abroad. *The Christian Science Monitor.*

Elliot, W. J. (1994). Compliance strategies. *Current Opinion in Nephrology & Hypertension, 3* (3), 271–278.

Fishbein, M., & Ajzen, I. (1975). *Belief, attitude, intention, and behavior: An introduction to theory and research.* Boston: Addison-Wesley.

Gallup Poll (2003). Why don't women take folic acid? Forgetfulness and denial, latest survey finds. Retrieved from http://search.marchofdimes.com/cgi-bin/MsmGo.exe?grab_id=41&page_id=8389376&query=GALLUP&hiword=GALLUP+March 1, 2004.

Hand, C. H., & Bradley, C. (1996). Health beliefs of adults with asthma: Toward an understanding of the difference between symptomatic and preventive use of inhaler treatment. *Journal of Asthma, 33* (5), 331–338.

Inglehart, R., Basanez, M., & Moreno, A. (1998). *Human values and beliefs:* A *cross-cultural sourcebook. Political, religious, sexual, and economic norms in 43 societies.* Ann Arbor: University of Michigan Press.

IOM (2003). Unequal treatment: Confronting racial and ethnic disparities in health care. http://books.nap.edu/catalogue/10260.html

Jennings-Dozier K. (1999). Perceptual determinants of Pap test up-to-date status among minority women. *Oncology Nursing Forum, 6,* 327–333.

Kalichman, S. C., Rompa, D., DiFonzo, K., Simpson, D., Austin, J., Luke W., Kyomugisha, F., & Buckles, J. (2001). HIV treatment adherence in women living with HIV/AIDS: Research based on the Information-Motivation-Behavioral Skills model of health behavior. *J Assoc Nurses AIDS Care 12* (4), 58–67.

Kloeblen, A. S., & Batish, S. S. (1999). Understanding the intention to permanently follow a high folate diet among a sample of low-income pregnant women according to the Health Belief Model. *Health Education Research, 14,* 27–38.

Levin, P. F. (1999). Test of the Fishbein and Ajzen models as predictors of health care workers' glove use. *Research in Nursing & Health, 22* (4), 295–307.

Marlatt, G. A., & Gordon, J. R. (1985). *Relapse prevention: Maintenance strategies in the treatment of addictive behaviors.* New York: Guilford Press.

Marlenga, B. (1995). The health beliefs and skin cancer prevention practices of Wisconsin dairy farmers. *Oncology Nursing Forum, 22* (4), 681–686.

Montgomery, A. J. (1996). AIDS education: Knowledge, sexual attitudes and sexual behavioral responses of selected college students. *ABNF Journal, 7* (2), 57–60.

Morris, W. (Ed.). (1993). *The American heritage dictionary.* Boston: American Heritage and Houghton Mifflin.

Morrison, D. M., Gillmore, M. R., & Baker, S. A. (1995). Determinants of condom use among high-risk heterosexual adults: A test of the theory of reasoned action. *Journal of Applied Social Psychology, 25* (8), 651–676.

Mudde, A. N., Kok, G., & Strecher, V. J. (1995). Self-efficacy as a predictor for the cessation of smoking: Methodological issues and implications for smoking cessation programs. *Psychology & Health, 10* (5), 353–367.

Pasket, E. D., Carter, W. B., Chu, J. E., & White, E. (1990). Compliance behavior in women with abnormal pap smears: Developing and testing a decision model. *Medical Care, 28* (7), 643–656.

Patel, S. C., & Spaeth, G. L. (1995). Compliance in patients with eyedrops for glaucoma. *Ophthalmic Surgery, 26* (3), 233–236.

Pellino, T. A. (1997). Relationships between patient attitudes, subjective norms, perceived control, and analgesic use following elective orthopedic surgery. *Research in Nursing and Health, 20,* 97–105.

Pender, N. J. (1996). *Health promotion in nursing practice.* Stamford, CT: Appleton & Lange.

Philis-Tsimikas, A., & Walker, C. (2001). Improved care for diabetes in underserved populations. *Journal of Ambulatory Care Management, 24* (1), 39–43.

Poss, J. E. (1999). Developing an instrument to study the tuberculosis screening behaviors of Mexican migrant farmworkers. *Journal of Transcultural Nursing, 10,* 306–319.

Prochaska, J. O., Velicier, W. E., Rossi, J. S., & Goldstein, M. G. (1994). Stages of change and decisional balance for 12 problem behaviors. *Health Psychology, 13* (1), 39–46.

Rexroth, R., & Davidhizar, R. (2003). Caring: Utilizing the Watson theory to transcend culture. *The Health Care Manager, 22* (4), 295–305.

Rosenberg, M. J., Burnhill, M. S., Waugh, M. S., Grimes, D. A., & Hillard, P. J. (1995). Compliance and oral contraceptives: A ...view. *Contraception, 52* (3), 137–141.

Rubel, A. J., & Ca... (1992). Social and cultural factors in successful contr... *...ublic Health Reports, 107*(6), 626–636.

Scherer, Y., K. & Bruce S... Knowledge, attitudes, and self-efficacy and complian... medical regimen, number of emergency department visi... hospitalizations in adults with asthma. *Heart & Lung, 30*...

Sheppard, B. H., Hartwick, J., & War... R. (1988). The theory of reasoned action: A meta-analy... past research with recommendations for modifications ...future research. *Journal of Consumer Research, 15* (3), 32...

Simons, M. R. (1992). Interventions related ...compliance. *Nursing Clinics of North America, 27* (2), 477–...

Somkin, C. P. (1993). Improving the effectivenes... breast self-examination in the early detection of breast canc... A selective review of the literature. *Nurse Practitioner Fo..., 4* (2), 76–84.

U.S. Census Bureau. (2001). *Statistical abstract of the United States.* Washington, DC: U.S. Government Printing Office.

van Balen, F., & Gerrits, T. (2001). Quality of infertility care in poor-resource areas and the introduction of new reproductive technologies. *Human Reproduction, 16* (2), 215–219.

Van Essen, G. A., Kuyvenhoven, M. M., & de Melker, R. A. (1997). Why do healthy elderly people fail to comply with influenza vaccinations? *Age and Aging, 26* (4), 275–297.

Wambach, K. A. (1997). Breastfeeding intention and outcome: A test of the theory of planned behavior. *Research in Nursing & Health, 20,* 51–59.

ADDITIONAL RESOURCES

Adamopoulos, J., & Kashima, Y. (1999). *Social psychology and cultural context.* Thousand Oaks, CA: Sage Publications.

Anderson, M.J., & Fienberg, S. E. (1999). *Who counts? The politics of census-taking in contemporary America.* New York: Sage Foundation.

Douglas, J. H. (1993). Issues in transcultural nursing highlighted in three international conferences. *Journal of Transcultural Nursing, 5* (1), 34.

Huntington, S.P., & Harrison, L.E. (2000). *Culture matters: How values shape human progress.* New York: Basic Books.

Matsumoto, D., Pun, K. K., Nakstani, M., Kadowaki, D., Weissman, M., McCarter, L., Fletcher, D., & Takeuchi, S. (1995). Cultural differences in attitudes, values, and beliefs about osteoporosis in first and second generation Japanese-American women. *Women & Health, 23* (4), 39–56.

Useful Web Pages with Information to Increase Cultural Competency

DiversityRx (www.diversityrx.org): **Mission:** Promoting language and cultural competence to improve the quality of

...nt, and ethnically diverse health care for minorit... communities.

Ethnomed (www.ethn... The EthnoMed site contains ...eliefs, medical issues and other information about ...he healthcare of recent immigrants related issues per... ...y of whom are refugees fleeing war-to Seattle or the... torn parts of th...

Transcultural Nursing Society (www.tcns.org): The mission of the global Transcultural Nursing Society is to ensure that the culture care needs of the people of the world will be met by nurses prepared in transcultural nursing.

ANA (2003). Position Statement: Cultural Diversity in Nursing Practice. American Nurses Association. Available at: http://nursingworld.org/readroom/position/ethics/etcldv.htm.

CHAPTER ❖ 6

REGULATORY CONTROL OF DRUGS

Gene White

THE FEDERAL FOOD DRUG AND COSMETIC ACT

The law that specifically defines the term "drug" and provides the legal basis for regulating the development, manufacture, marketing, and distribution of drugs in the United States is the Federal Food, Drug and Cosmetic Act (FDCA) that was enacted in 1938. The FDCA prohibits adulterated or misbranded drugs from being introduced into interstate commerce, or becoming adulterated or misbranded while in interstate commerce, or the receipt of such drugs after shipment in interstate commerce. Likewise, the Act provides that all drugs marketed after 1938 must prove that they are safe and effective for the conditions for which they are recommended before receiving the Food and Drug Administration's approval for marketing. After getting approval, manufacturers must establish a system for receiving information regarding the use of such drugs and report to the Food and Drug Administration (FDA) any adverse information that may call into question the drug's safety and effectiveness.

The Durham-Humphrey Amendment to the FDCA divides drugs into two categories. If the FDA determines that adequate directions for the safe and effective use of the drug by a layman for the conditions recommended cannot be written, then the drug must be dispensed only pursuant to a valid prescription. Therefore, the drug's immediate container must bear the label "Caution: Federal Law Prohibits Dispensing Without a Prescription." The drug is then called a *legend drug*. If the FDA determines that such directions can be written, a prescription is not needed to purchase the drug. It is then referred to as an *over-the-counter (OTC) drug*.

Persons regulated by the provisions of this law could be subjected to strict liability or liability without fault. This means that a person could be criminally convicted even though the violation was done unintentionally or without knowledge that the event had occurred. Those placing themselves under the provisions of this law should take it very seriously.

FEDERAL CONTROLLED SUBSTANCE ACT

In the late 1960s the United States found itself in the middle of a growing drug abuse problem. While illicit drugs were a large part of the problem, so were legal drugs. Some legend drugs that could only be legally dispensed pursuant to a prescription were being diverted for illegal use. It was determined that certain drugs needed to be under stricter regulation than that imposed by the FDCA. Therefore, in 1970 Congress enacted the Federal Controlled Substance Act (CSA).

The CSA places certain drugs into one of five schedules by using the following three criteria:

- Does the drug have a currently accepted medical use in the United States?

- Does the drug have a potential for abuse?
- What is the severity of dependence of the drug, both psychologically and physiologically?

The five schedules are designated as C-I, C-II, C-III, C-IV, and C-V, with the severity of controls decreasing as the numbers get larger. See Table 6–1 for a description of the schedules. In general, drugs in schedules C-II, C-III, and C-IV are legend drugs and require a prescription before they can be legally dispensed. Some preparations in Schedule C-V require a prescription. However, there are preparations in Schedule C-V that have acceptable directions for use and may be obtained without a prescription. These preparations may be sold over-the-counter in limited quantities within 48 hours to any one person. The pharmacist is required to keep a bound book showing the name of the C-V preparation, the quantity sold, the name and address of the purchaser, the date of the purchase, and the pharmacist's initials.

The appropriate schedule of controlled substances can usually be determined by reading the manufacturer's label attached to the immediate container of the drug. The schedule number will be shown in the upper right hand corner inside a C that is at least twice as large as any other printing on the label, or it will appear as background print over the entire label with other label requirements superimposed. All other legend drugs that are not in one of the five schedules are usually referred to as noncontrolled legend drugs. However, there are several states that have given these noncontrolled legend drugs the designation of C-VI drugs.

TABLE 6–1. Description of Drug Schedules

C-I	The only schedule of drugs that do not have a recognized medical use in the United States and therefore cannot be legally marketed. These drugs may be used for research purposes.
C-II	Drugs that have a currently accepted medical use in the United States and a high abuse potential, with severe psychological or physiological dependence. Examples: morphine, Demerol, cocaine, codeine, Methadone, amphetamine, Ritalin and the fast-acting barbiturates (amo-, pento-, and secobarbital).
C-III	Drugs that have a currently accepted medical use in the United States and an abuse potential below that of C-I and C-II. Abuse of these drugs may lead to moderate or low physical dependence or high psychological dependence. Examples: certain codeine products such as Empirin No. 3, Tylenol No. 4, paregoric, anabolic steroids, and certain barbiturates in combination with other active medicinal ingredients.
C-IV	The same as C-III except a lower abuse potential. Overuse of these drugs causes only a limited physical or psychological dependence. Examples: chloral hydrate, phenobarbital, and certain tranquilizers such as Librium and Valium.
C-V	The same as C-IV except there is a lower potential for abuse and less physical and psychological dependence than C-IV. Examples: preparations containing a limited quantity of a narcotic drug in combination with a non-narcotic active medicinal ingredient and used for anticough purposes. Also diphenoxylate in combination with atropine sulfate for antidiarrheal purposes.

PRESCRIPTIONS

ELEMENTS OF A PRESCRIPTION

Before a pharmacist can legally dispense a legend drug, it must be authorized by a valid prescription. It is the pharmacist's responsibility to be certain that the required tangible and intangible characteristics are present to constitute such a prescription.

Tangible (physical) characteristics:

1. Patient's full name and address.
2. Prescriber's full name and address.
3. Prescriber's DEA number if a controlled substance is prescribed.
4. Drug name.
5. Drug strength and dosage form, if appropriate.
6. Quantity to be dispensed.
7. Directions for use.
8. Refill instructions, if applicable.
9. Substitution rights.
10. Signed and dated by the prescriber on the day issued.

Intangible (nonphysical) characteristics:

> Federal regulations written pursuant to the CSA provide the following: "A prescription for a controlled substance to be effective must be issued *for a legitimate medical purpose* by an individual practitioner *acting within the usual course of his professional practice.* The responsibility for the proper prescribing and dispensing of controlled substances is upon the prescribing practitioner, but a corresponding responsibility rests with the pharmacist who fills the prescription." (Code of Federal Regulations, 1991)

If the pharmacist knows or should have known that the prescribed controlled drug will not be used for legitimate medical purposes, such as maintaining a patient's addiction to drugs or prescribing a central nervous system stimulant to assist a driver in sleep deprivation for extended periods of time, then the prescription is not a valid authorization to dispense medication. Likewise, if a dentist prescribes an antibiotic to treat a gunshot wound or a physician prescribes a tranquilizer to calm down a neighbor's hyperactive cat, the prescriber would not be acting within the usual course of his or her professional practice and the prescription would be invalid. Most states, either by statute or regulation, have applied these intangible characteristics to noncontrolled, legend drugs.

WHO MAY PRESCRIBE LEGEND DRUGS

The FDCA provides that legend drugs can be dispensed only upon the written or oral prescription of *a practitioner licensed by law* to administer such drugs. In general, it is state law that determines who can become a practitioner licensed by law to administer such drugs. This normally covers medical doctors (M.D.), dentists (D.D.S.), osteopaths (D.O.), podiatrists (D.P.M.), and veterinarians (D.V.M.). States have now begun to grant limited prescriptive authority to other health practitioners such as nurse practitioners, physician assistants, optometrists, and pharmacists. Among those states that have enacted such laws, the terms and conditions of the prescriptive authority vary greatly.

FILLING PRESCRIPTIONS

The general rule for C-II drugs is that the pharmacist must have a written prescription before the medication can be legally dispensed. There is an exception in an emergency situation if the proper procedure is followed. In this case, an emergency situation is defined as one in which:

1. The patient's health will be adversely affected without the medication.
2. No other medication will work.
3. The prescriber cannot reasonably be expected to get the pharmacist a prescription.

The pharmacist may then accept an oral prescription for a C-II drug and reduce it to writing showing all of the information needed except the prescriber's signature. An amount of drug sufficient to get a patient through the emergency situation up to a maximum three-day supply may be dispensed. If the pharmacist does not recognize the prescriber or has any reason to doubt the authenticity of the prescriber, the pharmacist must make a reasonable effort to determine that the oral order came from a bonafide practitioner. Within 72 hours from giving the oral order, the prescriber must send the pharmacist a written prescription for the medication already dispensed (postmarked within 72 hours). The written prescription must contain the phrase, "Authorization for emergency dispensing" and bear the date of the oral order. The written prescription from the prescriber must be attached to the order prepared by the pharmacist and kept on file. If the written order is not received (postmarked) from the prescriber within 72 hours, the pharmacist is required to report the prescriber to the Drug Enforcement Agency. Should the pharmacist fail to report the prescriber, then the statutory authority allowing the pharmacist to dispense a C-II drug on oral order is revoked and the pharmacist has illegally distributed a C-II drug.

Prescriptions for C-II drugs may not be refilled. It is permissible to partially fill a C-II prescription in several instances:

1. If the pharmacist does not have the full quantity prescribed; then the prescription may be partially filled. The remaining portion must be dispensed within 72 hours of the partial filling or it cannot be dispensed and the prescriber must be notified.
2. C-II prescriptions for patients in long-term care facilities (LTCF) may be partially filled in the following manner. The prescriber may write for up to a maximum 60-day supply of a C-II drug. The pharmacist may partially fill the prescription until the total quantity prescribed is dispensed or up to 60 days from the date of issuance, whichever comes first.
3. A prescription for a C-II drug may be partially filled for an ambulatory patient with a medical diagnosis documenting a terminal illness. The practitioner must classify the patient as terminally ill and the pharmacist must verify and record such notation on the prescription. The prescription may be partially filled for a maximum of 60 days from the date of issuance or until the total quantity of medication prescribed is dispensed, whichever comes first.

Prescriptions for C-III or C-IV drugs may be received from the prescriber either orally or in writing. If received orally, they must be promptly reduced to writing and show all of the necessary information except the prescriber's signature. If so authorized by the prescriber, C-III and C-IV prescriptions may be refilled up to five times or within six months from the date of issuance, whichever comes first. After this six-month period, these prescriptions may not be filled or refilled.

Prescriptions for noncontrolled legend drugs may also be received either in writing or orally and promptly reduced to writing. These prescriptions may be refilled as authorized by the prescriber on the face of the original prescription. The length of time in which these prescriptions can be filled or refilled varies among the states, but is usually around two years from the date of issuance.

FILING OF PRESCRIPTIONS

The CSA provides three methods for filing the hard prescription copy in a pharmacy:

1. Prescriptions may be kept in three separate files. One file for the C-II prescriptions; one for C-III, C-IV, and C-V prescriptions; and another file for noncontrolled legend prescriptions.
2. The file for C-II prescriptions and a separate file for C-III, C-IV, C-V, and noncontrolled legend prescriptions.
3. One file for C-II, C-III, C-IV, C-V prescriptions and a separate file for noncontrolled legend prescriptions.

When C-III, C-IV, and C-V prescriptions are mixed with any other prescriptions, they must be marked with a red C at least one inch high in the lower right-hand corner of the prescriptions. Some states require that C-II prescriptions always be filed by themselves and therefore only allow methods 1 and 2.

REFILL INFORMATION

When a prescription is refilled, the pharmacist must note, on the hard copy of the prescription or in a computer, the date of the refill, the amount dispensed if different from the quantity prescribed, and the pharmacist's initials. Most pharmacies maintain electronic records of prescriptions and quantities dispensed and refilled. Rules on how to maintain these records will vary depending on the state.

DISPENSING GUIDELINES

The Poison Prevention Act is a federal law that requires that prescription medication be dispensed in child-resistant containers unless it comes under one of the following exemptions.

1. The prescriber may request that the medication be dispensed in a container that is not child resistant. Such a request could cover all of the medication prescribed by the practitioner for one patient at a time, but not for all of the practitioner's patients at once.
2. The patient may request that his or her medication be dispensed in a non-childproof container. While the patient can give a blanket consent that all of his or her medication be dispensed in non-childproof containers, the pharmacist is required to check with the patient verbally each time medication is dispensed. While federal law does not require that the patient's consent be obtained in writing, it would certainly be prudent for the pharmacist to do so. Some state statutes provide immunity from civil liability when the pharmacist obtains a signed consent form from the patient.
3. Drugs dispensed to institutionalized patients may be packaged in non-childproof containers to be administered by institutional personnel.

Some OTC products such as aspirin, methyl salicylate, ibuprofen, and methyl alcohol are required to be in childproof containers. The manufacturer is allowed to select one size of this product other than the most popular size and package it in a non-childproof container. This is done for the convenience of the elderly and handicapped, and the package must bear a label stating that "This package is for households without young children."

REGISTRATION AND BIENNIAL INVENTORY

The CSA requires all pharmacies or pharmacists to register with the DEA every three years as a class 3 registrant. This registration allows pharmacists legally to possess and dispense schedule C-II through C-V drugs. Every pharmacy or pharmacist registrant must conduct a complete and accurate inventory of all controlled substances every two years. This inventory must be signed and dated by the pharmacist conducting the inventory. While not required by law, many pharmacists prefer to keep a perpetual inventory of controlled substances in order to detect shortages quickly. A complete and accurate record of all controlled substances received and dispensed or otherwise disposed of must be kept.

ELECTRONIC PRESCRIBING

Many states presently allow some form of electronic transmission of prescriptions. In this process, the prescription is electronically transmitted via a database exchange or email converted to fax to the patients' pharmacy. The database is usually a desktop/laptop computer or personal digital device (PDA). The prescription is then filled from the electronically transmitted order. The physician is required, in many of these states, to keep a written record of what is prescribed. With the passing of the federal Electronic Signatures in Global and National Commerce Act or E-SIGN in October 2000, the barrier of requiring paper records is lifted. However, other issues, such as the inability to transmit C-II pharmaceuticals, still hamper the process. Ensuring the security of confidential patient information when prescriptions are transmitted via these newer modalities is also a concern. It is likely that in the next decade, electronic prescribing will be standard practice (Hisle, 2001).

REFERENCES

Code of Federal Regulations. 21 CFR Sect. 1306.04 (2003), 71.

Hisle, J. M. (2001). Throw away the prescription pad? Debate over electronic prescription and fulfullment. *Medical Crossfire, 3,* 47–56.

Pharmacy Law Digest. St. Louis: Facts and Comparisons. Supplemented annually.

CHAPTER ❖ 7

PHARMACOTHERAPY RESOURCES FOR THE PROVIDER

Geneva Briggs

All healthcare practitioners need up-to-date, easy-to-use, and easy-to-find resources to answer questions about medications in everyday practice. Ideally, the information should be unbiased and cover more than might be available on an FDA label, if necessary. This chapter addresses the various options and resources currently available to help you find the medication information you need. Because computerized resources change rapidly, any specific products mentioned may have evolved or no longer be available. The examples of each kind of product discussed here should pique your interest in the range and depth of resources you can turn to for help in your practice.

PRINTED RESOURCES

Books and journals in printed and bound formats have been and still remain the primary resources for medication information. Although computerized information has exploded and has the advantage of being more current, not everyone has access to a computer or to either CD-ROM disk versions of texts and journals or to the Internet at their workplaces. Printed materials are widely available, are less costly, and allow the user to choose different versions so the information is most useful for a particular situation or practice. Their major disadvantage is the time lag between the date of writing and publication. Textbooks and handbooks are out of date as soon as they are published because new medications and new research information about the use of both older and new medications are being released as the books are in production. Even materials updated yearly may not contain the very newest medications. The most current *printed text* information can be found in two resources:

- *Drug Facts and Comparisons:* Can be obtained in either a hardcover book updated yearly or in a loose-leaf format that is available as a subscription service and updated monthly.
- *AHFS Drug Information:* Published yearly with new information sent quarterly in a softcover format. Also includes faxed updates.

The majority of written resources come in five major formats: textbooks, journals, newsletters, resource books, and handbooks (Shaughnessy, Slawson, & Bennett, 1994). Examples of all the formats are cited in Table 7–1. Textbooks often contain more information than the practitioner may want to read to find a quick answer to a simple question. And due to the publication time lag, newer medications and new uses for medications will not be addressed. Pharmacotherapy textbooks are valuable for an overall perspective on the treatment of a disease or condition with medications, but the user should ensure that he or she is using the most recent edition of a text for the most current information (Knott & Scott, 1994).

Journals provide the most recent information on medications, but the sheer number of journals can be daunting and can cause information overload for the

TABLE 7–1. Example Printed and Computerized Pharmacotherapy Resources

Pharmacotherapy Resource	Publisher	Description/Comments	Frequency of Publication and/or Updates
Textbooks			
Pharmacotherapy: A Pathophysiologic Approach	McGraw-Hill/Appleton & Lange 800-262-4729 *www.accessmedbooks.com*	Comprehensive text on pharmacotherapeutics	Most recent edition: 2002
Applied Therapeutics: The Clinical Use of Drugs	Applied Therapeutics, Inc. 360-253-7123	Comprehensive text on pharmacotherapeutics; presents information in case-study format	Most recent edition: 2003
Basic and Clinical Pharmacology	Lippincott Williams & Wilkins 800-638-0672 *www.lww.com3*	Complete, yet concise pharmacology text; focuses on not only the basic mechanisms of drug action but also the clinical use of drugs and monitoring of therapeutic and adverse effects	Most recent edition: 2004
Reference Books			
AHFS Drug Information	American Society of Health System Pharmacists 301-657-3000 *www.ashp.org*	Extensive drug monographs; includes non-FDA-approved indications and doses	Yearly with quarterly updates (available online)
Drug Facts and Comparisons	Facts and Comparisons 314-878-2515 *www.drugfacts.com*	Easy-to-use information on administration, brand and generic identification, and available dosage forms; lists inactive ingredients, such as alcohol and sugar and orphan drugs	Yearly with monthly updates
Drug Interaction Facts	Facts and Comparisons	Clinical significance, mechanisms, and management of drug-drug and drug-food interactions	Yearly updates
Handbook of Nonprescription Drugs	American Pharmaceutical Association 800-878-0729 *www.aphanet.org*	Although named as a handbook, this is really a hybrid textbook and medication resource, covers disease processes that are treated with OTC products, such as sunburn or poison ivy; information about selected OTC medications	Every three years; most recent: 2002
Nonprescription Drug Therapy	Facts and Comparisons	Monographs of OTC therapy that contain information on etiology, symptoms, treatment, and patient counseling	Quarterly
Drugs in Pregnancy and Lactation	Lippincott Williams & Wilkins	Covers fetal and neonatal (breast-feeding) risks of maternal drug ingestion, 1999 edition available on CD	Periodically; most recent edition: 2001
Physician's Desk Reference (PDR)	Medical Economics Data 800-232-7379 *www.medec.com*	Contains FDA-approved package insert labeling, inactive ingredients, pictures of some products, manufacturers' addresses and phone numbers, not comprehensive	Yearly: biannual supplements for additional cost
Herbal Medicine—Expanded Commission E Monographs	Lippincott Williams & Wilkins	Monographs include history, efficacy, safety, and quality standards for top selling herbs	Periodically; most recent edition: 2000
The Review of Natural Products	Lippincott Williams & Wilkins	Over 300 monographs that include botany, chemistry, pharmacology, medicinal uses, toxicology, documented drug interactions, and patient information	Periodically; most recent edition: 2002
Martindale: The Complete Drug Reference	Pharmaceutical Press *www.amazon.com*	Good for identifying foreign medications; British publication	Every five to six years; most recent edition: 1999

TABLE 7–1. Example Printed and Computerized Pharmacotherapy Resources *(continued)*

Pharmacotherapy Resource	Publisher	Description/Comments	Frequency of Publication and/or Updates
Drugs Available Abroad. A Guide to Therapeutic Drugs Available and Approved Outside the U.S.	Gale Research Inc. 800-877-4253 *www.amazon.com*	Lists drugs available in other countries	Periodically; most recent edition: 1991
USP DI, Volume I, Drug Information for the Health Care Professional	United States Pharmacopeial-Convention, Inc. 800-227-8772	Drug monographs; adverse effects organized by severity; orphan drug products	Yearly with monthly updates (available online)
Handbooks			
Geriatric Dosage Handbook	Lexi-Comp Inc. 800-837-LEXI *www.Ramex.com*	Brief monographs; dosage adjustments for patients with renal and hepatic failure	Yearly
Pediatric Dosage Handbook	Lexi-Comp Inc.	Brief monographs with pediatric dosing information	Yearly
Pocket Version—Drug Facts and Comparisons	Facts and Comparisons	Condensed version of Drug Facts and Comparisons; monographs have similar layout	Yearly
Red Book	Medical Economics Data	Average wholesale prices, manufacturers' addresses and phone numbers, and drug information center and poison control center numbers	Yearly with monthly average wholesale price updates
Newsletters			
Prescriber's Letter	Therapeutic Research Center 209-472-2440	Up-to-date information on drug interactions and new medication uses gleaned from current primary literature; referenced	Monthly
The Medical Letter	The Medical Letter, Inc. 800-211-2769 *www.medletter.com*	Reviews of new medications, drug classes, new indications; referenced and unbiased	Monthly (available online)
Journal Watch	Journal Watch 800-843-6356 *www.jwatch.com*	Reviews current primary literature; referenced	Bimonthly (available online)
Software—Drug Interactions			
The IBIS Guide to Drug-Herb and Drug-Nutrient Interactions	Integrative Medical Arts 877-526-IBIS *www.ibismedical.com*	Drug-herb and drug-nutrient interactions, patient education handouts	Periodically
Adverse Drug Interactions Program	The Medical Letter, Inc.	Searches interactions between two and up to fifty medications; allows user to list each medication patient is taking and then view possible interactions and reference citations	Biannually
CD-ROMs			
Drug Information Fulltext	American Society of Health System Pharmacists	Contains full text of AHFS Drug Information plus extra information and Handbook on Injectable Drugs; allows searching of database; network version is available	Yearly
Drug Facts and Comparisons	Facts and Comparisons	Contains same information as loose-leaf version	Yearly
International Pharmaceutical Abstracts (IPA)	American Society of Health System Pharmacists	Abstracts from 600 worldwide pharmaceutical, medical, and health care journals since 1970	Quarterly

(continued)

TABLE 7–1. Example Printed and Computerized Pharmacotherapy Resources *(continued)*

Pharmacotherapy Resource	Publisher	Description/Comments	Frequency of Publication and/or Updates
USP-DI	United States Pharmacopeia/ Micromedex, Inc.	Drug monographs; adverse effects organized by severity; orphan drug products	Quarterly
Clinical Pharmacology	Gold Standard Multimedia, Inc. 235 S. Main Street, Suite 206 Gainesville, FL 32601-6585 800-375-0943 *www.gsm.com*	Over 2000 drug monographs; can maintain patient profiles, generate reports, write prescriptions, check for drug interactions; color pictures of drug products; online subscription also available	Quarterly
Drug Interaction Facts	Facts and Comparisons	Can obtain information on interactions by single drug or multiple drugs (up to 20) and by severity	Quarterly

average practitioner. Newsletters summarize the latest developments in a particular field for a particular health care practitioner. Their targeted information can keep one abreast of significant findings of either current studies, which may or may not include medications (for example, *Journal Watch,* published by the New England Medical Association), or on medication issues (see *The Medical Letter,* published by *The Medical Letter, Inc.*).

Resource books contain medication information only, typically in monograph form. Monographs are detailed descriptions of drugs containing generic and brand names, indications, pharmacology, mechanisms of action, contraindications, precautions, adverse effects, drug interactions, dosage, administration, dosage forms, and patient information (Price & Goldwire, 1994). *Drug Facts and Comparisons* and *AHFS Drug Information* cover most medications marketed in the United States and contain FDA and non-FDA approved indications and dosing guidelines. Since *The Physician's Desk Reference* (PDR) contains FDA-approved package insert information about medications that a manufacturer chooses to pay to have published, it is not comprehensive (Cohen & Insel, 1996). Because the PDR contains only the FDA-approved labeling, the latest information about dosing and nonapproved indications is also not available (Cohen, 2001). Specialty resource books concentrate on a single area or topic, such as drug interactions, adverse effects of medications, or medication use in pregnancy. A *current* drug interactions resource book is a necessity for any healthcare practitioner who prescribes, dispenses, or administers medications because new drug interactions are constantly being discovered. Given the increasing use of herbal and alternative medications, a reference on these products is essential for most practitioners (Sweet, Gay, Leady & Stumpf, 2003). Practitioners who work with children and child-bearing-age women should have references on pediatric dosing and medications in pregnancy and lactation. Handbooks usually contain only selected information about a few medications or limited information about multiple medications and are common for specialty areas such as geriatrics or pediatrics. Handbooks can be useful for a practitioner in a specialty area if the specific medications usually used are covered in sufficient detail. Handbooks also tend to be smaller and more portable.

COMPUTER-BASED RESOURCES

In recent years the number of computer-based resources available has exploded. Many handbooks and reference books are available in both a printed and computer version (diskette or compact disk). The current compact disk read-only memory (CD-ROM) has storage capacity of over 600 megabytes of information (Millman & Lee, 1995). This is equivalent to 250,000 to 300,000 pages of text and more than 400 floppy disks. Because CDs can hold so much information, the CD version of a reference may contain such extras as pictures, graphs, or tables not found in the printed version.

For primary literature information, MEDLINE, covering over 3,700 international journals, is the most comprehensive database of citations for articles in medicine and bioscience. Many different CD-ROM products have evolved from the database: You can obtain the complete database from 1966 to the present, or only the most recent citations (3–5 years), or only citations from clinical journals. MEDLINE is also available from different online sources, discussed later.

Before making a significant investment in computer-based resource materials, the user should consider a few key points: computer accessibility, computer requirements, computer literacy of the end user, costs compared to the printed version if available, the frequency of upgrades and the associated costs, and the format of information obtained. A computer needs to be accessible at the time resource use is desired, and the user needs to be able to find the desired information quickly and efficiently. Consider the computer requirements for the program; given the space consumption and requirements of some programs, additional memory or a faster compact disk player may be needed. Some programs require multiple CD players or are cost-prohibitive for most single users; these versions are primarily intended for institution use and purchase. The information format in a program is also important. Some databases—*International Pharmaceutical Abstracts,* for example—are only bibliographic, providing only the citation and/or abstract of an article, whereas others contain the full text from an article. Consider how often a program is updated, if at all, and the costs of any updates or upgrades.

Carefully evaluate any software or compact disk program before buying to see that it meets identified needs. Many companies will allow a demonstration or trial period with their products. Look beyond the "bells and whistles" of a program to assess its true benefit to your practice.

The newest way to have portable resources at the point of patient care is the personal data assistant (PDA). Numerous drug and medical information resources are available for the PDA. Table 7–2 includes a web address listing available medical software for PDAs. PDA software must be examined like any other pharmacotherapy resource for breadth, clinical dependability, and ease of use (Enders, Enders, & Holstad, 2002, Keplar & Urbanski, 2003).

ONLINE RESOURCES

Online resources can connect you with many CD-ROM and printed materials, often for free. Connection to an online resource is usually through a personal computer or mainframe computer workstation. Online resources are available in several ways: access to large databases in remote locations through direct computer connection (university library), through a commercial online service (not specifically medically related), or electronic bulletin boards sponsored by professional organizations or schools. Online resources can conveniently answer questions quickly if you are computer literate and hardware is available for immediate use. Before committing to an online service, consider the amount of time you will likely use the service, its billing plan, and the format and quality of information obtained. Some services have an hourly use charge and are accessed through a long-distance telephone call, an additional charge. Also consider what additional computer equipment may be necessary to access an online service (i.e., modem or communications software).

Commercial online services such as CompuServe and America Online offer access to the Internet and have

TABLE 7–2. Websites for Pharmacotherapy Information

Site Name	Site Address	Comments
Medscape	*http://www.medscape.com/*	Offers peer-reviewed, practice-oriented information; full-text journal articles; MEDLINE; continuing education; drug monograph database from First DataBank and AHFS including patient education handouts; free but healthcare provider must register
RxList	*http://www.rxlist.com/*	Drug monograph database
NLM Gateway	*http:/gateway.nlm.nih.gov/gw/cmd*	National Library of Medicine (NLM) gateway; can search MEDLINE/PubMed (1966–present), Old MEDLINE (1958–1965) and other databases
FDA	*http://www.fda.gov/*	Information from FDA on drugs, medical devices, foods, biologics, toxicology, and cosmetics
World Health Organization	*http://www.who.int*	Statistical information, weekly epidemiologic record, world health report, and vaccination information for world travel
National Institutes of Health (NIH)	*http://www.nih.gov/*	NIH research news, grants and contracts, and health information
Centers for Disease Control (CDC)	*http://www.cdc.gov/*	Disease outbreaks, CDC recommendations, and vaccination information for world travel
Healthy Palm Pilot	*www.healthypalmpilot.com*	Lists over 700 medical resources available for use on a PDA

medically related discussion groups in which health professionals and nonprofessionals can participate. Consider answers to pharmacotherapy questions obtained from discussion groups of unknown reliability. Such groups might, in fact, be good resources for obtaining leads to information or finding out how someone else dealt with a particularly difficult patient or situation. Directing patients to computer discussion groups may help them deal with and understand their illnesses.

Internet-based technology has changed the way biomedical information is distributed. The result has been widespread availability of clinical, research, and educational resources through personal computers (Kramer & Cath, 1996). Table 7–2 lists some World Wide Web sites that contain or can assist practitioners in finding medication-related information on the Internet. Many additional professional organizations, government agencies, and pharmaceutical companies have their own websites, so be sure to browse to see what is new in your specialty. If you rely on the Web for information, you have to diligently and regularly validate content of the sites you use (Bergeron, 1999).

PATIENT MEDICATION INFORMATION

Medication information resources for patients also come in printed and computer formats (see Table 7–3). The same issues discussed previously should be considered when choosing a patient education resource. Additionally, consider the reading level of the information provided, customizability, and availability in multiple languages if applicable to a practice setting. The printed output of a computer program, for example, might not be legible for an elderly patient needing a larger-print format.

OTHER RESOURCES

Other sources of medication information that warrant discussion include pharmaceutical companies, drug information centers, and poison control centers.

Pharmaceutical companies provide medication information through two primary sources—manufacturer's sales representatives (MSRs) and in-house drug information centers. A pharmaceutical company is obviously a good source for basic product information (Shaughnessy, Slawson, & Bennett, 1994). Under current FDA regulations, the MSR can provide a health professional with information on FDA-approved and unapproved uses of a product (Wechsler, 1997). Additional information about nonapproved uses can be given to a health professional by a pharmaceutical company's in-house drug information center. The in-house drug information centers only provide information about an individual company's products, but may be able to assist your quest for information on various uses, adverse effects, and drug interactions with their products. One problem with obtaining information

TABLE 7–3. Patient Education Resources

Pharmacotherapy Resource	Publisher	Description/Comments	Frequency of Publication and/or Updates
Books			
USP DI, Volume II, Advice for the Patient	Medical Economics 800-232-7379 *www.medec.com*	Patient information on same products as in USP-DI, Volume I, Drug Information for the Health Professional; 12th grade reading level; also available on CD	Yearly with monthly updates (available online)
Patient Drug Facts	Facts and Comparisons 800-223-0554 *www.drugfacts.com*	Patient information on same products as in Drug Facts and Comparisons; color pictures for product identification	Yearly with quarterly updates
The Medication Teaching Manual: The Guide to Patient Drug Information, 7th edition	American Society of Health System Pharmacists 301-657-3000 *www.ashp.org*	One-page patient information sheets on over 600 medications; easy to read; available in Spanish	Periodically, most recent edition: 1998
Software			
MedTeach	American Society of Health System Pharmacists	Patient information sheets on over 500 medications; easy to read; available in Windows or MS-DOS versions; also available in Spanish; can customize printout	Quarterly (additional cost)
MedFacts	Facts and Comparisons	Patient information sheets on over 4,000 medications, derived from Patient Drug Facts; printouts can be customized in English or Spanish	Periodically; most recent edition: 2000

from a pharmaceutical company is that the information has the potential to be biased (Shaughnessy et al., 1994). And obtaining answers from manufacturer's in-house drug information centers can take 1 to 14 days (Price & Goldwire, 1994). A list of pharmaceutical companies' addresses and phone numbers is available in both the PDR and the Red Book.

Drug information centers, usually affiliated with a university and/or large medical center, sometimes can be a valuable resource for answering difficult questions. Unfortunately, not all centers take calls from the outside community. If you have access to a drug information center, consider the following prior to calling: Is there a fee for the service? Have all other resources been exhausted? How fast can the center respond with an answer? Usually a center will want to know what resources have already been used to avoid duplication.

Some drug information centers are available on the Internet. These sites vary in the types of services they provide, the populations they serve, and whether they charge a fee. Two sites that answer drug information questions from anyone for free are Ohio Northern University College of Pharmacy's Drug Information Center (*http://druginfo.onu.edu*) and the University of Maryland School of Pharmacy's Drug Information Service (*https://rxsecure.umaryland.edu/program/umdi*) (Belgado, 2001).

Most communities have access to a poison control center through a toll-free number. The centers assist both the general public with information and health professionals treating a potential poison ingestion. The number of the local center should be available in the telephone book under emergency numbers. Before calling, have the following information available: age of the patient, substance ingested or clues to the ingestion, amount ingested, time of ingestion, and patient signs and symptoms.

SUGGESTED MINIMUM PHARMACOTHERAPY LIBRARY

A suggested minimum pharmacotherapy library should contain the following:

- Pharmacotherapy reference text (most recent edition)
- Updated drug information resource program or book
- Updated drug interaction screening program or book
- Newsletter subscription for area of practice interest
- Handbook for area of practice interest
- Access to very current information or obscure information that may not be in any of these resources—through an online service, drug information center, or both (Mazza, 1994; Cauchon & Leduc, 2001)

CONCLUSION

All healthcare providers who prescribe, dispense, or administer medications need current and easily accessible medication information. This chapter has given a brief overview of the available resources and suggested a minimum library to have available in practice.

REFERENCES

Belgado, B. S. (2001). Drug information centers on the internet. *Journal of American Pharmaceutical Association, 41,* 631–632.

Bergeron, B.P. (1999) Where to find practical patient education materials. Empowering your patients without spending a lot of time and money. *Postgraduate Medicine, 105,* 35–38.

Cauchon, M., & Leduc, Y. (2001) Finding the right information at the right time. Part 1: Drugs, reference books, clinical practice guidelines. *Canadian Family Physician, 47,* 337–338.

Cohen, J. S. (2001). Adverse drug effects, compliance, and initial doses of antihypertensive drugs recommended by the Joint National Committee vs the Physician's Desk Reference. *Archives of Internal Medicine, 161,* 880–885.

Cohen, J. S., & Insel, P. A. (1996). The Physicians' Desk Reference: Problems and possible improvements. *Archives of Internal Medicine, 156,* 1375–1380.

Enders, S. J., Enders, J. M., Holstad, S. G. (2002). Drug-information software for palm operating system personal digital assistants: Breadth, clinical dependability, and ease of use. *Pharmacotherapy, 22,* 1036–1040.

Keplar, K. E. & Urbanski, C. J. (2003). Personal digital assistant applications for the healthcare provider. *Annals of Pharmacotherapy, 37,* 287–296.

Knott, T. L., & Scott, U. K. (1994). New perspectives in information retrieval. *Clinical Reviews in Allergy, 12,* 201–210.

Kramer, J. M., & Cath, A. (1996). Medical resources and the Internet: Making the connection. *Archives of Internal Medicine, 156,* 833–842.

Mazza, J. J. (1994). A library for internists, VIII: Recommendations from the American College of Physicians. *Annals of Internal Medicine, 120,* 699–720.

Millman A., & Lee, N. (1995). CD ROMs, multimedia, and optical storage systems. *British Medical Journal, 311,* 676–678.

Price, K. O., & Goldwire, M. A. (1994). Drug information resources. *American Pharmacy, NS34,* 30–39.

Shaughnessy, A. F., Slawson, D. C., & Bennett, J. H. (1994). Becoming an information master: A guidebook to the medical information jungle. *Journal of Family Practice, 39,* 489–499.

Sweet, B. V., Gay, W. E., Leady, M. A., Strumpf, J. L. (2003). Usefulness of herbal and dietary supplement references. *Annals of Pharmacotherapy, 37,* 494–499.

Wechsler, J. (1997). Final reform bill "modernizes" FDA, permits dissemination of off-label and economic data. *Formulary, 32,* 1254.

Zierler-Brown, S. (2001). How do herbal resources measure up? *Journal of the American Pharmaceutical Association, 41,* 896–897.

CHAPTER ❖ 8

ADVERSE DRUG EVENTS AND DRUG INTERACTIONS

Geneva Briggs

Responsible drug therapy requires knowing not only the efficacy of a particular drug in a particular disorder or disease state but also what combinations and conditions might actually aggravate a situation. It also requires knowing that unexpected reactions such as allergies may occur. This chapter covers both adverse drug events—those reactions or incidents that are not wished for—and drug interactions—some of which are indeed factored into the pharmacotherapy and some for which providers should be alert.

ADVERSE DRUG EVENTS

An adverse drug event is an unwanted or undesirable occurrence resulting from the use of a medication. An adverse drug event, as defined in this chapter, includes adverse drug reactions resulting from allergy, intolerance, drug interaction, or unknown mechanism and medication misadventures (hospitalization, death, etc.) caused by use of a medication. *Adverse drug event* is a more inclusive term than *adverse drug reaction,* but the terms are sometimes used interchangeably.

Information about adverse drug events with medications is gathered from clinical trials, spontaneous reporting by health professionals and occasionally by consumers to manufacturers and government agencies, and published case reports. The full extent of adverse events with medications is unknown because reporting of adverse drug events is a spontaneous, incomplete process. The majority of reports come from hospitals, yet the majority of drug use is in the outpatient setting. Minor gastrointestinal disturbances, rashes, itching, drowsiness, insomnia, weakness, headache, tremulousness, muscle twitches, and fever account for up to 71% of reported reactions (Atkin & Shenfield, 1995). It is estimated that 2 to 15% of all hospitalizations are the result of adverse medication events (Atkin & Shenfield, 1995; Johnstone, Kirking, & Vison, 1995; Nelson & Talbert, 1996). Studies have found an adverse drug event frequency of 4.2 to 6.6 per 100 admissions (Senst, Achusim, Genest, et al., 2001). Of these adverse events, approximately 30% are preventable (Kanjanarat, Winterstein, Johns, et al., 2003). Many events do not result in hospitalizations but cause significant morbidity. The treatment of adverse drug events is costly to both the healthcare system and society. Drug-related morbidity and mortality has been estimated to cost $76.6 billion annually in the United States (Johnson & Bootman, 1995).

WHAT IS AN ADVERSE DRUG REACTION?

Many definitions have evolved as to what constitutes an adverse drug reaction. The World Health Organization (WHO) defines an adverse drug reaction as any noxious, unintended, and undesired effect of a drug that occurs at a dose used in humans for prophylaxis, diagnosis, or therapy (WHO, 1975). The Food and Drug Administration (FDA) has broadened the definition of a reportable adverse drug reaction to include any adverse event associated with the use of a drug in humans, regardless of whether it is considered drug-related. These adverse events may occur in the course of the use of a drug product in professional practice; from drug overdose, whether accidental or intentional; from drug abuse; from drug withdrawal; and from any significant failure of expected pharmacological action (U.S. Department of Health and Human Services, 1985).

CLASSIFICATION

Adverse drug reactions are categorized into two groups: predictable and unpredictable. *Predictable reactions* are generally dose-dependent and related to the pharmacologic actions of the drug. These reactions include side effects, toxicity, drug interactions, and secondary effects related to pharmacologic properties but not the primary therapeutic properties (i.e., sedation from antihistaminic activity of a tricyclic antidepressant). *Unpredictable reactions* are usually dose-independent, are not always related to the pharmacologic actions of the drug, and are related to the individual's immunologic response or genetic differences (Gruchalla, 2001). Examples of unpredictable reactions include drug intolerance (exaggerated pharmacologic or toxic effects in vulnerable subsets of patients) and idiosyncratic, anaphylactoid, and allergic (immunologically mediated) reactions.

To evaluate whether a reaction is due to a medication, consider the temporal relationship of medication administration to the reaction, previous reports of the same or similar reaction, patient history of a similar reaction or reaction to a similar class of medication, and resolution of the reaction upon discontinuation of the substance (Kando, Yonker, & Cole, 1995). Also consider alternative causes for the reaction, presence of toxic drug concentrations, any positive dose-response relationship, and recurrence of the reaction when the drug is reintroduced (Kando et al., 1995). Rechallenge is seldom possible or ethical, but if attempted, discontinuation of the drug should be five times the elimination half-life before reintroduction to ensure that the drug has been eliminated completely from the body. Also, the reaction should have completely resolved symptomatically, and any abnormal laboratory values should be normalized. Most cases of rechallenge are by accident, which is why documentation of reactions is very important for prevention. Based on all these issues, reactions can be classified as definitely, probably, possibly, or indistinguishably caused by the suspected agent (Atkin & Shenfield, 1995).

A reaction can be considered mild if symptomatic treatment or dosage alteration is necessary but a change in medication is not required. Moderate reactions do require a change in medication. A severe reaction is defined as one that is unexpected or untoward or results in permanent disability or death (Kando et al., 1995).

Predictable Reactions

Predictable reactions usually are related to the pharmacologic properties of a medication. Several characteristics are risk factors for predictable reactions (Bates, Miller, Cullen, et al., 1999):

- Advanced age
- Female gender
- History of a previous adverse event
- Multiple medications
- Duration of hospital stay
- Liver disease
- Renal disease

Unpredictable Reactions

Unpredictable reactions include *anaphylactoid, allergic,* and *idiosyncratic* reactions. There are no predictive factors for anaphylactoid and idiosyncratic reactions. Some factors do impact the risk of developing allergic reactions, such as age, gender, genetics, associated illnesses, drug-related factors such as route of administration, and previous drug administration. Young children have a lower risk of allergic reactions because of limited prior exposure to medications. Women have higher rates of cutaneous reactions (Bigby, Jick, Jick, & Arndt, 1986). Patients with atopic dermatitis, allergic rhinitis, and asthma tend to have more severe allergic reactions than patients without these conditions (Van Arsdel, 1991).

Genetic ability to metabolize drugs also can affect the rate of allergic reactions. Patients who are slow acetylators, for example, are more likely to develop drug-induced lupus when treated with procainamide or hydralazine (Beringer & Middleton, 2001). Concomitant illnesses such as infectious mononucleosis, lymphocytic leukemia, and gout are associated with higher incidences of macropapular rashes with ampicillin (Van Arsdel, 1991). AIDS patients have higher incidences of cutaneous reactions with sulfonamides and amoxicillin-clavulanate (Van Arsdel, 1991).

Dose, frequency of exposure, and route of administration affect the frequency of some allergic reactions.

Some allergic reactions only occur with high doses, whereas others require intermittent exposure to a drug for a reaction to develop. Topical administration is most sensitizing followed by intramuscular, intravenous, and then oral (Van Arsdel, 1991). A history of an allergic reaction to a drug or chemically similar drug is the most reliable risk factor for development of a subsequent reaction (Beringer & Middleton, 2001).

REPORTING ADVERSE EVENTS

Reporting adverse drug events is a professional and legal obligation, so appropriate information on medication-related problems is communicated to the broader medical community. Within the United States, the FDA has primary responsibility for collecting, analyzing, and disseminating information on adverse drug events. Individual manufacturers have the responsibility to collect pre- and postmarketing information on their products. Postmarketing surveillance is important for several reasons. A medication is studied in limited numbers of patients prior to marketing, so reactions that occur rarely (i.e., 1 in 100,000 exposures) are often not detected. Dose-dependent reactions are usually discovered in premarketing studies, but idiosyncratic reactions may not be. Also, medications are not necessarily studied in patients with multiple diseases, complicating factors, or complicated medication regimens. Reactions are detected once a product reaches the general market and is given to complicated patients. Additionally, most drug interactions are not discovered until after a medication is marketed and given to many patients, because the inclusion criteria of premarketing studies usually limit the number of concomitant medications a study subject is receiving.

Lack of knowledge of all the risks associated with a new medication is attributable to deficiencies in the premarketing process, referred to as "the Five Toos" (Sills, Tanner, & Milstein, 1986):

- *Too few patients to detect rare events:* Thirty thousand people would have to take a medication to detect an adverse drug reaction that occurs in 1 in 10,000 exposures (McCloskey, 1996).
- *Too simple:* Patients who take multiple medications or have complicated medical conditions are excluded from clinical trials.
- *Too median-aged:* Most trials do not represent the very young and old.
- *Too narrow:* Indications for a newly approved drug are narrow based on premarketing clinical trials, but once marketed the drug may be used for other related but untested indications.
- *Too brief:* Most clinical trials are short; some adverse drug events may not appear for years.

Appropriate reporting often depends on where one is practicing. Hospitals and some other organized medical systems usually have an organization-specific process for reporting adverse drug events. An adverse drug event reporting system is mandated by the Joint Commission on Accreditation of Hospital Organizations (JCAHO). In these types of settings, reporting should follow the organizational process. The end result of health system reporting should be dissemination of the information within the organization and to the appropriate reporting body (i.e., FDA).

In a solo practice or clinic setting without a structured reporting system, reports should be filed directly with the FDA through the MedWatch program. The MedWatch program was initiated in 1993 to simplify and consolidate reporting of serious adverse drug events and medical device problems. Events are reported on the MedWatch form (Figure 8–1). The form can be mailed, faxed, or sent by modem to the FDA. Reactions to vaccines are reported on a different form (Vaccine Adverse Event Reporting System—VAERS), shown in Figure 8–2. The phone number for MedWatch is 800-FDA-1088; for VAERS it is 800-822-7967.

To get the most useful information, the FDA requests that only serious adverse events be reported through MedWatch. To be considered a *serious event,* the patient outcome is death, life-threatening, hospitalization (initial or prolonged), disability (significant, persistent, or permanent), or a congenital anomaly, or intervention is required to prevent permanent impairment or damage. Serious events that occur from medications (prescription or over-the-counter drugs or biologics), medical devices, nutritional products (dietary supplements, infant formulas), homeopathic remedies, or health food store products should all be reported. The actions the FDA can take on reported adverse drug reactions include labeling changes, letters to health professionals, requirement of further study by the manufacturer, or withdrawal of a drug from the market.

PREVENTION

It is estimated that 28 to 56% of all adverse drug events are preventable (Classen, Pestotnik, Evans, et al, 1997; Kanjanarat, Winterstein, Johns, et al, 2003; Kelly, 2001; Nelson & Talbert, 1996; Rothschild, Bates, & Leape,

MEDWATCH
THE FDA MEDICAL PRODUCTS REPORTING PROGRAM

For VOLUNTARY reporting
by health professionals of adverse
events and product problems

Page ___ of ___

Form Approved: OMB No. 0910-0291 Expires:12/31/94
See OMB statement on reverse

FDA Use Only

Triage unit
sequence #

A. Patient information

1. Patient identifier
In confidence

2. Age at time of event:
or
Date of birth:

3. Sex
☐ female
☐ male

4. Weight
___ lbs
or
___ kgs

B. Adverse event or product problem

1. ☐ Adverse event and/or ☐ Product problem (e.g., defects/malfunctions)

2. Outcomes attributed to adverse event
(check all that apply)
☐ death ________ (mo/day/yr)
☐ life-threatening
☐ hospitalization – initial or prolonged
☐ disability
☐ congenital anomaly
☐ required intervention to prevent permanent impairment/damage
☐ other: ________

3. Date of event (mo/day/yr)

4. Date of this report (mo/day/yr)

5. Describe event or problem

6. Relevant tests/laboratory data, including dates

7. Other relevant history, including preexisting medical conditions (e.g., allergies, race, pregnancy, smoking and alcohol use, hepatic/renal dysfunction, etc.)

C. Suspect medication(s)

1. Name (give labeled strength & mfr/labeler, if known)
#1
#2

2. Dose, frequency & route used
#1
#2

3. Therapy dates (if unknown, give duration)
from/to (or best estimate)
#1
#2

4. Diagnosis for use (indication)
#1
#2

5. Event abated after use stopped or dose reduced
#1 ☐yes ☐no ☐doesn't apply
#2 ☐yes ☐no ☐doesn't apply

6. Lot # (if known)
#1
#2

7. Exp. date (if known)
#1
#2

8. Event reappeared after reintroduction
#1 ☐yes ☐no ☐doesn't apply
#2 ☐yes ☐no ☐doesn't apply

9. NDC # (for product problems only)
– –

10. Concomitant medical products and therapy dates (exclude treatment of event)

D. Suspect medical device

1. Brand name

2. Type of device

3. Manufacturer name & address

4. Operator of device
☐ health professional
☐ lay user/patient
☐ other: ________

5. Expiration date (mo/day/yr)

6.
model # ________
catalog # ________
serial # ________
lot # ________
other #

7. If implanted, give date (mo/day/yr)

8. If explanted, give date (mo/day/yr)

9. Device available for evaluation? (Do not send to FDA)
☐ yes ☐ no ☐ returned to manufacturer on ________ (mo/day/yr)

10. Concomitant medical products and therapy dates (exclude treatment of event)

E. Reporter (see confidentiality section on back)

1. Name, address & phone #

2. Health professional?
☐ yes ☐ no

3. Occupation

4. Also reported to
☐ manufacturer
☐ user facility
☐ distributor

5. If you do NOT want your identity disclosed to the manufacturer, place an " X " in this box. ☐

FDA

Mail to: MEDWATCH
5600 Fishers Lane
Rockville, MD 20852-9787

or FAX to:
1-800-FDA-0178

FDA Form 3500 (6/93)

Submission of a report does not constitute an admission that medical personnel or the product caused or contributed to the event.

FIGURE 8–1. Sample form: MedWatch.

ADVICE ABOUT VOLUNTARY REPORTING

Report experiences with:
- medications (drugs or biologics)
- medical devices (including in-vitro diagnostics)
- special nutritional products (dietary supplements, medical foods, infant formulas)
- other products regulated by FDA

Report SERIOUS adverse events. An event is serious when the patient outcome is:
- death
- life-threatening (real risk of dying)
- hospitalization (initial or prolonged)
- disability (significant, persistent or permanent)
- congenital anomaly
- required intervention to prevent permanent impairment or damage

Report even if:
- you're not certain the product caused the event
- you don't have all the details

Report product problems – quality, performance or safety concerns such as:
- suspected contamination
- questionable stability
- defective components
- poor packaging or labeling

How to report:
- just fill in the sections that apply to your report
- use section C for all products except medical devices
- attach additional blank pages if needed
- use a separate form for each patient
- report either to FDA or the manufacturer (or both)

Important numbers:
- 1-800-FDA-0178 to FAX report
- 1-800-FDA-7737 to report by modem
- 1-800-FDA-1088 for more information or to report quality problems
- 1-800-822-7967 for a VAERS form for vaccines

If your report involves a serious adverse event with a device and it occurred in a facility outside a doctor's office, that facility may be legally required to report to FDA and/or the manufacturer. Please notify the person in that facility who would handle such reporting.

Confidentiality: The patient's identity is held in strict confidence by FDA and protected to the fullest extent of the law. The reporter's identity may be shared with the manufacturer unless requested otherwise. However, FDA will not disclose the reporter's identity in response to a request from the public, pursuant to the Freedom of Information Act.

The public reporting burden for this collection of information has been estimated to average 30 minutes per response, including the time for reviewing instructions, searching existing data sources, gathering and maintaining the data needed, and completing and reviewing the collection of information. Send your comments regarding this burden estimate or any other aspect of this collection of information, including suggestions for reducing this burden to:

Reports Clearance Officer, PHS
Hubert H. Humphrey Building,
Room 721-B
200 Independence Avenue, S.W.
Washington, DC 20201
ATTN: PRA

and to:
Office of Management and Budget
Paperwork Reduction Project
(0910-0230)
Washington, DC 20503

Please do NOT return this form to either of these addresses.

FDA Form 3500-back **Please Use Address Provided Below – Just Fold In Thirds, Tape and Mail**

Department of
Health and Human Services
Public Health Service
Food and Drug Administration
Rockville, MD 20857

Official Business
Penalty for Private Use $300

NO POSTAGE NECESSARY IF MAILED IN THE UNITED STATES OR APO/FPO

BUSINESS REPLY MAIL
FIRST CLASS MAIL PERMIT NO. 946 ROCKVILLE, MD

POSTAGE WILL BE PAID BY FOOD AND DRUG ADMINISTRATION

MEDWATCH
The FDA Medical Products Reporting Program
Food and Drug Administration
5600 Fishers Lane
Rockville, MD 20852-9787

FIGURE 8–1. *continued.*

2000). Although not all adverse drug events can be prevented, many can be avoided. Some simple things can be done to prevent or avoid reactions: appropriate dosing of medications based on gender, age, current literature, and concomitant medications and conditions; avoidance of drug interactions when possible; and labeling of patient records with prior reactions (Cohen, 1999). To prevent future reactions, any adverse drug reaction should be documented in detail in the patient's record. Patients should also be educated to communicate any reactions they have had to all health-care providers. Patients who have had serious reactions, such as anaphylaxis or angioedema,

VAERS

VACCINE ADVERSE EVENT REPORTING SYSTEM
24 Hour Toll-free information line 1-800-822-7967
P.O. Box 1100, Rockville, MD 20849-1100
PATIENT IDENTITY KEPT CONFIDENTIAL

For CDC/FDA Use Only
VAERS Number ______
Date Received ______

Patient Name:	Vaccine administered by (Name):	Form completed by (Name):
Last First M.I.	Responsible Physician ______	Relation to Patient ☐ Vaccine Provider ☐ Patient/Parent ☐ Manufacturer ☐ Other
Address	Facility Name/Address	Address *(if different from patient or provider)*
City State Zip	City State Zip	City State Zip
Telephone no. (____)______	Telephone no. (____)______	Telephone no. (____)______

1. State
2. County where administered
3. Date of birth __/__/__ (mm dd yy)
4. Patient age
5. Sex ☐ M ☐ F
6. Date form completed __/__/__ (mm dd yy)
7. Describe adverse event(s) (symptoms, signs, time course) and treatment, if any
8. Check all appropriate:
   - ☐ Patient died (date __/__/__ mm dd yy)
   - ☐ Life threatening illness
   - ☐ Required emergency room/doctor visit
   - ☐ Required hospitalization (____ days)
   - ☐ Resulted in prolongation of hospitalization
   - ☐ Resulted in permanent disability
   - ☐ None of the above
9. Patient recovered ☐ YES ☐ NO ☐ UNKNOWN
10. Date of vaccination __/__/__ (mm dd yy) Time ______ AM PM
11. Adverse event onset __/__/__ (mm dd yy) Time ______ AM PM
12. Relevant diagnostic tests/laboratory data
13. Enter all vaccines given on date listed in no. 10

	Vaccine (type)	Manufacturer	Lot number	Route/Site	No. Previous doses
a.					
b.					
c.					
d.					

14. Any other vaccinations within 4 weeks prior to the date listed in no. 10

	Vaccine (type)	Manufacturer	Lot number	Route/Site	No. Previous doses	Date given
a.						
b.						

15. Vaccinated at:
   ☐ Private doctor's office/hospital ☐ Military clinic/hospital
   ☐ Public health clinic/hospital ☐ Other/unknown
16. Vaccine purchased with:
   ☐ Private funds ☐ Military funds
   ☐ Public funds ☐ Other /unknown
17. Other medications
18. Illness at time of vaccination (specify)
19. Pre-existing physician-diagnosed allergies, birth defects, medical conditions (specify)
20. Have you reported this adverse event previously? ☐ No ☐ To health department ☐ To doctor ☐ To manufacturer
21. Adverse event following prior vaccination (check all applicable, specify)

	Adverse Event	Onset Age	Type Vaccine	Dose no. in series
☐ In patient				
☐ In brother or sister				

Only for children 5 and under

22. Birth weight ____ lb. ____ oz.
23. No. of brothers and sisters

Only for reports submitted by manufacturer/immunization project

24. Mfr. / imm. proj. report no.
25. Date received by mfr. / imm. proj.
26. 15 day report? ☐ Yes ☐ No
27. Report type ☐ Initial ☐ Follow-Up

Health care providers and manufacturers are required by law (42 USC 300aa-25) to report reactions to vaccines listed in the Table of Reportable Events Following Immunization. Reports for reactions to other vaccines are voluntary except when required as a condition of immunization grant awards.

Form VAERS -1

FIGURE 8–2. Sample form: Vaccine Adverse Event Reporting System (VAERS).

"Fold in thirds, tape & mail - DO NOT STAPLE FORM"

NO POSTAGE
NECESSARY
IF MAILED
IN THE
UNITED STATES
OR APO/FPO

BUSINESS REPLY MAIL

FIRST-CLASS MAIL PERMIT NO. 1895 ROCKVILLE, MD

POSTAGE WILL BE PAID BY ADDRESSEE

VAERS
P.O. Box 1100
Rockville MD 20849-1100

DIRECTIONS FOR COMPLETING FORM

(Additional pages may be attached if more space is needed.)

GENERAL

- Use a separate form for each patient. Complete the form to the best of your abilities. Items 3, 4, 7, 8, 10, 11, and 13 are considered essential and should be completed whenever possible. Parents/Guardians may need to consult the facility where the vaccine was administered for some of the information (such as manufacturer, lot number or laboratory data.)
- Refer to the Reportable Events Table (RET) for events mandated for reporting by law. Reporting for other serious events felt to be related but not on the RET is encouraged.
- Health care providers other than the vaccine administrator (VA) treating a patient for a suspected adverse event should notify the VA and provide the information about the adverse event to allow the VA to complete the form to meet the VA's legal responsibility.
- These data will be used to increase understanding of adverse events following vaccination and will become part of CDC Privacy Act System 09-20-0136, "Epidemiologic Studies and Surveillance of Disease Problems". Information identifying the person who received the vaccine or that person's legal representative will not be made available to the public, but may be available to the vaccinee or legal representative.
- Postage will be paid by addressee. Forms may be photocopied (must be front & back on same sheet).

SPECIFIC INSTRUCTIONS

Form Completed By: To be used by parents/guardians, vaccine manufacturers/distributors, vaccine administrators, and/or the person completing the form on behalf of the patient or the health professional who administered the vaccine.

Item 7: Describe the suspected adverse event. Such things as temperature, local and general signs and symptoms, time course, duration of symptoms diagnosis, treatment and recovery should be noted.

Item 9: Check "YES" if the patient's health condition is the same as it was prior to the vaccine, "NO" if the patient has not returned to the pre-vaccination state of health, or "UNKNOWN" if the patient's condition is not known.

Item 10: and 11: Give dates and times as specifically as you can remember. If you do not know the exact time, please indicate "AM" or "PM" when possible if this information is known. If more than one adverse event, give the onset date and time for the most serious event.

Item 12: Include "negative" or "normal" results of any relevant tests performed as well as abnormal findings.

Item 13: List ONLY those vaccines given on the day listed in Item 10.

Item 14: List any other vaccines that the patient received within 4 weeks prior to the date listed in Item 10.

Item 16: This section refers to how the person who gave the vaccine purchased it, not to the patient's insurance.

Item 17: List any prescription or non-prescription medications the patient was taking when the vaccine(s) was given.

Item 18: List any short term illnesses the patient had on the date the vaccine(s) was given (i.e., cold, flu, ear infection).

Item 19: List any pre-existing physician-diagnosed allergies, birth defects, medical conditions (including developmental and/or neurologic disorders) for the patient.

Item 21: List any suspected adverse events the patient, or the patient's brothers or sisters, may have had to previous vaccinations. If more than one brother or sister, or if the patient has reacted to more than one prior vaccine, use additional pages to explain completely. For the onset age of a patient, provide the age in months if less than two years old.

Item 26: This space is for manufacturers' use only.

FIGURE 8–2. *continued.*

should be told how to obtain bracelets or necklaces to wear that identify the problem medication and reaction. Prescribers should have knowledge of the drugs they prescribe, select them objectively, provide the patient with risk-versus-benefit information to enable the patient to make an informed decision as to whether to accept the therapy and warn about unwanted reactions and interactions (Day, 1995).

DRUG INTERACTIONS

Medications can interact with other medications, disease states, food, or the social habits of the patient. Such interactions frequently occur, but most are not clinically significant. Although usually thought of in a negative sense, interactions can be positive in nature and intentionally used to benefit the patient. This section will discuss the different types of interactions and give some common, significant examples for each type.

DRUG-DRUG INTERACTIONS

Drug-drug interactions can be classified as pharmacokinetic or pharmacodynamic. The drug whose action is altered by an interaction is termed the *object drug*, and the drug that alters the action is the *precipitant drug*.

Pharmacokinetic interactions include positive and negative effects on drug absorption, distribution, metabolism, and excretion (see Chapter 2 for explanation of these terms). Gastrointestinal absorption can be affected by drug binding in the GI tract, altered GI motility, altered intestinal flora, and altered gastrointestinal pH. Absorptive interactions can affect both the rate and extent of absorption. The most important interactions usually affect the overall extent of absorption (Hansten & Horn, 1996b). Sucralfate forming insoluble complexes with ciprofloxacin is an example of a binding interaction (Garrelts, Godley, Peterie, et al., 1990). Anticholinergics, which slow GI motility, and metoclopramide, which increases GI motility, can affect the rate of absorption of many medications, but changes in GI motility rarely affect the overall extent of absorption significantly (Hansten & Horn, 1996b). H_2 antagonists may markedly reduce absorption of drugs that require an acidic medium to dissolve adequately, such as ketoconazole (Lelawongs, Barone, Colaizzi, et al., 1988).

Distribution interactions occur when drugs compete for binding sites on plasma proteins or tissues. When this happens, the free or unbound serum concentration of one or both drugs may increase, which may result temporarily in increased drug response. Protein-binding interactions are usually important when the displaced drug is highly bound, has a limited body distribution, is slowly eliminated, and has a low therapeutic index. The enhanced pharmacologic effects of such a displaced drug usually only occur for a few days because more unbound drug is available for elimination by the liver and kidneys. For example, warfarin is a highly protein-bound drug susceptible to protein-binding drug-drug interactions. Chloral hydrate is one drug that can displace warfarin from protein-binding sites, resulting in an increase in hypoprothrombinemic effect that could last for up to a week (Hansten & Horn, 1996b). With continued combination therapy, the total plasma concentration of warfarin declines and the free warfarin concentration returns to preinteraction levels.

Liver metabolism can be increased by enzyme induction or decreased by enzyme inhibition. The onset of induction usually is gradual over one to two weeks. Dissipation of the reaction once the inducing agent is removed may take longer than two weeks (Fuhr, 2000). Some examples of liver enzyme inducers include barbiturates, carbamazepine, rifampin, and phenytoin (Fuhr, 2000). Enzyme inhibition usually occurs rapidly (within one or more doses of the inhibitor). An exception is erythromycin, whose effect may be delayed by several days. Examples of enzyme inhibitors include cimetidine, erythromycin, isoniazid, ketoconazole, and fluoxetine (Fuhr, 2000).

Renal elimination of drugs can be altered by many mechanisms, including alteration of urinary pH affecting passive tubular secretion, active tubular secretion, and glomerular filtration (nephrotoxicity) (Hansten & Horn, 1996b). Probenicid competes with penicillin to reduce active tubular secretion and renal clearance of the penicillin (Hansten & Horn, 1996b). The penicillin-probenicid interaction has been used to enhance the effect of the penicillin. An example of nephrotoxicity causing a drug-drug interaction is when a digitalized patient treated with gentamicin develops aminoglycoside-induced renal failure, which leads to digoxin toxicity.

A *pharmacodynamic interaction* occurs when a drug affects the outcome or toxicity of another drug without any change in the second drug's serum concentration. Pharmacodynamic effects of drugs can be additive or antagonistic. Pharmacodynamic interactions can be therapeutic (e.g., combinations of antihypertensives), can result in adverse effects (e.g., multiple anticholinergic drugs), or can result in negation of therapeutic effect (e.g., nonsteroidal antiinflammatory drugs [NSAID] blunting the antihypertensive effect of clonidine). These types of interactions occur commonly, but when anticipated, do not usually cause serious difficulties.

Table 8–1 lists selected important drug interactions. The reader is cautioned to always consult an updated drug interactions text and the package labeling for drug products prior to prescribing, dispensing, or administering any medication.

DRUG–DISEASE INTERACTIONS

Drug–disease interactions can occur when a medication adversely or positively impacts a disease. Drug–disease interactions are usually thought of in a negative sense because a positive impact on a disease would be viewed as a therapeutic effect of the medication. Medications can affect diseases in various ways, such as when hydrochlorothiazide increases glucose and impairs glycemic control in the diabetic (White & Campbell, 1995).

TABLE 8–1. Selected Clinically Significant Drug–Drug Interactions

Object Drug	Interacting Drug	Mechanism/Management
Fluoroquinolones	Aluminum- and magnesium-containing antacids, sucralfate	Aluminum, magnesium, and sucralfate can significantly reduce absorption of quinolone antibiotics. If concomitant use is necessary, give the quinolone 4 to 6 hours before or 2 hours after the other agents.
Monoamine oxidase inhibitors (MAOIs)	Meperidine	Meperidine blocks the neuronal uptake of serotonin, and MAOIs inhibit central nervous system (CNS) metabolism of serotonin. The combination of meperidine and MAOIs results in accumulation of CNS serotonin, leading to agitation, blood pressure increase, hyperpyrexia, and convulsions.
	Tricyclic antidepressants, selective serotonin reuptake inhibitors	Combination can result in excessive CNS serotonin, resulting in agitation, blood pressure increase, hyperpyrexia, and convulsions.
Lithium	Nonsteroidal antiinflammatory drugs (NSAIDs)	NSAIDs inhibit the renal clearance of lithium, resulting in increased serum lithium concentrations and potential toxicity. Lithium concentrations and patient symptoms should be monitored closely when NSAID therapy is initiated or discontinued.
	Thiazide diuretics	Thiazide diuretics increase serum lithium concentrations and potential toxicity. Concomitant use should be undertaken with caution. Lithium concentrations and patient symptoms should be monitored closely when thiazide therapy is initiated or discontinued.
Warfarin	Trimethoprim/sulfamethoxazole (Bactrim, Co-Trimoxazole)	Trimethoprim/sulfamethoxazole combinations inhibit the metabolism of warfarin and compete with warfarin for plasma protein-binding sites. These two factors result in increased hypoprothrombinemic response to warfarin. Warfarin dosage adjustment is necessary when the combination is used.
	Amiodarone	Amiodarone inhibits the metabolism of warfarin, resulting in excessive anticoagulation unless warfarin dosage is adjusted.
Theophylline	Erythromycin	Erythromycin can inhibit the metabolism of theophylline, resulting in increased serum concentrations of theophylline. If a combination is necessary, reduce the theophylline dose during erythromycin therapy.
Potassium-sparing diuretics, potassium supplements	Angiotensin-converting enzyme inhibitors	Angiotensin-converting enzyme inhibitors tend to increase serum potassium. Concurrent use of potassium supplements or potassium-sparing diuretics can result in hyperkalemia.

Sources: Finley, Warner, & Peabody (1995); Quinn & Day (1995); Anastasio, Cornell, & Menscer (1997); Fish (2001); Pai, Graci, & Amsden (2000); Wittkowsky (2000); and Seymor, & Routledge (1998).

Clinicians should be aware of the important drug–disease interactions for the diseases commonly seen in their patients. The reader is referred to Unit III for discussion of specific drug–disease interactions.

DRUG–FOOD INTERACTIONS

Interaction between drugs and food does not always get the attention it deserves. Since the frequency of ingestion of food with medications is far greater than the frequency of ingestion of two or more medications together, these interactions need to be considered. Nutrients may positively or negatively affect the bioavailability and ultimate efficacy of oral medications through many mechanisms. Negative effects to consider are binding with the medication to form nonabsorbable complexes and reduced absorption due to delayed gastric emptying, destruction by gastric acid, or altered ionization status of the medication (Maka & Murphy, 2000). Positive effects include increased absorption in the presence of certain types of food such as fat. Table 8–2 lists selected clinically significant drug-food interactions.

DRUG–HERB INTERACTIONS

The use of herbal medications has increased dramatically in recent years. As this use has increased, so have the reports of interactions between herbal medicines and vari-

TABLE 8–2. Selected Clinically Significant Drug-Nutrient Interactions

Medication	Interaction	Mechanism/Management
Decreased Absorption/Bioavailability		
Alendronate	Food and any liquids other than water	Must be taken with 6–8 oz of plain water 30 min before meal.
Penicillin G	Food, especially milk, and metal ions reduce absorption	May be due to binding; space 2 h apart.
Tetracycline	Dairy products (calcium), iron	Chelation can decrease absorption by > 50%; take tetracyclines 1 h before or 2 h after food.
Fluoroquinolones (ciprofloxacin, ofloxacin, lomefloxacin, enoxacin)	Iron, calcium, copper, magnesium, manganese, zinc	Binding can decrease absorption significantly; space 2 h apart or temporarily discontinue cation-containing products if possible.
Etidronate (Didronel)	Milk, iron, calcium, aluminum	Binding; separate by 2 h.
Didanosine	Food	Acid-labile drug that should be taken under fasting conditions because food stimulates acid secretion.
Zidovudine	Food	Reduced bioavailability; take on empty stomach.
Captopril	Food	Unknown mechanism; on empty stomach or at same time each day.
Azithromycin	Food	Food reduces absorption significantly; space 2 h apart.
Sucralfate	Food	Sucralfate binds with proteins in food; space 2 h apart.
Theophylline timed-release (Theo-Dur Sprinkle, Theo-24, Uniphyl)	Food	Rate of absorption can be affected, causing high theophylline concentrations; avoid taking with high-fat foods or take 1 h before eating.
Iron, folic acid, vitamin A, essential fatty acids	Cholestyramine, colestipol	Bile acid sequestrants can bind listed nutrients and prevent absorption.
Enteral feedings	Phenytoin suspension, carbamazepine suspension, warfarin	Binding to components in the enteral formulation decreases absorption. Adjust medication dose as needed.
Fat soluble vitamins (K, A, D, E)	Orlistat	Reduced absorption of fat soluble vitamins. Patients should take a multivitamin daily at least 2 h after orlistat or at bedtime.
Increased Absorption/Bioavailability		
Atovaquone	High-fat food	Enhances absorption.
Calcium channel blockers (felodipine, nifedipine)	Grapefruit juice	Flavonoid glycosides present in grapefruit juice inhibit the metabolism of these agents by the cytochrome P-450 (CYP1A2 and CYP3A4) enzymes in the liver.
Cyclosporine	Grapefruit juice	Inhibition of the hepatic and extrahepatic cytochrome CYP3A4 metabolism results in higher serum levels of cyclosporine.
Griseofulvin	Fatty food	Serum levels are double those of fasting state.
Lovastatin	Food	Increased absorption.
Nitrofurantoin	Food or milk	Increased absorption by 200–400%, most likely because of delayed gastric emptying, allowing increased time for dissolution.
Pharmacodynamic Interactions		
Warfarin	Food high in vitamin K	Exogenous vitamin K antagonizes the anticoagulant effect of warfarin.
MAOI (phenelzine, tranylcypromine)	Tyramine-containing foods and beverages	Combination can result in hypertensive crisis and death due to tyramine buildup.

Sources: Singh (1999); Alonso-Aoerte & Varela-Moreiras (2000); Seymor & Routledge (1998); Kirk (1995); Maka & Murphy (2000); and Fish (2001).

TABLE 8–3. Selected Clinically Significant Drug-Herb Interactions

Medications	Herb	Mechanism/Management
Warfarin	Ginkgo, garlic, danshen, St. John's wort, dong quai, kava-kava	Increased risk of bleeding. Avoid combination.
Cyclosprin, amitriptyline, digoxin, indinavir, theophylline, (e.g. antiretrovirals saquinavir)	St. John's wort	Lowered blood concentrations of these medications. Avoid combination.
Serotonin reuptake inhibitors	St. John's wort	Potential for syndrome of excessive serotonin with combination. Avoid combination.

Sources: Wittkowsky (2001); Fugh-Berman (2000); Izzo & Ernst (2001); Scott & Elmer (2002).

ous drugs. Table 8–3 lists selected clinically significant drug–herb interactions. Because little information is available about interactions with herbal medications, the reader is cautioned to always ask patients about their use of these medications and to be vigilant for changes in the patient that may signal a drug interaction.

DRUG—SOCIAL HABIT INTERACTIONS

Social habits, such as smoking tobacco or marijuana and alcohol consumption, can interact with medications. Polycyclic hydrocarbons from tobacco induce liver enzyme metabolism (Zevin, & Benowitz, 1999). Since cigarette smoke increases the metabolism of theophylline, tacrine, flecainide, propranolol, haloperidol, imipramine, pentazocine, and estradiol, smokers may require larger dosages (Zevin, 1999). There appears to be a relation between cigarettes smoked per day and the magnitude of many smoking–drug interactions. Heavy smokers (>25 cigarettes/day) are more likely to manifest interactions with drugs (Hansten & Horn, 1996a). Cigarette smoking is associated with a lesser magnitude of blood pressure and heart rate lowering during treatment with beta-blockers, less sedation from benzodiazepines, and less analgesia from some opioids, most likely reflecting the effects of the stimulant actions of nicotine (Zevin, 1999). Diabetics who smoke may require one-third the insulin of nonsmokers. This appears to be due to increased catecholamine and corticosteroid release caused by smoking and to reduced subcutaneous insulin absorption due to smoking-induced vasoconstriction (Hansten & Horn, 1996a).

Delta-9-tetrahydrocannabinol (THC), cannabidiol, and other cannabinoids found in marijuana can inhibit or increase metabolism of some drugs (Hansten & Horn, 1993a). Duration of marijuana smoking affects the direction of the interaction. Inhibition of metabolism occurs within hours of use, while induction requires ten to fourteen days of regular use to occur. The potency of the marijuana, additional smoking of cigarettes, and concurrent alcohol consumption can also impact the interaction of marijuana with medications. For instance, marijuana increases the metabolism of theophylline (Hansten & Horn, 1993a). Excessive marijuana use can impair glucose control in diabetics by an unknown mechanism. Combined use of alcohol with marijuana may result in additive perceptual, cognitive, and motor impairment.

Alcohol interacts with numerous medications. The combination of disulfiram with as little as 15 mL of alcohol can cause a disulfiram reaction (nausea, vomiting, headache, cutaneous flushing, vasodilation, respiratory difficulties, tachycardia, confusion, drowsiness, hypotension, shock, and even death). The combination of alcohol and metronidazole or oral sulfonylureas (primarily chlorpropamide) can cause a mild disulfiram-like reaction. Alcohol, even in limited daily quantities, potentiates the hepatotoxicity of acetaminophen (Zimmerman & Maddrey, 1995). Cases of fatal hepatotoxicity have been reported with usual doses of acetaminophen (3–4 g/day) and limited alcohol intake in the presence of illness and reduced nutrition intake. Hepatic metabolism of drugs is modified by ethanol intake (Weathermon & Crabb, 1999). Acute binges inhibit the microsomal oxidative enzyme systems, impairing metabolism of barbiturates, chloral hydrate, tolbutamide, and warfarin. Chronic ethanol ingestion stimulates the microsomal enzymes of the liver and thus accelerates metabolism of the same drugs that acute binge drinking inhibits. Patients with alcoholic liver disease will have impaired liver metabolism.

The effects of alcohol are additive with the pharmacodynamic effects of central nervous system depressants, including antihistamines, opiates, barbiturates, benzodiazepines, anti- psychotics, and antidepressants. Alcohol can increase the gastric mucosal damage from aspirin and other NSAIDs. Additive hypoglycemic effects occur when acute alcohol intake is combined with insulin and oral hypoglycemics.

CLINICAL OUTCOME

The outcome of a drug interaction is dependent on several factors: sequence of drug administration, duration of therapy with the combination, dose of the two drugs, other drugs taken by the patient, and the therapeutic index of the object drug (Pitscitelli, 2000). Adverse effects from a drug interaction are situational and may require a combination of factors to be present or occur at the same time. For example, a patient stabilized on cimetidine who is started on warfarin would not experience a problem unless the cimetidine dose was changed or the drug discontinued. Conversely, a patient on warfarin who is started on cimetidine without a decrease in warfarin dose may have a significant increase in prothrombin time due to metabolic inhibition of warfarin by the cimetidine.

AVOIDING DRUG INTERACTIONS

When deciding whether an interaction from a drug combination is possible, current drug interaction texts should be consulted (see Chapter 7 for information on resources). When new drugs come to market, the adverse effects problem described earlier occurs in a similar manner with drug interactions. Drug interaction studies are sometimes conducted premarketing with the most likely interacting drugs (e.g., a new drug is metabolized by a particular liver enzyme system; a study with known inhibitors of this system would be conducted). Unfortunately, the drug interaction studies are likely to have been conducted with healthy volunteers, which does not always reflect what will occur in patients. Also with new drugs, only drug-drug and possibly drug-disease interactions may be known prior to marketing. Drug-nutrient and drug–social habit interactions may not be discovered until a drug is in wide use.

Avoiding drug interactions begins with identifying patients at risk (i.e., the patient is receiving warfarin, which is known to have significant interactions). Patients receiving medications with known interactions should be (1) educated about what medications and/or nonprescription medications to avoid and (2) warned always to notify any healthcare practitioner that they are taking potentially problematic medication. Patient records should also contain a warning. Once a patient is identified as being at risk for a drug interaction, appropriate precautions should be taken to minimize adverse consequences. Management strategies will depend on the type of interaction:

- Some combinations are absolutely contraindicated: monoamine oxidase (MAO) inhibitors and selective serotonin reuptake inhibitors (SSRI).
- Alternatives should be used with other combinations: theophylline and erythromycin—use a different antibiotic.
- Most absorption interactions can be easily managed by appropriate spacing of medications: separate antacid from ciprofloxacin by 2 h.
- Other interactions may require monitoring, although the drug combination does not need to be avoided: an antihypertensive and TCA (tricyclic antidepressant)—both can cause orthostatic hypotension, but this can be monitored.

REFERENCES

Alonso-Aoerte, E., & Varela-Moreiras, G. (2000). Drugs-nutrient interactions: A potential problem during adolescence. *European Journal of Clinical Nutrition, 54* (Suppl.), S69–S74.

Anastasio, G. D., Cornell, K. O., & Menscer, D. (1997). Drug interactions: Keeping it straight. *American Family Physician, 56,* 883–895.

Atkin, P. A., & Shenfield, G. M. (1995). Medication-related adverse reactions and the elderly: A literature review. *Adverse Drug Reactions and Toxicological Reviews, 14,* 175–191.

Bates, D. W., Miller, E. B., Cullen, D. J., Burdick, L., Williams, L., Laird, N., Petersen, L. A., Small, S. D., Sweitzer, B. J., Vander Vliet, M., & Leape, L. L. (1999). Patient risk factors for adverse drug events in hospitalized patients. *Archives of Internal Medicine, 159,* 2553–2560.

Beringer, P. M., & Middleton, R. K. (2001). Drug allergies and anaphylaxis. In M. A. Koda-Kimble, L. E. Young, W. A., Kradjan & J. Guglielmo (Eds.), *Applied therapeutics: The clinical use of drugs.* Baltimore, MD: Lippincott Williams & Wilkins.

Bigby, M., Jick, S., Jick, H., & Arndt, K. (1986). Drug-induced cutaneous reactions. A report from the Boston Collaborative Drug Surveillance Program on 15,438 consecutive inpatients, 1975 to 1982. *Journal of the American Medical Association, 256,* 3358–3363.

Classen, D. C., Pestotnik, S. L., Evans, R. S., Lloyd, J. F., & Burke, J. P. (1997). Adverse drug events in hospitalized patients: excess length of stay, extra costs, and attributable mortality. *Journal of the American Medical Association, 277,* 301–306.

Cohen, J. S. (1999) Ways to minimize adverse drug reactions. Individualized doses and common sense are key. *Postgraduate Medicine, 106,* 163–168, 171–172.

Day, A. T. (1995). Adverse drug reactions and medical negligence. *Adverse Drug Reaction Bulletin, 172,* 651–654.

Finley, P. R., Warner, M. D., & Peabody, C. A. (1995). Clinical relevance of drug interactions with lithium. *Clinical Pharmacokinetics, 29,* 172–191.

Fish, D. N. (2001) Fluoroquinolone adverse effects and drug interactions. *Pharmacotherapy, 21,* 253s–272s.

Fugh-Berman, A. (2000). Herb-drug interactions. *Lancet, 355,* 134–138.

Fuhr, U. (2000). Induction of drug metabolising enzymes: Pharmacokinetic and toxicological consequences in humans. *Clin Pharmacokinet, 38,* 493–504.

Garrelts, J. D., Godley, P. J., Peterie, J. D., Gerlach, E. H., & Yakshe, C. C. (1990). Sucralfate significantly reduces ciprofloxacin concentrations in serum. *Antimicrobial Agents and Chemotherapy, 34,* 931–933.

Gruchalla, R. S. (2001). Drug metabolism, danger signals, and drug-induced hypersensitivity. *Journal of Allergy and Clinical Immunology, 108,* 475–488.

Hansten, P. D., & Horn, J. R. (1993a). Effects of marijuana smoking on drug interactions. *Drug Interactions Newsletter, 13,* 107–109.

Hansten, P. D., & Horn, J. R. (1996a). Cigarette smoking and drug interactions. *Drug Interactions Newsletter, 16,* 943–946.

Hansten, P. D., & Horn, J. R. (1996b). Drug interactions. *Drug Interactions Newsletter, 16,* 893–904.

Izzo, A. A., & Ernst, E. (2001) Interactions between herbal medicines and prescribed drugs: A systematic review. *Drugs, 61,* 2163–2175.

Johnson, J. A., & Bootman, J. L. (1995). Drug-related morbidity and mortality. A cost-of-illness model. *Archives of Internal Medicine, 155,* 1949–1956.

Johnstone, D. M., Kirking, D. M., & Vison, B. E. (1995). Comparison of adverse drug reactions detected by pharmacy and medical records departments. *American Journal of Health-System Pharmacy, 52,* 297–301.

Kando, J. C., Yonker, K. A., & Cole, J. O. (1995). Gender as a risk factor for adverse events to medications. *Drugs, 50*(1), 1–6.

Kanjanarat P., Winterstein A. G., Johns T. E., Hatton R. C., Gonzalez-Rothi R., Segal R. (2003). Nature of preventable adverse drug events in hospitals: A literature review. *American Journal of Health-System Pharmacy, 60,* 1750–1759.

Kelly, W. N. (2001). Potential risks and prevention, part 4: Reports of significant adverse drug events. *American Journal of Health-System Pharmacy, 58,* 1406–1412.

Lelawongs, P., Barone, J. A., Colaizzi, J. L., Hsuan, A. T., Mechlinski, W., Lejendre, R., & Guarnieri, J. (1988). Effect of food and gastric acidity on absorption of orally administered ketoconazole. *Clinical Pharmacy, 7,* 228.

Maka, D. A., & Murphy, L. K. (2000) Drug-nutrient interactions: a review. *AACN Clinical Issues, 11,* 580–589.

McCloskey, B. A. (1996, May). Improving adverse drug reaction reporting in the community setting. *Medical Interface,* 85–87.

Nelson, K. M., & Talbert, R. L. (1996). Drug-related hospital admissions. *Pharmacotherapy, 16,* 701–707.

Pai, M. P., Graci, D. M., & Amsden, G. W. (2000). Macrolide drug interactions: An update. *Annals of Pharmacotherapy, 34,* 495–513.

Pitscitelli, S. (2000). Preventing dangerous drug interactions. *Journal of the American Pharmaceutical Association, 40* (Suppl 1), S44–S45.

Quinn, D. I., & Day, R. O. (1995). Drug interactions of clinical importance. An updated guide. *Drug Safety, 12,* 393–452.

Rothschild, J.M., Bates, D.W., & Leape, L.L. (2000). Preventable medical injuries in older patients. *Archives of Internal Medicine, 160,* 2717–2728.

Senst, B.L., Achusim, L.E., Genest, R.P., Cosentino, L.A., Ford, C.C., Little, J.A., Raybon, S.J., & Bates, D.W. (2001). Frequency of adverse drug events in a health care network. *American Journal of Health-System Pharmacy, 58,* 1126–1132.

Seymor, R.M., & Routledge, P.A. (1998). Important drug-drug interactions in the elderly. *Drugs and Aging, 12,* 485–494.

Scott, G. N., & Elmer, G. W. (2002). Update on natural product-drug interactions. *American Journal of Health-System Pharmacy, 59,* 339–347.

Sills, J. M., Tanner, L. A., Milstein, J. B. (1986). Food and Drug Administration monitoring of adverse drug reactions. *American Journal of Hospital Pharmacy, 43,* 2764–2770.

Singh, B.N. (1999). Effects of food on clinical pharmacokinetics. *Clinical Pharmacokinetics, 37,* 213–255.

U.S. Department of Health and Human Services. (1985). New drug and antibiotic regulation: Section 314.80, post marketing reporting of adverse drug experiences. *Federal Register, 50,* 7500–7501.

Van Arsdel, Jr., P. P. (1991). Classification and risk factors for drug allergy. *Immunology and Allergy Clinics of North America, 11,* 475–480.

Weathermon, R., & Crabb, D. W. (1999). Alcohol and medication interactions. *Alcohol Research and Health, 23,* 40–54.

White, J. R., & Campbell, R. K. (1995). Drug/drug and drug/disease interactions and diabetes. *Diabetes Education, 21,* 283, 285–286.

Wittkowsky, A. K. (2001). Drug interactions update: Drugs, herbs, and oral anticoagulation. *Journal of Thrombosis and Thrombolysis, 12,* 67–71.

World Health Organization (WHO). (1975). *Requirements for adverse reaction reporting.* Geneva: Author.

Zevin, S., & Benowitz, N. L. (1999) Drug interactions with tobacco smoking: An update. *Clinical Pharmacokinetics, 36,* 425–438.

Zimmerman, H. J., & Maddrey, W. C. (1995). Acetaminophen (paracetamol) hepatotoxicity with regular intake of alcohol: Analysis of instances of therapeutic misadventure. *Hepatology, 22,* 767–773.

CHAPTER ❖ 9

EVALUATING PATIENT SELF-CARE AND OVER-THE-COUNTER DRUGS

Karen D. Rich

THE MEDICATION SELF-CARE MOVEMENT

Over the past several decades, individuals increasingly have looked first to self-care management when confronted with changes in health. It is estimated that self-care, without physician intervention, accounts for the management of 70 to 95% of all illnesses (Vuckovic & Nichter, 1997). Self-care includes a variety of activities performed by individuals to prevent disease, treat illness, and promote health. Use of nonprescription medications is just one facet of a variety of different methods including traditional medical practices, behavioral modifications, and alternative therapies, to name a few. The hallmark of the self-care movement is the patient as an active participant in the healthcare decision-making processes (Holt & Hall, 1993).

Most research on self-care has focused on prescription medication use, because the essentially unlimited access to nonprescription drugs leads to difficulties in obtaining solid data on over-the-counter (OTC) medication use. Roper Starch Worldwide conducted a survey on American self-care practices and attitudes in 2001 for the Consumer Healthcare Products Association (CHPA, formerly known as the Nonprescription Drug Manufacturer's Association). The survey was conducted via telephone and included 1,505 interviews with adult Americans. The survey found that nearly 80% of Americans reported using an OTC medication to deal with any of twelve common ailments in the past six months. Additionally, nearly three-fourths of those surveyed indicated the desire to treat themselves rather than seeing a doctor. Roughly 6 out of 10 people stated that they would like to diagnose and treat more of their conditions at home instead of seeing a doctor. Clearly, the trend towards self-care is strong (Self-Care in the New Millennium, 2001). Many of the factors contributing to the popularity of the self-care movement are listed in Table 9–1.

CONSUMER SOPHISTICATION AND DEMOGRAPHICS OF OTC DRUG USE

People turn to a variety of resources for health information including physicians, family and friends, newspapers, the Internet, television, medical reference books and pharmacists (Self-Care in the New Millennium, 2001; Phillips & Osborne, 2000). According to the Roper Starch 2001 survey, patient methods reported for dealing with common ailments in the previous 6 months were use of OTC medications (77%), waiting to see if the problem would go away on its own (69%), consulting a physician (43%), use of prescription medications (38%), use of dietary supplements (26%), and changing the diet (25%). Older Americans tend to rely much more on physicians for advice than do younger Americans, regardless of the seriousness of the health concern. Table 9–2 lists the most likely problems to be treated with a nonprescription drug.

According to the first report of the Slone survey, which focused on nearly 2,600 U.S. ambulatory adults,

TABLE 9–1. Factors Influencing the Trend Toward Self-Care

- Rising costs of medical care
- Increased individual responsibility
- Rising education level in the general population
- Lack of available medical services
- Skepticism of medical care
- Desire to exercise self-control
- Desire to avoid contact with health professionals or lack of relationship with health provider
- Medication availability
- Pharmaceutical advertising

Adapted from: Covington (2000); Vuckovic & Nichter (1997).

six of the ten most frequently used FDA-regulated drugs (prescription or OTC) during the 1998–1999 telephone survey were OTC drugs. The top four included acetaminophen, ibuprofen, aspirin, and pseudoephedrine hydrochloride (Kaufman, Kelly, Rosenberg, Anderson, & Mitchell, 2002). Providers may be at once supportive of patient self-medication for minor illness as a means of reducing office visits and lowering healthcare costs, while simultaneously being concerned about the patient's ability to accurately self-diagnose and use the medications appropriately in a manner that reduces risk of adverse events (Brass, 2001).

However, the 2001 Roper Starch survey reported that 96% of Americans are either somewhat or very confident about healthcare decisions they make for themselves. It also found that nearly 90% of Americans believe that OTC drugs are safe when used as directed. Ninety-five percent of those surveyed reported that they read directions prior to initial use of an OTC medication, 89% reportedly read package labels in order to choose an appropriate OTC drug, and 91% of those surveyed reported reading about potential side effects and interactions. The survey also indicates that in general the majority of Americans believe OTC drugs are effective and need to be used carefully, as you would a prescription medication (Self-Care in the New Millennium, 2001).

TABLE 9–2. Common Problems Consumers Are Most Likely to Treat with OTC Drugs

- Headache
- Common cold
- Muscle aches and pains
- Dermatologic conditions
- Minor wounds
- Premenstrual symptoms and menstrual symptoms
- Upset stomach
- Sleeping problems

Adapted from: Covington (2000).

Clearly delineating use of OTC drugs in population subsets is challenging due to the mass availability of OTC drugs and difficulty in accurately tracking their use. Past studies have produced conflicting results regarding predictors of OTC drug use. The Slone study reported the highest overall prevalence of medication use was among women aged 65 or older. However, this information included prescription as well as nonprescription drugs, vitamins, minerals, and herbal/supplement use (Kaufman et al., 2002). Data from the 2001 Roper Starch survey indicate that women are slightly more inclined than men to use OTC drugs, and that younger Americans are more inclined to use OTC medications than older Americans. Reportedly 80% of 18- to 34-year-olds had used an OTC product in the past 6 months compared to 67% of people ≥65 years of age. Another source reports that roughly one-third of all nonprescription medications in the United States are consumed by individuals aged 65 or older (Covington, 2000).

Children are also recipients of nonprescription medications. A U.S. population-based survey of OTC drug use by more than 8,000 preschool-age children was conducted by Kogan, Pappas, Yu, and Kotelchuck (1994). During the survey, 70% of mothers who identified their children as being ill during the previous 30 days reported giving their children OTC medications. Overall, 53.7% of 3-year-olds in this study had received an OTC medication in the past 30 days.

In clinical practice, practitioners are likely to find large variations in patient sophistication and health-related education. This patient-specific information should guide the clinician in working with the patient to identify the appropriate level of self-care versus health professional assistance needed.

ACCESSIBILITY AND ADVERTISING

Accessibility and effective marketing are key motivators in encouraging patient self-care with OTC medications. Because nonprescription drugs are not bound by the same constraints as prescription medications, it is relatively easy for patients to obtain them. The CHPA reports that over 100,000 OTC products are available in the United States marketplace today (CHPA, 2002a), often in nonpharmacy venues such as grocery stores, gas stations, or convenience stores.

Advertisements for OTC drugs can be found in nearly every communication medium—print, radio, Internet, television. While patients influenced by direct-to-consumer advertisements for prescription drugs must convince their physicians to prescribe a particular drug, the same constraints are not present when advertising OTC drugs. In essence, the "middle man" is taken out. Nonprescription drug manufacturers are urged to follow a voluntary code of advertising practices for nonsprescription medicines. The code stresses the importance of being truthful and honest in advertising the safety and efficacy of nonprescription medications. It also recommends that consumers be urged to read label information and follow directions (CHPA, 2002b). However, concern has been raised regarding potentially unbalanced presentations of efficacy claims versus safety warnings (Sheftell, Dodick, & Cady, 2001). Researchers investigated this issue further by conducting a small study where five clinical pharmacists reviewed fourteen print advertisements for OTC drugs found in common lay journals. The pharmacists reviewed the ads for accuracy of product claims, assessment of illustrations, information presented on side effects or contraindications, the educational value of the information presented, and overall information deficiencies regarding the drug product. The clinical pharmacist reviewers in this study found that half of the advertisements lacked accurate statements, and more than 50% lacked information considered essential for individuals to make informed decisions about product use. Additionally, the majority of advertisements lacked adequate information on safety, and only one addressed potential side effects. Overall, the reviewers felt the advertisements were mostly promotional and lacked substantial educational value (Sansgiry, Sharp, & Sansgiry, 1999). Clearly, patients need to seek more information than is often found in advertisements before using a particular OTC drug.

OTC DRUG USE AND HEALTHCARE COSTS

Probably the greatest driving force behind the promotion of self-care and OTC drug use is the desire to lower healthcare costs. The CHPA reports that OTC drugs accounted for less than 2% of total U.S. healthcare expenditures during 2000. Approximately $19 billion was spent on nonprescription drugs out of the estimated $1.2 trillion spent on healthcare (CHPA, 2002a). Data from independent researchers in 1997 suggest that OTC drugs save Americans approximately $20 billion per year in healthcare costs. This figure is attributed to savings on prescription costs, doctor visits, time lost from work, insurance costs, and travel (CHPA, 2002a). In 2001, the average OTC drug cost was reportedly about $4.75 as compared to the average prescription drug cost of $44.42. Adding an office visit charge of roughly $70 means that self-treatment with an OTC drug could save about $100 per episode (Perry, 2001).

Insurance coverage, or lack thereof, is an increasingly important determinant in patient access to healthcare. Patients without adequate insurance coverage or access to healthcare for other reasons may choose to self-treat with OTC drugs out of necessity. Additionally, encouragement of OTC drug use may benefit patients participating in healthcare plans with capitated prescription reimbursement. This is particularly true for patients with chronic conditions, where it is likely that the maximum limit will be reached during a coverage period.

On the other hand, most healthcare plans do not cover OTC medications. Patients with prescription drug insurance coverage may be reluctant to purchase OTC medications if the after-insurance cost of the prescription medication is lower than the price of an OTC drug (Gianfrancesco, Manning, & Wang, 2002). However, many managed care organizations have increased co-pays for prescription drugs so that in the current marketplace, the co-pay for a prescription medication is often more expensive than an OTC drug. This may influence patients to purchase more OTC drugs rather than paying the rising prescription drug co-pays (Levy, 1998). Additionally, health plans may look to increased coverage of OTCs in the future as a means of controlling costs. Likely candidates for coverage are those drugs that were previously available only by prescription. Some plans may consider adding selected OTC drug coverage as a means of encouraging preventive measures (e.g., calcium supplements for the prevention of osteoporosis) or as a competitive edge to attract or retain plan members (Beavers, 1999; Perry, 2001). Health plan coverage of at least selected OTC drugs or classes is likely to increase in the coming years.

REGULATION OF OTC DRUGS

FOOD AND DRUG ADMINISTRATION APPROVAL PROCESS

The 1938 federal Food, Drug and Cosmetic (FD&C) Act was the first legislation to require that manufacturers prove the safety of their products for humans (reference used in this section was Gilbertson, 1993). The act required that products be cleared through a new drug application (NDA) prior to marketing. The act also required proper labeling and instructions for use. This legislation had been under consideration for several years, but was finally enacted after the deaths of more than 100 people due to the use of the toxic solvent ethylene glycol in a newly formulated sulfanilamide elixir.

Several amendments were made to the 1938 FD&C Act. The 1951 Durham-Humphrey Amendment [*Federal Food, Drug and Cosmetic Act,* Section 503(b), 21 USC 353(b)] provided criteria for drugs that must be limited to prescription-only use, for separating prescription and nonprescription drugs into two distinct classes, and for requiring adequate labeling instructions. The 1962 Kefauver-Harris Amendment (*Federal Food, Drug and Cosmetic Act,* Section 505, 21 USC 355.32) was key in requiring manufacturers to prove effectiveness for intended uses as well as the safety of drugs prior to approval. It also required review of all drugs approved between 1938–1962 to ensure they met the efficacy standards set by the amendment. A review of prescription medications was conducted in the 1960s by a procedure called the Drug Efficacy Study Implementation (DESI). Near the end of that review, it was determined that nonprescription medications also needed extensive review. Due to the massive number of OTC products available (approximately 300,000), the FDA decided to evaluate OTC products by active ingredient (approximately 700), subdivided by therapeutic category (see Table 9–3). This review is formally known as the OTC drug review and was begun in 1972.

TABLE 9–3. Product Categories by which the FDA is Reviewing OTC Drug Ingredients

Acne	Hair grower/loss
Anorectal	Hexachlorophene
Antacid	Hormone (topical)
Anthelmintic	Hypo/hyperphosphatemia
Anticaries	Ingrown toenail relief
Antidiarrheal	Insect repellents (internal)
Antiemetic	Internal analgesic
Antiflatulent	Leg muscle cramps
Antifungal	Laxative
Diaper rash[a]	Menstrual products
Antimicrobials	Nailbiting/thumbsucking
Alcohol (topical)	deterrents
Antibiotics, first aid	Nighttime sleep-aid
Antiseptics (topical)	Ophthalmic products
Diaper rash[a]	Oral health care
Mercurials	Oral mucosal injury
Antiperspirant	Overindulgence remedies
Aphrodisiac	Ingredients intended to minimize
Benign prostatic hypertrophy	or prevent inebriation
Boil ointments	Pediculicides
Camphorated oil	Poison treatment
Cholecystokinetic	Antidotes—toxic ingestion
Corn/callus removers	Emetics
Cough/cold/allergy bronchodilator/	Relief of oral discomfort
antiasthmatic combinations	Salicylanilides (TBS)
Anticholinergic	Skin bleaching
Antihistamine	Skin protectant
Antitussive	Astringents (wet dressings)[b]
Bronchodilator	Diaper rash[a]
Expectorant	Fever blister/cold sore (external)[b]
Nasal decongestant	Insect bites and stings[b]
Dandruff/seborrhea/psoriasis	Poison (ivy/oak/sumac)
Daytime sedative	treatment/prevention[b]
Deodorants (int.)	Smoking deterrent
Digestive aids	Stimulant
Exocrine pancreatic insufficiency	Stomach acidifier
External analgesic	Sunscreen
Astringents (wet dressings)[b]	Sweet spirits of nitre
Diaper rash[a]	Topical otic (earwax)
Fever blister/cold sore (external)[b]	Topical otic (swimmer's ear)
Insect bites and stings	Vaginal contraceptive
Male genital desensitizers	Vaginal drug products
Poison (ivy/oak/sumac) treatment/	Vitamin/mineral
prevention[b]	Wart remover
Fever blister/cold sore (internal)	Weight control

[a]See also antimicrobials, external analgesics, and skin protectants.
[b]See also skin protectants.

Source: Gilbertson (1993).

THE OTC DRUG REVIEW

The OTC drug review is a three-phase process: (1) advisory panel review, (2) tentative final monograph publication, and (3) final monograph publication. The results of each phase are published in the *Federal Register.* Phases 2 and 3 are still ongoing. The ultimate goal of this rulemaking process is to establish standards for active ingredients (as opposed to new drug applications, which evaluate final dosage forms) and labeling OTC products in each therapeutic category.

Phase I

This phase lasted about one decade and involved over 300 individuals who served on advisory panels. The advisory panels classified active ingredients into one of three categories upon review:

- *Category I:* Generally recognized as safe and effective (GRASE) for the claimed therapeutic indication.
- *Category II:* Not generally recognized as safe and effective (NRASE) or having unacceptable indications.
- *Category III:* Insufficient data available to permit final classification.

The panels also recommended labeling instructions. In the end, the review panels summarized their recommendations and submitted 58 reports to the Food and Drug Administration (FDA). These were published in the

Federal Register to give notice of proposed rulemaking and to invite public comment.

Phase II

The second phase, tentative final monograph publication, is where the FDA reviews the recommendations from the review panels, public comment, or newly available data and then publishes a proposed rule in the *Federal Register.* Once again, time is allowed for public comments, hearings, or objections.

Phase III

The last phase, final monograph publication, is the point at which the FDA publishes its final rule after considering all new information since the tentative final monograph. The final rule is then published in the *Code of Federal Regulations.* Usually the rule is considered to be in effect 1 year after publication in the *Federal Register.* At this point, all manufacturers must comply with regulations. New OTC products do not require submission of an NDA if they meet the regulations of the final monograph for that particular active ingredient.

Impact of the Review

The OTC drug review has had a significant impact on the availability of some active ingredients. All in all, the OTC drug review examined 722 active ingredients. Counting multiple therapeutic claims for some ingredients, a total of 1454 ingredients promoted for specific uses were evaluated. Of the 1454 ingredients, the FDA first banned 233 substances as active ingredients across 19 different therapeutic classes as of May 7, 1991 (*Clinical Pharmacy,* 1991). In 1993 the FDA removed an additional 415 substances across seven different therapeutic classes (Gilbertson, 1993).

PRESCRIPTION-TO-OTC STATUS RECLASSIFICATION

The OTC drug review has been responsible for the reclassification of over forty prescription drugs to OTC status since the review began. The 1951 Durham-Humphrey Amendment defined three different criteria limiting drugs to prescription-only use [*Federal Food, Drug and Cosmetic Act,* Section 503(b), 21 USC 353(b)]:

- Habit-forming agents (listed specifically in the act)
- Drugs not safe for use except under the supervision of a licensed practitioner because of toxicity or other collateral measures necessary to use
- NDA that limits drug to prescription-only use

Currently, the second criterion probably has the most impact as agents are brought forward for potential reclassification. The criteria the FDA relies upon when considering a drug for prescription-to-OTC status switch include a high margin of safety (low potential for toxicity, low potential for misuse or abuse, low risk-to-benefit ratio), consideration of whether the condition is self-diagnosable and self-treatable, and adequate labeling (directions, warnings, ability of patient to comprehend instructions). There are currently four different mechanisms by which a drug may be reclassified as an OTC drug (as shown in Figure 9–1). The most common mechanism by which drugs are reclassified currently is through filing a supplemental NDA (mechanism 3).

- *Mechanism 1:* Filing a new NDA for a currently prescription-only drug
- *Mechanism 2:* "Switch regulation": filing a petition to exempt a prescription drug from prescription requirements
- *Mechanism 3:* Filing a supplemental NDA for OTC status for a drug currently restricted to prescription-only use
- *Mechanism 4:* OTC drug review process

Seventy-three ingredients, dosages, or indications have been switched from prescription to OTC status since 1976. This means that over 700 OTC products available today contain ingredients that were available by prescription only less than thirty years ago (CHPA, 2002a). Numerous parties stand to benefit from reclassification of prescription drugs to OTC status. Manufacturers benefit when a patent expiration is pending since reclassifying an agent to OTC status extends the life of the drug. Consumers benefit from a wider selection of agents to assist them in self-care as well as the potential cost savings for reasons discussed previously. Practitioners can spend less time treating less serious patient care problems and devote more time to serious problems (Brass, 2002; Reynolds, 2002). Third-party payers may also benefit from prescription-to-OTC drug switching by shifting the costs of drugs to the patient. A prime example of this is the petition to switch prescription second-generation antihistamines to OTC status. The petition was actually filed by Blue Cross of California. The antihistamine manufacturers were opposed to the switch. The FDA Nonprescription Drugs Advisory Panel recommended that the drugs be switched to OTC status in May 2001 (Newton, Benninghoff, Pray, & Popovich, 2002). Loratidine was approved for OTC use in November 2002. Table 9–4 lists

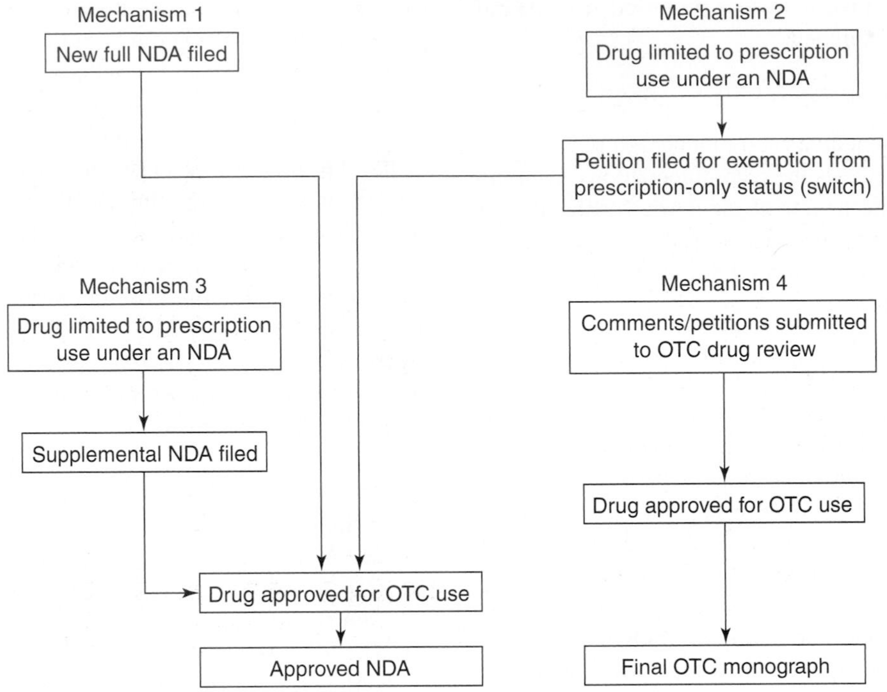

FIGURE 9–1. Mechanisms for reclassifying prescription drugs to OTC. *Source: Gilbertson (1993).*

the drugs switched from prescription to OTC status since 1975. As the OTC market grows, consideration of potential problems associated with OTC medication use must be considered.

POTENTIAL PROBLEMS WITH OTC DRUG USE

IMPROPER USE

Though OTC drug use has many positive aspects, most notably apparent reductions in healthcare costs and ease of access and availability to the patient, there are also potential drawbacks. Of greatest concern is that patients will use the drugs improperly or for improper indications. Improper drug use may potentially harm the patient, cause a delay in the patient's seeking treatment for a serious underlying condition, or interact adversely with other drugs or substances the patient is taking. Some argue that for these reasons OTC drug use may not be cost effective and may actually increase overall healthcare costs due to increased utilization of medical services (Gianfrancesco et al., 2002). The potential for harm is especially worrisome for the patient who perceives OTC medications as completely safe and without any potential for side effects or harm because of their nonprescription status. Although OTC medications are reviewed rigorously to ensure a high safety margin, even OTC medications can have severe side effects if used improperly (Brass, 2001). Rebound headache caused by chronic, improper OTC analgesic use is one example of the consequences of improper use (Sheftell et al., 2001).

LACK OF COUNSELING

A consumer survey in 1995 by the consulting firm Kline & Co. reported that 60% of individuals surveyed reported relying on professional advice to select an OTC product (Griffle, 1995). Although this indicates that a majority of patients request assistance in the selection of OTC drugs, there is still a large percentage who do not consult a healthcare professional about the use of OTC medications. For those patients who may rely solely on the manufacturer (via package labeling) for information about proper use, the necessary instructions may not be adequately communicated. Given their training and availability, pharmacists make ideal candidates for OTC medication consultation. Unfortunately, such counseling on OTC medications may not take place since the drugs are often

TABLE 9–4. Ingredients and Dosages Transferred from Rx-to-OTC Status (or New OTC Approvals) by the Food and Drug Administration since 1975 (as of July 3, 2003)

Ingredient	Adult Dosage	Product Category	Date of OTC Approval	Product Examples
1. brompheniramine maleate	4 mg/4–6 hours (oral)	antihistamine	September 9, 1976	Dimetane (A. H. Robins)
2. chlorpheniramine maleate	4 mg/4–6 hours (oral)	antihistamine	September 9, 1976	Allerest (Pharmacraft), Chlor-Trimeton (Schering), Contac (SmithKline), Sudafed Plus (Warner-Lambert)
3. oxymetazoline hydrochloride	0.05% aqueous solution (topical)	nasal decongestant	September 9, 1976	Afrin (Schering), Duration (Plough), Dristan Long Lasting (Whitehall), Neo-Synephrine-12 Hour (Bayer)
4. pseudoephedrine hydrochloride	60 mg/4 or 4–6 hours (oral) 240 mg max/24 hours	nasal decongestant	September 9, 1976	Sudafed (Warner-Lambert), Neo-Synephrinol (Bayer)
5. pseudoephedrine sulfate	60 mg/4 or 4–6 hours (oral)	nasal decongestant	September 9, 1976	Afrinol (Schering), Chlor-Trimeton (Schering)
6. xylometazoline hydrochloride	.01% aqueous solution (topical)	nasal decongestant	September 9, 1976	Orrivin (Ciba)
7. doxylamine succinate (NDA)	25 mg single dose only (oral)	sleep aid	October 18, 1978	Unisom (Pfizer)
8. hydrocortisone	0.25 to 0.50% (topical)	antipruritic (anti-itch)	December 4, 1979+	Cortaid (Upjohn), Lanacort (Combe)
9. hydrocortisone acetate	0.25 to 0.50% (topical)	antipruritic (anti-itch)	December 4, 1979+	Bactine (Miles), Caldecort (Pharmacraft)
10. acidulated phosphate fluoride rinse	0.02% fluoride in aqueous solution	dental rinse	March 28, 1980	
11. sodium fluoride rinse	0.05% aqueous solution (topical)	dental rinse	March 28, 1980	Flourigard (Colgate-Palmolive)
12. stannous fluoride gel	0.4% gel (topical)	anticaries gel	March 28, 1980	Gelkam Gel (Colgate-Palmolive)
13. stannous fluoride rinse	0.1% aqueous solution (topical)	dental rinse	March 28, 1980	Stan Care (Block)
14. ephedrine sulfate	0.1 to 1.25% (topical)	anorectal/vasoconstrictor	May 27, 1980	Pazo Ointment (Bristol-Myers)
15. epinephrine hydrochloride	0.005 to 0.01% (topical)	anorectal/vasoconstrictor	May 27, 1980	
16. phenylephrine hydrochloride	0.25% (topical)	anorectal/vasoconstrictor	May 27, 1980	
17. chlorpheniramine maleate (NDA)	12 mg/12 hours (oral timed-release)	antihistamine	July 23, 1981	Triaminic 12 (Sandoz)
18. phenylpropanolamine hydrochloride (NDA)	75 mg/12 hours (oral timed-release)	nasal decongestant	July 23, 1981	Triaminic 12 (Sandoz)
19. diphenhydramine hydrochloride (NDA)	25 mg/4 hours (oral)	antitussive	August 7, 1981	Benylin (Parke-Davis)
20. haloprogin	1.0% (topical)	antifungal	March 23, 1982	
21. miconazole nitrate	2.0% (topical)	antifungal	March 23, 1982	Micatin (Ortho)
22. diphenhydramine hydrochloride	50 mg single dose only (oral)	sleep aid	April 23, 1982	Sominex 2 (Beecham), Sleep-eze 3 (Whitehall)
23. diphenhydramine monocitrate	76 mg single dose only (oral)	sleep aid	April 23, 1982	Excedrin PM (Bristol-Myers)
24. dyclonine hydrochloride	0.05 to 0.1% solution or suspension, 1 to 3 mg as lozenge	oral anesthetic	May 25, 1982	Sucrets Maximum Strength (SmithKline)
25. dexbrompheniramine maleate (NDA)	6 mg/12 hours (oral timed-release)	antihistamine	September 3, 1982	Drixoral (Schering)
26. pseudoephedrine sulfate (NDA)	120 mg/12 hours (oral timed-release)	nasal decongestant	September 3, 1982	Afrinol Repetabs (Schering)
27. triprolidine hydrochloride	2.5 mg/4–6 hours	antihistamine	November 26, 1982	Actifed Capsules (Warner-Lambert), Actidil Syrup and Capsules (Warner-Lambert)
28. ibuprofen (NDA)	200 mg/4–6 hours (oral)	internal analgesic/ antipyretic	May 18, 1984	Advil (Whitehall), Nuprin (Bristol-Myers)
29. dexbrompheniramine maleate	2 mg/4–6 hours (oral)	antihistamine	January 15, 1985	
30. diphenhydramine hydrochloride	25–50 mg/4–6 hours (oral)	antihistamine	January 15, 1985	Benadryl 25 (Warner-Lambert)
31. pseudoephedrine hydrochloride (NDA)	120 mg/12 hours (oral timed-release)	nasal decongestant	June 17, 1985	Actifed (Warner-Lambert)
32. triprolidine hydrochloride (NDA)	5 mg/12 hours	antihistamine	June 17, 1985	Actifed 12-hour Capsules (Warner-Lambert)
33. oxymetazoline hydrochloride (NDA)	0.025% solution/drops (topical)	ocular vasoconstrictor	May 30, 1986	Ocuclear (Schering)
34. pyrantel pamoate	11 mg/kilo of body weight maximum dose 1 gram (oral)	antihelmintic	August 1, 1986	Pin-X (Effcon)
35. povidone iodine sponge (NDA)	10% (new dosage form)	antimicrobial	January 7, 1987	E-Z Scrub 241 (Deseret)
36. diphenhydramine hydrochloride	25–50 mg/4–6 hours (oral)	antiemetic	April 30, 1987	

(continued)

TABLE 9–4. Ingredients and Dosages Transferred from Rx-to-OTC Status (or New OTC Approvals) by the Food and Drug Administration since 1975 (as of July 3, 2003)

Ingredient	Adult Dosage	Product Category	Date of OTC Approval	Product Examples
37. dexbrompheniramine maleate (NDA)	3 mg/6–8 hours (oral)	antihistamine	May 22, 1987	Drixoral Plus (Schering)
38. chlophedianol hydrochloride	25 mg/6–8 hours (oral)	antitussive	August 12, 1987	
39. doxylamine succinate	7.5 mg – 12.5 mg/4–6 hours (oral)	antihistamine	August 24, 1987	Nyquil (Procter & Gamble)
40. loperamide (NDA)	4 mg then 2 mg, 8 mg/day (oral)	antidiarrheal	March 3, 1988	Imodium A-D (Johnson & Johnson)
41. hydrogenated soybean oil and lecithin	12.4 gm powder in 2–3 oz water 20 minutes before gall bladder x-rays	cholecystokinetic	February 28, 1989	Liposperse (Merck)
42. ibuprofen, pseudoephedrine HCl (NDA)*	200 mg ibuprofen, 30 mg pseudoephedrine HCl	analgesic/decongestant	September 19, 1989	Advil Cold and Sinus (Wyeth)
43. clotrimazole (NDA)	1% lotion and cream/2 times daily	antifungal	October 23, 1989	Lotrimin AF (Schering)
44. permethrin (NDA)	1% cream rinse	pediculicide (head lice)	May 5, 1990	Nix (Warner-Lambert)
45. clotrimazole (NDA)	1% cream and 100 mg inserts	anticandidal	November 30, 1990	Gyne-Lotrimin (Schering), Mycelex-7 (Miles)
46. miconazole nitrate	2.0% cream and 100 mg inserts	anticandidal	March 13, 1991	Monistat 7 (Ortho)
47. hydrocortisone	above 0.50% to 1.0%	antipruritic (anti-itch)	August 30, 1991+	
48. hydrocortisone acetate	above 0.50% to 1.0%	antipruritic (anti-itch)	August 30, 1991+	
49. clemastine fumarate (NDA)	1.34 mg/12 hours	antihistamine	August 21, 1992	Tavist-1 (Sandoz Consumer)
50. clemastine fumarate (in combination with phenylpropanolamine HCl (NDA)	1.34 mg/12 hours	antihistamine/ decongestant	August 21, 1992	Tavist-D (Sandoz Consumer)
51. dexchlorpheniramine maleate	2 mg/4–6 hours (oral)	antihistamine	December 9, 1992	(last monograph switch)
52. naproxen sodium (NDA)	220 mg/4–6 hours (oral)	internal analgesic/ antipyretic	January 11, 1994	Aleve (Bayer)
53. pheniramine maleate with naphazoline HCl (NDA)	0.3%; 0.025% in solution	ophthalmic antihistamine/ decongestant	June 8, 1994	Naphcon A (Alcon), Opcon A (Bausch & Lomb), Ocuhist (Akorn)
54. antazoline phosphate with naphazoline HCl (NDA)	0.5%; 0.05% in solution	ophthalmic antihistamine/ decongestant	July 11, 1994	Vasocon A (Ciba)
55. famotidine (NDA)	10 mg, up to 20 mg/day	acid reducer	April 28, 1995	Pepcid AC (J&J Merck)
56. ibuprofen suspension 100 mg/5 ml for pediatric use (NDA)	7.5 mg/kg up to 4 times a day	internal analgesic/ antipyretic	June 16, 1995	Children's Motrin (McNeil Consumer)
57. cimetidine (NDA)	200 mg up to twice per day	acid reducer	June 19, 1995	Tagamet HB (SmithKline)
58. ketoprofen (NDA)	12.5 mg every 4 to 6 hours	internal analgesic	October 16, 1995	Orudis KT (Whitehall-Robins), Actron (Bayer)
59. ranitidine (NDA)	75 mg up to twice per day	acid reducer	December 19, 1995	Zantac 75 (Warner Wellcome)
60. butoconazole nitrate (NDA)	2.0% cream and applicators (3 days)	anticandidal	December 26, 1995	Femstat 3 (Procter & Gamble)
61. minoxidil (NDA)	2.0% topical solution	hair grower	February 9, 1996	Rogaine (Pharmacia & Upjohn)
62. nicotine polacrilex (NDA)	2 mg and 4 mg gum	smoking cessation	February 9, 1996	Nicorette (SmithKline Beecham)
63. nizatidine (NDA)	75 mg up to twice daily	acid reducer	May 9, 1996	AXID AR (Whitehall-Robins Healthcare)
64. miconazole nitrate (NDA)	2.0% cream and 200 mg inserts	anticandidal	April 16, 1996	Monistat 3 (Ortho)
65. nicotine transdermal system (NDA)	15 mg patch	smoking cessation	July 3, 1996	Nicotrol (McNeil Consumer)
66. clotrimazole (NDA)*	1% cream & 200 mg inserts	anticandidal	July 29, 1996	Gyne-Lotrimin 3 (Schering-Plough)
67. nicotine transdermal system (NDA)	21, 14, & 7 mg patches	smoking cessation	August 2, 1996	Nicoderm CQ (SmithKline Beecham), Habitrol (Novartis)(Nov. 12, 1999)
68. bentoquatam (NDA)*	5% lotion	poison ivy protection	August 26, 1996	Ivy Block (EnviroDerm)
69. cromolyn sodium (NDA)	4% nasal solution	allergy prevention & treatment	January 6, 1997	Nasalcrom (McNeil Consumer)
70. tioconazole (NDA)	6.5% vaginal ointment	anticandidal	February 11, 1997	Vagistat-1 (Bristol-Myers Squibb), Monistat 1 (McNeil)

71. loperamide/simethicone (NDA)*	2 mg loperamide, 125 mg simethicone	antidiarrheal/antigas	June 26, 1997	Imodium Advanced (McNeil Consumer)
72. triclosan (dentifrice) (NDA)*	0.30% triclosan/0.243% fluoride	antigingivitis	July 11, 1997	Total (Colgate-Palmolive)
73. ketoconazole (NDA)	1% shampoo	dandruff shampoo	October 10, 1997	Nizoral (Johnson & Johnson Consumer Products)
74. minoxidil (NDA)*	5.0% topical solution	hair grower	November 17, 1997	Rogaine Extra Strength for Men (Pharmacia & Upjohn)
75. aspirin/caffeine/acetaminophen (NDA)**	250mg/65mg/250mg	migraine	January 14, 1998	Excedrin Migraine (Bristol-Myers Squibb)
76. miconazole nitrate (NDA)*	4.0% cream	anticandidal	March 30, 1998	Monistat 3 (Advanced Care Products)
77. terbinafine hydrochloride (NDA)	1.0% cream	antifungal	March 9, 1999	Lamisil AT (Novartis)
78. cimetidine suspension (NDA)*	suspension	acid reducer	July 9, 1999	Tagamet HB 200 (SmithKline Beecham)
79. naproxen Na, pseudoephedrine HCl (NDA)*	220 mg naproxen Na, 120 mg pseudoephedrine HCl	analgesic/decongestant	November 29, 1999	Aleve Cold & Sinus (Bayer Consumer Care)
80. ibuprofen (NDA)**	200 mg	migraine	February 25, 2000	Motrin Migraine Pain (McNeil Consumer Healthcare)
81. ibuprofen (NDA)**	200 mg	migraine	March 16, 2000	Advil Migraine Liqui-Gels (Whitehall-Robins)
82. docosanol (NDA)*	10% cream	cold sore/fever blister	July 25, 2000	Abreva Cream (Avanir Pharmaceutical)
83. famotidine, calcium carbonate, magnesium hydroxide (NDA)*	10 mg famotidine, 800 mg calcium carbonate, 165 mg magnesium hydroxide	heartburn, acid indigestion	October 17, 2000	Pepcid Complete (J & J/Merck)
84. butenafine hydrochloride (NDA)	1.0% cream	athlete's foot, jock itch, ringworm	December 7, 2001	Lotrimin Ultra (Schering-Plough)
85. ibuprofen, pseudoephedrine HCl, suspension for pediatric use (NDA)*	100 mg ibuprofen, 15 mg pseudoephedrine HCl/5 mL; 5 or 10 mL up to 4 times a day	analgesic/decongestant	April 18, 2002	Children's Advil Cold (Wyeth)
86. nicotine polacrilex troche/lozenge (NDA)*	2 mg and 4 mg	smoking cessation	October 31, 2002	Commit (Glaxo SmithKline)
87. loratadine (NDA)	10 mg/day	antihistamine	November 27, 2002	Claritin Tablets, Claritin Redi Tabs, Claritin Syrup (Schering-Plough)
88. loratadine, pseudoephedrine sulfate (NDA)	10 mg loratadine, 240mg pseudoephedrine sulfate daily	antihistamine/ decongestant	November 27, 2002	Claritin-D 12 Hour Extended Release Tablets, Claritin-D 24 Hour Extended Release Tablets (Schering-Plough)
89. omeprazole magnesium (NDA)	20 mg/day	acid reducer to treat frequent heartburn	June 20, 2003	Prilosec OTC (Procter & Gamble)

FDA approval for OTC marketing is on an interim basis pending adoption of a Final Monograph.
*New OTC NDA—Not previously Rx
**New OTC indication, product previously OTC

Source: Consumer Healthcare Products Association, July 2003. Used with permission.

physically separated from the prescription drug dispensing area and are available in a variety of nonpharmacy venues. Most discussions regarding OTC drugs in pharmacies are initiated by patients as opposed to pharmacists (Taylor, 2001). A study of drug-related problems with OTC medications in Swedish pharmacies revealed that the most common types of drug-related problems were uncertainty about the indication for a drug (e.g., choosing the wrong type of drug for treating a condition) and therapeutic failure. The most common types of interventions by pharmacy personnel were providing drug counseling, recommending switching to other drugs, and physician referral (Westerlund, Marklund, Handl, Thunberg, & Allebeck, 2001).

LABELING CONCERNS

While most Americans reportedly read the label of an OTC medication prior to initial use, this may not equate to comprehension of the intended instructions, warnings, and other included information. Historically, OTC medication labels have varied widely in the format and presentation of information. Due to the potential for confusion and in an effort to ensure safe and effective use of OTC medications, the FDA finalized a new rule in March 1999 establishing standardized content and a standardized format for all OTC drug product labeling. The new format is intended to significantly improve readability and comprehension by enhancing visual cues, familiarizing individuals to the location of key information on the label, using less complex terminology and shorter sentences, and decreasing "cognitive load" for the reader. In developing this rule, the agency researched literature, conducted several studies, and considered input from multiple interested parties including health professionals, students, professional organizations, trade associations, manufacturers, consumers, and consumer organizations. The new rule applies to all available OTC medications and will be implemented over a period of six years from the date of rule finalization (FDA, 1999).

Another hazard related to product labeling is the introduction of product line extensions. Expanding a product line capitalizes on the popularity of a particular product by using the same name in new products (i.e., Tylenol P.M. or Robitussin-DM). However, the new products do not always contain the main ingredient found in the original product. Patients and healthcare practitioners may inadvertently select an inappropriate agent for the patient because of this practice. Table 9–5 illustrates this point with one OTC product line. The products listed in the table represent only one-fourth of the variety of Robitussin products available on the market currently. Several suggestions have been made to decrease OTC selection confusion, such as that manufacturers limit product line extensions unless a specific patient need will be satisfied, restrict the use of brand names to products containing the active ingredients, and adopt a standard nomenclature for suffixes used in product line extensions (Covington, 2000).

TABLE 9–5. Selected Robitussin Products

Product	Active Ingredients
Robitussin	Guaifenesin 100 mg/5 mL
Robitussin-CF	Guaifenesin 100 mg/5 mL
	Pseudoephedrine HCl 30 mg
	Dextromethorphan hB 10 mg/5 mL
Robitussin-DM	Guaifenesin 100 mg/5 mL
	Dextromethorphan Hbr 10 mg/5 mL
Robitussin Night Relief	Pseudoephedrine Hcl 10 mg/5 mL
	Pyrilamine maleate 8.3 mg/5 mL
	Dextromethorphan Hbr 5 mg/5 mL
	Acetaminophen 108.3 mg/5 mL
Robitussin-PE	Guaifenesin 100 mg/5 mL
	Pseudoephedrine Hcl 30 mg/5 mL
Robitussin Pediatric	Dextromethorphan 7.5 mg/5 mL
Robitussin Allergy & Cough	Dextromethorphan 10 mg/5 mL
	Pseudoephedrine HCl 30 mg/5 mL
	Brompheniramine maleate 2 mg/5 mL

Source: Drug Facts & Comparisons (2002).

DELAY IN OBTAINING NEEDED TREATMENT

Delaying needed treatment may be caused by inaccurate patient self-diagnosis where the OTC drug may be totally ineffective, or in cases where the efficacy of the OTC medication is suboptimal and a prescription medication is warranted. Additionally, patients may be at risk for adverse effects associated with the drug, from which they have little chance of benefiting.

One example of potentially inaccurate self-diagnosis leading to a delay in obtaining needed medical treatment is the use of OTC antifungal agents for treatment of presumed vaginal candidiasis. A time-location study was done where symptomatic women presenting at local pharmacy/grocery stores with an OTC antifungal agent for purchase were offered entry into the study and were evaluated within 24 hours by clinical examination and the appropriate laboratory tests to confirm a diagnosis of candidiasis. Of the 95 women who elected to participate in the study, only one-third of them made the correct diagnosis of vaginal candidiasis. Another 20% had candidiasis coexisting with another type of vaginitis. Neither a previous clinically based diagnosis of vulvovaginal candidiasis or reading the package label were associated with improved accuracy of self-diagnosis. Half of the women in this study needed a prescription product for adequate treatment of coexisting infections. The consequence of delay in accurate diagnosis was considered to be minor in most of the cases, but was considered to be moderate to severe in about one-fifth of the cases (Ferris, Nyirjesy, Sobel, Soper, Pavletic, & Litaker, 2002).

GUIDELINES FOR APPROPRIATE USE OF OTC DRUGS

OTC medications are appropriate for many conditions, including to treat symptoms of minor, self-limiting illnesses; to prevent a disease or disorder (i.e., aspirin to prevent stroke); to manage chronic conditions [i.e., nonsteroidal anti-inflammatory drugs (NSAIDs) for arthritis]; or to cure certain conditions (i.e., vaginal yeast infections) (Holt & Hall, 1993). OTC medications may also significantly reduce healthcare costs. Self-care measures, particularly nonprescription drug use, should be recognized as an important part of the overall health status of the patient by both healthcare providers and patients alike. A thorough history of OTC drug use should be obtained during the patient visit. Patients may not deem OTC drugs as "real" medications because they may be obtained in so many different types of settings. Therefore, asking very specific questions regarding OTC drug use is important during the patient history and medication interview, something that is often forgotten. A study was conducted to ascertain patient-physician communication regarding OTC drug use during primary care office visits. It included data from 414 adult patient encounters involving 27 resident physicians. Data was gathered from audiotapes and transcripts of the visit encounters, as well as patient interviews by members of the research team immediately following the physician visit. Based on patient reported use of OTC medications during post-visit research team interviews, results showed that of patients reporting OTC medication use in the previous month, 58% did not tell the physician during the office visit. Only 14% of those not reporting OTC drug use to their physicians did not believe it was important for the physician to know. The remaining nonreporters either did not state a reason for not reporting use, did not tell because the physician did not ask, or simply forgot. Physicians specifically asked patients about OTC medication use in only a little more than a third of the visits. With the increased number of medications available OTC now and in the future, a more proactive approach to ascertaining OTC drug use is needed in order to avoid potential adverse events from duplicate therapy, interactions with other drugs, and potential contraindications to use of the drug. Physicians rarely or never stated information about or asked questions regarding these issues during the office visits in this study (Sleath, Rubin, Campbell,z Gwyther, & Clark, 2001). Additionally, with many generic versions of most OTC products available, practitioners can help reduce patient costs by suggesting an equivalent generic product in place of a branded one or recommend that the patient consult with the pharmacist when selecting a product.

Although the FDA has required changes to the format of OTC product labeling, patients will still benefit from verbal instructions on appropriate OTC drug use. According to a 1992 study by Holt et al., patients seemed to best interpret the correct responses to instructions that were given with specific hourly intervals (i.e., "every 12 hours" instead of "twice a day"). Although the profession of pharmacy has placed greater emphasis in recent years on increasing patient counseling both for prescription and OTC medications, the wide access of OTC medications to the patient may preclude a pharmacist-patient interaction. Thus, the healthcare provider needs to counsel the patient on recommended OTC use at the time of the visit. To maximize the benefits of OTC use and decrease the likelihood of adverse events, the following should be emphasized in the counseling process:

- Reason for self-treatment
- Description of drug or treatment
- Proper administration of drug or treatment
- Potential side effects and precautions
- Normal response time and what to do if the desired response does not occur

As with all other facets of healthcare, the practitioner must use discretion in the recommendation of OTC drugs based upon the perceived level of patient sophistication and education and the seriousness of the condition being treated.

REFERENCES

Beavers, H. (1999). If health plans are to cover OTCs, new controls should be set up. *Drug Topics, 143*(15), 41.

Brass, E.P. (2001). Changing the status of drugs from prescription to over-the-counter availability. *The New England Journal of Medicine, 345*(11), 810–816.

Clinical Pharmacy. (1991), *10,* 88, 93.

Consumer Healthcare Products Association (CHPA). (2003). Rx-to-OTC switches since 1976. (List updated July 3, 2003). Retrieved 3/19/04 from Consumer Healthcare Products Association Web site: www.chpa-info.org.

Consumer Healthcare Products Association (CHPA). (2002a). OTC facts and figures. Retrieved 5/9/02 from Consumer Healthcare Products Association Web site: www.chpa-info.org.

Consumer Healthcare Products Association (CHPA). (2002b). Voluntary codes and guidelines of the self-care industry: Code of advertising practices for nonprescription medicines. Retrieved 5/9/02 from Consumer Healthcare Products Association Web site: www.chpa-info.org.

Covington, T. R. (2000). Self-care and nonprescription pharmacotherapy. In L. V. Allen, R. R. Berardi, E. M. DeSimone, J. P. Engle, N. G. Popovich, W. M. Rosenthal, & K. J. Tietze (Eds.), *Handbook of nonprescription drugs* (12th ed.). Washington, DC: American Pharmaceutical Association.

Drug Facts & Comparisons. (2002). St. Louis: Facts & Comparisons.

Ferris, D.G., Nyirjesy, P., Sobel, J.D., Soper, D., Pavletic, A., & Litaker, M.S. (2002). Over-the-counter antifungal drug misuse associated with patient-diagnosed vulvovaginal candidiasis. *Obstetrics & Gynecology, 99*(3), 419–425.

Food and Drug Administration (FDA). (1999). Over-the-counter human drugs; labeling requirements. Retrieved 5/9/02 from FDA Web site: www.fda.gov/cder/otc/label/label-fr-reg.htm.

Gianfrancesco, F., Manning B., & Wang, R. (2002). Effects of prescription to OTC switches on out-of-pocket health care cost utilization. *Drug Benefit Trends, 14*(3), 13–30, 44.

Gilbertson, W. E. (1993). FDA's review of OTC drugs. In T. R. Covington, L. C. Lawson, & L. L. Young (Eds.), *Handbook of nonprescription drugs* (10th ed). Washington, DC: American Pharmaceutical Association.

Griffle, K. G. (1995). Opinions. *Drug Topics, 139*(18), 52–53.

Holt, G. A., Dorcheus, L., Hall, E. L., Beck, D., Ellis, E., & Hough, J. (1992). Patient interpretation of label instructions. *American Pharmacy, NS32,* 58–62.

Holt, G. A., & Hall, E. L. (1993). The self-care movement. In T. R. Covington, L. C. Lawson, & L. L. Young (Eds.), *Handbook of nonprescription drugs* (10th ed.). Washington, DC: American Pharmaceutical Association.

Kaufman, D.W., Kelly, J.P., Rosenberg, L., Anderson, T.E., & Mitchell, A.A. (2002). Recent patterns of medication use in the ambulatory adult population of the United States. *The Journal of the American Medical Association, 287*(3), 337–344.

Kogan M. D., Pappas G., Yu S. M., & Kotelchuck, M. (1994). Over-the-counter medication use among U.S. preschool-age children. *The Journal of the American Medical Association, 272*(13), 1025–1030.

Levy, S. (1998). Increased co-pays open door for wider usage of OTC drugs. *Drug Topics, 142*(23), 54.

Newton, G. D., Benninghoff, A.J., Pray, W. S., & Popovich, N. G. (2002). New OTC drugs and devices 2001: A selective review. *Journal of the American Pharmaceutical Association, 42,* 267–277.

Perry, L. (2001). More MCOs will use OTCs as first line of defense. *Drug Topics, 145*(11), 40.

Phillips, A.W., & Osborne, J.A. (2000). Survey of alternative and nonprescription therapy use. *American Journal of Health-System Pharmacy, 57,* 1361–1362.

Reynolds, T. (2002). Switching from prescription to over the counter. *Annals of Internal Medicine 136*(2), 177–180.

Sansgiry, S., Sharp, W.T., Sansgiry, S.S. (1999). Accuracy of information on printed over-the-counter drug advertisements. *Health Marketing Quarterly, 17*(2), 7–18.

Self-Care in the New Millennium, Roper Starch Worldwide for Consumer Healthcare Products Association, March 2001. Retrieved 5/9/02 from Consumer Healthcare Products Association Web site: www.chpainfo.org/pdfs/CHPA%20Final%20Report%20revised%20(03-20)_.pdf.

Sheftell, F., Dodick, D., & Cady, R. (2001). Direct-to-consumer advertising of OTC agents under current FTC regulations: Concerns and comment. *Headache, 41*(6), 534–536.

Sleath, B., Rubin, R.H., Campbell, W., Gwyther, L., & Clark, T. (2001). Physician-patient communication about over-the-counter medications. Social Science & Medicine, 53, 357–369.

Taylor, J. (2001). OTC counseling: Review of pharmacists' performance. *Medscape Pharmacists, 2*(2), accessed 5/9/02 at Medscape Web site: www.medscape.com/viewarticle/408580.

Vuckovic, N., & Nichter M. (1997). Changing patterns of pharmaceutical practice in the United States. *Social Science and Medicine, 44*(9), 1285–1302.

Westerlund, L.T., Marklund, B.R., Handl, W.H., Thunberg, M.E., & Allebeck, P. (2001). Nonprescription drug-related problems and pharmacy interventions. *The Annals of Pharmacotherapy, 35,* 1343–1349.

CHAPTER ❖ **10**

HERBAL THERAPIES FOR COMMON HEALTH PROBLEMS

Debra S. Israel ◆ Ellis Quinn Youngkin

In the nineteenth and prior centuries, herbal remedies for a wide variety of complaints were commonly found on pharmacy shelves. Then, in the twentieth century, such preparations took a back seat to prescription medicines, many of which had as their bases the very same herbs that had lost favor as the new century evolved. Now herbs (botanicals used to treat disease conditions, often chronic) and phytomedicinals (galenicals made by extracting herbs with various solvents) are back in a big way, conservatively estimated at $5 billion in the retail market in the United States (Bauer, 2000). Between 1994 and 2000, more than 158 million Americans used dietary supplements (Brodeur, 2002). It is estimated that up to 40% of Americans currently use alternative therapies (Gulla & Singer, 2000). A study of community-dwelling women 65 years of age and over found that 45.3% (39 of 86 subjects) had used an average of 2.5 herbal products (98 total herbal products) in the past year, and 85.4% of remedies were used on a continuous basis with a mean use of 348 months (Yoon & Horne, 2001). The herbal use was in addition to an average over the past year of 3.8 over-the-counter drugs and supplements and 3.2 prescription medications. Seventy-one of the 98 herbal products used were not reported to providers, and only 41% told their health providers at all about herbal use. As the country enters the new millennium, the herbs that were touted for their wonders hundreds, and even thousands, of years ago will continue to be in wide use, only they will have the advantage of modern scientific evaluation behind their use. The Office of Alternative Medicine was established in 1992 by the National Institutes of Heath (NIH) at the instruction of Congress to support research in the field. In 1998, this office became the National Center for Complementary and Alternative Medicine (NCCAM). The mission of NCCAM is to explore complementary and alternative healing practices by using rigorous science to train researchers in this field and to disseminate authoritative information to the public and professionals.

The safety and effectiveness of selected herbal therapies must be of concern to healthcare providers who are asked daily about such remedies by their patients. Thousands of people are planning to take or are already taking herbal preparations, and providers must be knowledgeable about their use. A survey of family practice patients indicated that half had used or were using alternative therapies, and only 53% had told their physician (Elder, Gillcrist, & Minz, 1997). Patients used the nontraditional therapies because they believed they would work. Physician factors like acceptance, open-mindedness, nonjudgmental attitudes, acknowledging the need for the person to be in control of his or her own care, the limits of traditional medicine, and "narrow-mindedness" were mentioned in the discussion of whether the patients told their physicians about the use of alternative therapies. Another study of family practice patients found supplement use (vitamins, minerals, herbs) was not related to age; use increased after one year; women used supplements more; younger people believed supplements were safer than prescribed drugs and were less likely to tell their physicians of use than those over 50 years old (Durante, Whitmore, Jones, & Campbell, 2001). A study of herb and supplement use (nonvitamin, nonmineral) of members of a large group health plan found that about 33% of the adults used one or more herb or supplement (Echinacea and Ginkgo biloba were most often used); and use was highest among women, whites, 45 to 65 year olds, graduates of college, and those with selected health conditions (Schaffer, Gordon, Jensen, and Avins, 2003). Another survey assessed the use of alternative therapies in patients presenting to a emergency department. Of 39 patients surveyed, 56% had tried alternative therapies in the past, and most patients (70%) did not inform their physicians of such usage (Gulla & Singer, 2000). A study of 142 emergency department children (mean age 5.3 years) found that 45% of caregivers had given the child one or more herbal remedies in the last year; most commonly aloe juice, echinacea, and sweet oil (Lanski, Greenwald, Perkins, & Simon, 2003). Less than half discussed giving the child such a remedy with a healthcare provider. A study of Hispanic and non-Hispanic white adults 65 and older found that 49% had used herbs in the last year for health care maintenance or a perceived problem (Zeilmann, Dole, Skipper, McCaabe, Dog, & Rhyne, 2003). For the provider to simply say to a patient, "There are no quality-controlled standards for production, or no double-blind, placebo-controlled clinical trials, so don't use them," is short-sighted and akin to telling the sexually active teen to "Just say no." People are going to use herbal remedies, so being informed is imperative. A better and more realistic provider approach is to know the answers to the questions in the following paragraph.

Which herbal therapies are effective and safe for common problems such as constipation, headache, dysmenorrhea, or head cold? What is the scientific support in the literature and where does it come from? What is the best dosage to use and for how long? In what form should the therapy be provided? Additionally, other questions to ask the patient are suggested by Tyler and Foster (1996): Has the patient used the product before and what happened? Are there any allergies to plant materials? Who is using or planning to use the product (the patient or someone else in the household, such as a child)? Does the patient understand the importance of closely following label instructions for use? Is the patient taking any other prescription or non-prescription medications (that could interact negatively with the herbal therapy)? Most importantly for women, are they pregnant or breast-feeding?

Some herbal preparations can be harmful. For example, the Food and Drug Administration (FDA) is removing ma huang (ephedrine or ephedra) from the marketplace in 2004. Ongoing reports of deaths and serious health problems (heart attack, stroke, seizure, and psychosis) for more than ten years have led to this decision (Chen, Biller, Willing, Lopez, 2004; Hurley, 1995; Schulman, 2003). The concern is that consumers will flock to other herbs, such as bitter orange, that are less studied than ephedra, to try to lose weight. Bitter orange contains a stimulant substance, synephrine, similar to ephedra that increases the blood pressure and causes vasoconstriction. A recent randomized double-blind, placebo-controlled, crossover study of the effects of an ephedra-caffeine dietary weight loss product found that the mean systolic blood pressure and maximal QTc interval were increased significantly in users (McBride, B.F., Karapanos, A.K., Krudysz, A., Kluger, J., Coleman, C., & White, C., 2004).

Thus, healthcare providers must carefully determine what herbal preparations their patients are taking, how much, and by what route, and what conventional drugs the patients are taking that may interact negatively with these herbal ingested substances in light of illness and/or symptoms. This chapter will provide the practitioner with some background information on selected acceptable herbal therapies for some commonly encountered complaints in primary care, as well as some general information.

SAFETY, EFFECTIVENESS, REGULATION, AND DANGERS

Over 1400 herbs are sold commercially, most as dietary supplements, and only a few are classified as safe and effective by the FDA. These include aloe, cascara, psyllium, senna, witch hazel, capsicum/cayenne pepper, and slippery elm. For the FDA to classify a substance as safe and effective, sufficient information has to be submitted for adequate evaluation (Tyler & Foster, 1996). That the FDA has not classified an herb as safe and effective does not mean the herbal preparation is automatically unsafe or ineffective; it means that a lack of data exists for Category I placement. Nevertheless, in 1994, the Dietary Supplement Health and Education Act ruled that herbs could be labeled with information on their effects in the body but must contain a disclaimer that the product has not received FDA review and is not intended for use as a drug but as a dietary supplement (Hurley, 1995). It is understandable why companies are not willing to invest huge sums to gain clinical evidence of safety and effectiveness since most herbs are not patentable (Tyler & Foster, 1996).

In other countries, especially in Europe and Great Britain, herbal therapies have been considered for treatment along with conventional medicines for years. Germany established the German Commission E, appointed by the Ministry of Health in 1978 to investigate the safety and efficacy of herbal therapies. This commission published more than 300 monographs on herbs through the German Federal Health Agency (now the Federal Institute for Drugs and Medical Devices) until 1995 (Blumenthal, 1998). Commission E's role significantly changed after that to be a commission for registration of phytomedicines to be sold as prescription drugs, as well as to make decisions about nonprescription herbal registration extensions. An English translation of the Commission E monographs was published in 1998 (Blumenthal, 1998). Since then, concern has arisen about the accuracy of the information contained in both the German and English monographs since the published monographs are not referenced. Thus, failing to reveal the sources of information the Commissioners used to form their recommendations is a severe limitation and falls outside the accepted standards for rigorous scientific publications (Bauer, 2000). The World Health Organization (WHO) has recommended adoption of regulations by member countries to deal with issues of safety, efficacy, and quality (Libster, 2002), and WHO began publishing monographs in 1998 with standards for herbal drugs (Blumenthal, 1998). Countries are responding to the concerns about safety by creating regulatory entities, such as the Complementary Medicines Evaluation Committee in Australia, the Natural Health Products Directorate in Canada, and the European Agency for the Evaluation of Medicinal Products (Rousseaux & Schachter, 2003).

Ernst (2002) notes that trials of herbal medicinal products have been too few, too small, and too short. It is encouraging that some of the best-selling herbal products have been examined in randomized clinical trials, including ginkgo, St. John's wort, saw palmetto, ginseng, echinacea, and kava. These trials, plus some systematic reviews, will be used in this chapter to help clinicians better understand these herbs. Even systematic reviews have limitations, but they are clearly needed in the field of herbal medicine. The NCCAM is currently recruiting patients for trials using a number of herbs, including garlic, ginkgo, ginseng, black cohosh, chamomile tea, and echinacea. The NCCAM website (*www.nccam.nih.gov*) can provide additional information.

Another issue is the lack of standardization of the herbal products currently on the market. Since there are no government oversights or industry standards for the quality of herbal preparations available in the United States, one cannot be sure exactly what part of the plant is being used (flowers, stem, root, seeds, fruit, or other). There is well-documented evidence of inaccurate labeling and intentional substitution by herbal manufacturers. Adulterated products are a particular problem, leading some manufacturers to develop and advertise standardized, pure doses in the hopes of preventing more restrictive legislation (Brodeur, 2002). In this type of environment, U.S. herbs should be viewed as a "buyer beware" situation (Bauer, 2000). A number of companies—such as Consumerlab.com, the U.S. Pharmacopoeia, and *Consumer Reports*—are conducting independent testing of supplements (Brodeur, 2002). Information on the testing of herbal products, if available, is provided in this chapter.

The regulation of teas falls in a "gray" area of regulation between food and drugs, according to the FDA (Snider, 1991). Herbal teas are not regulated since they are considered foods. Care is especially important in the use of imported teas or ones grown at home since the concentration may be very high, and thus dangerous, if consumed in excess (Youngkin & Israel, 1996). Further muddying the herbal waters, food manufacturers are adding herbs to food products, obviously to boost sales (Barnes & Winter, 2001). One example is the addition of ginkgo biloba to Snapple iced tea. The concern of health providers should be promises of benefits without supportive research, possible long-term harmful effects, need for safety advisories on labels, and no FDA oversight.

Miller (1996), a gerontological nurse specialist, advises patients to be sure they have no medical condition that might need treatment before taking nonprescription remedies; discuss such remedies with their provider; use products that contain just one ingredient; check warnings on labels and seek help if any untoward symptoms occur; understand that safety standards are not required of such products; and consider that if it sounds too good to be true, it most likely is not true. Interactions between herbs and other medicines, either prescription or over the counter, abound. It wasn't until reports of interaction effects between herbs like St. John's wort or Ginkgo biloba and prescription drugs became more common that the whole arena of interactions and potential interactions that can be life-threatening rose to prominence (Bond & Hanaford, 2003; Williamson, 2003). Herbs are generally taken long-term, thus, the risk for interaction effects on the cardiovascular, central nervous, immune and other systems become more likely. The provider must be more vigilant than ever in trying to find out if the patient is using herbs or other supplements. An analysis of herb-drug interactions indicated that most occurred due to an effect on the metabolism of the product through the cytochrome p450 enzymes (Brazier & Levine, 2003).

Many herbal preparations are mixtures of herbs, necessitating that the consumer be knowledgeable about a wide variety of herbs in order to separate information about each component for safety. Libster (2002) also advises the herbal user to employ all five senses and common sense in feedback about safety. A study of ingredients in 10 of the most commonly purchased herbs in retail stores found that the recommended daily dose (RDD) was consistent with a benchmark in ingredients and RDD in only 43% of the 880 products examined (Garrard, Harms, Eberly, & Matiak, 2003). In addition, Internet sources may be misleading, stating that an herbal therapy can prevent an illness, or treat, or cure a disease, even though regulations forbid this type of labeling claim (Morris & Avorn, 2003). The references at the end of this chapter provide some excellent resources to buy and keep on hand to evaluate herbal preparations. Many lay resources are not based on science, and although they may have accurate information, in many no or few references are given to help the consumer feel confident about safe and effective use. In addition, there are a number of sites on the World Wide Web that can provide accurate and updated information on herbs and herbal products. Some of these sites are: *www.herbmed.org*; *www.naturaldatabase.com*; *www.ncbi.nih.gov/pubmed*; *www.vm.cfsan.fda*; *www.usp.org*; *http://dietarysupplements.info.nih.gov*; *www.consumerlab.com*; *http://odp.od.nih.gov/ods/question.html*; *www.herbal-ahp.org/*

Last, for ultimate safety, no herbal therapies should be used by pregnant women, nursing mothers, or infants and young children until definitive data exist to prove safety (Tyler & Foster, 1996). An issue of great concern is the effect of herbal products on the embryo or fetus. Hormonal as well as interaction effects of the herb with other drugs are thought to cause most of the untoward effects rather than direct effects of the herb on the unborn child (Rousseaux & Schachter, 2003).

DOSAGE FORMS OF HERBAL THERAPIES

Herbs are prepared in different ways to get the most effective active ingredients from the specific herb. For instance, if some herbs are dried, such as St. John's wort or feverfew, properties are lost (Keville, 1996). For other herbs that contain a lot of water, like calendula or comfrey, drying is the best method of preparation. Table 10–1 gives an overview of various preparations of herbs for use internally or externally.

COMMON CONDITIONS AND HERBAL REMEDIES

Selected conditions commonly encountered in primary healthcare are presented in alphabetical order in this section. One or more herbal remedies that have scientific support for use and appropriate dose and form are given.

TABLE 10–1. Delivery Forms of Herbs and Phytomedicinals

- *Infusions (teas):* Herbs steeped in hot water; plant materials are in a coarsely comminuted form unless commercially cut extra fine for quick tea. Infusions can be cold; used for fragrant herbs that lose their essential oils if heated.
- *Decoctions:* Generally, roots and bark simmered gently for longer periods to produce the tea.
- *Poultices:* Fresh plants pounded, blended, or chewed into a sticky paste form, spread on an injury, and wrapped with a bandage. Another type of poultice is made from powder mixed with water to form the paste for external use.
- *Capsules or tablets:* Finely powdered herbs for oral ingestion; they release the active ingredient in the stomach. They may be enteric-coated to protect from inactivation in the stomach if the herb is damaged by acid.
- *Syrups:* Tinctures, liquid extracts, glycerites, or teas.
- *Extracts or galenicals:* Liquid or solid phytomedicinals that can be standardized more readily because the herb is extracted with solvents.
- *Tinctures:* Concentrated liquid herbal extracts diluted by adding to water or juice; alcohol is the solvent used for extracting the herb.
- *Vinegars:* Prepared like tinctures but with an infusion of herb into vinegar, not alcohol; herbal vinegars are not strong enough for medicinal use.
- *Body oils:* Made from herbs for massage or for external remedies, such as for sore muscles.
- *Skin salves:* Thickened herbal oils that adhere to the skin.
- *Compresses:* Can be hot or cold if the cloth is soaked in an herbal liquid preparation such as tea, diluted tincture, oil, or water.
- *Herbal bath:* Generally, a relaxation method, but herbal therapies can be combined with other therapies, such as aromatherapy, to accomplish a medicinal goal such as stimulation of circulation or muscle relaxation. Small baths for feet or hands can be prepared from teas or oils.
- *Glycerites:* Syrupy liquids made with glycerin without alcohol as an alternative to more potent tinctures.

Sources: Keville (1996) and Tyler & Foster (1996).

Any signs or symptoms of adverse effects that the patient develops require stopping the herbal therapy immediately and calling the healthcare provider or going to an emergency room if serious. Providers are reminded that herbs are drugs, despite patients' common misconception that they are "natural" and, therefore, "safe." As drugs, allergic responses and untoward effects can occur. Table 10–2 provides the common and scientific names of a selection of commonly used herbs.

TABLE 10–2. Common, Scientific, and/or Other Names of Selected Herbs

Aloe vera:	*Aloe barbadensis,* Barbados aloe, Curacao aloe
Angelica:	*Angelica archangelica,* garden angelica, European angelica
Bearberry:	*Arctostaphylos uva ursi,* uva-ursi, Ericaceae
Black cohosh:	*Cimicifuga racemosa,* black snake root, rattleweed, rattleroot, squawroot
Caffeine:	Contained in *Coffea arabic L.* or other *Coffea* (coffee); *Camellia sinensis (L.)* O. Kuntze (tea); *Cola nitida* (kola or cola); *Theobroma cacao* L. (Cocoa); *Paullinia cupana* H.B.K. (cuarana paste); *Ilex paraguariensis* St.Hil. (mate)
Caigua:	*Cyclanthera pedata,* wild cucumber, achojcha
Capsicum:	*Capsicum spp.,* cayenne pepper, chile pepper, red pepper
Chamomile:	*Matricaria recutia, Chamaemelum nobile,* German or Hungarian chamomile
Chaste tree berry:	*Vitex agnus-castus,* chaste tree, chaste berry, Vitex
Cranberry:	*Vaccinium macrocarpon,* cranberry juice
Echinacea:	*Echinacea angustifolia, E. purpurae, E. pallida,* Sampson root
Elder:	*Sambuccua canadensis nigra,* elderberry
Eleuthero:	*Eleutherococcus senticosus,* Siberian ginseng
Ephedra:	*Ephedra sinica,* ma huang, Ephedraceae
Evening primrose oil:	*Oenothera biennis,* black currant, borage seed oil
Feverfew:	*Tanacetum parthenium,* Chrysanthemum parthenium
Garlic:	*Allium sativum L.,* clove garlic
Ginger:	*Zingiber officinale Rosc.,* African ginger, black ginger, race ginger, gingerroot
Ginkgo biloba:	*Ginkgo biloba L.,* ginkgo tree
Ginseng:	*Panax ginseng* (Oriental), *Panax quinquefolius* (American), Asiatic ginseng, wonder-of-world (Chinese ginseng), five-fingers, five-leafed ginseng (American ginseng)
Goldenrod:	*Solidago virgaurea L.* (American), *S. serotina, S. Canadensis L.*
Hawthorn:	*Crataegus laevigata* (Pior) DC., *C. oxyacantha auct., C. monogyna Jacq.,* May bush, May tree, thorn-apple tree, whitehorn
Horehound:	*Marrubium vulgare L.,* marrubium
Kava:	*Piper methysticum*
Licorice:	*Glycyrrhiza glabra L.* (European), *G. uralensis Fisch.* (Chinese), licorice root, sweet licorice, sweet wood
Melissa:	*Melissa officinalis L.,* lemon balm
Nettle:	*Urtica diocia,* common nettle, stinging nettle, great stinging nettle
Peppermint:	*Menthax piperita L.,* mint
Plantago seed/husk:	*Plantago psyllium L.* (Spanish); *P. indica L.* (French); *P. ovata* Forskal (Blond Psyllium or Indian Plantago seed)
Pygeum:	*Pygeum africanum*
St. John's wort:	*Hypericum perforatum L.,* amber, goatweed, Johnswort, Klamath weed
Saw palmetto:	*Serenoa epens, Sabal serrulata*
Senna:	*Senna alexandrina, Cassia acutifolia, C. angustifolia*
Slippery elm:	*Ulmus rubra Muhl., U. fulva*
Tea tree oil:	*Melaleuca alternifolia, tea tree*
Valerian:	*Valeriana officinalis L., valerian*
Witch hazel:	*Hamamelis virginiana L., H. vernalis Sarg.*

Sources: Mindell (1992), Tierra (1990), Tyler (1994), Tyler & Foster (1996), and Youngkin & Israel (1996).

ANXIETY, STRESS, AND DEPRESSION

St. John's Wort

This herb comes from the dried flowering tops of a member of the St. John's wort family that grows in Europe, Asia, Africa, North America, and Australia (Leung & Foster, 1995). It has anxiolytic, antidepressant, and antiinflammatory properties, but its most important activity is said to be as a treatment for mild or moderate depression (Harrer & Sommer, 1994). Several active constituents have been identified. The two that are likely the most active are hypericin and hyperforin, with hyperforin the primary active constituent. Extracts of this herb inhibit the reuptake of serotonin, dopamine, and norepinephrine, which contributes to the antidepressant activity of St. John's wort (Butterweck, 2003; Jellin, Gregory, Batz, Hitchens, et al., 2002). Numerous trials have evaluated the activity of St. John's wort for the treatment of mild to moderate depression. One meta-analysis evaluated 28 randomized, double-blind clinical trials and concluded that St. John's wort is more effective than placebo and is similar in effectiveness to low-dose tricyclic antidepressants in the treatment of mild to moderate depression (Ernst, 2002). There is also data suggesting that St. John's wort is as effective as some selective serotonin reuptake inhibitors (SSRIs) (Jellin et al., 2002). Kasper and Dienel (2002) found that hypericum extract reduced all signs and symptoms of depression generally in mild to moderate disease similarly to the way SSRIs influence the disease. St. John's wort may not be as beneficial in the treatment of moderate to severe depression based on information from recent trials (Shelton et al., 2001; Hypericum Depression Trial Study Group, 2002). When used in combination with valerian, St. John's wort improves depression coexisting with anxiety more readily without significant side effects (Muller, Pfeil, & von den Driesch, 2003). St. John's wort is generally well tolerated. Side effects can include GI discomfort, anxiety, insomnia, headache, and dry mouth. The most common side effect is photosensitivity, and patients should be cautioned about taking appropriate protective measures to avoid direct sunlight (Jellin et al., 2002). Another concern with St. John's wort is that it may interact with other medications through activation of the cytochrome p450 system. St. John's wort can decrease the plasma levels of many prescribed drugs, including antiviral agents, anticoagulants, and oral contraceptives, to name a few (Ernst, 2002; Harris, Jang, & Tsunoda, 2003; Markowitz, Donovan, DeVane, Taylor, et al., 2003). Hubner (2003) found that although Staphylococcus aureus does acquire a resistance to hyperforin, a principle antibacterial component of hypericum, cross resistance against antibiotics generally used in practice did not occur, and the usual treatment dose daily of hypericum extract (900 mg daily), did not result in resistance of the organism. It is important to avoid concomitant use of St. John's wort and MAO inhibitors and other antidepressants because patients are at risk for the development of serotonin syndrome. Patients should not add St. John's wort to an already prescribed antidepressant regimen (Jellin et al., 2002, Ernst, 2002). St. John's wort is one of eight herbs advised for discontinuation prior to any surgery in which a possible induced increase in metabolism by St. John's wort of perioperative period drugs could create a hazard (Ang-Lee, Moss, & Yuan, 2001). The other seven herbs advised for discontinuation are echinacea, ephedra, garlic, ginkgo, ginseng, kava, and valerian. Although combining low-dose oral contraception (OC) with St. John's wort extract did not lead to evidence of ovulation, bleeding between cycles did increase, which might result in women not using OCs correctly, thus increasing risk of pregnancy (Pfrunder, Schiesser, Gerber, Haschek et al., 2003). Another study of a moderate dose OC concluded that the breakthrough bleeding was associated with increased CYP3A activity that could decrease effectiveness and suggested adding a barrier method for better protection (Hall, Wang, Huang, Hamman et al., 2003). Abebe (2003) warns that St. John's wort may cause xerostomia (Abebe, 2003). The practitioner is urged to review current literature on drug interactions of St. John's wort when prescribing this herb (Brazier & Levine, 2003).

Advised Dosage: For mild to moderate depression, the dose most commonly used in clinical trials was 300 mg three times a day, usually standardized to 0.3% hypericin content (Jellin et al., 2002). Other studies have used a 0.2% hypericin extract with the dosage at 250 mg two times a day. One cup of tea taken one to three times a day can also be used by steeping 2–4 grams of the dried herb in 150 ml boiling water for 5–10 minutes, then straining (Jellin et al., 2002). Libster (2002) suggests 1–2 teaspoons of the herb—dry or fresh—in a cup of water 1–2 times daily. Alternatively, a liquid extract (1:1 in 25% alcohol) is typically taken as 2–4 mls 2–3 times a day (Jellin et al., 2002; Libster, 2002). It may take several weeks for the clinical effects to be seen (Ernst, 2002). Patients should be cautioned not to abruptly discontinue St. John's wort due to the risk of adverse withdrawal effects (Jellin et al., 2002). The content of hypericin and hyperforin can vary widely in the products on the market. See next section for additional information (Draves & Walker, 2003; Garrard et al., 2003). St. John's wort is not advised for pregnant or lactating women.

Comments on Product Testing: In 2000, ConsumerLab.com purchased 21 brands of St. John's wort to test for quality of ingredients and levels of cadmium. Cadmium from the environment accumulates naturally in the plant as it grows. Cadmium is carcinogenic and though the amounts found in St. John's wort should not be enough to cause disease, it can add to a person's total exposure. It is, therefore, preferable to identify products with the lowest cadmium levels. One-third, or seven products, did not pass testing because they either did not have their stated label claim of hypericin, did not contain the minimum standard of hypericin needed to pass this review, or contained levels of cadmium that exceeded acceptable levels for this review. Readers are referred to the Consumerlab.com website for additional information on specific products.

Valerian

Some individuals use valerian to relieve anxiety and tension. However, this herb can act as a stimulant in some people, causing anxiety (see Insomnia section in this chapter for more information on valerian). Use valerian with caution for anxiety.

Kava

This herb comes from the underground root of the kava plant (a pepper plant, *Piper methysticum*) and is also called kava-kava or ava (Norton & Ruze, 1994; Tyler, 1997a). *Piper methysticum,* the scientific name, means intoxicating pepper. Kava was used as a ceremonial drink for thousands of years by Pacific Islanders (Fiji, Polynesia, Melanesia, Micronesia) to create a feeling of relaxation. There is recent concern that preparations containing kava can cause hepatotoxicity, including hepatitis, cirrhosis, and liver failure in patients ingesting relatively normal doses, short term. At least 25 documented cases of liver toxicity following kava use are reported; some patients needed liver transplantation after, using kava for only 1–3 months. In addition, there were several deaths reported (NCCAM Consumer Advisory, March 2002).

Canada and Germany have banned kava sales, but Great Britain and the United States have not (Mills, Singh, Ross, Ernst, et al., 2003; Schulze, Raasch, & Siegers, 2003; Stickel, Baumuller, Seitz, Vasilakis, et al., 2003). Controversy regarding the toxicity of kava exists, with the estimate of hepatotoxicity as comparable to reported cases of benzodiazepines (Schulze). Two studies in Germany found positive effects on sleep and anxiety with kava versus placebo when used in randomized trials for four weeks (Gastpar & Klimm, 2003; Lehrl, 2004). In the United States, the FDA is advising consumers of the potential risk of liver injury from the use of dietary supplements containing kava. Risk versus benefit must be assessed before recommending the use of kava. Patients with a history of liver problems or those that are regular alcohol consumers should avoid taking kava. Routine monitoring of liver function tests is recommended for those who continue to use this herb. Careful review of food products, such as teas, for addition of this herb is advised for safety. A veterans hospital in Oregon found that half of patients with fulminant hepatic failure had recently used or were currently using herbs or dietary supplements that were potentially hepatotoxic (Estes, Stolpman, Olyaei, Corless, et al., 2003).

BREAST TENDERNESS

Chaste Tree Berry

See *Premenstrual Symptoms.*

Evening Primrose Oil

See *Muscle/Joint Pain and Inflammation.*

BRONCHIAL ASTHMA

Ephedra

The aboveground (aerial) parts are used of the species, found in warm, dry areas of Asia, the Americas, and Europe (Tyler & Foster, 1996). It is commonly called *ma huang,* and the stem contains the active ingredients, primarily an alkaloid mixture of ephedrine and pseudoephedrine. Ephedra has been used to treat bronchial asthma for at least 5000 years, producing bronchodilation, vasoconstriction, and decreased bronchial edema (Hebel, 1996; Tyler, 1994). Ephedra, used for weight loss and to enhance athletic performance, has been banned. Ephedra is dangerous, with numerous case reports linking ephedra use to palpitations, insomnia, hypertension, myocardial infarction, psychosis, seizure, stroke, and death. In several of these reports, ephedra was shown to be harmful even with short-term use with relatively low doses (20 to 60 mg) (FDA, 2000; Haller & Benowitz, 2000). The addition of caffeine, as seen in some weight-loss products, further increases the risk. Contraindications to ephedra use include high blood pressure, heart disease, diabetes, glaucoma, enlargement of the prostate, and hyperthyroidism. (Given the safety concerns associated with this herb, its use is not recommended.)

COLDS AND FLU

Echinacea

This herb comes from aerial (aboveground) parts and/or roots of the purple coneflower, a member of the aster family found naturally in the midwestern United States (Tyler & Foster, 1996). There are three species of echinacea (*E. purpurea, E. angustifolia,* and *E. pallida*). Active ingredients vary with the source of the herb, but include a number of acids, essential oils, alkylamides, polysaccharides, and other constituents. It is used orally for the treatment of cold and flu symptoms and for its immunostimulating actions (Jellin, 2002). The data supporting the efficacy of echinacea are mixed. Most of the studies have been conducted in Germany, where echinacea is approved by the Federal Health Agency for use to support therapy for upper respiratory tract infections, wounds, and urogenital infections. Many of these studies had poor methodology, so conclusive results were difficult to obtain. For instance, treatment assignments were not randomized or blind in most studies, and some of the echinacea extracts contained additional ingredients that may have contributed to the effects (O'Hara, Keifer, Farrell, & Kemper, 1998). Ernst (2002) evaluated a summary of sixteen randomized clinical trials of echinacea for upper respiratory tract infection. Overall, the results from these trials were inconclusive. Several trials did suggest a beneficial effect, but there was concern that publication bias distorted the results of the reviews. Thus, it is difficult to make strong recommendations for the use of this herb. Available evidence is incomplete, but some data suggest a possible supportive role in treating infections (O'Hara et al., 1998). In addition, it is not clear if any particular formulation or echinacea species offers a greater benefit over the others. A recent study of echinacea as a cold treatment for children found that use did not shorten the time of the cold or decrease severity, and children treated with the herb had more rashes (Taylor, Weber, Standish, Quinn, et al., 2003). However, in a randomized, double-blind, placebo controlled study of adults in Canada, a standardized formulation of echinacea given at the onset of the first cold symptoms led to a reduction in the severity of symptoms (Goel, Lovlin, Barton, Lyon, et al., 2004).

Echinacea is generally well tolerated, though adverse reactions, such as fever, nausea vomiting, abdominal pain, allergic reactions, and sore throat have been reported (Jellin et al., 2002). Atopic patients, especially those with allergies to plants in the daisy family, appear to be at increased risk for allergic reactions. Caution should be used when recommending this herb to patients with autoimmune diseases (multiple sclerosis, lupus, plus others) and those with HIV/AIDS, since echinacea has immunostimulating properties (Jellin et al., 2002). A rapidly progressive case of nephritis has been reported as an adverse effect (Advisor Forum, 2002). If echinacea is given with drugs that depend upon CYP3A or CYP1A2 for elimination, the clearance of these drugs may be adversely affected (Gorski, Huang, Pinto, Hamman, et al, 2004).

Advised Dosage. A number of different doses have been used to treat the common cold and flu. If using tablets containing 6.78 mg of *Echinacea purpurea* crude extract (based on 95% herb and 5% root), a dose of two tablets three times daily is advised (Jellin et al., 2002). Blumenthal, Goldberg, and Brinckman (2000) suggests 0.3 ounce or 0.9 gram of root in 150 mL boiled water three times a day. Beginning use at the first sign of the infection and not taking it longer than suggested on the packaging is advised. In addition, an *Echinacea purpurea* herb juice, *Echinacea pallida,* root tincture, and freeze-dried plant dose have all been used (Jellin et al., 2002; Libster, 2002).

Comments on Product Testing. Consumerlab.com evaluated 25 echinacea products in October and November 2000. Only 14 products (56%) passed their review. Products failed for various reasons. Some products did not have detectable levels of the herb species claimed on the label, others exceeded label claims or had microbacterial contamination. Readers are referred to the Consumerlab.com website for additional information on specific products.

Elder

Berries of the elderberry tree have long been used as a folk remedy for the flu, colds, and neuralgia (Keville, 1996; Mindell, 1992). Elder is said to enhance the immune system as well as stop cold and flu viruses. Flowers from the elder plant may have diuretic and laxative properties, but these effects are not well established. Limited clinical data exist on the efficacy of elderberry in the treatment of the flu. One placebo-controlled, double-blind study evaluated a standardized elderberry extract (Sambucol) on a group of individuals living in a kibbutz during an influenza outbreak in 1993. The majority of patients receiving elderberry had improvement in symptoms within two days, whereas the control group showed improvement within six days (Zakay-Rones, Varsano, & Zlotnik, 1995). An Israeli study of five herbal remedies found that Sambucol black elderberry extact and two other Sambucol products increased production of inflammatory and anti-inflammatory cytokines, inferring that those suffering from influenza might benefit from use (Barak, Birkenfeld, Halperin & Kalickman, 2002). Reported side effects of elderberry juice include weakness, dizziness, and stupor. Raw and unripe fruit can cause GI side effects (Jellin et al., 2002).

Advised Dosage. In adults, four tablespoons of elderberry juice-containing syrup (Sambucol) each day for three days for the treatment of the flu has been used (Jellin et al., 2002). Blumenthal et al. (2000) suggests a tea of 1 teaspoon dry berries or flowers in 150 mL of hot water one to two times daily as hot as safe to drink.

Horehound

See *Coughs.*

CONSTIPATION

Plantago Seed and Husk

This herb is also called psyllium or plantain, and comes from cleaned, dried, ripened seeds grown in Europe, India, and Pakistan; seeds and seed husks contain insoluble (80%) and soluble (20%) fiber (Tyler & Foster, 1996). The components act as a bulk laxative as the seed coats swell, increasing intestinal volume and stimulation, and the mucilage from the seeds provides lubrication and increased transit time (European Scientific Cooperative, 1992; Plantaginis ovatae testa, 1990). There is also evidence that plantago seed lowers cholesterol and low-density lipoprotein (LDL) levels (Plantaginis ovatae testa, 1990; Sprecher et al., 1993). Psyllium also may be effective for irritable bowel syndrome (IBS) by helping to normalize bowel function and relieve symptoms of abdominal pain. Seeds from non-commercial preparations should not be chewed, crushed, or ground due to release of a pigment that may cause nephrotoxicity. Most commercial preparations of plantago do not contain this pigment. Side effects include GI symptoms, such as flatulence, abdominal pain, nausea, diarrhea, constipation, and dyspepsia. Psyllium may interact with a number of drugs, including some antiseizure medications, warfarin, digoxin, and oral hypoglycemics. It is recommended to administer oral drugs either one hour before or four hours after psyllium to avoid drug interactions (Jellin et al., 2002). Rarely, allergic reactions occur with use. Plantago seed should not be used in people with diabetes mellitus or GI obstructions.

Advised Dosage. The amount required to treat constipation can vary. It is recommended to start with small amounts and increase to desired response to decrease the unwanted side effects. The typical daily dose of psyllium is 7 to 40 grams, divided two to three times a day. Mix 7 grams of seed in at least 240 ml of water. For IBS, 7 grams one to three times daily can be used. Adequate fluid intake is important to avoid choking and esophageal or bowel obstruction (Jellin et al., 2002). The use of psyllium seed or husk is contraindicated with intestinal stenosis, bowel obstruction (real or possible), and poorly controlled diabetes (Libster, 2002).

Senna

The preparation is made from dried leaflets of Alexandria and Tinnevelly senna, from the Middle East and Asia primarily, that act as a cathartic (Leung & Foster, 1995; Tyler, 1994; Tyler, Brady, & Robbers, 1988). Senna can cause cramps, and chronic abuse causes potassium loss, electrolyte and fluid imbalance, and reduced effectiveness of other drugs such as cardiac glycosides. It can cause a potential for toxicity of such drugs, and its use is contraindicated in pregnancy or lactation. If senna is used for a prolonged period (more than one to two weeks), it can cause "laxative-dependency syndrome," which is characterized by diarrhea, poor gastric motility, and a colon that does not function (Jellin et al., 2002).

Advised Dosage. The usual dose is 15 to 30 mg of sennoside B daily (Jellin et al., 2002). As a tea, chopped senna leaf is steeped for 10 minutes in warm water (not boiling) and strained before drinking. Cold water may cause fewer GI symptoms. Directions on the label should be followed to use the smallest dose possible for a soft stool. Standardized over-the-counter senna preparations do improve control of dosing (Jellin et al., 2002). Use of this herb beyond one to two weeks is not recommended unless the patient is under the supervision of a healthcare practitioner (Tyler & Foster, 1996).

COUGH

Horehound

Horehound comes from the dried aerial flowering parts of a member of the mint family found in Europe and the United States (Tyler & Foster, 1996). The leaves contain a volatile oil and other active ingredients, especially marrubiinic acid, which has a strong choleretic activity (Tyler, 1994). Extracts of horehound are used to flavor foods and beverages and as an expectorant in lozenges and cough syrups. Horehound is possibly effective when used for coughs (Jellin et al., 2002). It should not be used in pregnancy or lactation.

Advised Dosage. The usual dose is one to two grams dried cut herb (use the aboveground parts) steeped in 150 ml boiling water during the day as an expectorant. Horehound-flavored candy is sold as a cough suppressant (Tyler, 1994).

Licorice

Licorice is reputed to calm coughs and have expectorant qualities. The extract is used in lozenges, candies, and teas (Tyler, 1994). However, in the United States, most licorice candy is flavored with anise oil and contains no real licorice. For upper respiratory tract mucus membrane inflammation, the usual dose of licorice (*Succus liquiritiae*) is 0.5 to 1 grams (Jellin et al., 2002). Glycyrrhizin, a constituent, has an expectorant effect. See Gastric Ulcers in this chapter for more information on licorice.

DYSMENORRHEA

Black Cohosh

Black cohosh (*Cimicifuga racemosa* or *Actaea racemosa*) comes from the dried rhizome and roots of a member of the buttercup family native to North America (Tyler & Foster, 1996). Black cohosh is approved by Germany's Commission E for use in treating menopause, dysmenorrhea, and PMS. Black cohosh contains many constituents, but its mechanism of action remains unknown and evidence of estrogenic activity from laboratory tests is mixed (Jellin et al., 2002). There are some reports that black cohosh has estrogenic activity in some tissues, which lends evidence to its possible activity when taken orally for symptoms of menopause (Jellin et al., 2002; Libster, 2002). However, researchers at the University of San Diego did not find measurable estrogen activity in black cohosh or chaste tree berry (Oerter, Janfaza, Wong, & Chang, 2003). It is suggested that *Cimicifuga racemosa* exerts a central, not hormonal effect (Borrelli, Izzo, & Ernst, 2003). In addition, black cohosh has not demonstrated estrogenic activity in assays that would promote breast cancer cell growth (Lupu, Mehmi, Atlans, Tsai, Pisha, et al., 2003). The North American Menopause Society finds that results of clinical trials are not sufficient to support or not support the efficacy of black cohosh for menopausal treatment although it lists the herb as one nonprescription therapy along with lifestyle as a beginning line of treatment (Treatment of menopause-associated, 2004). Currently, there is insufficient information available about effectiveness of black cohosh in the treatment of dysmenorrhea to recommend it for this condition. A double-blind study reported at the 84th annual meeting of The Endocrine Society noted that black cohosh and conjugated estrogen significantly decreased hot flashes daily over placebo (Barclay, 2002). The mechanism is thought to be related to a reduction in LH (Libster, 2002). Blood lipid and bone-specific alkaline phosphatase improved with black cohosh without endometrial thickening. Three months of black cohosh at 40 mg per day was used in the Endo 2002 study. The herb needs to be taken for at least four weeks before symptoms improve (Jellin et al., 2002). An analysis of randomized, controlled trials of complementary and alternative medicine therapies for menopausal symptoms showed that black cohosh may improve hot flashes but only short-term use is recommended since information about safety long-term is inadequate (Kronenberg & Fugh-Berman, 2003). Few adverse events and no known major drug interactions are reported with black cohosh and most adverse events (97%) are minor (Dog, Powell, & Weisman, 2003; Kligler, 2003). Common side effects include gastrointestinal upset; other reported side effects include dizziness, headache, weight gain, and cramping (Jellin et al., 2002). It is contraindicated during pregnancy, but has been used to facilitate labor (Libster, 2002).

Advised Dosage. For menopause and PMS, most studies have used a specific black cohosh extract (Remifemin, Enzymatic Therapy, and Phytopharmacia) standardized to contain 1 mg triterpene glycosides, calculated as 27-deoxyacetin, per 20 mg tablet. The dose used was 40 to 80 mg twice daily, to provide 4 to 8 mg triterpene glycosides. The manufacturer is now providing data that due to improvement in the extraction process, a lower dose of 20 mg twice daily is recommended, providing 2 mg triterpene glycosides, the active constituent (Jellin et al., 2002). Libster (2002) mentions a 500-mg capsule three times daily, as well as a 40-mg per day dried herb product to be taken in divided doses.

FLATULENCE

Chamomile

This popular herb comes from the dried flower heads of the German chamomile; Roman chamomile, grown mainly in Great Britain, is different chemically from the German variety (Tyler & Foster, 1996). An essential oil in the German variety has well over 100 components. The dried flower heads and the volatile oil have antiinflammatory, antispasmodic, and antimicrobial actions. Chamomile is used for GI spasms, inflammatory diseases, and as an anti-flatulent (Jellin, 2002; Libster, 2002). Persons allergic to ragweed, asters, or chrysanthemums should use it with caution (Tyler, 1993, 1994) since contact dermatitis and hypersensitivity reactions have occurred. The primary concern, though rare (five reported cases in nearly 100 years), is anaphylactic shock in the event of allergic reaction (Libster, 2002; Tyler, 1994). Vomiting can occur if tea that is highly concentrated is consumed. Pregnant and lactating women should avoid using chamomile (Jellin et al., 2002).

Advised Dosage. The usual dose is from dried flower heads, 2 to 8 grams three to four times daily. Alternately, a tea may be prepared. Steep 3 grams of the dried flower heads in 150 mL boiling water for 5 to 10 minutes and then strain (Jellin, 2002; Libster, 2002).

GASTRIC ULCERS

Licorice

The preparation is made from the dried rhizome and roots from European, Chinese, or other varieties of licorice (Tyler & Foster, 1996). Licorice contains constituents glycyrrhizin and glycyrrhetinic acid that block the metabolism of prostaglandins E and F2 alpha. The peptic ulcer–healing property of this herb may be due to this effect (Jellin et al., 2002). Glycyrrhizin, when taken in high amounts, can produce effects similar to the natural hormone aldosterone. This can lead to increases in blood pressure, fluid retention, and hypokalemia. Manufacturers have found a way to remove glycyrrhizin from licorice, producing a "deglycyrrhizinated licorice" or

DGL. Products containing DGL generally are not associated with the side effects associated with glycyrrhizin products, but it is not clear if DGL provides the same potential clinical benefits as whole licorice. Results from studies using DGL for ulcer treatments have been inconclusive (Jellin et al., 2002). Patients should be aware that many "licorice"-containing products in the United States actually do not contain licorices but rather anise oil. Products manufactured in Europe are more likely to contain authentic licorice and have the associated side effects previously listed. Contraindications for use include liver cirrhosis, cholestatic liver disease, hypertonia, hypokalemia, diabetes, congestive heart failure, and pregnancy and lactation (Jellin et al., 2002).

Advised Dosage. The usual dose of licorice (*Succus liquiritiae*) is 1.5 to 3 grams for gastric and duodenal ulcers. A tea, taken three times daily, may be prepared by simmering 1 to 4 grams of the powdered root in 150 mL boiling water for 5 to 10 minutes, then straining (Jellin et al., 2002).

Slippery Elm

See *Sore Throat and Laryngitis.*

GASTRITIS AND COLITIS

Slippery Elm

See *Sore Throat and Laryngitis.*

HAY FEVER

Nettle

See *Prostate Enlargement (Benign)* for a description of the herb and its primary use. The freeze-dried herb in capsules has been found to be helpful for sneezing and itching of hayfever (Bricklin, 1996b). Nettle and a placebo were used to treat 69 hayfever patients in Oregon. Of the nettle group 58% had moderate to excellent relief in a week versus only 37% of the placebo group. More research is indicated (Jellin et al., 2002). The bristly hairs of the plant can act like little needles to inject the substance under the skin, causing irritation (Bricklin, 1996b). When ingested, mild gastrointestinal effects have been reported (Anderson, Miller & Adams, 2003; Tyler, 1997b). Avoid the use of nettle in pregnant and lactating women (Jellin et al., 2002). It may decrease anticoagulant drug effects, increase blood glucose levels, depress CNS activity, and lower blood pressure (Jellin et al., 2002).

Advised Dosage. *Do not ingest uncooked plants; they may be poisonous.* For allergic rhinitis, a usual dose of stinging nettle extract is 300 mg two to three times daily, though higher doses have been used. Alternatively, a tea can be taken up to three times per day and is made by steeping 1.5 to 5 grams of aboveground parts in 150 mL boiling water for 10 minutes, followed by straining. Nettle is also available as a fresh juice, dried extract, and liquid extract (Jellin et al., 2002). Follow directions for appropriate dosing.

HEADACHES

Caffeine

A number of plants contain caffeine, such as coffee (dried ripe seeds from the madder family), tea leaves and buds, kola (dried cotyledon from the cola family), cocoa or cacao (roasted seed of the cocoa family), guarana (crushed seeds from a member of the soapberry family), and mate or yerba mate (dried leaves of a member of the holly family) (Tyler & Foster, 1996). Caffeine is a compound of methylxanthine and is metabolized in the liver to paraxanthine, theophylline, and theobromine. Caffeine acts to stimulate the central nervous system, heart, and muscles (Jellin et al., 2002). Studies show that when combinations such as caffeine/ibuprofen or caffeine/acetaminophen/aspirin were given to subjects with tension headaches, the subjects had significantly better relief from caffeine-containing analgesics than to placebo or the other agents alone (Diamond, Balm, & Freitag, 2000; Migliardi, Armellino, Freidman, et al., 1994). One study found that caffeine combined with indomethacin and prochlorperazine was significantly more effective in treating acute migraine that sumatriptan (DiMonda, Nicolodi, Aloisio, DelBianco, et al., 2003). Caffeine can cause numerous side effects, including nervousness, insomnia, tachycardia, diuresis, and gastric irritation. Caffeine-induced headache is seen when children and adolescents consume large amounts of caffeinated cola drinks daily (Hering-Hanit & Gadoth, 2003). Patients with cardiac conditions, diabetes, hypertension, peptic ulcer disease, and kidney disease should use caffeine with caution (Jellin et al., 2002). Caffeine interacts with numerous drugs, herbs, and supplements with the potential to cause serious consequences. Use routinely may lead to tolerance, and if discontinued abruptly, to headache, irritability, drowsiness, mood shifts, and fatigue (Paluska, 2003). Medication overuse headache is a risk for people who frequently take medications, including those combined with caffeine, to treat headaches (Fritsche & Diener, 2002).

Readers should consult a more comprehensive review for additional information. In beverages, caffeine has a short-lived, weak diuretic effect (Tyler, 1994).

Advised Dosage. For headaches, the usual dose of caffeine is up to 250 mg per day. One cup of coffee or tea contains approximately 75 to 200 mg and 50 mg of caffeine, respectively (Jellin et al., 2002). Espresso coffee (6 ounces) has 310 mg caffeine; boiled coffee (180 ml), 100 mg; and instant coffee (180 ml), 65 mg (Libster, 2002).

Feverfew

Feverfew comes from the dried leaves of a member of the aster family, native to Europe, and is grown as an ornamental flower in the United States (Tyler & Foster, 1996). Feverfew leaf has been found to have at least 39 constituents. It is unclear as to which specific constituents are responsible for feverfew's pharmacological effects. It has been previously suggested that at least 0.2% of parthenolide was needed for efficacy, but studies have not confirmed this finding (Jellin et al., 2002). Feverfew is used for preventing migraine headaches and, if taken prophylactically, this herb can significantly reduce the migraine headache frequency and the symptoms of migraines (pain, nausea, vomiting) if the headache does occur (Ernst & Pillter, 2000). Feverfew is recommended as a second-line preventive agent in the U.S. Headache Consortium 2000 Guidelines (Ramadan, Silberstein, Freitag, et al., 2002). A German study of a stable extract of feverfew found a decrease in frequency of migraine attacks that was dose-dependent, with a similar percentage of patients reporting one or more adverse event in both the treatment and the placebo groups (Pfaffenrath, Diener, Fischer, Friede, et al. 2002). There are currently not enough data to support the use of feverfew to treat or abort acute migraine headache (Jellin et al., 2002). Side effects may include gastric discomfort, mouth ulcers, loss of taste, and dermatitis (Jellin et al., 2002; O'Hara et al., 1998). If patients are chronically taking feverfew rebound headaches may occur if the herb is suddenly discontinued (O'Hara et al., 1998). Feverfew should be avoided in pregnant women and in those with coagulation problems (Jellin et al., 2002; O'Hara et al., 1998). No effect on lactation was noted (Libster, 2002), but Jellin et al. (2002) advise avoidance if breastfeeding.

Advised Dosage. Fifty to 100 mg of feverfew extract daily for migraine prophylaxis has been used in clinical studies. The dose of the freeze-dried leaf, taken with food or after eating, is 50 to 125 mg per day. Several references note that some feverfew products contain little or no feverfew (Jellin et al., 2002; O'Hara et al., 1998). This lack of standardization can lead to variable responses, though Jellin et al. (2002) note that standardization to 0.2% to 0.35% as has been seen in studies is not necessary for effectiveness.

HEMORRHOIDS

Plantago Seeds and Husk

See *Constipation.*

Witch Hazel

Witch hazel comes from twigs and leaves of a botanical native to North America, cultivated in Europe, and made commercially in the United States as a distilled extract (Tyler & Foster, 1996). Hydroalcohol extracts are used in Europe (Tyler, 1994). The tannins in witch hazel are believed to cause the astringent effect, but this effect is due to added alcohol in the commercially available steam distillate that does not contain tannins. Witch hazel is used as an antiinflammatory and astringent for hemorrhoids and skin and mucous membrane injuries (Jellin et al., 2002; Libster, 2002). This herbal preparation has no precautions. It is applied topically as needed.

HYPERLIPIDEMIA

Garlic

Dried or fresh bulbs from the lily family, garlic has been cultivated for 5000 years worldwide (Tyler & Foster, 1996). Garlic is an allium, and its active ingredients are a volatile oil containing many sulfur compounds. The most important of these is allicin, which when self-condensed into ajoene has antiplatelet aggregation and antibacterial activity. Allicin is produced when an amino acid derivative that contains sulfur, alliin, in the intact cells of garlic is released with crushing of the cells. Contact with an enzyme in neighboring cells, allinase, yields alliin, a very potent, odoriferous antibiotic (Tyler, 1994). Garlic is used for a multitude of conditions, including preventing coronary artery disease, treatment of hypertension and hyperlipidemia, and preventing vascular changes associated with atherosclerosis (Jellin et al., 2002; Libster, 2002; O'Hara et al., 1998). The use of garlic for hyperlipidemia is controversial. Study results are mixed, as some trials have shown no significant benefit and others show evidence that garlic can modestly improve total cholesterol, low-density lipoprotein cholesterol, and triglyceride levels (Alder, Lookinland, Berry, & Williams, 2003; Jellin et al., 2002). High-density lipoprotein cholesterol does not appear to be affected by garlic. Two meta-analyses found a 9 to 12% decrease in cholesterol in hyperlipidemic patients after one month of treatment with garlic tablets. Subsequent trials have been mixed, with most (4 of 7 trials) failing to find any significant changes in lipids, though three of the negative trials had small numbers of patients. Three trials that had positive findings showed a 6.1 to 11.5% reduction in cholesterol in the patients receiving garlic. This data was similar to that found in the previous meta-analyses (O'Hara et al., 1998). Libster (2002) notes that a 1998 study by Berthold, Sudhop, and von Bergmann in *JAMA* concluded that there was no evidence that garlic lowered blood lipid levels, but that the type of garlic used in that study did not contain allicin, the main lipid-lowering constituent. To prevent malodorous breath, patients can take enteric-coated garlic tablets. Garlic rarely may cause an allergic reaction, and the most common side effect is GI discomfort. It may lower blood glucose levels and increase blood insulin concentrations (Jellin et al., 2002).

Advised Dosage. Garlic extract 600 to 1200 mg in divided doses three times a day has been used for hyperlipidemia and hypertension (Jellin et al., 2002). Standardized garlic powder extract containing 1.3% allicin content is what most clinical trials used. Aged garlic extract, typically containing only 0.03% allicin, has also been used. One fresh garlic clove (3 to 4 grams) contains approximately 1% allicin (Jellin et al., 2002; O'Hara et al., 1998). The quality of commercial garlic preparations varies greatly, and some may not have enough active allicin to be effective. One analysis of "standardized" preparations revealed that 93% were lacking effective amounts of allicin (O'Hara et al., 1998). In addition, some odorless garlic products may not contain enough active compound (Jellin et al., 2002).

INSOMNIA

Valerian

Valerian is derived from the dried or fresh root of a member of the valerian family. It grows wild in temperate areas of the Americas and Euroasia (O'Hara et al., 1998). Valerian's sedative-hypnotic, anxiolytic, and antidepressant effects are said to be due to the constituents, valepotriates and volatile oils, though other unidentified constituents may be involved (Foster & Tyler, 1999; Jellin et al., 2002). These constituents bind, in vitro, to the same receptors as benzodiazepines, although with less similarity and milder clinical effects (O'Hara et al., 1998). In two randomized, placebo-controlled blinded studies, use of valerian resulted in improved sleep quality and decreased time to sleep onset. These results are comparable to low-dose benzodiazepines, though valerian may not relieve insomnia as quickly as benzodiazepines. It may take several days to weeks of valerian use to have effective relief (Jellin et al., 2002). A small study of children with intellectual deficits for serious sleep problems found that valerian reduced sleep latencies significantly and nocturnal awake time, particularly with hyperactive children (Francis & Dempster, 2002). Researchers suggested further long-term investigation. Another small study of valerian for insomniacs after benzodiazepine withdrawal found some subjective sleep quality improvement as compared to placebo (Poyares, Guilleminault, Ohayon, & Tufik, 2002). Valerian is generally thought to have low toxicity, but some adverse effects have been reported. Four cases of hepatotoxicity have been linked to valerian usage (MacGregor, Abernathy, Dahabra, Cobden, & Hayes, 1991). In addition, headaches, excitability, uneasiness, and cardiac changes have been reported in controlled clinical trials (Hebel, 1996). Valerian should only be used for short-term management of insomnia. Benzodiazepine-like withdrawal symptoms have occurred when treatment was discontinued after extended use. Those persons taking valerian long-term should taper it slowly when discontinuing (Jellin et al., 2002). Valerian should not be used by pregnant or lactating women, or by those in situations where alertness is required (Libster, 2002).

Advised Dosage. For insomnia, most studies have used 400 to 900 mg of valerian extract up to two hours before bedtime for up to 28 days (Jellin et al., 2002). Libster (2002) recommends taking the herb, regardless of form, no more than 30 to 60 minutes before bedtime; 300 to 500 mg per day is advised. Alternatively, one to two cups of valerian tea may consumed before bedtime, prepared from a teaspoon of the dried root (Bricklin, 1996a). The tea's unpleasant smell may make taking tablets or capsules more palatable.

Comments on Product Testing. In 2000, Consumerlab.com purchased eighteen valerian products. These products were analyzed for their total valerenic acid content to determine if they possessed the valerian type and amounts stated on the label. Only nine products passed the product testing. Four of the eight that failed testing had no detectable levels of expected valerenic acid and the other four had only about half the expected amounts claimed on their labels. Readers are referred to the

Consumerlab.com website for additional information on specific products.

IRRITABLE BOWEL SYNDROME

Peppermint

Peppermint comes from the dried leaves and flowering tops of a mint family member grown in Europe, Egypt, and the United States (Tyler & Foster, 1996). Several clinical trials indicate that peppermint may be effective in treating IBS (Liu, Chen & Yeh, 1997; Pittler & Ernst, 1998). However, a review of traditional and nontraditional therapies for IBS, including peppermint oil, concluded that the effectiveness of the treatments was not supported by available evidence and could not be recommended with any reliability (Fennerty, 2003). A review of treatments for recurrent abdominal pain in children 5 to 18 years old supported the belief that peppermint oil enteric-coated capsules are helpful and safe for IBS (Weydert, Ball & Davis, 2003). Peppermint oil can cause heartburn, esophageal sphincter relaxation, and allergic reactions (Jellin et al., 2002). It is considered unsafe in large amounts in pregnancy, but safe in the amounts found in foods. It should be avoided in children and infants because it may cause laryngeal and bronchial spasms (Jellin et al., 2002).

Advised Dosage. The usual dosage of peppermint for IBS is 0.2 to 0.4 mL three times a day. Enteric-coated capsules should be used, and it should be taken between meals (Jellin et al., 2002).

Plantago Seed and Husk

See *Constipation.*

MEMORY, CONCENTRATION, AND ALERTNESS PROBLEMS

Ginkgo Biloba

The extract comes from the dried leaves of the *Ginkgo biloba* (maidenhair tree) of the ginkgo family (only surviving member of this family or genus of plants). Ginkgo biloba is one of the top-selling herbal medicinal products in the United States with sales reaching $247 million in 1997 (O'Hara et al., 1998). The main constituents from the leaf of ginkgo biloba include flavonoids and terpene lactones. Studies suggest that ginkgo has antihypoxic, antiplatelet, and free radical scavenging effects that work together to protect tissue against ischemia (Jellin et al., 2002). Ginkgo biloba is most commonly used for memory impairment, dementia, tinnitus, and intermittent claudication (Ernst, 2002). In one review of studies of memory impairment but not dementia, eight were found to be sound methodologically, and all but one found that ginkgo had positive effects on cognitive function compared with placebo (Ernst, 2002). German health authorities have concluded that treatment with a standardized extract of ginkgo (EGb 761) is safe and effective for peripheral and cerebral circulatory disturbances, including memory impairment and claudication. In addition, efficacy of EGb 761 in decreasing symptoms of cerebrovascular insufficiency has been reported in several clinical trials (Jellin et al., 2002; O'Hara et al., 1998). Birks, Grimley, and Van Dongen (2002) concluded after analyzing relevant, unconfounded, randomized, double-blind controlled studies using comparison placebos that Gingko use may be associated with improved cognition and function, and seems to be as safe as placebo. Findings from a case-control study investigating cognitive function and subsequent impairment in community dwelling women over 75 years suggested that treatment with standardized Ginkgo biloba extracts may decrease the risk of Alzheimer's dementia development (Andrieu, Gillette, Amouyal, Nourhashemi, et al., 2003). A one-week trial of Ginkgo biloba treatment in postmenopausal women showed improved non-verbal memory, frontal lobe function, and sustained attention, but not in symptoms of menopause (Hartley, Heinze, Elsabagh, & File, 2003). However, a trial in patients with dementia and age-associated memory impairment did not show a significant Ginkgo treatment effect to support that this herb is beneficial for patients with these problems (van Dongen, van Rossum, Kessels, Sielhorst, et al., 2003). Persson et al. (2003) did not find that Ginkgo or Ginseng benefitted memory performance in adult volunteers who were healthy. Thus, findings are mixed for Ginkgo's efficacy. In a 52-week, randomized, double-blind, placebo-controlled, parallel group, multicenter study, researchers found that Egb 761, the extract of ginkgo biloba used in Europe for cognitive symptom disorders, was associated with modestly improved (statistically significant) cognitive performance and social functioning in patients suffering from mildly to severely demented Alzheimer disease or multi-infarct dementia (LeBars, Katz, Berman, Itil, Freedman, & Schatzberg, 1997). The use of the extract was safe in this study. The highly refined extract used was significantly different from gingko products available over the counter in the United States. There is not strong data currently to indicate if ginkgo biloba would improve mental alertness in healthy people. European studies are said to be small and flawed, leaving many unanswered questions (Is ginkgo biloba, 1998). Ginkgo may cause minor reversible gastric disturbances, and rarely, headache, dizziness, and vertigo (Jellin et al., 2002). Two cases of bleeding after long-term use have been reported (Is gingko biloba, 1998). It may interact with aspirin or other anticoagulant drugs. It is not advised in pregnancy or lactation.

Advised Dosage. Clinical trials with ginkgo used doses of 120 mg to 320 mg per day. The most common dose of ginkgo is 40 mg three times per day or 80 mg twice a day of an extract standardized to 22% to 27% flavone glycosides and 5% to 7% terpene lactones (Ernst, 2002; O'Hara et al., 1998).

Comments on Product Testing. Consumerlab.com purchased thirty leading brands of ginkgo biloba in August 1999 to determine whether they possessed proper amounts of flavonol glycosides and terpene lactones. Almost one-quarter of the thirty brands tested did *not* have the levels of chemical markers expected. While the ideal composition of ginkgo is not known, it is recommended that consumers seek products that are most similar to those used in clinical trials. The challenge in picking these standardized products is that label claims may not be accurate. Readers are referred to the Consumerlab.com website for additional information on specific products.

Ginseng

Three different herbs are commonly called ginseng: Asian or Korean ginseng (*Panax ginseng*), American ginseng (*Panax quinquefolius*) and Siberian "ginseng" (*Eleutherococcus senticosus*). The Siberian product is not true ginseng (O'Hara et al., 1998), and the Asian ginseng has been the focus of most research. Ginseng has been used for thousands of years for a variety of medical problems due to its alleged sedative, hypnotic, demulcent, aphrodisiac, and antidepressant activity. Ginseng is classified as an "adaptogen" that assists with various stress resistances through shorter reaction times, increased alertness, better concentration, improved stamina, and overall improved well-being (Ernst, 2002). The main constituents of Asian ginseng are triterpenoid saponins that are referred to as ginsenosides or panaxosides. A number of subtypes of ginsenosides have been identified, and they appear to have a wide range of pharmacological activity. For example, one ginsenoside is a CNS stimulant and raises blood pressure, while another acts as a CNS depressant and lowers blood pressure (Jellin, 2002). There is some evidence to suggest that Panax ginseng can improve cognitive function, but that ginseng alone does not improve memory. One study showed that a combination of Panax ginseng plus ginkgo leaf improved memory in otherwise healthy people ages 38 to 66 years (Jellin et al., 2002). The challenge with ginseng is finding results of well-designed trials that support its use. Vogler, Pittler, and Ernst (1999) undertook a systematic review of randomized clinical trials with ginseng. Sixteen trials were reviewed and included any type of ginseng extract for many diverse indications. These trials evaluated the use of ginseng for physical performance, psychomotor performance and cognitive function, immunomodulation, diabetes mellitus, and herpes simplex type-II infections. Volger et al. (1999) concluded that none of these sixteen trials showed efficacy of ginseng root for any of those indications evaluated. Ginseng is believed to be generally safe but side effects such as diarrhea, euphoria, headache, hypertension, hypotension, insomnia, mastalgia, nausea, and vaginal bleeding have been reported. There is controversy about the existence of a "ginseng abuse syndrome." Some authors describe this syndrome, which includes hypertension, nervousness, insomnia, increased libido, estrogenic effects, as one that occurs with prolonged use at high doses (Ernst, 2002). Others discount this syndrome as existing and note that many of these side effects occur even after short-term use of Panax ginseng (Jellin et al., 2002). Patients with diabetes should use American ginseng with caution since it has hypoglycemic activity (Jellin et al., 2002). Libster (2002) notes that ginseng has not been proven to be teratogenic and that there is not a contraindication for using it in pregnancy by German Commission E, but there are other sources that advise avoidance. Thus, use in pregnancy and lactation is not advised due to lack of known safety data.

Advised Dosage. If the cut or powdered root is used, the typical dose orally is 0.6 to 3 grams one to three times per day (Jellin et al., 2002). Capsules of 100, 250, and 500 mg doses are available, and 200 to 600 mg daily is a usual dosage. The usual dose for short-term treatment is 0.5 to 2 grams of dry ginseng root, which equates to 200 to 600 mg of extract daily (Ernst, 2002).

Comments on Product Testing. In 2000, Consumerlab.com purchased twenty-two brands of Asian and American ginseng and tested them for identity, quality, and purity. Only nine products tested met all of the standards. Seven products had less than the required concentration of ginsenosides. The other products failed due to high levels of either pesticides and/or heavy metals.

Readers are referred to the Consumerlab.com website for additional information on specific products.

MENOPAUSAL SYMPTOMS

Black Cohosh

See *Dysmenorrhea.*

Chaste Tree Berry

See *Premenstrual Symptoms.*

MOUTH ULCERS

Chamomile

See *Flatulence.*

MUSCLE/JOINT PAIN AND INFLAMMATION

Capsicum

This herb is also called cayenne, red pepper, or chili pepper; it comes from the dried ripe fruit of members of *Solanaceae* family (Tyler, 1994). Capsicum as a topical preparation has been found to be effective for the temporary pain relief of osteoarthritis, rheumatoid arthritis, shingles, and diabetic neuropathy (Halat & Dennehy, 2003; Jellin et al., 2002). It is FDA-approved for topical analgesia (Tyler, 1993, 1994). The active ingredient is capsaicin. When applied topically, capsaicin decreases arthritic joint pain (Fugh-Berman, 1996). In one double-blind, controlled study, tenderness and pain of osteoarthritis were decreased by 40%; however, no beneficial effects on rheumatoid arthritis were found (McCarthy & McCarty, 1992). Capsaicin is useful for fibromyalgia, herpes zoster pain and itching after the shingles have resolved, and cluster headache pain. Postmastectomy pain syndrome was found to respond significantly better than placebo to capsaicin. Capsaicin may also be safe and effective for treatment of diabetic neuropathy. It causes substance P, a neuropeptide that mediates pain impulse transmission from the peripheral nerves to the spinal cord, to be depleted (Tyler, 1994). This effect takes several weeks to occur. Hands must be thoroughly washed after application of these products to prevent transfer to eyes and mucous membranes. If the cream gets in eyes or on sensitive skin, it will cause burning.

Advised Dosage. Capsaicin cream is FDA approved in a cream base for over-the-counter (OTC) use. Follow the directions on the package. It can take from several days to a few weeks for the full analgesic effect (Jellin et al., 2002). Application three to four times daily for pain relief is recommended. The cream, which is not water soluble, can be removed with a diluted vinegar solution.

Evening Primrose (Black Currant, Borage Seed) Oil

Evening Primrose Oil (EPO) comes from seeds of the evening primrose, a member of the primrose family, native to eastern North America, but naturalized widely elsewhere (Tyler & Foster, 1996). Black currant and borage seeds are used similarly. The primary active component is a fixed oil containing *cis*-linoleic acid and *cis*-gamma-linolenic acid (GLA) (Leung & Foster, 1995). EPO is purported to be useful for many conditions, including premenstrual syndrome (PMS), mastalgia, endometriosis, eczema, acne, rheumatoid arthritis, multiple sclerosis, just to name a few (Dickerson, Mzyck, & Hunter, 2003; Libster, 2002; Jellin et al., 2002). GLA is thought to be responsible for the anti-inflammatory effects of EPO, and it is postulated that patients with PMS may have lower levels of GLA. Thus, by replenishing GLA, EPO may act to decrease some of the symptoms of PMS. Douglas (2002) concludes from an advanced MEDLINE search that calcium carbonate should be the first-line treatment for mild to moderate PMS, and that other therapies such as EPO could be tried but are unproven. Clinical data suggest that EPO may be effective for mastalgia and for some symptoms of PMS. However, evening primrose oil, fish oil, and a control oil offered no significant differences in benefit in treating breast pain (Blommers, de Lange-DeKlerk, Kuik, Bezemer, et al., 2002). Additionally, EPO may reduce the symptoms of rheumatoid arthritis (Leventhal, 1994; Zurier, Rossetti, Jacobson, et al., 1996). Side effects include nausea, indigestion, soft stools, and headache (Jellin et al., 2002).

Advised Dosage. For PMS, 2 to 4 grams daily are advised (Jellin et al., 2002). For mastalgia, 3 to 4 grams are recommended (Libster, 2002). For rheumatoid arthritis, 540 mg to 2.8 grams daily were effective (Belch & Hill, 2000). Four to 6 grams daily of EPO standardized to 8% is used with adults for the treatment of atopic eczema; 2 to 4 grams in children (Jellin et al., 2002; Libster, 2002).

NAUSEA AND MOTION SICKNESS

Ginger

The preparation comes from the dried or fresh rhizome of *Zingiber officinale Roscoe* (Tyler, 1994). Ginger had been used for many centuries for numerous medical conditions in which nausea and vomiting occur (Pettit, 2001). Currently, in the practice of Western alternative medicine, the primary uses of ginger include treatment of vertigo, prevention of motion sickness, and the prevention of the nausea associated with morning sickness (Grant & Lutz, 2000; Jellin et al., 2002; Libster, 2002; Lien, Sun, Chen, Kim, et al., 2003; Portnoi, Chng, Karimi-Tabesh, Koren, et al., 2003; Westfall, 2004). Ginger appears to be effective when used for vertigo, though there is limited clinical data supporting this use (Jellin et al., 2002). The clinical data on use of ginger for the prevention of motion sickness is mixed, with ginger reducing nausea in some but not all controlled human trials (Libster, 2002; O'Hara et al., 1998). The reasons for these discrepancies may be due to the types of ginger used or may reflect the difficulty in objectively measuring the symptoms of nausea. The safety of ginger in pregnancy is controversial. Blumenthal et al. (2000) note that the dose for nausea therapy is not harmful to the fetus, but concern about uterine bleeding with large doses leads many to advise not using it (Brinker, 1998). In a study with hyperemesis gravidarum sufferers, significant reduction in nausea resulted from 250 mg of ginger four times a day (O'Hara et al., 1998). An Australian randomized study of ginger for nausea in pregnancy versus a placebo found that nausea and retching were significantly reduced, and all the infants born of mothers using ginger had normal birthweight, gestational age, Apgar scores, and frequencies of congenital abnormalities comparable to the general population of infants born that year (Willetts, Ekangaki, & Eden, 2003). Both ginger and vitamin B_6 equally reduced nausea and vomiting of pregnancy in a Thai study (Sripramote & Lekhyananda, 2003). Ginger is well tolerated when used in recommended dosages.

Advised Dosage. For motion sickness prevention, 1 gram of dried powdered ginger root 30 minutes to 4 hours before travel is advised (Jellin et al., 2002). Alternatively, oral ginger capsules may be used. A ginger tea may be prepared by steeping 0.5 to 1 gram of dried root in 150 mL boiling water for 5 to 10 minutes and then straining. The usual dose for adults for nausea therapy is 250 mg to 1 gram powdered root two to three times a day (O'Hara et al., 1998). A piece of candied ginger 1 inch square and ¼ inch thick equal to about 1 gram of ginger can be obtained from Asian food stores. Canada Dry and Schweppes ginger ale contain the real ginger and 12 ounces is needed for a therapeutic dose.

OBESITY

A number of herbal fiber products, laxatives, diuretics, and proposed "herbal weight loss remedies" have received major attention since serious complications associated with two popular prescription medications for weight loss resulted in discontinuation of use. Some of the herbal therapies are not recommended, some are dangerous, and some have real application if used safely. See the earlier discussion of ephedra and Chapter 32 for further discussion of herbal therapies in the management of obesity.

PREMENSTRUAL SYMPTOMS

Black Cohosh

See *Dysmenorrhea.*

Chaste Tree Berry

This herb comes from fruits from a member of the verbena family, which grow as shrubs or trees in West Asia and southwestern Europe (Tyler & Foster, 1996). The primary active ingredients are flavonoids, but the fruits also contain an essential oil and glycosides (Jellin et al., 2002). Chasteberry is used for several menstrual-associated conditions including dysmenorrhea; abnormal bleeding patterns such as frequent periods, heavy prolonged periods, and infrequent periods; and symptoms associated with PMS and menopause ((Fugh-Berman & Kronenberg, 2003; Jellin et al., 2002; Wuttke, Jarry, Christoffel, Spengler, et al., 2003). There is evidence that chasteberry inhibits the secretion of prolactin, and this effect appears to be dose dependent. Chasteberry doses of 120 mg per day, considered a lower dose, may decrease estrogen and increase progesterone and prolactin levels through FSH and LH influence. Doses of chasteberry at approximately 480 mg per day, considered higher level, appear to bind to dopamine receptors and decrease release of prolactin (Yanni & Klein, 2000). Clinical studies demonstrate that chasteberry may be effective for PMS (Berger, Schaffner, Schrader, et al., 2000; Schellenberg, 2001). Patients should be cautioned that it may take 4 to 12 weeks before a significant improvement in symptoms is seen (Jellin et al., 2002). This herb should not be used by pregnant or lactating women. Side effects of GI upset, rash and urticaria, acne, intramenstrual bleeding, headache, and nausea occur in about 2 to 5% of patients (Jellin et al., 2002). It may cause GI side effects occasionally, and itching and rash rarely. Chaste tree berry possibly may interfere with dopamine-receptor antagonists, and it is contraindicated in pregnancy. Long-term effects are not known.

Advised Dosage. Doses of chasteberry used for PMS vary, depending upon the formulation (Jellin et al., 2002). One study using chasteberry extract (Ze440) used 20 mg per day (Berger et al., 2000) while another study, using a different chasteberry extract, used 4 mg per day. If using crude herb extracts, doses of 20 to 240 mg per day up to 1800 mg per day in two to three divided doses have been used (Jellin et al., 2002). Some suggest this herb is best taken on an empty stomach.

Evening Primrose Oil

See *Muscle/Joint Pain and Inflammation.*

PROSTATE ENLARGEMENT (BENIGN)

Nettle

This herb comes from aboveground plant leaves and root parts of the stinging nettle, a member of family Uricaceae (Tyler, 1994). Clinical studies support the use of the root to treat benign prostatic hypertrophy (BPH) (Dvorkin & Song, 2002; Fagelman & Lowe, 2002). Stinging nettle root contains hydroalcoholic extracts that may suppress prostatic cell metabolism, as well as constituents that influence the immune system and are weakly anti-inflammatory (Jellin et al., 2002). Several, but not all, clinical trials have shown increased urine output, decreased nocturia, and decreased urinary frequency. Potential side effects include gastrointestinal disturbances, allergic reactions, and sweating. Patients should be cautioned not to confuse stinging nettle with white dead nettle, which is used for gastrointestinal complaints (Jellin et al., 2002).

Advised Dosage. The dosage of stinging nettle depends upon the formulation used: dried hydroalcoholic extract (5:1 extracted with 20% methanol), 600 to 1200 mg per day; liquid extract (1:1 in 45% alcohol), 1.5 to 7.5 ml three times a day. For nettle tea, steep 1.5 grams dried powdered root in 150 ml boiling water for 5 to 10 minutes, strain; up to 4 to 6 grams/day can be consumed (Jellin et al., 2002).

Saw Palmetto

This herb is developed from the dried fruits from a member of the palm family growing in the wild in Georgia and Florida (Tyler & Foster, 1996). Saw palmetto is currently most widely used to improve signs and symptoms of BPH (Gerber, 2002). The exact mechanism by which saw palmetto works is not fully understood, though it does appear to act similarly to finasteride by inhibiting the enzyme 5-alpha-reductase, which blocks the conversion of testosterone to dihydroxytestosterone. Numerous clinical trials support the use of saw palmetto for BPH. These trials show that saw palmetto is likely as efficacious as finasteride, with fewer side effects (Gordon & Shaughnessy, 2003). The data on whether prostate size is reduced with saw palmetto is mixed (Ernst, 2002, Jellin et al., 2002, O'Hara et al., 1998). Patients should be warned that treatment with saw palmetto for one to two months may be needed before significant symptomatic improvement is seen (Jellin et al., 2002). Saw palmetto is well tolerated with generally mild adverse effects, though they may include GI complaints and headaches (Jellin et al., 2002). Prostate size and PSA levels may or may not be reduced by saw palmetto (Jellin et al., 2002; Libster, 2002). Study results are mixed.

Advised Dosage. The recommended dose is 160 mg twice daily or 320 mg once daily of the lipophilic (soft native) extract containing 80 to 95% fatty acids (Jellin et al., 2002; Libster, 2002). Alternately, one to two grams of whole berries or 0.6 to 1.5 ml of a liquid extract may be taken (Jellin et al., 2002), or 400 mg of dry normalized extract twice daily (Blumenthal et al., 2000; Libster, 2002).

Comments of Product Testing. In 1999, ConsumerLab.com purchased and tested 27 leading brands of saw palmetto to determine if they possessed the minimum amounts of specific fatty acids and sterols found in the products used in published clinical trials. Five products were eliminated from testing because their label claims were below a standardized level of fatty acid. Of the 17 that passed, the majority contained additional oils that may or may not provide additional clinical benefit. Only two products that passed contained the saw palmetto extract that was similar to that used in the clinical trials.

Readers are referred to the Consumerlab.com website for additional information on specific products.

Pygeum

This herb, *Pygeum africanum,* comes from an evergreen tree, *Prunus africana,* found in southern and central Africa (Keville, 1996; Tyler, 1997). Pygeum bark contains a number of constituents that are thought to be beneficial in the treatment of BPH (Dvorkin & Song, 2002; Fagelman & Lowe, 2002; Gerber, 2002). Data suggests that some of these constituents reduce inflammation in the prostate and also inhibit prostate growth factors, which are substances implicated in inappropriate prostate enlargement. Even though numerous clinical trials demonstrate that pygeum bark can improve some of the symptoms of BPH, saw palmetto is thought to be a better treatment. Pygeum is generally well tolerated with gastrointestinal distress the most common complaint (Jellin et al., 2002).

Advised Dosage. The lipophilic extract dose is 100 to 200 mg per day in six- to eight-week cycles. Alternatively, pygeum extract can be given as 50 mg twice daily or 100 mg once daily (Jellin et al., 2002).

SKIN PROBLEMS

Aloe Vera

Aloe vera is a mucilaginous gel that comes from the center of the leaf of the aloe vera, a lily family member (Tyler & Foster, 1996). The gel is used topically for first-degree burns, frostbite, and minor skin irritations for its anti-inflammatory, emollient, pain-lessening, and wound-healing features (Jellin et al., 2002; Libster, 2002; Mackay & Miller, 2003). The fresh gel is applied topically as needed, and it is considered safe.

Evening Primrose Oil

See *Muscle/Joint Pain and Inflammation.*

Melissa

The preparation is developed from leaves of lemon balm, a member of the mint family (Tyler & Foster, 1996). The ingredients are a volatile oil, a tannin, flavonoids, and other compounds (Leung & Foster, 1995). Melissa, also called lemon balm, has antibacterial, antiviral, sedative, and antiflatulent properties. It is also used topically to treat cold sores (herpes labialis) resulting in significant reduction in symptoms on the second day after lesions appear (Jellin et al., 2002; Libster, 2002). Its antiviral effects are due to tannin and polyphenol constituents. Side effects are rare though hypersensitivity reactions have occurred. It should not be used in the first trimester of pregnancy (Libster, 2002).

Advised Dosage. For cold sores, apply the cream or ointment that contains 1% of a 70:1 lyophilized extract two to four times per day at the first prodromal sign until lesions are healed, up to 14 days. Alternatively, a tea can be applied to the lesions. Prepare tea by steeping 2 to 3 teaspoons (2 to 3 grams) of finely cut leaf in 150 ml boiling water for 5 to 10 minutes, strain. Saturate cotton ball and apply to lesion several times daily (Jellin et al., 2002).

Tea Tree Oil

A steam-distilled volatile oil made from the leaves of a shrub or small tree, this is a member of the Myrtacea family found in swampy or wet areas in Australia (Tyler & Foster, 1996). The oil contains terpene hydrocarbons and other components and is bacteriostatic and germicidal if it contains high levels of terpinen-4-ol. Tea tree oil has been shown to be effective when used topically for acne vulgaris, tinea pedis (athlete's foot), and for onychomycosis (Jellin et al., 2002). A highly concentrated product seems to be most effective. The main constituent of tea tree oil, terpinen-4-ol, is antibacterial and antifungal. It should not be ingested or put in the ear as it is toxic. Reported local skin effects are irritation, contact dermatitis/eczema, and inflammation. Some people may be sensitive to the oil and develop a skin irritation or allergy, but it is generally not toxic (Jellin, et al. 2002).

Advised Dosage. For acne, apply a 5% tea tree oil gel daily; for athlete's foot, apply a 10% tea tree cream twice daily for one month; for onychomycosis, application of a 100% tea tree oil solution twice daily for six months has been shown to be comparable to clotrimazole 1% solution (Jellin et al., 2002).

SORE THROAT AND LARYNGITIS

Slippery Elm

The preparation comes from the dried inner bark of a member of the elm family found in eastern North America (Tyler & Foster, 1996). The inner bark contains mucilage, starch, and tannins. Its action is as a mucilaginous demulcent, emolient, and nutrient to soothe irritated mucous membranes (Jellin et al., 2002). As a soothing demulcent for sore throats, slippery elm has received FDA approval. It is safe, and no precautions are advised.

Use of whole bark is contraindicated in pregnancy (Jellin et al., 2002).

Advised Dosage. Powdered inner bark as a 1:8 decoction, 4 to 16 ml taken three times daily (Jellin et al., 2002). Commercially prepared tablets and troches may also be purchased.

URINARY INFECTION/ INFLAMMATION

Bearberry

Bearberry is made from the dried leaves of a plant that grows in cold regions of the northern hemisphere (Tyler & Foster, 1996). Bearberry has urinary antiseptic and astringent effects, and its constituents include a phenol called arbutin, tannins, and hydroquinone. Bearberry may be effective in treating urinary tract infections (Jellin et al., 2002). There is also data that bearberry in combination with dandelion can prevent urinary tract infections. Concern exits about using this herb long term because of the possible cytotoxic effects of hydroquinone. Patients should avoid using bearberry for more than one week at a time or for more than five times per year (Jellin et al., 2002). Bearberry can cause nausea and vomiting, and larger amounts can be very toxic. Avoid use in children and pregnant and lactating women. The antibacterial activity of bearberry can be decreased by foods that acidify the urine, including acidic fruits and juices like cranberry (Jellin et al., 2002).

Advised Dosage. Of dried herb, the typical dose is 1.5 to 4 grams daily. A tea can also be used; steep 3 grams dried leaf in 150 mL cold water for 12 to 24 hours, strain, drink four cups daily. Do not exceed recommended amounts. For urinary symptoms that last longer than 48 hours, medical advice should be sought (Jellin et al., 2002).

Cranberry

The juice or extract of the American cranberry is used to treat UTIs. In the 1920s, cranberry was recognized as having a bacteriostatic effect; now, action is thought to be due to prevention of adhesion of bacteria to mucosal cells (Jellin et al., 2002; Libster, 2002). There is evidence that daily consumption of cranberry juice (300 ml) can *prevent* recurrent UTIs in women. Currently, there is not enough evidence to show that encapsulated forms of concentrated cranberry will have the same preventive effect. There is also no conclusive evidence that cranberry juice works to treat UTI infections (Jellin et al., 2002), though a number of studies show positive response with use by individuals at high risk for UTIs (Libster, 2002). Pregnant women may use unsweetened cranberry juice. People who are at risk for oxalate and uric acid formation with more acidic urine may need to avoid medicinal use (Libster, 2002). No precautions are indicated, although ingestion of large amounts (more than 3–4 L/day) may result in gastrointestinal disturbances, including diarrhea (Hebel, 1996). It is useful for prophylaxis with diaphragm users, women who have coitally related UTIs, and elderly women (Fugh-Berman, 1996).

Advised Dosage. The ideal dose of cranberry juice that is needed to prevent UTIs is not known. References vary in advised daily amount from 1 to 10 ounces per day to 8 to 16 ounces daily (Jellin et al., 2002).

Libster (2002) advises 5 to 20 ounces daily, ½ cup of fresh cranberries daily, or one to two 250 mg tablets three times daily. Cranberry juice cocktail is approximately 26% to 33% pure cranberry juice, sweetened with either fructose or an artificial sweetener (Jellin et al., 2002).

Goldenrod

The preparation is from the dried flowering aboveground (aerial) parts of European or American species of the aster family (Tyler & Foster, 1996). Active ingredients include saponins, diterpenes, tannins, flavonoids, and other components. It is used to prevent or treat urinary calculi and kidney stones. It should be avoided if the user is allergic to aster family members and is contraindicated in impaired cardiac or kidney function.

Advised Dosage. One cup of tea, two to four times daily, between meals, is a usual dose of goldenrod. Prepare tea by steeping 1 to 2 teaspoons (3 to 5 grams) of dried herb in 150 ml boiling water for 5 to 10 minutes, then strain. Daily dose is generally 6 to 12 grams. Goldenrod may also be consumed as a tincture or liquid extract. Drink at least 2 liters of water per day when using this herb (Jellin et al., 2002).

REFERENCES

Abebe, W. (2003). An overview of herbal supplement utilization with particular emphasis on possible interactions with dental drugs and oral manifestations. *Journal of Dental Hygiene, 77*(1), 37–46.

Advisor Forum. (2002, March). Does echineacea help or harm the immune system? *The Clinical Advisor,* 75.

Alder, R., Lookinland, S., Berry, J., & Williams, M. (2003). A systematic review of the effectiveness of garlic as an antihyperlipidemic agent. *Journal of the American Academy of Nurse Practitioners, 15*(3), 120–129.

Andrieu, S., Gillette, S., Amouyal, K., Nourhashemi, F., Reynish, E., Ouseet, P., Albarede, J., Vellas, B., Grandjean, H.; EPIDOS study. (2003). Association of Alzheimer's disease onset with ginkgo biloba and other symptomatic cognitive treatments in a population of women aged 75 years and older from the EPISOS study. *The Jouranl of Gerontology. Series A, Biological Sciences and Medical Sciences, 58*(4), 372–377.

Ang-Lee, M.K., Moss, J., & Yuan, C.S. (2001). Herbal medicines and perioperative care. *Journal of the American Medical Association, 286,* 208–216.

Barak, V., Birkenfeld, S., Halperin, T., & Kalickman, I. (2002). The effect of herbal remedies on the production of human inflammatory and anti-inflammatory cytokines. *The Israel Medical Association Journal, 4*(11 Suppl), 919–922.

Barclay, L. (2002, June 24). Black cohosh controls menopausal symptoms. *Medscape Medical News.* Report from Endo 2002: Abstracts P3-333, P3-317. June 21, 2002.

Barnes, J.E., & Winter, G. (2001). Supplemental products growing. *The New York Times,* In *The Sun Sentinel,* May 27, 2001, p. 4A.

Bauer, B. A. (2000). Herbal therapy. What clinicians need to know to counsel patients effectively. *Mayo Clinic Proceedings 75*(8), 835–841.

Belch, J. F., & Hill, A. (2000). Evening primrose oil and borage oil in rheumatologic conditions. *American Journal of Clinical Nutrition,* (suppl), 325S–325S.

Berger, D., Schaffner, W., Schrader, E., Meier, B., & Brattstrom, A. (2000). Efficacy of Vitex agnus castus L. extract Ze 440 in patients with pre-menstrual syndrome (PMS). *Archives of Gynecology & Obstetrics, 264*(3), 150–153.

Birks, J., Grimley, E., Van Dongen, M. (2002). Ginkgo biloba for cognitive impairment and dementia. *Cochrane Database Systematic Review,* (4), CD003120.

Blommers, J., de Lange-De Klerk, E., Kuik, D., Bezemer, P., & Meijer, S. (2002). Evening primrose oil and fish oil for severe chronic mastalgia: A randomized, double-blind, controlled trial. *American Journal of Obstetrics & Gynecology, 187* (5), 1389–1394.

Blumenthal, M. (Ed.). (1998). *The complete German Commission E Monographs: Therapeutic guide to herbal medicines,* Austin, TX: American Botanical Council, and Boston, MA: Integrative Medicine Communications.

Blumenthal, M., Goldberg, A., & Brinckman, J. (2000). *Herbal medicine: Expanded Commission E monographs.* Newton, MA: Integrative Medicine Communications.

Bond, C. & Hannaford, P. (2003). Issues related to monitoring the safety of over-the-counter (OTC) medicines. *Drug Safety, 26*(15), 1065–1074.

Borrelli, F., Isso, A., Ernst, E. (2003). Pharmacological effects of Cimicifuga racemosa. *Life Sciences, 73*(10), 1215–1229.

Brazier, N. & Levine, M. (2003). Drug-herb interaction among commonly used conventional medicines: A compendium for health care professionals. *American Journal of Therapeutics, 10*(3), 163–169.

Bricklin, M. (1996a, January). Herbs that ease the mind. *Prevention,* 15, 16, 18.

Bricklin, M. (1996b, August). Healing plants around the world. *Prevention,* 21–22.

Brinkebor, R.M., Shah, D.V., & Degenring, F.H. (1999). Echinaforce and other Echinacea fresh plant preparations in the treatment of the common cold. A randomized, placebo controlled, double-blind clinical trial. *Phytomedicine,* 6, 1–6.

Brinker, F. (1998). *Herb contraindications and drug interactions.* Sandy, OR: Eclectic Medical Publications.

Brodeur, M. A. (2002). Understanding dietary supplement regulation. *AWONN, 6*(2), 106–109.

Butterwick, V. (2003). Mechanism of action of St. John's wort in depression: What is known? *CNS Drugs, 17*(8), 539–562.

Chen, C., Biller, J., Willing, S., & Lopez, A. (2004). Ischemic stroke after using over the counter products containing ephedra. *Journal of the Neurological Sciences, 217*(1), 55–60.

Diamond, S., Balm, T.K., & Freitag, G. (2000). Ibuprofen plus caffeine in the treatment of tension-type headache. *Clincial Pharmacology and Therapeutics, 68*(3), 312–319).

Dietlein, G. & Schroder-Bernhardi, D. (2003). Doctors' prescription behaviour regarding dosage recommendations for preparations of kava extracts. *Pharmacoepidemiology and Drug Safety, 12*(5), 417–421.

DiMonda, V., Nicolodi, M., Aloisio, A., DelBianco, P., Fonzari, M., Grazioli, I., Uslenghi, C., Vecchiet, L., & Sicurteri, F. (2003). Efficacy of a fixed combination of indomethacin, prochlorperazine, and caffeine versus sumatriptan in actue treatment of multiple migraine attachs: A multicenter, randomized, crossover trial. *Headache, 43*(8), 835–844.

Dog, T., Powell, K., & Weisman, S. (2003). Critical evaluation of the safety of Cimicifuga racemosa in menopause symptom relief. *Menopause, 10*(4), 299–313.

Douglas, S. (2002). Premenstrual syndrome. Evidence-based treatment in family practice. *Canadian Family Physician, 48,* 1789–17997.

Draves, A. & Walker, S. (2003). Analysis of the hypericin and pseudohypericin content of commercially available St. John's Wort preparation. *Canadian Journal of Pharmacology, 10*(3), 114–118.

Durante, K. M., Whitmore, B., Jones, C.A., & Campbell, N.R. (2001). Use of vitamins, minerals, and herbs: A survey of patients attending family practice clinics. *Clinical and Investigative Medicine, 24*(5), 242–249.

Dvorkin, L. & Song, K. (2002). Herbs for benign prostatic hyperplasia. *Annals of Pharmacotherapy, 36*(9), 1443–1452.

Elder, N. C., Gillcrist, A., & Minz, R. (1997). Use of alternative health care by family practice patients. *Archives of Family Medicine, 6*(2), 181–184.

Ernst, E. (2002). The risk-benefit profile of commonly used herbal therapies: ginkgo, St. John's wort, ginseng, echinacea, saw palmetto, and kava. *Annals of Internal Medicine 136,* 42–53.

Ernst, E., & Pillter, M.H. (2000). The efficacy and safety of feverfew (Tanacetum parthenium L.): An update of a systematic review. *Public Health Nutrition, 3(4A),* 509–514.

Estes, J., Stolpman, D., Olyaei, A., Corless, C., Ham, J., Schwartz, J., & Orloff, S., (2003). High prevalence of potentially hepatotoxic herbal supplment use in patients with fulminant hepatic failure. *Archives of Surgery, 138*(8), 852–858.

European Scientific Cooperative for Phytotherapy (ESCOP). (1990). *Proposal for European monographs* (Vol. 1). Bevrijdingslaan, The Netherlands: ESCOP Secretariat. Reported in Tyler and Foster, 1996.

European Scientific Cooperative for Phytotherapy (ESCOP). (1992). *Proposal for European monographs* (Vol. 2). Bevrijdingslaan, The Netherlands: ESCOP Secretariat. Reprinted in Tyler and Foster, 1996.

Fagelman, E. & Lowe, F. (2002). Herbal medications in the treatment of benign prostatic hyperplasia. *The Urologic Clinics of North America, 29*(1), 23–29.

Fennerty, M. (2003). Traditional therapies for irritable bowel syndrome: An evidence based appraisal. *Reviews in Gastroenterological Disorders, 3*(Suppl 2), S18–S24.

Foster, S. & Tyler, V. (1999). Tyler's honest herbal (4th ed.). New York: Haworth Herbal Press.

Francis, A. & Dempster, R. (2002). Effect of valeriana edulis, on sleep difficulties in children with intellectual deficits: Randomised trial. *Phytomedicine, 9*(4), 273–279.

Fritsche, G. & Diener, H. (2002). Medication overuse headaches—what is new? *Expert OpinDrug Saf, 1*(4), 331–338.

Fugh-Berman, A. (1996). *Alternative medicine: What works. A comprehensive, easy-to-read review of the scientific evidence, pro and con.* Berkeley, CA: Odouson Press.

Fugh-Berman, A. & Kronenberg, F. (2003). Complementary and alternative medicine (CAM) in reproductive-age women: A review of randomized controlled trials. *Reproductive Toxicology, 17*(2), 137–152.

Garrard, J., Harms, S., Eberly, L., & Matiak, A. (2003). Variations in product choices of frequently purchased herbs: Caveat emptor. *Archives of Internal Medicine, 163*(19), 2290–2295.

Gastpar, M. & Klimm, H. (2003). Treatment of anxiety, tension and restlessness states with Kava special extract WS 1490 in general practice: A randomized placebo-controlled double-blind multicenter trial. *Phytomedicine, 10*(8), 631–639.

Gerber, G. (2002). Phytotherapy for benign prostatic hyperplasia. *Current Urology Reports, 3*(4), 285–291.

Goel, V. Lovlin, R., Barton, R., Lyon, M., Bauer, R., Lee, T., & Basu, T. (2004). Efficacy of a standardized Echinacea preparation (Echinilin TM) for the treatment of the common cold: A randomized, double-blind, placebo-controlled trial. *Journal of Clinical Pharmacology and Therapeutics, 29*(1), 75–83.

Gordon, A. & Shaughnessy, A. (2003). Saw palmetto for prostate disorders. *American Family Physician, 67*(6), 1281–1283.

Gorski, J., Huang, S., Pinto, A., Hamman, M., Hilligoss, J., Zaheer, N., Desai, M., Miller, M., & Hall, S. (2004). The effect of Echinacea (Echinacea purpurea root) on cytochrome P450 activity in vivo. *Clincial Pharmacology and Therapeutics, 75*(1), 89–100.

Grant, K. L., Lutz, R. B. (2000). Ginger. *American Journal of Health-System Pharmacy, 57*(10), 945–947.

Gulla, J., & Singer, A. J. (2000) Alternative therapies among emergency department patients. *Annals of Emergency Medicine, 35*(3), 226–228.

Halat, K. & Dennehy, C. (2003). Botanicals and dietary supplements in diabetic peripheral neuropathy. *Journal of the American Board of Family Practice, 16*(1), 47–57.

Hall, S. Wang Z., Huang, S., Hamman, M., Vasavada, N., Adigun, A., Hilligoss, J., Miller, M., & Gorski, J. (2003). The interaction between St. John's wort and an oral contraceptive. *Clinical Pharmacology & Therapeutics, 74*(6), 525–535.

Haller, C. A., Benowitz, N. L. (2000). Adverse cardiovascular and central nervous system events associated with dietary supplements containing ephedra alkaloids. *New England Journal of Medicine, 342*(25), 1833–1838.

Harrer, G., & Sommer, H. (1994). Treatment of mild/moderate depression with hypericium. *Phytomedicine, 1,* 3–8.

Harris, R., Jang, G., & Tsunoda, S. (2003). Dietary effects on drug metabolism and transport. *Clinical Pharmacokinetics, 42*(13), 1071–1088.

Hartley, D., Heinze, L., Elsabagh, S. & File, S. (2003). Effects on cognition and mood in postmenopausal women of 1-week treatment with Ginkgo biloba. *Pharmacology, Biochemistry, and Behavior, 75*(3), 711–720.

Hebel, S. K. (Ed.). (1996). The Lawrence review of national products. St. Louis: Facts and Comparisons.

Hering-Hanit, R. & Gadoth, N. (2003). Caffeine-induced headache in children and adolescents. *Cephalagia, 23*(5), 332–335.

Hoffman, D. (1991). *The new holistic herbalist* (3rd ed.). New York: Element.

Huber, A. T. (2003). Treatment with Hypericum perforatum L. does not trigger decreased resistance in Staphylococcus aureaus against antibiotic and hyperforin. *Phytomedicine, 10*(2–3), 206–208.

Hurley, D. (1995, May). Pharmacists need to increase knowledge of herbal remedies as use skyrockets. *Pharmacy Practice News,* 24–25.

Hypericum Depression Trial Study Group. (2002). Effect of Hypericum perforatum (St. John's wort) in major depressive disorder. *Journal of the American Medical Association, 287,* (14), 1807–1814.

Is gingko biloba a memory booster? (1998, January). *University of California at Berkeley Wellness Letter, 14*(3), 1–2.

Jellin, J. M., Gregory, P. J., Batz, F., Hitchens, K., et al. (2002). *Pharmacist's Letter/Prescriber's Letter Natural Medicines Comprehensive Database* (4th ed.). Stockton, CA: Therapeutic Research Faculty.

Kasper, S. & Dienel, A. (2002). Cluster analysis of symptoms during antidepressant treatment with Hypericum extract in mildly to moderately depressed outpatients. A meta-analysis of data from three randomized, placebo-controlled trials. *Psychopharmacology, 164*(3), 301–308.

Kennedy, D. & Scholey, A. (2003). Ginseng: Potential for the enhancement of cognitive performance and mood. *Pharmacology, Biochemistry, and Behavior,* 75(3), 687–700.

Keville, K. (1996). *Herbs for health and healing.* Emmaus, PA: Rodale Press.

Kligler, B. (2003). Black cohosh. *American Family Physician, 68*(1), 114–116.

Kronenberg, F. & Fugh-Berman, A. (2003). Complementary and alternative medicine for menopausal symptoms: A review of randomized, controlled trials. *Annals of Internal Medicine, 137*(10), 805–813.

Lanski, S.L., Greenwald, M., Perkins, A., & Simon, H.K. (2003). Herbal therapy use in a pediatric emergency department population: Expect the unexpected. *Pediatrics, 111*(part 1 of 5), 981–985.

LeBars, P. L., Katz, M. M., Berman, N., Itil, T. M., Freedman, A. M., & Schatzberg, A. F. (1997). A placebo-controlled, double-blind, randomized trial of an extract of Ginkgo biloba for dementia. North American Egb Study Group. *Journal of the American Medical Association, 278*(16), 1327–1332.

Lehrl, S. (2004). Clinical efficacy of kava extract WS R1490 in sleep disturbances associated with anxiety disorders. Results of a multicenter, randomized, placebo-controlled, double-blind clinical trial. *Journal of Affective Disorders, 78*(2), 101–110.

Leung, A. Y., & Foster, S. (1995). *Encyclopedia of common natural ingredients used in foods, drugs, and cosmetics* (2nd ed.). New York: Wiley.

Leventhal, L. J. (1994). Treatment of rheumatoid arthritis with gammalinolenic acid. *Annals of Internal Medicine, 119*(9), 867–692.

Libster, M. (2002). *Delmar's integrative herb guide for nurses.* Albany, NY: Delmar.

Lien, H., Sun, W., Chen, Y., Kim, H., Hasler, W., & Owyang, C. (2003). Effects of ginger on motion sickness and gastric slow-wave dysrhythmias induced by circular vection. *American Journal of Physiology. Gastronintestinal and Liver Physiology, 284*(3), G481–489.

Liu, J. H., Chen, G. H., & Yeh, H. Z. (1997). Enteric-coated peppermint-oil capsules in the treatment of irritable bowel syndrome: a prospective, randomized trial. *Journal of Gastroenterology, 32*(6), 765–8.

Lupu, R., Mehmi, I., Atlas, E., Tsai, M., Pisha, E., Oketch-Rabah, H. Nuntanadorn, P., Kennelly, E., & Kronenberg, F. (2003). Black cohosh, a menopausal remedy, does not have estrogenic activity and does not promote breast cancer cell growth. *International Journal of Oncology, 23*(5), 1407–1412.

MacGregor, F., Abernathy, V., Dahabra, S., Cobden, I. & Hayes, P. (1991). Hepatotoxicity of herbal remedies. *British Medical Journal, 299,* 1156–1159.

Makay, D. & Miller, A. (2003). Nutritional support for wound healing. *Alternative Medicine Review, 8*(4), 359–377.

Markowitz, J., Donvan, J., DeVane, C., Taylor, R., Ruan, Y., Wang, J., & Chavin, K. (2003). Effect of St. John's wort on drug metabolism by induction of cytochrome P450 3A4 enzyme. *Journal of the American Medical Association, 290*(11), 1500–1504.

Mayo Clinic Special Report. (1999). Herbal diet pills: Do they work? *May Clinic Health Information.* Rochester, MN: Mayo Foundation for Medical Education and Research.

McBride, B.F., Karapanos, A.K., Krudysz, A., Kluger, J., Coleman, C., & White, C. (2004). Electrocardiographic and hemodynamic effects of a multicomponent dietary supplement containing ephedra and caffeine: A randomized controlled trial. *Journal of American Medical Association, 291*(2), 216–221.

McCarthy, G. M., & McCarty, D. J. (1992). Effects of topical capsaicin in the therapy of painful osteoarthritis of the hands. *Journal of Rheumatology, 19,* 604–607.

Migliardi, J.R., Armellino, J. J., Freidman, M., et al. (1994). Caffeine as an analgesic adjuvant in tension headache. *Clincial Pharmacology and Therapeutics, 56*(5), 576–586

Miller, C. A. (1996). Alternative healing products: Herbal and homeopathic remedies. *Geriatric Nursing, 17*(3), 145–146.

Mills, E., Singh, R. Ross, C., Ernst, E., & Ray, J. (2003). Sale of kava extract in some health food stores. *Canadian Medical Association Journal, 169*(11), 1163–1164.

Mindell, E. (1992). *Earl Mindell's herb bible.* New York: Fireside.

Morris, C. & Avorn, J. (2003). Internet marketing of herbal products. *Journal of the American Medical Association, 290*(11), 1519–1520.

Muller, D. Pfeil, T., & von den Driesch, V. (2003). Treating depression comorbid with anxiety–results of an open practice-oriented study with St. John's wort WS5572 and valerian extract in high doses. *Phtyomedicine, 10*(Suppl 4), 25–30.

Norton, S. A., & Ruze, P. (1994). Kava dermopathy. *Journal of the American Academy of Dermatology, 31*(1), 89–97.

O'Hara, M., Keifer, D., Farrell, K., & Kemper, K. (1998). A Review of 12 commonly used medicinal herbs. *Archives of Family Medicine, 7*(6), 523–536.

Oerter, K., Janfaza, M., Wong, J., & Chang R. (2003). Estrogen bioactivity in fo-ti and other herbs used for their estrogen-like effects as determined by a recombinant cell bioassay. *The Journal of Clinical Endocrinology and Metabolism, 88*(9), 4075–4076.

Paluska, S. (2003). Caffeine and exercise. *Current Sports Medicine Report, 2*(4), 213–219.

Persson, J., Bringlov, E., Nilsson, L., & Nyberg, L. (2003). The memory-enhancing effects of Ginseng and Ginkgo biloba in healthy volunteers. *Psychopharmacology, November* 25.

Pfaffenrath, V., Diener, H., Fischer, M., Friede, M. Henneicke-von Zepelin, H. (2002). The efficacy and safety of Tanacetum partenium (feverfew) in migraine prophylaxis–a double-blind, mulitcentre, randomized placebo-controlled dose-response study. *Cephalalgia, 22*(7), 523–532.

Pfrunder, A., Schiesser, M., Gerbver, S., Haschke, M., Bitzer, J., & Drewe, J. (2003). *British Journal of Clinical Pharmacology, 56*(6), 683–690.

Pettit, J.L. (2001). Alternative medicine: Ginger. *Clinician Reviews, 11*(11), 72, 75–76.

Pittler, M. H., & Ernst, E. (1998). Peppermint oil for irritable bowel syndrome: A critical review and meta-analysis. *American Journal of Gastroenterology, 93*(7), 1131–1135).

Plantaginis ovatae testa (Indische Flohsamenschalen); Plantaginis ovatae semn (Indische Flohsamen). Bundesanzeiger. 1990 Feb 1. Monograph in Tyler and Foster, 1996.

Portnoi, G., Chng, L., Karimi-Tabesh, L., Koren, G., Tan, M., & Einarson, A. (2003). Prospective comparative study of the safety and effectiveness of ginger for the treatment of nausea and vomiting of pregnancy. *American Journal of Obstetrics Gynecology, 189*(5), 1374–1377.

Poyares, D., Guillenminault, C., Ohayon, M., & Tufik, S. (2002). Can valerian improve the sleep of insomniacs after benzodiazepine withdrawal? *Progress in Neuropsychopharmacology & Biological Psychiatry, 26*(3), 539–545.

Ramadan, N. M., Silberstein, S.D., Freitag, F. G., Gilbert, T. T., & Frishberg, B. M. (2002) Evidence-based guidelines for migraine headache in the primary care setting: pharmacological management for the prevention of migraine. *U.S. Headache Consortium, Apr. 2000 www.aan.com/professionals/practice/pdfs/g10090.pdf* (Accessed 2 July 2002).

Rousseaux, C. & Schachter, H. (2003). Regulatory issues concerning the safety, efficacy, and quality of herbal remedies. *Birth Defects Research Part B Developmental Reproductive Toxicology, 68*(6), 505–510.

Schaffer, D.M., Gordon, N.P., Jensen, C.D., & Avins, A.L. (2003). Nonvitamin, nonmineral supplment use over a 12 month period by adult members of a large health maintenance organization. *Journal of American Dietetic Association, 103*(11), 1500–1505.

Schellenberg, R. (2001). Treatment for the premenstrual syndrome with agnus castus fruit extract: Prospective, randomized, placebo controlled study. *British Medical Journal, 322*(7279), 1134–1137.

Schulman, S. (2003). Addressing the potential risks associated with ephedra use: A review of recent efforts. *Public Health Report, 118*(6), 487–492.

Schulze, J., Raasch, W., & Siegers, C. (2003). Toxicity of kava pyrones, drug safety and precautions–a case study. *Phytomedicine, 10*(Suppl 4), 68–73.

Shelton, R. C., Keller, M. B., Gelenberg, A., Dunner, D.L., Hirschfeld, R., Thase, M. E., et al. (2001). Effectiveness of St. John's wort in major depression: A randomized controlled trial. *Journal of the American Medical Association, 285*(15), 1978–1986.

Snider, S. (1991). *Herbal teas and toxicity. FDA Consumer.* Rockville, MD: DHHS Publication No. 92–1185.

Sprecher, D. L. Harris, B. V., Goldberg, A. C., et al. (1993). Efficacy of psyllium in reducing serum cholesterol levels in hypercholesterolemic patients on high- or low-fat diets. *Annals of Internal Medicine, 119,* 545–554.

Sripramote, M. & Lekhyananda, N. (2003). A randomized comparison of ginger and vitamin B6 in the treatment of nausea and vomiting of pregnancy. *Journal of the Medical Association of Thailand, 86*(9), 846–853.

Stickel, F., Baumuller, H., Seitz, K., Vasilakis, D., Seitz, G., Seitz, H., & Schuppan, D. (2003). Hepatitis induced by Kava (Piper methysticum rhizoma). *Journal of Hepatology, 39*(1), 62–67.

Taylor, J., Weber, W., Standish, L., Quinn, H., Goesling, J., McGann, M., & Calabrese, C. (2003). Efficacy and safety of Echinacea in treating upper respiratory tract infections in children: A randomized controlled trial. *Journal of the American Medical Association, 290*(21), 2824–2830.

Tierra, M. (1990). *The way of herbs.* New York: Pocketbooks.

Treatment of menopause-associated vasomotor symptoms: Position statement of The North American Menopause Society. (2004). *Menopause, 11*(1), 11–33.

Tyler, V. E. (1993). *The honest herbal: A sensible guide to the use of herbs and related remedies* (3rd ed.). New York: Pharmaceutical Products Press.

Tyler, V. E. (1994). *Herbs of choice: The therapeutic use of phytomedicinals.* New York: Pharmaceutical Products Press.

Tyler, V. E. (1997a, October). Nature's stress buster. *Prevention,* 90–95.

Tyler, V. E. (1997b, December). Promising herbs for prostate problems. *Prevention,* 69–72.

Tyler, V. E., Brady, L. R., & Robbers, J. E. (1988). *Pharmacognosy* (9th ed.). Philadelphia, PA: Lea & Febiger.

Tyler, V. E., & Foster, S. (1996). Herbs and phytomedicinal products. In *Handbook of nonprescription drugs* (pp. 695–711). Washington, DC: American Pharmaceutical Association.

Van Dongen, M., van Rossum, E., Kessels, A., Sielhorst, H., & Knipschild, P. (2003). Ginkgo for elderly people with dementia and age-associated memory impairment: A randomized clinical trial. *Journal of Clinical Epidemiology, 56*(4), 367–376.

Vogler, B. K., Pittler, M.H., & Ernst, E. (1999). The efficacy of ginseng. A systematic review of randomised clinical trials. *European Journal of Pharmacology, 55,* 567–575.

Westfall, R. (2004). Use of anti-emetic herbs in pregnancy: Women's choices, and the question of safety and efficacy.

Complementary Therapies in Nursing and Midwifery, 10(1), 30–36.

Weydert, J., Ball, T., & Davis, M. (2003). Systematic review of treatments for recurrent abdominal pain. *Pediatrics, 111*(1), 1–11.

Willetts, K., Ekangaki, A., & Eden, J. (2003). Effect of a ginger extract on pregnancy-induced nausea: A randomized controlled trial. *Australia New Zealand Journal of Obstetrics Gynaecology, 43*(2), 139–144.

Williamson, E.M. (2003). Drug interactions between herbal and prescription medicines. *Drug Safety, 26*(150, 1075–1092.

Wuttke, W., Jarry, H., Christoffel, V., Spengler, B., & Seidlova-Wuttke, D. (2003). Chaste tree (Vitex agnus-castus)–pharmacology and clinical indications. *Phytomedicine, 10*(4), 348–357.

Yanni, L., & Klein, W. (2000). Alternatives to traditional hormone replacement therapy. *Women's Health in Primary Care, 3*(7), 477–489.

Yoon, S-J. L., & Horne, C.H. (2001) Herbal products and conventional medicines used by community-residing older women. *Journal of Advanced Nursing, 33*(1), 51–59.

Youngkin, E. Q., & Israel, D. (1996). A review and critique of common herbal alternative therapies. *Nurse Practitioner, 21*(10), 39–62.

Zakay-Rones, Z., Varsano, N., & Zlotnik, M. (1995). Inhibition of several strains of influenza virus in vitro and reduction of symptoms by an elderberry extract (*Sambucus nigra L.*) during an outbreak of influenza B Panama. *Journal of Alternative and Complementary Medicine, 1*(4), 361–369.

Zeilmann, C.A., Dole, E.J., Skipper, B.J., McCabe, M., Dog, T.L., & Rhyne, R.L. (2003). Use of herbal medicine by elderly Hispanic and non-Hispanic white patients. *Pharmacotherapy, 23*(4), 526–532.

Zurier, R. B., Rossetti, R. G., Jacobson. E. W., et al. (1996). Gamma-linolenic acid treatment of rheumatoid arthritis. A randomized, placebo-controlled trial. *Arthritis and Rheumatism, 39*(11), 1808–1817.

CHAPTER ❖ 11

IMMUNIZATIONS

Debra K. Hearington

Vaccination attempts to protect humans from disease have been reported since the seventh century, although the first written reports are from the eleventh century (Plotkin & Plotkin, 1999). The twentieth century has seen the practice develop and flourish, and the incidence of many diseases that once caused significant morbidity and mortality has dramatically declined. One such disease, smallpox, was declared eradicated from the world in 1980 (World Health Organization [WHO], 1980). Polio has been eradicated from the United States and Europe. Others, including measles in the Western Hemisphere and polio worldwide, probably will be eradicated within the next few years.

The threat of bioterrorism is causing the federal government to consider using the vaccines to protect the public against the potential threats. One of those vaccines, for smallpox, hasn't been used in nearly thirty years. This chapter will address two potiential agents of bioterrorism, smallpox and anthrax.

This chapter will also briefly discuss vaccine-controllable diseases, immunization schedules, and vaccines in development. The reader should refer to Plotkin and Orenstein (1999), the most current edition of the Centers for Disease Control (CDC) publication *Epidemiology & Prevention of Vaccine-Preventable Diseases* (The Pink Book), and the Centers for Disease Control publications, *Morbidity and Mortality Weekly Report* (MMWR), for more information.

SELECTED PRINCIPLES OF IMMUNITY

Vaccines confer active immunity to disease. *Active immunity* occurs following exposure and recovery from an infection in certain diseases. For example, recovery from chicken pox, *varicella* infection, confers active immunity to chicken pox so that individuals rarely suffer from that disease a second time. Active immunity also occurs following inoculation, ingestion, or inhalation of an altered form of an infectious organism or product of the organism (e.g., toxin) that has been modified to induce immunity but not produce disease (Sell, 1996). Conferring lifelong immunity to diseases against which immunizations are effective may require more than one dose of the vaccine. *Passive immunity* occurs when immune products are transferred from one living being to another.

Passive immunity is temporary, usually lasting several weeks to months. Newborn infants have immunity to specific infectious agents because antibodies have been transferred from the mother in utero. This immunity generally lasts 3 to 4 months (Sell, 1996). Humoral antibodies may also be transferred in human immunoglobulin and immunoglobulins from the serum of immunized animals. Pooled human immune globulin is useful in treating exposures to hepatitis A and measles, and specific human immune globulin may be given for exposures to hepatitis B, pertussis, rabies, tetanus, vaccinia (cowpox), and infection with varicella-zoster (Sell, 1996). Specific equine immune globulin may be given after bites by snakes and black widow spiders, and exposure to diphtheria and botulism toxins (Sell, 1996). Immune globulins must be given immediately following exposure to the infecting-organisms, and in some cases, must be repeated.

Once a large proportion of a population of people are immunized, other unimmunized people are indirectly protected because transmission of the infectious agent may be interrupted. This concept is called *herd immunity* (Orenstein, Hinman, Rodewald, 1999). Herd immunity is an important factor in the eradication of diseases against which immunizations are effective.

CHILDHOOD IMMUNIZATIONS

Immunization against diseases known to cause significant morbidity and mortality in the population is begun in infancy. Those diseases are pertussis, poliomyelitis, and meningitis caused by *Haemophilus* influenza type B (HIB), diphtheria, tetanus, rubeola, mumps, hepatitis B, chicken pox, and pneumococcal infections. Rubeola causes severe damage to fetuses, and the population is immunized to protect the unborn. Immunizations begun in infancy have been successful in protecting children from illnesses often fatal in the first year of life, such as pertussis and meningitis caused by *Haemophilus* influenza type B. Certain immunizations cannot be given in the first year of life because of limited efficacy or because of the high risk of an allergic reaction to a vaccine component, such as egg protein. Those immunizations include varicella and measles-mumps-rubella (MMR).

See the recommended childhood immunization schedule (Fig. 11–1) for the timing of childhood immunizations.

POLIOMYELITIS

The poliovirus is an enterovirus, with three serotypes, that replicates in the oropharynx and the intestinal tract. Often, the infection (viremia) following is asymptomatic. However, the infection may result in apparently minor illness with no sequelae or minor illness followed by severe illness—aseptic meningitis or paralytic poliomyelitis. Mild illness is characterized by fever, sore throat, headache, and/or gastrointestinal symptoms. Nonparalytic poliomyelitis is characterized by the appearance of meningitis symptoms 1 to 2 days following the onset of mild illness, and occurs in 1 to 2% of patients. Recovery is usually complete; however, in a small percentage of cases, mild muscle weakness or paralysis occurs. Paralytic poliomyelitis is characterized by sudden onset of muscle weakness and aches in the back and/or extremities and progresses to flaccid paralysis and loss of deep tendon reflexes. Paralytic poliomyelitis may occur with or without prodromal symptoms, and happens in less than 2% of all poliovirus infections. Paralysis generally does not progress after the temperature returns to normal, and recovery occurs gradually over several months. Some patients experience residual muscle weakness or paralysis for the rest of their lives. The death rate from paralytic poliomyelits is 2 to 10% of cases (CDC, 2000; Sutter, Cochi, Melnick, 1999).

A postpolio syndrome occurs in 25 to 40% of persons 30 to 40 years old following paralytic poliomyelitis. They experience muscle pain and may have an exacerbation of existing weakness or develop new weakness or paralysis (CDC, 2000; Sutter, Cochi, Melnick, 1999). Those who develop postpolio syndrome were infected in the 1940s and 1950s when wild poliovirus was circulating (CDC, 2000; Sutter, Cochi, Melnick, 1999).

The virus is transmitted by direct fecal-oral contact and indirectly by contaminated sewage and water and contact with infectious saliva or feces (CDC, 2000). Humans are the only reservoir, which is an advantage in the eradication effort. The Western Hemisphere was certified to be free of indigenous wild poliovirus in September 1994, because there is no evidence of any polio infection caused by circulating wild virus in this part of the world (CDC, 1994; CDC, 2000). The World Health Assembly adopted the goal of global eradication by the year 2000, however, cases of wild-type polio virus are still occurring. Transmission of serotype 2 has apparently been globally interrupted, with only 11 cases reported in SEAR in 1999. Zero cases were reported in 2000 (CDC, 2001a).

Areas with documented poliovirus transmission are targeted by local governments for increased acute flaccid paralysis (AFP) surveillance activities, improved stool collection techniques, and mass vaccination sweeps. The mass vaccination sweeps are typically door-to-door campaigns focusing on vaccinating children 0 to 6 years with OPV. Sweeps are repeated one to three times to ensure adequate immunization; however, some are hampered by the difficulties in reaching geographically remote locations. Wild-type poliovirus has been found in Bulgaria (determined to be imported), Southeast Asia, and several countries in the Africa region as recently as 2001 (CDC, 2001b, 2001e, 2001f, 2001g, 2001h). Despite the small number of cases (3000 in the year 2000), the CDC still anticipates global eradication of poliomyelitis in this decade (2000–2010) (CDC, 2001d). The issue currently

Recommended Childhood and Adolescent Immunization Schedule UNITED STATES • JULY–DECEMBER 2004

Vaccine ▼ / Age ▶	Birth	1 mo	2 mo	4 mo	6 mo	12 mo	15 mo	18 mo	24 mo	4–6 y	11–12 y	13–18 y
Hepatitis B[1]	HepB #1		HepB #2			HepB #3					HepB Series	
Diphtheria, Tetanus, Pertussis[2]			DTaP	DTaP	DTaP		DTaP			DTaP	Td	Td
Haemophilus influenzae type b[3]			Hib	Hib	Hib	Hib						
Inactivated Poliovirus			IPV	IPV		IPV				IPV		
Measles, Mumps, Rubella[4]						MMR #1				MMR #2	MMR #2	
Varicella[5]							Varicella				Varicella	
Pneumococcal[6]			PCV	PCV	PCV	PCV			PCV		PPV	
Influenza[7]						Influenza (Yearly)					Influenza (Yearly)	
Vaccines below red line are for selected populations												
Hepatitis A[8]											Hepatitis A Series	

This schedule indicates the recommended ages for routine administration of currently licensed childhood vaccines, as of April 1, 2004, for children through age 18 years. Any dose not given at the recommended age should be given at any subsequent visit when indicated and feasible. ▬ Indicates age groups that warrant special effort to administer those vaccines not previously given. Additional vaccines may be licensed and recommended during the year. Licensed combination vaccines may be used whenever any components of the combination are indicated and the vaccine's other components are not contraindicated. Providers should consult the manufacturers' package inserts for detailed recommendations. Clinically significant adverse events that follow immunization should be reported to the Vaccine Adverse Event Reporting System (VAERS). Guidance about how to obtain and complete a VAERS form can be found on the Internet: *www.vaers.org* or by calling 800-822-7967.

Range of recommended ages — Only if mother HBsAg(-) — Preadolescent assessment — Catch-up immunization

DEPARTMENT OF HEALTH AND HUMAN SERVICES
CENTERS FOR DISEASE CONTROL AND PREVENTION

The Childhood and Adolescent Immunization Schedule is approved by:
Advisory Committee on Immunization Practices *www.cdc.gov/nip/acip*
American Academy of Pediatrics *www.aap.org*
American Academy of Family Physicians *www.aafp.org*

Footnotes
Recommended Childhood and Adolescent Immunization Schedule UNITED STATES • JULY–DECEMBER 2004

1. Hepatitis B (HepB) vaccine. All infants should receive the first dose of hepatitis B vaccine soon after birth and before hospital discharge; the first dose may also be given by age 2 months if the infant's mother is hepatitis B surface antigen (HBsAg) negative. Only monovalent HepB can be used for the birth dose. Monovalent or combination vaccine containing HepB may be used to complete the series. Four doses of vaccine may be administered when a birth dose is given. The second dose should be given at least 4 weeks after the first dose, except for combination vaccines which cannot be administered before age 6 weeks. The third dose should be given at least 16 weeks after the first dose and at least 8 weeks after the second dose. The last dose in the vaccination series (third or fourth dose) should not be administered before age 24 weeks.

Infants born to HBsAg-positive mothers should receive HepB and 0.5 mL of Hepatitis B Immune Globulin (HBIG) within 12 hours of birth at separate sites. The second dose is recommended at age 1–2 months. The last dose in the immunization series should not be administered before age 24 weeks. These infants should be tested for HBsAg and antibody to HBsAg (anti-HBs) at age 9–15 months.

Infants born to mothers whose HBsAg status is unknown should receive the first dose of the HepB series within 12 hours of birth. Maternal blood should be drawn as soon as possible to determine the mother's HBsAg status; if the HBsAg test is positive, the infant should receive HBIG as soon as possible (no later than age 1 week). The second dose is recommended at age 1–2 months. The last dose in the immunization series should not be administered before age 24 weeks.

2. Diphtheria and tetanus toxoids and acellular pertussis (DTaP) vaccine. The fourth dose of DTaP may be administered as early as age 12 months, provided 6 months have elapsed since the third dose and the child is unlikely to return at age 15–18 months. The final dose in the series should be given at age ≥4 years. **Tetanus and diphtheria toxoids (Td)** is recommended at age 11–12 years if at least 5 years have elapsed since the last dose of tetanus and diphtheria toxoid-containing vaccine. Subsequent routine Td boosters are recommended every 10 years.

3. *Haemophilus influenzae* type b (Hib) conjugate vaccine. Three Hib conjugate vaccines are licensed for infant use. If PRP-OMP (PedvaxHIB or ComVax [Merck]) is administered at ages 2 and 4 months, a dose at age 6 months is not required. DTaP/Hib combination products should not be used for primary immunization in infants at ages 2, 4 or 6 months but can be used as boosters following any Hib vaccine. The final dose in the series should be given at age ≥12 months.

4. Measles, mumps, and rubella vaccine (MMR). The second dose of MMR is recommended routinely at age 4–6 years but may be administered during any visit, provided at least 4 weeks have elapsed since the first dose and both doses are administered beginning at or after age 12 months. Those who have not previously received the second dose should complete the schedule by the visit at age 11–12 years.

5. Varicella vaccine. Varicella vaccine is recommended at any visit at or after age 12 months for susceptible children (i.e., those who lack a reliable history of chickenpox). Susceptible persons age ≥13 years should receive 2 doses, given at least 4 weeks apart.

6. Pneumococcal vaccine. The heptavalent **pneumococcal conjugate vaccine (PCV)** is recommended for all children age 2–23 months. It is also recommended for certain children age 24–59 months. The final dose in the series should be given at age ≥12 months. **Pneumococcal polysaccharide vaccine (PPV)** is recommended in addition to PCV for certain high-risk groups. See *MMWR* 2000;49(RR-9):1-35.

7. Influenza vaccine. Influenza vaccine is recommended annually for children aged ≥6 months with certain risk factors (including but not limited to asthma, cardiac disease, sickle cell disease, HIV, and diabetes), healthcare workers, and other persons (including household members) in close contact with persons in groups at high risk (see *MMWR* 2004;53;[RR-6]:1-40) and can be administered to all others wishing to obtain immunity. In addition, healthy children aged 6–23 months and close contacts of healthy children aged 0–23 months are recommended to receive influenza vaccine, because children in this age group are at substantially increased risk for influenza-related hospitalizations. For healthy persons aged 5–49 years, the intranasally administered live, attenuated influenza vaccine (LAIV) is an acceptable alternative to the intramuscular trivalent inactivated influenza vaccine (TIV). See *MMWR* 2004;53;[RR-6]:1-40. Children receiving TIV should be administered a dosage appropriate for their age (0.25 mL if 6–35 months or 0.5 mL if ≥3 years). Children aged ≤8 years who are receiving influenza vaccine for the first time should receive 2 doses (separated by at least 4 weeks for TIV and at least 6 weeks for LAIV).

8. Hepatitis A vaccine. Hepatitis A vaccine is recommended for children and adolescents in selected states and regions and for certain high-risk groups; consult your local public health authority. Children and adolescents in these states, regions, and high-risk groups who have not been immunized against hepatitis A can begin the hepatitis A immunization series during any visit. The 2 doses in the series should be administered at least 6 months apart. See *MMWR* 1999;48(RR-12):1-37.

FIGURE 11–1. Recommended Childhood and Adolescent Immunization Schedule being addressed by the CDC is that of adequate containment of wild poliovirus in laboratories so that reintroduction of the virus to an essentially polio-free world doesn't happen (CDC, 2001d).

There are two vaccines currently available: oral polio vaccine (OPV) and inactivated polio vaccine (IPV). An inactivated, injectable vaccine was introduced in the United States in 1955 and was less potent than the most recent injectible IPV licensed for use in 1987. When the trivalent OPV, a live attenuated vaccine, became available in the early 1960s, use of IPV declined for all except immunocompromised persons (CDC, 1997f).

No adverse reactions to IPV have been documented, but a hypersensitivity reaction may occur in those sensitive to streptomycin, polymyxin B, and neomycin. There is a small risk of paralysis following administration of OPV (CDC, 1997f). The condition known as vaccine-associated paralytic poliomyelitis (VAPP) carries a risk of 1 case in 2.4 million doses of OPV administered and 1 case per 750,000 first doses administered (CDC, 1997f). VAPP occurs because persons vaccinated with OPV excrete live virus in their stools for up to 6 weeks following immunization, which may cause infection in susceptible (unimmunized and immunocompromised) persons. Since there are no more cases of wild poliovirus infection and an inactivated vaccine is available, the risk of VAPP occurring because of the oral vaccine is considered unacceptable. Therefore, the Advisory Committee on Immunization Practices (ACIP), the American Academy of Pediatrics (AAP), and the American Academy of Family Physicians (AAFP) recommends exclusive use of OPV vaccine in the United States (CDC, 2000a). The schedule appears in Figure 11–1.

OPV is the vaccine of choice for use in polio outbreaks because it induces antibodies in more recipients following administration. This is due to its replication in the intestinal tract (CDC, 2000). OPV may be used in the United States for unvaccinated children traveling in less than 4 weeks to regions where polio is endemic or children whose parents refuse IPV. In the latter case, OPV may be used for the third and/or fourth polio dose. Risks of VAPP must be discussed with parents or caregivers (CDC, 2000).

It is not recommended that adults 18 years and older residing in the United States be routinely immunized due to their low risk for exposure to polioviruses and some degree of immunity from childhood immunization. The CDC recommends vaccination for adults in the following circumstances: The adult is traveling to areas where poliomyelitis is endemic or epidemic; the adult is a member of a community or specific population group with disease caused by wild polioviruses; the adult is a laboratory worker who handles specimens that may contain polioviruses; the adult is a healthcare worker who may have contact with persons excreting wild polioviruses; or the adult has never been vaccinated and has children who will be receiving OPV. IPV only is recommended for adults who have never been vaccinated because of the higher risk of VAPP in adults. In this case, two doses of IPV should be administered at intervals of 4 to 8 weeks, with a third dose 6 to 12 months after the second. Adults who received primary immunization with OPV or IPV and are in the above risk categories may receive either OPV or IPV for their subsequent immunization. The CDC recommends that vaccination in pregnancy be avoided even though adverse effects of IPV or OPV on pregnant women or fetuses have not been documented. However, should a pregnant woman require immediate protection, she should be immunized according to the recommended schedule for adults (CDC, 2000).

For more information on the above information or immunization of people not covered in the above information, contact the CDC at 1-800-CDC-SHOT (1-800-232-7468).

PERTUSSIS

Pertussis, also known as whooping cough, is a disease characterized by severe, paroxysmal coughing spasms leading to cyanosis and vomiting. Complications include subconjunctival hemorrhages, epistaxis, facial edema, ulceration of the lingual frenulum, pneumonia, pneumothorax, dehydration, otitis media, hernias, rectal prolapse, encephalitis with seizures, and malnutrition (CDC, 2002; Edwards, Decker & Mortimer, 1999). The disease, caused by *Bordetella pertussis,* a gram-negative bacillus, initially appears to be a mild upper respiratory infection with low-grade fever and an occasional cough that increasingly becomes more spasmodic and paroxysmal (Edwards 1999). The disease is spread through close contact (respiratory route) and lasts 2 to 6 weeks. Erythromycin is the drug of choice, but generally it is not effective in ameliorating symptoms unless administered early in the course of illness (CDC, 2002). Erythromycin or trimethoprim-sulfamethoxazole should be given prophylactically to household and close contacts of the infected person for 14 days, regardless of age and vaccination history, to minimize or prevent transmission. In addition, close contacts under age 7 who have not completed the four-dose primary series should complete the series as soon as possible, and anyone who completed the series but has not received a pertussis-containing vaccine within 3 years of exposure should receive a booster dose (CDC, 2002a).

Studies have shown that adults may be the primary source of *Bordetella pertussis* transmission to children and other susceptible adults (CDC, 2002; Edwards et al., 1999; Herwaldt, 1991; Nelson, 1978; Nennig, Shinefield, Edwards, Blade, & Fireman, 1996; Red Book 2000, Schmitt; Wirsing, König, Neiso, Bogaerts, Bock, et al., 1996; Wright, Edwards, Decker, & Zeldin, 1995). The disease also has been recognized in adolescents with chronic cough (Cromer, Goydos, Hackell, Mezzatesta, Dekker, & 1993). This is thought to be due to declining immunity in adolescents and adults and the presence of *Bordetella pertussis* in the community (Cromer et al., 1993; Wright et al., 1995). Surveillance data from 1997 through 2000 demonstrated a 60% increase in pertussis cases among adults and 11% increase in infants as compared with data from 1994–1996. This trend may lead to a new recommendation that persons over age 7 years be given booster doses of acellular pertussis vaccine to reduce transmission to other adults and children (CDC, 2002).

Two forms of pertussis vaccine are available: whole-cell preparations and acellular preparations. Severe adverse reactions including high fever (>40.5°C or 105°F); persistent, inconsolable crying for longer than 3 hours; seizures, with and without fever; a hypotonic, hyporesponsive episode; and encephalopathy have been reported following administration of whole-cell preparations (CDC, 1997e, 2002; Edwards et al., 1999). They occur infrequently, and based on studies that showed a possible causal relationship between whole-cell pertussis vaccine and severe neurologic reactions and studies that did not demonstrate such a relationship, practitioners are somewhat divided on the issue of giving whole-cell pertussis vaccines. However, it has been documented that more adverse reactions, including severe local reactions, are reported following whole-cell pertussis vaccine than acellular pertussis vaccine (CDC, 1997e; Decker, Edwards, Steinhoff, Rennels, Pichichero, et al., 1995). This, combined with studies demonstrating equal, if not better, efficacy of acellular pertussis vaccines, has led to the ACIP recommendation to immunize infants and children with acellular pertussis vaccine (CDC, 1997e).

Acellular pertussis vaccine is available combined with diphtheria and tetanus vaccines. A preparation of pertussis vaccine combined with diphtheria, tetanus, and *Haemophilus* influenza type B (HIB) vaccines called Tri-Hibit also is available but may only be given for the fourth dose after 3 doses of DtaP and 3 doses of Hib vaccine (Red Book, 2000). Tripedia is currently the only licensed DtaP product approved for the fifth dose in the DtaP vaccine series (CDC, 2002a).. Other combination preparations of acellular pertussis and other vaccines are in research and development at the present time. See Figure 11–1 for the schedule for administering pertussis vaccine to children.

DIPHTHERIA

Toxigenic strains of *Corynebacterium diphtheriae,* a gram-positive bacillus, cause diphtheria, which usually is transmitted by close person-to-person contact (respiratory spread) and rarely by direct contact with skin lesions or materials contaminated with the discharge of skin lesions. The disease may involve any mucous membrane, and sites of infection include the nose, tonsils, and throat, larynx, conjunctiva, skin, and genitalia. A membrane forms that is white in the nose and bluish-white progressing to greyish-green and black if bleeding has occured in the mouth and throat. The membrane adheres to the tissue, and extensive membrane formation in the throat or larynx (depending on the site of disease) may lead to airway obstruction. Symptoms depend on the site of involvement, but include low-grade fever, mucopurulent nasal discharge (may be blood-tinged), sore throat, anorexia, hoarseness, and barking cough with laryngeal involvement; in severe disease, prostration, stupor, coma, and lymphadenopathy and marked edema in the neck are present. Cutaneous involvement is manifested by ulcers with clearly demarcated edges and membrane or a scaling rash, although any chronic skin lesion may contain toxigenic and nontoxigenic strains of *C. diphtheriae* (CDC, 2002a). Complications include myocarditis, neuritis, palatal, ocular, and diaphragmatic paralysis; and death (CDC, 2002a).

Treatment is with both diphtheria antitoxin and antibiotics—erythromycin PO or IM or procaine penicillin G IM, and the infected person should be isolated. The person is not contagious after 48 h of antibiotic administration. Diphtheria antitoxin is available in the United States only through an investigational drug protocol through the CDC (CDC, 2002a). Contacts should be given a diphtheria toxoid booster and IM benzathine penicillin G or oral erythromycin. Antitoxin should be given at the first sign of illness (CDC, 2000a). Having the infection does not appear to result in lifelong immunity; therefore, booster doses should be given at the appropriate intervals, even with a history of diphtheria illness.

Reporting of nontoxigenic strains of *C. diphtheriae* is no longer required, and contacts do not need to be investigated. All cases caused by toxigenic strains are reportable. Since 1980, most of the reported cases of diphtheria in the United States occurred in unimmunized or inadequately immunized persons. *C. diptheriae* continues to circulate in areas of the United States with previously endemic diphtheria and in other parts of the world (CDC, 2002a). Healthcare providers need to continue focusing on adequate immunization of children and adults against diphtheria.

Diphtheria toxoid is available in combination with tetanus toxoid and/or pertussis vaccine, and effectiveness is estimated to be >95% after the primary series is completed (three doses in adults and four doses in infants, spaced at the recommended intervals). Adults require a diphtheria toxoid booster every ten years to boost waning immunity (CDC 2002a). Multiple boosters at less than 10-year intervals should not be given as Arthus-type hypersensitivity reactions may occur. Anaphylaxis is rare. Mild illness, pregnancy, and immunosuppression are not contraindications to receiving diphtheria toxoid vaccine (CDC, 2002a).

See Figure 11–1 for the recommended schedule in children and Figure 11–3 for unimmunized adults.

TETANUS

Tetanus is not a communicable illness, but one that is often fatal. Therefore, protection by immunization is extremely important. It is caused by an exotoxin produced by *Clostridium tetani,* a gram-positive rod, and results in skeletal muscle spasm and rigidity first involving the jaw and neck. Humans and animals harbor the organism, which is found in the intestines and feces, and can also be found in soil, street dust, and manure. Spores may also be found on the skin and in contaminated heroin (CDC 2002a). The organism enters at wound sites and the spores germinate, producing toxins that are disseminated through the circulatory and lymphatic systems. Tetanus may be local, where muscle contraction and spasm is limited to the area of injury. Localized tetanus is unusual, but it may occur and precede the development of generalized tetanus (Wassilak, Orenstein, & Sutter, 1999). Cephalic tetanus is rare and may occur with otitis media when the organism is present in middle ear fluid or following head injuries. Neonatal tetanus may occur following infection of the unhealed umbilical stump. The most common form is generalized tetanus, beginning with jaw muscle rigidity (lockjaw) followed by neck stiffness and spasm of the facial muscles in some cases. Difficulty in swallowing, abdominal muscle rigidity, spasms of other muscles, fever, sweating, increased blood pressure, and periodic tachycardia also occur. Complications include laryngospasm, fractures, coma, pulmonary embolism, aspiration pneumonia, and death (CDC, 2002a;Wassilak et al., 1999).

Treatment includes administration of human tetanus immune globulin (TIG) at diagnosis. Other therapy may include administration of oral or intravenous metronidazole or alternatively parenteral penicillin G; and administration of agents to relieve muscle spasm, in addition to other supportive therapy (Red Book, 2000, pp. 564–565). Infection does not produce immunity, so those with a history of tetanus disease need to be immunized with tetanus toxoid according to the appropriate schedule for age and previous vaccination history (CDC, 2002a).

Tetanus toxoid is combined with diphtheria toxoid and/or pertussis vaccine. Following the primary series, immunity generally lasts 10 years. Therefore, persons should receive booster doses every 10 years following the primary series. A repeat dose of tetanus toxoid should be given when "dirty" wound injuries occur more than 5 years after a tetanus booster. When the injured are unsure of the date of last tetanus booster, a booster should be given. In the case of an injured person who has had two doses or less of tetanus toxoid, or who is uncertain of a prior history of tetanus immunization, tetanus immune globulin should be given in addition to the immunization (CDC, 2002a). Pregnancy, immunosuppression, or presence of minor illness is not a contraindication to tetanus immunization.

Local reactions, erythema, induration, and pain at the injection site are common. An abscess at the injection site may also occur, and local reactions are generally self-limited.

See Figure 11–1 for the recommended immunization schedule.

MEASLES

The measles virus belongs to the Paramyxoviridae family, genus *Morbillivirus.* Infection with this virus causes illness that begins with fever, up-per respiratory symptoms, and conjunctivitis. Koplik's spots appear on the buccal mucosa 1 to 2 days preceding the development of a red, maculopapular rash beginning at the hairline and proceeding downward. The lesions are discrete but may become confluent on the upper body and face, and initially they blanch with pressure. The rash then fades in the order it progressed, and desquamation may occur over severely involved areas. Other symptoms include malaise, anorexia, diarrhea, and generalized lymphadenopathy. Complications include diarrhea, otitis media, pneumonia, encephalitis, hepatitis, appendicitis, pericarditis, myocarditis, thrombocytopenia, laryngotracheobronchitis, ileocolitis, glomerulonephritis, hypocalcemia, and Stevens-Johnsons syndrome. Subacute sclerosing panencephalitis (SSPE) is a rare, severe complication of measles infection and may occur years after infection (1 month to 27 years). SSPE is a degenerative disease of the central nervous system resulting in behavioral and personality changes, seizures, coma, and death (Redd, Markowitz, & Katz, 1999). Measles in pregnancy may result in spontaneous abortion or premature birth, although there is no evidence that infection in the first trimester causes birth defects (unlike rubella) (Redd, et al., 1999).

Treatment is primarily supportive, although high doses of vitamin A seem to reduce morbidity and mortality in developing countries. No other forms of therapy for measles or SSPE have been shown to be effective. However, Ribaviron may decrease the duration of the illness (Redd et al., 1999). Immune globulin may be administered prophylactically to susceptible persons in whom the vaccine is contraindicated following exposure to the measles virus. Susceptible persons include children under 1 year of age, pregnant women, immunocompromised persons, and others with a contraindication to administration of a live vaccine (Redd et al., 1999).

Periodic measles outbreaks have occurred since the onset of mass immunization programs; however, the number of reported cases began declining in 1992 (CDC 2002a). There was a slight increase in 1994, from 312 confirmed cases in 1993 to 961 cases in 1994. The outbreaks were noted to be primarily among people in groups that oppose vaccination. In 1995, the number of cases dropped to 309, the lowest since national surveillance began (CDC, 1997c). Increasingly, the cases reported in the United States have been imported, and they often lead to an outbreak among children and adults who have not had a second measles vaccination. The data suggest that wild-type virus transmission in the United States has been interrupted numerous times, which favors the goal of eradication (CDC, 1997c, 2002a).

A live attenuated vaccine for measles is available alone or in combination with mumps and rubella vaccines. The recommended schedule has been changed several times, but it is now known that two doses are required to establish and maintain long-term immunity. The vaccine is ineffective in infants under 1 year of age because the presence of maternal antibody inhibits the immune response to the vaccine (CDC, 1997c). Children should receive the first dose at 12 to 15 months of age and a repeat dose at school entry. For those who are already in school and who have not received the second dose, the booster dose should be given at entry to middle or high school. College students should receive a second dose of measles vaccine if they have not previously had one or if they have no evidence of immunity. Healthcare workers and international travelers also need to get the vaccine if they have not been immunized with two doses of measles vaccine after the first birthday or they have no evidence of immunity (CDC, 2002a).

The vaccine contains a small quantity of egg protein because it is grown in chick culture; therefore, caution must be used in immunizing those with a history of severe hypersensitivity reactions to eggs. Extreme caution should also be used when immunizing those with a history of severe reactions to neomycin. Mild illness is not a contraindication to vaccination with measles vaccine. Pregnancy and immunosuppression are contraindications, although measles vaccine may be given to persons with HIV infection. In persons who have received blood products recently, measles vaccine should be delayed. Contact the CDC for information on when to immunize those who have received blood products (CDC, 2002a).

Adverse events following vaccination with live measles vaccine include fever, rash, and thrombocytopenia. The fever and rash occur 5 to 12 days postvaccination and occur because of replication of the measles vaccine virus. Fifteen percent or less experience fever; 5% or less experience rash (CDC, 2002a).

RUBELLA

Rubella is a generally mild, exanthematous disease caused by the rubella virus, a togavirus (genus *Rubivirus*). The disease is characterized by a maculopapular, erythematous rash beginning on the face and neck and progressing downward. In young children there is often no prodrome, but the prodrome in older children and adults consists of low-grade fever, malaise, mild conjunctivitis, upper respiratory symptoms, and lymphadenopathy. The rash may be pruritic, is fainter than the measles rash, and does not coalesce (CDC, 2002a). Arthralgia and arthritis occur in up to 70% of adult women and may last as long as 1 month. Complications include chronic arthritis, encephalitis, orchitis, neuritis, panencephalitis, and hemorrhages caused by thrombocytopenia. Congenital infection results in birth defects (up to 85% of infants infected in the first trimester of pregnancy), and the primary goal of immunization against rubella is to protect the unborn fetus. Congenital rubella syndrome can affect all organ systems, and damage occurs when infection is present in the first 20 weeks of pregnancy. After that, defects from rubella infection are rare (CDC, 2002a; Plotkin & Plotkin, 1999).

> *In recent years, more than one half of cases of congenital rubella syndrome occurred because of missed opportunities for vaccination in the mothers* (CDC, 1997i, p. 353). There have been 31 outbreaks of rubella in the United States since 1993, and 42 cases in 2003 (http://www.cdc.gov/mmwr/PDF/link/mm5313.pdf).

Treatment is supportive. Ordinary immune serum globulin and hyperimmune globulin have been used in an attempt to prevent fetal infection in pregnant women exposed to rubella, but this has not been shown to be effective (CDC, 2002a; Plotkin & Plotkin 1999). Red Book, 2000, p. 497. A rubella vaccine is available singly and mixed with mumps and measles vaccines, and it confers lifelong immunity. Adverse events following immunization include fever, lymphadenopathy, arthralgia, and occasionally, rash and acute arthritis. Rubella vaccine should not be administered to persons with moderate to severe illness (minor illness is not a contraindication), immunosuppressed persons, pregnant women, and persons with a recent history of receiving antibody-containing blood products. HIV infection is not a contraindication to immunization. Women who receive rubella vaccine should avoid pregnancy for 3 months. A vaccine virus has been isolated from the pharynx of vaccinees, and while they are not contagious to others, breastfeeding mothers may infect their infants. Those infants may develop a mild illness with rash, without serious effects. Therefore, breastfeeding is not a contraindication to rubella immunization (CDC, 2002a, Red Book, 2000, pp. 498–499).

MUMPS

The mumps virus is a paramyxovirus that is spread by respiratory droplets. Following replication in the nasopharynx and lymph nodes, the virus spreads to multiple tissues and glands, including the meninges, salivary glands, testes, ovaries, and pancreas. The most common manifestation is parotitis (inflammation of the salivary glands), which may be unilateral or bilateral. Thirty to forty percent of infected persons experience parotitis. A prodrome of myalgia, anorexia, malaise, headache, and low-grade fever may occur. Mumps may present as a lower respiratory infection in young children. Mumps infections may be asymptomatic in up to 20% of cases. Complications include meningoencephalitis (adults are at greater risk), orchitis, oophoritis, myocarditis, deafness, nephritis, pancreatitis, mastitis, arthropathy, and fetal death. Death may also result from mumps infection (CDC, 2002; Plotkin & Wharton, 1999). Mumps disease confers lifelong immunity.

Treatment is supportive. Postexposure prophylaxis with mumps immune globulin or immune globulin (IG) has not been shown to be effective.

Vaccination with live virus mumps vaccine is estimated to be 95% efficacious, and immunity is presumed to be lifelong (CDC, 2002). Adverse reactions to mumps vaccine are rare but include parotitis, low-grade fever, rash, pruritus, and purpura. Mumps vaccine is available singly, with rubella vaccine, and with measles and rubella vaccines.

Contraindications to vaccination include a history of severe allergy to eggs and neomycin, persons with moderate to severe illness, immunosuppressed persons, pregnant women, and those recently transfused with antibody-containing blood products. Women should not become pregnant for 3 months after receiving the vaccine. Protocols have been developed for immunizing those with egg allergy. Persons with HIV may receive the vaccine (CDC, 2002a).

HAEMOPHILUS INFLUENZA TYPE B

Haemophilus influenzae, a gram-negative coccobacillus, causes many types of infection in children under 5 years of age. The most common are meningitis, epiglottitis, pneumonia, arthritis, cellulitis, otitis media, and bronchitis. Otitis media and bronchitis may also be caused by nontypable strains of *H. influenzae.* Osteomyelitis and pericarditis also may occur. Most infections require hospitalization and treatment with antibiotics—chloramphenicol, cefotaxime, or ceftriaxone. Ampicillin-resistant strains are common in the United States; therefore, ampicillin should not be used to treat infections thought to be caused by HIB. Transmission is thought to be by respiratory droplet spread. Household contacts may be prophylaxed with rifampin to prevent disease spread and eliminate the carrier state (CDC, 2002a; Red Book, 2000; pp. 262, 284; Ward, Zangwill, 1999).

Immunization against HIB was first recommended in 1985 for all children at 24 months of age (Ward, Zangwill, 1999). With further vaccine development, immunization is now recommended beginning at 2 months of age. Several HIB vaccines are available singly or in combination with diphtheria, tetanus, and whole-cell pertussis vaccines; however, whole-cell pertussis vaccines are not recommended for use in the United States (CDC, 2002a). Healthcare personnel administering the vaccine should be sure to review the package insert of the vaccine to be sure the HIB vaccine chosen is appropriate for the age of the child being immunized.

Adverse events following HIB vaccination include swelling, redness, and pain at the injection site. Fever and irritability are infrequent. Previous anaphylactic reaction to HIB vaccine is a contraindication to receiving further doses. Minor illness is not a contraindication to vaccination (CDC, 2002a; Red Book, 2000, p. 267).

VARICELLA

Chickenpox is a common childhood disease, caused by the varicella-zoster virus, a herpesvirus. The virus is transmitted by respiratory droplets and is highly contagious. Viral replication occurs and can be transmitted to others before the characteristic skin rash appears. The rash may be preceded by a prodrome of malaise, headache, decreased appetite, and low-grade fever. Macular lesions then appear, beginning on the trunk and face and spreading to extremities. The lesions progress from macules to papules to vesicles, which may then be scratched open and ooze fluid. The vesicles eventually scab over. Lesions erupt in crops generally over a 3-day period and are present in various stages of progression all over the body at the same time. The disease is contagious from 48 h prior to eruption of the lesions until all lesions have scabbed over. The disease is transmitted by the respiratory droplet route and by direct contact with skin lesions.

Chickenpox is relatively benign in most healthy children, but severe complications can occur. Adults, children under 1 year, and immunocompromised children tend to have more serious disease and a higher rate of complications and death (CDC, 2002a, Gershon, Takahashi, & White, 1999). The most common complication of varicella infection is secondary bacterial infection of skin lesions. Other common complications include pneumonia, dehydration, and involvement of the central nervous system, including aseptic meningitis, encephalitis, and cerebellar involvement. Reye's syndrome has been reported in cases of children who took aspirin during the acute illness. More rarely, appendicitis, transverse myelitis, thrombocytopenia, hemorrhagic varicella, purpura fulminans, glomerulonephritis, arthritis, myocarditis, clinical hepatitis, orchitis, uveitis, iritis, and Guillain-Barré syndrome have been reported.

Uncomplicated cases of chickenpox are managed primarily with supportive therapies; antihistamines and oatmeal baths provide some relief for itching. If fever is present, acetaminophen may be prescribed. As with any acute illness, increased fluid intake is important.

Complicated cases and chickenpox in high-risk cases are managed according to the complications that appear. Therapy is directed at the specific symptoms that appear (for example, antibiotics for secondary bacterial infections and intravenous fluids for dehydration). Acyclovir is used orally or intravenously in higher-risk cases, such as immunocompromised clients and adults. Informed clients may request acyclovir, thinking that it will reduce the severity of illness. It has been shown to reduce numbers of lesions and number of days of fever, but not the course of the illness in otherwise healthy children (Gershon, et al., 1999). Acyclovir should be given within 24 h of the onset of rash. Famciclovir and valacyclovir have not been studied for the treatment of varicella (Gershon et al., 1999).

Varicella-zoster immune globulin (VZIG) is effective against chickenpox; however, it must be given within 96 h of exposure to be effective in preventing or modifying clinical varicella. Administration of VZIG should be considered for susceptible, unvaccinated children and adults, including immunocompromised persons, pregnant women, newborns whose mothers developed clinical disease 5 days before to 2 days after delivery, and preterm infants with postnatal exposure. VZIG is given intramuscularly, never intravenously.

Varivax, a live attenuated vaccine, is available and is recommended for routine vaccination of all children at 12 to 18 months of age, and by the thirteenth birthday for children never vaccinated with no history of actual disease. After age 13, varicella infections tend to be more severe, and two doses of vaccine are required to insure adequate immunity (CDC, 2002a). When two doses are given, they should be separated by 4 to 8 weeks. If more than 8 weeks have passed, the second vaccine may still be administered without starting the series over. Breakthrough disease may occur in some vaccinated individuals, although the disease is mild with fewer lesions and no fever in most cases. The rash tends to be maculapapular rather than vesicular with few lesions (Red Book, 2000, p. 633). If a patient does develop significant rash (greater than 100 lesions) and fever following vaccine administration, it could be due to wild-virus vaccine from a recent exposure. Clinicians should consider this probability in addition to considering the possibility of infection caused by the vaccine virus (Feder, La Russa, Steinberg, & Gershon, 1997; Red Book, 2000, p. 633).

Contraindications to varicella vaccine include previous history of severe allergic reaction to a vaccine component (the vaccine contains trace amounts of neomycin and gelatin) or following a previous dose of vaccine, moderate or severe illness, immunosuppression, HIV infection, and a history of receiving antibody-containing blood products in the previous 5 months (CDC, 2002a). The risk of varicella to the developing fetus is very low; however, in the absence of reliable data on varicella vaccination in pregnancy, pregnant women should not be immunized (CDC, 2002a, & Gershon et al., 1999). However, should a pregnant woman be inadvertently vaccinated, the clinician should report the case to the Varicella Vaccination in Pregnancy Registry established by the CDC and the varicella vaccine manufacturer. The registry collects data on maternal-fetal outcomes following varicella vaccination in pregnancy. The phone number is 1-800-986-8999 (CDC, 2002a).

Controversy initially surrounded the recommendation of routine varicella vaccination of children and reportedly one-third of physicians surveyed by the Merck Company were not recommending the vaccine (Watson & Haupt, 1997). Issues cited involve adding another injection to the childhood immunization schedule, especially for a disease that is relatively benign in healthy children; questions regarding the duration of immunity following vaccination; waning immunity among immunized children leading to the risk of varicella infection in adulthood; transmission of the virus from the vaccine itself; questions of increased risk of varicella-zoster in adults; and safety, efficacy, and storage issues (Watson & Haupt, 1997). Twenty-year studies in Japan and 10-year studies in the United States have indicated persistent immunity. This could be due to two factors: vaccine efficacy and/or persistent immunity secondary to natural "boosters" by continuing wild-virus circulation (Asano, Suga, Yoshikawa, Kobayashi, Yasaki, et al., 1994; Kuter, Weibal, Guess, Matthews, Morton, et al., 1991; Watson, Gupta, Randall, & Starr, 1994; Watson, Pierey, Plotkin, et al., 1993). Long-term followup studies are continuing, but if questions persist and if the evidence indicates, a recommendation to repeat the dose in adoglescence may be made (Plotkin, 1996, Red Book, 2000, p. 633). Breakthrough disease following immunization, another concern, is generally mild and occurs at a very low rate, 110 to 150 cases in 11,000 children vaccinated since 1981 (Watson & Haupt, 1997). When a rash develops following vaccination, the transmission of the virus to household contacts is approximately 17%. In those cases, the household contacts had direct contact with the vaccinee's rash. There is no documentation of airborne spread (Red Book, 2000, p. 633; Watson & Haupt, 1997).

Studies have shown the risk of varicella-zoster to be decreased in persons who have received the varicella vaccine, rather than increased as some have feared. During varicella virus infection, the virus descends from skin lesions to the dorsal root ganglia, entering a latent phase. Zoster occurs when the virus reactivates (Plotkin, 1996). Since some skin lesions may appear following varicella immunization, the virus may migrate to the dorsal root ganglia, leading to the potential for zoster infection; however, fewer ganglia would be infected than in the case of wild-virus infection. Also, the incidence of rash following immunization is low, less than 6% overall, so the long-term effect of the varicella vaccine may be a decrease in the incidence of zoster (Plotkin, 1996, Watson & Haupt, 1997). All cases of zoster reported to date (8 in more than 9000 vaccinated children and 1 case in more than 1500 adolescents and adults vaccinated) have been mild and not associated with complications, such as postherpetic neuralgia. The rate reported in children is four to five times less than occurs in zoster following natural varicella infection (CDC, 2002a).

The most compelling argument for widespread childhood vaccination is the effect of immunization on wild-virus transmission. If the majority of children are vaccinated, adults will have decreased exposure to wild virus. The net effect will be to decrease the incidence of disease in children and adults. The incidence will be further decreased if present recommendations to immunize susceptible adults and children over age 13 are followed (Plotkin, 1996).

The most common complications following immunization are injection-site complaints (pain, redness, and swelling) and fever. Less common are rash at the site and generalized rash (Red Book, 2000, p. 633; Watson & Haupt, 1997).

HEPATITIS B

The hepatitis B virus (HBV) is a hepadnavirus that can cause acute and/or chronic infection. The mortality rate of acute fulminant hepatitis, which occurs in 1 to 2% of those with acute hepatitis, is 63 to 93%. Chronic disease occurs in approximately 10% of acute hepatitis cases. Infants are much more likely to become HBV carriers after acquiring HBV infection from their mothers at birth (90%) than adults with acute hepatitis leading to the chronic carrier state (6–10%). Thirty percent to 50% of HBV-infected children become carriers. Twenty-five percent of carriers develop chronic active hepatitis, which often leads to cirrhosis, and the rate of liver cancer in persons with chronic infection is 12 to 300 times that of noncarriers. Dialysis patients and persons with certain immunodeficiency diseases (e.g., HIV) develop the chronic carrier state following acute hepatitis at a higher rate than previously healthy persons (CDC, 2002a; Mahoney & Kane, 1999; Red Book, 2000, p. 289–290).

HBV infection occurs more frequently in Pacific Islanders, Alaskan natives, persons receiving multiple transfusions of blood and blood products, persons engaging in high-risk behaviors (multiple sexual partners, intravenous drug abusers), and immigrants from other countries with high rates of hepatitis B infection (Africa, Asia, parts of the Middle East, and the Amazon Basin, in particular) (AAP Committee on Infectious Diseases, 1992; CDC 2002a; Krugman & Stevens, 1994). Four percent of cases occur secondary to household contact with a chronic carrier, and 2% of cases occur in healthcare workers. Twenty-five percent of cases have no identifiable risk factors (CDC, 2002a). The incidence in the United States peaked in 1985 with approximately 70 cases per 100,000 population; the rate was approximately 40 cases per 100,000 in 1992 (CDC, 2002a) and estimated total of 79,000 cases in 2001 (CDC, 2002b).

Acute hepatitis B is transmitted by parenteral or mucosal exposure to blood and blood products, contaminated needles and syringes, tattooing, hemodialysis, oral surgery, semen, intimate sexual contact, and perinatally. Hepatitis B may be transmitted through contact between broken skin and contaminated blood and saliva (bites). It does not appear to be transmitted by kissing or by contact with body fluids with a lower concentration of HBV, such as tears, sweat, urine, stool, or respiratory droplets. Also, touching contaminated surfaces and then touching skin lesions or mucous membranes may be a source of infection (CDC, 2002a).

Acute hepatitis B infection may be subclinical and virtually asymptomatic. The incubation period is from 6 weeks to 6 months postexposure. The prodromal phase is characterized by fever, headache, malaise, anorexia, nausea and vomiting, right upper quadrant pain, myalgia, arthralgia, arthritis and skin rashes, and dark urine. Diarrhea or constipation may occur. One to 2 days later, jaundice appears and the person develops hepatomegaly with tenderness and light or grey stools. This phase generally lasts 1 to 3 weeks. The convalescent phase lasts for weeks or months, and although jaundice, anorexia, and other symptoms disappear, malaise and fatigue may persist. Most cases result in complete recovery and immunity from reinfection (a function of anti-HBs antibody); however, chronic infection may also result. Complications of acute hepatitis B are fulminant hepatitis and chronic infection (CDC, 2002a; Mahoney & Kane, 1999).

Treatment is supportive. Interferon-α is used to treat chronic hepatitis B infection, with a success rate of 25 to 50% (CDC, 2002a). Clearly, prevention is the best option.

Two recombinant hepatitis B vaccines are available in the United States, Recombivax HB and Engerix-B. Both are safe and effective. Initially, immunization was recommended for high-risk groups but was unsuccessful because of the underidentification of risk and lack of preventive healthcare in identified high-risk groups. The present strategy for hepatitis B prevention recommended by the DHHS is fourfold: prenatal testing of all pregnant women for HbsAg, routine vaccination of all newborn infants, vaccination of adolescents, and vaccination of adults at high risk of infection. Prenatal testing of pregnant women will identify infants who need immunoprophylaxis for hepatitis B and household contacts who need vaccination (CDC, 2002a). All initimate and household contacts with carriers should also be immunized.

Since national recommendations were made, many states have mandated the practice and the rates of infant immunization with hepatitis B vaccine have increased. However, barriers still exist, such as the number of shots needed to complete the series, cost, resistance among providers, and the belief among parents that their child is not at risk (Woodruff, Stevenson, Yusuf, Todoroff, Kwong, Rodoroff, et al., 1996). However, the benefits have been documented: HBV transmission among Native American children in Alaska has been interrupted because of the infant immunization program, and preliminary studies indicate a decreased liver cancer rate among vaccinees in Japan (AAP Committee on Infectious Diseases, 1992; Cheng-Liang Lee & Ying-Chin Ko, 1997).

The present recommended schedule for infant immunization is a three-shot series with injections given at birth, 1 to 2 months, and 6 to 18 months of age or at 1 to 2 months, 4 months, and 6 to 18 months of age. The best time for giving preterm infants their first hepatitis B immunization has not been determined, (CDC, 2002a) but at least one study has shown immunization at hospital discharge with the series completed at the appropriate intervals to yield a response-to-immunization rate of 90%. Nonresponders in that study had higher birth weights and gestational ages and gained less weight before vaccine initiation than responders, but after a fourth dose, they responded with seroconversion (Kim, Chung, Hodinka, De Maio, West, et al., 1997). Other previous studies had shown suboptimal response rates that seemed to be somewhat dependent on weight at vaccine initiation, which led to an AAP recommendation to delay immunization in preterm infants until hospital discharge or 2 months of age (Kim et al., 1997). Kim et al. (1997) suggest that based on the present data, preterm infants receive anti-HBs serologies following immunization to determine seroconversion status and the need for a fourth shot. Infants (term and preterm) born to HbsAg-positive mothers need to receive immunoprophylaxis with hepatitis B immune globulin and hepatitis B vaccine at birth or as soon as possible thereafter (CDC, 2002a).

A combination vaccine of hepatitis B and *Haemophilus* influenza type B vaccines (COMVAX) is approved for use in children. It may be given at 2, 4, and 12 to 15 months of age (Clinician Reviews, 1997). TWINRIX is the combination hepatitis A and hepatitis B vaccine approved by the FDA in May 2001. It is administered at 0, 1, and 6 months, with the same dosing intervals as recommended for the hepatitis B vaccine. TWINRIX is approved for adults aged 18 and older (CDC, 2002a).

The recommended vaccine schedule for children and adults is a three-shot series, given at time 0, 1 month later, and then 2 to 12 months later. Dialysis patients and immunocompromised patients may require a fourth dose. Postvaccination testing for immunity may be useful in those groups and for persons at occupational risk for exposure to hepatitis B (CDC, 2002a). Postvaccination testing may also be useful in persons who are more likely to be nonresponders: aged over 40 years, male, obese, a smoker, those who suffer from chronic illness, those who received hepatitis B vaccine in the buttock, those who received incorrect doses of vaccine, and/or those who were not vaccinated according to the recommended intervals (CDC, 2002a).

The vaccine is always given intramuscularly, and the dose varies according to the vaccine selected. That information is available on the package insert supplied with the vaccine. Hepatitis B vaccine may be safely given at the same time as diphtheria, tetanus, and pertussis (DTP), diphtheria, tetanus, acellular pertussis (DtaP), HIB, polio, and MMR vaccines (AAP Committee on Infectious Diseases, 1992, CDC, 2002a).

For unimmunized persons exposed to hepatitis B, hepatitis B immune globulin should be given and hepatitis B vaccination initiated. HBIG should always be given as close as possible to the time of exposure, e.g., immediately after birth or a needlestick. When sexual contact is involved, HBIG should be given within 14 days of the last sexual contact. Household contacts of someone just diagnosed with hepatitis B should be prophylaxed if they are unimmunized infants or contacts that have had identifiable blood exposure such as with shared toothbrushes and razors (CDC, 2002a).

Pregnancy and immunosuppression are not contraindications to vaccination since the vaccine is made of noninfectious HbsAg particles. Data regarding the effects of hepatitis B immunization on the developing fetus are not available, but the risk of severe disease in the mother and chronic infection in the infant is great if the mother acquires hepatitis B in pregnancy. The only known contraindication is that of previous severe allergic reaction to hepatitis B vaccine or a component of the vaccine (CDC, 2002a; Mahoney Kane, 1999).

Adverse events are rare, but include pain at the injection site, fatigue, headache, irritability, and low-grade fever.

ELECTIVE IMMUNIZATIONS FOR SELECTED INFECTIOUS DISEASES

INFLUENZA

Influenza viruses (Orthomyxoviridae family) are highly contagious and cause serious and sometimes fatal illness, primarily in persons over age 65. There are three known basic antigen types—A, B, and C. Type A has three hemagglutinin subtypes (H1, H2, and H3) and two neuraminidase subtypes (N1 and N2). Influenza A causes moderate to severe illness in all age groups and can infect animals as well as humans. Influenza B, which is more stable antigenically than type A, causes milder disease and affects only humans, primarily children. Type C only affects humans, and most cases are subclinical. Type A demonstrates high antigenic variability (type B to a lesser extent), which leads to epidemics of new variants of influenza viruses each year. The mortality rate from influenza and related complications is high—an influenza A pandemic in 1918–1919 caused an estimated 20 million deaths and in nine U.S. epidemics from 1972–1973 to 1991–1992, more than 20,000 deaths occured in each season. In each of four of those epidemics, more than

40,000 deaths occurred; more than 90% of those deaths were among persons over age 65 (CDC, 1997g; Maassab, Herlocker & Brant 1999).

Influenza is manifested by sudden onset of fever, myalgia, sore throat, and nonproductive cough. Rhinorrhea, headache, chest burning, intestinal symptoms, and ocular symptoms may also occur. Influenza viruses A, B, and C are not the cause of the viral intestinal illnesses characterized by fever, vomiting, diarrhea, and myalgia that most refer to as the "flu" or the "intestinal flu." Various other infectious agents are involved in those illnesses. The healthcare provider needs to clearly communicate to clients the difference between the two types of illnesses and the prevention and treatment of each.

Complications of influenza include secondary bacterial pneumonia (most common complication) and primary influenza viral pneumonia, which is less common but carries a high fatality rate. Myocarditis and worsening of chronic pulmonary diseases are also complications. Reye's syndrome may occur in children and may be associated with type B influenza (CDC, 2002a).

Treatment is supportive; there is no known cure. The antivirals amantadine hydrochloride and rimantadine hydrochloride are available for treatment within 48 h of the onset of symptoms. They are not curative, but may reduce the duration of fever and other symptoms. When used prophylactically, they are 70 to 90% effective in warding off infection; however, they are only effective against influenza type A. Rimantadine generally causes fewer side effects in the elderly than amantadine (CDC, 2002a). Zanamivir and Oseltamivir are approved for the treatment of influenza A and B. As with amantidine & rimantadine, they should be given within 48 h of the onset of symptoms. Oseltamivir is also approved for influenza prophylaxis (CDC, 2002a).

Inactivated whole-virus and split-virus vaccines are available in the United States. The split-virus vaccine, also labeled as *subvirion* or *purified-surface-antigen* vaccine, has a lower potential for causing febrile reactions and therefore should be used for children less than 12 years of age. Adults may be given either the split-virus or whole-virus vaccine. Each year the vaccine is reformulated according to the strains that are thought to be likely to circulate in the upcoming year. The vaccine contains three strains, usually two type A and one type B, and is only good for the year for which it is formulated. For example, the vaccine for the 1997–1998 "flu season" contained A/Bayern/07/95-like (H1N1), A/Wuhan/ 359/95-like (H3N2), and B/Beijing/184/93-like hemagglutinin antigens. U.S. manufacturers used antigenically equivalent strains for the above antigens—A/Johannesburg/82/96 (H1N1), A/Nanchang/933/95 (H3N2), and B/Harbin/ 07/94 (CDC, 1997j). The strains are identified by virus type, A or B; geographic origin, eg, Johannesburg; strain number, eg, 82; year of isolation, e.g., 96; and virus subtype, eg, H1N1 (CDC, 1997j; 2002a). The vaccine should be given only in the year for which it is developed; otherwise, the vaccine will not confer adequate protection. The vaccine is 90% effective in healthy young adults when the vaccine strain is similar to the circulating strain. Efficacy in the elderly has been estimated to be 40 to 60%; however, it is 50 to 60% effective in preventing hospitalization and 80% effective in preventing death in immunized elderly who develop clinical illness (CDC, 2002a). A nasal inhalation influenza vaccine, cold-adapted influenza vaccine (CAIV) FluMist™, received FDA approval and became widely available for use in the Fall of 2003. The vaccine was approved for use in persons aged 5 to 49. Special considerations included cautioning recipients to avoid close contact with immunosuppressed or other vulnerable persons due to the risk of transmitted the weakened vaccine virus. On-going studies to determine whether CAIV is more or less effective in protecting against influenza infection than the injectable trivalent influenza vaccine are being conducted.

Persons targeted for immunization include persons aged 65 or older; persons over 6 months of age with chronic illnesses such as asthma, emphysema, cardiovascular disease, HIV disease, and immunosuppression; residents of long-term care facilities; and persons aged 6 months to 18 years receiving chronic aspirin therapy. Pregnant women should be immunized, preferably after the first trimester, unless high-risk conditions are present and the influenza season will begin during the first trimester. Because no major systemic effects are associated with the vaccine, the vaccine is not a live-virus vaccine, and data on more than 2000 pregnancies have not shown adverse fetal effects, it is thought to be safe during pregnancy. In addition, persons who have contact with the above high-risk populations, such as healthcare workers, caretakers, and household contacts, should receive influenza immunizations. The Advisory Committee on Immunization Practices recommends that children aged 6 to 23 months and their household contacts be immunized against influenza. This age group is at risk for hospitalization if infected with influenza (CDC, 2002a). Foreign travelers should also be immunized, since influenza viruses are present worldwide and may occur at different times of the year. Travelers may contact the CDC or local health department for information regarding influenza activity in the country or countries of interest (CDC, 2002a).

The influenza vaccine should be administered from October through mid-November, but may be given as early as September and at any time during the influenza season. October through mid-November is the optimal time because the influenza season usually peaks between late December and early March, and antibody levels in some vaccinated persons may begin to decline within a few months of vaccine administration. Therefore, the vaccine should be given 4 to 6 weeks prior to the date of anticipated outbreak (CDC, 1997g). One dose of the vaccine is sufficient; however, previously unvaccinated (against influenza) children aged 9 years or less should be given two doses 1 month apart to ensure adequate antibody response. The second dose should be given prior to December, if possible (CDC, 1997g).

Adverse effects are few, but include pain, redness, and induration at the injection site. Mild systemic effects, such as fever, malaise, and myalgia, have also been reported. Immediate hypersensitivity reactions are rare.

Contraindications to vaccination with influenza virus are severe egg allergy and allergy to other vaccine components, primarily thimerosal. The Murphy and Strunk (1985) protocol for influenza vaccination may be considered for those with severe egg allergy and medical conditions that place them at high risk for complications of influenza. Intradermal skin tests may be performed first to determine egg protein sensitivity. Those with negative skin tests results may receive the vaccine. Those with positive skin tests results may be immunized with small doses of diluted and then undiluted vaccine in 15-min intervals. Emergency equipment for immediate resuscitation in case of anaphylactic reaction must be available (Murphy & Strunk, 1985).

PNEUMOCOCCAL DISEASE

Streptococcus pneumoniae, also called pneumococcus, causes pneumococcal disease, most commonly manifested as pneumonia, bacteremia, and/or meningitis. It also causes 30 to 60% of episodes of acute otitis media in children. Pneumococcus is the most common cause of nursing home-acquired pneumonia, and it accounts for 50% of hospital-acquired pneumonia and up to 36% of community-acquired pneumonia (CDC, 1997d, 2002a). Children under 2 years of age and persons 65 years of age and older are at higher risk for developing pneumococcal infection. The elderly have a higher complication and fatality rate following pneumococcal infection than do previously healthy children and adults. Pneumococcal meningitis is seen more often in blacks, and pneumococcal disease occurs more often in males than females (CDC, 1997h, 2002a, p. 179)

Symptoms of pneumococcal pneumonia include sudden onset of fever and shaking chills, with cough, pleuritic chest pain, malaise, weakness, tachycardia, tachypnea, and dyspnea developing shortly thereafter. Sputum is mucopurulent and rusty in color. Symptoms of pneumococcal meningitis are similar to other forms of bacterial meningitis—fever, headache, lethargy, nausea, vomiting, nuchal rigidity, and irritability. Cranial nerve signs, seizures, and coma may follow. Pneumococcus is transmitted by droplets and by "autoinoculation" from the upper respiratory tract (CDC, 2002a).

Pneumococcal infections are treated with penicillin (drug of choice) or cephalosporins for penicillin-allergic people. Erythromycin may be prescribed for pneumonia and ceftriaxone or chloramphenicol (not the drug of choice) for meningitis. However, penicillin-resistant strains are emerging, and resistance to other antibiotics is also rising in the United States and in other parts of the world (CDC, 1997h; Fedson, Musher, & Eskola, 1999).

Two 23-valent polysaccharide pneumococcal vaccines are available in the United States, Pneumovax 23 and Pnu Immune 23. Eighty-five to ninety percent of the serotypes causing invasive pneumococcal disease in children and adults in the United States are represented in the 23-valent vaccines. Although studies have yielded inconsistent results regarding efficacy in preventing pneumonia, the 23-valent vaccines have been shown to be 60 to 70% effective in preventing invasive disease (CDC, 1997h, 2002a). Eighty percent or more of healthy young adults receiving the vaccine develop an antigen-specific antibody response; although how this response correlates with protection against disease hasn't been shown (CDC, 1997h). The vaccine generates poor antibody response to most of the serotypes in children less than 2 years of age. Children aged 2 to 5 years may have inconsistent responses to some of the common pediatric serotypes (CDC, 1997h); however, a study of a 5-valent pneumococcal vaccine given in three doses to children younger than 2 years with and without HIV infection demonstrated the vaccines to be safe and immunogenic for all children receiving the vaccine (King et al., 1997). A 7-valent pneumoccal conjugate vaccine, PREVNAR, is available and recommended for children aged 2 months to 2 years. It is administered following the same schedule as DtaP for the first 4 injections of the series. Recently, due to vaccine shortages, the AAP recommended with holding the 3rd & 4th doses of the vaccine in healthy, low-risk children. Children at high risk for complications of invasive pneumococcal disease should still receive the 4 shot series. (CDC, March 2, 2004) This is very important because 80% of childhood pneumococcal disease occurs in this age group (CDC, 2002a). Antibody response to the 23-valent vaccine also is poor or absent in immunocompromised individuals over age 2. More study involving repeated doses of vaccine in cases likely to be unresponsive to a single dose needs to be done.

The Advisory Committee on Immunization Practices (ACIP) of CDC recommends that the 23-valent vaccine be given to all persons aged 65 years and over, persons aged 2 years and over with chronic illness, persons aged 2 years and over with functional or anatomic asplenia, persons aged 2 years and over living in environments in which the risk for disease is high, and immunocompromised persons aged 2 years and over at high risk for developing infection (CDC, 1997h). Risk factors in otherwise immunocompetent individuals include chronic cardiovascular diseases, chronic pulmonary diseases, chronic liver diseases, diabetes mellitus, persons with functional or anatomic asplenia, and children with sickle cell disease. Asthma is not associated with increased risk for pneumococcal disease unless it occurs with other chronic pulmonary disease or long-term systemic corticosteroid use (CDC, 1997h).

Serotype-specific antibody levels decline 5 to 10 years following vaccination and decrease more rapidly in some groups than others. How this affects protection against disease is unknown (CDC, 1997h). One study demonstrated that protection may last for at least 9 years following initial vaccination (Butler, Breiman, Campbell, Lipman, Broome, et al., 1993), but more studies are needed. At the present time, ACIP recommends revaccination for those 2 years or older at greatest risk for serious pneumococcal infection "and for those who are likely to have a rapid decline in pneumococcal antibody levels, provided that 5 years have elapsed since receipt of the first dose of pneumococcal vaccine" (CDC, 1997h). Children aged 10 and younger considered to be at highest risk for severe pneumococcal disease should be revaccinated after 3 years. Persons 65 years old and older should be revaccinated if they received the first dose before age 65 and 5 years or more have passed since the first dose. Those at highest risk for rapid antibody decline after initial vaccination are those with functional or anatomic asplenia, nephrotic syndrome, renal failure, renal transplantation, leukemia, lymphoma, Hodgkin's disease, multiple myeloma, generalized malignancy, other conditions associated with immunosuppression, and those receiving immunosuppressive chemotherapy, including long-term systemic corticosteroids. If vaccination status is unknown, those in the above categories should receive the pneumococcal vaccine (CDC, 1997h).

Local reactions such as redness, pain, and swelling are the most common adverse reactions to vaccine. Very few experience fever, muscle aches, and severe local reactions. Severe allergic reactions are very rare—about 5 in every 1 million doses (CDC, 2002a).

A history of severe allergic reaction to a previous dose of pneumococcal vaccine or a vaccine component (phenol or thimerosal in pneumococcal vaccines) and moderate to severe illness are contraindications to vaccination. Pregnant women should not be given pneumococcal vaccine since the safety of pneumococcal vaccine in pregnancy has not been evaluated. Ideally, women at high risk for pneumococcal disease should be vaccinated before pregnancy (CDC, 2002a).

HEPATITIS A

Hepatitis A is a hepatovirus (Picornaviridae family) that generally causes mild disease in those infected. Infected children under age 5 are usually asymptomatic; those acquiring the disease after puberty usually exhibit clinical symptoms. The incubation period is about 1 month with a range of 15 to 45 days. Symptoms include sudden onset of fever (usually low-grade), malaise, nausea, headache, myalgia, and arthralgia. The disease is transmitted by contaminated food and water and is more common in countries with poor sanitation. Diagnosis depends upon laboratory testing to differentiate hepatitis A from other forms of viral hepatitis. Hepatitis A disease can be prolonged over several months, but never develops into chronic liver disease. Recovery from hepatitis A confers life-long immunity. Treatment is supportive (CDC, 2002a).

Passive immunization with standard, pooled human immune globulins is available and is about 85% effective; however, the duration of immunity is only 2 to 5 months, depending upon the dose given. An inactive hepatitis A vaccine is available for active immunization of those at risk for hepatitis A disease and for travelers. The vaccine is approximately 90% effective in adults following a single dose of the vaccine; however, immunity may wane after 1 year. Therefore, a booster shot 6 to 12 months after the first shot is recommended for adults, primarily those who are frequent travelers and/or those planning to stay abroad for extended periods. The recommended schedule for children aged 2 to 17 calls for a primary dose with a booster dose 6 to 12 months later. Immunity is thought to last for 10 years following a booster dose (CDC, 2002a; *Clinician Reviews,* 1996; Feinstein, & Gust, 1999; Nettleman, 1993).

It is unknown if the hepatitis A vaccine is harmful to a fetus; however, because it is an inactivated virus, the risk is thought to be low. The provider should evaluate the risk-benefit profile based on the individual client's situation. The vaccine may be safely given to immunocompromised persons because it is inactivated (CDC, 2002a).

Side effects include soreness at the injection site, headache, and malaise in adults and soreness or induration at the injection site, feeding problems, and headache in children. No serious adverse reactions have been reported (CDC, 2002a).

MENINGOCOCCAL DISEASE

Meningococcal disease is caused by *Neisseria meningitidis,* a gram-negative bacillus. It primarily manifests as meningitis and meningococcemia, although myocarditis, endocarditis, pericarditis, conjunctivitis, pharyngitis, urethritis, and cervicitis may also be seen. Meningococcemia begins with sudden onset of fever, malaise, myalgia, headache, and often vomiting and diarrhea. A maculopapular rash occurs in most cases, and it progresses to a petechial rash. Meningococcal septicemia may lead to hypotension, disseminated intravascular coagulation (DIC), and death. In cases of meningococcal meningitis, meningeal signs, vomiting, headache, and petechial rash are common (Lepow, Perkins, Hughes, & Poolman, 1999). The mortality rate for meningococcal meningitis is 13% and 11.5% for meningococcal septicemia (CDC, 1997b). *N. meningitidis* is transmitted by the respiratory system; carriers are asymptomatic.

The antibiotic of choice in managing meningococcal disease is aqueous penicillin G. Ceftriaxone also is highly effective; chloramphenicol and cefotaxime are other antibiotics that can be successfully used. Small doses of dexamethasone may be given in meningitis cases before antibiotic therapy is initiated and continued for 14 days to reduce the chance of deafness and to alleviate other central nervous system symptoms. Supportive therapy to manage shock and DIC may also be necessary (Lepow et al., 1999). Close contacts of persons with meningococcal disease should be prophylaxed as soon as possible after onset of disease in the primary patient with oral rifampin or intramuscular ceftriaxone. Ciprofloxacin is an acceptable alternative for prophylaxis in nonpregnant, nonlactating adults. Both rifampin and ciprofloxacin are contraindicated in pregnancy; ceftriaxone is not. Children should not be given ciprofloxacin unless no alternative is available (CDC, 1997b, 2002a).

Persons with underlying medical conditions, immunosuppressed persons, persons with immunocompromising disease, and persons with asplenia are at increased risk for meningococcal disease. The disease used to be common in military recruits, but the rates have decreased dramatically due to immunization of all military recruits (CDC, 1997b, 2002a). The rates of meningococcal disease are highest in children 3 to 12 months of age (CDC, 1997b, 2002a).

A quadrivalent polysaccharide vaccine, Menomune, is available in the United States and should be administered to those considered to be at high risk for disease, especially those with functional or anatomic asplenia and those with terminal complement component deficiency diseases. This vaccine contains the four serogroups known to cause meningococcal disease in humans—A, C, Y, and W-135. Serogroups B and C account for most of the meningococcal disease in the United States, although the proportion of cases caused by Y strains is increasing (CDC, 1997b, 2002a).

The vaccine is ineffective in children under 2 years of age, but may be given to children as young as 3 months of age in cases where the child is at high risk for infection. If given to infants and young children, two doses 3 months apart should be administered. Antibody levels in adults have been shown to decline in 2 to 3 years; therefore, revaccination may be considered if necessary within 3 to 5 years. The vaccine may be given in pregnancy.

Vaccines have been developed to target serogroups A and C, and serogroup B alone. New vaccines for serogroups A and C have yet to be evaluated. Serogroup B vaccines have been evaluated, and efficacy is estimated to be 57 to 83% in older children and adults. However, efficacy is poor in children under 4, who have the highest rate of disease. None of the serogroup B vaccines are licensed for use in the United States (CDC, 1997b, 2002a).

RABIES

Clinical rabies is rare in the United States, primarily because of the routine vaccination of dogs and cats. However, infected wild animals such as skunks, raccoons, bats, and foxes constitute a continuing source of human risk. Bites or scratches from those animals and infected, unvaccinated domesticated animals may transmit the rabies virus to humans, causing encephalitis and death in most cases. By 1994, there were only five known cases of survival from rabies infection, three of whom suffered long-term sequelae (Plotkin, Rupprecht, & Koprowski, 1999). Children are at high risk due to their animal-friendly behavior, although all age groups are equally at risk of contracting the disease with exposure. Raccoons are the primary reservoirs of rabies in the mid-Atlantic and southeastern states, skunks in the north and south central states and California, the gray fox in Arizona and Texas, the coyote in Texas, and the arctic fox and red fox in Alaska and upper New York state. Dogs along the U.S.-Mexico border are also likely to be infected (Phelps, 1997). Rodents, such as squirrels, hamsters, and guinea pigs, and lagomorphs (hares and rabbits) are generally not a source of infection, but groundhogs may be a source of infection (Phelps, 1997).

Corneal transplantation was a source of infection in six cases. Two cases were acquired from airborne exposure in the laboratory, and two were acquired from airborne exposure in bat-infested caves (Phelps, 1997). The clinician should ask about these potential sources of infection when attempting to rule out rabies disease.

Rabies has an incubation period of 20 to 90 days (range 4 days to 19 years) and initial clinical manifestations are relatively nonspecific (Phelps, 1997). If the initial injury is in the head or face, the incubation period is shorter. The initial symptoms in humans include headache, malaise, anorexia, fatigue, fever, and pain or paresthesia at the site of exposure (Phelps, 1997; Plotkin et al., 1999). Anxiety, apprehension, irritability, insomnia, and depression also may occur. Following the prodrome, hyperactivity, disorientation, hallucinations, seizures, bizarre behavior, nuchal stiffness, and paralysis develop and may occur intermittently and be associated with stimulation. Hydrophobia occurs in most cases. Other manifestations that may appear are hyperventilation, muscle fasciculations, and hypersalivation (Phelps, 1997; Plotkin et al., 1999). In some cases, the patient may not exhibit the hyperactivity and other irritable CNS signs. Instead, paralysis appears and the disease progresses to stupor and coma (Phelps, 1997). The course of illness is rapid, less than 2 weeks. Death may occur suddenly after cardiac and respiratory arrest, or more gradually following the development of coma and use of intensive life support (Phelps, 1997; Plotkin et al., 1999).

Preexposure prophylaxis with three intramuscular doses of 1 mL of human diploid cell vaccine (HDCV) or rabies vaccine adsorbed (RVA) on days 0, 7, and 21 or 28 or three intradermal doses of 0.1 mL of HDCV on days 0, 7, and 28 may be initiated in persons at high risk for exposure. Those persons include anyone who works with domestic or wild animals such as veterinarians, animal handlers, animal control workers, and wildlife workers; spelunkers who are exposed to bat-infested caves; those who handle live rabies virus in laboratories, and travelers to countries where rabies is endemic in dogs (CDC, 1999a, Phelps, 1997). If the person must also take antimalarials before traveling to a rabies-enzootic area, the intradermal HDCV therapy should be initiated at least 1 month prior to traveling, or the intramuscular route used, because chloroquine phosphate (and perhaps other antimalarials) interferes with the antibody response to intradermal HDCV (CDC, 1999a). Booster doses must be given if exposure to rabid animals occurs or if immunity has waned as determined by serologic tests of antibody levels (CDC, 1999a, Phelps, 1997).

Postexposure treatment is available and must be initiated as soon as possible following exposure. The challenge is to identify the exposure and match clinical symptoms with the possible cause, because in some cases no known exposure can be documented. Then the risk that the animal was infected must be considered. In two cases identified by Phelps (1997), a bite or scratch apparently did not occur. In one case, a bat was found in a child's bedroom, and in another, a man opened the mouth of a dead bat to examine the teeth. Once a bite or scratch has occured and the risk for infection is determined to be high, the wound should be washed thoroughly with soap and water. Human rabies immune globulin (HRIG) should be administered immediately, one-half dose directly in the wound and the remainder injected intramuscularly in the gluteal area. Human diploid cell vaccine (HCDC) must also be administered intramuscularly in the deltoid or anterior thigh in small children (never in the buttocks in any client) on days 0, 3, 7, 14, and 28 (CDC, 1999; Phelps, 1997). Protocols for intradermal injection have been developed and also are effective, as well as less expensive. Treatment may be delayed for up to 48 h while awaiting laboratory test results (if the animal causing the injury was caught), when the risk of infection is determined to be low as in the case of a dog bite when the vaccination status of the dog is unknown (Phelps, 1997). However, when in doubt, treat. Treatment may be halted if laboratory tests show the animal was not infected with rabies.

When a person has been previously treated with HDCV, either as preexposure or postexposure prophylaxis, a two-dose schedule may be followed with HDCV given on days 0 and 3, without HRIG (CDC, 1999). If other rabies vaccines were used for previous vaccination and antibody response has been documented, the two-dose schedule with HDCV may be followed. If antibody response has not been documented, the full postexposure schedule with HDCV and HRIG must be followed (Plotkin et al., 1999).

Pain, redness, swelling, and itching at the injection site are the most common reactions seen. Systemic reactions, such as headache, nausea, muscle aches, dizziness, and abdominal pain may also occur. Immune-complex-like reactions, including itching, arthralgia, arthritis, allergic edema, nausea, vomiting, malaise, and fever may occur after booster doses. Guillain-Barré-like illness has been reported in three cases, it resolved without sequelae (Phelps, 1997). If an allergic reaction to HDCV is observed, an alternative vaccine such as RVA may be given since it has a different tissue origin. Prophylactic antihistamines may be used for those with a history of severe allergies, and epinephrine should be available if needed when those persons are vaccinated. Those receiving steroids or other immunosuppressive medications should have antibody levels checked following vaccination. Pregnancy is not a contraindication to rabies vaccination (Plotkin et al., 1999).

Contact the local or state health department or the rabies section of the Centers for Disease Control (404-639-1050 or 1075) for more information and advice on diagnosis and treatment.

TUBERCULOSIS

Tuberculosis (TB) disease, caused by *Mycobacterium tuberculosis,* accounts for most death and disease in the world. It causes serious illness in those who develop active disease. Many are asymptomatic at the onset of infection and develop symptoms from months to years after primary infection with *M. tuberculosis.* This is referred to as reactivation, postprimary, adult-type, or reinfection tuberculosis. Initially, symptoms are mild and include mild cough, night sweats, malaise, weight loss, fatigue, irritability, and low-grade fever. The disease may ultimately progress to severe pulmonary disease, disseminated tuberculosis, and/or tuberculous meningitis leading to death if untreated. Early detection often is difficult because in both of those manifestations of TB, tuberculin skin tests may be negative and chest radiographs may be normal (Smith & Starke, 1999).

In Europe and the United States, improving sanitation, living conditions, and socioeconomic conditions led to the decline in deaths from tuberculosis. Conditions that favor transmission of the disease are crowded living and working conditions, war, famine, and population displacement (as in refugee situations). There is also an association between the development of tuberculosis and infection with human immunodeficiency virus (HIV).

Treatment is available with antibiotics; however, drug-resistant strains of *M. tuberculosis* are proliferating, especially among the population infected with HIV. While the available vaccine, bacille Calmette-Guérin (BCG), has never been used in the United States, its use may be considered now because of the rapid development of drug resistance. Unfortunately, studies regarding the efficacy of the BCG vaccine have yielded widely varying results, probably because of the nature of tuberculosis disease and the lack of reliable serological markers for immunity to mycobacteria. The effects on tuberculous disease of nontuberculous mycobacteria, which are prevalent in the environment, are unknown. Their immunologic effects on humans may contribute in some way to the prevention and control of tuberculosis (Smith & Starke, 1999). Studies done in areas in which the prevalence of environmental mycobacteria is low have yielded high vaccine efficacy rates. Conversely, studies done in areas of high mycobacteria prevalence have yielded the lowest efficacy rates (Smith & Starke, 1999).

The primary method of controlling tuberculosis disease spread in the United States is by skin-testing children at 12 months of age, school entry (age 4 or 5), and other significant events such as college entry or at the time of employment in certain companies; aggressive investigation of known case contacts; and prophylactically treating those with positive skin tests and/or chest radiographs without clinical evidence of disease. BCG vaccine is recommended only in cases where the risk of transmission of TB from intimate and prolonged exposure is high and the noninfected person cannot be removed from the environment, and in groups with high TB infection rates. BCG vaccine causes local reactions, including scarring and lymphadenitis. It should not be given to immunocompromised individuals, those with HIV infection, or those who are pregnant. More research into the use of BCG in HIV-infected persons and into the development of new, more effective tuberculosis vaccines is needed if we hope to more adequately protect people from and eliminate tuberculosis disease (Smith & Starke, 1999).

See Chapter 22 for more information on diagnosing and treating tuberculosis.

TRAVELER'S IMMUNIZATIONS

Persons traveling abroad are at risk of contracting selected diseases based on the prevalence of those diseases in the country of destination. Persons traveling to developing countries are at increased risk of common diseases generally not seen in the more developed countries with appropriate sanitation and food and water controls. This section will briefly review some of the diseases for which a traveler may be at risk and available vaccines for prevention.

DISEASES ASSOCIATED WITH CONTAMINATED FOOD AND WATER

Cholera, hepatitis A, typhoid fever, and traveler's diarrhea are all associated with ingestion of contaminated food and water and are more prevalent among travelers to developing countries than the developed world. Primary emphasis is placed on prevention by cautioning travelers to avoid eating raw vegetables and fruits and raw or partially cooked shellfish, fish, and meat and to avoid drinking tap water and unpasteurized milk. Ice should be avoided, but beverages made from boiled water are safe. Bottled carbonated beverages are safe; however, the lips of bottles with metal caps may be a source of contamination. Boiling water is the most reliable way to purify it, but using iodine and portable water purifiers is also effective (Nettleman, 1993, 1996).

The majority of persons contracting *cholera* are asymptomatic or experience mild diarrhea for a few days. The cholera vaccine efficacy is approximately 50%, and two doses must be given 1 month apart. Immunity lasts 6 months or less. Because of the inadequate effectiveness of the vaccine, vaccine side effects, and the very low risk of contracting cholera, vaccination is no longer recommended (Nettleman, 1993, 1996; Red Book, 2000, pp. 638–640).

The *hepatitis A* vaccine is safe and efficacious for many years when given in two doses, as noted previously. All travelers to developing countries, especially those who will not be staying in tourist areas, who will be eating in local restaurants, and/or who will stay for an extended period of time, should get the vaccine. Immune globulin is approximately 85% effective in preventing hepatitis A infection when given within 2 months prior to the exposure, and it is another option for travelers. If travel is to occur within 1 month of receiving the first hepatitis A vaccine, the traveler should also receive immune globulin (Barnett, Chen, & Rey, 1999; Nettleman, 1993, 1996).

An inactivated parenteral vaccine and a live attenuated oral vaccine are available for protection against *typhoid fever;* however, neither is 100% effective. Therefore, as with cholera, prevention of exposure is of utmost importance. Studies have shown the efficacy of parenteral typhoid vaccine to be 51 to 77% and 67% or better with oral vaccine. The parenteral vaccine is given in two doses, 4 weeks apart. The oral vaccine is given in four doses, 1 dose every other day. Booster doses are needed every 3 years for the parenteral vaccine and every 5 years for the oral vaccine, although long-term followup data on the oral vaccine are lacking. There is a high incidence of adverse effects with the parenteral vaccine; fewer adverse effects are seen with the oral vaccine. The oral vaccine should not be given to immunocompromised persons and children under 6 years of age; the parenteral vaccine may be given to immunocompromised persons and children over 6 months of age. Safe use of either vaccine in pregnancy has not been established (Barnett, et al., 1999; Levine, 1999; Nettleman, 1996).

Traveler's diarrhea can be caused by a variety of bacteria, most commonly enterotoxigenic *Escherichia coli, Salmonella, Shigella,* and *Campylobacter.* There are no available vaccines for prevention; however, the traveler should have antibiotics available in case diarrhea develops. Adults may take fluoroquinolones or trimethoprim-sulfamethoxazole to treat the diarrhea. Short-term travelers may wish to take daily ciprofloxacin to prevent diarrhea. Antimotility agents, such as Pepto-Bismol, loperamide, or diphenoxylate hydrochloride, may also be used. If bloody diarrhea, severe abdominal pain, or high fever is present, the traveler should not take antimotility agents and should seek medical attention (Nettleman, 1993, 1996; Red Book, 2002, p. 504).

MALARIA, JAPANESE ENCEPHALITIS, AND YELLOW FEVER

Malaria is transmitted by the female *Anopheles* mosquito, *Japanese encephalitis* by the *Culex* mosquito, and yellow fever by the *Aedes* mosquito. Travelers to areas where the above diseases are endemic should take the appropriate precautions to minimize exposure, such as using insect repellants, protective clothing, and mosquito netting. Chloroquine may be taken to reduce the likelihood of acquiring malaria. In areas of chloroquine resistance, mefloquine may be taken; however, it should not be taken by those also taking antiarrhythmics or beta blockers. When these drugs cannot be taken, or when the traveler is going to an area of mefloquine resistance, daily doxycycline may be taken. For travel to areas of chloroquine and mefloquine resistance, or when mefloquine cannot be taken, travelers may take a treatment supply of pyrimethamine-sulfadoxine (Fansidar) with them in case symptoms of illness develop. Primaquine should be given prophylactically to travelers who have had extended stays and significant mosquito exposure in areas where *Plasmodium vivax* or *P. ovale* malaria is endemic. Primaquine is usually taken during the last 2 weeks of chloroquine chemoprophylaxis (Barnett et al., 1999; Nettleman, 1996; Sears & Sack, 1995).

Contact the local or state health department or the CDC for the most current information on areas where malaria is present, and whether the malarial strains are known to be resistant to chloroquine or mefloquine.

An inactivated-virus vaccine is available to protect against *Japanese encephalitis,* prevalent in much of Asia. It should be given to travelers expecting to stay in endemic areas during the seasons in which disease transmission is most likely (May through October) for longer than 1 month. The vaccine is given in three doses (Barnett et al., 1999; Nettleman, 1993, 1996).

Yellow fever occurs in South America and Africa. Travelers to areas with known infected mosquito populations should receive the live attenuated vaccine (Barnett et al., 1999). Some countries require proof of yellow fever vaccination before they will allow travelers to enter. The CDC licenses official vaccination centers where the traveler may receive the vaccine and the International Certificate of Vaccination documenting vaccination against yellow fever (Nettleman, 1996).

MENINGOCOCCAL DISEASE

Travelers to areas where meningococcal disease is prevalent should receive the available polysaccharide capsular vaccine. Meningococcal disease is endemic in sub-Saharan Africa and epidemics have been reported in Brazil, Kenya, Tanzania, and Saudi Arabia. Outbreaks also have occurred in New Delhi and Nepal. Immunization is recommended for travelers to Burundi and northern India (Lepow et al., 1999; Sears & Sack, 1995). The type B serotype causes most of the cases of meningococcal disease in the United States and was the cause of the outbreak in Brazil. Types A and C predominate in other countries. The vaccine is effective against types A, C, Y, and W135. No vaccine against type B is available (Lepow et al., 1999). See the section on elective immunizations for selected infectious diseases for more information about meningococcal disease.

PLAGUE

The average traveler is at very low risk of acquiring human plague (transmitted by fleas on rodents); however, those who will be working or living in close contact with rodents should be immunized (Nettleman, 1996; Sears & Sack, 1995; Tithall, Eley, Williamson & Dennis, 1999).

POLIOMYELITIS

Because poliomyelitis still exists in developing countries, the CDC recommends that travelers to those countries be immunized. If more than 10 years have passed since the primary series was completed, a booster dose of OPV or IPV may be given. In adults who were never immunized, IPV should be given according to the appropriate primary series schedule (CDC, 2002a). See the section on childhood immunizations for more information about polio vaccines.

Travelers should be sure their "routine" immunizations are up-to-date, including diphtheria/ tetanus and rubeola. Influenza and pneumococcal vaccines should be administered to those at risk for those infections (see the section on elective immunizations for selected infectious diseases). Travelers should also be aware of diseases endemic in the countries of destination and precautions that should be taken to avoid exposures. Insect-borne diseases, such as dengue fever, leishmaniasis, filariasis, and Lyme disease, have no available vaccines for protection, therefore, precautions with repellants, appropriate clothing, and netting should be taken. Also, schistosomiasis may be contracted by wading or swimming in fresh water so travelers should swim only in chlorinated pools and salt water, upstream from sewage dumps (Nettleman, 1996; Sears & Sack, 1995).

Healthcare providers should refer questions regarding recommendations for vaccination and precautions for travelers to foreign countries to local or state health departments or the CDC. Additionally, when travelers return from foreign countries with unidentified illness or when illness defying diagnosis presents in patients who have traveled to other countries, healthcare providers should consult with experts in travel medicine and/or infectious diseases and the CDC. Many diseases may appear months to years after exposure, and others are difficult to diagnose because they are uncommon in the United States. Prompt consultation and referral, if necessary, are crucial to ensure appropriate treatment and to prevent complications.

For current information regarding requirements and recommendations for travelers, call the CDC at 404-332-4559. This service is available 24 hours a day, 7 days a week.

BIOTERIORISM

The events of September 11, 2001, brought a renewed, or least a reinvigorated, interest in addressing the risk of bioterrorism. While it is impossible to review all agents that may be used in a biological assault, there are agents of bioterrorism whose spread would be hampered or thwarted by vaccines. Two such agents are smallpox and anthrax. The Centers for Disease Control, in collaboration with other governmental and healthcare agencies, are actively working on increasing vaccine efficacy, safety, and availability for smallpox and anthrax vaccines. They are also developing plans for emergency use of such vaccines and treatments for the diseases should outbreaks occur. Several large-scale meetings involving numerous experts and interested parties were held in May and June 2002 to address what should be done in anticipation of a smallpox attack. There were several recommendations ranging from vaccinating every person to using vaccine only after an outbreak occurs. The most current information on preparedness for an attack is available at www.partnersforimmunization.org. Eventually, hearings will be held regarding developing action plans for other forms of biological assaults. This chapter will focus on the two forms of attack that appear most likely. In fact, the United States has already experienced an anthrax attack, and experts are using lessons learned from that attack to address future possible attacks.

SMALLPOX

Smallpox, also referred to as variola, is caused by the variola virus and is carried only by humans. It is closely related to cowpox, which afflicts cows most often but may also be found in humans. Those infected with cowpox are immune to smallpox. Variola is an Orthopoxvirus. Transmission is by direct droplet contact with nasal and/or orophyngeal membranes. Transmission also occurs through direct contact with linens used by infected persons. Very close contact may also result in alveolar inoculation. Indirect transmission through aerosols or a fomite vector is uncommon but possible (CDC, 2001c).

The initial presentation of smallpox is much like the flue (influenza). Approximately 7 to 17 days following exposure, an individual may experience a 2- to 3-day prodrome of high fever, extreme fatigue, headache, and backache. Following this prodome a maculopapular rash develops on the oral mucosa, face, and forearms and quickly progresses to popular, vesicular, then pustular by the seventh day. Scabbed lesions have formed by the end of 2 weeks. After beginning in the mouth and on the forearms, the rash spreads to the trunk and legs. The period of contagion lasts until all of the scabs have separated, but the individual is most contagious while the oral lesions are active (CDC, 2001c).

The mortality rate of smallpox was approximately 30%; however, it was about 96% for the more severe forms of the disease. One form, the flat-type smallpox is characterized by velvety, flat, confluent lesions, and severe toxemia. The lesions do not become pustular. There is also an hemorrhagic form of smallpox that is virtually always fatal (CDC, 2001c).

The vaccinia vaccine is the vaccine used to immunize the population against smallpox. The vaccine used during the time of active immunization programs was a live-virus vaccine derived from calf lymph. The vaccine presently licensed, Dryvax, contains live vaccinia virus. The vaccinia vaccine is cross-protective for the Orthopoxviruses. Immunity wanes after 5 years but may persist for 10 or more years. Revaccination boosts immunity. The vaccine may be given within the first few days of exposure to smallpox and result in the prevention of the disease or reduced severity of symptoms (CDC, 2001c). This fact has led many investigators to recommend that a "ring-type" vaccination program be implemented should smallpox be reintroduced through bioterrorism. However, the vaccine has serious side effects, particularly among those with immunodeficiency diseases and those with eczema. For this reason, the vaccine is contraindicated for persons with HIV infection, those immunosuppressed by chemotherapeutic agents, those with eczema or other skin conditions, infants, children and pregnant women. VIG (immunoglobulin derived from the plasma of those immunized against vaccinia) is useful in treating severe reactions to the vaccin 2001c).

The United States kept a stockpile of the vaccine following the conclusion of all vaccination programs (the general public in 1972 and the military in 1980) (CDC, 2001c). It has been determined that present stockpiles may be diluted, making fewer doses available than previously thought. Acambis in Cambridge, UK, is manufacturing additional vaccine doses (www.partnersforimmunization.org)

ANTHRAX

Anthrax, a zoonotic disease caused by *Baccillus anthracis,* was first used in a bioterrorist attack in the United States in 2001. Prior to that time, the last reported case of naturally occurring anthrax in a human in United States was reported in 1992 (CDC, 2002a). *B. anthracis* is a gram-positive, spore-forming bacterium whose spores can exist in soil for decades. The spores germinate when they come in contact with a glucose and protein rich environment such as blood and tissue of mammals. The three clinical forms of anthrax, cutaneous, gastrointestinal and inhalational, may all be fatal. Infection with *B. anthracis* results in the production of lethal and edema toxins that lead to tissue necrosis. Infection may result in overwhelming septicemia and meningitis as the bacteria invade the lymphatic system causing necrosis leading to the release of the bacteria into the blood stream and central nervous system. Cutaneous anthrax occurs when the bacterium invades an abrasion or cut in the skin and ultimately results in eschar formation as the lesion progresses from popular to vesicular then ulcerates. Vesicles may develop around the original lesion and adjacent lymph nodes may swell. Fever, malaise, and headache may also be present. The lesions are initially pruritic but painless. Death may occur in up to 20% of cases without antibiotic treatment (CDC, 2002a).

Gastrointestinal transmission of *B. anthracis* occurs following the ingestion of contaminated meat. Pharyngeal lesions and bowel inflammation occur, resulting in sore throat, dysphagia, nausea, vomiting, abdominal pain, hematemesis, and hematochezia. The death rate of GI anthrax is estimated to be 25 to 60% (CDC, 2002a). No gastrointestinal cases of anthrax have been reported in the United States (CDC, 2000b).

Inhalation anthrax results from the inhalation of spores from the air. This may occur from the direct (primary) aerosolization occurring from working with skin or hair from an infected animal or bioterrorist attack. Spores that settle on surfaces may become agitated, yielding a secondary aerosolization of inhalable spores. Larger spores (>5 microns in diameter) settle on surfaces and may become agitated enough to re-enter the air but require a great deal of energy to be aerosolized. Those spores are too large to reach the lower respiratory tract. Smaller particles, >5 microns in diameter, remain in the atmosphere without settling; therefore, secondary aerosolization would not be a threat. The smaller particles are small enough to reach the lower respiratory tract and cause infection (CDC, 2000b, 2002a).

Symptoms of inhalation anthrax are nonproductive cough, myalgia, fatigue, fever, progressing to severe dyspnea, cyanosis, high fever, and shock. Nasal congestion and rhinorrhea are not features of anthrax. Chest X-rays demonstrate pleural effusion and mediastinal widening (from lymphadenopathy). Meningitis may occur. Ten of 11 patients affected by the bioterrorist attack in 2001 experienced profound, drenching sweating. Death may occur within hours of onset of symptoms (CDC, 2002a).

Inhalation anthrax yields the greatest fatality rate, up to 97% without antibiotics. Even with antibiotic treatment, death occurs in up to 75% of cases, however, the fatality rate from the bioterrorist was 45%. The lower death rate is attributed to aggressive, intensive therapy and the use of multiple antibiotics (CDC, 2002a).

The vaccine currently licensed for use in the United States is Anthrax Vaccine Adsorbed (AVA). It does not contain the actual bacteria but cellular products and toxin components adsorbed to aluminum hydroxide. The vaccine is administered subcutaneously in 6 doses; the first 3 at 0, 2, and 4 weeks followed by 3 more doses at 6, 12, and 18 months. Annual boosters are recommended as there is no data on the duration of immunity following the initial vaccine series.

DECISION MAKING REGARDING IMMUNIZATIONS

Special consideration must be given to children, immunocompromised persons, the elderly, and pregnant and lactating women. In addition, those not immunized in childhood according to the routine schedule require special consideration in getting "caught up." Timing and administration of multiple vaccines must also be considered, as well as efficacy when antibody-containing blood products have been administered prior to immunization. Figure 11–2 lists a catch-up schedule for childhood vaccines, and Figure 11–3 is a recommended schedule for adult vaccines by age and medical condition. Whenever a question arises about specific circumstances, such as whether to give a vaccine after an individual has received blood products, when the next dose of a vaccine should be given or if the series needs to be started over, and dosing information, the provider should refer to the package inserts or call the state or local health department or the Centers for Disease Control.

Risks and benefits of vaccine administration must be carefully considered when administering elective vaccines. Most of the more commonly given vaccines yield more benefits than risks and therefore should be administered to those at risk for the diseases prevented by the vaccine. The risk-benefit profile is one of the reasons

For Children and Adolescents Who Start Late or Who Are >1 Month Behind

The tables below give catch-up schedules and minimum intervals between doses for children who have delayed immunizations. There is no need to restart a vaccine series regardless of the time that has elapsed between doses. Use the chart appropriate for the child's age.

Catch-up schedule for children age 4 months through 6 years

Dose 1 (Minimum Age)	Minimum Interval Between Doses			
	Dose 1 to Dose 2	**Dose 2 to Dose 3**	**Dose 3 to Dose 4**	**Dose 4 to Dose 5**
DTaP (6 wk)	4 wk	4 wk	6 mo	6 mo[1]
IPV (6 wk)	4 wk	4 wk	4 wk[2]	
HepB[3] (birth)	4 wk	8 wk (and 16 wk after first dose)		
MMR (12 mo)	4 wk[4]			
Varicella (12 mo)				
Hib[5] (6 wk)	**4 wk:** if first dose given at age <12 mo **8 wk (as final dose):** if first dose given at age 12-14 mo **No further doses needed:** if first dose given at age ≥15 mo	**4 wk**[6]**:** if current age <12 mo **8 wk (as final dose)**[6]**:** if current age ≥12 mo and second dose given at age <15 mo **No further doses needed:** if previous dose given at age ≥15 mo	**8 wk (as final dose):** this dose only necessary for children age 12 mo–5 y who received 3 doses before age 12 mo	
PCV[7]: (6 wk)	**4 wk:** if first dose given at age <12 mo and current age <24 mo **8 wk (as final dose):** if first dose given at age ≥12 mo or current age 24-59 mo **No further doses needed:** for healthy children if first dose given at age ≥24 mo	**4 wk:** if current age <12 mo **8 wk (as final dose):** if current age ≥12 mo **No further doses needed:** for healthy children if previous dose given at age ≥24 mo	**8 wk (as final dose):** this dose only necessary for children age 12 mo–5 y who received 3 doses before age 12 mo	

Catch-up schedule for children age 7 through 18 years

Minimum Interval Between Doses		
Dose 1 to Dose 2	**Dose 2 to Dose 3**	**Dose 3 to Booster Dose**
Td: 4 wk	Td: 6 mo	Td[8]: **6 mo:** if first dose given at age <12 mo and current age <11 y **5 y:** if first dose given at age ≥12 mo and third dose given at age <7 y and current age ≥11 y **10 y:** if third dose given at age ≥7 y
IPV[9]: 4 wk	**IPV**[9]: 4 wk	**IPV**[2,9]
HepB: 4 wk	**HepB: 8 wk** (and 16 wk after first dose)	
MMR: 4 wk		
Varicella[10]: 4 wk		

1. **DTaP:** The fifth dose is not necessary if the fourth dose was given after the fourth birthday.
2. **IPV:** For children who received an all-IPV or all-oral poliovirus (OPV) series, a fourth dose is not necessary if third dose was given at age ≥4 years. If both OPV and IPV were given as part of a series, a total of 4 doses should be given, regardless of the child's current age.
3. **HepB:** All children and adolescents who have not been immunized against hepatitis B should begin the HepB immunization series during any visit. Providers should make special efforts to immunize children who were born in, or whose parents were born in, areas of the world where hepatitis B virus infection is moderately or highly endemic.
4. **MMR:** The second dose of MMR is recommended routinely at age 4 to 6 years but may be given earlier if desired.
5. **Hib:** Vaccine is not generally recommended for children age ≥5 years.
6. **Hib:** If current age <12 months and the first 2 doses were PRP-OMP (PedvaxHIB or ComVax [Merck]), the third (and final) dose should be given at age 12 to 15 months and at least 8 weeks after the second dose.
7. **PCV:** Vaccine is not generally recommended for children age ≥5 years.
8. **Td:** For children age 7 to 10 years, the interval between the third and booster dose is determined by the age when the first dose was given. For adolescents age 11 to 18 years, the interval is determined by the age when the third dose was given.
9. **IPV:** Vaccine is not generally recommended for persons age ≥18 years.
10. **Varicella:** Give 2-dose series to all susceptible adolescents age ≥13 years.

Reporting Adverse Reactions
Report adverse reactions to vaccines through the federal Vaccine Adverse Event Reporting System. For information on reporting reactions following immunization, please visit www.vaers.org or call the 24-hour national toll-free information line (800) 822-7967.

Disease Reporting
Report suspected cases of vaccine-preventable diseases to your state or local health department.

For additional information about vaccines, including precautions and contraindications for immunization and vaccine shortages, please visit the National Immunization Program Web site at www.cdc.gov/nip or call the National Immunization Information Hotline at 800-232-2522 (English) or 800-232-0233 (Spanish).

FIGURE 11–2. "Catch-up" immunization schedule for children and adults not previously immunized according to the routine childhood schedule.

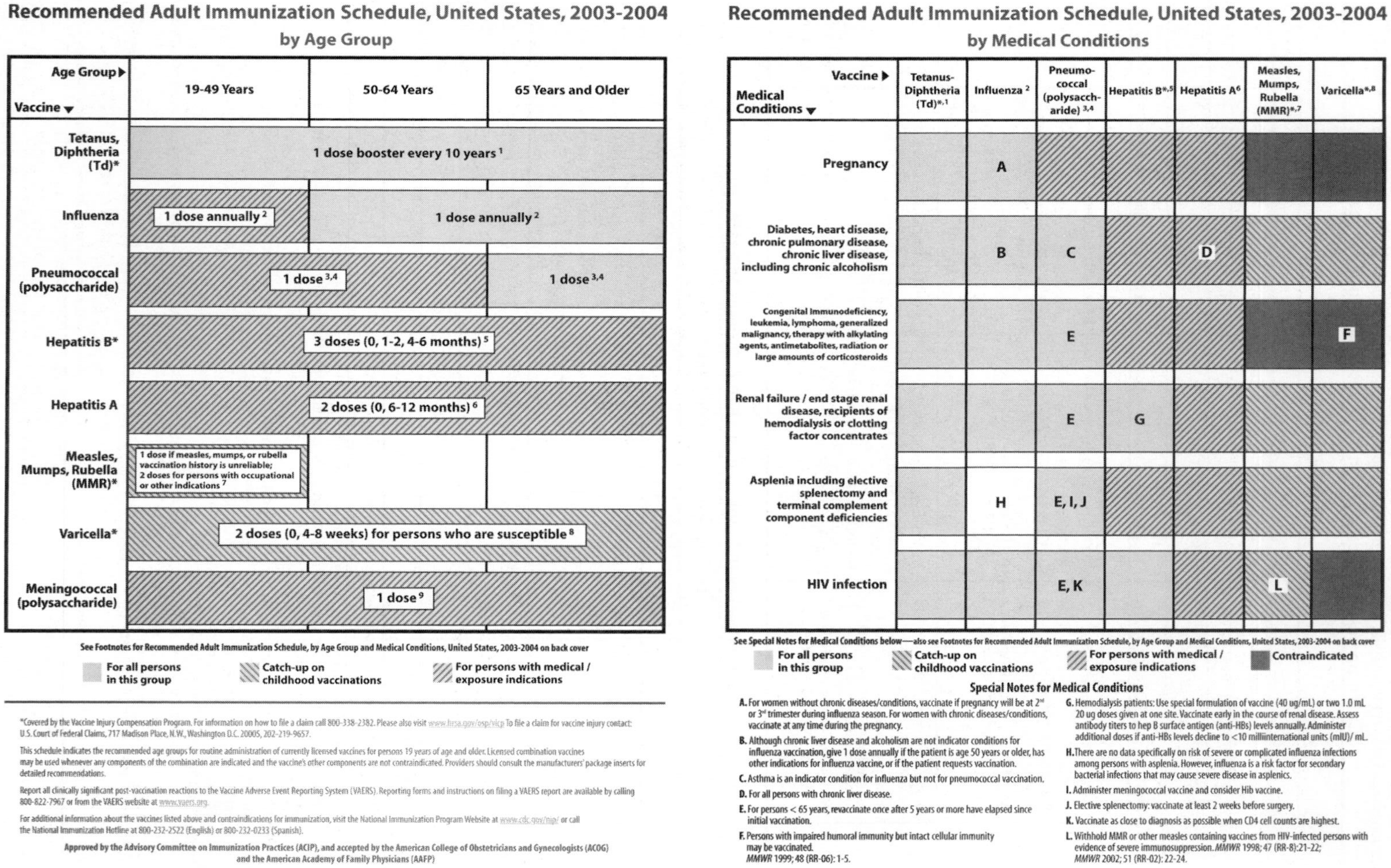

Recommended Adult Immunization Schedule, United States, 2003-2004
by Age Group
Age Group ▶
Vaccine ▼
19-49 Years
50-64 Years
65 Years and Older
Tetanus, Diphtheria (Td)*
1 dose booster every 10 years 1
Influenza
1 dose annually 2
1 dose annually 2
Pneumococcal (polysaccharide)
1 dose 3,4
1 dose 3,4
Hepatitis B*
3 doses (0, 1-2, 4-6 months) 5
Hepatitis A
2 doses (0, 6-12 months) 6
Measles, Mumps, Rubella (MMR)*
1 dose if measles, mumps, or rubella vaccination history is unreliable; 2 doses for persons with occupational or other indications 7
Varicella*
2 doses (0, 4-8 weeks) for persons who are susceptible 8
Meningococcal (polysaccharide)
1 dose 9
See Footnotes for Recommended Adult Immunization Schedule, by Age Group and Medical Conditions, United States, 2003-2004 on back cover
For all persons in this group
Catch-up on childhood vaccinations
For persons with medical / exposure indications
*Covered by the Vaccine Injury Compensation Program. For information on how to file a claim call 800-338-2382. Please also visit www.hrsa.gov/osp/vicp To file a claim for vaccine injury contact: U.S. Court of Federal Claims, 717 Madison Place, N.W., Washington D.C. 20005, 202-219-9657.
This schedule indicates the recommended age groups for routine administration of currently licensed vaccines for persons 19 years of age and older. Licensed combination vaccines may be used whenever any components of the combination are indicated and the vaccine's other components are not contraindicated. Providers should consult the manufacturers' package inserts for detailed recommendations.
Report all clinically significant post-vaccination reactions to the Vaccine Adverse Event Reporting System (VAERS). Reporting forms and instructions on filing a VAERS report are available by calling 800-822-7967 or from the VAERS website at www.vaers.org.
For additional information about the vaccines listed above and contraindications for immunization, visit the National Immunization Program Website at www.cdc.gov/nip/ or call the National Immunization Hotline at 800-232-2522 (English) or 800-232-0233 (Spanish).
Approved by the Advisory Committee on Immunization Practices (ACIP), and accepted by the American College of Obstetricians and Gynecologists (ACOG) and the American Academy of Family Physicians (AAFP)
Recommended Adult Immunization Schedule, United States, 2003-2004
by Medical Conditions
Vaccine ▶
Medical Conditions ▼
Tetanus-Diphtheria (Td)*,1
Influenza 2
Pneumococcal (polysaccharide) 3,4
Hepatitis B*,5
Hepatitis A 6
Measles, Mumps, Rubella (MMR)*,7
Varicella*,8
Pregnancy
A
Diabetes, heart disease, chronic pulmonary disease, chronic liver disease, including chronic alcoholism
B
C
D
Congenital immunodeficiency, leukemia, lymphoma, generalized malignancy, therapy with alkylating agents, antimetabolites, radiation or large amounts of corticosteroids
E
F
Renal failure / end stage renal disease, recipients of hemodialysis or clotting factor concentrates
E
G
Asplenia including elective splenectomy and terminal complement component deficiencies
H
E, I, J
HIV infection
E, K
L
See Special Notes for Medical Conditions below—also see Footnotes for Recommended Adult Immunization Schedule, by Age Group and Medical Conditions, United States, 2003-2004 on back cover
For all persons in this group
Catch-up on childhood vaccinations
For persons with medical / exposure indications
Contraindicated
Special Notes for Medical Conditions
A. For women without chronic diseases/conditions, vaccinate if pregnancy will be at 2nd or 3rd trimester during influenza season. For women with chronic diseases/conditions, vaccinate at any time during the pregnancy.
B. Although chronic liver disease and alcoholism are not indicator conditions for influenza vaccination, give 1 dose annually if the patient is age 50 years or older, has other indications for influenza vaccine, or if the patient requests vaccination.
C. Asthma is an indicator condition for influenza but not for pneumococcal vaccination.
D. For all persons with chronic liver disease.
E. For persons < 65 years, revaccinate once after 5 years or more have elapsed since initial vaccination.
F. Persons with impaired humoral immunity but intact cellular immunity may be vaccinated. MMWR 1999; 48 (RR-06): 1-5.
G. Hemodialysis patients: Use special formulation of vaccine (40 ug/mL) or two 1.0 mL 20 ug doses given at one site. Vaccinate early in the course of renal disease. Assess antibody titers to hep B surface antigen (anti-HBs) levels annually. Administer additional doses if anti-HBs levels decline to <10 milliinternational units (mIU)/ mL.
H. There are no data specifically on risk of severe or complicated influenza infections among persons with asplenia. However, influenza is a risk factor for secondary bacterial infections that may cause severe disease in asplenics.
I. Administer meningococcal vaccine and consider Hib vaccine.
J. Elective splenectomy: vaccinate at least 2 weeks before surgery.
K. Vaccinate as close to diagnosis as possible when CD4 cell counts are highest.
L. Withhold MMR or other measles containing vaccines from HIV-infected persons with evidence of severe immunosuppression. MMWR 1998; 47 (RR-8):21-22; MMWR 2002; 51 (RR-02): 22-24.

FIGURE 11–3. Immunization schedule for adults, by age and medical condition.

Footnotes for
Recommended Adult Immunization Schedule by Age Group and Medical Conditions, United States, 2003-2004

1. **Tetanus and diphtheria (Td)**—Adults including pregnant women with uncertain histories of a complete primary vaccination series should receive a primary series of Td. A primary series for adults is 3 doses: the first 2 doses given at least 4 weeks apart and the 3rd dose, 6-12 months after the second. Administer 1 dose if the person had received the primary series and the last vaccination was 10 years ago or longer. Consult *MMWR* 1991; 40 (RR-10): 1-21 for administering Td as prophylaxis in wound management. The ACP Task Force on Adult Immunization supports a second option for Td use in adults: a single Td booster at age 50 years for persons who have completed the full pediatric series, including the teenage/young adult booster.
Guide for Adult Immunization. 3rd ed. ACP 1994: 20.

2. **Influenza vaccination**—Medical indications: chronic disorders of the cardiovascular or pulmonary systems including asthma; chronic metabolic diseases including diabetes mellitus, renal dysfunction, hemoglobinopathies, or immunosuppression (including immunosuppression caused by medications or by human immunodeficiency virus [HIV]), requiring regular medical follow-up or hospitalization during the preceding year; women who will be in the second or third trimester of pregnancy during the influenza season. Occupational indications: health-care workers. Other indications: residents of nursing homes and other long-term care facilities; persons likely to transmit influenza to persons at high-risk (in-home care givers to persons with medical indications, household contacts and out-of-home caregivers of children birth to 23 months of age, or children with asthma or other indicator conditions for influenza vaccination, household members and care givers of elderly and adults with high-risk conditions); and anyone who wishes to be vaccinated. For healthy persons aged 5-49 years without high risk conditions, either the inactivated vaccine or the intranasally administered influenza vaccine (Flumist) may be given.
MMWR 2003; 52 (RR-8): 1-36; *MMWR* 2003;53 (RR-13): 1-8.

3. **Pneumococcal polysaccharide vaccination**—Medical indications: chronic disorders of the pulmonary system (excluding asthma), cardiovascular diseases, diabetes mellitus, chronic liver diseases including liver disease as a result of alcohol abuse (e.g., cirrhosis), chronic renal failure or nephrotic syndrome, functional or anatomic asplenia (e.g., sickle cell disease or splenectomy), immunosuppressive conditions (e.g., congenital immunodeficiency, HIV infection, leukemia, lymphoma, multiple myeloma, Hodgkins disease, generalized malignancy, organ or bone marrow transplantation), chemotherapy with alkylating agents, anti-metabolites, or long-term systemic corticosteroids. Geographic/other indications: Alaskan Natives and certain American Indian populations. Other indications: residents of nursing homes and other long-term care facilities.
MMWR 1997; 46 (RR-8): 1-24.

4. **Revaccination with pneumococcal polysaccharide vaccine**—One time revaccination after 5 years for persons with chronic renal failure or nephrotic syndrome, functional or anatomic asplenia (e.g., sickle cell disease or splenectomy), immunosuppressive conditions (e.g., congenital immunodeficiency, HIV infection, leukemia, lymphoma, multiple myeloma, Hodgkins disease, generalized malignancy, organ or bone marrow transplantation), chemotherapy with alkylating agents, anti-metabolites, or long-term systemic corticosteroids. For persons 65 and older, one-time revaccination if they were vaccinated 5 or more years previously and were aged less than 65 years at the time of primary vaccination. *MMWR* 1997; 46 (RR-8): 1-24.

5. **Hepatitis B vaccination**—Medical indications: hemodialysis patients, patients who receive clotting-factor concentrates. Occupational indications: health-care workers and public-safety workers who have exposure to blood in the workplace, persons in training in schools of medicine, dentistry, nursing, laboratory technology, and other allied health professions. Behavioral indications: injecting drug users, persons with more than one sex partner in the previous 6 months, persons with a recently acquired sexually-transmitted disease (STD), all clients in STD clinics, men who have sex with men. Other indications: household contacts and sex partners of persons with chronic HBV infection, clients and staff of institutions for the developmentally disabled, international travelers who will be in countries with high or intermediate prevalence of chronic HBV infection for more than 6 months, inmates of correctional facilities. *MMWR* 1991; 40 (RR-13): 1-19.
(www.cdc.gov/travel/diseases/hbv.htm)

6. **Hepatitis A vaccination**—For the combined HepA-HepB vaccine use 3 doses at 0, 1, 6 months). Medical indications: persons with clotting-factor disorders or chronic liver disease. Behavioral indications: men who have sex with men, users of injecting and noninjecting illegal drugs. Occupational indications: persons working with HAV-infected primates or with HAV in a research laboratory setting. Other indications: persons traveling to or working in countries that have high or intermediate endemicity of hepatitis A.
MMWR 1999; 48 (RR-12): 1-37. (www.cdc.gov/travel/diseases/hav.htm)

7. **Measles, Mumps, Rubella vaccination (MMR)**—Measles component: Adults born before 1957 may be considered immune to measles. Adults born in or after 1957 should receive at least one dose of MMR unless they have a medical contraindication, documentation of at least one dose or other acceptable evidence of immunity. A second dose of MMR is recommended for adults who:
   - are recently exposed to measles or in an outbreak setting
   - were previously vaccinated with killed measles vaccine
   - were vaccinated with an unknown vaccine between 1963 and 1967
   - are students in post-secondary educational institutions
   - work in health care facilities
   - plan to travel internationally

   Mumps component: 1 dose of MMR should be adequate for protection. Rubella component: Give 1 dose of MMR to women whose rubella vaccination history is unreliable and counsel women to avoid becoming pregnant for 4 weeks after vaccination. For women of child-bearing age, regardless of birth year, routinely determine rubella immunity and counsel women regarding congenital rubella syndrome. Do not vaccinate pregnant women or those planning to become pregnant in the next 4 weeks. If pregnant and susceptible, vaccinate as early in postpartum period as possible.
MMWR 1998; 47 (RR-8): 1-57; *MMWR* 2001;50: 1117.

8. **Varicella vaccination**—Recommended for all persons who do not have reliable clinical history of varicella infection, or serological evidence of varicella zoster virus (VZV) infection who may be at high risk for exposure or transmission. This includes, health-care workers and family contacts of immunocompromised persons, those who live or work in environments where transmission is likely (e.g., teachers of young children, day care employees, and residents and staff members in institutional settings), persons who live or work in environments where VZV transmission can occur (e.g., college students, inmates and staff members of correctional institutions, and military personnel), adolescents and adults living in households with children, women who are not pregnant but who may become pregnant in the future, international travelers who are not immune to infection. Note: Greater than 95% of U.S. born adults are immune to VZV. Do not vaccinate pregnant women or those planning to become pregnant in the next 4 weeks. If pregnant and susceptible, vaccinate as early in postpartum period as possible.
MMWR 1996; 45 (RR-11): 1-36; *MMWR* 1999; 48 (RR-6): 1-5.

9. **Meningococcal vaccine (quadrivalent polysaccharide for serogroups A, C, Y, and W-135)**—Consider vaccination for persons with medical indications: adults with terminal complement component deficiencies, with anatomic or functional asplenia. Other indications: travelers to countries in which disease is hyperendemic or epidemic ("meningitis belt" of sub-Saharan Africa, Mecca, Saudi Arabia for Hajj). Revaccination at 3-5 years may be indicated for persons at high risk for infection (e.g., persons residing in areas in which disease is epidemic). Counsel college freshmen, especially those who live in dormitories, regarding meningococcal disease and the vaccine so that they can make an educated decision about receiving the vaccination. *MMWR* 2000; 49 (RR-7): 1-20.
Note: The AAFP recommends that colleges should take the lead on providing education on meningococcal infection and vaccination and offer it to those who are interested. Physicians need not initiate discussion of the meningococcal quadrivalent polysaccharide vaccine as part of routine medical care.

why sequential IPV/OPV schedules are now recommended for childhood polio immunization.

The provider should take advantage of every opportunity to immunize. Numerous reports of outbreaks of certain illnesses note that there were missed opportunities to immunize those who were ultimately stricken with disease. Some opportunities are missed because the provider is concentrating on other aspects of care and may not focus on the need for immunization if the client does not ask. Others are missed because providers may elect not to immunize if the client has a mild illness. Some of the barriers to immunization of children (and adults, in some cases) include the cost of vaccines, the access to care, the number of vaccine injections that must be given at each visit, and the number of visits required to ensure adequate immunization. *The provider should review the client's immunization status at every preventive healthcare visit or every sick visit if the client does not make and/or keep appointments for primary, preventive care visits.* This is especially true for the elderly, who are at high risk for acquiring influenza and pneumococcal disease, among others. Adults over age 50 are also at risk for tetanus and diphtheria as immunity wanes. Sixty-seven percent of cases of tetanus reported in the United States each year are among adults over age 50, and studies have shown that up to 40% of adults have inadequate levels of antitoxin antibodies. Additionally, up to 60% of adults lack a protective level of antibodies against diphtheria (Clinical Guidelines, 1997). Every effort should be made to see that adults and children are adequately immunized. See Figure 11–3 for an adult immunization schedule.

Providers also should assist clients to seek immunizations at reduced or no cost by referring them to sites that offer immunizations required by law to those who are unable to pay, as in the case of the local health department. Elective immunizations may also be obtained at reduced cost at local health departments in most cases. Providers should also strive to educate clients on the importance and necessity of immunization. Many people have forgotten, or simply do not know, how severe certain diseases are, and therefore they may not be as motivated to be adequately immunized. It is very important that parents understand the necessity of child immunizations at the appropriate time. It often is helpful to review the schedule and the rationale for immunization with them. Pointing out that most of the injections are given in the first 15 to 18 months of life, and that "catching up" an older child is frightening and painful because of the number of injections required at such frequent intervals, may gain the reticent parent's compliance with an immunization schedule.

REPORTING OF ADVERSE EVENTS AND THE NATIONAL VACCINE INJURY COMPENSATION PROGRAM

The Department of Health and Human Services established the Vaccine Adverse Event Reporting System (VAERS) in 1990 to comply with conditions specified in the National Childhood Vaccine Injury Act of 1986. Prior to that time, the CDC and the FDA monitored reports of adverse events. Adverse effects after administration of vaccines purchased with public money were reported to the CDC, and adverse effects of vaccines purchased with private money were reported to the FDA. The agencies worked together to create VAERS. Those responsible for vaccine administration are required to report anaphylaxis, encephalitis, residual seizure disorders, paralytic poliomyelitis, and acute complications or sequelae of these events to VAERS. Additionally, providers are encouraged to report any clinically significant adverse event following administration of U.S. licensed vaccines in case those events may later be causally associated with vaccine administration. Copies of forms for reporting adverse events are mailed to physicians in the United States likely to administer vaccines and state health departments that, in turn, distribute forms to public health clinics (CDC, 2002a).

The VAERS 24-hour phone number is 800-822-7967. Callers may receive assistance in completing the forms, obtaining additional reporting forms, and answering questions about VAERS. The website is www.vaers.org. Reports may be filed by mail, fax, or the Internet. VAERS receives reports from health professionals, vaccine manufacturers, and the general public (CDC, 2002a).

The Vaccine Injury Compensation Program (VICP) was established as a result of the National Childhood Vaccine Injury Act of 1986 and went into effect in October 1988. Claims for injuries or death resulting from DTP, DtaP, diphtheria/tetanus (DT), tetanus toxoid (TT), tetanus/diphtheria (Td), MMR or individual component vaccines, IPV, and OPV may be made. For more information on this program, write or call the program:

National Vaccine Injury Compensation Program
Health Resources and Services Administration
Parklawn Building, Room 8-05
5600 Fishers Lane
Rockville, MD 20857
Telephone 301-443-6593

Persons needing specific information on how to file a claim may call 800-338-2382 toll-free. The website is <www.hrsa.gov/osp/vicp/index.htm> (CDC, 2002a).

NEW HORIZONS

Vaccines for many diseases are in the process of research and development. Such diseases include hepatitis C and E, cytomegalovirus, rotavirus, and HIV. Adenovirus vaccines are used in military recruits, but are not available for general use. Improvements are sought in vaccines currently used—such as for pertussis and meningococcus—to increase efficacy and decrease adverse events. Additionally, many different combination vaccines are in development so that the number of immunizations given in a routine childhood visit may be decreased. New technologies will expand the scope of traditional vaccination from prevention of disease to changing the physiology of disease and for immunological treatment of disease. Diseases and conditions that would ultimately be affected include allergy, infertility, cancer, and AIDS (Ellis, 1994).

Human rotavirus causes severe diarrhea, abdominal cramping, and vomiting, leading to dehydration and death if untreated. It is a leading cause of death in children in developing countries (approximately 1 million children per year). In the United States, approximately 100,000 children are hospitalized and 125 die annually. Treatment is directed at managing hydration status until the disease resolves. There is no cure. A vaccine, shown to reduce severe diarrheal illness and resultant dehydration in several clinical trials, was approved by the FDA on December 12, 1997, and routine vaccination of full-term infants was recommended by the CDC's Advisory Committee on Immunization Practices (Getting rid, 1998). The vaccine, RotaShield, marketed by Wyeth-Lederle, was be given in 3 oral doses at 2, 4 and 6 months of age (CDC panel, 1998). However, the vaccine was pulled from the market due to its association with intussusception (CDC, 1999b). RotaTeg (Merck) and Rotarix (GlaxoSmithKline) are new rotavirus vaccinations currently in clinical trials (Rosenthal, 2004).

PROGRAMS FOR IMPROVING IMMUNIZATION RATES

Many local, regional, state, and national programs have been developed to address the continuing problem of underimmunization of preschool children. The president of the United States initiated the Childhood Immunization Program in 1993 to "(1) eliminate indigenous cases of 6 vaccine-preventable diseases (i.e., diphtheria, HIB disease [among children aged less than 5 years], measles, poliomyelitis, rubella, and tetanus [among children aged less than 15 years]) by 1996; (2) increase vaccination coverage levels to at least 90% among 2-year-old children by 1996 for each of the vaccinations recommended routinely for children (for hepatitis B, the objective is set for 1998); and (3) establish a vaccination-delivery system that maintains and further improves high coverage levels." (CDC, 1994). Activities to meet those goals include efforts to improve quality and quantity of vaccination delivery services, increase community participation and education, reduce vaccine cost for parents by implementing the Vaccines for Children program (begun October 1, 1994), improve surveillance for coverage and disease, form and strengthen partnerships, and improve vaccines (CDC, 1994). The "National Infant Immunization Week" was established in 1993, and each year materials are sent to health careproviders and related professional organizations and to various community organizations and leaders across the country to facilitate activities to increase public awareness. August is National Immunization Awareness Month and localities nationwide plan educational activities to raise public awareness. For more information refer to the CDC website on the Internet <www.cdc.gov/nip/home.html>.

Contact your local or state health department for information on programs to improve immunization rates in your area.

SUMMARY

Tremendous progress has been made in vaccine development in the last 40 years. However, many diseases for which vaccines are available are still prevalent even though they are now, for the most part, preventable. It is important to remember that although no vaccine is 100% safe or 100% effective, immunizing the population is successful in achieving herd immunity and controlling or eliminating disease. Smallpox has been declared eradicated from the world; polio is soon to follow and then, with continued diligent immunization efforts, perhaps measles. Hepatitis B immunization may be instrumental in decreasing the numbers of people with hepatocarcinoma (Cheng-Liang Lee & Ying-Chin Ko, 1997; Mahoney & Kane, 1999).

The provider must convey to clients the importance of receiving all necessary immunizations on time and when circumstances necessitating immunization arise, such as traveling or when at high risk for contracting a vaccine-preventable illness. The provider should also be able to explain to clients what the diseases look like to facilitate understanding of why the vaccines are so important. Third, providers must take advantage of every opportunity to immunize their clients. Many cases of vaccine-preventable diseases occur in cases in which opportunities to vaccinate were missed by providers.

New vaccines are in development; some are improvements of existing vaccines, some are combinations of existing vaccines, some are new forms of vaccines, such as the new influenza nasal inhalation vaccine preparation, and others are being developed for diseases for which there are no current vaccines. Up-to-date information is available from the Centers for Disease Control via the World Wide Web: www.cdc.gov/nip/home.html. To find out the location of immunization clinics in your area and answers to commonly asked questions, call 1-800-232-2522. See Chapter 37 for immunization issues specific to children and HIV infection.

REFERENCES

American Academy of Pediatrics Committee on Infectious Diseases. (1992). Universal hepatitis B immunization. *Pediatrics, 89,* 795–800.

Asano, Y., Suga, S., Yoshikawa, T., Kobayashi, I., Yasaki, T., Shibata, M., Tsuzuki, K., & Ito, S. (1994). Twenty year follow-up of protective immunity of the Oka strain live varicella vaccine. *Pediatrics, 94*(4, Pt 1), 524–526.

Barnett, E.D., Chen, R.T., & Rey, M. (1999). Vaccines for interantional travel. In S.A. Plotkin & W.A. Orenstein (eds.), *Vaccines* (3rd ed.). Philadelphia: W.B. Saunders.

Butler, J. C., Breiman, R. F., Campbell, J. F., Lipman, H. B., Broome, C. V., & Facklam, R. R. (1993). Pneumococcal polysaccharide vaccine efficacy. An evaluation of current recommendations. *JAMA, 270,* 1826–1831.

CDC panel calls for use of rotavirus vaccine. (1998). Newstand @thrive.

Centers for Disease Control (CDC). (1994, February 4). Reported vaccine-preventable diseases—United States, 1993, and the Childhood Immunization Initiative. *MMWR, 43*(4), 57–60.

Centers for Disease Control (CDC). (1997a, May 2). Availability of diphtheria antitoxin through an investigational new drug protocol. *MMWR, 46*(17), 380.

Centers for Disease Control (CDC). (1997b, February 14). Control and prevention of meningococcal disease: Recommendations of the Advisory Committee on Immunization Practices (ACIP). *MMWR, 46*(#RR-5).

Centers for Disease Control (CDC). (1997c, June 13). Measles eradication: Recommendations from a meeting cosponsored by the World Health Organization, the Pan American Health Organization, and CDC. *MMWR, 46*(#RR-11).

Centers for Disease Control (CDC). (1997d, January 24). Outbreaks of pneumococcal pneumonia among unvaccinated residents in chronic-care facilities—Massachusetts, October 1995, Oklahoma, February 1996, and Maryland, May—June 1996. *MMWR, 46*(3), 60–62.

Centers for Disease Control (CDC). (1997e, March 28). Pertussis vaccination: Use of acellular pertussis vaccines among infants and young children. *MMWR, 46*(#RR-7).

Centers for Disease Control (CDC). (1997f, January 24). Poliomyelitis prevention in the United States: Introduction of a sequential vaccination schedule of inactivated poliovirus vaccine followed by oral poliovirus vaccine. *MMWR, 46*(#RR-3).

Centers for Disease Control (CDC). (1997g, April 25). Prevention and control of influenza: Recommendations of the Advisory Committee on Immunization Practices (ACIP). *MMWR, 46*(#RR-9).

Centers for Disease Control (CDC). (1997h, April 4). Prevention of pneumococcal disease: Recommendations of the Advisory Committee on Immunization Practices (ACIP). *MMWR, 46*(#RR-8).

Centers for Disease Control (CDC). (1997i, April 25). Rubella and congenital rubella syndrome—United States, 1994–1997. *MMWR, 46*(16), 350–354.

Centers for Disease Control (CDC). (1997j, April 18). Update: Influenza activity—United States and worldwide, 1996–97 season, and composition of the 1997–98 influenza vaccine. *MMWR, 46*(#RR-15).

Centers for Disease Control (CDC). (1999a, January 8). Human rabies prevention—United States, 1999. *MMWR, 48* (#RR-1).

Centers for Disease Control (CDC). (1999b, November 5). Withdrawal of rotavirus vaccine recommendations. *MMWR, 48*(43).

Centers for Disease Control (CDC). (2000, May 19). Poliomyelitis prevention in the United States. Updated Recommendations of the Advisory Committee on Immunization Practices (ACIP). *MMWR, 49* (RR05).

Centers for Disease Control (CDC). (2001a, March 30). Apparent global interruption of wild poliovirus type 2 transmission. *MMWR, 50* (12).

Centers for Disease Control (CDC). (2001b, June 15). Progress toward poliomyelitis eradication—West and Central Africa, 1999–2000. *MMWR, 50*(23).

Centers for Disease Control (CDC). (2001c, June 22). Vaccine (smallpox) vaccine. *MMWR, 50*(RR-10).

Centers for Disease Control (CDC). (2001d, July 27). Global progress toward laboratory containment of wild polioviruses, June 2001. *MMWR, 50* (29).

Centers for Disease Control (CDC). (2001e, August 31). Progress toward poliomyelitis eradication—Southeast Asia, January 2000–June 2001. *MMWR, 50*(34).

Centers for Disease Control (CDC). (2001f, September 28). Progress toward poliomyelitis eradication—Angola. Democratic Republic of Congo, Ethopia & Nigeria, January 2000–June 2001. *MMWR, 50*(38).

Centers for Disease Control (CDC). (2001g, October 5). Public Health dispatch: Update: Outbreak of poliomyelitis—Dominican Republic & Haiti, 2000–2001. *MMWR, 50*(39).

Centers for Disease Control (CDC). (2001h, November 23). Imported wild poliovirus causing poliomyelitis—Bulgaria, 2001. *MMWR, 50*(46).

Centers for Disease Control (CDC). (2002a). *Epidemiology and prevention of vaccine preventable diseases (The pink book)*. www.

Centers for Disease Control (CDC). (2002b, June 28). Achievements in public health; Hepatitis B vaccination—United States, 1982–2002. *MMWR, 51*(25).

Chen, R. T., Rastogi, S. C., Mullen, J. R., Hayes, S. W., Cochi, S. L., Donlon, J. A., & Wassilak, S. G. (1994). The Vaccine Adverse Event Reporting System (VAERS). *Vaccine, 12,* 542–550.

Cheng-Liang Lee, & Ying-Chin Ko. (1997). Hepatitis B vaccination and hepatocellular carcinoma in Taiwan. *Pediatrics, 99,* 351–353.

Clinical Guidelines. (1997). Tetanus and diphtheria immunization/prophylaxis in adults and older adults. *The Nurse Practitioner, 22*(3), 116–120.

Clinician Reviews. (1996). New vaccine for hepatitis A prevention. *Clinician Reviews, 6*(5), 32.

Clinician Reviews. (1997). Infant and adolescent immunizations: New guidelines reflect latest policy changes. *Clinician Reviews, 7*(2), 67–77.

Cromer, B. A., Goydos, J., Hackell, J., Mezzatesta, J., Dekker, C., & Mortimer, E. A. (1993). Unrecognized pertussis infection in adolescents. *American Journal of Diseases of Children, 147,* 575–577.

Decker, M. D., Edwards, K. M., Steinhoff, M. C., Rennels, M. B., Pichichero, M. E., Englund, J. A., Anderson, E. L., Deloria, M. A., & Reed, G. F. (1995). Comparison of 13 acellular pertussis vaccines: Adverse reactions. *Pediatrics, 96*(3), 557–566.

Edwards, K. M., Decker, M. D., Graham, B. S., Mezzatesta, J., Scott, J., & Hackell, J. (1993). Adult immunization with acellular pertussis vaccine. *Journal of the American Medical Association 269,* 53–56.

Edwards, K. M., Decker, M. D., Mortimer, E.A. (1999). Pertussis vaccine. In S.A. Plotkin & W.A. Orenstein (eds.), *Vaccines* (3rd ed.). Philadelphia; W.B. Saunders.

Ellis, R. W. (1994). New technologies for making vaccines. In S. A. Plotkin & E. A. Mortimer, Jr., *Vaccines* (2nd ed.). Philadelphia: W. B. Saunders.

Feder, H. M., LaRussa, P., Steinberg, S., & Gershon, A. (1997). Clinical varicella following varicella vaccination: Don't be fooled. *Pediatrics, 99,* 897–899.

Fedson, D.S., Musher, D.M., & Eskola, J (1999). Pneumococcal vaccine. In S.A. Plotkin & W.A. Orenstein (Eds.), *Vaccines* (3rd ed.). Philadelphia: W.B. Saunders.

Feinstein, S.M., & Gust, I.D. (1999). Hepatitis A vaccine. In S.A. Plotkin & W.A. Orenstein (Eds.), *Vaccines* (3rd ed.). Philadelphia: W.B. Saunders.

Gershon, A.A., Takahashi, M., & White, C.J. (1999). Varicella vaccine. In S.A. Plotkin & W.A. Orenstein (Eds.), *Vaccines* (3rd ed.). Philadelphia: W.B. Saunders.

Getting rid of rotavirus. (1998). *Environmental Health Perspectives, 106*(3).

Herwaldt, L. (1991). Pertussis in adults: What physicians need to know. *Archives of Internal Medicine, 151,* 1510–1512.

Hull, H. F., Ward, N. A., Hull, B. P., Milstien, J. B., & de-Quadros, C. (1994). Paralytic poliomyelitis: Seasoned strategies, disappearing disease. *Lancet, 343,* 1331–1337.

Kim, S. C., Chung, E. K., Hodinka, R. L., DeMaio, J., West, D. J., Jawad, A. F., & Watson, B. (1997). Immunogenicity of hepatitis B vaccine in preterm infants. *Pediatrics, 99,* 534–536.

King, J. C., Vink, P. E., Farley, J. J., Smilie, M., Parks, M., & Lichenstein, R. (1997). Safety and immunogenicity of three doses of a five-valent pneumococcal conjugate vaccine in children younger than two years with and without human immunodeficiency virus infection. *Pediatrics, 99,* 575–580.

Krugman, S., & Stevens, C. E. (1994). Hepatitis B vaccine. In S. A. Plotkin & E. A. Mortimer, Jr., *Vaccines* (2nd ed.). Philadelphia: W. B. Saunders.

Kuter, B. J., Weibal, R. E., Guess, H. A., Matthews, H., Morton, D. H., Neff, B. J., Provost, P. J., Watson, B. A., Starr, S. E., & Plotkin, S. A. (1991). Oka/Merck varicella vaccine in healthy children: Final report of a two-year efficacy study and seven-year follow-up studies. *Vaccine, 9,* 643–647.

Lepow, M.L., Perkins, B. A., Hughes, P.A., & Poolman, J.T. (1999). Meningococcal vaccines. In S.A. Plotkin & W.A. Orenstein (Eds.), *Vaccines* (3rd ed.). Philadelphia: W.B. Saunders.

Levine, M.M. (1999). Typhoid fever vaccines. In S.A. Plotkin & W.A. Orenstein (Eds.), *Vaccines* (3rd ed.). Philadelphia: W.B. Saunders.

Mahoney, F.J., & Kane, M. (1999) Hepatitis B vaccine. In S.A. Plotkin & W.A. Orenstein (Eds.), *Vaccines* (3rd ed.). Philadelphia: W.B. Saunders.

Mortimer, E.A., Jr., & Wharton, M. (1999). Diptheria toxoid. In S.A. Plotkin & W.A. Orenstein (Eds.), *Vaccines* (3rd ed.). Philadelphia: W.B. Saunders.

Murphy, K. R., & Strunk, R. C. (1985). Safe administration of influenza vaccine in asthmatic children hypersensitive to egg proteins. *Journal of Pediatrics, 106,* 931–933.

Nelson, J. D. (1978). The changing epidemiology of pertussis in young infants: The role of adults as reservoirs of infection. *American Journal of Diseases of Children, 132,* 371–373.

Nennig, M. E., Shinefield, H. R., Edwards, K. M., Black, S. B., & Fireman, B. H. (1996). Prevalence and incidence of adult pertussis in an urban population. *JAMA, 275,* 1672–1674.

Nettleman, M. D. (1993). *Emporiatrics: An introduction to travel medicine.* Iowa City, IA: College of Medicine, University of Iowa.

Nettleman, M. D. (1996). Preparing the international traveler. *Gastroenterology Clinics of North America, 25,* 451–469.

Orenstein, W.A. Hinman, A.R. & Rodewald, L.E. (1999). In S.A. Plotkin & W.A. Orenstein (Eds.), *Vaccines* (3rd ed.). Philadelphia: W.B. Saunders.

Peters, S. (1997, February). The state of pediatric immunizations today. *ADVANCE for Nurse Practitioners,* 43–49.

Phelps, R. (1997). Rabies: Confronting the continuing threat. *Contemporary Pediatrics, 14*(7), 136–150.

Plotkin, S. A. (1996). Commentary: Varicella vaccine. *Pediatrics, 97,* 251–253.

Plotkin, S. A. (1999). Rubella vaccine. In S.A. Plotkin & W.A. Orenstein (Eds.), *Vaccines* (3rd ed.). Philadelphia: W.B. Saunders.

Plotkin, S.A., & Orenstein, W.A. (Eds.). (1999). *Vaccines* (3rd ed.). Philadelphia: W.B. Saunders.

Plotkin, S.A., Rupprecht, C.E., & Koprowski, H. (1999) Rabies vaccine. In S.A. Plotkin & W.A. Orenstein (Eds.), *Vaccines* (3rd ed.). Philadelphia: W.B. Saunders.

Plotkin, S.A., & Wharton, M. (1999) Mumps vaccine. In S.A. Plotkin & W.A. Orenstein (Eds.), *Vaccines* (3rd ed.). Philadelphia: W.B. Saunders.

Plotkin, S.L., & Plotkin, S.A. (1999). A short history of vaccination. In S.A. Plotkin & W.A. Orenstein (Eds.), *Vaccines* (3rd ed.). Philadelphia: W.B. Saunders.

Red Book, 25th edition. (2000). Elk Grove Village, IL: Committee on Infectious Diseases, American Academy of Pediatrics.

Redd, S.C., Markowitz, L.E. & Katz, S.L. (1999). In S.A. Plotkin & W.A. Orenstein, *Vaccines* (3rd ed.). Philadelphia: W.B. Saunders.

Rosenthal, M. (2004). Research on rotavirus vaccines continues as need remains pressing. *Infection Diseases in Children, 17*(3).

Schmitt, H.-J., Wirsing von König, C. H., Neiss, A., Bogaerts, H., Bock, H. L., Schulte-Wissermann, H., Gahr, M., Schult, R., Folkens, J. U., Rauh, W., & Clemens, R. (1996). Efficacy of acellular pertussis vaccine in early childhood after household exposure. *JAMA, 275*(1), 37–41.

Sears, S. D., & Sack, D. A. (1995). Medical advice for the international traveler. In L. R. Barker, J. R. Burton, & P. D. Zieve (Eds.), *Principles of ambulatory medicine* (4th ed.). Baltimore: Williams & Wilkins.

Sell, S. (1996). *Immunology, immunopathology, and immunity* (5th ed.). Stamford, CT: Appleton & Lange.

Smith, K.C., & Starke, J.R. (1999). Bacille Calmette-Guerin vaccine. In S.A. Plotkin & W.A. Orenstein (Eds.), *Vaccines* (3rd ed.). Philadelphia: W.B. Saunders.

Sutter, R.W., Cochi, S.L., & Melnick, J.L. (1999). Live attenuated poliovirus vaccines. In S.A. Plotkin & W.A. Orenstein (Eds.), *Vaccines* (3rd ed.). Philadelphia: W.B. Saunders.

Titball, R.W., Eley, S., Williamson, E.D., & Dennis, D.T. (1999). Plague. In S.A. Plotkin & W.A. Orenstein (Eds.), *Vaccines* (3rd ed.). Philadelphia: W.B. Saunders.

Ward, J.I., & Zangwill, K.M. (1999). Haemophilus influenzae vaccines. In S.A. Plotkin & W.A. Orenstein (Eds.), *Vaccines* (3rd ed.). Philadelphia: W.B. Saunders.

Wassilak, S.G.F., Orenstein, W.A., & Sutter, R.W. (1999). Tetanus toxoid. In S.A. Plotkin & W.A. Orenstein (Eds.), *Vaccines* (3rd ed.). Philadelphia: W.B. Saunders.

Watson, B., Gupta, R., Randall, T., & Starr, S. (1994). Persistence of cell-mediated and humoral immune responses in healthy children immunized with the live attenuated varicella vaccine. *Journal of Infectious Diseases, 169,* 197.

Watson, B., & Haupt, R. M. (1997). Varicella vaccine: Removing the roadlocks. *Contemporary Pediatrics, 14*(5), 166–181.

Watson, B., Pierey, S., Plotkin, S. A., et al. (1993). Modified chickenpox in children immunized with the Oka/Merck varicella vaccine. *Pediatrics, 91,* 17.

Woodruff, B. A., Stevenson, J., Yusuf, H., Kwong, S. L., Todoroff, K. P., Hadler, J. L., Connecticut Hepatitis B Project Group, Hoyt M. A., & Mahoney, F. J. (1996). Progress toward integrating hepatitis B vaccine into routine infant immunization schedules in the United States, 1991 through 1994. *Pediatrics, 97,* 798–803.

World Health Organization (WHO). (1980, May 2). Smallpox declared eradicated. *MMWR.*

Wright, S. W., Edwards, K. M., Decker, M. D., & Zeldin, M. H. (1995). Pertussis infection in adults with persistent cough. *JAMA, 273,* 1044–1046.

III ❖ Special Issues and Patient Populations

CHAPTER ❖ 12

PEDIATRIC ISSUES

Katharine A. Gracely-Kilgore

Several factors influence the choice and administration of medications to pediatric and adolescent patients. These factors include the pharmacokinetics and physiologic differences of childhood, the developmental stage of the child, practical needs of the child and family, safety issues, and pediatric patients' response to pain. Since the focus of this book is on ambulatory care, this chapter will not address IV or emergency drugs.

USE OF DRUGS IN CHILDREN—HISTORICAL PERSPECTIVE AND CURRENT CONTROVERSIES

Up until the period following World War II children were simply given smaller adult doses with no relation to weight or age (Lucey, 1992). Then a "series of therapeutic disasters" from 1950 to 1970 (Lucey, 1992, p. xiii), helped awaken pediatric providers to the dangers of haphazard medication administration and the need for more careful and precise dosing.

- In the early 1950s, it was discovered that delivering a high percentage of oxygen for long periods of time to premature infants caused retinopathy of prematurity and possible subsequent blindness (Phelps, 1993).
- In the 1960s, several neonates died when given chloramphenicol because their natural low levels of the liver enzyme glucuronyl transferase were unable to conjugate the drug (Nahata, 1993). The infants developed hypotension, hypoxemia, and eventually shock and death, and had an ashen gray color, thus the name "Gray-baby" syndrome (Smith, 1992).
- In the 1970s, it was reported that premature babies who were repeatedly bathed in 3% hexachlorophene (Phisohex) suffered vacuolar encephalopathy of the brainstem (Ghadially & Shear, 1992).

The Food and Drug Administration (FDA) is the agency that oversees the safety and efficacy of drugs used in the United States. Before 1962, there were no assurances that pediatric drugs were tested in the pediatric population. Then, in 1997, Congress passed the FDA Modernization Act, which allows the FDA to issue a written request for pediatric data for compounds that are, or may be, used in pediatric patients and allows for a patent extension for companies that are successful in conducting studies for pediatric labeling. The FDA's final ruling, in 1998, requires pediatric studies for certain new and already marketed drugs. (Berlin, 2000, p. S125).

As of 2000, approximately 30% of the drugs available in the United States have been shown to be safe and effective for children (Handbook of Pediatric Drug Therapy, 2000, pp. vii–viii). Lack of testing by the pharmaceutical companies may be due to a perceived lack of market share (Miller & Fioravante, 1997, p. 1), lower profits in relation to cost of research and development, as well as a smaller number of drugs required for pediatric patients, who comprise a smaller percentage of the life span (Blumer, 1999). The term *therapeutic orphan* (Yaffe & Aranda, 1992, p. 5) refers to the situation in which a pediatric patient is deprived of the use of a drug because it has only been approved for use in adults. However, some providers may choose to use an unapproved drug for a patient if they feel that the benefits outweigh the risks (Blumer, 1999). This "off label" drug use is controversial (Wilson, Kearns, Murphy, & Yaffe, 1994). There is the potential for the healthcare provider to be caught in a situation where a drug unapproved by the FDA might be considered. For legal reasons, the provider is strongly encouraged to only use FDA-approved drugs.

A recent controversy is the recommendation of the American Academy of Pediatrics for mandatory labeling by pharmaceutical companies of the inactive ingredients contained in prescription and over-the-counter medications. Oral medications are not required to have inactive ingredients listed, yet some of them can cause adverse reactions in children, including bronchospasm, headache, seizures, cross-sensitivity reactions, diarrhea, hyperosmolality and lactic acidosis. There are more than 773 of these ingredients, and they can include sweeteners, dyes, and preservatives. Also, fragrances and flavoring agents are not required to be listed (Pediatrics, 1997).

PHARMACOKINETICS: PEDIATRIC VARIATIONS

Physiologically, children's and adolescents' bodily systems develop at different rates, with some systems maturing much sooner than others. The ways that drugs are absorbed, distributed, metabolized, and excreted varies with the maturity of various body systems (see Table 12–1). Conversely, some medications may affect the development process itself and the results will not be readily apparent for many years (Yaffe & Aranda, 1992).

This section will address these four pharmacokinetic areas by age, following FDA groupings. The FDA categorized children into groups according to age because it was felt that some age-dependent factors may affect the safety and efficacy of drugs used in children (Yaffe & Aranda, 1992). The FDA groups referred to in this chapter are neonate (birth to 1 month), infant-toddler (1 month to 2 years), child (2 years to onset of puberty), and adolescent (onset of adolescence to adult life) (Yaffe & Aranda, 1992). The discussion will not include premature infants because of the specialized nature of the care of this population.

NEONATE

Absorption

The skin of neonates has a thinner dermis, epidermis, and stratum corneum layers (Bindler & Howry, 1991; *Handbook of Pediatric Drug Therapy,* 2000), thus resulting in greater permeability. Neonates' large skin surface in relation to body weight (Blumer & Reed, 1992; *Handbook of Pediatric Drug Therapy,* 2000) causes systemic availability to be 2.7 times that of adults (Blumer & Reed, 1992). Because of these factors, the weakest strength of any medication must be ordered and used sparingly. Hexachlorophene, lindane (see Drug Table 806), and strong steroids (see Drug Table 807) are to be avoided, and healthcare providers and caregivers must be cautious with the use of over-the-counter (OTC) preparations (Cetta, Lambert, & Ros, 1991). Fluorinated steroids should never be applied to the face at any age. Inflamed, burned, or denuded skin (Blumer & Reed, 1992) or skin covered with disposable diapers or occlusive dressings (Pagliaro, 1995) absorbs medication to a greater degree (Blumer & Reed, 1992; Pagliaro, 1995). Therefore, when treating severe diaper rash, medications need to be applied sparingly.

Drugs can easily pass into the nasolacrimal duct of the eye, thus causing increased systemic absorption, especially of anticholenergics (Pagliaro, 1995). One or two drops of any medication is sufficient. If necessary to impede absorption, the caregiver can practice nasolacrimal obstruction (NLO), which is gentle external pressure at the inner canthus to close the drainage system. Increased production of tears causes decreased absorption (Pagliaro, 1995), so the caregiver must not give eyedrops if the neonate is crying.

A major factor in drug absorption is the gastrointestinal (GI) tract. A variable and prolonged gastric emptying time and prolonged transit time and peristalsis contribute to increased absorption of oral medications and the potential for overdose if too large a dose is given. Higher gastric pH is also a factor (Blumer & Reed, 1992; *Handbook of Pediatric Drug Therapy,* 2000). Medications given via the lower rectum have greater systemic absorption (Kauffman, 1992), so the healthcare provider must be cautious of overdosage. However, suppositories are erratically absorbed, especially if feces are present (*Handbook*

TABLE 12–1. Pediatric Pharmacokinetic Differences as Compared to Adults

	Neonate	Infant	Child
Absorption			
Gastric acidity	Achlorhydria at 10–30 days after birth	Reaches adult levels at 1–2 years	
Gastric emptying time	Prolonged 6 to 8 h; irregular peristalsis	Reaches adult levels at 6–8 months; irregular peristalsis	Same as adult
GI motility intestinal transit time	Highly variable; influenced by the presence/absence of food		
Pancreatic enzyme activity	Decreased	Full activity capacity dependent on specific enzyme	
GI surface area	More sensitive to chemicals that may cause more nausea, vomiting, and diarrhea		
Dietary components	Acidic/alkaline foods will alter gastric pH		
Skin permeability	Thinner stratum corneum; more surface area/body weight	Thinner stratum corneum	
Distribution			
Total body water	Increased		Same as adult
Albumin	Lower, concentrations (3.0–4.0 g/dL); lower binding affinity	Plasma proteins reach adult levels by 1 year	
Blood-brain barrier	More permeable	Similar to adult	
Fat composition	Lower than adult (15–20% of TBW); lipid-soluble drugs stored to a lesser degree	21–26% TBW	Adolescent boys lose fat (12% of TBW); adolescent girls accumulate fat (25% of TBW)
Metabolism			
Liver	Some hepatic enzymes reduced; most metabolize drugs at a rate several times lower than adult		Most enzyme systems mature by 2–4 years of age
Excretion			
Renal blood flow	Reduced	9 months reaches adult levels	
Glomerular filtration	Decreased	9 months reaches adult levels	
Tubular function	Decreased	>9 months reaches adult levels	Decrease in renal tubular clearance with the onset of adolescence

TBW = total body weight.

Source: Niederhauser, V.P. (1997), Prescribing for children: Issues in pediatric pharmacology. Nurse Practitioner, 22(3), p. 18.

of Pediatric Drug Therapy, 2000), so other routes are preferred over the rectal route.

Other considerations in this age group include the fact that infants are nose breathers until 3 months of age, so drops should be instilled to one side of the nose at a time. Also, tooth discoloration has been associated with the use of ciprofloxacin (Lumbiagannon, Pengsaa, & Sookpranee, 1991). The neonate has many immature body systems, so the healthcare provider must be alert to the risk of toxicity with the use of *any* drug because of increased absorption and must monitor the patient carefully.

Distribution

Peripheral circulation is poorly developed, and vasoconstriction occurs in response to cold, causing decreased absorption (Bindler & Howry, 1991). A decreased muscle mass (25% of body weight versus 40% in adults) provides a smaller area for absorption of intramuscular medications (Bindler & Howry, 1991), so intramuscular or subcutaneous routes are not the best choices for the neonate. The oral route is preferred unless the infant is very ill, in which case medication is given intravenously.

Immature myelinization of the central nervous system (CNS) until age 2 years (Bindler & Howry, 1991; Lehne, Moore, Crosby, & Hamilton, 1990) enables drugs to pass the blood-brain barrier more easily (Miller & Fioravanti, 1997). Encephalopathy is more commonly seen as a toxic side effect (Bindler & Howry, 1991). The risk of CNS depression is great in the neonate (Lehne et al., 1990), so one must monitor the patient carefully if CNS drugs such as phenobarbital are prescribed (see Drug Table 308.1).

Metabolism

The liver affects drug metabolism in neonates and infants because of their immature enzyme systems. There is variability in this impact since enzyme systems mature at different rates (Skaer, 1991). Most drugs are metabolized slower in neonates, but in some there may be an increased metabolism. Most enzyme systems mature between 2 and 4 years of age. Fewer total plasma proteins (Sagraves, 1995) and less albumin (Niederhauser, 1997), along with the lower binding affinity of albumin, allow for more free drug to be available for absorption (Sagraves, 1995), especially phenobarbital, phenytoin, and salicylates (Nahata, 1993). Also, maternal hormones and a large amount of free and fatty acids bind with plasma proteins, thus restricting the binding of drugs with plasma proteins (Bindler & Howry, 1991). Drugs such as sulfonamide antibiotics can compete with albumin-binding sites (see Drug Table 102.9; 102.10) and can cause increased risk of kernicterus in the neonate (Siberry & Iannone, 2000; Skaer, 1991).

Excretion

Due to the smaller number of tubular cells, shorter tubules, and decreased renal flow in neonates (Bindler & Howry, 1991), their glomelular filtration rate is decreased (Behrman & Vaughan, 1987; Merenstein & Gardner, 1989; Reed & Besunder, 1989). This results in drugs having a longer half-life and increased absorption, especially digoxin, penicillins, aminoglycosides, salicylates, and thiazide diuretics (see Drug Tables 102.6, 207, 208.4, 307) (Niederhauser, 1997). Dosage intervals of drugs, especially those mentioned above, may have to be increased (Wink, 1991).

INFANTS

Absorption

The GI emptying time reaches adult levels at 6 to 8 months (Blumer & Reed, 1992), and greater small intestine surface area (Kauffman, 1992), increases absorption of oral medications. Because body surface area doubles by 1 year of age (Kauffman, 1992), topical agents are still greatly absorbed. As an example, Maswoswe, Egbunike, Stewart, et al. (1994) discuss a 6-month-old child with varicella who died from diphenhydramine toxicity (see Drug Table 705) from application of Caladryl to its entire body for several days. Because of increased absorption, transdermal patches are not FDA-approved for pediatric patients (Pagliaro, 1995). Certain drugs are contraindicated at this age. Oil-based nasal sprays can cause aspiration and lipid pneumonia (Pagliaro, 1995), and accurate dosages of opioid drugs can cause respiratory depression in children under 1 year of age (Kauffman, 1992).

As with neonates, muscle mass is decreased and peripheral circulation is variable, thus decreasing absorption (*Handbook of Pediatric Drug Therapy,* 2000). Although most immunizations and their booster doses are given intramuscularly during infancy and childhood, the oral route is preferred for ill young children. Acutely ill children may need intravenous medication.

Distribution

Infants have a greater percentage of fluid to solid body weight, which increases the distribution area, requiring higher dosages of water soluble drugs per body weight (*Handbook of Pediatric Drug Therapy,* 2000; Miller & Fioravante, 1997).

Metabolism

As the neonate matures into infancy, "Both hepatic and renal function not only equal, but in some cases exceed normal adult function between one year and puberty" (Kauffman, 1992, p. 213).

Excretion

By 9 months of age most excretion functions have reached adult levels (Niederhauser, 1997).

CHILDREN

Absorption

For the child, maturing systems are still vulnerable. Fluoroquinolones have been found to be toxic to cartilage (see Drug Table 102.4) (Todd, 1995) and are therefore not recommended for children under the age of 12 years. Tetracycline has been found to cause tooth staining in children under 8 years of age. Acetaminophen can lead to liver toxicity if overdosed (Kiebler & Mowry, 1994). A shorter GI transit time in the young child decreases absorption of sustained-release drugs (Pederson & Moller-Peterson, 1984; Rogers, Kalisker, Weiner, & Szafler, 1985), so these types of drugs should not be used. Gastric emptying time exceeds or equals adult levels (Kauffman, 1992), which results in increased absorption (Green & Mirkin, 1984; Kearns & Reed, 1989), especially of liquid medications (Kauffman, 1992).

Distribution

By childhood most distribution functions reach adult levels.

ADOLESCENTS

Absorption

Inflammatory bowel disease (Yaffe & Aranda, 1992) or any condition associated with diarrhea and/or vomiting, such as an eating disorder or viral gastroenteritis, can cause decreased absorption of oral medications, including oral contraceptives. With oral contraceptives, the use of a back-up method of birth control must be reinforced during an acute illness. For a chronic condition, a different method of birth control, such as medroxyprogesterone (Depo-Provera), may need to be chosen (see Drug Table 603.6).

DEVELOPMENTAL STAGES AND ADMINISTERING MEDICATIONS

When administering medications, or more likely, when counseling caregivers on how to administer medications, the healthcare provider always must consider the developmental level of the child. For example, the approach to giving medications to toddlers is very different from the approach to school-aged children. The reader is referred to Erik Erikson's and Jean Piaget's theories of child development for background information.

NEONATES

Since separation from parents is one of the biggest issues for neonates, it is recommended that caregivers hold the neonates securely when administering any medication. And even though it may seem silly, caregivers should also tell the neonates that they are getting medicine to make them feel better. In this way the caregivers will be in the habit of explaining the reason for the medication to the children, and this matter-of-fact explanation to children will help increase compliance when children are older. It is sometimes difficult to open neonates' eyes, so drops must be applied quickly. When giving oral medications, it is best to put the medicine in a nipple or special device, so the infants can suck the medicine. Do not put it in a bottle of formula or other liquids, because the infants may not finish the bottle. The caregiver also can give very small amounts of the medicine slowly to the inside of the cheek with an oral syringe. The neonates' taste has not developed, so the medicine should not be spit out, and the infants will take the medicine better if they are hungry (Bindler & Howry, 1991). To help encourage neonates or infants to swallow, the caregiver can stroke the throat or blow a puff or air into the face, which is called the *Santmyer swallow reflex* (Pagliaro, 1995). Masks are used to deliver nebulizer treatments for lung conditions. Rectal suppositories are sometimes given to neonates, e.g., glycerin suppositories for constipation. The suppositories should never be cut because the medication is not evenly dispersed (Pagliaro, 1995).

INFANTS

Administration of eye medication is seen as frightening and as an intrusion to infants (Pagliaro, 1995). Infants and toddlers do not like nose sprays because of the tickling sensation, taste, and difficulty in breathing; they feel that it is an invasion of their bodies (Pagliaro, 1995). Therefore, they should be told what to expect, that it will last only a short time, and that they can have a drink of their favorite liquid after accepting the spray; infants should be held gently during the administration.

Giving oral medications can be a challenge. Infants under 3 months can turn away from oral medications, and when the sense of taste develops, they can spit out a medication that they do not like. To help disguise medication, mix it with small amounts of certain soft foods, such as applesauce, yogurt, or pudding, unless the medication becomes unstable in these foods (Chater, 1993). Do not add medications to formula or other liquids. Infants may refuse it because of the taste, and in addition to not getting the full dose of medication, they may subsequently refuse the liquid. Stranger anxiety develops around 9 months, so let the caregivers give the medication. If strangers must do it, they can play games such as peek-a-boo with the infants first to gain their trust before administering medications. Infants also can reach for and grasp the medication cup and crawl away if not held.

TODDLERS

Certain characteristics are unique to toddlers. The first is negativism. Toddlers' favorite word is "NO," so expect that as an answer to any question you ask. Do not ask them if they are ready to take their medication; state that it is time for their medication. Only give choices for those things that you want as the result: which cup to use, the choice of Band-Aid or sticker, which arm to use first, etc. Do not get into a power struggle; set limits and do what you have to do quickly, especially with procedures or injections. Tell toddlers JUST before giving medication or an injection that you are going to give it. Do not discuss what will happen in the future; they are concerned with the present (Pagliaro, 1995). Ignore negative behavior and praise positive behavior.

Toddlers like routine and having things done in the same way (Wong, 1993a). It gives them a sense of control and security. They may want the same cup or the same drink after taking medicine or insist upon taking the medicine a certain way. Place a desired sticker where the children tell you to.

Toddlers are egocentric. They see illness, medication, and painful procedures as being their fault and a form of punishment (Dixon, 1992). Reinforce that they are not at fault. To help them gain a sense of control, let them play with the equipment, such as a mask, beforehand if possible, and definitely afterwards. Let them hold the cup if you know they are going to take the medication. Let them give it to a doll or stuffed animal first, if that will help them cooperate. Give short and simple explanations. "This medicine is to help your ear infection go away so you can get better," is sufficient. Let the caregivers help hold the children if they wish to. Praise the children for cooperating and cuddle them afterwards. Allow for outlet of aggression in a play situation (Pagliaro, 1995), especially after an unpleasant procedure, such as an injection.

If toddlers absolutely refuse oral medication, another route may have to be chosen (Pagliaro, 1995). However, an effective method of administering oral medication to a resisting child is to place the oral syringe diagonally across the tongue while delivering the medication into the inside of the cheek (Bindler & Howry, 1991). Toddlers should never be told that medication is candy (*Handbook of Pediatric Drug Therapy,* 2000; Miller & Fioravante, 1997).

Rectal medication is to be avoided because of the possible negative feelings associated with toilet training (*Handbook of Pediatric Drug Therapy,* 2000) as well as fear of body entry.

PRESCHOOLERS

Preschoolers are more cooperative than toddlers. They like to help (Pagliaro, 1995). Let them hold or play with the equipment; this gives them a sense of control. Children will usually take medication willingly if given a simple, truthful explanation: "This will help you get better." If expected to take a medication, they usually will cooperate (Pagliaro, 1995). Reinforce their cooperation by praising positive behaviors.

Other characteristics of preschoolers are animism and magical thinking (Dixon, 1992; Wong, 1993a). When explaining things, choose words carefully. They see things in a concrete sense. Objects in their world seem to be alive. "Germs in your throat" may seem to them to be unseen alive objects. They also think that all their blood will come out after receiving an injection, and that a Band-Aid will stop the blood loss. It helps to show the site and show that there is no blood loss. They will understand better if a procedure is demonstrated on a doll or stuffed animal and/or with a drawing (Pagliaro, 1995).

Their time concept is limited (Wong, 1993b). Explain each time a medication is given why they must take it (Pagliaro, 1995). Also, associate times for medication with events in their life: lunch, dinner, and bedtime (Pagaliaro, 1995).

When prescribing oral medications, order liquids unless the child can tolerate chewable tablets. The taste of the medication may need to be disguised. Do not call the medication candy. The caregiver may need to give medication to an imaginary friend first before giving it to the child. For inhalation medications, nebulizers are increasingly being used, as are dry powder inhalers (PDIs). See Chapter 22.

SCHOOL-AGERS

School-agers want to feel a sense of accomplishment (Selekman, 1993). If possible, let them help, e.g., by shaking the bottle of medication (Martin, 1992). Let them decide which liquid to take with the medication or whether to have a tablet, capsule, chewable tablet, or liquid. They can assume some responsibility in remembering to take their medication. They agree even when not understanding (Pagliaro, 1995), so explain carefully and ask them to explain the information to you. Use drawings to explain how the body works, the need to take medication, and how medications work. Reassure them that medication is not punishment. Use the word "medication," not "drug" (Martin, 1992). They are learning about drug abuse in school and that drugs are bad.

Five- or six-year-olds may be able to take a tablet or a capsule, depending upon the size. The healthcare provider must be certain of the children's ability to swallow tablets before ordering them. Chewable tablets are a good choice at this age, since they do not require refrigeration. Some chewable tablets have a tart taste and may be refused. Tablets can be crushed, and some capsules can be opened and put in food.

ADOLESCENTS

Adolescents may alternate between cooperation and negativism. They should be encouraged to take part in the decision making regarding their medication (Khunti, 1996). They are able to give themselves medication, but may not always remember or want to. Having a chart to mark the dose taken instead of constant verbal questions or reminders is a better way to keep track of medications taken. Once-a-day dosing is best; twice-a-day dosing is also good.

Adolescents want to be treated like adults, but may still need to be treated like children. They may not ask for help in administering eye- or eardrops. They should be able to tolerate tablets, but may still prefer liquids. Most older adolescents have abstract thinking and can understand reasons for illness and the necessity of needing medication. *Truthfully* explain the facts to adolescents. Communicate with them in an honest, understanding, and nonjudgmental way so the adolescents will feel comfortable in talking with the provider and disclosing needed information. Ask what other drugs they are taking, over-the-counter as well as illicit (Hein, 1992). Adolescents may use alcohol or illegal drugs that can interact with prescription drugs (Hein, 1992).

Adolescents do not like to feel different. With a chronic illness, they may feel different, and refuse to take their medication. A support group or meeting or talking on the phone with just one other person with the same illness may help alleviate this feeling of alienation or isolation. Also, pointing out some of their favorite celebrities with the same condition may help. The healthcare provider should explain things in such a way as to make compliance "cool."

Adolescents are concerned with the present. They will want an "instant" cure for acne, and may be frustrated with the slow progress of treatment.

Female adolescents may need vaginal medication for the first time. Explain how it works and use a diagram to show how it is inserted. Be sensitive to their feelings and embarrassment or lack of embarrassment.

Adolescents may be modest if needing an injection in the hip. They may still be afraid of needles (Schichor, Bernstein, Weinerman, et al., 1994). Adolescents may need reminders or charts to rotate sites for insulin injections.

PRACTICAL TIPS FOR PRESCRIBING MEDICATIONS

When prescribing medications, there are only two acceptable methods for calculating doses. These are milligrams of drug per kilogram of body weight (mg/kg) and milligrams of drug per square meter of body surface (mg/m^2). The surface area is a relationship between the height and weight and is the most accurate. However, not all drug doses are calculated by the body surface area formula by the manufacturers; most have been calculated in milligrams per kilogram. If there are questions regarding pediatric dosing, the American Academy of Pediatrics indicates that the manufacturer's packets are the official source of medication dosages (American Academy of Pediatrics Committee on Drugs, 1978).

Easy reference tables now are produced by drug companies for their products. They list age, weight, and dose, and may also state the size of the container to order. If tables do not exist, providers are encouraged to create their own tables of frequently used medications. Several examples of some of the most common antibiotic drugs are included in Table 12–2 and common over-the-counter medications in Table 12–3. Although some providers are weighing children in kilograms, the prevalent practice is to weigh in pounds. Thus the practice guides (see Table 12–2) in this chapter will cite pounds, not kilograms.

The provider's choice of medication needs to reflect understanding of ease of dosing, cost, efficacy with present and newer schedules, potential to develop resistance, as well as caregiver/patient preference. For example, many

TABLE 12–2. Practical Tips: Doses of Common Antibiotics for Children

Drug	Weight, lb	Dosage	Youngest Age Medication Safely Given
Amoxicillin; 40 mg/kg/d; q 8 h		125 mg/5 ml (1 tsp)	3 months
	6	1/4 tsp	
	10	1/2 tsp	
	16	3/4 tsp	
Amoxicillin; 45 mg/kg/d; q 12 h		400 mg/5 ml (1 tsp)	
	20	1/2 tsp	
	30	3/4 tsp	
	40	1 tsp	
	60	1 1/2 tsp	
Amoxicillin/clavulanate		400 mg/5 ml (1 tsp)	3 months
potassium (Augmentin);	11	1/4 tsp	[increased incidence of diarrhea
45 mg/kg/d; q 12 h	22	1/2 tsp	if used under 1 year of age]
	33	4/5 tsp	
	44	1 tsp	
	55	1 1/3 tsp	
	66	1 2/3 tsp	
	77	2 tsp	
Amoxicillin/clavulante potassium		600 mg/5 ml (1 tsp)	3 months
(Augmentin ES-600)	20	3/4 tsp	[increased incidence of diarrhea
90mg/kg/d; q 12 h	30	1 tsp	if given under 1 year of age]
	35	1 1/4 tsp	
	40	1 1/2 tsp	
	50	1 3/4 tsp	
Azithromycin (Zithromax);		100 mg/5 ml (1 tsp)	6 months
10 mg/kg; 5 mg/kg/d; q 24 h	22	1 tsp on day one	
		1/2 tsp next 4 days	
		200 mg/5 ml (1 tsp)	
	44	1 tsp on day one	
		1/2 tsp next 4 days	
	66	1 1/2 tsp on day one	
		3/4 tsp next 4 days	
Cefadroxil (Duricef);		250 mg/5ml (1 tsp)	1 month
30 mg/kg/d; q 12 h	10	1/4 tsp	
	20	1/2 tsp	
	30	3/4 tsp	
	40	1 tsp	
	50	1 1/4 tsp	
	60	1 1/2 tsp	
Cefdinir (Omnicef) 7 mg/kg/d;		125 mg/5 ml (1 tsp)	6 months
q 12 h x 5d–10d	20	1/2 tsp	
	40	1 tsp	
	60	1 1/2 tsp	
	80	2 tsp	
or			
14 mg/kg/d; q d x 10 d	20	1 tsp	
	40	2 tsp	
	60	3 tsp	
	80	4 tsp	
Cefpodoxine proxetil (Vantin);		50 mg/5 ml (1 tsp)	5 months
10 mg/kg/d; q 12 h	14	1/2 tsp	
	18	3/4 tsp	
		100 mg/5 ml (1 tsp)	5 months
	25	1/2 tsp	
	36	3/4 tsp	
	49	1 tsp	

(*continued*)

TABLE 12–2. Practical Tips: Doses of Common Antibiotics for Children (*Continued*)

Drug	Weight, lb	Dosage	Youngest Age Medication Safely Given
Cefprozil (Cefzil); 30 mg/kg/d;		125 mg/5 ml (1 tsp)	6 months
q 12 h	10	1/2 tsp	
	15	3/4 tsp	
		250 mg/5 ml (1 tsp)	
	20	1/2 tsp	
	30	3/4 tsp	
	40	1 tsp	
Cefuroxime axetil (Ceftin);		125 mg/5 ml (1 tsp)	3 months
30 mg/kg/d; q 12 h	9	1/2 tsp	
	13	3/4 tsp	
	18	1 tsp	
	22	1 1/4 tsp	
	26	1 1/2 tsp	
	33	1 3/4 tsp	
	37	2 tsp	
Clarithromycin (Biaxin);		125 mg/5 ml (1 tsp)	6 months
15 mg/kg/d; q 12 h	20	1/2 tsp	
	37	1 tsp	
		250 mg/5 ml (1 tsp)	
	55	3/4 tsp	
	73	1 tsp	
Erythromycin;		200 mg/5 ml (1 tsp)	Neonate
30–50 mg/kg/d; q 6 h	15	1/4 tsp	
	25	1/2 tsp	
	50	1 tsp	
	100	1 1/2 tsp	
	>100	2 tsp	
Bicillin L-A (Penacillin	Neonate	50,000 units/kg	Neonate
G Benzathine)	<2 years	300,000 units	Never give IV; give IM only
	>2 years;	600,000 units	
	<60 lb		
	>60 lb	1,200,000 units	
Nitrofurantoin (Macrodantin)		25 mg/5 ml (1 tsp)	1 month
5–7 mg/kg/d; q 6 h	22	1/2 tsp	
	44	1 tsp	
	66	1 1/2 tsp	
Penicillin V potassium	18	1/2 tsp of 125 mg/5 ml	Neonate
(Pen-Vee K); 25–	35	1 tsp of 125 mg/5 ml	
50 mg/kg/d; q 6 h	>35	1 tsp of 250 mg/5 ml	
Trimethoprim (8 mg/kg/d);	22	1 tsp	2 months
sulfamethoxazole	44	2 tsp	
(Co-Trimoxazole)	66	3 tsp	
(40 mg/kg/d) (Bactrim,	88	4 tsp	
Septra) q 12 h			

Source: Adapted from Gennrich & Chan (1996), Physician's Desk Reference (2004). Taketomo, Hodding, & Krause (1993), and tables produced by manufacturers of medications.

TABLE 12–3. Practical Tips: Pediatric Doses of Common Over-the-Counter Medications

Drug	Weight/Age	Dosage	Youngest Age Medication Safely Given
Acetaminophen (Tylenol):	11 lb	1/4 tsp of 160 mg/5 ml (1 tsp) (0.4 mL of 80 mg/mL)	Neonate
10 mg/kg/dose; q 4 h	17 lb	1/2 tsp of 160 mg/5 cc (0.8 mL of 80 mg/mL)	
		160 mg/5 ml (1 tsp)	
	23 lb	3/4 tsp	
	35 lb	1 tsp	
	47 lb	1 1/2 tsp	
	59 lb	2 tsp	
	71 lb	2 1/2 tsp	
	95 lb	3 tsp	
	>95 lb	4 tsp	
Chlorpheniramine (Chlor-		2 mg/5 ml (1 tsp)	
Trimeton): 1–2 mg/dose;	3 months-2 years	1/4 tsp	3 months
q.i.d.	2–6 years	1/2 tsp	
	6–12 years	1 tsp	
	>12 years	2 tsp	
Guaifenesin (Robitussin):		100 mg/5 ml (1 tsp)	
12 mg/kg/day; q.i.d.	6 months-1 year	1/4 tsp	6 months
	1–6 years	1/2 tsp	
	6–12 years	1 tsp	
	>12 years	2 tsp	
Ibuprofen (Advil, Motrin):		100 mg/5 ml(1 tsp)	
7.5 mg/kg/dose; q 6-8h	17 lb	1/2 tsp	6 months
	23 lb	3/4 tsp	
	35 lb	1 tsp	
	47 lb	1 1/2 tsp	
	59 lb	2 tsp	
	71 lb	2 1/2 tsp	
	95 lb	3 tsp	
Pseudoephedrine (Sudafed):		15 mg/5 ml(1 tsp)	
4 mg/kg/d; tid	17 lb	1/2 tsp	4 months
	23 lb	3/4 tsp	
	35 lb	1 tsp	
	47 lb	1 1/2 tsp	
	59 lb	2 tsp	
	71 lb	2 1/2 tsp	
	95 lb	3 tsp	
Pseudoephedrine		7.5 mg/0.8 ml	
(PediaCare): tid	11 lb	0.4 ml	3 months
	17 lb	0.8 ml	
	23 lb	1.2 ml	
	35 lb	1.6 ml	
Combinations			
Dimetapp: tid[a]	6–11 months	1/4 tsp	6 months
	1–2 years	1/2 tsp	
	2–6 years	1 tsp	
	6–12 years	2 tsp	
	> 12 years	4 tsp	
Triaminic (all products):	4 months-1 year	1/4 tsp	4 months
tid[b]	1–2 years	1/2 tsp	
	2–6 years	1 tsp	
	6–12 years	2 tsp	
	> 12 years	4 tsp	

[a]Contains brompheniramine maleate and pseudoephedrine HCl.

[b]Ingredients differ; may include pseudoephedrine HCl, chlorpheniramine maleate, dextromethorphan HBr, acetominophen, or guaifenesin.

Sources: Adapted from Gennrich & Chan (1996), Physician's Desk Reference for Nonprescription Drugs & Dietary Supplements (2003), and tables produced by manufacturers of medications.

providers may consider using second- and third-generation broad spectrum antibiotics for the treatment of otitis media. Yet recent studies still show that amoxicillin is the first drug of choice for the initial treatment of otitis media (Berman, Byrns, Bondy, et al., 1997; Rosenfeld & Bluestone, 1999). Some studies have shown that older children can be treated for uncomplicated otitis media with only 5 days of medication (Gooch, Blair, Puopdo, et al., 1996; Hoberman, Paradise, Burch, et al., 1997; Kozyrskyj, Hildes-Ripstein, Lougstaffe, et al., 1998; Paradise, 1995a), taking into account other conditions, such as season of the year, severity of the episode, previous history of otitis, and the child's response to current treatment (Paradise, 1995b). In addition, the recent use of ceftriaxone (Rocephin) as a one-time intramuscular injection has also been found to be equally effective as the traditional 10-day course (Barnett, Teele, Klein, et al., 1997; Bauchner, Adams, Barnett, & Klein, 1996; Chamberlain, Boenning, Waisman, et al., 1994; Green & Rothrock, 1993). In one of these studies (Bauchner et al., 1996), parents overwhelmingly indicated a preference for a one-time injection for their child's next case of otitis media. However, some authors warn against its use because of increasing bacterial resistance (Goldfarb & Medendorp, 1994; Rosenfeld & Bluestone, 1999).

Currently, high-risk populations, such as persons who are homeless or migrant workers (see Chapter 15) or some emergency room patients, might be candidates for the one-time intramuscular medication for specific bacterial infections (Rosenfeld & Bluestone, 1999; Varsano, Volvitz, Horev, et al., 1997). Other special circumstances, particularly in cases where the ability to tolerate or absorb oral drugs is compromised, or in children unable to take oral medication, might also lead the provider to consider using an injection (Varsano et al., 1997). Yet if one is assured that the caregiver will be able to administer the complete course of medication, the narrowest spectrum antibiotic is still preferred, taking into account the cost and caregiver preference for frequency of administration. Parents not in a high-risk group who request one-time injections need to have information about the risk of developing resistant organisms discussed with them in a respectful manner.

There are many practical tips for writing prescriptions, teaching, and safety that have been generated from providers experienced in pediatric care that may be helpful to those less familiar with this population. Tips for medication writing are summarized in Table 12–4, teaching tips for parents and families in Table 12–5, and safety issues in Table 12–6.

TABLE 12–4. Practical Tips: Prescription Writing

1. Always get a **weight** at **every** pediatric visit. A child can lose weight easily with an illness. Even if the infant or child was seen 3 days ago, today's weight is critical to calculate correct medication dosage.
2. **Do not go above the recommended adult doses** when ordering for adolescents. If drugs were ordered by milligram per kilogram, too high a dose would be ordered.
3. As a rule, **start** with the **smallest dose** or the **weakest strength,** especially if treating a neonate. For example, topical gel preparations, such as tretinoin for acne, are stronger than lotions or creams.
4. "**Round up**" the dose if it falls between the given choices **unless it is a toxic drug or has severe side effects,** since compliance is not usually 100%.
5. With **acetaminophen** products, **calculate** the dose by **weight,** not age.
6. It has been difficult to dose patients **under 2 years of age** for OTC preparations. If a schedule does not exist, a provider can use the milligram per kilogram value of at least one of the ingredients to calculate the dose needed if there is a compelling reason to use a specific medication and no other practical options exist. See Table 12–2.
7. In **writing a prescription,** be very explicit in your terminology. It is best to write out numbers. State "chewable" tabs if that is what is desired. State "suspension," especially for Cortisporin otic medication. Be consistent in writing "tsp," "cc," or "ml," and tell the caregiver the term that you are writing. If you write "5 ml," tell the caregiver to give "5 ml," not "one teaspoon." This also helps remind them to use a measuring device and not a household teaspoon. Write a zero preceding decimals (Burg & Bourret, 1994), but not after. Print or type if your handwriting is not legible (Burg & Bourret, 1994). Order the exact amount needed. If more is given, the caregiver may be tempted to use more than is needed or use the remainder for another sick child. Write the patient's weight on the prescription, especially for antibiotics, and write the mg/kg if you are ordering a dose that is different than normal.
8. You may write the reason for the antibiotic on the prescription. For example: "for ear infection" (J. M. Shalf, Personal Communication, July 15, 1996).
9. An example of a written prescription:
   Amoxicillin susp 125 mg/5 ml
   150 ml
   5 ml PO tid × 10 days for ear infection
   No refills
10. If medication needs to be sent to **school** or **day care,** write on the prescription for two bottles and have the pharmacist split the amounts according to the number of days needed. Some school systems require a special form that includes the name of the medication, dosage, and time and duration to be given.
11. **New schedules** and drugs are frequently introduced, including lower age limits. Review the literature on the proposed change and/or consult with collaborating physicians and/or pharmacists for efficacy or side effects of proposed changes. For example, cefpodoxime proxetil and cefdinir (Adler, McDonald, Trostmann, et al., 2000) can now be given once a day.

TABLE 12–5. Practical Tips: Teaching

1. Always **explain** the name of the medication (brand and generic), the class of drug, what it is for, why it was chosen, and any side effects (Martin, 1992; Wink, 1991). This will help to increase compliance by increasing the caregiver's or patient's understanding.
2. If ordering an **extended-release** tablet or capsule, teach the caregiver or the patient the terms associated with these drugs: CR (controlled-release or continuous-release), DUR (duration), LA (long-acting), SA (sustained-action), SR (sustained-release or slow-release), TD (time-delay), and XR (extended-release) (Pagliaro, 1995, p. 19). Reinforce **not crushing or opening** these tablets or capsules (Pagliaro, 1995; Sagraves, 1995).
3. Give **verbal and written** instructions reinforcing any special instructions about medications—e.g., decreasing doses of prednisone or when to stop a medication if different from the usual time period.
4. Reinforce the idea of **proper storage.** Most antibiotics need refrigeration, and caregivers and patients need to be reminded of this. If traveling, order a medication that does not need to be refrigerated, such as cefixime, cefuroxime axetil, or trimethoprim-sulfamethoxazole or chewable if available (see Drug Tables 102.2, 102.3, and 102.10).
5. Have the caregivers or patient read back to you any instructions you have given them. By having them read the instructions back to you, you screen for understanding and reading level. Having written instructions is helpful, because listening and retention are decreased when someone is distracted by worry about a sick child, a crying baby, or other children in the room. The healthcare provider can give preprinted instructions with appropriate blanks to be filled in for various situations or alternate forms of instruction, such as audio- or videotape, if the patient's or the caregiver's vision and/or reading is not optimal. Copies of written instructions can be placed in the chart to facilitate communication. Check for understanding of key information by stressing important items.

PAIN IN CHILDREN AND ADOLESCENTS

Pain from injections and blood tests seems to be expected in pediatrics. Sometimes adults become immune to the reactions of children and adolescents to painful procedures. On the other hand, some adults have not forgotten their experience as children and are still afraid of needles as adults.

In pediatrics, painful procedures are caused by vaccinations, other injections, and the taking of blood through a fingertip or vein. To help the child cope, for the neonate and small infant, it is best to cuddle them after the injection. Beginning at 8 to 12 months, infants associate pain with the needle and syringe, so the healthcare provider must keep the syringe out of sight just until time to give the injection (Bindler & Howry, 1991). Toddlers should be told that the injection will hurt, but only for a short time. They need to be held securely and be given the injection quickly. For older infants and children, providers can try diversionary measures: blowing when receiving the injection, closing eyes, wriggling toes, counting to 10 (Pagliaro, 1995), tapping another part of the body, and looking the other way. McCaffery and Beebe (1989) have advocated pinching and grasping the deltoid muscle when giving an injection there, ice massage, use of hot and cold, imagery, singing, listening to music, tapping a rhythm, rhythmic massage, and slow rhythmic breathing.

A newer method of pain relief is the use of EMLA cream that contains 2.5% lidocaine and 2.5% prilocaine (Farrington, 1993; Goode & Betcher, 1994). It must be applied to intact skin 1 to 2 hours before the procedure, depending upon the depth of penetration desired, with the maximum depth of approximately 5 mm being achieved at 2 hours (Farrington, 1993). Although numerous studies have shown that EMLA reduces pain associated with venipuncture, lumbar punctures, or intravenous insertion, the data on its use to reduce injection pain is scarce and conflicting. Three studies (Morris, Hughes, Hardy, et al., 1994; Raveh, Weinberg, Sibirsky, et al., 1995; Taddio, Nulman, Goldbach, et al., 1994) support the ability of EMLA to reduce pain of injections. Only one of these studies (Taddio et al., 1994) involved children. In contrast, a Danish study found EMLA did not reduce pain in MMR immunizations in older children (Hansen & Sorensen, 1993). The provider needs to monitor future research developments to determine the advisability of EMLA use for immunizations in children.

Several studies have explored the use of diversionary methods in a clinical setting, and two studies found that having children blow was the easiest and most effective (French, Painter, & Coury, 1994; Geldmaker, 1994). Children can blow against a mobile, a pinwheel, or imaginary birthday candles. For older children, it is best to explain that they will experience pain for a short time, but the pain will end. Be sensitive to their psychological level; they may respond at a more immature level than their chronological age. An analgesic can be given for the pain if necessary. The reader is referred to the literature for more detailed information about pain.

SUMMARY

Prescribing and administering medications to children can be challenging but not insurmountable. Important information as well as practical guidelines have been highlighted in this chapter. The provider should consult Chapter 5 for further considerations helpful in working

TABLE 12–6. Practical Tips: Safety Issues

1. Reinforce using a **measuring device** for giving medications, not the household teaspoon, which can hold anywhere from 2 to 10 ml (Madlon-Kay & Mosch, 2000).
2. Advise patients to drink plenty of **fluids** when taking pills (Martin, 1992) and to only take one pill at a time if more than one is ordered (Pagliaro, 1995).
3. **Avoid liquid oil formulations** such as **castor oil or mineral oil** in infants/toddlers due to the risk of aspiration and lipid pneumonia (Pagliaro, 1995).
4. Aminoglycoside eardrops should **not** be instilled if there is a risk of eardrum perforation; or P.E. tubes; hearing loss or deafness can occur (Livingstone & Livingstone, 1989). Auralgon eardrops are also contraindicated if the eardrum is perforated (Barone, 1996) (see Drug Table 402.2).
5. Beware of "compounding pharmacists": those who make their own drugs or change already manufactured ones (Perrin, 1996). Adding flavors to antibiotics by a pharmacist is permissible.
6. Granting refills on a prescription depends upon many factors. If one would like to see a patient back, it is best not to write prescriptions with refills. Certain medications should never have refills (controlled substances and usually antibiotics). It is permissible to order refills on medicines that might be necessary in an emergency situation—for example, albuterol for asthmatics. It is also a good idea not to order refills until you are better acquainted with the patient.
7. Caregivers should understand **drops** versus dropperfuls. Several medications for neonates and infants are ordered in drops, and overdoses have occurred because the caregiver mistakenly gave dropperfuls instead of drops (Rudy, 1992). Many caregivers also use one dropper—for example, one that comes with acetaminophen drops—for different medications. They need to be taught to use only the dropper that comes with the medication. It is a good idea to have samples of different medication droppers available so parents can be shown the one that belongs with the medication ordered (Pagliaro, 1995).
8. **Reinforce followup.** Caregivers should know to call or return to the clinic if there is no improvement in 48 hours with antibiotics, or whenever deemed necessary. Caregivers may tend to give more of a medication if they see no improvement. You as the healthcare provider also need to see how the child is tolerating the medication. A phone call from you in a few days can be very helpful.
9. **Always explain allergic symptoms and the possibility of an allergic reaction with any medication ordered.** Allergic symptoms in children can include rash, hives, vomiting, diarrhea, anaphylaxis, or any other unusual symptoms (Cochran, 1991). Neomycin is a common allergen and is contained in Cortisporin otic suspension and Neosporin (see Drug Tables 402.1 and 805). Caregivers may not realize that a certain medication is in a certain class. They may only know the brand name. That is why you should state the brand name as well as the class when giving a prescription. For example, "I'm ordering amoxicillin, which is a penicillin. Is your child allergic to penicillin?" **Always ask more than once about allergies.** Caregivers may forget in their anxiety about their child.
10. **Allergies should be displayed in a prominent place in the chart.**
11. Check with African American patients about their ability to take **acetaminophen, aspirin,** or **sulfa.** Glucose-6-phosphate dehydrogenase (G6PD) deficient patients will have a hemolytic anemic reaction if given these drugs (Siberry & Iannone, 2000, p. 616) (see Drug Tables 301, 307, 102.9, 102.10).
12. **Be explicit in charting** any medications given, including dosage, frequency, and duration. Ask at each visit the current medications, along with the dose given, including OTCs. Ask about herbal use.
13. **Storage** of medications at home should be in a safe place, not in the bathroom, but in a locked box on a high shelf. Medication in the refrigerator should be on a high shelf and in a box that is difficult to open. When visiting relatives, caregivers should remind them to keep their medications out of the reach of children, especially purses, where many people keep medicines. Most medications for the elderly do not have child-resistant packaging (Rodgers, 1996).
14. Reinforce **not sharing** medications or putting them in other unlabeled containers, especially when sending a child to camp (Lishner & Busch, 1994).
15. Have the **poison control phone number** handy in case of accidental poisoning.
16. Advise caregivers to check labels for **additives** such as alcohol, sugars, sodium (Pagliaro, 1995), food dyes, and preservatives (Sagraves, 1995).
17. Use the **clinical rule** to double-check doses chosen. The average 12-year-old gets 100% of the adult dose, a 6-year-old gets approximately one-half of the adult dose, and a 2- to 3-year-old gets approximately one-quarter of the adult dose. If these approximations do not match calculated doses, check your calculations.

with families. In addition issues for pediatric rehabilitation are addressed in Chapter 14.

The author would like to express her thanks to the following for their input to this chapter: Jerome M. Shalf, MD; Christie Lessels, RN, MS, CFNP; David Ballowe; Janet Younger, Ph.D., CPNP; and Elizabeth Builta RN, M.S, CPNP, for their reviews of an earlier draft of this manuscript.

REFERENCES

Adler, M., McDonald, P.J., Trostmann, U., Keyserling, C., & Tack, K. (2000). Cefdinir vs. amoxicillin/clavulanic acid in the treatment of suppurative acute otitis media in children. *Pediatric Infectious Disease Journal, 19*(12), S166-170.

American Academy of Pediatrics Committe on Drugs. (1978). Unapproved uses of approved drugs: The physician, the packaging insert, and the PDR. *Pediatrics, 62* (2), 262–264.

Barnett, E. D., Teele, D. W., Klein, J. O., Cabral, H. J., & Kharasch, S. J. (1997). Comparison of ceftriaxone and trimethoprim-sulfamethoxazole (sulfamethoxozole) for acute otitis media. *Pediatrics 99*(1):23–28.

Bauchner, H., Adams, W., Barnett, E., & Klein, J. (1996). Therapy for acute otitis media. *Archives of Pediatric and Adolescent Medicine, 150,* 396–399.

Behrman, R. E., & Vaughan, V. C. (1987). *Nelson's textbook of pediatrics* (13th ed.) (pp. 231–237). Philadelphia: WB Saunders. Cited in Wink (1991).

Berlin, C. M., Jr. (2000). Challenges in conducting pediatric pediatric drug trials. *Journal of Allergy and Clinical Immunology, 106*(3), S125-127.

Berman, S., Byrns, P. J., Bondy, J., Smith, P.J., & Lezotte, D. (1997). Otitis media–related antibiotic prescribing patterns, outcomes, and expenditures in a pediatric medicaid population. *Pediatrics, 100*(4), 585-592.

Bindler, R. M., & Howry, L. B. (1991). *Pediatric drugs and nursing implications* (pp. 1–45). Norwalk, CT: Appleton & Lange.

Blumer, J. L. (1999). Off-label uses of drugs in children. *Pediatrics, 104*(3), 598–602.

Blumer, J. L., & Reed, M. D. (1992). Principles of neonatal pharmacology. In S. J. Yaffe & J. V. Aranda (Eds.), *Pediatric pharmacology: Therapeutic principles in practice* (2nd ed.) (pp. 164–177). Philadelphia: W. B. Saunders.

Burg, F. D., & Bourrett, J. A. (1994). *Current pediatric drugs.* Philadelphia: W. B. Saunders.

Cetta, F., Lambert, G. H., & Ros, S. P. (1991). Newborn chemical exposure from over-the-counter skin care products. *Clinical Pediatrics, 30,* 286–289.

Chamberlain, J. M., Boenning, D. A., Waisman, Y., Ochsenschlager, D. W., & Klein, B. L. (1994, November). Single-dose ceftriaxone versus 10 days of cefaclor for otitis media. *Clinical Pediatrics,* 642–646.

Chater, R. W. (1993). Pediatric dosing: Tips for tots. *American Pharmacy, NS33,* 55–56.

Cochran, F. B. (1991). Hypersensitivity to carbamazepine mimicking infection. *Clinical Pediatrics, 30,* 95–96.

Dixon, S. D. (1992). Two years: Learning the rules—Language and cognition. In S. D. Dixon & M. T. Stein, *Encounters with children: Pediatric behavior and development* (p. 248). St. Louis: Mosby–Year Book.

Farrington, E. (1993). Lidocaine 2.5%/prilocaine 2.5% EMLA cream. *Pediatric Nursing, 19,* 484–486, 488.

French, G. M., Painter, E. C., & Coury, D. L. (1994). Blowing away shot pain, a technique for pain management during immunization. *Pediatrics 93* (3), 384–388.

Geldmaker, B. (1994). *Pediatric pain interviews* (Video). Richmond, Virginia Commonwealth University.

Gennrich, J. L. & Chan, P. D. (1996). *Pediatric Drug Reference* (pp. 23, 38, 55). Fountain Valley, CA: Current Clinical Strategies Publishing.

Ghadially, R., & Shear, N. H. (1992). Topical therapy and percutaneous absorption. In S. J. Yaffe & J. V. Aranda (Eds.), *Pediatric pharmacology: Therapeutic principles in practice* (2nd ed.) (pp. 72–77). Philadelphia: W. B. Saunders.

Goldfarb, J., & Medendorp, S. (1994, November). New therapies for otitis media. *Clinical Pediatrics,* 647–648.

Gooch, W. M. III, Blair, E., Puopolo, A., Paster, R. Z., Schwartz, R. H., Miller, H C., Smyre, H. L., Yetman, R., Giguere, G. G., & Collins, J. J. (1996). Effectiveness of five days of therapy with cefuroxine axetil suspension for treatment of acute otitis media. *Pediatric Infectious Disease Journal, 15*(2), 157–164.

Goode, I. A., & Betcher, D. L. (1994). EMLA. *Journal of Pediatric Oncology Nursing 11,* 38–41.

Green, S. M., & Rothrock, S. G. (1993). Single-dose intramuscular ceftriaxone for acute otitis media in children. *Pediatrics, 91* (1), 23–30.

Green, T. P., & Mirkin, B. L. (1984). *Clinical pharmacokinetics: Pediatric considerations.* In L. Z. Benet, N. Massoud, & J. G. Gambertoglio, (Eds.), *Pharmacokinetic basis for drug treatment* (pp. 269–282). New York: Raven Press. Cited in Kauffman (1992).

Handbook of pediatric drug therapy. (2000). Springhouse, PA: Springhouse (pp. vii-viii, 1–4, 804).

Hansen, B. W., & Sorensen, P. V. (1993). The EMLA cream versus placebo in MMR vaccination of older children in general practice. *Ugeskr Laeger, 155*(29):2263–2265.

Hein, K. (1992). Drug therapeutics in the adolescent. In S. J. Yaffe & J. V. Aranda (Eds.), *Pediatric pharmacology: Therapeutic principles in practice* (2nd ed., pp. 220–233). Philadelphia: W. B. Saunders.

Hoberman, A., Paradise, J.L., Burch, D. J., Valinski, W. A., Hedrick, J. A., Aronovitz, G. H., Drehobl, M. A., & Rogers, J. M. (1997). Equivalent efficacy and reduced occurrence of diarrhea from a new formulation of amoxicillin/clavulante potassium (Augmentin R) for treatment of acute otitis media in children. *Pediatric Infectious Disease Journal, 16*(5), 463–420.

Kauffman, R. E. (1992). Drug therapeutics in the infant and child. In S. J. Yaffe & J. V. Aranda (Eds.), *Pediatric pharmacology: Therapeutic principles in practice* (2nd ed.) (pp. 212–219). Philadelphia: W. B. Saunders.

Kearns, G. L., & Reed, M. D. (1989). Clinical pharmacokinetics in infants and children: A reappraisal. *Clinical Pharmacokinetics, 17,* 29–67. Cited in Kauffman (1992).

Khunti, K. (1996, February). Issues in adolescent asthma: Compliance. *Maternal and Child Health,* 36–38.

Kiebler, B., & Mowry, J. B. (1994). Acetaminophen's potential for morbidity and mortality. *Pediatric Nursing, 20,* 491–494.

Kozyrskyj, A. L., Hildes-Ripstein, G. E., Longstaffe, S.E.A., Wincott, J. L., Sitar, D. S., Klassen, T. P., Moffatt, M.E.K. (1998). Treatment of acute otitis media with a shortened course of antibiotics. *Journal of American Medical Association, 279*(21), 1736–1742.

Lehne, R. A., Moore, L. A., Crosby, L. J., & Hamilton, D. B. (1990). *Pharmacology for nursing care* (pp. 29–84). Philadelphia: W. B. Saunders. Cited in Wink (1991).

Lishner, K., & Busch, K. (1994). Safe delivery of medications to children in summer camps. *Pediatric Nursing, 20,* 249–253.

Livingstone, C., & Livingstone, D. (1989). Drug delivery. Part 6: Formulations for the eye, nose, and ear. *The Pharmaceutical Journal, 242,* 688–689. Cited in Pagliaro (1995).

Lucey, J. F. (1992). Forward to the second edition. In S. J. Yaffe & J. V. Aranda (Eds.), *Pediatric pharmacology: Thera-*

peutic principles in practice (2nd ed). Philadelphia: W. B. Saunders.

Lumbiagannon, P., Pengsaa, K., & Sookpranee, T. (1991). Ciprofloxacin in neonates and its possible adverse effect on teeth. *Pediatric Infectious Disease Journal, 10,* 619–620.

Madlon-Kay, D. J., & Mosch, F. S. (2000). Liquid medication dosing errors. *Journal of Family Practice, 49*(8), 741–744.

Martin, S. (1992). Catering to pediatric patients. *American Pharmacy, NS32,* 47–50.

Maswoswe, J. J., Egbunike, I., Stewart, K. R., et al. (1994). Suspected fatal diphenhydramine toxicity by application to the skin of an infant with varicella. *Hospital Pharmacy, 29,* 26, 28–30, 53. Cited in Pagliaro (1995).

McCaffery, M., & Beebe, A. (1989). *Pain: Clinical manual for nursing practice* (pp. 133, 143, 146, 155, 173, 176, 177, 213). St. Louis: C. V. Mosby.

Merenstein, G. B., & Gardner, S. L. (1989). Handbook of neonatal intensive care (2nd ed.) (pp. 141–159). St. Louis: C. V. Mosby. Cited in Wink (1991).

Miller, S., & Fioravante, J. (1997). *Pediatric medications: A handbook for nurses* (pp. 1–10). St. Louis, MO: Mosby.

Morris, K. P., Hughes, C., Hardy, S. P., Matthews, J. N., & Coulthard, M. G. (1994). Pain after subcutaneous injection of recombinant human erythropoietin: does Emla cream help? *Nephrology Dialysis and Transplant, 9*(9): 1299–1301.

Nahata, M. C. (1993, August). Therapeutic considerations in pediatric patients. *Pharmacy and Therapeutics,* 752–762.

Niederhauser, V. P. (1997). Prescribing for children: Issues in pediatric pharmacology. *Nurse Practitioner, 22* (3), 16–30.

Pagliaro, A. M. (1995). Administering drugs to infants, children, and adolescents. In L. A. Pagliaro & A. M. Pagliaro (Eds.), Problems in pediatric drug therapy (3rd ed., pp. 3–101). Hamilton, IL: Drug Intelligence Publications.

Paradise, J. L. (1995a). Managing otitis media: A time for a change. *Pediatrics, 96*(4), 712–715.

Paradise, J. L. (1995b). Treatment guidelines for otitis media: The need for breadth and flexibility. *Pediatric Infectious Disease Journal, 14*(5), 429–435.

Pediatrics (1997). Inactive ingredients in pharmaceutical products: Update (Subject review) 99 (2) 268–278.

Perrin, J. H. (1996). Pediatrician and compounding pharmacist: A dangerous liaison. *Archives of Pediatric and Adolescent Medicine, 150,* 224–226.

Phelps, D. L. (1993). Retinopathy of prematurity. *Pediatric Clinics of North America, 40,* 705–714.

Physician's Desk Reference (58th ed.) (2004). pp. 408–417, 456–458, 503–507, 980–983, 1045–1048, 1079–1080, 1427–1431, 1435–1438, 1441–1444, 1463–1467, 2149–2151, 2178–2180, 2682–2687, 2793–2797.

Physician's Desk Reference for Nonprescriptive Drugs & Dietary Supplements (24th ed.) (2003). pp. 677, 686–688, 705–707, 741, 747–749, 778–779, 781–782, 785–793.

Raveh, T., Weinberg, A., Sibirsky, O., et al. (1995). Efficacy of the topical anesthetic cream, EMLA, in alleviating both needle insertion and injection pain. *Annals of Plastic Surgery, 35*(6), 576–579.

Reed, M. D., & Besunder, J. B. (1989, October). Developmental pharmacology: Ontogenic basis of drug disposition. *Pediatric Clinics of North America, 36,* 1053–1074. Cited in Wink (1991).

Rodgers, G. B. (1996). The safety effects of child-resistant packaging for oral prescription drugs. *Journal of the American Medical Association, 275,* 1661–1665.

Rosenfeld, R.M., & Bluestone, C.D. (1999). Clinical pathway for acute otitis media. In R.M. Rosenfeld & C.D. Bluestone (Eds.), *Evidence-based otitis media* (pp. 240–258). Hamilton, Ontario: B.C. Decker, Inc.

Rudy, C. (1992). A drop or a dropper: The risk of overdose. *Journal of Pediatric Health Care, 6,* 40, 51–52.

Sagraves, R. (1995, November/December). Pediatric dosing information for health care providers. *Journal of Pediatric Health Care,* 272–277.

Schichor, A., Bernstein, B., Weinerman, H., Fitzgerald, J., Yordan, E., & Schechter, N. (1994). Lidocaine as a diluent for ceftriaxone in the treatment of gonorrhea. *Archives of Pediatric and Adolescent Medicine, 148,* 72–75.

Selekman, J. (1993). Health promotion of the school-age child and family. In D. L. Wong, *Whaley & Wong's essentials of pediatric nursing* (4th ed.) (p. 425). St. Louis: C. V. Mosby.

Siberry, G. K., & Iannone, R. (Eds.). (2000). *The Harriet Lane handbook* (15th ed.); pp. 669–670, 679, 805. St. Louis: Mosby.

Simon, R. E. (1996). Ibuprofen suspension: Pediatric antipyretic. *Pediatric Nursing, 22,* 118–120.

Skaer, T. L. (1991). Dosing considerations in the pediatric patient. *Clinical Therapeutics, 13,* 526–544.

Smith, A. L. (1992). Chloramphenicol. In S. J. Yaffe & J. V. Aranda (Eds.), *Pediatric pharmacology: Therapeutic principles in practice* (2nd ed.) (pp. 276–286). Philadelphia: W. B. Saunders.

Taddio, A., Nulman, I., Goldbach, M., Ipp, M., & Koren, G. J. (1994). Use of lidocaine-prilocaine cream for vaccination pain in infants. *Journal of Pediatrics 124*(4):643–648.

Taketomo, C.K., Hodding, J.H., & Kraus, D.M. (1993). *Pediatric dosage handbook* (pp. 414–415). Cleveland: Lexi-Comp, Inc.

Todd, J. K. (1995). Antimicrobial therapy of pediatric infections. In W. W. Hay, Jr., J. R. Groothuis, A. R. Hayward, & M. J. Levin (Eds.), *Current pediatric diagnosis and treatment* (12th ed.) (pp. 1012–1016). Norwalk, CT: Appleton & Lange.

Varsano, I., Volvitz, B., Horev, Z., Robinson, J., Laks, Y., Rosenbaum, I., Cohen, A., Eilam, N., Jaber, L., Fuchs, C., & Amir, J. (1997). Intramuscular ceftriaxone compared with oral amoxicillin-clavulante for treatment of acute otitis media in children. *European Journal of Pediatrics 156*(11), 858–863.

Wilson, J. T., Kearns, G. L., Murphy, D., & Yaffe, S. J. (1994). Paediatric Labeling Requirements. *Clinical Pharmacokinetics, 26,* 308–325.

Wink, D. M. (1991). Giving infants and children drugs: Precision + caution = safety. *Maternal Child Nursing, 16,* 317–321.

Wong, D. L. (1993a). Health promotion of the toddler and family. In D. L. Wong, *Whaley & Wong's essentials of pediatric nursing* (4th ed.) (pp. 345, 347). St. Louis: C. V. Mosby.

Wong, D. L. (1993b). Health promotion of the preschooler and family. In D. L. Wong, *Whaley & Wong's essentials of pediatric nursing* (4th ed.) (p. 369). St. Louis: C. V. Mosby.

Yaffe, S. J., & Aranda, J. V. (1992). Introduction and historical perspective. In S. J. Yaffe & J. V. Aranda (Eds.), *Pediatric pharmacology: Therapeutic principles in practice* (2nd ed.) (pp. 3–9). Philadelphia: W. B. Saunders.

CHAPTER ❖ 13

GERIATRIC ISSUES

Geneva Briggs

Much of current U.S. healthcare practice is concerned with the needs of the older adult. As the vanguard of the "baby boomer" generation now advances from middle into old age, that demographic bulge is going to require even more attention and resources. At this time, the elderly—those over 65 years of age—consume approximately 30% of prescription and 40% of nonprescription medications (Cohen, 2000). Age-related changes, the increased number of chronic diseases, and healthcare professionals' varying levels of knowledge and skill contribute to some of the significant issues in geriatric pharmacotherapy: adverse drug events, excessive and inappropriate medications, and nonadherence (Cohen, 2000). The goals of pharmacotherapy for the elderly client should include obtaining maximal benefit with minimal harm.

The following discusses age-related changes in medication handling and response. Most of the research on this subject has been conducted in the young-old (55–65 years) and not the middle-old (65–85) or the old-old (>85). Because no one ages at the same rate, it is best to individualize your approach with each patient.

PHARMACOKINETIC CHANGES WITH AGING

The four phases of pharmacokinetics are absorption, distribution, metabolism, and excretion. The effects of aging on those phases are summarized in Table 13–1. In brief, although there are changes in drug absorption with aging, none of these are clinically significant or affect how medications are given to the elderly (Vestal, 1997). Conditions common to the elderly—achlorhydria, malabsorption, constipation, or diarrhea—can reduce drug absorption (Lee, 1996). Drug distribution is altered in the elderly because of changes in body composition. These changes include a decrease in lean body mass, increased body fat, and decreased total body water (Vestal, 1997). The increase in body fat can lead to excess storage of fat-soluble drugs, such as diazepam, a long-acting benzodiazepine. Water-soluble drugs, such as aminoglycosides and alcohol, can reach higher serum levels in the elderly due to reduced total body water (Vestal, 1997).

With aging there can be a decline in plasma albumin levels (Grandison & Boudinot, 2000). Since many drugs are bound to serum albumin, this change can mean an increase in unbound drug in the system and, potentially, an increase in adverse effects (Grandison & Boudinot, 2000). Alterations in protein binding that occur in the elderly are generally not attributed to age, but rather to physiological and pathophysiological changes or disease states that occur more frequently in the elderly (Grandison & Boudinot, 2000). Changes in protein binding are important for drugs that are highly bound to albumin, such as phenytoin and salicylates.

With aging there is a decrease in liver mass, volume, and blood flow (Vestal 2000). These declines are important because the liver is a major route of drug elimination.

TABLE 13–1. Pharmacokinetic Phases and Changes with Aging

Pharmacokinetic Parameter	Physiologic Change with Aging
Absorption	Increased gastric pH Increased GI transit time Decreased blood flow to muscles Decreased skin hydration Increase in keratinized cells
Distribution	Decreased lean body mass Decreased total body water Increased total body fat Decreased albumin levels
Renal elimination	Decreased glomerular filtration rate Decreased secretion
Metabolism	Decreased liver mass and volume Decreased liver blood flow Diminished enzyme activity

Sources: Vestal (2000); Grandison & Boudinot (2000).

Liver metabolic activity declines 1% per year after the age of 40 (Vestal, Norris, Tobin, Cohen, Shock, & Andres, 1975). Liver metabolism can be divided into two broad phases: oxidative (phase I) and conjugative (phase II). Phase I metabolism is impaired the most in the elderly (Vestal, 2000). A group of drugs that undergo significant phase I metabolism are the long-acting benzodiazepines, such as diazepam, flurazepam, and chlordiazepoxide. The elimination half-life of the long-acting benzodiazepines is significantly prolonged in the elderly versus a younger population. The half-life of diazepam in an elderly person is 82 h versus 37 h in a younger person (Ray, Griffen, & Downey, 1989). Aging does not appear to affect phase II metabolism.

Kidney function declines in two-thirds of the population at a rate of 1% per year beginning after age 50 (Vestal, 2000). This decline affects pharmacotherapy significantly because the kidney is also a major organ for drug elimination. The decreased glomerular filtration rate leads to the prolongation of the half-life of renally eliminated drugs and can lead to accumulation of these drugs within the body. Most dosage adjustments in the elderly are due to decreases in renal function.

Age-related changes in renal function are not necessarily reflected in an increase in serum creatinine because of the concurrent decrease in muscle mass (Smythe, Hoffman, Kizy, & Smuchowski, 1994). Renal function can be estimated using numerous equations, some of which are more accurate than others. Although not necessarily the most accurate, the Cockcroft-Gault equation is the most commonly used because it is easy to calculate (Cockcroft & Gault, 1976; Smythe et al., 1994):

$$\text{CrCl}\,(\text{mL/min}) = \frac{(140 - \text{age})(\text{wt})}{72 \times (\text{SCr})} \times 0.85\,(\text{for women})$$

$$\text{CrCl} = \text{creatinine clearance}$$

$$\text{SCr} = \text{serum creatinine in mg/dL}$$

$$\text{wt} = \text{kgs}$$

PHARMACODYNAMIC CHANGES WITH AGING

Pharmacodynamics is the study of what a drug does to the body. When a change in body response occurs with a drug, finding the cause is difficult and may include such reasons as altered pharmacokinetics, diminished homeostatic responses, or true changes in receptor interaction. The elderly are known to have a decreased response to beta-adrenergic receptor stimulators and blockers (Vestal, 2000). Whether this change is due to aging, disease, or both is unknown, and this change is probably not clinically significant. Studies have also supported the commonly held belief that the elderly have an increased sensitivity to benzodiazepines, narcotic analgesics, warfarin, diltiazem, verapamil, and alcohol even when pharmacokinetic changes are taken into account (Vestal, 2000).

ALTERATIONS IN HOMEOSTATIC MECHANISMS THAT AFFECT MEDICATIONS

With aging, homeostatic mechanism changes alter an elderly patient's response to medications. One well-described change is a decrease in baroreceptor sensitivity (Vestal, 2000). This can cause orthostatic changes alone, and is compounded by medications that lower blood pressure, such as antihypertensives, antipsychotics, and levodopa. Orthostatic hypotension can result in falls and subsequent hip fractures and head injuries.

The elderly are also sensitive to the anticholinergic effects of many medications (Moore & O'Keefe, 1999). With aging, a cholinergic deficit in the brain may occur that is thought to account for the benign forgetfulness the elderly may experience (Tune, 2001). The primary medication classes with anticholinergic properties are tricyclic antidepressants, antipsychotics, and antihistamines. Beyond the usual adverse effects of dry mouth, constipation, and urinary retention, these medications can cause confusion in the elderly (Moore & O'Keefe, 1999). Patients with dementia are especially prone to the adverse effects of such medications.

The use of flurazepam, diazepam, chlordiazepoxide, amitriptyline, doxepin, imipramine, thioridazine, or haloperidol significantly increases an older person's risk of having a hip fracture or an automobile accident (Ray et al., 1989). The reason for this increased risk is not known, but it may be due to alterations in pharmacokinetics (benzodiazepines), changes in homeostatic mechanisms (tricyclic antidepressants and antipsychotics), or changes in pharmacodynamics that have not been identified.

MEDICATION ISSUES

POLYPHARMACY

The elderly take more prescription and nonprescription medications than the average population (Yang, Tomlinson, & Naglie, 2001). Studies indicate the elderly take a range of 2.5 to 5.3 prescription and 0 to 4 over-the-counter medications daily (Golden, Preston, Barnett, et al., 1999; Hanlon, Schmader, Rudy, & Weiberger, 2001; Yang et al., 2001). Because of the complexity of medication regimens, concerns about compliance, and costs of medications, try to streamline your patient's medication regimen. Reasons to target the regimens of the elderly include the high rate of medication use; changes in pharmacokinetics, pharmacodynamics, and homeostatic mechanisms; the high rate of adverse drug events in this age group; and the often limited incomes of the elderly (Hanlon et al., 2001).

ADVERSE DRUG EVENTS

The over-65 population is prone to adverse drug events because of alterations in the body's handling of medications and the number of medications they take, but probably not age itself. It is estimated that 10 to 17% of hospital admissions among the elderly are due to adverse drug events (Cohen, 2000). In addition, the elderly do not tolerate or recover from adverse events as well as younger people (Atkin & Shenfield, 1995). Diseases can present atypically in the elderly and confusion, falls, or incontinence may actually be the result of an adverse drug event. Be extra vigilant when starting an elderly person on a new medication, both to identify new problems that may occur and to ensure new problems are not dismissed by the patient or practitioner as simply part of the aging process.

ADHERENCE

Adherence is a problem in all age groups, not just the elderly. Fifty percent of all patients are estimated to be nonadherent with medications (Cohen, 2000). In one study, 30% of elderly patients took less than 70% of at least one prescribed medication and 18% took 120% of at least one prescribed medication (Gray, Mahoney, & Blough, 2001). The elderly are especially at risk because (Salzman, 1995):

- They take increased numbers of medications.
- They may have acquired disabilities that make taking or remembering medications difficult (stroke, arthritic changes, dementia).
- They may have limited incomes to pay for costly medications.
- They may be illiterate or have trouble seeing to read.

Healthcare providers should be particularly alert for adherence problems. Some strategies for improving adherence are medication and disease education, written information to supplement verbal education, and devices such as pillboxes or non-child-resistant tops. Be conscious of patients' hearing deficits that can impair their understanding of verbal instructions.

TOXICITY/POISONINGS

Accidental poisoning in the elderly accounted for 25% of calls to a state poison control center in one study (Kroner, Scott, Waring, & Zanga, 1993). The elderly are more likely to require hospitalization and to die from poisonings. The most frequently implicated drugs in fatal poisonings in the elderly are analgesics, cardiovascular medications, theophylline, and antidepressants (Haselberger & Kroner, 1995). Remind patients about dosages, proper storage, and what to do when doses are missed. Advise them to read the label each time and take medications in a well-lit area. This simple recommendation will prevent them from accidentally taking the wrong medication or ingesting a nonmedicinal substance. For patients with visual impairment, strategies such as specific medication bottle placement for easier and safer use are necessary. All medications should be kept out of reach of children *and* confused adults.

STEPS TO HEALTHY PRESCRIBING

To summarize all the issues highlighted in this chapter, the following are suggested steps for healthy prescribing of medications for the elderly. These tips are not only helpful for the elderly, but make good sense for any patient.

1. Take a careful medication history (prescription, over-the-counter, homeopathic, etc.).
2. Have patients bring all items they regularly take to visits for review.
3. Prescribe only for a specific and rational indication.
4. Consider the patient's overall condition, including mental status, quality of life, and nutritional status, before prescribing.
5. Define the goal of therapy.
6. Begin with lowest available dose and increase doses slowly.
7. Use the fewest drugs and simplest regimen possible.
8. Talk with the patient and/or caregivers about the treatment plan.
9. Reinforce verbal education with written materials (at the appropriate educational level and in large type).
10. Consider the cost of medications to patients.
11. Periodically review and "weed out" outdated or no longer needed medications.
12. Have the patient maintain a medication list to show to all healthcare providers.
13. Alert the patient and caregivers about potential adverse effects and have them monitor for these.
14. Maintain a high index of suspicion regarding adverse events and drug interactions.
15. Exercise caution with newly marketed medications; the effects in the elderly may not be known.
16. Avoid problem medications or use with extreme caution (see Table 13–2).

REFERENCES

Atkin, P. A., & Shenfield, G. M. (1995). Medication-related adverse reactions and the elderly: A literature review. *Adverse Drug Reactions and Toxicology Reviews, 14,* 175–191.

Beers, M. H. (1997). Explicit criteria for determining potentially inappropriate medication use by the elderly. An update. *Archives of Internal Medicine, 157,* 1531–1536.

Beers, M. H., Ouslander, J. G., Rollingher, I., Reuben, D. B., Brooks, J., & Beck, J. C. (1991). Explicit criteria for determining inappropriate medication use in nursing home residents. *Archives of Internal Medicine, 151,* 1825–1832.

Cockcroft, D. W., & Gault, M. H. (1976). Prediction of creatinine clearance from serum creatinine. *Nephron, 16,* 31–41.

Cohen, J. S. (2000). Avoiding adverse reactions. Effective lower-dose drug therapies for older patients. *Geriatrics, 55,* 54–64.

Fick, D. M., Cooper, J. W., Wade, W. F., Waller, J. L., Maclean, J. R., Beers, M. H. (2003). Updating the Beers criteria for potentially inappropriate medication use in older adults. *Archives of Internal Medicine, 163,* 2716–2724.

TABLE 13–2. Medications to Avoid or Use with Caution in the Elderly

High likelihood of severe outcome if used in the elderly
Alprazolam > 2mg/day
Amiodarone (Cordarone)
Amitriptyline (Elavil)
Barbiturates (except phenobarbital)
Belladonna alkaloids (Donnatal and others)
Carisoprodol (Soma)
Chlorazepate (Tranxene)
Chlordiazepoxide (Librium)
Chlorpheniramine (Chlor-Trimeton)
Chlorpropamide (Diabinese)
Clidinium and chlordiazepoxide (Librax)
Cyclobenzaprine (Flexaril)
Cyproheptadine (Periactin)
Diazepam (Valium)
Dicyclomine (Bentyl)
Diphenhydramine (Benadryl)
Disopyramide (Norpace)
Doxepin (Sinequan)
Flurazepam (Dalmane)
Halazepam (Paxipam)
Hydroxyzine (Atarax)
Hyoscamine (Levsin)
Indomethacin (Indocin)
Ketoralac (Toradol)
Lorazepam > 3 mg/day
Meperidine (Demerol)
Meprobamate (Miltown)
Methylcarbamol (Robaxin)
Methyldopa (Aldomet)
Mineral oil
Oxazepam (Serax) > 60 mg/day
Pentazocine (Talwin)
Promethazine (Phenergan)
Propantheline (Pro-Banthine)
Quazepam (Doral)
Temazepam (Restoril) > 15 mg/day
Thioridazine (Mellaril)
Ticlopidine (Ticlid)
Triazolam (Halcion) > 0.25 mg/day
Trimethobenzamide (Tigan)
Lower likelihood of severe outcome if used in the elderly
Cimetidine (Tagamet)
Digoxin (Lanoxin) > 0.125 mg/day
Dipyridamole (Persantine)
Ergoloid mesylates (Hydergine)
Ethacrynic acid (Edecrin)
Ferrous sulfate > 325 mg/day
Phenylbutazone (Butazolidin)
Propoxyphene (Darvon)
Reserpine > 0.25 mg/day

Sources: Beers (1997); Beers, Ouslander, Rollinger, Reuben, Brooks, & Beck (1991); Fick, Cooper, Wade, Waller, Maclean, Beers (2003).

Golden, A. G., Preston, R. A., Barnett, S. D., Llorente, M., Hamdan, K., & Silverman, M.A. (1999). Inappropriate medication prescribing in homebound older adults. *Journal of the American Geriatrics Society, 47,* 948–953.

Grandison, M. K., & Boudinot, F. D. (2000). Age-related changes in protein binding of drugs. Implications for therapy. *Clinical Pharmacokinetics, 38,* 271–290.

Gray, S. L., Mahoney, J. E., & Blough, D. K. (2001). Medication adherence in elderly patients receiving home health services following hospital discharge. *Annals of Pharmacotherapy, 356,* 539–545.

Hanlon, J. T., Schmader, K. E., Ruby, C. M., & Weinberger, M. (2001). Suboptimal prescribing in older inpatients and outpatients. *Journal of the American Geriatrics Society, 49,* 200–209.

Haselberger, M. B., & Kroner, B. A. (1995). Drug poisoning in older patients. Preventative and management strategies. *Drugs and Aging, 7,* 292–297.

Kroner, B. A., Scott, R. B., Waring, E. R., & Zanga, J. R. (1993). Poisoning in the elderly: Characterization of exposures reported to a poison control center. *Journal of the American Geriatrics Society, 41,* 842–846.

Lee, M. (1996). Drugs and the elderly: Do you know the risks? *American Journal of Nursing, 96,* 25–31.

Moore, A. R., & O'Keefe, S. T. (1999). Drug-induced cognitive impairment in the elderly. *Drugs and Aging, 15,* 15–28.

Ray, W. A., Griffen, W. R., & Downey, W. (1989). Benzodiazepines of long and short half-life and the risk of hip fractures. *Journal of the American Medical Association, 262,* 3303–3307.

Salzman, C. (1995). Medication compliance in the elderly. *Journal of Clinical Psychiatry, 56* (Suppl. 1), 18–22.

Smythe, M., Hoffman, J., Kizy, K., & Smuchowski, C. (1994). Estimating creatinine clearance in elderly patients with low serum creatinine concentrations. *American Journal of Hospital Pharmacy, 51,* 198–204.

Tune, L. E. (2001) Anticholinergic effects of medication in elderly patients. *Journal of Clinical Psychiatry, 62* (Suppl 21), 11–14.

Vestal, R. E. (1997). Aging and pharmacology. *Cancer, 80,* 1302–1310.

Vestal, R. E., Norris, A. H., Tobin, J. D., Cohen, B. H., Shock, N. W., & Andres, R. (1975). Antipyrine metabolism in man: Influence of age, alcohol, caffeine and smoking. *Clinical Pharmacology and Therapeutics, 18,* 425–432.

Yang, J. C., Tomlinson, G., & Naglie, G. (2001) Medication lists for elderly patients: Clinic-derived versus in-home inspection and interview. *Journal of General Internal Medicine, 16,* 112–115.

CHAPTER ❖ 14

INDIVIDUALS WITH DISABILITIES

Stephanie G. Metzger

A holistic approach to pharmacotherapeutic interventions will ensure that individuals with disabilities are not treated only as a medical condition. Health care and health maintenance issues for individuals with disabilities provide a unique challenge and opportunity for primary healthcare providers. Although it is essential to have a firm understanding of each diagnosis, the physical, cognitive, and emotional considerations of the individual cannot be lost within the diagnosis. The conceptual issues that arise are globally explored in this chapter, and implications for the pediatric population are included. Specific health issues and common health problems for individuals with disabilities are also reviewed. Since the scope of pharmacotherapy management for this population is broad, this chapter focuses on the information needed by the generalist primary care provider. The provider must also be aware of the individual's functional abilities in order to make effective pharmacotherapy choices.

Legislative reform during the last decades has helped to equalize life opportunities for individuals with disabilities. The Americans with Disabilities Act (ADA) of 1990 encompasses civil rights protection so that no individual with a disability can be discriminated against in opportunities for employment, public services, public accommodations, or health care. Unfortunately, social prejudices and misconceptions continue to make life needlessly difficult for such individuals. Society has not completely realized that challenged individuals strive for the same roles in life fulfillment, relationships, and meaningful employment as their nondisabled peers. The healthcare provider must be sensitive to each unique individual to obtain complete, accurate information on which to base pharmacotherapeutic options. All too often, the level of disability is determined not by physical or cognitive limitations but by the attitude of healthcare workers and architectural barriers within healthcare settings (Boetaavia, 2001; Hahn & Beaulaurier, 2001).

PRIMARY HEALTHCARE ISSUES AND PHARMACOTHERAPY

The Chinese culture uses two symbols to illustrate crisis, one meaning danger and one meaning opportunity. An opportunity exists in the primary care setting to provide comprehensive care in an atmosphere of normalcy for individuals with disabilities. The primary care needed involves health maintenance and anticipatory guidance, managing common conditions associated with the disability and monitoring specialized pharmacotherapeutic treatment related to the disability. The control of healthcare delivery rests with each individual, and physiologic management is enhanced by integrating treatment into the routine. Individuals with disabilities, their families, and their support systems have the same developmental needs and tasks all of us have. Active participation in life experiences is critical to the attainment of developmental milestones.

Primary care providers generally do not initiate major drug therapies for individuals with disabilities. However, the provider is often responsible for monitoring the efficacy and side effects of any special pharmacotherapy and therefore should be aware of possible interactions with commonly prescribed medications. Effective primary care for individuals with disabilities mandates interdisciplinary collaboration. It is essential that each team member coordinate his or her specialties to address the unique needs of each individual with a disability. For the pediatric population, a family-centered approach that fosters communication and collaboration between the family and the team is stressed. This approach also is useful with the adult population.

The primary care provider may serve as a consultant to the individual with a disability to help with decision making. Recognize and appreciate that the individual or family members may be more knowledgeable than you are about specific issues relating to the disability. In an atmosphere of teamwork, this does not have to be an uncomfortable position for you. For example, asking an individual who has recurrent urinary tract infections to collaborate regarding self-catheterization will foster communication and empower the individual. The provider and the individual must synchronize to ensure complete and unbiased information about treatment, interventions, and outcomes.

To promote health in individuals with a disability, primary healthcare needs must be addressed. Pharmacotherapeutic treatment and routine healthcare management, coupled with medical and psychosocial anticipatory guidance, must not be fragmented by the healthcare delivery system. The provider should collaborate with subspecialists to address any unique complexities. Each disability, whether congenital or acquired, has its own trajectory and uses rehabilitation services at various points along the healthcare continuum. Rehabilitation, which is a custom-designed, educational, problem-solving process, helps the individual minimize the effects of the disability and promotes functional outcomes. The primary care provider does not abdicate care but works with subspecialists to enhance organization and problem solving to achieve effective symptom management and to monitor treatment modalities. The provider may not be an expert on the individual's disability but may be an expert on the individual. This allows the provider to give maximal support and advocacy, which is essential if the individual is not to be lost within a sea of subspecialists and pharmacotherapeutic interventions.

Primary health care for children with disabilities involves developmental assessment, health maintenance screening, and immunization procedures that may be neglected or overlooked. Caring for a child with a disability involves caring for the entire family. Families often may feel that they struggle for control over the care of their child and must be recognized as experts (Nelson, 2002). Families of children with disabilities have 24-hour daily responsibility for the coordination and care of their children; involvement with the healthcare team fluctuates. Since each family is unique, the family's perception of the disability is more important than the severity of the disability or the intensity of the caregiver demands. Whether a child has a congenital or acquired disability, family expectations are altered. All families grieve for the loss of their perfect child and make life adjustments that tend to characterize their disabled child as an asset or as a liability. Families of children with disabilities question emancipation and the ability to master self-care skills. Cognitive abilities and the social implications of being disabled often leave children poorly prepared for adulthood and unable to make the transition to independence. Primary care providers may find themselves ill-prepared to help an adult attain independence, especially when community supports are sparse. Interdisciplinary collaboration with rehabilitation specialists is necessary from the onset of the disability to promote self-care activities and independence.

The age of onset of the disability shapes life experiences and self-definition. A progressive disability such as multiple sclerosis requires periodic self-concept adjustments as the symptoms determine functional abilities. A sudden disability means that stages of grief and acceptance will be influenced by developmental stage. For example, a 14-year-old with a disability has a different adolescent experience than an adult who acquires a disability and has experienced adolescence as an individual without a disability. Family and social support systems, financial resources, and access to the healthcare system, combined with individual personality, influence functional outcomes regardless of the disability or the developmental age when the disability is acquired.

SPECIFIC ISSUES IN PHARMACOTHERAPY

COGNITIVE ISSUES

The goal of the provider is for the individual to adhere to the pharmacotherapeutic plan. Deviation from the prescribed treatment plan may be intentional or not. Detailed assessment of cognitive and functional abilities may be necessary to determine reasons for noncompliance. Assessment of cognitive ability is essential since pharmacotherapeutic interventions require such abilities and strategies. For example, an individual who sustained a brain injury through trauma or cerebral vascular accident may recover functional self-care abilities but have long-term memory storage and retrieval deficits. Prescribing a medication with the least number of daily dosages may help ensure that the medication is taken.

Bear in mind that there is a clear distinction between traumatic and nontraumatic spinal cord injury. Traumatic spinal cord injury usually does not hinder cognitive abilities, unless accompanied by brain injury. Congenital spinal cord injury often has a central nervous system component and possibly associated decreased cognitive capabilities. An individual with a spinal cord injury may require either cognitive considerations or adaptations in packaging, or both. Individuals with impaired cognition, for whatever reason, will benefit from the least number of medications possible, with the fewest dosage requirements. Individuals with epilepsy, for example, may have memory problems and, without specific memory strategies, may be unable to maintain a pharmacotherapeutic schedule. Dose schedules can be modified to coincide with physical cues such as setting a watch alarm, meal times, or the availability of a support person for administration. Daily or weekly medication containers may be helpful in an environment free of children. Color-coded bottles, charts, and calendars—along with written dosage schedules and instructions for what to do in case of a missed dose—can ensure that pharmacotherapeutic treatment is successful. Remember to update written instructions even for minor changes.

SEXUALITY ISSUES

All humans are sexual beings, although individuals with a disability are often viewed as less than whole and assumed to be asexual or devoid of feelings and desires. Try to get a clear understanding of the medical aspects of the disability and its relation to sexuality prior to initiating pharmacotherapeutic intervention. Individuals with a disability may be homosexual or heterosexual; however expressed, it is important to recognize sexual preference and to include partners in sexual counseling. The literature has few studies relating to female sexuality, since it has been falsely assumed that females are less interested or are passive participants in sexual activities (Gilson, Cramer, & DePoy, 2001). For example, research on female sexuality after a spinal cord injury is scarce compared with male sexuality research, due in part to the traditional asexual myth, as well as the greater number of males with spinal cord injury (Gilson, Cramer & Depoy, 2001; Nosek, Howland, Rintala, et al., 2001). Research interest has centered on pregnancy and complications of pregnancy in spinal-cord-injured females, bracketing women's sexuality with the act of childbearing.

Acquired neurologic injury—such as a traumatic brain or spinal cord injury or a cerebral vascular accident—often results not only in physical disabilities but also influences sexuality. Injuries may cause impairment to motor and sensory areas, limiting mobility or balance and changing or depleting sensory areas. For example, aphasia may limit speech, thereby decreasing communication, and apraxia may limit voluntary movements. Neurologic injury may change emotions, affect, social response, perception, and cognition. Timing sexual activity to coincide with peak concentrations of analgesic or antispasmodic medications may enhance sexual function. The serum level of sex hormones may be altered by tricyclic antidepressants, such as imipramine, and medications such as calcium channel blockers may produce sexual dysfunction. When assessing sexual concerns, it is important to remember that difficulty in sexual expression and activity may be caused by physical factors, such as mobility or genital function, or environmental or situational factors, as well as pharmacotherapeutic interventions.

Development of a sexual identity is different for individuals who have been disabled from birth compared to those who become disabled as adults (Nosek et al., 2001). Children and adolescents with a disability may not have the opportunity to understand their bodies, changes within them, and how to appropriately channel emerging sexual feelings. Parents of children with disabilities can be so devoted to the physical management of their child and the accompanying dependency issues that sexuality is denied. Parents may also view their disabled child as a child for life or question lifespan and therefore not foster attainment of a sexual identity. Providers can help parents to develop a specific plan for sexuality education based on functional ability, not chronological age. Children with disabilities are sexually maltreated at a rate 1.7 times higher than their nondisabled peers, and education is the most effective protection from such abuse (Advocacy in Action, 2002; American Academy of Pediatrics, 1996). Education and information are often absent in the care of adolescents with a disability. Thirty percent of adolescents with spina bifida reported no useful source of information regarding spina bifida and sexuality (Sawin, Buran, Brei, & Fastenau, 2002). Feelings of sexual inadequacy and undesirability may foster vulnerability to sexual exploitation, and primary care providers must use careful assessment techniques to detect possible abuse or exploitation (Nosek et al., 2001).

WOMEN'S HEALTH ISSUES

Physical inaccessibility is often the reason cited by women with disabilities for delay or avoidance of gynecological care. There is also a dearth of healthcare providers—generalists or specialists—who are willing to help and are knowledgeable in gynecological care for women with disabilities. Research has shown that in a barrier-free environment, healthcare providers can positively influence the maintenance of women's health. This environment allows women to learn about reproductive health as well as preventive health measures, such as breast self-examination. Women with disabilities not only face healthcare issues related to their disability but also specific issues related to sensuality and sexuality.

Pelvic examinations are an integral part of women's healthcare. A physically accessible examination table must lower to 19 inches to allow for independent transfer and have arm support for safe and comfortable positioning. Women with decreased range of motion and spasticity may require adaptations of the gynecological examination. Spasticity is often exacerbated by examination positioning, which may trigger adductor spasms. Use the knee-chest position or side-lying position to decrease positional spasticity. Warming the speculum or reversing the speculum to use a handle-up position may also decrease spasticity. If a Pap smear is not indicated, Xylocaine gel may be applied to the speculum to decrease the potential for spinal-cord-induced autonomic dysreflexia as well as spasticity. The examination should be scheduled to coincide with the maximum concentration of antispasmodic medication. Women who use intrathecal Lioresal for control of severe spasticity may require a bolus of medication to be delivered prior to examination. Both spasticity and spinal cord injury will be discussed later in this chapter.

Contraceptive options for women with disabilities involve discussion and consideration of many factors. Although safe sex is paramount, the risk of pregnancy and the risks associated with the contraceptive method must be considered. Latex allergies, mobility issues, manual dexterity, and cognitive issues factor into the choices offered. For example, the physiological risks of thrombosis associated with oral contraceptives, impaired sensation for use of the IUD, and dexterity issues related to barrier methods must be openly discussed and evaluated in women with spinal cord injury. Norplant, which does not employ estrogen, may provide an option for women with motor issues who are not physiologically at risk for hormonal contraception. Depo-Provera may be an option if time and transportation are available for quarterly administration. Contraceptive issues must be approached with the same level of comfort and commitment used with all activities of daily living.

Pregnancy, labor and delivery, and parenting are lifestyle choices for women with disabilities that may require routine healthcare considerations or complex interventions. Health issues such as neurogenic bowel and bladder, skin management, and thrombosis may be intensified with pregnancy and labor and delivery. Women with disabilities may also need referral to specialists for issues related to fertility. No matter what the level of the intervention, the primary care provider will be involved with a team of specialists to ensure maximal health. For a comprehensive discussion of healthcare for women with disabilities, refer to Sawin & Horton (2003).

NEUROGENIC BOWEL AND BLADDER ISSUES

Neurogenic bowel and bladder are common health maintenance issues for individuals with disabilities that often become a silent secondary disability, limiting both social and sexual opportunities. These issues can be assessed by the primary care provider to initiate treatment or referred to an advanced practice nurse or rehabilitation specialist if complex interventions and management are required.

Urinary incontinence may be the result of a spinal cord injury, multiple sclerosis, cerebral vascular accident, or spinal dysraphism. It causes embarrassment, decreases therapy and mobility options, causes skin breakdown and urinary tract infection, and may be the deciding factor between social functioning and long-term care. Before initiating pharmacotherapeutic management, the reason for the incontinence must be established. The mnemonic DIAPPERS—D(delirium), I(infection), A(atrophic vaginitis), P(pharmaceuticals), P(psychosocial), E(endocrine), R(reduced mobility), and S(stool impaction) (Resnick & Yalla, 1985)—may help assess the reversible causes of incontinence. Reversible causes must be corrected before pharmacotherapeutic treatment is given. A neurogenic bladder may result in an inability to store urine, an inability to empty urine, or both. Urodynamic evaluation guides pharmacotherapeutic treatment and is necessary to determine if the neurogenic bladder is due to causes within the bladder, such as coordination of bladder contraction and bladder pressure, or to causes related to the bladder outlet or the external sphincter.

Although various pathophysiologies may contribute to a neurogenic bladder, the goal of treatment is to prevent upper urinary tract deterioration and to provide socially acceptable continence (Sturman, 2002). The general principles of urinary management are the same for both the pediatric and adult populations, and continence is sought through catheterization and pharmacotherapeutic agents. However, psychosocial factors and compliance vary among age groups. The young child will be dependent on parental intervention and possibly uninterested in management, whereas the adolescent may be very socially motivated to become continent. Clean intermittent catheterization is the treatment of choice to preserve upper urinary tract function in the presence of a neurogenic bladder. Latex-free catheters are used, and the individual is taught the technique based on cognitive ability, dexterity, and mobility. Depending on cognitive ability, a child as young as 6 can begin to participate in catheterization by naming the supplies and may be independent between the ages of 8 and 12 (Peterson, Rauen, Brown, & Cole, 1994). Similarly, an individual with a high-level spinal cord injury may direct an attendant in this procedure. Those who are unable to perform urethral catheterization may need to be evaluated for surgical options, such as to create an abdominal reservoir that can be self-catheterized. It is important to realize that a urine culture from an individual who is self-catheterizing may contain flora and fauna suggestive of a urinary tract infection. However, if the individual is asymptomatic, without fever, pain, or altered urinary pattern, antibiotic treatment is not initiated as the flora and fauna are due to colonization, not active infection. Instead, fluids are increased along with the maintenance of a strict catheterization procedure and schedule. Only when symptoms of an infection are present is treatment initiated with culture-sensitive antibiotics (Schryvers & Nance, 1999). In addition, a meta-analysis of adults found that antimicrobial prophylaxis for most individuals with neurogenic bladder was not supported. They did recommend, however, further study with those who had frequent UTIs that limited daily functioning and well being (Morton et al., 2002).

Pharmacotherapeutic treatment is initiated based on the prominent cause of the neurogenic bladder as determined by the urodynamic evaluation. Anticholinergic agents are frequently used to relax the smooth muscle of the bladder. Oxybutynin is the first-line drug of choice to decrease intravesicular pressure and increase bladder capacity. It may be instilled intravesically if the anticholinergic side effects produced by oral administration are intolerable. If oxybutynin fails, a favorable response may result from a trial with propantheline and dicyclomine, both anticholinergic medications with differing sites of action. Imipramine, a tricyclic antidepressant, is used in the treatment of neurogenic bladder to suppress bladder contractions and increase bladder capacity. Alpha blockers such as phenylpropanolamine or ephedrine also may be employed to improve urinary storage.

The ability to maintain bowel continence is based on rectal compliance and capacity and the autonomic and somatic nervous systems' ability to coordinate defecation. Treating neurogenic bowel is based on maintaining a regular emptying pattern that does not allow stool to accumulate, thereby minimizing the complications of constipation and diarrhea. Constipation may lead to impaction when hardened fecal material obstructs the rectum. Paradoxical diarrhea or frequent watery stools may be a result of constipation, causing a dilated colon. Diarrhea may be interchanged with stool accumulation. Constipation may also exacerbate the symptoms of neurogenic bladder by decreasing bladder capacity.

A bowel training program prevents constipation and diarrhea by complete elimination of formed or semi-formed stools. Elements of a bowel program may include adequate fluid intake, adequate dietary fiber, exercise to increase peristalsis, medications or techniques to stimulate evacuation, and timed evacuation. A reasonable goal is to have a pattern of regular soft stools at least every two days and to have no more than one bowel accident per month. The time involved in a bowel program should be between 30 and 45 minutes. The ability to maintain continence is not voluntary, and factors such as medical condition and pharmacotherapeutic treatment, functional ability to participate in a bowel training program, financial resources, diet, lifestyle, and emotional desire for continence must all be evaluated. Every bowel program is customized, and the establishment of a successful bowel training program is labor-intensive for the individual as well as the provider and may take weeks to months to establish.

Pharmacotherapeutic interventions are based on the two distinct issues of stool motility through oral medication and stool evacuation through mechanical intervention. Preparations that affect motility include stool softeners, osmotic agents, and stimulants. For example, Colace, lactulose, and mineral oil are used for softening the stool. Lactulose, a nonabsorbable sugar, is often used for infants and young children. Miralax, a synthetic osmotic agent made from polyethylene glycol, is being used for periods of up to 14 days followed by a two- to four-week non-use holiday. Safety studies regarding stimulants such as senna and bisacodyl are currently in progress. Products containing cascara, casanthra, and aloe have been taken off of the market (Gastroenterology, 2002). Bulking the stool through preparations such as psyllium (Metamucil) allows stool passage by changing consistency.

Stool evacuation techniques include digital stimulation, suppositories, and enemas. Digital stimulation and suppositories trigger the colon to empty. Suppositories may be mild, such as glycerin, or may provide contact irritation, such as bisacodyl. Enemas also trigger evacuation of stool and may be used as part of a routine bowel program or may be used to relieve constipation. Enemas vary in amount of expansion used from very small, such as Therevac and Babylax enemas, to Fleet and bisacodyl enemas. Specialists in the treatment of neurogenic bowel also use preparations and techniques such as the Magic Bullet suppository, enema continence catheter, and biofeedback.

MOBILITY ISSUES

Immobilization is a major consideration for some individuals with disabilities. The multi-system involvement of immobility causes metabolic and regulatory alterations. Nutritional recommendations as well as pharmacotherapeutic interventions must be considered, since obesity severely limits functional ability.

Medications that increase appetite or require food intake to decrease gastrointestinal distress may not be the most efficacious. Metabolic changes due to immobilization include loss of body protein and expansion of extracellular water volume, which alters drug kinetics. For example, gentamicin clearance is increased, which requires an increased dosage to maintain therapeutic levels. Cardiac complications are prevalent since a sedentary lifestyle lowers levels of high-density lipoprotein cholesterol. Orthostatic hypotension may be problematic, and sodium and fluid intake must be monitored since supplementary sodium chloride tablets may be necessary.

Since alpha-adrenergic blockers such as phenoxybenzamine potentiate orthostatic hypotension, they may not be the best choice for individuals with a spinal cord injury. A spinal cord injury also results in increased calcium excretion due to bone reabsorption of the paralyzed portion of the body. Kidneys unable to excrete all the increased calcium can lead to hypercalcuria and hypercalcemia. Hypercalcemia may cause nausea, vomiting, dehydration, lethargy, polydypsia, and polyuria. As part of the differential consideration, obtain a serum calcium level. Limiting oral calcium intake and vitamin D intake may decrease gastrointestinal absorption. Long-term control involves corticosteroids and oral phosphates. Increased calcium reabsorption also places the individual at risk for osteoporosis and urinary tract calculi.

Immobility and the lack of muscular pumping allow blood to pool in the calf, placing the individual at risk for deep venous thrombosis and of the complication of pulmonary embolism. The overall incidence of deep venous thrombosis in this adult population is 16.3%, with the highest incidence occurring in the first two weeks after injury, although deep venous thrombosis can occur beyond this time frame (Green, Chen, Chmiel, et al, 1994). Note also that acute subclinical pulmonary embolism may be present in as many as 14% of individuals with spinal cord injury (Weingarden & Belen, 1992). The incidence of venous thrombosis in the pediatric population is poorly documented, and risk assessment is based on Tanner stage of physical maturity. Prophylactic treatment is questioned in the prepubertal population, but if diagnosed, treatment is recommended to decrease the risk of a pulmonary embolism (Radecki & Gaebler-Spira, 1994).

Prophylaxis management of deep venous thrombosis is beyond the scope of this chapter, and there is debate over the safety and efficacy of various prophylactic approaches. However, individuals with a spinal cord injury may be maintained on anticoagulation therapy for up to six months with various dosing and laboratory evaluation schedules monitored by the primary care provider. Remember too that the presence of a device to prevent blood clots from traveling, such as a Greenfield filter, does not exclude venous thrombosis from differential considerations. Clinical signs and diagnosis may be complicated by the alteration in, or absence of, sensation owing to changes in the neurologic system. Therefore, all complaints of pleuritic chest pain require a diagnostic evaluation.

HETEROTOPIC OSSIFICATION

Heterotopic ossification is the abnormal formation of new bone in periarticular soft tissue areas of individuals who have sustained such traumatic injuries as a spinal cord injury, brain injury, or burns. Heterotopic ossification has been reported in 16–53% of individuals with spinal cord injury, most commonly between months 1 and

4 and rarely after month 12 postinjury. Presenting findings are swelling, heat, loss of range of motion, and possibly fever. For individuals with a spinal cord injury, the hip is the most common site, followed by the knee, shoulder, and elbow. Differential considerations include deep vein thrombosis, cellulitis, joint sepsis, tumor, and fracture. Roentgenograms may be negative during the early weeks because of insufficient ossification, and a triple-phase bone scan will be necessary for diagnosis. Laboratory evaluation will reveal an increase in the serum alkaline phosphatase level during the acute phase.

Early diagnosis and treatment of heterotopic ossification are essential to preserve function. Aggressive and regular passive range of motion is the treatment modality of choice. In the adult population, disodium etidronate may be used to attempt to limit or prevent the extent of ossification by inhibiting bone matrix mineralization. Although the ideal treatment length has not been established, the overall goal is to use the lowest effective dose for the shortest duration. An initial dosage of 5 mg/kg per day may be used for up to six months, with severe instances requiring dosages of 10 mg/kg per day for up to three months. Dosage above 20 mg/kg per day is contraindicated. Pharmacologic research on the prophylactic use of disodium etidronate is being undertaken. Disodium etidronate is used cautiously in the pediatric population because of possible interference with bone metabolism in the developing skeleton (Molnar & Alexander, 1999).

AUTONOMIC DYSREFLEXIA

Autonomic dysreflexia is a life-threatening phenomenon of elevated blood pressure caused by reflex activity of the sympathetic and parasympathetic nervous systems when a spinal cord lesion is above the sympathetic splanchnic outflow. Individuals with a spinal cord injury proximal to thoracic level 6 are at risk for a sudden uninhibited sympathetic response causing hypertension. The sudden paroxysmal hypertension may elevate systolic pressure as high as 200 mm Hg and diastolic pressure as high as 100 mm Hg. At any point, an increase in the baseline pressure of 20 mm Hg is considered autonomic dysreflexia. This condition may be constant, subside within three years of the spinal cord injury, or may be subject to remissions and exacerbations.

Autonomic dysreflexia can be triggered by noxious events to the body below the level of the spinal cord injury. Symptoms include a sudden onset of headache, hypertension, sweating, nasal congestion, and piloerection. Immediate removal of the noxious stimuli is essential. If this treatment is not effective, pharmacotherapy intervention is imperative (see Table 14–1). Prevention of noxious stimuli is accomplished through bowel, bladder, and skin management programs. Although the symptoms of mild autonomic dysreflexia are uncomfortable, severe hypertension associated with dysreflexia may lead to cerebral hemorrhage. Close monitoring is manditory. Severe hypertension is an emergency, and immediate pharmacotherapy must be initiated. Associated hemodynamic changes also place the individual at risk for heart failure. Older individuals with spinal cord injury are at the greatest risk for such life-threatening consequences.

SPASTICITY

Spasticity is one of the most common health problems for individuals with disabilities and is often associated with cerebral palsy, traumatic brain injury, spinal cord injury, and multiple sclerosis. Spasticity is easy to recognize, complex to characterize, and difficult to treat. It is characterized as an abnormally increased and prolonged muscle contraction in response to rapid movements or rapid changes in position. Spasticity is often recognized by hyperactive deep tendon reflexes; Babinski's sign; increased resistance to passive movement; clonus, flexor, or extensor spasms; and abnormal voluntary movements. The amount and degree of spasticity fluctuate, and therefore multiple clinical assessments are necessary.

Evaluating spasticity revolves around the question of whether it interferes with functional ability. Ask the individual to demonstrate the functional activity affected by spasticity. Spasticity alters the ability to make smooth voluntary movements. Sitting or transferring may be affected, or it can alter cosmesis, cause skin breakdown or pain, disturb sleep, or interrupt sexual function. Conversely, spasticity may have a salubrious affect by providing muscle tone useful in gait, promoting limb repositioning, and improving circulation, thereby decreasing the risk of deep venous thrombosis (Kita & Goodkin, 2002).

When an individual who is neurologically stable exhibits increased spasticity, precipitating factors must be evaluated. Any noxious physical stimuli—a urinary tract infection or kidney stone, pressure sore, acute infectious process or bowel or bladder distension—or psychological stimuli—such as stress—may exacerbate spasticity. Management of spasticity begins with physical and rehabilitative therapy to eliminate nociceptive stimuli. There are several pharmacotherapeutic agents available to treat

TABLE 14–1. Autonomic Dysreflexia: Causes, Symptoms, and Treatments

Symptoms	Causes	Interventions	Medication	Prevention
Hypertension Headache Flushing **above** lesion Sweating **above** lesion Pallor **below** lesion Nasal congestion Blurred vision Dilated pupils Bradycardia Increased spasticity		Monitor heart rate Monitor blood pressure Raise head of bed Lower legs Remove tight clothes Remove equipment	*Sublingual* Nifedipine *PO* Dibenzyline Minipress Procardia *IV* Hydralazine Hyperstat Nipride	Educate family, caregivers, coworkers, and professional colleagues.
Bladder	Blocked/kinked catheter	Catheterize with Pontocaine Drain slowly Irrigate Foley catheter Unkink tubing Empty bag		Establish and maintain effective bladder program.
Bowel	Impaction Distention Digital stimulation Suppository Enema Hemorrhoids	Rectal exam and disimpaction with Xylocaine gel		Establish and maintain effective bowel program.
Integumentary	Lesion Pressure Ingrown toenail Positioning Tight clothing Tight straps on equipment ↑/↓ temperature Sunburn	Topical anesthetic to skin lesion		Establish and maintain effective skin monitoring program.
External or painful stimuli	Medical instrumentation Sexual activity Labor and delivery Menstruation Fracture Infection Urinary tract infection Renal calculi Epididymitis			Use anesthetic agents before procedures and painful conditions. Prompt treatment of symptomatic infections.

spasticity. The frequency of doses and adverse effects may make control of severe spasticity difficult. If the agent improves the symptoms but fails to improve functional abilities, it is unlikely that another agent will be beneficial. The goals of treatment are to diminish spasticity without causing voluntary muscle weakness, to maintain the positive effects of spasticity, and to limit sedation caused by the medication. No standard pharmacotherapeutic intervention can be recommended since spasticity may be either spinal or cerebral in origin, and the site of origination guides pharmacotherapeutic treatment decisions. Flexor spasms in a complete spinal cord injury differ from severe spasticity associated with multiple sclerosis, which is markedly different from spastic diplegia in children with cerebral palsy (Nance, 2001).

The primary care provider may begin treatment of spasticity but is more often involved in the monitoring of treatment initiated by a specialist. Medications must be closely monitored since abrupt withdrawal by the individual or the provider may yield potentially serious consequences. General muscle relaxants such as methocarbamol are not effective in the treatment of spasticity and should not be initiated. Lioresal, a gamma-aminobutyric acid agonist, was previously the first-line pharmacotherapeutic treatment of choice but is being replaced by tizanidine hydrochloride. Both agents are more beneficial in spinal cord injury and multiple sclerosis than in cerebrally originated spasticity. Lioresal has a wide dose range and experts in the treatment of spasticity may far exceed the maximum recommended dose range of 80 mg per day. Adverse effects of both medications may be drowsiness, weakness, fatigue, confusion and headache. These side effects are more common with Lioresal and usually dissipate within several days of initiation. These effects can be reduced by starting with a low dose and increasing dosage at a seven-day interval instead of the usual four-day interval. Lioresal may decrease seizure threshold, a consideration for individuals with epilepsy. It may also have an additive central nervous system depressant effect if used with other depressants. A withdrawal syndrome that may include psychosis, hallucinations, or seizures as well as rebound spasticity is likely if Lioresal is abruptly discontinued without slowly weaning the dose (Gelber & Jozefczyk, 1999).

Both clonazepam and diazepam may be useful as combination therapy with Lioresal and are often used to decrease nocturnal spasms. Sedative effects may be problematic for daytime use. Diazepam is used for spasticity that originates in the spinal cord and also has some efficacy in individuals with cerebral palsy. The side effects of decreased cognitive ability and motor control often render diazepam an unacceptable choice. True physiologic addiction may take place, and abrupt withdrawal can include seizures. A paradoxical reaction of insomnia, anxiety, hostility, hallucinations, and increased spasticity has been reported with long-term use.

Clonidine has shown marked improvement in spasticity, particularly after a cerebral vascular accident. However, such side effects as hypotension and constipation may be unacceptable in individuals with spinal cord injury. Clonidine may induce bradycardia that dissipates when the medication is discontinued (Elovic, 2001).

Dantrolene may be effective in treating spinal cord spasticity and spasticity with a cerebral origin, but it has fallen out of favor since other pharmacotherapeutic options are available. Hepatotoxicity is a concern, and it should not be used in individuals with severe hepatic disease. Before initiating therapy, baseline liver function tests must be obtained and then monitored at routine intervals. A clinically apparent response to treatment may not be noticed until one week after dose adjustment. If a response is not seen within two weeks at a maximum dosage level, discontinue use because of the hepatic risks. The adverse effect of weakness makes dantrolene an unacceptable choice for individuals with multiple sclerosis.

The oral agents used to treat spasticity have sedating properties, and the dose required to adequately decrease severe spasticity may impair cognition and functional abilities (Kita & Goodkin, 2002). Referrals may be necessary for treatment options aside from or in conjunction with oral pharmacotherapeutic agents. Experts in the management of spasticity may use botulinum toxin injections into the neuromuscular junction to weaken spastic muscles. Dosage is dependent on the desired effect. For example, the dose required for precise control of a fine motor muscle is lower than the dose to control painful spasms in a nonfunctional limb. The average duration of response to injection is two to six months depending on the dose and the size and activity of the muscle (Gelber & Jozefczyk, 1999). Ablative surgery, the selective dorsal root rhizotomy, may be used for severe spasticity. Ideal candidates for this procedure are between the ages of 2 and 6 years, and an extensive rehabilitation program is required afterward.

For severe spasticity, a new treatment uses intraspinal drug therapy to precisely deliver the antispasmodic agent directly to the receptors within the spinal cord. A surgically implanted, externally programmable pump is used to deliver intrathecal Lioresal. Intraspinal drug therapy has resulted in improvement in functional abilities as well as lifestyle activities such as sleep, bladder management, and relief of discomfort. Such practical issues as cost, surgical risk, refilling intervals, individual commitment, and available expertise must be considered prior to pump implantation (Stempien & Tsai, 2000).

LATEX ALLERGY

Awareness of latex sensitivity and allergy has increased over the past decade. This is due in part to a 1991 recall of latex enema tips by the Food and Drug Administration (FDA) as well as the establishment of universal precautions that require repeated exposure to latex for healthcare providers. Latex is a natural material found in the milky sap of the *Hevea brasiliensis* plant, the rubber tree. Individuals at risk for developing an allergy are those who are repeatedly exposed to products containing latex, such as healthcare providers and individuals with spina bifida, spinal cord injury, or congenital genitourinary tract anomalies, as well as those undergoing multiple surgeries. Identify at-risk individuals and treat an allergic reaction promptly.

During an allergy history, explore allergies to tropical fruit, chestnuts, and avocados that have all been associated with latex sensitivity. A history of an allergic reaction to a glove or balloon is also crucial. Individuals with spina bifida have an 18 to 40% incidence of latex sensitivity (Buhr, 2000; NIOSH, 2002). Individuals with spinal cord injury have a lower incidence of latex allergy as compared to individuals with spina bifida. Specific guidelines for dealing with latex in the primary care environment are available to guide office practices (Fisher & Sawin, 1998). This higher incidence is thought to be due to exposure to latex from birth in individuals with spina bifida (Gunther, Nelitz, Parsch, Puhl, 2000). It can be extrapolated that individuals with congenital genitourinary anomalies will also have a higher incidence of latex allergy due to exposure from birth. The second largest risk group is healthcare workers, with estimates ranging from 2.6% to 16.9%. More than 1,000 episodes of anaphylaxis and 15 deaths were reported to the FDA (Sussman, 1998).

Symptoms of a local allergic response to latex include watery eyes, itching, sneezing, and hives, whereas a systemic reaction results in anaphylaxis. Reactions occur when latex touches the skin or mucous membranes or enters the bloodstream. Sensitivity may become so great that opening a package of latex gloves can trigger a reaction due to the airborne particles. Definitive evidence for latex allergy is difficult because each test—the skin prick, intradermal, or radioallergosorbent—measures only the amount of the reaction at that particular point in time (Becker, 2000). A "latex alert" should be used as a safeguard for those who are in a high-risk group but who have not had any symptoms of an allergic reaction. The identification of "latex allergy" is for individuals who have displayed latex sensitivity either locally or systemically and who must have a latex-free environment. All children at risk of latex allergy must be identified, particularly before undergoing surgical procedures (Sussman, 1998). A medic alert bracelet and autoinjectable epinephrine are essential for high-risk individuals.

It is both difficult and time-consuming to know all the products that contain latex since there are no current labeling requirements. An individual with a latex sensitivity or allergy is at greatest risk from gloves, catheters, balloons, balls (Koosh and tennis), condoms, dental dams, nipples, pacifiers, tape, Chux, rubber bands, and Band-Aids. The Spina Bifida Association maintains a current website at www.sbaa.org with up to date information regarding items with latex. Latex allergy must be considered when injecting medications in the office or in the hospital. Do not draw up medications into a syringe through the rubber cap on a medication vial or inject medications into latex ports on intravenous tubing.

At-risk individuals require preassessment by anesthesia, and dental and surgical procedures should be scheduled for the first case in the morning in a latex-free environment. Same-day procedures are not appropriate because of intensive postoperative monitoring requirements. Patients with a history of latex allergy are treated 24 hours preoperatively and postoperatively with IV or oral diphenhydramine and methylprednisolone 1 mg/kg per dose and cimetidine 5 mg/kg per dose every 6 h. Individuals at high risk are treated every 12 h preoperatively with oral diphenhydramine 1 mg/kg per dose, followed by prednisone 0.5 mg/kg per dose every 12 h. In the case of anaphylaxis, treatment includes the above medications as well as epinephrine and airway support (Kwittken, Becker, Oyefara, et al., 1992).

PRESCRIPTIVE CONSIDERATIONS

A unique issue for individuals with disabilities is the appropriate use of nonpharmacologic prescriptions. Individuals with disabilities see many specialists and use specialized equipment and therapy resources to maximize their functional abilities. Technological advances offer a myriad of options and therapies that must be wisely assessed by the primary care provider. The goals for therapeutic interventions as well as the health/dollar benefits should be known before providing the prescription.

Equipment ranges from the simple—a reacher or bath seat—to the complex—orthotic intervention for ambulation or powered mobility. The prescribing provider must really understand what models, brands, and vendors are most appropriate for the individual and the disability. For example, a standard, prefabricated orthosis may be prescribed when a hinged, custom-made orthosis would allow for more dorsiflexion and improve functional gait. If the funding for the prefabricated orthosis is used, there may not be funding options for the customized orthosis. Similarly, prescribing a child's wheelchair that cannot be adjusted as the child grows or ordering a nonadjustable axle plate that does not allow the wheels to be moved to the most optimal pushing position is disastrous. A team approach allows the provider, individual, therapists, rehabilitation specialist, and reimbursement source to coordinate and prescribe proper fitting and functioning assistive devices and therapies to increase functional abilities. A suboptimal choice is a major negative outcome; therefore, a standard prescription for therapeutic equipment or a blanket request for therapy does not exist.

In addition, unique teaching needs for medication or equipment must be considered in this population. Evaluate the learning needs of your patients and alter education as appropriate. For example, individuals with visual impairments may need a special system devised for safety and instructions that are accessible in an audiotape. The practitioner will need to know if patients have access to a Kerzler reader and would prefer written instructions. If learning disabilities are an issue, a multiple approach, such as visual and auditory, might be optimal for complex regimes.

SUMMARY

Primary care for individuals with disabilities is the crux of health maintenance. The unique complexities presented by the disability allow the provider to address issues related to pharmacotherapeutic intervention, routine health care, common health conditions, and health issues related to the disability. The primary care provider does not abdicate care, but can both provide care and guide and direct care provided by subspecialists. Pharmacotherapeutic interventions must be customized for the disability and the combined effects on the body systems. A holistic view of the individual by the primary care provider forms the basis of collaboration and partnership, which is essential to maximize health. All too often, it is forgotten that an individual with a disability is an ordinary person who does ordinary things in extraordinary ways.

REFERENCES

Advocacy in Action: Health Professionals Response to the Abuse and Neglect of Children with Disabilities. *Teleconference,* April 2002.

American Academy of Pediatrics. (1996). Sexuality education of children and adolescents with developmental disabilities. *Pediatrics, 97*(2), 275–278.

Bataavia, A. (2001). The new paternalism: Portraying people with disabilities as an oppressed minority. *Journal of Disability Policy Studies, 12*(2), 107–113.

Becker, H.S. (2000). Research utilization. An analysis of the epidemiology of latex allergy: Implications for primary prevention. *Medsurg Nursing, 9*(3), 135–143.

Buhr, V. (2000) Screening patients for latex allergies. *Journal American Academy Nurse Practitioner, 12*(11):466.

Elovic, E. (2001). Principles of pharmaceutical management of spastic hypertonia. *Physical Medicine and Rehabilitation Clinics of North America, 12*(4), 793–816.

Fisher, D., & Sawin, K. (1998). Latex allergy: Pearls for practice in the primary care setting. *Journal of the American Academy of Nurse Practitioners, 10*(5), 203–208.

Gastrointerology (2002). *The Prescribers Letter, 9*(610), 32.

Gelber, D.A., & Jozefczyk, P.B. (1999). Therapeutics in neurorehabilitation: Therapeutics in the management of spasticity. *Journal of Neurologic Rehabilitation, 13*(1), 5–14.

Gilson, S.F., Cramer, E.P., & DePoy, E. (2001). Redefining abuse of women with disabilities: A paradox of limitation and expansion. *Affila-Journal of Women and Social Work,* 16(2), 220–235.

Green, D., Chen, D., Chmiel, J. S., Olsen, N. K., Berkowitz, M., Novick, A., Alleva, J., Steinberg, D., Nussbaum, S., & Tolotta, M. (1994). Prevention of thromboembolism in spinal cord injury: Role of low molecular weight heparin. *Archives of Physical Medicine and Rehabilitation, 75,* 290–292.

Gunther, K.P., Nelitz, M., Parsch, K., Puhl, W. (2000). Allergic reactions to latex in myelodysplasia: A review of the literature, 9(3):180–4.

Hahn, H., & Beaulaurier, R.L. (2001, Summer). Attitudes toward disabilities: A research note on activists with disabilities. *Journal of Disability Policy Studies, 12*(1), 40–46.

Kita, M., & Goodkin, D.E. (2002). Drugs used to treat spasticity. *Drugs, 59*(3), 487–495.

Kwittken, P. L., Becker, J., Oyefara, B., Danziger, R., Pawlowski, N. A., & Sweinberg, S. (1992). Latex hypersensitivity reactions despite prophylaxis. *Allergy Proceedings, 13*(3), 123–127.

Molnar, G.E., & Alexander, M.A. (1999). Head injury. In *Pediatric Rehabilitation* (3rd ed.). Philadelphia: Hanley and Belfus.

Morton, S.C., Shekelle, P.G., Adams, A.L., Bennett, C., Dobkin, B.H., Montgomerile, J. & Vickrey, B.G. (2002). Antimicrobial prophylaxis for urinary tract infections in persons with spinal cord dysfunction. *Archives of Physical Medicine & Rehabilitation, 83,* 129–138.

Nance, P.W. (2001). Alpha adrenergic and serotonergic agents in the treatment of spastic hypertonia. *Physical Medicine and Rehabilitation Clinics of North America, 12*(4), 889–905.

Nelson, A.M. (2002). A metasynthesis: Mothering other-than-normal children. *Qualitative Health Research, 12*(4), 515–530.

NIOSH (National Institute of Occupational Safety and Health). (2002). *Preventing reactions to natural rubber latex in the workplace.* NHHS Publication No. 97–135. Washington, DC: U.S. Government Printing Office.

Nosek, M.A., Howland, C.A, Rintala, D.H., Young, M.E., & Chanpong, G.F. (2001). National Study of Women with Physical Disabilities: Final report. *Sexuality and Disability, 19*(1), 5–39.

Peterson, P. M., Rauen, K. K., Brown, J., & Cole, J. (1994). Spina bifida: The transition into adulthood begins in infancy. *Rehabilitation Nursing, 19*(4), 229–238.

Radecki, R. T., & Gaebler-Spira, D. (1994). Deep vein thrombosis in the disabled pediatric population. *Archives of Physical Medicine and Rehabilitation, 75,* 248–250.

Resnick, N. M., & Yalla, S. V. (1985). Current concepts: Management of urinary incontinence in the elderly. *New England Journal of Medicine, 313*(13), 800–805.

Sawin, K.J. & Horton, J. (2003). Health care concerns for women with physical disability and chronic illness. In E. Youngkin & M. Davis (Eds.), *Women's health: A primary care clinical guide* (3rd ed.). Stamford, CT: Appleton & Lange.

Sawin, K. J., Buran, C. F., Brei, T.J., & Fastenau, P.S. (2002). Sexuality issues in adolescents with chronic neurological conditions. *Journal of Perinatal Education, 11*(1), 22–34.

Schryvers, O., & Nance, P.W. (1999). Urinary and gastrointestinal systems medications. *Physical Medicine and Rehabilitation Clinics of North America, 10*(2), 473–492.

Stempien, L., & Tsai, T. (2000). Intrathecal baclofen pump use for spasticity: A clinical survey. *American Journal of Physical Medicine and Rehabilitation, 79*(6), 536–41, 547–550, 564.

Sturman, G. (2002). The bladder and the bowel: The pharmacology of continence. *Nursing and Residential Care, 4*(3), 112, 114–6, 140–141.

Sussman, G.L. (1998). Latex allergy in surgical and nonsurgical children. *Or Reports, 7*(1), 2p.

Weingarden, S. I., & Belen, J. G. (1992). Clonidine transdermal system for treatment of spasticity in spinal cord injury. *Archives of Physical Medicine and Rehabilitation, 73,* 876–877.

CHAPTER ❖ 15

MIGRANT AND HOMELESS POPULATIONS

J. Claire Whiting

The provision of quality primary care to migrant workers and homeless clients poses significant challenges. Since lifestyle and environmental issues compound their situations, the pharmacotherapeutic considerations in the care of these two vulnerable populations are addressed in this chapter within the context of those variables. Pediatric implications for migrants and the homeless also are included.

THE MIGRANT FARM WORKERS POPULATION

The size of the population of migrant farm workers and their dependents is currently estimated to be slightly more than 4 million people (Go & Baker, 1995). For the purpose of this chapter, a migrant farm worker is defined as one who travels over 75 miles to engage in employment in agriculture. Fifty-six percent of farm workers migrate; 80% of these individuals are Latino. Of the Latino workers, 77% are from Mexico, 2% from other countries, and 9% are U.S. born. Caucasians make up 7% of all migrant farm workers. Only 1% are African American. This is a major shift in population over the last two decades from African American to Latino. Of the Latino population, 22% are U.S. citizens, 24% have legal permits to work in the United States, and 52% have no work authorization. The average age of a migrant farm worker is 31; 80% are male, 20% are female. Fifty-two percent are married, and of the married only 50% are accompanied by their family. The greater the number of children a worker has, the more likely the migrant worker is separated from the family (U.S. Department of Labor, 2000).

COMMON HEALTH PROBLEMS OF MIGRANT WORKERS

Significant gaps in information exist concerning the health status of the migrant worker populations. The common health problems of migrants may be classified into occupational, lifestyle, and generic conditions. The occupational health problems include pesticide exposure and poisoning, injury, or trauma. In Arcury, Quandt, Cravey, Elmore, and Russell (2001), it was noted that cultural beliefs conflicted with safety practices for hand washing. Latinos believe if cold water is applied to a hot body, illness will occur. Therefore, hand washing and hydration factors may pose problems for both the migrant and owner if the latter is not culturally competent. On-the-job trauma or injuries are the most likely to be addressed, since these most directly affect productivity. Nonemergent, generic, and lifestyle health problems are likely to go unaddressed due to cultural differences.

The Latino culture is primarily patriarchal on issues concerning use of money and decision making. Time lost from the job, lack of money and transportation, and limited access to healthcare prevent many from getting their health needs met. The common health problems often neglected may be diabetes, hypertension, dental disorders, dermatological problems, anemia, and infections. Bechtel, Shepherd, and Rogers (1995) noted that women suffer more from urinary tract infections, lack of prenatal care, and anemia. Two lifestyle illnesses are of great significance. One-third of this population has positive PPDs, due to inadequate housing or crowding (Bechtel et al., 1995). Second, hepatitis A, transmitted through fecal-oral routes under poor sanitary conditions, is spread quickly in endemic areas. For children, by the age of 10, there has been greater than 70% anti-HAV prevalence in areas similar to migrant camps. HAV immunization has been considered for children from ages 2 to 10 living under these conditions (Dentiger, Heinrich, Bell, Fox, Katz, Culver, & Shapiro, 2001).

Major health problems of migrant workers' children aged 5 through 15 were found to be communicable diseases, such as pediculosis and upper respiratory infections, ear/eye/nose/throat problems, dental problems, anemia, and injuries (Go & Baker, 1995). A study by Bechtel et al. (1995) also found that children of migrant and seasonal farm workers were exposed to extreme levels of violence: Fifty-two percent of the children surveyed had been exposed to the results of some type of violence. Of these children exposed to violence, 46% witnessed someone being beaten, mugged, shot at, and/or murdered, and 19% had been victims of violence themselves. This exposure to violence, compounded by the issues of poverty and a transient lifestyle, may be reflected in these children's higher risk for emotional and behavioral problems.

MIGRANT RESOURCES

In an attempt to fill in gaps for migrant healthcare and safety, new resources have developed to connect this population to healthcare providers. These resources address the issue of frequent relocation before healthcare treatment has been completed or before continuity of care can be given The new resources are as follows:

Migrant Clinicians Network at *http://www.migrantclinicians.org/services* provides many services such as TB Net (for tracking TB and latent tuberculosis infection [LTB]), Diabetes, Environmental Health, and more. Providers may register migrants for medical record assistance for continuity of care.

ERIC Clearinghouse on Rural Education and Small Schools at *http://aeliot.ael.org/~eric/digests/edorc947.html* provides information about migrants and politics.

THE HOMELESS POPULATION

Documentation of the homeless population depends on definition and method of counting, thus true numbers may only be estimated. Homeless individuals in this chapter will be considered those living on the streets, places not intended for human habitation, shelters, or temporary or inconsistent night-time residences provided at no cost. This excludes persons in treatment facilities, prisons, or places where an individual is detained. This definition includes single-room occupancy hotels rooms paid with vouchers, but not doubled-up persons (Gelberg, Andersen, & Leake, 2000; National Coalition for the Homeless [NCH], 2002b). The way the homeless are counted is critical, be it "point prevalence," or one location and one date check, versus several episodic counts. It is estimated on any one given night there are about 3.5 million homeless individuals (NCH, 2002a). Reasons for the increasing numbers are blamed on decreased affordable rental housing (reducing the number of flop houses, demolishing substandard housing, and building upgraded housing), increased poverty, changes in employment practices, deindustrialization, increased competing needs for social services, and increased substance abuse, and poor health (Gelberg et al., 2000; Martens, 2001; U.S. Conference of Mayors, 2002, 2003).

Interesting but not surprising, a list of risk factors for becoming homeless includes poor health, financial crisis, poor credit, unemployment, imprisonment, a history of being in a foster home as a child, a victim of child abuse (physical or sexual) or domestic violence, mental illness, and substance abuse (Martens, 2001; NCH, 1999a & b). The fastest rising population is families with children (40%). Children make up 25% of the homeless population. The remaining population is 41% single males, 13% single females, and 5% unaccompanied children. By ethnicity, 50% are African American, 35% are Caucasian, 12% are Hispanic, 2% are Native American, and 1% are Asian, as reported by the U.S. Conference of Mayors (2001; NCHb, 2002). Most studies have covered metropolitan areas due to the sheer volume and lack of community services. Rural areas differ by having a more homogeneous population by race and ethinicity, and communities tend to "take care of their own" (Wagner, Menke, & Ciccone, 1995).

COMMON HEALTH PROBLEMS OF THE HOMELESS

It is generally known that the homeless have a higher rate of physical morbidity and mortality. The most common health problems by age are: (0–1) dermatologic, infection, and anemia; (1–11) infection, asthma, behavior problems, missed immunization, anemia, and depression; (12–19) behavior problems, acute infections, STDs, muscle-skeletal problems, pregnancy, and drug and/or alcohol abuse. Adults' health problems include infections, drug and alcohol abuse, HBP, DM, STDs, eye, dental, arthritis, cancer, liver, renal, and trauma (Amarasingham et al., 2001; Crane & Warnes, 2001). Salit, Kahn, Hartz, Vu, and Mosso (1998) show that homeless individuals stayed an extra 4.1 days longer in the hospital (36%) than any other population, primarily due to mental illness, substance abuse, AIDS, and placement problems. It has been said that medical care for the homeless is more crisis management than adequate care (Crane & Warnes, 2001).

Communicable diseases are a significant problem among the homeless. The greatest risk factor for TB is homelessness (Martens, 2001). Risk factors in this population include being of advancing age, African American descent, an IV drug user; duration of homelessness; and living in single-room occupancy hotels (SROH). SROH occupants are three times more likely to convert to latent TB infection (LTBI) due to poor ventilation and high contact situations (Zolopa, Hahn, Gorter, Miranda, Wlodarczyk, Peterson, Pilote, & Moss, 1994). A profound finding by Gelberg, Panarites, Morgenstern, Leake, Andersen, and Koegel (1997) is that when homeless people found out about their LTBI, nearly 80% sought medical care. This is a dramatic difference in behavior than was once thought (Gelberg et al., 2000; Gelberg et. al, 1997). Previously, the general belief was this population would seek medical help only if symptomatic.

Just as TB is higher in the homeless population, so HIV has a seroprevalance of 19%. The risk factors for being HIV positive multiply even more with being female, a crack user, an IV drug user; sharing "works"; using in a "shooting gallery"; having multiple sex partners (this was an even greater predictor than unprotected sex in this population); selling sex; homosexuality, and African American ethnicity (Martens, 2001; Smereck, Hockman, 1998; Zolopa et al., 1994). These two major communicable diseases take their toll on their own; multidrug resistance strains of TB compound the problem.

Mental health disorders and substance abuse are major problems for the homeless. Approximately 22% of homeless adults have some degree of severe, persistent, disabling mental illness. Only 7% require institutionalization (NCH, 2002b). Sixty-six percent of the homeless meet the criteria for chronic substance abuse. Seventy-seven percent have a dual diagnosis (Belcher, Greene, McAlpine, & Ball, 2001). This population is difficult and disruptive. Many shelters' policies exclude intoxicated/drugged individuals. These individuals are even more vulnerable to victimization. They are also less eligible for treatment programs due to their homelessness (Belcher et al, 2001), a no win situation.

Homeless children are the most vulnerable of all, needing stability for proper growth and development. Families many times are separated when they arrive at shelters. Fathers are not considered part of the family unit and go to a separate single men's shelter. Family units are mostly mothers with children. If substance abuse or mental illness is a part of the problem, then the children are often taken to foster homes. The system is unprepared for conventional families or families headed by a single male. Disruption of the family unit, if it was not the cause of homelessness, becomes a part of homelessness too many times. Children experience developmental delays, anxiety, depression, poor school attendance, and undue achievement (NCH, 1999a). Many children start alcohol and drugs by the age of 13 to 15 (Belcher et al., 2001). Youth trying to make it on the streets face extraordinary pressures. To survive, they exchange sex for food, clothing, and shelter. As a consequence 2.3% of persons under 25 are HIV positive (NCH, 1999a). It is clear that lifestyles chosen by the homeless to survive create or produce many of their health problems.

MEDICATION AND TREATMENT CONSIDERATIONS FOR MIGRANT WORKERS AND THE HOMELESS

Significant similarities exist between migrants and the homeless concerning medication and treatment considerations. Both populations perceive barriers between them and the services actually available to them, and neither are frequently able to comply fully with management plans. Given the presenting complaints most commonly seen in a primary care setting, the clinician is confronted with significant issues. (Table 15–1 highlights selected issues for the clinician who provides care to these populations). The client may present with a more advanced stage of illness. For migrants, this could reflect the varied

TABLE 15–1. Considerations in Choosing Medication for Migrant and Homeless Populations

Consideration	Action	Example*
Stage of illness—clients seek care when in more advanced stage.	Treat more aggressively with more broad-spectrum antibiotic.	Treat pneumonia with a macolide if it is available in clinic.
Clinic location and structure; appointment schedule and hours	If client lives a distance from clinic or cannot return to clinic, treat more aggressively.	Treat child with borderline otitis media with whatever acceptable antibiotic is available in the clinic. If once-a-day medication (i.e., Cipro) is available, use it.
Lack of acceptance in community or lack of translators	Avoid problematic community settings. If a pharmacy is known to treat migrant or homeless people with disrespect, find other alternatives. Develop a list of well-respected volunteers for translation and transportation and to assist with community relations issues.	Women who have a yeast infection could be treated by over-the-counter Monistat. Clinic either provides the medicine or finds escort to the pharmacy to facilitate optimum outcome.
Difficulty in filling prescriptions	Provide medication rather than prescription.	Provide worker with low back pain with nonsteroidal anti-inflammatory in appropriate doses with gastric-sparing teaching information.
Difficulty with multiple doses and medications requiring storage	Treat when possible with as few doses per day as available. If practical, give daily dose to patient at homeless shelter.	Give once-a-day medication to child with acute otitis media if clinic samples or voucher if program exists. First-line choice of medication is determined more by what's available, the budget of the clinic, and community resources. Although amoxicillin may be the drug of choice in non-complicated situations, Cipro or another daily medication should be used if available. A recently approved single injection of ceftriaxone would be another available option.
Noncompliance	Avoid rebound medications.	For HBP provide either *an inexpensive* generic diuretic or a combination low-dose diuretic with ACE-inhibitor.

**These are clinical examples that reflect the chapter references and the clinical experiences of the author/editors.*

cultural interpretation of the significance of the illness or injury. They may be hesitant to seek care given the possible impact on their employment.

Clinic location and appointment schedules are very important. Utilization of a clinic will depend on clinic hours being coordinated with other services that the populations utilize and limited waiting times.

These clients may also confront significant attitudinal barriers on the part of the healthcare provider or resource used. The practitioner must have both the interest and the skill to address the complex needs of the migrant or homeless client. The need for specialty referral or hospitalization may be "overlooked" even if required. Translation resources are often quite limited, making the investigation of the presenting complaint, the delineation of the differential diagnosis, and the development of the management plan flawed. The homeless population rarely trusts the traditional healthcare delivery system, so development of nonthreatening relationships is essential.

Medication should be given to both the homeless and migrant workers rather than using prescriptions because of problems in their getting a prescription filled. Also consider the storage requirements of any medications. Nyamathi and Shuler (1989) completed a retrospective study of the factors affecting medication compliance of 61 homeless males sheltered at the Union Rescue Mission in Los Angeles. The study examined those factors that positively or negatively impacted the compliance with the medication regime as well as those that impacted perception of health. The most common reasons negatively affecting compliance with medication usage included the lack of privacy, lack of a storage area, the increased risk of medication being stolen, and the difficulty in obtaining medication. Refrigeration is frequently not available. Pills often are ground to powder while being carried. Consider also providing only enough medication to cover the individual until the next visit, as loss or sale of medication is quite common. Once-a-day dosing is the best option when possible (Brickner et al., 1993).

Decisions regarding antibiotics for treatment of acute infections must include consideration of the cost of medication, the frequency of dosing, and the patient's ability to understand the use of the drug. For migrant workers particularly, considerations also include the worker's time in the fields, access there to food and water, and the risk of side effects related to sun exposure. Bear in mind that with some viral conditions there is great risk of a secondary bacterial infection. Since monitoring conditions and modifying lifestyle in terms of increased fluids and rest are difficult at best, antibiotics are often more frequently prescribed. The following clinical situation highlights some of the challenges faced by the clinician.

> Anthony was a 37-year-old Caucasian male who presented at the clinic complaining of the "flu." He had noted nasal congestion and an intermittent productive cough for approximately four days. He described the sputum as white. He had not felt well but did not believe he had a fever. He was a one-pack-per-day smoker. He was sleeping at one of the temporary shelter sites and had been working the day labor pool. His physical exam was normal although an intermittent cough was noted. A chest x-ray was not easily available. The decision was made to use an oral antibiotic, as well as to administer a PPD (purified protein derivative).

Dermatologic conditions pose a real challenge with regard to pharmacotherapeutic intervention for the migrant population. Depending on the etiology of the condition, ongoing exposure to the irritant is a given. The availability of medication and the frequency of the dosage is a struggle. Adequate hygiene and appropriate dressing or protection from the elements may not be feasible.

As previously noted, the prevalence of untreated or undertreated chronic illness in both populations is quite high. Therefore, it is important to assess for chronic conditions whenever the client makes contact with the delivery system. The treatment of chronic conditions in both populations frequently does not reflect textbook standards because those guidelines are unrealistic.

Diabetes mellitus and hypertension are examples of this point. Treatment of these diseases requires continuity of care, monitoring, and lifestyle modifications to manage the conditions. The American Diabetic Association guidelines for diagnosis and treatment of diabetes requires monitoring of blood sugars and a stable living situation. As noted by Fleischman and Farnham (1992) and by Usatine et al. (1994), attempting to control a diabetic homeless person is a dangerous goal since there is significant instability in eating and activity patterns. Syringes, alcohol swabs, and medication may be subject to theft or sale. Learning to inject oneself, monitoring one's condition, etc., require frequent visits and the development of a trusting relationship. Therefore, the goal is often moderate control of blood glucose without hypoglycemia, using oral hypoglycemics as much as possible.

With regard to hypertension, as noted by the Seventh Report of the Joint National Committee on Prevention, Detection, Evaluation, and Treatment of High Blood Pressure (U.S. Department of Health and Human Services, 2003), recommendations for followup of an elevated initial set of blood pressure measurements range from immediate intervention to confirming an elevation within two months, depending on the initial reading. In the homeless population, there is an increased frequency of hypertension in younger individuals, and it is therefore wise to check blood pressure on all adults. Of course, several blood pressure readings at more frequent intervals are optimal for a more accurate assessment. Decisions about when to implement drug therapy must be carefully individualized in light of the increased risk of noncompliance, limited followup, and difficulty in modifying lifestyle in terms of diet, stress, and substance abuse. The choice of a drug should reflect the following considerations: once-a-day dosing if possible, limited need for laboratory monitoring (use diuretics or combination low-dose ACE-inhibitors), and drugs without rebound (Hall, 1999).

Use of any medication in the vulnerable migrant or homeless populations needs understanding of culture, lifestyle, environment, literacy level, and wider scope of possible hazards or complications. Clients believe if a little is good, more is better. Informing clients of the serious nature of proper use of medication indicates better followup of instructions (Gelberg et al., 2000). Use every method available to help ensure safe, simple medication administration, find a coding system for bottles to aid in scheduling of proper doses, use medicine boxes to help facilitate medication compliance, and use appropriate language for instructions (Travena, Simpson, & Nutbeam, 2003).

In treating persons with TB or LTBI (previously called TB chemoprophylaxis), one must stay current with standards of care. The *Morbidity and Mortality Weekly Report* (MMWR), published by the Centers for Disease Control and Prevention (CDC), provides the newest recommendations (2000). This may be obtained by phone (888-232-3228). New guidelines recommend nine months of treatment instead of the previous six. When it is possible, use *directly observed therapy* with twice weekly dosing. Recommended scheduling and dosing may vary for HIV-positive clients. There are recommendations for BCG/Bacillus of Calmette and Guerin vaccination for controlling TB in the United States in the MMWR of April 26, 1996 (Volume 45/No. RR-4). BCG is not without its complications, but in some instances such as this population, it may be beneficial. It is not recommended for persons positive for HIV (CDC, 1996).

OTHER HELPFUL RESOURCES

Homelessness

Health Care for the Homeless: *http://www.hchirc.com*

National Homeless: *http://www.nationalhomeless.org*

National Coalition for the Homeless: *http://www.nch.ari.net*

TB

Center for Disease Control: *http://www/cdc.gov/nchstp/tb*

TB Net: *http://www.migrantclinician.org*

HIV

HIV/AIDS and Homeless: *http://www.migrantclinician.org*

Diabetes

American Diabetes Association: *http://www.diabetes.org/default.htm/*

Diabetes Track II: *http://www.migrantclinican.org*

Children

American Academy of Pediatrics: *http://www.aap.org*

REFERENCES

Amarasingham, R., Spalding, S.H., & Anderson, R.J. (2001). Disease conditions most frequently evaluated among the homeless in Dallas. *Journal of Health Care for the Poor and Underserved,* 12 (2), 162–175.

Arcury, T.A., Quandt, S.A., Cravey, A.J., Elmore, R.C., & Russell, G.B. (2001). Farmworker reports of pesticide safety and sanitation in the work environment. *American Journal of Industrial Medicine,* 39, 487–498.

Baumohl, J. (1996). (Ed.). *Homeless in America.* National Coalition for the Homeless, Phoenix, AZ: Onyx Press.

Bechtel, G.A., Shepherd, M.A., & Rogers, P.W. (1995). Family, culture, and health practices among migrant farmworkers. *Journal of Community Health Nursing,* 12(1), 15–22.

Belcher, J.R., Greene, J.A., McAlpine, C., & Ball, K. (2001). Considering pathways into homelessness: Mothers, addictions, and trauma. *Journal of Addictions Nursing,* 13(3–4), 199–208.

Brickner, P. W., McAdam, J. M., Torres, R. A., Vicic, W. J., Conanan, B. A., Detrano, T., Piantieri, O., Scanlan, B., & Scharer, L. K. (1993). Providing health services for the homeless: A stitch in time. *Bulletin of the New York Academy of Medicine, 70*(3), 146–170.

Centers for Disease Control. (1996, April 26). The role of BCG vaccine in the prevention and control of tuberculosis in the United States. Joint Statement for the Elimination of Tuberculosis and the Advisory Committee on Immunization Practices. *MMWR, 45* (RR-4), 1–18.

Centers for Disease Control. (2000, June 9). Targeted tuberculin testing and treatment of latent tuberculosis infection. ATS/CDC Statement Committee on Latent Tuberculosis Infection. *MMWR, 49* (RR-6), 1–51.

Crane, M., & Warnes, A.M. (2001). Primary health care services for single homeless people: Defects and opportunities. *Family Practice,* 18, 272–276.

Dentinger, C.M., Heinrich, N.L., Bell, B.P., Fox, L.M., Katz, D.J., Culver, D.H. & Shapiro, C.N. (2001). A prevalence study of hepatitis A virus infection in a migrant community: Is hepatitis A vaccine indicated? *The Journal of Pediatrics, 138*(5), 705–709.

Fleischman, S., & Farnham, T. (1992). Chronic disease in the homeless. In D. Wood (Ed.), *Delivering health care to homeless persons.* New York: Springer.

Gelberg, L. (1992). Health of the homeless: Definition of problem. In D. Wood (Ed.), *Delivering health care to homeless persons.* New York: Springer.

Gelberg, L., Andersen, R.M., & Leake, B.D. (2000). The behavioral model for vulnerable populations: Application to medical care use and outcomes for *Homeless people. Health Services Research, 34*(6), 1273–1302.

Gelberg, L., Panarites, C.J., Morgenstern, H., Leake, B., Andersen, R.M., & Koegel, P. (1997). Tuberculosis skin testing among homeless adults. *Journal of General Internal Medicine, 12,* 25–33.

Go, V., & Baker, T. (1995). Health problems of Maryland's migrant farm laborers. *Maryland Medical Journal, 44*(8), 605–608.

Hall, DW.D. (1999). A Rational Approach to the Treatment of Hypertension in Special Populations. American Family Physician, 60(1), 156–162.

Lewis, J.H., Andersen, R. M., & Gelberg, L. (2003). Health Care for Homeless Women. *Journal of General Internal Medicine,* 18, 921–928.

Martens, W.H.J. (2001). A review of physical and mental health in homeless persons. *Public Health Reviews, 29,* 13–33.

National Coalition for the Homeless. (1999c, June). Health care and homelessness. NCH Fact Sheet #8. *http://nch.ari.net/health.html.*

National Coalition for the Homeless. (1999b, June). Homeless families with children. NCH Fact Sheet #7.

National Coalition for the Homeless. (1999a, April). Homeless youth. NCH Fact Sheet #11.

National Coalition for the Homeless. (2001, July) Education of homeless children and youth. NCH Fact Sheet #10.

National Coalition for the Homeless (2002a, September) How many people experience homelessness? NCH Fact Sheet #2.

National Coalition for the Homeless. (2002b, September). Who is homeless? NCH Fact Sheet #3.

Nyamathi, A., & Shuler, P. (1989). Factors affecting prescribed medication compliance of the urban homeless adult. *Nurse Practitioner, 14*(8), 47–54.

Salit, S.A., Kuhn, E.M., Hartz, A.J., Vu, J.M., & Mosso, A.L. (1998). Hospitalization costs associated with homelessness in New York City. *New England Journal of Medicine, 338*(24), 1734–1740.

Smereck, G.A.D & Hockman, E.M. (1998). Prevalence of HIV infection and HIV risk behaviors associated with living place: On-the-street homeless drug users as a special target population for public health intervention. *Journal of Drug and Alcohol Abuse, 24*(2), 229–319.

Trevena, L.J., Simpson, J.M. & Nutbeam, D. (2003) Soup kitchen consumer perspectives On the quality and frequency of health service interactions. *International Journal For Quality in Health Care,* 15(6), 495–500.

Usatine, R. P., Gelberg, L., Smith, M. H. & Lesser, J. (1994). Health care for the homeless: A family medicine perspective. *American Family Physician, 49*(1), 139–146.

U.S. Conference of Mayors. (2002, December). *Hunger homelessness on the rise in major U.S. cities.* Washington, DC: Author (www.usmayors.org).

U.S. Conference of Mayors (2003, December). Sodexho Hunger and Homelessness Survey 2003, Washington, D.C.

U.S. Department of Health and Human Services (2003). *The Seventh Report of the Joint National Committee on Prevention, Detection, Evaluation, and Treatment of High Blood Pressure.* Washington, DC: National Institutes of Health.

U.S. Department of Labor. (2000). *Findings from the National Agricultural Workers Survey (NAWS) 1997–1998.* San Mateo, CA: National Coalition for the Homeless.

Wagner, J.D., Menke, E.M., & Ciccone, J.K. (1995). What is known about rural homeless families? *Public Health Nursing,* 12(6), 400–408.

Zolopak, A.R., Hahn, J.A. Gorter, R., Miranda, J., Wlodarczyk, D., Peterson, J., Pilote, L. & Moss, A.R. (1994). HIV and tuberculosis infection in San Francisco's homeless adults. *Journal of the American Medical Association, 272*(6), 455–461.

CHAPTER ❖ 16

INDIVIDUALS WITH PAIN

Cynthia J. Simonson

Each year, millions of Americans seek medical assistance for the relief of intolerable pain. Despite major medical and scientific advances, the undertreatment of pain remains a major public health problem in the United States (Dahl, Bennett, Bromley, & Joranson 2002). Pain is the most common reason that patients seek care. One adult in five suffers from chronic pain. Pain is the third leading reason for absence from work in the United States, which represents an annual expenditure of at least $50 billion (Katz, 2002). Despite the widespread prevalence of pain and the abundance of analgesic therapies, pain generally ranks low on the medical treatment priority list, (but remains high on the list of concerns of the public. Respondents to a survey commissioned by *Modern Maturity* magazine in 2000 said that they feared dying in pain more than they feared death itself (Dahl et al., 2002; Redford, 2002). The reasons for undertreatment of pain have been well documented and remain unchanged. They include inadequate knowledge and inappropriate attitudes of healthcare professionals, patient and family fears and misconceptions, barriers in the drug regulatory system, problems within the system of the delivery of care such as poor access to opioids in minority pharmacies, and inadequate reimbursement for drugs and other therapies (Dahl et al., 2002; Morrison, Wallenstein, Natale, Senzel, & Huang, 2000; Pargeon & Hailey, 1999; Stieg, Lippe, & Shepard, 1999).

The issue of cultural sensitivity is also becoming a more important factor in delivering effective pain management. In the past decade, the United States has witnessed immigration rates second only to the peak years before World War I. Within each ethnic group, individuals come from all walks of life with differing religious, educational, occupational, and economic statuses. The design of effective healthcare interventions to alleviate pain for culturally diverse patients presents a complicated task for healthcare professionals (Lasch, 2000). In an effort to establish better treatment of pain, the Agency for Health Care Policy and Research (AHCPR) of the Public Health Service developed evidence-based guidelines for the treatment of acute low back pain, acute pain, cancer pain (Acute Low Back Problems in Adults Clinical Practice Guideline Panel, 1994; Acute Pain Management Guideline Panel, 1992; and Management of Cancer Pain Guideline Panel, 1994). Since that time at least six other major organizations have published pain management guidelines that relate to specific disorders or populations (Sanders, 2000).

Clearly, there remains a need for better pain management. The Joint Commission on Accreditation of Healthcare Organizations has issued new standards for pain assessment and treatment that will formally acknowledge pain control as a patient right and an organizational responsibility (Chapman, 2000). Hopefully, these, along with the other evidenced-based guidelines and many professional organizations focused on pain, will help move the healthcare system on toward adequate and appropriate management of pain.

This chapter includes subsections describing the four types of pain, the use of pain assessment tools, various nonpharmacologic analgesic interventions, and the pharmacologic treatments used in managing pain. A chronic pain treatment guideline is also presented. Although many of the concepts described can be used in the treatment of most other painful conditions, this chapter focuses primarily on the management of patients with chronic pain.

PAIN TYPES

ACUTE VERSUS CHRONIC PAIN

Pain can be classified as either acute or chronic, depending on its onset and duration. Acute pain has an easily defined onset and is transient, occurring only between the time of tissue injury and tissue recovery. Acute pain serves a major medical function by alerting patients and clinicians that tissue damage may exist (American Pain Society [APS], 2003; Marcus, 2000).

Although acute pain is a symptom of another medical condition, chronic pain is a syndrome in its own right (Marcus, 2000; Weisberg & Clavel, 1999). Chronic pain persists or recurs over an extended period of time and interferes with the patient's functioning. The personality changes that can occur in patients experiencing chronic pain include feelings of helplessness, hopelessness, and meaninglessness (Marcus, 2000; Weisberg & Clavel 1999). Patients become increasingly depressed and dysfunctional, and may suffer a diminished quality of life (Chang, 1999; Marcus, 2000; Weisberg & Clavel, 1999).

Unlike acute pain, the goals of treating chronic pain are not to eliminate the pain completely, but to teach the patient coping mechanisms, increase the patient's level of functioning, and attempt to reduce pain to its most tolerable level. This can be a challenging process involving numerous trials of different pharmacologic and nonpharmacologic interventions (Cherny, 2000; Marcus, 2000; Weisberg & Clavel, 1999).

NOCICEPTIVE VERSUS NEUROPATHIC PAIN

Pain also can be classified by its source; it is either nociceptive or neuropathic. Nociceptive pain is the result of stimulation of pain receptors, called nociceptors, located throughout the body. (Portenoy, 2001) Nociceptive pain can be further subdivided into somatic and visceral pain. Somatic nociceptive pain originates from the skin or skin structures and is dull and aching in quality. This type of pain is well localized to a specific area of the body. Tendinitis, postsurgical pain, and musculoskeletal pain are examples of somatic nociceptive pain. Visceral nociceptive pain originates from the internal organs as a result of infiltration, compression, or stretching of these tissues. Visceral nociceptive pain is difficult to localize and is often referred to sites distant from the site of origin. Myocardial infarction pain, referred to the arm and shoulder, is a classic example of visceral nociceptive pain. Nociceptive pain of either subgroup responds well to nonsteroidal antiinflammatory agents and opioids alone or in combination (AGS Panel, 2002; Chang, 1999; Weisberg & Clavel, 1999).

Neuropathic pain originates from compression or injury to a peripheral nerve fiber or the central nervous system. Patients describe this type of pain as shooting, electrical, or burning in nature. Postherpetic neuralgia, trigeminal neuralgia, and diabetic neuropathy are examples of neuropathic pain syndromes. In general, neuropathic pain is less responsive to commonly used analgesic medication classes. Adjunct analgesics including antidepressants, and anticonvulsants may be required in the treatment of this type of pain (AGS Panel, 2002; Belgrade, 1999).

Although the four previously mentioned pain types are distinct, all may be present in a patient simultaneously. This is particularly true in patients with cancer pain or geriatric patients with multiple health problems. To provide maximal pain relief, combinations of interventions may be necessary, particularly when different pain types coexist (AGS Panel, 2002; Chang, 1999; Marcus, 2000).

It is also now known that psychosocial factors can precipitate or exacerbate organic disorders such as chronic pain (Gallagher, 1999a; Weisberg & Clavel, 1999). Research in psychoneuroimmunology suggests some of the neurohormonal and neuroimmune pathways by which psychological factors impact on pathophysiology in pain (Weisberg & Clavel, 1999). The complexity and diversity in presentation of chronic pain symptoms can be explained by the interrelationships among pathophysiologic changes, psychological functioning, and the social and cultural factors that affect a patient's perception of and response to distress. Multidisciplinary assessment and management of the psychosocial factors operating in each complex chronic pain patient are recommended (Gallagher, 1999b; Weisberg & Clavel, 1999).

PAIN ASSESSMENT

Since pain is experiential, the best way to assess pain is to listen to and believe the patient. The AHCPR Cancer Pain Management Guideline recommends the following assessment guidelines:

- Health professionals should ask about pain and believe the patient's report.
- The initial evaluation of pain should include a detailed history, including an assessment of pain intensity and characteristics, a physical assessment emphasizing the neurologic examination, and a psychosocial assessment.
- Pain should be assessed with easily administered rating scales and should document the efficacy of management plans.
- Changes in pain patterns or the development of new pain should trigger a diagnostic evaluation and modification of the treatment plan.

Additional assessment strategies include:

- On initial presentation of any older person to any healthcare service, a healthcare professional should assess the patient for evidence of chronic pain (AGS Panel, 2002).
- A cultural assessment should be part of pain assessment. If language is a barrier, it is important and appropriate to involve an interpreter who will convey the meaning of the patient's words (Lasch, 2000).
- Many patients utilize complementary therapies and are sometimes reluctant to report their use. Assessment should include careful questioning on use of alternative and complementary therapies as well as use of lay healers.

NONPHARMACOLOGIC ANALGESIC THERAPIES

Many nonpharmacologic analgesic treatments are available and can be very useful in the treatment of chronic pain. It is recommended that because of the many misconceptions about pain and its treatment, education for patients and their families should be a part of all management strategies. Information should be given about the ability to effectively control pain, and myths about opioids should be corrected. It is also recommended that psychosocial interventions be included early in the course of pain management, but that they not be used as substitutes for analgesics. Information about support groups, community resources, and spiritual support should be included. Patients should be encouraged to report the occurrence of new pain to their healthcare practitioner before seeking palliation from modalities such as acupuncture, massage therapy, and healing touch therapy.

Nonpharmacologic therapies include treatments such as massage, chemicals applied to the skin, cold, heat, transcutaneous electrical nerve stimulation (TENS), vibration, acupuncture, distraction, imagery, meditation, relaxation, art or music therapy, hypnosis, biofeedback, cognitive-behavioral therapy, psychodynamic therapies and energies such as healing touch therapy (AGS Panel 2002; Langenfeld, Cipani & Borckardt, 2002; Lyne, Coyne & Watson, 2002; Van Fleet, 2000).

These nonpharmacologic treatments sometimes can be adequate alone. They are most often used in conjunction with analgesics and other nonpharmacologic treatments. Not all patients find these treatments beneficial, but they almost always should be given a trial.

PHARMACOLOGIC ANALGESIC THERAPIES

ASPIRIN, SALICYLATES, AND NONSTEROIDAL ANTIINFLAMMATORY DRUGS

Nonsteroidal antiinflammatory drugs (NSAIDs) are among the most frequently prescribed analgesic medications (Bell & Schnitzer, 2001). NSAIDs inhibit the enzyme cyclooxygenase to prevent prostaglandin and thromboxane synthesis. Prostaglandins sensitize nociceptors and decrease the pain threshold to pain mediators such as bradykinin, substance P, and histamine. By suppressing the actions of prostaglandins, NSAIDs produce analgesia and have antiinflammatory properties (APS, 2003; Bell & Schnitzer, 2001).

NSAIDs are generally used for the treatment of mild to moderate pain (APS, 2003). They are considered first-line therapy in most rheumatic disorders (Rehman & Lane, 1999). NSAIDs are commonly used in combination with other analgesic medications, such as opioids. Combining opioids and NSAIDs produces greater pain relief than when either modality is used alone. In addition, NSAIDs have an opiate sparing effect that allows lower doses of opioids to be used (Bell & Schnitzer, 2001).

Over 20 NSAIDs are commercially available. Many are now available in less costly over-the-counter or generic forms (see Drug Table 306). Thus far, no study has shown one NSAID to be more efficacious than another (Chang, 1999). However, there is a significant interpatient variability in response (APS, 2003). If an NSAID of one structural class is not effective at maximally tolerable doses, a trial of a second NSAID of a different structural class may be beneficial (APS, 2003) (see Drug Table 306).

By inhibiting the synthesis of these prostaglandins, use of NSAIDs can lead to gastrointestinal upset and ulceration, compromised renal function, and platelet inhibition. Bronchospasm may also occur with the use of NSAIDs because of the inhibition of bronchodilating leukotrienes (Chang, 1999).

Dermatitis, central nervous system effects, hepatitis, acute interstitial nephritis, and hepatotoxicity are a few of the idiosyncratic reactions that have been reported by patients receiving NSAIDs (Bell & Schnitzer, 2001). The incidence of allergic reactions to NSAIDs is small. Aspirin-sensitive patients should also avoid NSAIDs due to the possibility of cross-reactions (APS, 2003).

A new group of NSAIDs, the coxibs, has been developed in an effort to reduce the side effects from the prostagladin suppression of the NSAIDs. Both groups of drugs inhibit prostaglandin synthase, but NSAIDs inhibit the two recognized forms, cyclooxygenase-1 and cyclooxygenase-2; the coxibs are selective to cyclooxygenase-2. The inhibition of cyclooxygenase-2 has been more directly implicated in relieving inflammation, and the inhibition of cyclooxygenase-1 has been more directly implicated in adverse effects in the gastrointestinal tract. The coxibs (celecoxib, rofecoxib, and valdecoxib) offer patients a safer alternative to standard NSAIDs by providing comprable analgesic and antiinflammatory efficacy with significantly reduced GI toxicity (Bell & Schnitzer, 2001; FitzGerald & Patrono, 2001). These agents are similar in most respects except for one limiting factor with celecoxib. It is metabolized by the cytochrome P-450 system and carries the potential for drug interactions when combined with other inhibitors of the P-450 system (Lucas & Lipman, 2002).

NSAIDs have a ceiling effect. Each NSAID has a maximum dose beyond which there is no additional analgesic benefit (APS, 2003) (see Drug Table 306). Within the dosing range, the dose required to produce analgesia is generally smaller than that needed for the NSAIDs' antiinflammatory effects (Bell & Schnitzer, 2001).

NSAIDs are an integral part of the management of mild to moderate pain and should be used unless there is a contraindication (APS, 2003). Efficacy being equal, over-the-counter availability, generic availability, cost, adverse effect profiles, and pharmacokinetic differences become the primary determinants in drug selection.

ACETAMINOPHEN

Acetaminophen is widely used for the relief of mild to moderate pain (APS, 2003). Acetaminophen works centrally, through inhibition of the cyclooxygenase enzyme (Cherny, 2000). The analgesic potency of acetaminophen, aspirin, and NSAIDs is comparable (Rehman & Lane, 1999). However, unlike aspirin and the NSAIDs, acetaminophen has no antiinflammatory properties (APS, 2003).

Acetaminophen produces very few adverse reactions (see Drug Table 301). Unlike aspirin and the NSAIDs, it does not cause gastrointestinal adverse effects and does not affect platelet function (APS, 2003). Acetaminophen may be used in aspirin-sensitive patients (APS, 2003). Because of the association between aspirin and Reye's syndrome, acetaminophen is the analgesic and antipyretic of choice in children. The most serious adverse effect of acetaminophen is dose-related hepatotoxicity. Acetaminophen undergoes a saturable metabolic process. Beyond the saturation point, an alternative hepatotoxic metabolite is formed. To avoid hepatotoxicity, the manufacturer recommends limiting the maximum daily acetaminophen dose to 4 g. Patients with chronic alcoholism or liver disease are more susceptible to hepatotoxicity and may experience liver damage at lower acetaminophen doses (APS, 2003).

Acetaminophen is available over the counter in a variety of generic formulations. It is available in both oral and rectal preparations (see Drug Table 301). Because of its attractive adverse effect profile, relatively low cost, and comparable analgesic efficacy, acetaminophen is an acceptable first-line treatment for many painful conditions (AGS Panel, 2002).

OPIOIDS

Opioids are used in the treatment of moderate to severe pain (Liter, 2002). Opioids are commonly used in the postoperative and malignant pain settings. Although the routine use of opioids in nonmalignant pain is controversial, opioids are an acceptable alternative for other analgesic interventions that have been ineffective (Belgrade, 1999).

Opioids produce their pharmacologic and adverse effects through binding to opioid receptors throughout the central nervous system and peripheral tissues. There are three types of opioid receptors: mu, kappa, and delta. The mu receptor is considered the prototypical opioid receptor (Lucas & Lipman, 2002). When stimulated, the mu receptor produces analgesia, miosis, euphoria, reduced gastrointestinal motility, respiratory depression, urinary retention, sedation, nausea, tolerance, and physical dependence (Cherny, 2000). Kappa receptor stimulation produces analgesia, dysphoria, psychotomimetic effects, miosis, and respiratory depression. Stimulation of the delta opioid receptor produces analgesia without respiratory depression (Cherny, 2000).

Opioids are classified as controlled substances by the Food and Drug Administration (FDA). As such, there is a known potential for abuse. When prescribing, monitoring, and counseling patients about opioid therapy, it is important to differentiate between the terms tolerance, physical dependence, and psychological dependence. Tolerance and physical dependence are normal physiologic changes that occur in most patients who receive opioids for more than one month (APS, 2003). Tolerance is defined as the need for a higher dose, after repeated administration, to maintain the same effect (Chang, 1999). Physical dependence occurs when the body becomes accustomed to receiving opioids. If the opioids are withdrawn, the body will exhibit withdrawal symptoms within 6 to 72 h. To avoid opioid withdrawal, the dose of opioids should be slowly tapered (25% reduction in dose every other day) upon drug discontinuation (APS, 2003). Psychological dependence, or addiction, indicates that the patient is taking the medication for reasons other than its intended use. This occurrence is not a characteristic of the drug class alone, but is a combined effect of biochemical, societal, and psychological factors affecting the patient (APS, 2003).

Opioids are classified by their ability to stimulate or block opioid receptors (Lucas & Lipman, 2002). Pure agonists include morphine, codeine, dihydrocodeine, hydrocodone, oxycodone propoxyphene, hydromorphone, methadone, meperidine, oxymorphone, levorphanol, and fentanyl. These medications exert their action primarily by stimulation of the mu opioid receptor. Unlike NSAIDs, pure opioid agonists do not have a ceiling effect; additional analgesia may be obtained by increasing the opioid dose (Cherny, 2000; Savage, 1999).

Buprenorphine is the only commercially available partial agonist. It is a partial agonist at the mu opioid receptor, but an antagonist at the kappa receptor (Cherny, 2000). Compared to the pure agonists, buprenorphine is less effective and has an analgesic ceiling effect (Management, 1994). If given to a patient receiving high doses of a pure opioid agonist, withdrawal symptoms may occur (APS, 2003). This is due to buprenorphine's relatively lower analgesic potency and its displacement of the pure agonist at the opioid receptor sites (Cherny, 2000).

Mixed agonist-antagonists include pentazocine, butorphanol, dezocine, and nalbuphine. These agents are agonists at the kappa receptor and weak antagonists at the mu receptor (Cherny, 2000). Patients who are opioid-tolerant should not be given a mixed agonist-antagonist. The mu antagonism of the mixed agents risks opioid withdrawal symptoms. Similar to partial agonists, mixed agonist-antagonists have an analgesic ceiling effect. Because of their primary kappa receptor stimulation, these agents are known to produce psychotomimetic effects (Cherny, 2000). The role of these agents in the treatment of severe pain and chronic pain is limited.

Naloxone and naltrexone are opioid antagonists. All opioid receptor types are blocked by these agents. The primary role of the opioid antagonists is to displace opioid agonists from their receptor sites to reverse opioid-induced adverse effects (Cherny, 2000).

Opioids can also be grouped by the severity of pain in which they are used. Codeine, dihydrocodeine, hydrocodone, and propoxyphene are less potent and are used in the treatment of moderate pain (Liter, 2002). Although a few of these agents are available as single-entity preparations, most are combined with aspirin or acetaminophen. The acetaminophen content in the combination products limits the ability to escalate the dose (APS, 2003). These agents are short-acting and must be dosed frequently (i.e., every 2 to 4 h) (Cherny, 2000).

Opioids used for severe pain can be grouped by their duration of action. Morphine, oxycodone, oxymorphone, hydromorphone, meperidine, and fentanyl are short-acting agents (Cherny, 2000). Morphine is the prototypical opioid. It is used as a standard of comparison for all other opioids. Hydromorphone is more potent than morphine. Because of its high solubility and potency, hydromorphone is often used for subcutaneous administration of relatively high opioid doses (APS, 2003). Meperidine is considerably less potent than morphine and is converted to a neurotoxic metabolite. This agent has no role in the treatment of chronic pain (APS, 2003). Of the short-acting opioids, morphine (MS Contin, Kadian, Oramorph SR), oxycodone (OxyContin), and fentanyl (Duragesic Patches) are formulated in sustained-release preparations to increase patient convenience and to provide a constant level of pain relief (Cherny, 2000).

Fentanyl is also available in an oral transmucosal formulation (Actiq). It is a short-acting form indicated for the treatment of breakthrough pain in patients who are already receiving and are tolerant of opioid therapy (Lucas & Lipman, 2002).

Methadone and levorphanol are potent, long-acting, pure opioid agonists. Methadone is used in the prevention of opioid withdrawal for patients who are physically dependent on opioids. When used in this capacity, methadone is usually given once daily. Patients receiving methadone for analgesic purposes may require dosing every 4 to 8 h. These medications are not considered first-line agents because of the difficulty in rapidly titrating to an effective dose (Cherny, 2000; Gouldin, Kennedy & Small; 2000).

Methadone, however, is considered a second choice drug in the management of cancer pain. Methadone has a number of unique characteristics, including excellent oral and rectal absorption, no known active metabolites, high potency, low cost, and longer administration intervals, as well as an incomplete cross-tolerance with respect to other mu-opioid receptor agonist drugs (Gouldin, et al., 2000). However, its use is limited by the remarkably long and unpredictable half-life, large interindividual variations in pharmacokinetics, the potential for delayed side effects, and the limited knowledge of correct administration intervals and the equianalgesic ratio with other opioids when administered chronically (APS, 2003; Gouldin et al., 2000). Serious adverse effects can be avoided if the initial titration is done on an as-needed basis. When a steady state of pain control with tolerable side effects has been reached, an around-the-clock schedule can be established based on the 24h dose needed for good pain control (Cherny, 2000).

Adverse effects that may occur with the use of opioid medications include nausea and vomiting, sedation, constipation, urinary retention, pruritus, and respiratory depression (APS, 2003). Nausea, vomiting, and sedation occur early in therapy or immediately after a dosage increase. Tolerance develops quickly to these effects (Cherny, 2000). Patients who have a history of experiencing opioid-induced nausea and vomiting may require scheduled antiemetics for the first several days of opioid therapy until tolerance occurs. If sedation is problematic, smaller, more frequent doses may be used (Cherny, 2000). Stimulant medications, such as caffeine and methylphenidate, have been administered to counteract sedation in cancer pain patients receiving high doses of opioids, (APS, 2003; Cherny, 2000).

Constipation is the most frequently reported adverse effect with the chronic use of opioids (Cherny, 2000). Unlike other opioidinduced adverse effects, tolerance does not develop to constipation (Cherny, 2000). Patients should be given a stimulant laxative (senna, bisacodyl, or phenolphthalein) and possibly a stool softener (docusate) on a routine basis (Cherny, 2000). Osmotic laxatives (lactulose, magnesium citrate) or bowel preparations, such as Golytely, may be needed intermittently. Oral naloxone can be given for refractory constipation. Naloxone is not well absorbed by the oral route; therefore, the risk of precipitating opioid withdrawal is small. If patients experience nausea, early satiety, and bloating, these may be signs of delayed gastric emptying and the use of metoclopramide or cisapride may be helpful (Cherny, 2000).

Urinary retention and pruritus are more commonly seen when opioids are administered by the epidural or intrathecal route. Bear in mind that antidepressants also cause urinary retention and may be a contributing factor when opioids and antidepressants are combined. Pruritus may also be treated with antihistamines (APS, 2003).

The most serious and most feared opioid-induced adverse reaction is respiratory depression. Clinically significant respiratory depression is rare when opioids are given to patients who are experiencing acute pain. Patients receiving opioids chronically rarely experience this effect since tolerance develops to respiratory depression (APS, 2003). Signs of central nervous system depression accompany respiratory depression and include somnolence, unarousability, mental confusion, and slowed respiratory rate. Since its use will precipitate withdrawal in the opioid-dependent patient, naloxone should be reserved for potentially life-threatening situations (Cherny, 2000). When naloxone is required, the dose should be titrated slowly to response (0.4 mg diluted with 10 mL saline given intravenously in 0.5-cc increments every 2 min) (APS, 2003).

Opioids may be administered by many routes, including subcutaneous, intramuscular, intravenous, epidural, intrathecal, oral, buccal, sublingual, transnasal, transdermal, rectal, and by inhalation (Cherny, 2000). Patients who are unable to take oral medications to reach a tolerable dose have many available options. The least invasive, most cost-effective method should be tried before moving to more invasive techniques. In general, the oral route of administration is preferred because of its convenience and lower cost (Liter, 2002). Intramuscular injections should be avoided; they are painful and the medication is erratically absorbed from the site of administration (Cherny, 2000).

Fortunately, unlike other analgesic classes, opioids have well-accepted equianalgesic doses, which allows the clinician to convert between agents and between routes of administration. Most opioids require a dosage increase when converting from the parenteral to the oral route. Close monitoring after an opioid conversion or dosage change is required to evaluate the need for further dosage adjustments (Cherny, 2000).

A method commonly used after titrating to a relatively stable opioid dose is to prescribe one long-acting agent and one "as needed" short-acting agent. The long-acting opioid (sustained-release morphine, oxycodone, methadone, or levorphanol) should be used on a scheduled basis, with "as needed" short-acting medications prescribed for pain that is not relieved by the scheduled dose (APS, 2003). The "as needed" or breakthrough dose should be approximately 15 to 50% of the total daily scheduled medication dose. Patients who routinely require frequent breakthrough doses within a dosing interval (e.g., more than two doses in 4 h or more than six doses in 24 h) need an increase in their scheduled medication. The goal of this technique is to maintain a constant level of pain relief with the scheduled medication, while only occasionally requiring the breakthrough medication (Cherny, 2000).

ANTIDEPRESSANTS

Antidepressants have been used in a variety of chronic pain conditions including cancer pain, fibromyalgia, tension and migraine headache, postherpetic neuralgia, diabetic neuropathy, arthritis, and low back pain. Although antidepressants have been used in treating many painful conditions, they are most effective in treating burning neuropathic pain states (Lucas & Lipman, 2002).

The precise mechanism of the analgesic action of antidepressants is not understood. Initially, antidepressants were thought to provide analgesia simply by relieving depression. Subsequent studies found antidepressants produced analgesia in nondepressed patients, demonstrating that antidepressants possess an analgesic activity independent of their antidepressant action. Antidepressants are believed to produce analgesia by inhibiting the reuptake of serotonin and norepinephrine, neurotransmitters involved in the descending inhibitory pain pathway (Sumpton & Moulin, 2001).

Other suggested mechanisms of action include enhanced endorphin secretion, sodium channel blockade, inhibition of substance P, a neuropeptide involved in both pain and depression, and NMDA receptor antagonism (King, 2003).

Many antidepressants are marketed today. The first-generation, older agents have cyclic structures. Cyclic antidepressants are categorized as either tertiary or secondary amines. In general, compounds with tertiary amine structures (e.g., amitriptyline, imipramine, and doxepin) possess more serotonergic activity than noradrenergic activity. Conversely, secondary amines (e.g., nortriptyline, desipramine, and protriptyline) preferentially affect norepinephrine to a greater extent than serotonin (Vaillancourt & Langevin, 1999).

Second-generation, newer antidepressants (e.g., trazodone, nefazodone, bupropion, and the selective serotonin reuptake inhibitors, such as fluoxetine, paroxetine, sertraline, and fluvoxamine) are structurally unrelated to the cyclic antidepressants and are more selective in the receptors and neurotransmitters they affect. Antidepressants that affect both the serotonergic and noradrenergic systems appear to provide the most analgesia. The tricyclic antidepressants, which block the reuptake of both serotonin and norepineprine, are generally much more effective as analgesics than the selective serotonin reuptake inhibitors.

A newer class of antidepressants, serotonin and noradrenergic reuptake inhibitors (SnaRI), have shown equivalent efficacy on mood disorders with a significant reduction in side effects. Venlafaxine, the most investigated of these new drugs, has been shown to be the most effective in the treatment of different kinds of pain (Mattia, Paoletti, Coluzzi, & Boanelli, 2002; King, 2003). Venlafaxine causes fewer adverse effects since it does not bind to muscarinic-cholinergic, histaminic, or adrenergic receptors. The most common adverse effect seen is nausea. Elderly patients may experience an increase in blood pressure that may require a decrease in dosage (Sumpton & Moulin, 2001).

Adverse effects caused by antidepressants include anticholinergic, cardiovascular, and central nervous system effects (APS, 2003). In general, tertiary amines appear to produce more adverse effects than secondary amines, and the second-generation antidepressants are better tolerated (Lucas & Lipman, 2002).

Anticholinergic adverse effects are the most common and also the most bothersome produced by this medication class. These include blurred vision, constipation, urinary retention, and dry mouth. Sugarless gum or candy may help relieve dry mouth. Pharmacologic interventions, including pilocarpine eye drops (blurred vision), hydration and bulk laxatives (constipation), and bethanechol (urinary retention) may be required to counteract these effects (APS, 2003).

Orthostatic hypotension caused by alpha receptor blockade can be a significant problem. Less orthostasis has been reported with the use of nortriptyline (APS, 2003).

Because of their interactions with histamine receptors, certain antidepressants (e.g., amitriptyline, imipramine, doxepin, and trazodone) can cause central nervous system sedation. This "adverse reaction" may be beneficial in the patient with pain and insomnia. Conversely, the selective serotonin reuptake inhibitor fluoxetine produces central nervous system stimulation and may lead to insomnia (APS, 2003).

Seizures are one of the more serious central nervous system adverse effects seen in patients receiving antidepressants. Antidepressants lower the seizure threshold. Patients at risk for experiencing seizures (i.e., patients with epilepsy or head injuries, patients who receive concomitant seizure-threshold–reducing medications such as phenothiazines, substance abusers, or patients who experience withdrawal from alcohol or sedatives/hypnotics) should be monitored closely (Vaillancourt & Langevin, 1999).

Other adverse reactions produced by antidepressants include weight changes and sexual dysfunction. Weight gain may occur with tricyclic antidepressants, whereas weight loss is more common with fluoxetine and other selective serotonin reuptake inhibitors. Sexual dysfunction has been reported with all antidepressant classes (APS, 2003).

Doses of antidepressants for pain management are lower than those used for depression. Small doses should be started initially (i.e., 10 to 25 mg of amitriptyline or doxepin) and then increased in small increments (10 to 25 mg) at 2- to 4-day intervals to an effective dose (approximately 75 to 150 mg). When used for their analgesic properties, most antidepressants should be given as a single bedtime dose, taking advantage of the sedating properties while minimizing bothersome anticholinergic properties that peak during sleep. Often, early morning oversedation will subside in the first weeks of treatment. Be cognizant of the potential for nocturnal orthostatic hypotension, especially in elderly patients, when the entire daily dose is given at bedtime (APS, 2003).

The onset of analgesic action is variable, occurring from a few days to several weeks after therapy is initiated. If a patient has a therapeutic failure with an antidepressant of one structural class, a medication in another class may be tried (Vaillancourt & Langevin, 1999).

Matching the medication to the patient is somewhat of a challenge because of the many intolerable adverse effects of these medications. Antidepressants used as analgesic adjuvants generally are not completely effective and are rarely used as single drug therapy. However, antidepressants have an alternative mechanism of action that when combined with other analgesic medication classes, may provide additional pain relief. (Lucas & Lipman, 2002; King, 2003).

ANTICONVULSANTS

Most anticonvulsants appear to provide analgesia and are used in the treatment of many neuropathic pain syndromes (APS, 2003; King, 2003). Overall, these agents are more effective in treating neuropathic pain that is shooting or electrical in quality (APS, 2003).

Anticonvulsants are believed to exert their analgesic activity by inhibiting aberrant nerve firing, leading to neural membrane stabilization. However, the specific mechanism by which each anticonvulsant provides membrane stabilization differs (Laird & Gidal, 2000; King, 2003).

Gabapentin is a novel antiepileptic agent, originally developed as a gamma-aminobutyric acid-mimetic compound to treat spasticity. It has been shown to be a potent anticonvulsant. Although its exact mode of action is not known, gabapentin appears to have a unique effect on voltage-dependent calcium ion channels at the postsynaptic dorsal horns and may interrupt the series of events that possibly leads to the neuropathic pain sensation. Gabapentin has been clearly demonstrated to be effective for the treatment of neuropathic pain in diabetic neuropathy and postherpetic neuralgia (Rose & Kam, 2002). With its low side effect profile and low profile of drug interactions, it is becoming the anticonvulsant of choice for treatment of neuropathic pain (Laird & Gidal, 2000). Gabapentin has been shown to be effective at dosages of 300 to 3600 mg/day; however, dosages of at least 900 mg/day were most effective. The optimal dosage appears to be 1800 to 2400 mg/day in divided doses (Laird & Gidal, 2000). The literature indicates that other new anticonvulsants, lamotrigine and oxcarbazeine, can also provide significant analgesia (Ross, 2000). Because the new anticonvulsants have more benign side-effect profiles, they have generally replaced the anticonvulsants such as phenytoin, carbamazepine and valproate sodium for pain management. One exception is that trigeminal neuralgia usually responds better to carbamazepine than to any other medication (King, 2003).

The recommended starting dose of carbamazepine is 100 mg twice daily. Due to rate-limiting sedation, the dose must be gradually increased to effect. A dose range of 200 to 1600 mg daily is generally effective. Carbamazepine induces its own metabolism. After a few weeks of therapy, an increase in carbamazepine dosage may be required because of increased drug clearance (APS, 2003).

If phenytoin is used, the initial dose is 300 mg of the sustained-release preparation, given once daily. Symptoms that occur at a concentration near the upper limit or above the therapeutic range include nystagmus, slurred speech, ataxia, and confusion. To avoid toxicity, small incremental dosage adjustments of phenytoin are required, especially when nearing the upper limit of the therapeutic range (Whitaker, Kennedy & Small, 1999).

In rare instances, carbamazepine and phenytoin have caused hepatic dysfunction, neutropenia, and thrombocytopenia. Liver function tests and complete blood counts should be monitored at baseline and intermittently for the first few months of therapy. Patients should be instructed to contact their primary care practitioner or pharmacist if they experience fever, sore throat, flu-like symptoms, bruising, or jaundice. Since chronic use of phenytoin can lead to gingival hyperplasia, patients receiving phenytoin should be encouraged to use good oral hygiene (APS, 2003).

ANTIARRHYTHMICS

The lidocaine patch is useful in the treatment of localized pain such as postherpetic neuralgia, low back pain, diabetic neuropathy and complex regional pain syndrome (Paice, 2002; King, 2003). Lidocaine patches are applied at the site of pain and are left on for twelve hours per day. Up to 3 patches can be applied at a time (King, 2003). Because of it local effect, the side-effect profile is benign and is a good choice for patients who may have difficulty tolerating other analgesics (King, 2003) or as an addition to other forms of analgesia.

CORTICOSTEROIDS

Corticosteroids have antiinflammatory properties that make them useful in the management of many painful conditions. Corticosteroids exert their antiinflammatory properties through inhibiting leukotriene and prostaglandin synthesis. The most common use of corticosteroids is in the treatment of nerve compression pain in patients with cancer (APS, 2003).

GENERAL TREATMENT GUIDELINES

The following points describe strategies used in the management of patients with chronic pain.

- Always believe your patient's report of pain and communicate that belief.
- Keep the regimen as simple and as cost-effective as possible.
- Use the oral route of administration whenever possible because of its convenience and lower cost (Acute Pain Management, 1999).
- Individualize the analgesic regimen for each patient.
- Maximize the dose of each medication before declaring it a therapeutic failure.
- Analgesic medication should be given on a scheduled basis. It is easier to prevent pain than to control pain of a higher intensity (King, 2003).
- For patients with chronic, nonmalignant pain, maximize all other therapies before opting for an opioid (Belgrade, 1999).
- For mild pain, patients should receive either acetaminophen, aspirin, or NSAID (Liter, 2002).
- For moderate pain, or if mild pain persists or increases, a pure opioid analgesic used to treat moderate pain (e.g., codeine or hydrocodone) should be added to the previous step (Liter, 2002).
- For severe pain, or if moderate pain persists or increases, the dosage of the opioid should be increased or the patient should be converted to a more potent opioid agonist (e.g., morphine or oxycodone) (Cherny, 2000).
- An analgesic adjuvant (e.g., antidepressant or anticonvulsant) can be used at any point in therapy, if appropriate (Cherny, 2000).

REFERENCES

Acute Low Back Problems in Adults Clinical Practice Guideline Panel. (1994). *Acute Low Back Problems in Adults. Clinical Practice Guideline.* AHCPR Pub. No. 95-0643. Rockville, MD: Agency for Health Care Policy and Research, Public Health Service, U.S. Department of Health and Human Services.

Acute Pain Management Guideline Panel. (1992, February) *Acute pain management: Operative or medical procedures and trauma. Clinical practice guideline.* AHCPR Pub. No. 92-0032. Rockville, MD: Agency for Health Care Policy and Research, Public Health Service, U.S. Department of Health and Human Services.

American Geriatrics Society (AGS) Panel on Persistent Pain in Older Persons. (2002). The management of Persistent pain in older persons—*Journal of American Geriatrics Society, 50* (Suppl 6), 5205–224.

American Pain Society. (2003). *Principles of analgesic use in the treatment of acute pain and cancer pain* (5th ed.). Glenview, IL: Author.

Bell, G. M., & Schnitzer, T. J. (2001). Cox-2 inhibitors and other nonsteroidal anti-inflammatory drugs in the treatment of pain in the elderly. *Clinics in Geriatric Medicine, 17*(3), 489–503.

Belgrade, M. J. (1999). Opioids for chronic nonmalignant pain: Choosing suitable candidates for long-term therapy. *Postgraduate Medicine, 106*(6), 115–124.

Chang, M. C. (1999). Cancer pain management. *The Medical Clinics of North America: Chronic Pain, 83*(5), 711–736.

Chapman, C. R. (2000). New JCAHO standards for pain management. Carpe diem. *APS Bulletin, 10*(4).

Cherny, N. I. (2000). The management of cancer pain. *CA: A Cancer Journal for Clinicians, 50,* 70–116.

Dahl, J. L., Bennett, M. E., Bromley, M.D., & Joranson, D.E. (2002). Success of the state pain initiatives: Moving pain management forward. *Cancer Practice, 10* (Suppl 1), S9–13.

FitzGerald, G. A., & Patrono, C. (2001). The coxibs, selective inhibitors of cyclooxygenase-2. *New England Journal of Medicine, 345*(6), 433–442.

Gallagher, R. M. (1999a). Treatment planning in pain medicine: Integrating medical, physical, and behavioral therapies. *The Medical Clinics of North America: Chronic Pain, 83*(5), 823–849.

Gallagher, R. M. (1999b). Primary care and pain medicine: A community solution to the public health problem of chronic pain. *The Medical Clinics of North America: Chronic Pain, 83*(5), 555–583.

Gouldin, W. M., Kennedy, D. T., & Small, R. E. (2000). Methadone: History and recommendations for use in analgesia. *APS Bulletin, 10*(5).

Katz, W. A. (2002). Musculoskeletal pain and its socioeconomic implications. *Clinical Rheumatology, 21* (Suppl 1), S2–4.

King, S. A. (2003). Chronic pain control: What's adequate—and appropriate? 10 Questions Physicians Often Ask. Consultant, 43(13), 1558–1573.

Laird, M. A., & Gidal, B. E. (2000). Use of gabapentin in the treatment of neuropathic pain. *The Annals of Pharmacotherapy, 34,* 802–807.

Langenfeld, M. C., Cipani, E., & Borckardt, J. J. (2002). Hypnosis for the control of HIV/AIDS-related pain. *International Journal of Clinical Experimental Hypnosis, 50*(2), 170–180.

Lasch, K. E. (2000). Culture, pain, and culturally sensitive pain care. *Pain Management Nursing, 1*(3, Suppl 1), 16–22.

Liter, M.E. (2002). Cancer pain management. *Oncology Special Edition, 5,* 37–41.

Lucas, L. K., & Lipman, A. G., (2002). Recent advances in pharmacotherapy for cancer pain management. *Cancer Practice, 10* (Suppl 1), S14–20.

Lyne, M.E., Coyne, P. J., & Watson, A. C. (2002). Pain management issues for cancer survivors. *Cancer Practice, 10* (Suppl 1), S27–32.

Management of Cancer Pain Guideline Panel. (1994, March). *Management of cancer pain. Clinical practice guidelines.* AHCPR Publication No. 94–0592. Rockville, MD: Agency for Healthcare Policy and Research, U.S. Department of Health and Human Services, Public Health Service.

Marcus, D. A. (2000). Treatment of nonmalignant chronic pain. *American Family Physician, 61,* 1331–1338, 1345–1346.

Mattia, C., Paoletti, F., Coluzzi, F., & Boanelli, A. (2002). New antidepressants in the treatment of neuropathic pain. A review. *Minerva Anestesiologica, 68*(3), 105–114.

Morrison, R. S., Wallenstein, S., Natale, D. K., Senzel, R. S., & Huang, L. L. (2000). "We don't carry that"—failure of pharmacies in predominatly nonwhite neighborhoods to stock opioid analgesics. *New England Journal of Medicine, 342,* 1023–1026.

Paice, J. A. (2002). Treating postherpetic neuralgia with lidocaine patch. *Clinical Journal of Oncology Nursing, 6*(1), 58.

Pargeon, K. L., & Hailey, B. J. (1999). Barriers to effective cancer pain management: a review of the literature. *Journal of Pain and Symptom Management, 18,* 358–368.

Portenoy, R. K. (2001). *Three step analgesic fadder for management of cancer pain* (pp. 6–22). New York: McMahon Publishing Group.

Redford, G.D. (2002). Their final answers: An exclusive modern maturity survey. *Modern Maturity, 43W,* 66, 68.

Rehman, Q., & Lane, N. E. (1999). Getting control of osteoarthritis pain: An update on treatment options. *Postgraduate Medicine, 106*(4), 127–134.

Rose, M. A., & Kam, P. C. A. (2002). Gabapentin: Pharmacology and its use in pain management. *Anaesthesia, 57,* 451–462.

Ross, E. L. (2000). The evolving role of antiepileptic drugs in treating neuropathic pain. *Neurology, 55* (Suppl 1), S41–46.

Sanders, S. H. (2000). Integrating practice guidelines for chronic pain: From the Tower of Babel to the Rosetta Stone. *APS Bulletin, 10*(6).

Savage, S. R. (1999). Opioid use in the management of chronic pain. *The Medical Clinics of North America: Chronic Pain, 83*(5), 761–786.

Stieg, R. L., Lippe, P., & Shepard, T. A. (1999). Roadblocks to effective pain treatment. *The Medical Clinics of North America: Chronic Pain, 83*(5), 809–821.

Sumpton, J. E., & Moulin, D. E. (2001). Treatment of neuropathic pain with venlafaxine. *The Annals of Pharmacotherapy, 35,* 557–559.

Vaillancourt, P.D., & Langevin, H. M. (1999). Painful peripheral neuropathies. *The Medical Clinics of North America: Chronic Pain, 83*(5), 627–642.

Van Fleet, S. (2000). Relaxation and imagery for symptom management: Improving patient assessment and individualizing treatment. *Oncology Nursing Forum, 27*(3), 501–514.

Weisberg, M. B., & Clavel, Jr., A. L. (1999). Why is chronic pain so difficult to treat? Psychological considerations from simple to complex care. *Postgraduate Medicine, 106*(6), 141–64.

CHAPTER ❖ 17

PREGNANCY AND LACTATION

Laurie A. Buchwald

The fact that pregnancy is a natural event does not preclude the need for occasional medication use. Whether an over-the-counter preparation or a prescription drug is used, most women will find it necessary to take some kind of medication during a 40-week gestation. The same is true for the woman who is lactating. One study of pregnant women revealed that on the average, each woman took four drugs, 25% took five or more, almost 10% took eight or more, and only 4% took none (Niebyl & Kochenour, 1999). Epidemiological studies have determined that between one- to two-thirds of all pregnant women take at least one medication during pregnancy (Loebstein, Lalkin, & Koren, 2001). Given this, providers who care for pregnant and lactating women must have an understanding of the changes that occur in maternal physiology and pharmacokinetics. This chapter addresses these changes as well as highlights positive pharmacotherapeutics during the preconception period. Drug management of common illnesses and discomforts of pregnancy are also discussed.

PHYSIOLOGIC CHANGES DURING PREGNANCY

Pregnancy induces a number of physiologic changes (see Table 17–1). The tone and motility of the gastrointestinal (GI) tract—including the stomach, the small bowel, and the colon—are decreased. The smooth muscle–relaxing effects of progesterone are thought to be the cause and result in a 30 to 50% increase in gastric and intestinal emptying time (Loebstein, Lalkin, & Koren, 2001). Estrogen and progesterone levels rise, as do the levels of triglycerides, cholesterol, and phospholipids, resulting in an increased competition for protein-binding sites. Simple diffusion leads to equality of serum concentrations between the mother and fetus (McCombs & Cramer, 1999). However, blood proteins that bind with drugs in the fetus are lower than in the mother so more free concentration of a drug may exit in the fetus. This is especially true of drugs that are bound highly in the mother's blood. The liver does not enlarge, and there is no significant increase in hepatic blood flow (Cunningham, MacDonald, Gant, et al., 1997; Murray & Seger, 1994). Total body water increases by as much as 8 L, and total body fat and weight are also significantly increased (Cunningham et al., 1997; Hedstrom & Martens, 1993). Maternal cardiac output increases by 30 to 50% during pregnancy, and plasma volume also increases by 50% (Cruikshank, Wigton, & Hays, 1996; Cunningham et al., 1997). It nears 70% in twin pregnancies (Hacker & Moore, 1998). The glomerular filtration rate is 50% higher than in the nonpregnant woman, and causes a decrease in blood-urea-nitrogen (BUN) and creatinine levels.

Changes also occur in the respiratory, integumentary, skeletal, and endocrine systems, but it is beyond the scope of this chapter to review those changes that do not significantly affect drug response during pregnancy.

TABLE 17–1. Maternal Physiologic Changes Affecting Pharmacokinetics

- Increase in total body water: approximately 8 L
- Increase in total body fat and weight gain: 3–4 kg
- Decreased tone and motility of the GI tract
- Increased glomerular filtration rate: 50%
- Increased cardiac output: 30–50%
- Increased blood volume: 50%
- Increased plasma protein production
- Decreased plasma albumin concentration
- Increased competition for plasma protein binding sites

Sources: Baer & Williams (1996); Cunningham et al. (1997); Forney (1996); Loebstein et al. (2001); Murray & Seger (1994).

CHANGES IN PHARMACOKINETICS DURING PREGNANCY

The properties of pharmacokinetics are discussed in Chapter 2. The following sections review those properties that are affected by the changes in maternal physiology.

ABSORPTION

The absorption of medications during pregnancy is affected by several factors. The decrease in GI tone and motility due to progesterone influence may cause the drug to remain in the stomach longer, leading to increased absorption of drugs that are slowly absorbed and delayed absorption of those that are easily absorbed (Gutierrez, 1999). Nausea and vomiting, symptoms commonly experienced by women in the first trimester, often alter the eating habits of pregnant women and may ultimately reduce the amount of drug available for absorption (Forney, 1996). Acidity is reduced in pregnancy, increasing basic drug absorption and decreasing acidic drug absorption (Gutierrez, 1999).

DISTRIBUTION

Of the four kinetic properties, distribution is affected most by maternal physiologic changes. The increase in plasma volume results in an increased volume for distribution and can lead to a prolonged drug elimination half-life (Murray & Seger, 1994). Drugs that are water soluble can be diluted from the increased extracellular fluid in pregnancy (Gutierrez, 1999). Drugs that are fat soluble, in association with a 3 to 4 kg increase in body fat in pregnancy, may stay longer in the body (Gutierrez, 1999; Murray & Seger, 1994). Higher free fatty acids alter distribution of some drugs also. Drugs that have high protein binding and lower lipid solubility, such as anticonvulsants, are influenced to have a longer half-life and slower elimination by the increase in volume of distribution (Gutierrez, 1999). Decreased albumin levels result in a limited number of receptor or binding sites. Hormones, which are strongly protein-bound, compete for the available sites, leaving fewer sites available for binding drugs. Ultimately, this results in a wide distribution of free, unbound drug in the body (Forney, 1996).

BIOTRANSFORMATION

The liver is the primary site for metabolism of drugs. Since blood flow through the liver is relatively unchanged during pregnancy, this property of kinetics is essentially unchanged (Hansen & Yankowitz, 2002). Drugs cleared only by the liver are eliminated in pregnancy similarly to the nonpregnant woman (Gutierrez, 1999). Progesterone intensifies drug biotransformation in pregnancy. Along with higher levels of hepatic enzymes, more rapid clearance in the liver and faster elimination occur, shortening drug half-life (Gutierrez, 1999).

EXCRETION

The elimination of drugs from the body through the kidneys is the most important route of excretion. The serum level of a drug in the mother must fall to allow diffusion of that drug from the fetus's circulation and ultimate clearance (Gutierrez, 1999). Renal blood flow increases by 25 to 50%, and glomerular filtration increases by 50% (Forney, 1996). As a consequence, those drugs that have substantial renal excretion have increased rates of clearance (Murray & Seger, 1994). The fetus can eliminate drugs, also, through its liver drug-biotransforming enzymes (Gutierrez, 1999). However, excreted drug and metabolites from fetal urine in the aminiotic fluid may lead to additional exposure as the fetus swallows amniotic fluid.

PLACENTAL TRANSFER

Medications that cross through the placenta must pass through the syncytiotrophoblast, the stroma of the intervillous space, and the fetal capillary wall (Cunningham et al., 1997). This histological barrier is not an actual physical barrier, and throughout pregnancy, a wide range of substances pass to the fetus. Placental transfer mechanisms include: (1) *simple diffusion,* where the molecular size and available surface area may or may not permit transfer; (2) *active transport,* where concentrations of substances are higher in the fetus and transported back to the mother against the concentration gradient; (3) *pinocytosis,* where soluble molecules, such as viruses, cross the placental membrane in small vesicles as particles and are released; (4) *facilitated diffusion,* where glucose is transferred to the fetus more rapidly than with simple diffusion; and (5) *leakage,* when fetal cells enter the mother's cirulation through small membrane breaks such as with Rh sensitization (Gutierrez, 1999). In essence, the ease of movement of a drug from the maternal to fetal circulation is influenced by such factors as molecular size/weight/configuraton, lipid solubility, physiochemical composition, distribution of the drug selectively in the body or widely, and whether it is nonprotein bound and nonionized (Gutierrez, 1999; Niebyl & Kochenour, 1999). Medications that have a small molecular size, are nonprotein bound, nonionized, and lipophilic readily cross the placenta and may negatively impact the developing fetus. The maternal blood pressure and position affect drug availability to the fetus, with left lateral position promoting blood flow across the placenta and standing or supine interfering (Gutierrez, 1999). Drugs with molecular weights of 250 to 500 d can cross the placenta easily (Cohen, 1992). Most drugs used therapeutically have molecular weights lower than 600 d and, therefore, cross the placenta without difficulty (Murray & Seger, 1994). Protein binding of drugs to maternal plasma proteins causes transfer to be slow.

GUIDELINES FOR MEDICATION USE IN PREGNANCY

The Food and Drug Administration (FDA) has developed a drug classification system designed to guide providers as they choose medications for their pregnant clients (see Table 17–2). Risk factors have been assigned to all drugs based on the level of risk that the drug poses to the developing fetus. One of the problems with developing this classification system is that controlled drug trials to determine safety, efficacy, and pharmacokinetic alterations in pregnancy are rare. Because of the lack of data, many agents are given a category C designation. This category includes a statement that the drug should be given only if potential benefits justify potential risks to the fetus. Healthcare providers should know that complete reliance on the FDA classification system is inadequate for clinical decision making (Tillett, Kostich, VandeVusse, 2003). A review of available malformation reports in comprehensive sources such as Drugs in Pregnancy and Lactation, 6th ed. 2002 allows for more complete decision making.

TABLE 17–2. Food and Drug Administration Pregnancy Risk Classification

Category A

Controlled studies in women fail to demonstrate a risk to the fetus in the first trimester, nor is there evidence of a risk in later trimesters, and the possibility appears remote. Prenatal vitamins are an example.

Category B

Either animal reproduction studies have not demonstrated a fetal risk (there are no controlled studies in pregnant women) or animal reproduction studies have shown an adverse effect (other than a decrease in fertility) that was not confirmed in controlled studies in women in the first trimester (and there is no evidence of a risk in later trimesters). The penicillins are an example.

Category C

Either studies in animals have revealed adverse effect on the fetus (teratogenic or embryocidal effects or other) and there are no controlled studies in women, or studies in women and animals are not available. Drugs should be given only if the potential benefit justifies the potential risk to the fetus. Many drugs fall into this category.

Category D

There is positive evidence of human fetal risk, but the benefits from use in pregnant women may be acceptable despite the risk (e.g., if the drug is needed in a life-threatening situation or for a serious disease for which safer drugs cannot be used or are ineffective). An appropriate statement should be included in the "warnings" section of the labeling. An example is Carbamazepine.

Category X

Studies in animals or human beings have demonstrated fetal abnormalities or there is evidence of fetal risk based on human experience, or both, and the risk of the drug in the pregnant women clearly outweighs any possible benefit. The drug is contraindicated in women who are or may become pregnant. An appropriate statement must be included in the "contraindications" section of the labeling. Isotretinoin for acne is an example.

Sources: Baer & Williams (1996); Briggs, Freeman, & Yaffe (1996); Cunningham et al. (1999); Larimore & Petrie (2000).

DRUG TERATOGENESIS

The FDA is now proposing changes in the pregnancy labeling system for drugs because of the difficulty in using and understanding the old classification system (Hansen & Yankowitz, 2002). The latest information can be obtained online (*www.fda.gov*; search the site for "pregnancy" and "labeling").

A teratogen is any substance, agent or process capable of causing abnormal development (Sever & Mortensen, 1996; Gutierrez, 1999). The variables responsible for teratogenic effects are 1) timing, specifically the organogenesis period; 2) the particular agent and its characteristics; 3) the chronicity and dosage of the drug; 4) cellular damage due to the mechanism of the drug's action through secondary cell effects; 5) the susceptibility of the specific fetus, which can vary widely; and 6) the way the effect manifests itself, such as death, malformation, functional deficit, or retarded growth (Conover, 1994; Gutierrez, 1999). Concurrent exposure to other agents, individual maternal metabolism and route of administration also must be evaluated (Kochenour, 1995). The "classic" teratogenic period is between day 31 and 71 after the first day of the last menstrual period. Niebyl (1996) notes that drugs administered early in this classic period will affect the organs developing at that time, such as the heart or neural tube. The ear and palate are forming at the end of the teratogenetic period and may be affected by drugs administered during that time. It should be remembered that drug exposure occurring more than 10 weeks after the last menses will not generally cause congenital malformations (Yaffe & Briggs, 2003). It is reassuring to note that "the dose required to cause embryo/fetal dysfunction is less than or equal to the dose that causes intrauterine growth restriction (IUGR), which is less than the dose that causes malformation, which in turn is lower than the lethal dose (Yaffe & Briggs, 2003). Providers must weigh the untreated disease risks of the mother against potential risks to the developing fetus if a drug is used. Ideally, preconceptional counseling for women with diseases, such as epilepsy, will aid in decision making. Table 17–3 lists some medications suspected or proven to be teratogens.

DRUG THERAPY DURING LACTATION

The past two decades have seen a significant increase in the number of women who breastfeed. Considering this, clinicians must understand how drugs are excreted into breast milk.

TABLE 17–3. Known or Suspected Teratogens/Significant Adverse Effects on the Fetus[a]

Angiotensin-converting enzyme (ACE) inhibitors (D)	Diethylstilbestrol (X)
Accutane (X)	Disulfuram (C)
Alcohol	Estrogens (X)
Aminopterin (X)	Etretinate (X)
Aminoglycosides	Haloperidol (C)
Androgenic hormones	Hydroflumethiazide (D)
Busulfan (D)	Isotretinoin (X)
Carbamazepine (C)	Lithium (D)
Chlorambucil (D)	Methimazole (D)
Chloramphenicol (C)	Methotrexate (D)
Chlordiazepoxide (D)	Penicillamine (D)
Chlorpropamide (D)	Phencyclidine (X)
Clomiphene (X)	Phenytoin (D)
Clomipramine (C)	Propylthiouracil (D)
Cocaine (C)	Radioactive iodine
Cortisone (D)	Tetracycline (D)
Coumarins (D)	Thalidomide
Cyclophosphamide (D)	Thioguanine (D)
Cytarabine (D)	Trimethadione (D)
Danazol (X)	Vaccines, e.g., MMR (X), Varicella (X)
Dextroamphetamine (C)	Valproic acid (D)
Diazepam (D)	Warfarin (D)

[a] FDA pregnancy designation in parentheses.

Sources: Cohen (1992); Cunningham et al. (1997); Little & Gilstrap (1998); Loebstein et al., (2001); Niebyl & Kochenour (1999); Reeder, Martin, & Koniak-Griffin (1997); Remich (1998); Sherwin, Scoloveno, & Weingarten (1995).

THE TRANSMISSION OF DRUGS THROUGH BREAST MILK

Drug ingestion by a breastfeeding infant is usually less than 1 to 2% of the total maternal dose (Gutierrez, 1999). Those drugs that have wide distribution throughout the body usually have a low concentration in breast milk, and, only the free or unbound portion of the drug is available for diffusion into breast milk.

A drug must first be absorbed into the maternal circulation for it to be excreted into the breast milk. Many of the same factors that influence placental transfer of drugs also influence drug excretion into breast milk (see Table 17–4).

TABLE 17–4. Factors Influencing Drug Transfer Through Breast Milk

- Absorption of drug by the mother's body: half-life, absorption rate, route of administration
- Movement of drug from maternal plasma to breast milk
- Molecular size and weight: smaller size = greater transfer
- pH of the drug: nonionized drugs = greater transfer
- Lipid solubility: increased solubility = greater transfer
- Protein binding: non-protein-bound = greater transfer
- Drug distribution: wide distribution = low concentration

Sources: Akridge (1998); Gutierrez (1999); Murray & Seger (1994); O'Dea (1992).

Most drug molecules pass into breast milk by passive diffusion, but some are moved by pinocytosis, facilitated diffusion, and active transport (Forney, 1996). The ease of movement of a drug into maternal circulation is influenced by such factors as small molecular size, high lipid solubility, and whether it is nonprotein bound and nonionized (Murray & Seger, 1994).

CLASSIFICATION OF DRUGS USED DURING LACTATION

The Committee on Drugs of the American Academy of Pediatrics (AAP) has reviewed drugs in lactation and categorized them as follows:

1. Contraindicated (see Table 17–5A)
2. Requires temporary cessation of breastfeeding
3. Effects unknown but may be of concern
4. Use with caution
5. Usually compatible (Silberstein, 1993, p. 535).

The following questions and options should be considered when prescribing drug therapy to lactating women:

1. Is the drug therapy really necessary?
2. Use the safest drug.
3. Could a sustained-release or long-acting drug be used?
   The AAP Guidelines for use of prescription and nonprescription drugs by nursing mothers are available online at *http://www.aap.org/policy/0063.html* (Montauk & Rheinstein, 2002). Acetaminophen and NSAIDs are deemed safe for breastfeeding mothers to use. First-generation antihistamines are considered to be potentially risky for the newborn or premature infant, causing sedation, irritability, crying, sleep disturbances, problems with feeding, and paradoxical stimulation. Long term use is not advised. Aspirin should not be used because it can increase the risk for rashes and bleeding abnormalities in the infant (Montauk & Rheinstein, 2002). No safety data for guaifenesin is available, and little is available on antitussives that act centrally. The level of alcohol found in most medications is not thought to pose a safety hazard to the nursing baby. Safety measures advised are: (1) Use an alternative to medication if possible; (2) take medications before period of longest sleep for the infant or after nursing; (3) do not use extra-strength, long-acting, or combination medications; and (4) observe the infant for side effects (Montauk & Rheinstein, 2002).
4. If there is a possibility that a drug may present a risk to the infant, consider measuring the blood level in the nursing infant.
5. Drug exposure to the nursing infant may be minimized by having the mother take the medication just after completing a breastfeeding and/or just before the infant is due a lengthy sleep period. (Akridge, 2004; Dillon, Wagner, Wiest, & Newman, 1997; Eisenstat & Carlson, 1995; Ito, 2000; Murray & Seger, 1994; Sherwin, et al., 1996). For a more complete listing refer to Committee on Drugs (2001).
6. Is the infant showing signs of a drug reaction? (Committee on Drugs, 2001, p. 777; Gutierrez, 1999).

Drugs usually considered compatible with lactation are shown in Table 17–5B.

TABLE 17–5A. Drugs That Are Contraindicated During Lactation

Alcohol	Iodine
Aminoglycosides	Lithium
Amphetamines	Marijuana
Bromocriptine	Methotrexate
Chronic aspirin use	Minor tranquilizers
Cocaine	Narcotics
Chloramphenicol	Nicotine/tobacco
Cimetidine	Phencyclidine (PCP)
Cyclophosphamide	Phenindione
Cyclosporine	Quinolones
Doxorubicin	Radioactive isotopes
Ergotamine	Tetracycline
Gold salts	Thiouracil
Heroin	Vancomycin

Sources: Akridge (1998); Dillon, Wagner, Wiest, & Newman (1997); Eisenstat & Carlson (1995); Ito (2000); Murray & Seger (1994); Sherwin et al. (1996). For more complete listing refer to Committee on Drugs (2001).

TABLE 17–5B. Drugs That are Usually Compatible During Lactation

Acetominophen	Mexilitine
Amoxicillin	Minoxidil
Azithromycin	Oral contraceptives
Beta adrenergic agonists	Penicillins
Cephalosporins	Piroxicam
Cisplatin	Procainamide
Cromolyn	Propranalol
Dicloxacillin	Suprafen
Diltiazem	Terbutaline
Erythromycin	Theophylline
Ibuprofen	Ticarcillin
Ipratropium (Altrovent)	Tolmetin
Labetalol	Trimethoprim-sulfamethoxazole
Methimazole	Valproic acid
Metronidazole	Verapamil

Sources: Akridge (1998); Eisenstat & Carlson (1995); Ito (2000). This listing is not exhaustive.

PRECONCEPTION CARE

The concept of identifying and reducing a woman's reproductive risks before conception is known as *preconception care.* Such care ideally begins a year before a planned pregnancy (Yeong, 2004). Promoting optimum health for mother and infant is the aim. Assessment should identify risks that will allow the provider to intervene to prevent problems or to counsel the parents about potential problems that might be reduced. Is the woman engaging in any high-risk behaviors, such as tobacco, alcohol, or illicit drug use? Are there pre-existing medical conditions that may cause potential damage to mother and baby? This is the time for the promotion of healthy lifestyle behaviors, such as nutrition and exercise, and avoidance of teratogens. Interventions during the preconception period include changing medications if necessary, referrals to high-risk clinics or substance abuse treatment centers, and making sure that immunizations are current. The goal of preconception care is to maximize the health of the woman and to give prospective parents the opportunity to make lifestyle adjustments to improve their chances of a successful outcome in pregnancy (Yeong, 2004).

SCREENING FOR SUBSTANCE USE AND ABUSE

Tobacco, alcohol, illicit drugs, and caffeine can adversely affect pregnancy. Substance abuse occurs in approximately 10% of all pregnancies (Cunningham et al., 1997). One factor to consider when assessing for substance abuse is that illicit drug users seldom abuse only one drug. Specific questions should be asked about each substance to obtain an accurate history. Another factor to consider is that many illegal substances contain impurities and contaminants. These impurities have adverse effects on both the mother and the fetus (Cunningham et al., 1997). Providers should be aware of the various screening tools available to aid in the assessment of substance abuse.

Alcohol

The use of alcohol during pregnancy has been implicated in mental retardation, intrauterine fetal demise, growth retardation, low birth weight, central nervous system abnormalities, behavioral deficits, spontaneous abortions, and abruptio placentae (Cefalo & Moos, 1995; Cunningham et al., 1997; Yatte & Briggs, 2003.) What is arresting about this is that all of these conditions—known to have been caused by alcohol use—are preventable. Fetal alcohol syndrome (FAS) is the most common environmental cause of mental retardation in developed countries (Sokol & Martier, 1996). The research is unclear as to whether alcohol use in any amount is safe, but as little as 1 oz of alcohol per day has been implicated (Cunningham et al., 1997; Remich, 2004). Assess each patient for the use of alcohol. Counsel her about the known detrimental effects of alcohol, and encourage her to stop using it during the preconception period and pregnancy. Refer the patient to an appropriate program if she is unable to limit her intake on her own.

Tobacco

Associations have been found between smoking and infertility, spontaneous abortions, ectopic pregnancies, placental complications (abruptio placentae, placenta previa), low birth weight, preterm birth, lags in developmental milestones, and infant mortality (Cunningham et al., 1997; Hacker & Moore, 1998; Kuczkowski, 2003; Remich, 2004). Providers should encourage women who smoke to reduce or quit the habit by providing appropriate education and literature, support, and referrals to smoking cessation programs if necessary. Use of nicotine-inhibiting products, such as the transdermal patch, may need to be considered for the woman who smokes more than one pack a day and is unable to stop smoking (Kuczkowski 2003; Remich, 2004). The risks to the fetus of the other toxic substances in smoke may far outweigh the risks from the medical nicotine. Bupropion hydrochloride (Zyban), an FDA Pregnancy Category B drug, may need to be considered if nondrug efforts to stop smoking fail. Risks versus benefits with pregnant and lactating women must be weighed for all drug therapies.

Illicit Drugs

Illicit drug use during pregnancy has been correlated with fetal addiction, prematurity, low birth weight, placental abruption, stillbirth, growth retardation, congenital anomalies, and behavioral and learning disabilities (Cefalo & Moos, 1995; Cunningham et al., 1997; Niebyl, 1996; Remich, 2004). Commonly abused drugs include cocaine, heroin, marijuana, and methamphetamines. Cocaine exposure increases fetal risk for physical anomalies, death, and behavioral abnormalities. Polydrug use is frequent, and women who abuse illicit drugs often use alcohol and nicotine as well (Cohen & Keith, 1994; Hacker & Moore, 1998). All patients, regardless of socioeconomic background, should be evaluated for illicit drug use. Those with identified problems should be referred to a substance abuse treatment program. Although it is important to emphasize the detrimental side effects of substance abuse of any kind, doing so in a guilt-provoking manner will not encourage women to stop. In fact, this approach will only serve to alienate substance-abusing patients.

Caffeine

In small oral amounts, caffeine in pregnancy may be safe (Jellin, Gregory, Batz, et al., 2000, p. 200). More than 200 mg orally per day (more than 1 to 2 cups of tea or coffee daily) may cause caffeine withdrawal signs in the infant. Premature delivery, spontaneous abortion, and low birth weight are associated with high doses of caffeine in pregnancy. The caffeine in breast milk is approximately half of that in the mother's blood, but it may accumulate in the infant since it is excreted slowly, thus small or no amounts are safest (Jellin et al., 2000). Signs of caffeine in the infant are irritability, sleep problems, and increased bowel activity. Prior to pregnancy, advise women of this information and that caffeine use may cause increased diuresis and worsen mood swings (Remich, 2004).

GUIDELINES FOR MEDICATION USE IN THE PRECONCEPTION PERIOD

The following general guidelines for preconception counseling regarding medication use should be considered:

- It is impossible to state with complete assurance that any medication used during pregnancy is completely safe, but there are relatively few drugs that are definitely known to be teratogenic in humans.
- All medications, including over-the-counter remedies, should be reviewed and assessed for their risk-to-benefit ratio.
- Many variables interact to determine the effect of a drug on the developing fetus.
- Category X drugs should be avoided for all women likely to become pregnant, and, when possible, avoid category D drugs as well (or use the lowest possible dose).
- Women who require medication for their own health needs should be made aware that although the general rule is to avoid medications, drug therapies are beneficial to pregnancy outcome in some circumstances, and in those cases, the safest choice is to take the prescribed medication (Cefalo & Moos, 1995).

POSITIVE PHARMACOTHERAPEUTICS DURING THE PRECONCEPTION PERIOD

Vitamins and Minerals

Vitamins are not produced in the body and must be supplied by the diet. In the United States, it is rare to find women who have a vitamin deficiency because so many foods are enriched or fortified. A well-balanced diet can provide most of the nutrients for optimal maternal and fetal health, except for iron and folic acid. Several studies, including the Medical Research Council and the Budapest trial, have shown conclusively that a woman's risk for having a pregnancy affected by neural tube defects can be substantially reduced by taking folic acid periconceptually (Daly, Kirke, Molloy, Weir, & Scott, 1995). This research has prompted the Centers for Disease Control (CDC), the Committee on Genetics of the American Academy of Pediatrics, and the American College of Obstetricians and Gynecologists to recommend that all women of reproductive age take 0.4 mg of folic acid per day. The greatest benefit is if the woman takes the folic acid for at least one month prior to conception and during the first trimester (McCombs & Cramer, 1999).

Prenatal Vitamin

A prenatal vitamin is generally prescribed for all pregnant women. The dosage of vitamins in most prenatal supplements reflects the increased recommended daily allowance (RDA) for pregnancy (Cefalo & Moos, 1995). Each tablet should contain at least (Remich, 2004, p. 469):

30 mg of elemental iron
15 mg of zinc
2 mg of copper
250 mg of calcium (not as calcium phosphate)
2 mg of vitamin B_6
1.0 mg of folic acid
50 mg of vitamin C
200 I.U. of vitamin D
Administration: One tablet by mouth each day.
Side effects: Constipation, nausea, GI upset.
Client education: Take the tablet on an empty stomach with a drink that is high in vitamin C (avoid taking with coffee, tea, or milk)
FDA designation: Category A.

Iron Supplement

The recommended intake of elemental iron to prevent iron deficiency anemia (IDA) is 30 mg per day (the amount generally found in one prenatal vitamin). See Table 17–6. Treatment for IDA is one of the following orally (Wheeler, 2002, p. 234):

- 60 to 120 mg elemental iron daily, and a multivitamin and mineral supplement with 15 mg zinc, 2 mg copper, 250 mg or less calcium, 25 mg or less magnesium. Calcium and magnesium can interfere with iron absorption. Iron should be taken separately from the prenatal vitamin for best absorption.
- 200 mg elemental iron daily.
- 320 mg ferrous sulfate and 500 mg ascorbic acid one to three times daily.

Side effects: Constipation and nausea.

Client education: Take on an empty stomach with a drink high in vitamin C (avoid taking with coffee, tea, or milk). If nausea is present, a slow-release preparation with meals may decrease symptoms (Wheeler, 2002).

FDA designation: Category A

IMMUNIZATIONS DURING PREGNANCY AND LACTATION

The preconception period is the time to determine if all childhood immunizations have been given and to ensure that immunity has been conferred. Ideally, all immunizations should be completed well before three months prior to conception. However, administration of vaccines to women seeking prenatal care is an opportunity for preventive intervention (Glezen, 2001). Live-virus vaccines in pregnancy are contraindicated due to potential fetal risk, but termination of pregnancy is not usually indicated if the pregnant woman receives a live-virus vaccine by mistake or if she becomes pregnant in the first three months after vaccination (CDC Advisory Committee on Immunization Practices, 1998, p. 1). Counseling as to the risk is necessary if this happens. Inactivated vaccines, though not shown to be teratogenic in the first trimester, should not be given until the second trimester (Wells, DiPiro, Schwinghammer, & Hamilton, 2000). Table 17–7 summarizes immunization recommendations during pregnancy. In 1997, the Centers for Disease Control recommended that all women in their second and third trimesters of pregnancy be offered the influenza vaccine. Decisions about immunization during pregnancy require thoughtful consideration of the probable and potential severity of the disease for both mother and fetus, the significance of the exposure, the incubation period of the disease, the maternal immune status for the infection in question, the allergic history, and the availability of immunization agents, as well as the efficacy, toxicity, and side effects of such agents (Faix, 2002). The entire Advisory Committee on Immunization Practices (ACIP) report is available at the CDC's National Immunization Program Web site at *http://www.cdc.gov/nip*.

TABLE 17–6. Percentage of Elemental Iron in Common Iron Preparations

Preparation	Percentage of Elemental Iron (%)	Elemental Iron (mg)
Ferrous sulfate (325 mg)	20	60–65
Ferrous gluconate (325 mg)	12	37–39
Ferrous fumarate (100 mg)	33	100

Source: Sproat (1999).

RUBELLA

A resurgence of rubella infection occurred between 1988 and 1991, and the greatest incidence affected individuals over the age of 15 years (Cefalo & Moos, 1995). The major cause of this resurgence was the failure to immunize children. For this reason, a second measles-mumps-rubella (MMR) vaccine was added to the immunization schedule. Women of reproductive age are at risk for being nonimmune to rubella, and in fact, 6 to 11% remain seronegative for the rubella antibody (Remich, 1998). When a pregnant woman contracts this highly contagious disease, there is up to a 54% chance that the fetus will become infected if exposed before week 15 of pregnancy (Wheeler, 2002). Congenital rubella syndrome may lead to a wide variety of manifestations: intrauterine growth re-

TABLE 17–7. Summary of Immunization Recommendations During Pregnancy*

Immunization	Recommendation in Pregnancy
Tetanus-diptheria	Give in second and third trimesters
Rabies	Give anytime in pregnancy
Hepatitis B, oral polio (eIVP), influenza, pneumococcal	Give if indicated**
Measles, mumps, rubella, and varicella	Contraindicated in pregnancy
Hepatitis A	Safety in pregnancy not determined

*Note contraindications for any person receiving vaccines such as an allergy to eggs.

**Give influenza vaccine to those women who are nearing flu season or who are at risk for complications of influenza.

Sources: Bertino & Casto (1999); Wells, et al. (2000); Wheeler (2002).

tardation, cataracts, glaucoma, deafness, patent ductus, septal defects, CNS defects, anemia, TCP, hepatitis, and bone and chromosomal abnormalities (Wheeler, 2002). All women of reproductive age should have documented evidence of immunity to rubella. If a woman is seronegative prior to pregnancy, she should be given the rubella vaccine and counseled to wait three months before becoming pregnant. However, if a woman is found to be seronegative during prenatal testing, she should not be given the vaccine and should be cautioned to avoid anyone with a rash or viral illness (Gall, 2003; Remich, 2004).

HEPATITIS B VIRUS

Hepatitis B infection is a major cause of acute hepatitis and its more serious sequelae: chronic hepatitis, cirrhosis, and hepatocellular carcinoma (Cunningham et al., 1997). Transfer of the infection from the hepatitis B-positive mother to the fetus is thought to be by ingestion of infected material during delivery or exposure subsequent to birth. Transplacental transmission is uncommon. Of 18,000 infants born to mothers who test positive for hepatitis B, 4,000 will become chronically infected (Cunningham et al., 1997). Hepatitis B is transferred from mother to infant in 80 to 90% of cases in which the mother contracted the disease in the third trimester but will be transferred in only 10% of the cases when the virus is contracted during the first trimester (ACOG, 1998b). The infant whose mother is positive for hepatitis B surface antigen (HbsAG) is treated with the first dose of HBV vaccine within 12 hours after birth and hepatitis B immune globulin within 24 hours after birth (Wheeler, 2002). All women should be screened for hepatitis B during the prenatal period. Women at high risk for infection and a negative surface antigen should be counseled and vaccination strongly considered. Vaccination will protect them and their infants from the many acute and chronic complications of hepatitis B (Faix, 2002).

VARICELLA

Complications are serious for the fetus and the mother if she contracts varicella during pregnancy, including congenital varicella syndrome (eye and limb abnormalities, microcephaly), scarring of the skin, premature delivery, neonatal death from lack of immunity, or varicella pneumonia in the mother (Wheeler, 2002). If the delivery can be delayed for at least five to seven days after the mother first becomes ill, passive immunity is transferred. If not, the baby should be given varicella zoster immune globulin. Having had the disease confers immunity. As with other live-virus vaccines, pregnancy should be delayed until three months after receiving varicella immunization.

DRUG MANAGEMENT OF COMMON DISCOMFORTS IN PREGNANCY AND LACTATION

This section addresses the pharmacotherapeutic management of the discomforts that commonly accompany pregnancy. The more serious illnesses such as migraine headaches, pyelonephritis, or hyperemesis gravidarum are not addressed. Refer to other sources for discussions of more complicated illnesses during pregnancy, and for nonmedication management of common discomforts. The healthcare provider is encouraged to try conservative measures first where appropriate before resorting to the use of medications.

HEADACHE

Diagnosis

Tension headache is a frequent complaint during pregnancy. The pain often starts in the back of the neck and head and progresses to feeling a tight "rubberband" pressure around the head. The pain is often bilateral, dull, and steady. The headache may begin in the morning, but will usually worsen throughout the day. Photophobia and gastrointestinal distress are uncommon. Women with previously diagnosed migraine with aura may find that the frequency and intensity of headaches worsens with pregnancy. Others with menstrual or tension type headaches may experience improvement during the gestation (Unger, 2002).

Drug Management

Acetaminophen is the preferred medication for headache pain during pregnancy (Wheeler, 2002). There is no evidence of teratogenic effect. Aspirin and ibuprofen may increase the bleeding time and have undesired harmful effects on the pregnancy, especially during the third trimester (Wheeler, 2002). Women should be instructed to avoid aspirin and non-steroidal anti-inflammatory drugs (NSIADs) during pregnancy. They should be cautioned to read labels carefully because many over-the-counter combination medications may contain these ingredients (Tillett, Kostich, & Vandevusse, 2003). When over-the-counter measures fail to control pain in the pregnant woman, the use of prescription narcotics is sometimes employed. This use, of course, depends on the licensure and prescriptive authority of the healthcare provider and the severity of symptoms in the patient. Narcotics do cross the placental barrier and while no studies in humans have shown an association between narcotic use in the first trimester and structural birth defects, all narcotics can cause CNS suppression (Norton & Vargas, 2003). Prescription narcotics should be used on a limited basis and only in consultation with a physician. In regard to migraine headaches, limited experience and data are available regarding the use of serotonin receptor agonists, and pregnant women should be counseled that based on this lack of information, no clear risk has been established (Hansen & Yankowitz, 2002). The use of sumatriptan may be acceptable in select pregnant women (those who have a clear history of migraine headaches and a known positive response to sumatriptan, especially when other class B medications fail) (Wald & Walling, 2002). Acetaminophen is excreted into breast milk in small concentrations only and is considered compatible with breastfeeding (Briggs, Freeman, & Yaffe, 1994). Use of ibuprofen is associated with premature closure of the fetal ductus arteriosus and persistent pulmonary hypertension in the infant (Wheeler, 2002).

URINARY TRACT INFECTION

Pregnancy increases a woman's risk for developing urinary tract infections (UTIs). Several physiologic changes occur that promote these infections, including increased glomerular filtration rate and urinary volume, loss of ureteral tone leading to urinary stasis, and changes in the chemical composition of the urine (Cunningham et al., 1999).

Diagnosis

Asymptomatic bacteriuria is the most common urinary tract infection encountered during pregnancy, occurring in 2 to 7% of all pregnant women (Gilstrap & Ramin, 2001). It is defined as 100,000 organisms per ml of urine in a woman without symptoms. The significance of asymptomatic bacteriuria is that it can cause pyelonephritis and its possible association with preterm labor, low birth weight infants, PIH, and anemia (Cunningham et al., 1997; Wheeler, 2002). The majority of upper UTIs occur as a result of undiagnosed or untreated lower UTIs.

Acute cystitis affects 1 to 3% of pregnant women and is diagnosed when the urinalysis shows white cells and bacteria. Nitrites and red blood cells may also be present. Often, the client is symptomatic for dysuria, frequency, hesitancy, and urgency. *Escherichia coli* accounts for 80 to 90% of UTIs in obstetric clients. *Klebsiella, Enterobacter, Proteus, Enterococcus faecalis,* and group B streptococcus account for most of the rest of the cases (Lucas & Cunningham, 1993).

Drug Management

Clients with asymptomatic bacteriuria and acute cystitis are best treated with a short course of antibiotics: a three-day course of nitrofurantoin 100 mg twice a day is appropriate (ACOG, 1998a; Duff, 2002). Gilstrap and Ramin (2001) agree, noting that therapy should generally be given for three days for the initial infection with longer courses used only in the case of recurrent infection. Providers often err on the side of overtreatment in that a seven- to ten-day course of therapy is commonly given (Wheeler, 2002). Several authors recommend that ten- to fourteen-day treatment be reserved for recurrent infections only (Duff, 2002; Lucas & Cunningham, 1993; Vercaigne & Zhanel, 1994). Another medication alternative for recurrent infection would be the continuous use of 50 mg of nitrofurantoin at bedtime. With nitrofurantoin (a category B drug), use may be a concern with African American women with G6PD deficiency, though rare (Wheeler, 2002). Amoxicillin and ampicillin are not recommended, since 33% of organism-causing UTIs are resistent to them (ACOG, 1998a). While there have been some reports of problems with the use of nitrofurantoin and sulfonamides near term, these drugs have been widely used, and there have been no increased reports of fetal abnormalities. (Dasche & Gilstrap, 1997; Duff, 2002; Hodgman, 1994). See Table 17–8. The AAP recommends that exposure to sulfonamides via breast milk

TABLE 17–8. Medications for Urinary Tract Infections

Drug/Dosage	FDA Designation	AAP Category
Sulfisoxazole: 2 g, then 1 g qid	B	Compatible
Sulfamethoxazole-Trimethoprim DS: 800 mg then 160 mg bid	C	Compatible
Nitrofurantoin: 100 mg bid	B	Compatible
Ampicillin: 250 mg qid	B	No category[a]
Amoxicillin: 500 mg tid	B	Compatible
Cephalosporin (first): 250 mg qid	B	No category[a]

[a]Ampicillin and cephalexin are not assigned a category, but both are excreted into breast milk in low concentrations.

Sources: ACOG (1998b); Cunningham et al. (1997); Duff (1993); Gutierrez (1999); Reilly & Clemenson (1993).

should be avoided in the ill, stressed, or premature infant, and in infants with hyperbilirubinemia or G6PD deficiency (Murray & Seger, 1994).

NAUSEA AND VOMITING

Nausea and vomiting often represent the first signs of pregnancy, and usually resolve by 12 to 14 weeks gestation (McCombs & Cramer, 1999). Nausea and vomiting develop in approximately 40 to 80% of women in early pregnancy (Wheeler, 2002). Although the etiology of nausea and vomiting is unclear, high levels of circulating hormones have been implicated, along with upper gastrointestinal dysmotility, dietary, and emotional factors (Broussard & Richter, 1998). Hyperemesis gravidarum—pernicious vomiting of pregnancy—is a severe form of nausea and vomiting often associated with weight loss, ketonuria, electrolyte imbalance, and dehydration (Eliakim, Abulafia, & Sherer, 2000).

Drug Management

After ensuring that more serious conditions such as hyperemesis gravidarum have been ruled out, nonpharmacologic measures should be attempted first to alleviate the nausea and vomiting. If dietary and lifestyle changes have proven ineffective, initiation of the medications may hasten the resolution of the problem. Pharmacologic therapy should be reserved for women with persistent symptoms and should be used after discussion of the risks and benefits of the medication to be initiated (Broussard & Richter, 1998). The following drugs may be considered: vitamin B6 (pyridoxine) 10 to 25 mg tid or qid; or vitamin B6 with doxylamine 12.5 mg tid or qid. This is equivalent to one-half of a 25 mg Unisom Sleep tablet (Wheeler, 2002, p. 203). Other drugs (category B) that may be considered for more persistent symptoms are meclizine (Antivert), promethazine (Phenergan), diphenhydramine (Benadryl); dimenhydrinate (Dramamine), and metoclopramide (Reglan). While unfortunately expensive, ondasetron (Zofran) has proven to very effectively reduce the symptoms of nausea and vomiting when taken twice daily. Prochlorperzine (Compazine) is not recommended, but if nausea and vomiting persist, use may be necessary. Discuss with the physician.

INDIGESTION/HEARTBURN

Pregnancy causes relaxation of the lower esophageal sphincter and decreased peristalsis and motility. These changes in the GI tract often cause reflux indigestion and esophagitis in the pregnant woman. Dietary and lifestyle modifications are the cornerstone of treatment for indigestion and should be the first interventions recommended (elevation of the head of the bed, avoiding meals within three hours of going to sleep, avoiding large meals, and avoiding foods that are esophageal irritants) (Katz & Castell, 1998). If these suggestions are unsuccessful in relieving the indigestion, the following medications may be recommended.

Drug Management

Aluminum, magnesium, and calcium antacids are safe if taken in therapeutic doses in the second and third trimesters of pregnancies (Gutierrez, 1999). Calcium has a very short duration of action (McCombs & Cramer, 1999). Antacids may be considered a first-line therapy, keeping in mind that those containing sodium bicarbonate can lead to excessive edema and should be avoided (Cunningham et al., 1997). Antacids can also interfere with iron absorption. H2 receptor agonists have long been proven to reduce the symptoms of indigestion in the non-pregnant patient and may be used during pregnancy if other methods have failed. Hansen and Yankowitz (2002) found no evidence to associate the use of ranitadine and cimetidine with fetal malformations.

CONSTIPATION

The slowing of the GI tract in pregnancy, compounded by the addition of iron in the prenatal vitamin, often leads to constipation. The expanding uterus may also act as a mechanical obstacle to normal bowel evacuation. Forty percent of women complain of constipation at some time during pregnancy, with 20% doing so in the third trimester (Cunningham et al., 1997).

Drug Management

The first approach to treating constipation is to encourage a diet high in fiber and fluids. Exercise also increases peristalsis and can reduce the incidence of constipation. If dietary and lifestyle modifications are not effective, then the clinician may recommend bulk-forming laxatives, such as Metamucil, or stool-softening agents, such as docusate sodium (Colace). Harsh stimulant and osmotic laxatives and purgatives, such as castor oil, should be avoided (Gutierrez, 1999; Larimore & Petrie, 2000). Pregnant women should also avoid nonabsorbable oil preparations such as mineral oil because they may interfere with the absorption of lipid-soluble vitamins (Cunningham et al., 1997).

UPPER RESPIRATORY INFECTIONS AND ALLERGIC RHINITIS

Pregnancy does not predispose women to upper respiratory infections (URIs) or allergic rhinitis, but the symptoms of a URI may be exaggerated by the normal vascular congestion that often occurs during pregnancy. Gestational rhinitis affects 30% of pregnant women. Estrogen and progesterone have been linked to nasal mucosal swelling, cyclic changes in female nasal mucus, and increased activity of nasal mucosal glands (Schatz & Zeiger, 1997). URI symptoms may include rhinorrhea, rhinitis, cough, and sore throat. The challenge for the provider will be to determine whether the URI is viral or bacterial in origin, or if the symptoms may be associated with seasonal allergies.

Drug Management

Recommend conservative, nonpharmacologic measures first, but know which medications are safe for the patient to use (see Table 17–9). Although pseudoephedrine (Sudafed, Novafed, Drixoral, Afrin) is commonly used to alleviate symptoms of rhinitis, sinusitis, colds, and allergies, it acts by vasoconstriction and shrinking swollen membranes, thus care must be advised to the pregnant woman. Overuse topically (more than 3 to 5 days) can lead to rebound and increased congestion and dependence. It is best to suggest saline nose drops initially and save this type of remedy for worsening symptoms. Studies have revealed a potential for increased risk of gastroschisis associated with the use of pseudoephedrine to 2 to 6 in 10,000 births in women who used pseudoephedrine in the first trimester from 1 to 2 per 10,000 births in the general population (Schatz & Zeiger, 1997).

TABLE 17–9. Medications for URIs and Allergic Rhinitis

"Cold" Medications	FDA Designation	AAP Category
Pseudoephedrine	C	Compatible
Dextromethorphan	C	No known category
Guaifenesin	C	No known category
Allergic Rhinitis	**FDA Designation**	**AAP Category**
Loratadine	B	
Cetirizine	B	
Diphenhydramine	C	No category[a]
Chlopheniramine	B	No data available
Brompheniramine	C	Compatible
Cromolyn	B	No data available

[a]The drug manufacturer considers the drug to be contraindicated in breastfeeding because of the increased sensitivity of newborns or premature infants to antihistamines. Change drug name from Claritin to loratadine.

Werler, Sheehan, and Mitchell (2002) note that use of pseudoephedrine alone did not increase the risk, but the combination of pseudoephedrine with other drugs, such as acetaminophen, was associated with increased risk of small intestinal atresia as well as gastroschisis and small intestinal atresia. Women should be counseled about this potential risk and use of the medicines may be deferred during the first trimester. The best treatment for cough is increased intake of water, but dextromethorphan (an antitussive) and guaifenesin (an expectorant) may be used should the cough be refractive to fluids. Antihistamines, such as diphenhydramine, chlorpheniramine, and brompheniramine, are helpful in relieving allergy symptoms (rhinorrhea, itchy and watery eyes, postnasal drip). Neither the Collaborative Perinatal Project nor the Boston Collaborative Drug Surveillance Program identified any significant difference in frequency of congenital anomalies among children of mothers who took any of these "cold" medicines (Murray & Seger, 1994). Newer, nonsedating antihistamines, such as loratadine and cetirizine, are considered to be safe during pregnancy and lactation and may be used to treat the symptoms of allergic rhinitis (Larimore & Petrie, 2000). The use of first- and second-generation antihistamines is not advised in the first trimester (Montauk & Rheinstein, 2002). Fexofenadine is a category C drug and needs more testing before use in pregnancy. Intranasal cromolyn or beclomethasone may be better for chronic symptoms (Schatz & Zeiger, 1997). These drugs are not recommended for use in the treatment of URIs.

ANTIBIOTIC USE DURING PREGNANCY AND LACTATION

Infection is the most common problem in pregnancy, and healthcare providers are often called upon to use antibiotics to treat UTIs, vaginitis, STDs, and URIs. It is imperative that the provider have a thorough knowledge of antibiotic therapy as all antibacterials cross the placenta in varying degrees. Maternal physiologic changes alter the pharmacodynamics of antibiotics with the increases in blood volume and creatinine clearance typically leading to lower serum concentrations. Antibiotics passively diffuse into breast milk. The ingestion of antibiotics through breast milk is generally considered to have neither a beneficial nor a harmful effect on the infant (Edwards, 1997). Of greatest concern during lactation is that antibiotics can modify the gastrointestinal flora of the nursing infant and can lead to diarrhea or other GI upset (Dillon et al., 1997).

Breastfeeding does not usually need to be interrupted when maternal antimicrobials are prescribed, but the provider should refer to current guidelines when in doubt.

PHARYNGITIS/SINUSITIS/ OTITIS MEDIA

Should the URI symptoms lead to diagnosis of a bacterial infection, the appropriate antibiotic must be selected. Knowing the latest recommendations for diagnosing and treating bacterial infections is mandatory. For the pregnant woman, the antibiotic must also be effective against the maternal infection and cause no harm to the developing fetus.

Drug Management

In general, it is safe to prescribe penicillins and cephalosporins during pregnancy, turning to erythromycin as an alternative when an allergy to penicillin or cephalosporin exists (see Table 17–10) (Edwards, 1997). No reports of animal or human teratogenicity have been associated with the use of penicillins or cephalosporins. The same is true of erythromycin. The drugs are excreted into breast milk in low concentrations, and there have been no reports of adverse effects in the nursing infant (Dillon et al., 1997). *Tetracyclines should never be used during pregnancy.* Taken after the fourth month in pregnancy, tetracycline can cause deciduous teeth to be stained and use in pregnancy is associated with a toxic hepatic response (Gutierrez, 1999). Fluoroquinolones are not recommended in pregnancy, lactation, or with persons under age 18 years (Gutierrez, 1999).

TABLE 17–10. Medications for Bacterial Infections

Infection	Antibiotic	FDA Designation	AAP Category
Pharyngitis	Penicillin V	B	Compatible
	Amoxicillin	B	No category[a]
	Erythromycin	B	Compatible
Sinusitis or otitis media	Ampicillin	B	No category[a]
	Amoxicillin	B	No category[a]
	Bactrim	C	Compatible
	Cefuroxime	B	No category[a]
Otitis media	(Same as listed for sinusitis)		

[a]These antibiotics are excreted into the breast milk in low concentrations; adverse effects are rare, but three potential problems exist for the nursing infant: modification of bowel flora, direct effects on the infant (allergic response/sensitization), and interference with interpretation of culture results (Briggs, Freeman, & Yaffe, 1998).

VAGINITIS

Vaginal infections are a common complaint during pregnancy. The most frequent infections are bacterial vaginosis (BV), *Trichomonas vaginalis,* and vulvovaginal candidiasis (VVC).

Bacterial Vaginosis

BV is responsible for 40 to 50% of vaginal infections and has been associated with preterm delivery, premature rupture of membranes, intraamnionic infection, and postpartum infection. (Hanson, 2002). Benefits of therapy include reducing the risk for infectious complications associated with BV, reducing the risk for other STDs, and possible reduction in the risk for preterm delivery in the high-risk woman (Morbidity and Mortality Weekly Report, 2002). BV results from an overgrowth of anaerobic bacteria. Clients may complain of vaginal discharge, odor, and mild lower abdominal discomfort, or they may be asymptomatic. The presence of homogeneous discharge, vaginal pH of greater than 4.5, positive amine "whiff" test, and clue cells support the diagnosis of BV.

Drug Management. Metronidazole (250 mg PO tid for 7 days) is the treatment of choice for BV in the pregnant woman. No consistent association between metronidazole use during pregnancy and teratogenic or mutagenic effects in newborns has been demonstrated with numerous studies and meta-analyses (MMWR, 2002). The CDC provides no recommendation in the new 2002 guidelines regarding waiting until the second trimester to use metronidazole. Screening and treatment of high-risk women for preterm birth is advised for the initial prenatal visit. Another treatment option is Clindamycin 300 mg PO bid for 7 days. The use of topical agents during pregnancy is not supported by available research (MMWR, 2002). Partners do not need to be treated. The American Academy of Pediatrics recommends using metronidazole with caution during lactation (see Table 17–11).

Trichomonas Vaginalis

About 15 to 20% of symptomatic vaginitis is caused by *Trichomonas vaginalis* (Hanson, 2002). *Trichomonas* has been found in 20% of women during prenatal examinations and is associated with an increased incidence of premature rupture of membranes, preterm delivery, and low birthweight (MMWR, 2002). Women complain of yellow-green, foul-smelling, frothy discharge, and not uncommonly, of intermittent vaginal spotting and dyspareunia. Some women have few or no symptoms. The

TABLE 17–11. Medications for Vaginitis

Drug	FDA Designation	AAP Category
Bacterial Vaginitis		
Metronidazole 250 mg PO tid × 7d	B	Use with caution
Clindamycin 300 mg PO bid × 7d	B	Compatible
Trichomonas Vaginalis		
Metronidazole 2 gm single dose	B	Discontinue drug for 12 to 24 hours to allow for drug excretion
Vulvovaginal Candidiasis[a]		
Miconazole topical × 7d	C[b]	No data available
Clotrimazole topical × 7d	B	No data available
Butoconazole topical × 7d	C[b]	No data available
Terconazole topical × 7d	C[b]	No data available

[a]Only topical azole creams are recommended by the CDC (MMWR, 2002).
[b]Used topically, no association has been found between this drug and congenital malformations (Briggs, Freeman, & Yaffe, 1998).

diagnosis is made by the identification of motile trichomonads on microscopy, although they may only be identified 60 to 70% of the time. The most sensitive method for diagnosis is culture, but cost is a factor.

Drug Management. Metronidazole is the only trichomonacidal drug available in the United States, and it is quite effective in eradicating *T. vaginalis* (MMWR, 2002). Initial treatment should be a single dose of 2 g for both partners, with a 7-day course of 500 mg bid initiated if first treatment is unsuccessful. Please refer to the discussion regarding metronidazole use during pregnancy in the Bacterial Vaginasli section.

Vulvovaginal Candidiasis

VVC accounts for 20 to 30% of vaginal infections in pregnant women. The *Candida* species are considered to be part of the normal vaginal flora, and symptoms of infection are thought to develop when an overgrowth of these organisms occurs (Duff, 1993). *Candida albicans* accounts for 85 to 90% of the cases (Hanson, 2002). Symptoms include vaginal and vulvar pruritis and irritation and a white, curd-like discharge. The wet mount reveals hyphae, pseudohyphae, and/or budding yeast. *C. glabrata* only presents with budding yeast (Hanson, 2002).

Drug Management. Oral agents, designated as category C, are not recommended in pregnancy. Only topical azole therapies for 7 days are recommended for use among pregnant women (MMWR, 2002). Table 17–11 lists several topical agents of proven value in the treatment of VVC. Candidiasis is not considered to be sexually transmitted, therefore the partner does not need to be treated, although this may be considered if repeated episodes occur.

SEXUALLY TRANSMITTED DISEASES

Sexually transmitted diseases (STDs), of which there are many, are common during pregnancy. Some STDs are uncomplicated and easily treated; others are associated with preterm labor, premature rupture of membranes, chorioamnionitis, and postpartum endometritis. Potential infections in the neonate include sepsis, conjunctivitis, and pneumonitis. Risk factors for STDs include low socioeconomic status, urban status, multiple sexual partners, illicit drug use, and youth. Since it is neither possible nor appropriate to assume which women will have STDs, all pregnant women should be asked about STDs, counseled about the possibility of perinatal infections, and ensured access to treatment as needed (MMWR, 2002). Recommended prenatal screening should include testing for gonorrhea, chlamydia, hepatitis B, syphilis, HIV, and hepatitis C for the high-risk woman. All women should be counseled and a consent form signed prior to being tested for HIV. It is recommended that the most current copy of the *CDC Treatment Guidelines* for STDs be available. For a more in-depth discussion of STDs, refer to Chapter 36. Table 17–12 provides medication managment for uncomplicated STDs in pregnancy. More complex disorders should be managed in consultation with, or referred to, an obstetrician or infectious disease specialist.

DEPRESSION

Women may seek consultation regarding antidepressant use prior to pregnancy, but more often than not, they present for the initial prenatal appointment having discontinued medications that have been prescribed for mental health reasons. Pregnancy can cause women to experience a worsening of their symptoms of depression and can in fact cause some women to experience a new onset of symptoms. Considering the negative sequelae of depression during pregnancy, many providers are continuing to prescribe antidepressants to their pregnant clients. While more studies are needed, and long-term data is not available, the selective serotonin reuptake inhibitors (SSRIs) do not seem to increase the risk for congenital malformations (Larimore & Petrie, 2000). Hansen and Yankowitz (2002) and Niebyl and Kochenour (1999) agree and note that sertraline, paroxetine, and fluoxetine

TABLE 17–12. Medications for Uncomplicated STDs in Pregnancy

STD	Drug	FDA Designation	AAP Category
Gonorrhea	Ceftriaxone 125 mg IM[a]	B	Compatible
	plus		
	Azithromycin 1g PO single dose	B	Compatible
Chlamydia	Erythromycin 500 mg qid × 7d[b]	B	Compatible
	OR		
	Amoxicillin 500 mg tid × 7d	B	Compatible
	OR		
	Azithromycin 1g PO single dose	B	Compatible
Syphilis (primary, secondary, and early latent of less than 1 year's duration)	Penicillin G[c] benzathine 2.4 million u IM × 1	B	No category
Syphilis (late latent)	Penicillin G benzathine 7.2 million u divided in three doses of 2.4 million u IM, at 1-week intervals	B	No category
HPV (human papillomavirus)	Cryotherapy with trichloracetic acid (TCA) 80–90%; repeat weekly if necessary up to 3–4 weeks, then refer.	N/A	N/A
	• Lesions have a tendency to proliferate during pregnancy		
	• Podophyllin, imiquimod, podofilox are contraindicated during pregnancy		
HSV (herpes simplex virus)	Acyclovir[d]	B	
Pediculosis pubis	Permethrin 1% lotion applied to affected areas and washed off after 10 min or pyrethrins with piperonyl butoxide applied to affected areas and washed off after 10 min; repeat 1 week as needed; *lindane should not be used*	B	
Scabies	Permethrin 5% lotion applied to all areas of the body from the neck down; wash off after 8–14 h; *lindane should not be used*	B	

[a]Cephalosporin-intolerant women should be treated with one dose of spectinomycin 2 gm IM.
[b]Amoxicillin 500 mg tid × 7 days may be used if erythromycin cannot be tolerated.
[c]Women who are allergic to penicillin should be treated with penicillin after desensitization, as there are no proven alternatives. Referral to an obstetrican for desensitization is indicated.
[d]The safety of acyclovir, pamciclovir, and valacyclovir in pregnancy has not been established. See the current CDC Treatment Guidelines for a discussion of use in pregnancy.

Source: Morbidity and Mortality Weekly Report (2002).

do not appear to be associated with teratogenic effect. Some studies do suggest that SSRI use is associated with earlier delivery and consequent lower birth rate (Simon, Cunningham, & Davis, 2002). In that depression has also been linked to lower birth weight and preterm delivery, ob/gyn healthcare providers must weigh the risk of medication use against the high risk of relapse that occurs when pregnant women with mental health disorders discontinue medications. Gjere (2001) recommends that non-pharmacologic treatments be utilized initially if depression is not severe (light therapy, cognitive behavioral therapy, psychotherapy and nutrition). Collaboration with a mental health therapist, while ideally established prior to pregnancy, should be initiated and continued through the gestation.

While experience with lactation is limited, these drugs appear in low concentrations in milk after maternal ingestion. The American Academy of Pediatricians has placed these drugs in the category of Effects Unknown But May Be of Concern (Committee on Drugs, 2001). Consultation with an obstetrician is indicated when deciding to use SSRIs or other medications used to treat mental health disorders.

REFERENCES

Akridge, K. M. (2004). Postpartum and lactation. In E. Q. Youngkin & M. S. Davis (Eds.), *Women's health: A primary care clinical guide* (3rd ed.; pp. 613–676). Upper Saddle River, NJ: Prentice Hall.

Altshuler, L. & Yonkers, K. (2004). What ob/gyns need to know about drug therapy in bipolar gravidas. *OBG Management, 16*(1), 27–38.

American Academy of Pediatrics Committee on Drugs. (1994). The transfer of drugs and other chemicals into human milk. *Pediatrics, 93*(1), 137–150.

American College of Obstetricians and Gynecologists. (1998a). *Antimicrobial therapy for obstetric patients* (ACOG Education Bulletin No. 245). Washington, DC: Author.

American College of Obstetricians and Gynecologists. (1998b). *Viral hepatitis in pregnancy* (ACOG Education Bulletin No. 248). Washington, DC: Author.

Baer, C. L., & Williams, B. R. (1996). *Clinical pharmacology and nursing.* Springhouse, PA: Springhouse.

Barron, W. M., Lindheimer, M. D., & Davison, J. M. (Eds.). (2000). *Medical disorders in pregnancy* (3rd ed.). St. Louis: Mosby–Year Book.

Bertino, J. S., & Casto, D. T. (1999). Vaccines, toxoids, and other immunologies. In J. T. Dipiro, R. L. Talbert, G. C. Yee, G. R. Matzke, et al. (Eds.), *Pharmacotherapy: A pathophysiologic approach* (4th ed.). Stamford, CT: Appleton & Lange.

Briggs, G. G., Freeman, R. K., & Yaffe, S. J. (1998). Drugs in pregnancy and lactation (5th ed.). Philadelphia: Lippincott Williams & Wilkins.

Broussard, C. N., & Richter, J. E. (1998). Nausea and vomiting of pregnancy. *Gastroenterology Clinics of North America, 27*(1), 123–151.

Cefalo, R. C., & Moos, M. K. (1995). *Preconceptional health care: A practical guide.* St. Louis: Mosby–Year Book.

Centers for Disease Control and Prevention (CDC) Advisory Committee on Immunization Practices. (1998). In L. Wheeler, *Nurse-midwifery handbook: A practical guide to prenatal and postpartum care.* Philadelphia, PA: Lippincott Williams-Wilkins.

Cohen, M. S. (1992). Special aspects of perinatal and pediatric pharmacology. In B. G. Katzung (Ed.), *Basic and clinical pharmacology* (pp. 853–861). Norwalk, CT: Appleton & Lange.

Cohen, L. S., & Keith, L. G. (1994). Drug abuse in pregnancy. In F. P. Zuspan & E. J. Quilligan (Eds.), *Current therapy in obstetrics and gynecology* (pp. 241–242). Philadelphia: W. B. Saunders.

Committee on Drugs. (2001). The transfer of drugs and other chemicals into human milk. *Pediatrics, 108*(3), 776–789.

Cruikshank, D. P., Wigton, T. R., & Hays, P. M. (1996). Maternal physiology in pregnancy. In S. G. Gabbe, J. R. Niebyl, & J. L. Simpson (Eds.), *Obstetrics: Normal and problem pregnancies* (pp. 91–110). New York: Churchill Livingstone.

Cunningham, F. G., MacDonald, P. C., Gant, N. F., Leveno, K. J., Gilstrap, L. C., Hankins, G. D. V., & Clark, S. L. (1997). *Williams obstetrics* (19th ed.). Stamford, CT: Appleton & Lange.

Daly, L. E., Kirke, P. N., Molloy, A., Weir, D. G., & Scott, J. M. (1995). Folate levels and neural tube defects. *The Journal of the American Medical Association, 274*(21), 1698–1702.

Dasche, J. S., & Gilstrap, L. C. (1997). Antibiotic use in pregnancy. *Obstetrics and Gynecology Clinics of North America, 24*(3), 617–629.

Dillon, A. E., Wagner, C. L., Wiest, D., & Newman, R. B. (1997). Drug therapy in the nursing mother. *Obstetrics and Gynecology Clinics of North America, 24*(3), 675–694.

Duff, P. (1993). Antibiotic selection for infections in obstetric patients. *Seminars in Perinatology, 17*(6), 367–378.

Duff, P. (1996). Maternal and perinatal infections. In S. G. Gabbe, J. R. Niebyl, & J. L. Simpson (Eds.), *Obstetrics: Normal and problem pregnancies* (pp. 1193–1246). New York: Churchill Livingstone.

Duff, P. (2002). Antibiotic selection in obstetrics: Making cost-effective choices. *Clinical Obstetrics and Gynecology, 45*(1), 59–72.

Edwards, M. S. (1997). Antibacterial therapy in pregnancy and neonates. *Clinics in Perinatology, 25*(1), 251–266.

Eisenstat, S. A., & Carlson, K. J. (1995). Use of medication in pregnancy and lactation. In K. J. Carlson & S. A. Eisenstat (Eds.), *Primary care of women.* St. Louis, MO: Mosby.

Eliakim, R., Abulafa, O., & Sherer, D. M. (2000). Hyperemesis gravidarum: A current review. *American Journal of Perinatology, 17*(4), 207–218.

Faix, R. G. (2002). Immunization during pregnancy. *Clinical Obstetrics and Gynecology, 45*(1), 42–58.

Forney, S. L. (1996). Drug therapy in childbearing and breastfeeding clients. In N. L. Pinnell (Ed.), *Nursing pharmacology* (pp. 100–109). Philadelphia: W. B. Saunders.

Gall, S. A. (2003). A realistic vaccination program for all patients, including gravidas. *OBG Management, 15*(12), 37–47.

Gilstrap, L. C., & Ramin, S. M. (2001). Urinary tract infections during pregnancy. *Obstetrics and Gynecology Clinics of North America, 28*(3), 581–591.

Gjere, N. A. (2001). Psychopharmacology in pregnancy. *Journal of Perinatal and Neonatal Nursing, 14*(4), 12–25.

Glezen, W. P. (2001). Maternal vaccines. *Primary Clinics in Office Practice, 28*(4), 791–806.

Gutierrez, K. (1999). *Pharmacotherapeutics: Clinical decision-making in nursing.* Philadelphia: W.B. Saunders Co.

Hacker, N. F., & Moore, J. G. (1998). *Essentials of obstetrics and gynecology* (3rd ed.). Philadelphia: W. B. Saunders Co.

Hanson, V. (2002, June 25). *It's a bug's life.* Presentation at the AWHONN 2002 Convention, Boston, MA.

Hansen, W. F., & Yankowitz, J. (2002). Pharmacologic therapy for medical disorders during pregnancy. *Clinical Obstetrics and Gynecology, 45*(1), 136–152.

Hedstrom, S., & Martens, M. G. (1993). Antibiotics in pregnancy. *Clinical Obstetrics and Gynecology, 36*(4), 886–892.

Ito, S. (2000). Drug therapy for breastfeeding women. *New England Journal of Medicine, 343*(2), 118–127.

Jack, B. W., & Culpepper, L. (1991). Preconception care. *Journal of Family Practice, 32*(3), 306–313.

Jellin, J. M., Gregory, P., Batz, F., Hitchens, K., et al. (2000). *Pharmacist's Letter/Prescriber's Letter natural medicines comprehensive database* (3rd ed.). Stockton, CA: Therapeutic Research Faculty.

Katz, P. O., & Castell, D. O. (1998). Gastroesophageal reflux disease during pregnancy. *Gastroenterology Clinics of North America, 27*(1), 153–167.

Kochenour, N. (1994). Medications in early pregnancy. In J. T. Queenan (Ed.), *Management of high-risk pregnancy* (4th ed.; pp. 36–42). Boston: Blackwell Scientific.

Kuczkowski, K. M. (2003). Tobacco and ethanol use in pregnancy: Implications for obstetric and anesthetic management. *The Female Patient, 28*(4), 16–22.

Larimore, W. L., & Petrie, K. A. (2000). Drug use during pregnancy and lactation. *Primary Care, 27*(1), 35–53.

Little, B. B., & Gilstrap, L. C. (1998). Human teratology principles. In L.C. Gilstrap & B. B. Little (Eds.), *Drugs and pregnancy* (2nd ed.; pp. 7–24). New York: Chapman & Hall.

Loebstein, R., Lalkin, A., & Koren, G. (2001). Pharmacokinetic changes during pregnancy and their clinical relevance. In G. Koren (Ed.), *Maternal-fetal toxicology: A clinician's guide* (3rd ed.; pp.1–21). New York: Marcel Dekker.

Lucas, M. J., & Cunningham, F. G. (1993). Urinary infection in pregnancy. *Clinical Obstetrics and Gynecology, 36*(4), 855–867.

McCombs, J., & Cramer, M. (1999). Pregnancy and lactation: Therapeutic concerns. In J. T. Dipiro, R. L. Talbert, G. C. Yee, G. R. Matzke, et al. (Eds.), *Pharmacotherapy: A pathophysiologic approach* (4th ed.). Stamford, CT: Appleton & Lange.

Montauk, S. L., & Rheinstein, P. H. (2002). Appropriate use of common OTC analgesics and cough and cold medications. An *American Family Physician* mongraph.

Morbidity and Mortality Weekly Report (MMWR). (2002, May 10). *2002 Guidelines for treatment of sexually transmitted diseases, 51*(No. RR-6), Atlanta, GA: U.S. Department of Health and Human Services, PHS, Centers for Disease Control and Prevention.

Murray, L., & Seger, D. (1994). Drug therapy during pregnancy and lactation. *Emergency Medicine Clinics of North America, 12*(1), 129–149.

Niebyl, J. R., & Kochenour, N. K. (1999). Medications in pregnancy and lactation. In J. T. Queenan (Ed.), *Management of high risk pregnancy* (pp. 43–51). Oxford, UK and Malden, MA: Blackwell Science.

Norton, M. E. & Vargas, J. E. (2003). When a pregnant patient needs analgesics. *Contemporary OB/GYN, 48*(12), 37–51.

O'Dea, R. F. (1992). Medication use in the breastfeeding mother. *NAACOG's Clinical Issues, 3*(4), 598–604.

Reeder, S. J., Martin, L. L., & Koniak-Griffin, D. (1997). *Maternity nursing: Family, newborn, and women's health care.* Philadelphia: Lippincott.

Reilly, K., & Clemenson, N. (1993). Infections complicating pregnancy. *Primary Care, 20*(3), 665–684.

Remich, M. (2004). Promoting a healthy pregnancy. In E. Q. Youngkin & M. S. Davis (Eds.), *Women's health: A primary care clinical guide* (3rd ed.; pp. 461–504). Upper Saddle River, NJ: Pearson/Prentice Hall.

Schatz, M., & Zeiger, R.S. (1997). Asthma and allergy in pregnancy. *Clinics in Perinatology, 24*(2), 407–432.

Sever, L. E., & Mortensen, M. E. (1996). Teratology and the epidemiology of birth defects: Occupational and environmental perspectives. In S. G. Gabbe, J. R. Niebyl, & J. L. Simpson (Eds.), *Obstetrics: Normal and problem pregnancies* (pp. 185–213). New York: Churchill Livingstone.

Sherwin, L. N., Scoloveno, M. A., & Weingarten, C. T. (1995). *Nursing care of the childbearing family.* Norwalk, CT: Appleton & Lange.

Silberstein, S. D. (1993). Headaches and women: Treatment of the pregnant and lactating migraineur. *Headache, 33,* 533–540.

Simon, G. E, Cunningham, M. L, & Davis, R. L. (2002). Outcomes of prenatal antidepressant exposure. *American Journal of Psychiatry,* 159:2055–2061.

Sokol, R. J., & Martier, S. (1996). High risk pregnancy: Alcohol. *Contemporary OB/GYN, 12,* 19–23.

Sproat, T. T. (1999). Anemias. In J. T. Dipiro, R. L. Talbert, G. C. Yee, G. R. Matzke, et al. (Eds.), *Pharmacotherapy: A pathophysiologic approach* (4th ed.). Stamford, CT: Appleton & Lange.

Tillett, J., Kostich, L. M., & VandeVusse, L. (2003). Use of over-the-counter medications during pregnancy. *Journal of Perinatal and Neonatal Nursing, 17*(1), 3–18.

Unger, J. (2002). Headache disorders in women. *Women's Health, 2*(7), 395–403.

Vercaigne, L. M., & Zhanel, G. G. (1994). Recommended treatment for urinary tract infection in pregnancy. *Annals of Pharmacotherapy, 28,* 248–250.

Wells, B. G., DiPiro, J. T., Schwinghammer, T. L., & Hamilton, C. (2000). *Pharmacotherapy handbook* (2nd ed.). Stamford, CT: Appleton & Lange.

Wendel, P. J., & Wendel, Jr., G. D. (1993). Sexually transmitted diseases in pregnancy. *Seminars in Perinatology, 17*(6), 443–451.

Werler, M. M., Sheehan, J. E., & Mitchell, A. A. (2002). Maternal medication use and risks of gastroschisis and small intestinal atresia. *American Journal of Epidemiology, 155*(1), 26–31.

Wheeler, L. (2002). *Nurse-midwifery handbook: A practical guide to prenatal and postpartum care.* Philadelphia: Lippincott Williams-Wilkins.

Yaffe, S. J. & Briggs, G. G. (2003). "Is this drug going to hurt my baby?" *Contemporary OB/GYN, 48(1)*57–68.

Yeong, K. L. C. (2004). Assessing health during pregnancy. In E. Q. Youngkin & M. S. Davis (Eds.), *Women's health: A primary care clinical guide* (3rd ed.; pp. 427–459). Upper Saddle River, NJ: Pearson/Prentice Hall.

CHAPTER ❖ 18

CONTRACEPTIVES

Catherine Berardelli

This chapter, which explores the full spectrum of contraceptive alternatives available to patients today, would have been otherwise impossible to write had it not been for the undaunting activist work of women such as Margaret Sanger (Caufield, 2003; Lynaugh, 1991). A women's rights activist, pioneer in family planning, and a nurse (Yasunari, 2000), Sanger braved governmental condemnation and imprisonment in order to answer the pleas of women in her care to "Please tell me the secret. . ." (Lynaugh, 1991, p. 124) of preventing unwanted pregnancies. It was Margaret Sanger who, among other contributions, introduced the diaphragm in the United States and fought for women's reproductive rights through her early work in the family planning movement. It is our hope that this chapter will assist clinicians in providing thoughtful, sensitive, thorough information to patients, enabling them to be informed decision makers about their own reproductive health.

Contraception, or fertility control, has been defined as the deliberate management of conception or childbirth. This control and management may be achieved using a variety of devices, chemicals, surgical procedures, fertility awareness methods, and postcoital methods. Thus, choosing a contraceptive method is an important decision involving the ability to anticipate and plan for the occurrence of sexual intercourse. It has been reported, however, that "Nearly half (48%) of the 6 million pregnancies that occur each year in the US are unintended" (FDA approval of mifepristone, 2000, p. 4), suggesting that planning has either been ineffective or nonexistent. Norris (1988, p. 135) has suggested that one's "ability to anticipate and prepare for intercourse is contingent on the ability to think about sexual intercourse, contraception, and the negative impact on one's life of an unplanned pregnancy." This notion has important implications for clinicians in practice, especially as it relates to patient education. The clinician's mission is to assist patients in choosing contraceptive methods best fitting their personal lifestyles while taking into consideration the feelings and attitudes of the patient and the patient's partner. To that end, this chapter will discuss all currently available forms of contraception and also provide information about methods on the horizon. A compilation of perfect use and typical use failure rates from various contraceptive methods is provided in Table 18–1.

FACTORS AFFECTING REPRODUCTIVE CHOICE

The reproductive life span of a woman may encompass forty or more years, and for men the production of sperm is continuous throughout life. Therefore, it is natural to expect that a variety of contraceptive methods may be used. As family planning needs change, it is necessary for sexual partners to acquire accurate information about the factors that may affect their contraceptive needs in order to more accurately reevaluate their pregnancy prevention choices.

TABLE 18–1. Percentage of Accidental Pregnancy During First Year of Use Associated with Contraception Methods

Method	Perfect Use Failure Rate %	Typical Use Failure Rate %
No method	85	85
Withdrawal	4	19
Periodic abstinence		25
Spermicide alone	6	26
Cervical cap with spermicide	9	20
Diaphragm with spermicide	6	20
Condom:		
Male	3	14
Female	5	21
IUD:		
Progestasert	1.5	2
ProGard Copper T	0.6	0.8
LNg20	0.1	0.1
Oral contraceptives:		
Combined	0.1	5
Progestin only	0.5	5
Depo-Provera	0.3	0.3
Lunelle		0.1
Norplant & Norplant-2	0.05	0.05
Transdermal contraceptive patch	0.4	0.7
NuvaRing		0.65
Female sterilization	0.4	0.4
Male sterlization	0.1	0.15

Sources: Hatcher, Nelson, Zieman, et al. (2001); Hatcher, Trussell, Stewart, et al. (1998); Kubba, Guillebaud, Anderson & MacGregor (2000); Likis (2002).

Caufield (2003) enumerates a number of factors influencing the selection of birth control methods. These factors, listed in Table 18–2, mandate the existence of a true collaborative effort between the patient and healthcare provider to determine the method that best fits into the tapestry of people's reproductive lives.

SEXUAL HISTORY TAKING

Developing the skills necessary to complete a thorough sexual history enhances the clinician's ability to effectively counsel patients regarding their choice of contraceptive method. Sexual history taking is a skill requiring the clinician to become comfortable with sexual language, including the straightforward jargon with which the patient may be more familiar (Alexander, 1996; Nusbaum & Hamilton, 2002). In addition, clinicians need to be skilled in a wide variety of therapeutic communication techniques to facilitate information gathering. The single most important therapeutic communication technique at the clinician's disposal is that of attentive, active listening.

TABLE 18–2. Factors Influencing Selection of Birth Control Methods

Age and maturity	Stage of reproductive life
Relationship status	Health history
Cultural and religious beliefs	Presence of physical/mental limitation
Motivation/degree of cooperation	Individual locus of control
Comfort with one's own body	Monogamous versus multiple sexual partners
Cost and effectiveness of method	Method characteristics
Previous method experience	Noncontraceptive benefits
Frequency of intercourse	Access to healthcare

Source: Caufield (2003).

Empowering the patient to provide information that may feel embarrassing and uncomfortable to them requires a private place for taking a sexual history. This is essential so that the sharing of intimate information can be done in relative comfort and safety. In addition, a warm greeting and a genuinely respectful attitude will help initiate rapport at the outset of the interview. It also is important that the patient be fully aware of the nature of the interview, the type of information being requested, and the purpose for which the information is being obtained. Table 18–3 includes a listing of skills and techniques that often help in gathering sensitive information from patients.

SEXUALLY TRANSMITTED DISEASE RISK RELATED TO CONTRACEPTIVE CHOICES

Both men and women bear responsibility for making contraceptive decisions and seeking birth control methods reflecting their reproductive needs. Consideration must also be given to how effective each method is in preventing sexually transmitted diseases (STDs). As part of the clinician's sexual history taking, and within the context of contraceptive decision making, a full assessment regarding the patient's risk of contracting STDs should be conducted.

TABLE 18–3. Techniques in Sensitive Information Gathering

- Patient modesty and privacy is of paramount importance
- Assure patient confidentiality
- Clearly state what information can and cannot be held in confidence
- Develop attentive listening skills
- Ask questions in nonjudgmental manner
- Ask questions about specific behaviors instead of lifestyle issues
- Never assume sexual orientation
- Use open-ended questions
- Allow time, including periods of silence, for patients to elaborate
- Pay attention to verbal and nonverbal cues
- Never prejudge

Sources: Adapted from Alexander (1996), Caufield (2003) & Nusbaum & Hamilton (2002).

Even though abstinence is the one best method for both preventing pregnancy and STDs, it is simply not a viable contraceptive alternative for many. Therefore, when counseling a patient about contraception, it is important to discuss disease transmission and risk reduction strategies as well. O'Connell (1996, p. 476) states, "[A woman] has a much higher risk of contracting an infection than of becoming pregnant. Even on the day a woman's risk of pregnancy is highest, the day before ovulation, the risk of contracting gonorrhea from an infected man is four times greater than the risk of pregnancy." Youngkin (1995, p. 743) poignantly notes that "sexually transmitted diseases are like a huge runaway train" with an estimated 15 million new STD cases occurring yearly in the United States (Finer, Darroch, & Singh, 1999). Thus, in addition to discussing the effectiveness in preventing pregnancy and the safety, cost, and convenience of a particular contraceptive method, clinicians must also discuss the method's protection effectiveness against contracting STDs.

BARRIER METHODS

Barrier methods have been providing a mechanical barricade to advancing sperm since the seventeenth century (Hatcher et al., 1998), and they provide effective protection from pregnancy and STDs if they are used correctly and consistently. These methods include male and female condoms, diaphragms, cervical caps, vaginal sponges, and spermicides, including vaginal contraceptive films. The mechanism of action, effectiveness, advantages, disadvantages, and patient education requirements of each are discussed below.

MALE CONDOMS

Historians have identified several uses for the condom throughout history (Himes, 1963). Egyptian men in 1350 B.C. are said to have worn them as decorative covers for their penises, and in the 1560s Fallopius, an Italian anatomist, described a protective linen sheath used to cover the penis during intercourse. However, it was not until the 1700s when penile sheaths made from animal intestines were given the name *condom* and were used to protect men from STDs and to prevent pregnancy (Frezieres & Walsh, 2000).

Condoms currently on the market are made from latex rubber, polyurethane, and the nonsynthetic intestinal tissue of certain animals. They come in a wide variety of colors, shapes, sizes, textures, and thicknesses; (Hatcher et al., 1998; Kubba et al., 2000) preventing pregnancy by blocking sperm from entering the vagina and cervix. Some contain spermicidal lubrication, most commonly nonoxynol-9, which is used to immobilize and kill sperm following ejaculation. (See section on spermicides for discussion of disadvantages.)

Latex condoms help prevent transmission of STDs, including herpes virus, hepatitis B, and HIV by preventing direct contact with body fluids. Current research has shown the nonsynthetic condom to be more porous than the latex condom, thereby lessening its effectiveness in preventing the transmission of STDs (Hatcher et al., 1998). Individuals with latex allergies now have the option of using a polyurethane condom that is nonallergenic, stronger than the latex condom, and more effective in controlling the transmission of STDs than those condoms made of animal intestine (Hatcher et al., 1998; Kubba et al., 2000). A nonallergenic condom made of latex-free natural rubber, called Tactylon by Sensicon Corp. is not widely available (Caufield, 2003). This condom, made from a synthetic thermoplastic elastomer, is made from FDA-approved material for synthetic nonallergenic gloves (Caufield, 2003; Frezieres & Walsh, 2000).

Effectiveness is directly related to consistent and correct usage (Caufield, 2003; Hatcher et al., 1998; Workowski & Levine, 2002). Current statistics measure pregnancy prevention effectiveness in terms of failure rate for typical versus perfect use. Caufield (2003) suggests that failure rates vary between 12% (typical use) and 3% (perfect use) while Hatcher et al. (1998) and Kubba et al. (2000) suggest failure rates of 14% (typical use) and 3% (perfect use). Failure rates increase dramatically if patients use petroleum-based lubricants. Advantages and disadvantages of condoms are provided in Table 18–4.

TABLE 18–4. Advantages and Disadvantages of Male Condoms

Advantages	Disadvantages
• Easily accessible (no prescription needed) • Cost-effective • Significant STD protection (latex or polyurethane) • Male participation in contraception • Enhances erection • Can be used during lactation	• Allergic reaction to latex or lubrication • Slippage/breakage • Unwillingness of male partner to use • Interferes with sexual spontaneity • Decreased pleasure and/or sensation • Skin condoms ineffective protection against STDs including HIV • Heat may weaken rubber condoms

Sources: Adapted from Caufield (2003) and Hatcher et al. (1998).

Condom users should be cautioned regarding the use of oil-based or petroleum-based lotions or lubricants. Products such as shortening, whipped cream, massage oils, vegetable oils, and vaginal yeast suppositories or creams are not safe to use with latex condoms but may be used with polyurethane condoms (Hatcher et al., 2001).

Patient education needs to stress the importance of checking the expiration date on condoms prior to use and that they can only be used once. In addition, patients need to understand that condoms must be placed on the penis before contact with perineal area, they need to be rolled all the way on, and they should be held tight when removing to avoid spillage. It is advisable to use a second method, such as spermicide, to enhance effectiveness.

FEMALE CONDOMS

In 1993, the FDA approved the Reality female condom for distribution in the United States in response to increased demand for an easily reversible, easily accessible, woman-controlled method of contraception that also addressed concerns regarding the increase of STDs among women (Boston Women's Health Collective, 1998, Gollub, 2000). Made of thin polyurethane approximately 17 cm long with one closed and one open flexible end, the female condom completely shields the vagina and cervix and partially covers the perineal area. When properly inserted, the condom prevents sperm from entering the vagina and cervix and provides a protective barrier against most STDs, including HIV (Caufield, 2003; Gollub, 2000).

The effectiveness of female condoms in preventing unwanted pregnancy varies from a 21% failure rate with typical use to a 5% failure rate with perfect use. Its effectiveness is similar to those of the diaphragm and cervical cap in the United States (Caufield, 2003; Kubba et al., 2000). The manufacturer currently suggests that the Reality condom can be left in place for up to 8 hours and should be used only once, and then discarded. Hollander (2001, p. 155), however, describes a recent study concluding that "the female condom can be washed and reused several times and still meet structural standards set by the FDA." Table 18–5 lists the advantages and disadvantages of female condoms.

Proper insertion technique is an important teaching consideration. The inner ring of the closed end should be squeezed together and inserted until the ring is past the pubic bone, completely covering the cervix. It is important to check to make sure the pouch has not become twisted during insertion since this would make penile insertion very difficult. The pouch should then extend along the vagina and on to the perineum.

TABLE 18–5. Advantages and Disadvantages of Female Condoms

Advantages	Disadvantages
• Easily accessible • Easily reversible • Requires no prescription • Protective against STDs and HIV • Can be used during lactation • Can be inserted well before intercourse • Can be removed immediately after intercourse	• Three times as costly as male condoms • Can only be used once • Cumbersome to insert • Slippage can occur • May be esthetically unpleasing (noise with use, ring dangles outside vagina)

Sources: Adapted from Boston Women's Health Collective (1998), Caufield (2003), and Hatcher et al. (1998).

DIAPHRAGMS

Used since the late 1800s in Europe, the diaphragm gained acceptance in the United States during the 1920s. It is a dome-shaped cup with a flexible spring-like rim made of heavy latex rubber, which, when combined with a spermicidal cream or jelly, provides both a mechanical barrier to shield the cervix and a chemical to kill sperm. To be effective, the diaphragm must be inserted into the vagina prior to intercourse so that the posterior rim rests in the posterior fornix and the anterior rim fits snugly behind the pubic bone. It must remain in this position for at least 6 h after intercourse but should not be worn longer than 24 h because of the possible increased risk of developing toxic shock syndrome.

Diaphragms are available in four styles and a range of sizes indicating the cup size in millimeters (see Table 18–6). To ensure effectiveness with proper usage, any diaphragm must be properly sized and fitted.

Proper fitting of a diaphragm requires a vaginal examination. An estimate of the diagonal length of the vaginal canal from the posterior vaginal fornix to the symphysis pubis provides the measurement necessary for determining the appropriately sized diaphragm. This estimated measurement is accomplished by inserting the middle and index fingers into the vagina until the middle finger touches the posterior vaginal wall. Mark the point on the clinician's hand that touches the symphysis pubis, and then select a diaphragm diameter corresponding to the length between the middle finger and the point where contact was made with the symphysis pubis. When inserted, the diaphragm should fit snugly against the pubic bone, should completely cover the cervix, and should touch the

TABLE 18–6. Comparison of Diaphragms

Diaphragm Type	Sizing	Special Considerations
Coil spring rim	Koromex (latex): 50–95 mm Ortho coil (latex): 50–95 mm Ramses (gum rubber): 50–95 mm	Has sturdy rim with firm spring strength; well suited for woman with average vaginal musculature and average pubic arch depth
Arcing spring rim	Koroflex (latex): 60–95mm Ortho All-Flex (latex): 55–95 mm Ramses Bendex (gum rubber): 65–95 mm	Sturdy rim with firm arching spring strength eases insertion; well suited for most women; can be retained in presence of rectocele or cystocele and in women with relaxed muscle tone
Flat spring rim	Ortho-White (latex): 55–95 mm	Thin gentle spring strength especially useful in women with firm musculature, in women with a shallow notch behind the pubic bone, or in nulliparous women; can be inserted with plastic introducer
Wide seal rim	Milex Wide-Seal (latex: 60–95 mm; comes in either arcing or spring coil	Flexible flange on inside rim of dome keeps spermicide in place and enhances seal between rim and vaginal wall

Adapted from Allen (2004); Caufield (2003); Hatcher et al. (1998).

lateral vaginal walls. Movement by the patient, such as walking, sitting, or squatting, should not displace the diaphragm and should not cause discomfort. Table 18–7 lists the advantages and disadvantages of diaphragms.

Women with chronic urinary tract infections, a history of toxic shock syndrome, a severely displaced uterus or vaginal cystocele, scoliosis, or spina bifida should be counseled to use another form of birth control.

Once the diaphragm has been fitted, the patient will need to practice insertion and removal. Teaching should include timing of diaphragm insertion (within 6 h before intercourse) and how to check for proper placement (the patient should be able to feel the outline of the cervix through the soft rubber cup, and the rim of the diaphragm should fit snugly behind the pubic bone). Like condoms, diaphragms react to oil- and petroleum-based products, producing a birth control product that is ineffective due to destruction of the rubber. Therefore, if lubricants are being used, the patient should be warned to use only water-soluble products (Allen, 2004; Caufield, 2003; Hatcher et al., 1998).

TABLE 18–7. Advantages and Disadvantages of Diaphragms

Advantages	Disadvantages
• Cost-effective • Can be used 3 years with proper care • Good method for women needing contraception on irregular basis • Easily reversible • Can use during lactation • Provides some protection against STDs • Does not require partner involvement • Protects against cervical neoplasia • Controlled by the woman	• Requires accurate fitting • Initial cost for fitting may be high • May interfere with sexual spontaneity • Increased incidence of UTIs, especially with arcing spring • Allergic reactions to latex/rubber or spermicide • Takes time to learn insertion and removal • Requires refitting for loss or gain of weight or after pregnancy, abortion, or miscarriage

Adapted from Boston Women's Health Collective (1998) Caufield (2003); Hatcher et al. (2001).

CERVICAL CAPS

This barrier method, resembling a small version of a diaphragm with a deep cup, is made of soft rubber (Caufield, 2003) and is meant to fit snugly over the cervix, creating a seal between the soft flexible rim and the outer edge of the cervix. It provides a barrier against advancing sperm, and when spermicide is put inside the dome prior to insertion, the chemical aids in killing sperm, thereby achieving dual pregnancy and some STD prevention.

Approved for distribution by the FDA in 1988, the Prentif cavity rim cervical cap maintains effectiveness ratings similar to the diaphragm: 9% failure rate with perfect use and 20% failure rate with typical use. (Caufield, 2003; Kubba et al., 2000). Parous women have an unintended pregnancy rate of 40% in the first year of typical use with the cervical cap (Caufield, 2003).

Approved for U.S. distribution in March 2002, the Lea's Shield is a reusable elipitically shaped cervical cap with an anterior loop that aids removal. Its failure rate at 9% for perfect use and 14% for typical use will vary by parity (FDA approves Lea's Shield, 2002).

Like the diaphragm, the cervical cap must be fitted by a properly trained healthcare provider and manifests similar advantages and disadvantages. It provides continuous protection for up to 48 h and may be left in place without adding additional spermicide for no more than 48 h.

Women with cervical erosion or laceration should not be fitted with a cervical cap, and women with a long or irregularly shaped cervix may be unable to wear the cervical cap. Other contraindications for use include allergy to latex or rubber. Some early concern about the cap increasing the risk of abnormal Pap smear has not been supported by research (Hatcher et al., 1998). The FDA does advise a 3-month Pap after insertion.

It is important for a woman to understand how much spermicide to use in conjunction with the cervical cap: enough to fill about one-third of the cap, which is then spread around the inside of the cap without applying any to the rim. Too much spermicide can cause a break in the suction of the cap to the cervix. The cap should be washed with soap and water, rinsed thoroughly, air dried and stored at room temperature. The manufacturer recommends the cap be replaced annually (FDA approves Lea's Shield, 2002; Hatcher et al., 1998). To prevent odors, the cervical cap can be soaked for approximately 20 min in a solution of one cup of water to one tablespoon of either cider vinegar or lemon juice. The cap should then be thoroughly rinsed and dried before use.

FemCap, a silicone rubber cap used as a barrier contraceptive, received FDA approval for distribution in the United States in March 2003. The device comes in three sizes: 22 mm size for nulliparous women, 26 mm size for parous women who have not had vaginal deliveries and 30 mm size for parous women who have delivered full term newborns (Summary of safety and effectiveness data, 2003). The FemCap carries the same instructions as the other cervical caps for insertion, use of spermicide, length of "leave-in" time, and care and handling.

VAGINAL CONTRACEPTIVE SPONGE

First FDA-approved in 1983, the Today Sponge was removed from distribution in 1995 and recently reintroduced to the United States market (Greydanus, Patel, & Rimsza, 2001; Hatcher et al., 1998). It is a safe and effective over-the-counter concave-shaped sponge containing nonoxynol-9 as its spermicidal agent (Greydanus et al., 2001). In addition, the Protectaid Sponge is available in some markets. This sponge contains "3 spermicides with a polydimethylsiloxane dispersing agent;. . ." (Greydanus et al., 2001, p. 568). The combination of spermicidal agents has both antiviral and antimicrobial effects. The sponge may fall out with straining in parous women, and should be reintroduced if protruding (Caufield, 2003). Instructions for use should be followed carefully, calling for thorough wetting and squeezing before introducing, with the dimple against the cervix. It is left in place for 6 hours after last intercourse; no more than 30 total hours is advised.

VAGINAL CONTRACEPTIVE RING

NuvaRing, a 2001 FDA approved flexible vaginal ring used for pregnancy prevention, releases a continuous low dose of the hormones etonogestrel and ethinyl estradiol (First hormonal vaginal, 2001; NuvaRing, 2001). On average the released levels of etonogestrel and ethinyl estradiol are 0.120 mg/d and 0.015 mg/d respectively. Recent clinical trials demonstrate efficacy at "1 to 2 preganancies per 100 women-years of use" (NuvaRing, 2001, p. 777). An advantage of this method is that it avoids the first-pass effect on the liver and provides blood levels that are fairly constant (Brach, Mishell, Lahteenmaki, et al., 2001; Caufield, 2003). Available only through prescription, the device is inserted into the vagina by the woman herself between days 1 and 5 of the menstrual cycle and left in place for 3 weeks. At the end of the third week the device is removed and discarded. No ring is inserted for one week, during which time menstruation should occur (First hormonal vaginal, 2001). A new ring must be inserted "1 week to the day after the previous ring's removal even if menstrual bleeding is not finished" (NuvaRing, 2001, p. 777). Side effects include increased vaginal discharge, vaginitis and leukorrhea. In addition, the vaginal ring carries "the hormonal class warning about possible risk of thromboembolism, stroke, and myocardial infarction, as well as the warning against concurrent cigarette smoking" (NuvaRing, 2001, p. 777). A back-up method is needed for 7 days if the ring is removed for 3 hours or more (Caufield, 2003).

TRANSDERMAL CONTRACEPTIVE PATCH

November 2001, the FDA approved the first hormone contraceptive transdermal contraceptive system (patch), Ortho-Evra. It contains a combination of ethinyl estradiol and norelgestromin (the primary active metabolite of norgestimate) and delivers a sustained daily dose of 20 μg and 150 μg respectively to the systemic circulation (Abrams, Skee, Natarajan, et al., 2001; Wysocki & Moore, 2002). Its mechanism of action is the same as the combined oral contraceptives (COC's). One advantage is that the patch can be worn on different body locations including the abdomen, buttock, upper outer arm and upper torso. It should not be worn on the breasts. It is worn continuously for one week and then replaced with a new patch for a total of three weeks of patch wear. During the fourth week, no patch is worn. Withdrawal bleeding is expected to begin during this patch-free week (Caufield,

2003; First contraceptive skin patch, 2002; Wysocki & Moore, 2002). Efficiacy from clinical trials is 99%, similar to that of COCs. Caution should be used when considering the transdermal system for obese women. Holt, Cushing-Haugen, and Daling (2002), noted a 33% failure rate among women with a baseline body weight of ≥ 198 pounds at the start of treatment. These authors have noted that among COC users, women weighing ≥ 150 pounds are 1.6 times more likely to experience COC failure than those weighing < 150 pounds. Table 18-8 lists the advantages and disadvantages of this new method of contraception. Side effects include those commonly associated with COCs. In addition the patch has been associated with a higher occurrence of breast discomfort and breakthrough bleeding during the first two cycles (Elliott & Chan, 2001).

SPERMICIDES

Distributed as foams, jellies, creams, suppositories, and films, spermicide must be inserted into the vagina prior to intercourse and works by immobilizing and killing sperm (Caufield, 2003). When used as the sole protective device, a spermicide provides protection for one episode of sexual intercourse and is effective for approximately 1 h after insertion. The most common active spermicidal ingredients are nonoxynol-9 and octoxynol. Both are equally effective in preventing pregnancy; the failure rate with typical use is 26% versus 6% with perfect use (Hatcher et al., 1998).

Although spermicides have appeared to have some use in decreasing STD transmission such as with gonorrhea and chlamydia (Cook & Rosenberg, 1998; Greydanus et al., 2001), Roddy, Zekeng, Ryan, et al. (2002) found that the use of condoms plus nonoxynol-9 spermicidal gel was associated with higher rates of both gonorrhea and chlamydia than was the condom use alone. The CDC does not recommend a spermicide for STD/HIV prevention (Workowski & Levine, 2002). Possible increased HIV transmission secondary to vaginal inflammation and lesions from nonoxynol-9 use has been demonstrated (Fichorova, Tucker, & Anderson, 2001; Workowski & Levine, 2002). See Table 18–9 for advantages and disadvantages of spermicides.

Timing is everything when using spermicides. Spermicides that come in the form of foams, jellies, or creams should be applied no more than 15 min before vagina-to-penis contact is anticipated. If the patient chooses suppositories or vaginal contraceptive film, she needs to follow package instructions and wait the appropriate amount of time before intercourse to allow the adequate dispersement of the spermicide. No matter what type of spermicide is used, patients need to be cautioned about the need to reapply the spermicide prior to each episode of intercourse in order to maintain effectiveness of the method. Patients should be advised to keep a supply on hand and to make sure they check the expiration date before use. In addition, use of a second method, such as one of the barrier methods, is recommended to enhance effectiveness. Finally, should irritation or burning occur with use, the patient is advised to discontinue use (Boston Women's Health. Collective, 1998; Caufield, 2003; Hatcher et al., 1998).

INTRAUTERINE DEVICES

A well-liked contraceptive method in the 1960s and 1970s, the intrauterine device (IUD) declined in popularity during the 1980s (Hatcher et al., 1998). It is used frequently as a method of birth control world-wide, but is the method of choice for less than 1% of women of childbearing age in the United States (Burkman & Shulman,

TABLE 18–8. Advantages and Disadvantages of Transdermal Contraceptive Patch

Advantages	Disadvantages
• Easy to use • Cost similar to COCs • Allows for sexual spontaneity • Highly effective • Considered immediately effective if begun on day 1 of menstrual cycle	• Potential for minor skin irritation at application site • Potential adherence problems • May be less effective in women weighing ≥ 198 pounds

Adapted from Elliott & Chan (2001); Wysocki & Moore (2002).

TABLE 18–9. Advantages and Disadvantages of Spermicides

Advantages	Disadvantages
• Widely available without prescription or examination • Cost effective • Easily available as a backup method • Completely reversible • Can provide lubrication during intercourse	• May interfere with spontaneity • Must be on hand at or near time of intercourse • Skin irritation of vulva or penis • Reports of higher rates of STDs • Inability to learn correct insertion technique • Abnormal vaginal anatomy interfering with placement

Adapted from Caufield (2003) and Hatcher et al. (1998).

2001; Cheng, 2000; Thonneau, Goulard, & Goyaux, 2001). The decrease in popularity of the IUD is commonly attributed to the high incidence of pelvic infections and septic abortions brought about by the use of one particular type of IUD, the Dalkon shield (Cheng, 2000).

Currently, three IUDs are commercially available in the United States; the Progestasert, the ParaGard Copper T380A, and the Levonorgestrel-releasing IUD (LNg20) (Burkman & Shulman, 2001; FDA gives green light, 2001; Kaunitz, 2001b). The Progestasert has been on the market continuously since 1976 and contains 38 mg of progesterone in a delivery system releasing 65 μg daily (Cheng, 2000). This product must be replaced yearly and has been found to decrease menstrual flow and cramping as a result of the slow release of progesterone.

The ParaGard Copper T380A, a copper-bearing IUD containing barium sulphate to facilitate x-ray visibility, has been on the market since 1988. This T-shaped polyurethane device has a very fine copper wire wound around it and a white polyethylene string attached to the end to facilitate removal (Caufield, 2003). The LNg-20 (trade name Mirena) became FDA-approved for distribution in the United States in 2001. This device, which "consists of a polyethylene T frame surrounded by a levonorgestrel-containing cylinder" (Burkman & Shulman, 2001, p. 1), releases 20 μg per 24 h of levonorgestrel and remains effective for 5 years (Scott, 2000). Berlex Laboratories distributes this IUD in the United States.

The mechanism of action for the IUD is mainly by preventing fertilization of the ova by the sperm (Caufield, 2003). Fertilization is rare in IUD users. If it does occur, the foreign body effect of the IUD on the enometrium (white blood cells, enzymes, and prostaglandins released) further interferes with sperm mobility toward the fallopian tubes as well as preventing implantation and causing blastocyte lysis. Copper ions released from the ParaGard Copper T 380A have a debilitating effect on the sperm. Progestasert's daily release of progesterone and LNg20's daily release of levonorgestrel suppresses the endometrium, thereby inhibiting sperm migration, while ParaGard Copper T380A appears to interfere with the uptake of estrogen by the uterine mucosa (Burkman & Shulman, 2001; Caufield, 2003; Dickey, 2002; Hatcher et al., 1998). In addition, LNg-20 and Progestasert thicken the cervical mucus, decreasing sperm penetrability, and eventually thin the endometrium to a state of atrophy (Caufield, 2003). In some instances, ovulation is prevented.

Hatcher et al. (1998) note a variation in the effectiveness of the three types of IUDs with the LNg-20 being most effective. Typical use rates vary from 2 (Progestasert), to 0.8 (ParaGard Copper T), to a low of 0.1 (LNg-20). Caufield (2003) notes effectiveness can be influenced by the size and shape of the IUD, as well as by the rate of expulsion and the age and parity of the woman.

All potential IUD users must be carefully screened for contraindications prior to insertion of the device. The suggested patient profile is a woman without a history of pelvic inflammatory disease or ectopic pregnancy, who is in a mutually monogamous relationship, has had one full-term pregnancy, and desires reversible, long-term contraception (Caufield, 2003; Kaunitz, 2001b). It should be noted that contrary to most beliefs, diabetes is not a contraindication to IUD use as noted by the World Health Organization (Medical eligibility criteria for contraceptive use, 3rd edition, 2003). Table 18–10 enumerates the manufacturer-specific contraindications to IUD use.

After a thorough health history is taken, the physical examination should include a bimanual pelvic examination with particular attention to the size, shape, consistency, and position of uterus. In addition the following laboratory studies should be completed: a Pap smear,

TABLE 18–10. Contraindications to IUD Use

Progestasert/Mirena	ParaGard T380A
• History of pelvic surgery that may be associated with increased risk of ectopic pregnancy • Presence or history of STDs • Untreated cervicitis or vaginitis • Conditions associated with immunosuppression • Incomplete involution after abortion or birth • Current DVT/PE; breast cancer, liver neoplasia, a history of ischemic heart diseases, migranial with focal neuro symptoms	• Known allergy to copper • Diagnosed Wilson's disease • Untreated cervicitis or vaginitis • Conditions associated with increased susceptibility to infections, eg, AIDS, leukemia, chronic steroid therapy • Previously inserted IUD not removed
General Contraindications	
• History of pelvic inflammatory disease • Intravenous drug abuse • Non-mutually monogamous relationship • Genital bleeding of unknown etiology • Pregnancy or suspected pregnancy • Abnormality of uterus resulting in distortion of uterine cavity • Genital actinomycosis • Trophoblast disease	

Sources: Caufield (2003); Prescribing information for Mirena (Berlex), ParaGard Cu T380A (Ortho), Progestasert (ALZA).

STD screen, vaginal wet mount, hematocrit, and pregnancy test in absence of menses or in cases of irregular menses. Thorough counseling regarding the advantages and disadvantages of the method should be included during the preinsertion visit. Time during this preinsertion visit should be sufficient to clarify information and obtain a prior written consent. Any preexisting condition such as anemia or vaginal infection should be treated prior to insertion of the IUD.

Scott (2000) highlights the current controversy regarding the relative merits of prophylactic antibiotic use at the time of IUD insertion. Some clinicians prescribe either 200 mg of doxycycline, administered 1 h prior to insertion, or 500 mg of erythromycin, administered 1 h prior and 6 h following insertion, to decrease the chance of uterine infection following insertion. Scott (2000, p. 87) notes that "many experts believe this [prophylactic antibiotic use] is unnecessary, . . . nevertheless a woman who is at increased risk of subacute bacterial endocarditis needs to be covered." The current American Heart Association protocol suggests a 2 g dose of oral amoxicillin be given 1 h prior to insertion for low-to-moderate risk patients; for patients considered high risk, a combination of IV amoxicillin and garamycin should be used. If the patient is allergic to penicillin, vancomycin is the drug of choice (Scott, 2000). Advantages and disadvantages of the IUD are listed in Table 18–11.

An IUD may be inserted at any time during the menstrual cycle as long as the woman is not pregnant. Caufield (2003) suggests that mid-cycle insertion, when the cervix is softer, may cause less discomfort. Hatcher et al., (1998) note an increased incidence of IUD expulsion and higher infection rate when IUDs are inserted during menses. All phases of IUD insertion require the practitioner to use a slow, steady, and gentle movement. It will be necessary to redetermine uterine position with bimanual examination prior to insertion. Methods of insertion vary slightly with the type of IUD; therefore, the healthcare provider should always read and follow the manufacturer's instructions for insertion.

Patient education should include a thorough explanation of what to expect during and after IUD insertion. Women should be instructed how and when to check for the IUD string, how to recognize the signs and symptoms of infection, and how to monitor for danger signs using the acronym PAINS: P = period, late or with abnormal spotting or bleeding; A = abdominal pain and/or pain with intercourse; I = infection symptoms or exposure; N = not feeling well, i.e., experiencing fever, chills, or pelvic pain; S = string is either missing or shorter or longer than normal (Caufield, 2003).

TABLE 18–11. Advantages and Disadvantages of IUDs

Advantages	Disadvantages
• Requires no continuing action, once inserted	• Insertion requires trained health provider
• Allows for sexual spontaneity	• Must regularly check for presence of IUD string
• Continuously effective	
• Cost effective, once inserted	• May increase risk for pelvic infections
• Progesterone IUD may decrease menstrual flow and dysmenorrhea	• Does not decrease risk of contracting STDs
• Can be used during lactation	• May cause increased dysmenorrhea and menstrual flow

Sources: Caufield (2003); Hatcher et al. (1998); Scott (2000).

STERILIZATION

Voluntary surgical contraception for either the man or woman continues to be one of the most widely used methods of family planning worldwide. "More than 220 million couples worldwide" (ACOG practice bulletin #46, 2003, p. 287) use this as their contraceptive method. In the United States approximately 11 million women rely on this form of contraception with "approximately 700,000 tubal sterilizations and 500,000 vasectomies . . . performed . . . annually" (ACOG practice bulletin #46, 2003, p. 287).

Defined as the surgical interruption or closure of pathways for sperm or ova, this method of contraception is considered permanent. However, surgical procedures have been developed to successfully reverse this contraceptive method.

Sterilization methods available through laparoscopy are (1) occlusion with partial resection by unipolar electrosurgery, (2) occlusion with transection by unipolar electrosurgery, (3) occlusion by bipolar electrocoagulation, and (4) occlusion with clips or silastic rings (ACOG practice bulletin #46, 2003). Failure of sterilization is higher than once thought, being about 1.85% in a ten-year period, with 30% of these being ectopic pregnancies (Baill, Cullins, & Patti, 2003). The bipolar method is considered to be safer than the unipolar, but fails more often (Gordon & Speroff, 2002). Three ways of occluding the tubes with clips or a ring are the Hulka-Clemens clip, the Filshie clip, and the Falope (Yoon) ring. The Hulka-Clemens clip has the highest failure rate over ten years but offers good reversibility. The ring has the best ten-year failure rate of the three (ACOG practice bulletin #46, 2003).

Clinicians need to have the most current information available for the patient and her partner so they can make the best choice about sterilization.

As part of the ten-year CDC study, the CREST study (Peterson, 1996) found that approximately 6% of the women in the study consulted a healthcare provider regarding the possibility of reversal at some point during the five years following their sterilization procedure. The study found that women under 30 made up the largest percentage of women seeking information about reversal. Other factors influencing possible regret included changes in marital status, death of a child, socioeconomic status, and whether the sterilization was performed in conjunction with cesarean section (Baill, Cullins, & Patti, 2003). Wilcox, Chu, and Peterson (1990) have identified the following characteristics that make patients ideal candidates for tubal reanastomosis: (1) younger than 43, (2) documented ovulation, (3) of average weight for height, (4) at least 4 cm of healthy tubal tissue remaining.

As with all other forms of fertility control, voluntary surgical sterilization is a personal decision best made after reviewing all the options and carefully weighing the risks and benefits. Areas to be included when providing presterilization counseling to patients are outlined in Table 18–12. Advantages and disadvantages of sterilization are listed in Table 18–13.

November 2002 the FDA approved a new, nonsurgical, female sterilization device: Essure System (manufactured by Conceptus, Inc). It is a small expanding microcoil which, when placed in the fallopian tubes, causes occlusion of the tubes thus preventing fertilization of the egg by the sperm (FDA approves new female, 2003; FDA may soon consider, 2002; New female sterilization device, 2003). One microcoil is inserted by a special catheter inserted through the vagina, into the uterus and then into each fallopian tube.

TABLE 18–12. Presterilization Counseling Guidelines

- Stress the probable permanency of the method for women
- Include both partners and discuss both male and female procedures
- Provide full discussion of all fertility control options
- Provide information about failure rates, both 1-year and cumulative
- Reinforce risk reduction activities related to sexually transmitted infections
- Be aware of factors that may lead to poststerilization regret
- Advise that sexuality is not affected negatively
- Explain that menses may or may not be affected
- Provide full complement of information on all patient-appropriate surgical procedures

Sources: ACOG practice bulletin #46 (2003); Pollack (1996).

TABLE 18–13. Advantages and Disadvantages of Sterilization

Advantages	Disadvantages
• Provides permanent fertility control	• Inherent risks of any surgical procedure
• Highly effective, convenient, one-time decision	• Difficult to reverse
• Long term: low cost, low risk	• Cost initially high
• Certain techniques can be done immediately after abortion or childbirth	• Vasectomy not immediately effective
• Considered immediately effective	• Not protective against HIV/AIDS or other STDs

Sources: Adapted from Kubba et al. (2000); Peterson (1996).

The device consists of three components: (1) a stainless steel inner coil which attaches the device to the special catheter used for placement, (2) an outer coil made from Nitinol which anchors the device in the fallopian tube, and (3) polyethelene terephthalate fibers which form a mesh between the two coils causing a moderate inflammatory reaction with fibrosis resulting in permanent occlusion of the tube (FDA may soon consider, 2002). For three months following insertion of the device, the woman must use an alternate form of contraception and at the end of the third month must return for a follow-up x-ray to determine proper placement (FDA approves new female, 2003). This device is contraindicated under the following circumstances: is uncertain about desire for permanent sterilization, has a history of previous tubal ligation, is pregnant or suspected of being pregnant, had delivery or termination of pregnancy less than 6 weeks before device placement, has active or recent pelvic infection, has allergy or hypersensitivity to nickel (Essure summary prescribing information, 2002). No adverse effects have been reported in clinical trials and no pregnancies were reported after 24 months in a study of 439 women between the ages of 21 and 40 (New female sterilization device, 2003). Healthcare providers are required to complete a training program prior to prescribing the device.

FERTILITY AWARENESS METHODS

There are a variety of techniques women can use to determine fertile from infertile periods during the menstrual cycle (Weschler, 2001). These fertility awareness methods (FAMs) help women determine their fertile period by learning to "read" the expected physiological changes caused by hormonal fluctuations occurring during the normal menstrual cycle (Caufield, 2003; Hatcher et al., 1998; Weschler, 2001). Correct use of FAMs provides 97 to 99% effectiveness (Fehring, 2004).

Women who become attuned to and learn to recognize the measurable body changes that occur around the time of ovulation can use this information to effectively manage their fertility over time without the need to rely on other devices. A FAM's main mechanism of action as a contraceptive method, avoidance of unprotected intercourse during the woman's fertile period, is based on the following factors: (1) An ovum is usually released each cycle; (2) the ovum is released 14 days before menstruation; (3) the ovum lives for approximately 24 h; and (4) sperm may live for 5 days in a woman's body. Therefore, women may be fertile for as long as 5 days before ovulation, because of sperm life, and for up to 3 days after ovulation, because of ova life.

The two most common FAMs include monitoring a woman's basal body temperature (BBT) on a daily basis and checking cervical mucus changes daily. Using the two methods together, called the *symptothermal method*, provides important confirmatory information for patients who choose this method of fertility control.

A woman's basal body temperature, the lowest temperature reached by the body of a healthy person during waking hours, fluctuates with the ovulatory cycle as much as 0.8°F (Weschler, 2001). Using this method requires a thermometer that measures in tenths of a degree and a BBT chart. BBT should be taken daily before rising, eating, or drinking and charted to observe ovulatory patterns over time.

Ovulation occurs at a point in the menstrual cycle at which progesterone levels increase as a result of the surge in luteinizing hormone. Concomitantly, there is a rise in the BBT of 0.4°–0.8°F. This temperature increase continues until menstruation, at which point there will be a return to preovulation BBT. If conception has occurred, the BBT will remain elevated.

Over the course of several months, patterns should emerge, providing valuable information as to fertile and infertile periods, enabling the patient to predict the end of the fertile period and the beginning of the luteal (nonfertile) phase (Caufield, 2003). If using this method alone, women should be counseled to refrain from unprotected intercourse from day 4 of the menstrual cycle until after BBT has been elevated for 3 days (Weschler, 2001), unless pregnancy is desired.

Determining ovulatory patterns by observing changes in the cervical mucus was first developed in the early 1960s by Billings (Boston Women's Health Collective, 1998), who sought a method of contraceptive protection in compliance with the teachings of the Catholic Church.

Secreted by the exocrine glands lining the cervical canal, cervical mucus changes character in response to hormonal changes throughout the menstrual cycle (Caufield, 2003). In order to determine the time of ovulation, a patient is instructed to assess the vaginal area for level of wetness or dryness on a daily basis and also to note changes in color and consistency of the mucus. It is normal for women to experience several days of dryness immediately following menstruation. Then there will be a period when the mucus will appear milky white, translucent yellow, or clear and slightly sticky. Corresponding to a peak in estrogen, which occurs immediately before ovulation, the amount of mucus increases and it becomes clear and slippery to touch, similar in consistency to egg whites. Mucus with this consistency facilitates the movement of sperm toward the awaiting ova.

After ovulation has occurred, the amount of mucus decreases, and it returns to a milky white, sticky consistency. Before ovulation, dry days when no cervical fluid is present are the days considered safe (Caufield, 2003). A daily record should be kept noting the cervical mucus changes.

The symptothermal method combines the BBT and cervical mucus methods along with noting other physiological changes such as breast tenderness, change in libido, and mittelshmerz. Experts contend that combining FAMs offers patients the highest degree of effectiveness in pregnancy protection versus using each method independently. The failure rate with perfect use ranges between 1% and 3%. Some experts add an optional sign of fertility: the position of the cervix and its openness. The cervix is usually deeper/higher in the vagina, softer, open, and wet close to ovulation (Caufield, 2003). Advantages and disadvantages of FAMs are listed in Table 18–14.

Preparation for using this method of fertility control and understanding how to accurately interpret the charts requires thorough and ongoing education. Kits and monitors to use at home to predict ovulation are in development for couples who wish to prevent pregnancy (Caufield, 2003). Table 18–15 describes the content areas essential for FAMs. These should be incorporated into the teaching plan for patients choosing to use FAMs.

COITUS INTERRUPTUS (WITHDRAWAL)

This method of fertility control has been used throughout history and was "a natural response to the discovery that ejaculation into the vagina caused pregnancy" (Hatcher et

TABLE 18–14. Advantages and Disadvantages of Fertility Awareness Methods

Advantages	Disadvantages
• Increases user knowledge of reproductive cycle • Acceptable to most religious groups • Actively involves both partners • No side effects • Cost effective • Provides information about potential fertility problems • Does not interrupt normal body functions • Uses no devices or chemicals	• Does not provide protection against HIV/AIDS/STDs • Mandates cooperation between partners • Not reliable if cycle is irregular, lactating, or perimenopausal • Perceived lack of sexual spontaneity • Many factors alter cycle, decreasing reliability

Source: Adapted from Caufield (2003); Weschler (2001).

al., 1998, p. 303). It involves having the man remove his penis from the vagina and perineal area before ejaculation in an effort to keep sperm and ova separate. Although few statistical data exist to accurately determine effectiveness, most contraceptive experts suggest that the failure rate with perfect use in the first year is about 4% and 19% with typical use (Caufield, 2003; Hatcher et al., 1998). Fertility awareness methods and withdrawal are often used together (Caufield, 2003). Advantages and disadvantages of coitus interruptus are listed in Table 18–16.

ORAL CONTRACEPTIVES

Oral contraceptives (OCs) are the most popular method of birth control and are used by nearly 20 million women in the United States (Caufield, 2003). This popularity is due to several factors including high efficacy, simplicity of use, rapid reversal in effects after discontinuation, and menstrual cycle benefits (Dickey, 2002). After oral contraceptives were synthesized in the 1950s, many formulation changes were made in the hopes of ameliorating potential complications and adverse effects (Greydanus et al., 2001). These changes include a reduction in the doses of estrogen and progestin, timing of the progestin in the cycle, and third-generation progestins that differ in pharmacologic activity from other progestins.

TABLE 18–15. Essential Content Areas in Preparation for Using FAMs

- Normal menstrual cycle
- Mechanics of the method
- Required equipment
- Method selection
- Charting the data
- Determining fertile period
- Alternative sexual activity during fertile periods

Sources: Weschler, 2001

TABLE 18–16. Advantages and Disadvantages of Coitus Interruptus

Advantages	Disadvantages
• Does not cost anything • Involves no artificial devices or chemicals • Can be used during lactation • It is always available	• Requires control on the part of the man • Not protective against STDs, HIV/AIDS • Diminished sexual pleasure • Premature ejaculation

Sources: Boston Women's Health Collective (1998); Caufield (2003), Hatcher et al. (1998).

The first pill marketed, Enovid 10, contained constant doses of both estrogen and progestin; however, doses were much higher than those used today and resulted in an increased risk of thromboembolism. Today, doses of estrogen and progestin are 5 to 7 and 25 times lower, respectively, than those used in the initial formulations. Sequential formulations were introduced in the 1960s, but are no longer marketed. These pills contained estrogen given during the first 2 weeks; then progestin was added during the third week of the cycle. Sequential OCs were shown to be less effective and associated with an increased risk of endometrial cancer (Bucci & Carson, 1997).

CURRENT FORMULATIONS

The majority of women taking OCs receive combination pills, a mixture of synthetic estrogen and one of several progestins. Combination pills are marketed as fixed, biphasic, or triphasic OCs, depending on whether the hormone dose varies throughout the 21-day cycle. Most OCs contain a "fixed" amount of estrogen and progestin in each pill; therefore, every pill in the 21-day active-pill cycle is the same. Biphasic OCs, introduced in 1982, are composed of two pill strengths. Estrogen remains constant throughout the cycle; however, the progestin dose is lower during the first 10 days of the cycle. Triphasic OCs initially were developed to decrease the total monthly dose of progestin, potentially leading to a reduction in adverse effects. (Greydanus et al., 2001). Estrostep contains three strengths that vary in estrogen content, gradually increasing the dose throughout the cycle and resulting in lower monthly estrogen doses. A new combination OC, Cyclessa (desogestrel/ethinyl estradiol), provides a very low estrogen dose per triphasic tablet of 25 μg. Progestin only pills are known as "minipills" and are primarily used in women who have contraindications to estrogen or do not tolerate combination pills. Minipills will be discussed in more detail in the section on progestin-only contraceptives. Table 18–17 lists selected OCs with their respective formulation types. Several OC formulations are in some phase of study for FDA approval and are expected to be marketed in the coming months (The Research Pipeline, 2000). One such newly approved (September 2003) oral contraceptive is Seasonale (Barr Laboratories). This monophasic COC has 84 "active" pills and 7 placebo pills. "Under Seasonale's dosing regimen the number of expected menstrual periods that a woman usually experiences are reduced from once a month to about once every three months" (FDA approves seasonale oral contraceptive, 2003). Data from recent clinical trials demonstrates a higher incidence of break-through bleeding during the "first few cycles of use" (FDA approves seasonale oral contraceptive, 2003).

MECHANISM OF ACTION AND EFFICACY

As previously discussed, OCs are comprised of estrogen and progestin or progestin only (mini-pills). OCs prevent pregnancy by a variety of mechanisms and have a wide range of effects, resulting in a myriad of potential symptoms. Estrogenic effects that prevent conception include: (1) inhibition of ovulation by suppression of follicle-stimulating hormone (FSH) and luteinizing hormone (LH), which occurs because the pituitary gland "thinks" a woman is already pregnant; and therefore, hormones that would normally stimulate the ovary are not released; (2) inhibition of implantation with high doses of estrogen alters uterine secretions and endometrial cellular structure; (3) acceleration of ovum transport; and (4) degeneration of the corpus luteum (luteolysis), which prevents normal implantation and placental attachment. Progestins are thought to (1) inhibit ovulation by suppression of LH; (2) produce thick cervical mucus, which hampers sperm transport; (3) inhibit the enzymes that allow sperm to penetrate the ovum (capacitation); (4) slow ovum transport; and (5) inhibit implantation due to atrophic changes in the endometrium.

As a result of these varied mechanisms, OCs are an extremely effective method of birth control with perfect use failure rate within the first year of 0.5% and 0.1% for progestin-only and combined OCs, respectively. With typical use, it is estimated 5% of women will become pregnant within the first year of use with either progestin-only or combination OCs (Hatcher et al., 2001; Katzung, 2001).

TABLE 18–17. Selected Oral Contraceptive Formulations

Formulation	Drug	Estrogen	Amount (μg)	Progestin	Amount (mg)
Monophasic	Alesse	Ethinyl (E.) Estradiol	20	Levonorgestrel	0.1
	Brevicon/Modicon	E. Estradiol	35	Norethindrone	0.5
	Demulen 1/35	E. Estradiol	35	Ethynodiol Diacetate	1.0
	Desogen/Orthocept	E. Estradiol	30	Desogestrel	0.15
	Loestrin 1.5/30	E. Estradiol	30	Norethindrone acetete	1.5
	Lo/Ovral	E. Estradiol	30	Norgestrel	0.3
	Levlen/Nordette	E. Estradiol	30	Levonorgestrel	0.15
	Seasonale	E. Estradiol	30	Levonorgestrel	0.15
	Ortho-Cyclen	E. Estradiol	35	Norgestimate	0.25
	Ortho Novum 1/50	Mestranol	50	Norethindrone	1.0
	Ovcon 50	E. Estradiol	50	Norethindrone	1.0
	Zovia 1/35	E. Estradiol	35	Ethynodiol Diacetate	1.0
	Yasmin*	E. Estradiol	30	Drospirenone	3.0
Multiphasic	Cyclessa	E. Estradiol	25	Desogestrel	1.0/1.25/1.5
	Estrostep	E. Estradiol	20/30/35	Norethindrone Acetate	1.0/1.0/1.0
	Jenest	E. Estradiol	35/35	Norethindrone	0.5/1.0
	Ortho-Novum 10/11	E. Estradiol	35/35	Norethindrone	0.5/1.0
	Ortho-Novum 7/7/7	E. Estradiol	35/35/35	Norethindrone	0.5/0.75/1.0
	Ortho Tri-Cyclen	E. Estradiol	35/35/35	Norgestimate	0.180/0.215/0.250
	Ortho Tri-Cyclen Lo	E. Estradiol	25	Norgestimate	0.180/0.215/0.250
	Triphasil/Tri-Levlen/Trivora	E. Estradiol	30/40/30	Levonorgestrel	0.05/0.075/0.125
Minipill	Micronor/Nor-QD	None		Norethindrone	0.35
	Ovrette	None		Norgestrel	0.075

*Yasmin contains a progestin-mild diuretic in combination with estrogen.

Adapted from Caufield, (2003); Dickey (2002); News flash: Add new 25 mcg Cyclessa (2001); Seasonale prescribing information (2003).

COMPONENTS AND BIOLOGICAL ACTIVITY OF ORAL CONTRACEPTIVES

In the United States, OCs contain one of either two synthetic estrogens, ethinyl estradiol or mestranol. These compounds differ from one another in terms of potency. Mestranol is an inactive form of estrogen that must be converted by the liver to the pharmacologically active form of estrogen, ethinyl estradiol. It is thought that mestranol is approximately 67% as potent as ethinyl estradiol. Therefore, Ortho-Novum 1/50, which contains 50 μg of mestranol, has roughly the same estrogenic effects as Ortho-Novum 1/35, which contains 35 μg of ethinyl estradiol (Dickey, 2002; Hatcher et al., 1998; Katzung, 2001). Both mestranol and ethinyl estradiol only produce estrogenic activity.

In contrast, the eight progestins currently available in the United States for use in OC formulations differ in progestational, androgenic, estrogenic, and endometrial (prevalence of spotting and breakthrough bleeding) activity. These progestins, along with their respective biological activities, are listed in Table 18–18. Estrogenic effects occur with certain progestins secondary to their metabolism to estrogenic substances. Additionally, antiestrogenic effects may be present. Androgenic effects are due to the structural similarity between progestins and testosterone. Norgestimate, desogestrel, and gestodene (an investigational progestin in the United States) are considered third-generation progestins and, when compared with levonorgestrel, are associated with reduced androgenic effects. Moreover, estrogenic effects do not occur with several progestins, including norgestimate, desogestrel, gestodene, and levonorgestrel. Interestingly, levonorgestrel has higher androgenic activity than norethindrone. (Bucci & Carson, 1997; Coenen, Thomas, Borm, et al., 1996; Likis, 2002; Stone, 1995).

TABLE 18–18. Biologic Activity of Oral Contraceptive Progestins

Progestin	Progestational Activity	Estrogenic Activity	Androgenic Activity
Desogestrel	9.0	0	3.4
Ethynodiol Acetate	1.4	3.4	0.6
Gestodene	12.6	0	8.6
Levonorgestrel	5.3	0	8.3
Norethindrone	1.0	1.0	1.0
Norethindrone Acetate	1.2	1.5	1.6
Norethynodrel	0.3	8.3	0
Norgestimate	1.3	0	1.9
Norgestrel	2.6	0	4.2

Adapted with permission from Dickey (2002).

Since progestins vary in their propensity for causing estrogenic, progestational, androgenic, and endometrial activity, understanding the differences between the progestins is essential for selecting appropriate OCs and managing adverse effects. Pharmacological differences between OCs result from the type of progestin used and the estrogen and progestin dose in the formulation. For example, Ortho-Novum 7/7/7, containing norethindrone and ethinyl estradiol 35 μg, has greater estrogenic activity than Tri-Cyclen, containing norgestimate and the same dose of ethinyl estradiol, because of the added estrogenic effect from norethindrone being converted, in vivo, to estrogen. Table 18–19 compares the relative pharmacologic effects of selected OCs. Using information from this table will allow the practitioner, in a logical, systematic manner, to choose the most appropriate OC and switch OCs if adverse effects develop. Table 18–20 describes potential adverse effects associated with each type of activity.

MANAGING ADVERSE EFFECTS

As discussed previously, adverse effects from OCs may be classified by the type of activity responsible for them (Table 18–20). In most cases, management involves switching patients to an OC with a different estrogenic, progestational, androgenic, or endometrial activity level, depending on which adverse effect is present (see Table 18–19 for pharmacologic activity of respective OCs).

In addition to pharmacologic activity, the time framework in which the adverse effect develops is important to management. Adverse effects from OCs may be worst in the first several months, constant over time, worse over time, or worse after pill discontinuation (Dickey, 2002; Hatcher et al., 1998). By determining when the adverse effect occurred and if it is worse upon starting OCs, it may be possible to continue therapy for at least 3 months instead of switching pills. Side effects that normally dissipate after the first 3 months include nausea, dizziness, cyclic weight gain, edema, breast fullness and tenderness, and breakthrough bleeding. Conversely, some side effects such as acne, depression, and decreased libido may be constant over time. Table 18–21 reviews management strategies for commonly occurring OC adverse effects.

Rarely, serious side effects may occur with OCs and patients should be instructed to contact their provider if the following warning signs (ACHES) develop: A = abdominal pain (severe); C = chest pain (severe), shortness of breath, or coughing up blood; H = headaches; E = eye problems such as blurred vision, flashing lights, or blindness; and S = severe leg pain (calf or thigh). These signs

TABLE 18–19. Activity of Selected Oral Contraceptives[a]

Oral Contraceptive	Endometrial Activity[b]	Estrogenic Activity	Progestational Activity	Androgenic Activity
50 μg Estrogen				
Ovral	4.5	42	1.3	0.8
Ortho-Novum 1/50	10.6	32	1.0	0.34
Ovcon 50	11.9	50	1.0	0.34
Demulen 50	13.9	26	1.4	0.21
Sub-50 μg Estrogen (monophasic)				
Lo-Ovral	9.6	25	0.8	0.46
Desogen/Orthocept	13.1	30	1.5	0.17
Levlen/Nordette	14.0	25	0.8	0.46
Brevicon/Modicon	24.6	42	0.5	0.17
Loestrin 1.5/30	25.2	14	1.7	0.8
Alesse	26.5	17	0.5	0.31
Zovia 1/35	37.4	19	1.4	0.21
Sub-50 μg Estrogen (multiphasic)				
Ortho Novum 7/7/7	14.5	48	0.8	0.25
Tri-Levlen/ Triphasil/Trivora	15.1	28	0.5	0.29
Ortho Tri-Cyclen	17.7	35	0.3	0.15
Estrostep	26.2	16	1.2	0.53
Progestin-only				
Ovrette	34.9	0	0.08	0.13
Micronor/Nor-QD	42.3	1	0.12	0.13

[a]OCs cannot be precisely compared because activity rates are from different noncomparative studies in distinct patient populations.
[b]Percentage of spotting and breakthrough bleeding.

Adapted with permission from Dickey (2002).

may signal gallbladder disease; hepatic adenoma; a blood clot in the lungs or myocardial infarction; stroke, hypertension, or migraines; other temporary vascular problems; or a blood clot in the legs (Caufield, 2003; Likis, 2002).

BENEFITS, RISKS, AND UNCERTAINTIES ASSOCIATED WITH OCs

In the majority of cases, OCs are a safe and reliable method of birth control for women under 50 who do not smoke. Surprisingly, women who use combination OCs are at a lower risk for development of endometrial and ovarian cancer. OCs may also benefit women at risk for pelvic inflammatory disease and ectopic pregnancies and those who have ovarian cysts, benign breast disease, severe dysmenorrhea, iron deficiency anemia, endometriosis, hirsutism, and acne (Burkman, 2001a; Dickey, 2002; Hatcher et al., 1998). Jensen and Speroff (2000) report that combination OCs have been associated with a lower rate of PID, most likely due to the thickened cervical mucus and subsequent lowered rates of ascending infections. AWHONN recommended adding folic acid to OCs to help reduce neural tube birth defects (Commentary, 2004).

Although many benefits have been documented with OCs, caution should be exercised when deciding to use OCs in certain women because of the potential for exacerbation of a variety of conditions. Table 18–22 lists absolute and relative contraindications to OC use.

CARDIOVASCULAR COMPLICATIONS AND METABOLIC CHANGES

With the availability of third-generation progestins and the reduction in dosage of estrogen in combination OCs, the risks for cardiovascular disease, including effects on lipid metabolism, hypertension, glucose tolerance, venous thromboembolism, myocardial infarction, and stroke, have been reduced compared with the increased risk for cardiovascular disease associated with older OC formulations. The Oxford Family Planning Association Contraceptive Study published in 1977 demonstrated an increase in the risk of death from cardiovascular disease of 4.7-fold in women, taking OCs containing 50 μ g of estrogen (Vessey, McPherson, & Johnson, 1977). No evidence suggests that OCs containing low doses of estrogen place women at an increased risk for developing cardiovascular disease, although certain patient-specific characteristics

TABLE 18–20. Selected Adverse Effects Associated with Hormonal Activity

System	Estrogen Excess	Progestin Excess	Androgen Excess	Estrogen Deficiency	Progestin Deficiency
General	Chloasma Chronic nasal pharyngitis Allergic rhinitis	Appetite increase Depression Fatigue Hypoglycemia symptoms Libido decrease Neurodermatitis Weight gain (noncyclic)	Acne Cholestatic jaundice Hirsutism Libido increase Oily skin and scalp Rash and pruritus Edema	Nervousness Vasomotor symptoms	N/A
Cardiovascular	Capillary fragility CVA DVT Telangiectasias Thromboembolic disease	Hypertension Leg vein dilation	N/A	N/A	N/A
Reproductive	Breast cystic changes Dysmenorrhea Hypermenorrhea Increase in breast size	Cervicitis Flow length decrease Moniliasis	N/A	Absence of withdrawal bleeding Bleeding and spotting during pill days 1–9 Continuous bleeding and spotting Flow decrease Vaginitis (atrophic)	Breakthrough bleeding and spotting during pill days 10–21 Delayed withdrawal bleeding Dysmenorrhea Heavy flow and clots
Premenstrual	Bloating Dizziness, syncope Edema Headache (cyclic) Irritability Leg cramps Nausea, vomiting Visual changes (cyclic) Weight gain (cyclic)	N/A	N/A	N/A	Bloating Dizziness, syncope Edema Headache (cyclic) Irritability Leg cramps Nausea, vomiting Visual changes (cyclic) Weight gain (cyclic)

N/A = not applicable.

Sources: Caufield (2003); Dickey (2002), and Hatcher et al. (1998).

may place a woman at an increased risk. (Endrikat, Klipping, Cronin, et al., 2002; Lawrenson & Farmer, 2000; Spitzer, 2000; Westhoff, 2000; Winkler, 2000).

Hypertension

Hypertension is a relative contraindication to OC use even if a woman's blood pressure is well controlled on antihypertensive medications (Narkiewicz, Graniero, D-Este, et al., 1995). Both estrogen and progestin may cause mild elevations in blood pressure in approximately 5% of normotensive women and 9 to 16% of hypertensive women. Monitoring blood pressure in women taking OCs is recommended, and if it is elevated, switching to an OC with a lower progestational activity or discontinuing therapy should result in a normalization of blood pressure within 3 months. Women are more likely to develop hypertension with increasing age, longer duration of OC use, and family history of hypertension. However, hypertension may occur in women without risk factors and at any time while receiving OCs (Bucci & Carson, 1997; Dickey, 2002; Kaunitz, 2001a).

Lipid Metabolism

OCs may alter lipid metabolism. Estrogen has beneficial effects on the lipid profile. Conversely, progestins, especially those with appreciable androgenic activity, may raise LDL-cholesterol and lower HDL-cholesterol. Differences among OC formulations in the propensity to affect the lipid profile have been demonstrated in various clinical studies. Some studies suggest that third-generation progestin formulations containing desogestrel, gestodene, and norgestimate have resulted in beneficial effects on the lipid profile, raising HDL-cholesterol and reducing LDL-cholesterol, and suggest a potential cardioprotective effect with long-term use (Endrikat, et al., 2002; Kaunitz, 2001a; Lobo, Skinner, Lippman, & Cirillo, 1996; Wiegratz, Lee, Kutschera, Bauer, et al., 2002). Regardless of the lipid profile changes resulting from OCs, the detrimental cardiovascular effects (stroke, venous thromboem-

TABLE 18–21. Management Strategies for Commonly Occurring Adverse Effects

Adverse Effect	Causal Factors	Management Strategies
Menstrual Disorders		
Absence of withdrawal menses	• Insufficient estrogen to develop endometrium and vessels • Most common in women taking low-dose estrogen OCs • May appear after OCs have been taken for several months	• Rule out pregnancy • Continue same OC without menses • Continue same OC and add exogenous estrogen for 1 mo. • Switch to OC with same amount estrogen but increased endometrial activity
Dysmenorrhea	• Rare in anovulatory cycles unless there is passage of blood clots • Endometriosis	• Switch to OC with more progestin/androgen activity and less estrogen activity • Use an NSAID
Heavy menstruation	• Insufficient progestin activity or excess estrogen activity	• Rule out pathological causes • Switch to OC with more progestin/androgen activity or less estrogen activity
Breakthrough bleeding (BTB) and spotting	• Early BTB: insufficient estrogen activity, associated with failure to menstruate during off days • Late BTB: insufficient progestin activity • Most common with low-dose OCs • Most common reason for discontinuation	• Rule out pathological condition, inconsistent pill-taking and pregnancy; reassure • Allow three cycles for patient to adjust to OC • Switch to OC with more endometrial activity
Sensory-Nervous System		
Dizziness	• Associated with fluid retention • Usually disappears after third cycle	• Switch to OC with less estrogen activity
Headache	• May be due to estrogen • Usually associated with fluid retention or vascular spasm	• Switch to OC with less estrogen activity • May have to discontinue OC if headache persists; stop if severe visual symptoms, or aura
Depression	• May be due to progestin • Characterized by apathy, listlessness, feelings of dejection, anorexia, insomnia, and restlessness	• Switch to OC with less progestin activity • Consider discontinuing OC if depression occurs in patients with history of depression, or depressive severe • Vitamin B_6 (pyridoxine) may be used
Other Side Effects		
Acne and hirsutism	• Associated with androgenic activity • Low-dose pills improve acne	• Switch to OC with more estrogen activity • Switch to OC with less androgen activity
Nausea and vomiting	• Associated with estrogen dose • Most severe with initial cycles	• Take with food or at bedtime • Switch to OC with less estrogen activity
Weight change	• Associated with both estrogen and progestin depending if cyclic or noncyclic weight gain • Studies do not find association between weight gain and OC use	• Switch to OC with less progestin and less androgen if appetite increases hypoglycemic symptoms • Switch to OC with less estrogen activity if cyclic weight gain in breast, hips, and thighs

Sources: Caufield (2003); Dickey (2002); Hatcher et al. (1998).

TABLE 18–22. Contraindications to OC Use

Absolute	Relative
Cardiovascular: thrombophlebitis, thromboembolic disorders, cerebral vascular disease	Migraine or vascular headaches
Breast cancer: known or suspected	Hypertension
Endometrical cancer: known or suspected	Recent hepatitis
Estrogen-dependent neoplasia: known or suspected	Diabetes mellitus or history or gestational diabetes
Hepatic ademoma, carcinoma or benign liver tumors	Obesity >20% of ideal body weight
Impaired liver function	History or cardiac or renal dysfunction
Pregnancy: known or suspected	Hyperlipidemia
Undiagnosed abnormal vaginal bleeding	Psychic depression
	Age over 50
	Age over 35 for smoker
	Sickle-cell or sickle-C disease
	Ulcerative colitis
	Use of drugs known to interact with OCs

Adapted from Caufield (2003); Dickey (2002); Hatcher et al. (1998); Hatcher et al. (2001); Speroff (2000).

bolism, and myocardial infarction) demonstrated with OC use are thought to be caused by the thrombogenic properties of OCs, and are not related to lipid alterations.

Glucose Intolerance/Insulin Insensitivity

Most women without diabetes do not experience glucose intolerance or changes in insulin sensitivity while taking low-dose OCs, although high-dose older OC formulations have resulted in increased glucose levels, increased plasma insulin levels, and decreased glucose tolerance. (Nelson, 2001; Speroff, 2000). Diabetes mellitus increases with new low-dose pills have not been shown (Gaspard, Scheen, Endrikat, Buicu, et al., 2003). Norgestimate and desogestrel are not thought to alter glucose metabolism. If an OC is prescribed to a woman who has a history of glucose intolerance, it would be advisable to choose one containing a third-generation progestin to minimize adverse carbohydrate effects and to monitor glucose tolerance on a periodic basis (Hatcher et al., 1998; Speroff, 2000). Please refer to the special populations section in this chapter for information on the use of OCs in women with diabetes.

Venous Thromboembolism and Pulmonary Embolism

Venous thromboembolism and pulmonary embolism are rare, yet serious, complications of OCs. For this reason OCs should not be used in women with a history of deep venous thrombosis (DVT). The estrogen component of OCs has been shown to increase the hepatic synthesis of selected vitamin K–dependent clotting factors and fibrinogen, decrease the activity of antithrombin III and protein S (endogenous inhibitors of clotting), and increase platelet aggregation. These effects lead to an increased propensity for thrombosis, especially in women who smoke. The incidence of venous thromboembolism was reported in early studies to be 3 to 11 times higher in women who used OCs compared to nonusers. (Heinemann, 2000; Lawrenson & Farmer, 2000; Wiegratz et al., 2002; Winkler, 2000).

Studies with second-generation progestins have been "associated with an unfavorable effect on lipid profile [leading to a] potential risk of arterial disease" (Westhoff, 2000, p. 1). Third-generation progestins, with weak androgenic activity, "may have the potential to reduce the risk of adverse arterial events" (Westhoff, 2000, p.1).

Taking a careful family and personal history for increased risk of venous thromboembolism is highly recommended. Risk factors for venous thromboembolism include hereditary thrombophilia, lupus anticoagulant, malignancy, immobility or trauma, obesity, and varicose veins (Katzung, 2001). It may be advisable for women who have risks for venous thromboembolism not to be initially started on OCs and, if started, to obtain a signed informed consent. A close family history of thrombophlebitis or thromboembolic disorder should be an absolute contraindication to OC use since this suggests an inherited susceptibility (Dickey, 2002).

Myocardial Infarction

In addition to an increased risk for venous thromboembolism, women who receive OCs have a greater relative risk for myocardial infarction (MI), primarily if other cardiovascular risks are present. The risk of MI increases with advancing age and cigarette smoking. Women who smoke and are over 35 years old are at an increased risk for MI and other cardiovascular conditions, such as stroke and venous thromboembolism. For this reason, OCs should not be used in women older than 35 years of age who smoke. Data indicate OCs with less than 50 μg of estrogen may be used in healthy, nonsmoking women up to 50 years old (Dickey, 2002; Hatcher et al., 1998). However, the lowest dosage possible in an OC for safety and efficacy should always be used.

Risk for MI also may vary depending on the type of progestin in the OC formulation. Heinemann (2000) and Lewis, Spitzer, Heinemann, et al., (1996) report that third-generation progestins are associated with a reduction in MI risk or with no difference in risk compared to second-generation OCs. Women taking OCs containing less than 50 μg of estrogen and a second-generation progestin had a significantly increased odds ratio of acute MI of 3.1 compared to nonusers of OC. In those women receiving third-generation OCs the odds ratio was 1.1, indicating no increase in MI risk compared to women not receiving OCs. The risk of MI with second-generation OCs is still considered low when compared to results of studies published in the 1970s with higher-dose OCs. Age is a major factor, as is smoking. A recent meta-analysis (Spitzer, Faith, & MacRae, 2002, p. 2307) "confirms that third-generation OCs do not convey harm in regard to MI compared with non-users of OCs." However, other authors (ACOG practice bulletin #18, 2000; Keeling, 2003; Tanis, van den Bosch, Kemmeren, Cats, et al., 2001) caution clinicians about prescribing oral contraceptives to smokers over 35 years old.

Stroke

Another complication associated with OCs is stroke, either thrombotic (ischemic) or hemorrhagic. Early data with higher dose pills suggested the risk of stroke was 5 times greater in pill users versus nonusers, with even greater risk in those women who smoked (Bucci & Carson, 1997; Heinemann, 2000). The World Health Organization [WHO] Collaborative Study (1996a) demonstrated that the risk of hemorrhagic stroke was not increased in younger women and was only slightly increased in older women when receiving currently prescribed low-dose OCs. Another study examining the risk of thrombotic and hemorrhagic stroke has also concluded that new, low-dose OCs do not place healthy women of childbearing age at any greater risk for stroke (Endrikat et al., 2002; Heinemann, 2000). Women with diabetes and hypertension generally were not given OCs in this study. Another study (WHO Collaborative Study, 1996b) evaluated ischemic stroke and combined oral contraceptives and found the incidence of ischemic stroke to be low in women of reproductive age. Furthermore, the risk can be reduced if users are younger and do not smoke or have a history of hypertension. After age 40 women who use OCs have a greater risk of thrombotic stroke (Dickey, 2002).

NEOPLASTIC EFFECTS

The association between OC use and breast cancer has been evaluated in many epidemiologic reports (Hawley, Nuevo, DeNeef, & Carter, 1993; Herbst & Berek, 1993; Nelson, 2001). A meta-analysis (Collaborative Group, 1996) using data from 54 epidemiologic studies, including a total of 53,297 women with breast cancer and 100,239 women without breast cancer, was conducted. This meta-analysis concluded that in women currently taking OCs and within 10 years of discontinuing OCs, there was a small increase in the risk of contracting breast cancer. Current OC users had a 24% greater risk of breast cancer compared to nonusers. The risk was greater in higher dose OCs and decreased progressively after OC discontinuation. If diagnosed, breast cancer in OC users was less clinically advanced than breast cancer diagnosed in non-OC users. Moreover, a slightly decreased risk of breast cancer was found in those women who had stopped using OCs for more than 10 years. It is unclear whether these findings were due to earlier diagnosis of breast cancer, to biological hormonal effects, or to a combination of these factors. Results of the Women's Contraceptive and Reproductive Experiences (Women's CARE) Study demonstrate no significant association between OC use and breast cancer (Marchbanks, McDonald, Wilson, Folger, et al., 2002). These study results confirm the earlier Cancer and Steroid Hormone (CASH) study conducted in 1986.

The effect of OCs on cervical cancer remains unclear because of the many variables other than OC use that may influence the risk of cervical cancer (Katzung, 2001). These variables include number of sexual partners and age at first coitus, exposure to human papillomavirus, use of barrier contraceptives, and smoking. Because the risk of cervical cancer is unknown, periodic cervical screening should be performed.

As briefly discussed earlier, women who use combination OCs are at a lower risk for development of endometrial and ovarian cancer. Epidemiologic studies (Jensen & Speroff, 2000; Likis, 2002) demonstrate the ability of combination oral contraceptives to provide a substantial protective effect against ovarian and endometrial cancers. These contraceptives offer between a 40 and 80% risk reduction against ovarian cancer with risk decreasing the longer OCs are used. In addition, OC users enjoy an approximate 50% decreased risk of endometrial cancer. The risk reduction begins within the first year of use, and protection endures for at least 15 years after OCs have been discontinued. This decreased risk is thought to involve the maintenance of regular withdrawal bleeding (Centers for Disease Control, 1987a, 1987b; Contraception for Women, 2001).

Although extremely rare, an increase in hepatocellular adenomas has been associated with OC use. These benign tumors, occurring in 1.3 per million women between 31 and 44 years of age using OCs, may lead to rupturing of the liver capsule and death. Ongoing, severe abdominal pain is a sign of this complication (Hatcher et al., 1998).

DRUG INTERACTIONS

Obtaining an accurate medication history is essential to ensure that drug interactions do not go unnoticed or compromise patient care. Medication history taking may be complicated in OC users because many women do not consider the pill to be a "drug"; therefore, they may not disclose taking OCs when asked about current medications (Likis, 2002). Additionally, multiple physicians may be involved, one prescribing the OC and another prescribing a potentially interacting medication. Many medications have the potential to reduce the efficacy of OCs, thereby putting a woman at risk for pregnancy. Breakthrough bleeding may be a sign that a drug interaction has occurred (Dickey, 2002). Mechanisms by which drugs may interact with OCs include interference with gastrointestinal absorption, alteration in gastrointestinal bacterial flora, and pharmacokinetic changes. Additionally, OCs may interfere with other medications or exacerbate various disease states, thereby reducing the effectiveness of drug therapy. Aspirin and aceptaminophen users may need higher doses (Dickey, 2002). Table 18–23 provides information on drug interactions with oral contraceptives along with management strategies.

In addition to medications altering the serum concentration of OCs, grapefruit juice and vitamin C may increase the bioavailability of ethinyl estradiol. The clinical importance of this interaction has not yet been demonstrated; however, if estrogen concentrations are elevated significantly, a woman may be at risk for cardiovascular complications (Bucci & Carson, 1997; Weber et al., 1996).

Women should also be asked about their use of over-the-counter herbal products. Products such as the herb St. John's wort, commonly used for depression, may decrease

TABLE 18–23. Selected Drug Interactions with Combined Oral Contraceptives and Management Strategies

Drug Class	Generic Name (Trade)	Effect	Patient Management
Drugs That May Reduce Effectiveness of Oral Contraceptives			
Antibiotics	Erythromycin Penicillins Tetracycline	No evidence found that OC efficacy is reduced by antibiotics.	Use second method of contraception during the treatment course and for at least 1 week after discontinuing the antibiotic (1 month for rifampin).
		Antibiotics may eliminate GI bacteria, thereby disturbing the enterohepatic circulation of estrogen, which results in lower serum estrogen concentrations. GI transport may increase or diarrhea may also decrease absorption of estrogen.	
	Griseofulvin Rifampin	Griseofulvin or rifampin may increase estrogen metabolism.	
Antivirals	Ritonavir (Norvir) Nevirapine (Viramune)	Ritonavir may lower estrogen levels by about 40%; nevirapine may lower serum levels of OCs.	Use alternative method of contraception.
Anticonvulsants (including barbiturates)	Carbamazepine (Tegretol) Felbamate (Felbatol) Phenobarbital Phenytoin (Dilantin) Primidone (Mysoline)	Induction of liver microsomal enzymes (increases metabolism), leading to decreased OC effect.	Use alternative method of contraception or consider a higher-dose product (50 µ g ethinyl estradiol; monitor for signs of estrogenic side effects). Valproic acid does not appear to interact with OCs.
Effect of Oral Contraceptive on Other Drugs or Disease States			
Anticoagulants	Warfarin (Coumadin)	OCs increase vitamin-K–dependent clotting factors, decrease efficacy of anticoagulant.	Do not use OCs in patients who require anticoagulation.
Antidiabetic agents	Insulin; oral hypoglycemics	High-dose OCs may impair glucose tolerance.	Use low-dose estrogen and progestin OC or alternative method.
Antihypertensives		OCs may increase blood pressure.	Use alternative method in patients with hypertension or switch to low-dose OC.
Beta blockers	Acebutolol (Sectral) Metoprolol (Lopressor) Propranolol (Inderal)	OCs lower metabolism of some beta blockers, thereby increasing their effects.	Increase dose of beta blocker if needed; monitor cardiovascular status.
Bronchodilators	Theophylline	Increase effect of theophylline.	Use with caution.
Corticosteroids	Prednisone	OCs raise serum levels.	May need to lower dose of steroid.
Tricyclic antiepressants	Amitriptyline (Elavil) and others	OCs may increase the metabolism of tricyclic antidepressants (TCAs), thereby increasing their effects.	Monitor for TCA toxicity and lower dose if necessary.
Anxiolytics	Diazepam (Valium) Chlordiazepoxide (Librium)	OCs may increase the effects.	Monitor for overdose and lower dose if necessary.
Antibiotics	Troandomycin	Increase risk of cholestasis.	Use alternative method of contraception.

Source: Caufield (2003); Dickey (2002); Hatcher et al. (1998); Novir, Rezulin, and Viramune package inserts.

the effectiveness of oral contraceptives, therefore, women should be advised to refrain from concomitant use or to use a second method of birth control (Likis, 2002).

CHOOSING AN ORAL CONTRACEPTIVE AND INITIATING THERAPY

Before deciding to place a woman on an OC, the clinician needs to address several issues such as contraindications, drug interactions, patient lifestyle, compliance, acceptance, hormone sensitivity, and cost. According to an economic study on contraception, the most cost-effective forms of contraception are the copper-T IUD, vasectomy, and injectable and implantable contraceptives. Although oral contraceptives cost just under $2,000 over 5 years, based on a 1995 study, the cost savings related to prevented pregnancies is almost $15,000, making the method quite cost effective for women wishing to postpone pregnancy (Burkman, 2001b). Reevaluation of economic cost/benefits should be undertaken to include new contraceptive methods including Lunelle, NuvaRing, Mirena, and the transdermal patch. Additionally, advantages and disadvantages of OCs should be discussed with patients.

Once it has been determined to use an OC, many formulations are available, each with differences in potential side effects and tolerability. Since high-dose OCs are associated with increased risks, the clinician should initiate OC therapy with the lowest estrogen dose that is effective: E. Estradiol level of 35 μg or less (Caufield, 2003; Dickey, 2002). In addition, Caufield (2003) suggests initiating low-dose monophasic combined OCs such as Alesse, Levlite, or LoEstrin 1/20 with older women.

Patients may have inherent sensitivities to the estrogenic, progestational, androgenic, or endometrial effects of OCs. If a woman appears more sensitive to a certain type of activity, initial OC selection should minimize this effect. For example, a woman who is more sensitive to estrogenic effects may have a history of migraine, severe nausea, vomiting, or hypertension during pregnancy; large or fibrocystic breasts; and heavy menses. An OC with lower estrogenic activity would be an appropriate choice for this patient. A woman would be considered to be progestin-sensitive if she has a history of toxemia, excessive weight gain, tiredness, or varicose veins during pregnancy; depression; and excessive premenstrual edema. Androgen sensitivity is associated with irregular heavy menses, acne, hirsutism, and oily skin. An OC with high progestational activity and low androgenic activity would be appropriate in this setting. Tables 18–19 and 18–20 also may be used to guide a practitioner in OC selection (Dickey, 2002; Hatcher et al., 1998).

Before a woman is placed on an OC, a complete medical history and physical examination should be conducted and repeated at least once a year while using OCs. The physical examination may be deferred by the physician if requested by the patient. The physical examination should include blood pressure, breasts, abdomen, and pelvic organs. Cervical cytology and any pertinent laboratory tests should also be checked.

PATIENT INSTRUCTIONS AND COMPLIANCE ISSUES

Although the annual failure rate is 0.1% with perfect OC use, typical users have an annual failure rate averaging 5%, and higher failure rates may occur in certain populations. The primary reason for this discrepancy between perfect and typical failure rates is lack of compliance. As many as one half of women discontinue OCs within the first year of use, primarily due to fear of potential side effects and actual side effects such as breakthrough bleeding (Nelson, 2001). Those OC users who discontinue therapy may not adopt alternate means of birth control, placing themselves at an additional risk for pregnancy. Providing adequate counseling is crucial in improving compliance and enhancing OC effectiveness (Burkman, 2001a; Likis, 2002; Nelson, 2001). Table 18–24 provides counseling suggestions for providers to use with their patients in the hopes of improving patient correct OC use.

Specific directions for taking OCs should be discussed and provided to patients in writing along with the package insert and product information required for estrogen products. Patients should be instructed to read all directions and take the pill at approximately the same time every day, which promotes compliance and consistent plasma concentrations. There are 21-day and 28-day pill packs, each containing 21 "active" pills. The 28-day pill packs contain seven placebo pills taken during the last week. There is also a 91-day extended use pack, recently approved by the FDA for use in the United States. It contains 84 "active" pills and 7 placebo pills (FDA approves Seasonale, 2003). The woman with unpleasant symptoms during the hormone-free interval benefits from extended-cycle OCs with reduced symptoms and bleeding, without loss of safety (Arias, 2003; Darney, 2003). Taking a pill daily with no off days may be easier for some women to remember. OCs are started on the

TABLE 18–24. Suggestions for Improving Correct OC Use

Recommendation	Comment
What women should know before starting OCs	1. How OCs work and how to take them. 2. What to do if they miss a pill or pills. 3. Common, transient, and serious side effects.
Dispel OC misinformation	Also discuss health benefits from OCs; put in proper perspective.
Instructions	Verbal and written instructions given to all patients, discussed point by point; each followup visit should offer another copy of instructions. If questions arise at a later point, make sure the patient knows how to get additional information.
Demonstrate use of pill pack	All users, especially first-time users. Proper use enhanced with 28-day pack.
Time of day to take OC	Help select specific time; may want to briefly discuss daily schedule to identify optimal time; taking after dinner or with a bedtime snack may cause nausea.
Extra refills	Include extra cycle in prescription for missed pills or lost packets.
Missed pills procedure	Discuss backup method.
STDs	Discuss prevention of STDs. Provide condoms and discuss proper use.
Followup visits; inquire about problems	A nonjudgmental approach to uncover and solve problems with taking pills. Ask what was done if a pill was missed. Schedule followup in 1–2 months.
Repeated compliance problems	Counsel women about using another method if OC user has repeated difficulty remembering to take OC.

Sources: Caufield (2003); Hatcher et al. (1998).

first day of menses or on the first Sunday after the onset of menses. If menses begin on Sunday, the women should start taking the OC that same Sunday. Initiating OCs on Sunday will usually avoid menses during the weekend. Those patients starting OC on the first day of menses will not require any backup contraceptive method; however, Sunday starters need to use an alternate contraception method as a backup for 7 days (Dickey, 2002). The patient's next menses will begin during the 7 placebo tablets if using a 28-day or 91-day pill pack. If using a 21-day pill pack, the patient should be instructed to start the next pack 1 week after finishing the last, even if she is still menstruating (Hatcher et al., 1998).

Missing scheduled pills is a common occurrence in both adolescents and older women. Greydanus et al. (2001) note that while the typical use failure rate for adults is 5%, for the adolescent population the failure rate varies between 5 and 15%. These authors suggest lack of compliance, ambivalence, worries about side effects, and ability to stick to a regimen of taking the pill once a day at the same time every day as the four major areas leading to the increased failure rate among adolescents. In addition to providing patient education to improve taking OCs correctly and reduce the incidence of missing pills, it is equally important to make sure patients understand what to do if an active pill or pills have been missed. If an inactive pill has been missed, the patient should be instructed to throw away the missed pills and start the next pill pack on the regularly scheduled day. Since these are placebo tablets, missing one of the last seven pills in a 28-day or 91-day OC pack will not put a woman at risk for pregnancy. Data suggest that the most critical times to miss pills are directly prior to or after the 7-day hormone-free period (Dickey, 2002). Table 18–25 provides guidelines for missed "active" pills. Other reasons to use an alternate form of contraception in addition to missed pills include diarrhea, vomiting, and administration of interacting drugs that might reduce the effectiveness of OCs. Diarrhea or vomiting may reduce the amount of estrogen and progestin absorbed. Table 18–23 provides a list of drugs that may reduce the efficacy of OCs. A backup method should be used in these situations for the remainder of the cycle. OCs do not protect against STDs, including HIV. For this reason, consistently and correctly using latex or polyurethane condoms is highly recommended. Some practitioners recommend using an alternate method during the first pill pack, although FDA guidelines state a backup method is only required for the first 7 days in those patients starting on Sunday (Dickey, 2002; Hatcher et al, 1998).

Return to fertility may be delayed after OCs have been discontinued. Some practitioners suggest that women wait two to three normal menstrual periods before becoming pregnant to allow for reestablishment of ovulation and menses. No increase in birth defects has been shown in women who conceived in the month after OC discontinuation (Bucci & Carson, 1997).

Some patient conditions, such as endometriosis, suggest use of OCs continuously without a break for a period of 3 months or longer (Hatcher et al., 2001).

TABLE 18–25. Guidelines for Missed "Active" Pills

Pills Missed	Time in Cycle	Patient Interactions
1	Anytime	• Take pill as soon as you remember. Take the next pill at your regular time (you may take 2 pills in one day). • Backup method of contraception is not necessary
2	First 2 weeks	• Take 2 pills on the day you remember and 2 pills the next day. • Then take 1 pill a day until you finish the pack. • You MAY BECOME PREGNANT if you have intercourse in the 7 days after you miss pills. You MUST use another contraceptive method for those 7 days.
2	Third week	• Day 1 starter: Throw out the pill pack and start a new pack that same day. • Sunday starter: Keep taking 1 pill every day until Sunday; on Sunday, throw out pill pack and start a new pack that same day. • It is expected that you will not have a period this month. However, if you miss your period 2 months in a row, call your doctor or clinic because you may be pregnant. • You MAY BECOME PREGNANT if you have intercourse in the 7 days after you miss pills. You MUST use another contraceptive method for those 7 days.
3	Anytime	• Day 1 starter: Throw out the pill pack and start a new pack that same day. • Sunday starter: Keep taking 1 pill every day until Sunday; on Sunday, throw out pill pack and start a new pack that same day. • It is expected that you will not have a period this month. However, if you miss your period 2 months in a row, call your doctor or clinic because you may be pregnant. • You MAY BECOME PREGNANT if you have intercourse in the 7 days after you miss pills. You MUST use another contraceptive method for those 7 days.

Sources: Caufield (2003); Dickey (2002); Hatcher et al. (1998).

LONG-ACTING INJECTABLE COMBINED HORMONAL CONTRACEPTIVE

Approved by the FDA for distribution in the United States in October 2000, Lunelle is a monthly combination hormone injection for contraception (Kaunitz, 2001c; Wysocki, 2001). The product contains 25 mg of medroxyprogesterone acetate (MPA) and 5 mg of estradiol cypionate (E_2C), which, in combination, provide "pharmacologic properties of nearly pure progesterone and natural estrogen, thereby minimizing the potential for adverse effects" (Wysocki, 2001, p. 56). This injectable contraceptive inhibits ovulation, which is its primary mechanism of action. Lunelle has been studied worldwide by the World Health Organization since 1981 (Kaunitz, 2001c; Shulman, 2000), with pregnancy rates reported to range from "0–2 pregnancies per 1000 women-years of use" (Shulman, 2000, p. 726). Recommended dose is 0.5 mL, injected intramuscularly every 28 to 30 days. Initial injection should be administered within 5 days of the onset of a normal menstrual period, within 7 days following a first-trimester abortion, or between 3 and 6 weeks postpartum (Kaunitz, 2000). Lunelle carries the same contraindications as those listed for combination oral contraceptives. These include known or suspected pregnancy, past or present history of thrombophlebitis or thomboembolic disorders, cerebral vascular or coronary artery disease, liver dysfunction, breast or endometrial cancer, or undiagnosed abnormal vaginal bleeding.

PROGESTIN-ONLY CONTRACEPTIVES

Estrogen is not an essential component to pregnancy prevention. Progestin-only compounds provide contraceptive protection to women who are unable to take combined OCs because of their side effects and risks. Mechanism of action includes suppression of LH and FSH, which inhibits ovulation; decreased and thicker cervical mucus, which inhibits sperm motility; and atrophic changes in the endometrium (Hatcher et al., 1998; Schnare, 2002). Progestin-only contraceptives are considered safe for women who have contraindications to estrogen-containing contraceptives (World Health Organization, 2000).

The "Minipill"

The minipill is a progestin-only pill that delivers the same dose of progestin every day (see Table 18–17 for a list of minipill OCs). Minipills are prescribed to a minority of women. They are not used as frequently as combination OCs because of decreased efficacy and a propensity for untoward side effects such as breakthrough bleeding or spotting. However, in certain patients, mini-pills may offer advantages over combination OCs. Reasons to choose a minipill include a contraindication to the estrogen component of combined OC (i.e., thromboembolism); risk for estrogen-related side effects such as hypertension, headache, and varicose veins; previous patient experiences of intolerable side effects from estrogen in combination OC; smokers older than 35 years of age; and breastfeeding mothers. Estrogen suppresses lactation, and since this effect is not present with progestin-only OCs, the minipill is an excellent choice for a breastfeeding mother. Starting on the first day of menses, patients take the minipill every day without a 7-day pill-free interval. A backup method of contraception is not necessary during the initial cycle because effects on cervical mucus appear immediately; however, it may be prudent to use an alternate method during this time because of the potential to forget pills or take them late during the initial cycle. Table 18–26 provides additional information on progestin-only pills (Dickey, 2002; Hatcher et al., 1998; Schnare, 2002).

Long-Acting Progestin Contraceptives

Medroxyprogesterone Acetate. Depot-medroxy-progesterone acetate (DMPA) (Depo-Provera) inhibits ovulation by suppression of FSH and LH levels and by eliminating the LH surge. Additionally, DMPA produces an atrophic endometrium and thick cervical mucus, decreasing sperm penetration. DMPA is administered as a 150-mg deep IM injection given in the gluteal, deltoid, or quadricep muscle within 5 days after the onset of menstrual bleeding and repeated every 3 months. Initially, administration during the first few days of the menstrual cycle ensures an immediate contraceptive effect, improves efficacy, and avoids administration in pregnancy. Vials contain 150 mg/mL. Prior to injection, the vial should be shaken to produce an even dispersion of the suspension. Massaging the injection site is not recommended because this is associated with higher initial serum levels but lower levels after 90 days. Although DMPA should be administered every 3 months, there is a 2-week "grace period" in which the patient may be late in receiving the next injection yet still be protected from becoming pregnant (Bucci & Carson, 1997; Hatcher et al, 1998; Hatcher et al., 2001).

Advantages and disadvantages of DMPA are listed in Table 18–27. Fertility may be delayed after discontinuation of DMPA for up to 24 months. After 15 and 24 months from the last injection, 75% and 95% of women conceive, respectively. Therefore, if a woman is planning on conceiving within the next year, DMPA is not an appropriate method. Bone density may be negatively affected due to the fact that DMPA inhibits the secretion of pituitary gonadotropin, which suppresses estrogen production (American Academy of Pediatrics, 1999). Studies (Cundy, Cornish, Roberts, et al., 1998; Gbolade, Ellis, Murby, et al., 1998; Scholes, LaCroix, Ichikawa, et al., 1998) have found lower bone density in long-term DMPA users with effects being most pronounced in younger women. These effects appear to be reversible, and the clinical significance of bone density changes remains unknown.

TABLE 18–26. Progestin-Only Pills (Minipills)

Mechanism	• Inhibit ovulation by suppression of LH. • Produce thick cervical mucus, which hampers sperm transport. • Inhibit the enzymes that allow sperm to penetrate the ovum (capacitation). • Slow ovum transport. • Inhibit implantation due to atrophic changes in the endometrium.
Effectiveness	• Low failure rate: 0.5% per year. • Typical failure rate: 3% per year.
Major adverse effects	• Menstrual cycle disturbance.
Advantages	• No adverse effects related to estrogen. • Safer than combined OCs. • Nursing mothers: Does not reduce lactation. • May use in women who cannot receive estrogen (refer to estrogen contraindications) or in women who are experiencing intolerable adverse effects from estrogen. However, according to FDA requirements, package insert information for minipills lists contraindications related to estrogen.
Disadvantages	• May be less effective than combined OC. Compliance with minipills is essential. • Timing is critical to ensure effectiveness. Must be taken no more than 27 hours between doses. • Slightly higher risk for ectopic pregnancy and functional ovarian cyst.
Precautions	• A backup contraceptive method during the initial 7 to 28 days on minipills should be used. • If a minipill is taken over 3 h late, another contraceptive method should be used for 48 h. • If a minipill is missed, a backup method should be used until the woman restarts or until her next period.

Sources: Dickey, 2002; Hatcher et al., 1998; Schnare, 2002.

TABLE 18–27. Advantages and Disadvantages of Depot-Medroxyprogesterone Acetate (DMPA)

Advantages	Disadvantages
• Safe, effective, reversible, long-acting method • Decreased dysmenorrhea and blood loss • Does not require medical personnel to remove (unlike Norplant) and is simple to administer • Ectopic pregnancy risk reduced • Privacy maintained • Patient memory only required for followup injections every 3 months (does not need to remember daily or with intercourse) • May give to patients for whom estrogen is contraindicated; may reduce ovarian/endometrial cancer risk • Drug interactions not reported with use • Will not suppress lactation; increases milk • Reduces iron-deficiency anemia, sickle-cell anemia; may decrease number and severity of sickle crises • Considered immediately effective; fear of pregnancy lessened • May improve endometriosis	• Menstrual disturbance: occurs in the majority of women with irregular unpredictable spotting or continuous heavy bleeding (uncommon); amenorrhea after 1 year of use develops in 33–50% of women; primary reason for discontinuation • Delayed fertility—average 10 months; 25% 1 year • Risk of osteoporosis: decreased bone mineral density • Weight gain; increased appetite • Depression • Breast cancer risk: may enhance the growth of preexisting tumors • Condoms needed for STD protection • Some experience decreased libido • Headaches • Possible elevation of LDL; lowered HDL • If allergic, cannot discontinue • Breast tenderness

Sources: Caufield (2003); Gordon & Speroff (2002); Hatcher et al. (1998); Hatcher et al. (2001).

Other adverse effects include weight gain (1 to 4 kg per year on average, depending on the study), depression, headache, abdominal bloating, asthenia, dizziness, nervousness, mild elevations in serum triglycerides, decreases in HDL-cholesterol, and increases in LDL-cholesterol and total cholesterol (Bucci & Carson, 1997; Frederiksen, 1996; Hatcher et al., 1998; Hatcher et al., 2001; Sangi-Haghpeyka, Poindexter, Bateman, & Ditmore, 1996; Westoff, 1996). One study evaluating the use of DMPA in an urban setting noted a low continuation rate at 1 year of 28.6%. Patients discontinued therapy because of intolerable side effects and changes in their menstrual cycle (Sangi-Haghpeykar et al., 1996).

DMPA had been used in other countries for several decades prior to approval for use in the United States by the FDA in 1993. The reason for this delay was concern over the potential for an increased risk for breast cancer, documented in studies on beagle dogs given prolonged exposure to high-dose DMPA. Subsequently, two large, retrospective case-controlled studies have evaluated the risk for breast cancer in women treated with DMPA (Paul, Skegg, & Spears, 1989; WHO Collaborative Study, 1991). In DMPA users, the overall risk of breast cancer is no higher than in nonusers; however, the risk in certain populations is higher. One study found a slight increase in risk in the first 4 years of use (WHO Collaborative Study, 1991). The risk did not increase over time. Another study showed that women under 35 years of age at diagnosis who had ever received DMPA were at elevated risk. Women between ages 25–34 were observed to have a relative risk of 2.0, and those who had been given DMPA for more than 2 years before age 25 had an even higher relative risk of 4.6 (Paul et al., 1989). Findings from these studies suggest that DMPA may enhance the growth of preexisting tumors, and the risk for breast cancer appears to be similar to the risk found with oral contraceptives (Kaunitz, 1996).

The effect of DMPA on other types of reproductive cancers has also been studied. DMPA is associated with a reduction of 80% in endometrial cancer. Ovarian cancer may be reduced, and cervical cancer appears to be unaffected by the use of DMPA (Hatcher et al., 2001; Kaunitz, 1996; Thomas, Ray, & WHO, 1995).

Levonorgestrel Implant. In December 1990, the Food and Drug Administration approved the long-acting levonorgestrel implant (Norplant). Levonorgestrel is the synthetic progestin contained in the 6 flexible, nonbiodegradable, hollow silastic (silicon rubber) tubes that are inserted under the skin of the upper arm. The progestin slowly diffuses into systemic circulation for 5 years, and serum levels of levonorgestrel gradually decline over this time. The level of progestin is lower than that found in combination OCs. Norplant (6-capsule) was removed from the market by the manufacturer due to a concern that some lots might release insufficient levonorgestrel to maintain adequate contraception (Lunelle use rises, 2001; Schnare, 2002). However, it was reinstated for use in 2002, stating backup methods had been determined not to be needed (Update on advisory for norplant, 2002). In a letter to health care professionals, Weyth acknowledges that the 6-capsule Norplant system will no longer be manufactured so that as clients reach the 5-year expiration date, other contraceptive options will be needed (2002 safety alert—Norplant, 2002). Norplant-2, also a levonorgestrel long-acting implant, was approved by the FDA in November 1996 for distribution in the United States. It consists of 2 silastic rods, each containing 70 mg of the progestin hormone released at a steady rate over a 2-year period (Brache, Faundes, Alvarez, & Cochon, 2002; Croxatto, 2002; Glasier, 2002; Qin, Goldber, & Hao, 2001). The mechanism of action for both Norplant and Norplant-2 is similar to the mechanism of Depo-Provera.

Heavier women have a larger volume of distribution with lower serum concentration of levonorgestrel, leading to an increased risk of pregnancy. Hatcher et al. (1998, p. 471) notes the pregnancy risk is "2.4% after 5 years among women weighing more than 154 pounds and 1.5% among women weighing 131 to 153 pounds." Insertion is recommended during the first 7 days of the menstrual cycle to ensure ovulation is inhibited. If insertion is delayed past this time, a backup method of contraception is recommended (Schnare, 2002).

Norplant has side effects that are similar to other progestin-only contraceptive methods. The most common adverse effect is irregular menstrual bleeding, occurring during the first year in about 40% of women (Erskine, Shinewi, Pollard, & Kubba, 2000). Table 18–28 shows selected common adverse effects that may occur in women using Norplant. Other side effects include headache, nausea, dizziness, depression, acne, weight gain, and hirsutism (Brache et al., 2002).

TABLE 18–28. Selected Common Adverse Effects from Norplant

Adverse Effect	Incidence, %
Many bleeding days or prolonged bleeding	27.6
Spotting	17.1
Amenorrhea	9.4
Irregular bleeding	7.6
Frequent bleeding onsets	7
Removal difficulties	6.2
Scanty bleeding	5.2
Breast discharge	≥ 5
Cervicitis	≥ 5
Musculoskeletal pain	≥ 5
Abdominal discomfort	≥ 5
Leukorrhea	≥ 5
Vaginitis	≥ 5
Pain or itching near implant site	3.7

Source: Norplant package insert.

Drug interactions with phenytoin, phenobarbital, carbamazepine, primidone, and rifampin may occur due to the increase in hepatic metabolism of levonorgestrel. Unlike DMPA, fertility returns quickly, within 1 month after removal of the implant. Before deciding to insert Norplant, it is important to consider absolute and relative contraindications to use. Absolute contraindications are genital bleeding of unknown cause, pregnancy, acute liver disease, thromboembolic disease, breast cancer, or liver tumors. Relative contraindications include drugs that interact with Norplant, mental depression, breastfeeding in women less than 6 weeks postpartum, severe acne, chronic disease, hypercholesterolemia, smoking, ectopic pregnancy history, hypertension, diabetes mellitus, gallbladder disease, cardiovascular disease, and severe vascular headaches.

Continuation rates for Norplant and Norplant-2 have been reported to be between 87 to 91% after one year of use. Menstrual disturbances, including irregular uterine bleeding and amenorrhea, are the most common reasons given for discontinuing the implants (Glasier, 2002). Patient counseling continues to play an important role in maintaining patient satisfaction and improving long-term use of this method. Hatcher et al. (1998) and Hatcher et al. (2001) provide a thorough discussion of insertion and removal techniques.

CONTRACEPTIVES IN SPECIAL PATIENT POPULATIONS

Women with either insulin-dependent or non-insulin-dependent diabetes mellitus can be prescribed progestin-only OCs or low-dose OCs if tissue damage and serious vascular complications are not present and if they are followed closely by their provider (Hatcher et al., 1998). Before starting therapy, weight, blood pressure, glucose control, and fasting lipids should be evaluated and checked every 3 to 4 months thereafter. Microalbuminuria should also be determined. Depo-Provera and Norplant may be used in diabetic women; however, these contraceptives have been shown in some studies to result in statistically, but not clinically, significant negative effects on glucose tolerance and lipid levels (Betschart, 1996; Kjos, 1996; Womack & Beal, 1996).

Women with epilepsy are usually treated with anticonvulsants such as phenobarbitol, carbamazepine, phenytoin, and ethambutol, which may lower serum concentrations of OCs, thereby increasing risk for pregnancy. High-dose (i.e., 50 μg of ethinyl estradiol) OCs may be used in these situations, but poor cycle control and lack of reliability are possibilities. Breakthrough bleeding indicates the OC is less effective in this instance (Sawin, 2003). Therefore, other contraceptive methods are recommended.

Women with disabilities have special needs related to fertility management (Sawin, 2003). Moreover, in many cases, contraception information is not provided to women who have disabilities. Spinal cord injury patients, because of decreased mobility, are at an increased risk for deep vein thrombosis; therefore, estrogen-containing OCs augment this potential risk. Women with spinal cord injuries may still become pregnant and may give birth without complications. Hormonal therapy may affect the course of multiple sclerosis, and OCs are contraindicated in women who are paralyzed or who have restricted mobility. There are conflicting data regarding the use of OCs in women with cystic fibrosis. Bronchial mucus may become scant, and endocervical polyps may develop. However, one small study found that pulmonary function and respiratory symptoms were not affected in young women treated with OCs (Sawin, 2003).

EMERGENCY CONTRACEPTION (EC)

Major women's health organizations are recommending that Plan B be an over-the-counter drug (AWHONN News and Views, 2004). Having EC available does not appear to change sexual behavior or the use of contraception (Nelson, Linn, Derman, & Strickland, 2004).

In 1998 the World Health Organization placed the "morning-after" pill on its List of Essential Drugs. Two alternatives are currently marketed in the United States: Plan-B and Preven. Neither should be confused with the more controversial French drug, RU 486 or mifepristone, which can induce abortion up to 7 weeks gestation (Avery, 2002; Schaff & Mawson, 2001). Plan-B contains two 0.75 mg tablets of levonorgestrel taken 12 hours apart within 72 hours of unprotected intercourse (Apgar, 2000; Grimes, Hanson, & Sondheimer, 2001). Preven contains 4 tablets, each possessing a combination of 50 mg of ethinyl estradiol and 0.25 mg of levonorgestrel. Two tablets are taken twice, 12 hours apart within 72 hours of unprotected intercourse. Costs are comparable for both at approximately $20. Studies of both methods have found that while they are equally effective, the progestin-only Plan-B is better tolerated than the combination Preven. Side effects include nausea and vomiting, breast tenderness, low abdominal pain and menstrual changes. Preven carries the same contraindications for use as combination OCs (Apgar, 2000, Emergency contraception update, 2000; Grimes et al., 2001). There are a number of combination OC regimens available for EC, such as taking 4 pills initially of an OC such as Lo-Ovral or Nordette, then 12 hours later taking another 4 pills. Number of pills vary with the formulation. Please consult a contraceptive reference, such as Hatcher et al. (2001), for more information. Side effects of using the combined estrogen-progestin OC regimens have made the progestinonly regimen, Plan-B much more acceptable for use (Hatcher et al., 2001).

In addition to Preven and Plan-B, in September 2000 the FDA approved the use of mifepristone and misoprostol for medical abortion up to 7 weeks gestation (Schaff & Mawson, 2001). Mifepristone acts to stop the effects of progesterone, causing shedding of the uterine lining. It also increases production of prostaglandins, thereby increasing uterine contractility and causes the cervix to soften and dilate (Schaff & Mawson, 2001; Emergency contraception update, 2000). Misoprostol is a synthetic prostaglandin that causes increased uterine contractility. The two medications taken 2 days apart provide between 92 and 98% effectiveness ". . . for pregnancies up to 49 days gestation. In pregnancies longer than 49 days gestation the mifepristone plus oral misoprostol regimen has an efficacy rate of 77–88%" (Schaff & Mawson, 2001, p. 2). The protocol for administration requires an initial visit during which time the 600 mg mifepristone is administered. A second visit is required on day 3 for administration of 400 μg misoprostol, and a third visit for followup is required on or before day 14 to substantiate completion of the termination. Use of this method requires confirmation of pregnancy ≤ 49 days without evidence of ectopic pregnancy. Women should be screened for Rh blood type and, if negative, given a 50 g dose of Rh immune globulin on day 1 of the protocol.

No matter what form of emergency contraception is used, it is essential for the clinician to provide thorough counseling regarding alternatives, the benefits and risks of each method, the costs, side effects and warning signs of possible complications, and who to contact in case of emergency (FDA approval of mifepristone, 2000; Schaff & Mawson, 2001).

FUTURE CONTRACEPTIVES

No perfect contraceptive method exists. The methods described in the preceding sections vary in efficacy, adverse effects, and other characteristics. Future contraceptive methods should be acceptable, effective, easy to use, free of long- and short-term adverse effects, affordable, suitable for different times of the reproductive cycle, and suitable in different age groups.

Currently under investigation are several contraceptives (both oral and patch) using a new progestin, trimegestone. Because of its potency, it can be given in smaller doses thereby causing fewer progestin-related side effects. It has also been shown to have lower androgenic properties and is therefore less likely to produce side effects such as acne and excess body hair (The Research Pipeline, 2000).

The FDA has also recently approved phase I clinical trials of quinacrine pellets for use as a nonsurgical form of female sterilization (Lippes, Brar, Gerbracht, Neff, & Kokkinakis, 2003). This drug, which has been on the market as a treatment for malaria, has been used in pellet form for female sterilization in a number of countries around the world with a greater than 98% protection rate at 2 years of use (Zipper & Kessel, 2003).

Immunocontraceptives are also under clinical trials. These are vaccines causing the body to produce antibodies against hCG. Contraceptive protection is said to be reversible, since without vaccination boosters, antibody production will decrease. Problems with this form of contraception include potential development of auto-antibodies (Evolution and revolution, 2000).

Several microbicide gels are under investigation. They work to maintain the normal acidic pH of the vagina. Sperm and microorganisms are destroyed when they come in contact with the acidic area (The Research Pipeline, 2000).

A number of multinational male contraception clinical trials have been studying the potential contraceptive efficacy of steroids including the use of androgens alone, androgens with estrogen and progestins, and androgens with GnRH antagonists (Christensen, 2000; Handelsman, 2000; Lyttle & Kopf, 2003; McLachlan, MacDonald, Rushford, et al., 2000; Meriggiola, Costantino, & Cerpolini, 2002; Shafik, 2000). The primary aim of these potential contraceptives is to "produce reversible suppression of sperm output to reduce the number of ejaculated sperm to levels that reliably prevent fertilization" (Handelsman, 2000, p. 8).

REFERENCES

Abrams, L., Skee, D., Natarajan, J., Wong, F., & Lasseter, K. (2001). Multiple-dose pharmacokinetics of a contraceptive patch in healthy women participants. *Contraception, 64*, 287–294.

ACOG practice bulletin #18. (2000). *2004 Compendium of Selected Publications*. Washington, D.C.: Author.

ACOG practice bulletin #46. (2003). *2004 Compendium of Selected Publications*. Washington, D.C.: Author.

Alexander, L. (1996). Taking a sexual history to help patients prevent STDs. *Contraception Report, 7*, 12–14.

Allen, R. (2004). Diaphragm fitting. *American Family Physician, 69*, 97–100.

American Academy of Pediatrics, Committee on Adolescence. (1999). Contraception and adolescents. *Pediatrics, 104*, 1161–1166.

Apgar, B. (2000). Plan-B contraception decreases risk of pregnancy. *American Family Physician, 61*, 3425–3426.

Arias, R. (2003, December). Extended-cycle oral contraception—clinical experiences. *The Female Patient,* Supplement, 10–17.

Avery, C. (2002). One last chance. *Canadian Business, 75*, 15.

AWHONN News and Views. (2004). AWHONN urges approval of OTC emergency contraception. *AWHONN Lifelines,* 8(1), 65–66.

Baill, I., Cullins, V., & Patti, S. (2003). Counseling issues in tubal sterilization. *American Family Physician, 67*, 1287–1294.

Betschart, J. (1996). Oral contraception and adolescent women with insulin-dependent diabetes mellitus: Risks, benefits, and implications for practice. *Diabetes Educator, 22*, 374–378.

Boston Women's Health Collective. (1998). *Our bodies ourselves for the new century*. New York: Simon & Schuster.

Brache, V., Mishell, D., Lahteenmaki, P., Alvarez, F., Elomaa, K., Jackanicz, T., & Faundes, A. (2001). Ovarian function during use of vaginal rings delivering three different doses of nestorone. *Contraception, 63*, 257–261.

Brache, V., Faundes, A., Alvarez, F., & Cochon, L. (2002). Nonmenstrual adverse events during use of implantable contraceptives for women: Data from clinical trials. *Contraception, 65*, 63–74.

Bucci, K., & Carson, D. (1997). Contraception. In J. T. Dipero (Ed.), *Pharmacotherapy: A pathophysiologic approach* (3rd ed.) Stamford, CT: Appleton & Lange.

Burkman, R. (2001a). Current perspectives on OC's. *Dialogues in Contraception, 6*, 1–3.

Burkman, R. (2001b). Economic issues and contraception. *Dialogues in Contraception, 6*, 1–3, & 8.

Burkman, R., & Shulman, L. (2001). The levonorgestrel IUD. *Dialogues in Contraception, 7*, 1–3 & 8.

Caufield, K. A. (2003). Controlling fertility. In E. Q. Youngkin & M. S. Davis (Eds.), *Women's health: A primary care clinical guide* (3rd ed.) Stamford, CT: Appleton & Lange.

Centers for Disease Control, National Institute of Child Health and Human Development. (1987a). Combination oral contraceptive use and the risk of endometrial cancer. *Journal of the American Medical Association, 257*, 796–800.

Centers for Disease Control, National Institute of Child Health and Human Development. (1987b). The reduction in risk of ovarian cancer associated with oral-contraceptive use: The cancer and steroid hormone study. *New England Journal of Medicine, 316*, 650–655.

Cheng, D. (2000). The intrauterine devise: Still misunderstood after all these years. *Southern Medical Journal, 93*, 859–864.

Christensen, D. (2000). Male choice: The search for new contraceptives for men. *Science News, 158*, 222–223.

Coenen, C., Thomas, C., Borm, G., Hollanders, J., & Rolland, R. (1996). Changes in androgens during treatment with four low-dose contraceptives. *Contraception, 53*, 171–176.

Collaborative Group on Hormonal Factors in Breast Cancer. (1996). Breast cancer and hormonal contraceptives: Further results. *Contraception, 54*, 1S–106S.

Commentary (2004). Fortifying oral contraceptives with folic acid. *AWHONN Lifelines, 8*(1), 12–13.

Contraception for women in the perimenopause. (2001). *The Contraception Report, 12*, 4–12.

Cook, R., & Rosenberg, M. (1998). Do spermicides containing nonoxynol-9 prevent sexually transmitted infections? *Sexually Transmitted Diseases, 25*, 144–151.

Croxatto, H. (2002). Progestin implants for female contraception. *Contraception, 65*, 15–19.

Cundy T., Cornish, J., Roberts, H., Elder, H., & Reid, R. (1998). Spinal bone density in women using depot medroxyprogesterone contraception. *Obstetrics and Gynecology, 92*, 569–573.

Darney, P. (2003, December), Current trends in contraception: Extended-cycle options. *The Female Patient,* Supplement.

Dickey, R. (2002). *Managing contraceptive pill patients (11th ed.)*. Durant, OK: Essential Medical Information Systems, Inc.

Elliott, W., & Chan, J. (December, 2001). Norelgestromin/ethinyl estradiol transdermal system—Ortho Evra—Ortho pharmaceuticals. *Internal Medicine Alert*, 190–191.

Emergency contraception update. (2000, August). *Clinical Proceedings*, Retrieved 7/2/02 from http://www.arhp.org/CPAugust_2000/emergencyconupdate.htm.

Endrikat, J., Klipping, C., Cronin, M., Gerlinger, C., Ruebig, W., Schmidt, W., & Dusterberg, B. (2002). An open label, comparative study of the effects of a dosereduced oral contraceptive containing 20 μg ethinyl estradiol and 100 μg levonorgestrel on hemostatic, lipids, and carbohydrate metabolism variables. *Contraception, 65*, 215–221.

Erskine, M., Shinewi, F., Pollard, L., & Kubba, A. (2000). Tolerability and reasons for discontinuation of Norplant in an inner city population. *Journal of Obstetrics and Gynaecology, 20*, 180–182.

Essure summary precribing information. (2002). *Conceptus Incorporated.* Retrieved 3/10/04 from http://www.essure.com/static/hcp/prescribing/pdf.

Evolution and revolution . . . (2000). *The Contraception Report, 10*, 15–25.

FDA approval of mifepristone: An overview. (2000). *The Contraception Report, 11*, 4–10.

FDA approves Lea's Shield. (2002). *The Contraception Report, 13*, 4–5 & 11.

FDA approves new female sterilization device. (2003, March). *Biomedical Safety & Standards*, 31–32.

FDA approves seasonale oral contraceptive. (2003, September). *FDA Talk Paper*. Retrieved 3/8/04 from http://www.FDA.gov/BBS/topics/ANSWERS/ANSO1251.html

FDA gives green light to berlex's mirena intrauterine system. (2001). *Contraceptive Technology Update, 22*, 13–15.

FDA may soon consider new female sterilization device. (2002). *The Contraception Report, 13*, 12–13, 15.

Fehring, R. J. (2004). The future of professional education in natural family planning. *Journal of Obstetric, Gynecologic, & Neonatal Nursing, 33*(1), 34–43.

Fichorova, R., Tucker, L., & Anderson, D. (2001). The molecular basis of nonoxynol-9-induced vaginal inflammation and its possible relevance to human immunodeficiency virus type 1 transmission. *Journal of Infectious Diseases, 184*, 418–429.

Finer, L., Darroch, J., & Singh, S. (1999). Sexual partnership patterns as a behavioral risk factor for sexually transmitted diseases. *Family Planning Perspectives, 31*, 228–236.

First contraceptive skin patch. (2002). *FDA Consumer*, 4.

First hormonal vaginal contraceptive ring. (2001). *FDA Consumer*, 4.

Frederiksen, M. (1996). Depot medroxyprogesterone acetate contraception in women with medical problems. *Journal of Reproductive Medicine, 41 (Suppl.)*, 414–418.

Frezieres, R., & Walsh, T. (2000). Acceptability evaluation of a natural rubber latex, a polyurethane, and a new non-latex condom. *Contraception, 61*, 369–377.

Gaspard, U., Scheen, A., Endrikat, J., Buicu, C., Lefebvre, P., Gerlinger, C., & Heithecker, R., (2003). A randomized study over 13 cycles to assess the influence of oral contraceptives containing ethinylestradiol combined with drospirenon or desogestrel on carbohydrate metabolism. *Contraception, 67*, 423–430.

Gbolade, B., Ellis, S., Murby, B., Randall, S., & Kirkman, R. (1998). Bone density in long term users of depot medroxyprogesterone acetate. *British Journal of Obstetrics and Gynecology, 105*, 790–795.

Glasier, A. (2002). Implantable contraceptives for women: Effectiveness, discontinuation rates, return of fertility, and outcome of pregnancies. *Contraception, 65*, 29–37.

Gollub, E. (2000). The female condom: Tool for women's empowerment. *American Journal of Public Health, 90*, 1377–1381.

Gordon, J. & Speroff, L. (2002). *Handbook for clinical gynecologic endocrinology & infertility.* Philadelphia, PA: Lippincott, Williams & Wilkins.

Greydanus, D., Patel, D., & Rimsza, M. (2001). Contraception in the adolescent: An update. *Pediatrics, 107*, 562–573.

Grimes, D., Hanson, V., & Sondheimer, S. (2001, March). New approaches to emergency contraception. *Patient Care for the Nurse Practitioner*, 44–54.

Handelsman, D. (2000). Hormonal male contraception. *International Journal of Andrology, 23, Suppl.*, 8–12.

Hatcher, R., Nelson, A., Zieman, M., Darney, P., Creinin, M., & Stosur, H. (2001). *A pocket guide to managing contraception: 2001–2002 edition*. Tiger, GA: Bridging the Gap Foundation.

Hatcher, R., Trussell, J., Stewart, F., Stewart, G., Kowal, D., Guest, F., Cates, W., & Policar, M. (1998). *Contraceptive technology* (17th rev. ed.). New York: Irvington.

Hawley, W., Nuovo, J., DeNeef, C., & Carter, P. (1993). Do oral contraceptive agents affect the risk of breast cancer? A meta-analysis of the case-control reports. *Journal of the American Board of Family Practice, 6*, 123–135.

Heinemann, L. (2000). Emerging evidence on oral contraceptives and arterial disease. *Contraception, 62*, 29S–36S.

Herbst, A., & Berek, J. (1993). Impact of contraception on gynecologic cancers. *American Journal of Obstetrics and Gynecology, 168*, 1980–1985.

Himes, N. (1963). *Medical history of contraception*. New York: Gamut Press.

Hollander, D. (2001). Female condoms remain structurally sound after being washed and resused as many as seven times. *International Family Planning Perspectives, 27*, 155–156.

Holt, V., Cushing-Haugen, K., & Daling, J. (2002). Body weight and risk of oral contraceptive failure. *Obstetrics and Gynecology, 99*, 820–827.

Jensen, J., & Speroff, L. (2000). Health benefits of oral contraceptives. *Obstetrics and Gynecological Clinics of North America, 27*, 705–721.

Katzung, B. (2001). *Basic & Clinical Pharmacology* (8th ed.). New York: Lange Medical Books/McGraw-Hill.

Kaunitz, A. (1996). Depot medroxyprogesterone acetate contraception and the risk of breast and gynecologic cancer. *Journal of Reproductive Medicine 41, (Suppl.)* 419–427.

Kaunitz, A. (2000). Injectable contraception: New and existing options. *Obstetrics and Gynecology Clinics of North America, 27*, 741–780.

Kaunitz, A. (2001a). Transition from OC's to HRT. *Dialogues in Contraception, 6*, 4.

Kaunitz, A. (2001b). The levonorgestrel intrauterine system: An effective new contraceptive option. *Contraceptive Technology Report, BB #458*, 1–7.

Kaunitz, A. (2001c). Lunelle: Evaluation of a new monthly contraception injection for U.S. women. *Contraceptive Technology Reports*, 1–4.

Keeling, D. (2003). Combined oral contraceptives and the risk of myocardial infarction. *Annals of Medicine, 35*, 413–418.

Kjos, S. (1996). Contraception in diabetic women. *Obstetrics and Gynecology Clinics of North America, 23*, 243–257.

Kubba, A., Guillebaud, J., Anderson, R., & MacGregor, E. (2000). Contraception. *The Lancet, 356*, 1913–1919.

Lawrenson, R., & Farmer, R. (2000). Venous thromboembolism and combined oral contraceptives: Does the type of progestogen make a difference? *Contraception 62*, 21S–28S.

Lewis, M., Spitzer, W., Heinemann, L., et al. (1996). Third generation oral contraceptives and risk of myocardial infarction: An international case-control study. *British Medical Journal, 312*, 88–90.

Likis, F. (2002). Contraceptive applications of estrogen. *Journal of Midwifery & Women's Health, 47*, 139–156.

Lippes, J., Brar, M., Gerbracht, K., Neff, P., & Kokkinakis, S. (2003). An FDA phase I clinical trial of quinacrine sterilization (QS). *International journal of gynaecology and obststrics, 83, Supp. 2*, S45–49.

Lobo, R., Skinner, J., Lippman, J., & Cirillo, S. (1996). Plasma lipids and desogestrel and ethinyl estradiol: A meta-analysis. *Fertilization and Sterilization, 65*, 1100–1109.

Lunelle use rises, Norplant use drops. (2001). *Contraceptive Technology, 22*, 102–104.

Lynaugh, J. (1991). The death of Sadie Sachs. *Nursing Research, 40*, 124–125.

Lyttle, C., & Kopf, G. (2003). Status and future direction of male contraceptive development. *Currently Opinion in Pharmacology, 3*, 667–671.

Marchbanks, P., McDonald, J., Wilson, H., Folger, S., Mandel, M., Daling, J., Bernstein, L., Malone, K., Ursin, G., Strom, B., Norman, S., Wingo, P., Burkman, R., Berlin, J., Simon, M., Spirtas, R., & Weiss, L. (2002). Oral contraceptives and the risk of breast cancer. *New England Journal of Medicine, 346*, 2025–2032.

McLachlan, R., McDonald, J., Rushford, D., Robertson, D., Garrett, C., & Baker, G. (2000). Efficacy and acceptability of testosterone implants, alone or in combination with a 5-reductase inhibitor, for male hormonal contraception. *Contraception, 62*, 73–78.

Medical eligibility criteria for contraceptive use, 3rd edition. (2003, October). *Working Group Meeting, World Health Organization*, Geneva. Retrieved on 3/14/04 from http://www.WHO.int/reproductive-health/publications/MEC_3/index/htm.

Meriggiola, M., Costantino, A., & Cerpolini, S. (2002). Recent advances in hormonal male contraception. *Contraception, 65*, 269–272.

Narkiewicz, K., Graniero, G., D-Este, D., Mattarie, M., Zonzin, P., & Palatini, P. (1995). Ambulatory blood pressure in mild hypertensive women taking oral contraceptives: A case-control study. *American Journal of Hypertension, 8*, 249–253.

Nelson, A. (2001). Perceived and actual side effects of oral contraception. *Dialogues in Contraception, 6*, 1–4.

Nelson, A., Lin, E., Derman, R., & Strickland, J. (2004). Contraceptive update: Part 2. *The Female Patient, 29*(1), 19–23.

New female sterilization device. (2003, Jan/Feb). *FDA Consumer*, 6.

News flash: Add new 25-mcg cyclessa to triphasic oral contraceptive options. (2001). Contraceptive Technology Update, 22, 85–87.

Norris, A. (1988). Cognitive analysis of contraceptive behavior. Image: Journal of Nursing Scholarship, 20, 135–140.

Nusbaum, M., & Hamilton, C. (2002). The proactive sexual health history. *American Family Physician, 66*, 1705–1712.

NuvaRing. (2001). *Formulary, 36*, 777.

O'Connell. M. (1996). The effect of bith control methods on sexually transmitted disease/HIV risk. *Journal of Obstetric, Gynecologic and Neonatal Nursing, 25*, 476–480.

Paul, C., Skegg, D., & Spears, G. (1989). Depot medroxyprogesterone (Depo-Provera) and risk of breast cancer. *British Medical Journal, 299*, 759–762.

Peterson, H. (1996). Update on female sterilization: Failure rates, counseling issues, and post-sterilization regret. *Contraception Report, 7*, 4–11.

Pollack, A. (1996). Guidelines for pre-sterilization counseling. *The Contraception Report, 7*, 12–14.

Qin, L., Goldberg, J., & Hao, G. (2001). A 4-year follow-up study of women with Norplant-2 contraceptive implants. *Contraception, 64*, 301–303.

The Research Pipeline. (2000, September). *Contemporary OB/GYN, 98*, 101.

Roddy, R., Zekeng, L., Ryan, K., Tamoufe, U., & Tweedy, K. (2002). Effect of Nonoxynol-9 gel on urogenital gonorrhea and chlamydial infection: A randomized controlled trial. *Journal of the American Medical Association, 287*, 1117–1123.

Sangi-Haghpeykar, H., Poindexter, A., Bateman, L., & Ditmore, J. (1996). Experiences of injectable contraceptive users in an urban setting. *Obstetrics and Gynecology, 88*, 227–233.

Sawin, K. (2003). Issues for women with physical disability and chronic illness. In E. Q. Youngkin & M. S. Davis (Eds.), *Women's health: A primary care clinical guide* (3rd ed.). Stamford, CT: Appleton & Lange.

Schaff, E., & Mawson, J. (2001, February). Gauging the effectiveness of mifepristone and misoprostol. *Contraceptive Technology Reports*, 1–8.

Schnare, S. (2002). Progestin contraceptives. *Journal of Midwifery & Women's Health, 47*, 157–166.

Scholes, D., LaCroix, A., Ichikawa L., Ott, S., & Barlow, W. (1998). Two-year rates of bone loss associated with initation of depot medroxyprogesterone acetate contraception. *Bone, 23*, 1095.

Scott, P. (2000). Inserting an intrauterine device. *JAAPA, 13*, 87–92.

Seasonale prescribing information. (2003). *Duramed Pharaceuticals, Inc.* Retrieved 3/11/04 from http://www.seasonale.com/pdfs/Seasonale_prescribing_info.pdf.

Shafik, A. (2000). Advances in male contraception. *Archives of Andrology, 45*, 155–167.

Shulman, L. (2000). Contraception 2000: Lunelle, an injectable combination contraceptive option. *Journal of Women's Health & Gender-Based Medicine, 9*, 725–729.

Speroff, L. (2000). Oral contraceptives and carbohydrate metabolism. *Dialogues in Contraception, 6*, 1–3, 7–8.

Spitzer, W. (2000). Oral contraceptives and cardiovascular outcomes: Cause or bias? *Contraception, 62*, 3S–9S.

Spitzer, W., Faith, J., & MacRae, K. (2002). Myocardial infarction and third generation oral contraceptives: Aggregation of recent studies. *Human Reproduction, 17*, 2307–2314.

Stone, S. (1995). Desogestrel. *Clinical Obstetrics Gynecology, 38*, 821–828.

Summary of safety and effectiveness data. (2003). *FDA Recent Device Approvals*. Retrieved 3/9/04 from http://www.FDA.GOV/CDRH/PDF2/P020041.html.

Tanis, B., van den Bosch, M., Kemmeren, J., Cats, V., Helmerhorst, F., Algra, A., van der Graff, Y., & Rosendaal, F. (2001). Oral contraceptives and the risk of myocardial infarction. *New England Journal of Medicine, 345*, 1787–1793.

Thomas, D., Ray, R., and the WHO Collaborative Study of Neoplasia and Steroid Contraceptives. (1995). Depot-medroxyprogesterone acetate (DMPA) and risk of invasive adenocarcinomas and adenosquamous carcinomas of the uterine cervix. *Contraception, 52*, 307–312.

Thonneau, P., Goulard, H. & Goyaux, N. (2001). Risk factors for intrauterine device failure: A review. *Contraception, 64*, 33–37.

2002 safety alert—Norplant. (7/26/02). *Medwatch: The FDA Safety Information and Adverse Event Reporting Program*. Retrieved 3/11/04 from http://www.FDA.gov/medwatch/SAFETY/2002/norplant.htm

Update on advisory for norplant. (7/26/02). *FDA Talk Paper*. Retrieved 3/11/04 from http://www.FDA.gov/BBS/Topics/ANSWERS/2002/ANSO1161.html

Vessey, M., McPherson, K., & Johnson, B. (1977). Mortality among women participating in the Oxford Family Planning Association Contraceptive Study. *Lancet, 2*, 727–731.

Weber, A., Jager, R., Borner, A., et al. (1996). Can grapefruit juice influence ethinylestradiol bioavailability? *Contraception, 53*, 41–47.

Weisberg, E. (1995). Prescribing oral contraceptives. *Drugs, 49*, 224–231.

Weschler, T. (2001). *Take charge of your own fertility: The definitive guide to natural birth control, pregnancy achievement, and reproductive health, revised edition.* New York: HarperCollins.

Westhoff, C. (1996). Depot medroxyprogesterone acetate contraception metabolic parameters and mood changes. *Journal of Reproductive Medicine, 41 (suppl.)*, 401–406.

Westhoff, C. (2000). Oral contraceptives and cardiovascular risk: An end to the debate? *Contraception, 62*, 1S–2S.

WHO Collaborative Study of Neoplasia and Steroid Contraceptives. (1991). Breast cancer and depot-medroxyprogesterone acetate: A multinational study. *Lancet, 338*, 833–838.

WHO Collaborative Study of Cardiovascular Disease and Steroid Hormone Contraception. (1996a). Haemorrhagic stroke, overall stroke risk, and combined oral contraceptives: Results of an international, multicentre, case-control study. *Lancet, 348*, 505–510.

WHO Collaborative Study of Cardiovascular Disease and Steroid Hormone Contraception. (1996b). Ischaemic stroke and combined oral contraceptives: Results of an international, multicentre, case-control study. *Lancet, 348*, 498–505.

World Health Organization. (2000). *Improving access and quality of care in family planning: Medical eligibility criteria for contraceptive use*, 2nd ed. Geneva: World Health Organization.

Wiegratz, I., Lee, J., Kutschera, E., Bauer, H., von Hayn, C., Moore, C., Mellinger, U., Winkler, U., Gross, W., & Kuhl, H. Effect of dienogest-containing oral contraceptives on lipid metabolism. *Contraction, 65*, 223–229.

Wilcox, L., Chu, S., Peterson, H. (1990). Characteristics of women who considered or obtained tubal reanastomosis: Results from a prospective study of tubal sterilization. *Obstetrics and Gynecology, 75*, 661–665.

Winkler, U. (2000). Hemostatic effects of third- and second-generation oral contraceptives: absence of a causal mechanism for a difference in risk of venous thromboembolism. *Contraception, 62*, 11S–20S.

Womack, J., & Beal, M. (1996). Use of Norplant in women with or at-risk for noninsulin-dependent diabetes. *Journal of Nurse-Midwifery, 41*, 285–296.

Workowski, K., & Levine, W. (2002, May). CDC sexually transmitted diseases treatment guidelines - 2002. *MMWR Recommendations and Reports, 51(RR06)*, 1–20. Retrieved 7/2/02 from http://cdc.gov/mmwr/preview/mmwrhtml/rr5106al.htm.

Wysocki, S. (2001). Lunelle: A new contraceptive alternative. *The Nurse Pactitioner, 26*, 55–59.

Wysoki, S., & Moore, A. (2002). New developments in contraception: The first transdermal contraceptive system. *Women's Health Care, 1*, 9–15.

Yasunari, K. (2000). Peace profile: Margaret Sanger. *Peace Review, 12*, 619–626.

Youngkin, E. (1995). Sexually transmitted diseases: Current and emerging concerns. *Journal of Obstetric, Gynecologic, and Neonatal Nursing, 24*, 743–758.

Zipper, J., & Kessel, E. (2003). Quinacrine sterilization: A retrospective. *International Journal of Gynaecology and Obstetrics, 83, Supp. 2*, S7–11.

CHAPTER ❖ 19

MENOPAUSE AND CURRENT MANAGEMENT

Susan Rawlins ◆ Adrianne K. Tillmanns

Menopause is not a disease and pharmacologic intervention is not required for "cure." Menopause is better conceptualized as a developmental achievement. Occurring between the ages of 45 and 55 in most women, it is the culmination of a variety of universally occurring physiologic events. Understanding these menopausal physiologic events allows the provider to anticipate and support the woman during the varied presentations of normal menopause. While pharmacologic intervention is not universally required to manage the normal menopause, relief of symptoms will improve feelings of wellbeing in many symptomatic women.

Menopause, by commonly accepted definition, is the last episode of menstrual bleeding experienced by a woman and is therefore a retrospective assessment (Executive summary, 2001). The climacteric or perimenopause is the time of transition surrounding the actual menopause. During the early climacteric period of natural menopause, most women experience declining ovarian follicular function with anovulation, alternating periods of hyperestrogenism and hypoestrogenism, decreased serum progesterone, and increased serum gonadotrophins (Santoro, Brown, Adel, & Skurnick, 1996). Testosterone levels also decline, but in natural menopause the decline is very gradual. The anovulatory cycles produce irregular, unpredictable vaginal bleeding for several years before amenorrhea eventually develops. Vasomotor instability and alterations in mood, memory, and sexual functioning accompany the changes in the menstrual cycle in some women. Over the course of several years, the low serum estrogen levels lead to progressive urogenital atrophy, rapid demineralization of the bones, and unfavorable lipoprotein changes. Although the function of androgens in women is not completely understood, and low serum testosterone levels after bilateral salpingo-oophorectomy have been associated with decreased libido (Hoeger & Guzick, 1999; Laughlin, Barrett-Conner, Kritz-Silverstein, & von Muhlen, 2000). The hormonal milieu of the climacteric places perimenopausal women at increased risk for endometrial cancer (Santoro et al., 1996). Although most women experience symptoms related to their changing hormonal profile, less than 30% report major psychologic distress during the perimenopausal transition (Bromberger, Meyer, Kravitz, et al. 2001; von Muhlen, Soroko, Kritz-Silverstein, & Barrett-Conner, 2000).

Pharmacologic management of the climacteric is not directed toward curing this natural condition; the goal is relief of distressing symptoms without increasing long-term morbidity or premature mortality. During the early years of this century, most women died shortly before or soon after menopause, so the physiologic consequences of menopause were of little concern. Due to improvements in public health and medical science, most women today successfully achieve menopause and many can expect to live more than 30 years thereafter (McKinlay, Brambilla, & Posner, 1992). The consequences of menopause are now a concern of all women and society as well, for long life without good health is a burden, not a blessing. This chapter presents the most current recommendations for pharmacologic management of symptomatic peri- and postmenopausal women. The conditions most commonly associated with menopause such as unpredictable anovulatory bleeding, vasomotor instability, and urogenital atrophy improve with hormone therapy. Osteoporosis and colorectal cancer may be prevented with hormone therapy, but other therapeutic options should be considered first in asymptomatic women. The benefit of hormone therapy for other conditions reported by aging women such as impaired memory, altered psychological functioning, and reduced sexual responsiveness are less clear. And finally, hormone therapy should not be prescribed for the primary prevention of cardiovascular disease.

The anovulatory cycles that occur during perimenopause result in unpredictable vaginal bleeding that can be quite distressing to most women. This problem is amenable to hormone therapy. The alterations in psychological functioning that occur in some women during the climacteric can have their roots in many areas other than hormonal decline. However, poor sleep—a common problem of perimenopausal women—may be directly related to hormonal and vasomotor changes. Changes in libido, also, may be multifactoral in cause, but one influencing factor may be hormonal declines in estrogen and androgen. Hormone therapy (HT) has been reported to have both positive and negative effects on conditions such as rheumatoid arthritis, Parkinson disease, and stroke. Additional studies are needed to confirm the actual benefits and risks in these conditions. Osteoporotic fractures, symptomatic urogenital atrophy, and colorectal cancers are prevented with HT (Goldstein, Newcomb, & Stampfer, 1999; Liang & Karlson, 1996; Paganini-Hill & Barreto, 2001; Tsang, Ho, & Lo, 2000; Writing Group for WHI, 2002). All pharmacologic interventions are associated with potential risks, and HT is no exception. The known risks of estrogen therapy (ET) include increases in endometrial cancer, venous thromboembolism, and, most recently, stroke (National Institutes of Health, 2004). EPT, the addition of a progestin—in the case of the Women's Health Initiative, medroxyprogesterone acetate—to estrogen, is associated with small but significant increases in breast cancer, pulmonary embolism, and coronary heart disease (Writing Group for WHI, 2002). A discussion of the potential risks and benefits associated with EPT is presented later in this chapter. A discussion of the potential risks associated with HT is presented later in the chapter. These risks vary from life-threatening, such as breast and endometrial cancer, to nuisance problems, like breast tenderness and unpredictable uterine bleeding.

In keeping with the North American Menopause Society's recommendation for uniform and consistent terminology, throughout this chapter, the following terminology will be used: ET refers to estrogen therapy; EPT refers to combination estrogen and progestogen therapy; and HT refers to both ET and EPT (NAMS, 2003a).

CONDITIONS ASSOCIATED WITH MENOPAUSE

DYSFUNCTIONAL UTERINE BLEEDING

Menstrual cycle changes begin early in the perimenopausal transition in response to decreased numbers of primordial follicles as well as decreased sensitivity of the remaining follicles to gonadotropins. Rising FSH levels shorten the follicular phase of the cycle, resulting in more frequent cycles with heavier bleeding in the early transition years. As women approach the final menstrual period, anovulation becomes more common, cycles lengthen, and bleeding tends to be lighter in volume. Ovulation occurs unpredictably, and pregnancy is possible. In addition to cycle changes, many women experience spotting the day or two before menses. Heavy, prolonged bleeding or intermenstrual bleeding should be evaluated by endometrial biopsy to rule out endometrial cancer. Menstrual cycle dysfunction can be managed with low-dose oral contraceptives, progestins alone, or HT (Kaunitz, 2001; Nachtigall, 1998; Santoro et al., 1996; Taffe & Dennerstein, 2002).

VASOMOTOR INSTABILITY

Vasomotor instability, commonly called a *hot flash* or *flush,* is commonly associated with the perimenopause transition and the menopause but occurs quite frequently in reproductive-aged women and in up to 30% of older reproductive-aged women with regular menstrual cycles (Freeman, Grisso, Berlin, et al., 2001). Up to 85% of perimenopausal women experience hot flashes, night sweats, and/or sleep disturbances as a result of vasomotor instability (Santoro et al., 1996). In one recent cross-sectional survey of community women 45 to 54 years old, 65% experienced hot flashes, 56% night sweats, 45% trouble sleeping, 49% mood swings, and 44% memory problems (Bosworth, Bastian, Kuchibhatla, et al., 2001). In a longitudinal study of hot flashes over 25 years, the maximal prevalence of hot flashes was at 52 to 54 years of age, decreasing progressively in older age groups reaching a prevalence of 9% by age 72. In this study, 20% of women sought treatment for symptoms (Rodstrom, Bengtsson, Lissner, et al., 2002). Hot flash intensity and frequency varies not only between women, but also in any given woman over time. Some women are almost incapacitated with their symptoms, while others report only occasional hot flashes that are barely noticeable (Nachtigall, 1998). Several studies report no difference in hot flash rates between African American and Caucasian women (Freeman, Sammel, Grisso, et al., 2001; Phan, Freeman, & Grisso, 1997). Earlier studies (Schwingl, Hulka, & Harlow, 1994) suggested thin women experience more hot flashes than heavier women; newer data indicate women with higher BMI experience more hot flashes than thin women (Freeman, Sammel, et al., 2001; Wilber et al., 1998). Other factors associated with an increased incidence of hot flashes are lower education, sedentary lifestyle, alcohol intake, smoking, and a history of maternal hot flashes (Avis, Crawford, & McKinlay, 1997; Gold, Sternfeld, Kelsey, et al., 2000; Ivarsson, Spetz, & Hammar, 1998; Staropoli, Flaws, Bush, & Moulton, 1998). It is important to note that conditions other than menopause are associated with hot flash symptoms, including hyperthyroidism, pheochromocytoma, carcinoids, leukemia, pancreatic tumors, and panic attack (NAMS, 2000a). The menopausal hot flash results from instability in the thermoregulatory centers of the brain in response to the decline in estrogen.

DISTURBANCES OF PSYCHOLOGICAL AND COGNITIVE FUNCTIONING

Women in the perimenopausal transition experience mood and cognitive disturbances including irritability, anxiety, mood swings, and memory loss/forgetfulness (Bosworth et al., 2001). In spite of these symptoms, most women have neutral or positive feelings about the menopausal transition (Olofsson & Collins, 2000; Sommer et al., 1999). It has been reported that women have a lifetime risk for major depressive disorder of 20 to 25% with a mean age of onset of 40 (Nachtigall, 1998) and that the perimenopausal transition is associated with a high rate (30%) of depressive symptoms (Bosworth et al., 2001). Analysis of confounding variables demonstrates that the depressive symptoms are not related to the menopausal state itself but to the presence of menopausal symptoms such as hot flashes, night sweats, insomnia, and inability to concentrate (Avis, Crawford, Stellato, & Longcope, 2001). Other conditions associated with increased depressive mood are negative mood earlier in life, sedentary lifestyle, inadequate income, personal stress, history of premenstrual complaints, and smoking (Bosworth et al., 2001; Dennerstein, Lehert, Burger, et al., 1999). With the high rate of depression in U.S. women, it is important for the clinician to differentiate major depression from depressive symptoms related to menopausal changes so that appropriate therapy can be selected. Estrogen replacement therapy is associated with improvements of perimenopause-related depression and improved mood (Boyle & Murrihy, 2001; Schmidt, Nieman, Danaceau, et al., 2000). In a recent analysis of WHI data, depression was significantly related to cardiovascular disease (CVD) risk and was an independent predictor of CVD death even after adjustment for known confounding variables. Whether treatment for depression will lower CVD risk is unknown (Wassertheil-Smoller, Shumaker, Ockene, et al., 2004).

Cognitive functioning declines with aging and rates of Alzheimer's disease increase after menopause when estrogen declines. Women have three times the risk of Alzheimer's disease as men. High estrogen levels are associated with some aspects of improved cognition (Drake, Henderson, Stanczyk, et al., 2000). Estrogen is thought to protect brain function through a variety of mechanisms including increased cerebral blood flow, anti-inflammatory effects, enhanced activity at neuronal synapses, as well as others as discussed in a recent review by Shepherd (2001). In small studies, estrogen therapy has been shown to improve cognitive functioning, but this effect may depend upon the specific parameter of cognition studied, tests used, type of HT, duration of treatment, and specific areas of the brain studied (Fluck, File, & Rymer, 2002; Smith, Giordani, Lajiness-O'Neil, & Zubieta, 2001). In one study, improvement was noted only when menopausal symptoms were alleviated (LeBlanc, Janowsky, Chan, & Nelson, 2001). Cognitive function is maintained in surgically menopausal women when estrogen is initiated soon after surgery (Verghese et al., 2000). In contrast, the Rancho Bernardo study showed no benefit on cognition from long-term estrogen use (Barrett-Conner & Kritz-Silverstein, 1993). In the HERS study, HRT was not associated with cognition. Reanalysis of data from the HERS study indicated that women with elevated total and LDL-C had an increased likelihood of cognitive impairment; lowering the total and LDL-C levels over the 4 years of the study decreased the odds of cognitive impairment. Statin use was associated with a lower likelihood of cognitive impairment (Yaffe et al., 2002). Estrogen use has been associated with a delay in the onset and may prevent the occurrence of Alzheimer's disease (Paginini-Hill, 1996; Tang et al., 1996; Waring et al., 1999).

Analysis of the estrogen plus progestin arm of the Women's Health Initiative Memory Study (WHIMS) revealed that when hormone therapy is initiated in generally healthy, asymptomatic women age 65 or older, the risk of probable dementia increased, mild cognitive impairment was not prevented and cognitive functioning was not improved (Rapp, Espeland, Shumaker, et al., 2003; Shumaker, Legault, Rapp, et al, 2003). Similar findings were reported for the estrogen-only arm (National Institutes of Health, 2004). The effect of hormone therapy on cognition and dementia in women younger than 65 was not studied.

Alterations in sleep are associated with decreased cognitive functioning and depressed mood. Estrogens have been shown to improve sleep (Antonijevic, Stalla, & Steiger, 2000; Hays, Ockene, Brunner, et al., 2003; Polo-Kantolo, Erkkola, Helenius, et al., 1998). Micronized progesterone has been shown in one small study to improve sleep efficiency over medroxyprogesterone acetate (Montplaisir, Lorrain, Denesle, & Petit, 2001).

UROGENITAL ATROPHY

The genital and urinary tracts arise from a common embryonic precursor cell line and both contain abundant estrogen receptors. After several years of diminished estrogen, the urogenital tract begins to atrophy (Hextal & Cardozo, 2001). The vulvar epithelium thins, and the collagen and adipose tissue supporting structures diminish (Hammond, 1996). The vagina shortens, loses elasticity, and thins. Vaginal secretions decrease in volume and become more alkaline with a corresponding change in vaginal flora. (Garcia-Closas, Herrero, Bratti, et al., 1999). The urethra and trigone of the bladder also atrophy with estrogen loss. These alterations of the physiology of the urogenital tract increase the likelihood of trauma, infection, and pain (Hammond, 1996). Not surprisingly, menopausal women experience dyspareunia, cystitis, stress, and urge incontinence. Many women accept incontinence as a consequence of aging and do not report this condition unless specifically asked by their provider. Urinary incontinence may affect up to 35% of women aged 60 and older. Incontinence leads to decreased quality of life in up to 44% of affected women (Sherburn et al., 2001; Vinker et al., 2001). Good vaginal health, an essential component of high-level wellness in women, is enhanced by estrogen therapy. Studies indicate that local estrogen, but not oral estrogen, decreases urinary tract infections in menopausal women (Brown, Vittinghoff, Kanaya, et al., 2001; Eriksen, 1999; Raz & Stamm, 1993).

REDUCED SEXUAL RESPONSIVENESS

In spite of the physical changes of the vulva and vagina, most women continue to be sexually active throughout their lives and place great value on this aspect of their relationships. Of those who report not being sexually active, the most common reason for lack of sexual activity is the absence of a functional partner (Lindgren, Berg, Hammar, & Zuccon, 1993). In a large, demographically representative survey of U.S. adults, 43% of women reported sexual dysfunction (Laumann, Paik, & Rosen, 1999). These problems include decreased libido, arousal, and orgasm. One contributing factor to a decline in sexual functioning may be the disruption of the rapid eye movement (REM) phase of sleep, which commonly occurs during menopause. Both men and women experience nocturnal genital congestion during REM sleep, which helps maintain the ability to mount a sexual response (Graziottin, 1996). The pathophysiology of female sexual dysfunction is poorly understood but is believed to involve psychosocial, hormonal, and physiological components. It is associated with normal aging and is not directly related to serum testosterone levels. Berman and colleagues provide a thorough review of this condition (Berman, Berman, Werbin, & Goldstein, 1999). Androgen replacement improves sexual functioning more than estrogen alone in oophorectomized women and in women dissatisfied with estrogen alone (Sarrel, Dobay, & Wiita, 1998; Shifren et al., 2000). The risks of androgen therapy are discussed later in the chapter.

OSTEOPOROSIS

Osteoporosis is a preventable and treatable disorder that currently affects 30 million women in the United States. It is characterized by decreased bone mass, compromised structural integrity of the skeleton, and increased fracture risk. For white women, 1 out of 2 will experience an osteoporotic fracture during their lifetime. The economic burden of osteoporosis and associated fractures in the United States is estimated to be $13.8 billion. Postmenopausal white women have the greatest risk for osteoporosis, but this condition affects all races and men. Prevention, detection, and treatment of osteoporosis are achievable goals in all practice settings. A variety of pharmacologic and nonpharmacologic treatments are available (NOF, 2000).

CARDIOVASCULAR DISEASE

Cardiovascular disease is discussed in detail in Chapter 20. It is the leading cause of death in women, and increased risk of cardiovascular disease has been linked to the loss of estrogen that accompanies menopause (Minino & Smith, 2001). As women enter the climacteric, they experience changes in serum lipoproteins, including increased cholesterol and LDL-C and decreased HDL-C that increased their risk for heart disease. Older epidemiologic studies indicated that HT reduced cardiovascular death rates in menopausal women by as much as 50% (Grady, Rubin, & Petitti, 1992). Estrogen replacement therapy improves lipoprotein profile, endothelial function, and coronary blood flow (Godsland, 2001; Hall, Collins, Csemiczky, & Landgren, 2002; Higashi, Sanada, Sasaki, et al., 2001; Hirata, Shimada, Watanabe, et al., 2001). Recently published studies indicate that HT may not prevent the progression of established CVD and is in fact associated with an increased risk of venous thromboembolism (VTE), and a possibly a small increased risk coronary heart disease and pulmonary embolism. Data from the HERS trial indicate that neither conjugated equine estrogen (CEE) nor CEE plus medroxyprogesterone acetate (MPA) reduce mortality or morbidity in older women with established coronary artery disease (Hulley, Grady, Bush et al., 1998). This lack of benefit of HT in established coronary heart disease persisted through 6.8 years of follow-up (Grady, Harrington, Bittner, et al., 2002). In the ERA study, HT had no effect on coronary atherosclerosis progression (Herrington, Reboussin, Brosnihan, et al., 2000). In a randomized, controlled primary prevention trial (Women's Health Initiative), a specific formulation of HT (CEE plus MPA) was found to increase the incidence of coronary heart disease by 7 cases per 10,000 women; increase the risk of VTE by 18 cases per 10,000 and increase the risk pulmonary embolism by 8 cases per 10,000, and increase the risk stroke by 8 per 10,000. No increase in deaths from any cause was observed (Writing group for WHI, 2002). Final analysis of the WHI data on CHD risk revealed that while there were an increased number of cardiovascular events in the HT group; it was not statistically different from placebo except for the increased risk of CHD in the first year of use and VTE through-out the study. In addition, women with high baseline LDL levels (> 242 mg/dl) who received HT had twice the rate of CHD than those in the placebo group. The study authors concluded that HT does not provide cardiac protection and may increase risk in the first year of use (Manson, Hsia, Johnson, et al., 2003). In contrast, Sanderson and colleagues demonstrated that a 17 β estradiol and norethisterone acetate combination reduced myocardial ischemia and increased exercise tolerance in postmenopausal women with established angina pectoris (Sanderson, Haines, Yeung, et al., 2001). Haines and colleagues reported an anti-ischemic action of HT in postmenopausal women with established angina pectoris (Haines, Yeung, Yip, et al., 2001). Further studies are needed to clarify the effect of different formulations, delivery routs, timing of initiation, and dose of HT and the effect of estrogen alone on the incidence of cardiovascular disease in women. The estrogen-only arm of the WHI found no significant increase or decrease in coronary heart disease with ET (National Institutes of Health, 2004). The best evidence available indicates that while HT is not associated with significant cardiovascular risk, it should not be prescribed for the primary or secondary prevention of cardiovascular disease.

SPECIFIC CONSIDERATIONS FOR PHARMACOTHERAPY

WHEN DRUG THERAPY IS NEEDED

Menopause is a time of physical, emotional, and developmental change and, as such, many women seek advice and guidance from healthcare providers. This is an optimal time to reinforce healthy lifestyle behaviors such as appropriate diet, physical activity, controlling serum lipids, no smoking, moderate alcohol intake, and stress reduction. For women experiencing decreased quality of life due to menopausal symptoms, many treatments are available, but a discussion of options should not be limited to symptomatic women. Therapeutic options should be discussed with all women during the perimenopausal transition and postmenopausal years. Women younger than 40 who have had natural or induced (surgical or pharmacologic) menopause are of special concern, and this group in particular will benefit from estrogen therapy. The physiologic and psychologic manifestations of menopause can be treated with a variety of interventions including lifestyle modification, nonpharmacologic management, and pharmacologic (hormonal and nonhormonal) therapy (NAMS, 2000b; NAMS, 2004).

Decisions concerning treatment are based upon an assessment of presenting symptoms, disease risk profile, presence of contraindications, and the personal preferences of the individual woman. No intervention is risk-free, but with careful analysis, a therapeutic option with the desired benefits and acceptable risks can be formulated. Recent studies continue to document that vasomotor symptoms respond to a variety of estrogen-containing treatments as well as nonhormonal therapies such as the antidepressants, venlafaxine, and fluoxetine (Barton, Loprinzi, & Ko, 2002; Gambacciani, Ciaponi, Cappagli, Genazzani, 2001; NAMS, 2004; Notelovitz, Cassel, et al., 2000; Notelovitz, Lenihan, et al., 2000; Rebar, Trabal, & Mortola, 2000; Shulman, Yankov, & Kerstin, 2002). Urogenital atrophy responds to systemic or local estrogen therapy (Eriksen, 1999; Hammond, 1996; Hextal & Cardozo, 2001; Rioux, Devlin, Gelfand, et al., 2000). Although estrogen improves mood and depressive symptoms, antidepressants are the appropriate therapy for major depression (Boyle & Murrihy, 2001; Schmidt et al., 2000). Interestingly, in one preliminary study, older depressed women taking estrogen and sertraline had greater global improvement and quality of life than women on sertraline alone (Schneider, Small, & Clary, 2001).

Duration of therapy depends upon the persistence of symptoms, individual risk factors, occurrence of adverse events, response to therapy, and personal preference. Young, surgically menopausal women should benefit from estrogen therapy at least until the average age of menopause. Most women seeking treatment for control of vasomotor symptoms need treatment for 5 years or less, but some women with persistent hot flashes request treatment for longer periods to maintain an acceptable quality of life. The safety of estrogen therapy has been documented for at least 5 years (Kaunitz, 2002). Long-term studies of the use of antidepressants for vasomotor symptoms are not available. Though antidepressants are considered safe, recent concerns regarding possible increased suicide risks with SSRIs are being studied. The long-term safety of herbal therapies has not been studied.

Estrogen, bisphophonates, calcitonin, and raloxifene have been shown to increase bone density and decrease fractures due to osteoporosis (NAMS, 2002; NOF, 2000; Writing Group for WHI, 2002). In a woman at high risk for breast cancer, the risks of estrogen appear to outweigh the benefits for osteoporosis prevention (NAMS, 2000b; Writing Group for WHI, 2002). While a number of observational studies have documented prevention of death from or delay in developing cardiovascular disease in menopausal women taking estrogen, recent randomized controlled trials have demonstrated no benefit in preventing the onset or progression of cardiovascular disease by HT (Ettinger, Friedman, Bush, & Quesenberry, 1996; Grady et al., 1992; Grodstein, Manson, Colditz, et al., 2000; Grodstein, Mason, & Stampfer, 2001; Herrington et al., 2000; Hulley et al., 1998; National Institutes of Health, 2004; Writing Group for WHI, 2002). Since only one estrogen and one combination HT were studied, it is unknown if other estrogens or combinations of estrogen/progestin or estrogen/progesterone might yield other results. Until randomized clinical trials using other formulations of ET or HT show benefit, Et or HT should not be prescribed for the sole purpose of preventing or treating cardiovascular disease. The prevention and management of established cardiovascular disease is discussed in Chapter 20.

The role for ET or HT in the prevention and the delay of the onset of Alzheimer's disease is in question (Grodstein, Newcomb, & Stampfer, 1999; National Institutes of Health, 2004; Writing Group for WHI, 2002).

SHORT-TERM AND LONG-TERM GOALS OF PHARMACOTHERAPY

Short-term goals of pharmacotherapy include the relief of vasomotor symptoms, control of dysfunctional uterine bleeding, improved sleep quality, improved psychological and cognitive functioning, and overall improvement in perceived quality of life by decreasing the frequency and severity of symptoms during the perimenopause transition and early menopause. Long-term therapy is designed to protect women from osteoporosis without increasing the incidence of other causes of mortality or morbidity. (NAMS, 2000b) Research is ongoing to determine the best way to achieve these long term goals.

NONPHARMACOLOGIC THERAPY FOR CONTROL OF MENOPAUSAL SYMPTOMS

1. *Hot flashes:* The following are nonpharmacologic suggestions for managing hot flashes offered by Barton and colleagues (Barton et al., 2002). (They are not as effective as HT and offer no protection for bones or urogenital atrophy.)
   - Cool ambient room temperatures, especially at night while sleeping
   - Avoid alcohol
   - Personal dietary triggers (if known) for avoidance
   - Vitamin E (800 mg PO daily)
   - Relaxation and deep, abdominal breathing (6–8 per minute)
   - Layering clothing
2. *Vaginal dryness*
   - *Lubricant use:* Over-the-counter moisturizers such as Replens or Gyne-Moistrin can increase vaginal comfort (Scharbo-DeHaan, 1996).

- *Sexual intercourse:* Although formal studies are lacking, sexual intercourse encourages genital vascular congestion and may improve vaginal moisture and suppleness (Scharbo-DeHaan, 1996).
- *Masturbation:* Autoerotic activities have been recommended by some authors to improve vaginal lubrication (Lichtman, 1996).

3. *Urinary incontinence:* These therapies are effective in some women, but do not reverse urogenital atrophy. For a general review of incontinence therapy, see O'Shaughnessy, (2003).
   - *Kegel exercises:* Kegels improve pelvic floor muscle tone and involve alternating contraction and relaxation of the pubococcygeus muscle. Women should begin with ten alternating 3-s contractions and relaxations per day and gradually increase to 10-s contractions and relaxations 80–150 times per day (Walsh, Scura & Whipple, 1997).
   - *Bladder retraining:* Patients gradually increase the time between voiding by 15 min weekly until they are voiding every 3 to 4 h (Walsh, Scura & Whipple, 1997).
   - *Diuretics avoidance:* Incontinence therapy is enhanced if prescribed drugs and dietary compounds that induce diuresis can be avoided (Hurt, 1996).
   - *Surgical intervention:* For a review of surgical interventions, see Mostwin, Genadry, Sanders, and Yang, 1996.
4. *Osteoporosis prevention:* The following are recommendations of the National Osteoporosis Foundation (NOF, 2000). (These therapies are more effective when combined with pharmacotherapy.)
   - *Weight-bearing exercise:* Walking, jogging, stair climbing, dancing, and tennis.
   - Calcium intake of 1200 mg/day from a combination of diet and supplementation; 1500 mg/day is recommended by the NIH Consensus Statement of Optimal Calcium Intake (1994). Calcium should be taken in divided doses, such as 500 mg three times daily for best absorption.
   - Vitamin D 400–800 IU/day or at least 15 min of direct sunlight daily. Supplementation is recommended for those at risk for deficiency such as elderly, chronically ill, housebound, or institutionalized individuals.
   - *Variable-resistance weight training:* One successful regimen is 20-min sessions, three times per week (Notelovitz et al, 1997).
   - Avoid smoking and refrain from taking more than two drinks each of caffeine or alcohol per day.
5. *Cardiovascular disease:* These recommendations to prevent cardiovascular disease are from the *Guide to Preventive Cardiology for Women* developed by the American Heart Association and the American College of Cardiology (Chobanian, Bakris, Black, et al., 2003; Mosca, Grundy, Judelson, et al., 1999).
   - Stop smoking
   - Be physically active each day Accumulate >30 minutes of activity each day
   - Maintain blood pressure <130/80
   - Reduce high blood cholesterol
   - Aim for a healthy weight, BMI between 18.5 and 24.8; waist circumference <35″
   - Improve nutrition: lower fat, limit sodium, include high fiber
   - Use positive coping mechanisms for stress
   - Manage diabetes

TIME FRAME FOR INITIATING PHARMACOTHERAPY

Pharmacotherapy may be initiated when a woman expresses a desire for symptomatic relief and has no contraindications. Therapy should be directed toward controlling the presenting complaint, for example, hot flashes, vaginal dryness, or irregular menstrual cycles. In asymptomatic menopausal women, treatment is geared toward prevention of long-term morbidity and mortality associated with osteoporosis. Non-hormonal therapies should be the first choice for prevention and treatment of osteoporosis (non-severe) in asymptomatic menopausal women. The best time frame for initiating pharmacotherapy to prevent osteoporotic fractures and duration of therapy are not clearly defined. Bone loss is accelerated in early years after menopause and HT intervention during the first 5 years postmenopause helps maintain bone mass and prevent fracture (Eastell, 1998; Writing Group for WHI, 2002). Bone mineral density (BMD) testing should be considered for all postmenopausal women who are undecided or have chosen not to initiate bone-preserving therapy. The National Osteoporosis Foundation (NOF) recommends BMD measurement for all women <65 with at least one risk factor and all women over age 65 regardless of risk factors. For osteoporosis prevention, the NOF recommends initiating pharmacologic treatment in all women who have a BMD T-score below −2, even in the absence of risk factors, and in women with BMD T-scores below −1.5, if they have one or more additional fracture risk factors. In addition, all postmenopausal women who present with vertebral or hip fractures are considered candidates for pharmacologic treatment without BMD measurement (NOF, 2000). HT is thought to increase the incidence of breast cancer if continued beyond 5 years, so the use of HT for longer periods of time to prevent osteoporosis is questionable (Writing Group for WHI, 2002). The alternatives to HT for prevention and treatment of osteoporosis include bisphophonates (alendronate and risedronate), calcitonin, and selective estrogen receptor modulators (raloxifene) (NOF, 2000). Postmenopausal women with osteoporosis were followed for 10 years comparing alendronate and placebo. Alendronate provided therapeutic results that were gradually lost when stopped (Bone, Hosking, Devogelaer, et al., 2004). Decisions should be based on risk/benefit analysis and patient preference after appropriate counseling. See Table 19–1 for an overview of the drug classes used for the pharmacologic management of the climacteric.

TABLE 19–1. Overview of Drug Classes for Pharmacological Management of the Climacteric

Combination oral contraceptives
Estrogens
Natural estrogens
Conjugated equine estrogens
Esterified estrogens
Micronized estrogens
Estropipate
Synthetic estrogens
Diethylstilbestrol
Ethinyl estradiol
Quinesterol
Progestins
Natural progesterone
Progesterone derivatives
Medroxyprogestrone acetate
Megace
19-nortestosterone derivatives
Norethindrone
Norethindrone acetate
Norgestimate
Androgens
Natural testosterone
Dehydroepiandrosterone
Synthetic testosterone
Estrogen–androgen combinations
Estrogen–progestin combinations
Bone resorption inhibitors
Alendronate sodium
Calcitonin
Risedronate sodium
Calcium supplements
Calcium carbonate
Calcium citrate
Calcium lactate
Calcium gluconate
Selective estrogen receptor modulators
Raloxifene

HISTORY AND PHYSICAL EXAMINATION PRIOR TO THERAPY

Before initiating any therapy, a thorough history and complete physical examination are required. The history should focus on identifying any contraindications for hormone use as well as risk factors for heart disease (Table 19–2), breast cancer (Table 19–3), osteoporosis (Table 19–4) and thromboembolism.

In addition, determine the woman's perception of the need for and risks of hormone therapy so that these issues can be addressed during counseling. Any current herbal or alternative therapies she may be using must be identified because they can have an additive effect with estrogen. A complete physical examination with special emphasis on breast and pelvic findings should be conducted.

The contraindications to the use of the estrogen in combination oral contraceptive pills are discussed in Chapter 18. Contraindications to the low doses of estrogen used in menopausal hormone replacement therapy are similar but not identical. The accepted contraindications are (1) undiagnosed abnormal vaginal bleeding, (2) active liver disease, (3) current or recent thrombophlebitis or thromboembolic disease, (4) breast cancer, and (5) endometrial cancer (NAMS, 2000b). Coronary heart disease is a contraindication based on recent studies (Penckofer, Hackbarth, & Schwertz, 2003). In addition to the absolute contraindications listed above, other conditions are considered relative contraindications and require careful consideration of the benefits and risks before initiation of and careful, frequent monitoring while using therapies that include estrogen. These conditions are (1) migraine headaches, (2) familial mixed hyperlipidemia or hypertriglyceridemia, (3) history of gallbladder disease and no

TABLE 19–2. Risk Factors for Heart Disease

Cigarette smoking
Physical inactivity
High fat, low fiber diet
Obesity, waist circumference >35″
Life stress
High blood pressure
Elevated lipids, lipoproteins
Diabetes

Source: Adapted from Mosca et al., 1999.

TABLE 19–3. Risk Factors for Developing Breast Cancer

Female gender
Aging
Genetic risk factors
First-degree relative with breast cancer
Personal history of breast cancer
Atypical hyperplasia on breast biopsy
Caucasian race
Early menarche < age 12
Late menopause > age 50
Exogenous hormones
Alcohol intake of more than 1 drink per day
Obesity
Not breastfeeding
Nulliparity
First full-term pregnancy after 30
Physical inactivity
Environmental pollution

Source: Adapted from the American Cancer Society (2002).

cholecystectomy, (4) history of endometriosis, (5) history of leiomyomas, and (6) seizure disorders (NAMS, 2000b).

Once abnormal vaginal bleeding has been diagnosed and treated, cardiovascular disease, thromboembolism, and cancer ruled out, HT may be initiated. Although a general consensus has not been achieved, some physicians will consider hormone replacement therapy for long-term survivors of breast and endometrial cancer (Dew, Eden, Beller, et al., 1998; DiSaia & Brewster, 2002; Peters, Fodera, Sabol, et al., 2001; Suriano et al., 2001) as well as for women with resolved thromboembolic disease or liver disease (NAMS, 2000b). Although controversial, consideration may be given to a nonoral form of estrogen for women with elevated triglycerides (>300 mg/dL) or gall bladder dysfunction after cholycystectomy (NAMS, 2000b). Because of the steady state delivery of transdermal estrogen, it may be more beneficial for women who develop headaches with fluctuations in estrogen levels (Lufkin, & Ory, 1994).

TABLE 19–4. Key Risk Factors for Osteoporotic Fracture (Demonstrated in large, ongoing, prospective study)

Personal history of fracture as an adult
History of fracture in first-degree relative
Current cigarette smoking
Low body weight (<127 lbs)
Other Risk Factors for Fracture
Caucasian race
Advanced age
Female sex
Estrogen deficiency
Lifelong low calcium intake
Inadequate physical activity
Health-Related Risk Factors for Fracture
Alcoholism
Dementia
Poor health/frailty
Impaired eyesight
Recurrent falls

Source: Adapted from National Osteoporosis Foundation (NOF, 2000).

Common conditions that are not contraindications for estrogen therapy are cervical cancer, diabetes, and controlled hypertension. It is notable that the Postmenopausal Estrogen/Progestin Interventions (PEPI) trial (Writing Group, 1995) found no change and possibly a decrease in blood pressure with women on hormone therapy. Currently healthy women with risk factors for osteoporosis or colorectal cancer could reap the most benefits from hormone therapy.

Laboratory Tests

For many women, the age of onset and characteristic symptoms and physical findings allow the diagnosis of menopause without laboratory confirmation. In other women, laboratory data may provide critical information to help the clinician select the appropriate treatment. The following laboratory tests can be used to identify problems associated with the climacteric.

Gonadotropin Measurements

If the diagnosis of menopause cannot be made with confidence from the history and physical examination findings, measurement of gonadotropins may help establish the diagnosis. Elevated levels of gonadotropins (FSH > 30 IU/L) (NAMS, 2000a; Burger, Dudley, Hopper, et al., 1996) indicate menopausal status. Because FSH increases before and to a greater extent than LH, it is the preferred measurement and it is seldom necessary to measure LH. Many women, during the early transition years, will be symptomatic and have normal gonadotropins. After eliminating pathologic causes of symptoms, a symptomatic woman with normal gonadotropins can be started on a trial of hormone therapy or low-dose oral contraceptives (Kaunitz, 2001; Santoro et al, 1996).

Mammography

The U.S. Preventive Services Task Force recommends screening mammography, with or without clinical breast examination, every 1 to 2 years for women aged 40 and older (screening for breast cancer, 2002). Because estrogen may play a role in tumor progression in some breast cancers, mammograms should be obtained before initiating estrogen therapy and annually thereafter.

Endometrial Biopsy

Any woman experiencing abnormal vaginal bleeding should be evaluated for endometrial cancer. Either transvaginal sonography or endometrial biopsy is a safe, effective first diagnostic procedure. Endometrial biopsy with one of the slender cannula biopsy instruments is a simple, usually atraumatic, office procedure that reliably identifies cancer when sufficient tissue is obtained. A transvaginal sonography finding of ≥ 5 mm is considered abnormal and needs further evaluation. The choice of procedure depends upon assessment of patient risk, clinician skills, availability of high-quality sonography, and patient preference (Goldstein, Bree, Benson, et al., 2001).

Bone Density Measurements

For women with increased risk factors for osteoporosis, a measurement of bone density will monitor bone integrity and help predict fracture risk. The most precision is obtained with dual energy x-ray absorptimetry (DEXA), but cost-effective screening can be obtained with single-photon absorptiometry (SPA) of the radius or calcaneus. Alternative testing techniques include quantitative computed tomography (QCT), which can be used as an alternative to DEXA for vertebral measurements, or ultrasound densitometry, which is not as precise as DEXA or SPA but appears to be a good predictor of fracture risk (NOF, 2000).

CLIENT INFORMATION

All perimenopausal women need to be counseled on how to achieve and maintain a healthy lifestyle. Older women tend to be given unacceptably low rates of clinical preventive services (Bergman-Evans & Walker, 1996). Counseling should include information on nutrition, exercise, sexual health, rest and recreation, stress reduction, immunizations, dental health, smoking cessation, alcohol and drug use/abuse, and injury and violence prevention (American College of Obstetricians and Gynecologists [ACOG], 1995). In addition to the general counseling, women need specific information about the risks and benefits of any treatment regimen selected.

Oral Contraceptives

Oral contraceptives (OCs) appear to be a safe, effective therapeutic choice to manage perimenopausal symptoms in healthy, nonsmoking women without contraindications to OC use. They provide contraception, regulate menstrual bleeding, control vasomotor symptoms, decrease future fracture risk, and decrease endometrial and ovarian cancer risk (Kaunitz, 2001). Many perimenopausal women are unaware of their risk of pregnancy and fail to use effective contraception. As a result, 51% of pregnancies in women over 40 are unintended, and 65% of these pregnancies end in abortion (Henshaw, 1998). In nonsmoking women, OCs appear to have fewer health risks than pregnancy. Counseling should be aimed at increasing women's knowledge of their life stage risks and the benefits and risks of OCs to meet their needs. Placing perimenopausal women on OCs has only been considered an option in recent years. As large numbers of women begin using OCs in the perimenopause, unique risks may emerge that are currently unknown. It will be important for clinicians to monitor the literature for evidence of currently unknown risks such as increased risk of breast cancer or unusually high rates of VTE or cardiovascular events.

Hormone Therapy

Women beginning hormone therapy should be informed about the benefits and risks as well as prepared for the expected side effects with thorough and appropriate counseling. Each woman must decide if the benefits of therapy outweigh the combination of risks (genetic and biologic) and inconvenient side effects (environmental, lifestyle, and personal characteristics) that accompany hormone therapy. A thorough history will identify the particular symptoms and risks an individual woman may face as she ages.

Hormone Therapy Risks. The most serious risks associated with hormone therapy include the development or promotion of reproductive tract cancers. Breast cancer is known to be estrogen-dependent in many women and is a concern of women taking exogenous estrogen. A multitude of studies have investigated the impact of estrogen on the development of breast cancer with varying and often conflicting results. All women in this age group have an increased risk of breast cancer, and the effect of estrogen on that risk is not absolutely known. Mahavni and Sood (2001) provide an excellent review of hormone therapy and cancer risk. While two observational studies suggest a decreased risk of breast cancer in HT users, the majority of studies reviewed showed a small but statistically significant increase of breast cancer in HT users, and estrogen-progestin use may increase cancer risk more than estrogen alone (Ross, Paganini-Hill, Wan, & Pike, 2000; Schairer, Lubin, Troisi, et al., 2000). The increased risk of breast cancer is small, with an estimated increase of 6 excess breast cancers above the estimated 63 per 1000 expected in this population (Clavel-Chapelon & Hill, 2000). In the Women's Health Initiative, a randomized clinical trial that addressed the effects of CEE plus MPA in otherwise healthy menopausal women, a small (8 extra cases per 10,000 women) increase in breast cancer incidence was noted. Although this increase was not statistically different from placebo, the trial was stopped because the combined increase of all risks moved beyond a predetermined safety boundary. The estrogen-only arm of this trial was stopped due to increased stroke risk, not breast cancer risk. In the WHI, there were no increased deaths in the HT group due to any cause, including cancer (Writing Group for WHI, 2002). In one small, randomized, controlled study that lasted 22 years, HT was associated with a reduced risk of breast cancer (Nachtigall, Smilen, Nachtigall, et al., 1992). In one study that looked at mortality from breast cancer, women on HT when breast cancer was diagnosed had better survival rates than women not on estrogen (Schairer, Gail, Byrne, et al., 1999). To clarify the risk and benefits of ET, the WHI in the United States will continue until 2005.

The effect of HT on the development of ovarian cancer is also noted for conflicting results. While Coughlin and colleagues (Coughlin, Giustozzi, Smith, et al., 2000) reported that ET had no association with the development of ovarian cancer in a meta-analysis of 15 case-controlled studies, Rodriguez and colleagues (Rodriguez, Patel, Calle, et al., 2001) reported an increase risk for ovarian cancer mortality in postmenopausal women who used estrogen for 10 or more years. The mortality rate for women not using estrogen was 26.4 per 100,000 women compared to 64.4 age-adjusted deaths from ovarian cancer per 100,000 women who used estrogen for 10 years or more (Rodriguez et al., 2001). Lacey and colleagues (Lacey, Mink, Lubin, et al., 2002) investigated the effects of HT on breast cancer incidence in 44,241 women who participated in the Breast Cancer Detection Demonstration Project. In this study, a small but statistically significant increase in epithelial ovarian cancer occurred with ET use for 10 to 19 years (an estimated 2 additional ovarian cancers per 10,000 women-years of use). Although HT was not associated with a statistically significant increase in epithelial ovarian cancer, only 18 women using HT developed ovarian cancer (Lacey et al., 2002). In another recent study, investigators reported an increased risk of ovarian cancer among women who took estrogen plus sequential progestins, but not among those who used continuous combination estrogen-progestin regimens. The greatest risk was seen with greater than 10 years of use (Riman, Dickman, Nilsson, et al., 2002).

Further studies are needed to delineate the impact of postmenopausal estrogen on the development of ovarian cancer.

In addition, it is well documented that there is an increased risk of endometrial hyperplasia and cancer in women with a uterus who take estrogen alone (Hill, Weiss, Beresford, et al., 2000; Persson, Weiderpass, Bergkvist, et al., 1999; Writing Group, 1995). Most, but not all, of the endometrial cancer experienced by women during estrogen replacement therapy tends to be well differentiated with an excellent cure rate (Woodruff & Pickar, 1994). The risk for endometrial cancer can be significantly reduced but not totally eliminated by adding a progestin to the estrogen therapy in women who have a uterus. (Hill et al., 2000; Persson et al, 1999; Writing Group, 1995).

Finally, HT is associated with an increased risk of gallbladder disease requiring surgery (Grodstein, Colditz, & Stampfer, 1994) as well as deep vein thrombosis (Hulley et al., 1998, Writing Group WHI, 2002).

Hormone Therapy Side Effects. A woman should be given anticipatory guidance to prepare her for the most common nuisance side effects. Make her a partner in establishing the appropriate therapy. She needs to monitor and report side effects to allow optimal titration of the dosage. Unpredictable bleeding for the first 4 to 6 months of therapy is common. Nuisance side effects involve both the estrogen and progestin components of HT. The estrogen component has been associated with complaints of nausea, edema, breast tenderness, contact lens intolerance, headache, and aggravation of porphyria. The progestin component can create premenstrual syndrome symptoms, such as fatigue, depression, edema, breast tenderness, insomnia, or chloasma (Wich & Carnes, 1995).

Bone Resorption Inhibitors

Alendronate sodium and risedronate sodium are bisphosphonates approved for the prevention and treatment of osteoporosis. Both drugs have been shown to improve bone density and reduce fracture rates of the spine and hip (Bone, Hosking, Devogelaer, et al., 2004; Geusens & McClung, 2001; Liberman, Weiss, Broll, et al., 1995; Marcus, Wong, Heath, & Stock, 2002; Watts, 2001). Alendronate dosage is 5 mg/day or 35 mg once weekly for prevention and 10 mg/day or 70 mg once weekly for treatment. Risedronate dosage is 5 mg/day or 35 mg once weekly for prevention and treatment. Although risedronate appears to cause fewer GI problems than alendronate (Taggart et al., 2002), both drugs have a risk of esophagitis (and rarely, esophageal ulcers) and patients should be strongly counseled as follows:

1. To take the drug in the morning at least 30 minutes before any food, drink, or other medication and with a large (6 to 8 oz) glass of water.
2. Not to lie down for at least 30 minutes after taking the medication.
3. To contact her healthcare provider if heartburn or difficulty swallowing develops, since this may herald esophageal ulcerations.

Calcium interferes with the absorption of bisphophonates and should be taken at least 30 min after the morning dose.

Calcitonin also inhibits bone resorption. In a large randomized clinical trial, salmon calcitonin nasal spray at a dose of 200 IU/day significantly reduced the risk of new vertebral fractures in postmenopausal women with osteoporosis (Chestnut, Silverman, Andriano, et al., 2000). One unique aspect of calcitonin is that it has an analgesic effect and relieves pain associated with vertebral fractures (Lyritis & Trovas, 2002).

Selective estrogen receptor modulators (SERMs) are bone resorption inhibitors. Raloxifene is the only SERM approved for osteoporosis prevention and treatment. Data from the MORE trial (Ettinger, Black, Mitlak, et al., 1999) indicate raloxifene 60 mg/day reduces fracture rates of the spine but not at the hip or other appendicular sites. In addition, raloxifene has been shown to decrease breast cancer risk and increase hot flashes, leg cramps, and risk for deep vein thrombosis.

OUTCOMES MANAGEMENT

SELECTION OF THE APPROPRIATE AGENT

Pharmacologic management of the climacteric is an art as well as a science. You must balance the personal preferences and characteristics of the individual with the known medical risks and benefits of any drug intervention. The most difficult management decisions usually occur during the perimenopausal period. After thorough evaluation and consideration of the contraindications to each therapy, the clinician has the pharmacologic options for management discussed below.

Oral Contraceptives

During the perimenopausal years (ages 40–50), women will often present with unpredictable anovulatory vaginal bleeding, hot flashes, or both. Low-dose oral contraceptives are ideal first-line drugs for this group of women. They prevent pregnancy; induce regular, predictable menstrual bleeding; and reduce the risk of ovarian and endometrial cancer while providing the estrogen to maintain bone health, prevent hot flashes and improve quality of life (Davis, Godwin, Lippman, et al., 2000; Kaunitz, 2001). The woman who is having anovulatory bleeding but not having hot flashes also is a candidate for low-dose OCs once endometrial cancer has been ruled out.

Women should stop OCs at menopause. Woman who are symptomatic and request treatment can be transitioned to an appropriate therapeutic regimen. Traditional indications of menopause (amenorrhea and elevated FSH) are not applicable to women on OCs because they will continue to have withdrawal menses as long as they take the pill, and the estrogen in the pill will suppress FSH even for several weeks after discontinuing the pill (Crenin, 1996; Kaunitz, 2001). The current recommendation is to continue OCs until the expected time of menopause, with one author suggesting age 55 or older as an appropriate age to switch healthy, nonsmoking women from OCs to HT (Kaunitz, 2001). One study found that most menopausal women have an FSH/LH ratio >1 and/or serum $E_2 < 20$ pg/mL (Crenin, 1996). If the woman does not desire hormone therapy, an appropriate nonhormonal regimen can be selected to address her particular set of symptoms or physical risks—for example, an antidepressant for vasomotor symptoms or bisphosphonate for low bone mass.

Progestin

If the perimenopausal woman with irregular anovulatory bleeding prefers to not take OCs, cyclic withdrawal to oral progestin is an appropriate alternative therapy. Medroxyprogesterone acetate (MPA) 10 mg daily for the first 14 days of the month will prevent endometrial hyperplasia. Estrogen may be started when the woman fails to have withdrawal bleeding from the progestin (Gambrell, 1997). If a woman does not want systemic hormones, or if contraception is required, the levonorgestrel-releasing intrauterine system (LNG-IUS) has been shown to control dysfunctional uterine bleeding in many women (Varila, Wahlstrom, & Rauramo, 2001).

Hormone Therapy

The symptomatic menopausal woman has a variety of options that will control symptoms and improve quality of life. The most common menopausal symptoms (vasomotor instability, urogenital atrophy, sleep disturbances and the related mood and cognitive disruptions) are caused by the decline in estrogen and improve with hormone therapy. Because of the high efficacy and relative safety with less than 5 years of use, hormone therapy may be offered to symptomatic women who have no contraindications, whose quality of life is decreased by the symptoms, and who request therapeutic intervention. The lowest effective dose for the shortest time is advised. If hormones are contraindicated or not desired for personal reasons, nonhormonal options such as venlafaxine 75 mg/day or fluoxetine 20 mg/day are an option. Although not FDA approved for this indication, both agents have been shown to be effective in reducing hot flashes in clinical trials (Barton et al., 2002). If hormone therapy is chosen, estrogen plus a progestin (EPT) (NAMS, 2003B) should be used in women with a uterus and estrogen alone (ET) used in women without a uterus. HT therapy can be initiated in a variety of ways. It can be given with individual doses of estrogen and progestin, which allows greater flexibility to titrate each individual hormone to the woman's needs, but requires the woman to take two separate pills a day or a progestin pill with estrogen given by vaginal ring or transdermal gel or patch. The risk of this regimen is that the woman could stop the progestin while continuing to take the estrogen and be at risk for endometrial cancer. Estrogen can be given with the LNG-IUS providing the progestin. This is not an FDA approved use of the LNG-IUS, but it has several advantages over oral progestin: (1) It provides contraception if the woman is perimenopausal; (2) local effect limits systemic side effects of the progestin; and (3) it induces amenorrhea in most women (Varila, Wahlstrom, & Rauramo, 2001). The LNG-IUS may be too large to use in women many years postmenopausal who have experienced the normal uterine involution. Finally, there are a variety of estrogen/progestin combination products formulated with a variety of progestins for use in the postmenopausal woman. The advantages of combination products are convenient dosing in a single pill or patch and the fact that the progestin dose has been balanced to the estrogen dose and is known to prevent endometrial hyperplasia. Speroff, Glass, and Kase (1999, p. 739) recommend use of combined estrogen/progestin after hysterectomy in the following special circumstances: (1) history of endometriosis, (2) supracervical hysterectomy, (3) after treatment of endometrial cancer, (4) history of endometroid tumors of the ovary, (5) in the presence of significant osteoporosis, (6) with elevated triglycerides. In the United States, the most thoroughly studied oral estrogen is conjugated equine estrogen (CEE) Premarin, which contains ten different estrogenic compounds. Recent studies have linked CEE, when combined with medroxyprogesterone acetate (MPA), to small increases in risk for cardiovascular disease and breast cancer (Writing Group for WHI, 2002). Esterified estrogens (Estratab), micronized estradiol (Estrace), transdermal estrogens (Estrogel, Estraderm, Climara, and Vivelle) and vaginal estrogen (Femring) are not identical compounds to conjugated estrogens, and whether these compounds will have the same adverse effects on cardiovascular disease and breast cancer is unknown. Clinicians should assume the same risks occur until studies provide evidence of safety. Few comparative studies exist of the various estrogens (Ansbacher, 2001). The traditional starting dose for estrogen is 0.625 mg of CEE or equivalent estrogen formulations for preventing osteoporosis and control of vasomotor symptoms. Recent studies indicate that low-dose estrogen (0.3 mg estrone, 0.25 mg micronized estradiol oral; 25 mg estradiol transdermal), especially in conjunction with calcium and vitamin D, could be effective treatments for osteoporosis in older women (Prestwood, Kenny, Unson, & Kulldorff, 2000; Prestwood, Thompson, Kenny, et al., 1999). The lower doses of estrogen appear to control vasomotor symptoms and prevent osteoporosis (Gallagher, 1999; Schneider & Gallagher, 1999). It is unknown whether the lower doses of estrogen carry the same risk of breast cancer and cardiovascular events as the higher doses that have been studied. In younger women taking oral contraceptives, lowering the estrogen dose has resulted in fewer cardiovascular events. For the young, surgically menopausal woman, a higher initial dose may be required to control hot flashes. With higher doses of estrogen, a higher dose of progestin may be needed for endometrial protection (Nand, Webster, & Wren, 1995). Over time, the dose should be titrated downward to the lowest dose to control symptoms.

Transdermal estrogen systems are available for nonoral delivery of hormones. The 0.05-mg patch is the usual starting dose and is thought to be approximately equivalent to 0.625 mg of oral conjugated estrogen. The transdermal patch offers very stable serum levels of estradiol and may control symptoms in women who are sensitive to the fluctuations in serum levels of estrogen that occur during oral therapy. Some women may prefer a nonoral estrogen. Transdermal estrogen, in conjunction with oral progestin has been shown to be comparable to oral estrogen in some parameters but not others. For example, it has been shown to decrease total cholesterol, LDL-C, and triglycerides, but not raise HDL-C in short-term studies (Erenus, Karakoc, & Gurler, 2001; Vehkavaara et al., 2000; Vehkavaara et al., 2001; West et al., 2001.) In longer-term studies, transdermal estrogen has been shown to improve BMD in a manner similar to oral estrogen (Cetinkaya, Kokcu, Yanik, et al., 2001). Long-term, randomized, controlled, comparison trials are needed to distinguish the unique benefits of individual estrogen preparations and delivery routes. Injectable estrogen is not appropriate for menopausal hormone therapy.

Once the agent and starting dose have been selected, a regimen must be chosen. There is no one "right" way to prescribe hormone therapy; rather, appropriate options should be tailored to the particular woman's symptoms, needs, and preferences. Adherence to therapy depends heavily on the client's thorough understanding of the short-term and long-term benefits and preparation for the anticipated side effects. Women who have undergone a hysterectomy should be prescribed estrogen alone, in doses sufficient to control symptoms. Women who have retained their uteruses are at increased risk for developing endometrial hyperplasia if they take estrogen alone. For these women, a progestin is added to the regimen to inhibit endometrial growth (Writing Group, 1995). There are three regimens for HT: sequential, continuous combined, and pulsed progestin. In the sequential regimen, estrogen is taken every day and progestin for at least 14 consecutive days each month. Bleeding will occur a few days after the last dose of progestin in almost all women (Writing Group, 1995). In the continuous combined regimen, estrogen and progestin are taken daily. Unpredictable bleeding occurs for the first few months, then amenorrhea develops in most women (Nand et al., 1995). Continued successful use may be improved with continuous combined therapy (Eiken & Kolthoff, 2002). In the pulsed regimen, estrogen is given daily and progestin is given cyclically 3 days on then 3 days off. The pulsed regimen has only been studied with the proprietary formulation by Monarch Pharmaceuticals. Bleeding profiles of the pulsed regimen are similar to the continuous combined regimen. The types of estrogens for menopausal treatment include estrone (conjugated equine estrogens, esterified estrogens, and estropipate), micronized estradiol, and ethinyl estradiol. The progestogens for menopausal treatment include local therapy with the LGN-IUS, vaginal progesterone gel, oral medroxyprogesterone acetate (MPA), norethindrone (NET), and micronized progesterone. Several companies offer prepackaged combined HT that has the advantage of a single daily pill or a patch. There is one formulation for sequential HT, Premphase (CEE 0.625 mg daily and MPA 5 mg daily for the last 14 days). There are a variety of continuous combined formulations available. Prempro (CEE 0.625 mg and MPA 2.5 mg daily), Activella (E_2 1 mg and norethindrone acetate [NETA] 0.5 mg), and FemHRT (EE 5 μg and NETA 1 mg) are oral regimens and CombiPatch (0.05 mg E_2 and either 0.14 or 0.025 mg NETA) is a transdermal regimen. Finally, the one pulsed regimen is Prefest (E_2 1 mg daily and 0.09 mg norgestimate pulsed 3 days on and 3 days off). For all regimens, unpredictable bleeding is common in the first few months of treatment. Any continued bleeding after 6 months or increase in amount, duration, or frequency of bleeding requires evaluation.

For most of the past forty years, only limited options existed for the hormonal management of menopause, and most research has been done on doses, formulations, and treatment regimens not favored today. Most new formulations for HT contain micronized estradiol rather than CEE. No new formulation contains MPA for the progestin. The Women's Health Initiative halted the study arm that used the combination of CEE and MPA due to increased incidence of cardiovascular disease and breast cancer. Increased risk of ischemic stroke and dementia have also been shown (Wassertheil-Smoller, Hendrix, Limacher, et al., 2003). The increased risks are also thought to be associated with other formulations of estrogen and progestin/progesterone. Research is needed on these new formulations and delivery methods to identify unique benefits and risks. With the number of preparations now available, clinicians have the opportunity to tailor therapy to individual needs. If a woman is on OCs during the perimenopause transition, it may be possible to transition to menopausal HT regimens using the same progestin. Novel delivery options exist, such as a transdermal estrogen/progestin patch or estrogen combined with the LNG-IUS (Varila, Wahlstrom, & Rauramo, 2001) or vaginal natural progesterone (de Ziegler, Ferriani, Moraes, & Bulletti, 2000). In one study, women who were willing and able to try different types of HT had longer duration of HT use than women who made no changes in formulations (Gavin, Thorp, & Ohsfeldt, 2001).

In the years to come, more products and formulations will become available for managing menopausal symptoms and the consequences of aging. Readers are urged to keep abreast of current drug therapies and supporting scientific evidence for use as these drugs and devices come on the market. Standards of practice are changing rapidly and safe clinical practice will depend upon clinicians closely monitoring research findings and published national guidelines.

Startup problems should be anticipated, and women should be prepared for breast tenderness, vaginal bleeding, and the inconvenience of daily dosing. Frequent contact between women and their providers will facilitate improved treatment adherence. Problems can be identified, and changes in dosages or drugs, can be initiated before the woman becomes discouraged and electively discontinues treatment. A suggested followup schedule is: (1) telephone contact during the first month of treatment, (2) an office visit every 3 months until a suitable dose and regimen have been established, and (3) yearly visits thereafter. Annual physical examination and laboratory studies are required for continued hormone therapy.

Bone Resorption Inhibitors

For those who are unable to take estrogen, bisphophonates (alendronate and risedronate), calcitonin, and raloxifene are bone resorption inhibitors approved for postmenopausal women with osteopenia or established osteoporosis (NOF, 2000). Each of these therapeutic options offers unique benefits. The bisphophonates appear to provide the best fracture prevention at all sites but have strict dosing requirements and are associated with esophagitis and, rarely, esophageal ulceration (Geusens & McClung, 2001; Liberman et al., 1995). Calcitonin has analgesic properties for severe osteoporosis and osteoporotic fractures but appears to lose effectiveness for fracture prevention after a few years (Chestnut et al., 2000; Lyritis & Trovas, 2002). Raloxifene, a SERM, appears to reduce the risk of vertebral fracture and breast cancer but increases vasomotor symptoms, leg cramps, vaginal atrophy, and risk of venous thromboembolism (Ettinger et al., 1999). Studies on the effectiveness of each of these options included calcium supplementation and vitamin D. New options for osteoporosis treatment are on the horizon—for example, a once-a-year injection and development of bone formation stimulators.

Calcium Supplementation and Vitamin D

Because intake of adequate calcium is vital to maintaining bone mass regardless of whether hormonal or nonhormonal therapies are chosen, try to ensure that appropriate dietary and supplemental sources of calcium are taken by menopausal women. All adult women and menopausal women should obtain 1200 to 1500 mg of elemental calcium daily either through diet or a combination of diet and calcium supplementation. In addition, an intake of 400 to 800 IU of vitamin D per day is recommended for anyone at risk of deficiency such as people > 70 and chronically ill, housebound, or institutionalized women (NOF, 2000). Daily calcium intake of greater than 2 g/day should be avoided. Several formulations of calcium are available for supplementation: Calcium carbonate contains the highest proportion of elemental calcium by weight, but calcium chelates such as citrate may be more effective for promoting bone formation (Chung & Maroulis, 1996). Calcium citrate is also more appropriate for women on proton-pump inhibitors.

Excess dietary calcium may induce unfavorable calcium-mineral interactions, particularly with iron, zinc, and magnesium. Since calcium inhibits iron absorption, encourage women with low dietary iron intake to consume their calcium between or after meals. A zinc deficiency could develop in women with low levels of dietary zinc on high-calcium diets, so zinc may need to be supplemented. Finally, excess calcium can cause magnesium deficiency in special circumstances such as diabetes or alcoholism. To prevent magnesium deficiency, 100 mg of magnesium for every 500 mg of calcium is recommended for these situations. Most cases of calcium-induced mineral deficiency occur with calcium intake of greater than 2 g/day (Whiting, Wood, & Kim, 1997).

MONITORING FOR EFFICACY

Efficacy is demonstrated by resolution of presenting symptoms and continued adherence to the treatment regimen. When a woman has multiple symptoms, it is not unusual for one or more symptoms to be relieved but not all. For example, hot flashes may be controlled, but genital atrophy continues. If the woman is otherwise asymptomatic, supplementation with vaginal estrogen (vaginal cream, tablet, or silastic ring) is preferred to increasing the dose of oral estrogen. Some women experience decreased sexual desire and increased sexual dysfunction that is unresponsive to HT. After several months of HT trial, if decreased libido continues to be a problem, a trial of an estrogen/androgen combination therapy can be tried. The most appropriate androgen and the best delivery route in menopausal women are not currently known. There is one estrogen/androgen combination approved for use in menopausal women that contains methyl-testosterone. Other androgens, such as dehydroepiandrosterone

(DHEA) and its sulfate (DHEAS) as well as transdermal testosterone are being investigated (Hoeger & Guzick, 1999). It is important to note that the oral estrogen/androgen combination prevents the favorable changes in lipoproteins seen with estrogen alone and careful monitoring is advisable (Watts et al., 1995). A progestin should still be used for endometrial protection with estrogen/androgen combination therapy.

Relief of symptoms provides more information on therapy efficacy than laboratory tests, but laboratory studies are available.

1. *Vaginal cytology:* The maturation index supplies information about local tissue response to estrogen. Adequate estrogen therapy produces abundant superficial cells, whereas a high percentage of parabasal cells indicates low estrogen.
2. *Bone density measurements:* In untreated postmenopausal women, repeat DEXA testing is recommended at 3- to 5-year intervals (NAMS, 2002). In treated postmenopausal women, repeat DEXA before 2 years of therapy may not be clinically useful (Cummings, Palermo, Browner, et al., 2000).
3. *Serum estrogen levels:* In women who continue to be symptomatic on estrogens, including nonoral routes, measuring serum estradiol will differentiate estrogen deficiency from other causes of symptoms. Serum estradiol levels of 40 to 100 pg/mL are adequate for menopausal symptom control. Because conjugated equine estrogens are compounds with many estrogenic substances, monitoring estradiol is more effective when estradiol-containing compounds are used (Notelovitz, 2002). With adequate serum estradiol levels and continuing symptoms, a thorough search must be made for other causes.

MONITORING FOR TOXICITY

All pharmacologic interventions have risks, and monitoring for safety is essential. Antidepressants have shown utility in decreasing the frequency of hot flashes. The monitoring of these drugs is discussed in Chapter 33. Bisphosphonates, calcitonin, and raloxifene are all FDA-approved treatments for osteoporosis. The selection and monitoring of these agents in presented in Chapter 26. Hormone therapy risks include an increased incidence of endometrial cancer, breast cancer, cardiovascular disease (CHD, VTE, pulmonary embolism, and stroke), ovarian cancer, and gallbladder disease. For any given woman these risks are small and appear to be related to dose and duration of therapy. Important considerations are to use the lowest dose that controls symptoms and duration of therapy to last only as long as symptom severity requires intervention. The benefit of long-term use of hormones to prevent cognitive decline is unproven at this time. Women who develop hip or lower extremity fracture or cancer, who are hospitalized, or who have surgery or long periods of immobility are at increased risk of VTE and should stop HT. Other known risk factors for VTE include hypertension and high BMI. Monitoring for these risks involves cooperation between provider and patient. Any unexpected abnormal vaginal bleeding must be evaluated by endometrial biopsy. With cyclic administration of a progestin, bleeding is expected to occur during the last few days of progestin or the week after the progestin is stopped. A high index of suspicion is indicated and a biopsy should be performed if heavy bleeding occurs at any time, if bleeding persists over time, or if bleeding occurs at unexpected times. Vaginal probe sonography can be used to evaluate endometrial status. If the endometrium measures <5 mm in double-wall thickness, endometrial cancer is very unlikely (Goldstein et al., 2001). Endometrial biopsy is recommended when the endometrial thickness is ≥ 5 mm. The woman should be informed of the need to return for evaluation if any of the above bleeding patterns occur.

HT increases the risk of developing breast cancer. Surviving breast cancer in the long term is improved with early detection and treatment. Therefore, providers must carefully evaluate each woman if she suspects a breast abnormally or at least annually for suspicious changes in the breast. Diagnostic mammograms and biopsies should be performed as needed, and screening mammograms should be done annually.

Women taking HT should be counseled to return for evaluation of any unusual abdominal pain. Gallbladder disease should be considered and investigated when appropriate symptoms are present in women who are taking HT.

Estrogen/androgen combination therapy is not associated with the favorable changes in lipoproteins seen with estrogen alone and should be used with caution in women with elevated blood lipids or other cardiovascular disease risks (Speroff, 1999, p. 740; Watts et al., 1995).

FOLLOWUP

The duration of hormone therapy for optimal health promotion is unknown. For control of hot flashes, hormone therapy is needed for only a few months to a few years; for prevention of urogenital atrophy osteoporosis, longer therapy is needed. The duration of systemic hormone therapy for most women should be no more than 5 years. For continuing vaginal atrophy, local therapy with estrogen is associated with improvement of symptoms and minimal systemic effect of estrogen. The long-term safety of local estrogen has not been studied. For continuing osteoporosis therapy, women should be switched to an alternative nonhormonal treatment.

Peri- and postmenopausal women should have annual health assessments that focus on evaluation of annoying side effects, risks, benefits, and continuing need for any pharmacologic intervention; the development of age-related complications; and the use of preventive health practices (dental health, immunizations, etc.). An assessment of satisfaction with sexual intimacy issues is an important part of the healthcare visit. A complete physical exam and lab work are recommended based on age and health status. Selected monitoring includes annual mammogram, blood pressure check, height measurement, periodic lipid screening, bone density measurement, and other studies as needed. In addition, a generally healthy lifestyle should be encouraged, involving regular exercise, a low-fat, high-fiber diet, and adequate calcium intake as well as avoiding smoking and excessive alcohol and caffeine.

There is much to learn about the optimal management of women's health during the midlife years. In the coming years, data from ongoing studies will provide a wealth of information to guide clinical decisions. With the results of these and future studies, a more desirable management regime may be developed that creates fewer side effects and risks for women and accrues greater benefits.

REFERENCES

American Cancer Society. (2002). *What are the risk factors for breast cancer?* [Internet: *http://www.cancer.org/eprise/main/docroot/CRI/content/CRI_2_4_2X_What_are_the_risk_factors_for_breast_cancer_5?sitearea=CRI*].

American College of Obstetricians and Gynecologists (ACOG). (1995, August). *Health maintenance for perimenopausal women.* ACOG Technical Bulletin, No. 210 Washington, DC: Author.

Ansbacher, R. (2001). The pharmacokinetics and efficacy of different estrogens are not equivalent. *American Journal of Obstetrics and Gynecology, 184*(3), 255–263.

Antonijevic, I., Stalla, G., & Steiger, A. (2000). Modulation of the sleep electroencephalogram by estrogen replacement in postmenopausal women. *American Journal of Obstetrics and Gynecology, 182*(2), 277–282.

Avis, N., Crawford, S., & McKinlay, S. (1997). Psychosocial, behavioral, and health factors related to menopause symptomatology. *Women's Health, 3*(2), 103–120.

Avis, N., Crawford, S., Stellato, R., & Longcope, C. (2001). Longitudinal study of hormone levels and depression among women transitioning through menopause. *Climacteric, 4*(3), 243–249.

Barrett-Conner, E., & Kritz-Silverstein, D. (1993). Estrogen replacement therapy and cognitive function in older women. *Journal of the American Medical Association, 269*(20), 2637–2641.

Barton, D., Loprinzi, C., & Ko, M. (2002). Managing hot flashes: Findings on alternatives to traditions hormonal therapy. *Menopause Management, 11*(3), 15–19.

Bergman-Evans, B., & Walker, S. N. (1996). The prevalence of clinical preventive services utilization by older women. *Nurse Practitioner, 21*(4), 88–106.

Berman, J., Berman, L., Werbin, T., & Goldstein, I. (1999). Female sexual dysfunction: Anatomy, physiology, evaluation and treatment options. *Current Opinion in Urology, 9*(6), 536–568.

Bone, H., Hosking, D., Devogelaer, J., et al. (2004). Ten years experience with alendronate for osteoporosis in postmenopausal women. *New England Journal of Medicine,* 350(12),1189–1199.

Bosworth, H., Bastian, L., Kuchibhatla, M., Steffens, D., McBride, C., Sugg Skinner, C., Rimer, B., & Siegler, I. (2001). Depressive symptoms, menopausal status, and climacteric symptoms in women at midlife. *Psychosomatic Medicine, 63*(4), 603–608.

Boyle, G., & Murrihy, R. (2001). A preliminary study of hormone replacement therapy and psychological mood states in perimenopausal women. *Psychological Reports, 88*(1), 160–170.

Bromberger, J., Meyer, P., Kravitz, H., Sommer, B., Cordal, A., Powell, L., Ganz, P., & Sutton-Tyrrell, K. (2001). Psychologic distress and natural menopause: A multiethnic community study. *American Journal of Public Health, 91*(9) 1435–1442.

Brown, J., Vittinghoff, E., Kanaya, A., Agarwal, S., Hulley, S., & Foxman, B. (2001). Urinary tract infections in postmenopausal women: Effect of hormone therapy and risk factors. *Obstetrics and Gynecology, 98*(6), 1045–1052.

Burger, H., Dudley, E., Hopper, J., Shelley, J., Green, A., Smith, A., Dennerstein, L., & Morse, C. (1996). The endocrinology of the menopausal transition: A cross-sectional study of a population-based sample. *Journal of Clinical Endocrinology and Metabolism, 80*(12), 3537–3545.

Cetinkaya, M., Kokcu, A., Yanik, F., Basoglu, T., Malatyalioglu, E., & Alper, T. (2001). Comparison of the effects of transdermal estrogen, oral estrogen, and oral estrogen-progestogen therapy on bone mineral density in postmenopausal women. *Journal of Bone and Mineral Metabolism, 20*(1), 44–48.

Chesnut, C., Silverman, S., Andriano, K., Genant, H., Gimona, A., Harris, S., Kiel, D., LeBoff, M., Maricic, M., Miller, P.,

Moniz, C., Peacock, M., Richardson, P., Watts, N., & Baylink, D. (2000). A randomized trial of nasal spray salmon calcitonin in postmenopausal women with established osteoporosis: The prevent recurrence of osteoporotic fractures study. PROOF Study Group. *American Journal of Medicine, 109*(4), 267–276.

Chobanian, A., Bakris, G., Black, H., et al. (2003). The Seventh report of the Joint National Committee on prevention, detection, evaluation, and treatment of high blood pressure: The JNC 7 Report. *Journal of the American Medical Association, 289*(19), 2560–2572.

Chung, P. H., & Maroulis, G. B. (1996). Osteoporosis: An update on prevention and treatment. *Female Patient, 21,* 39–50.

Clavel-Chapelon F., & Hill, C. (2000). Hormone replacement therapy in menopause and risk of breast cancer. *Presse Medicale, 29*(31), 1688–1693.

Coughlin, S., Giustozzi, A., Smith, S., & Lee, N. (2000). A meta-analysis fo estrogen replacement therapy and risk of epithelial ovarian cancer. *Journal of Clinical Epidemiology, 53*(4), 367–375.

Crenin, M. (1996). Laboratory criteria for menopause in women using oral contraceptives. *Fertility and Sterility, 66*(1), 101–104.

Cummings, S., Palermo, L., Browner, W., Marcus, R., Wallace, R., Pearson, J., Blackwell, T., Eckert, S., & Black, D. (2000). Monitoring osteoporosis therapy with bone densitometry: Misleading changes and regression to the mean. Fracture Intervention Trial Research Group. *Journal of the American Medical Association, 283*(10), 1318–1321.

Davis, A., Godwin, A., Lippman, J., Olson, W., & Kafrissen, M. (2000). Triphasic norgestimate/ethinyl estradiol oral contraceptive for treating dysfunctional uterine bleeding. *Obstetrics and Gynecology, 96*(6), 913–920.

Dennerstein, L., Lehert, P., Burger, H., & Dudley, E. (1999). Mood and menopausal transition. *The Journal of Nervous and Mental Disease, 187*(11), 685–691.

Dew, J., Eden, J., Beller, E., Magarey, C., Schwartz, P., Crea, P., & Wren, B. (1998). A cohort study of hormone replacement therapy given to women previously treated for breast cancer. *Climacteric, 1*(2), 137–142.

de Ziegler, D., Ferriani, R., Moraes, L., & Bulletti, C. (2001). Vaginal progesterone in menopause: Crinone 4% in cyclical and constant combined regimens. *Human Reproduction, 15*(Suppl 1), 149–158.

DiSaia, P., & Brewster, W. (2002). Hormone replacement therapy for survivors of breast and endometrial cancer. *Current Oncology Reports, 4*(2), 152–158.

Drake, E., Henderson, V., Stanczyk, F., McCleary, C., Brown, W., Smith, C., Rizzo, A., Murdock, G., & Buckwalter, J. (2000). Asociations between circulating sex steroid hormones and cognition in normal elderly women. *Neurology, 54*(3), 599–603.

Eastell, R. (1998). Drug therapy: Treatment of postmenopausal osteoporosis. *The New England Journal of Medicine, 338* (11), 736–746.

Eiken, P., & Kolthoff N. (2002). Compliance with 10 years of oral hormonal replacement therapy. *Maturitas, 41*(2).

Erenus, M., Karakoc, B., & Gurler, A. (2001). Comparison of effects of continuous combined transdermal with oral estrogen and oral progestogen replacement therapies on serum lipoproteins and compliance. *Climacteric, 4*(3), 228–234.

Eriksen, B. (1999). A randomized, open, parallel-group study on the preventive effect of an estradiol-releasing vaginal ring (Estring) on recurrent urinary tract infections in postmenopausal women. *American Journal of Obstetrics and Gynecology, 180*(5), 1072–1079.

Ettinger, B., Black, D., Mitlak, B., Knickerbocker, R., Nickelsen, T., Genant, H., Christiansen, C., Delmas, P., Zanchetta, J., Stakkestad, J., Gluer, C., Krueger, K., Cohen, J., Eckert, S., Ensrud, K., Avioli, L., Lips, P., & Cummings, S. (1999). Reduction of vertebral fracture risk in postmenopausal women with osteoporosis treated with raloxifene: Results from a 3-year randomized clinical trial. Multiple Outcomes of Raloxifene Evaluation (MORE) Investigators. *Journal of the American Medical Association, 282*(7), 637–645.

Ettinger, B., Friedman, G. D., Bush, T., & Quesenberry, C. P., Jr. (1996). Reduced mortality associated with long-term postmenopausal estrogen therapy. *Obstetrics and Gynecology, 87*(1), 6–12.

Executive summary: Stages of Reproductive Aging Workshop (STRAW). (2001) *Menopause,* 8(6), 402–407.

Fluck, E., File, S., & Rymer, J. (2002). Cognitive effects of 10 years of hormone-replacement therapy with tibolone. *Journal of Clinical Psychopharmacology, 22*(1) 62–7.

Freeman, E., Grisso, J., Berlin, J., Sammel, M., Garia-Espana, B., & Hollanger, L. (2001). Symptom reports from a cohort of African American and white women in the late reproductive years. *Menopause, 8*(1), 33–42.

Freeman, E., Sammel, M., Grisso, J., Battistini, M., Garcia-Espana, B., & Hollanger, L. (2001). Hot flashes in the late reproductive years: Risk factors for African American and Caucasian women. *Journal of Women's Health and Gender-Based Medicine, 10*(1), 67–76.

Gallagher, J. (1999). Moderation of the daily dose of HRT: Prevention of osteoporosis. *Maturitas, 33*(Suppl 1), S57–S63.

Gambacciani, M., Ciaponi, M., Cappagli, B., & Genazzani, A. (2001). Effects of low-dose continuous combined conjugated estrogens and medroxyprogesterone acetate on menopausal symptoms, body weight, bone density, and metabolism in postmenopausal women. *American Journal of Obstetrics and Gynecology, 185*(5), 1180–1185.

Gambrell, R. (1997). Strategies to reduce the incidence of endometrial cancer in postmenopausal women. *American Journal of Obstetrics and Gynecology, 177*(5), 1196–1204.

Garcia-Closas, M., Herrero, R., Bratti, C., Hildesheim, A., Sherman, M., Morera, L., & Schiffman, M. (1999). Epidemiologic determinants of vaginal pH. *American Journal of Obstetrics and Gynecology, 180*(5), 1060–1066.

Gavin, N., Thorp, J., & Ohsfeldt, R. (2001). Determinants of hormone replacement therapy duration among postmenopausal women with intact uteri. *Menopause, 8*(5), 377–383.

Geusens, P., & McClung, M. (2001). Review of risedronate in the treatment of osteoporosis. *Expert Opinion on Pharmacotherapy, 2*(12), 2011–2025.

Godsland, I. (2001). Effects of postmenopausal hormone replacement therapy on lipid, lipoprotein, and apolipoprotein(a) concentrations: Analysis of studies published from 1974–2000. *Fertility and Sterility, 75*(5), 898–915.

Gold, E., Sternfeld, B., Kelsey, J., Brown, C., Mouton, C., Reame, N., Salamone, L., & Stellato, R. (2000). Relation of demographic and lifestyle factors to symptoms in a multiracial/ethic population of women 40–55 years of age. *American Journal of Epidemiology, 152*(5), 463–473.

Goldstein, F., Newcomb, P., & Stampfer, M. (1999). Postmenopausal hormone therapy and the risk of colorectal cancer: A review and meta-analysis. *American Journal of Medicine, 106*(5) 574–82.

Goldstein, R., Bree, R., Benson, C., Benacerraf, B., Bloss, J., Carlos, R., Fleischer, A., Goldstein, S., Hunt, R., Kurman, R., Kurtz, A., Laing, F., Parsons, A., Smith-Bindgam, R., & Walker, J. (2001). Evaluation of the woman with postmenopausal bleeding: Society of Radiologists in Ultrasound–sponsored consensus conference statement. *Journal of Ultrasound in Medicine, 20*(10), 1025–1036.

Grady, D., Herrington D., Bittner V., Blumenthal R., Davidson M., Hlatky M., Hsia J., Hulley S., Herd A., Khan S., Newby L., Waters D., Vittinghoff E, Wenger N., HERS Research Group. (2002). Cardiovascular disease outcomes during 6.8 years of hormone therapy: Heart and Estrogen/progestin Replacement Study follow-up (HERS II). *JAMA,* 288(1):49–57.

Grady, D., Rubin, S., & Petitti, D. (1992). Hormone therapy to prevent disease and prolong life in postmenopausal women. *Annals of Internal Medicine, 117*(12), 1016–1037.

Graziottin, A. (1996). HRT: The woman's perspective. *International Journal of Gynaecology and Obstetrics, 52*(Suppl. 1), S11–16.

Grodstein, F., Colditz, G. A., & Stampfer, M. J. (1994). Post menopausal hormone use and cholecystectomy in a large prospective study. *Obstetrics and Gynecology, 83,* 5–11.

Grodstein, F., Manson, J., Colditz, G., Willett, W., Speizer, F., & Stampfer, M. (2000). A prospective, observational study of postmenopausal hormone therapy and primary prevention of cardiovascular disease. *Annals of Internal Medicine, 133*(12), 933–941.

Grodstein, F., Manson, J., & Stampfer, M. (2001). Postmenopausal hormone use and secondary prevention of coronary events in the nurses' health study: A prospective, observational study. *Annals of Internal Medicine, 135*(1), 1–8.

Grodstein, F., Newcomb, P., & Stampfer, M. (1999). Postmenopausal hormone therapy and the risk of colorectal cancer: a review and meta-analysis. *American Journal of Medicine, 106*(5), 574–582.

Haines, C., Yeung, L., Yip, G., Tang, K., Yim, S., Jorgensen, L., & Woo, J. (2001). Anti-ischemic action of estrogen-progestogen continuous combined hormone replacement therapy in postmenopausal women with established angina pectoris: A randomized, placebo-controlled, double-blind, parallel-group trial. *Journal of Cardiovascular Pharmacology, 38*(3), 372–383.

Hall, G., Collins, A., Csemiczky, G., & Landgren, B. (2002). Liproproteins and BMI: a comparison between women during transition to menopause and regularly menstruating healthy women. *Maturitas, 41*(3), 177–185.

Hammond, C. B. (1996). Menopause and hormone replacement therapy: An overview. *Obstetrics and Gynecology, 87*(Suppl. 2), 2S–15S.

Hargrove, J. T., & Eisenberg, E. (1995). Menopause. *Medical Clinics of North America, 79*(6), 1337–1356.

Hays J., Ockene J., Brunner R., Kotchen J., Manson J., Patterson R., Aragaki A., Shumaker S., Brzyski R., LaCroix A., Granek I., Valanis B., Women's Health Initiative Investigators. (2003). Effects of estrogen plus progestin on health-related quality of life. *New England Journal of Medicine,* 348:1839–1854.

Henshaw, S. (1998). Unintended pregnancy in the United States. *Family Planning Perspectives, 30*(1), 24–29, 46.

Herrington, D., Reboussin, D., Brosnihan, B., Sharp, P., Shumaker, S., Snyder, T., Furberg, C., Kowalchuk, G., Stuckey, T., Rogers, W., Givens, D., & Waters, D. (2000). Effects of estrogen replacement on the progression of coronary-artery atherosclerosis. *The New England Journal of Medicine, 343*(8), 522–529.

Hextal, A., & Cardozo, L. (2001). The role of estrogen supplementation in lower urinary tract dysfunction. *International Urogynecology Journal, 12*(4), 258–261.

Higashi, Y., Sanada, M., Sasaki, L., Nakagawa, K., Goto, C., Matsuura, H., Ohama, K., Chayma, K., & Oshima, T. (2001). Effects of estrogen replacement therapy on endothelial function in peripheral resistance arteries in normotensive and hypertensive postmenopausal women. *Hypertension, 37*(2), 651–657.

Hill, D., Weiss, N., Beresford, S., Voigt, L., Daling, J., Stanford, J., & Self, S. (2000). Continuous combined hormone replacement therapy and risk of endometrial cancer. *American Journal of Obstetrics and Gynecology, 183*(6), 1456–1461.

Hirata, K., Shimada, K., Watanabe, H., Muro, T., Yoshiyama, M., Takeuchi, K., Hozumi, T., & Yoshikawa, J. (2001). Modulation of coronary flow velocity reserve by gender, menstrual cycle, and hormone replacement therapy. *Journal of the American College of Cardiology, 38*(7), 1879–1884.

Hoeger, K., & Guzick, D. (1999). The use of androgens in menopause. *Clinical Obstetrics and Gynecology, 42*(4), 883–894.

Hulley S., Furberg C., Barrett-Connor E., Cauley J., Grady D., Haskell W., Knopp R., Lowery M., Satterfield S., Schrott H., Vittinghoff E., Hunninghake D.; HERS Research Group. (2002). Noncardiovascular disease outcomes during 6.8 years of hormone therapy: Heart and Estrogen/progestin Replacement Study follow-up (HERS II). *JAMA, 288*(1):58–66.

Hulley, S., Grady, D., Bush, T., Furberg, C., Herrington, D., Riggs, B., & Vittinghoff, E. (1998). Randomized trial of estrogen plus progestin for secondary prevention of coronary heart disease in postmenopausal women. Heart and Estrogen/progestin Replacement Study (HERS) Research Group. *Journal of the American Medical Aassociation, 280*(7), 605–613.

Hurt, W. G. (1996). Urinary incontinence in older women. *Menopausal Medicine, 4*(3), 1–4.

Ivarsson, T., Spetz, A., & Hammar, M. (1998). Physical exercise and vasomotor symptoms in postmenopausal women. *Maturitas, 29*(2), 139–146.

Kaunitz, A. (2001). Oral contraceptive use in the perimenopause. *American Journal of Obstetrics and Gynecology, 185*(Suppl 2), S32–37.

Kaunitz, A. (2002). Use of combination hormone replacement therapy in light of recent data from the Women's Health Initiative. *Medscape Women's Health eJournal, 7*(4).

Lacey, J., Mink, P., Lubin, J., Sherman, M., Troisi, R., Hartge, P., Schatzkin, A., & Schairer, C. (2002). Menopausal hormone replacement therapy and risk of ovarian cancer. *JAMA, 288*(3), 334–341.

Laughlin, G. A., Barrett-Conner, E., Kritz-Silverstein, D., & von Muhlen, D. (2001). Hysterectomy, oophorectomy, and endogenous sex hormone levels in older women: The Rancho Bernardo Study. *Journal of Clinical Endocrinology and Metabolism, 85*(2), 645–651.

Laumann, E., Paik, A., & Rosen, R. (1999). Sexual dysfunction in the United States: Prevalence and predictors. *Journal of the American Medical Association, 281*(6), 537–544.

LeBlanc, E., Janowsky, J., Chan, B., & Nelson, H. (2001). Hormone therapy and cognition: A systematic review and meta-analysis. *Journal of the American Medical Association, 285*(11), 1489–1499.

Liang, M., & Karlson, E. (1996). Female hormone therapy and the risk of developing or exacerbating systemic lupus erythematosus or rheumatoid arthritis. *Proceedings of the Association of American Physicians, 1008*(1), 25–28.

Liberman, U. A., Weiss, S. R., Broll, J., Minne, H. W., Quan, H., Bell, N. H., Rodriguez-Portales, J., Downs, R. W., Jr., Dequeker, J., Favus, M., Seeman, E., Recker, R. R., Capizzi, T., Santora, A. C., II, Lombardi, A., Shah, R. V., Hirsch, L. J., Laurence, J., & Karpf, D. B. (1995). Effect of oral alendronate on bone mineral density and the incidence of fractures in postmenopausal osteoporosis. *New England Journal of Medicine, 333*(22), 1437–1443.

Lichtman, R. (1996). Perimenopausal and postmenopausal hormone replacement therapy–Part 2: Hormonal regimens and complementary and alternative therapies. *Journal of Nurse-Midwifery, 41*(3), 195–210.

Lindgren, R., Berg, G., Hammar, M., & Zuccon, E. (1993). Hormonal replacement therapy and sexuality in a population of Swedish postmenopausal women. *Acta Obstetrica et Gynecologica Scandinavica, 72,* 292–297.

Lufkin, E., & Ory, S. (1994). Relative value of transdermal and oral estrogen therapy in various clinical situations. *Mayo Clinic Proceedings, 69*(2), 131–135.

Lyritis, G., & Trovas, G. (2002). Analgesic effects of calcitonin. *Bone, 30*(5 Suppl 1), 71–74.

Marcus, R., Wong, M., Heath, H., & Stock, J. (2002). Antiresorptive treatment of postmenopausal osteoporosis: Comparison of study designs and outcomes in large clinical trials with fracture as an endpoint. *Endocrine Reviews, 23*(1), 16–37.

Mahavni, V., & Sood A. (2001). Hormone replacement therapy and cancer risk. *Current Opinion in Oncology, 13*(5), 384–389.

McKinlay, S., Brambilla, D., & Posner, (1992). The normal menopause transition. *Maturitas, 14*(2), 103–115.

Minino, A., & Smith, B. (2001). Deaths: Preliminary data for 2000. *National Vital Statistics Reports, 49*(12), 1–40.

Mosca, L., Collins, P., Herrington, D., Mendelsohn, M., Pasternak, R., Robertson, R., Schenck-Gustafsson, K., Smith, S., Taubert, K., & Wenger, N. (2001). Hormone replacement therapy and cardiovascular disease. *Circulation, 104*(4), 499–503.

Mosca, L., Grundy, S., Judelson, D., King, K., Limacher, M., Oparil, S., Pasternak, R., Pearson, T., Redberg, R., Smith, S., Winston, M., & Zinberg, S. (1999). Guide to preventive cardiology in women. *Circulation, 99*(18), 2480–2484.

Mostwin, J. L., Genadry, R., Sanders, R., & Yang, A. (1996). Anatomic goals in the correction of female stress urinary incontinence. *Journal of Endourology, 10*(3), 207–212.

Montplaisir, J., Lorrain, J., Denesle, R., & Petit, D. (2001). Sleep in menopause: Differential effects of two forms of hormone replacement therapy. *Menopause, 8*(1), 3–4.

Nachtigall, L. (1998). The symptoms of perimenopause. *Clinical Obstetrics and Gynecology, 41*(4), 921–927.

Nachtigall, M., Smilen, S., Nachtigall, R., Nachtigall, R., & Nachtigall, L. (1992). Incidence of breast cancer in a 22-year study of women receiving estrogen-progestin replacement therapy. *Obstetrics & Gynecology, 80*(5), 827–830.

Nand, S. L., Webster, M. A., & Wren, B. G. (1995). Continuous combined piperazine oestrone sulphate and medroxyprogesterone acetate hormone replacement therapy: A study of bleeding pattern, endometrial response, serum lipid and bone density changes. *Australian and New Zealand Journal of Obstetrics and Gynaecology, 35*(1), 92–96.

National Institutes of Health (2004). NIH asks participants in Women's Health Initiative estrogen-alone study to stop study pills, begin follow-up phase. [Online.] Accessed March 25, 2004: www.nhlbi.nih.gov/new/press/04-03-02.htm.

National Osteoporosis Foundation (NOF). (2000). *Physician's guide to prevention and treatment of osteoporosis.* Washington, DC: Author.

North American Menopause Society (NAMS). (2000a). Clinical challenges of perimenopause: Consensus opinion of the North American Menopause Society. *Menopause, 7*(1), 5–13.

North American Menopause Society (NAMS). (2000b). A decision tree for the use of estrogen replacement therapy or hormone replacement therapy in postmenopausal women: Consensus opinion of the North American Menopause Society. *Menopause, 7*(2), 76–86.

North American Menopause Society (NAMS). (2002). Management of postmenopausal osteoporosis: Position statement of the North American Menopause Society. *Menopause, 9*(2), 84–101.

North American Menopause Society (NAMS) (2003a). Estrogen and progestogen use in peri- and postmenopausal women: September 2003 position statement of The North American Menopause Society. *Menopause, 10*(6)497–506.

North American Menopause Society (NAMS) (2003b). Role of progestogen in hormone therapy for postmenopausal women: position statement of The North American Menopause Society. *Menopause, 10*(2)113–132.

North American Menopause Society (NAMS). (2004). Treatment of menopause-associated vasomotor symptoms: Position statement of the North American Menopause Society. *Menopause, 11*(1),11–33.

Notelovitz, M. (1997) Osteoporosis: Alternatives for keeping bones strong. *Contemporary Nurse Practitioner, 2*(1), 7–19.

Notelovitz, M. (2002). Why individualizing hormone therapy is crucial: Putting the results of the WHI into perspective. *Medscape Women's Health eJournal, 7*(4).

Notelovitz, M., Cassel, D., Hille, D., Furst, K., Dain, M., Vande-Pol, C., & Skarinsky, D. (2000). Efficacy of continuous sequestial transdermal estradiol and norethindrone acetate in relieving vasomotor symptoms associated with menopause. *American Journal of Obstetrics and Gynecology, 182*(1 pt 1), 7–12.

Notelovitz, M., Lenihan, J., McDermott, M., Kerber, I., Nanavati, N., & Arce, J. (2000). Initial 17beta-estradiol dose for treating vasomotor symptoms. *Obstetrics and Gynecology, 95*(5), 726–731.

Olofosson, A., & Collins, A. (2000). Psychosocial factors, attitude to menopause and symptoms in Swedish perimenopausal women. *Climacteric, 3*(1), 33–42.

Optimal Calcium Intake. NIH Consensus Statement Online 1994 June 6–8; 12(4):1–31

O'Shaughnessy, Michael (2003). Incontinence, Urinary: Comprehensive Review of Medical and Surgical Aspects. Emedicine. *www.emedicine.com/med/topic2781.htm.* Last updated 11/21/2003.

Paganini-Hill, A. (1996). Oestrogen replacement therapy and Alzheimer's disease. *British Journal of Obstetrics and Gynaecology, 103*(S13), 80–86.

Paganini-Hill, A., & Perez, B. (2001). Stroke risk in older men and women: aspirin, estrogen, exercise, vitamins, and other factors. *Journal of Gender-Specific Medicine* 4(2), 18–28.

Penckofer, S., Hackbarth, D., & Schwertz, D. (2003). Estrogen plus progestin: The cardiovascular risks exceed the benefits. *The Journal of Cardiovascular Nursing, 18*(5), 347–355.

Persson, I., Weiderpass, E., Bergkvist, L., Bergstrom, R., & Schairer, C. (1999). Risks of breast and endometrial cancer after estrogen and estrogen-progestin replacement. *Cancer Causes and Control, 10*(4), 253–260.

Peters, G., Fodera, T., Sabol, J., Jones, S., & Euhus, D. (2001). Estrogen replacement therapy after breast cancer: A 12 year follow-up. *Annals of Surgical Oncology, 8*(10), 828–832.

Phan, K., Freeman, E., & Grisso, J. (1997). Menopause and hormone replacement therapy: Focus groups of African American and Caucasian women. *Menopause, 4*(1), 71–79.

Polo-Kantolo, P., Erkkola, R., Helenius, H., et al. (1998). When does estrogen replacement therapy improve sleep quality? *American Journal of Obstetrics and Gynecology, 178*(5), 1002–1009.

Prestwood, K., Kenny, A., Unson, C., & Kulldorff, M. (2000). The effect of low dose micronized 17ss-estradiol on bone turnover, sex hormone levels, and side effects in older women: A randomized, double blind, placebo-controlled study. *Journal of Clinical Endocrinology and Metabolism, 85*(12), 4462–4469.

Prestwood, K., Thompson, D., Kenny, A., Seibel, M., Pilbeam, C., & Raisz, L. (1999). Low dose estrogen and calcium have an additive effect on bone resorption in older women. *Journal of Clinical Endocrinology and Metabolism, 84*(1), 179–183.

Rapp S., Espeland M., Shumaker S., Henderson V., Brunner R., Manson J., Gass M., Stefanick M., Lane D., Hays J., Johnson K., Coker L., Dailey M., Bowen D.; WHIMS Investigators. (2003). Effect of estrogen plus progestin on global cognitive function in postmenopausal women: the Women's Health Initiative Memory Study: a randomized controlled trial. *JAMA, 289*:2663–2672.

Raz, R., & Stamm, W. (1993). A controlled trial of intravaginal estriol in postmenopausal women with recurrent urinary tact infections. *New England Journal of Medicine, 329*(11), 753–756.

Rebar, R., Trabal, J., & Mortola, J. (2000). Low dose esterified estrogens (0.3 mg/day): Long-term and short-term effects on menstrual symptoms and quality of life in postmenopausal women. *Climacteric, 3*(3), 176–182.

Riman, T., Dickman, P., Nilsson, S., Correia, N., Nordlinder, H., Magnusson, C., Weiderpass, E., & Persson, I. (2002). Hormone replacement therapy and the risk of invasive epithelial ovarian cancer in Swedish women. *Journal of the National Cancer Institute, 94*(7), 497–504.

Rioux, J., Devlin, C., Gelfand, M., Steinberg, W., Hepburn, D. (2000). 17beta-estradiol vaginal tablet verses conjugated equine estrogen vaginal cream to relieve menopausal atrophic vaginitis. *Menopause, 7*(3), 156–161.

Rodriguez, C., Patel, A., Calle, E., Jacob, E., & Thun, M. (2001). Estrogen replacement therapy and ovarian cancer mortality in a large prospective study of U.S. women. *Journal of the American Medical Association, 285*(11), 1460–1465.

Rodstrom, K., Bengtsson, C., Lissner, L., Milsom, I., Sundh, V., & Bjorkelund, C. (2002). A longitudinal study of the treatment of hot flushes: The population study of women in Gothenburg during a quarter of a century. *Menopause, 9*(3), 156–161.

Ross, R., Paganini-Hill, A., Wan, P., & Pike, M. (2000). Effect of hormone replacement therapy on breast cancer risk: Estrogen versus estrogen plus progestin. *Journal of the National Cancer Institute, 92*(4), 328–332.

Sanderson, J., Haines, C., Yeung, L., Yip, G., Tang, K., Yim, S., Jorgensen, L., & Woo, J. (2001). Anti-ischemic action of estrogen-progestogen continuous combined hormone replacement therapy in postmenopausal women with established angina pectoris: A randomized, placebo-controlled, double-blind, parallel-group trial. *Journal of Cardiovascular Pharmacology, 38*(3), 372–383.

Scharbo-DeHaan, M. (1996, December). Hormone replacement therapy. *Nurse Practitioner,* 1–15.

Santoro, N., Brown, J. R., Adel, T., & Skurnick, J. H. (1996). Characterization of reproductive hormonal dynamics in the perimenopause. *Journal of Clinical Endocrinology and Metabolism, 81*(4), 1495–1501.

Sarrel, P., Dobay, B., & Wiita, B. (1998). Estrogen and estrogen-androgen replacement in postmenopausal women dissatisfied with estrogen-only therapy. Sexual behavior and neuroendocrine responses. *Journal of Reproductive Medicine, 43*(10), 847–856.

Schairer, C., Gail, M., Byrne, C., Rosenberg, P., Sturgeon, S., Brinton, L., & Hoover, R. (1999). Estrogen replacement therapy and breast cancer survival in a large screening study. *Journal of the National Cancer Institute, 91*(3), 264–270.

Schairer, C., Lubin, J., Troisi, R., Sturgeon, S., Brinton, L., & Hoover, R. (2000). Menopausal estrogen and estrogen-progestin replacement therapy and breast cancer risk. *Journal of the American Medical Association. 283*(4), 485–91.

Schmidt, P., Nieman, L., Danaceau, M., Tobin, M., Roca, C., Murphy, J., & Rubinow, D. (2000). Estrogen replacement in perimenopause-related depression: A preliminary report. *American Journal of Obstetrics and Gynecology, 183*(2), 414–420.

Schneider, H., & Gallagher, J. (1999). Moderation of the daily dose of HRT: Benefits for patients. *Maturitas, 33*(Suppl 1), S25–9.

Schneider, L., Small, G., & Clary, C. (2001). Estrogen replacement therapy and antidepressant response to sertraline in older depressed women. *American Journal of Geriatric Psychiatry, 9*(4), 393–399.

Schwingl, P. J., Hulka, G. S., & Harlow, S. D. (1994). Risk factors for menopausal hot flashes. *Obstetrics and Gynecology, 84*(1), 29–34.

Shepherd, J. (2001). Effects of estrogen on congnition, mood, and degenerative brain diseases. *Journal of the American Pharmaceutical Association, 41*(2), 221–8.

Sherburn, M., Guthrie, J., Dudley, E., O'Connell, H., & Dennerstein, L. (2001). Is incontinence associated with Menopause. *Obstetrics & Gynecology, 98*(4), 628–633.

Shifren, J., Braunstein, G., Simon, J., Casson, P., Buster, J., Redmond, G., Burki, R., Ginsburg, E., Rosen, C., Leiblum, S., Caramelli, K., & Mazer, N. (2000). Transdermal testosterone treatment in women with impaired sexual dysfunction after oophorectomy. *New England Journal of Medicine, 343*(10), 68208.

Shulman, L., Yankov, V., & Kerstin, U. (2002). Safety and efficacy of continuous once a week 17β-estradiol/levonorgestrel transdermal system and its effects on vasomotor symptoms and endometrial safety in post menopausal women: the result of two multicenter, double-blind, randomized, controlled trials. *Menopause, 9*(3), 195–207.

Shumaker S., Legault C., Rapp S., Thal L., Wallace R., Ockene J., Hendrix S., Jones B. 3rd, Assaf A., Jackson R., Kotchen J., Wassertheil-Smoller S., Wactawski-Wende J., WHIMS Investigators. (2003). Estrogen plus progestin and the incidence of dementia and mild cognitive impairment in postmenopausal women: the Women's Health Initiative Memory Study: a randomized controlled trial. *JAMA, 289:*2651–2662.

Sit, A., Modugno, F., Weissfeld, J., Berga S., & Ness, R. (2002). Hormone replacement therapy formulations and risk of epithelial ovarian carcinoma. *Gynecologic Oncology, 86*(2): 118–23.

Smith, Y., Giordani, B., Lajiness-O'Neill, R., & Zubieta, J. (2001). Long-term estrogen replacement is associated with improved nonverbal memory and attentional measures in postmenopausal women. *Fertility & Sterility, 76*(6), 1101–7.

Sommer, B., Avis, N., Meyer, P., Ory, M., Madden, T., Kagawa-Singer, M., Mouton, C., Rasor, N., & Adler, S. (1999). Attitudes toward menopause and aging across ethnic/racial groups. *Psychosomatic Medicine, 61*(6), 868–75.

Speroff, L., Glass, R., & Kase, N. (1999). Postmenopausal hormone therapy. *Clinical gynecology endocrinology and infertility* (6th ed.). Baltimore: Lippincott Williams & Wilkins.

Staropoli, C., Flaws, J., Bush, T., & Moulton A. (1998). Predictors of menopausal hot flashes. *Journal of Women's Health, 7*(9), 1149–55.

Suriano, K., McHale, M., McLaren, C., Li, K., Re, A., DiSaia, P. (2001). Estrogen replacement therapy in endometrial cancer patients: a matched control study. *97*(4), 555–560.

Taffe, J., & Dennerstein, L. (2002). Menstrual patterns leading to the final menstrual period. *Menopause, 9*(1), 32–40.

Taggart, H., Bolognese, M., Lindsay, R., Ettinger, M., Mulder, H., Josse, R., Roberts, A., Zippel, H., Adami, S., Ernst, T., & Stevens, K. (2002). Upper gastrointestinal tract safety of risedronate: a pooled analysis of 9 clinical trials. *Mayo Clinic Proceedings, 77*(3), 262–70.

Tang, M-X., Jacobs, D., Stern, Y., Marder, K., Schofield, P., Gurland, B., Andrews, H., & Mayeux, R. (1996). Effect of oestrogen during menopause on risk and age at onset of Alzheimer's disease. *Lancet, 348,* 429–432.

Tsang, K., Ho, S., & Lo, S., (2000) Estrogen improves motor disability in parkinsonian postmenopausal women with motor fluctuations. *Neurology, 54*(12):2292–8.

Varila, E., Wahlstrom, T., & Rauramo, I. (2001). A 5-year follow-up study on the use of a levonorgestrel intrauterine system in women receiving hormone replacement therapy. *Fertility & Sterility, 76*(5), 969–73.

Vehkavaara, S., Hakala-Ala-Pietila, T., Virkamaki, A., Bergholm, R., Ehnholm, C., Hovatta, O., Taskinen, M., & Yki-Jarvinen, H. (2000). Differential effects of oral and transdermal estrogen replacement therapy on endothelial function in postmenopausal women. *Circulation, 102*(22), 2687–93.

Vehkavaara, S., Silveira, A., Hakala-Ala-Pietila, T., Virkamaki, A., Hovatta, O., Hamsten, A., Taskinen, M., & Yki-Jarvinen, H. (2001). Effects of oral and transdermal estrogen replacement therapy on markers of coagulation, fibrinolysis, inflammation and serum lipids and lipoproteins in postmenopausal women. *Thrombosis & Haemostasis, 85*(4), 619–25.

Verghese, J., Kuslansky, G., Katz, M., Sliwinski, M., Crystal, H., Buschke, H., & Lipton, R. (2000). Cognitive performance in surgically menopausal women on estrogen. *Neurology, 55*(6), 872–4.

Vinker, S., Kaplan, B., Nakar, S., Samuels, G., Shapira, G., & Kitai, E. (2001). Urinary incontinence in women: prevalence, characteristics and effect on quality of life. A primary care clinic study. *Israel Medical Association Journal, 3*(9), 663–6.

von Muhlen, D., Soroko, S., Kritz-Silverstein, D., & Barrett-Conner, E. (2000). Vasomotor symptoms are not associated with reduced bone mass in postmenopausal women: the Rancho Bernardo Study. *Journal of Women's Health & Gender-based Medicine, 9*(5):505–11.

Walsh Scura, K., & Whipple, B. (1997). How to provide better care for the postmenopausal woman. *American Journal of Nursing, 97*(4), 36–43.

Waring, S., Rocca, W., Peterson, R., O'Brien, P., Tangalos, E., & Kokmen, E. (1999). Postmenopausal estrogen replacement therapy and drisk of AD: a population based study. *Neurology, 52*(5), 965–70.

Wassertheil-Smoller, S., Hendrix, S., Limacher, M., et al. (2003). Effect of estrogen plus progestin on stroke in postmenopausal women. *Journal of the American Medical Association, 289,* 2673–2684.

Wassertheil-Smoller, S., Shumaker, S., Ockene, J., Talavera, G., Greenland, P., Cochrane, B., Robbins, J., Aragaki, A., Dunbar-Jacob, J. (2004). Depression and Cardiovascular Sequelae in Postmenopausal Women. *Archives of Internal Medicine, 164:*289–298.

Watts, N. (2001) Risedronate for the prevention and treatment of postmenopausal osteoporosis: results from recent clinical trials. *Osteoporosis International, 12*(Suppl 3), S17–22.

Watts, N. B., Notelovitz, M., Timmons, M. C., Addison, W. A., Wiita, B., & Downey, L. J. (1995). Comparison of oral estrogens and estrogens plus androgen on bone mineral density, menopausal symptoms, and lipid-lipoprotein profiles in surgical menopause. *Obstetrics and Gynecology, 85*(4), 529–537.

West, S., Hinderliter, A., Wells, E., Girdler, S., & Light, K. (2001). Transdermal estrogen reduces vascular resistance and serum cholesterol in postmenopausal women. *American Journal of Obstetrics & Gynecology, 184*(5), 926–33.

Whiting, S. J., Wood, R., & Kim, K. (1997). Calcium supplementation. *Journal of the American Academy of Nurse Practitioners, 9*(4), 187–192.

Wich, B. K., & Carnes, M. (1995). Menopause and the aging female reproductive system. *Endocrinology and Metabolism Clinics of North America, 24*(2), 273–295.

Wilber, J., Miller, A., Montgomery, A., & Chandler, P. (1998). Sociodemographic characteristics, biological factors, and symptom reporting in midlife women. *Menopause, 5*(1), 43–51.

Woodruff, J., & Pickar, J. (1994). Incidence of endometrial hyperplasia in postmenopausal women taking conjugated estrogens (Premarin) with medroxyprogesterone acetate or conjugated estrogen alone. *American Journal of Obstetrics and Gynecology, 170,* 1213–1223.

Writing Group for the PEPI Trial. (1995). Effects of estrogen or estrogen/progestin regimes on heart disease risk factors in postmenopausal women. The Postmenopausal Estrogen/Progestin Interventions (PEPI) trial. *JAMA, 273*(3), 199–208.

Writing Group for the Women's Health Initiative Investigators. (2002). Risks and benefits of estrogen plus progestin in healthy postmenopausal women: principal results From the Women's Health Initiative randomized controlled trial. *JAMA, 288*(3):321–33, 2002.

Yaffe, K., Barrett-Connor, E., Lin, F., & Grady, D. (2002). Serum lipoprotein levels, statin use, and cognitive function in older women. *Archives of Neurology, 59*(3), 378–84.

IV ❖ Pharmacotherapy for Common Primary Care Disorders

CHAPTER ❖ 20

CARDIOVASCULAR DISORDERS

Ruth McCaffrey ◆ Michael Crouch ◆ Sharon Thrush

Cardiovascular disease (CVD) is the leading cause of death in the United States and other developed countries. It is the second most frequent cause of death in developing countries. More than 60 million Americans, greater than 1 in 5, have some form of cardiovascular disease, including high blood pressure, coronary heart disease, stroke, and congestive heart failure. Each year about one million deaths in the United States are due to cardiovascular disease. Approximately 500,000 of these deaths are attributed to heart attack and 150,000 to stroke. One-sixth of cardiovascular deaths occur in persons younger than 65 years old. While the rate of cardiovascular mortality has declined over the past 35 years, it is unclear whether this decline is due to preventive measures or improvements in medicine, which have caused a decline in all case mortality. The effects of CVD on family resources, productivity, and caregiver burden after stroke and myocardial infarction are great. In 2001 cardiovascular disease cost the U.S. healthcare system $358 billion in expenditures and lost productivity (American Heart Association, 2002).

An important goal in treating CVD is prevention. The goals of prevention are to assist the patient to establish healthy lifestyle changes that promote cardiovascular health. In order to be effective, life style changes must be suggested with consideration of the person's history, ethnicity, culture, genetics, and motivation for change. These issues can present a challenge for the nurse practitioner.

Various organizations, including the American Heart Association, publish guidelines that provide evidence-based recommendations for drug therapy. There remain, however, sharp differences in patient commitment to hypertension treatment, and the utilization of a tailored approach to hypertension management is inherent to achieving control. It remains a challenge for practitioners to keep up with the new cardiovascular agents. Despite these obstacles, the practitioner can help patients through education and treatment. Working together, the practitioner and patient can improve longevity and quality of life while decreasing the cost of CVD to society.

This chapter will discuss the diagnosis and treatment of hypertension, heart failure, arrhythmias including atrial fibrillation, peripheral vascular conditions, coronary artery disease, ischemic heart disease and angina, mitral valve prolapse, and hyperlipidemia.

HYPERTENSION

BLOOD PRESSURE REGULATION

Hypertension occurs in 25% of all adults in the United States; 60% of those adults over 65 years old. High blood pressure is a major cause of stroke, renal failure, and coronary heart disease. Research has demonstrated that cardiovascular mortality doubles for participants with high normal blood pressures when compared to persons with optimal blood pressures. Another study showed a twofold and threefold increase in the risk of congestive heart failure in hypertensive men and women when compared to normotensive persons in the population. Advances in diagnosing and treating hypertension have reduced the rate of coronary heart disease by 49% and stroke by 58% (Goldman & Bennett, 2000).

Under normal conditions, blood pressure (BP) is regulated by a complex system of neurohumoral and renal feedback loops. These feedback loops control cardiac output and total peripheral resistance. When the balance between cardiac output (CO) and total peripheral resistance (TPR) is disturbed, changes in blood pressure occur ($BP = CO \times TPR$).

Cardiac output is the heart rate (HR) times the stroke volume (SV). Heart rate and stroke volume have sympathetic and parasympathetic control mechanisms. Stroke volume is also determined by cardiac contractility, preload, and afterload. Peripheral resistance is determined by venous and arterial forces and opposition to the forces. Peripheral resistance is, therefore, the vascular reactivity—vasodilatation and vasoconstriction in response to various neural and humoral impulses. Of importance in the humoral regulation is the renin-angiotensin-aldosterone (RAA) system.

Renin is released by the juxtaglomerular cells of the kidney. Renin changes angiotensinogen from the liver into angiotensin I, an inactive decapeptide. Angiotensin I is converted to angiotensin II by the angiotensin-converting enzyme (ACE). Angiotensin II, a powerful vasoconstrictor, increases peripheral resistance, thereby increasing blood pressure. Angiotensin II also stimulates the secretion of aldosterone from the adrenal cortex and release of antidiuretic hormone (ADH), which in turn promotes sodium and water retention in the kidney. Again, under normal conditions, this system is activated when arterial blood pressure drops, thereby increasing blood pressure by increasing cardiac output and peripheral resistance.

ETIOLOGY

The etiology of primary hypertension remains a mystery. Blood pressure normally increases in response to both internal and external forces. Continued elevation of blood pressure results in thickening of the arteries and arterioles from constant vasoconstriction and the high force exerted in the vessels. As the blood pressure continues to be elevated, hypertrophy and hyperplasia in the blood vessels occur and arterioles become permanently narrowed.

Early in the development of hypertension, it is thought that cardiac output increases. Although not proven, the increase in cardiac output may be accompanied by or may stimulate peripheral resistance. The hemodynamic theory postulates that there is an increase in retention of sodium and water that increases cardiac output. As the extracellular fluid volume increases, the regulatory mechanisms compensate by stimulating vasoconstriction. Blood volume remains high, total peripheral resistance continues to increase, and hypertension results (Elliot & Black, 2002).

In the early stages, there is no damage to blood vessels. If the condition is recognized and the cardiac output is decreased, the arterioles return to the normal tone. However, in some susceptible individuals the cardiac output may decrease, but the vascular tone does not return to normal. In this case, blood pressure remains high and vascular damage starts.

A second theory regarding the mechanisms that promote hypertension lays the blame on a defect in the autoregulatory mechanisms that determine vasoconstriction and vasodilatation. As with the hemodynamic theory, there is an increase in cardiac output. The autoregulatory mechanisms react by causing vasoconstriction. The kidneys respond by increasing the excretion of sodium and water, and the cardiac output and blood volume return to normal; however, the autoregulatory mechanisms do not return the vascular system tone to normal. Rather, it is thought that the autoregulatory system establishes a new blood pressure baseline that is hypertensive and that it works to maintain (Dunphy & Winland-Brown, 2000).

A third theoretical approach to the etiology of hypertension involves sodium. Sodium and the accompanying water retention seem to be the stimulus for the increased cardiac output that the other theories identify as the beginning of hypertension. There may be two mechanisms causing this phenomenon. First, there may be an inherited defect in the kidney for sodium excretion. An intake of sodium of more than 50 mEq/day places a strain on the kidney and activates the defect.

The second possible mechanism may be an inability of the sodium-potassium pump to work properly. Normally, the sodium-potassium pump moves sodium and potassium across the cell membrane. It is possible that a hormone may inhibit sodium release from the cells. Intracellular sodium increases as does intracellular calcium. Intracellular calcium enhances contractility, particularly of the smooth muscles of the vascular tree. The resulting vasoconstriction and increased peripheral resistance lead to hypertension (Haak, Richardson, Davey, & Parker-Cohen, 1994). In long-standing hypertension, patients have normal or decreased cardiac output and hypertension is maintained through peripheral resistance (Elliot & Black, 2002).

In light of the above theories, there are four factors that are important for determining the best treatment:

1. At first, *cardiac output increases* possibly because of sodium and water retention caused by either an inherited defect and moderate to high sodium intake or a defect in the sodium-potassium pump.
2. *Peripheral resistance increases* possibly because of a response to increased cardiac output, a response to inappropriate autoregulation, or a response to increased calcium in the cells.
3. *Renin and angiotensin activation* causes vasoconstriction, sympathetic activation, and aldosterone secretion, which in turn promotes retention of sodium and loss of potassium.
4. *Peripheral resistance increases* with normal or low CO, which maintains high blood pressure in longstanding hypertension.

Isolated systolic hypertension (ISH) is an important type of hypertension that was once thought insignificant. Elevations in systolic hypertension are due to either increased cardiac output or peripheral resistance, or both. ISH is often associated with aortic valvular insufficiency, arteriovascular (AV) fistulas, thyrotoxicosis, and Paget's disease. The cause is a rigidity of the aorta and is most common among the elderly. As the aorta becomes less responsive, total peripheral vascular resistance increases, and cardiac output increases to maintain systemic circulation. ISH is associated with a high risk for cardiovascular morbidity and mortality and therefore requires treatment (Basile, 2002; Elliott & Black, 2002; Joint National Committee, 2003; Mulrow, Lau, Cornell, & Brand, 2002).

SPECIFIC CONSIDERATIONS FOR PHARMACOTHERAPY

When Drug Therapy Is Needed

Early recognition and treatment of hypertension has long been considered important in the prevention of end-organ failure. Consequences of untreated or inadequately treated hypertension include:

- *Cardiovascular complications,* such as left ventricular hypertrophy with heart failure, coronary artery disease, myocardial infarction, and sudden death
- *Peripheral vascular complications,* such as intermittent claudication and gangrene
- *Renal complications,* such as parenchymal damage, nephrosclerosis, renal arteriosclerosis, renal insufficiency, and renal failure
- *Cerebrovascular complications,* such as transient ischemia, cerebrovascular accident (CVA), cerebral thrombosis, aneurysm, and hemorrhage
- *Retinal complications,* such as retinal vascular sclerosis, exudation, and hemorrhage

Short- and Long-Term Goals of Pharmacotherapy

The primary goal of pharmacotherapy is to return the blood pressure to normal levels using the least expensive, least complex form of therapy. Maintaining the blood pressure within a normal range will decrease morbidity and mortality and promote better quality of life.

Nonpharmacologic Therapy

Treatment of hypertension has been proven to reduce morbidity and mortality (Arauz-Pacheco, Parrott, & Raskin, 2002; Leonetti & Zanchetti, 2002; Niskanen, Hedner, Hansson, Lanke, & Nikolas, 2001). Blood pressure must be considered in the context of total risk factors since attempts to reduce blood pressure without working to alter total risk frequently meets with failure. Lifestyle interventions are initiated prior to or in conjunction with pharmacologic therapy and are a lifelong process of change.

Recommended changes that have been shown effective in some individuals include smoking cessation, weight reduction if appropriate, dietary sodium restriction to less than 2.3 g/day, relaxation techniques, decrease or elimination of caffeine, and discontinuance of certain pressure drugs (oral contraceptives, adrenal steroids, sodium-containing antacids, nonsteroidal antiinflammatory drugs [NSAIDs], and some antidepressants). Other possibly effective nonpharmacologic treatments include potassium, calcium, and magnesium supplements, alcohol restriction, regular aerobic activity, and a vegetarian and/or low-saturated-fat diet (Greenlund, Giles, Keena, Croft, & Mensah, 2002; Kinsella, 2002; Moore, Conlin, Ard, & Svetkay, 2002; Strazzullo, 2002).

Lifestyle change is always approached gradually with all age groups, particularly the elderly. Research in elders 60 to 85 years of age has found a combined program of decreased sodium intake, loss of weight (as appropriate), and increased physical activity to significantly decrease blood pressure by the end of a 6-month period (JNC VII, 2003). An exercise program starting slowly and increasing to 30 min three to five times a week will result in less muscle strain and use of NSAIDs. The exercise program will help a reasonable weight reduction program. An increase in fiber and fruit will help decrease calories and increase potassium and calcium. The increase in fiber also will help decrease constipation. The effectiveness of any program for the elderly will not be demonstrated for 3 to 6 months (JNC VII, 2003; Karmazyn, Noble, & Florez, 2002).

Time Frame for Initiating Pharmacotherapy

If lifestyle modifications have not lowered blood pressure to the desired range, the practitioner must decide whether to begin pharmacologic interventions. The Joint National Committee (JNC VII) guidelines direct the practitioner to individualize the patient's drug therapy, giving consideration to the severity of blood pressure elevation, and the compelling indications. Compelling indications include heart failure, post-myocardial infarction, high coronary disease risk, diabetes, chronic kidney disease, and recurrent stroke prevention. The practitioner should also include in the decision-making process such factors as the cost of medication, metabolic and subjective side effects, and drug-drug interactions. Refer to Table 20–1 (JNC VII, 2003).

Although controversy still exists, treatment of ISH decreases the risk of a stroke by three times. Treatment should be initiated at systolic blood pressures of 160 or greater even though the diastolic pressure is less than 90 (Systolic Hypertension in the Elderly Program [SHEP] Cooperative Research Group, 2001).

The JNC VII report lists systolic blood pressure as the most important component in all patient types. It also states that diastolic blood pressure will reach goal in most patients once systolic pressure has been controlled. Treatment should be initiated if systolic blood pressure > 120 mm/Hg if compelling conditions are present regardless of diastolic pressure.

Overview of Drug Classes for Treatment

The treatment of hypertension includes drugs from a variety of classes which can be used as monotherapy or in combination. See Drug Table 205.

Assessment Needed Prior to Therapy

The goals of the assessment are to determine if the person really has hypertension, to search for secondary (treatable) causes, to assess end-organ damage, to identify risk factors, and to assess comorbidity. When diagnosing the severity of hypertension, risk factors and end-organ disease must be taken into consideration so that the most appropriate therapeutic measures are taken.

Determination of Hypertension. The established criteria for hypertension come from the JNC. Hypertension is not diagnosed on the basis of a single blood pressure reading. It is generally defined as sustained elevation of systolic and/or diastolic blood pressure. In general, a high blood pressure reading at three different visits constitutes hypertension. The immediacy of confirmation of the elevated blood pressure and treatment are dependent on the blood pressure level. Table 20–2 indicates levels and stages of hypertension (JNC VII, 2003).

Clinical Assessment. The history-taking part of the examination should include the following:

- Age, sex, race, and family history.
- Hypertensive history including severity, duration, symptoms, precipitating events, comorbid factors, and prior treatment and response to treatment.
- Symptoms of transient ischemic attack (TIA), CVA, coronary artery disease (CAD), angina, premature ventricular contraction (PVC), and congestive heart failure (CHF).
- Symptoms of periodic headaches, palpitations, perspiration (pheochromocytoma), muscular weakness,

TABLE 20–1. Therapeutic Approach using Blood Pressure, and Compelling Indications

Category	Systolic BP mm/Hg	Diastolic BP mm/Hg	Lifestyle Modification	Without Compelling Indications	With Compelling Indications
Normal	<120	And <80	Encourage		
Prehypertension	120–139	Or 80–89	Yes	No antihypertensive drug indicated	Drugs for compelling indications
Stage I Hypertension	140–159	Or 90–99	Yes	Thiazide diuretic; May consider ace inhibitors, ARB, beta blockers, Ca channel blockers, or combinations	Drugs for compelling indications Other antihypertensive drugs (diuretics, ace inhibitors, ARB, beta blockers, calcium channel blockers, or combinations
Stage II Hypertension	>160	Or > 100	Yes	2-drug therapy for most. Usually including a thiazide diuretic	Same as stage I

Adapted from JNC VII Guidelines (2003)

Nml narrow pp = compliant aorta
pulse pressure
systolic − diastolic

TABLE 20–2. Compelling Indications for Individual Drug Classes

High-Risk conditions with compelling indication	Diuretic	Beta-Blocker	ACE Inhibitor	ARB	Calcium Channel Blocker	Aldosterone antagonist
Heart Failure	X	X	X	X		X
Post MI		X	X			X
High Coronary Disease Risk	X	X	X		X	
Diabetes	X	X	X	X	X	
Chronic Kidney Disease			X	X		
Recurrent Stroke Prevention	X		X			

Adapted from JNC VII (2003).

cramps, polyuria (primary aldosteronism), intermittent claudication, and headaches (coarctation of the aorta, PVC).

- Risk/lifestyle factors including family history, smoking, alcohol use, stress, obesity, diabetes, lack of exercise, and high sodium intake.
- Medications including oral contraceptives, steroids, thyroid hormone, cocaine, licorice, and OTC medications such as cold medications, diet pills, and nasal sprays. NSAIDs are linked to the development of hypertension as well as having an adverse effect on the action of antihypertensive medications (JNC VII, 2003).

The physical examination should include the following:

- Vital signs and weight. Check BP in both arms, and check postural hypotension.
- Funduscopic evaluation of arteriosclerotic and hypertensive changes (AV nicking, arteriolar narrowing, exudates, papilledema).
- Neck: distended veins, bruits, or thyroid enlargement.
- Cardiac and chest: evidence of hypertrophy and heart failure, valvular disease, murmurs, or gallops.
- Abdominal: masses and bruits, especially over renal arteries.
- Peripheral arteries: palpate and auscultate for bruits.
- Neurologic evaluation.
- Evidence of gout, thyroid disorder, or Cushing's syndrome.

Laboratory studies help determine risk factors, end-organ failure and secondary etiology and should include:

- CBC
- Urinalysis
- Serum sodium, potassium, calcium, uric acid, and glucose to screen for secondary hypertension from hyperparathyroidism, hyperaldosteronism, renal insufficiency, diabetes, gout, or nephrosclerosis
- Lipids
- Serum creatinine and creatinine clearance
- Electrocardiogram, chest x-ray, and echo cardiogram

The following are additional clues that may identify the physiologic mechanism involved in hypertension and therefore the most appropriate treatment regimen.

1. Edema, weight gain, chronic renal failure = *increased extracellular volume.*
2. Decreased weight, orthostatic hypotension, diuretic effect creating an increase in BUN = *decreased extracellular volume.*
3. Narrow pulse pressure, high diastolic pressure, cold extremities = *increased vascular resistance.*
4. Wide pulse pressure, orthostatic hypotension, warm extremities = *decreased vascular resistance.*
5. Tachycardia, wide pulse pressure = *increased cardiac output.*
6. Increased BUN, S_3 gallop = *decreased cardiac output.*

The Elderly and Hypertension. The pathophysiology of hypertension in the elderly is different from that found in younger individuals. The elderly generally have:

- Lower plasma volumes
- Decreased aortic compliance
- Decreased plasma-renin activity
- Decreased aldosterone levels
- Reduced baroreceptor sensitivity
- Decreased renal clearance
- Higher likelihood of salt sensitivity

Cardiac function in the older person changes. Maintaining cardiac output becomes a function of increased left ventricular volume and increased stroke volume. However, the older person with hypertension actually has a decreased cardiac output. The predominant vascular abnormality is the reduced arterial distensibility due to rigidity of the vessels (Arauz-Pacheco et al., 2002).

Patient/Caregiver Information

Although most lifestyle changes promote health and well-being, the outcome for treatment of hypertension remains equivocal. Pharmacologic therapy has proved effective in reducing morbidity and mortality in large populations. Patient compliance in the treatment of hypertension represents a major key to success.

Patients should be educated on the reduced effect of their antihypertensive therapy caused by various over-the-counter preparations such as NSAIDs and ibuprofen and diet aids that contain phenylpropanolamine or ephedra (herbal fen-phen). Some patients will experience an increase in blood pressure with oral nasal decongestants such as pseudoephedrine.

OUTCOMES MANAGEMENT

Selecting an Appropriate Agent

The JNC VII (2003) guidelines direct the practitioner to individualize each patient's drug therapy, giving consideration to the severity of blood pressure elevation, target organ damage, and the presence of other conditions and risk factors. In addition to these, consideration must be given to cost, the ease in following the treatment regimen, the potential for drug-drug interactions, and the profile of side effects including sexual, psychological, and cognitive functions.

Initiation of pharmacotherapy has been guided by the step-care approach, and yet individualization and consideration of coexisting conditions may enhance clinical as well as patient compliance and desired outcomes. The variety of agents permits tailoring of the therapy to the individuals and the physiologic mechanism of their hypertension. Whatever therapy is chosen, the blood pressure should be decreased slowly over 2 to 6 months (Mulrow et al., 2002).

The JNC VII treatment algorithm recommends thiazide diuretics as the preferred agent for initial treatment of hypertension since they lower morbidity and mortality. Ace Inhibitors, Angiotension II antagonists, beta blockers, and calcium channel blockers are also acceptable.

About 50 to 60% of patients with hypertension will respond to any agent used as monotherapy. The guidelines continue with recommendations if the response from the initial agent is inadequate. The practitioner either can increase the drug dose, substitute another agent, or add a second agent from a different drug class. If with moderate doses of monotherapy, the BP is higher than desired, the practitioner may wish to try another agent particularly if the patient is experiencing adverse effects. If the moderate doses of monotherapy have lowered the BP but not yet to the desired level, a patient with Stage 1 HTN may need to try another agent, whereas a patient with Stage 2 would benefit from the addition of a second agent from a different class. If a second drug, primarily a diuretic, is added to any other antihypertensive agent, then about 80% of patients will respond (Mulrow et al., 2002). If the response is again inadequate, continue to add agents from another drug class or refer to a hypertension specialist.

It is important also to consider contraindications or coexisting conditions when deciding upon an agent of choice. A goal could be to treat these patients with hypertension and a coexisting condition with monotherapy.

The JNC VII report gives information on drug therapy that might be considered when there are compelling indications or there may be a favorable effect on a comorbid condition. Table 20–2 lists the drugs with the compelling indication.

- Compelling Indications
  - Diabetes mellitus (type 1) with proteinuria: ACE I
  - Heart failure: ACE I, angiotensin II receptor antagonist, diuretics
  - ISH (older patients): diuretics (preferred), calcium antagonists (long-acting dihydropyridine)
  - MI: beta blockers (non-intrinsic sympathomimetic activity), ACE I (with systolic dysfunction)
- Favorable Effects on Comorbid Conditions
  - Angina pectoris: beta blockers, calcium channel blockers
  - Atrial tachycardia and fibrillation: beta blockers, calcium antagonists (non-dihydropyridines)
  - Cyclosporine-induced hypertension (caution with the dose of cyclosporine): calcium antagonists
  - Diabetes mellitus (type 1 and 2) with proteinuria: ACE I (preferred), calcium antagonists
  - Diabetes mellitus (type 2): low dose diuretics
  - Dyslipidemia: alpha blockers
  - Essential tremor: beta blockers (non-cardioselective)
  - Heart failure: carvedilol, losartan potassium
  - Hyperthyroidism: beta blockers
  - Migraine: beta blockers (non-cardioselective), calcium antagonists (non-dihydropyridine)
  - Myocardial infarction: diltiazem, verapamil
  - Osteoporosis: thiazides
  - Preoperative hypertension: beta blockers
  - Prostatism (BPH): alpha blockers
  - Renal insufficiency (caution in renovascular hypertension and creatinine level ≥ 3 mg/dL): ACE I
- Situations in which drug therapy may have an unfavorable effect on comorbid conditions
  - Bronchospastic disease: beta blockers
  - Depression: beta blockers, central alpha antagonists, reserpine
  - Diabetes mellitus (type 1 and 2): beta blockers, high dose diuretics

- Dyslipidemia: beta blockers (non-intrinsic sympathomimetic activity), diuretics (high dose)
- Gout: diuretics
- Second or third degree heart block: beta blockers, calcium antagonists (non-dihydropyridine)
- Heart failure: beta blockers (except carvedilol metoprolol XL,) calcium antagonists (except amlodipine, felodipine)
- Liver disease: labetalol, methyldopa
- Peripheral vascular disease: beta blockers
- Pregnancy: ACE I, angiotensin II receptor blockers
- Renal insufficiency: potassium sparing agents
- Renovascular disease: ACE I, angiotensin II receptor blockers

Monotherapy for the control of hypertension is useful in stage 1 hypertension (JNC VII, 2003; Weir, Maibach, & Bakin, 2000). The most effective choice for monotherapy in treating stage 1 hypertension is made using gender, race, and age as criteria. Young Caucasian males respond well to an ACE or angiotension II antagonist because the cause of hypertension in young white males is often increased rennin production. Beta blockers, calcium channel blockers, chlorthalidone, and clonidine are also effective; however, these drugs may have unwanted or unacceptable side effects in this population. In young male patients diuretics have proven to be the least effective. In elderly Caucasians diuretics, beta blockers, ACE inhibitors, angiotensin II antagonists, and calcium channel blockers are effective. Chlorthalidone and clonidine are effective in this group but the side effect of syncope and dizziness means that more care must be taken when prescribing these to elders. Young African Americans respond to calcium channel blockers, while older African Americans respond to calcium channel blockers, diuretics, and clonidine.

More women than men have hypertension, but until recently, women have been relatively underrepresented in clinical trials. Studies suggest that, although differences exist, women benefit significantly when they receive therapy to normalize blood pressure (Hayes & Taler, 1998). In general, thiazide diuretics work well as monotherapy to reduce blood pressure in women. Beta blockers, ACE inhibitors, angiotesin II antagonists, and calcium channel blockers also are effective in lowering blood pressure in women.

In stage one hypertension:

- Young African American: calcium channel blocker
- Young Caucasian: ACE inhibitor or beta blocker
- Older African American: calcium channel blocker, or diuretic
- Older Caucasian: calcium channel blocker, or diuretic; ACE inhibitor, or beta blocker
- Women: thiazide diuretics, ACE I, angiotensin II antagonists

If the initial response with the lowest possible dose is inadequate, then either increase the dose, change to an alternative drug, add a thiazide diuretic, or add a second drug at a low dose.

If adding a second drug, consider the following combinations:

- Thiazide diuretics with any of the nondiuretic drugs
- ACE inhibitor plus a calcium channel blocker
- Alpha blocker plus a beta blocker
- ACE inhibitor plus an alpha blocker (monitor for hypotension)

In severe hypertension begin with diltiazem and a dihydropyridine calcium channel blocker (edema is an adverse effect).

In resistant hypertension determine if the patient is taking and absorbing the drug(s). Add an adequate dose of a diuretic or add a loop diuretic, especially if there is renal failure.

Recent studies have demonstrated the benefit of treating isolated systolic hypertension. Several studies concluded that low-dose chlorthalidone as a first-step medication could reduce the incidence of total stroke by 36% along with a 32% decrease in major cardiovascular events. Atenolol at 25 mg/day or reserpine at 0.05 mg/day are used if the systolic blood pressure was not reached with first-step drug therapy (Leonetti & Zanchetti, 2002; Mulrow et al., 2002). The results of several studies assisted the members of the previous JNC V to make their recommendations for thiazide diuretics and beta blockers as first choice in the treatment of hypertension (Tobian, Brunner, Cohn, et al., 1994). Kostis, Davis, and Cutler (1997) performed an analysis on the data from the SHEP study to determine if heart failure, which is often preceded by ISH, was reduced by a diuretic-based antihypertensive stepped-care treatment. They concluded that a low-dose chlorthalidone regimen produced an 80% risk reduction in patients with a prior myocardial infarction and exerted a strong protective effect in preventing heart failure.

Other large studies such as the Multiple Risk Factor Intervention Trial and the European Working Party on Hypertension in the Elderly Trial evaluated the incidence of morbidity and mortality in patients with either or both elevations of systolic and diastolic blood pressure (Lapalio, 1995). The Swedish Trial in Old Patients with Hypertension (STOP-Hypertension) evaluated the benefits of treating hypertension in older patients (70–84 years). Patients included in the study had systolic blood pressure of 180 to 230 mm Hg with a diastolic pressure of at least 90 mm Hg, or a diastolic pressure of 105 to 120 mm Hg irrespective of systolic pressure. The authors concluded that treatment of hypertension in patients, both men and women, in this age range resulted in reduction in cardiovascular morbidity and mortality (Elliot & Black, 2002). The drug therapy used in this study included atenolol 50 mg and hydrochlorothiazide 25 mg plus amiloride 2.5 mg, metoprolol 100 mg, or pindolol 5 mg. All the medications were given once a day.

These studies focused on the use of diuretics and/or beta blockers in the treatment of hypertension. As such, they were the only pharmacotherapy that could be shown to reduce morbidity and mortality. The Systolic Hypertension in Europe (SYST-EUR) trial group presented their findings on the results of starting with the dihydropyridine calcium antagonist nitrendipine in a stepwise antihypertensive regimen. Enalaril and/or hydrochlorothiazide were added if the sitting systolic blood pressure remained above 150 mm Hg. The group reported 42% fewer strokes and 26% fewer cardiac endpoints (CHF, MI) when compared with placebo recipients.

It is important to remember that elderly patients are more susceptible to developing orthostatic hypotension resulting from antihypertensive treatment. There also is some degree of autonomic dysfunction in the elderly, so treatment should not be aggressive. Initiating pharmacotherapy with half the usual recommended dose and increasing slowly should help prevent incidences of cerebral or cardiac hypoperfusion.

The Antihypertensive and Lipid-Lowering Treatment to Prevent Heart Attack (ALLHAT) trial evaluated chlorthalidone, amlodipine, lisinopril, and doxazosin for lowering blood pressure. One arm of the study demonstrated that there was a higher risk of stroke, CHD death, nonfatal revascularization, angina, and CHF in those patients taking doxazosin. The other treatment arms of the study are continuing. Implications thus far are that for step 1 treatment monotherapy, chlorthalidone appears to be a better choice than doxazosin (ALLHAT Officers and Coordinators for ALLHAT Collaborative Research Group, 2000).

Monitoring for Efficacy and Toxicity

Diuretics. Diuretics are considered first-line therapy for the treatment of hypertension in patients without cautionary/contradictory comorbid conditions. When not used as monotherapy, diuretics are often used to augment the initial therapy of calcium channel blockers, ACE inhibitors, or beta blockers. The pharmacodynamics of thiazide diuretics are inhibition of sodium and water reabsorption and arterial vasodilation. The initial drop in blood pressure is from a decreased cardiac output that is later followed by a reduction in peripheral resistance.

The thiazide diuretic hydrochlorothiazide (HCTZ) is the most widely prescribed. In the past, HCTZ was often used as monotherapy and at much larger doses per day. Patients experienced such adverse events as hyperglycemia and hyperlipidemia. A lower dose of 12.5 to 25 mg/day reduces the likelihood of these adverse events while decreasing the systolic blood pressure in the range of 15–20 mm Hg and diastolic blood pressure 8–15 mm Hg (Klungel, Heckbert, Longstreth, Furberg, & Kaplan, 2001). The more potent loop diuretics (furosemide, butamide) have the disadvantage of requiring more frequent dosing but are advantageous in patients with creatinine clearances of < 30 mL/min. However, loop diuretics are rarely chosen for the management of hypertension. The loop diuretic torsemide has the unique pharmacokinetic property of a longer half-life and can be prescribed once a day (Puschett, 2000). The potassium-sparing diuretics should be used in patients who develop hypokalemia while on low-dose thiazide treatment and are unable to take potassium supplements or express a desire to avoid multiple drug regimens.

Beta Blockers. There are data to support beta blockers' ability to reduce morbidity and mortality, making them first-line therapy according to the JNC VII guidelines (JNC, 2003). Beta blockers have been shown to be an effective single-drug therapy in young and middle-aged patients, as well as in patients with coronary artery disease. Beta blockers decrease the rate, myocardial contractility, and conduction velocity of the heart, resulting in a decreased cardiac output. In addition, inhibition of renin release and a reduction of sympathetic nervous system activity centrally contribute to the antihypertensive effect.

The agents do vary in their cardioselectivity (atenolol, betaxolol, bisoprolol, metoprolol), intrinsic sympathomimetic activity (ISA-acebutolol, cartelol, penbutolol, pindolol), penetration of the blood brain barrier (lipid solubility—propranolol, timolol, metoprolol), and additional alpha blockade (labetalol).

The nonselective beta blockers without ISA are associated with the adverse events of hyperglycemia and hyperlipidemia. However, these changes may be temporary and the exact clinical significance is minimal. The patient should be monitored for the occurrence. Other adverse events to consider when prescribing beta blockers include a tendency to cause peripheral vasoconstriction, have a negative inotropic and chronotropic action on the heart, bronchoconstriction, and accentuation of insulin resistance. Beta blockers may be counterproductive in patients who must lose weight or increase exercise. A paradoxical increase in BP in volume-dependent patients may occur. On the other hand, beta blockers are well suited in treating hypertension in patients who also have angina, arrhythmias, or migraines. Beta blockers without ISA are indicated in patients following myocardial infarction since they have been shown to prevent the recurrence of infarction and sudden death.

Like most antihypertensive therapy, doses of beta blockers are started at the low end of the range and increased or augmented with another agent such as a diuretic to achieve outcome. Longer dosing intervals can successfully treat hypertension (HTN) and should assist in patient compliance.

Alpha Blockers. The $alpha_1$ blockers (prazosin, doxazosin, terazosin) can lower blood pressure along with reducing cholesterol, improving glucose tolerance, and increasing insulin sensitivity. These agents will not induce reflex increases in cardiac output and renin release. Although these are very beneficial aspects, the adverse events of hypotension and tachyphylaxis limit the usefulness of these agents. These agents are not recommended as first line or monotherapy based on the results of the ALLHAT trial. They are reasonable treatments for hypertension when patients also have BPH, so long as there is another antihypertensive being used concomitantly.

It is important to advise patients about first-dose or reinstituted-dose orthostatic hypotension and reflex tachycardia. Educate patients to take the first dose, or one that is missed after one or two doses, at bedtime or at a time when they can recline for a few hours.

$Alpha_2$ Agonists and Adrenergic Blocking Agents. The two currently prescribed agents are clonidine and reserpine. Clonidine may be effective in patients with severe HTN or renin-dependent disease. Although clonidine lowers BP without reflex tachycardia or metabolic changes in the patient, it does cause CNS sedation, partial tachyphylaxis, and interference with sexual function. Rebound hypertension may occur in some individuals with the discontinuation of clonidine. Concomitant administration with a beta blocker or in the presence of peripheral neuropathy may enhance the alpha activity, leading to a paradoxical increase in BP.

ACE Inhibitors. The cardioprotective and renoprotective effects of ACE inhibitors make these agents useful in patients with reduced left ventricular function (CHF), established or high risk of CAD, and proteinuria (Culy & Jarvis, 2002). ACE inhibition causes suppression of the vasoconstrictor angiotensin II and potentiation of the vasodilator bradykinin. The suppression of angiotensin II results in suppression of aldosterone secretion. Together there is decreased vasoconstriction, sodium and water retention, along with vasodilation via bradykinin. Bradykinin also enhances insulin sensitivity. ACE inhibitors appear consistently and effectively to decrease left ventricular mass in hypertensive patients.

An estimation of the renin state of a patient should be attempted to avoid profound hypotension with the initiation of the ACE inhibitor. High-renin states occur in patients with dehydration, reduced salt intake, renovascular hypertension, CHF, liver disease, or diuretic-therapy-induced volume contraction. To reduce the chance of hypotension, begin at lower doses (one-half normal or at the bottom of dosage range) and titrate slowly to the desired outcome. The ACE inhibitors have a slow onset and a long duration of action, allowing for once-a-day dosing. Assessment of activity should be 3 to 4 weeks after initiating therapy.

ACE inhibitors are known to occasionally result in a dry, hacking cough, which may subside with continued treatment. Renal insufficiency may occur with ACE inhibitors, especially in predisposed patients (e.g., volume depleted). There is no way to predict the occurrence of renal insufficiency; however, the patient's serum creatinine should be followed for several weeks. Many patients will have a slight increase in their serum creatinine during the initiation of an ACE inhibitor, although this will resolve with continued treatment.

Because of the blockade of aldosterone, the patient is susceptible to hyperkalemia. The practitioner should routinely monitor for this possible electrolyte abnormality with initiation of therapy, albeit it rarely necessitates discontinuation of therapy. The patient should be educated on the avoidance of potassium-containing supplements or salt substitutes.

Suspect noncompliance, NSAID use, or excessive salt intake whenever there is an increase in the patient's blood pressure. The teratogenic effects of ACE inhibitors precludes the use of these agents during pregnancy.

Calcium Channel Antagonists. Calcium channel antagonists are numerous but may be divided into two groups: L-type and T-type. The only T-type calcium channel antagonist approved for use in the United States was mibefradil, and it was subsequently removed due to drug-drug interactions and lack of an advantage over other marketed calcium channel antagonists. The L-type agents are categorized into two subgroups. The first subgroup contains verapamil and diltiazem. The second group contains nifedipine and the other dihydropyridines. Overall, the L-type channels are found in the plasma membrane, sinoatrial node, and atrioventricular node. By blocking the voltage-dependent L-type channels, these calcium channel blockers contribute to pacemaker activity, regulate AV conduction, vasodilate coronary and peripheral arteries, and, in some cases, have a negative inotropic effect on the heart. The second subgroup (nifedipine and other dihydro-pyridines) has a greater vasodilatory effect, whereas diltiazem and verapamil (first subgroup) affect the heart rate and contractility to a greater degree.

Concerns for using nifedipine include cardiac ischemia, proteinuria, glucose intolerance, and the development of peripheral edema. Psaty, Heckbert, Koepsell, et al. (1995) suggested that patients with no preexisting cardiac disease appear to be at higher risk for coronary events when using short-acting calcium channel antagonists. Research regarding calcium channel antagonists shows that short-acting agents (e.g., nifedipine) should be avoided and long-acting agents are reasonable to use where concomitant disease states with hypertension support their implementation. For instance, verapamil and diltiazem may reduce diabetic proteinuria, whereas amlodipine is safe for use in the management of hypertension in patients with heart failure (LVEF <40%) (Basile, 2002).

Vasodilators. The direct-acting vasodilators hydralazine and minoxidil are considered second- or even third-line agents because of the side effects of reflex tachycardia and water and sodium retention. Consequently, a diuretic, beta blocker, or alpha agonist should be prescribed concurrently. In turn, vasodilators may improve the efficacy of beta-blocker and diuretic therapy.

Minoxidil is also considered a potassium channel opener (Hubler, 2000). Through this mechanism, minoxidil acts as an indirect calcium channel antagonist. When the potassium channels are opened, the influx of calcium is inhibited.

Angiotensin II Blockers. The newest additions to the antihypertensive lineup are the angiotensin II inhibitors (losartan, valsartan, irbesartan, candesartan, telmisartan). These agents block the effects of angiotensin II, with no effect on the metabolic pathway of bradykinin. Without angiotensin II there is limited vasoconstriction and secretion of aldosterone. With no disruption of the normal inactivation of bradykinin, there is less incidence of cough and allergic reactions.

There are two types of angiotensin II receptors: AT_1 and AT_2. At this time only the functions of the AT_1 type are known and manipulated pharmacologically. The AT_1 receptors are found on vascular endothelium and are responsible for vasoconstriction, stimulation of thirst, and sodium reabsorption. These receptors are involved in vascular and myocardial restructuring and remodeling. The AT_2 receptors are found in the adrenal medulla and the uterus and in fetal tissues (Weir, 1996).

In summary, there are several approaches to the treatment of hypertension and a plethora of agents. The future will bring more large studies, and even more new agents along with commercial combination products. The recent addition of the combination of an ACE I and calcium channel blocker has been shown to be effective and increases compliance compared to both drugs given separately. This combination therapy joins others such as ACE inhibitors and diuretics and beta blockers and diuretics to simplify treatment regimens and increase patient compliance.

Followup Recommendations

The goal of therapy is to maintain the blood pressure within normal limits and prevent end-organ failure. If the treatment is appropriate treatment and blood pressure becomes stable, management becomes relatively routine. The provider should consider consultation with a physician for any patient with a stage III or IV hypertension.

A followup physical examination will include funduscopic examination, symptoms of dizziness or syncope, heart size, heart sounds, symptoms of shortness of breath, palpitations, chest pain, lung sounds, peripheral pulses, bruits, temperature, and sensation. Diagnostic studies should include creatinine, lipids, blood sugar, electrolytes, and an EKG. Other diagnostic procedures should be conducted as indicated by the history and physical.

The JNC VII summarizes the recommended followup time frame based on the classification.

With unstable blood pressure:

1. Refer to a physician and then follow frequently. This may be three times a week or more depending on the severity of the BP readings and the need for ongoing education and monitoring of effects of medications. Unstable blood pressure is best followed in consultation with a cardiologist or physician.

2. During followup visits, try to ascertain the degree of compliance with nonpharmacologic and pharmacologic treatments. Lack of compliance continues to be a major problem in management of hypertension.
3. Assess the number and degree of side effects of medications.
4. Continue to assess other medications, especially over-the-counter medications the patient may be taking.
5. Continue patient education.

With stable blood pressure:

1. Recheck every 3 to 6 months. The frequency depends on needs of the patient for education, ongoing monitoring, and compliance. Telephone followup or more frequent visits may improve compliance with treatment plan.
2. Always assess signs and symptoms of adverse reactions to medication(s), compliance with the treatment plan, and effectiveness of therapy.
3. Conduct an annual physical examination with focus on risk factors and end-organ involvement.
4. Consult a physician when there are signs and symptoms of additional cardiovascular problems or a change in response to the medication.

HEART FAILURE

Heart failure, a frequent complication of hypertension and ischemic heart disease, is a common diagnosis in clinical practice. In fact, it is the only cardiovascular disease state that is increasing in prevalence, especially in the elderly. Heart failure is associated with limitation of activity and decrease in quality of life. Limitation of activity varies from minimal limitation to inability to carry out any physical activity. One-year survival after the diagnosis varies from 57% for men and 64% for women. However, the 5-year survival drops to 25% for men and 38% for women. The more severe the disease, the lower the 1- and 5-year survival rates. The death rate for heart failure in 1990 was almost 38,000. Also, the people with a diagnosis of heart failure have a higher likelihood of succumbing to a sudden cardiac death than the overall population (Konstam, Dracup, et al., 1994).

DEFINITION

Heart failure occurs when the myocardium is unable to pump enough blood to meet the metabolic demands of the body. Heart failure is a problem of volume overload and poor tissue perfusion. The result is a constellation of symptoms that limit functional abilities. Heart failure can be either a systolic or diastolic dysfunction.

PATHOPHYSIOLOGY

The problem inherent in heart failure is the ineffective functioning of the myocardium due to systolic and/or diastolic dysfunction. The myocardium loses muscle mass often because of ischemia. Decreased muscle mass leads to dilated cardiomyopathy, resulting in a decrease in cardiac output and therefore ineffective tissue perfusion. The result of myocardial changes is an alteration in myocardial contractility, preload, afterload, and heart rate. Decreased contractility and increased preload and afterload increase pressure in the associated cardiac chamber. As the pressure increases, the myocardial fibers lengthen. Ventricular dilatation and elevation of diastolic pressure results. Hemodynamically, when the heart is unable to meet the demands of the body and is considered in failure, two factors account for the clinical presentation: decreased cardiac output and elevation of ventricular diastolic pressures.

In an attempt to compensate for the loss of myocardial effectiveness, the body sets into motion a complex system of neurohormonal mechanisms. These reflexes attempt to restore blood pressure through increasing peripheral resistance, altering the left ventricular function, and increasing sodium and water retention. The heart rate is increased with sympathetic stimulation. This may lead to arrhythmias and additional ischemia. Although compensatory and protective mechanisms take place, in someone with heart failure they act to increase cardiac afterload, which in turn continues to decrease cardiac performance and increase volume overload (Figure 20–1).

- increased capillary pressure ---► pulmonary or systemic edema
- decreased cardiac output ---► neurohormonal responses: decreased renal blood flow ---► activation of renin-angiotensin-aldosterone system ---► sodium and water retention ---► increased peripheral resistance and left ventricular afterload, and increased preload
- increased sympathetic activity ---► stimulation of myocardial contractility, heart rate, venous tone ---► increase in preload, tachycardia, ischemic attacks, increased pulmonary edema
- increased peripheral resistance ---► reduction in renal blood flow, left ventricular afterload
- increased arginine vasopressin ---► vasoconstriction, inhibits water excretion

FIGURE 20–1. The compensatory mechanisms in heart failure (from Haak et al., 1994; Kloner & Dzau, 1990; Kradjan, 1993; Massie, 1996).

In the early stages of heart failure, the compensatory mechanisms may be successful in maintaining the needs of the body. As failure of the myocardium progresses, however, the physiologic needs of the body are not met and the clinical symptoms become apparent.

TYPES OF HEART FAILURE

The New York Heart Association developed a functional system for classifying heart failure. Class I patients have no symptoms of heart failure, Class II patients have mild heart failure, Class III have moderate heart failure, and Class IV have severe heart failure. Symptoms experienced by persons diagnosed with Class I or II heart failure can be relatively minor and easily mistaken as signs of natural aging. Many people in these two mild functional categories may not even be aware of having heart failure. Class III and Class IV, or advanced heart failure, however, is often seriously debilitating, deeply affecting quality of life. The etiology of heart failure can be classified as systolic or diastolic. Clinical manifestations of systolic and diastolic heart failure are similar, and it is difficult to differentiate between the two prior to echocardiography.

Systolic Dysfunction

The most common form of heart failure is left ventricular systolic dysfunction. The mechnisms of systolic dysfunction are decreased cardiac output → decreased ejection fraction → increased left ventricular end-diastolic pressure → increased ventricular preload → decreased contractile force → decreased blood pressure → compensatory responses.

The etiology is coronary artery disease, myocardial infarction, chronic hypertension, and valvular abnormalities.

Symptoms include dyspnea on exertion, fatigue, weakness, orthopnea, peripheral edema, and chronic cough. The patient also may complain of restlessness, insomnia, nocturia, anorexia, memory loss, and confusion.

Diastolic Dysfunction

The mechanisms of diastolic dysfunction are reduced ventricular compliance (ventricles rigid and unable to relax enough to accept all blood) → increased ventricular diastolic pressure → increased atrial pressures → increased pressure in pulmonary and systemic venous systems. Normal ventricular function and ejection fraction are indicative of diastolic dysfunction.

The etiology is left ventricular hypertrophy due to hypertension, hypertrophic or restrictive cardiomyopathy, diabetes, and pericardial disease.

Many of the same symptoms of left ventricular systolic dysfunction apply, particularly dyspnea and peripheral edema.

Possible symptoms of right heart failure include peripheral edema, ascites, weakness, mental confusion, hepatic congestion, right upper quadrant abdominal pain, anorexia, constipation, bloating, nausea, vomiting, splenomegaly, jugular venous distension (JVD), and hepatojugular reflux (HJR).

Possible symptoms of left heart failure include dyspnea, orthopnea, paroxysmal nocturnal dyspnea, inability to exercise, weakness, fatigue, nocturia, mental confusion, cough, hemoptysis, basilar crackles, pleural effusions, pulmonary edema, S_3 heart sound.

SPECIFIC CONSIDERATIONS FOR PHARMACOTHERAPY

When Drug Therapy Is Needed

Heart disease is a progressive chronic condition that may severely limit functional abilities. Prevention is a major factor. Management of hypertension and other cardiovascular diseases as well as diabetes may decrease the incidence of heart failure. Evaluation for a drug-induced cause is important. Once it is determined that there is no other etiology for the presentation of congestive heart failure, the practitioner will need to initiate pharmacotherapy. The choice of agents and the aggressiveness of treatment will be based on the patient's signs and symptoms. Untreated CHF can progress to further disability, more hospitalizations, and decreased quality of life.

Short- and Long-Term Goals of Pharmacotherapy

The goals of therapy are to control the symptoms of CHF so that the patient may continue with as many activities of daily living as possible, and to reduce mortality. Short-term therapy is directed at decreasing fluid congestion in the periphery and lungs while assisting the heart's contractility. By breaking the vicious cycle of CHF, long-term pharmacotherapy can be directed towards maintaining cardiac function while slowing the progression of the disease.

Quality-of-life considerations may vary depending on the severity of the disease. If the patient has mild symptoms, then survival is primary followed by exercise capacity and then symptom management. With moderate symptoms, the patient may desire more exercise capacity, with survival followed by symptom control. The patient with severe symptoms may express control of symptoms as primary, followed by exercise capacity and last, survival.

Nonpharmacologic Therapy

Nonpharmacologic treatment involves lifestyle modifications, particularly diet and activity. Dietary changes include a moderate (2g) sodium restriction. This usually is achieved by teaching the patient to add no salt during cooking or at the table. Sodium restriction is often difficult for patients to follow, and a more severe restriction results in noncompliance (Massie, 1996). The American Heart Association has many helpful publications for patients and families, including a cookbook that uses alternate spices to improve flavor.

Because of the depressant effect of alcohol, it is recommended that it be either eliminated or restricted to one drink a day. Caffeine should be limited because of the stimulatory effect on the heart. Finally, fluid intake needs to be assessed and limited when necessary (Kinsella, 2002).

When heart failure symptoms are severe, resting the heart through a decrease in activity may facilitate recompensation of the myocardium. Activity restriction during the acute phase is needed to reduce symptoms. Limited activity along with pharmacologic therapy may promote copious diuresis. A semireclined position promotes increased renal profusion, leading to increased diuresis. However, after the acute phase, patients are encouraged to begin an exercise program. In most cases, an exercise program that emphasizes a gradual increase in activity is beneficial in reducing symptoms and improving endurance.

Time Frame for Initiating Pharmacotherapy

Pharmacotherapy should be initiated along with lifestyle modifications. The type of pharmacotherapy for CHF will depend on the presenting symptomology of the patient. Hospitalization and aggressive treatment will be necessary for patients who present in acute or severe failure. Additional treatments will be based upon resolution of acute symptoms and the desired functional level.

See Drug Tables 205.1, 205.7, 207, 208.

Assessment Prior to Therapy

The history and physical examination concentrate on the signs and symptoms of heart failure, which relate to the alteration in function of the heart. Left-sided heart failure is the most common and involves systolic left ventricular dysfunction. The most helpful classification is according to functional limitations (see Table 20–3).

TABLE 20–3. New York Heart Association Classification of Heart Failure

- Class I: No limitation on activity. No fatigue, dyspnea, or palpitations with physical activity.
- Class II: Slight limitation on activity. Comfortable at rest but fatigue, palpitations, and dyspnea with ordinary physical activity.
- Class III: Marked limitation of activity. Comfortable at rest but fatigue, palpitations, and dyspnea, during ordinary physical activity.
- Class IV: Unable to carry out any physical activity without discomfort. Fatigue, palpitations, and dyspnea at rest.

Using the functional classification, a patient may present without any symptoms; therefore, it is important to perform a complete history and physical examination. Because systolic and diastolic and left and right dysfunction may occur together, the assessment needs to include information on all manifestations of the disease.

Areas of Focus

History. Previous medical history includes hypertension, myocardial infarction, congenital heart problems, untreated streptococcal infection, and coronary artery disease. Symptoms include onset and severity, ability to perform activities of daily living including instrumental activities, usual exercise, and changes in ability, sleep patterns, and mental status.

Respiratory. Commonly, the patient will complain of shortness of breath with exertion. As the syndrome progresses, the symptoms increase. Be sure to ascertain symptoms of a nonproductive cough, often worse when lying down. Patients may be comfortable at rest but have dyspnea when changing clothes or during assessment of gait and balance. Observe the patient during conversation. Note the ability to complete sentences without distress. Inquire about the number of pillows or if able to sleep lying down.

Gastrointestinal. Assess appetite, nausea, vomiting, and pain.

Pain. Check for angina, chest pain, right upper quadrant pain caused by right heart failure and the resultant congestion in the liver, loss of appetite, nausea, and peripheral edema.

Urinary. Assess for nocturia.

Precipitating Events and Conditions. Assess for previous myocardial infarction, hypertension, use of NSAIDs (sodium-retaining), pulmonary embolism, infection, anemia and use of certain calcium channel antagonists (diltiazem and verapamil), beta blockers, and other negative inotropic drugs.

Weight. With severe heart failure, weight loss with cachexia may be apparent. Weight gain over a short period of time is indicative of fluid overload.

Color. Assess for cyanosis.

Vital Signs. Check for tachycardia, hypotension, and decreased pulse pressure.

Neck. Check height of pulsations of jugular veins, jugular distention, and carotid pulses. Evaluate pulse pressure, the presence of atrial stenosis, and hepatojugular reflux. Thyroid examination is important. Hyperthyroidism and hypothyroidism represent two treatable causes of heart failure.

Lungs. Check for crackles at the bases, dullness to percussion (pulmonary effusion), expiratory wheezes, and rhonchi.

Heart. Check enlargement of the heart, downward and lateral displacement of the point of maximal impulse (PMI) and diffuse PMI, parasternal lift, diminished first heart sound, S_3 gallop (heard just after S_2) that may start in the left ventricle, and a fourth heart sound that may be heard. Murmurs could indicate valvular disease or dilated ventricles.

Abdomen. Hepatic enlargement, tender or nontender, may occur with right-sided failure. Pressure on the liver may produce a positive hepatojugular reflux. Also assess ascites and upper right quadrant tenderness.

Extremities. Pitting edema of the legs may be in the lower legs and extend to the thighs and abdomen. Assess temperature and color of extremities.

Laboratory. A CBC should be done to check for anemia, one sign in high-output cardiac failure. With severe heart failure, polycythemia may occur.

Chemical Profile. Azotemia, low sedimentation rate, respiratory alkalosis, elevated liver enzymes, and elevated bilirubin and BUN may occur. Do a thyroid profile and check thiamine level if high output is suspected.

Urinalysis. Proteinuria and high specific gravity may be present.

Electrocardiogram. This helps define possible etiologies such as secondary arrhythmias, valvular disease, myocardial infarction, coronary artery disease, and ventricular hypertrophy. A stress test electrocardiogram is indicated if ischemia is suspected.

Echocardiogram. The echocardiogram is preferred and justified because it helps differentiate between systolic and diastolic dysfunction. An ejection fraction of less than 40% indicates systolic dysfunction. The normal ventricular function and ejection fraction are indicative of diastolic dysfunction. The echocardiogram also reveals the size and function of the ventricles and atria and is able to detect valvular problems, old myocardial infarctions, and other possible etiologies of heart failure.

Chest X-ray. Examine the x-ray for the size and shape of the heart. Typically, the chest x-ray shows cardiomegaly. Interstitial edema, alveolar fluid, dilation of the veins of the upper lobe, and perivascular edema may indicate pulmonary venous hypertension. The chest x-ray may also show pleural effusion, common with heart failure.

Patient/Caregiver Information

It is important that the patient and the patient's family be informed and understand the diagnosis, including the prognosis, and symptoms of worsening heart failure and actions to take in the event these symptoms occur. Information should be provided on activity and dietary recommendations. The effects of medications, dosing, side effects, and mechanisms to enhance compliance should be discussed.

OUTCOMES MANAGEMENT

Selecting an Appropriate Agent

The American Heart Association/American College of Cardiology has recently published revised guidelines for the management of heart failure. These guidelines can be reviewed in detail for management descriptions. In summary, for the ambulatory setting, general treatment includes four agents:

1. Diuretics
2. ACE I
3. Digoxin
4. Beta blockers.

Diuretics are reserved for patients who require treatment for volume overload. ACE inhibitors are indicated for all patients with LVEF less than 40% due to significant reduction in mortality in these individuals. Digoxin is indicated in all patients with systolic dysfunction (LVEF <40%) and symptoms; the drug decreases symptoms of heart failure and hospitalization for the disease, but has no effect on reducing mortality. Beta blockers should be used early in the management of heart failure, given the positive effect on survival. Therapy with beta blockers should be started at a low dose and increased slowly to minimize or prevent exacerbation of the heart failure symptoms. A final drug that can be added to the above four agents is spironolactone—however, it is reserved for patients who are in severe heart failure (NYHA class IV). Spironolactone has been shown to decrease mortality in patients with severe heart failure in combination with standard care. The website for the full guidelines is http://216.185.112.5/downloadable/heart/5360_HFGuidelineFinal.pdf

Monitoring for Efficacy and Toxicity

Diuretics. Diuretics (thiazides, potassium-sparing, and loop) are the drugs of choice for reducing the symptoms of volume overload and the accompanying pulmonary and/or peripheral edema. To date, diuretics have not been shown to decrease the mortality of CHF. Diuretics, through their reduction of atrial and ventricular diastolic pressure, may inhibit the progression of ventricular hypertrophy. However, in patients without signs and symptoms of volume overload, diuretics may be harmful because of induction of neurohormonal activation (Hayes & Taler, 1998; Klungel et al., 2001).

Thiazide diuretics (hydrochlorothiazide, indapamide, metolazone), whose site of action is the early distal convoluted tubule, can manage mild volume overload. Thiazide diuretics become less effective when the glomerular filtration rate is less than 30 mL/min.

Loop diuretics (furosemide, bumetanide, torsemide) remove a greater percentage of sodium and water and are favored when volume overload is more severe. Loop diuretics act in the ascending limb of the loop of Henle, induce a prostaglandin-mediated increase in renal blood flow, and maintain their activity in renal impairment. Loop diuretics maintain their effectiveness as glomerular filtration rates decrease, but are reduced with concurrent administration of nonsteroidal antiinflammatory drugs (Basile, 2002; Goldman & Bennett, 2000).

Furosemide is the most commonly prescribed loop diuretic, primarily based on drug cost and familiarity with its use in clinical practice. Among the three loop diuretics, torsemide has several unique features (White & Chow, 1997). Torsemide produces less potassium loss because of less action at the proximal convoluted tubule. Its bioavailability is similar to bumetanide but greater than furosemide. Torsemide's half-life is longer than the other two and permits true once-a-day dosing. About 25% of torsemide is excreted unchanged in the urine; for bumetanide this fraction is 50% and for furosemide 50 to 80%. Torsemide does not interact with cimetidine and warfarin. A helpful dosage equivalence scale is 10–20 mg of torsemide = 1 mg of bumetanide = 40 mg of furosemide.

The effectiveness of diuretics can be assessed by the following:

- Increase in exercise tolerance
- Decrease in pulmonary congestion and rales
- Weight loss
- Less edema (using these first four parameters, the practitioner and the patient may develop criteria for self-adjustment of diuretic pharmacotherapy to maintain desired weight)
- Less neck vein distention (more aggressive diuretic pharmacotherapy may be needed if the patient has an elevated pressure in the internal jugular vein or evidence of hepatojugular reflux)
- Disappearance of S_3 gallop

If the activity of the loop diuretic diminishes, the addition of a thiazide diuretic (metolazone or hydrochlorothiazide) provides a synergistic effect. The rationale is that the loop diuretic is increasing the delivery of sodium to the distal convoluted tubule, resulting in an increased amount removed by the thiazide diuretic. The possibility of an edematous gastrointestinal tract may be the cause of decreased efficacy since there is diminished rate of absorption, with lowered peak concentrations (Brater, 1985).

It should be noted that diuretics can increase the activity of renin, thus decreasing their efficacy. With chronic use, the patient needs to be monitored for the onset of hypokalemia, hyponatremia, hypomagnesemia, hypochloremic alkalosis, hyperglycemia, and hyperuricemia. Hypokalemia occurs in 10 to 36% of patients receiving diuretics, primarily occurring with loop agents. There is an average decrease of between 0.5 and 0.7 mmol/L of serum potassium with long-term use of diuretics. The decrease is dose-related and more likely to occur in patients who have unrestricted sodium intake. Hypokalemia should be treated with potassium replacements to decrease the likelihood of hypochloremic alkalosis and persistent hypokalemia. Hypokalemia can also exacerbate digitalis intoxication in patients receiving digoxin.

Alternatively, potassium-sparing diuretics (amiloride, spironolactone, triamterene) may be used to minimize potassium loss with diuresis since they are more potent natriuretic agents. Their site of action is the late distal convoluted tubule and collecting ducts. It is important to monitor closely the serum potassium level whenever these agents are used in treatment. This is especially important in patients receiving potassium supplements (don't forget about the potassium salts used by patients vs. table salt) or an ACE inhibitor (which reserves potassium at the kidney). Serum magnesium needs to be evaluated in patients with refractory hypokalemia.

If the patient becomes fatigued or hypotensive or has azotemia in the presence of a normal jugular venous pressure, excessive diuresis is the likely cause. The dose of the agent should be reduced or discontinued. In patients with diastolic dysfunction, diuretics need to be used cautiously to avoid volume depletion, orthostatic hypotension, and aggravation of the CHF.

ACE Inhibitors. ACE inhibitors reduce preload and afterload by arterial and venous dilation. The pharmacodynamics of these agents involve inhibition of angiotensin II (afterload reduction) and the resultant inhibition of aldosterone secretion (preload reduction). In addition, ACE inhibitors prevent the breakdown of the vasodilator bradykinin. Because of the evidence demonstrating increased survival, these agents are considered first-line therapy, versus digoxin, for mild to moderate CHF and especially in patients with symptomatic CHF associated with reduced systolic ejection or left ventricular remodeling. Current ACE inhibitors indicated to treat CHF are captopril, enalapril, fosinopril, lisinopril, quinapril, ramipril, perindopril, and trandolapril. There are differences among these agents in regards to their pharmacokinetics; however, the outcome is comparable. Captopril and lisinopril are not prodrugs and therefore do not need to be converted by the liver to an active form. Fosinopril is 50% fecally and 50% renally eliminated (as is trandolapril for HTN), whereas the others are 90% renally eliminated. Ramipril and quinapril are not removed by hemodialysis as are the others, except lisinopril, which is unknown.

The desired response to ACE inhibitors requires several weeks of administration. This time period probably is due to the adjustment needed by the body's various hormonal responses. The plasma renin activity is not indicative of the long-term success of these medications (Packer et al., 1993). Doses need to be started low and can be adjusted upwards about every 2 to 3 days, though weekly is more realistic, until symptomatic relief occurs. The target doses are captopril 50 mg tid, enalapril 10 mg bid, fosinopril 20 mg daily, lisinopril 20 mg daily, perindopril 4 mg daily, quinapril 10 mg bid, ramipril 5 mg bid, and trandolapril 4 mg daily, unless the patient develops intolerable side effects.

Special attention should be given to the patient's fluid and sodium status before initiating an ACE inhibitor in order to prevent hypotension and renal insufficiency. If the patient is on diuretic therapy or has recently had an increase in his or her diuretic dose, the starting doses of ACE inhibitors should be reduced (captopril 6.25–12.5 mg tid, enalapril 2.5 mg one or two times per day, lisinopril 5 mg/day, and quinapril 5 mg/day) to help prevent hypotension. A reduction in diuretic doses or an increase in sodium intake should minimize the chance of renal insufficiency. A helpful parameter is if the serum sodium concentration is less than 135 mmol/L, the patient probably will have a high level of plasma renin activity and thus increased sensitivity to the ACE inhibitors (Cohn, 1996).

Retention of potassium is another possible adverse effect. Although hyperkalemia rarely develops, other sources of potassium (diet, salt substitutes, potassium supplements) should be discussed with the patient.

Other patient complaints include rash, dysgeusia, reflex tachycardia, hypotension, and a dry, hacking cough. Up to 40% of the population get a cough independent of ACE inhibitor therapy, although the incidence is greater when an ACE inhibitor is prescribed.

Cardiac Glycosides: Digoxin. Digoxin has a positive inotropic and a negative chronotropic effect on the heart. The mechanism of action for digoxin is inhibition of the NaK-ATPase, which results in its positive inotropic effect increased vagal tone, and some evidence of blunting of excessive neurohumoral activation. The net effects are an increase in cardiac index, a decrease in systemic vascular resistance and pulmonary capillary wedge pressure (PCWP), and little change in arterial blood pressure.

In recent years the therapeutic efficacy of digoxin has been disputed for patients with heart failure and normal sinus rhythm. However, the withdrawal of digoxin can have an adverse effect (McMurray & Pfeffer, 2002). In the Digitalis Investigation Group (DIG) study, it was noted there was no significant effect of digoxin on mortality, as with ACE inhibitors, but there was a reduction in the hospitalization rate and improvement in patient symptoms. (McMurray & Pfeffer, 2002). Digoxin should be used in patients along with diuretics and an ACE inhibitor early in the course of the disease. Its use, however, should not supplant the initiation of beta blocker therapy.

Special pharmacokinetic considerations of digoxin include its large volume of distribution and predominantly renal elimination. Because of a significant distribution phase, serum levels should be collected at least after the oral dose, but ideally just before the next dose. Therapeutic serum levels are generally in the range of 0.5 to 2.0 ng/mL, although the goal concentration in heart failure is about 1 ng/mL, based on the results of the Digitalis Investigation Group (DIG) study (Haji & Movahed, 2000).

A serum level must be evaluated in conjunction with any adverse signs and symptoms the patient may exhibit since there is not a good correlation between serum levels and the presence of signs and symptoms of toxicity. The half-life of digoxin normally is 1.5 h in a patient with normal renal function, but is extended to 5 days in anuric patients.

Patients with heart failure and normal sinus rhythm should be started on digoxin without a loading dose. In this setting dosing should be either, 0.125 or 0.25 mg daily. Dosing of digoxin is based on ideal body weight and the patient's estimated creatinine clearance. As emphasized by the Heart Failure Society of America Guidelines, doses of digoxin should be 0.125 mg daily for the management of heart failure. Rarely should a dose of 0.25 be used (HFSA Guidelines, 1999). The half-life of digoxin is 36 to 48 hours in patients with normal renal function but is extended markedly in patients with decreased renal function.

Adverse effects may be noncardiac (nausea, vomiting) or cardiac (dysrhythmias). Additionally, hypokalemia, hypomagnesemia, and hypercalcemia will predispose the patient to cardiac manifestations.

Beta Blockers. Recent evidence suggests that in stable heart failure, patients benefit from the addition of a beta blocker (e.g., metoprolol, carvedilol), with gradual titration over 4 to 6 weeks to higher doses. This is based on the neurohormonal model of heart failure in which activation of the sympathetic nervous system and the reninangiotensin-aldosterone system contributes to the hemodynamic and clinical abnormalities. Currently, beta blockers may be useful in patients with idiopathic dilated cardiomyopathy. Dosing guidelines for successful outcomes include:

1. Start slowly titrating the dose every 1 to 4 weeks.
2. Improvements may not be seen for 3 to 12 months.
3. Effectiveness may be greater in patients with high adrenergic activity, resting tachycardia, and depressed left ventricular function.
4. Nonselective agents with peripheral vasodilating properties may be better because of an increase in $beta_2$ and $alpha_1$ receptors from continual adrenergic stimulation.

Two currently available agents are metoprolol and carvedilol. Metoprolol is a selective beta blocker with peripheral vasodilatory effects. Carvedilol is a nonselective beta blocker with vasodilating action via alpha-adrenergic blockade. Carvedilol also has calcium channel blocking activity at high doses. Although this action does not provide additional benefits in blood pressure reduction, it may be responsible for local vascular bed vasodilation. The cardioprotective effect of carvedilol may be due to its antioxidant properties. Carvedilol prevents the generation of oxygen free radicals and the oxidation of LDL and uptake into coronary vasculature (Chen & Chow, 1997; Hubler, 2000). Carvedilol carries an FDA indication for the treatment of mild or moderate heart failure of ischemic or cardiomyopathic origin when used in combination with digoxin, diuretics, and ACE inhibitors. When carvedilol was compared to placebo in patients with chronic heart failure, the risk of death and hospitalization for cardiovascular causes was reduced by 65% when used in combination with digoxin, diuretics, and an ACE inhibitor.

Other Agents. In addition to the standard of care for heart failure (diuretics, ACE inhibitors, digoxin, and beta blockers), various other drugs have been evaluated in this disease state. Spironolactone has shown very promising results in patients with severe heart failure (Class IV). In fact, this agent added to diuretics, ACE inhibitors, with or without digoxin significantly decreases mortality. At this point, its use is reserved for severe heart failure until additional data are published.

Angiotensin II receptor antagonists also have been evaluated in heart failure and show promising benefit. Their action is similar to that of ACE inhibitors, but they do not interfere with the metabolism of bradykinin. As such, there should be less potential to induce cough. Investigations with losartan and valsartan demonstrate these agents are reasonable alternatives in patients intolerant to an ACE inhibitor (e.g., cough). Despite a lower incidence of angioedema with angiotensin II receptor antagonists, case reports of angioedema have been published, and caution should be exercised in those with a history of this disorder with an ACE inhibitor.

The calcium channel blockers amlodipine and felodipine have both been evaluated in heart failure. Neither agent has a benefit as it relates to reducing mortality. In those with heart failure who require additional antianginal therapy, these agents can be safely used in heart failure. One should note that the FDA-approved indications for these agents differ, and only amlodipine is approved as both an antianginal and antihypertensive.

The calcium channel blockers felodipine and amlodipine have been studied in the treatment of CHF. These two agents have an action more restricted to the vascular walls and may augment vasodilation induced by

ACE inhibitors (Cohn, 1996). More recently it has been proposed that in CHF the cells are programmed for cell death by tissue necrosis factor alpha and interleukin-6, leading to decreased myocardial contractility. The beneficial effects of amlodipine may be the result of its inhibition of interleukin-6.

The angiotensin II type 1 receptor blockers may also prove useful in the treatment of CHF. Their action is similar to that of the ACE inhibitors, but they do not interfere with the metabolism of bradykinin. As such, there should be less potential to induce cough. Another advantage may be the local inhibition of angiotensin II effects when compared to the ACE inhibitors. However, the effect of angiotensin II receptor blockers on mortality is unknown. These agents should be reserved for patients who cannot tolerate the ACE-inhibitor-induced cough or the side effects of hydralazine–isosorbide dinitrate therapy (Dunphy & Winland-Brown, 2001; Goldman & Bennett, 2000).

Followup Recommendations

There is no standard frequency of followup. After the initial diagnosis and treatment and once the patient is stabilized, visits to the provider may be as frequent as every 2 to 3 weeks or every 3 to 6 months. Patient education and evaluation of effectiveness of therapy are needed during early stages.

Each visit includes the patient's perception of symptoms discussed previously as well as vital signs and heart and lung sounds. Always reevaluate using the New York Heart Association classification (Table 20–4).

Closely follow electrolytes, chest x-rays, and electrocardiograms, as well as renal (BUN and creatinine) and liver function tests.

If diuretics are being used, observe for signs of excessive diuresis: weight change, orthostatic hypotension, dry mouth, thirst, weakness, oliguria, nausea, vomiting, dizziness, confusion, falls, cramps, restlessness, and drowsiness.

TABLE 20–4. Phases of Depolarization and Repolarization

- Phase 0: Depolarization and rapid movement of calcium or sodium into the cell; referred to as upstroke
- Phase 1: Early repolarization; slow influx of calcium into the cell
- Phase 2: Plateau; continuation of repolarization with slow influx of sodium and calcium into the cells
- Phase 3: Repolarization; potassium moves outside cell; repolarization but not quite resting
- Phase 4: Return to resting potential via the sodium/potassium ATPase pump with magnesium serving as a catalytic enzyme

If ACE inhibitors are part of the regimen, check for cough, rash, swelling of the face, eye, lips, or tongue, sore throat, fever, hypotension, dehydration, vomiting, diarrhea, potassium level, and renal function.

Monitor steady-state blood levels of digitalis just prior to next dose or in the presence of signs of toxicity (confusion, nausea, vomiting, dizziness, arrhythmias, headaches, visual disturbances, weakness).

Always ask about other medications including over-the-counter medications, especially NSAIDs, since these agents promote sodium and water retention and decrease renal function in the elderly.

ARRHYTHMIAS

Arrhythmia, or dysrhythmia, is a disturbance in cardiac rhythm. The conduction system of the heart begins in the sinoatrial (SA) node of the heart. The SA impulse activates the atria and AV node. The AV node transmits the impulse across the septum to the bundle of His in the ventricles. The impulse then moves through the ventricles by way of the right and left bundle branches and the Purkinje system. Disturbances in rate and rhythm are due to disturbances in this electrophysiologic system and are most frequently caused by reentry problems or disturbances in automaticity (Dunphy & Winland-Brown, 2001; Goldman & Bennett, 2000).

Some definitions of the mechanisms of arrhythmias follow (Dunphy & Winland-Brown, 2001; Goldman & Bennett, 2000).

- *Impulse conduction:* Impulse conduction is altered at the SA or AV node, in the ventricular conduction system, or within the atria or ventricles. It is associated with the development of reentry circuits.
- *Reentry:* When the normal pathway for depolarization is blocked, the impulse seeks another route. The alternate pathway is unidirectional and causes a delay in depolarization and impulse conduction. This delay causes another impulse to be initiated at the original site. Reentry circuits may be at the SA or AV nodes or may be alternate pathways that circumvent either node. Reentry mechanisms may be the most important in arrhythmias.
- *Automaticity:* The capacity of special cells in the cardiac muscle to automatically generate depolarization is known as automaticity. Spontaneous depolarization or pacemaker activity normally occurs in the SA and AV nodes as well as the bundle of His. However, the SA node works at a faster rate and usually prevents

the slower pacemakers in the AV node and Purkinje system from firing unless it is dysfunctional.

- *Abnormal impulse formations* are arrhythmias caused by problems with automaticity. As described, the SA node is the normal pacemaker. Ectopic pacemakers (nonnormal pacemakers) are outside the SA node. Abnormal rhythms occur when the ectopic pacemaker cells reach threshold before the SA node discharges the impulse, thus initiating a beat before the SA node. The ectopic pacemaker continues to generate impulses after repolarization.

Pharmacotherapy for arrhythmias is organized according to electrophysiological effects. Therefore, to understand pharmacotherapy for arrhythmias, it is important to examine the electrophysiologic properties of the cardiac muscle and to define commonly used terms.

- *Depolarization:* Change in the voltage at the cell membrane caused by the initiation of the action potential; electrical activation of cells. Allows movement of sodium, calcium, and potassium across the cell membrane.
- *Repolarization:* Deactivation of the electrical activity at the cell membrane. The depolarization and repolarization can be described in phases (Table 20–4).
- *Action potential:* The first step in contraction is when the cardiac cells are excited, changing the distribution of ions at the cell membrane. Ions move through channels into the myocardial cells. The movement of ions causes changes in membrane voltage. Channels in each cell allow the action potential to move through cells, causing depolarization of the cell.
- *Resting membrane potential:* Describes the voltage difference at the cell membrane. The resting membrane potential indicates a higher negative charge outside the cell membrane and is noted as −60 to −80 mV (millivolts) depending on the location. This value is an important determinant of the speed of impulse conduction. At the SA node (pacer) the resting membrane potential is less negative. Therefore, it is able to be receptive to new impulses sooner than other cardiac cells with a more negative resting membrane potential. Resting potential in the cardiac cells is the time of repolarization.
- *Fast channel:* Rapid conduction of impulses. The channel opens, allowing the rapid influx of sodium or calcium ions into the cell depending on the cardiac tissue. The movement of sodium into the cell causes depolarization of the cell.
- *Slow channel:* After the rapid influx of sodium, the channel allows the slow influx of calcium. Conduction of impulses at this time is slow.
- *Action potential duration* (APD): Time from the beginning of the action potential to the return of the resting potential; phases 0 to 4.
- *Refractory period:* Time from the start of depolarization through contraction.
- *Effective refractory period* (ERP): Time from the beginning of the action potential to the beginning of repolarization when no new action potential can be initiated. It is the time needed to open the sodium and calcium channels; phases 0 to 3.5.
- *Relative refractory period:* Short time from the end of the ERP to the end of repolarization when the membrane potential is beginning to be negative; able to depolarize but a stronger than usual stimulus is needed.

There are many cardiac arrhythmias. The usual classifications are supraventricular, ventricular, and conduction arrhythmias.

SPECIFIC CONSIDERATIONS FOR PHARMACOTHERAPY

When Drug Therapy Is Needed

Cardiac arrhythmias can be divided into two categories: those related to abnormal impulse formation and those due to abnormal conduction. Arrhythmias that arise from the sinus node can range from respiratory sinus arrhythmia to pathological sinus pauses and sinus arrest. Cardiac impulses originating from areas other than the sinus node are referred to as ectopics. These may arise from other areas in the atria, at the atrioventricular junction, along the Purkinje system or in the ventricles. Abnormalities in conduction can occur at any site within the heart. Impulses may be blocked or fail to leave the area of initiation. The AV node is the most common site at which an abnormality may occur in conduction that causes a rhythm disturbance. Conduction blocks range from a minor prolongation in transmission time to complete blockage of conduction that results in asystole. The atria can also have abnormalities in conduction that result in atrial flutter or fibrillation. The most common arrhythmia seen in clinical practice is atrial fibrillation. The concern is twofold with these types of arrhythmias. First, there is a concern for the possibility of thrombus formation and subsequent occlusion of arteries in the brain. Second is the ventricular response rate to the atrial impulses.

When evaluating a patient with symptoms suggestive of a rhythm disturbance, or with a documented arrhythmia, a determination needs to be made whether the arrhythmia is simple and benign or potentially dangerous. The rhythm may suggest the presence of an underlying problem such as hyperthyroidism or a drug reaction. Careful analysis of underlying disease states and drug reactions should be evaluated along with pharmacological treatment for the actual arrhythmia.

There are many types of arrhythmias, ranging from common, to asymptomatic, to life-threatening. Antiarrhythmic pharmacotherapy has not been proved completely effective, and many medications have side effects that are more harmful than the arrhythmia. Therefore, the value of using pharmacotherapy is evaluated by the potential mortality or morbidity of the arrhythmia and the associated side effects of the medications. Treatment is most often based on the history and symptoms of the patient, potential side effects of medications, and provider comfort with a particular agent.

Short- and Long-Term Goals of Pharmacotherapy

Pharmacotherapy and the associated short- and long-term goals are dependent on the condition being treated and the underlying disease state. Pharmacotherapy is often used in symptomatic patients until a pacemaker or permanent correction of the arrhythmia is possible. These types of arrhythmias include bradycardia and second- and third-degree heart blocks. Drugs may be used in conjunction with permanent pacing such as with acute ventricular block or an MI with ventricular block. Finally, pacing may be instituted followed by pharmacotherapy.

As with any disease state, the goals of therapy are to prevent mortality and morbidity, prevent complications, and promote quality of life. Pharmacologic therapy is used to restore the rate and force of contraction, change thresholds, change refractory periods, decrease myocardial demand, prevent reentry, and alter repolarization and depolarization. The goals include:

1. *Prevention of sudden death.* Sudden cardiac death is most often associated with ventricular fibrillation. Prior to fibrillation, the patient usually demonstrates ventricular tachycardia, complete heart block, or sinus node arrest. Correction of the arrhythmia and underlying disease, using pharmacotherapy as well as other interventions, is crucial for the prevention of sudden death.
2. *Correction of life-threatening arrhythmias.* Ventricular standstill, tachycardia, fibrillation, and premature beats may be precursors of sudden death. Acute paroxysmal supraventricular tachycardia in the presence of heart disease requires termination of the attack as well as prevention of future attacks. Aggressive treatment with pharmacotherapy and mechanical interventions is essential.
3. *Prevention of complications.* The elderly, in particular, may experience syncope associated with an arrhythmia, increasing their chance of falling. The falls may result in hip, wrist, and other fractures. These in turn limit functional abilities and decrease quality of life. Arrhythmias with a higher incidence of syncope include AV block, automaticity problems as found with sick sinus syndrome, ventricular and supraventricular tachycardia, and heart disease. Atrial fibrillation and paroxysmal supraventricular tachycardia are highly correlated with thromboembolitic stroke (Hayes & Taler, 1998; Klungel et al., 2001), as well as other embolic problems. Because of the strong association with CVA, converting the rhythm to normal sinus rhythm is essential. Treatment includes anticoagulants and aspirin plus medications to control the ventricular rate.

Nonpharmacologic Therapy

Some arrhythmias respond to nonpharmacologic interventions. Treatment begins with identification of the cause and treatment of any reversible conditions.

- *Atrial premature beats:* May disappear if heart rate is increased.
- *Paroxysmal supraventricular tachycardia:* The Valsalva maneuver, lowering the head below the body, stretching the arms and trunk, coughing, or holding the breath are methods that the patient can use to try to terminate the attack. Carotid sinus pressure over one carotid sinus and then the other is often successful in interrupting an attack. However, this should be performed only by professionals, in patients without a bruit or history of transient ischemic attacks. An ECG or auscultation should be used to monitor the heart rate during the procedure.
- *Symptomatic bradycardia, Moritz II AV block, or complete heart block:* Require a permanent pacemaker.
- *Ventricular arrhythmia:* Automatic implantable cardiac defibrillator (AHCD).

Time Frame for Initiating Pharmacotherapy

Initiation of pharmacotherapy is based on the patient's tolerance of the arrhythmia and whether any correctable cause is identified. Factors that must be considered in evaluating the patient's ability to tolerate the arrhythmia include the heart rate, duration of the arrhythmia, and any underlying cardiac disease and its severity. Arrhythmias that should be treated and are responsive to pharmacotherapy include atrial fibrillation or flutter, paroxysmal supraventricular tachycardia, automatic atrial tachycardias, and ventricular tachycardia.

For specifics regarding drug therapy, refer to Drug Table 202. Overall, the use of antiarrhythmic agents in the United States is declining for three reasons: First is the significant proarrhythmic adverse effect; the second reason is the increased mortality associated with the use of antiarrthmics in certain clinical situations; finally, the increased use of nondrug therapies (e.g., ablation and AICD) have decreased the need for antiarrythmic drugs overall. When choosing a drug, one should always consider the uniqueness of each compound. Some of these agents have unusual pharmacokinetic parameters and many have multiple drug-drug interactions and adverse effects. Most notably, the Class I and Class III antiarrhythmic agents may prolong the QT interval on the ECG, potentially leading to proarrhythmia (e.g., torsades de pointes).

Assessment Needed Prior to Therapy

History and Physical Examination

- *Symptoms:* Inquire about onset and duration of symptoms such as dizziness, syncope, lightheadedness, fatigue, confusion, and falls in the elderly population and palpitations or sensations of skipped beats or a racing heart. Inquire about chest pain, angina, shortness of breath, and dyspnea.
- *Risk factors:* Explore coronary artery disease (CAD), previous myocardial infarction, cardiac surgery, inflammatory heart disease, cardiomyopathies, valvular disease, hypertension, previous CVA, alcohol or drug abuse, and rheumatic heart disease.
- *Medication history:* Review medications, including OTC and herbal, for anticholinergic and sympathomimetic effects. Examples to consider include digoxin, beta blockers, calcium channel blockers, antiarrhythmic medications, tricyclic antidepressants, antipsychotics, cold remedies, and diet aids.
- *Physical examination of the heart:* Always auscultate heart sounds and observe the rate, rhythm, pulse deficit, pattern (such as regularity of irregular heart rate), variations in first heart sound, intensity of heart sounds, response to exercise, and changes in heart sounds with position or respirations. Examine for orthostatic hypotension.

Diagnostic Testing

- *Electrocardiogram:* This is best done when the patient is experiencing a symptom; therefore, ambulatory monitoring is important for diagnosing arrhythmia. If symptoms accompany exercise or stress, an exercise ECG is useful. Frequent syncope may require inpatient monitoring.
- *Electrophysiologic testing:* An intracardiac ECG with programmed atrial and/or ventricular stimulation is good for complex arrhythmias. It is used after the initial ECG and ambulatory ECG prove inconclusive to evaluate the effectiveness of pharmacotherapy in people with life-threatening arrhythmias or accessory pathway arrhythmias, as a differential diagnostic tool for ventricular or supraventricular arrhythmias, and for evaluation of pacing devices.
- *Laboratory:* CBC, chemistry profile, thyroid profile, and digoxin level (if appropriate).

Patient/Caregiver Information

Educate the patient regarding the role of stress, lack of sleep, chocolate, and alcohol in increasing vulnerability of the heart to electrophysiologic induction of atrial flutter and fibrillation. If the patient also is taking digoxin therapy, the heart rate during exercise should be kept below 140–150 beats per minute.

Patients should be aware that the resting heart rate may be elevated during time of illness.

OUTCOMES MANAGEMENT

Selecting an Appropriate Agent and Monitoring for Efficacy and Toxicity

Atrial Fibrillation or Flutter. Pharmacotherapeutic management of symptomatic patients is first directed at restoring and maintaining the sinus rhythm or controlling the ventricular rate, and then to preventing thromboembolism. Heart rate control is a requirement for all patients. Direct-current cardioversion (DCC) is the most commonly used and successful treatment in the restoration of sinus rhythm. Drug therapies to control ventricular rate include digoxin, calcium channel blockers such as verapamil and diltiazem, and beta blockers. Anticoagulants such as warfarin and aspirin are prescribed to reduce the risk of a thromboembolic event. The type I antiarrhythmics (quinidine, procainamide, flecainide) and type III antiarrhythmics (amiodarone, sotalol) are often prescribed in an attempt to sustain sinus rhythm. The Class III antiarrhythmics are the preferred agents. One should always consider concomitant disease states when choosing antiarrhythmics. Flecainide is contraindicated in patients with any type of heart disease (e.g., CAD, CHF).

In managing a patient with atrial fibrillation or flutter (Bauman, Parker, & McCollam, 1995), the practitioner needs to evaluate the onset or duration of the arrhythmia and the severity of symptoms. The treatment algorithms differ for atrial fibrillation onset of less than 48 h or greater than 48 h and then if either acute (<12 months) or chronic (>12 months).

If atrial fibrillation onset is less than 48 hours, therapy is as follows (Goroll & Mulley, 2002):

Step 1: Control ventricular rate, consider antithrombotic therapy, and observe for spontaneous conversion
Step 2: Prompt electrical or pharmacologic conversion
Step 3: Need for antiarrhythmic therapy—yes, if unstable hemodynamics or frequent recurrences; no, if stable hemodynamics, infrequent recurrences, or first episode

The duration of the atrial fibrillation is the best predictor of the success of either electrical or pharmacologic conversion and the probability of maintaining sinus rhythm. Often about 50% of the patients with new-onset atrial fibrillation of short duration will spontaneously convert to sinus rhythm within 24 to 48 h. If atrial fibrillation has been present for longer than 1 year, restoring sinus rhythm is more difficult. Occasionally long-standing atrial fibrillation will spontaneously convert and appears to be a result of left atrial fibrosis.

DCC has a success rate of greater than 80% in restoring sinus rhythm. However, there are adverse effects associated with cardioversion. These include embolic events, hypotension, pulmonary edema, depressed left ventricular contractility, and arrhythmias. Even so, cardioversion is an effective treatment modality.

If atrial fibrillation has been present for longer than 48 h, use the following algorithm (Goroll & Mulley, 2002):

Step 1: Control ventricular rate and start antithrombotic therapy (heparin and/or warfarin or aspirin)
Step 2: Duration of atrial fibrillation <1 year Warfarin therapy for 3–4 weeks or determine by transesophageal echocardiography the presence of intracardiac thrombi—if none present, proceed to cardioversion.
- Cardioversion or pharmacologic conversion
  - Need for antiarrhythmic therapy—yes, unstable hemodynamics or frequent recurrences; no, stable hemodynamics, infrequent recurrences, or first episode
  - Continue warfarin 1–2 months and monitor for recurrences
- Duration of atrial fibrillation >1 year
- Chronic antithrombotic therapy; ensure control of ventricular rate (this approach can also be considered for duration <1 year instead of cardioverting the patient)

Drugs that may be beneficial in pharmacological conversion include disopyramide, procainamide, quinidine, flecainide, propafenone, sotalol, amiodarone, and dofetilide. The choice of one of these agents depends on whether the patient has concomitant heart diseases. If heart disease is not present, agents to consider include flecainide, propafenone, or sotolol. The other agents listed above serve as alternatives. On the other hand, for the patient with heart failure, amiodarone or dofetilide are the only treatment advocated. For patients who have concomitant coronary artery disease, sotalol is preferred, with amiodarone, dofetilide, disopyramide, procainamide, and quinidine listed as alternatives. Finally, if a patient has hypertension, one should choose amiodarone if there is established LVH > 1.4 cm (Fuster, ACC/AHA/ESC Guidelines, 2001).

The type IC agents flecainide and propafanone have been successful in converting atrial fibrillation to sinus rhythm in patients with recent onset. If the arrhythmia is of less than 7 days duration, flecainide 200 mg or propafanone 600 mg as a single dose has shown similar efficacy in conversion to sinus rhythm (Golzari, Cebul, & Bahler, 1996). Flecainide should be avoided in the post–myocardial infarction setting because of increased mortality. Both of these agents via their pharmacodynamics allow more atrial impulses to be conducted through the AV node, which may result in a faster ventricular rate. Propafanone may prove to be of value in treating paroxysmal atrial fibrillation; however, the hematologic adverse effects have limited its widespread use in this setting.

Sotalol has both type II (beta-blocker) and type III (cardiac action potential duration prolongation) properties. The efficacy of this agent has yet to be well established. Current studies suggest conversion to sinus

Amiodarone & Digoxin

rhythm with sotalol is no better than a placebo and less than quinidine (Golzari et al., 1996) in maintaining sinus rhythm in more than 50% of the patients (Prystowsky, Benson, Fuster, et al., 1996).

Amiodarone may have the greatest potential for converting and maintaining sinus rhythm even with its slow onset. Almost two thirds of patients remained in sinus rhythm for up to 1 year while receiving amiodarone (Prystowsky et al., 1996). A low dose of 200 mg of amiodarone per day is often successful in maintaining sinus rhythm while minimizing the adverse effects seen in 75% of the patients when ≥ 400 mg per day is prescribed (Fuster, ACC/AHA/ESC Guidelines, 2001). Because amiodarone has a long half-life, loading doses (e.g., 400 mg tid) are typically necessary to achieve conversion or maintain normal sinus rhythm. Amiodarone's place in treatment may be in symptomatic patients with drug-refractory, recurrent atrial fibrillation. Also, amiodarone appears to have the lowest proarrhythmic effect of all the above-mentioned agents.

Even with the use of antiarrhythmics, reversion to atrial fibrillation within 1 year occurs in almost half of the patients. This reflects the limited efficacy of these drugs and the high incidence of treatment cessation caused by adverse effects.

Concomitant ventricular rate control therapy can be accomplished with the use of digoxin, a calcium channel blocker (verapamil, diltiazem), or a beta blocker. In patients with severe symptoms these medications may be administered intravenously, whereas in the less symptomatic patients they may be given orally to control the ventricular rate.

By enhancing vagus nerve activity on the heart, digoxin decreases conduction through the AV node with a slowing of the ventricular response. The adequacy of the dose can be judged by a ventricular rate goal of 70–90 beats per minute. Remember that digoxin does not convert patients out of atrial fibrillation and cannot adequately control ventricular response during exercise. Digoxin, either alone or in combination with other agents, works best in the management of atrial fibrillation in patients who are minimally symptomatic (mild palpitations) and/or who have heart failure related to impaired systolic ventricular function. In the latter, beta blockers and calcium channel blockers are undesirable because of their negative inotropic effects.

Daily maintenance doses of digoxin range from 0.125 to 0.375 mg. Patients with impaired renal function will need their dosage adjusted accordingly. Measurement of serum levels will help in determining patient compliance and to rule out digoxin toxicity. However, the patient should be evaluated for symptoms of digoxin toxicity such as nausea, vomiting, weakness, and visual disturbances since there is not always a correlation between serum level and toxicity. A therapeutic serum level of digoxin is 0.8 to 2.0 μg/mL. Blood sampling should occur at steady state (7 to 14 days depending on renal function) and at least 6 h after an oral dose or just before the next scheduled dose. The practitioner should also monitor potassium and magnesium serum levels and maintain electrolytes within normal levels to reduce the incidence of digoxin toxicity.

To assist digoxin in the control of the acute and long-term ventricular rate, especially during exercise-related increases, metoprolol, verapamil, or others of these drug categories may be added. Metoprolol, a beta blocker, is a type II antiarrhythmic that decreases conduction through the AV node, prolonging the PR interval. It also has a direct slowing effect on the sinus rate. The calcium channel blocker verapamil is a type III antiarrhythmic that slows calcium flux across the slow channels of vascular smooth muscle and cardiac cells. Verapamil depresses the AV node and has a negative chronotropic effect on the SA node. Diltiazem, also a calcium channel blocker, has a similar effect but to a lesser degree. None of the calcium channel blockers will convert patients to a sinus rhythm. A benefit of verapamil and diltiazem is that their effect on rate control is not diminished during exercise or stress. A limitation to the use of beta blockers or calcium channel blockers is coexisting heart failure. Calcium channel blockers may inhibit the nonrenal clearance of digoxin.

Although evidence for long-term antiarrhythmics is unclear, recent studies reveal the value of antithrombotic therapy in patients with atrial fibrillation to prevent stroke either prior to cardioversion or with chronic atrial fibrillation (Akhtar, Reeve, & Movahed, 1998; Jacobson, Makowski, & Heywood, 2000). The patient most likely to benefit is one who is over 60 years of age; has valvular, ischemic, or hypertensive heart disease; has respiratory or systemic disease; and has no contraindications to warfarin therapy. In patients with no identified risk factors, atrial fibrillation alone, or who are noncompliant, the use of 325 mg of aspirin per day should be considered (Huffman, 1999). Dosing warfarin to achieve international normalizing ratio (INR) values of 2.0 to 3.0 is recommended (see Table 20–5).

In the past, loading doses of warfarin have been advocated to achieve adequate coagulation levels faster. Warfarin, however, has unique pharmacokinetic parameters (e.g., half-life of 36 hours), and inhibition of the co-

TABLE 20–5. Anticoagulation Recommendations for Patients with Atrial Fibrillation

Age	Risk Factors[a] Present	
<65	None	ASA 325 mg/day or no therapy
<65	Yes	Warfarin INR 2–3 or ASA 325 mg/day in patients with significant bleeding risk factors
65–75	None	Warfarin INR 2–3 or ASA 325 mg/day in patients with significant bleeding risk factors
65–75	Yes	
>75		

[a]Risk factors are hypertension, previous stroke or TIA, heart failure, diabetes mellitus, coronary artery disease, mitral valve disease, prosthetic heart valve, and thyrotoxicosis.

agulation cascade with warfarin takes days, irrespective of the patient's initial INR. Hence, the most prudent method of dosing is initiating a dose that is reasonable for long-term anticoagulation (e.g., 3 to 5 mg q day) and monitoring the INR for adjustment. This is especially important given the increased use of amiodarone. Amiodarone increases the activity of warfarin by twofold, and this interaction is delayed, making it difficult to identify onset. If hospital discharge is the rationale for warfarin loading (because a therapeutic INR is desired before discharge), the practitioner can initiate anticoagulation therapy with low molecular weight heparin while waiting for a therapeutic warfarin level.

Chronic atrial fibrillation or flutter greater than 12 months is managed by blocking the AV node as in acute scenarios. However, DCC is not attempted unless the patient has severe symptoms. In both situations, long-term anticoagulation is warranted.

Paroxysmal Supraventricular Tachycardia. The treatment of PSVT is governed by the severity of symptoms and/or width of the ARS complex and possible arrhythmias. In patients with severe symptoms, DCC is the primary treatment. If the patient is experiencing mild symptoms, pharmacotherapy is directed by the width of the QRS complex. When the QRS complex is narrow and regular, suggesting AV node reentrant tachycardia, the treatments consist of verapamil, diltiazem, or adenosine. Adenosine has emerged as the drug of choice, given its safety profile and short half-life. If the QRS complex is wide and regular, suggesting VT, the treatment is adenosine or procainamide. Finally, if the QRS complex is wide and irregular, suggesting AF with an accessory pathway, procainamide is the treatment of choice (Akhtar et al., 1998; Jacobson et al., 2000).

If PSVT is frequent or if there are symptoms of decreased cardiac output and perfusion, such as shortness of breath, lightheadedness, or chest pressure, electrophysiologic studies such as radiofrequency ablation are called for. This treatment removes the pathway of reentry and therefore stops the PSVT. Drug therapy is rarely used for long-term management of this condition if the patient is a candidate for ablation. If ablation is not an option, trials of agents such as verapamil, dioxin, aquinidine, procainamide, beta blockers, flecainide, propafanone, or amiodarone may be undertaken.

Ventricular Arrhythmias. Because of the life-threatening nature of many of the ventricular arrhythmias, a cardiology consultation or referral is recommended. Therapy is probably best initiated by the cardiologist with maintenance and followup care, in many instances, by the primary care provider.

Ventricular Premature Beats. In patients without appreciable heart disease, pharmacotherapy may be warranted if the palpitations significantly interfere with the patient's life. If this is the situation, metoprolol, a beta blocker, has been successful.

In patients with heart disease, the decision to use pharmacotherapy is not as apparent. The results of the cardiac arrhythmia suppression trial (CAST) studies indicate that while ectopy was suppressed, the risk of death was increased (Echt, Liebson, Mitchell, et al., 1991). Currently, patients who are post–myocardial infarction with complex ventricular ectopy remain at risk for death, and therapies besides beta blockers designed to reduce this risk need further evaluation. Low-dose amiodarone, after sufficient loading doses, has emerged as the standard long-term antiarrhythmic in this situation.

Ventricular Tachycardia. VT is often precipitated by electrolyte disturbances, ischemia, organic heart disease, or drug toxicity. As such, initial management should be directed toward detection and correction of the condition.

In acute episodes of VT in which the patient is severely symptomatic, DCC should be performed. Again, the possibility of an underlying cause such as myocardial infarction should be investigated.

Intravenous amiodarone (with hospitalization) may be necessary in patients with transient VT as seen in acute myocardial ischemia. Once the underlying cause is identified and treated, further antiarrhythmic therapy is unlikely.

Advanced cardiac life support (ACLS) guidelines should be used in the management of a patient with asymptomatic or mild symptoms associated with an acute episode of VT (AHA/Emergency Cardiac Care Committee, 2000). See Table 20–6.

TABLE 20–6. Recommendations for the Use of Antiarrythmics

Antiarrythmic	Classification	Comments
Amiodarone	IIB	ARREST study showed significant increase in live admissions as compared to placebo; for VF/pulseless VT. In stable monomorphic and polymorphic ventricular tachycardia.
Lidocaine	Indeterminate	Lack of studies in humans demonstrating its effectiveness for shock-resistant ventricular fibrillation. Previous studies revealed no significant increase in survival.
Magnesium	IIB	Only indicated when a patient has hypomagnesemia or the patient has torsades de pointes and hypomagnesemia. Routine use in patients post MI is no longer recommended.
Procainamide	IIB	Indicated for intermittent or recurrent ventricular fibrillation or ventricular tachycardia; however, requires long infusion time and there is a lack of clinical studies or reliable retrospective studies to support use during cardiac arrest.

Source: AHA/ECC: ACLS Guidelines 2000 ACLS Guidelines (2000).

Management of chronic, recurrent sustained VT is important since these patients are at risk for sudden death and should be directed by an experienced practitioner or cardiologist. An electrophysiologic study performed in the hospital can assist in the selection of effective pharmacotherapy and the possible role of automatic implantable cardiac defibrillator (AICD) therapy in patients not responsive to drug therapy (Mohammed, Lauer, Homoud, Wang, & Estes, 2002).

Various antiarrhythmics can be used for the treatment of ventricular tachycardia, although their role has been minimized with the advancement of nondrug therapies such as AICD.

The treatment of sustained ventricular arrhythmias is best handled by an experienced practitioner or cardiologist. Electrophysiologic studies, surgical excision of the focus, and implantable automatic cardioverter defibrillators may be necessary in patients who are unable to tolerate drug therapy or who are resistant to pharmacologic management.

Followup Recommendations

Followup is based on the problem, etiology, symptoms, possible complications, and medications. Unfortunately, because there are many types of arrhythmias that may or may not be associated with symptoms and may or may not be life-threatening, prescribed times for followup vary.

However, when initiating pharmacotherapy, the pharmacodynamics of the medication may help identify the frequency of visits. During the initial treatment phase, visits every day may be appropriate to observe for adverse reactions. Keep the following suggestions in mind for the followup:

1. *History and physical examination:* Always auscultate heart sounds, and check vital signs, including orthostatic hypotension. Inquire about nausea and other GI disturbances, symptoms of CNS disturbance, palpitations, and shortness of breath or wheezing.
2. *ECG:* Observe for new arrhythmias, heart block, and left ventricular function.
3. *Laboratory:* Appropriate tests are determined by the common side effects of the medications prescribed. Included are thyroid function, electrolytes, renal function, liver function, and CBC.
4. If the patient is placed on an anticoagulant for atrial fibrillation, obtain a prothrombin time reported as an INR to eliminate laboratory variation.

PERIPHERAL ARTERIAL DISEASE

Peripheral arterial disease (PAD) is commonly seen in patients with systemic atherosclerosis. The most frequent symptom of PAD is intermittent claudication, which is due to the poor oxygenation of the muscles of the lower extremities. Typical symptoms the patient may exhibit are an aching pain; cramping; or numbness in the calf, buttock, hip, or arch of the foot. These symptoms are exacerbated by walking or exercise and are relieved by rest. Progression of PAD can result in limb ischemia, causing gangrene, requiring amputation in 3 to 8% of patients (see Table 20–7).

SPECIFIC CONSIDERATIONS FOR PHARMACOTHERAPY

When Drug Therapy Is Needed

Many arterial aneurysms and occlusive diseases require surgical intervention. Conditions such as aneurysm, aortic dissection, occlusion of major arteries, and other acute manifestations of arterial disease may either be treated with or without medications until surgical intervention. In most cases, medication in combination with nonpharmacologic therapy is needed to promote the optimal level of function and quality of life.

TABLE 20–7. Peripheral Vascular Disease

	Process	Signs/Symptoms
Occlusive Disease		
Aorta/iliac arteries	Aorta: starts distal to bifurcation. Iliac: starts proximal to bifurcation. Atherosclerosis that eventually occludes one or both iliac arteries and aorta just below renal arteries.	Intermittent claudication in calf muscles, thighs, and buttocks. Pain is usually bilateral. Leg weakness, especially when walking. Impotence in men common. Pulses: femoral pulses absent or weak. Distal pulses often absent. Bruit: possibly aorta or over iliac or femoral arteries. Skin: atrophic changes. Color and temperature changes not necessarily apparent unless distal arteries involved.
Femoral/popliteal arteries	Occlusion of superficial arteries in area of knee and thigh. Atherosclerosis starts in distal part of superficial femoral artery and may extend to popliteal artery. The superficial femoral artery slowly becomes completely occluded.	Intermittent claudication in calf and foot. Atrophic changes of lower leg: hair loss, thin skin, loss of subcutaneous tissue and muscle mass. Dependent rubor, blanching of skin with elevation of extremity, foot cool to touch. Pulses: absence of popliteal and pedal.
Lower leg/foot	Atherosclerotic changes in tibial and common peroneal arteries; pedal arteries most common.	Development of collateral circulation may create a stable or slowly progressive disease process. Symptoms may be minimal to severe. Intermittent claudication. Aching and fatigue during exercise or exertion, usually first in calf muscles. With progression of disease, pain may be constant or walking a minimal distance will cause cramping. May have pain at rest, especially at night. Pulses: pedal absent. Skin: dependent rubor, cool to touch, hairless, atrophic.
Thromboangiitis obliterans (Buerger's disease)	Affects both arteries and veins. Inflammatory as well as thrombic processes involved. The inflammatory process is intermittent with characteristic exacerbations and remissions. Process occurs in segments with exacerbations producing occlusions in new areas. Thrombic process occurs in distal arteries, usually in lower extremities in the foot and lower leg, but also in fingers.	Most common in men <40 who smoke. History of frequent episodes of superficial thrombophlebitis in different areas of extremity with resulting small tender bands along superficial veins. Intermittent claudication, rest pain, numbness, tingling, burning, or other changes in sensation. Affected part: cold and pale or rubor that may be pronounced with dependent position and may not change color when elevated; asymmetric changes in toes; possible ulcerations around nail beds. Pulses: dorsalis pedis, posterior tibial, ulnar, or radial may be diminished or absent.
Raynaud's disease	Digital arteries involved. Etiology unknown: probably due to sympathetic nervous system abnormality. Arteries sensitive to vasospastic stimuli causing paroxysmal digital cyanosis. Progressive. Raynaud's phenomenon: same process but associated with disorders such as rheumatoid arthritis, systemic lupus erythematosis, and other connective tissue disease, and in conjunction with thromboangiitis obliterans and thoracic outlet syndrome.	Most common in women ages 15–45. Attacks are paroxysmal, bilateral, and usually precipitated by cold. They typically start with pallor or cyanosis of one or two fingertips followed by rubor and sometimes pain, throbbing, sensory changes, and edema. Warming creates termination of attack. Raynaud's phenomenon: unilateral, nonprogressive.
Venous Disease		
Varicose veins	Superficial veins, usually of lower extremities, become dilated, elongated, and tortuous. Etiology: may be inherited, fundamental weakness in walls, or valvular incompetence.	May be asymptomatic. Usual: dull, aching, heavy feeling or easy fatigue from standing. Vessels dilated, tortuous, visible beneath skin in leg and thigh. Skin: may have brown discoloration and thinning above ankle.
Thrombophlebitis (general)	Occlusion of vein, either partial or complete, accompanied by inflammation. Results in platelet aggregation on the vein wall followed by thrombus formation. Trauma to wall of vein most frequent cause. From beginning of process to inflammatory changes is 7–10 days. Fibroblasts attack the thrombus, causing scarring of the vessel and valvular destruction.	
Thrombophlebitis (specific) deep vein	Usually starts in calf but may be in pelvis. Process extends up popliteal and femoral veins. Etiology: post surgical, oral contraceptives especially in women who smoke and are over 30, hypercoagulability as seen in some cancers.	May be asymptomatic until embolus occurs. Frequently complain of aching, tightness or pain in calf. Most noticeable when walking. Signs not always present: swelling of calf, fever, tachycardia, positive Homan's sign (leg pain with dorsiflexion of foot).
Superficial	Most common site in saphenous vein of legs, but may be in any superficial vein. Unknown etiology or post trauma; early sign of cancer of the pancreas, associated with other cancers.	Tenderness, erythema and edema along vein, warm to touch, fever. Changes linear rather than circular.
Chronic insufficiency	Result of inadequate venous return over a period of time. Blood pools in lower legs; circulation sluggish to the point that waste products not removed. Etiology: usually due to deep vein thrombophlebitis and the resulting destruction of walls and valves of vessels. Also may be due to trauma, neoplastic obstruction in pelvic veins or varicose veins.	Skin: hyperpigmentation of lower legs especially the skin over the feet and ankles, shiny, thin. Edema of the leg. Itching, discomfort in legs when standing. Stasis dermatitis and recurrent ulcer formation com mon.

Short- and Long-Term Goals of Pharmacotherapy

When treating the peripheral vascular disorders of occlusive (PVD) or Raynaud's phenomenon, the goal is symptom relief. Pharmacotherapy is directed at relief of the symptoms of intermittent claudication and nocturnal leg cramps. Ideally, the long-term goals of therapy are to slow the progression of the disease, which should improve blood flow and relieve pain. With improved blood flow, ulcerations and progression to gangrene may be prevented. If the symptom of severe pain persists, then a pain care plan should be initiated.

Nonpharmacological Therapy

In management of PAD, any lifestyle change that reduces the risk factors for PAD is beneficial. To this end smoking cessation, weight loss, lowering of lipid levels, and exercise are essential.

Smoking is the most significant risk factor for developing PAD. Patients with intermittent claudication who smoke have 3 times the risk of needing an amputation or death, compared to those patients who do not smoke. The 5-year mortality rate for patients with intermittent claudication who continue to smoke is 40 to 50%.

Walking daily promotes the development of collateral circulation and improves function. Patients should have an exercise/walking routine set for them. If the patient experiences intermittent claudication, instruct him or her to stop for about 3 minutes, then resume exercise/walking for the remainder of the allotted time.

Protection of the involved extremity(ies) prevents accidental injury that could result in major complications. With circulation compromised, normal healing processes are slow to nonexistent. Generally, the involved extremity should be kept warm and not exposed to either cold or hot temperatures. Keep the extremity clean and moisturized but not moist.

Varicose veins are usually managed with nonpharmacologic treatment or surgery. Varicose veins with minimal symptomatology are frequently managed with elastic stockings if the patient does not want surgery. The medium or heavy stockings give support to the veins of the lower leg and should be worn during times when the patient is standing. However, the patient should avoid standing for long periods of time or wearing constrictive clothing. When the stockings are not worn, elevation of the legs is recommended. Using stockings and elevation of the extremities, in addition to managing symptoms, may also prevent progress of the condition.

Specific conditions requiring a cardiology or surgical consult include: aortic abdominal aneurysm, popliteal and femoral aneurysm, aortic dissection, occlusive disease, arterial thrombus or embolism, varicose veins (depending on the extent of the condition), and thromboangiitis obliterans.

Time Frame for Initiating Pharmacotherapy

Pharmacotherapy should be initiated simultaneously with exercise and lifestyle modifications in patients who remain symptomatic.

Assessment Needed Prior to Therapy

History and Physical Examination

- *Medical:* Check chronic conditions associated with atherosclerosis, neoplasms, previous surgical procedures, diabetes, liver, kidney disease, and trauma.
- *Social:* Assess occupational history, smoking habits, and alcohol use.
- *Symptoms:* Check pain location, quality, duration, aggravating factors, relief measures (what and effectiveness), and frequency (including pain at rest); presence of intermittent claudication; ability to walk before symptoms: two blocks (mild arterial occlusion); less than one block (moderate to severe occlusion); and discomfort when standing. Skin symptoms include changes in skin color, temperature, texture, and hair and presence of numbness, tingling, and burning sensations. Check heart sounds, murmurs, arrhythmias, vital signs, bruits, and BP both arms (observe difference). Check pulses, temperature and color of extremities, atrophic changes, ulcerations, and dermatitis. Color changes with dependent positioning. In the abdomen check bruits, pain, and organomegaly.
- *Diagnostic studies:*
  - *Electrocardiogram:* for aortic aneurysm or aortic dissection.
  - *Ultrasound:* for abdominal aneurysm or peripheral artery aneurysm.
  - *Arteriogram:* for thromboangiitis obliterans.
  - *Aortography:* for occluded aorta or iliac arteries.
  - *Ankle-Brachial Index:* An ankle-brachial index is performed to quantify the degree of limb ischemia. The ankle-brachial index is the ratio of the ankle systolic pressure to the brachial artery systolic pressure. An ankle-brachial index greater than 0.90 is considered normal; 0.70–0.89 mild disease; 0.50–0.69 moderate disease; and less than 0.50 severe disease.

In order to measure the ankle-brachial index, the practitioner first takes two standard blood pressure readings in both arms. Then, using a standard blood pressure cuff and Doppler ultrasound, take two blood pressure readings in both legs using the dorsalis pedis or posterior tibial arteries. To calculate the index, divide the highest systolic ankle pressure by the highest systolic brachial pressure for each limb.

- Doppler ultrasound: for deep vein thrombosis.
- *Laboratory:* CBC and chemical profile will assist in differential diagnosis of hypercoagulation, pancreatic disease, liver disorders, and infectious processes.

Patient/Caregiver Information

Patients should be advised to stop smoking and keep walking. Graduated pressure elastic stockings should be worn when standing, and legs should be elevated whenever possible. Constrictive clothing around the legs, such as tight socks, stockings, or garters, should be avoided. Although elastic stockings are the nonpharmacologic treatment of choice, they are made of thick, heavy material and are difficult to get on. Therefore, patients often do not wear the stockings as regularly as necessary for full benefit. Teaching the importance of pressure to prevent symptoms and additional problems plus techniques to assist in dressing may promote compliance with treatment strategies.

OUTCOMES MANAGEMENT

Selecting an Appropriate Agent

Treatment begins by minimizing risk factors and controlling coexisting conditions such as diabetes, hypertension, and smoking. Managing hyperlipoproteinemia can slow the progression of the disease (see the section on treatment of hyperlipidemias for additional information).

Monitoring for Efficacy and Toxicity

Intermittent Claudication

Pentoxifylline. Pentoxifylline has several mechanisms that have proven beneficial in the treatment of intermittent claudication (IC) and is approved by the FDA. Overall, pentoxifylline reduces blood viscosity and improves blood flow. This is accomplished by increasing red blood cell deformability, while decreasing platelet adhesiveness and blood fibrinogen. Pentoxifylline may be more effective when used early in the disease state when the patient presents with moderately severe ischemia without rest pain, ischemic ulcers, or severe claudication.

Treatment with pentoxifylline (Trental) in early small trials has shown improvement in maximum walking distance of patients with intermittent claudication, though more recent and larger trials have shown pentoxifylline to be only minimally effective in improving intermittent claudication.

Antiplatelet Agents. Cilostazol (Pletal), a phosphodiesterase III inhibitor, was approved by the FDA in 1999 for the treatment of intermittent claudication. Cilostazol has antiplatelet properties as well as improving vasodilation, increasing plasma HDL-cholesterol levels, and decreasing plasma triglyceride levels. Cilostazol is contraindicated in patients with NY Class III or IV heart failure.

Aspirin alone has no effect on intermittent claudication symptoms but in combination with dipyridamole, it may decrease the progression of peripheral vascular disease.

Ticlopindine (Ticlid) blocks the activation of platelets by adenosine diphosphate (ADP). Studies have shown that ticlopindine treatment has decreased the number of strokes and myocardial infarctions in patients with intermittent claudication, though ticlopindine is not FDA approved for the treatment of intermittent claudication.

Clopidogrel (Plavix), a new thienopyridine derivate whose actions are similar to that of ticlopindine, is indicated for the secondary prevention of ischemic events in patients who have had a recent myocardial infarction, stroke, or symptomatic PAD. The CAPRIE study demonstrated that when clopidogrel was compared to aspirin those patients on clopidogrel had a 23.8% risk reduction of stroke, myocardial infraction, or other vascular death in the PAD group. Clopidogrel is not indicated for the treatment of intermittent claudication (Scheinfeld, 2001).

Beta Blockers. Beta blockers are often prescribed for patients with coronary artery disease and hypertension. Concern surrounds the use of these agents if the patient also has concomitant PVD. Studies are equivocal, showing no difference, a worsening of symptoms, and an improvement in symptoms (Wallingford, 2000). In theory, beta blockers inhibit $beta_2$-induced vasodilation during exercise. This, coupled with reduced systemic blood flow through stenotic arteries or collateral vessels, suggests these agents would be detrimental. At this time beta blockers should be used cautiously in patients with intermittent claudication. Begin with low doses and titrate slowly while monitoring for increased PVD symptoms.

Investigational Agents. Several antiplatelet drugs are currently being evaluated for their use in PVD. These include prostaglandin E_1 and I_2, which are potent vasodilators and inhibitors of platelet aggregation (Wallingford, 2000).

Presently these agents are only available as intravenous infusions. Other agents in clinical evaluation, or not available in the United States, include naftidrofuryl, levcarnitine, and propionyl levocarnitine (Haitt, 2001).

Defibrotide, a calcium channel blocker, has been shown to improve symptoms and treadmill exercise time in approximately half the patients. It has been demonstrated that defibrotide increases tissue plasminogen activator production and release, PGI_2 formation, and inhibition of platelet activation (Schlant, Applegate, Boden, & Piephro, 2002). L-carnitine, an amino acid which improves muscle metabolism, improved walking distance in studies that supplied 2 g twice a day for 3 weeks (Haitt, 2001).

ACE inhibitors may be an alternative in patients with hypertension and IC. These agents may preserve collateral blood flow.

Raynaud's Phenomenon

Calcium Channel Blockers. Nifedipine is the drug of choice for patients with Raynaud's disease who continue to experience symptoms after nonpharmacologic management is implemented. The peripheral vasodilating effects of this calcium channel blocker may be able to prevent the vascular response caused by cold exposure and $alpha_2$-receptor-mediated activity. Other calcium channel blockers have variable benefits. Doses of 30 to 120 mg three times a day of diltiazem showed benefit but not to the extent of nifedipine. Diltiazem may be preferred in patients who do not tolerate the side effects of nifedipine. Verapamil, with fewer peripheral vasodilating properties, showed no subjective or objective benefit. The remainder of the calcium channel blockers (nicardipine, isradipine, felodipine, and amlodipine) have reportedly shown some benefit in patients but not conclusively (Haitt, 2001).

$Alpha_1$-Adrenergic Antagonists. Prazosin at doses of 1 mg three times a day has shown moderate benefit in a majority of patients. Compliance may be an issue since this agent has significant side effects, especially if the dose is increased. Older agents, such as reserpine, guanethidine, methyldopa, phentolamine, and phenoxybenzamine should be avoided because of significant side effects. Dosage recommendations continue to be made in the literature for reserpine 0.125 to 1.0 mg/day, guanethidine 10 to 50 mg/day, and phenoxybenzamide 10 mg qid. Research continues on a superior agent, but to date none have exceeded nifedipine's action. When applied to the hands, nitroglycerin ointment resulted in fewer and less severe attacks (Coffman, 1991; Roath, 1989); however, the side effects may decrease usefulness. Other medications that have or are being evaluated include niacin, serotonin receptor antagonists, ACE inhibitors, and thymoxamine, an $alpha_1$ antagonist.

Nocturnal Leg Muscle Cramps. With the FDA's removal of quinine from over-the-counter distribution and the deletion of leg cramps as an indication for use, the mainstay of treatment is nonpharmacologic. However, if the practitioner believes the benefit of quinine therapy exceeds the risks, careful monitoring of the patient is necessary. In addition, the dose should not exceed the prescribed amount of 200 to 300 mg taken at bedtime with an additional dose taken earlier in the evening if necessary. The patient may find it helpful to keep a diary of the number and extent of leg cramps during therapy.

Followup Recommendations

Appropriate followup of patients is dependent on severity of condition and treatment regimen.

- For arterial disease, followup should include investigation of new symptoms and monitoring of blood pressure, pulses, and bruits. Providers must be alert to symptoms of any atherosclerotic or arteriosclerotic conditions.
- For venous disease, always check pulses, color, temperature, and atrophic changes in the skin. Observe and treat stasis ulcers.
- Monitor PTT if the patient is on anticoagulant therapy.
- Question the patient about exercise and smoking and alcohol use.
- Continue education about dietary modifications and protection of the involved part.
- Question the patient about new medications, including over-the-counter medications and birth control pills.

CORONARY HEART DISEASE

Coronary heart disease includes coronary artery disease (CAD) and ischemic heart disease. The underlying problem is the deprivation of oxygen to the heart muscle caused by atherosclerosis of the coronary arteries. As the coronary arteries become occluded, the decreased blood supply injures cells with ischemia as a result. Angina pectoris is the result of myocardial ischemia.

CORONARY ARTERY DISEASE

The development of ischemic heart disease begins with CAD. A major factor in the development of CAD is atherosclerosis. It is likely that atherosclerosis is associated with hyperlipidemia and the accumulation of LDL cholesterol.

Atherosclerosis

Atherosclerosis, a form of arteriosclerosis, is a chronic abnormal thickening and hardening of the arteries. This condition is due to deposits of fat in the form of cholesterol and fibrin in the arterial wall.

Although the exact mechanism is unknown, changes occur within the arterial wall. The vascular smooth muscle cells move close to the basement membrane. It is thought the cells secrete enzymes that attack the basement membrane, allowing the formation of atherosclerotic lesions. Atherosclerotic lesions are classified as a fatty streak, fibrous plaque, or complicated lesion. A fatty streak lesion is a smooth muscle cell filled with lipid material and appears flat and yellow. Fatty streaks are found in the aorta of children less than 1 year of age. The lesion does not cause narrowing or obstruction, may be reversible, and appears regardless of gender, race, or environment. Fatty streak lesions may give rise to fibrous plaque lesions.

Fibrous plaque lesions indicate advancing atherosclerotic processes. The lesion is a smooth muscle cell that is full of lipid material and encircled with a matrix of collagen, elastic fibers, and mucoprotein. The white, elevated lesion begins the occlusive process by invading the walls of the artery and then protruding into the artery lumen. The fibrous plaque is most often found where arteries bifurcate or curve or in areas of narrowing.

Complicated lesions are calcified fibrous plaques. As the lesions grow and become hard, there is ulceration or disintegration of the lining of the artery. The complicated, advanced lesions are the most frequent cause of occlusion of the artery.

Collateral circulation develops in response to the decreasing blood supply. Because the atherosclerotic process is slow, new arteries may form around the area of potential occlusion, thereby minimizing the symptoms experienced. However, the collateral vessels also develop atherosclerotic plaques and in turn become occluded. Symptoms may not appear for 40 to 50 years after the beginning of the disease process.

Neither arteriosclerosis nor atherosclerosis is isolated in a single vessel nor unique to a single disease. The major arteries are most frequently affected. The manifestations of atherosclerosis are dependent on the extent of the pathologic process, the number of vessels involved, location of the involved vessels, age, genetic predisposition, physiologic status, and other risk factors. Symptoms are not noted by the individual until about 60% of the vessel is occluded. In addition to the narrowing and occlusion, arteries may lose structural components of the vessel wall, leading to aneurysms.

Additional Risk Factors

In addition to atherosclerosis and hyperlipidemia, the development of CAD is associated with:

- *Hypertension:* Continuous pressure on the walls of the arteries causes damage to the walls and either precipitates or exacerbates the process of atherosclerosis.
- *Cigarette smoking:* The mechanism is unknown, but the release of epinephrine and norepinephrine caused by nicotine increases BP by an increase in heart rate and peripheral vascular resistance. The catecholamines may also release fatty acids, resulting in higher LDL cholesterol. Other possible mechanisms include an increase in adhesiveness of the platelets, causing increased clot formation in the arteries, or hypoxemia, which may result in atherosclerosis caused by increased permeability of the arterial walls.
- *Diabetes mellitus:* This condition is associated with hyperlipidemia, hypertension, and obesity.
- *Genetic factors:* CAD is more likely to occur if there is a familial history of a myocardial event, especially before the age of 50. This genetic predisposition is usually associated with hyperlipidemia and occurs more often in men than women.
- *Hypoestrogenemia:* Women with low estrogen levels are more at risk for the development of CAD than women with normal estrogen levels. However, oral contraceptives (OCs) are associated with increased triglyceride and total cholesterol levels, increased platelet aggregability, and altered prothrombin and clotting factors, leading to possible MI in premenopausal women. Although OCs were once thought contraindicated for women 35 to 50, they have been found safe for nonsmoking women. Present data do not indicate an increased risk of CAD and years taking OCs. The relationship between estrogen and CAD continues to be investigated.
- *Lifestyle/personality:* A sedentary lifestyle and Type A personality have been associated with a high incidence of coronary heart disease; however, research has not verified this relationship.

Myocardial Ischemia

Myocardial ischemia begins with inadequate blood flow to supply the needs of the myo-cardium. The first signs occur when the demand for oxygen increases, such as during exercise, increased systolic blood pressure, stress, hyperthyroidism, and anemia. An ischemic attack occurs when a major artery is narrowed by 50%.

If the attack lasts up to 20 minutes, the cells lose their ability to contract and therefore decrease the function of the myocardium. Deprived of oxygen, the cells are unable to use glucose through aerobic metabolism and turn to anaerobic metabolism. The result is an accumulation of lactic acid.

Clinically, the individual will have symptoms of chest pain (angina pectoris), arrhythmias, and electrical abnormalities on an ECG.

Angina pectoris is the most common presenting symptom of myocardial ischemia. The patient presents with precordial chest pain that is transient and frequently associated with exertion or stress. See Table 20–8 for a listing of the types of angina.

Angina has been classified by the Canadian Cardiovascular Society according to severity during activity, which may be helpful for the provider and patient in assessment of the problem (see Table 20–9).

SPECIFIC CONSIDERATIONS FOR PHARMACOTHERAPY

When Drug Therapy Is Needed

Pharmacotherapy is directed at reducing myocardial oxygen consumption, improving coronary artery blood flow, slowing the progression of the disease process, and preventing morbidity and mortality associated with CHD. The initiation of drug therapy should be considered in any patient who experiences symptoms. Drug therapy should be used in conjunction with lifestyle modifications. In addition, early recognition and treatment of hyperlipidemia, hypertension, and diabetes mellitus is important.

TABLE 20–8. Types of Angina Pectoris

Type of Angina	Description
Stable angina	Exertional, classic angina. Discomfort is predictable, precipitating factors known, and the pattern of discomfort the same for each episode. Usually brought on by exertion and relieved with rest.
Unstable angina	Between stable angina and a myocardial infarction. It is also known as preinfarction angina and acute coronary insufficiency. Onset and characteristics of pain differ for each episode. There is an increasing frequency, duration, and severity of attacks. May occur at rest.
Prinzmetal angina	Variant angina. Discomfort occurs at rest and is unpredictable. It is associated with vasospasms of coronary arteries. When pain occurs during sleep, it is associated with REM sleep. It may have a transient ST elevation.
Syndrome X	Typical presentation of angina but no evidence of coronary artery disease or spasm. Myocardial ischemia due to disease of coronary microcirculation.

Adapted from Abrams (1991) and Massie (1996).

TABLE 20–9. Canadian Cardiovascular Society Classification System

- Class I: No limits to normal activity, but angina occurs with prolonged exertion
- Class II: Slight limitation on normal activity; angina with walking >2 blocks
- Class III: Marked limitation in normal activity; angina with walking <2 blocks
- Class IV: Severe limitation in normal activity; angina with little activity or at rest

Short- and Long-Term Goals of Pharmacotherapy

The long-term goal is to ensure that the supply of oxygen and nutrients to the myocardium equals the demand. Therefore, the immediate goal of pharmacotherapy is the prevention of angina and restoration of cardiovascular function. Long-term drug therapy is directed at reducing the risk of further cardiovascular or cerebral incidents.

Nonpharmacologic Therapy

Prevention through diet, exercise, and smoking cessation, as discussed in the sections on hypertension and hyperlipidemia, is applicable to the treatment of CHD. Early detection and treatment of diabetes and hypertension will help decrease the progress of atherosclerosis and the development of CAD.

Time Frame for Initiating Pharmacotherapy

The initiation of pharmacotherapy should be individualized and based on the history and physical examination, as well as any presenting signs and symptoms of angina (see the assessment section for differential diagnosis). If the patient is experiencing angina, determination of the type and classification will direct the course of action:

1. If the patient meets the definition of unstable angina, hospitalization or a cardiology consult is required.
2. In the patient with chronic stable, severe angina pectoris, the presenting circumstances will direct whether the patient can be treated in the outpatient setting or require hospitalization. If the patient is experiencing more than five episodes of chest pain daily with minimal exertion, hospital evaluation is recommended.

3. In the patient with chronic stable, mild angina pectoris, an outpatient evaluation and initiation of pharmacotherapy when indicated is recommended.

   See Drug Tables 205.5, 205.6, 205.7, 206.

Assessment Needed Prior to Therapy

History. The practitioner should cover the following items with the patient (Arnstein, Buselli, & Rankin, 1996; Brown & Kloner, 1990; Massie, 1996; O'Keefe, 1995):

- *What precipitates discomfort:* Cover activities that bring on discomfort such as walking up stairs or hills, or other forms of exercise or exertion; past infectious disease with fever; and stress, anxiety, meals, cold air, or smoking. Ask the patient the number of times a week, day, or month the discomfort occurs.
- *Description of discomfort:* This is usually described as discomfort, pressure, heaviness, or even burning or squeezing and may radiate to the left neck, jaw, or epigastrium. Discomfort typically moves from the sternum, to the left shoulder, to the upper arm, and down the forearm to the wrist and fourth and fifth fingers. Radiation of pain may also be to the right in the same pattern, but this is not as frequent as the left. Discomfort lasts 15 s or up to 15 min. Characteristically, the pain is relieved by rest. Pain that can be pointed to with one finger is usually not angina. Levine's sign is the patient describing discomfort using a fist over the sternum. Angina during sleep may be due to increased venous return in the supine position.
- *Measures tried and measures effective in relieving pain:* Angina is suspected if relief of pain occurs within ½–2 min of taking nitroglycerin. Angina is also suspected if nitroglycerin is taken prior to anticipated exertion and no discomfort occurs with the exertion. Relief of esophageal spasm, however, may also occur with nitroglycerine. Relief when leaning forward is more indicative of pericarditis than angina. Discomfort lasting only a few seconds is not usually angina.
- *Risk factors:* Cigarette smoking or a family history of hyperlipidemia, hypertension, heart attacks, and diabetes puts the patient at risk. Additional factors include catecholamines, oral contraceptives, age and gender.
- *Any previous diagnostic tests.*

Differential Diagnosis

- *Neuromuscular origin:* Pain is increased with inspiration and herpes rash; pain occurs with palpation.
- *Gastrointestinal origin:* esophageal involvement, peptic ulcer disease, or gastritis, or gallbladder disease. Pain is usually not related to exertion. Food may decrease or make pain worse. Pain may be relieved with antacids. Pain is often in lower chest.
- *Psychogenic origin:* Pain not related to exertion; hyperventilation present.
- *Pulmonary origin:* Dyspnea, cough, and pleuritic pain of sudden onset, sharp, and exacerbated by inspiration; may or may not be associated with exertion or signs of right ventricular failure. May mimic angina.
- *Cardiovascular origin:* Complete assessment of discomfort is necessary to differentiate types of angina or sharp pain; pain is worse in supine position or pain that is sharp or tearing, often in the back, indicative of pericarditis or dissecting aortic aneurysm.

Physical Examination. Because of the multiple causes of chest pain, the physical examination is not always conclusive. Therefore, the examination must include many different areas of assessment.

Cardiovascular Examination. Elevated systolic and diastolic blood pressure; heart sounds show gallop, apical systolic murmur, S_4 heart sound, and arrhythmias, which are typical during an attack. Vital signs, heart sounds, presence of bruits, quality of pulses, and heart size are important parameters for examination.

Chest and Respiratory Examination. Breath sounds, friction rubs, and signs of hyperinflation are evident with percussion. Perform palpation of anterior ribs, especially at intercostal junctions.

Spinal Examination. Palpation of the cervical or thoracic spine may produce severe pain similar to angina. Pain usually occurs on the outer arm and thumb rather than fourth and fifth fingers.

Abdominal Examination. Check for epigastric tenderness and right upper quadrant pain.

Funduscopic Examination. Examine for changes associated with hypertension or atherosclerosis.

Laboratory Examination. Any patient suspected of having CAD needs additional studies to both diagnose CHD and rule out other causes of chest pain (Abrams, 1991; Massie, 1996).

Hematologic Examination. Obtain CBC, chemical profile including lipids, and thyroid profile. Make sure diabetes, hyperlipidemia, anemia, polycythemia, and thyroid abnormalities are not causative factors.

Other Tests. Myocardial ischemia is associated with electrical changes. However, the ECG may be normal or may show an old myocardial infarction, ST or T changes, conduction defects, or left ventricular abnormalities. Ischemia may be noted with depressed ST segments, T wave inversion, or ST elevation. These changes occur during an attack. An exercise ECG is the most helpful and noninvasive test. ST depression or chest pain is precipitated by exercise. Exercise testing is indicated for confirmation of angina, to determine the activity limitation and its severity, to assess the prognosis of those with diagnosed CHD, and to evaluate therapeutic response. Ambulatory ECG monitoring may detect silent ischemia. Possible additional tests are stress thallium, coronary angiography, and echocardiogram.

Patient/Caregiver Information

The most important information for a patient with CHD is recognition of symptoms requiring emergency care. The patient should be instructed to have available sublingual nitroglycerin tablets and to use them when experiencing chest pain. The tablets may or may not produce a stinging sensation under the tongue, but additional doses at 5-min intervals should be based on the continuation of chest pain. The patient should keep the nitroglycerin tablets in the original container and replace them approximately every 6 months if the container is opened or if tablets are exposed to excessive environmental or body heat.

The patient should be instructed about those activities that may precipitate angina. These include activity that places strain on the thoracic or upper extremity muscles such as lifting, walking uphill, and physical activity. The patient may also experience angina without exertion such as following meals or exposure to cold, upon awakening, after strong emotions, and following carbon monoxide inhalation. If sexual intercourse causes discomfort, it should be avoided; patients need to be assured that without discomfort it is perfectly safe. If the patient knows that such an activity will result in chest pain, then the patient can use sublingual nitroglycerin prior to that activity.

OUTCOMES MANAGEMENT

Selecting an Appropriate Agent

Selection of drug therapy is made on an individualized basis. The degree and type of angina will direct the need for monotherapy or a combination of beta blocker, nitrate, or calcium channel antagonist. An aspirin is always added to therapy, not for antianginal effects, but for the reduction in platelet activity and risk reduction for myocardial infarction. Beta blockers are the preferred treatment for stable angina combined with nitrates and calcium channel antagonist, as necessary (Fuster, 2000; ACC/AHA/ACP-ASIM Guidelines, 1999).

Monitoring for Efficacy and Toxicity

Nitrates. Nitrates are effective in treating all forms of angina. The site of action is the peripheral vascular tree, especially the venous and coronary blood vessels. Nitrates can dilate severely atherosclerotic vessels as well. The vasodilation lowers blood pressure, which in turn reduces myocardial wall tension, a major determinant of myocardial oxygen need. This results in a more favorable balance of myocardial oxygen supply and demand.

The sublingual dosage form is effective in treating acute episodes of angina, whereas the long-acting preparations are effective in preventing the development of angina. Monotherapy with sublingual nitroglycerin can be given in patients with less severe and occasional anginal attacks (less than one per day). The dose of sublingual nitroglycerin that decreases blood pressure by 10 mm Hg or heart rate by 10 beats per minute provides an optimum hemodynamic effect. The patient will often experience the adverse effects of dizziness, lightheadedness, and headache, but these can be reduced by teaching the patient to sit while taking the nitroglycerin. Headache pain can be managed with acetaminophen. Pain relief should begin in 3 to 5 min and lasts approximately 30 min. The patient should repeat the dose every 5 min for a total of three doses if pain is not relieved. If the patient is still experiencing angina after three doses or if the patient must repeat the dose every 30 to 60 min, he or she should be instructed to seek emergency care.

Longer-acting preparations should be considered in patients experiencing more severe and frequent anginal attacks. A variety of dosage forms (ointment, patches, tablets, capsules) are available. Nitrate tolerance can develop with all these forms of nitrates. Therefore, a nitrate-free period of a minimum of 8 to 12 h each day is necessary to maintain efficacy. Eight hours appears to be sufficient for nitroglycerin, while isosorbide may need 12 h of nitrate-free time. The nitrate-free period depends on the time of day the patient experiences the least number of anginal attacks. When an oral preparation such as isosorbide dinitrate is prescribed, the last dose of the day should not be later than 5:00 P.M. if taking three times a day. If taking twice a day, the doses should be at 7:00 A.M. and 2:00 P.M.

Beta Blockers. Beta blockers are the preferred first-line treatment for stable angina. By blocking the $beta_1$ receptors in the heart, beta blockers decrease heart rate, blood pressure, and contractility, with the net effect of reducing myocardial oxygen demand and increasing exercise tolerance. Beta blockers are useful as monotherapy treatment of chronic exertional stable angina or in combination with nitrates and calcium channel blockers. Beta blockers and nitrates can work in a complementary fashion. The beta blockers can block the reflex tachycardia induced by nitrate therapy, and the nitrates can reduce the left ventricular volume created by the beta blockers. Beta blockers can reduce the risk of postmyocardial reinfarction.

Dosing of beta blockers is titrated upward until the resting heart rate is 50 to 60 beats per minute. When the patient exercises, the maximal heart rate is either limited to 100 beats per minute or no more than 20 beats per minute or 10% over resting heart rate. Most beta blockers are effective in the treatment of angina when dosed no more than twice a day.

Adverse effects of beta blockers are numerous and are an extension of their pharmacodynamics. Beta blockers can produce additional cardiovascular changes of heart failure, bradycardia, heart block, hypotension, and peripheral vasoconstriction with intermittent claudication. Those beta blockers that are not cardioselective or lose this selectivity at higher doses can cause bronchospasm and alteration in glucose metabolism. The lipophilic beta blockers can cause CNS problems such as fatigue and depression.

Patients need to be educated about not abruptly stopping their beta blocker therapy since a buildup of catecholamines can result in an increased load on the heart to the point of myocardial infarction. This is especially critical in patients with severe atherosclerosis or unstable angina. When a beta blocker needs to be discontinued, a downward reduction in the dose is required. There is no set rate for this reduction, but two alternatives are (1) to reduce the dose by half every 3 to 4 days, decrease the frequency to daily every 3 to 4 days, and hold at daily for 3 to 4 days before stopping; or (2) decrease the dose over 2 days while using the patient's heart rate as a guideline.

Calcium Channel Antagonists. These agents can be divided into the dihydropyridines and non-dihydropyridine agents. The non-dihydropyridines consist of verapamil and diltiazem. These agents are quite effective for stable angina since they result in vasodilatation as well as slow the heart rate. The dihydropyridines consist of nifedipine, amlopdipine, felodipine, among others. These agents do not affect heart rate, but result in marked vasodilatation. Immediate release nifedipine is not recommended due to extensive vasodilatation, large fluctuation in serum peak and trough concentrations, and potential increased mortality in coronary artery disease.

The type II agents are preferred because of their vascular selectivity, peripheral and coronary, when compared to the type I agents verapamil and diltiazem, and their minimal activity on myocardial conduction and contractility. Of the type II agents, nicardipine has the most vasoselectivity followed by nifedipine, isradipine, and amlodipine with slightly less. Felodipine has the least vasoselectivity of this group. Not all of these agents have a FDA-approved indication (refer to Drug Table 205.6).

Calcium channel blockers can be added to nitrates and/or beta blockers (cautiously with verapamil or diltiazem) for additional benefit in patients remaining symptomatic. A calcium channel blocker is especially beneficial in patients with coexisting hypertension. Calcium channel blocker adverse events of concern are heart block, left ventricle dysfunction, bradycardia, and hypotension.

Aspirin. Because of aspirin's ability to bind irreversibly to platelets and decrease aggregation, it prevents the genesis of unstable angina and myocardial infarction. The daily dose of 80–325 mg may be given prophylactically in patients with coronary artery disease.

The following summarizes the pharmacotherapy care plans for each type of angina:

- *Stable angina:* Begin with nitroglycerin SL monotherapy in patients with less frequent angina. If the anginal attacks increase in frequency and severity, then the addition of a long-acting nitrate and/or beta blocker therapy is indicated. Beta blockers are preferred, especially if a patient has had a myocardial infarction. Nitrates are the alternative when beta blockers are contraindicated, or a long-acting nitrate and a beta blocker can be considered for their synergistic activity as well as the fact that each offsets the adverse effects of the other. The nitrate will have to be dosed to avoid the development of tolerance. If the patient continues to be symptomatic, then maximizing the doses of the current agents is indicated until they are effective or until side effects prevent further escalation of the dose. Alternatively, additional drug therapy such as a calcium channel blocker can be started. Aspirin therapy (325 mg/day—enteric-coated in patients experiencing gastrointestinal irritation) should be given to patients who have a history of myocardial infarction. If the patient is intolerant to aspirin, then clopidogrel (or ticlopidine) can be given. All therapy is titrated to the desired hemodynamic effect while minimizing the incidence of side effects.

- *Unstable angina:* If a patient presents to an ambulatory clinic with symptoms of unstable angina, initiate treatment with sublingual nitroglycerin and aspirin and then refer either to a cardiologist if low risk (new onset, <20 min in length, no pain at rest, normal or unchanged ECG) or transfer to an emergency room.
- *Variant angina:* Nitrates and calcium channel blockers appear to be effective in the treatment of variant (Prinzmetal's or vasospastic) angina. Sublingual nitroglycerin can provide symptomatic relief and should be encouraged.
- *Syndrome X:* Syndrome X is also known as microvascular ischemia. There appears to be an imbalance between the inherent vasoconstrictor and vasodilator responses of the vessel. It is thought that there may be a link between this type of ischemia and mental stress.

No drug therapy is especially effective in the treatment of syndrome X. The calcium channel blockers and nitrates may provide some benefit but are not always successful. Although the beta blockers are less effective and may actually aggravate the condition through unopposed alpha stimulation, they may be able to block the norepinephrine release caused by the stress. The current recommendation is to use SL nitroglycerin for acute pain relief along with a calcium channel blocker while avoiding environmental and dietary stimulants.

Followup Recommendations

Frequency of monitoring depends on the individual and the severity of the CHD. Consultation with a cardiologist is important to establish a treatment plan. Patients at high risk should be seen as frequently as every 2 weeks.

If a patient has unstable angina, hospitalization is necessary. When it is deemed safe to treat on an outpatient basis, followup within 72 h is generally essential. During followup, an ECG, evaluation of vital signs, another physical examination including heart sounds, and a hematocrit level should be done.

Education is important for anyone with angina and should cover the following items:

1. When to seek medical intervention for changes in pain frequency, intensity, and duration.
2. Importance of following the medical regimen.
3. Importance of smoking cessation and positive reinforcement for successes.
4. Exercise plan.
5. Diet.
6. Activities including driving, sexual relations, and exertion.
7. Use of nitroglycerin. Use when angina present, and repeat twice every 5 min if needed. If there is still no relief, seek medical intervention.
8. Stress reduction techniques.

Frequency of followup is individualized according to patient symptoms and the need for professional supportive management. At each followup visit:

1. Evaluate exercise, diet, smoking cessation, and stress reduction.
2. Discuss the medical regimen and the patient's ability to comply with the program.
3. Discuss medications and explore possible side effects.
4. The use of an ECG for monitoring is controversial. If the patient is having an asymptomatic MI (silent), the management strategies are the same as previously stated. If there is an acute MI, the ECG is indicated by the symptoms.
5. Do a blood chemistry and CBC.
6. Do a prothrombin time with INR if the patient is taking warfarin.
7. Monitor vital signs and heart and lung sounds.
8. Assess for development of additional risk factors, and inquire about any additional medications including over-the-counter drugs.

MITRAL VALVE PROLAPSE

Mitral valve prolapse, also called floppy mitral valve, is a very common abnormality, particularly in young women. Although it was once thought to be the result of rheumatic heart disease, research indicates that it is likely of genetic origin and associated with other congenital connective tissue abnormalities such as Marfan's syndrome or simply an isolated abnormality. Abnormal volume regulation, autonomic nervous system function, and neuroendocrine function may accompany mitral valve prolapse.

Mitral valve prolapse is present when the anterior and posterior leaflets (cusps) of the mitral valve bulge or balloon into the atrium during systole. The abnormal function is due to thickened, enlarged, scalloped, and sometimes elongated leaflets. Mitral regurgitation, the most common physical finding, occurs when the abnormality is sufficient to allow blood to leak into the atrium.

Although the condition is common, symptoms are either nonexistent or vague. Most patients have no limit on physical function and frequently are more troubled psychologically by the diagnosis. Symptoms include nonspecific chest pain, palpitations, light-headedness, syncope, fatigue (particularly in the morning), lethargy, weakness, panic attacks, and anxiety. The variety of symptoms and the number seem unrelated to the extent of the prolapse. However, palpitations, chest pain, syncope, fatigue, and dyspnea are associated with altered autonomic function. The condition is usually nonprogressive. Complications occur if there is significant mitral regurgitation or secondary disease states. If there is progressive mitral regurgitation, it is usually due to dilatation of the mitral annulus or rupture of the chordal structures (Fortuin, 1996).

SPECIFIC CONSIDERATIONS FOR PHARMACOTHERAPY

When Drug Therapy Is Needed

Pharmacotherapy for mitral valve prolapse may be indicated for the following medical reasons: (1) preventing recurrence of rheumatic fever, (2) preventing infective endocarditis, (3) preventing thromboembolism, and (4) managing atrial arrhythmias.

Although the incidence of bacterial endocarditis is not positively known, the best medical treatment when infection occurs still has a 3 to 40% mortality rate (Chenoweth & Burket, 1997). Therefore, prophylactic antibiotic coverage is warranted in patients who have mitral valve prolapse. However, the American Heart Association recommends antibiotics in patients with regurgitation and not in the absence of regurgitation. Individuals who have a mitral valve prolapse associated with thickening and/or redundancy of the valve leaflets may be at increased risk for bacterial endocarditis, particularly men ≥45 years of age.

The AHA (American Heart Association, 2002) recommends antibiotic prophylaxis for the following cardiac conditions and medical procedures:

- Cardiac conditions (high risk):
  - Prosthetic cardiac valves, including bioprosthetic and hemograft valves
  - Previous infective endocarditis
  - Complex cyanotic congenital heart disease including single ventrical states, transposition of the great arteries, and tetralogy of Fallot
  - Surgically constructed pulmonary shunts or conduits
- Cardiac conditions (moderate risk):
  - Most other congenital cardiac malformations, including patent ductus arteriosus, ventricular septal defect, and coarctation of the aorta
  - Rheumatic and other acquired valvular dysfunctions, even after surgical repair
  - Mitral valve prolapse with valvular regurgitation and/or thickened leaflets
  - Hypertrophic cardiomyopathy
- Medical procedures:
  - Dental procedures known to induce gingival or mucosal bleeding, including routine professional cleaning
  - Tonsillectomy and/or adenoidectomy
  - Surgical operations that involve intestinal or respiratory mucosa
  - Bronchoscopy with a rigid bronchoscope
  - Sclerotherapy for esophageal varices
  - Esophageal dilation
  - Endoscopic retrograde cholangiography with biliary obstruction
  - Biliary tract surgery
  - Urethral dilation or cystoscopy
  - Urinary tract surgery, including prostate surgery

Short- and Long-Term Goals of Pharmacotherapy

The immediate benefit of prophylactic antibiotics is the prevention of bacterial endocarditis in susceptible individuals since bacterial endocarditis is associated with significant mortality and long-term morbidity. The use of pharmacotherapy in the prevention of thromboembolism or management of atrial arrhythmias needs to be individualized based on the overall status of the patient.

Nonpharmacologic Therapy

Most patients are asymptomatic and do not require treatment. Complications usually occur after age 50, at which point surgery may be indicated. There generally is no restriction on activity. Vigorous exercise and sports are only restricted if there is another associated abnormality or if there is a decrease in intravascular volume associated with the prolapse and the person may experience syncope with exercise.

Adequate salt intake is indicated in patients with associated intravascular volume depletion, any abnormal renin-aldosterone response to volume depletion, or alterations in the autonomic nervous system (the patient has symptoms of chest pain, palpitations, fatigue, dyspnea, anxiety, or panic attacks).

Caffeine, alcohol, and cigarettes should be avoided by patients with mitral valve prolapse to decrease the risk of palpitations (American Heart Association, 2001).

Time Frame for Initiating Pharmacotherapy

For prophylactic antibiotics to have a beneficial effect, serum and tissue levels must have reached peak levels prior to the dental or surgical procedure. All of the oral antibiotic regimens are given 1 h prior to the procedure. When designed to prevent thromboembolism, therapy should be started in patients with documented systemic embolism or chronic or paroxysmal atrial fibrillation. Management of atrial arrhythmias may be necessary when paroxysms are frequent or reversion to normal sinus rhythm cannot be attained (Hancock, 1996b).

See Drug Tables 102, 202.

Assessment Needed Prior to Therapy

History. Because many patients often are asymptomatic and any symptoms are vague and may not indicate a problem of cardiovascular origin, the history may be inconclusive. Inquire about functional limitations. Younger patients may experience palpitations, effort intolerance, or light-headedness due to hyperresponsiveness to an endogenous sympathetic stimulus (Fortuin, 1996). Inquire about any family history of valvular disease or disorders of connective tissue.

Physical Examination. Cardiac auscultation will be the key to diagnosis because valvular disease causes murmurs. Listen for the characteristic midsystolic click. Clicks may be multiple and may be followed by a midsystolic murmur or a late systolic crescendo murmur. The click and/or murmur may vary from one examination to another, from one position to another, and with temperature, respirations, and time of day. Multiple clicks are possible and may indicate a higher degree of prolapse and regurgitation. Auscultate in the standing position because the abnormal sounds are accentuated when standing. A pansystolic murmur may indicate significant mitral regurgitation possibly caused by a ruptured chordae tendineae.

In checking the skeletal system, observe for long arms (longer than usual for height) and thoracic narrowing or other chest wall abnormalities (typical of Marfan's syndrome).

Diagnostic Measures. The ECG may be normal. The chest x-ray will be normal. The echocardiogram is the most useful test to confirm physical findings and will also evaluate other valves. It should not be used as a routine screen since most mitral valve prolapses are benign.

Patient/Caregiver Information

Any patient with mitral valve prolapse will need to take precautions prior to dental and surgical procedures (outlined in the previous section). Written instructions should include the types of procedures and the importance of informing the provider of the presence of mitral valve prolapse.

Regular exercise and activities usually should be encouraged. If the patient experiences syncope with exercise or if there is another limiting factor, exercise should not be vigorous and competitive sports limited.

OUTCOMES MANAGEMENT

Selecting an Appropriate Agent

The American Heart Association (AHA, 2002) recommends the following prophylaxis regimens for the prevention of infective endocarditis:

Dental, Upper Respiratory Tract, or Esophageal Procedures

- Routine
  Amoxicillin:
    Adults: 2 g PO 1 h before procedure
    Children: 50 mg/kg PO 1 h before procedure
- Penicillin-allergic patients
  Clindamycin:
    Adults: 600 mg PO 1 h before procedure
    Children: 20 mg/kg 1 h before procedure
  OR
  Cephalexin or cefadroxil:
    Adults: 2 g PO 1 h before procedure
    Children: 50 mg/kg PO 1 h before procedure
  OR
  Azithromycin/clarithromycin:
    Adults: 500 mg PO 1 h before procedure
    Children: 15 mg/kg PO 1 h before procedure
- Patients unable to take oral medications
  Ampicillin:
    Adults: 2 g IM or IV 30 min before procedure
    Children: 50 mg/kg IM or IV 30 min before procedure

- Penicillin-allergic patients unable to take oral medications
  Clindamycin:
    Adults: 600 mg IV 30 min before procedure
    Children: 20 mg/kg IV 30 min before procedure
  OR
  Cefazolin:
    Adults: 1 g IM or IV 30 min before procedure
    Children: 25 mg/kg IM or IV 30 min before procedure

Genitourinary/Gastrointestinal Procedures (Excluding Esophageal Procedures)

- High-risk patients
  Adults: Ampicillin 2 g IV or IM plus gentamicin 1.5 mg/kg (maximum 120 mg) IV 30 min before procedure; amoxicillin 1 g PO or ampicillin 1 g IV 6 h after initial dose
  Children: Ampicillin 50 mg/kg IM or IV (maximum 2 g) plus gentamicin 1.5 mg/kg 30 min before procedure; 6 h later, ampicillin 25 mg/kg IV or IM or amoxicillin 25 mg/kg PO
- High-risk penicillin-allergic patients
  Adults: Vancomycin 1 g IV over 1–2 h plus gentamicin 1.5 mg/kg (maximum 120 mg) IV or IM; complete injection/infusion 30 min before procedure
  Children: Vancomycin 20 mg/kg IV over 1–2 h plus gentamicin 1.5 mg/kg IV or IM; complete injection/infusion 30 min before procedure
- Moderate-risk patients
  Adults: Amoxicillin 2 g PO 1 h before procedure or ampicillin 2 g IM or IV 30 min before procedure
  Children: Amoxicillin 50 mg/kg PO 1 h before procedure or ampicillin 50 mg/kg IM or IV 30 min before procedure
- Moderate-risk penicillin-allergic patients
  Adults: Vancomycin 1 g IV over 1–2 h; complete infusion 30 min before procedure
  Children: Vancomycin 20 mg/kg IV over 1–2 h; complete infusion 30 min before procedure
  NOTE: Total pediatric dose should not exceed adult dose.

Warfarin pharmacotherapy should be prescribed whenever the patient has had a previous episode of embolism or atrial fibrillation of paroxysmal or chronic nature and either rheumatic mitral valve disease, mitral annular calcification, or mitral valve prolapse. Warfarin should be dosed to achieve an INR of 2.0 to 3.0 (warfarin-dosing algorithms are presented in the section on arrhythmias). Patients who have experienced a transient ischemic attack (TIA) of unknown etiology are candidates for 325 mg/day of aspirin or clopidogrel (ticlopidine is an alternative). If the TIAs continue, long-term anticoagulation with warfarin should be prescribed. In patients in whom warfarin is not tolerated, aspirin doses of 975 mg/day or ticlopidine 250 mg bid can be prescribed (Hancock, 1996).

The most common arrhythmia is atrial fibrillation. The atrial fibrillation may be paroxysmal or become chronic and as such is often permanent. During paroxysmal episodes, counter-shock or antiarrhythmic therapy may cause reversion to normal sinus rhythm. Long-term therapy with antiarrhythmic agents may help maintain sinus rhythm, whereas many patients may have permanent fibrillation (Hancock, 1996).

Monitoring for Efficacy and Toxicity

Refer to the anti-infective agents in Drug Table 102 for a description of pharmacodynamics and pharmacokinetics and symptoms of toxicity and adverse reaction.

Followup Recommendations

1. Repeat echocardiograms yearly if the patient has mitral systolic murmurs, increased left ventricular size, or thickening of the leaflets (cusps) because these complications are most common. Echocardiograms are indicated as the person ages since clinically significant regurgitation occurs with age.
2. Yearly visits include a complete history of symptoms associated with mitral valve prolapse and cardiac auscultation to detect additional clicks or new murmurs.
3. With age, more complications may occur, especially in males over 50. History and physical examination should update information on the following conditions: TIA, stroke, CHF, syncope, and arrhythmias.

HYPERLIPIDEMIA

In order to understand both coronary artery disease and peripheral vascular disease, it is important to understand lipids, lipid metabolism, and the relationship between lipids and atherosclerosis (refer to section on coronary artery disease). Abnormalities in lipoproteins can result in a predisposition to premature coronary artery disease, pancreatits (from elevated triglycerides), and cerebrovascular accident.

Lipoproteins are divided into four major classes, based on density, composition, and electrophoretic mobility:

1. Chylomicrons
2. Very Low Density Lipoproteins (VLDL)
3. Low Density Lipoproteins (LDL)
4. High Density Lipoproteins (HDL)

Cholesterol is essential for the manufacture and repair of plasma proteins; it is part of all cell membranes, bile salts, and steroid hormones. Cholesterol originates exogenously through dietary intake or endogenously through synthesis in the liver. Dietary cholesterol comes only from foods of animal origin. Triglycerides are the main component of VLDL. Triglycerides are derived from dietary fat and are needed to transfer food energy to cells. The majority of triglycerides are stored in tissues as glycerol, fatty acids, and monoglyceroids. The liver is responsible for converting them back into triglycerides. Thus, triglycerides are considered stored energy.

LDL is considered a precursor to atherosclerosis. HDL is considered protective, but the exact mechanism is still unknown. The density of the lipoproteins is synonymous with the content of triglyceride. This is an inverse relationship where the higher the triglyceride levels the lower the density of the lipoprotein.

Testing for adults should begin at age 20, and a fasting lipoprotein profile should be obtained once every 5 years. (National Cholesterol Education Program: ATPIII Guidelines, 2001). Refer to Table 20–10 for classification of values.

TABLE 20–10. ATP III Lipoprotein Profile

Lipoprotein	Range/Value (in mg/dL)	Classification
Total Cholesterol		
	< 200	Desirable
	200–239	Boderline high
	> 240	High
LDL		
	< 100	Optimal
	100–129	Near optimal/above optimal
	130–159	Borderline high
	160–189	High
	> 190	Very high
HDL		
	< 40	Low
	> 60	High
Triglycerides		
	< 150	Normal
	150–199	Borderline high
	200–299	High
	> 500	Very high

After obtaining a fasting lipoprotein panel the patient's risk factors must be examined to determine a LDL-lowering therapy. These risk factors include:

- Cigarette smoking
- Hypertension (BP > 140/90 mmHg or on hypertensive medication)
- Low HDL (< 40 mg/dL), family history of premature CHD (CHD in male first-degree relative <55 year; CHD in female first-degree relative <65 years old)
- Age (men >45; women >55 years old)

The ATP III identifies three categories of risk that modify the goals and modalities of LDL-lowering therapy, refer to the Table 20–11.

A 10-year risk factor is calculated using the Framingham scoring system. The system is very easy to use as it assigns a point score to each of the 5 risk factors: age, total cholesterol, smoking, HDL, and systolic blood pressure. A table is then used to assign the percentage of risk of developing CHD with in 10 years based on the patient's point score. Refer to Figure 20–2. This is an example of calculating a patient's 10-year risk for CAD using the Framingham risk assessment tool.

> Mr. Hughes is a 46-year-old male with a history of smoking 1 pack of cigarettes a day for the past 20 years. He recently had a fasting lipid profile drawn at his family doctor's office. His total cholesterol was 211, and HDL cholesterol was 32. His blood pressure was 148/90 on no antihypertensive medications.
>
> Using the Framingham tool Mr. Hughes gets 3 points for his age, 5 points for his total cholesterol, 5 points for being a smoker, 2 points for his HDL, and 1 point for his blood pressure. His total point score is 16. His 10-year risk is 25%.

Anyone with hyperlipidemia should be assessed to rule out secondary dyslipidemia before starting lipid-lowering therapy. Some causes of secondary dyslipidemia include diabetes, hypothyroidism, obstructive

TABLE 20–11. Modified LDL Goal According to Risk Category

Risk Category	LDL Goal (mg/dl)
CHD and CHD Risk Equivalents*	<100
Multiple (2+) Risk Factors	<130
Zero to One Risk Factor	<160

*CHD risk equivalents consist of:

1. Peripheral vascular disease, abdominal aortic aneurysm, and symptomatic carotid artery disease
2. Diabetes
3. A 10-year risk factor for CHD > 20%.

Estimate of 10-Year Risk for Men

Age	Points
20–34	−9
35–39	−4
40–44	0
45–49	3
50–54	6
55–59	8
60–64	10
65–69	11
70–74	12
75–79	13

	Points by Age				
Total Cholesterol	20–39	40–49	50–59	60–69	70–79
< 160	0	0	0	0	0
160–199	4	3	2	1	0
200–239	7	5	3	1	0
240–279	9	6	4	2	1
>280	11	8	5	3	1

	Points by Age				
	20–39	40–49	50–59	60–69	70–79
Nonsmoker	0	0	0	0	0
Smoker	8	5	3	1	1

HDL(mg/dl)	Points
>60	−1
50–59	0
40–49	1
<40	2

Systolic BP(mm/Hg)	Treated	Untreated
<120	0	0
120–129	0	1
130–139	1	2
140–159	1	2
>160	2	3

Point Total	10 yr Risk %
<0	<1
0	1
1	1
2	1
3	1
4	1
5	2
6	2
7	3
8	4
9	5
10	6
11	8
12	10
13	12
14	16
15	20
16	25
17 or >	>30

Estimate of 10-Year Risk for Women

Age	Points
20–34	−7
35–39	−3
40–44	0
45–49	3
50–54	6
55–59	8
60–64	10
65–69	12
70–74	14
75–79	16

	Points by Age				
Total Cholesterol	20–39	40–49	50–59	60–69	70–79
<160	0	0	0	0	0
160–199	4	3	2	1	1
200–239	8	6	4	2	1
240–279	11	8	5	3	2
>280	13	10	7	4	2

	Points by Age				
	20–39	40–49	50–59	60–69	70–79
Nonsmoker	0	0	0	0	0
Smoker	9	7	4	2	1

HDL (mg/dl)	Points
>60	−1
50–59	0
40–49	1
<40	2

Systolic BP (mm/Hg)	Treated	Untreated
<120	0	0
120–129	1	3
130–139	2	4
140–159	3	5
>160	4	6

Point Total	10 yr Risk %
<9	<1
9	1
10	1
11	1
12	1
13	2
14	2
15	3
16	4
17	5
18	6
19	8
20	11
21	14
22	17
23	22
24	27
25 or >	>30

FIGURE 20–2. Framingham 10-Year Risk Assessment

liver disease, chronic renal failure, and drugs that elevate LDL and lower HDL (progestins, anabolic steroids, and corticosteroids).

In summary, cholesterol, in the form of VLDL, LDL, and HDL, has major implications for the development of heart disease, particularly coronary artery disease. Lowering total cholesterol, and particularly LDL, decreases the incidence of coronary heart disease, may slow the progression of atherosclerosis, and may even reverse atherosclerotic changes. (Gotto, 2001; La Rosa, 2002; Wierzbicki & Mikhailidis, 2002). Lowering LDL and raising HDL are significant in reducing risk factors in the development of coronary heart disease.

SPECIFIC CONSIDERATIONS FOR PHARMACOTHERAPY

When Drug Therapy Is Needed

Lifestyle modifications should be the first line of management although drug therapy may be the best option for patients. Practitioners are fully aware that treatment of hyperlipidemia can result in a reduced risk of coronary heart disease death and nonfatal MI. Lowering the LDL using whatever strategies that produce the best outcome is the goal. However, the dietary restrictions of decreasing fats may prove unpalatable for some. Others may be compliant with dietary and exercise measures, yet continue to have elevated lipid levels. The practitioner's role must include educating the patient and the patient's family about the importance of lowering LDL and increasing HDL levels.

Short- and Long-term Goals of Pharmacotherapy

The long-term goal of therapy is to prevent the progression of the atherosclerotic process, thereby decreasing morbidity and mortality from coronary heart disease and arterial peripheral vascular diseases.

Short-term goals must be aimed at identification of populations at risk and primary prevention. Individuals with high cholesterol, high LDL, and low HDL, but with no indication of coronary heart disease, need to be treated to try to prevent onset of disease. In addition, individuals with manifestations of CHD need to begin treatment to prevent the progression of the atherosclerotic process.

The goal of therapy is to bring LDL and HDL to within normal limits as well as to lower total cholesterol to within normal limits. LDL should be reduced to as low as possible, and in patients with established coronary heart disease this means no less than 100 mg/dL. Although numerical goals are set, a 1% reduction in total cholesterol is associated with a 2–3% reduction in CHD, and any reduction in LDL is a positive step (Gotto, 2001; La Rosa, 2002; Wierzbicki & Mikhailidis, 2002). One additional factor to consider when developing a therapeutic plan is the ratio of cholesterol to HDL. Generally, the higher the cholesterol: HDL ratio, the higher the risk for development of atherosclerosis and coronary heart diseases. Therefore, it is important to decrease the ratio between total cholesterol and HDL.

Nonpharmacologic Therapy

Diet. Therapeutic lifestyle changes should be implemented in all patients considered at risk for hyperlipidemia. Because the majority of cholesterol enters the system via the diet, dietary changes may decrease cholesterol and LDL. Dietary management is delineated as a Step I or a Step II diet. The Step I recommendation is to decrease the dietary fat intake to less than 30% of the total calories. In addition, daily saturated fat intake is to be less than 10% of the calories with no more than 300 mg of cholesterol. Polyunsaturated fats, once thought more acceptable, are now found to decrease HDL and are therefore also restricted. Olive oil and canola oil do not decrease HDL, and their use should be promoted (Wierzbicki & Mikhailidis, 2001).

The Step II diet is more restrictive. It should be started in anyone with established coronary heart disease or when the Step I diet has less than desired benefit. In the Step II diet, fat is restricted to 20% of calories, limiting saturated fat to 7%, and 200 mg of cholesterol per day.

Fiber is also implicated in the reduction of cholesterol. Soluble fiber, as found in oat bran, broccoli, apples, beans, and grapefruit, has been found modestly effective in decreasing cholesterol. Psyllium powders are also a source of soluble fiber. Although soluble fiber may be useful as part of the dietary management of hyperlipidemia, it must be approached with caution. If oat bran is used in baked goods containing oils and eaten with butter, the value of the oat bran is lost. Also, psyllium and high-fiber foods cause abdominal bloating and flatus, which may decrease adherence to dietary changes.

Alcohol, in moderation, is slightly effective in raising the HDL level. However, it is important to advise patients about the detrimental effects of alcohol such as obesity and alcohol abuse.

Exercise. Exercise in conjunction with weight loss may decrease LDL and increase HDL (Gotto, 2001).

Time Frame for Initiating Pharmacotherapy

The decision to proceed to drug therapy and the desired goals are based on the National Cholesterol Education Program (NCEP) guidelines (Expert Panel on Detection, Evaluation, and Treatment of High Blood Cholesterol in Adults, 2001) (see Table 20–12).

Assessment Needed Prior to Therapy

Patients with hyperlipidemia are asymptomatic until pathologic changes associated with high cholesterol and high LDL occur. Therefore, it is important to assess risk factors for cardiovascular disease (Expert Panel on Detection, Evaluation, and Treatment of High Blood Cholesterol in Adults, 2001).

History

Genetic Predisposition. A family history of cardiovascular events is an important factor in hyperlipidemia and coronary heart disease.

Smoking. This is a definite risk factor in all cardiovascular problems. In addition, smoking cessation may raise the HDL level.

Diet. The ATP III guidelines recommend a therapeutic lifestyle change that consists of reduced dietary intake of:

- Saturated fat to less than 7% of total calories
- Polyunsaturated fat up to 10% of total calories
- Monounsaturated fat up to 20% of total calories
- Total fat as 25 to 35% of total calories
- Carbohydrates as 50 to 60% of total calories
- Fiber at 20 to 30 grams/day
- Protein as 15% of total calories
- Cholesterol at less than 200 mg/day
- Total calories: Balance calorie intake and expenditure to maintain desirable body weight (National Cholesterol Education Program: ATP Guidelines, 2001).

Exercise. A sedentary lifestyle contributes to lower HDL. The patient should be asked about type, duration, and frequency of exercise.

Secondary Causes. Other causes may be responsible for the hyperlipidemia and therefore should be assessed. Included are:

- Obesity
- Diabetes
- Hypothyroidism
- Nephrotic syndrome
- Renal insufficiency
- Obstructive liver disease
- Cushing's disease
- Medications such as estrogen, oral contraceptives, steroids, thiazide, and beta blockers without ISA

Physical Examination. Unless the individual has diagnosed heart disease, there are few physical findings related to hyperlipidemia. A complete physical examination may reveal cardiovascular disease. However, laboratory testing probably is the best screening and diagnostic technique available.

Hypothyroid Profile. Hypothyroidism may cause hyperlipidemia.

CBC and Chemical Profile. These tests identify liver function and kidney function, as well as screening for diabetes.

Patient/Caregiver Information

Patient compliance is a definite factor. During the asymptomatic period, the patient may not be able to justify changes in diet and activity or the expense of antilipidemic medications. Education on lifestyle modification techniques to minimize the side effects of medication and utilization of allied health professionals such as dieticians and pharmacists to reinforce the information is critical for patient understanding and compliance. As with many chronic problems, a case manager may be helpful to as-

TABLE 20–12. LDL Cholesterol Goals and Cut Points for Therapeutic Lifestyle Changes (TLC) and Drug Therapy in Different Risk Categories

Risk Category	LDL-C Goal	LDL Level at Which to Initiate Therapeutic Lifestyle Changes (TLC)	LDL Levels at Which to Consider Drug Therapy
CHD or CHD Risk Equivalents (10-year risk > 20%)	<100 mg/dL	> 100 mg/dL	> 130 mg/dL (100–129 mg/dL: drug optional)
2+ Risk Factor (10-year risk > 20%)*	<130 mg/dL	>130 mg/dL	10-year risk 10–20% >130 mg/dL 10-year risk <10% >160 mg/dL
0–1 Risk Factor **	<160 mg/dL	>160 mg/dL	>190 mg/dL (160–189 mg/dL: LDL-lowering drugs optional

*Some authorities recommend use of LDL-lowering drugs in this category if an LDL cholesterol <100 cannot be achieved by therapeutic lifestyle changes. Others prefer use of drugs that primarily modify triglycerides and HDL, e.g., nicotinic acid or fibrate. Clinical judgment also may call for deferring drug therapy in this subcategory.

**Almost all people with 0-1 risk factor have a 10-year risk <10%, thus risk assessment in people with a 0-1 risk factor is not necessary.

Adapted from Expert Panel (2001).

sist the practitioner in coordination of resources to reinforce education.

OUTCOMES MANAGEMENT

Selecting an Appropriate Agent

Pharmacotherapy for hyperlipidemia involves matching the lipid disorder with the best agent. Other considerations include the existence of concomitant disease states. Several treatment algorithms are available to assist the practitioner along with the NCEP guidelines. The NCEP guidelines recognize bile acid sequestrates, nicotinic acid, and statins as the major drug categories in the treatment of hyperlipidemias (Expert Panel, 2001). A simple treatment algorithm consists of the following:

- *Hypercholesterolemia:* bile acid resins (BAR), niacin, or statins
- *Mixed hyperlipidemia:* niacin or statins; possibly fibric acids
- *Hypertriglyceridemia:* niacin or fibric acids

If the response is inadequate, then a second agent is added or an alternative agent is used.

Statin therapy is commonly used as a first-line therapy for patients with dyslipidemias, and niacin, bile acid dequesterants, and fibric acid derivatives are used in combination, as necessary. The reader is referred to the most recent NCEP guidelines. Most importantly, the first goal of therapy is reduction of LDL-C, as long as there is not a marked elevation in triglycerides.

Monitoring for Efficacy and Toxicity

Statins. The statins (atorvastatin, fluvastatin, lovastatin, pravastatin, simvastatin rosuvastatin) are HMG-CoA reductase inhibitors. The inhibition of this enzyme reduces the biosynthesis of cholesterol. This results in lowered LDL and triglyceride (TG) levels and elevated HDL levels. The effects of the statins are dose-dependent. Dosage adjustments can be made every 4 weeks with laboratory studies performed just prior to next possible adjustment. To improve the efficacy of all the statins except atorvastatin, the patient should take the dose in the evening. The serum levels of the statins coincide with the nighttime increase in cholesterol biosynthesis. Atorvastatin appears to have equal efficacy whether taken in the morning or evening.

Atorvastatin has a greater LDL cholesterol-lowering potential than the other agents at the lowest daily dose. Atorvastatin 10 mg has lowered LDL cholesterol by 39% compared to lovastatin 20 mg at 24%, simvastatin 5 mg at 24%, pravastatin 10 mg at 22%, and fluvastatin 20 mg at 25%. At the upper dose per day, atorvastatin lowered LDL by 60% compared to 34 to 40% for the others and triglycerides by 37% compared to 11 to 24% for the others. The effect on HDL was very similar. If switching to atorvastatin is considered, begin with 10 mg per day regardless of the dose of the current HMG-CoA reductase inhibitor.

The statins are shown to slow progression of atherosclerotic lesions, resulting in fewer CHD events along with a good safety profile. Although side effects are uncommon, patients may complain of GI symptoms and headache. Hepatotoxicity and myopathy are more serious side effects. Baseline LFTs should be performed and repeated every 6 to 8 weeks during the first year or if patient is symptomatic to screen for elevations in transaminase enzymes. Recently, the FDA approved monitoring for simvastatin of baseline LFTs and then semiannually only for the first year of treatment or until 1 year after the last elevation in dose. Levels three times the upper normal limit may occur and appear to be dose-dependent. However, LFTs return to normal when the statin is discontinued. Myopathy is suspected when a patient complains of muscle aches, soreness, or weakness and is confirmed when the CPK is greater than 10 times the upper limit of normal.

Patients should be educated on the need for lovastatin to be taken with the evening meal to increase bioavailability, whereas pravastatin, simvastatin, and fluvastatin should be taken at bedtime. Again, atorvastatin can be taken without regard to meals or time of day.

Safety Concerns. The safety of lipid-lowering drugs is of major concern for the practitioner and the patient alike. Muscle toxicity, especially rhabdomyolysis, is of particular concern. From October 1997 to December 2000, 772 cases of rhabdomyolysis were reported to the U.S. Food and Drug Administration (FDA). Included in these 772 cases were 72 deaths. The actual number of rhabdomyolysis cases is unknown as the FDA uses a voluntary reporting system.

387 of these same 772 reported cases were patients who were receiving cerivastatin (Baycol), 31 of which died. In 12 of these 31 deaths the patient was also receiving gemfibrozil therapy. Cerivastatin was voluntarily withdrawn from the U.S. market in August 2001.

Several clinical trials have shown statins to be safe. These trials include the PPP (Pravastatin Pooling Project) study where investigators observed treatment with provastatin 40 mg/day and found no cases of severe myopathy. Another such trial, the Air Force/Texas Coronary

Atheroscelerosis Prevention Study, examined lovastatin usage over a 5-year period. Two cases of rhabdomyolsis were reported in the placebo group and 1 case in the lovastatin group, though this occurred when the patient was not receiving the lovastatin.The outcomes of these and other clinical trials have shown that the benefits of statin drugs outweigh the risk of rhabdomyolysis due to the low incidence of occurrence.

Bile Acid Resins (sequestrates). The three BARs are cholestyramine, colestipol, and colesevelam. These medications are anion exchange agents that bind bile acids, interrupting the recycling of bile acids through the enterohepatic circulation. The hepatocytes are stimulated to convert cholesterol into bile acids. The reduced concentration of cholesterol stimulates LDL receptor synthesis, which leads to the removal of circulating LDL, and thus reduced blood levels. The BAR mechanism is synergistic with other medications of different actions.

The BARs have numerous gastrointestinal side effects, such as nausea, bloating, epigastric fullness, constipation, and flatulence, that may affect patient compliance. Patient education on the importance of increased fluid intake (not waiting for the thirst stimulus) and fiber intake are important. A technique of mixing the powder with pulpy juices and swallowing with minimal air intake may help reduce the GI problems.

Because the BARs are exchange resins, there is an increased chance for drugs and vitamins to bind if taken within 4 h of the resin. Therefore, such drugs as niacin, digoxin, warfarin, thyroxine, thiazide diuretics, beta blockers, and any other anionic drugs need to be taken 1 hour before or 4 hours after the resin.

Ezetimibe's (Zetia) mechanism of action is different than other lipid lowering agents. Ezetimibe works at the brush borders in the small intestine to block absorption of cholesterol. The recommended usage is in addition to a statin drug but it may be used alone. When used in conjunction with statins it lowered total cholesterol and LDL, increased HDL, and lowered triglycerides. At this time it is contraindicated in use with fibrates.

Niacin. Niacin lowers all serum lipids when administered in high doses because it reduces the production of VLDL particles by the liver. This reduction of VLDL, and consequently LDL, is a result of inhibition of lipolysis with decreased free fatty acids in plasma, decreased hepatic esterification of TG, a possible direct effect on the hepatic production of apolipoprotein B, and a reduction in the synthesis of apolipoprotein A [Lp(A)].

Doses of 1200 to 1500 mg/day are necessary to reduce TG and raise HCL. Doses of niacin often are 2000 to 3000 mg/day to lower LDL levels (McKenney, Proctor, Harris, et al., 1994). Doses of niacin should be started low and titrated slowly. Begin with a dose of 200 to 250 mg per day in divided dosages, and then increase by 200 to 250 mg per day every 3 to 7 days. A newer formulation Niaspan® may be dosed once daily in the evening. At the large amounts, the majority of patients will experience at least one of the side effects of vasodilation, flushing, itching or headache. A 325 mg aspirin tablet given 30 min prior to the morning dose of niacin can reduce the symptoms. It is thought the side effects are mediated through prostaglandins. To minimize any GI side effects, the niacin may be taken with food.

The greatest concern with the use of niacin is hepatoxicity. This side effect is almost exclusively associated with sustained-release products and appears to be dose-dependent at doses greater than 1500 mg/day. The use of a crystalline form of niacin is associated with a lower incidence of hepatoxicity. Liver function tests should be performed at baseline and then every 6 to 8 weeks the first year or whenever the patient is symptomatic. The new niacin formulation Niaspan® does not result in a higher incidence of hepatotoxicity associated with the sustained-release products. Of note, the sustained-release products are classified as dietary supplements, not as drugs under the watchful eye of the FDA. Many patients may already be taking a form of niacin on their own, and the possibility should be explored when taking a medication history.

Fibric Acids. The fibric acids, clofibrate, fenofibrate, and gemfibrozil, lower triglyceride levels by increasing the enzymatic action of lipoprotein lipase. Gemfibrozil has been the single agent available to treat elevated triglycerides for some time since clofibrate has been associated with increased mortality and fenofibrate was recently released.

The fibric acid derivatives share similar adverse effects of myalgias, elevated liver enzymes, and gastrointestinal distress and rashes. The one concerning side effect is an increase in gallstone formation because of the increased concentration of cholesterol in the bile caused by these drugs.

Estrogen Replacement Therapy. Estrogen replacement therapy (ERT) has historically been considered as an alternative for treating lipid disorders in postmenopausal women at high risk. This recommendation was based on epidemiological data, not well-controlled trials (Barrett-Conner & Bush, 1991; Grady, Rubin, Rettiti, et al., 1992). This approach has changed since the publication of the HERS trial. This investigation demonstrated that initiating estrogen therapy in patients with established CAD could be detrimental and increase the risk of myocardial infarction during the first year of therapy, possibly due to its procoagulant effects. This adverse effect did not persist after the first year, but it certainly calls into question the use of estrogen for secondary treatment of dyslipidemia. Whether this is true for primary prevention is unknown; however, for patients with established CAD, one should not start estrogen for dyslipidemia treatment. If estrogen is used for another indication (e.g., osteoporosis prevention or vasomotor symptoms), another agent for lipid management such as the statin drugs should be initiated instead of estrogen (Hulley, Grady & Bush, 1999).

In summary, statins provide the greatest LDL lowering and are the most likely to achieve LDL goals. They are the easiest for patients to take and maximize compliance. Additionally, the statins have clear data that they decrease morbidity and mortality as both primary and secondary prevention.

A BAR should be used when additional LDL reduction is needed.

Niacin should be used for the management of triglyceride elevations, low HDL concentrations, and in patients with pattern B dyslipidemia.

Gemfibrozil should be used when niacin is contraindicated, or as a specific treatment for elevated triglycerides.

Followup Recommendations

It is important to individualize the plan of care. Motivation for long-term changes and medications may prove difficult for some patients. Followup must allow time to discuss compliance with the plan, modify medications, and consider relaxing some restrictions on diet.

General followup on each visit should include investigation of risk factors for the development of possible complications including coronary heart disease, cerebrovascular disease, and peripheral vascular disease. Weight, vital signs, and discussion about diet and the long-term plan must be part of each visit.

Laboratory measurements should include cholesterol and LDL levels in 4 to 6 weeks and then again at 3 months following the institution of dietary changes. If LDL is lowered to between 100 and 130 mg/dL with dietary changes, check in 3 months and then every year. When the patient is on medications as well as a diet, lipid profiles should be done 2 to 4 times a year.

Liver function tests should be performed at baseline and periodically for up to 1 year to monitor for hepatotoxicity associated with the statins; however, clinicians should realize that monitoring varies greatly, as listed in the package insert, from one agent to the next.

REFERENCES

Abrams, J. (1991). Angina pectoris: Mechanisms, diagnosis, and therapy. *Cardiology Clinics, 9*(1), 1.

Akhtar, W., Reeves, W., & Movahed, A. (1998, July 29). Indications for anticoagulation in atrial fibrillation. *American Family Physicians.*

ALLHAT Officers for ALLHAT Collaborative Research Group. (2000). ALLHAT results. *Journal of the American Medical Association, 283*(15), 1967–1975.

American Heart Association. (2002). Biostatistical fact sheet. *International Cardiovasuclar Disease Statistics.* http://www.americanheart.org

American Heart Association/Emergency Cardiac Care Committee. (2000). 2000 ACLS Guidelines: Primary Goal of AHA/ECC. Circulation, 102, 1–3.

Arauz-Pacheco, C., Parrott, M., & Raskin, P. (2002). Morbidity and mortality in patients with hypertension. *Diabetes Care, 25*(1), 134–142.

Arnstein, P., Buselli, E., & Rankin, S. (1996). Women and heart attacks: Prevention, diagnosis, and care. *Nurse Practitioner, 21*(5), 57–69.

Barrett-Connor, E., & Bush, T. L. (1991). Estrogen and coronary heart disease in women. *JAMA, 265,* 1861–1867.

Basile, J.N. (2002). Analysis of recent papers in hypertension. *Journal of Clinical Hypertension, 8*(23), 235–46.

Bauman, J. L., Parker, R. B., & McCollam, P. L. (1995). *Tachycardias. Pharmacotherapy self-assessment program* (2nd ed.). American College of Clinical Pharmacy, Kansas City, MO.

Brater, D. C. (1985). Resistance to loop diuretics. Why it happens and what to do about it. *Drugs, 30,* 427–443.

Brown, E. J., & Kloner, R. (1990). Angina pectoris. In R. Kloner (Ed.), *The guide to cardiology* (2nd ed.) (pp. 173–198). New York: LeJacq Communications.

Chen, B. P., & Chow, M. S. (1997). Focus on carvedilol: A novel beta adrenergic blocking agent for the treatment of congestive heart failure. *Formulary, 32*(8), 795–805.

Chenoweth, C. E., & Burket, J. S. (1997). Antimicrobial prophylaxis: Principles and practice. *Formulary, 32,* 692–713.

Coffman, J. D. (1991). Raynaud's phenomenon: An update. *Hypertension, 17,* 593.

Cohn, J. N. (1996). The management of chronic heart failure. *New England Journal of Medicine, 335,* 490–498.

Culy, C.R., & Jarvis, B. (2002). Quinapril: A further update of its pharmacology and therapeutic use in cardiovascular disorders. *Drugs, 62*(2), 339–385.

Dunphy, L., & Winland-Brown, J. (2000). *Primary care: The art and science of advanced practice nursing.* Philadelphia: F.A. Davis.

Elliott, W., & Black, H. (2002). Treatment of hypertension in the elderly. *American Journal of Geriatric Cardiology, 11*(1), 11–21.

Echt, D. S., Liebson, P. R., Mitchell, B., et al. (1991). Mortality and morbidity in patients receiving encainide, flecainide, or placebo. The cardiac arrhythmia suppression trial. *New England Journal of Medicine, 324,* 781–788.

Expert Panel on Detection, Evaluation, and Treatment of High Blood Cholesterol in Adults. (2001). Executive summary of the Third Report of the National Cholesterol Education Program (NCEP) Expert Panel on Detection, Evaluation, and Treatment of High Blood Cholesterol in Adults (Adult Treatment Panel III). NIH 01-3670 2001. National Institute of Health: National Heart, Lung & Blood Institute.

Fortuin, N. J. (1996). Valvular heart disease. In J. D. Stobo, D. B. Hellmann, P. W. Landenson, et al. (Eds.), *The principles and practice of medicine* (23rd ed.) (pp. 59–67). Stamford, CT: Appleton & Lange.

Fuster, J. (2001). ACC/AHA/ESC Guidelines for the management of atrial fibrillation. *Journal of the American College of Cardiology, 38,* 1266–87.

Goldman, L., & Bennett, J. C. (2000). *Cecil textbook of medicine.* Philadelphia: W.B. Saunders Co.

Golzari, H., Cebul, R. D., & Bahler, R. C. (1996). Atrial fibrillation: Restoration and maintenance of sinus rhythm and indications for anticoagulation therapy. *Annals of Internal Medicine, 125,* 311–323.

Goroll, A., & Mulley, A. (2000). *Primary care medicine: Office evaluation and management of the adult patient.* Philadelphia: Lippincott, Williams and Wilkins.

Gotto, A.M. (2001). Contemporary diagnosis and management of lipid disorders. (2nd ed.). Newton, PA: *Handbooks in Health Care Co.*

Grady, D., Rubin, S. M., Pettiti, D. B., et al. (1992). Hormone therapy to prevent disease and prolong life in postmenopausal women. *Annals of Internal Medicine, 117,* 1016–1037.

Greenlund, K., Giles, W., Keenan, N., Croft, J., & Mensah, G. (2002). Prevention of stroke through diet and exercise. *Stroke, 33*(2), 565–571.

Haak, S., Richardson, S., Davey, S., & Parker-Cohen, P. (1994). Alterations of cardiovascular function. In K. McCance & S. Huether, *Pathophysiology: The biologic basis for disease in adults and children* (2nd ed.) (pp. 1000–1084). St. Louis: C. V. Mosby.

Haitt, W. (2001). Medical treatment of peripheral arterial disease and claudication. *New England Journal of Medicine, 344,* 1608–1621.

Haji, S., & Movahed, A. (2000, July). Update on digoxin therapy in congestive heart failure. *American Family Physician.*

Hancock, E. (1996). Valvular heart disease. In D. Dale & D. Federman (Eds.), *Scientific American medicine* (1 Card XI 1–16). New York: Scientific American.

Hayes, S., & Taler, S. (1998). Hypertension in women: Current understanding of gender differences. *Mayo Clinic Proceedings, 73*(2), 157–165.

HFSA Guidelines. (1999). Management of patients with heart failure caused by left ventricular systolic dysfunction—pharmacological approaches. *Journal of Cardiac Failure, 5,* 357–382.

Hubler, J. (2000). The 2000 Canadian hypertension working group recommendations: A summary. *Canadian Journal of Cardiology, 17*(5), 535–538.

Huffman, G. B. (1999). Stroke prevention in patients with atrial fibrillation. *The Journal of Cardiology, 27*(9), 334–350.

Hulley, S., Grady, D., & Bush, T. (1999). Hormone replacement therapy and secondary prevention of cardiovascular heart disease. *JAMA, 281* (9), 794–797.

Jacobson, S., Markowski, B., & Heywood, L. (2000). Heart disease: Pharmacologic management. *Annals of Internal Medicine, 113*(7), 549–554.

Joint National Committee on Prevention, Detection, Evaluation, and Treatment of High Blood Pressure. (2003). The seventh report of the joint national committee on prevention, detection, evaluation, and treatment of high blood pressure (JNC VII). *Hypertension, 42*(Dec. 2003), 1206–1252.

Karmazyn, A., Noble, T., & Florez, M. (2002). Management of hypercholesterol. *Drugs, 61*(3), p. 20-8 375–389.

Kinsella, A. (2002). American Heart Association issues and dietary guidelines. *Home Health Nursing, 20*(2), 86–88.

Kloner, R., & Dzau, V. (1990). Heart failure. In R. Kloner (Ed.), *The guide to cardiology* (2nd ed.) (pp. 359–381). New York: LeJacq Communications.

Klungel, O. H., Heckbert, S. R., Longstreth, Jr. W. T., Furberg, C. D., & Kaplan, R. C. (2001, January 8). Antihypertensive drug therapies and the risk of ischemic stroke. *Archives of Internal Medicine, 161,* 37–43.

Konstam, M., Dracup, K., et al. (1994). *Heart failure: Evaluation and care of patients with left-ventricular systolic dysfunction. Clinical practice guideline no. 11.* AHCPR publication no. 94-0612. Rockville, MD: Agency for Health Care Policy and Research, Public Health Service, U.S. Department of Health and Human Services.

Kostis, J. B., Davis, B. R., & Cutler, J. (1997). Prevention of heart failure by antihypertensive drug treatment in older persons with isolated systolic hypertension. *JAMA, 278,* 212–216.

Kradjan, W. (1993). Congestive heart failure. In M. Koda-Kimble & L. Young (Eds.), *Applied therapeutics* (5th ed.). Vancouver, WA: Applied Therapeutics.

Lapalio, L. R. (1995). Hypertension in the elderly. *American Family Physician, 52,* 1161–1165.

Leonetti, G., & Zanchetti, A. (2002). Results of antihypertensive treatment trials in the elderly. *American Journal of Geriatric Cardiology, 11*(1), 41–57.

Massie, B. (1996). Heart. In L. Tierney, S. McPhee, & M. Papadakis (Eds.), *Current medical diagnosis and treatment* (35th ed.) (pp. 295–403). Stamford, CT: Appleton & Lange.

McKenney, J. M., Proctor, J. D., Harris, S., et al. (1994). A comparison of the efficacy and toxic effects of sustained- vs. immediate-release niacin in hypercholesterolemia patients. *JAMA, 271,* 672–677.

McMurray, J., & Pfeffer, M. A. (2002). New therapeutic options in congestive heart failure: Part II. *Circulation, 105*(18), 2223–2228.

Moore, T., Conlin, P., Ard, J., & Svetkay, L. (2002). DASH diet is effective treatment for stage 1 isolated systolic hypertension. *Hypertension, 38*(2), 155–158.

Mulrow, C., Lau, J., Cornell, J., & Brand, M. (2002). Pharmacotherapy for hypertension in the elderly. *Chrane Abstract Review.*

National Cholesterol Education Program: Third report of the expert panel on detection, evaluation, and treatment of high blood cholesterol in adults (Adult treatment panel III). National Heart, Lung, and Blood Institute, Bethesda, MD. NIH Publication No. 01–3305.

Niskanen, L., Hedner, T., Hansson, L., Lanke, J. & Nikolas, A. (2001). Reduced cardiovascular morbidity and mortality. *Diabetic Care, 24*(12), 2091–2096.

O'Keefe, J. H. (1995). Insights into the pathogenesis and prevention of coronary artery disease. Treatment of mild hypertension study research group. *Mayo Clinic Proceedings, 70,* 69.

Packer, M., Narahara, K. A., Elkayam, U., et al. (1993). Double blind, placebo controlled study of the efficacy of flosequinan in patients with chronic heart failure. Principal investigators of the REFLECT Study. *Journal of the American College of Cardiology, 22,* 65.

Prystowsky, E. N., Benson, D. W., Fuster, V., et al. (1996). Management of patients with atrial fibrillation. A statement for healthcare professionals from the Subcommittee on Electrocardiograph and Electrophysiology, American Heart Association. *Circulation, 93,* 1262–1277.

Psaty, B. M., Heckbert, S. R., Koepsell, T. D., et al. (1995). The risk of myocardial infarction associated with antihypertensive drug therapies. *JAMA, 274,* 620–625.

Puschett, J. B. (2000). Diuretics and the therapy of hypertension. *American Journal of the Medical Sciences, 319*(1).

Roath, S. (1989). Management of Raynaud's phenomenon. Focus on new treatments. *Drugs, 37,* 700–712.

Scheinfeld, R. M. (2001). Management of peripheral arterial disease and intermittent claudication, *Journal American Board of Family Practice, 14*(6), 443–445.

Schlant, P., Applegate, E., Broder, M., & Piephro, T. (2002). *Calcium channel blockers revisited. Monograph.* Atlanta, GA: Emory University.

Strazzullo, P. (2002). Salt in hypertension. *Journal of Hypertension, 20*(4), 561–563.

The seventh report of the Joint National Committee on Prevention, Detect, Evaluation, and Treatment of High Blood Pressure: The JNC VII Report. (2003). *JAMA, 289:* 2560–2572.

Systolic Hypertension in the Elderly Program Cooperative Research Group. (1993). Implications of the systolic hypertension in the elderly program. *Hypertension, 21,* 335–343.

Tobian, L., Brunner, H. R., Cohn, J. N., et al. (1994). Modern strategies to prevent coronary sequelae and stroke in hypertensive patients differ from the JNC V consensus guidelines. *American Journal of Hypertension, 7,* 859–872.

Wallingford, A. (2000). Beta blockers and heart disease. *Lancet, 35*(4), 1751–1756.

Weir, M. R. (1996). Angiotensin-II receptor antagonists: A new class of antihypertensive agents. *American Family Physician, 53,* 589–594.

Weir, M.R., Maibach, E. W., & Bakin, G. L. (2000). Implications of a health lifestyle and medication analysis for improving hypertensive control. *Archives of Internal Medicine, 160*(4), 481–490.

White, C. M. & Chow, M. S. (1997). Pharmacologic management of congestive heart failure. *U.S. Pharmacist, 22,* 117–125.

Wierzbicki, A. S., & Mikhailidis, D. P. (2002). Beyond LDL-C the importance of raising HDL-C. *Current Medical Research and Opinion, 18*(1), 36–44.

CHAPTER ❖ 21

UPPER RESPIRATORY DISORDERS

Jill E. Winland-Brown

Many patients seen by primary care providers on a daily basis present with some form of upper respiratory disorder. Patient education can help prevent or reduce the severity of some of these disorders as well as ameliorate their condition during the course of the illness. These disorders collectively result in millions of hours lost from school or work and millions of dollars paid out for remedies good and ill-advised. Patient distress is real, whether the cause is a relatively benign common cold or a life-threatening attack of epiglottitis. Signs and symptoms can be difficult to differentiate initially because multiple conditions can result in rhinorrhea, aches, fatigue, and coughs. Meticulous history taking, a comprehensive physical examination, and/or diagnostic testing can help determine if these symptoms are indicative of allergic rhinitis, the common cold, sinusitis, pharyngitis, or croup, the subjects of this chapter.

ALLERGIC RHINITIS

Allergic rhinitis is the most common chronic nasal problem in the United States, affecting approximately 20 to 40 million people. While 10 to 30% of all adults, most commonly between 30 to 40 years of age, are affected, up to 40% of children, typically beginning around age 10, are also affected (Dunphy & Porter, 2001; Kaiser, Mellon & Elder, (2001). Symptoms often lead to discomfort, absenteeism from school and work, daytime fatigue due to sleep loss, reduced ability to concentrate, decreased quality of life, and expenditure of billions of dollars for healthcare (Dunphy & Porter, 2001; Kaiser, Mellon, & Elder, 2001).

Allergic rhinitis is an immunologically mediated condition stimulated by a type 1 antigen-antibody reaction (Kaiser et al., 2001). When an individual, often with a genetic predisposition to an allergy, is exposed to a specific antigen, allergen-specific IgE molecules are produced and then bind to mast cells in the respiratory epithelium. Reexposure to offending allergic stimuli results in degranulation of mast cells and basophils, which triggers the release of histamines, kinins, prostaglandins, and esterases, causing an immediate local vasodilation, mucosal edema, and increased mucous production. About half of all patients with allergic rhinitis develop a late phase reaction 4 to 6 hours later with an additional release of histamine and cellular infiltration of eosinophils, basophils, neutrophils, and mononuclear cells. This late-phase reaction results in hyperresponsiveness to antigenic and nonantigenic stimuli and has been linked to the development of chronic disease (Kaiser et al., 2001).

The most common form of allergic rhinitis has a seasonal pattern and is mainly associated with inhalant pollen allergens from trees, grass, and ragweed. The year-round, perennial type of allergic rhinitis is caused by dust mites, cockroaches, molds, and animal dander. A variety of other irritants aggravate allergic rhinitis such as tobacco, fires, cold, polluted air, and perfumes. In addition to environmental sources, genetic factors play an important role. Persons with allergic rhinitis often have a positive family history of the condition (Kaiser et al., 2001).

A triad of nasal congestion, sneezing, and clear rhinorrhea is most characteristic of allergic rhinitis. Coughing, itching of the nose, throat, and eyes, complaints of postnasal drip, puffiness, red watery eyes, and a sense of fullness in the ears may occur. The onset of symptoms is usually between the ages of 10 and 20 years. Chronic allergic rhinitis is a predisposing factor for the development and exacerbation of asthma, sinusitis, nasal polyposis, and otitis media (Kaiser et al., 2001).

SPECIFIC CONSIDERATIONS FOR PHARMACOTHERAPY

When Drug Therapy Is Needed

When allergen avoidance is ineffective or impractical, drug therapy is indicated. Antihistamines, decongestants, nasal cromolyn, and/or nasal corticosteroids are all effective in reducing or preventing symptoms.

Antihistamines control symptoms of sneezing, rhinorrhea, nasal pruritis, and conjunctivitis by blocking the effects of histamine on end organs (Kaiser et al., 2001). First-generation oral antihistamines are inexpensive and considered first-line therapy. Second-generation antihistamines such as loratadine and fexofenadine do not readily cross the blood-brain barrier, resulting in minimal sedation, and have minimal anticholinergic properties. Cetirizine, considered a second-generation antihistamine, is an active metabolite of hydroxyzine and possesses mild sedative properties. Desloratadine is an active metabolite of loratadine and is nonsedating. (Kaiser et al., 2001). See Drug Table 705.

Levocabastine and azelastine are topical antihistamines that are effective in reducing allergic ocular symptoms.

Because antihistamines do not relieve nasal congestion, decongestants are sometimes required. Decongestants are sympathomimetics that cause vasoconstriction by stimulating alpha-adrenergic receptors in the nasal mucosa. Decongestants decrease tissue edema and nasal congestion, and they improve nasal airway patency and ventilation. Decongestants can be administered in oral or topical forms. Oral decongestants are often given in combination products with antihistamines to improve compliance, enhance effectiveness, and counterbalance the sedative effects of antihistamines. Topical decongestants are indicated for short-term use in patients with severe nasal congestion who need rapid relief. They may also be used prior to application of intranasal corticosteroids to reduce turbinate swelling and facilitate delivery and action of the steroid. See Drug Table 703.

Although the exact mechanism of action is unknown, topical intranasal corticosteroids reduce nasal vasodilation, edema, and inflammation. Intranasal corticosteroids may be combined with antihistamines for enhanced effectiveness in reducing allergic reactions. Using corticosteroids intranasally can achieve high drug concentrations at receptor sites in the nasal mucosa with minimal risk of systemic effects (Kaiser et al., 2001). In contrast, systemic corticosteroids can cause numerous and possibly serious adverse reactions. Thus, oral corticosteroids are reserved for short-term therapy in patients with severe, debilitating rhinitis. See Drug Table 706.

Intranasal cromolyn sodium may also be effective in treating some patients with allergic rhinitis, particularly patients with high immunoglobulin E (IgE) levels. Cromolyn sodium interferes with the degranulation of sensitized mast cells and is effective in relieving itching, sneezing, and rhinorrhea, but is less efficacious in treating nasal obstruction than other therapies.

Intranasal ipratropium bromide is effective for symptomatic relief of rhinorrhea associated with allergic and nonallergic perennial rhinitis or symptomatic relief of rhinorrhea associated with the common cold in patients ≥12 years of age. Intranasal anticholinergics have an excellent safety profile and cause few side effects. Although these drugs reduce rhinorrhea, they have a minimal effect on nasal congestion as compared to intranasal corticosteroids.

Short-Term and Long-Term Goals of Pharmacotherapy

The short-term goal of pharmacotherapy is to eliminate, control, or reduce the symptoms arising from allergen triggers and inflammation while simultaneously minimizing the adverse side effects of therapy. The long-term goal is to prevent the onset of symptoms of allergic rhinitis and mimimize complications. Patients should be educated in the ways they can help themselves prevent and treat their own symptoms. See Table 21–1.

Time Frame for Initiating Pharmacotherapy

Patients who have seasonal allergic rhinitis should begin pharmacological therapy 1 to 2 weeks before the anticipated season of sensitivity and onset of symptoms. In contrast, perennial allergic rhinitis is treated year-round. Medications should be taken regularly rather than intermittently after symptoms have developed. See Drug Table 705.

TABLE 21–1. How Patients Can Help Themselves Prevent and Treat Allergic Rhinitis

Prevention	
Control the Home Environment	
	Frequent vacuuming, damp mopping, and dusting with damp cloth
	Preferably have someone else clean, or wear facemask for 10–15 minutes after cleaning
	Use vacuum cleaner with double filtration system
	Use air conditioning during summer months
	Change air conditioner filter monthly
	Use dehumidifier in damp areas
	Keep doors and windows closed to decrease in flux of pollen and mold
	Eliminate carpets
	Avoid upholstered furniture
	Eliminate unwashable toys
	Cover mattresses and pillows with bacteria reducing cloth barriers
	Keep pets out of bedroom
	If allergic to cats and insist on keeping them, wipe cats with damp cloth every night
Reduce other Allergens and Irritants	
	Wear protective mask when outside or mowing lawn
	Wear long-sleeve shirts and pants when gardening
	Determine what triggers allergic reactions and avoiding offenders
	Stop smoking or avoiding second-hand smoke and other irritants
Treatment	
	Exercise regularly
	Use nasal saline sprays

Assessment Prior to Therapy

A *history* of onset, characteristics, duration, progression, and pattern of the symptoms should be obtained. Explore potential triggers such as exposure to animal dander, newly mown grass, pollen, dust, or mold, and ask about family history, other atopic diseases, and previous self-treatments.

In the *physical examination,* inspect the eyes for signs typical of allergic rhinitis: tearing, lid swelling, periorbital edema, conjunctival injection, and darkening under the eyes (i.e., allergic shiners). The nasal mucosa of patients with allergic rhinitis is pale and boggy, with a clear discharge. The pharynx should be observed for postnasal drip, tonsilar enlargement, and mild erythema (Kaiser et al., 2001). The lymph nodes, sinuses, nasal cavity, ears, and lungs should be carefully assessed to assist in differential diagnoses that may include vasomotor rhinitis, persistent infectious rhinitis, chronic sinusitis, rhinitis of pregnancy, hypothyroidism, adverse drug reactions, rhinitis medicamentosa, and mechanical obstruction (Kaiser et al., 2001). While empiric therapy is usually tried initially, diagnostic testing may be helpful.

Diagnostic testing is needed when the patient's symptoms are severe and do not respond to allergen avoidance and medications or when immunotherapy is being considered. A nasal smear positive for eosinophils may assist in the diagnosis of allergic rhinitis. Skin testing, either epicutaneous or intradermal, is the preferred means for confirming a diagnosis of allergic rhinitis, although it is time consuming and expensive. A blood test, radioallergosorbent testing (RAST), is an in vitro assay of specific IgE molecules, but is expensive and only covers specific allergens.

Patient/Caregiver Information

Antihistamines have many side effects. Warn patients of the possibility of drowsiness and decreased ability to perform certain skills such as driving and use of machinery when taking sedating antihistamines (occurs in about 40% of patients taking first-generation antihistamines). Inform patients that some antihistamines have strong anticholinergic properties, which may cause dry mouth, constipation, and urinary retention (Kaiser et al., 2001). These untoward effects may be reduced by starting with low doses and gradually increasing the dosage over several days or advising the patient to take initial doses at bedtime. Remind patients to take antihistamines regularly to prevent symptoms and to allow the body time to adjust to unwanted sedation.

Patients should inform their healthcare provider that they are taking antihistamines. Sedating antihistamines can potentiate the effects of agents that cause central nervous system alterations such as alcohol, antianxiety agents, antipsychotics, and narcotic analgesics. First-generation antihistamines may have additive anticholinergic activity when administered concurrently with tricyclic antidepressants, antispasmodics, and antiparkinsonian medications (Ferguson, 1997).

Patients should be taught to read drug labels before taking any over-the-counter medication since many cold products and sleep aids contain antihistamines.

Advise patients that intranasal decongestants may cause rebound congestion and should therefore be used for only 3 days. Teach patients that intranasal corticosteroids often have a delayed onset of activity and that symptoms may not improve for 1 to 2 weeks after starting therapy. Remind patients to take these drugs daily rather than sporadically or on an as-needed basis.

Because cromolyn nasal spray is ineffective in reducing allergic symptoms that are already present, advise patients that relief of symptoms may be delayed as long as 3 to 4 weeks when therapy is initiated. Addition of an antihistamine may be necessary until cromolyn reaches its full effect.

Intranasal medications must come in contact with the entire nasal mucosa to be effective. Therefore, nasal passages should be cleared prior to administering medications. Spray the medication quickly and firmly into the nostril while keeping the head upright. Spray each nostril separately and wait at least 1 min before the second spray. If possible, avoid sneezing or blowing the nose for 5 to 10 min after using an intranasal inhaler. Cleanse the medicine canister device after each use to reduce the chance of contamination. Medications that are delivered intranasally may cause irritation and bleeding of the nasal mucosa, sneezing, epistaxis, and headache (Kaiser et al., 2001).

OUTCOMES MANAGEMENT

Selecting Appropriate Agents

Antihistamines. Antihistamines are classified into two groups: first-generation and second-generation antihistamines. First-generation antihistamines include agents such as the alkylamines: brompheniramine, chlorpheniramine, and dexbrompheniramine; and ethanolamines: clemastine and diphenhydramine. Second-generation antihistamines include cetirizine, fexofenadrine, loratadine, and desloratadine. While all antihistamines tend to be effective, the second-generation ones are usually preferred due to their nonsedating effect. Selection of an agent should be based more upon duration of action, side-effect profile, risk of drug interactions, and cost. Patient noncompliance may be the largest predictor of treatment failure. Antihistamine therapy for allergic rhinitis should be initiated with the least expensive first-generation antihistamine. The most commonly used agent is diphenhydramine. Although sedation is an undesirable adverse effect of these agents, it may be minimized by slow dosage titration beginning with administration at bedtime only. After several days of bedtime dosing, a small morning dose may be added and increased based on symptom control and adverse effects. Tolerance to the sedative effects generally occurs after 1 to 2 weeks of continued dosing.

Because of the cost, second-generation antihistamines should be reserved for those patients unable to tolerate the traditional agents. These agents may be dosed once daily for enhanced patient compliance, with the exception of fexofenadine, which requires either once or twice daily administration depending on the dose. Decongestants may be added separately or in combined preparations with antihistamines to relieve nasal congestion not mediated by histamine receptors. See Drug Table 705.

Decongestants. Decongestants may be administered topically or orally to patients with nasal congestion as a symptom of allergic rhinitis. For short-term relief of nasal congestion or to enhance the delivery of an intranasal corticosteroid spray, topical phenylephrine, naphazoline, or oxymetazoline may be used for 3 to 5 days. Further use may be complicated by rebound congestion known as rhinitis medicamentosa. Pseudoephedrine is the most effective oral decongestant available. Oral decongestants may increase blood pressure, pulse rate, intraocular pressure, and urinary sphincter constriction. Therefore, these agents should be used with caution in patients with arrhythmias, coronary heart disease, hypertension, hyperthyroidism, glaucoma, diabetes, and prostatic hypertrophy. Dizziness and palpitations from the decongestant might be misinterpreted as a loss of glycemic control, which is why they are used with caution in patients with diabetes mellitus (Kaiser et al., 2001).

Contraindications to decongestant use include concomitant use of other sympathomimetic drugs, monoamine oxidase inhibitors, or tricyclic antidepressants. Their combined use may result in an additive effect with a resultant hypertensive crisis (Kaiser et al., 2001). See Drug Table 703.

Corticosteroids. Intranasal corticosteroids are effective in controlling all symptoms of allergic rhinitis. Available products include beclomethasone, budesonide, flunisolide, fluticasone, triamcinolone, and mometasone. Budesonide, fluticasone, triamcinolone, and mometasone are effective if administered on a once-daily regimen. Budesonide, triamcinolone, and flunisolide contain solvents that may be irritating to the nasal mucosa of some patients. Aqueous formulations of beclomethasone, triamcinolone acetonide, budesonide, and fluticasone are available and better tolerated. The relative cost of these agents varies, with triamcinolone and beclomethasone being the least expensive. Emphasis should be placed on regular use of these products versus on an as-needed basis. These agents should be added to antihistamine therapy as an adjunct to control nasal congestion or if antihistamine therapy fails to control symptoms (Dunphy & Porter, 2001: Kaiser et al., 2001).

Cromolyn sodium and ipratropium. Cromolyn sodium is a mast-cell stabilizer that may have utility in perennial allergic rhinitis if other therapies prove unsuccessful. It should be used to prevent symptoms from starting and not on an as-needed basis, for which it is generally ineffective. Mast-cell stabilizers should be reserved for those patients with chronic or severe symptoms. Cromolyn sodium has no known drug interactions, a good safety profile, and is available as a metered dose inhaler over the counter (Kaiser et al., 2001).

Ipratropium bromide is an anticholinergic agent that has no effect on histamine or other mediators of allergic rhinitis. While it is effective for relieving rhinorrhea, it does not help with nasal pruritis, congestion, sneezing, or ocular symptoms. This prescription-only drug should not be ordered for patients with closed angle glaucoma or patients with prostatic hypertrophy, especially if they are already taking an anticholinergic agent (Kaiser et al., 2001).

Leukotriene Modifiers. While leukotriene modifiers are used to manage asthma, their use in allergic rhinitis is being explored because of the role that leukotrienes play in this condition. Zafirlukast is being used in several studies to test the efficacy of its use in allergic rhinitis. This drug should not be routinely used for this purpose until the studies show evidence of its efficacy.

Monitoring for Efficacy

Antihistamine. Symptomatic relief begins to occur within several hours of administration but may take 2 to 4 weeks to reach its maximum effect. All antihistamines should be administered for 2 to 3 weeks prior to switching to an agent of another class.

Decongestants. An oral decongestant may be added if nasal congestion is not relieved by an antihistamine. Symptomatic improvement should occur within several hours of oral administration. Topical decongestants have a very rapid onset of action, usually relieving nasal congestion within minutes.

Corticosteroids. Most patients achieve moderate to significant symptomatic improvement within 2 to 4 weeks of initiating intranasal corticosteroid therapy, provided it is used on a continuous and regular basis. A trial of 8 weeks may be necessary for assessing efficacy. Patients are generally started on the maximum recommended dose. If nasal symptoms are controlled, the dose may be gradually reduced to the lowest effective dose. Each new dose should be continued for at least 1 week before any subsequent changes are made. Oral corticosteroids may be used for a "jump start" for a short 3 to 7 day period if symptoms are severe or if nasal polyps are present and refractory to other therapy. By then, symptomatic relief from intranasal corticosteroids should occur. Long-term oral corticosteroid therapy is not recommended due to the adverse effects of steroid therapy.

Cromolyn Sodium. Mast-cell stabilizers are used to prevent the symptoms of allergic rhinitis from initiating. Mast-cell stabilizers are expensive and require frequency of dosing, which can create compliance problems. Two or more weeks may be required before the beneficial effects of therapy are achieved.

Monitoring for Toxicity

Antihistamines. The adverse-effect profile of first-generation antihistamines includes anticholinergic as well as histamine-blocking effects. Antagonism of central histamine receptors may result in sedation, dizziness, and paradoxical excitation in children and the elderly. Anticholinergic effects may include dry mouth, urinary retention, constipation, and blurred vision. Second-generation antihistamines are devoid of or have minimal sedative properties because of their reduced lipophilicity compared to first-generation agents.

Decongestants. Adverse effects from decongestants result from central nervous system (CNS) stimulation caused by sympathomimetic effects. These include nervousness, restlessness, insomnia, tremor, dizziness, and headache. These adverse effects may counteract the sedative effects of antihistamine therapy. Tachycardia, palpitations, and elevations of blood pressure have been known to occur.

Corticosteroids. Intranasal corticosteroids are generally well tolerated. Nasal stinging and burning may occur and are more common with beclomethasone and flunisolide because of propellants. Aqueous formulations of beclomethasone and fluticasone are available and better tolerated. Improper administration of these agents can result in rare complications such as hemorrhagic crusting, ulceration, and perforation. See Drug Table 706.

Cromolyn Sodium. Adverse effects occur in less than 10% of patients. Common adverse effects associated with the use of intranasal mast-cell stabilizers include sneezing, nasal stinging and burning, and head-aches.

COMMON COLD

The common cold is the leading cause of acute morbidity as well as absenteeism from work and school. Children have approximately six to eight colds annually, whereas adults generally have two to four colds per year. Although colds are the most frequent reason for visiting healthcare providers, most colds can be effectively self-treated at home with over-the-counter medications and home remedies.

Common colds may be caused by multiple viruses. Rhinoviruses and corona-viruses are the most common viruses causing colds. In young children respiratory syncytial virus (RSV) is a common pathogen. Viral invasion of the upper respiratory tract inflames all or part of the mucosal membranes from the nose to the oropharynx. Transmission of the virus occurs through direct contact with infectious secretions on skin and environmental surfaces, brief transportation of large particles of respiratory secretions in the air, and airborne droplets (Dunphy & Porter, 2001).

Symptoms are usually self-limiting, lasting approximately 5 to 7 days. Patients typically complain of nasal discharge, congestion or obstruction, sneezing, coughing, postnasal discharge, sore throat, and hoarseness. Low-grade fever, headache, malaise, and inflamed, watery conjunctivae may be present. Complications of the common cold are unusual, other than transient middle ear effusion, although secondary bacterial infections may occur. These may lead to otitis media, sinusitis, pneumonia, and asthmatic bronchitis (Jackler & Kaplan, 2002).

SPECIFIC CONSIDERATIONS FOR PHARMACOTHERAPY

When Drug Therapy Is Needed

Decongestants are useful agents for the relief of cold symptoms and are beneficial in preventing sinus and eustachian tube obstruction that may lead to sinusitis and otitis media. Decongestants cause vasoconstriction and reduce nasal secretions and congestion, thereby improving nasal airway patency and ventilation. Although topical decongestants are effective for short-term therapy and provide a rapid decrease in nasal airway resistance, they have the potential to produce rebound congestion if used for more than 3 to 5 days (Jackler & Kaplan, 2002). Oral decongestants are best when treatment is needed for more than 3 to 4 days.

Cough suppressants such as codeine or dextromethorphan are beneficial when patients are unable to sleep or rest due to hacking, nonproductive coughs. However, suppression of a productive cough may lead to serious complications such as pneumonia because the body is unable to clear the lungs and airways of unwanted material.

Antihistamines and expectorants are available in many over-the-counter medications. Antihistamines are not effective because nasal congestion in colds is not mediated by histamine receptors. Therefore, antihistamines have no role in the management of the common cold. Antihistamines have anticholinergic effects that dry mucous membranes, which may be beneficial; but antihistamines can also exacerbate symptoms and increase upper airway obstruction by impairing the flow of mucus. While expectorants may work for some people in assisting them to clear their airways of mucus, the most cost-effective way is by being well hydrated with water.

Other pharmacological therapies that may prove helpful for the common cold include vitamin C and zinc echinacea lozenges.

Short-Term and Long-Term Goals of Pharmacotherapy

The goals are to relieve symptoms, reduce the risk of developing complications, and reduce the transmission of viral infection to others. Educate your patients in the ways they can help themselves prevent and treat their own symptoms; see Table 21–2.

Time Frame for Initiating Pharmacotherapy

Pharmacotherapy is needed for comfort and should be initiated only when cold-related symptoms are intolerable. Topical decongestants should be used for no longer than 3 to 5 days. See Drug Tables 703–707.

TABLE 21–2. How Patients Can Help Themselves Prevent and Treat Upper Respiratory Infections

Prevention
- Wash hands frequently to reduce spread of microorganisms
- Try to avoid people with colds or being in congested areas, especially during peak infectious seasons
- Stop smoking or avoid second-hand smoke and other irritants
- Avoid allergens and excessively dry heat
- Use a disinfectant spray occasionally on telephone mouthpieces, TV remote controls, and doorknobs
- Buy new toothbrushes for all family members every three months

Treatment
- Humidair
- Increase fluid intake
- Rest
- Regular nasal hygiene with a saline irrigation
- Steam inhalation and warm compresses if patient has sinus pressure
- Elevate head of bed when sleeping to facilitate sinus drainage
- In younger children with nasal congestion, clear the nose with bulb syringe
- Hard candy, lozenges, or warm saline gargles for sore throats
- Tylenol for aches and pains

Assessment Prior to Therapy

Obtain a *history* of the course and characteristics of symptoms. Assess for complications by questioning the patient about fevers, headaches, facial pain, severe sore throat, persistent cough, wheezing, and chest pain.

The *physical examination* should focus on the nose, pharynx, and lungs. In addition, the sinuses should be percussed and transilluminated. The ears should be examined, and lymph nodes should be palpated.

Diagnostic testing is not indicated unless complications are suspected.

Patient/Caregiver Information

Tactfully discuss the use and abuse of over-the-counter cold remedies. Explain that most colds are self-limited and resolve without any drug treatment. Emphasize that cold remedies are used to relieve symptoms and prevent complications rather than cure the infection. Teach patients to read labels on all medications bought for self-treatment. Most over-the-counter medications contain a combination of ingredients such as decongestants, antihistamines, analgesics, and expectorants that are usually ineffective in relieving symptoms and may cause adverse effects. A nasal spray such as oxymetazoline or phenylephrine may be rapidly effective but only for a few days. If symptoms are intolerable, suggest the patient use a single-ingredient cold medicine containing a decongestant. Warn patients with diabetes, hypertension, glaucoma, and benign prostatic hypertrophy to use decongestants cautiously and only after consultation with their health care provider (Jackler & Kaplan, 2002).

OUTCOMES MANAGEMENT

Selecting Appropriate Agents

Decongestants. Topical decongestants such as phenylephrine and oxymetazoline nasal sprays are currently recommended to relieve symptoms of nasal congestion and promote drainage of nasal secretions in patients with the common cold. They have a rapid onset of action and are devoid of drug–disease state interactions of oral decongestants. Oral decongestants are preferred if therapy continues longer than 3 to 5 days. Pseudoephedrine is a suitable first-line agent and is present in many over-the-counter cough and cold preparations. Some authorities recommend use of name brand pseudoephedrine products. Bioequivalence is not uniform between slow-release pseudoephedrine preparations and immediate-release products. Because of the age of this agent, it is exempt from regulation by the Food and Drug Administration. Phenylephrine is not useful as an oral decongestant because of its extensive first-pass metabolism, resulting in poor bioavailability. Children typically do not respond to over-the-counter antihistamine-decongestant combinations and their routine use is not recommended. See Drug Table 703.

Antitussives. Dextromethorphan and codeine may be helpful in suppressing a cough. A nonproductive cough should generally be suppressed only if it interferes with sleep. See Drug Table 704.

Expectorants. Maintaining an adequate fluid intake through the liberal consumption of water may prove to be the best expectorant. Guaifenesin, an ingredient in many over-the-counter cough and cold preparations, does not reduce cough frequency and provides no benefit as an expectorant. Coughs beginning after an upper respiratory infection usually respond to treatment with an antihistamine-decongestant combination (Chesnutt & Prendergast, 2002). See Drug Table 707.

Antipyretics/Analgesics. Nonsteroidal antiinflammatory agents (NSAID) such as indomethacin and naproxen are effective in reducing cough and relieving headache and fever. Aspirin and acetaminophen are effective analgesics and antipyretics. Aspirin should not be used in children or adolescents because of the risk of Reye's syndrome.

Anticholinergic Agents. Ipratropium bromide nasal spray may aid in the symptomatic relief or reduction of rhinorrhea and sneezing associated with the common cold. Because ipratropium is more expensive, oral decongestants should be tried initially.

Vitamin C. Vitamin C has long been used in the prevention and treatment of the common cold. The dosage remains controversial, but most authorities recommend 1000 mg 3 times per day for a slight decrease in the duration and severity of cold symptoms. Further research needs to be done in this area along with other vitamin and herbal remedies for viral rhinitis.

Zinc Gluconate. Zinc gluconate lozenges or zinc lozenges with echinacea also lack sufficient evidence regarding their effectiveness in treating the common cold. Usually one 15 mg lozenge is recommended every 3 hours while awake for 3 days. Use of these lozenges seem to reduce the severity of sore throat and hoarseness. The main adverse effects noted are nausea and a bad taste in the mouth.

Monitoring for Efficacy

Resolution of symptoms is the goal of all treatment modalities. If decongestants are not effective in relieving symptoms, addition of intranasal ipratropium bromide may prove useful. Cough suppression with dextromethorphan or codeine may be beneficial. If symptoms such as cough persist for longer than 1 week or are accompanied by high fever, rash, or persistent headache, the patient should be reevaluated for complications.

Monitoring for Toxicity

Refer to the Allergic Rhinitis section of this chapter for a detailed adverse-effect profile of decongestants and intranasal ipratropium bromide.

Dextromethorphan. The potential for toxic effects of dextromethorphan is very low. Adverse effects are rare. Nausea, drowsiness, and dizziness have been reported. Signs of acute toxicity may include blurred vision, nystagmus, ataxia, and shallow respirations.

Codeine. With oral antitussive doses of codeine, the frequency of adverse effects is low, but they include nausea, vomiting, constipation, dizziness, sedation, and palpitations. Codeine may be habit-forming. Respiratory depression with oral antitussive doses of codeine seldom occurs. Patients with asthma or pulmonary emphysema should be monitored closely for signs of respiratory insufficiency.

INFLUENZA

Influenza is a viral infection that occurs in epidemics lasting about 5 to 6 weeks. Persons over 70 years of age are affected four times more than persons under 40 years of age. Influenza viruses are of three antigenic types: A, B, and C. Although all three types can cause infections in humans, only types A and B can cause severe illness. Influenza is highly contagious and is transmitted by droplet nuclei rather than by fomites or large particle aerosols such as in respiratory synctial virus (RSV) or rhinoviruses. While scattered cases do occur, epidemics and pandemics appear typically during the fall or winter (Bouckenooghe & Shandera, 2002). Children are typically infected first and then transmit the virus to adults.

Characteristic symptoms include abrupt onset of fever, myalgia, sore throat, and nonproductive cough. In contrast to other upper respiratory infections, persons with influenza often suffer severe malaise that may last for several days. Complications include pneumonia, myositis, and central nervous system conditions. Elderly persons and individuals with chronic health problems are at increased risk for complications. Individuals over age 65 account for approximately 90% of the influenza-associated deaths in the United States, which is the reason for recommending flu shots annually in this age group.

SPECIFIC CONSIDERATIONS FOR PHARMACOTHERAPY

When Drug Therapy Is Needed

In the United States, two approaches are available to minimize the deleterious effects of influenza: immunoprophylaxis with inactivated vaccine and therapy with an antiviral drug. See Chapter 11 for discussion of the influenza vaccine.

Amantadine is approved for prophylaxis and treatment of influenza A in adults and children over 1 year of age. Rimantadine is approved for prophylaxis and treatment in adults, but only prophylaxis in children over the age of 1 year. Pharmacotherapy with amantadine and rimantadine is particularly important for unvaccinated elderly patients or patients with underlying medical problems who are at increased risk for complicated influenza infection Type A.

Other antiviral agents have been helpful in patients with severe cases of influenza A or B but are more costly. These are neuraminidase inhibitors such as inhaled zanamivir, given for 3 to 7 days, or oral oseltamivir. These agents are ordered within the first 48 hours of the appearance of symptoms in patients over 12 years of age. Antibacterial antibiotics are not effective in influenza unless there are bacterial complications. In febrile children, acetaminophen rather than aspirin should be administered (Bouckenooghe & Shandera, 2002).

Short-Term and Long-Term Goals of Pharmacotherapy

Goals of pharmacotherapy are to prevent influenza infections when used prophylactically and to reduce the duration and severity of symptoms in infected individuals. Patients should be advised that the best way to help themselves, once symptoms have begun, is to increase bed rest and fluid intake. See Table 21–2.

Time Frame for Initiating Pharmacotherapy

For reduction of signs and symptoms, pharmacotherapy should be started within 48 hours of illness onset or as soon as possible after symptoms are recognized. Pharmacotherapy should be discontinued as soon as clinically warranted or approximately 24 to 48 hours after the disappearance of signs and symptoms because of possible induction of antiviral resistance.

Assessment Prior to Therapy

During the history taking, question the patient about onset, characteristics, and duration of symptoms. Specifically inquire about myalgias and malaise, which are characteristic of influenza but are not typical in other upper respiratory infections. Determine whether the patient had an annual influenza vaccine. To identify possible complications of influenza, questions regarding chest pain, hemoptysis, severe muscle pain, and central nervous system problems such as confusion should be asked. Explore whether household members or close contacts of the patient are experiencing similar symptoms.

Observe for general appearance of lassitude and distress. Particularly in elderly patients and young children, assess hydration status. Thoroughly examine sinuses, ears, nose, throat, and chest. In severe cases, perform a complete abdominal and neurologic examination.

Diagnosis can usually be made from epidemiologic data obtained from a local or state health department that confirms influenza infection in a particular region or community. Typically, if an outbreak of influenza is in the area, diagnostic testing is not necessary but providers will treat the symptoms. The diagnosis may also be confirmed by viral culture, immunofluorescence staining, enzyme immunoassay, and/or rapid diagnostic testing of nasopharyngeal (nasal or throat) swab specimens, or blood tests (Uyeki & Winquist, 2001).

Patient/Caregiver Information

Remind the patient that these medications are only for those who have been symptomatic for less than 48 hours. It should be stressed that these are not a substitute for influenza vaccination.

OUTCOMES MANAGEMENT

Selecting Appropriate Agents

Amantadine-resistant and rimantadine-resistant viruses have been identified and are cross-resistant; therefore, switching to the other agent is of no benefit. Either agent may be chosen as first-line therapy for treatment or prophylaxis of influenza A in adults and prophylaxis in children. Only amantadine should be selected for treatment of influenza in children. The neuraminidase inhibitors, inhaled zanamivir and oral oseltamivir, are effective against both influenza Type A and B. All these antiviral agents have been shown to reduce the duration of influenza symptoms by about one day (Uyeki & Winquist, 2001).

Monitoring for Efficacy

When used as prophylaxis, efficacy is determined by the presence or absence of type A influenza illness. Outcomes of treatment are based on resolution of signs and symptoms including fever, myalgia, sore throat, and cough. Patients should be monitored for any adverse effects as well as any worsening of underlying respiratory disease.

Monitoring for Toxicity

Mild adverse effects such as nausea and anorexia occur with both amantadine and rimantadine and will usually subside with continued administration. More serious effects include behavioral changes, delirium, hallucinations, agitation, and seizures. Amantadine has been shown to have a higher incidence of central nervous system effects compared to rimantadine. These adverse effects of amantadine appear to be more common in patients with renal or hepatic dysfunction, seizure disorders, and certain psychiatric disorders and in the elderly. Reducing the dose of amantadine may prevent or reduce these adverse effects. The dose of amantadine and rimantadine should be reduced in patients with renal and/or hepatic dysfunction.

Both inhaled zanamivir and oral oseltamivir have been shown to have common GI adverse effects such as nausea and vomiting. Use of zanamivir has been associated with bronchospasm and worsening of underlying respiratory disease, so it should not be recommended in patients with asthma or COPD. Both of these neuraminidase inhibitors may have CNS adverse reactions, e.g., headache, insomnia, and vertigo.

RHINOSINUSITIS

The term sinusitis has been changed by the American Academy of Otolaryngology—Head and Neck Surgery (AAOHNS) to rhinosinusitis to accurately reflect the inflammation of the mucous membranes lining the paranasal sinuses. With the close proximity of the nose and sinuses, it is difficult to distinguish problems in one area from the other. In addition, acute sinusitis usually begins with rhinitis (Casiano, 2001).

With more than 17 million office visits in one year, rhinosinusitis surpassed that of asthma by 6 million. Rhinosinusitis is the most common reason for visiting the physician or nurse practitioner, while asthma is the second. Rhinosinusitis may be classified as infectious or noninfectious. Viral, bacterial, and fungal agents are included in the infectious types of rhinosinusitis. Noninfectious types include environmental sources (pollutants), allergies, physiologic factors such as vasomotor rhinitis, or age-related causes such as hormonal changes. It is possible that one type of rhinosinusitis may exacerbate another type. A comprehensive history and physical can usually distinguish between the types (Casiano, 2001).

Typically, rhinosinusitis is divided into five types based on duration of symptoms and extent of mucosal damage:

- Acute rhinosinusitis has an abrupt onset with a total resolution of symptoms within 4 weeks.
- Subacute rhinosinusitis has persistent nasal discharge despite therapy and resolves in 4 to 12 weeks with no permanent mucosal damage.
- Recurrent acute rhinosinusitis involves 4 or more episodes per year, with resolutions between attacks.
- Chronic rhinosinusitis occurs with episodes of prolonged inflammation and or repeated or inadequately treated acute infections. Symptoms persist for longer than 12 weeks despite appropriate therapy, and there is often permanent damage to the mucosa.
- Acute exacerbation of chronic rhinosinusitis involves a sudden worsening of chronic sinusitis, with a return to baseline after treatment (Casiano, 2001).

The pathogenesis of all types of rhinosinusitis is similar. The main etiologic factor is obstruction of the osteomeatal unit, which leads to lower levels of oxygen within the paranasal sinuses, decreased clearance of foreign material, and mucous stasis resulting in infection. Any factor or condition that blocks the flow of secretions can lead to the development of rhinosinusitis. For example, in acute rhinosinusitis, upper respiratory infections are important predisposing factors (Dunphy & Porter, 2001). Anatomical abnormalities such as a deviated nasal septum and nasal polyps are important antecedents to chronic rhinosinusitis. Other less common predisposing factors are extension of dental infections, barotrauma, neoplasm, trauma, and foreign bodies (Casiano, 2001).

Pathogens involved in rhinosinusitis depend on the duration of symptoms. In acute rhinosinusitis, common pathogens are *Streptococcus pneumoniae, Haemophilus influenzae,* and *Moraxella catarrhalis.* There has also been an increase in the incidence of beta-lactamase-producing and other resistant forms of bacteria. Pathogens involved in chronic rhinosinusitis usually include a mixture of aerobic and/or anaerobic flora. These include *Pseudomonas spp.*, staphylococci, peptostreptococci, and *Propionibacterium spp.* (Casiano, 2001).

Children with acute rhinosinusitis tend to have subtle symptoms of cough, rhinorrhea, periorbital puffiness, fatigue, and malaise. A daytime cough is an important predictor of chronic rhinosinusitis in children. In patients of all ages, a diagnosis of rhinosinusitis should be considered when a patient has persistent overall nasal/sinus symptoms lasting longer than 10 days and/or worsening symptoms or purulent rhinorrhea for more than five days (Casiano, 2001). Patients with allergic rhinosinusitis present with clear nasal discharge, generalized nasal obstruction, generalized headache or facial pain, a dry cough, sneezing, nasal and/or eye pruritis, and usually a personal history of allergies. Patients with bacterial rhinosinusitis present with purulent nasal discharge, focal or generalized nasal obstruction, focal or generalized headache/facial pain, and a purulent cough. In addition, these patients may have hyposmia or anosmia, fever, halitosis, dental pain, and fatigue (Casiano, 2001).

All types of rhinosinusitis may exacerbate asthma or otologic symptoms. Without appropriate medical therapy, both intracranial and extracranial complications may develop. Extracranial complications include ocular cellulitis, the most common complication, and frontal subperiosteal abscess. Intracranial complications include meningitis, cavernous sinus thrombosis, subdural empyema, and brain abscesses (Casiano, 2001; Hayes, 2001).

SPECIFIC CONSIDERATIONS FOR PHARMACOTHERAPY

When Drug Therapy Is Needed

Antibiotics are not recommended for cases of viral rhinosinusitis unless purulent rhinorrhea is present, symptoms worsen after more than 5 days, or total symptoms last longer than 10 days. Antibiotic therapy is always indicated for a minimum of 2 weeks in all cases of bacterial rhinosinusitis. In areas that have a low incidence of sinusitis due to beta-lactamase–producing strains of *H. influenzae* and *M. catarrhalis,* patients may be initially treated with an inexpensive, safe antibiotic such as amoxicillin. On the other hand, trimethoprim-sulfamethoxazole (TMP-SMX) is effective against beta-lactamase–producing organisms and thus may be used as first-line therapy; it is less effective against *S. pneumoniae.* Other first-line antibiotics besides amoxicillin and TMP-SMX may include amoxicillin/clavulanate, cefpodoxime, and cefuroxime, and for beta-lactam agents, macrolides. For patients with more persistent symptoms who have already had a course of antibiotic therapy that has been ineffective, amoxicillin/clavulanate, cefpodoxime, cefixime, clindamycin, and the respiratory quinolones should be tried. For patients with chronic sinusitis, the causative agents are usually a combination of aerobic and/or anaerobic flora. Most of these patients will respond to TMP/SMX, clindamycin, ciprofloxacin, or combination therapy. Respiratory quinolones should only be prescribed for adults (Casiano, 2001). For chronic sinusitis, the course of therapy should be for 30 days.

Other pharmacological approaches should be used to correct the underlying obstruction of the osteomeatal unit. Irrigation of the nose with saline is effective in shrinking the edematous mucosa, improving mucociliary flow, and clearing nasal debris. In addition, an intranasal corticosteroid should be prescribed. A trial of short-term oral steroids may be tried, as well as an oral decongestant. If the problem persists longer than a month, nasal saline irrigations and intranasal corticosteroid therapy should continue. If there is evidence of asthma, eosinophilia, or extensive hyperplastic sinusitis, a trial period of leukotriene modifiers may be prescribed (Hayes, 2001). Mucolytics are often recommended to liquify secretions and facilitate evacuation of sinus contents. Oral antihistamines and cromolyn sodium should be used only if the patient has allergies.

Short-Term and Long-Term Goals of Pharmacotherapy

Short-term goals of therapy include eradication of infection, reduction of tissue edema, and facilitation of sinus drainage. Long-term goals are maintenance of patency of the osteomeatal complex and prevention of recurrent infections and complications. Patients should be educated to help themselves prevent and treat their symptoms. See Table 21–1.

Time Frame for Initiating Pharmacotherapy

Sinusitis should be treated at the time of diagnosis to prevent life-threatening complications. Acute sinusitis is typically treated for 10 days in uncomplicated cases, whereas treatment of chronic sinusitis usually lasts 30 days.

Medications to reduce obstruction in the osteomeatal unit, such as topical and oral decongestants or oral antihistamines, also should be initiated at the time of diagnosis. Topical corticosteroids and/or cromolyn sodium sprays may be ordered with the knowledge that they may take at least 1 week to be effective.

Assessment Prior to Therapy

The *history* should focus on identifying symptoms consistent with rhinosinusitis such as purulent nasal discharge, headache that increases with bending, and a positive response to decongestants. Risk factors for developing rhinosinusitis should be explored. Past medical history should include questions concerning previous episodes and treatments of rhinosinusitis, ear infections, allergies, and asthma. Questions regarding high fevers, periorbital edema, severe headaches, and visual complaints should be included to explore the possibility of complications from rhinosinusitis.

The *physical examination* should focus on the nasal cavity. The frontal and maxillary sinuses should be transilluminated and percussed. The ears, pharynx, mouth, teeth, and chest should be examined for signs of infection. To assess for complications of rhinosinusitis, look for periorbital swelling and perform a neurologic examination.

The first episode of acute rhinosinusitis is usually treated empirically with antibiotics. The most reliable and cost-effective procedure for diagnosing and evaluating patients with rhinosinusitis is by fiberoptic examination of the nose and paranasal sinuses. X-rays of the paranasal sinuses have been found to be inaccurate and do not provide any additional information. While the computerized tomography (CT) is the radiologic examination of choice, due to its cost, it is reserved for management of recalcitrant cases and in patients needing surgical procedures.

The optimum way to confirm the diagnosis of maxillary and frontal rhinosinusitis and identify the causative pathogen is to obtain sinus aspirates by antral puncture. However, that procedure is impractical in most primary care settings (Hayes, 2001).

Patient/Caregiver Information

It is important to teach patients the proper use of nasal sprays (see patient information under Allergic Rhinitis). Education on strategies to prevent future bouts of rhinosinusitis should be part of the management plan. For example, some patients should be taught to avoid certain environmental irritants and allergens. Patients with recurrent episodes of rhinosinusitis should be instructed to begin decongestants at the first sign of symptoms to facilitate sinus drainage and prevent mucus stasis, which often leads to infection.

OUTCOMES MANAGEMENT

Selecting Appropriate Agents

Antimicrobial Treatment of Acute Rhinosinusitis. Antimicrobial selection for both adults and children is similar and should be based on the most likely pathogens involved. Inexpensive, safe antibiotics such as amoxicillin and TMP-SMX are good initial choices. However, amoxicillin is not effective against beta-lactamase–producing strains of *H. influenzae* and *M. catarrhalis,* and TMP-SMX is less effective against *S. pneumoniae.* In geographic areas where a high percentage of beta-lactamase–producing pathogens are known, other agents such as amoxicillin-clavulanate, cefuroxime, cefixime, and the macrolide antibiotics may be effective, but these agents are more costly. Rhinosinusitis caused by penicillin-resistant *S. pneumoniae* is treated with high-dose amoxicillin (60–80 mg/kg per day) or high-dose beta-lactamase–stable antibiotics. Treatment of acute rhinosinusitis thought to originate from dental infection should include an agent such as amoxicillin-clavulanate that is effective against anaerobic organisms. Rhinosinusitis in patients not responding to the above therapy may be due to *Chlamydia pneumoniae.* In this small percentage of patients (<10%), alternative therapy with a tetracycline, clarithromycin, or azithromycin should be initiated.

Antimicrobial Treatment of Chronic Rhinosinusitis. Patients with chronic rhinosinusitis are likely to have acute exacerbations of disease. Compared to acute sinusitis, acute infections associated with chronic sinusitis are more likely caused by gram-positive and gram-negative anaerobic bacteria. Therefore, antimicrobial selection should include coverage against these pathogens as well as the typical pathogens of acute disease. Single agents or combinations, such as amoxicillin-clavulanate, clindamycin, dicloxacillin-metronidazole, cefuroxime-metronidazole, or clarithromycin may be effective.

Adjunctive Therapy for Acute and Chronic Rhinosinusitis. Topical decongestants such as oxymetazoline nasal spray, as well as oral decongestants such as pseudoephedrine, are recommended to improve maxillary ostial function. Because of rebound congestion and tolerance, decongestant nasal sprays should be used only for 3 days. Topical corticosteroids such as beclomethasone dipropionate, flunisolide, triamcinolone acetonide, and fluticasone may prove useful in the management of rhinosinusitis. Intranasal corticosteroid sprays work after about 1 week. If used on a long-term basis, they should be discontinued for several weeks every 3 to 4 months to prevent nasal mucosal atrophy or minor epistaxis. When corticosteroid sprays are used, an oral or topical antihistamine spray may be used on the rare day when symptoms worsen. Any of the nonsedating oral antihistamines may offer the same efficacy without any of the anticholinergic side effects (Casiano, 2001; Hayes, 2001).

Monitoring for Efficacy

The efficacy of antimicrobial therapy is based on resolution of signs and symptoms of the illness. If symptoms do not begin to resolve within 5 to 7 days of initiating antimicrobial therapy, noncompliance, inappropriate drug selection, atypical pathogens, or resistant organisms must be considered.

Monitoring for Toxicity

Antimicrobial therapy with TMP-SMX has been associated with rash, including Stevens-Johnson syndrome, crystalluria, and photosensitivity. The most frequently reported adverse effects of penicillins or cephalosporins include rash and urticaria. Amoxicillin-clavulanate has also been associated with increased gastrointestinal complicants, including diarrhea. Hypersensitivity reactions such as hives, laryngeal edema, and anaphylactic shock pose an immediate threat and warrant medical attention. Gastrointestinal complaints such as nausea, vomiting, and diarrhea are the most frequently reported adverse effects of macrolide therapy.

PHARYNGITIS

Pharyngitis (inflammation of the pharynx and tonsils) is responsible for over 10% of all office visits and 50% of all outpatient antibiotic prescriptions (Jackler & Kaplan, 2002). Although most patients who seek care are concerned about streptococcal pharyngitis, other etiologic agents are often involved. Approximately 20 to 65% of all cases of pharyngitis result from noninfectious causes, such as postnasal drip or irritation due to allergies, or smoking. Viruses (i.e., adenoviruses, Epstein-Barr virus, herpesviruses, influenza viruses) are the most frequent pathogens causing pharyngitis. The most important pathogen to identify is group A beta-hemolytic streptococci (GABHS), also known as *S. pyogenes.*

Pharyngitis caused by GABHS may seem similar to infections caused by *Corynebacterium diphtheriae* (in the unimmunized patient) anaerobic streptococci, and *Corynebacterium haemolyticum* (Jackler & Kaplan,

2002). Other bacteria causing pharyngitis include *Mycoplasma pneumoniae* and *Chlamydia pneumoniae.* Pharyngitis caused by *N. gonorrhea, T. pallidum,* chlamydia, or herpes is typically a result of oral intercourse with an infected sexual partner (Dunphy & Porter, 2001).

Streptococcal pharyngitis occurs in approximately 30% of all children and 10% of all adults complaining of sore throat. It is predominantly an infection of school-aged children (ages 5–10) and is rare in children younger than 3 years of age. The typical clinical course is short-lived with mild symptoms and signs of tonsillopharyngeal erythema, enlarged anterior cervical nodes, and soft palate petechiae. On the other hand, some patients do experience severe throat pain, headaches, chills, abdominal pain, high fever, an edematous uvula, and a thick exudate covering the pharynx and tonsils. Infections with certain strains of GABHS produce an erythrogenic toxin and result in scarlet fever or scarlatina with a characteristic rash (Dunphy & Porter, 2001). Other suppurative (i.e., direct extension from the pharyngeal infection) complications such as peritonsillar abscess, cervical lymphadenitis, mastoiditis, and rhinosinusitis can occur.

Nonsuppurative complications that can arise from immune responses to the acute infection are a dangerous sequela of streptococcal pharyngitis. Acute glomerulonephritis may appear 1 to 3 weeks postinfection and usually is not prevented by appropriate antibiotic treatment. In contrast, antibiotic treatment can prevent the other significant nonsuppurative complication, acute rheumatic fever.

While the incidence of rheumatic fever has remained relatively low in the United States, with an evolution of more virulent strains of *S. pyogenes,* there will be an increase in GABHS complications (Dunphy & Porter, 2001).

SPECIFIC CONSIDERATIONS FOR PHARMACOTHERAPY

When Drug Therapy Is Needed

Although there are various etiologies of pharyngitis, healthcare providers especially want to identify and treat those patients with GABHS to prevent rheumatic fever, acute glomerulonephritis, and suppurative complications; as well as decrease contagion, and relieve symptoms (Cooper, Hoffman, Bartlett et al., 2001).

While drug therapy is not needed in most cases, antibiotics are ordered about 75% of the time for pharyngitis, both due to patient insistence and the healthcare provider's lack of time to discuss why other treatments may work as well (Cooper et al., 2001). To decrease the high rate of unnecessary antibiotic prescriptions for pharyngitis, it is recommended that the following strategies be used to select which patients should be treated with antibiotic therapy:

1. Determine the presence of four criteria: history of fever, tonsillar exudates, no cough, and tender anterior cervical lynphadenopathy.
2. Do not treat patients with one or none of the above criteria as they are unlikely to have a GABHS infection.
3. Test patients with two or more criteria with a rapid antigen test and prescribe antibiotics for those patients who test positive (Coopoer et al., 2001).

Other drug therapies relieve the symptoms of pharyngitis. Acetaminophen or ibuprofen are helpful in reducing fevers and discomfort. Throat lozenges and topical anesthetic throat sprays may be beneficial for adults and older children.

Short-Term and Long-Term Goals of Pharmacotherapy

The short-term goals of treatment for pharyngitis caused by GABHS are to resolve the infection, promptly relieve the symptomatic complaints, and prevent the transmission of the bacteria to others. The long-term goals of treatment are to prevent complications such as acute rheumatic fever. Patients should be instructed to increase fluid intake and use hard candy, cold drinks, or warm saline gargles to soothe throat pain. See Table 21–2 for additional information.

Time Frame for Initiating Pharmacotherapy

Antimicrobial therapy should be started immediately in those patients with a positive rapid antigen test. Controversy exists as to initiation of antimicrobial treatment in those individuals with a negative rapid antigen test when a strong clinical suspicion of streptococcal pharyngitis still exists.

The *history* and *physical examination* should be aimed at determining whether the patient has streptococcal pharyngitis or another type of pharyngitis. For example, pharyngitis due to coxsackievirus is accompanied by lesions in the mouth and on the hands and feet. Patients with infectious mononucleosis have exudative pharyngitis as well as fever and fatigue (see Chapter 37 for further discussion of infectious mononucleosis). The severity of the pharyngitis and the risk the patient has for developing complications should also be assessed.

The physical assessment should focus on the skin, head, nose, throat, mouth, chest, and abdomen. For example, inspection and palpation of the skin can reveal circumoral flushing, Pastia's lines, and a fine pinpoint exanthem in patients who have scarlet fever. Examination of the head, nose, and mouth can identify signs suggestive of viral pharyngitis, such as a clear nasal discharge and mouth ulcers. Neck, chest and abdominal assessments can rule out signs of complications that may occur with lymphadenitis, pneumonia, and splenomegaly in infectious mononucleosis. Examining the pharynx is crucial in determining the likelihood of streptococcal pharyngitis and to rule out complications such as a peritonsillar abscess, which occurs with asymmetric tonsillar swelling (Cooper et al., 2001; Dunphy & Porter, 2001).

A Rapid (10-minute) Strep Test is used in cases of exudative pharyngitis to detect GABHS. These tests are highly specific (90%) and sensitive (80 to 90%). In the summer, however, the Rapid Strep Test has a false-positive rate that approaches 50%. Because the likelihood of GABHS is minimal during that time, testing might not be done unless the patient is in a high-risk group for streptococcal infection (such as immunocompromised patients, patients with diabetes, or a history of rheumatic fever). The current "gold standard" remains a throat culture, which is considered appropriate for any patient with pharyngitis, a fever above 101 degrees, tonsillar exudate, and anterior cervical lymphadenopathy. Immunofluorescence staining or viral throat swab cultures may be used if a herpes infection is suspected (Dunphy & Porter, 2001).

Patient/Caregiver Information

Patients should be advised to take the full 10-day course of antibiotics even though they are likely to be asymptomatic within 24 to 48 hour. If patients do not feel significantly better in 2 to 3 days, they should return for further evaluation. Stress should be placed on informing the patient that the pharmacological treatment is aimed at resolving the acute infection as well as preventing the complications, particularly rheumatic fever. Side effects of medications and supportive home treatments should be discussed.

OUTCOMES MANAGEMENT

Selecting Appropriate Agents

Although numerous etiologies of pharyngitis have been described, antimicrobial treatment is aimed at eradication of GABHS from the pharynx to prevent rheumatic fever. Several factors should be considered when selecting the most appropriate antimicrobial treatment regimen. These factors include bacteriologic and clinical efficacy, compliance, cost, spectrum of activity, and potential side effects.

Antimicrobial Treatment of Streptococcal Pharyngitis. Although several classes of antimicrobial agents have been shown to eradicate group A streptococci from the pharynx, penicillin remains the drug of choice because of its proven efficacy and cost. The current recommended treatment for streptococcal pharyngitis consists of penicillin given as a 10-day, twice daily, oral regimen of penicillin V or a one-time dose of intramuscular penicillin G benzathine for patients expected to be noncompliant (Jackler & Kaplan, 2002). See Table 21–3 for treatment options. Warm penicillin G benzathine to room temperature before administering to reduce the pain of intramuscular injection. Ampicillin and amoxicillin offer no clinical advantage and an increased cost over penicillin.

Drug of Choice in Penicillin-allergic Patient. Patients with immediate (anaphylactic-type) hypersensitivity to penicillin should receive erythromycin ethyl succinate for 10 days. Cephalosporins should be avoided as <20% of penicillin allergic patients can also be allergic to these agents.

TABLE 21–3. Treatment of Streptococcal Pharyngitis

Agent	Dose	Mode	Duration
Penicillin G Benzathine	600,000 U for patients ≤ 30 lbs; 900,000 U for patients 30–60 lbs; 1.2 million U for patients > 60 lbs	Intramuscular	Once
Penicillin V	Children: 250 mg 3 times/day; Adolescents and adults: 500 mg 2 times/day	Oral	10 days
For Individuals allergic to penicillin			
Erythromycin: Ethyluccinate	Children: 40 mg/kg/day divided 3–4 times dly (maximum 3.2 g/day)	Oral	10 days
	Adults: 400 mg 4 times/day	Oral	10 days

Adapted from Cooper, Hoffman, & Bartlett, et al (2001); Jackler & Kaplan (2002)

Alternative Antimicrobial Agents. Antimicrobial agents, including azithromycin, clarithromycin, cefadroxil, and cephalexin, have been shown to effectively eradicate group A streptococci from the pharynx, although penicillin remains the only drug proven to prevent rheumatic fever. Advantages of azithromycin include less gastrointestinal irritation compared to erythromycin and a convenient dosing regimen; a 5-day course of once-daily administration is currently indicated.

Drug of Choice for Patients Whose Treatment Fails and Chronic Carriers of GABHS. In those patients who continue to harbor group A streptococci in the pharynx, a second course of antimicrobial should only be considered in symptomatic individuals or those who are asymptomatic with a previous history of rheumatic fever. Some studies suggest the presence of beta-lactamase–producing organisms in the upper respiratory tract may interfere with the activity of penicillin. Amoxicillin-clavulanate, clindamycin, or a combination of penicillin with rifampin given concurrently during the last 4 days of the regimen is recommended (Bisno, Gerber, Gwaltney, et al., 1997).

Individuals who are chronic carriers of group A streptococci (positive throat culture without illness) are at low risk for development of rheumatic fever. However, when these individuals develop an acute upper respiratory tract infection, it may be difficult to distinguish infection from colonization. Therefore, a single course of antimicrobial therapy is indicated in this patient population.

Monitoring for Efficacy

Signs and symptoms of streptococcal pharyngitis usually resolve several days after the initiation of antimicrobial therapy. Those patients who remain symptomatic or develop recurring symptoms and those who have had rheumatic fever and are at unusually high risk for recurrence should receive a throat culture 2 to 7 days after completion of the antimicrobial regimen (Dunphy & Porter, 2001). Patients are considered noncontagious following 24 hours of antimicrobial therapy.

Monitoring for Toxicity

The most frequently reported adverse effects of penicillin or cephalosporins include rash and urticaria. Hypersensitivity reactions such as hives, laryngeal edema, and anaphylactic shock pose an immediate threat and warrant medical attention. Gastrointestinal complaints are the most frequently reported adverse effects of macrolide therapy.

CROUP

Croup, or acute laryngotracheobronchitis, is a viral infection that produces inflammation and narrowing of the entire respiratory tract. The airway obstruction is greatest at the subglottic level. It is the most common cause of acute upper airway obstruction in children between the ages of 3 months and 6 years, with a peak occurrence in the second year of life. Croup is commonly caused by parainfluenza virus, although influenza, respiratory syncytial virus, rhinovirus, and *M. pneumoniae* may be causative pathogens. (Hill & Sullivan, 1999; Wright, Pomerantz, & Luria, 2002).

Croup is characterized by fever, inspiratory stridor, hoarseness, and a barking cough that is worse at night. Children typically exhibit symptoms of the common cold one to several days before the onset of stridor. The symptoms usually resolve within 3 to 7 days, although the cough may last for a longer period (Ball & Bindler, 1999).

Most children with croup have mild symptoms and are not brought in for medical attention. Of the children who present to the emergency department, approximately 20% have severe disease with cyanosis, hypoxemia, retractions, rales, and rapid respiratory rates and require hospitalization. Few children have respiratory failure that necessitates intubation. (Ball & Bindler, 1999; Hill & Sullivan, 1999).

Some children have repeated episodes of inspiratory stridor and are diagnosed with spasmodic croup. Spasmodic croup primarily occurs in children who have a history of atopy. With the control of *H. influenzae* type B through immunizations with the HIB vaccine, croup is now caused almost exclusively by viruses (parainfluenza, respiratory synctial, and rhinovirus), along with allergic and emotional influences.

Other conditions have characteristic symptoms that resemble those of croup and must be included in the differential diagnosis. These include foreign body aspiration, epiglottitis, and peritonsillar abscess. Epiglottis is caused by *H. influenza* (Hill & Sullivan, 1999).

SPECIFIC CONSIDERATIONS FOR PHARMACOTHERAPY

When Drug Therapy Is Needed

Initially, treatment consists of supportive care and reassurance by parents. At home, parents usually try humidification with cool air before the child presents to the emergency department (ED). Children with moderate to severe croup are treated in the ED. The use of oral steroids has been found to result in clinical improvement with mild to moderate croup and reduces the need for hospitalization. A nebulized steroid may also be used (Wright et al., 2002).

Nebulized racemic epinephrine and nebulized L-epinephrine appear equally effective in reducing airway obstruction. These agents stimulate alpha-adrenergic receptors, resulting in local vasoconstriction and a reduction in subglottic inflammation. After administration, patients can usually be discharged safely from the ED after a 3-hour observation period (Wright et al., 2002).

Corticosteroids with their antiinflammatory effects improve the clinical course of croup in children (Griffin, Ellis, Fitzgerald-Barron, et al., 2000). They may be given alone or in conjunction with or after nebulized epinephrine. Current data suggests that all children with croup who demonstrate dyspnea should be treated with corticosteroids, and children with more severe croup should be treated with nebulised adrenaline (Powell & Stokell, 2002; Wright et al., 2002). A review of randomized controlled trials found that children treated with nebulised steroids in the ED were significantly more likely to have an improvement in their condition and significantly less likely to need hospital admission (Griffin et al., 2000).

Short-Term and Long-Term Goals of Pharmacotherapy

The goals are to reduce airway obstruction, shorten the course of disease, and prevent hospitalization and intubation. Caregivers should be educated to help treat their children's symptoms.

Time Frame for Initiating Pharmacotherapy

As croup is mainly a self-limited condition, caregivers should initially try supportive care along with cool air humidification before bringing the child to the ED. The use of steroids in an oral preparation has shown to result in a clinical improvement of outpatients with mild to moderate croup and reduces the need for hospitalization. In addition, nebulized steroids may also be used (Wright et al., 2002). Caregivers need education as to when to administer these.

Assessment Prior to Therapy

If a child is in respiratory distress, plan for immediate transfer to a hospital and quickly question parents regarding onset of symptoms, fluid intake, voiding, and level of alertness. For children with mild to moderate symptoms, take the time to gather a *history* of pattern, duration, characteristics, and severity of symptoms. Explore the presence of associated symptoms such as high fever and production of purulent sputum, which is more characteristic of bacterial tracheitis than croup (Ball & Bindler, 1999). Inquire about immunization status to eliminate the likelihood of epiglottitis, since epiglottitis may be life-threatening, whereas croup is not.

During the *physical examination,* rapidly assess vital signs and respiratory status including respiratory rate, retractions, use of accessory muscles, nasal flaring, and cyanosis. Assess hydration status and decreased response to stimuli. Observe for signs of drooling and difficulty swallowing, which are characteristic of epiglottitis, an emergent problem requiring immediate transfer to a hospital. *Never attempt to examine the pharynx of a patient with signs and symptoms consistent with epiglottitis.* Perform a complete lung and heart examination (Ball & Bindler, 1999).

The *diagnosis* of croup is usually based on clinical presentation without diagnostic tests. If epiglottitis is suspected, a lateral inspiratory and expiratory chest x-ray and an anterior-posterior x-ray of the neck are recommended. If bacterial tracheitis is suspected, a culture of the sputum—for staphylococcus can confirm the diagnosis (Ball & Bindler, 1999).

Laboratory tests are usually not indicated. If there is clinical deterioration, an RSV titer, arterial blood gases, and a CBC should be done. If the RSV titer is positive, it will indicate that the coughing is probably not related to croup, but rather RSV infection. The CBC will determine dehydration, and the blood gases will indicate the need for aggressive therapy with supplemental oxygen (Hill & Sullivan, 1999).

Patient/Caregiver Information

Teach caregivers to carefully and frequently assess their child's hydration status, level of alertness, and respiratory rate. In particular, caution them that the effects of nebulized epinephrine are often short-lived and the child may have additional episodes of stridor and respiratory distress. Children treated with corticosteroids must be frequently monitored as well, even though the effects of these drugs are longer in duration. Since corticosteroids are only to be used for a short period of time, children should not experience adverse effects that occur with extended use of these agents.

OUTCOMES MANAGEMENT

Since croup is a predominately viral condition, antibiotics are only indicated in patients with fever for more than 5 to 7 days and showing deterioration of the condition. This is an attempt to manage bacterial superinfection.

Selecting Appropriate Agents

Epinephrine. Nebulized racemic epinephrine has been used with success in the management of moderate to severe symptoms of croup. Local vasoconstriction and decreased subglottic inflammation account for its clinical benefit in relieving stridor. Rebound mucosal vasodilation and dyspnea may occur with discontinuance; therefore, close observation is necessary. Nebulized racemic epinephrine also has been shown to reduce the number of children requiring intubation for severe croup. Current recommendations are for 0.25 mg in 2.5 mL normal saline nebulization every 2 hours for the hospitalized patient (Hill & Sullivan, 1999). The levorotatory form of epinephrine (L-epinephrine) has been shown to be equally effective compared to racemic epinephrine and is less expensive; it may be a suitable alternative (Wright et al., 2002).

Corticosteroids. The use of oral corticosteroids results in clinical improvement of outpatients with mild to moderate croup and reduces the need for hospitalization. The dosage for oral dexamethasone, as well as IV dexamethasone, is 0.75 to 9.0 mg/d. Nebulized budesonide may be used as well (Griffin et al., 2000; Wright et al., 2002).

Monitoring for Efficacy

A significant decrease in airway obstruction should occur 10 to 30 min after administering nebulized epinephrine and continue for 1 to 2 hours. Frequent administration may be necessary because of this. Patients should be monitored for rebound congestion. Patients treated with epinephrine and corticosteroids should be monitored for up to 12 hours prior to release.

Monitoring for Toxicity

Toxicity from single doses of corticosteroids has not been reported in clinical trials. Racemic epinephrine given on a routine basis may result in tachycardia, restlessness, anxiety, and tremor.

REFERENCES

Ball, J., & Bindler, R. (1999). *Pediatric nursing: Caring for children.* Stamford, CT: Appleton & Lange.

Bisno, A.L., Gerber, M.A., Gwaltney, J.M., Kaplan, E.L., & Schwartz, R.H. (1997). Diagnosis and management of Group A streptococcal pharyngitis: A practice guideline. *Clinical Infectious Diseases, 25,* 574–583.

Bouckenooghe, A.R., & Shandera, W.X. (2002). Infectious diseases: Viral & rickettsial. In L.M. Tierney, S.J. McPhee, & M.A. Papadakis (Eds.), *Current medical diagnosis and treatment* (pp. 1355–1396). New York: McGraw-Hill.

Casiano, R.R. (2001). A rational approach to treating rhinosinusitis. In Update on the management of respiratory tract infections. *Supplement to The Clinical Advisor,* Sept., 17–24.

Chesnutt, M.S., & Prendergast, T.J. (2002). Lung. In L.M. Tierney, S.J. McPhee, & M.A. Papadakis (Eds.), *Current medical diagnosis and treatment* (pp. 269–362). New York: McGraw-Hill.

Cooper, R.J., Hoffman, J.R., Bartlett, J.G., Besser, R.E., Gonzales, R., Hickner, J.M., & Sande, M.A. ((2001). Principles of appropriate antibiotic use for acute pharyngitis in adults: Background. *Annuals of Emergency Medicine, 37*(6), 711–719.

Dunphy, L.M., & Porter, B.O. (2001). Eyes, ears, nose & throat problems. In L.M. Dunphy & J.E. Winland-Brown (Eds.), *Primary care—The art and science of advanced practice nursing* (pp. 345–352). Philadelphia: F.A. Davis.

Ferguson, B. J. (1997). Allergic rhinitis: Options for pharmacotherapy and immunotherapy. *Post-graduate Medicine, 101,* 117–131.

Griffin, S., Ellis, S., Fitzgerald-Barron, A., Rose, J., & Egger, M. (2000). Nebulised steroid in the treatment of croup: A systematic review of randomized controlled trials. *British Journal of General Practice, 50*(451), 135–141.

Hayes, R.O. (2001). Pediatric sinusitis—when it's not just a cold. *Clinician Reviews, 11*(10), 53–58.

Hill, N.L., & Sullivan, L. (1999). Management guidelines for pediatric nurse practitioners. Philadelphia: F.A. Davis.

Jackler, R.K., & Kaplan, M.J. (2002). Ear, nose & throat. In L.M. Tierney, S.J. McPhee, & M.A. Papadakis (Eds.), *Current medical diagnosis & treatment* (pp. 227–268). New York: McGraw-Hill.

Kaiser, H.B., Mellon, M.H., & Elder, M.A. (Eds.). (2001, Fall). Allergic rhinitis and asthma: One airway, one disease Supplement to *Patient Care for the Nurse Practitioner,* 4–17.

Powell, C.V., & Stokell, R.A. (2000). Changing hospital management of croup. What does this mean for general practice? *Australian Family Physician, 29*(10), 915–919.

Uyeki, T., & Winquist, A. (2001). Influenza. In S. Barton (Ed.), *Clinical evidence* (pp. 550–556). London: BMJ.

Wright, R.B., Pomerantz, W.J., & Luria, J.W. (2002). New approaches to respiratory infections in children. Bronchiolitis and croup. *Emergency Medicine Clinics of North America,* 20(1), 93–114.

INTERNET RESOURCES

Allergy & Asthma Network/Mothers of Asthmatics: www.aanma.org

Alliance for the Prudent Use of Antibiotics: www.healthsci.tufts.edu/apua/apua.html

American Academy of Allergy, Asthma, & Immunology: www.aaaai.org

American Academy of Family Physicians: www.aafp.org

American Academy of Pediatrics: www.aap.org

American College of Allergy, Asthma & Immunology: www.allergy.mcg.edu

American Lung Association: www.lungusa.org

Antimicrobial Resistance: Prevention Tools: www.cdc.gov/drugresistance/technical/prevention_tools.htm (click for "Prescription Pad")

National Asthma Education and Prevention Program: www.nhlbi:nih.gov/about/naepp/index.htm

CHAPTER ❖ 22

LOWER RESPIRATORY DISORDERS

Kathleen M. Tauer ◆ Glen E. Farr

Lower respiratory tract infections have become a constant and increasingly prevalent part of primary care practice. The incidence of asthma across the life span has become commonplace even as pharmacotherapeutic modalities have made management easier. Pharmacotherapies have made advances in the management of cystic fibrosis, allowing these patients both longer and better quality lives. Incidences of pneumonia are higher with a concomitant range of drugs available to treat the various types of the illness. And tuberculosis, once thought to be almost eliminated, is turning up with renewed regularity, even in new drug-resistant versions, especially among immune-suppressed patients. This chapter reviews causes and treatment options for asthma in adult, pediatric, and pregnant populations; bronchiolitis in children; chronic obstructive pulmonary disease (COPD); cystic fibrosis; pneumonia in adult, pediatric, and pregnant populations; and tuberculosis.

ASTHMA

The incidence of asthma has risen significantly since the early 1980s, from approximately 6 million people then to the current estimate of > 15 million people. (Centers for Disease Control and Prevention [CDC], 1996a; Yang, Changgeng, & Xue, 2000). Asthma affects approximately 4.8 million children in the United States today, making it one of the most common chronic diseases of childhood (CDC, 1996a). Hospitalization rates are the highest among African Americans and children, with death rates from asthma highest among African Americans aged 15 to 24 years (NAEPP, 2002).

There are several theories as to why this significant increase in asthma is currently being seen:

1. There a gene on chromosome 11q13 that is strongly linked to maternal inheritance of asthma and possibly changes the IgE receptor. This suggests that certain air pollutants PLUS other allergens PLUS susceptible genes may promote increased IgE production, leading to allergic reactions and the development of asthma in certain individuals. Thus, asthma is probably not a single gene disorder but a multifactorial interaction between the gene and the environment (Yang, 2000).
2. When exposed to environmental insults, the T-lymphocyte cells normally answer an infection and provide protective antibodies. However, it is postulated that in children and adults who receive routine vaccines, multiple antibiotics, and other therapies to prevent/treat illnesses, their T-lymphocytes are poorly stimulated and do not respond appropriately when needed. This may allow other T-lymphocyte cells that produce cytokines and inflammatory mediators to overact and produce an intense response, leading to allergic sensitization (Landau, 1996).

   Two of the most significant risk factors for developing asthma are lower viral respiratory infections and and atopy (Lemanske, 2001).

3. Passive tobacco smoke exposure during infancy and childhood.
4. Family history of allergies and atopy (NAEPP, 2002).

The current working definition of asthma developed by the National Heart, Lung and Blood Institute in its 2002 Expert Panel Report (National Asthma Education and Prevention Program [NAEPP], 2002) reads:

> Asthma is a chronic inflammatory disorder of the airways in which many cells and cellular elements play a role, in particular, mast cells, eosinophils, T-lymphocytes, macrophages, neutrophils, and epithelial cells. In susceptible individuals, this inflammation causes recurrent episodes of wheezing, breathlessness, chest tightness, and coughing, particularly at night or in the early morning. These episodes are usually associated with widespread but variable airflow obstruction that is often reversible either spontaneously or with treatment. The inflammation also causes an associated increase in the existing bronchial hyperresponsiveness to a variety of stimuli. (p. 11)

Recent studies indicate that the inflammation of asthma can be categorized into phases. The acute symptoms of asthma give rise to bronchospasms which responds to bronchodilators. Both the acute and chronic inflammation affects the airway diameter and airflow as well as the underlying bronchial hyperresponsiveness, increasing the risk of bronchospasm. The treatment consists of anti-inflammatory medications which can reverse some of the processes, but some patients have "persistent airflow limitations" (NAEPP, 2002) and/or airway remodeling.

Variability between morning and evening peak expiratory flow (PEF) may reflect airway hyperresponsiveness and therefore serve to measure asthma instability and severity (NAEPP, 2002).

Children between 5 to 12 years of age have shown that early treatment of mild-to-moderate persistent asthma with ICS (inhaled corticosteroids) provides control and prevents progression of lung changes. However, in other pediatric age groups, lung function declines in the first 5 years after diagnosis occuring more rapidly than in the adult (Finder, 1999).

Airway diameters change and enlarge as the infant grows to adulthood, with peak size occurring at 16–23 years of age (Burrows, 1987). After 30 years of age, the forced expiratory volume (FEV_1) declines normally at a steady rate of about 30 mL/year; an accelerated decline is seen in smokers (Burrows, 1987; Hanson & Midthun, 1992). In the person without lung obstruction few problems are noted, but in those with asthma and COPD the normal changes are compounded with already diminished airflow secondary to the disease process, thus changing the morbidity of the illness and potentially making the quality of life poorer (Hanson & Midthun, 1992).

The NAEPP 1997 recommendations were organized around four components:

1. Use of objective measures of lung function to assess the severity of asthma and to monitor the course of therapy.
2. Environmental control measures to avoid or eliminate factors that precipitate asthma symptoms or exacerbations.
3. Comprehensive pharmacologic therapy for long-term management designed to reverse and prevent the airway inflammation characteristic of asthma as well as pharmacologic therapy to manage asthma exacerbations.
4. Patient education that fosters a partnership among the patient, his or her family, and clinicians.

The following sections discuss asthma assessment and monitoring; factors contributing to severity; pharmacologic therapy for daily management and acute exacerbations; and patient education for asthma in children, during pregnancy, and in adults based on the pathophysiology presented.

ADULT ASTHMA

The onset of asthma usually occurs in childhood and adolescence, but increasingly asthma has its onset or recurrence in adults and the elderly. Many otherwise healthy adults often ignore and/or rationalize some of the common presenting symptoms of asthma, resulting in their asthma remaining undiagnosed for a long time. In older adults and the elderly, the classic asthma symptoms of cough, wheezing, chest tightness, and shortness of breath can mimic many other medical conditions: congestive heart failure, pulmonary embolism emphysema, chronic bronchitis, pneumonia, and/or tracheobronchial tumor (Braman, 1993). It has been estimated that about 50% of adults with asthma had their initial onset in childhood, followed by a period of remission and then a resurgence in midlife (Oswald, Phelan, Lanigan, et al., 1997; NAEPP, 2002).

In adult onset asthma, allergens play a major role, but some patients have no family history or IgE antibodies to allergens. The mechanism of nonallergic asthma is not fully understood, although there is an inflammatory process that is similar but not identical to that of atopic asthma (Finder, 1999). Several other triggering factors can be gastroesophageal reflux, occupational pollutants, tobacco smoke, pollutants, and beta blockers (Chan-Yeung & Malo, 1994).

Asthma management in the adult can require aggressive daily pharmacotherapy primarily using inhaled steroids, long-acting beta$_2$ agonists, and now the new leukotriene antagonists. All persons with mild persistent, moderate persistent, and severe persistent asthma must be on daily medications. Asthma also can be an unrelenting disease in the elderly and require oral systemic steroids (NAEPP, 2002).

In addition to the usual goals for the management of asthma in the adult, make sure that the daily asthma medications used do not exacerbate other coexisting medical conditions and lead to deleterious health effects.

Specific Considerations for Pharmacotherapy

When Drug Therapy Is Needed. Because asthma is a chronic disease characterized by airway inflammation and bronchial hyperresponsiveness, daily medication is needed to control the symptoms, maintain normal activity levels, prevent recurrent exacerbations, optimize pharmacotherapy with minimal or no adverse effects, and prevent further irreversible lung changes (NAEPP, 2002).

Daily medications for those with mildly persistent to severe asthma have been shown to significantly reduce and control symptoms so individuals can lead fully normal functioning and healthy lives (NAEPP, 2002). Without adequate treatment of acute exacerbations and chronic symptoms, morbidity and mortality are increased, especially among African Americans and Hispanics. The highest death rates for these groups are 3 to 5.5 times higher than for Caucasians (NAEPP, 1997). It is estimated that about 80% of asthma patients in the United States may be receiving suboptimal treatment for their asthma, while asthma patients in Europe are more aggressively treated. In Sweden about 50% of asthma patients are now treated with inhaled steroids compared to about 15% of U.S. patients (Rachelefsky, 1995a). The NAEPP (2002) Expert Panel recommends more aggressive treatment for asthma patients of all ages. Their recommendations are as follows:

1. Identify factors that exacerbate asthma.
2. Monitor daily PEF with a symptom control record.
3. Write instructions on how to manage a decline in PEF.
4. Write instructions on managing an acute asthma exacerbation.
5. Intensive and extensive education should be given about asthma and its management.
6. Regular office visits with the healthcare provider can be combined with appropriate referral to a specialist.
7. Develop a partnership with the healthcare provider so that the decision making regarding asthma management is a joint effort between patient and provider.

Short- and Long-Term Goals of Pharmacotherapy. The short-term goals of asthma pharmacotherapy are to recognize a decline in the PEF and/or change in the diurnal pattern of the PEF, institute early treatment that may prevent an acute asthma exacerbation, aggressively treat an acute asthma flare (decrease bronchospasms, increase bronchodilation, and reduce inflammation), and return the person to his or her previous level of functioning (NAEPP, 2002).

The long-term goals of asthma management are to control symptoms, prevent daily exacerbations, recognize and manage triggering factors that exacerbate asthma, control nocturnal symptoms, prevent EIB (exercise-induced bronchospasms) through preventive medications, use daily medications regularly if necessary, decrease or ameliorate the long-term airway remodeling leading to irreversible lung changes, and reduce morbidity and mortality (NAEPP, 2002).

Nonpharmacologic Therapy

- Assess and avoid triggering factors that can provoke an asthma flare.
- Exercise regularly.

Time Frame for Initiating Pharmacotherapy. Once the diagnosis of asthma is established and the severity is determined, treatment must begin immediately with the appropriate agent(s). The goal is to resolve the symptoms as quickly as possible and restore normal lung function. In acute exacerbations the acute symptoms should resolve rapidly, but complete resolution of all symptoms may take several days to weeks, depending on the severity of the flare and other comorbid illnesses. Symptoms should continue to improve and not remain the same or decline.

See Drug Table 701.2.

Assessment Needed Prior to Therapy. See Tables 22–1, 22–2, and 22–3 for important history markers, physical examination findings, assessment parameters, and common diagnostic tests needed.

TABLE 22–1. History and Physical Examination for Asthma

Pertinent Baseline History Markers

- Childhood symptoms
- Current symptoms suggestive of wheezing, shortness of breath, chest tightness, breathlessness during play or exercise
- Asthma diagnosed in childhood
- Three episodes of wheezing lasting > 1 day and sleep disturbances
- Diagnosed with atopic dermatitis, allergic rhinitis, wheezing without colds, and elevated blood eosinophils
- Symptom description: seasonal pattern, limitation of ADL, sleep disturbance
- Hospitalizations for respiratory problems
- Current medications
- Associated health problems that could aggravate: nasal polyps, sinusitis, allergic rhinitis, eczema, gastroesophageal reflux disease (GERD), COPD, heart disease, hypertension, glaucoma, psychiatric problems
- Positive family history
- Occupation
- Hobbies, animals in the house

Physical Examination and Possible Findings

- Eyes: lens cloudiness, glaucoma
- Nose: purulent rhinorrhea, polyps
- Sinuses: pain
- Throat: posterior pharyngeal hypertrophied lymphoid tissue
- Chest: change in shape
- Heart: murmurs, S_3/S_4
- Lungs: wheezing, rhonchi, prolonged expiratory phase, use of accessory muscles, decreased breath sounds
- Abdomen: hepatosplenomegaly
- Neurologic: mental confusion, change in cerebellar function, change in motor coordination from baseline

Adapted from: Braman (1993), Martin (1996), NAEPP (2002).

Patient/Caregiver Information. All persons with asthma need to know how to use a peak flow meter and inhaler (see below).

1. Discuss the following with patients:
   - Patients need to have a complete health evaluation to find out if there are other health problems that could affect or be affected by asthma.
   - They need to be encouraged to discuss all symptoms and physical problems that make taking medication difficult.
2. In addition, patients need to understand that it is important for them to get help from a support group, family, friends, or a counselor when they feel stressed or depressed. Any life changes can increase the risk of having an asthma episode (NAEPP, 2002).

TABLE 22–2. Common Diagnostic Tests for Asthma and Their Possible Findings

Diagnostic Tests	Possible Findings
Spirometry	Decreased FEV_1, FVC
Chest x-ray	Hyperinflation, rule out lung masses, cavities
Nasal smears	Eosinophils
Allergy tests	+/−[a] dust mites, animal dander, mold, pollen
Special Tests as Indicated	
Bronchoprovocation challenge	
Sinus films	
EKG	
Other pulmonary tests	
Liver function tests	
Prothrombin time	
Upper GI series	

[a]+/− means finding may be either present or absent.

Adapted from NAEPP (2002), and Roncolli & Dempster (1996).

How to Use an Inhaler. Inhalers can be used by all asthma patients who are 5 years of age and older. Infants and young children will benefit most from a holding chamber and/or a face mask attached to the inhaler. These devices can also be useful to elderly patients.

With the ban on chlorofluorocarbons (CFCs) by 2005, dry-powder inhalers (DPIs) are common. Clients who have used MDIs previously may encounter difficult-to-master differences in administration technique.

Several different types of inhalers are currently on the market:

Metered dose inhaler without a spacer

1. Remove the cap and shake the inhaler.
2. Breathe out.
3. Put the mouthpiece in your mouth and at the start of a slow, deep inspiration, press the canister and continue to inhale deeply. Always hold the inhaler horizontal to the floor.
4. Hold your breath for 10–15 s.
5. Exhale into room air.
6. Wait 30–60 s and repeat steps 1 through 5.

Using a spacer is always preferred. It increases the amount of medication that is delivered to the lung and less is deposited on the tongue and in the back of the mouth. It also decreases the cough reflex, voice changes, and the risk of a yeast infection in the mouth. There are many models of spacers available, so ask your healthcare provider which one is right for you.

TABLE 22–3. Assessment Parameters for the Adult and Elderly on Asthma

Medications	Disease State	Adverse Reactions in Asthma
Beta blockers[a]	Hypertension Glaucoma	Can cause bronchospasms
$Beta_2$ agonist	CHF	Increases heart rate Potentiates heart failure
		Excess use (dose-dependent effect) can cause decrease in K+ and increase in QT interval on EKG
		$Beta_2$ receptor function decreases with age
Systemic steroids		Exacerbate TB, hypertension, peptic ulcer disease
		Cause/aggravate/accelerate osteoporosis, DM, loss of attention span, myopathy, increased skin fragility, memory and mood swings
Methylxanthine[b,c] (theophylline)	CHF, cirrhosis	Decreased clearance
	Cholestasis	
	BPH	Difficulty voiding
	Peptic ulcer disease, GERD	Relaxes the cardiac sphincter
NSAIDS/aspirin	Arthritis	Increased risk of bronchospasms, angioedema, urticaria
	Heart disease	
	Nasal polyps	
Nonallergic rhinitis	Hypertension	Cough
ACE inhibitors	CHF, diabetic nephropathy	

[a] Use of propanolol with zileuton can increase propanolol levels leading to increased $beta_2$ activity.

[b] Risk of seizures, cardiac arrhythmias, and death from methylxanthine toxicity increases with age; 16-fold greater risk of death.

[c] Erythromycin, cimetidine, allopurinal, ciprofloxacin, and zileuton increase methylxanthine levels; zafirlukast decreases theophylline levels.

Adapted from: Braman (1993) and NAEPP (2002).

When using a spacer:

1. Remove the cap and shake the inhaler.
2. Put the inhaler either into the back of the spacer or insert only the canister into the appropriate holder in the spacer.
3. Breathe out.
4. Press on the canister, breathe in deeply and slowly.
5. Hold your breath for 10–15 s.
6. Exhale back into the spacer, inhale again without pressing the canister, and exhale into room air.
7. Wait 30–60 s and repeat steps 1 through 6.

If using a steroid inhaler, always rinse your mouth after using the inhaler.

Turbuhaler/DPI

1. Unscrew and lift off the cover.
2. Hold the turbuhaler upright and twist the blue grip backward and forward twice if this is the first time the turbuhaler has been used. This "primes" the turbuhaler. For subsequent uses you need to twist the turbuhaler backward and then forward only once.
3. DO NOT SHAKE THE TURBUHALER.
4. Breathe out, put the mouthpiece between your lips, and breathe in as deeply and rapidly as possible—"suck the dry powder in."
5. Hold your breath for 10–15 s.
6. Exhale into room air.
7. DO NOT EXHALE back into the spacer.
8. Repeat steps 1 through 7 immediately after the first inhalation—you don't need to wait between inhalations.

If using a steroid inhaler, always rinse your mouth after using to prevent oral candidiasis ("thrush"). The new "Diskus" inhalers (Singulair, Advair) follow steps 3–7 above.

Autohaler

1. Remove the protective cover from the canister by pulling down the lip on the back of the cover.
2. Hold the inhaler upright, push the lever up, and then shake the canister.
3. Breathe out. Hold the canister upright, put the mouthpiece in the mouth, and close the lips around it securely. Hold the canister so that the air vents at the bottom aren't blocked.
4. Inhale slowly and continue breathing when the inhaler "clicks."
5. Hold your breath for 10–15 s.
6. Exhale into room air.
7. Hold the canister upright and press the lever down. Wait 1 min between inhalations.
8. After finishing, the lever must be pushed up ("on") before using the inhaler again. The inhaler won't operate if you don't follow these directions.

How to Use a Peak Flow Meter. A peak flow meter is a device that measures how well air moves out of your lungs. When an asthma episode is occurring, the airways of the lung begin to narrow slowly. By taking your peak flow measurement daily, you can often detect early airway narrowing, sometimes hours or days before you have any asthma symptoms.

If medicine is started before symptoms, you may be able to halt an asthma flare quickly and before it becomes severe.

A peak flow meter is most important for patients who use daily asthma medication. Patients who are 4 to 5 years of age and older can usually use a peak flow meter accurately.

The following five steps are necessary in order to obtain an accurate peak flow:

1. Move the indicator (usually a small red tab) to the bottom of the scale.
2. Stand up.
3. Take a very deep breath.
4. Holding the peak flow meter horizontal to the floor, place the mouthpiece in your mouth and close your lips securely around it.
5. Blow into the meter as hard and fast as you can (for children, it is like blowing out birthday candles).

Obtaining the Results

1. Write down the number you get. If you cough or make a mistake, don't write that number down. Repeat it.
2. Repeat steps 1 through 5 one or two more times and write down the best of the three numbers.
3. FIND YOUR BEST PERSONAL PEAK FLOW NUMBER. Your best personal peak flow number is the highest peak flow you can obtain over a 2 to 3 week period when your asthma is under good control. Good control is when you feel good, can do your regular activitis, and have no asthma symptoms.

Your personal best peak flow number may be higher or lower than someone else who is your age, height, or sex. Everyone's asthma is different so you need to find your personal best number. Your asthma treatment plan will be based on your personal best number. To find your personal best peak flow number, take your peak flow:

1. Twice daily for 2 to 3 weeks.
2. In the morning when you wake up and between 12 noon and 2 P.M. The early afternoon may not be possible for everyone, so late afternoon or early evening is acceptable.
3. As per instructions by your healthcare provider.

Outcomes Management

Selecting an Appropriate Agent. The NAEPP2 (2002) has developed four categories to classify asthma severity: mild intermittent, mild persistent, moderate persistent, and severe persistent. Table 22–11 shows the clinical features associated with these asthma severity classification categories.

Two strategies are recommended for managing therapy in the newly diagnosed asthmatic patient and/or the poorly controlled asthmatic patient, both involving step therapy. The first strategy is to begin at a level consistent with the patient's disease and "step up" therapy to achieve control of the symptoms. The second strategy is to initiate therapy at a higher level than the patient's severity to achieve rapid control of symptoms. After control is achieved, "step down" therapy to a level consistent with the patient's disease (NAEPP, 2002). The NAEPP recommends the latter approach, which usually achieves control of symptoms with a short burst of oral corticosteroids.

Step 1: Mild intermittent asthma. The individuals in this category often have EIB, or exacerbations that can be severe, separated by long periods of normal lung function and no symptoms. These exacerbations can be associated with viral respiratory infections and/or expose to allergens. In the elderly who experience symptoms of EIB, bronchospasms with a respiratory infection, or an allergen exposure, 50% resolve quickly with the standard treatment but the rest continue to have persistent symptoms (Braman, 1993). Table 22–4 lists the recommended treatment plan.

Step 2: Mild persistent asthma. Individuals in this category require daily medication. If the asthma is poorly controlled or symptoms at diagnosis are consistent with the criteria in this category, follow the treatment recommendations in Table 22–4.

Anti-inflammatory medications diminish airway inflammation and airway hyperresponsiveness (Lemanske, 2001; NAEPP, 2002; Robinson & Geddes, 1996). A good choice for an inhaled steroid is triamcinolone acetonide or beclomethasone. These inhaled steroids can be used two to four times a day, but if the frequency is problematic then consider flunisolide, fluticasone or budesonide, which might be dosed at once daily because of increased potency (Pincus, 2001), but usually requires twice daily dosing. A spacer should be used with all non-turbulator or DPI inhalers. It increases medication deposition in the lung, decreases oropharyngeal deposition, and may help improve pulmonary function (NAEPP, 2002). The elderly

TABLE 22–4. Stepwise Approach for Managing Asthma in Adults and Children Older Than 5 Years of Age: Treatment

Classify Severity: Clinical Features Before Treatment or Adequate Control			Medications Required To Maintain Long-Term Control
	Symptoms/Day / ***Symptoms/Night***	***PEF or FEV_1*** / ***PEF Variability***	***Daily Medications***
Step 4 **Severe Persistent**	Continual / Frequent	$\leq$60% / >30%	• Preferred treatment: –High-dose inhaled corticosteroids AND –Long-acting inhaled $beta_2$-agonists AND, if needed, –Corticosteroid tablets or syrup long term (2 mg/kg/day, generally do not exceed 60 mg per day). (Make repeat attempts to reduce systemic corticosteroids and maintain control with high-dose inhaled corticosteroids.)
Step 3 **Moderate Persistent**	Daily / >1 night/week	>60% – <80% / >30%	• Preferred treatment: –Low-to-medium dose inhaled corticosteroids and long-acting inhaled $beta_2$-agonists. • Alternative treatment (listed alphabetically): –Increase inhaled corticosteroids within medium-dose range OR –Low-to-medium dose inhaled corticosteroids and either leukotriene modifier or theophylline. If needed (particularly in patients with recurring severe exacerbations): • Preferred treatment: –Increase inhaled corticosteroids within medium-dose range and add long-acting inhaled $beta_2$-agonists. • Alternative treatment (listed alphabetically): –Increase inhaled corticosteroids within medium-dose range and add either leukotriene modifier or theophylline.
Step 2 **Mild Persistent**	>2/week but < 1x/day / >2 nights/month	$\geq$80% / 20–30%	• Preferred treatment: –Low-dose inhaled corticosteroids. • Alternative treatment (listed alphabetically): cromolyn, leukotriene modifier, nedocromil, OR sustained release theophylline to serum concentration of 5–15 mcg/mL.
Step 1 **Mild Intermittent**	$\leq$2 days/week / $\leq$2 nights/month	$\geq$80% / <20%	• No daily medication needed. • Severe exacerbations may occur, separated by long periods of normal lung function and no symptoms. A course of systemic corticosteroids is recommended.
Quick Relief All Patients	• Short-acting bronchodilator: 2–4 puffs short-acting inhaled $beta_2$-agonists as needed for symptoms. • Intensity of treatment will depend on severity of exacerbation; up to 3 treatments at 20-minute intervals or a single nebulizer treatment as needed. Course of systemic corticosteroids may be needed. • Use of short-acting $beta_2$-agonists >2 times a week in intermittent asthma (daily, or increasing use in persistent asthma) may indicate the need to initiate (increase) long-term control therapy.		

- The stepwise approach is meant to assist, not replace, the clinical decisionmaking required to meet individual patient needs.
- Classify severity: assign patient to most severe step in which any feature occurs (PEF is % of personal best; FEV_1 is % predicted).
- Gain control as quickly as possible (consider a short course of systemic corticosteroids); then step down to the least medication necessary to maintain control.
- Provide education on self-management and controlling environmental factors that make asthma worse (e.g., allergens and irritants).
- Refer to an asthma specialist if there are difficulties controlling asthma or if step 4 care is required. Referral may be considered if step 3 care is required.

may need an assistive device other than a spacer because of arthritis, musculoskeletal problems, and other factors that limit coordination. The VentEase is one such device. It is an adapter that facilitates activation of the MDI (metered dose inhaler) and bypasses deformities and coordination problems (Newman & Clarke, 1993). Newer assisted spacer devices are in the testing stage and appear greatly improved.

In the younger and middle-aged adult, bronchodilators are very effective; the elderly have a decreased beta-adrenergic response in the airways (NAEPP, 2002). The cholinergic bronchoconstrictive reflexes are intact and do not diminish with age (Davis & Bayard, 1988). Ipratropium bromide might be the preferred bronchodilator of choice for those over 60 years (NAEPP, 2002).

There is controversy regarding the use of sustained-release low-dose theophylline to control nocturnal symptoms. In NAEPP (2002) page 3-a3 states that "sustained release theophylline is an alternative but not preferred long-term-control medication." The healthcare provider in conjunction with the patient must make a decision whether to use theophylline after weighing the pros and cons. In the elderly, theophylline is not a safe drug to use because of concomitant diseases that may alter theophylline pharmacokinetics, multiple drug interactions, and often the inability to tolerate the medication (NAEPP, 2002).

In the elderly, obstructive lung disease, chronic bronchitis, and emphysema can coexist with asthma, making diagnosis difficult. Often a 2 to 3 week trial of oral systemic steroids can help determine the reversibility of the airflow obstruction and the extent of the therapeutic benefit of the steroids (Bousquet, Chanez, Vignola, & Michel, 1996; NAEPP, 2002).

Consider the step-up therapy if control deteriorates or the step-down therapy if control is maintained for several months.

Step 3: Moderate persistent asthma. Many adults with asthma also have nocturnal symptoms. The use of a long-acting $beta_2$ agonist relieves nocturnal symptoms and improves overall asthma control, especially when used in conjunction with inhaled steroids. Those with nocturnal symptoms should have an evaluation to rule out other treatable problems that could be causing or aggravating the nighttime symptoms. The long-acting $beta_2$ agonist is helpful in the elderly patient, too, but these patients must be warned that this is not a rescue medication (DuBuske, 1994).

If the asthma is poorly controlled or symptoms at diagnosis are consistent with criteria in this category, follow the treatment recommendations in Table 22–4 (Step 3). Improved asthma control has been noted with both a long-acting $beta_2$ agonist and a medium-dose inhaled steroid compared to doubling the dose of the current inhaled steroid (Woolcock, Lundbeck, Ringdal, & Jacques, 1996; NAEPP, 2002). Another option is to increase the potency of the medium-dose inhaled steroid. Fluticasone and budesonide are more potent than either triamcinolone or flunisolide on a per-puff basis, require fewer inhalations, and may more effectively inhibit the inflammatory process in the airways (Okamoto, Noonan, DeBoisblanc, & Kellerman, 1996; NAEPP, 2002) (see Tables 22–5 and 22–6).

Other therapeutic drugs are the leukotriene modifiers zileuton, zafirlukast, and montelukast. They are inhibitors of the metabolic pathway that activates the leukotrienes, which produce bronchoconstriction, airway inflammation, and bronchial hyperresponsiveness (Chanarin & Johnston, 1994; Henderson, 1994). Zileuton is a specific inhibitor of 5-lipoxygenase, thus inhibiting certain leukotrienes responsible for the effects of airway inflammation, edema, mucous secretion, and bronchoconstriction. Zileuton can be considered as a third line drug in the treatment of mild and moderate persistent asthma—first is ICS, then the addition of a long-acting $beta_2$ agonist (NAEPP, 2002). Zafirlukast is a selective leukotriene receptor antagonist of the components that cause anaphylaxis. Zafirlukast interferes with the development of airway edema, smooth muscle contraction, and altered cell activity associated with the inflammatory process in the lungs (Drug Facts and Comparisons, 2002; Wenzel & Kamada, 1996). The leukotrienes have demonstrated some selected anti-inflammatory effects, but their usefulness is limited (NAEPP, 2002). Because asthma is a disease of airway inflammation, the leukotrienes are considered adjunct therapy only. The inhaled steroids still remain the first-line therapy.

Montelukast inhibits the physiologic activity at the cysteinyl leukotriene receptor (CYSLT). This leukotriene inhibitor, similar to zileuton and zarfirlukast, interferes with airway inflammation. Montelukast may be considered for monotherapy in the treatment of mild, persistent asthma. This drug has been approved for use in children aged 2 years and older (Drug Facts & Comparisons, 2003).

Early recognition of declining PEFs is important for immediate action to be initiated. It is imperative that elderly adults monitor PEF daily as their perception of bronchoconstriction is blunted, allowing deterioration for longer periods, which then necessitates hospitalization rather than outpatient treatment (Connolly, Crowley, Charan, Nielson, & Vestal, 1992). In the elderly with moderate persistent to severe asthma with frequent exacerbations and wheezing, it is unlikely that symptoms will improve over time. Almost all elderly with these symptoms will require chronic oral systemic steroids. Persistent airflow obstruction demonstrated by spirometry testing is common in this group (Braman, 1993; Braman & Davis, 1986). For the management of an acute asthma exacerbation, refer to Table 22–7.

Every effort should be made to determine the etiology of the flare and correct the problem. It is important at the followup visit that the healthcare provider review daily medications, inhaler technique, and changes in the home or work environment. Consultation with a pulmonary specialist is necessary if the current asthma treatment plan repeatedly fails.

TABLE 22–5. Usual Dosages for Long-Term-Control Medications

Medication	Dosage Form	Adult Dose	Child Dose*
Inhaled Corticosteroids *(See Estimated Comparative Daily Dosages for Inhaled Corticosteroids).*			
Systemic Corticosteroids	*(Applies to all three corticosteroids.)*		
Methylprednisolone	2, 4, 8, 16, 32 mg tablets	• 7.5–60 mg daily in a single dose in a.m. or qod as needed for control	• 0.25–2 mg/kg daily in single dose in a.m. or qod as needed for control
Prednisolone	5 mg tablets, 5 mg/5 cc, 15 mg/5 cc	• Short-course "burst" to achieve control: 40–60 mg per day as single or 2 divided doses for 3–10 days	• Short-course "burst": 1–2 mg/kg/day, maximum 60 mg/day for 3–10 days
Prednisone	1, 2.5, 5, 10, 20, 50 mg tablets; 5 mg/cc, 5 mg/5 cc		
Long-Acting Inhaled Beta$_2$-Agonists *(Should not be used for symptom relief or for exacerbations. Use with inhaled corticosteroids.)*			
Salmeterol	MDI 21 mcg/puff DPI 50 mcg/blister	2 puffs q 12 hours 1 blister q 12 hours	1–2 puffs q 12 hours 1 blister q 12 hours
Formoterol	DPI 12 mcg/single-use capsule	1 capsule q 12 hours	1 capsule q 12 hours
Combined Medication			
Fluticasone/Salmeterol	DPI 100, 250, or 500 mcg/50 mcg	1 inhalation bid; dose depends on severity of asthma	1 inhalation bid; dose depends on severity of asthma
Cromolyn and Nedocromil			
Cromolyn	MDI 1 mg/puff Nebulizer 20 mg/ampule	2–4 puffs tid-qid 1 ampule tid-qid	1–2 puffs tid-qid 1 ampule tid-qid
Nedocromil	MDI 1.75 mg/puff	2–4 puffs bid-qid	1–2 puffs bid-qid
Leukotriene Modifiers			
Montelukast	4 or 5 mg chewable tablet 10 mg tablet	10 mg qhs	4 mg qhs (2–5 yrs) 5 mg qhs (6–14 yrs) 10 mg qhs (> 14 yrs)
Zafirlukast	10 or 20 mg tablet	40 mg daily (20 mg tablet bid)	20 mg daily (7–11 yrs) (10 mg tablet bid)
Zileuton	300 or 600 mg tablet	2,400 mg daily (give tablets qid)	
Methylxanthines *(Serum monitoring is important [serum concentration of 5–15 mcg/mL at steady state]).*			
Theophylline	Liquids, sustained-release tablets, and capsules	Starting dose 10 mg/kg/day up to 300 mg max; usual max 800 mg/day	Starting dose 10 mg/kg/day; usual max: • < 1 year of age: 0.2 (age in weeks) + + 5 = mg/kg/day • ≥ 1 year of age: 16 mg/kg/day

* Children ≤ 12 years of age

Step 4: Severe persistent asthma. Severe persistent asthma requires collaboration with a pulmonary specialist. If the patient requires oral steroids, use the lowest dose for the shortest time possible. For the elderly needing oral steroids, monitor closely for adverse effects, especially if comorbid illnesses are present.

If the asthma is poorly controlled or symptoms at diagnosis are consistent with the criteria in this category, follow the recommendations in Table 22–4 (step 4).

Monitoring for Efficacy. At each visit, ask the patient about any change in symptoms (cough with laughing, exercise, weather changes, environmental or work exposure), nocturnal symptoms, frequency of the beta$_2$ agonist use, PEF readings, changes in exercise tolerance, subjective symptoms, chest tightness, shortness of breath, wheezing, degrees of cough, and limitation of activities of daily living. The daily medications should be reviewed and inhaler use demonstrated to ensure correct technique and use of relief medications. The patient should be fully active with minimal to no symptoms and feel that asthma is not limiting his or her life. Elderly patients should be active and healthy and experience minimal symptoms secondary to their asthma and comorbid illnesses.

During the physical examination, check the following:

- Change from baseline
- Nose: purulent rhinorrhea
- Sinuses: pain
- Lungs: wheezing, crackles, rhonchi, decreased breath sounds, prolonged expiratory phase, respiratory rate
- Heart: murmurs, S_3 and/or S_4
- Skin: eczema
- Pulmonary function tests: FEV_1, FVC (if not available, use a PEF)

The examination may be more extensive but must be tailored to the patient's symptoms, age, other comorbid ill-

TABLE 22–6. Estimated Comparative Daily Dosages for Inhaled Corticosteroids

	Low Daily Dose		Medium Daily Dose		High Daily Dose	
Drug	**Adult**	**Child***	**Adult**	**Child***	**Adult**	**Child***
Beclomethasone CFC						
42 or 84 mcg/puff	168–504 mcg	84–336 mcg	504–840 mcg	336–672 mcg	> 840 mcg	> 672 mcg
Beclomethasone HFA						
40 or 80 mcg/puff	80–240 mcg	80–160 mcg	240–480 mcg	160–320 mcg	> 480 mcg	> 320 mcg
Budesonide DPI						
200 mcg/inhalation	200–600 mcg	200–400 mcg	600–1,200 mcg	400–800 mcg	> 1,200 mcg	> 800 mcg
Inhalation suspension for nebulization (child dose)		0.5 mg		1.0 mg		2.0 mg
Flunisolide 250 mcg/puff	500–1,000 mcg	500–750 mcg	1,000–2,000 mcg	1,000–1,250 mcg	> 2,000 mcg	> 1,250 mcg
Fluticasone						
MDI: 44, 110, or 220 mcg/puff	88–264 mcg	88–176 mcg	264–660 mcg	176–440 mcg	> 660 mcg	> 440 mcg
DPI: 50, 100, or 250 mcg/inhalation	100–300 mcg	100–200 mcg	300–600 mcg	200–400 mcg	> 600 mcg	> 400 mcg
Triamcinolone acetonide 100 mcg/puff	400–1,000 mcg	400–800 mcg	1,000–2,000 mcg	800–1,200 mcg	> 2,000 mcg	> 1,200 mcg

* Children ≤ 12 years of age

nesses, state of health, frequency of beta_2 agonist use, exacerbations, and any visits to the emergency room or healthcare provider's office for asthma flares.

The laboratory tests are based on the history and physical examination. For an acute exacerbation, a WBC and chest x-ray may be required, but more lab tests are necessary if the patient is elderly and/or has a comorbid illness. If the patient is on theophylline, levels should be obtained periodically. In the elderly, theophylline levels should be checked more often, especially if a sudden onset of mental changes occurs. Numerous medications and other factors can interfere with theophylline metabolism. Theophylline levels should be checked if the following conditions exist: change in medication dosing, stop-

TABLE 22–7. Management of an Acute Asthma Exacerbation

Initial Assessment

History, physical examination (heart rate, respiratory rate, wheezing, decreased breath sounds, use of accessory muscles), PEF

↓ ↓

Assess Severity

PEF: 50–80% of predicted or personal best | PEF <50% of predicted or personal best

↓ ↓

Initial Treatment

Inhaled short-acting beta_2 agonist: 2–4 puffs every 20 min three times or one nebulizer treatment

Inhaled short-acting agonist and an anticholinergic via nebulizer every 20 min or continuously for 1 h

↓

Repeat Assessment

Symptoms, physical examination, PEF

↓ ↓ ↓

Good Response	Incomplete Response	Poor Response
PEF >80% of predicted or personal best and increased from original PEF; no wheezing or shortness of breath; response to beta_2 agonist is sustained; continue beta_2 agonist q 3–4 h for 2–3 days; if on inhaled steroids, double dose for 7–10 days; +/− short burst of steroids, call clinician in 24 h.	PEF 50–80% of predicted or personal best and no change from original PEF; persistent wheezing and shortness of breath; continue beta_2 agonist; add oral steroids and taper; contact clinician immediately.	PEF <50% of predicted or personal best, marked wheezing and/or shortness of breath; repeat inhaled beta_2 agonist or nebulizer; add oral steroids and taper; if distress is increasing, severe, and/or unresponsive, send to the ER.

Adapted from NAEPP (2002).

ping or starting a medication that interferes with theophylline metabolism, a change in smoking frequency, and patients on zileuton or zafirlukast (*Drug Facts and Comparisons,* 2003). Levels should be drawn every 2 to 3 months, if the patient is elderly and/or taking medication that interferes with theophylline metabolism or the history or physical examination are suggestive of problems. An ALT/AST should be checked on patients at baseline if adding zileuton is considered. LFTs are checked once a month for 3 months, then q 6 to 12 months afterwards (*Drug Facts and Comparisons,* 2003), unless symptoms develop consistent with liver dysfunction. If liver elevations do occur, they can remain unchanged, resolve, or progress with continued zileuton therapy (Costello, Meltzer, & Bleecker, 1994; *Drug Facts and Comparisons,* 2003). Elevated liver enzymes occur in approximately 3 to 4% of people on zileuton and usually occur within 3 months of starting the medication.

Prothrombin time is monitored in those patients taking zileuton or zafirlukast and warfarin. Zileuton and zafirlukast can interact with warfarin and cause a significant increase in prothrombin time (PT) and international normalized ratio (INR). PT and INR need to be monitored periodically (*Drug Facts and Comparisons,* 2003).

Montelukast has not been shown to inhibit the P-450 cytochrome. Therefore there are no clinically significant changes in the pharmacokinetics of theophylline, warfarin, terfenadine, or oral contraceptives with norethindrone/ethinyl estradiol or prednisone. It has been reported equally safe at the recommended dose for the elderly as well as younger adults but some elderly may experience greater sensitivity to this medicine than others taken for asthma.

The most common adverse reactions are headache, influenza-like symptoms, abdominal pain, cough, and approximately a 2% risk of an increased ALT level. It is recommended that a baseline LFT level be drawn. In patients with mild to moderate hepatic insufficiency, the metabolism of montelukast was decreased. Currently, the developing drug company, Merck, does not recommend a dosage adjustment. However, appropriate clinical monitoring is warranted. At present, no safety data exist using montelukast in patients with severe hepatic insufficiency.

Montelukast is available in a 5 mg chewable tablet designed to be taken daily by children 6 to 14 years old and a 10 mg oral tablet for adolescents older than 15 years old and adults.

Monitoring for Toxicity. Patients should be questioned about any adverse reactions to their medications. Refer to the Drug Tables for the common toxicities and how to monitor them. In addition to the commonly discussed toxicities, the following adverse reactions need to be considered:

- *Beta$_2$ agonists:* Excessive use of inhaled beta$_2$ agonists must be discouraged, and the prescription for any beta$_2$ agonist should limit the adult from obtaining more than one inhaler per month unless a true athlete.
- *Oral steroids:* Because women on oral steroids are at risk for trabecular bone loss they should be encouraged to participate in weight-bearing exercises to the best of their ability, eliminate smoking and alcohol, and maintain adequate calcium intake (Braman, 1993; NAEPP, 2002).

  Daily elemental calcium intake of 1200 to 1500 mg and 400 to 800 units of vitamin D are essential. Avoid medications that can induce bone loss—i.e., antacids with aluminum, tetracyclines, furosemide, anticonvulsants. It may be impossible to avoid using these medications, but if they are used, close monitoring is required. If a patient is on long-term oral steroids, a bone densitometry evaluation is necessary because approximately 30% of bone is lost before there are changes on an x-ray (Braman, 1993; Grossman, 1998; Spahn & Kamada, 1995). Cataracts can occur with oral prednisone use, even with a dose as low as 7.5 mg/day or greater. Annual eye examinations are advised. Inhaled steroids do not seem to cause the same risk of developing cataracts that oral steroids do (Kamada & Szefler, 1995).

  Suppression of the adrenal axis can be caused by oral steroids at doses of 7.5 mg/day or more of prednisone and in those who receive frequent "bursts" of high-dose steroids. Complete recovery of adrenal suppression from long-term use or frequent "bursts" can take from 6 months to 1 year (Spahn & Kamada, 1995).
- *Leukotriene modifiers:* The leukotriene modifiers zileuton and zafirlukast can have some adverse reactions. Zileuton can cause a transient rise in liver enzymes, bloating, abdominal discomfort or pain, and diarrhea. The abdominal complaints are usually dose-dependent and can be decreased by adjusting the medication dose to two or three times per day. (*Drug Facts and Comparisons,* 2003). The efficacy of zileuton dosed at 3 times a day is very equivalent to 4 times a day; the efficacy decreases if dosed at 2 times a day but is still moderately effective (Wenzel & Kamada, 1996). Zileuton is metabolized by cy-

tochrome P-450, so use caution when prescribing a medication that inhibits these enzymes. When taking zileuton, concurrent use causes an increase in propanolol, theophylline, and warfarin levels, and these should be monitored carefully. Zileuton has not been shown to decrease the effectiveness of prednisone, oral contraceptives, digoxin, or phenytoin. Zileuton is contraindicated in patients with active liver disease or ALT/AST levels more than three times normal. The elderly and those with renal impairment do not need a dose adjustment (*Drug Facts and Comparisons,* 2003). This drug is only indicated in patients 12 years and older.

Zafirlukast must be taken on an empty stomach and dosed one tablet twice a day. The most common side effects are headache and nausea. Mild to moderate respiratory infections are reported in patients older than 55 who are also using inhaled steroids (*Drug Facts and Comparisons,* 2003). Zafirlukast does not increase liver enzymes. In the elderly (>65 years) and those with hepatic impairment, there is an increase in the plasma levels of zafirlukast, and thus a dose adjustment may be necessary (*Drug Facts and Comparisons,* 2003).

Followup Recommendations. Patients with mildly persistent to severe asthma who are stable can be seen every 6 to 12 months. The frequency of the office visits will depend on the patient's age, comorbid illness, medication use (especially theophylline and zileuton), and frequency of asthma flares and their severity. Spirometry should be done on all asthma patients once a year, and more often if there have been severe exacerbations. Other tests may be required, based on the patient's history, physical examination findings, and medication use.

PEDIATRIC ASTHMA

Underdiagnosis of asthma in infants and children younger than 12 years is a frequent problem because many of the classic signs and symptoms seen in adolescents and adults may be absent in this age group. The diagnosis of asthma should always be considered if any of the following indicators are present (although these are not diagnostic by themselves, multiple indicators do increase the possibility of asthma):

- More than 3 episodes of wheezing in an infant/young child lasting > 1 day, interfering with sleep, and risk factors: parent history of asthma, diagnosed atopic dermatitis, or if 2 of the following exist: allergic rhinitis, wheezing apart from colds, and peripheral blood eosinophilia. However, the absence of wheezing does not rule out asthma, since some children have significant airflow variability and obstruction yet don't wheeze (Lipworth, Fowler, & Wilson, 2002; NAEEP, 2002).
- Atopy is a strong predictor of asthma development in children. Atopy is the genetic susceptibility to produce IgE directed toward common environmental allergens, including house-dust mites, animal proteins, and fungi, etc. (NAEPP, 2002). This production of IgE sensitizes mast cells and potentially other lung cells so that future exposure to specific antigens can activate these cells.
- Chronic cough triggered by exercise or viral infections. Can also be triggered by a constellation of nighttime factors: changes in body temperature, humidity levels, and recumbent position and decreases in cortisol and epinephrine levels and increase in endogenous PAF (platelet-activating factor), resulting in increased bronchoconstriction and reflux problems. (NAEPP, 2002).
- Symptoms occur or worsen when exposed to smoke, menses, changes in weather, airborne chemicals or dust, or strong emotions (NAEPP, 2002).
- Chest pain or stomachache with no other obvious etiology (Li & O'Connell, 1996).
- Chronic rhinitis and sinusitis (NAEPP, 2002).

Specific Considerations for Pharmacotherapy

When Drug Therapy Is Needed. "Pharmacologic therapy is utilized to prevent and control the symptoms of asthma, reduce the frequency and severity of asthma exacerbations, and reverse airflow obstruction" (NAEPP, 2002). Because asthma is recognized as a chronic disorder with bronchial constriction that is at least partially reversible, chronic inflammation, and bronchial hyperresponsiveness, and in some patients airway remodeling, medications must be taken daily. The medications used for long-term control are anti-inflammatory agents that attenuate inflammation by reducing the markers of inflammation in airway tissues and blocking mediator release in the early and late phases of antigen response and long-acting bronchodilators for control of noctural symptoms and exercise-induced bronchospasm (NAEPP, 2002).

Immediate-relief medications, the short-acting bronchodilators, relax the airway smooth muscles and rapidly increase airflow, which reduces acute asthma exacerbations (NAEPP, 2002). There are two patterns of wheezing in children who wheeze with acute viral upper respiratory infections; those who have a remission of their symptoms in the preschool age and those who have persistent symptoms throughout childhood. In infants and young children < 5 years of age who wheeze frequently (> 3 episodes in a year lasting > 1 day and affecting sleep), risk factors associated with persistent asthma at 6 years of age were: parental history of asthma or an M.D. diagnosis of atopic dermatitis or two of the following—physician-diagnosed allergic rhinitis, a peripheral blood eosinophilia or wheezing without a viral infection (Castro-Rodriguez, Holberg et al, 2000.) Studies show that approximately "50 to 80% of children with asthma develop symptoms before their fifth birthday." (NAEPP, 2002, p.26.)

Further studies have shown that ICS (inhaled corticosteroids) in children > 5 years of age with mild-to-moderate persistent asthma, improved the pre-bronchodilator FEV_1, reduced bronchial hyper-responsiveness, decreased symptoms, decreased the frequency of $beta_2$ agonist use, had fewer courses of oral steroids and fewer hospitalizations. In children < 4 years of age, the limited studies showed similar results. (CAMP, 2000.) Other studies done on children with wheezing and asthma suggest that absolute lung growth may be suboptimal, especially during adolescence, and that lung function may never return to normal even though asthma becomes asymptomatic (Finder, 1999; Martinez, Wright, Taussig, et al., 1995). A number of other studies looked at childhood asthma and found, all those with persistent wheezing and asthma had airflow limitation in mid-life (Godden et al., 1994; Gold, Wypy, Wang, et al., 1994). The new, NAEPP (2002) report states that early intervention with low dose ICS has the potential to reduce a downward spiral in loss of lung function and preserve the quality of life.

A Finnish study evaluated the use of inhaled budesonide among subjects that were divided into six groups based on the duration of their symptoms, ranging from less than 6 months to over 10 years. Inhaled budesonide use was evaluated after 3 months, and the most improvement was seen in the group with asthma present for 6 months or less. The subjects were reevaluated again 2 years after initiating treatment, with the least benefit seen in the group whose asthma was present for 10 years or more before treatment was initiated. These data suggest that early introduction of anti-inflammatory agents could interrupt some of the irreversible component of the inflammatory process (Selroos, Pietinalho, Lofroos & Riska, 1995) (see Table 22–6). As more is learned regarding the pathophysiology of asthma, airway remodeling, and its long-term sequelae and more studies than examine the early use of inhaled steroids in children, the issue of when to initiate inhaled steroids in those with asthma may be resolved. However, aggressively treating children with moderately persistent or severe asthma with inhaled steroids may be prudent based on several studies that have been done showing less favorable long-term outcomes in those without inhaled steroids.

Short- and Long-Term Goals of Pharmacotherapy. The short-term goals of treatment are to provide prompt relief of bronchoconstriction and the accompanying symptoms of chest tightness, wheezing, shortness of breath, and cough (NAEPP, 2002). Systemic steroids are also necessary in the treatment of moderately persistent and severe exacerbations to prevent progression, hurry recovery, and prevent a relapse during recovery (NAEPP, 2002).

The long-term goals of treatment are to prevent or reduce the severity and frequency of exacerbations, control the symptoms of asthma, reverse airflow obstruction, and perhaps reduce airway remodeling (Murphy & Kelly, 1996; NAEPP, 2002).

Nonpharmacologic Therapy. The child's caregivers will need to control environmental factors that trigger an exacerbation.

Time Frame for Initiating Pharmacotherapy. Early recognition of declining PEF is important, and immediate action is required. At diagnosis, medication(s) will be started, depending on the asthma classification designation. It is imperative that they begin immediately.

The following guidelines developed by the NAEPP (2002) utilizes a "stop light" approach to management. This makes it easier for children to know how to manage and intervene in their own asthma. Table 22–8 describes this plan. Patient education is vital along with clearly written management instructions for long-term care (NAEPP, 2002).

Assessment Needed Prior to Therapy. Refer to the section on asthma in adults. Only the differences in children will be discussed here. In young children less than 4 to 5 years, the medical history, physical examination, and empiric pharmacologic therapy may be the only diagnostic tools available to the clinician because the age of the child prohibits spirometry testing. In the older child, spirometry testing is an important diagnostic tool, especially if the symptoms are atypical. Refer to Table 22–9

TABLE 22–8. Asthma Control Plan: The "Stop Light" Approach

Green Zone: All Clear

80–100% of your personal best PEF[a] signals good control.

No asthma symptoms so continue taking your medications as usual. Able to do normal activities and sleep without symptoms.

Yellow Zone: Caution

50–80% of your personal best PEF signals caution.

Asthma symptoms may be mild to moderate and keep you from doing your usual activities.

Use an inhaled short-acting $beta_2$ agonist immediately either as a metered dose inhaler or nebulizer with cromolyn and follow the treatment regimen prescribed by your healthcare provider for managing your yellow zone.

Red Zone: Medical Alert

50% or less of your personal best signals a medical alert.

Asthma symptoms are serious.

You must use a short-acting inhaled $beta_2$ agonist immediately, either as a metered dose inhaler or nebulizer with cromolyn. Call your healthcare provider immediately and/or go directly to the ER.

[a]Normative standards are based on height, age, and sex for Caucasians. Differences exist for African Americans, Native Americans, Hispanics, and Asians. Lung function varies across racial and ethnic populations so that the standards cannot be extrapolated to them. The most clinically useful standard then will be the child's personal best.

Adapted from NAEPP (2002).

TABLE 22–9. History and Physical Examination of Children With Asthma

Pertinent History Markers

- Family history of asthma, allergies, eczema
- Classic symptoms of wheezing, shortness of breath, chest tightness, sputum production, cough worse at night
- Precipitating factors that aggravate asthma-like symptoms: viral infections, exercise, environmental changes (cold air, weather changes, strong emotions, parent smoking), animals, menses, house-dust mites (mattresses, pillows, carpets)
- Pattern of symptoms: perennial, seasonal, episodic, continuous, or continuous with acute exacerbations
- History of frequent upper respiratory infections, chronic recurring rhinorrhea, sinusitis, otitis
- Effect of symptoms on activity level, schoolwork, sleep, and appetite
- Progression of symptoms
- Regular medications used, any relationship to exacerbations and medication use
- NSAID/aspirin sensitivity reflux symptoms

Physical Examination Needed and Possible Findings

- Vital signs: height and weight plotted on growth chart; may be <50% for age
- Skin: eczematous rash
- Eyes: vision, lens cloudiness
- Nose: rhinorrhea, allergic turbinates
- Oropharynx: posterior pharynx cobblestoning, mucus
- Heart: murmurs
- Lungs: wheezing, decreased breath sounds, use of accessory muscles
- Abdomen: tenderness

Adapted from NAEPP (2002), and Shuttari (1995).

for the history and physical examination. Refer to Table 22–10 for the diagnostic tests used in children.

Patient/Caregiver Information

1. Discuss parent's anxiety regarding an asthma flare and review at each visit the clearly written instructions on "how to" manage a flare.
2. Role playing scenarios of an asthma flare at home and in school can help a parent gain more control and confidence in managing an asthma flare.
3. Teach all parents and children to use MDI, spacers, and peak flow meters.
4. The following need to be discussed with parents of infants and young children:
   - It is important to keep all healthcare appointments, even if the infant is well.
   - It is important to act quickly with asthma symptoms.
   - Signs that indicate the need to seek immediate emergency care include:
     - Breathing rate increases to over 40 breaths/minute
     - Sucking or feeding stops
     - Skin between the infant's ribs is pulled in and tight
     - Chest gets bigger
     - Coloring changes; blue fingers, nails, or lips; pale or red face
     - Cry changes in quality
     - Nostrils widen; grunting

TABLE 22–10. Diagnostic Tests for Children With Asthma

Diagnostic Tests	Possible Findings
Spirometry if the child is older than 3 to 6 years	Decreased FEV_1 and FVC
Bronchoprovocation challenge	FEV_1 after a $beta_2$ agonist challenge. If asthma, 12% improvement should be seen in FEV_1
Nasal eosinophil smear	Positive
CBC	Eosinophilia
Skin testing	Usually positive for the common allergens; house-dust mites, fungi, animal protein (cat/dog hair)
Sweat test	Negative
Sinus x-ray	+/− sinusitis
Chest x-ray	+/− lung masses, infection, heart size, thoracic abnormalities
Selected GI tests	Changes in gastric emptying, esophagitis, pH changes suggestive of GERD

+/− means finding may be either present or absent.

Adapted from Luskin (1994) and NAEPP (2002).

- During an acute asthma episode parents should be warned NOT TO DO THE FOLLOWING:
  - Give large volumes of fluids; just give normal amounts
  - Rebreath in a paper bag
  - Give OTC antihistamines and/or cold medicines
  - Breathe warm moist air from a shower (NAEPP, 2002)

Outcomes Management

Selecting an Appropriate Agent. Determining an agent to use in the pharmacologic management of pediatric asthma depends on severity and age. The same asthma classification categories developed by the NAEPP Expert Panel (2002) are used for children as well as adults to make therapeutic decisions.

Step 1: Mild intermittent asthma. Table 22–11 lists the long-term control and quick-relief medications for children less than 5 years of age. See Table 22–4 for children older than 5. Patients in this category often experience symptoms with exercise (EIB), viral respiratory infections, and occasionally other triggering factors. A beta$_2$ inhaled agonist is the drug of choice, used on a prn basis for relief of symptoms; if pulmonary functions are normalized, then continued intermittent use is acceptable. If a beta$_2$ agonist is needed more than twice a week (except for exercise) and/or significant symptoms occur between exercise episodes, then the child should be reevaluated and/or moved to the next step of care. EIB can be present in healthy athletes without an asthma history (Busse & Lemanske, 2001). In all asthma patients, however EIB should be anticipated. EIB is a "bronchospastic event that is caused by a loss of heat, water or both from the lung during exercise because of hyperventilation of air that is cooler and drier than that of the respiratory tree" (McFadden & Gilbert, 1994, p. 1364). EIB usually occurs during or immediately after an activity, reaches its peak 5 to 10 min after stopping the activity and usually has resolved completely in another 20 to 60 min (Virant, 1991). In some, especially children, EIB may be the only precipitant of asthma. These children should be monitored regularly to ensure that they have no symptoms or reduction in their PEF in the absence of exercise. EIB can also be a marker of inadequate asthma management (NAEPP, 2002). Recommended management strategies include:

- A beta$_2$ agonist metered dose inhaler (MDI) used approximately 20 to 30 min before exercise can be helpful for 3 to 4 h (deBenedictis, Martinati, Solinas, Tuteri, & Boner, 1996; NAEPP, 2002).
- In young children, an albuterol nebulizer can be used.
- Cromolyn or nedocromil used 20 to 30 min before exercise can prevent EIB also (NAEPP, 2002).
- A lengthy warmup prior to exercise can be helpful and may preclude the need for medication or repeated medication.
- Long-term control of asthma symptoms with anti-inflammatory medication will reduce airway responsiveness and is associated with a decrease in the frequency and severity of EIB (NAEPP, 2002).

Step 2: Mild persistent asthma. The NAEPP Expert Panel recommends that children with persistent asthma—whether mild, moderate, or severe—receive daily long-term anti-inflammatory medications.

In children younger than 5 years, a spacer/holding chamber and face mask is useful.

Children who experience an acute asthma attack, need to followup with their primary care provider (PCP) or their pulmonary specialist. Monitoring regularly, twice daily, until the peak flow is between 80 to 100% of the child's personal best is important. The Albuterol MDI/nebulizer should be continued for approximately 3 to 5 days in moderate exacerbations and +/− tapered depending on the response to discontinuation of the beta$_2$ agonist. In those with a severe exacerbation, the short-acting beta$_2$ agonist is usually tapered over 5 days so no rebound asthma flare occurs.

Most children with asthma will be on a short course of either liquid/tablet form of prednisone. Prednisone is given in two divided doses of 1 to 2 mg/kg/day for the shortest time necessary, usually 3 to 5 days. Occasionally longer dosing is required but that increases the adverse effects experienced (NAEPP, 1997).

Assessment of the cause of the exacerbation should be undertaken. If no cause is found, then continue the medications as before; if a trigger is identified, then reduce, modify, or eliminate the trigger. PEF should be measured once daily, preferably in the morning since the level is at its nadir then; however, if the child's asthma is not stable, PEFs can be checked twice daily, in the morning, early afternoon or evening (NAEPP, 2002).

Step 3: Moderate persistent asthma. If symptoms persist despite the treatment measures instituted in Step 2, more aggressive therapy is required. As the severity of asthma increases, so does the potential for more side effects from the medications used. Consultation and/or referral to a pulmonary specialist is advisable. Table 22–11 (Step 3) lists the long-term control and quick-relief medications. Nocturnal asthma is often a feature of moderate or severe

TABLE 22–11. Stepwise Approach for Managing Infants and Young Children (5 Years of Age and Younger) with Acute or Chronic Asthma

Classify Severity: Clinical Features Before Treatment or Adequate Control	*Symptoms/Day* / *Symptoms/Night*	Medications Required to Maintain Long-Term Control: *Daily Medications*
Step 4 Severe Persistent	Continual / Frequent	• Preferred treatment: –High-dose inhaled corticosteroids AND –Long-acting inhaled beta$_2$-agonists AND, if needed, –Corticosteroid tablets or syrup long term (2 mg/kg/day, generally do not exceed 60 mg per day). (Make repeat attempts to reduce systemic corticosteroids and maintain control with high-dose inhaled corticosteroids.)
Step 3 Moderate Persistent	Daily / >1 night/week	• Preferred treatments: –Low-dose inhaled corticosteroids and long-acting inhaled beta$_2$-agonists OR –Medium-dose inhaled corticosteroids. • Alternative treatment: –Low-dose inhaled corticosteroids and either leukotriene receptor antagonist or theophylline. If needed (particularly in patients with recurring severe exacerbations): • Preferred treatment: –Medium-dose inhaled corticosteroids and long-acting beta$_2$-agonists. • Alternative treatment: –Medium-dose inhaled corticosteroids and either leukotriene receptor antagonist or theophylline.
Step 2 Mild Persistent	>2/week but < 1x/day / >2 nights/month	• Preferred treatment: –Low-dose inhaled corticosteroid (with nebulizer or MDI with holding chamber with or without face mask or DPI). • Alternative treatment (listed alphabetically): –Cromolyn (nebulizer is preferred or MDI with holding chamber) OR leukotriene receptor antagonist.
Step 1 Mild Intermittent	≤2 days/week / ≤2 nights/month	• No daily medication needed.
Quick Relief All Patients	• Bronchodilator as needed for symptoms. Intensity of treatment will depend upon severity of exacerbation. - Preferred treatment: Short-acting inhaled beta$_2$-agonists by nebulizer or face mask and space/holding chamber –Alternative treatment: Oral beta$_2$-agonist • With viral respiratory infection - Bronchodilator q 4–6 hours up to 24 hours (longer with physician consult); in general, repeat no more than once every 6 weeks - Consider systemic corticosteroid if exacerbation is severe or patient has history of previous severe exacerbations • Use of short-acting beta$_2$-agonists >2 times a week in intermittent asthma (daily, or increasing use in persistent asthma) may indicate the need to initiate (increase) long-term control therapy.	

- The stepwise approach is intended to assist, not replace, the clinical decisionmaking required to meet individual patient needs.
- Classify severity: assign patient to most severe step in which any feature occurs.
- There are very few studies on asthma therapy for infants.
- Gain control as quickly as possible (a course of short systemic corticosteroids may be required); then step down to the least medication necessary to maintain control.
- Provide parent education on asthma management and controlling environmental factors that make asthma worse (e.g., allergies and irritants).
- Consultation with an asthma specialist is recommended for patients with moderate or severe persistent asthma. Consider consultation for patients with mild persistent asthma.

Source: NAEPP, 2002 (Reference in the public domain)

asthma and is probably related to diurnal variations in airway responsiveness (Jarjour, Gelfand, McGill, & Busse, 1996).

The use of low-dose sustained-release theophylline is controversial. Theophylline has been demonstrated to have only *modest* clinical effectiveness as a bronchodilator but at low doses has been shown to have some anti-inflammatory properties (Johnson, 2001; Streetman, Bhatt-Mehta, & Johnson, 2001). It has been hypothesized that children younger than 7 years may have an increased sensitivity to theophylline and therefore increased side effects as well. Many children cannot tolerate the taste of theophylline and will vomit, and have subtle changes in memory, hand tremors, and anxiety. A comparison of

TABLE 22–11B. Stepwise Approach for Managing Asthma in Adults and Children Older Than 5 Years of Age: Treatment

Classify Severity: Clinical Features Before Treatment or Adequate Control			Medications Required To Maintain Long-Term Control
	Symptoms/Day / ***Symptoms/Night***	***PEF or FEV_1*** / ***PEF Variability***	***Daily Medications***
Step 4 **Severe Persistent**	Continual / Frequent	$\leq$60% / >30%	• Preferred treatment: –High-dose inhaled corticosteroids AND –Long-acting inhaled $beta_2$-agonists AND, if needed, –Corticosteroid tablets or syrup long term (2 mg/kg/day, generally do not exceed 60 mg per day). (Make repeat attempts to reduce systemic corticosteroids and maintain control with high-dose inhaled corticosteroids.)
Step 3 **Moderate Persistent**	Daily / >1 night/week	>60% – <80% / >30%	• Preferred treatment: –Low-to-medium dose inhaled corticosteroids and long-acting inhaled $beta_2$-agonists. • Alternative treatment (listed alphabetically): –Increase inhaled corticosteroids within medium-dose range OR –Low-to-medium dose inhaled corticosteroids and either leukotrriene modifier or theophylline. If needed (particularly in patients with recurring severe exacerbations): • Preferred treatment: –Increase inhaled corticosteroids within medium-dose range and add long-acting inhaled $beta_2$-agonists. • Alternative treatment (listed alphabetically): –Increase inhaled corticosteroids within medium-dose range and add either leukotriene modifier or theophylline.
Step 2 **Mild Persistent**	>2/week but < 1x/day / >2 nights/month	$\geq$80% / 20–30%	• Preferred treatment: –Low-dose inhaled corticosteroids. • Alternative treatment (listed alphabetically): cromolyn, leukotriene modifier, nedocromil, OR sustained release theophylline to serum concentration of 5–15 mcg/mL.
Step 1 **Mild Intermittent**	$\leq$2 days/week / $\leq$2 nights/month	$\geq$80% / <20%	• No daily medication needed. • Severe exacerbations may occur, separated by long periods of normal lung function and no symptoms. A course of systemic corticosteroids is recommended.
Quick Relief **All Patients**	• Short-acting bronchodilator: 2–4 puffs short-acting inhaled $beta_2$-agonists as needed for symptoms. • Intensity of treatment will depend on severity of exacerbation; up to 3 treatments at 20-minute intervals or a single nebulizer treatment as needed. Course of systemic corticosteroids may be needed. • Use of short-acting $beta_2$-agonists >2 times a week in intermittent asthma (daily, or increasing use in persistent asthma) may indicate the need to initiate (increase) long-term control therapy.		

- The stepwise approach is meant to assist, not replace, the clinical decisionmaking required to meet individual patient needs.
- Classify severity: assign patient to most severe step in which any feature occurs (PEF is % of personal best; FEV_1 is % predicted).
- Gain control as quickly as possible (consider a short course of systemic corticosteroids); then step down to the least medication necessary to maintain control.
- Provide education on self-management and controlling environmental factors that make asthma worse (e.g., allergens and irritants).
- Refer to an asthma specialist if there are difficulties controlling asthma or if step 4 care is required. Referral may be considered if step 3 care is required.

Source: NAEPP, 2002

standardized scholastic achievement test scores showed no differences between children taking theophylline and their sibling controls (Milgrom & Bender, 1995). With the advent of newer and less toxic drugs, theophylline is generally not used as a primary drug for asthma treatment. Many researchers do not recommend the use of theophylline for nocturnal asthma in children because of the potential toxicity profile, significant drug interactions, and the added expense of monitoring serum levels. Some healthcare providers have used a single dose of theophylline in the early evening as a way to control nighttime symptoms.

However, absorption and bioavailability changes with age, febrile viral illnesses, diet, and certain medications. This is a consideration when using theophylline. (Finder, 2001; NAEPP, 2002; Niederhauser, 1997; Roncolli & Dempster, 1996). A long-acting inhaled beta$_2$ agonist may be a better choice for nocturnal symptoms.

Step 4: Severe persistent asthma. Consultation with and/or referral to a pulmonary specialist is highly recommended for children in this category. Table 22–11 (Step 4) lists the long-term control and quick-relief medications. Management of oral systemic steroids consists of:

- Giving the lowest possible daily dose or preferably an alternate-day dose
- Monitoring closely for steroid side effects
- When control is achieved, stepping down to minimal doses of oral steroids and then to inhaled high-dose steroids because they have fewer side effects than oral systemic steroids (NAEPP, 2002; Niederhauser, 1997).

Oral systemic prednisone is dosed at 1 to 2 mg/kg per day in two to three divided doses and then tapered slowly once the child is symptom-free and the PEF returns to the child's personal best (*Drug Facts and Comparisons,* 2003; Grant, Duggan, Santosham, & DeAngelis, 1996).

Monitoring for Efficacy. Selection of a medication to use should be guided by the child's symptoms, severity of the asthma, safety profile of the medications, lowest effective daily dose, fewest number of medications on a daily basis, and reassessment of effectiveness and quality of daily life.

Each child must be taught to recognize symptom patterns that might indicate inadequate asthma control and maintain a symptom history record. He or she should check PEF once daily unless symptomatic and follow a detailed written action plan developed by the healthcare provider in the event of an exacerbation; this is a must for those with moderate to severe asthma and anyone with a history of severe exacerbations (NAEPP, 2002). The frequency of asthma exacerbations should be assessed at each visit. They may not be related to a triggering event but rather adherence to the treatment regimen, inhaler technique, side effects of the medications, incorrect level of medication usage for the activity, and an inappropriate diagnosis of the correct step classification and, therefore, incorrect pharmacotherapy (NAEPP, 2002). Each of these factors needs to be assessed regularly during office visits and after an acute asthma exacerbation. Quality of life should be periodically assessed for the child, which includes missed school days and disturbances in sleep and/or regular activities (NAEPP, 2002).

At each visit, assess the following changes from the baseline physical examination:

- Skin: eczema, other rashes
- Lungs: quality of breath sounds, change from last visit, wheezing, diminished breath sounds, respiratory rate, use of accessory muscles
- Heart: murmurs, rate
- PEF: FEV$_1$; if spirometry is used, then check FVC also

The rest of the examination depends on the complaint if it is other than respiratory and if this is a followup from an asthma exacerbation.

No consistent laboratory values are drawn unless the asthma exacerbation was secondary to pneumonia or the child is on long-term oral steroids. A blood glucose should be checked; consider a WBC with differential and other levels as appropriate.

Monitoring for Toxicity. For a description of the most common adverse reactions to inhaled and oral beta$_2$ agonists, theophylline, and inhaled and oral steroids, refer to the Drug Tables at the end of the book.

Cromolyn/nedocromil. The most common side effects of using cromolyn or nedocromil are coughing and wheezing during nebulization, but they are less bothersome when used with a short-acting beta$_2$ agonist. Serious adverse reactions are rarely reported with cromolyn sodium or nedocromil.

Oral steroids. Children on oral systemic steroids have far more serious side effects than those on inhaled steroids, but the risks still exist, especially on the higher inhaled doses. High-dose inhaled ICS potentially causes decreased adrenocortical reserves rather than clinical hypoadrenal symptoms. This may be a problem if there is significant stress to the body or a sudden cessation of the high dose ICS. Decreased adrenal reserves parallels other systemic changes occurring related to high-dose ICS such as decrease in bone density. The beneficial effects of ICS flatten out above 400 to 500 mcg/day in children and 800 mcg/day in adults while the adverse effects increase sharply (Lipworth et al., 2002; Agertoft, Pedersen, 2000).

Low-to-medium dose ICSs don't cause irreversible vertical growth. Children on the low-to-medium dose ICSs have a decreased growth velocity in the first year of treatment of approximately 1 cm or less. This decrease in growth is not sustained in the remaining years and is reversible. Studies ten years from the onset of treatment indicate that children will attain their final predicted height, and studies out six years indicate that there is no evidence of bone mineral density loss on the low-to-medium dose ICSs (Kalister, 2001 & Camp, 2000; Lipworth, 1999).

The doses of ICS that caused no adrenal suppression were budesonide and triamcinolone < 400 mcg/day and fluticasone < 200 mcg/day. In some children with severe persistent asthma, higher doses of ICSs may be necessary. However, the benefits of high-dose ICSs versus oral steroids are significant, and the risks of side effects less. The child/adolescent should be on the lowest effective dose of ICSs as soon as possible. A slow "step-down" trial should be tried as early as warranted with careful monitoring (Pincus et al., 2000).

The new recommendations based on these studies are:

Moderate to severe persistent asthma
< 5 years: low-to-medium dose ICS AND long-acting beta$_2$ agonist OR a medium dose ICS only
5 years: low-to-medium dose ICS AND a long-acting beta$_2$ agonist

This combination improves lung function, decreases symptoms, and decreases the need for a regular short-acting beta$_2$ agonist. It may also decrease the need for oral steroids, thus preserving bone density, normal growth, and HPA function. Adding a leukotriene antagonist, theophylline, or doubling the ICS is not as significant as an ICS and a long-acting beta$_2$ agonist (Lipworth, 2000; NAEPP, 2002).

Poorly controlled asthma can delay growth and has its own associated risks, balancing out the potential risks of inhaled steroids. Even high-dose inhaled steroids have significantly less potential for serious side effects than oral systemic steroids (NAEPP, 2002). With careful daily monitoring and a symptom control record, the number and severity of asthma flares in many children may be reduced. This can reduce the need for higher dose inhaled steroids and/or oral systemic steroids. One study of children during steroid treatment found that they were more sad, irritable, tired, and argumentative and manifested both visual and verbal memory deficits while taking oral steroids, but not 24 or 48 h after discontinuing them. The development of posterior subcapsular cataracts is seen with oral systemic steroids, but no association has been seen during the use of inhaled steroids (Allen, Bronsky, et al, 1998). The development of cataracts from oral steroids is dose-dependent (>7.5 mg/day) and cumulative over time (Toogood, 1993).

Followup Recommendations. Recommendations for monitoring children's asthma are:

1. Children with asthma should have regular health visits every 1 to 6 months, depending on the severity of the asthma, age of the child, and frequency of exacerbations.
2. At each office visit:
   a. Assess PEF and ensure correct PEF and inhaler technique.
   b. Review the symptom record and the daily PEF.
   c. Review current medications and if symptoms have been controlled for the past 2 to 3 months, consider a step-down approach, decreasing the last medication added by 25%. Continue this step-down therapy until the lowest possible dose is achieved that is effective.
   d. Most children with persistent asthma will always need a daily anti-inflammatory to suppress underlying airway inflammation and will relapse if all anti-inflammatory medications are withdrawn (Lipworth, 2001).
   e. Reassess the written instructions for the home management of acute exacerbations and verbally review any questions regarding management concerns.
   f. Discuss participation in sports and daily activities. Strongly encourage regular sports participation. A written plan should be given to the coach if the child participates on a sports team (NAEPP, 2002).
3. A written management plan should be prepared for the school with the input of the child and parent and must include: rescue medications that *must be readily available for the child to use during an acute asthma exacerbation* and a plan for the child to self-administer these medications if old enough; factors in school that may trigger an asthma flare and ways to help the student avoid exposure; administration of long-term medications, when appropriate; and use of a short-acting beta$_2$ agonist or cromolyn to prevent EIB.
4. If the child is old enough, spirometry should be done every 6 to 12 months.

ASTHMA IN PREGNANCY

With the increase in the incidence of asthma over the past 10 years in all age groups, there is a significant risk that asthma will be a complicating health problem of pregnancy. It is one of the most common pregnancy-related illnesses, affecting approximately 4% of all pregnancies (National Institutes of Health [NIH]/National Heart, Lung and Blood Institute [NHLBI], 1993). Asthma may occur either for the first time during a pregnancy or worsen during pregnancy. About one-third of pregnant women with asthma have adverse health problems, one-third will improve, and one-third will remain stable (NIH/NHLBI, 1993; Schatz 1999, 2001). Those patients whose asthma worsens during the first trimester and continues to be difficult to control will usually follow the same course in subsequent pregnancies. In those women with severe asthma at the start of the pregnancy, severity peaks after 26 weeks of gestation (ACAAI, 2002).

Because of the potential risk of uncontrolled asthma adversely affecting both the mother and fetus, NIH's National Heart, Lung and Blood Institute issued an Executive Summary on the Management of Asthma during Pregnancy (1993; Schatz 1999, 2001) recommending aggressive therapy. The pharmacologic therapy must be just as aggressive as if the woman were not pregnant. All pregnant women with moderate or severe asthma and those with frequent and/or severe asthma flares, should be assessed and followed by consultations with a pulmonologist.

Throughout pregnancy there are hormonal and anatomic changes that alter the respiratory, cardiovascular, and circulatory systems. These changes alter the pregnant woman's normal breathing pattern, leading to hyperventilation and dyspnea, which decreases the PCO_2 but is compensated for by a rise in Po_2. Hormonal increases, especially estrogen, leads to tissue edema, capillary congestion and hyperplasia of mucous glands which causes hypersecretion and increased mucosal friability. Forced vital capacity (FVC) decreases by 10 to 20% at the end of pregnancy with decreased expiratory reserve volume but residual volume (RV) and lung compliance remain unchanged (Sharma, 2003). With hyperventilation and mouth breathing, bronchospasms are more common because cool dry air may be delivered further down into the respiratory tree than usual (Shulman, Alderman, Ewig, & Bye, 1996). Physiological dyspnea occurs in about 60% of pregnant women during exertion and 20% of the time at rest. The physiological dyspnea of pregnancy occurs early in pregnancy and doesn't interfere with the usual ADL (activities of daily living). Exercise tolerance is usually minimally affected (ACOG/ACAAI, 2002). The physiological dyspnea of pregnancy must be distinguished from other more serious medical problems involving the pulmonary and cardiovascular systems.

In mild asthma, hypoxia is compensated for by hyperventilation, which keeps the PO_2 normal and the PCO_2 slightly decreased. As the airways become more constricted, ventilation-perfusion mismatching occurs. The result is arterial hypoxia. In severe obstruction, Po_2 continues to decrease while the PCO_2 rises to normal, signaling that the mother and especially the fetus are in the danger zone. Immediate treatment is required to prevent serious fetal and maternal complications.

With uncontrolled asthma, the risks to the fetus include increased possibility of oral clefts in the first trimester, intrauterine growth retardation, increased perinatal mortality, preterm delivery, neonatal hypoxia, and low birth weight (NIH/ACAAI 2002). The mother is at risk for preeclampsia, toxemia, hypertension, hyperemesis gravidarum, and vaginal hemorrhage (Kaliner, 1995). There have been no observational cohort data to show an association of increased fetal malformations, pre-eclampsia, preterm births, and low birth weight with maternal use of ICS, $beta_2$ agonists or theophylline. (Schatz, 2001). When respiratory status decline occurs, consider the following as triggers for the asthma flare: allergies, sinusitis, gastroesophageal reflux disease (GERD), occupational exposure, and rarely, a pulmonary embolus (Sharma, 2003).

Specific Considerations for Pharmacotherapy

When Drug Therapy Is Needed. All pregnant women with asthma must be aggressively treated to control symptoms, prevent exacerbations, maintain normal pregnant lung function and activity levels, avoid or reduce the adverse effects from asthma therapy, and avoid complications of uncontrolled asthma flares to the fetus and the mother.

Since the majority of inhaled medications are safe to use during pregnancy, there is no rationale for withholding treatment. The use of antihistamines, OTC (over-the-counter) cold remedies, large volumes of fluid, steam, and breathing into a paper bag are *not* recommended. These home treatments delay the onset of immediate appropriate therapy and can increase the risk of hypoxia to the mother and fetus (NIH/NHLBI, 1993).

Short- and Long-Term Goals of Pharmacotherapy. The short-term goals during an acute exacerbation are to dilate the bronchi, reverse the bronchospasms, and reduce airway inflammation. It is preferable to use only inhaled medications and not systemic steroids, but that may not be feasible. Because hypoxic complications $Po_2 < 95\%$, to the fetus can occur rapidly, therapy must provide a quick response and sustain that improvement.

The long-term goals are to prevent an asthma exacerbation, avoid environmental triggers (smoke, pollen, mold, animal protein, house dust mites, etc.) to greatly reduce the risk of symptoms and need for additional medication, maintain the mother's normal lung function and blood oxygenation, maintain the fetus's well-being and adequate oxygenation (NIH/NHLBI, 1993), and use the least amount of medication to maintain normal lung function but enough to control symptoms. The ultimate outcome is a well-oxygenated and healthy baby and mother.

Nonpharmacologic Therapy

1. Check PEFs once daily, preferably at the same time.
2. Use a spacer every time an inhaler is used.
3. Avoid or reduce exposure to triggering factors at home and work.
4. Use fetal monitoring.
5. Measure PO_2 and PCO_2.
6. Exercise appropriately since exercise can improve vasomotor rhinitis of pregnancy.
7. If symptoms of allergic rhinitis, sinusitis, or gastroesophageal reflux disease (GERD) occur, initiate the necessary preventive management.

Time Frame for Initiating Pharmacotherapy. Immediate recognition of declining PEF, quick early intervention, aggressive therapy, and slowly tapering the medications to the lowest effective dose are the goals. For the treatment of an acute asthma exacerbation, see Table 22–12.

In the pregnant woman if the asthma exacerbation becomes severe, fetal kick count decreases, $Po_2 < 95\%$ then intensive monitoring of the mother and fetus is critical. Medical treatment should be sought immediately to avoid further compromise.

Assessment Needed Prior to Therapy. For complete history and physical examination findings, refer to Table 22–1. Additional history items address specific pregnancy-related experiences. A comprehensive asthma assessment in the pregnant woman includes evaluation of fetal size, fetal heart rate, and fetal movement (see Table 22–13).

Patient/Caregiver Information

1. Every patient should keep a daily PEF diary.
2. All patients need a written care plan for an acute exacerbation and it should be reviewed regularly.
3. All patients need a short-acting $beta_2$ agonist inhaler with a spacer and/or a nebulizer.
4. Pregnant women need to know:
   - Asthma symptoms will become worse for about one-third of pregnant women.
   - Asthma symptoms may be the most severe between 24–36 weeks.
   - Uncontrolled asthma may affect the health of the baby. Not getting the baby oxygen, due to uncontrolled asthma, is a far greater risk than taking asthma medications.
   - Avoid the following during pregnancy: decongestants, some antibiotics such as tetracycline, live virus vaccines (killed are allowed), allergy shots (do not begin but may be continued if initiated prior to pregnancy), and medicines such as brompheniramine, epinephrine, phenylephrine, and phenylpropanolamine.
5. All common asthma triggers need to be avoided.

TABLE 22–12. Management of Acute Asthma During Pregnancy

Assess Severity

PEF is 50–80% of personal best or predicted value; note symptoms suggestive of an asthma flare: cough, breathlessness, wheezing, chest tightness, and shortness of breath; the degree of symptoms correlates poorly with severity of exacerbation	PEF <50% of personal best or predicted value especially in third trimester; improvement not sustained; "kick" count decreases; proceed to emergency room immediately.

↓

Initiate Treatment

Inhaled terbutaline two to four puffs q 20-min intervals for treatments or if unresponsive to terbutaline, use a single nebulizer treatment of albuterol

↓ ↓ ↓

Good Response	Incomplete Response	Poor Response
PEF >80% of personal best or predicted value; sustained response to $beta_2$ agonist for 4 h; continue $beta_2$ agonist q 3–4 h for 2–4 days; if on inhaled steroids, can double the dose for 7–10 days; contact the healthcare provider within 24 h	PEF 50–80% of personal best or predicted value; persistent chest tightness, shortness of breath, wheezing; continue $beta_2$ agonist; may need to begin oral prednisone, but call the clinician immediately for instructions and/or proceed to emergency room	PEF <50% of personal best or predicted value; proceed to emergency room immediately

Adapted from NAEPP (2002) and ACOG, ACAAI, 2002.)

TABLE 22–13. Diagnostic Tests for the Pregnant Woman with Asthma

Ultrasound at 12 to 20 weeks, depending on asthma severity
Sequential ultrasounds in second and third trimesters to evaluate fetal growth
Electronic fetal heart monitoring in third trimester to assess fetal well-being; more often if necessary
PEFs at each visit
Spirometry as baseline, but more often if repeat exacerbations

Adapted from NIH/NHLBI (1993).

6. Reassure patients that wheezing during labor and delivery is rare.
7. Breastfeeding is possible while taking asthma medications (NAEPP, 2002).

Outcomes Management

Selecting an Appropriate Agent. Consideration must be given to the safety of the drug used during pregnancy, utilizing the least amount of drug that will maintain control of symptoms, preventing an asthma exacerbation, and rapidly resolving an asthma flare in order to prevent maternal and fetal hypoxia. For an in-depth discussion on selecting an appropriate agent, refer to Outcomes Management in the Adult Asthma section.

Bronchodilators. In the pregnant patient, the only bronchodilator that is a Category B and approved for use is terbutaline. Since no $beta_2$ agonist has been shown to increase fetal mortality, decrease Apgar scores/birth weight or cause malformations, any $beta_2$ agonist that the pregnant woman has been using prior to her pregnancy can be continued. All pregnant women who require ICS and/or long-acting $beta_2$ agonists should continue all medications because not to do so has the potential to endanger the life of the mother and fetus (ACOG/ ACAAI, 2002). Symptom management, however, outweighs the risk of using any medications because of the greater risk of hypoxia to the fetus (*Drug Facts and Comparisons,* 2003). For further details refer to Drug Table 700.

Inhaled steroids. Inhaled ICS will be necessary in all pregnant women with mildly persistent to severe persistent asthma. According to ACOG/ACAAI (2002), they recommend using either inhaled beclomethasone or budesonide but if the pregnant woman's symptoms are stable on another ICS then that should be continued not changed. However, as in the non-pregnant woman, the lowest effective dose of ICS should be used. The pregnant woman requires careful monitoring because asthma severity can change quickly.

The leukotrienes that are used are; zileuton, montelukast and zarfirkulast. Zileuton is not to be used during pregnancy as animal studies have shown an adverse effects on the fetus' of pregnant mice. Montelukast and zarfirkulast can be used safely during pregnancy as there have been no problems detected in the fetus. However, these leukotrienes should only be used if the pregnant woman has recalcitrant asthma or is on these medications at the time of pregnancy and found to be effective (ACOG/ACAAI, 2002).

For information on drugs to avoid, refer to Outcomes Management in the Adult Asthma section.

Monitoring for Efficacy. At each visit the clinician should obtain a symptom history suggestive of an asthma flare: cough (occurs at rest, upon laughing, with tobacco smoke or noxious fumes, etc.), shortness of breath, chest tightness, breathlessness, nighttime awakening with cough, change in exercise tolerance, wheezing, and any respiratory infections. Assess the frequency of use of the bronchodilator and if the patient is using the steroid inhaler correctly (NAEPP, 2002).

Physical examination findings should assess:

- *Lungs:* Same as for the adult but focus on lung sounds at bases and wheezing with forced expiration.
- *Heart:* Murmurs.

The remainder of the examination is appropriate for the number of weeks of pregnancy. Fetal monitoring should be used as appropriate for gestational age, severity of asthma, and frequency of severe asthma episodes. Pulmonary function studies should include FEV_1 and FVC.

At each visit assess the lungs and heart, changes in the patient's own baseline, the PEFs, and other tests as appropriate for patient's pregnancy and asthma condition.

No laboratory tests are done routinely for asthma followup unless an acute illness occurs or monitoring for a coexisting condition is necessary.

Monitoring for Toxicity. A study of 180 pregnancies in which $beta_2$ agonists were used during the first trimester demonstrated no increased teratogenic risk to the fetus (ACOG/AAAAI, 2000; Schatz, 2001). $Beta_2$ agonists can cause tremors and tachycardia, and frequent use can lead to tolerance and paradoxical worsening of symptoms. Occasional use is not harmful, but constant use can mask worsening disease and prevent prompt action that can correct impending fetal hypoxia.

The adverse effects of using ICS are thrush in the mouth and dysphonia if the mouth isn't rinsed and water swallowed after ICS inhaler use. High dose ICS has the potential to cause some adverse effects (see Asthma Management in the Adult/Elderly). If oral steroids must be used, the shortest course and the lowest effective dose should be used to stabilize the patient and then taper as quickly as possible without adversely affecting the asthma. Oral steroids always have more side effects than inhaled steroids but are necessary for recovery from an acute attack.

For complete information on the bronchodilators and steroid inhalers, refer to Drug Tables 701 and 702.

Followup Recommendations. Asthma care should be incorporated as part of routine pregnancy care with special attention to:

- Symptom control
- Nocturnal symptoms
- Frequency of asthma flares, regardless of severity
- Frequency of $beta_2$ agonist use
- Daily medications
- Correct use of the spacer/inhaler
- PEF results
- Kick counts

The frequency of monitoring depends on the woman's pregnancy and asthma health; the more frequent and severe the exacerbations, the more frequent and intensive the monitoring.

BRONCHIOLITIS

Bronchiolitis is one of the most common respiratory infections seen in infants and young toddlers. An inflammation of the bronchioles—ciliated epithelial cells that increases mucous production, leading to cell death, and sloughing, leading to airway edema, narrowing, and obstruction. Previous bronchiolitis does not confer immunity and repeat infections are seen (Louden, 2001). RSV accounts for about 85% of all cases of bronchiolitis with 11% caused by adenoviruses. Parainfluenza virus usually begins earlier than RSV or adenoviruses (November) and occurs on an every other year basis (Louden, 2001). This disease is self-limited in most healthy young infants and toddlers, but in those with comorbid illnesses—heart disease, chronic lung disease (CLD), formerly called bronchopulmonary dysplasia (BPD), CF (cystic fibrosis) those who are premature, have had recent transplants, are immunosuppressed, or are on chemotherapy, the disease can be quite severe and requires more intensive health intervention (AAP, 2000; Meissner, Long & AAP, 2003). Risk factors for developing RSV are listed in Table 22–14. All infants and toddlers with RSV risk factors need close followup and attention. Even many healthy infants and toddlers who develop RSV can become so severely ill that treatment in a pediatric intensive care unit is required. See Tables 22–15, 22–16, and 22–17 for additional information on RSV in infants and toddlers.

TABLE 22–14. Respiratory Syncytial Virus Risk Factors

Infants in smoking environments
Males
Attendance at any child care facility during high-risk RSV season
Age: healthy infant < 6 months old, in the months between November and April **or** high-risk infant/toddler < 24 months old, in the months between November and April
Poor hand hygiene

Source: AAP Revised Statement on Treating RSV (2003).

The decision to treat as an outpatient versus an inpatient depends on many factors. The very young and preterm infants are at increased risk for apnea, whereas older infants and young toddlers are at risk for respiratory failure and/or dehydration. The nurse practitioner or physician's assistant who first encounters the acutely ill infant or toddler with bronchiolitis will rarely manage the case alone, but in collaboration with the physician.

Specific Considerations for Pharmacotherapy

When Drug Therapy Is Needed. Bronchodilators are controversial but the mainstay of management. They only improve reversible airway bronchospasm. There is some thought that the $beta_2$ agonists may improve oxygenation and minimally reduce airway resistance. ICS or oral steroids have no benefit on the outcome and have not been shown to decrease long-term wheezing associated with bronchiolitis or the later risk of developing asthma (Kimpen, 2001; Schindler, 2002). They are, however, effective in treating infants/toddlers with comorbid asthma.

The American Academy of Pediatrics Committee on Infectious Diseases and Committee on the Fetus and Newborn (Dec. 2003) revised their recommendations on the use of Palivizumab and RSV-IGIV, as well as the high-risk group that should receive the medication in prevention of severe lower respiratory infection with RSV.

The high-risk groups identified by the AAP are children under 24 months of age with chronic lung disease (CLD); certain preterm infants; and infants with congenital heart disease (CHD, both cyanotic and acyanotic). There are other conditions that may qualify for treatment prevention (Table 22-14A).

The two medications that have been approved for prevention of RSV in the high-risk group are Palivizumab and RSV-IGIV. Palivizumab is given intramuscularly at

Table 22-14A RSV-IGIV and Palivizumab Treatment Guidelines

Group 1
< 32 weeks gestation without CLD*
CHD^
CLD*
+/- in the following conditions: neurologic disease in VLBW#, number of siblings, childcare center attendance, pending cardiac surgery, distance to available hospital care for severe respiratory disease

Group 2
32–35 weeks gestation: prophylaxis for infants at greatest risk for severe RSV who are < 6 months old at start of the RSV season
Increased risk of RSV: childcare center attendance, school-age siblings, exposure to environmental air pollutants, congenital abnormalities of airways, severe neuromuscular disease

Group 3
< 2 years old with CLD who required supplemental oxygen, bronchodilator, diuretic, or corticosteroid therapy

Group 4
28 weeks gestation: may benefit from treatment during their first RSV season occurring in the first 12 months of life

Group 5
29–32 weeks gestation: may benefit from prophylaxis up to 6 months of age

*chronic lung disease; ^ congenital heart disease; # very low birth weight

Source: AAP Revised Policy on RSV Treatment (2003)

15 mg/kg, beginning at the start of the RSV season (November to April). The first dose is given on November 1 and the last dose on March 1. Palivizumab, but **not** RSV-IGIV, has been approved in children with hemodynamically congenital heart disease. RSV-IGIV may have been associated with an alteration in the blood viscosity in those children with CHD and an elevated hematocrit, which studies have shown to increase mortality rate (Meissner & Long, AAP Technical Report, 2003). There has been no associated interference with vaccine administration using Palivizumab. In studies, Palivizumab given monthly during RSV season has been associated with a

TABLE 22–15. History of the Infant/Toddler with RSV

- Begins with a URI
- 1-2 days later develops paroxysmal cough and dyspnea
- Poor feeding or anorexia
- Vomiting, especially post-tussive
- Grunting
- Irritable
- Audible wheezing
- Noisy breathing

Louden (2001).

TABLE 22–16. Physical Examination of an Infant/Toddler with RSV

- tachypnea 50-60/min
- tachycardia
- fever
- diffuse expiratory wheezing
- nasal flaring
- intercostal retractions
- inspiratory crackles
- mild conjunctivitis/pharyngitis
- apnea, < 6 weeks
- palpable liver/spleen secondary to hyperinflation of lungs and depres sion of diaphragm
- otitis media

AAP (2003) and Louden (2001).

decrease of 45 to 55% in hospitalization attributable to RSV (Meissner & Long, 2003).

RSV-IGIV has also been shown to decrease the severity of RSV infection in high-risk infants and toddlers. RSV-IGIV can be administered during RSV season to all high-risk infants and toddlers *without* hemodynamically congenital heart disease. It is given intravenously on the same dates as Palivizumab. If RSV-IGIV is given, immunization with MMR (measles, mumps, rubella) and varicella vaccines should be deferred for 9 months after the last dose of RSV-IGIV.

There has been no data in children with cystic fibrosis (CF) to indicate if there is an increased incidence of RSV, nor have there been trials of Palivizumab or RSV-IGIV in immunocompromised children (AAP Revised Policy for RSV Treatment, 2003).

Early ribavarin in the previously healthy infant with RSV significantly decreased airway reactivity and nonwheezing URIs (Dean & Khoshoo, 1999).

In infants and toddlers who are at increased risk for RSV, immunization for influenza is reasonable and prudent.

Short- and Long-Term Goals of Pharmacotherapy. The short-term goals are to shorten the ER visit and to prevent and/or shorten the hospital stay.

The long-term goals are to (1) decrease mortality in high-risk infants and toddlers; (2) decrease the incidence of lower respiratory tract infections, RSV-associated hospitalizations, and intensive care stays; and (3) prevent postbronchiolitis reactive airway disease and abnormal PFTs in later childhood (Meissner, Long & AAP, 2003).

TABLE 22–17. Diagnostic Tests for Infants/Toddlers with RSV

- CBC with differential
- CXR - hyperinflation and patchy infiltrates (non-specific)
- RSV culture
- RSV antibodies by immunofluorescence or ELISA
- RSV antigen nasal swabs

Kimpen (2001) and Louden (2001).

Nonpharmacologic Therapy

1. Give plenty of fluids for rehydration.
2. Use oxygen as needed.
3. Prevent airway reactivity and nonwheezing URIs (Dean & Khoshoo, 1999).

Time Frame for Initiating Pharmacotherapy. Early diagnosis of RSV is essential to institute pharmacologic therapy if the infant or toddler meets the criteria established by the AAP (2003) for its use.

Assessment Needed Prior to Therapy. A thorough history and physical examination with appropriate diagnostic tests is crucial. Refer to Tables 22–18 and 22–19 for the history, physical, and diagnostic information needs.

The criteria for outpatient/inpatient treatment and which medication to use is based on the history, physical exam, age of the infant, chronic medical conditions, severity of the illness, $PaO_2 < 90\%$, increased CO_2, inability to suck and breathe at the same time, and hydration status (Louden, 2001).

Patient/Caregiver Information

1. If the infant is managed as an outpatient, provide specific written instructions regarding changes to monitor, such as respiratory rate, ability to eat, playfulness, and lip color; worsening of other symptoms; and when to call the healthcare provider.
2. Palivizumab and RSV-16IU

TABLE 22–18. History and Physical Examination for Bronchiolitis

Pertinent History Markers
- Birth history
- Medical problems in the nursery: any treatments, followup needed
- Health status since home from the hospital
- Respiratory infection history since birth, symptoms, treatment, any hospitalizations, diagnosis
- Symptom presentation: URI symptoms and in 1-2 days paroxysmal cough, fever, wheezing, often posttussive vomiting, irritability, grunting, noisy breathing, poor feeding, +/− cyanosis
- Change in quality of eating and play

Physical Examination and Possible Findings

Tachypnea, common	Cyanosis
Tachycardia	Inspiratory crackles
Fever	Apnea, especially < 6 weeks
Mild conjunctivitis/pharyngitis	Otitis Media
Diffuse expiratory wheezing	Palpable liver/spleen secondary to hyperinflation of lungs and depression of diagraphm
Nasal flaring	
Intercostal retractions	

May present with some or most of these symptoms, depending on severity of the disease, age, and other comorbid illnesses

+/− means finding may be either present or absent.
Adapted from Louden (2001), Meissner, Long, & AAP (2003).

TABLE 22–19. Assessment of the Patient with Acute Bronchitis

Check vital signs - fever,* tachypnea
Auscultate lung fields - wheezing, rhonchi, prolonged expiratory phase^
Peak flow - may be low secondary to the inflammatory lung process

*high fever suggests assessment for pneumonia or influenza
^absence of breath sounds or crackles should prompt an assessment for pneumonia, bronchietasis, pneumothorax, etc
Knutson & Braun (2002) and MacKay (1996).

Outcomes Management

Selecting an Appropriate Agent. Supportive therapy is the mainstay of treatment for the healthy infant without risk factors who develops bronchiolitis. Usually rehydration and oxygen are all that is needed. If there is a moderately severe infection, it can be treated with a short hospital stay. Those with very mild disease and no other comorbid illness older than 6 weeks can be managed at home, with fluids, close monitoring, and frequent calls and visits to the healthcare provider.

The bronchodilator most beneficial for RSV-infected infants or toddlers is racemic epinephrine. Nebulized racemic epinephrine has been shown to have greater effectiveness in decreasing the respiratory rate and pulmonary resistance than nebulized albuterol. Clinical symptoms and oxygenation have been shown to be better using either racemic or subcutaneous epinephrine than albuterol.

Antibiotics, and oral or intravenous glucocorticoids, have no place currently in the management of acute bronchiolitis. The research to date demonstrates that these treatment modalities are ineffective.

Monitoring for Efficacy. Recovery is usually complete within several days if no major complications occur. When using nebulized racemic epinephrine or subcutaneous epinephrine, improvement in the clinical scores has been seen in about 30 min and in oxygenation in 60 min, and the heart rate decreased in 90 min. In those infants or toddlers treated as outpatients, improvement is noted within 48 to 72 h. The symptoms (respiratory rate, lip color, use of accessory muscles, ability to take fluids, etc.) should remain the same or improve but not worsen.

At each visit during the acute illness, check the following physical signs:

- Temperature: normal or elevated
- Respirations: rate, use of accessory muscles

- Lungs: wheezing, crackles, decreased breath sounds
- Heart: rate
- Abdomen: Palpable Liver/Spleen

Pulse oximetry should be checked if possible. If the infant or toddler looks toxic or the physical examination findings are deteriorating, then hospitalization is required. Other laboratory tests should be ordered as needed.

Monitoring for Toxicity. Epinephrine, used in appropriate doses, lowers heart and respiratory rate rather than increases it because of better oxygenation and decreased workload of the heart, and it probably provides some dilating effect on the alveoli (*Drug Facts and Comparisons,* 2003).

Followup Recommendations. In healthy infants and toddlers, a regular well-child visit can assess lungs, both at rest and after exercising, to ensure there is no wheezing. PFTs cannot be assessed in this age group. A good history from the parent may indicate any postbronchiolitis reactive airway problem.

In viral infections, bronchial hyperreactivity is common especially in boys and those with a family history of atopy and allergic disease. These patients must be treated with a bronchodilator during an acute exacerbation. In those infants and toddlers with a comorbid illness, more frequent office visits are needed. The frequency is determined by age, complications while hospitalized, status after hospitalization, and nature of the comorbid illness. In preterm infants and those less than 2 months, there is about a 10% risk of apnea. These infants must be closely monitored and may need home apnea monitoring.

ACUTE BRONCHITIS

Acute bronchitis is one of the most common diagnoses in ambulatory care. Cough is the predominant feature that brings people to the healthcare provider's office. The cough occurs within about 2 days of the onset of other symptoms, namely malaise, low-grade fever, and mild systemic symptoms. The cough is often harsh and none to minimally productive. If the cough is productive, the sputum color can range from clear to yellow/green. Sputum color is not indicative of a bacterial infection, since perioxadase released by the leukocytes causes the color changes (Knutson & Braun, 2002). Other symptoms may include wheezing, chest pain, dyspnea and hoarseness. The symptoms may be present in varying degrees or can be totally absent (Knutson & Braun, 2002). Most patients will have a cough for < 2 weeks, occasionally it can last 2 to 8 weeks (Chestnutt, 2002). If the cough fits the general pattern, then strongly suspect acute bronchitis. Bronchitis is almost always viral, rarely bacterial.

SPECIFIC CONSIDERATIONS FOR PHARMACOTHERAPY

When Drug Therapy Is Needed

Since acute bronchitis is viral and usually self-limiting, symptomatic relief is all that is generally needed.

Short- and Long-Term Goals of Pharmacotherapy

The short-term goals are to relieve the symptoms, control the cough or make it more effective, allow the patient to get the necessary undisturbed sleep at night, reduce the fever and/or alleviate the muscle aches and pains.

The long-term goals are to treat the lingering cough if needed and encourage adequate hydration and rest.

Nonpharmacologic Therapy

Nonpharmacologic therapy of acute bronchitis is mainly supportive: fluids, rest, and intensive education regarding the benign viral nature of this illness. If the patient smokes, this is an excellent opportunity to counsel regarding smoking cessation. The patient should stop smoking during at least the acute illness phase. The patient may need to return to the office for further smoking cessation instruction and/or medications.

Time Frame for Initiating Pharmacotherapy

Once the infection occurs, then the symptomatic treatment should start.

Assessment Needed Prior to Therapy

Generally, the patient with bronchitis is rarely acutely ill. If he or she is ill-appearing, then a more thorough history, physical, and appropriate lab/diagnostic work-up is required. Patients with comorbid illnesses, asthma, advanced age, malignancy, tuberculosis, immunocompromised state, COPD, and heart failure might require a more extensive workup: chest x-ray, CBC with a differential, office spirometry, and/or pulse oximetry. However, in the adult without comorbid illnesses, the history and routine physical should be sufficient to make the diagnosis. See Table 22–19 for patient assessment information.

PATIENT/CAREGIVER INFORMATION

Patients need to understand that bronchitis is a viral infection, similar to a cold virus, that will resolve on its own with symptomatic treatment. Antibiotics are not indicated for this illness. A clear and concise explanation of the natural disease course is helpful. The patient can expect that the cough may linger for 2 weeks or more. If it interferes with sleep, an inhaler may be beneficial. The patient should be aware of when to return to the healthcare provider: if the cough lasts > 1 month, if the patient has chest pain or is very short of breath, coughs up blood, develops a fever of > 101, and is continually weak and sick (Knutson & Braun, 2002).

OUTCOMES MANAGEMENT

Selecting an Appropriate Agent

Antitussives. Antitussive therapy is helpful to prevent and control the cough. If the cough is primarily nonproductive and/or minimally productive in an otherwise healthy adult and will not interfere with airway healing, then suppression would be beneficial. Selecting an antitussive drug is based on the etiology of the cough:

1. Antihistamines—allergic rhinitis
2. Decongestant/antihistamine—postnasal drainage with nasal congestion
3. Bronchodilator—asthma, reactive airway secondary to virus, etc
4. Nonspecific antitussives (dextromethorphan, tessalon, codeine, hydrocodone, carbetapentane, hydromorphone)—cough suppression only (Irwin et al., 1998)

Antibiotics. Because of the increasing resistance to antibiotics, antibiotics are not warranted or recommended for acute bronchitis. In the vast majority of studies examining the clinical effectiveness of antibiotics in the treatment of bronchitis, none were found to improve the course of bronchitis (Fahey, Stocks, & Thomas, 1998; Knutson & Braun, 2002).

Monitoring for Efficacy

The patient needs to return to the healthcare provider only if symptoms worsen or linger > 1 month. See Patient/Caregiver Information section for further details.

Monitoring for Toxicity

Instructions need to be given regarding when and how much narcotic cough syrup to take. The patient needs to be instructed regarding operating a motor vehicle, heavy machinery, and/or potentially dangerous equipment and drinking alcohol while using a narcotic-based cough medication. The narcotic cough medication should be reserved only for nighttime use to avoid any daytime problems.

Followup Recommendations

Healthy adults with acute bronchitis don't need to return to the healthcare provider unless symptoms persist or worsen. In patients with comorbid illnesses with acute bronchitis, followup is appropriate to monitor their progress and ensure that the comorbid illness is stable. These patients should be reevaluated in 1 week, sooner if increased symptoms related to the acute or chronic illness occur.

CHRONIC OBSTRUCTIVE LUNG DISEASE

Chronic obstructive lung disease has been defined by the Global Initiative for COPD as "a disease state characterized by airflow limitation that is not fully reversible. The airflow limitation is usually both progressive and associated with an abnormal inflammatory response of the lungs to noxious particles or gases" (Pauwels, Busit, Claverley, et al., 2001). The characteristics of the chronic airflow limitation of COPD is caused by a mix of small airway disease and parenchymal destruction (emphysema). Chronic inflammation leads to airway remodeling and narrowing of the airways. Destruction of the lung parenchyma by inflammation leads to the loss of alveolar attachment to the airway wall, decreased lung elastic recoil, an increase in the size of the mucus-secreting glands and ciliary dysfunction (de Boer, 2002; Pauwels et al., 2001). These changes produce hypersecretions in the lung, the inability of the airways to remain open during expiration, and eventually gas exchange abnormalities. In an adult without COPD, an inflammatory episode is normally followed by a repair process, but this process is thought to be deficient in the COPD patient (Stockley, 2002). The inflammatory changes and altered production of airway secretions and mucus in the lung increases the predisposition to airway infections. This in turn is associated with the acute exacerbations seen in COPD, which are characterized by cough, dyspnea, and excess secretions (Rennard & Farmer, 2002).

The "pathogenetic processes" (Rennard & Farmer, 2002) of COPD lead to important systemic effects as well: muscle-wasting affecting primarily the lower extremities, weight loss, tissue depletion, reduced capacity for exercise, and significant cardiovascular impairments (Petty, 2002; Rennard & Farmer, 2002). These systemic effects are not directly related to the airway flow limitation but need to be assessed in order to prevent worsening of the COPD (Rennard & Farmer, 2002).

COPD includes chronic bronchitis, chronic obstructive bronchitis or emphysema or a combination of these conditions and is the fourth leading cause of death in the United States today, and by the year 2020, it is expected to be the third leading cause of death and the fifth leading cause of disability (Rennard & Farmer, 2002). The death rate among men from COPD has remained steady, but the death rate among women has steadily climbed. This could be attributable to the fact that since the "liberation of women" more women now smoke (Mannino, 2002).

Identifying the risk factors for COPD is the first step in elucidating new strategies for prevention and treatment of this disease. See Table 22–20 for a summary of the risk factors for COPD.

In Table 22–20, COPD is a result of the interaction between the host and exposure factors. Only approximately 15 to 20% of smokers develop clinically significant COPD, which may be secondary to different genetics, inhaled environmental exposures, and a person's "total burden of inhaled particles" (Pauwels et al., 2001). However, a high proportion of those who smoke will develop abnormal lung function if they continue to smoke, even if not frank COPD. Tobacco smoke and occupational dusts/chemicals appear to act additively to increase a person's risk of acquiring COPD. The natural course of COPD is variable from person to person. COPD, however, is a progressive disease, especially if exposure to the noxious agent continues. If the exposure is halted, lung function may improve, the progression of COPD may continue at a slower decline but still continues due to the normal decline in lung function with age (Pauwels et al., 2001). Healthy nonsmokers have an age-related decline in their FEV_1 of about 30 ml/yr starting in the mid-30s. This decline is accelerated to 75 ml/year in smokers (Hanson & Midthum, 1992)

A diagnosis of COPD should be highly suspect in any patient who meets the criteria in Table 22–21.

The diagnosis is confirmed by spirometry. A post-bronchodilator $FEV_1 < 80\%$ of the predicted value and an $FEV_1/FVC < 70\%$ confirms there is airflow limitation that is only partially reversible (Pauwels et al., 2001; Sethi, 2002).

COPD can be classified into four stages of disease severity. See Table 22–22.

Stage 0, at risk for COPD, is often characterized by a chronic cough and sputum production with normal lung function as measured by spirometry. Stage I, mild COPD is characterized by a chronic cough and sputum production, which is often present for many years before the development of airflow limitation. In Stage II, moderate COPD, the patients often experience dyspnea, which can interfere with their routine daily activities. The impetus to seek healthcare in this stage is an inability to do their routine daily activities or a respiratory infection that worsens their lung function. Some patients, however, experience NO symptoms. As airflow limitations worsen, the patient enters Stage III, severe COPD. The symptoms of cough and sputum production continue, the dyspnea worsens, and additional symptoms suggestive of complications may emerge (Pauwels et al., 2001).

SPECIFIC CONSIDERATIONS FOR PHARMACOTHERAPY

When Drug Therapy Is Needed

COPD patients will need drug therapy specific to their disease state as well as other medications to help with smoking cessation. This will help prevent a more rapid deterioration in the lungs, control symptoms, reduce the

TABLE 22–20. Risk Factors for COPD

Host Factors	Genes ($alpha_1$ antitrypsin deficiency)
	Airway hyperresponsiveness
	Lung growth (maximal lung function)
Exposures	Smoking
	Occupational dusts and chemicals
	Indoor/outdoor pollution
	Infections (hx of severe respiratory infections as a child increases adult respiratory symptoms)
	Low socioeconomic status

Pauwels et al., (2001).

TABLE 22–21. Diagnosis of COPD

Cough
≥ 50 yrs of age
≥ mucoid sputum production
Dyspnea
History of exposures to the risk factors for the disease

Pauwels et al., (2001) and Sethi (2002).

TABLE 22–22. Classification of Severity: Stages of COPD

Stage	Characteristics
0 At risk	Normal spirometry Chronic symptoms (cough, sputum production)
I Mild COPD	$FEV_1/FVC < 70\%$ $FEV_1 > 80\%$ With/without chronic symptoms
II Moderate COPD	$FEV_1/FVC < 70\%$ $30\% < FEV_1 < 80\%$ predicted (IIA 50%, $FEV_1 < 80\%$ predicted); IIB $30\% < FEV_1 < 50\%$ predicted) With/without chronic symptoms
III Severe COPD	$FEV_1/FVC < 70\%$ $FEV_1 < 30\%$ predicted or $FEV_1 < 50\%$ predicted PLUS respiratory failure or clinical signs of Right-sided heart failure

Pauwels et al (2001).

frequency and severity of symptoms, improve exercise tolerance, and improve the overall health status.

SHORT AND LONG TERM GOALS OF PHARMACOTHEAPY

For maintenance of COPD, the short-term goals of pharmacotherapy are to intervene in the early stages of COPD to educate and provide medications for smoking cessation, control symptoms, improve exercise tolerance and to treat infections early and effectively. The long-term goals are to retard the progression of airflow limitation, prevent infection, reduce the need for hospitalization, improve and maintain exercise tolerance, maintain satisfactory nutritional status, optimize functional capabilities and identify effective medication compliance regimens (Pauwels, Busit et al., 2001; Hunter, King et al, 2001).

For acute exacerbations of COPD, the short-term goals of pharmacotherapy are to resolve the infection rapidly, maintain the person as an outpatient during treatment, if possible, choose the most appropriate antibiotic with the least side effects and most favorable compliance regimen. The long-term goals are to maintain an infection-free interval for as long as possible and encourage medical regimen compliance.

Nonpharmacologic Therapy

Nutrition is extremely important because weight loss negatively affects COPD prognosis. Numerous studies indicate that BMI is critical for long-term survival in COPD patients. Landbo, Prescott, Lange et al (1999) report that BMI and decreased mortality differed significantly depending on the Stage of COPD; Stage I and II had the lowest risk of mortality if the COPD patients had normal to slightly higher BMI's and even Stage III patients had improved survival rates with a higher BMI. A balanced diet that includes enough protein, carbohydrates, monounsaturated fats, omega-3 fats and low amounts of trans-hydrogenated fats, fruits, vegetables and dairy products is vital to overall health and survival without raising cholesterol/triglyceride levels. Supplemental high calorie and energy drinks may also need to be given to maintain and increase weight. Enough calories also helps strengthen respiratory effort which decreases dyspnea and improves overall symptoms. A nutritional consultation is important, especially in the elderly who may lack many essential components of a healthy diet. It is estimated that about 30% of patients with COPD may be malnourished (Wouters Creutzberg, & Schols, 2002). Improving the nutritional status of patients can lead to improved respiratory muscle strength.

Exercise programs, which could include weight training, especially the quadriceps, walking with specific heart rate targets, and bicycle/treadmill workouts, are tailored to the severity of the COPD stage. This exercise training may improve the patients' respiratory status, decrease dyspnea on exertion, and improve the general sense of well-being, even if there is no objective improvement of pulmonary function (Pauwels et al., 2001). Education about the disease process, compliance with the medicine regimen, smoking cessation, and exercising every day are important to review with the patients.

Oxygen is one of the principal nonpharmacologic therapies in COPD patients in Stage III. Long-term administration of oxygen has been shown to improve long-term survival in patients with respiratory failure. It also has a beneficial impact on mental status, exercise capacity, lung mechanics, and hemodynamics (Pauwels et al., 2001).

Patients who are on long-term oxygen therapy for chronic respiratory failure should use the oxygen if they fly. They should increase the O_2 flow by 1–2 L/min during the flight, which should maintain their PaO_2 of a least 6.7 kPa(50 mm Hg) (Gong, 1992). Patients who have a resting PaO_2 of > 9.3kPa(70 mm Hg) at sea level may be able to safely fly without supplemental oxygen, but could still develop severe hypoxemia. Any associated comorbidity—i.e., anemia, cardiovascular problem, etc.—that impairs oxygen flow to the tissues can lead to hypoxemia. Even walking down the aisle of the plane can profoundly aggravate hypoxemia (Christensen, Ryg, Refrem, & Skjonsberg, 2000).

Time Frame for Initiating Pharmacotherapy

A stepwise increase in treatment is required in patients with COPD, depending on the severity of the disease. A step-down approach is not applicable in COPD, due to the chronic progressive nature of the disease. In the early stages of COPD, smoking cessation is vital and, if appropriate, a change in environment if exposure to noxious gases/pollutants is occurring. Smoking cessation is the primary therapy to retard progression of airway disease and should be discussed at each patient visit with appropriate medications/support programs, etc. Therapy is begun as early as the patient needs for symptomatic relief and stepped up as needed.

Assessment Needed Prior to Therapy

See Tables 22–23, Table 22–24, and Table 22–25 for the appropriate history, physical assessment, and baseline pulmonary function tests required.

Patient/Caregiver Information

Patients need to be as well educated as possible about their disease state and strongly encouraged to participate in their own care. It may take several days for patients to notice subjective improvement from their medication. For patients who are on regularly scheduled medication, emphasize to the patient/caregiver that the medications need to be taken regularly even if they do not notice immediate benefit. Also periodically review the onset and duration of action and expected effects of the patient's medication regimen.

As with all medications, write down the patient's current medication regimen (including OTCs, alternative medications, and nutritional supplements) at each visit if changes are necessary and give a copy to the patient to carry with him or her. For example, suggest the patient carry a small notebook/calendar the size of a wallet or checkbook. The patient could also add notes and questions to this notebook.

Patients who smoke should be encouraged to quit at every clinician visit. Patients should be educated about the benefits of smoking cessation and that smoking cessation has been proven to slow the progression of COPD.

There are numerous drug interactions if theophylline is indicated in treatment. All patients need to clearly understand the potential for interactions and be instructed never to change their dose on their own, discontinue their medication, use another OTC/prescription/herbal therapy without letting the healthcare provider know they are on theophylline. Inhaler technique needs to be reviewed periodically and impress on them that using a spacer will be beneficial in delivering the medication further into the lungs.

TABLE 22–23. History of the Patient with COPD

Exposures to risk factors: smoking, occupational/environmental exposures
Past medical history: Childhood respiratory illnesses, asthma, sinusitis, nasal polyps, etc.
Family history of COPD
Pattern of symptom development: Coughing, sputum production, frequent respiratory infections, limited activities, and dyspnea
Previous hospitalizations for respiratory problems: Periodic episodes where symptoms worsen
Comorbidities: Cardiac, rheumatological, and hematological diseases
Current medications: Are they helping, what are the daily or prn medications
Social and family support

Pauwels et al. (2001).

TABLE 22–24. Assessment of the COPD Patient

There may be no physical signs evident on the physical exam until significant airflow limitation is present.
+/− bluish discoloration of the mucus membranes
+/− chest wall deformities reflects pulmonary hyperinflation; "barrel-shaped" protruding abdomen and/or relatively horizontal ribs
+/− paradoxical in-drawing of the lower ribcage on inspiration
+/− reduced cardiac dullness
Increased respiratory rate, often > 20 breaths/min
Usually pursed-lip breathing
Often resting muscle activation
Reduced breaths sounds
+/− wheezing during quiet breathing, inspiratory crackles

Pauwels et al. (2001).

OUTCOMES MANAGEMENT

Selecting an Appropriate Agent

Figure 22–1 shows a recommended treatment algorithm for the outpatient treatment of COPD (ATS, 2000; Pauwels et al., 2001).

TABLE 22–25. Common Diagnostic Tests in COPD

Spirometry—the hallmark for diagnosis*
Chest x-ray
Arterial blood gases, especially in advanced disease
Alpha-1 antitrypsin deficiency screening in COPD patients ≤ 45 yrs

* Refer to Table 22–24 for expected results in COPD patients.

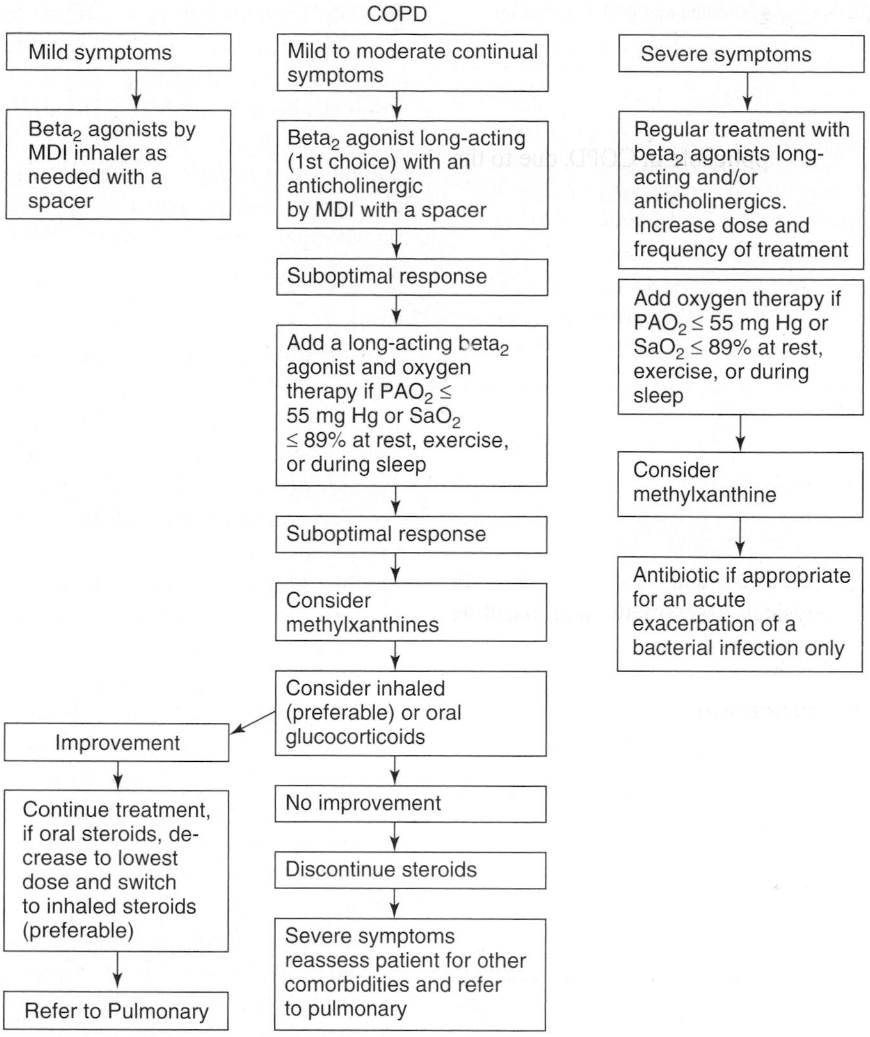

FIGURE 22–1. Algorithm for pharmacologic therapy in COPD. *Source: Pauwels, 2001; ATS Guidelines, 2000.*

Beta$_2$-Receptor Agonists. There are numerous inhaled beta$_2$-receptor agonists available in the United States. They include albuterol, bitolterol, isoetharine, metaproterenol, pirbuterol, salmeterol, and terbutaline. Inhaled beta$_2$ agonists cause bronchodilation via relaxation of the smooth muscles of the bronchial tree. They also decrease airway resistance in those patients with reversible airway obstruction, improve emptying time of the lungs, and reduce hyperinflation at rest and at exercise. Regular use of beta$_2$ agonists does not modify the decline in lung function in Stage I COPD nor the prognosis of the disease (Pauwels et al., 2001, *Drug Facts and Comparisons,* 2003).

Inhaled long-acting beta$_2$ agonists are central to the symptomatic management of COPD. Short-acting beta$_2$ agonists are either used on an as-needed basis "for relief of persistent or worsening symptoms or a long-acting beta$_2$ agonist on a regular basis to prevent or reduce symptoms" (Pauwels et al., 2001). They are often used in conjunction with anticholinergics for an additive brochodilatory long-acting effect. Inhaled beta$_2$ agonists are the preferred route because adverse effects are less likely and resolve more rapidly than the oral agents (*Drug Facts and Comparisons,* 2003). When the treatment is by inhaler, a spacer should always be used. Teaching the cor-

TABLE 22–26. Antibiotic Use and Depending on COPD Risk Factors

	Appropriate Antibiotic
Stage 2 and 3 (modeate and severe)	
underlying severe airflow obstruction	Augmentin
FEV_1 < 50% of predicted	Moxifloxacin
cormorbid illness	Levofloxacin
frequent exacerbations > 4/yr	Gatifloxacin
Stage 1 (low risk)	
none of the above risk factors	Azithromycin, Clarithromycin 3rd generation cephlasporin Moxifloxacin

**See Antibiotic Table 22–28 for further information; Sethi, 2002*

rect method of using the inhaler with a spacer is essential. COPD patients may find it more difficult to use these devices, so consider alternative breath-activated or spacer devices. Dry powders may be easier to use as well. In COPD with airflow limitation and poor inspiratory flow rates medication deposition will be more central and less lower lung (Kim et al., 1997).

Toxicity is dose related, so care needs to be taken when prescribing for a COPD patient with comorbidities as short-acting $beta_2$ agonists have the potential to precipitate cardiac arrhythmias (Pauwels et al., 2001). Short-acting inhaled $beta_2$ agonists have a rapid onset of bronchodilating effect but the onset is slower in COPD than asthma. Long-acting inhaled $beta_2$ agonists, salmeterol and formoterol, have a duration of effect of about 12 h or longer with no loss of effectiveness in COPD patients (Boyd et al, 1997). Nebulizers require more maintenance and may not be a good choice for an elderly COPD patient.

The long-acting $beta_2$ agonists have demonstrated improvement over ipatropium and theophylline in the management of COPD. They have improved clinical symptoms and spirometry, decreased exacerbations and improved the quality of life (Dougherty, Didur, Aboussouan, 2003). This seems logical then to start with a long-acting $beta_2$ agonist and as needed to add or to start simultaneously an ipatropium inhaler.

Anticholinergics. The bronchodilatory effects of the anticholinergics lasts longer than the short-acting $beta_2$ agonists, up to approximately 8 h. Inhaled ipratropium bromide is the primary anticholinergic used in the treatment of COPD and is considered a second-line agent. It is available as both an oral multidose inhaler (MDI) and as a solution for nebulization. Anticholinergic drugs are poorly absorbed, which limits the adverse side effects. Use of a nebulizer with a face mask and the anticholinergics has been shown to precipitate an acute glaucoma attack. This may be secondary to a direct effect of the solution on the eyes (Pauwels, Busit et al., 2001). Ipratropium produces bronchodilation by inhibiting the vagal stimulation of the tracheobronchial tree (Skorodin, 1993). For patients who require the regular use of an inhaled anticholinergic and an inhaled $beta_2$-receptor agonist, a Combivent inhaler (ipratropium and albuterol) may be a useful aid in compliance.

Methylxanthines. Controversy about the use of methylxanthines—the two most common are theophylline and aminophylline—remains. Theophylline has the ability to improve inspiratory muscle and diaphragmatic function but is potentially toxic and associated with serious side effects (Heath & Mongia, 1998).

Fragoso and Miller (1993) state that theophylline has been shown to improve spirometry and dyspnea. Theophylline may also improve mucociliary clearance, respiratory muscle performance, cardiovascular function, central respiratory drive, gas exchange, and exercise capacity. Its main value is in improving respiratory muscle performance. However, with close monitoring and attention to the side effects and when they are likely to occur, methylxanthines might have a place in the treatment of COPD (Pauwels et al., 2001; Heath & Mongia, 1998).

Patient dosing for theophylline needs to be individualized. Some patients may benefit from serum levels as low as 5 to 10 mg/L, but some patients may require serum levels in the range of 15 to 17 mg/L to show benefit (Heath & Mongia, 1998). It is important to assess the patient's response at each dosage. Since theophylline toxicity increases with increasing levels, it is important to monitor patients carefully and to educate them regarding drug interactions and signs and symptoms of toxicity. Some patients may benefit from theophylline administered once daily in the evening to improve nocturnal bronchospasms.

In general, patients should be prescribed sustained-release forms of theophylline to maintain adequate blood levels, to minimize peak and trough differences, and to aid in patient compliance.

Oxygen. Oxygen therapy is recommended for those patients who have $PaO_2 \leq 55$ mm Hg or $SaO_2 \leq 89\%$ at rest, with exercise, or during sleep. (Hunter & King, 2001).

Mucolytics and Expectorants. Guaifenesin is an expectorant that increases respiratory tract fluid and decreases the viscosity of secretions (*Drug Facts and Comparisons,* 2003). There are no strong studies to date supporting its use in the treatment of COPD. However, some clinicians support its use anecdotally.

In a number of studies mucolytics were not shown to provide significant relief. However, some patients may feel that the viscosity of their sputum is decreased using the mucolytics (Wallings, 2001).

Antibiotics. Antibiotics are indicated in acute exacerbations of chronic bronchitis and COPD when there is evidence of bacterial infection, especially in those patients who exhibit increased cough and dyspnea, increased sputum production, and purulent sputum. The treatment of an acute bacterial exacerbation of chronic obstructive pulmonary disease (ABE/COPD) is extremely challenging in the office setting. The assessment requires a multifactorial examination of the history, clinical and laboratory parameters that are specific for each individual patient. Some factors to consider that may predict possible treatment success/failure significantly are: age, previous hospitalizations and need for mechanical ventilation, severity of previous exacerbations and response to medical therapy, bacterial colonization status of the patient, general overall function of pulmonary status, patient's ability to tolerate treatment failure given his/her respiratory status and local antimicrobial resistance patterns (Eller, Ede, Schaberg et al, 1998).

Antibiotics are indicated *only* for an acute exacerbation of chronic bronchitis and COPD when there is evidence of a bacterial infection. Patients with a bacterial component to their illness often exhibit symptoms of increasing dyspnea and cough, and thickened, purulent, and increasing sputum.

The most current pathogens that are responsible for the "common and typical" bacterial infections of moderate-to-severe ABE/COPD are *S. pneumoniae, H. influenzae, M. catarrhalis, Haemophilus parainfluenzae* and *Staphylococcus aureus.* Because it is often difficult to identify a specific organism, antibiotic coverage should provide coverage for all anticipated organisms. In COPD patients with advanced disease and multiple risk factors, Klebsiella sp., Pseudomonas aeruginosa and other gram negative species may be the cause of their exacerbations. Wilson, 1998.

The treatment of mild* and moderate-to-severe ABE/COPD infections:

Initial Antibiotics:

Advanced generation of macrolides: Azithromycin 500mg po qd × 3 days; Clarithromycin 500 mg po qd × 7 days

Alternative Antibiotics:

Fluoroquinolones: Moxifloxacin 400 mg po qd × 5 days; Gatifloxacin 400 mg po qd × 7 days; Levofloxacin 500 mg po qd × 7 days Amoxicillin-clavulanate 875 mg po q 12 hours × 10 days

The treatment of severe and/or frequent recurrences:

Initial Antibiotics:

Fluoroquinolones: Moxifloxacin 400 mg po qd × 5 days; Gatifloxacin 400 mg po qd × 7 days; Levofloxacin 500 mg po qd × 7 days

Alternative Antibiotics:

Amoxicillin-clavulanate 875 mg po q 12 hours ¥ 10 days Ciprofloxacin is not recommended if S. pneumoniae is suspected (Grossman, 1998; DebAbate, Matthew, Warner et al, 2000)

Because of the increasing overuse of antibiotics and the rise of drug-resistant *S. pneumoniae* (DRSP) to fluroquinolones, the recommendations are to use an advance generation of macrolides as initial therapy and use the fluroquinolones as an alternative choice if patients fail the macrolides and/or there is a strong suspicion of a gram-negative organism. If patients fail therapy with one antibiotic, reassess the patient risk factors and then retreat with another antibiotic that provides coverage for other organisms (Wilson, 1998). When reinfection occurs, the antibiotic of choice should be one that has been effective in the previous exacerbations.

The same day that the patient sees the health care provider, the antibiotic prescription should be filled and started. The earlier the antibiotics are started the greater the chance of earlier improvement.

Nicotine Replacement. COPD patients who smoke should be strongly encouraged to quit smoking. Specific recommendations for nicotine replacement therapy and other smoking cessation strategies should be considered. See Drug Table 1003.

Immunizations. COPD patients should receive annual influenza vaccines. They should also receive an initial pneumococcal vaccine. Pneumococcal antibody titers may fall after several years, and it is recommended that re-vaccination with pneumococcal vaccine be done every 6 years (Pauwels, Busit et al., 2001). Annual influenza vaccines may increase theophylline levels acutely. Pa-

*Mild COPD with ABE, the health care provider can use Doxycycline 100mg po bid 7–14 days or Trimethoprim-sulfamethoxazole DS po bid 7–14 days.

tients receiving theophylline therapy should be monitored for theophylline toxicity when they receive their annual influenza vaccine. Some clinicians recommend decreasing the dose or holding theophylline for 24 h after vaccine administration (Drug Facts and Comparisons, 2003). Consult Chapter 11 for further information on immunizations.

Corticosteroids. Inhaled and oral steroids are much less effective and dramatic in COPD than in asthma and their role in managing patients is just beginning to be understood. In studies, Fluticasone proprionate inhaler has been shown to have some selective effect on the inflammatory cells in the bronchial mucosa which over time has stabilized the mast cells and shown improvement in clinical symptoms (Gizyycki, Hattotuwa, Barnes, Jeffery, 2002). Other studies have shown less favorable improvement in clinical symptoms and probably do not modify long-term decline in lung function (Highland, Strange, Heffner, 2003). Pauwels, Busit et al., (2001) report that the Lung Health Study (2000) recommend inhaled steroids regularly only for COPD patients who are symptomatic with FEV1 < 50% of predicted, in Stage III severe COPD and in those with frequent exacerbations or requiring treatment with oral steroids/antibiotics.

There is insufficient evidence to show that oral steroid are beneficial in COPD treatment unless there is a lung function response to them. Because of the potentially serious side effects of using oral steroids, their use should be curtailed to a pulmonary specialist (Pauwels, Busit et al., 2001; Sutherland, 2003).

Spiriva. Spiriva® HandiHaler® (tiotropium bromide inhalation powder) was approved in 2004 for the long-term, once-daily, maintenance treatment of bronchospasm associated COPD and is considered an important advance and first-line treatment for COPD. The medication is delivered by HandiHaler®, which uses a single capsule inserted into the device, and primed by the dispense button. This medication causes more dry mouth than Atrovent® but is one-third of the cost. Those who use it are cautioned to suck on sugarless candy to combat dryness. This medication is only for maintenance therapy, not for rapid relief of exacerbations (*Medical letter,* 2004).

Zileuton. Zileuton is a 5-lipoxygenase inhibitor used in the treatment of asthma. To date there are no studies on its use in COPD. It may, however, be useful in those patients who have an asthmatic component to their COPD.

Drugs to Avoid. Patients who have an asthmatic component to their COPD should avoid beta blockers, including oral and ophthalmic products, because they may cause bronchoconstriction. Patients with severe COPD need to avoid benzodiazepines because of their respiratory depressant effects and avoid antussives as they have a protective role in stable COPD (Drug Facts and Comparisons, 2003). Patients with underlying cardiovascular disease need to be cautious in their use of theophylline and oral $beta_2$ agonists.

Monitoring for Efficacy

At each visit the clinician should question the patient regarding subjective symptoms such as cough (frequency and severity), sputum production (quality and quantity), dyspnea, and wheezing. The patient should also be questioned regarding the quality of sleep (i.e., if he sleeps better or worse; need for inhalation therapy at night; several pillow orthopnea). Subjective assessment should include the patient's exercise tolerance (e.g., the number of flights of stairs or city blocks he can handle).

A patient daily diary may be useful to record signs and symptoms and medication use. A chart may be useful to aid in consistency of reporting symptoms and to minimize the time it takes a patient to record symptoms (and therefore increase compliance). Keep in mind the age and visual acuity of the patient, and make the charts with big enough print and dark enough copies.

At each visit, assess the following changes from the baseline physical examination:

- Lung: breath sounds, crackles, rhonchi, rales, respiratory rate, use of accessory muscles, pursed lip breathing, shortness of breath (SOB) while speaking
- Cardiac: gallop, S_3 or S_4, distant heart sounds, JVD, six- and 12-min walking distance
- Pulmonary function tests: FEV_1, FVC
- Weight & BMI measurement

An $alpha_1$-antitrypsin level should be measured for those COPD patients who develop the disease at less than 45 years of age, when there is a family history of $alpha_1$-antitrypsin deficiency, or when emphysema occurs without a significant smoking history (Ingram, 1994). Arterial blood gas determinations are not usually needed for stage I patients, but are indicated for stage II and stage III patients (Pauwels, Busit et al., 2001).

For patients taking theophylline, levels should be determined periodically. Initially, levels should be determined after a few days of therapy and after any change in dosage and during acute illness. There are numerous medications that interact with theophylline. Levels may need to be determined if a patient starts or stops any chronic medication. Smoking also influences theophylline metabolism. If a patient stops smoking, theophylline dosage may need to be adjusted. Patients requiring a single daily low dose of theophylline do not need frequent monitoring.

Monitoring for Toxicity

Patients should be questioned regarding adverse effects of medications at each visit. Patients should be educated regarding common and serious side effects of their medication when it is initially prescribed. Patients should be advised to seek immediate care when serious adverse effects occur. Table 22–27 shows common toxicities and how to monitor them. FEV_1 and FVC should be monitored at each visit to determine if the patients' COPD is worsening.

Follow Up Recommendations

Certain high risk patients who have been treated with an antibiotic for an acute exacerbation of their COPD will need followup within 72 hours in the office: the elderly; those with a significantly low FEV_1; co-morbid illnesses and those who have difficulty understanding how to take their medicines or those who will have difficulty with medication compliance (Wilson, 1998). Other non-high risk patients can either be contacted by telephone or be seen in the clinic within 3 to 5 days after starting the antibiotics. Those who must be seen more urgently will have increasing symptoms like dyspnea, fever, tachypnea and other systemic symptoms.

Once patients are stable after an acute exacerbation or on their regular medications, the patient with COPD may be able to go several months between clinician visits. COPD is a chronic progressive disease. Patients will need continuing care over their lifetime once the diagnosis of COPD is made.

CYSTIC FIBROSIS

Cystic fibrosis (CF) is one of the most common genetically inherited diseases of Caucasians, occurring in 1 of 2500 live births. Because of better drug treatments and a coordinated team approach to care by major medical centers, the survival rate has increased to 30 years plus. Approximately one-third of CF survivors are currently over the age of 18 (Yankaskas, Marshall, Sufian, et al., 2004). CF is a result of a mutation of the gene on the long arm of chromosome 7 that encodes the CF transmembrane conductance regulator (CFTR) (Boucher, 1996). CFTR acts as a channel for chloride in the membranes of the airways and gut, which is one means of hydrating the airway and the intestinal tract. If the CFTR is defective, this may limit mucous hydration. Dehydrated airways lead to decreased mucociliary clearance, which encourages bacterial colonization and repeated infections (Puchelle, de Bentzmann, & Zahm, 1995). All body areas are affected by the lack of mucous hydration as well, i.e., cervical glands, synovial cavities, bile ducts, etc. (Finder, 1999).

The defective CFTR also leads to failure to secrete sodium bicarbonate ($NaHCO_3$) and water by the pancreatic ducts, causing retention of the enzymes in the pancreas, and ultimately destroying the pancreatic tissue. The secretions are thickened, and over time this leads to destruction of the beta cells resulting in diabetes, generally manifesting in the adolescent or young adult (Brunzell & Schwarzenberg, 2002). CF patients can secrete almost a normal volume of sweat into the sweat glands but cannot absorb the NaCl from that sweat. Thus, the definitive test

TABLE 22–27. Selected Adverse Reaction Monitoring for Drugs used for COPD

Drug	Signs/Symptoms of Toxicity	Physical Examination Indicators of Toxicity	Laboratory Indicators of Toxicity
Inhaled ipratropium	Dry mouth, tachycardia, difficult urination	Tachycardia	
Inhaled $beta_2$ agonists	Tachycardia, tremors, nervousness, tolerance, paradoxical worsening	Tachycardia, tremors	
Oral $beta_2$ agonists	Tachycardia, tremors, nervousness, tolerance, paradoxical worsening	Hypertension, tachycardia, tremors	Hypokalemia
Theophylline	Nausea, vomiting, heartburn, nervousness, insomnia, tremors, seizure, tachycardia	Hypertension, tachycardia, tremors	Blood levels >20 mg/L, hypoglycemia
Oral corticosteroids	Symptoms of diabetes (polydipsia, polyphagia, polyuria), mental status changes	Hypertension, striae, skin thinning, purpura, cataracts, weight gain	Hypokalemia, hyperglycemia
Inhaled corticosteroids	Hoarseness, dysphonia, thrush	Thrush	

Adapted from Drug Facts & Comparisons, 2003

for the diagnosis of CF still remains the sweat chloride test (Finder, 1999).

Most patients with CF present with the signs and symptoms of the disease in childhood, but a significant number are not diagnosed until their 20s (Finder, 1999). The common presenting symptoms are (Finder, 1999):

- Failure to thrive/malnutrition
- Persistent respiratory problems, i.e. persistent wet cough with yellow/green sputum, chronic bronchitis, pulmonary infiltrates on x-ray, chronic purulent rhinorrhea, and sinusitis
- Malabsorption
- Family history of CF
- Meconium ileus
- Noisy breathing

(Brunzel & Schwarzenberg, 2002)

The most common complications that result from CF are

- Gallstones
- Diabetes
- Pneumothorax
- Abdomen problems—appendicitis, rectal prolapse
- Sinusitis
- Nasal polyps
- Cor pulmonale
- Recurrent lung infections with eventual loss of lung function
- Delayed onset of puberty in both males and females
- Intestinal obstruction
- Liver disease
- Elevated triglycerides
- Iron deficiency anemia
- BMD (bone mineral density) loss, increasing bone fracture risk and osteoporosis
- Sleep disorders

(Finder, 1999; Rigby, Pirzada, Taylor, et al., 2000):

SPECIFIC CONSIDERATIONS FOR PHARMACOTHERAPY

When Drug Therapy Is Needed

Drug therapy is the mainstay for the patient with CF to live a relatively comfortable and productive life and slow the progression of the disease. Infections should be treated rapidly and vigorously to restore the patient to the previous level of functioning. Without the appropriate nutrition, drug therapy, chest physiotherapy, and healthcare from a coordinated team, the CF patient's life would be limited to months rather than years. Drug therapy to maintain the associated complications is necessary as well to maintain an optimum level of health.

Short- and Long-Term Goals of Pharmacotherapy

The short-term goals are to treat any lung infections, resolve intestinal obstructions, and improve hydration and nutrition. The long-term goals include:

- Prevention of lung infections.
- Control the infection and restore the patient to his/her former state of well-being, if unable to eradicate.
- Promote mucociliary clearance and reduce the number of lung infections.
- Maintain normal absorption and nutrition through pancreatic enzyme replacement.
- Early recognition, intervention, and management of complications.
- Improve quality of life.

(Finder, 1999; Susan et al., 2002)

Nonpharmacologic Therapy

Breathing exercises, chest physiotherapy, exercise training, and adequate hydration and nutrition are the main nonpharmacologic treatments available today.

Breathing exercises must be done once or twice daily and are always followed by chest physiotherapy. To obtain the maximum benefit, the patient takes two deep breaths and exhales fully and forcefully so the mucus can be cleared. After exhaling, chest physiotherapy is performed. The sequence is repeated until mucus is expectorated (Brennan & Geddes, 2002).

Exercise tolerance and cardiopulmonary response to exercise are impaired in the patient with CF. Exercise training has been shown to be beneficial by improving both aerobic fitness and cardiopulmonary efficiency (Nixon, 1996). Every CF patient should be evaluated through exercise testing so an individualized program can be initiated.

Adequate daily hydration and nutrition are crucial to overall pulmonary health. Research has demonstrated that undernutrition secondary to an energy imbalance is the result of three primary factors: (1) reduced energy intake because of dietary insufficiency and/or anorexia from respiratory disease, abdominal symptoms, and/or clinical depression; (2) increased energy loss secondary to maldigestion, and (3) increased energy expenditure from advanced lung disease (Brennan & Geddes, 2002; Durie

& Pencharz, 1992). Every child with CF needs approximately 120–150% of the caloric requirements that a child without CF of the same sex and age requires. Some children even require caloric supplementation up to 200%. After periods of poor nutritional intake, the child with CF who increases his/her caloric intake significantly, can experience "catch-up" growth. The child with CF requires increased protein and the appropriate fats (conversion of fat to energy requires more oxygen consumption than converting either protein or carbohydrates) every day. Increased sodium without excessive intake is also needed every day. All infants, children, and adults with CF need daily vitamins; children and adults > 8 years old need 1 to 2 tablets daily (Powers and Patton, 2003).

Often getting in all the calories required daily can be problematic. Sometimes increasing the portion sizes, adding snacks and/or mini meals as well as high calorie dietary supplements are helpful. It is vital, therefore, to ensure that all CF patients regardless of duration of disease have a dietary consultation at every visit.

Time Frame for Initiating Pharmacotherapy

Treatment should be initiated as soon as the diagnosis is established, whether the patient is 1 day old or 20 years old. The earlier the treatment is started, the better the short-term outcome will be. *Pseudomonas aeruginosa* is a common invasive pathogen of the respiratory tract of CF patients. Studies have shown that early recognition and treatment can eradicate or successfully treat nonmucoid *P. aeruginosa* from the lungs before it can cause irreversible lung damage. Early treatment of lung infections can decrease the associated malnutrition states that can be a persistent pattern in CF (Susan et al., 2002). The long-term outcome is ultimately death, but the quality of life can be significantly improved with prompt treatment and frequent followup care by a CF medical healthcare team. Studies reveal that care delivered by a comprehensive CF team at a major medical center not only improves the quality of life but that patients with CF experience fewer hospitalizations and more prompt and earlier recognition and treatment of infections. This improved quality of life is due to a more holistic approach because an entire team has the updated knowledge required to manage these patients (Boucher, 1996).

Assessment Needed Prior to Therapy

The appropriate history and physical assessment as well as diagnostic test findings are described in Tables 22–28 and 22–29.

Patient/Caregiver Information

Chest Physiotherapy

1. All patients need written instructions regarding their chest physiotherapy.
2. The proper chest physiotherapy technique should be reviewed.

Nutrition

1. Patients need to keep a diary of their food intake so it can be reviewed at each visit with a nutritionist.
2. Monitor weight regularly.
3. Teach patients to adjust enzyme replacement for special events, ie, birthday parties, holidays.
4. Teach patients to increase calories, fat, vitamins, and minerals during periods of rapid growth, ie, infancy and adolescence.

General Information

1. Directions for taking medications should be written, since most CF patients are on multiple drugs.
2. Patients should be cautioned to *never* stop taking the enzyme replacement, change brands, or adjust the dose themselves until first talking with their health care provider (Drug Facts and Comparisons, 2003).
3. Review the subtle signs of a respiratory infection so quick action can be initiated.
4. Encourage regular exercise.

OUTCOMES MANAGEMENT

The daily management of the patient with CF is complicated and complex. The best healthcare should be delivered by a team of pulmonary specialists in CF. Data shows that healthcare by a medical center specializing in CF improves and prolongs the quality of life. Knowledge of CF is growing daily and only trained specialists can expertly manage their care. This section will focus on the necessary information that a primary healthcare provider will need to provide care.

Selecting an Appropriate Agent

Bronchodilators. Bronchodilators are used in patient with CF to cause dilation of the smooth muscle of the lung, which decreases airway resistance in patients with reversible airway obstruction (*Drug Facts and Comparisons,* 2003). See Drug Tables for the common side effects.

In the CF patient, nebulization is the preferred administration route because it provides a mist that can help wet secretions (Frederiksen, Lanng, Koch, & Hoiby,

TABLE 22–28. Significant History and Physical Examination Needed and Possible Findings for the CF Patient

Pertinent History	Possible Findings
Neonate	
• First stool passed	Abdomen: may have distension
• Vomiting	Rectal: possibly impacted stool
• Crying pattern	
Infant/Toddler	
• Failure to gain weight despite hunger and increased food	Height and weight plotted on chart
• May have foul-smelling, foamy, bulky stools	Abdomen: distention, tenderness
• Increased frequency but can be constipation (no BMs)	
• Wheezing, paroxysmal nonproductive cough	Lungs: wheezing, crackles, rhonchi
• Frequent respiratory infections	
• Nails	Heart: sound change
	Clubbing by the age of 3 years
School-Age/Adolescent	
• Growth delay	Tanner stage: delay
	Decreased bone mineral density (BMD)
	Should check regularly
• Delayed onset of puberty in girls and boys	
• Chronic respiratory problems: wheezing, productive cough, night cough, chest pain or hemoptysis, rhinorrhea	Lungs: wheezing, rhonchi, crackles Chest: becoming barrel-shaped
• Fatigue, change in energy level	Nails: clubbing
• Decrease in exercise tolerance	CBC with differential, serum ferritin, IBC
• Purulent rhinorrhea	Elevated blood glucose
• Stool pattern	Nose: purulent rhinorrhea
	Abdomen: tenderness, distention, hepatosplenomegaly
	Elevated liver enzymes
• Frequency of chest physiotherapy	
• Exercise plan adherence	
• Review daily diet, calorie intake, energy expenditure	Triglycerides, low cholesterol
	Heart: sound changes
• Check CBC with differential, blood glucose, lipid panel, BMD, and liver enzymes	
Adults	
• Symptom progression, especially at rest and night, more frequent and intractable pulmonary infections	Lungs: significant change in breath sounds, increased respiratory rate, shortness of breath Heart: sound changes, pulses
• Increasing hemoptysis, chest pain	Weight: every visit
• Weight loss	Extremities: changes in sensations

Adapted from Aris, Renner, Winders, et al. (1998); Boucher (1996); Figueroa, Carlos, Parks, et al. (2002); Reid, Withers, Francis, Wilson, & Kotsimbos (2002); Rigby et al. (2000).

1996). Albuterol and metaproterenol are the only $beta_2$ agonists that can be nebulized. Albuterol is the recommended $beta_2$ agonist of choice for nebulization. Pirbuterol, isoetharine, terbutaline, and bitolterol are not available to use in a nebulizer and safety has not been established in children <12 years (*Drug Facts and Comparisons,* 2003).

A $beta_2$ agonist is important in the treatment of CF. The first of the lung changes that occur in children is an increased RV/TLC (residual volume/total lung capacity), implying that the small airways are involved. As the disease progresses over years, there are reversible and nonreversible changes in FEV_1 and FVC in about 40 to 60% of patients. The reversible changes (airway relaxation can occur after constriction) might reflect either increased mucus in the lumen of the airway and/or airway reactivity, whereas the nonreversible changes (airways less flexible, more rigid, and damaged so relaxation is less possible) usually reflect chronic destruction and/or bronchiolitis (Boucher, 1996; Frederiksen et al., 1996).

Salmeterol, a long-acting bronchodilator, has not been utilized in the CF population.

Mucus Liquifying Agents. Dornase alfa is a purified solution of human recombinant DNA. CF patients accumulate very viscous and purulent mucus, making expectora-

TABLE 22–29. Pertinent Diagnostic Tests for Cystic Fibrosis

Diagnostic Tests	Possible Findings
Sweat chloride	Positive
Flat plate of abdomen	Impacted stool, intussusception
Stool specimen	Positive for fat
Chest x-ray	Pneumonia or atelectasis
Liver function tests	Elevated; amylase low or absent
Sputum culture	*S. aureus, H. influenzae,* and/or *Pseudomonas*
Pulse oximetry	Decreased arterial Po_2 levels
Spirometry	Decreased FEV_1 and FVC Increased TLV and RLV
Blood glucose	Increased in prediabetic and diabetic state
WBC	Results depend on health state
Special Tests	
B_{12} levels	
Levels of oto- and nephrotoxic drugs	Low, if enzyme replacement inadequate
Vitamin K levels	CF patients have altered pharmacokinetics

Adapted from Boucher (1996).

tion extremely difficult. This contributes to decreased pulmonary function and infection exacerbations (Puchelle et al., 1995). The following precautions must be adhered to when using this medication (AHFS, 1997; *Drug Facts and Comparisons,* 2003):

1. Store in the refrigerator.
2. Do not mix or dilute with any other medication in the nebulizer because it can alter the property of dornase and cause a physiochemical change in the patient.
3. Use immediately after opening the ampule.

Vitamins and Pancreatic Enzymes. It has been recognized that the degree of malnutrition correlates with the severity of the pulmonary disease and mortality (Yankaskas, Marshall, Sufian, et al 2004). It is vital to aggressively prevent or treat a malnutrition state in order to promote the patient's well-being, allow catchup growth, decrease lung infections, improve exercise tolerance, slow the deterioration of lung function, and perhaps prolong life. Dietary recommendations include: (1) a high-calorie diet, (2) liberal fat intake, and (3) vitamin and mineral supplements. Nutrition and vitamin and mineral supplementation are revised based on the state of health, periods of growth, illnesses, antibiotic use, and advancing disease (Patton, Byars, Powers et al., 2002).

CF patients, regardless of age, are prone to hyponatremic dehydration during periods of exercise, hot weather, and vomiting due to high losses of sodium sweat. These patients must be supplemented with sodium chloride, based on 1 mmol/kg/day (MacDonald, 1996).

Pancreatic enzyme replacement is required for all CF patients with pancreatic deficiency. The supplements must be given with each milk feeding, meal, and snack. Special consideration must be given to taking the pancreatic enzyme replacement correctly (see Table 22–30). The enteric-coated microcapsules *must not* be chewed, only swallowed. In the infant and toddler contents of the capsules can be sprinkled onto pureed fruit and fed.

Antibiotics. Use of both inhaled and oral antibiotics is common among this population. The choice of the antibiotics depends on the organism suspected and the severity of the lung infection. Chronic inhaled use of aminoglycosides and other drugs with antipseudomonal activity is to prevent/eradicate colonization of pseudomonas aeruginosa, thus decreasing the incidence of lung destruction. Susan et al, 2002.

Azithromycin orally 3 times a week has been shown to decrease hospitalization rates by 50%, increase weight gain and minimally affect improvement in lung function as measured by FEV_1 (Rubin and Henke, 2004).

The management of the CF patient should be at a medical center by a CF specialist because of the ever changing nature of treatment modalities and all the specialty care needed.

H_2 Blockers. Inadequate neutralization of gastric acid can result in inactivation of the pancreatic lipase enzyme. It is theorized that the H_2 blockers could improve digestion and absorption when given as adjunctive therapy with the pancreatic enzyme replacement (Forstner & Durie, 1996). Any of the H_2 blockers can be used effectively to enhance pancreatic enzyme absorption.

Insulin. Both regular and intermediate-acting insulin may be required when the blood glucose reaches consistent levels higher than 180 to 200. The diabetes of CF

TABLE 22–30. Pancreatic Enzyme Replacement Recommendation for Cystic Fibrosis

Infants

- 1000–2000 units lipase/120 mL of formula
- Increase as needed

Children to Adults

- 5000 units lipase/snack and meal
- Dosage should be increased in a stepwise manner
- If the requirement is > 2000 units lipase/kg per meal and snack, then further investigation is imperative
- If the child has a larger than usual snack or meal, the child will need another one or two capsules

Adapted from MacDonald (1996) and Ramsey, Farrell, Panchary, & The Consensus Committee (1992).

tends to be mild. Ketoacidosis is rare, but there have been retinal, kidney, and other vascular complications noted. It has been discovered that in CF patients the onset of microvascular complications occurs 10 years after the onset of hyperglycemia (Hayes, O'Brien, O'Brien, Fitzgerald, & McKennon, 1995). Diabetic complications occur but have not been a significant issue since most CF patients died prior to the onset of major sequelae. With the increase in life expectancy, more serious complications will present new challenges to the healthcare provider (Hayes et al., 1995).

Very tight glucose control is not recommended because ketoacidosis is rarely encountered and the blood glucose remains relatively stable. Decreased weight, body mass index (BMI), FEV_1, and FVC and an increase in the daily intake of pancreatic enzyme replacement can herald the onset of a prediabetic state. This change is insidious and affects overall health for years prior to diagnosis. It is important that attention is given to this constellation of changes so early intervention can be instituted. It has been shown that insulin therapy can improve lung function even in the prediabetic state (Brunzell, & Schwarzenberg, 2002; Lanng, Thorsteinsson, Nerupo, & Koch, 1992).

Liquid Supplements. The CF patient often requires an extremely high daily calorie intake to maintain normal pulmonary and overall health. It can be difficult to consume the number of calories required, so liquid supplements can be used. They are calorie-dense without being overwhelmingly filling (Powers et al., 2002). Both prescription and over-the-counter liquid supplements are equally effective.

Drugs to Avoid. Patients who have a reversible airway component to their pulmonary disease should avoid excessive $beta_2$ agonist use. Tolerance can develop and render the agonist minimally effective when needed, but time without the inhaler will render it effective again (AHFS, 1997).

Hypertriglyeridemia Medications. Hypertriglyeridemia is often first seen in the adolescent age group as isolated elevated triglycerides. The etiology may be secondary to a chronic low-grade inflammation and/or dietary imbalance in which there is an increased ratio of simple carbohydrate absorption to fat absorption (Figueroa et al., 2002). Drug therapy intervention may be needed. Consideration should be given to the niacins and the fibric acids. Niacin is metabolized in the gastrointestinal tract, while the fibric acids are metabolized by the liver. CF patients can have liver disease, which may require an adjustment in the medicine (Figueroa et al., 2002).

Iron Deficiency Anemia Medications. Iron deficiency anemia (IDA) occurs in about 75% of patients with CF, usually in women. The mechanism for the anemia is directly related to the underlying severity of the lung disease. Sputum contains high iron and ferritin concentrations and is related to the lung function. The higher the concentrations of iron and ferritin in the sputum, the more severe is the lung disease. The *P. aeruginosa* organism has the ability to obtain iron from the host airway and by stimulating an inflammatory cascade can divert iron away from hemoglobin synthesis. IDA may be a prognostic indicator of severe airway disease. Currently, there is no evidence to show that IDA results from pancreatic supplementation (Reid et al., 2002). Treatment consist of iron replacement therapy judiciously and perhaps in early disease using iron-binding agents and treatment to eradicate *P. aeruginosa* (Reid et al., 2002).

Bisphosphonates. There is an increased rate of bone fractures, especially the spine, in advanced CF. The bone mineral density (BMD) is often 2 SD below the mean. Both men and women had twice the rate of fractures than the general population. In those with spinal fractures, there was considerable loss of height, > 5 cm for men and women. The risk factors for increased fractures were cumulative prednisone doses, body mass index, and age of puberty (Aris et al., 1998). Osteoporosis is common in children and adults. Supplemental vitamin D doses of 400 to 800 IU were ineffective in maintaining normal vitamin D stores in the body. Everyone must be screened. How often depends on age and lung disease severity (Arch et al., 2001). Bisphosonates and calcitonin may be helpful in restoring bone mass.

Vaccines. It is imperative that CF patients receive their immunizations as close to the regular age as possible. The influenza vaccine should be given annually unless there is a severe allergy to eggs.

- Vaccines: Influenza, given yearly
- Pneumococcal, given every 3 to 5 years
- Metamune, given as a freshman entering college
- Hepatitis A, given to prevent any liver damage from the disease
- Hepatitis B, if not given as an infant, then vaccinate as soon as possible

Monitoring for Efficacy

At each visit, the clinician needs to obtain a detailed history regarding the following: decreased appetite, weight loss or failure to gain weight, decrease in regular exercise tolerance pattern, fatigue, increased cough and/or night sweats, increase in respiratory rate, abdominal distention or discomfort, change in character of stools (bulky, greasy, foul-smelling), and personality changes (i.e., irritability, signs of depression, anxiety, and eating disorders), back pain, fatigue and polyuria, polydipsia, and polyphagia (Finder, 1999). Review the medication list with the patient, correct the mixing of the nebulizer solutions, check frequency of chest physiotherapy, note any subtle changes that the patient may have noticed, and review if any pancreatic enzymes needed to be adjusted. Fever is rarely encountered in the CF patient, so careful assessment is important.

Possible physical examination findings to watch for include:

- Growth: height, weight, and head circumference in infants; height/weight throughout the age span
- Tanner stage: age-appropriate
- Nose: purulent rhinorrhea
- Lungs: wheezing, crackles, rhonchi
- Heart: murmurs, S_3, S_4
- Abdomen: distention, tenderness, pain, hepatosplenomegaly
- Nails: clubbing
- Pulmonary function tests (declining levels can signal an acute pulmonary exacerbation): FEV_1, FVC, TLV, RV

(Boucher, 1996)

The examination should be generally inclusive at each visit and even more detailed if a problem is detected during the history. It is important to be attuned to subtle changes, since 95% of CF patients die from complications of their lung infections (Boucher, 1996).

Laboratory data may need to be obtained, depending on the history, physical examination findings, and comorbid illnesses. These may include blood glucose, WBC with differential, stool for fat content, chest x-ray, LFTs, chemistry 18, blood gases, sputum cultures, and/or pulse oximetry.

Monitoring for Toxicity

It is imperative that the patient and/or parents be questioned about any adverse reactions experienced. All the common adverse effects of each medication should be written down and reviewed when initially prescribed. It has been noted that CF patients do not develop gastric ulcers on either oral steroids or high-dose NSAIDs. It is speculated that the viscous stomach secretions may confer protection.

Followup Recommendations

CF patients need to be seen by the healthcare team regularly because preventive care is crucial. The change from a chronic problem to an acute problem can be subtle. If the patient is seen regularly, every 6 to 8 weeks, and monitored frequently, any change in condition can be detected earlier. Intensive treatment can be initiated on an outpatient basis with fewer hospitalizations, less decline in function, and a more rapid return to activities of daily living. The tests that need to be performed will depend on the findings of the history and physical examination (Boucher, 1996).

PNEUMONIA

COMMUNITY-ACQUIRED PNEUMONIA IN ADULTS AND THE ELDERLY

Community-acquired pneumonia (CAP) annually affects approximately 5 to 6 million adults, hospitalizing almost 2 million, the 6th leading cause of mortality among the elderly in the United States today and of increasing concern as the baby-boomers age (NIAID, 1998). CAP is increased among African Americans as well as infants < 1 year of age but declines in the preschooler, school-age, adolescent and young adult. Despite the ready availability of both the influenza and pneumococcal vaccines, they are underutilized in the infant > 6 months, the elderly and minorities. Pneumonia tends to be more virulent in the elderly for a variety of reasons, including:

- decrease in mucociliary clearance
- decrease in lung recoil and chest wall compliance
- impairment of cough reflex
- decrease in production of antibodies to foreign antigens
- impaired macrophage microbial response
- impaired neutrophil migration
- changes in the entire immune system (use of NSAIDs masks symptoms and reduces immune response)
- nutritional deficits
- environmental risk, which is highest if in a nursing home, followed by those with semiskilled care and those at home
- greater adherence of microorganism to the oropharynx
- increased gram negative bacteria in the mouth (File, Tan & Plouffe, 2001)

Perhaps an explanation of why CAP in the elderly may carry a higher mortality rate is the difficulty in establishing a diagnosis. The elderly rarely present with the "classic" pneumonia symptoms. Instead, they often present with a minor cough, weakness, lethargy, mental status changes, new and/or increased falls, worsening of their underlying medical illness, metabolic derangement, new incontinence, failure to thrive and general deterioration. If a family member/friend/nursing care provider detects these symptoms in an elderly person for more than 1 day, it is imperative that health care is sought immediately (Krieger, 1996; Mouton, Bazaldua, Pierce, & Espino, et al, 2001). Unless the appropriate questions are asked or a family member is the historian, the pneumonia may be missed initially. When the pneumonia is finally diagnosed, the elderly person can be acutely ill, requiring hospitalization with a significantly greater risk of dying. The risk of severe pneumonia can be environment-related in the elderly. The frail, bedridden elderly in nursing homes or recently discharged from the hospital have the greatest risk of gram-negative and gram-positive organisms, such as *S. pneumoniae,* drug-resistant *S. pneumoniae* (DRSP). *H. influenzae, Klebsiella, Staphylococcus aureus,* gram-negative rods (GNR), and active tuberculosis. Atypical organisms that were once thought to be a rare cause of pneumonia in the elderly actually account for approximately 20% of the pneumonia cases today (Mouton et al., 2001). Consider mouth anaerobes if the elderly have teeth because anaerobic bacteria exist between teeth (Krieger, 1996).

While viral pneumonias are common across all age spans, adults often have a more mixed viral/bacterial pattern. *S. pneumoniae* is still the most common pathogen in those beyond the neonatal period and increasingly becoming drug-resistant. *H. Influenza,* once a major player in the etiology of pneumonia, has become less common in young adults as infants are now being immunized. (Pennachio, 2002).

Certain subgroups of adults, whether elderly or not, are at increased risk of pneumonia: smokers, alcohol abusers, users of immunosuppressive agents (NSAIDs and steroids, which the elderly tend to use regularly for the normal osteoarthritic pain), those with cardiac/COPD/neoplastic/HIV/TB, neurologic disease, military recruits and college students (ATS, 2001).

In the young and middle-aged healthy nonsmoker and non-alcohol abusing adult who develops pneumonia, the most likely etiology is *S. pneumoniae* and Legionella, then atypical bacteria and in the winter months, viral. In persons who are immunocompromised, consider *pneumocystis carinii, H. influenza, S. aureus,* viruses (CMV, adenoviruses, HSV, varicella) gram negative bacteria, fungal and tuberculosis (Mandell, Bartlett, Dowell, et al, 2003). In the IVDA, consider as causes of their pneumonia other than *S. pneumoniae, Klebsiella, H. Influenza,* anaerobes, fungal and gram negative whereas in the alcoholic think *Klebsiella, H. Influenza* and other bacteria associated with aspiration pneumonia (ATS, 2001; Bernstein and Locksley, 1997).

Table 22–31 summarizes the common pathogens and the clinical situations in which they are encountered.

The atypical pneumonias, mycoplasma and chlamydophilia (formerly called Chlamydia pneumonia), commonly occur throughout the lifespan. They rarely occur before age 6 years, increase during school-age, adolescents, continue to occur through young adulthood but decline in incidence during middle-age. Chlamydophilia accounts for about 10% of pneumonia in all age groups. If this pneumonia occurs in the elderly it can cause severe disease. (McIntosh, 2002).

Table 22–32 lists the common atypical pneumonias and their clinical manifestations.

Other less common pneumonias should be considered if the person works with/exposed to animals like cattle, sheep, pigs, horses, birds, cats, where they have lived and traveled in the past 6 weeks and exposure to fungal infections. This increases the risk for Q-fever, coccodioidomycosis, histoplasmosis, brucellosis, tularemia, *Chlamydia psittaci,* hantavirus and hypersensitivity pneumonitis. (Cunha & Ortega, 1996; Gales & McClain, 1997).

TABLE 22–31. Clinical Situations And Common Pathogens In Community-Acquired Pneumonia

Clinical Situations	Pathogens
Alcoholism	a,b,c,e,i
(If homeless add)	g
COPD/CLD	a,b,f,h
Diabetes	a,h
Episodic	a,d,e
IVDA	a,c,e,i
(If homeless add)	g
School-age children, adolescents, young adults, college students, military recruits	a,d,j
Non-lung chronic illness	a,e,h
Immunosuppressive state (using NSAIDs & steroids)	a,b,c,e,g,h,i,j
Smokers	b,e
Elderly	
Non-Nursing Home	a,b,d,i
Nursing Home	a,b,c,f,h,i

Legend: a = *S. pneumonia;* b = *H. influenzae;* c = *Klebsiella;* d = *M.* or *C. pneumoniae;* e = *Legionella;* f = *M. Catarrhalis;* g = TB; h = GNR (gram-negative rods); i = anerobes; j = *Nisseria-meningitides;* k = viruses

Mandell, Bartlett, Dowell, File et al. (2003) and Bartlett, Dowell, Mandell et al. (2000).

TABLE 22–32. Common Atypical Pneumonias and Clinical Manifestations

Atypical Pneumonia	Clinical Manifestations
Mycoplasma pneumoniae	Malaise, myalgias, arthralgias, low-grade fever +/− headache Nonproductive cough, after several days +/− productive cough that persists +/− OM, pharyngitis, tracheobronchitis Extrapulmonary symptoms: cardiac, gastrointestinal, liver/spleen enlargement, elevation of LFTs; neurologic changes, hematologic abnormalities
Chlamydophilia pneumonia	Biphasic course; erythematous, nonexudative pharyngitis with hoarseness first, then 1 week later cough begins; may be productive with bronchospasms and wheezing +/− fever, cervical adenopathy +/− eye involvement
Legionella pneumophila	Abrupt onset of myalgia, malaise, weakness, and headache; 24 h later fever, intermittent chills Nonproductive cough; eventually 50% develop thin mucoid purulent, copious volume; hemoptysis in 30% Diarrhea, nausea, vomiting, abdominal pain Altered mental status

+/− means finding may be either present or absent

Adapted from Bernstein & Locksley (1997); Cunha & Ortega (1996).

If an uncommon pneumonia or pneumonitis is suspected, a consultation or referral is warranted. Very specific testing may be necessary, and several of these diseases can become chronic with significant sequelae and result in death.

SARS has become a world-wide disease as mankind moves closer together through travel for business and pleasure. SARS should be suspected when a person has a fever, shortness of breath (SOB), +/− dry cough, difficulty breathing in the absence of radiographic pneumonia (respiratory symptoms usually appear 2 to 7 days after the onset of the illness), rhinorrhea, sore throat, diarrhea, has traveled to China, Taiwan, Hong Kong or has close contact with someone who has traveled there. Those who are employed in a laboratory that works with the live SARS virus or healthcare workers providing care to a SARS patient are also at increased risk. (CDC, 2004). Because the symptoms of SARS mimics so many other diseases, the history of travel and employment is crucial. A SARS-CoV test is available. If the healthcare provider suspects SARS, the Health Department should be notified immediately.

Laboratory abnormalities have been associated with SARS but are not diagnostic. They include the following: 1) lymphopenia with normal or low WBC 2) elevated transaminases 3) elevated creatinine phosphokinase 4) elevated lactic dehydrogenase 5) elevated C-reactive protein and 6) a prolonged PTT (partial thromboplastin time) (CDC, 2004).

SARS in the elderly often presents with little to no symptoms so an elderly person if has traveled to the high prevalence areas consider SARS as a diagnosis. Little is known about SARS in children as only a very small percentage have ever been diagnosed with the disease. A more likely diagnosis is RSV. (CDC, 2004).

Specific Considerations for Pharmacotherapy

When Drug Therapy Is Needed. Because of the increased mortality of all pneumonias in the elderly, complicated usually by other comorbid illnesses, there is universal agreement that antibiotic therapy and/or hospitalization is the norm.

Short- and Long-Term Goals of Pharmacotherapy. The short-term goals of treatment are to resolve the pneumonia, reduce the associated symptoms within 24 to 36 h, and reduce or prevent hospitalization.

The long-term goals are to reduce mortality; restore the person to the previous level of functioning; prevent recurrent episodes of pneumonia through adequate dental care, nutrition, hydration, and appropriate vaccination; and prevent or minimize an exacerbation of their comorbid illness during the acute pneumonia (File, Tan, & Plouffe, 1996; Musher, 1998).

Nonpharmacologic Therapy. This can include the use of oxygen, plenty of hydration, and rest.

Time Frame for Initiating Pharmacotherapy. Pneumonia must be treated as soon as possible in order to decrease the risk of mortality, especially in the elderly. All patients are strongly encouraged to start their antibiotics the same day they are seen in the office for their pneumonia evaluation. The ideal time to start the antibiotics is within 8 hours of the diagnosis. It has been shown in hospitalized patients that if IV antibiotics are started within 8 hours, mortality is significantly decreased, which might be extrapolated to the outpatient setting as well. Medication adherence is very important and the patient must be instructed regarding taking and finishing all their medicine even if they feel well.

The choice of treatment setting for the elderly with pneumonia is a decision based on the stability of the comorbid illness, vital sign abnormalities, hypoxemia on room air, severe electrolyte and/or hematological abnormalities- a WBC count of < 4000 or > 30,000, an absolute neutrophil count of < 1000, elevated BUN and creatinine, decreased platelet count, elevated protime (PT) or partial thromboplastin time (PTT) and radiographic evidence of multi-lobar involvement and bilateral infiltrates (ATS, 2001; Marrie, Lau, Wheeler et al, 2000). In the nonhospitalized nonacute elderly, close followup is essential if the person lives alone. Usually the younger and middle-aged otherwise healthy adult can be safely treated as an outpatient.

Assessment Needed Prior to Therapy. See Table 22–33 for baseline history information and physical examination criteria and Table 22–34 for findings specific to the common bacterial pneumonias.

Table 22–35 summarizes the common diagnostic tests to consider if the clinician suspects one of the community-acquired pneumonias.

Patient/Caregiver Information

- Clear information must be given regarding signs and symptoms that indicate a worsening of the pneumonia.
- Review common side effects of the medication.
- In the elderly, supply written directions or when to call and/or a relative/neighbor/friend to check on them daily.
- Do a close follow-up, if the patient is elderly; otherwise follow up in 48 to 72 h.

TABLE 22–34. History Specific to the Common Bacterial Pneumonias

Previous history of a URI	a, b, e
Fever:	
Sudden onset of high fever	a, c
Rare	d
Sudden shaking chills	a, c
Pleuritic chest pain	a, b, c
Productive cough:	
Rusty-colored sputum	a
Purulent sputum	b
Thick, tenacious, purulent	c
Dyspnea	a, b, c, d, e
Pleuritic chest pain	a, b, c
Possibility of:	
Vomiting/diarrhea	b, c, e
Hypotension	b, d
Mental confusion, asthenia	d
Cyanosis, jaundice	c
Falls, new incontinence	d
Anorexia, failure to thrive	d
Worsening of comorbid illness	d

Legend: a = *S. pneumoniae;* b = *H. influenzae;* c = *Klebsiella;* d = elderly; e = viral or mixed

Adapted from (Pennacho, 2001).

Outcomes Management

Selecting an Appropriate Agent. Selection of an appropriate antibiotic depends on age and comorbid illnesses; other factors that can change the usual pathogen such as smoking, alcohol, and drug abuse; cost; broad-based coverage for the usual pathogens; and a single therapy if possible.

TABLE 22–33. History and Physical Examination for Bacterial Pneumonias

History Information

- Risk factors: alcohol, smoking, chronic lung disease, immunologic deficiency, IVDA, homelessness, age
- Nutrition, anorexia, weight loss
- Recent hospitalizations
- Recent pneumococcal/influenza vaccines
- Symptoms: initial onset of symptoms, progression of symptoms, self-treatment, worsening of other illnesses
- Daily medications: prescribed, OTC, and other self-medications
- Comorbid illnesses
- Living environment
- Immunosuppressive drugs; NSAIDs, and/or steroids
- Recent travel

Physical Examination

- Generally ill-appearing
- Vital signs:
- Increased respiratory rate, labored, use of accessory muscles
- Increased heart rate (increased 10–15 beats/min/temp degree)
- Fever, often absent or low-grade, if > 38.3 (101), often indicates severe infection
- If heart rate is up significantly, need to consider CHF
- Hypotension in elderly
- Neck: JVD changes
- Skin: color, hydration
- Lips/teeth: cyanosis, cavities
- Lungs: dull percussion, + egophany, may/may not have consolidation or tactile fremitus, bronchial or tubular breath sounds, crackles; in elderly unable to breathe deeply, no crackles will be heard
- Abdomen: tenderness, hepatosplenomegaly
- Neurologic: change in mental status, cognition impairment, functional decline, cerebellar changes (frequent falls)

Adapted from Bartlett, Breiman, Mandell, & File (1995); Fraser (1997); Mouton et al. (2001); Norman (1999). Marrie, Lau, Wheeler et al, (2000)

TABLE 22–35. Diagnostic Tests to Consider and Expected Results for Community-Acquired Pneumonias

Pneumonia	Chest x-ray	WBC with Differential	Chemistry 18	Other Tests
S. pneumoniae	Homogeneous Usually LLL Can be bilateral	>12,000 with left shift (increased neutrophils and more immature white cells)	Changes based on age, comorbid illness	Sputum: rare to obtain without oral flora contamination; 50% positive
H. influenzae	Lobar/bronchopneumonia	Usually increased	Usually normal	Sputum: depends on comorbid illnesses
Klebsiella	Lesion in URL +/− multiple lobes; lobar consolidation +/− necrotizing	Decreased in alcoholics secondary to folate deficiency/poor bone marrow function Others: 12,000–20,000 WBC	Usually normal	
M. pneumoniae	Patchy infiltrates in lower lobes	Normal-low; check if elderly	Normal but check if elderly/ comorbid illness	
C. pneumoniae	Patchy broncho-pneumonia			
Legionella	Diffuse patchy infiltrates and poorly defined nodular densities; bilateral infiltrates 50%	+/− abnormal	Low sodium Low serum phosphorus levels	

+/− means finding could be either present or absent

Adapted from Areno, San Pedro, & Campbell (1996); ATS (2001); Cunha & Ortega (1996); Moroney (1996).

In 2001 the ATS formulated a set of guidelines that would treat community-acquired pneumonia using an empiric, not a syndrome-based, approach. The guiding principle behind this departure from the standard was to establish a diagnosis of pneumonia and a therapeutic plan employing an empiric regimen that takes into account the impact of age and comorbid illness on the risk for pneumonia. One of the most controversial decisions was to recommend that the Gram stain of the sputum, and culture not be used routinely as a diagnostic tool. There are multiple diagnostic tests to assist in identifying the offending pathogen, but there is *no one* test available to make the diagnosis. Therefore, history becomes extremely important (Niederman, 2002a, 2002b). There is considerable debate regarding this treatment approach, but these guidelines are to direct clinical practice only, so the clinician can still individualize treatment. Table 22–36 summarizes the ATS categories for the treatment of CAP. The Infectious Diseases Society of America (IDSA) recommends a clinical approach to community-acquired pneumonia (CAP). The Society's recommendations are similar but minor differences do exist. The differences are primarily concerning diagnostic testing in the outpatient setting and the significance of age with risk (ATS, 2000; Bartlett et al., 1998).

Adult Without Comorbid Illness. In the young or middle-aged adult without comorbid illness, CAP Group I, the most common pathogen responsible for CAP is *S. pneumoniae, Mycoplasma pneumoniae* and *chlamydophilia*

TABLE 22–36. Likely Pathogens Causing Community-Acquired Pneumonia and Empiric Treatment

Group I: CAP Outpatients with No Cardiopulmonary Disease, No Modifying Factors	Group II: CAP Outpatients with Cardiopulmonary Disease and/or Modifying Factors
Organisms *S. pneumoniae* *Mycoplasma pneumoniae* *Chlamyeophilia pneumoniae* *Haemophilis iinfluenza* Respiratory viruses Miscellaneous Legionella species *Mycobacterium tuberculosis* Endemic fungi Excludes patients at risk for HIV	**Organisms** *S. pneumoniae* *Mycoplasma pneumoniae* *Chlamydia pneumoniae* Mixed infection (bacteria plus a typical pathogen or virus) *Haemophilus influenza* Enteric gram-negative bacteria Respiratory viruses Miscellaneous *Moraxella catarrhalis, Legionella*, species, aspiration-related pathogens, (anaerobe), *Mycobacterium tuberculosis*, endemic fungi
Therapy - no recent antibiotics Recent antibiotic therapy Respiratory fluroquinolone along an advanced macrolide plus high dose beta-lactnamose penicillin inhibitor (ie., augmentin) Advanced-generation macrolide or Doxycycline	**Therapy** Beta-lactam, oral cefpodoxime, cefuroxime, high-dose amoxicillin (1gram q 8 hrs), or amoxicillin-clavulanate; or parenteral ceftriaxone followed by oral cefpodoxime PLUS Macrolide or doxycycline or respiratory fluoroquinolone OR Antipncumococcal fluoroquinolones as monotherapy

Source: ATS (2001). Mandell, Partlett, Dowell, et al, 2003 pneumonia is seen, especially in smokers. Legionella and mycobacterium tuberculosis must also be considered in the diagnosis. The recommendation is to treat with an advanced macrolide, such as azithromycin or clarithromycin, or doxycycline. Resistant pneumococci would be unusual in younger and healthier population (ATS, 2000). Clarithromycin can cause considerable gastrointestinal side effects, but if it is taken with food, avoiding caffeine and spicy and greasy foods, most people can tolerate the medication. The medication leaves an "aluminum" or "tinny" taste in the mouth, but this can be decreased by having a small piece of chocolate immediately after. Azithromycin can be taken on an empty stomach or with food without changing the bioavailability (*Drug Facts and Comparisons,* 2003).

The newer fluorquinolones—gatifloxacin, levofloxacin, moxifloxacin, and levofloxacin—are available to use as monotherapy and have the advantage of once-a-day dosing (ATS, 2001; Niederman, 2002a, 2002b). See Drug Table 102 for additional information.

Use of the older fluoroquinolones has been limited due to two problems: the rapid development of multiple bacteria resistance and numerous drug interactions. The future of the newer fluoroquinolones may be in question as they potentially could be rendered ineffective as well (Musher, 1998).

The recommendations by the ATS (2000) is that *Chlamydophilia pneumonia* and *Mycoplasma pneumoniae* be treated with the advanced-generation macrolides and not erythromycin in order to provide better coverage for *S. pneumoniae.*

Many clinicians still use the pencillins and first-generation cephalosporins, but with increasing resistance to *S. pneumoniae,* the advanced-generation macrolide or doxycycline is a more appropriate choice. Consideration of the risk factors for potential drug and pathogen resistance should warrant use of the newer macrolides or doxycycline.

The modifying factors that increase the risk of infection with a specific pathogen are:

Penicillin-resistant and drug-resistant pneumococci are more likely in individuals who are/have had:

- 65 years of age
- A history of alcoholism
- Beta-lactam treatment in past 3 months
- Immunosuppressive therapy, including steroids
- Multiple medical comorbidities
- Exposure to a child in daycare

Enteric gram-negative bacteria are found in individuals who are/have:

- Residence in a nursing home
- Underlying cardiopulmonary disease
- Multiple medical comorbidities
- Recent antibiotic therapy

Pseudomonas aeruginosa are found in individuals with or undergoing:

- Structural lung disease
- Corticosteroid therapy (> 10 mg/day)
- Broad spectrum antibiotic therapy for > 7 days in past month
- Malnutrition

(ATS, 2000)

Adult With Comorbid Illness

The ATS (2001) guidelines for the management of CAP Group II: outpatients with cardiopulmonary disease and the following modifying factors:

- Organisms
  - *S. pneumoniae* (including drug-resistant)
  - *Mycoplasma pneumoniae*
  - *Chlamydia pneumoniae*
  - Mixed infection (bacteria plus atypical or viral pathogen)
  - *H. influenza*
  - Enteric gram-negative
  - Respiratory viruses
  - Miscellaneous; moraxella, catarrhalis, Legionella sp., aspiration-related pathogens (anaerobic), mycobacterium tuberculosis, endemic fungi
- Excludes patients with HIV

Therapy

- Beta lactam, oral cefpodoxime, cefuroxime, high-dose amoxicillin (1 gram every 8 hours)
- or amoxicillin/clavulanate or parenteral ceftriazone followed by cefpodoxime

PLUS

- Macrolide or doxycycline

OR

- Antipneumococcal fluoroquinolone used alone like moxifloxacin, levofloxacin, or gatifloxacin

The use of trimethoprim-sulfamethoxazole is no longer recommended because of the resistant pneumococci pathogen. Because of the incidence of co-infection with an atypical pathogen, a macrolide is warranted. For some patients, monotherapy with a fluoroquinolone is more cost effective than two medications and easy once-a-day dosing.

The Elderly Patient. The elderly patient in a long-term care facility usually has a comorbid illness, often with mental confusion, difficulty swallowing, dehydration, etc, which makes taking oral antibiotics almost impossible. The nursing home patient may require inpatient management initially until symptoms improve. Hospitalization depends on the following parameters: fever < 95° and > 104°, significant tachycardia, $PaO_2 < 60$ mmHg, hypotension, WBC < 4000 per mm^3 or > 13000 per mm^3, tachypnea, BUN > 30 mg/dl, hematocrit < 30%, radiographic evidence of progressing infiltrates, sodium < 130 mEq/L and O_2 saturation <90% (Norman, 1999).

Less Common Pneumonias. Q fever and psittacosis, the less common pneumonias, can be treated on an outpatient basis with "cyclines" such as doxycycline, tetracycline, and minocycline. The other less common pneumonias may need consultation and/or hospitalization because all can have serious sequelae (Niederman, 2002a, 2002b).

Patients with HIV infections are usually treated as inpatients, but it depends on the organism, severity of the infection, positive or negative dissemination, status of the HIV infection, effectiveness of the protease inhibitors and the antibiotics, and other factors. These patients require the care of and consultation with infectious disease specialists (Yu & Maurer, 1996).

Monitoring for Efficacy. The usual course of treatment for the bacterial pneumonias is 10 to 14 days and for the atypical pneumonias 14 days; the course for the less common pneumonias depends on the etiologic agent (Niederman, 2002a, 2002b). Clinical signs and symptoms should be improving within 24 to 48 h; the maximum is 72 h unless deterioration occurs earlier. The WBC and fever should be normal or lower than at initial diagnosis within 48 h. The young patient and the patient without comorbid illness or other factors influencing pneumonia resolution will resolve symptoms the fastest. The history should be reviewed with each patient to ensure that the original positive history data related to the pneumonia symptoms are resolving. In the elderly, the neurologic examination and questions regarding improvement in behavioral changes will provide some of the best clues to the resolution of the pneumonia.

In slowly or nonresolving pneumonia always consider other factors that can influence the delay: the patient not taking the medication correctly; significant side effects so the patient discontinues the antibiotic; the antibiotic too expensive so the prescription never filled, etc.; as well as other coexisting problems (Bartlett et al., 1998; Mandell, 2003).

The follow-up examination must include all the same systems that were examined at the baseline physical to make the diagnosis of pneumonia. In the young adult and those without comorbid illness, examine:

- Vital signs: respiratory rate, heart rate, BP
- Lungs: tactile fremitus, egophany, tubular breath sounds, crackles, rhonchi, use of accessory muscles

If there were any extrapulmonary symptoms, then recheck them.

In the elderly and those with comorbid illnesses, the physical exam must be more inclusive:

- Vital signs: respiratory rate, heart rate, B/P
- Skin: color, cyanosis
- Neck: JVD
- Heart: arrhythmias, murmurs, S_3/S_4
- Lungs: change in breath sounds from initial examination, tactile fremitus, egophany, crackles, rhonchi, wheezing (breath sounds can get worse in the elderly from baseline as rehydration recurs)
- Abdomen: hepatosplenomegaly, tenderness
- Neurologic: alertness, degree of confusion, balance, gait, CN I–XII, sensory, motor

Chest x-rays (CXRs) always lag behind clinical improvement so followup CXRs should not be repeated for at least 6 to 8 weeks after initiating treatment. CXRs often worsen once treatment is started, especially in the elderly, because dehydration can minimize the pulmonary infiltrates, but with rehydration the infiltrates are amplified (Castro-Rodriguez, & Fine, 1996). Legionella infections may require up to 20 weeks to clear radiographically, whereas *M. pneumoniae* usually clears within 2 to 4 weeks (Fein, 1996; Mouton et al., 2001). A study done by Mittl, Schwab, Duchin, et al. (1994) found that radiologic resolution was most influenced by age and the number of lobes involved. Multilobar pneumonia resolved more slowly than unilobar, and clearing decreased by 20% per decade. Most *S. pneumoniae* radiographically cleared by 12 weeks, whereas those with bacteremia still had some radiograph changes even at 3 months. Complete resolution did not occur until 18 weeks (Fein, 1994). Refer to Figure 22–2 for the management of unresolved pneumonia.

In the elderly and those with renal impairment, a creatinine clearance calculation is necessary. Medication dosage is adjusted, depending on the degree of renal im-

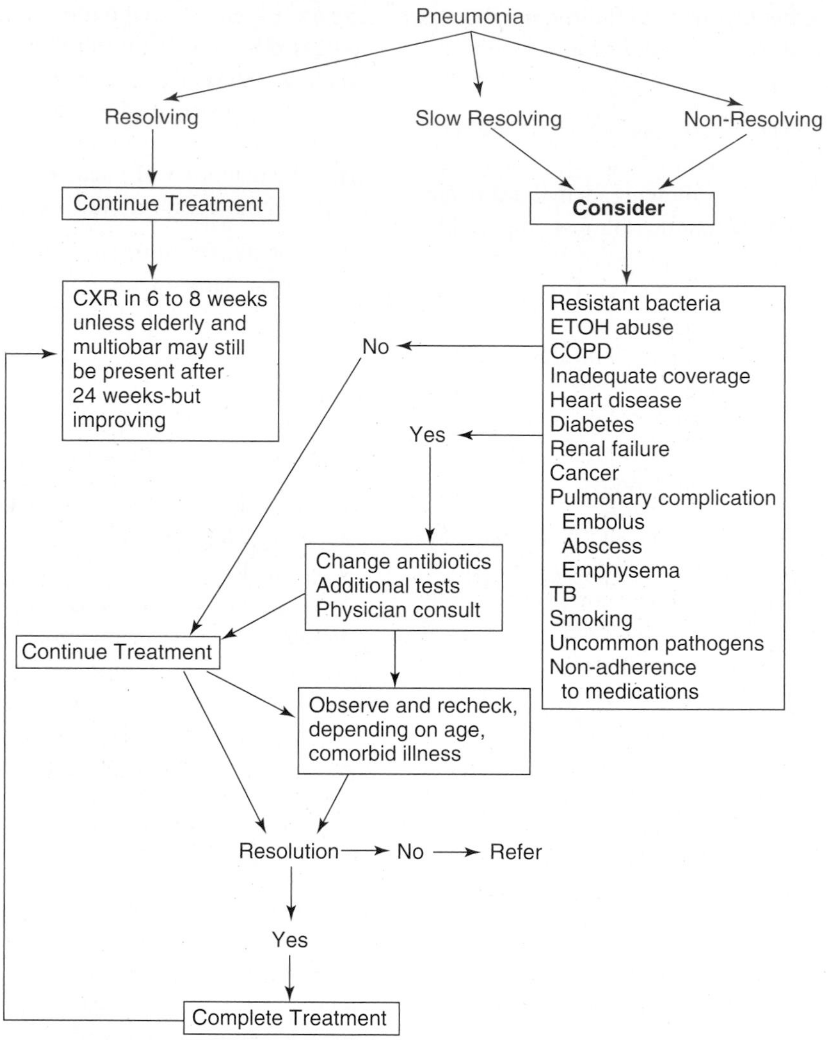

FIGURE 22–2. Algorithm for management of unresolved pneumonia. *Adapted from Fein (1996); Mandell, Bartlett Dowell et al. 2003; Moroney (1996).*

pairment: mild, moderate, or severe. If only serum creatinine is available, then convert to creatinine clearance using the following formula (PDR Generics, 2002).

$$\text{Males: } \frac{\text{Weight (kg)} \times (140 - \text{age})}{72 \times \text{serum creatinine}}$$

Females: $0.85 \times$ the value above

In those whose WBC with differential is >15,000, a repeat WBC should be redrawn at the followup visit. Other laboratory tests will be drawn as dictated by the history, physical, routine medications the patient is taking, potential interactions between the medications, and comorbid illnesses.

Monitoring for Toxicity. The penicillins and cephalosporins can cause skin rashes and an anaphylactic reaction. Cefaclor can produce a serum-like sickness, but symptoms usually resolve 3 to 4 days after discontinuing the drug. These two categories of drugs rarely cause other major adverse side effects (*Drug Facts and Comparisons,* 2003).

Doxycycline, as with all the "cyclines," increases the risk of phototoxicity and erosive esophagitis, especially if taken at bedtime on an empty stomach. These are not the drugs of choice for an elderly patient, those with a history of a peptic or active ulcer, an adult who works outside, or someone with risk factors such as alcoholism and IV drug abuse (*Drug Facts and Comparisons,* 2003).

Because the cephalosporins, fluoroquinolones, and penicillins are excreted through the kidney, a dose adjustment is usually necessary in the elderly and those with renal impairment. The fluoroquinolones may cause damage to growing cartilage and should not be used in anyone less than 16 years of age (*Drug Facts and Comparisons,* 2003). The most frequent side effects, as with the majority of antibiotics, are gastrointestinal.

For a complete listing of antibiotic side effects, refer to the Drug Tables.

Followup Recommendations. The young or middle-aged adult with pneumonia can be followed up in the clinic within 48 to 72 hrs unless symptoms are worsening. At that visit the WBC and other laboratory values can be repeated based on original values and the patient's response to therapy. If the patient appears toxic at the followup visit or fails to respond to treatment, then consultation with the physician is necessary.

A CXR is repeated as described above. The older or elderly adult with pneumonia and/or comorbid illnesses should be followed up in 24 h, if not hospitalized, and then as often as necessary. The WBC and other appropriate tests are repeated based on the results of the original tests, comorbid illness, type and severity of pneumonia, the patient's response to therapy, and the patient's living environment (Mouton et al, 2000).

PNEUMONIA IN CHILDREN AND ADOLESCENTS

Pneumonia occurs more commonly in the preschool-aged child and decreases in incidence in school-aged children and adolescents (Thompson, 1997). In developing countries though, pneumonia still remains a major health problem with a high incidence of mortality (Thompson, 1997). Pneumonia is caused by a variety of organisms: bacterial, viral, atypical, and other less common organisms. The principal organism will vary with the age of the child and season of the year, with males having a higher incidence of pneumonias (Prober, 1996). There is an increased incidence of pneumonia in children with altered local lung defenses and increased vulnerability. These are children with cystic fibrosis, prematurity, ciliary dyskinesia, and so on as well as those who live in homes with parents who smoke, with a lower socioeconomic environment, and with multiple children (Thompson, 1997).

Viral infections are the most common cause of pneumonia during the first several years of life, whereas atypical pneumonias are more common in the school-aged child and adolescents. Bacterial pneumonias are less common but do occur and tend to be more severe than those caused by nonbacterial infections (Prober, 1996).

Specific Considerations for Pharmacotherapy

When Drug Therapy Is Needed. It is generally accepted that all bacterial pneumonias are treated with the appropriate antibiotics to prevent complications or metastatic spread of the bacteria and empyema (Prober, 1996). Viral infections, however, are not treated with antibiotics; only supportive therapy is needed since the infection is self-limited and usually without complications. The most common viral organism is RSV, and it is only treated in certain circumstances. Refer to the section on Bronchiolitis for more details.

The atypical pneumonias, depending on severity, may be treated to shorten the course and prevent complications (Prakash, 1996).

Short- and Long-Term Goals of Pharmacotherapy. The short-term goals of therapy are to resolve the infection and to recognize and intervene in early extrapulmonary symptoms. The long-term goals are to prevent recurrent episodes of pneumonia and complications (lung abscesses, bacteremia) especially if patients have associated comorbid illnesses such as cystic fibrosis, asthma, or prematurity (Prober, 1996).

Nonpharmacologic Therapy. Encourage increased fluids, rest, and adequate nutrition.

Time Frame for Initiating Pharmacotherapy. Bacterial pneumonia should be treated at the time of diagnosis preferably within 8 hours of diagnosis in order to prevent the condition from worsening and exacerbating a comorbid illness. A complete course of antibiotics for 2 weeks is required with improvement noted in 24 to 36 h.

Viral pneumonias are managed with supportive care and, if comorbid illnesses exist, close followup is necessary (Green, 1997).

Atypical pneumonias are treated depending on the age, severity, length of illness, and extrapulmonary manifestations. Once the diagnosis is established, treatment is begun immediately. Improvement should be seen in 36 to 72 h (Hammerschlag, 1996; Powell, 1996).

Assessment Needed Prior to Therapy. Bacterial and viral pneumonias have great overlap in their signs and symptoms, so a careful history and physical exam can give valuable clues to the etiology of the pneumonia. Table 22–37 describes the history needed and potential examination findings in the child or adolescent with pneumonia. The above findings differ based on the pneumonia etiology and age of the patient. Table 22–38 summarizes common tests to diagnose pneumonia in children.

Concomitant disease states and contraindications include the following:

- Cystic fibrosis: The patient will need to be covered for *Pseudomonas* with two or three high-dose antibiotics for at least 3 to 4 weeks. Monitor for drug interactions.
- Asthma: Theophylline has multidrug interactions that can decrease or increase theophylline clearance.
- Heart disease: Can cause more strain on the heart secondary to increased heart rate and mismatch in ventilation-perfusion quotient.

TABLE 22–37. History and Physical Examination of Children with Pneumonia

Pertinent History Markers

- Age
- Season of year
- Past history: birth history and course in hospital, chronic illness, previous illness, hospitalizations, surgeries, frequent respiratory infections
- Onset of symptoms: rapid vs gradual
- Symptoms: laryngitis, malaise, chills, fever, tachypnea, grunting, post tussive vomiting, chest pain, noisy breathing, otalgia/otitis, chest pain, wheezing, body aches, cough (nonproductive/productive), headaches, vomiting, lethargy, anorexia, abdominal pain, sore throat, hoarseness
- Progression of symptoms: change in eating, playing, sleeping habits
- Others in family ill
- Daily medications, if any
- Where stays during day: daycare, private, family
- Self-treatment
- Reason for visit

Physical Examination and Possible Findings

- Vital signs:
  - Temperature: increased in bacterial/viral infections (younger the child, higher the temperature), usually normal to low-grade in atypical pneumonia
  - Respiratory/heart rate: increased in bacterial/viral pneumonia, usually normal in atypical
- Skin: maculopapular rashes
- Nose: nasal flaring, rhinorrhea
- Mouth: circumoral cyanosis
- Oropharynx: erythema of posterior pharynx
- Neck: cervical nodes, stiffness
- Lungs: intercostal, substernal, supraclavicular retractions, grunting, breath sounds on the opposite side may be exaggerated and tubular, inspiratory/expiratory wheezing, crackles*, not all children with pneumonia have crackles, rhonchi, listen for nature of cough: staccato, dry, paroxysmal, productive
- Heart: murmurs
- Abdomen: distention, tenderness
- Neurologic: ability to arouse if lethargic

Adapted from Schidlow & Callahan (1996).
*Margolis & Gadomski. (1998); Uirkku, Ruuskarem, 2002

Patient/Caregiver Information

1. Explain what signs and symptoms to monitor that would indicate a deterioration in the pneumonia.
2. Explain the common adverse effects of the antibiotics and how to minimize the symptoms.
3. Discuss important nonpharmacologic strategies.
4. Remind parents and patients to continue to give or take regular medications unless instructed otherwise.
5. For the older infant or toddler to age 12 years, follow the directions for taking Tylenol Elixir and Suspension liquid correctly. Take *only* every 4 to 6 h, *not to exceed* five doses in 24 h. *Use the special measuring cup provided only (no substitutions).* If needed for fever relief longer than 36 to 48 h, a call to the healthcare provider is necessary.
6. For young infants, follow the directions for taking Infant Tylenol Drops and Suspension Drops correctly.

TABLE 22–38. Common Diagnostic Tests for Children with Pneumonia

Diagnostic Tests	Possible Findings
Chest x-ray*	Nothing or patchy infiltrates, lobar consolidation, bilateral interstitial infiltrates, hyperinflation, pneumatoceles, effusions, nodular shadowing or enlargement of hilar lymph nodes (x-ray findings are variable depending on the type of pneumonia and from child to child)
WBC with differential	Usually >12,000 in bacterial pneumonia; normal/low in viral/atypical pneumonia
Mycoplasma pneumoniae PCR (polymerase chain reaction)	Positive
Viral specific-Ab tests	RSV, other viruses
Streptococcus pneumoniae Pneumococcal urinary antigen assay***	Positive
Chlamydophilia pneumoniae IgM titer using a Micro-immunofluorescence serologic test	> 1:16
PCR assay of respiratory secretions	Positive

Adapted from Prober (1996); Schidlow & Callahan (1996), Mandell, Bartlett, Dowell, 2003.
*bacterial pneumonia if lobar infiltrates
*viral pneumonia if interstitial infiltrates but can also be seen in a bacterial pneumonia
***not effective in infants <1 year old

Dose exactly every 4 to 6 h, *not to exceed* four doses in 24 h. *Use the special measuring dropper only (no substitutions).* If fever persists longer than 36 h, call the healthcare provider. *Infant Tylenol Drops are more potent per dose than the Suspension so exact measuring is imperative.*

7. Children's ibuprofen oral suspension can be used. Follow the directions exactly. *Use the calibrated dosage cup only (no substitutions).* Dose every 6 to 8 h but *do not exceed* four doses in 24 h. If the fever lasts longer than 36 h, call the healthcare provider (*Drug Facts and Comparisons,* 2003; PDR Generics, 2002).
8. Refer to Chapter 12 for correct administration techniques for giving medications to children.

Outcomes Management

Selecting an Appropriate Agent. The most common cause of pneumonia in the newborn (birth to 1 month) age group is group B streptococcus, *Listeria monocytogenes, E. coli* and other gram negative organisms like *S. aureus* (Thompson, 1997). Group B streptococcal pneumonia generally appears within the first 6 to 12 h after birth and can progress to fulminant disease rapidly if not detected early (Schidlow & Callahan, 1996). Any newborn, 1 month or less, who is ill-appearing, symptomatic, and/or diagnosed with pneumonia must be hospitalized for a complete sepsis workup. These newborns are never treated as outpatients. The nurse practitioner who examines an ill newborn will always seek consultation with the physician (Prober, 1996; Schidlow & Callahan, 1996).

The common offending organisms that cause pneumonia in the infancy and early childhood age group, in order of frequency, are (1) viruses, (2) *S. pneumoniae,* (3) RSV (4) pertussis, and (5) *H. influenzae* in unimmunized children.

Table 22–39 reviews the organisms, history, clinical manifestations, and recommended treatment for infants and young children, and Table 22–40 summarizes these issues in children older than 5 and adolescents.

Febrile infants who experience difficulty eating, respiratory distress, and hypoxemia should be hospitalized, whereas afebrile infants without any of the previously mentioned symptoms, well-appearing, with no other associated illnesses, and having a parent who can monitor the infant closely can be treated as outpatients. The febrile infant should be hospitalized because the pneumonia course is more variable and complications more frequent.

When bacterial pneumonia is suspected, use ceftriaxone IM, a third-generation cephalosporin that covers both gram-negative and gram-positive organisms. When the infant or young child is able to tolerate oral fluids and the respiratory and heart rates approach normal, treatment can be changed to an oral antibiotic or a second- or third-generation cephalosporin, amoxicillin/clavulanic acid, or an advanced macrolide (Klein, 1997; Prober, 1996).

Azithromycin and clarithromycin, available in suspension, have more coverage against Mycoplasma, Chlamydophilia pneumoniae, and non-drug-resistant strains of S. pneumoniae than erythromycin. The medication tastes bad, and most children will not take it. In children, azithromycin is equally as effective against the same organisms as clarithromycin, but easier to take: only one dose/day for 5 days in pill forms, so taste is not an issue or as an oral suspension.

Erythromycin can abort or eliminate pertussis if it is started in the catarrhal phase but will not shorten the paroxysmal phase if started then. Relapse occurs if treatment in children is for less than 14 days. The dose is 40 mg/kg per day divided qid orally for 14 days. An alternate drug for the treatment of pertussis is azithromycin or TMP-SMX (trimethoprim-sulfamethoxazole) (*Drug Facts and Comparisons,* 2003; Long, 1997; Niederhauser, 1997).

All the medications are given in either liquid or chewable preparations for the young infant, toddler, or preschooler. Dosages must be accurate as the young infant or child varies in drug absorption, distribution, metabolism, and excretion (Niederhauser, 1997).

Monitoring for Efficacy. The bacterial pneumonias tend to resolve rapidly after antibiotics are initiated. Improvement is noted within 24 to 48 h. The atypical pneumonias tend to resolve more slowly, but improvement should be noted after several days of antibiotics. In any child who remains symptomatic or whose symptoms resolve and then recur again, a reassessment is needed. In persistent symptoms always think cystic fibrosis, AIDS, foreign body, tracheobronchial anomalies, asthma, or systemic disease (Schidlow & Callahan, 1996). Also when resolution is slow, consider the possibility that the medication is given incorrectly, in an inaccurate dose or there is a change in the absorption of the medication (Niederhauser, 1997).

Chest x-ray resolution usually occurs in about 6 to 10 weeks after onset of antibiotics. If the chest x-ray fails to clear, then consider the above-cited medical conditions.

TABLE 22–39. Pneumonias in Infancy and Early Childhood

Organism	Significant History	Clinical Signs	Recommended Antibiotics
Respiratory syncytial virus	Refer to the section on bronchiolitis		
Parainfluenza	Season of year, other illness in family or community < 5 years of age Gradual onset +/− fever, URI symptoms for several days, then +/− productive cough	Tachypnea Tachycardia Rarely fever, +/− rhonchi, rales, inspiratory/expiratory wheezing with prolonged expiratory phase	No treatment necessary unless secondary infection, rare in healthy children
S. pneumoniae 1) Infants:	Usually starts with a stuffy nose, decreased appetite, fretfulness for several days, then abrupt onset of high fever, restlessness, and respiratory distress Infants may also have nausea, vomiting, diarrhea, +/− convulsions Increased risk if HIV, sickle cell anemia, nephrotic syndrome, renal failure, splenectomy, transplant (for all ages)	Ill-appearing Air hunger +/− cyanosis Nasal flaring +/− retractions +/− grunting +/− diminished breath sounds, fine crackles on affected side, but these findings are less common in infant/young child Breath sounds on the opposite side may be enhanced and tubular +/− abdominal distention secondary to increased air swallowing +/− palpable liver secondary to downward displacement of the diaphragm; consider CHF If lower lobe pneumonia, may be referred to abdomen, cause pain; if in upper lobes, can cause neck pain, nuchal rigidity	Usually hospitalized
2) Children:	Brief URI, develops shaking chills then high fever, restlessness, drowsiness, increased respirations, anxiety; can begin as dry hacky but productive-sounding cough in the young child who rarely expectorates Child may splint the affected side and/or lie on side with knees drawn up to chest	Tachypnea Tachycardia +/− circumoral cyanosis Retractions, nasal flaring Dullness to percussion, diminished tactile and vocal fremitus Decreased breath sounds and fine crackles on affected side Symptoms change as illness progresses; consolidation signs appear on days 2 to 3 and with resolution comes an increased productive cough of blood-tinged mucus	For outpatient treatment in children over 1 year of age: ceftriaxone I.M macrolides Augmentin/cephalosporins—if culture and sensitivities indicate
Pertussis	Usually < 12 mos but increasing in adults and elderly Three stages of illness: 1. Catarrhal phase: Often starts with coryza, conjunctivitis (1–2 weeks) 2. Paroxysmal phase: Followed by paroxysms of cough with posttussive vomiting (2–4 weeks) 3. Convalescence (1–2 weeks)	Conjunctivitis Low-grade fever Leukocytosis especially in young children Tachypnea	Treatment is only effective if begun in the catarrhal phase • ≥ 2 weeks: erythromycin delayed-release tabs 333 mg po tid × 14 days or erythromycin estolate 40–50 mg/kg/day × 14 days • ≤ 2 wks: intolerant to erythromycin, azythromycin 10–12 mg/kg/d for 5–7 days or a Z-pack or clarithromycin 15–20 mg/kg/d bid 10–14 days • intolerance to macrolides, use TMP/SMX = 8 mg/kg/d/40 mg/kg/d bid × 14 days Relapse occurs if treatment less than 14 days

+/− = findings could be either present or absent.

Adapted from Klein (1997); Prober (1996); Rubin & O'Hanley (1996); Schidlow & Callahan (1996), Red Book (2002).

TABLE 22–40. Pneumonias in Children Older Than 5 Years and Adolescents

Organism	History Information	Clinical Symptoms	Recommended Antibiotics
M. and *C. pneumoniae*	Wide array of presenting symptoms, but common is headache, abdominal pain, and vomiting Onset is insidious; malaise, myalgias Cough may begin as nonproductive and then progresses to productive cough with +/− chest pain that persists In those with *C. pneumoniae,* usually starts with nonexudative pharyngitis and hoarseness, then 1 week later productive cough begins May present as an exacerbation of a chronic illness, ie, asthma, undiagnosed reactive airway disease	+/− fever +/− erythematous TMs +/− sinus face pain Scattered or localized crackles, tubular breath sounds over affected area, +/− wheezing Paucity of clinical findings	Macrolides azithromycin clarithromycin erythromycin
S. pneumoniae	History and clinical manifestations as described in Table 22–33		Macrolides azithromycin clarithromycin erythromycin Third generation cephalosporins Augmentin (if cultures and sensitivities indicate)

Adapted from Klein (1997); Prakash (1996); Prober (1996); Schidlow & Callahan (1996).

During the physical examination, look for:

- Vital signs: temperature, respiratory and heart rates
- Nose: flaring
- Lungs: wheezing, crackles, diminished breath sounds, rhonchi, use of accessory muscles
- Heart: murmurs
- Abdomen: hepatosplenomegaly

The physical examination is based on the patient's age, type of pneumonia, severity, and physical examination at diagnosis.

Monitoring for Toxicity. The most common side effects are gastrointestinal and occasionally a rash. Diarrhea, if it occurs, can change the absorption rate of the medication. A change in medication may be necessary. Refer to Drug Table 102 for further information.

Followup Recommendations. The young infant or child needs to be seen daily until the symptoms are resolved and improvement noted. If deterioration occurs, then the patient needs to be hospitalized and/or the diagnosis reconsidered. In the older child or adolescent with a bacterial pneumonia followup is recommended within 48 h. If symptoms are improving, repeat followup is at the clinician's judgment. In those who do not respond as expected, reconsider the diagnosis and other factors that could prevent resolution: other coexisting disease states, parental smoking, not giving the medication correctly, incorrect medication, resistant organism, etc. In those with an atypical pneumonia, follow up in 3 to 5 days unless deterioration occurs (Klein, 1997; Prober, 1996).

In any patient with a comorbid illness, follow-up must be daily or every 2 days and the patient examined by the consulting physician if not hospitalized.

PNEUMONIA IN PREGNANCY

Pneumonia during pregnancy is an infrequent problem but has the potential to cause serious maternal and fetal distress. The fetus does not tolerate hypoxia, acidosis, fever, and tachycardia well, thus increasing the risk for preterm birth. Pneumonia is the most frequent cause of nonobstetric infection and the third leading cause of nonobstetric death (Munn, Atterbury, & Groome 1999). The incidence of pneumonia and complications is increased in pregnant women with underlying lung disease (especially asthma), renal failure, chronic liver disease, diabetes, postsplenectomy, cigarette smoking, chronic alcohol abuse and illicit drug use, anemia, and HIV infection (Pulmonary disorders, 1997; Lim, MacFarlane, & Colthorpe, 2001).

The most common causative organisms are the same as for the nonpregnant woman. *S. pneumoniae, M. pneumoniae,* and viruses. In pregnant women with HIV, coccidioidomycosis is the most common, but *P. carinii* can be the cause and is almost always fatal (Saade, 1997).

It is vital, therefore, to recognize the disease process and initiate prompt effective treatment, close observation, and follow-up. Pregnant women should be treated aggressively since an infectious pneumonitis can result in fetal complications and preterm labor (Saade, 1997).

Specific Considerations for Pharmacotherapy

When Drug Therapy Is Needed. In the pre-antibiotic era, maternal mortality was high. Fineland and Dublin's study done in 1939 showed a 32% mortality rate among 212 pregnant women with pneumonia. The studies done recently all demonstrated a significant decline in maternal and fetal morbidity and mortality with early diagnosis and appropriate antibiotic treatment (Lim, MacFarlane, Colthorpe, 2001). With the onset of antibiotic treatment, the incidence of preterm labor was also decreased (Lim, MacFarlane, Colthorpe, 2001).

Clearly, there is unanimous agreement that all pregnant women must be treated with the appropriate antibiotic whenever pneumonia is diagnosed. Depending on the coexisting illness, severity of the pneumonia symptoms, and trimester, the pregnant woman may be hospitalized and treated with IV antibiotics. For the noncritical pregnant woman with pneumonia, outpatient treatment with intensive followup is recommended.

Short- and Long-Term Goals of Pharmacotherapy. The short-term goals of therapy are to direct the antibiotic therapy at the most likely organism(s), choose an antibiotic that is safe and effective during pregnancy, and resolve the pneumonia. The long-term goals of therapy are to prevent maternal and fetal complications through rapid diagnosis, aggressive treatment, and prevention of a recurrence.

Nonpharmacologic Therapy. Urge hydration, rest, respiratory support, if needed, and cessation of smoking if warranted.

Time Frame for Initiating Pharmacotherapy. A high index of suspicion should be maintained whenever an upper respiratory infection does not resolve within the usual time frame. An appropriate workup should be done and treatment begun immediately. Rapid improvement will be noted if there is no uncontrolled coexisting illness and/or an organism causing atypical pneumonia. Close followup is necessary.

Assessment Needed Prior to Therapy. Refer to Table 22–33 for detailed history and physical examination findings for pneumonia in adults and the elderly. However, the additional history and physical findings in the pregnant woman may alert the clinician to a possible pneumonia; see Table 22–41. Additional tests are noted in Table 22–42.

There are no disease states where antibiotics cannot be used, but in certain diseases the antibiotics may have a Category C safety profile, cause oto- or neurotoxicity, and/or need dosage changes because of renal and liver disease, chemotherapy, alcohol or drug abuse, immunocompromise, and/or diabetes. If this occurs, consultation is necessary.

Patient/Caregiver Information

- Alert the pregnant woman to signs and symptoms of upper respiratory infections that do not resolve.
- Discuss if the woman has increased rate of breathing, and then call the healthcare provider.
- Discuss smoking cessation and drug and alcohol avoidance.
- If the woman has a coexisting illness, manage carefully and if signs or symptoms flare, seek medical care immediately.

Outcomes Management

Selecting an Appropriate Agent. Antibiotics are the mainstay of treatment for community-acquired pneumonia, but which organism is most likely the causative agent depends on smoking status, age, and comorbid illnesses. Since community-acquired pneumonia is most frequently caused by *S. pneumoniae,* atypical and viral pathogens in the relatively healthy pregnant woman, treatment must be directed at providing coverage for these organisms. Selec-

TABLE 22–41. History and Physical Examination for the Pregnant Woman with Pneumonia

History Markers
- Time of the year/area of the country: coccidioidomycosis occurs in drier months of the year and in endemic areas; Southwestern United States
- Other family members ill
- Nonspecific complaints: anorexia, headache, cough, and fever may be the initial symptoms for coccidioidomycosis
- Unresolved upper respiratory infection for 2 weeks or longer
- Smoking, alcohol, or illicit drug use
- Risk factors for HIV infection

Physical Findings
- Increased respiratory rate; may be earliest sign of infection
- +/− crackles at lung bases
- Tachypnea
- Cough
- Change in pulse oximetry
- Dyspnea

Adapted from NIH/NHLBI (1993); Lim, MacFarlane, Colthorpe, 2001.

TABLE 22–42. Diagnostic Tests for the Pregnant Patient with Pneumonia

Fetal ultrasound	12–20 weeks, depending on severity and type of pneumonia
Sequential ultrasound	Done during the second and third trimester to evaluate fetal growth depending on type of pneumonia and its chronicity
Electronic fetal heart monitoring	Considered in third trimester to assess fetal well-being or if fetal problems suspected

Adapted from Rigby & Pastorek (1996)

tion of an agent to treat pneumonia during pregnancy necessitates consideration of drug hypersensitivity, safety during pregnancy, dose frequency, cost and other associated factors, chronic illnesses, and smoking and alcohol use. Table 22–43 lists the most common pathogens and appropriate pharmacotherapy for pneumonia in pregnant women (Pulmonary Disorders, 1997).

Antibiotics. For the pregnant woman, high dose, amoxicillin, or azithromycin are safe drugs to use. Other excellent choices are the first- and second-generation cephalosporins, but the first-generation cephalosporins cephalexin and cephradine are inactivated by beta-lactamase-producing organisms. Several of the second-generation cephalosporins such as cefaclor are very stable in the presence of beta-lactamase enzymes, as is the third-generation cephalosporin cefpodoxime proxetil. Therefore, many organisms resistant to penicillins and some of the cephalosporins are susceptible to these second-and third-generation cephalosporins (*Drug Facts and Comparisons,* 2003). The pharmacokinetics of the cephalosporins change during pregnancy. They have (1) a shorter half-life, (2) lower serum levels, and (3) increased clearance (*Drug Facts and Comparisons,* 2003).

Amoxicillin/clavulanic acid will provide coverage for *S. pneumoniae* and *H. influenzae* but has more side effects than either azithromycin or the cephalosporins. Erythromycin can also be used but produces more side effects and at four-times-a-day dosing can be impractical. The estolate salt of erythromycin should be *avoided* during pregnancy as it can induce hepatotoxicity. The liver enzymes usually return to normal levels after discontinuing the drug (*Drug Facts and Comparisons,* 2003). Clarithromycin, another newer macrolide, is a Category C drug and therefore *not approved* for use during pregnancy (*Drug Facts and Comparisons,* 2003). Unfortunately, resistance to the "mycins" is also increasing, and cross-resistance to all the agents in this group is usual all fluoroquinolones are contra-indicated during pregnancy (Lim, MacFarlane, & Colthorpe, 2001).

Antiviral agents. Influenza A is seen during epidemics and can cause pneumonia in pregnancy. Amantadine is the drug of choice for prophylaxis but is a Category C, so a consultation is necessary. The drug must be given within 48 h of symptom onset, at a dose of 200 mg/day for 3 to 5 days or up to 48 h after symptoms resolve. This treatment can prevent or ameliorate the disease. Most of the complications of influenza are due to secondary bacterial infection, often *S. aureus, S. pneumoniae, H. influenzae,* and some gram-negative bacteria, which must be treated aggressively to prevent fulminant respiratory failure in the mother and fetal prob-

TABLE 22–43. Common Offending Organisms and Antibiotic Therapy in Pregnant Women with Pneumonia

Organism	Treatment Duration	Antibiotic
S. pneumoniae	Initial treatment for 14–21 days	Azithromycin,[a] high dose amioxicillin[b], augmentin
	Treatment failure probably secondary to resistant organism; treat for 14 days, may need longer duration	Augmentin, first- and some second-generation cephalosporins are not recommended[c]: (cefaclor, cefpodoxime proxetil, loracarbef), azithromycin
H. influenzae (smokers, ETOH abusers, immunocompromised)	Treat for 14–21 days	Second- and third-generation cephalosporin, advanced generation macrolides
M. pneumoniae	Treat for 10–14 days; some recommend 21 days	Azithromycin
Influenza A	Treatment for 5–7 days or 2 days after symptoms resolve	Amantidine[d] (possible hospitalization)
Varicella		Acyclovir (usually hospitalized)
Coccidioidomycosis		Hospitalize
P. carinii		Hospitalize

[a]Macrolides are the first-line drug therapy recommended by the ATS for treatment of Group I: CAP outpatients with no cardio-pulmonary disease, modifying factors. Refer to section under adult CAP for further information.

[b]10 to >30% penicillin resistance.

[c]Increasing resistance to cephalosporins is 10 to 30%; second- and third-generation cephalosporins have more gram-negative coverage.

[d]Amantadine is a Category C drug; consultation is needed.

Adapted from ATS, (2002); Bartlett & Mundy (1995), Drug Facts and Comparisons (2003); Fein (1996); Levison (1998).

lems (Lim, MacFarlane, Colthorpe, 2001). During epidemics, amantadine, or other antiviral medications as prophylaxis may be highly recommended for the pregnant woman who is at risk.

Varicella is a rare infection in pregnant women. It is estimated that about 95% of women of childbearing age have antibodies to varicella. If the primary infection of varicella occurs during pregnancy, there seems to be an increased incidence and virulence of varicella pneumonia. This can lead to a more complicated infection and higher mortality rate, up to 35 to 40%, than in the nonpregnant state (Nathwani, MacClean, & Conway, 1998). If the varicella infection occurs in the first trimester, there is an increased risk of fetal malformations so these women should be hospitalized and treated (Broussard, Payne, & George, 1991). Table 22–44 lists the typical symptoms of varicella.

The chest examination can be unimpressive and correlates poorly with the severity of the varicella infection, showing diffuse changes with the maximum changes occurring at the height of the skin eruption (Rigby & Pastorek, 1996). Administration of varicella-zoster immunoglobulin (VZIG) can prevent or attenuate the varicella infections in exposed individuals if given within 96 h. Early recognition is imperative (Pulmonary Disorders, 1997).

In HIV-related infections, coccidioidomycosis is becoming an increasingly common infection both in the endemic and nonendemic areas. The areas where the spores mostly live are semiarid with hot dry summers, mild winters, and moderate rainfall (Saage, Greybill, & Larsen et al., 2000). The spores are hardy and can easily be transported outside the endemic area. An index of suspicion for this disease should be maintained if the pregnant woman presents with a suggestive history of recent travel to the Southwest, and/or signs of extrapulmonary manifestations. A coccidioidomycosis infection in the second and third trimester carries a high risk of mortality (Galgiani, Ampel, & Catanzaro, 2000). Approximately 35 to 50% who develop coccidioidomycosis have nonspecific complaints such as flulike symptoms that appear 7 to 28 days after exposure and may also have eye, joint/muscle, skin, and pulmonary findings (Gales & McClain, 1997). The physical examination findings are often absent or very minimal with symptoms mimicking tuberculosis, cancer, pneumonia, and pleurisy (Gales & McClain, 1997). Pregnant women are usually at greater risk for dissemination of the coccidioidomycosis infection (Galgiani, Ampel, & Catanzaro, 2000). Because of the high mortality rate, early identification is imperative so that the pregnant woman can be hospitalized and treatment begun quickly.

TABLE 22–44. Common Symptoms of Varicella

Signs and Symptoms of Varicella	Symptoms of Varicella Pneumonia
• Persistent fevers, malaise • Myalgia occurs 2–5 days after onset of symptoms • Maculopapular/vesicular rash • Headaches	• Cough with dyspnea • Tachypnea +/− pleuritic chest pain, hemoptysis • Hypoxemia

+/− means finding can be either present or absent.

Adapted from Pulmonary Disorders (1997); Rigby & Pastorek (1996); Nathwani, MacClean, Conway, 1998

P. carinii pneumonia (PCP) can also occur during pregnancy and requires a high index of suspicion in women who are at increased risk. This is a life-threatening illness and is characterized by a dry cough, fever, tachypnea, dyspnea, a decrease in arterial Po_2, and respiratory alkalosis (Rigby & Pastorek, 1996). These women must be referred immediately to a specialist in HIV treatment.

Drugs to avoid. Any antibiotic that is a Category A or B is considered safe to use during pregnancy. The drugs that are in Category C are not considered first-line medications to use, but there are exceptions. The exceptions could include the case in which the drug is the only drug approved to treat severe infection and a chronic life-threatening infection, such as HIV, where toxic drugs are required. The nurse practitioner in these cases would be collaborating with and transferring care to the physician specialist in the management of the pregnant woman and not directing the care alone (*Drug Facts & Comparisons,* 2003).

Monitoring for Efficacy. The followup visit should be within 36 to 48 h after diagnosis. The pregnant woman needs to be questioned about symptom worsening or resolution, especially fever, cough, chest tightness, and dyspnea; associated nonpulmonary symptoms such as eye, skin, joint, and muscle problems; and smoking, alcohol, and illicit drug use.

Antibiotic therapy for atypical pneumonia is 10 to 21 days. Symptoms should begin to improve several days after initiating treatment. Refer to Table 22–32 for complete clinical manifestations of atypical pneumonia. A typical course of antibiotic therapy for bacterial pneumonia is 14 to 21 days. Improvement is seen in streptococcal pneumonia within 48 to 72 h after initiating treatment with the temperature, pulse, respiration, and pleuritic chest pain beginning to subside (Niederman, 2002a, 2002b). *H. influenzae* infection, if noninvasive, will respond to oral antibiotics rapidly, usually within 36 to 48 h. Antibiotics are given for 14 to 21 days as well. If the pregnant woman is not responding to the antibiotics as expected, reassess the diagnosis. Several causes should be considered:

- The organism is resistant to the antibiotic, especially penicillin- and/or macrolide-resistant.
- The patient is not taking the antibiotic or not taking it correctly.
- The diagnosis is incorrect.
- A comorbid illness or other associated factors, such as smoking, alcohol, or drug use, is influencing the disease course.

If all the causes have been taken into account, then most likely the organism is resistant and an antibiotic change is essential. Consider using augmentin, cefaclor, cefpodoxime, or azithromycin (Levison, 1998). Refer to Table 22–43 for a complete discussion of bacterial pneumonia treatment in this population.

Patients with varicella pneumonia and the HIV-related pneumonias are treated as inpatients so prompt recognition is important.

Monitoring for Toxicity. Some antibiotics can cause gastrointestinal upset, pseudomembranous colitis, rash, and serum-like illnesses. If the gastrointestinal symptoms are mild to moderate or an allergic reaction occurs, discontinuation of the drug is all that is usually needed. A change of antibiotics will be needed with attention to the cross-reactivity that can occur using either the penicillins or cephalosporins. Followup is needed to ensure that all allergic symptoms resolve and that the patient's pneumonia is resolving.

Followup Recommendations. In the pregnant woman with pneumonia, close followup is necessary to ensure the safety of the woman and the fetus. Followup in the office should be within 36 to 48 h after diagnosis. The symptoms should be significantly better; temperature, pulse, and respiratory rate should be within the normal range or slightly elevated. The physical examination should indicate an improvement in the chest symptoms, unchanged fetal kick counts, and a normal WBC count. In many patients, the temperature may remain elevated for about 4 days. This does not indicate a change of antibiotics; however, if the temperature remains significantly above normal for longer than 48 to 72 hrs, then a reevaluation is warranted. The chest x-ray is repeated in approximately 6 to 8 weeks if all symptoms have resolved or sooner if there is no response to the antibiotics (NIH/NHLBI, 1993; Niederman, 2002a, 2002b).

TUBERCULOSIS

Tuberculosis (TB) is an infection caused by Mycobacterium tuberculosis. TB is spread primarily by airborne transmission via inhalation of aerosolized lung secretions (droplets) of an individual infected with active pulmonary tuberculosis disease through coughing or sneezing.

The larger droplets mostly lodge in the upper airways where an active infection is unlikely. Some smaller droplets containing the tubercle bacilli can descend into the alveolar area where the majority are engulfed by alveolar macrophages, allowing the body's defense system to isolate and wall off the bacilli, thus preventing the spread and development of active disease. The body's defense system, neutrophils and macrophages, walls off the bacilli forming a granulomatous lesion, called a tubercle. From the inhalation of the droplets to granulomatous formation to a positive PPD is 2 to 10 weeks (CDC, 2000). Once the bacilli is walled off and isolated completely, immunity develops to prevent multiplication of the bacilli, so the tuberculosis can lie dormant for years (CDC, 2000). Those who have a responsive immune system can halt the multiplication of and wall off the tubercle thus preventing additional spread of the bacilli. Infection with the M. tuberculosis without disease, called latent tuberculosis infection (LTBI), can not be spread. In some individuals, the TB bacilli overwhelms the immune system or through endogenous reactivation in the elderly because of poor nutritional status, diabetes, drugs that suppress the immune system and debilitating disease, the bacilli can escape, multiply and become active disease. The likelihood that the TB bacilli will be transmitted depends on: the infectiousness of the person with TB; the environment where the exposure occurred; length of exposure and organism virulence (CDC, 2000).

Those at highest risk for developing TB are close contacts and HIV-positive individuals (100 times > risk of infection) but also many other groups of people. See Table 22–45. In fact, persons who are HIV-positive and infected with the M. tuberculosis have a risk of developing active disease at the rate of 7 to 10%/year (CDC, 2000). Since HIV is the strongest known risk factor for progression of latent tuberculosis infection (LTBI) to active disease, it is important that health care providers know the HIV status of their patients, if at all possible (CDC, 1998).

In the U.S., approximately 5% who have been infected with *M. tuberculosis* bacteria will develop active disease in the first 1 to 2 years after exposure while another 5% will develop active disease many years later. In all, approximately 10% of people with intact immune systems who develop a TB infection will progress to active disease at some time. 75–80% of the time the *M. tuberculosis* is a pulmonary infection. Extra-pulmonary TB infection more often occurs in imunosuppressed individuals and young children (CDC, 2000).

The incidence of multi-drug resistant tuberculosis (MDR-TB) is on the rise. MDR-TB is defined as *M. tuberculosis* organisms resistant to multiple drugs, usually two or more. MDR-TB is transmitted in the same manner as drug-susceptible TB. MDR-TB has two types: primary and secondary. Primary drug resistance occurs when the individual is initially infected with the resistant organism and secondary resistance occurs when the individual is non-adherent to prescribed anti-tuberculosis medications or initial inadequate therapy (CDC, 2000).

A PPD should be standard assessment for all persons who are at risk of developing tuberculosis. The PPD response is a delayed-type "cellular hypersensitivity" reaction not just to the *M. tuberculosis* but also to other non-tuberculosis mycobacterium or vaccines, like the BCG (CDC, 2000). Because BCG can cause a "false positive" tuberculin test, most experts believe that if the BCG vaccine was given > 1 year ago and the induration is > 10 mm or if it is > 5 mm induration and the 5mm group meets the appropriate criteria for tuberculin positivity by risk group (see Table 22–46), then they should be treated for LTBI (latent tuberculosis infection) (Horsburgh, Feldman, & Ridzon, 2000; ATS, 1999). The best time to read a PPD is 48 to 72 hours after placement. It should always be read by a health care provider as self-reading is inaccurate (ATS, 1994; U.S. Department of Health and Human Services [USDHHS], 1994).

Specific Considerations for Pharmacotherapy

When Drug Therapy Is Needed. When a PPD is positive and the person is diagnosed with LTBI, treatment is recommended and effective in preventing active TB disease. This is especially true if the person is at high risk for developing active disease either in the next two (2) years. Refer to Table 22–45 and Table 22–46.

Those with suspected active disease (+ PPD, + CXR, +/− systemic symptoms) need to be referred to the local Health Department/TB specialist for further work-up. The local Health Department should be called prior to sending the individual as they will not want the person to sit in the waiting room if high risk of active disease (CDC, 2000).

TABLE 22–45. Persons at High Risk for Tuberculosis

- Foreign-born persons from high-prevalence countries (Asia, Africa, Oceania, Latin America)
- Low-income and medically underserved populations, including minorities at high risk (eg, African Americans, Hispanics, Native Americans)
- Injecting drug users
- Alcoholics
- Persons with HIV infection
- Residents and personnel of correctional institutions, long-term care facilities, hospitals, and mental institutions
- Elderly
- Close contacts to infectious cases
- Migrant workers
- Persons with other medical risk factors, such as diabetes, malnutrition, postgastrectomy, end-stage renal disease, malignancies (leukemia, lymphoma), prolonged corticosteroid therapy, silicosis
- Children < 4 years of age
- Fibrotic changes on chest radiograph consistent with prior TB, especially if received no or inadequate treatment
- Recent infection with *M. tuberculosis* (+ PPD conversion within the last 2 years)
- < 10% of IDBW (ideal body weight)

Adapted from ATS (2001) and CDC (2001).

Short- and Long-Term Goals of Pharmacotherapy. The short-term goals of pharmacotherpay are to prevent progression to active disease in those who are infected, to prevent the spread of disease, educate regarding medication taking and; and to provide the safest and most effective therapy possible. Another goal is to provide the safest and most effective therapy in the shortest period of time. The long-term goals are to prevent development of drug-resistant TB and to prevent death from complications of TB.

Nonpharmacologic Therapy. Contagious individuals must practice good hygiene until they become noninfectious. They must always cover their mouths when coughing, cough into tissues or handkerchiefs, and dispose of them properly. Good handwashing is also extremely important. Usually patients with active disease are isolated until their sputum cultures are negative. Nutritional status should also be assessed because many patients maintain a poor caloric intake with weight loss while in the acute active phase of their illness. Good nutrition is important to maintain their immune function.

Time Frame For Initiating Pharmacotherapy. Persons who convert from a negative to a positive PPD or whose previous PPD status is unknown and is now positive, a negative CXR and no active disease, has LTBI (latent tuberculosis infection) and should be considered for preventive treatment. The decision to treat preventively is based on age, pregnancy status, high risk factors and con-

TABLE 22–46. Recommended Criteria for Tuberculin Positivity by Risk Group

Mantoux Test Induration Size	Group Considered to Be PPD-Positive
≥ 5 mm	HIV-infected persons
	Injecting drug users with unknown HIV status
	Close contacts of a person with infectious TB
	Persons with chest x-ray suggestive of old, healed TB
	Patients with organ transplants and other immune-suppressed patients receiving > 15 mg/day of prednisone for > 1 month or more
≥ 10 mm	Injecting drug users known to be HIV-negative
	Immigrants to the U.S. within the last 5 years from a high prevalence country
	Residents and employees of the following: Prisons, jails, nursing home, long-term care facility for the elderly, hospitals, health care facilities and residential facilities
	HIV + patients
	Homeless shelters
	Persons with the following conditions:
	Diabetes
	Silicosis
	Chronic renal failure
	Leukemia/lymphoma, cancers of the head & neck
	Weight loss > 10% of ideal body weight
	Gastrectomy
	Jejunoileal bypass
	Children < 4 years old
	Infants, children and adolescents exposed to high-risk adults
	Mycobacterial lab employees
≥ 15 mm	No risk factors

Adapted from CDC (2001).

tact with a person with active disease. However, because a person with LTBI is non-infectious and not able to spread the disease, the decision to start preventive therapy can be made over the course of several days (CDC, 2000).

Persons with highly suggestive indicators of active disease need to be referred to the local Health Department/TB specialist immediately. Because of the highly infectious nature of tuberculosis, the agency must be called to make the appropriate arrangements for immediate follow-up. If the clinician is going to treat the active TB in the office, a consultation with the Health Department is advisable.

Assessment Needed Prior to Therapy. Several important factors to remember when doing PPD testing and interpreting the results: 1) if no wheal is seen after placing the PPD then a repeat PPD is required, 2) if no induration, the PPD is read as "0" mm not as negative, 3) vaccination with live-attentuated vaccines (MMR, oral polio, varicella, oral typhoid or yellow fever) can cause suppression of the PPD response (a false-negative reading) 4) prednisone dose > 15 mg/day for more than 2 to 4 weeks suppresses the PPD response (a false-negative reading), 5) a false-positive occurs in persons infected with other mycobacteria infections, 6) higher false negative rates occurs in patients with poor nutrition, debilitating health, overwhelming acute illnesses or immunosuppression and 7) persons who know they have been exposed to someone with active disease need to have a PPD at time of exposure and repeated in 10 weeks (CDC, 2000).

Patients who have a + PPD and a CXR without active disease should also be assessed for any co-morbid illnesses, chronic medication use, pregnancy status, HIV status, liver disease, alcohol and drug use, country of origin and how long in the U.S. and any other high risk factors. Everyone should have baseline LFTs before starting therapy and any additional tests based on history (CDC, 2000).

Patients who are suspected of having active disease should have a thorough history and physical examination. The history should include the following:

- night sweats
- chest pain
- hemoptysis
- lethargy
- low-grade fever, usually late afternoon
- loss of appetite
- weight loss
- chills
- fatigue
- cough producing purulent sputum develops slowly, becoming more frequent over weeks and months
- dyspnea

Also ask about: patient's TB exposure, previous infection and any treatment, history of compliance with previous TB treatment, history of which drugs were used to treat the TB, follow-up after treatment, HIV status, potential/current pregnancy status, co-morbid medical conditions, especially renal/liver/vestibular/neurological disease, alcohol and drug use, home situation, place of employment, country of origin and length of time in the U.S. and other current medications.

The physical exam and diagnostic studies should include (CDC, 2000; Horsburgh, Feldman & Ridzon, 2000):

- CXR, abnormal but not 100% diagnostic of active TB
  Children need a PA and lateral

Adults need a PA, additional views at the health care provider's discretion

- Sputum smears (acid fast bacilli [AFB] not diagnostic of *M. tuberculosis* as can indicate presence of other mycobacteria)
- Sputum cultures (positive culture for *M. tuberculosis* confirms diagnosis) or nucleic acid amplification test (faster results)
- Hearing (may include audiogram and vestibular testing)* and vision screen with color discrimination^
- Urinalysis
- HIV test
- Pregnancy test, if appropriate
- Comprehensive Metabolic Panel, including creatinine and BUN^^
- CBC with differential and platelets#
- TSH and thyroid panel^
- Height and weight
- Exam of chest, heart, abdomen and neurological assessment
- Neuropsychiatric exam**

* if prescribing Streptomycin, amikacin, kanamycin, capreomycin
^ if using Ethambutol (EMB)
\# if prescribing P-aminosalicylic acid (PAS)
** if prescribing Cycloserine
^^amikacin, kanamycin, capreomycin, PAS, INH, rifampin

HIV infected persons require special consideration since their response is often different than someone with an intact immune system. HIV infected persons may have a + PPD, respiratory symptoms but a negative CXR. Three (3) sputum cultures should always be obtained. They can have negative sputum cultures but with respiratory symptoms, can still have active disease. HIV infected persons should always be referred to the local Health Department/TB specialist as their care can be very involved and may require other specialized testing (CDC, 2000).

Patient/Caregiver Information. All patients and caregivers should be educated about tuberculosis in clear language. Educate them about the difference between latent TB infection and active TB disease. They should also understand the modes of transmission and their drug regimens (dosing, frequency, adverse effects, and when to report adverse effects). Adherence to the medication regimen needs to be strongly emphasized, especially since patients will be on therapy for many months and may not feel sick. All information should be provided verbally as well as in writing and should be reviewed at each clinician visit.

SELECTING AN APPROPRIATE AGENT

Treating LTBI

The following persons should receive treatment for LTBI (CDC, 2000).

> 5mm induration:	HIV + individuals HIV + persons who are close contacts of persons with active disease Unknown HIV status and IVDA Close contacts of active TB persons Pulmonary fibrotic lesions on CXR from prior untreated or inadequately treated TB Adolescents exposed to adults in high risk groups Prednisone dose > 15 mg/day for > 1 month Organ transplant persons
> 10 mm induration:	IVDA PPD converter from negative to positive within past 2 years Recent immigrants from high-prevalence countries in past 5 years Residents and employees of prisons, long-term care facilities, hospital workers and homeless shelters Certain medical conditions; DM (2–4 fold increased risk), silicosis (30 fold increased risk), chronic renal failure (if dialysis, 10–25 fold in creased risk), cancers of head/neck, leukemia/lymphoma, wt loss > 10% ideal body wt, Children < 4 years
> 15 mm induration:	Persons with no risk factors

The treatment of LTBI is summarized in Table 22–47. The combination of rifampin (RIF) and pyrazinamide (PZA) is no longer an option for the treatment of LTBI because of the increased risk of hepatotoxicity resulting in liver deaths. The American Thoracic Society and the CDC issued these new recommendations regarding the use of this drug combination in 2003. There are certain special situations when this combination can be used but should be done only by the Health Department/TB specialist because of the risk.

INH penetrates well into all body fluids and is bactericidal against TB. INH is contraindicated in those patients with a drug allergy, history of INH-associated he-

TABLE 22–47. Drug Regimen for the Treatment of Latent Tuberculosis

	Oral dose mg/kg (maximum dose)			
	Daily		*Twice Weekly*^^	
Drug	***Adults***	***Children****	***Adults***	***Children***
Isoniazid × 9 mos^	5 mg (300mg)	10–20 mg (300mg)	15 mg (900mg)	20–40 mg (900mg)
Isoniazid × 6 mos+	5 mg (300mg)	10–20 mg (300mg)	15 mg (900mg)	20–40 mg (900mg)
Rifampin	10 mg (600mg)	10–20 mg (600mg)	10 mg (600mg)	— —
Rifampin and Pyrazinamide NO LONGER RECOMMENDED FOR LTBI TXMT**				

^^must be DOT (direct observation therapy)

* if children > 15 years and weigh more than 40 kg, then treat as an adult

^ preferred regimen for < 18 years and pregnant women

+ can be used for pregnant women but not for HIV+ persons, those with fibrotic lesions on CXR or children < 18 years

** increased liver cellular injury leading to liver death

Source: ATS & CDC, 2003

patitis and severe adverse reaction to INH. In those patients with underlying liver disease, a referral to the Health Department/TB specialist is indicated if this is the drug of choice. INH has a low incidence of hepatitis and is almost negligible prior to the age of 20 years. Studies show that even at age 50 to 64 years the risk of hepatitis is < 2%. The risk of INH hepatitis increases with a history of heavy alcohol use, current alcohol consumption and the immediate postpartum period, especially in the Hispanic women (CDC, 2000). INH can also cause peripheral neuropathies/neuritis. These neuropathies are more common in persons with diabetes mellitus, alcoholics, malnutrition, HIV + persons, pregnant patients and certain seizures disorders. They can be greatly reduced by concurrently giving 50 mg of pyrioxidine (vitamin B_6) 50mg/day (CDC, 2000). INH can be given with antiretroviral medications without drug-drug interactions. If a person is taking phenytoin and INH both medications are increased, so a reduction in the phenytoin level may be necessary (CDC, 2003).

In those persons who can't take INH, rifampin (RIF) is available. See Table 22–47. Rifampin is bactericial against organisms dividing rapidly and semi-dormant bacteria. This is an essential drug for short course treatment. Rifampin can also cause hepatotoxicity, its incidence is low by itself but increases when combined with INH. Rifampin, part of the rifamycin class, is a potent inducer of hepatic microsomal enzymes and accelerates the metabolism of numerous medications thus decreasing the effectiveness of the following drugs: *OCPs, warfarin* (may need a 2–3 fold increase), "*azoles*"—*ketaconazole, itraconazole* etc, *levothyroxine, glucocorticoids, oral steroids* (may need a 2–3 fold increase), *anti-convulsants, beta blockers, losartan, digoxin, sulfonylureas, nortriptyline, benzodiazopenes, dapsone, protease inhibitors (PI), non-nucleoside reverse transcriptase inhibitors (NNRTI)* and interferes with *verapamil* action (CDC, 2003; Drug Facts and Comparisons, 2003).

Other adverse effects are gastrointestinal discomfort, pruritis and orange discoloration of sputum, urine, sweat and tears.

Active Disease

Four different treatment options exist for active pulmonary TB. See Figure 22–3 for the Treatment Algorithm for TB. Because active TB is a serious health problem in the U.S., adequate treatment, compliance with the drug regimen and followup is essential. Effective treatment must be accomplished through the use of multiple drugs. Monotherapy should never be employed as it contributes to the emergence of multi-drug resistance tuberculosis (MDR-TB). (CDC, 2000). The treatment consists of daily or twice weekly medication which must always be DOT (direct observation therapy). Any regimen's success is based on the number of doses taken NOT the number of weeks/months that the medication is taken and must be completed within a certain time frame in order to consider the therapy completed (CDC, 2000).

There are two categories of anti-tuberculosis drugs that may be used; first-line and second-line agents. These drugs are listed in Table 22–48 but briefly described here.

First-Line Agents. Isoniazid (INH), Rifampin (RIF), Ethambutol (EMB), Pyrazinamide (PZA), Rifabutin and Rifapentine. Isoniazid and rifampin have been discussed for the treatment of LTBI earlier in this section.

Ethambutol (EMB) is thought to be bacteriostatic at lower doses and bactericidal at the higher intermittent doses. The recommended dose in children and adults is 15 to 20 mg/kg/day, and in retreatment the dose is started at 25 mg/kg/day for 60 days and then decreased for the remainder of the treatment to 15 mg/kg/day. The most common and serious adverse effect is retro-bulbar neuritis which is manifest by decreased visual acuity and/or decreased red/green color discrimination in one or both eyes. This effect is dose related. Occasionally skin rashes occur and the drug must be discontinued (Drug Facts and Comparisons, 2003; CDC 2000).

Pyrazinamide (PZA) is active against dormant or semi-dormant organisms within the macrophages. The usual adult dose is 15 to 20 mg/kg/day with a maximum dose of 2 gm. The most common serious adverse effect is

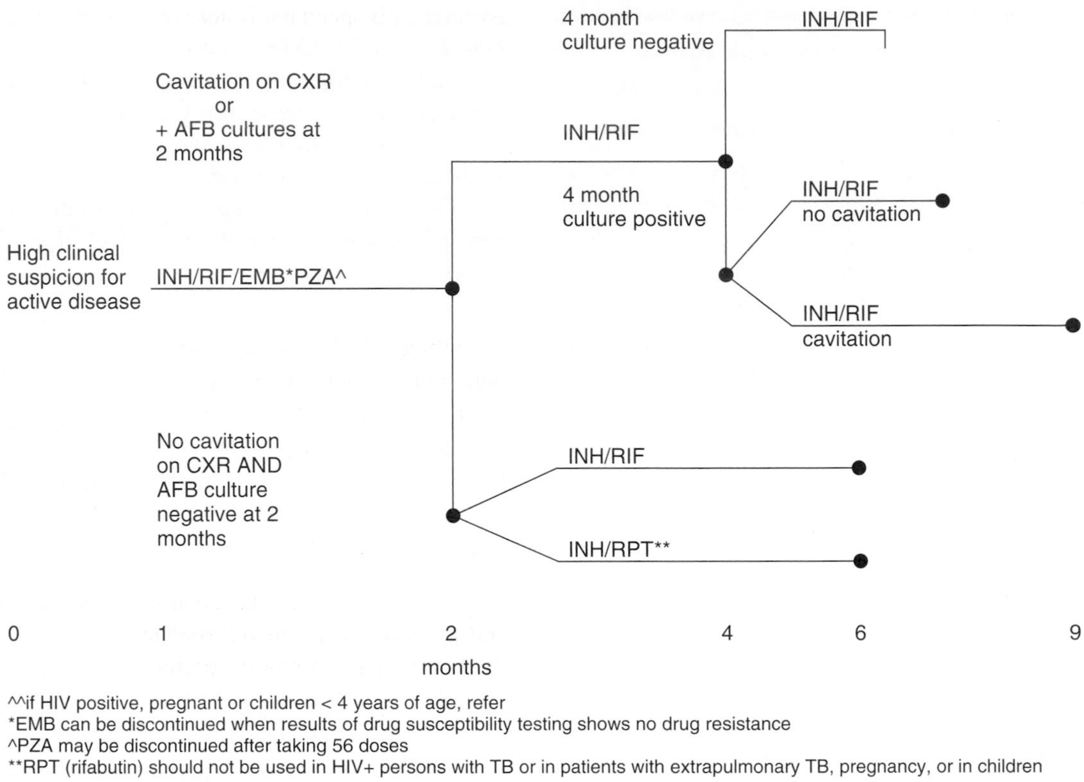

FIGURE 22–3. Treatment Algorithm for Tuberculosis^^ *Source: CDC, 2000.*

hepatotoxicity which is dose related and can occur at any time during therapy. Non-gouty polyarthralgias may occur in up to 40% of persons and asymptomatic hyperuricemia. Acute gout is uncommon. A transient mobilliform rash is common and self-limited and no reason to discontinue the drug. Photosensitivity is common so sunscreen protection is important (CDC, 2000).

Rifabutin is useful in persons who can't take Rifampin. Rifabutin is a less potent inducer of the hepatic microsomal enzymes but care still needs to taken if administered with a CYP-3A4 inhibitor, like clarithromycin, as it can decrease the clearance of Rifabutin thus increasing the risk of adverse effects. The adverse effects include gastrointestinal distress, polyarthralgias, hepatotoxicity (elevated ALT/AST), pseudo-jaundice (skin discoloration with a normal bilirubin) which is self-limited and resolves with discontinuation of the drug, rash and the orange discoloration of all the body fluids. If the person wears soft contact lenses and is taking any of the rifamycins, the lenses can be stained permanently.

Rifapentine (RPT) is an anti-tuberculosis drug used in the continuation phase of treatment of active disease. This drug is only used for HIV negative adults with no cavitation, negative sputum cultures and drug susceptible pulmonary TB. It has the same adverse effects as rifampin. (Drug Facts and Comparisons, 2003).

Second-Line Agents. The second-line agents should only be used by a TB specialist because they are less effective against the TB organism and more toxic.

Cycloserine can have serious CNS adverse effects ranging from headache to restlessness to psychosis and seizures which can affect up to 30% of persons taking the drug. The neurotoxic effects can be decreased with the addition of pyridoxine 100 to 200 mg/day. Patients with underlying psychiatric disorders are more likely to experience the CNS effects from this drug (CDC, 2000).

Ethionamide is bacteriostatic against the TB bacilli. The most common adverse effects are gastrointestinal distress, especially a metallic taste in the mouth, nausea, vomiting which can be severe, loss of appetite and abdominal pain. Many persons can not tolerate the full therapeutic dose initially and may need to be started at a lower dose and gradually increased to full dosage. Because of the severe vomiting, an anti-emetic may need to be administered along with ethionamide (CDC, 2000).

Streptomycin can be used in persons who are not immigrants from a high incidence country where drug resistant TB is common. There is increasing TB resistance to streptomycin. The most serious adverse effect is ototoxicity which manifests itself as a decreased hearing and vestibular changes. The vestibular changes are increased if on loop diuretics, like furosemide. Cicumoral parasthesias occur immediately after the injection but resolves. Nephrotoxicity can occur but is rare and presents as renal insufficiency.

Amikacin and Kanamycin are aminoglycoside antibiotics and are susceptible to most streptomycin resistant TB strains. These drugs have serious adverse effects of ototoxicity and nephrotoxocity. The drugs can cause deafness which is increased if on diuretics and renal impairment which is greater if the person already has underlying renal disease (CDC, 2000).

Capreomycin is an aminoglycoside antibiotic and used in TB resistant strains. This drug has a high incidence of nephrotoxicity and ototoxicity. The drug can cause depletion of potassium and magnesium, decreases creatinine clearance and leads to proteinuria. Vestibular disturbances and tinnitus are common with an increased incidence of deafness in the elderly with renal disease.

P-aminosalicylic acid (PAS) is bacteriostatic against TB and is used for resistant TB. This drug has multiple adverse effects; hepatoxicity, gastrointestinal distress, a malabsorption syndrome leading to steatorrhea and low serum folate levels, hypothyroidism with prolonged administration and doubling of prothrombin time (Drug Facts and Comparisons, 2003).

Flouroquinolones have been used to treat resistant TB. They produce a variety of adverse effects; nausea and bloating, dizziness, insomnia, headache tremulousness, rash, pruritus and photosensitivity. Any type of antacids can decrease the absorption of these drugs (CDC, 2000).

Drug-Resistant TB

Persons whose sputum cultures show multi-drug resistant strains must be referred to the Health Department/TB specialist for further evaluation and appropriate therapy. Those with MDR-TB often are candidates for the second line drug therapy which because of significant adverse effects are best managed by the experts.

If there are any questions regarding the treatment regimen for active tuberculosis or if a problem arises during the course of treatment, then a consult with the Health Department/TB specialist is necessary. A referral is also warranted when the PPD is positive, the patient is in a high risk group, AFB cultures are negative and the CXR shows upper lobe fibro-nodular infiltration (consistent with prior TB) and all other diagnoses have been ruled out.

SELECTING AGENTS FOR CHILDREN

The first-line agents for children, Isoniazid and Rifampin, are safe but care needs to be taken when giving either ethambutol (EMB) or pyrazinamide (PZA). Children with underlying renal/hepatic disease should be seen by the Health Department/TB specialist. Because of the significant adverse effects of the second-line agents, referral is warranted.

Treatment of LTBI

Infants exposed to active TB disease should have a PPD and a chest x-ray and referred immediately. Even if the PPD and chest x-ray are negative, infants can be anergic up until 6 months of age so treatment must be a serious consideration which is best evaluated by a specialist.

For children $>$ 4 years of age, TB testing and the work-up for a positive PPD is the same as for adults and the treatment regimen without active disease, is described in Table 22–47. All children $<$ 18 years old must be treated for 9 months. Children and adolescents $<$ 18 years old with underlying liver disease must have a consult with a specialist prior to using isoniazid, rifampin or pyrazinamide. Monthly evaluation of adverse effects and examining for hepatomegaly every 3 months to recheck LFTs remains the same as for adults (CDC, 2000).

Active Disease

If children $<$ 4 years of age are suspected of active TB or documented to have active TB, starting treatment is paramount. Children in this age group are at increased risk of disseminated TB. The treatment regimen for children is the same as for adults except for rifapentine (RPT). This drug is contraindicated in children.

There is a "decreased bacilliary burden in childhood-type TB" which lessens the likelihood of acquired drug resistance (CDC, 2000). However, it is still important to obtain an adequate sputum specimen and isolate the *M. tuberculosis.* Often this is extremely difficult so the presumed source's drug susceptibility is used. If the organism is drug-resistant, the child/adolescent is HIV positive and/or extrapulmonary TB, a referral is required.

Children and adolescents can develop "adult-type" TB (cavitation, upper lobe infiltrates and productive sputum). All of these children/adolescents should be started on the four-drug regimen (same as the adult regimen) until the susceptibility studies are completed. A regimen that is very effective (> 95% with < 2% adverse effects) for non drug-resistant TB is 6 months of isoniazid and rifampin with an initial 2 months of pyrazinamide (CDC, 2000). Even though ethambutol has serious adverse effects of retro-bulbar neuritis, it can be safely used if the dosage of 15–20 mg/kg/day is not exceeded, even though assessing visual acuity and color discrimination is very difficult in children < 6 years of age; however, it is best to refer to a pulmonary specialist.

Selecting Agents during Pregnancy and Lactation

PPD testing is not contraindicated during pregnancy. All women who are in a high-risk group should be tested like non-pregnant women.

Treatment for LTBI

All pregnant women who have a positive PPD, must have a chest x-ray with abdominal shielding and sputum cultures if appropriate. Isoniazid and rifampin are safe in pregnancy and both are considered compatible with breastfeeding but the drugs can be excreted in breast milk. Infant monitoring for any hepatitis or peripheral neuritis is necessary and any additional concerns should be addressed by a specialist. All pregnant women on isoniazid should also be on pyridoxine 50 mg to prevent the peripheral neuropathies. Pregnant women who are HIV positive or high risk medical conditions, should be referred to the Health Department/TB specialist (Rigby, 2000).

Active Disease

The treatment of active TB disease should begin promptly and usually consists of isoniazid, rifampin, ethambutol and pyridoxine daily while drug susceptibility tests are conducted. The actual care of the pregnant patient with active TB disease should be handled by the specialist. If an infant is born to a mother with active disease on anti-tuberculosis drugs and negative sputum cultures, the infant is unlikely to develop active TB disease. However, all infants should be closely assessed at birth and rechecked at 3 and 6 months. If the mother's sputum cultures were positive, then the infant must be checked closely because of an increased risk of active TB (Rigby, 2000).

MONITORING FOR EFFICACY

Treatment for LTBI

All patients who are treated for LTBI should be assessed monthly. It is important to ascertain that the medication is taken as prescribed. For anyone at risk of not completing self-administered medication, DOT (direct observation therapy) can be employed. It is important to explain the rationale for completing 9 months of therapy even though there is no active disease and the person feels well. The emphasis for medication adherence is especially vital in children < 4 years old.

Treatment for Active Disease

All patients who have active disease should be assessed weekly, every other week or monthly, depending on age, symptoms, medical conditions, adverse effects, language problems and risk of non-adherence. The medications should be reviewed at each visit and no more than a 1 month supply should be given. Some providers like the patient to bring all their pill bottles in at each visit so all the pills can be counted to assist in assessing medication compliance (CDC, 2000). In patients where adherence to the prescribed regimen is a problem, DOT (direct observation therapy) will be needed. DOT reduces the spread of TB and prevents the emergence of MDR-TB. DOT requires that the patient is observed taking their medication by a healthcare provider, public health worker or a responsible community/family member.

All patients should be assessed for improvement of any TB symptoms, ie late afternoon fevers, night sweats, weight loss, cough, fatigue, hemoptysis, etc. The patients should be weighed monthly and nutritional counseling provided if appropriate. A brief physical exam should include the lung and abdominal exam and any other assessment deemed appropriate.

Patients with positive sputum smears initially, should have sputum smears repeated every 2 weeks until 3 consecutive smears are negative. Sputum smears are best obtained early in the morning on at least 3 separate days. Newer testing methods, such as direct amplification tests and high-performance liquid chromatography, can identify the *M. tuberculosis* but cultures are still required for susceptibility testing. A patient is considered to be *mostly* non-infectious when 1) the patient is on an effective drug regimen, 2) clinical improvement is seen, and 3) there are 3 negative sputum acid-fast smears obtained on 3 different days. To determine absolute lack of infectiousness, it requires that sputum cultures be done every month until 2 consecutive sputum cultures are negative. However, this is often impractical as the results from the culture specimens can take up to 6 weeks to obtain so the smears are used. Technically a very low risk of infectiousness still remains using the smears (Horsburgh, Feldman, & Ridzon, 2000).

Smears and cultures usually become negative by 3 months. If the sputum smears and cultures remain positive at 3 months, a CXR is done and a reevaluation is needed by a TB specialist. If the bacilli are MDR-TB, then a referral is also required to a TB specialist. Chest x-rays should be done at 3 months if the sputum cultures are positive and then repeated at the completion of therapy (Horsburgh, Feldman, & Ridzon, 2000).

If the treatment of the initial phase is interrupted, assess the following:

- < 14 days, continue treatment to finish the course in 3 months, if not completed in 3 months, restart from the beginning
- > 14 days, restart treatment from the beginning

If the treatment of the continuation phase is interrupted, assess the following:

- < 80% of the anti-tuberculosis medication is finished in 3 months, recheck sputum smears and cultures. If negative, continue drug therapy to complete within 9 months of the original start date. If the sputum smears/cultures are positive, check drug susceptibility and restart the 4 drug regimen with DOT and consult with the Health Department.
- < 80% of the anti-tuberculosis medication is finished and > 3 months has lapsed, then check sputum smears/cultures and drug susceptibility and restart the 4 drug regimen while waiting for the test results and consult with the Health Department.
- > 80% of the planned doses have been completed then additional treatment is not necessary unless the initial AFB smears/cultures were positive.

The completion of therapy is based on the number of doses completed within 3 months for the initial phase of treatment not the number of weeks being treated. In the continuation phase, the number of doses should be completed within 4 months but it is acceptable to finish the doses within 6 months. A 6 month regimen must be completed within 9 months and for LTBI the doses must be completed within 12 months. When the doses are completed within the time frame allowed, the therapy is considered to be successfully completed.

Monitoring for Toxicity

LTBI Treatment

- INH—check LFTs at baseline, then every 3 months while on medication
- Check for paresthesias of hands/feet, fever > 3 days, rash, RUQ abdomen pain, anorexia, arthralgias, nausea/vomiting, persistent fatigue, icterus, dark colored urine
- RIF—check LFTs at baseline, then 2, 4, 8 weeks while on medication
- Check for drug-drug interactions
- Check for orange fluid discoloration in the sweat, urine, tears, sputum

Anyone who is at high risk for developing hepatotoxicity (pregnancy, history of alcohol abuse and currently drinking, chronic liver disease, IVDA) should have their LFTs drawn every month.

Active TB Treatment

- PZA—check LFTs at baseline, then at 2, 4, 8 weeks while on medication
  - Check blood sugars (DM more difficult to control)
  - Check skin for rashes
  - Check joints for polyarthralgias
  - Check for GI distress, encourage to take med with a full glass of water
  - Check baseline uric acid levels and then periodically
- EMB—check baseline visual acuity/red-green color discrimination
  - Check for ocular toxicity at each visit by questioning regarding decreased
  - Visual acuity, scotomas and loss of red-green color discrimination
  - Check visual acuity by the Snellen chart and color discrimination by the Ishihara test—if changes refer to ophthmalogtist
  - May need to check renal function, BUN and creatinine, and adjust dose based on creatinine clearance
- Aminoglycosides—check baseline hearing with an audiogram and vestibular function
  - Monitor for ototoxicity, vestibular dysfunction, and hearing loss

- Check for renal function, BUN and creatinine
- P-aminosalicyclic—check TSH levels as prolonged administration leads to hypothyroidism every 3 months
  - Check weight—causes a malabsorption syndrome
  - Check LFTs—causes hepatotoxicity every 2 months
  - Assess for GI distress
- Cycloserine—assess headache profile
  - Check a neuro status exam regularly as has CNS adverse effects
  - Check BUN and serum creatinine, increases risk of renal damage
- Ethionamide—check LFTs at baseline, then every 2 months
  - Check weight, appetite as can have severe nausea and vomiting

(Drug Facts & Comparisons, 2003)

Monitoring for Toxicity. Patients should be monitored monthly for signs and symptoms of drug toxicity. They should also be instructed to monitor themselves at home for toxicity and to report any symptoms immediately.

Patients being treated for TB disease should have pretreatment baseline measurements of LFTs (AST, ALT, bilirubin), renal function tests (serum creatinine and BUN), and CBC with platelets. If PZA is used, patients should have baseline serum uric acid levels measured. For patients being treated with EMB, a baseline visual acuity examination should be performed. For patients receiving streptomycin or any other aminoglycoside, baseline and periodic audiometry should be performed (USDHHS, 1994).

Patients at high risk for hepatotoxicity should have monthly LFTs assessed. Patients at higher risk of renal toxicity caused by aminoglycosides should have BUN and serum creatinine levels periodically assessed.

Followup Recommendations. Patients who were infected with INH- and RIF-sensitive strains of TB and who satisfactorily completed a 6- or 9-month course of therapy that included INH and RIF do not need routine followup. They should, however, be educated to report the subsequent development of any symptoms of TB (e.g., prolonged cough, fever, weight loss).

Patients who were infected with strains of TB resistant to INH and/or RIF need individualized followup (USDHHS, 1994).

Monthly followup visits should be done on everyone who has LTBI to ensure adherence to the medication regimen and assessment of any adverse effects of the medicine. Lab monitoring as appropriate for the medication.

Followup for active TB is usually weekly until the sputum smears/cultures are negative. Closer followup is warranted for those who have comorbid illnesses, adherence issues, age-related problems, pregnant women and children, especially infants, HIV positive and those who have a MDR-TB.

Once treatment is completed within the designated time frame and the TB was susceptible to the standard drug regimens, then no further routine followup is necessary. Everyone should be educated about reporting the development of TB symptoms with their PCP.

For those patients infected with MDR-TB, individualized follow-up is needed (CDC, 2000).

Patients with pulmonary TB disease are considered infectious if they are coughing, if their sputum smears contain acid-fast bacilli, if they are not receiving therapy or have just started therapy, or if they have a poor clinical or bacterial response to drug therapy. Patients are not considered infectious if they have received adequate therapy for 2 to 3 weeks, *and* they have a favorable clinical response (e.g., resolution of fever, night sweats, dyspnea, fatigue, and hemoptysis), *and* they have three consecutive negative sputum smears on samples from different days. Infectiousness may last several weeks to several months in patients with drug-resistant TB disease. Patients with drug-resistant TB disease need to be isolated until they are noninfectious. Patients infected with MDR-TB should be considered for isolation throughout their hospitalization (ATS, 2001; CDC 2000).

REFERENCES

Agertoft, L, Pedersen, S. (2000). Effects of long-term treatment with inhaled budesonide on adult height in children with asthma. *New England Journal of Medicine,* 343(15): 1064–1069.

AHFS Drug Information. (1997). G. K. McEvoy (Ed.). Bethesda: American Society of Health-System Pharmacists.

Allen, D. B., Bronsky, E. A., LaForce, C. F., Nathan, R. A., Tinkelman, D. G., Vandewalker, M. L., Konig, P. (1998). Growth in asthmatic children treated with fluticasone proprionate. *Fluticasone Proprionate Asthma Study Group,* 132(3 Pt1): 472–477.

Allen, D. B., Sharek, O. J., & Bergman, D. A. (2001). Effect of inhaled corticosteroids on growth. *Pediatrics, 108,* 1234 +.

American College of Obstetrics and Gynecology (ACOG) and the American College of Allergy, Asthma and Immunology (ACAAI) (2000). Joint statement on management of the pregnant female with asthma. *Annals of Allergy, Asthma and Immunology, 84,* 475–480.

American Academy of Pediatrics (AAP) Committee on Infectious Diseases. (2002). *Red book: Report of the Committee on Infectious Diseases.* Elk Grove Village, II: American Academy of Pediatrics.

American Thoracic Society (ATS). (1994). Treatment of tuberculosis and tuberculosis infection in adults and children. *American Journal of Respiratory and Critical Care Medicine, 149,* 1359–1374.

American Thoracic Society (ATS). (1995). Standards for the diagnosis and care of patients with chronic obstructive pulmonary disease. *American Journal of Respiratory and Critical Care Medicine, 152,* S77–S120.

American Thoracic Society (ATS). (2001). Guidelines for the management of ambulatory patients with community-acquired pneumonia: Diagnosis, assessment of severity, antimicrobial therapy and prevention. *Am J Resp Crit Care, 163,* 1730–1754.

American Thoracic Society website (2000): www.thoracic.org.statements

ATS & IDSA. (2003). Treatment of TB. Morbidity and Mortality Weekly Report. June 20:52(RR11); 1–77.

Areno, J., San Pedro, G., & Campbell, G. D. (1996). Diagnosis and prognosis in community-acquired pneumonia: When and where should the patient be treated. *Seminars in Respiratory and Critical Care Medicine, 17*(3), 231–236.

Aris, R., Renner, J., Winders, A. et al. (1998). Increased rate of fractures and severe kyphosis: Sequelae of living with cystic fibrosis into adulthood. *Archives of Int Med, 128*(3), 186–209.

Arunabh, M. D., & Niederman, M. (1996). Prevention of community-acquired pneumonia. *Seminars in Respiratory and Critical Care Medicine, 17*(3), 273–280.

Barbato, A., Turato, G., Baraldo, S., Bazzan, E., Callabrese, F., Tura, M., Zuin, R., Beghe, B., et al. (2003). Airway inflammation of childhood asthma. *American Journal of Respiratory Critical Care Medicine,* 168; 798–803.

Bartlett, J., & Mundy, L. (1995). Communityacquired pneumonia. *New England Journal of Medicine, 333*(24), 1618–1623.

Bartlett, J. G., Dowell, S. F., Mandell, L. A., et al (2000). Practice guidelines for the management of community-acquired pneumonia in adults. *Clin Inf Dis,* 31, 347–382.

Bernstein, M. S., & Locksley, R. M. (1997). Infections due to gram-positive bacilli. Infectious disease. *Scientific American, 51.*

Boucher, R. (1996). Cystic fibrosis. In *Nelson's Textbook of Pediatrics* (15th ed.). Philadelphia: WB Saunders.

Bousquet, J., Chanez, P., Vignola, A. M., & Michel, F. B. (1996). Asthma and chronic bronchitis: Similarities and differences. *Respiratory Medicine, 90,* 187–190.

Boyd, G., Moice, A. H., Poundsford, J. C., Siebert, M., Peslis, N., & Crawford, C. (1997). An evaluation of salmeterol in the treatment of chronic obstructive pulmonary disease (COPD). *European Respiratory Journal,* 10: 815–821.

Bozzoni, M., Radice, L., Frosi, A., Vezzoli, S., Cuboni, A., & Vezzoli, F. (1995). Prevalence of pneumonia due to *Legionaella pneumophila* and *Mycoplasma pneumoniae* in a population admitted to a Department of Internal Medicine. *Respiration, 62,* 331–335.

Braman, S. S. (1993). Asthma in the elderly patient. *Pulmonary Diseases in the Elderly Patient,* 14(3): 413–422.

Braman, S. S., & Davis, S. M. (1986). Wheezing in the elderly. Asthma and other causes. *Clinics in Geriatric Medicine, 2*(2), 269–283.

Brennan, A. L, & Geddes, D. M. (2002). Cystic fibrosis. *Current Openion Infectous Disease, 15*(2), 175–182.

Briggs, G. G., Freeman, R. K., & Yaffe, S. J. (1994). *Drugs in pregnancy and lactation: A reference guide to fetal and neonatal risk* (4th ed.). Baltimore: Williams and Wilkins.

Briggs, R. G., Mahre, W. C., & Sibai, B. M. (1996). Community acquired pneumonia in pregnancy. *American Journal of Obstetrics and Gynecology, 174,* 389 +.

Broussard, R. C., Payne, D. K., & George, R. B. (1991). Treatment with acyclovir in varicella pneumonia in pregnancy. *Chest, 99*(4), 1045–1047.

Brunzell, S., & Schwarzenberg, S. (2002). Cystic fibrosis-related diabetes and abnormal glucose tolerance: Overview and medical nutrition therapy. *Diabetes Spectrum, 15*(2), 124–128.

Burrows, B. (1987). The natural history of asthma. *Journal of Allergy and Clinical Immunology, 3* (Pt 2), 373–377.

Busse, W. W., & Lemanske, R. F. (2001, February 1). Asthma. *New England Journal of Medicine, 344*(5), 350–362.

Cassiere, H., Rodrigues, J. C., & Fein, A. M. (1996). Delayed resolution of pneumonia. *Postgraduate Medicine, 99*(1), 151–158.

Castro-Rodriguez, J. A., Holberg, C. J., Wright, A. L., Martinez, F. D. (2000). A clinical index to define risk of asthma in young children with recurrent wheezing. *American Journal of Respiratory Critical Care Medicine,* 162 (4 Pt 1): 1403–1406.

Catanzaro, A. (1984). Pulmonary mycosis in pregnant women. *Chest, 86,* 145–195.

Centers for Disease Control and Prevention. (1996a). Control and prevention. Asthma mortality and hospitalizations among children and youth—United States. *MMWR, 45,* 350–353.

Centers for Disease Control and Prevention. (1996b). The role of BCG vaccine in the prevention and control of tuberculosis in the United States: A joint statement by the Advisory Council for the Elimination of Tuberculosis and the Advisory Committee on Immunization Practices. *MMWR, 45,* RR4.

Centers for Disease Control and Prevention. (2000, June 9). The diagnosis and treatment of active tuberculosis. *MMWR.*

Centers for Disease Control and Prevention. (2001). *New estimates for asthma tracked.* Retrieved from: http://www.cdc.gov/nchs/releases/01facts/asthma.htm. 23 July 2002.

CDC. (2004). Clinical guidance on the identity and evaluation of possible SARS-CoV disease among persons presenting with community-acquired pneumonia. Accessed Jan 8, 2004 at website www.cdc/gov/ncidod/sars

Chanarin, N., & Johnston, S. L. (1994). Leukotrienes as a target in asthma therapy. *Drugs, 47*(1), 12–24.

Chan-Yeung, M. & Malo, J. L. (1994). Aetiological agents in occupational asthma. *European Respiratory Journal, 7*(2), 346–371.

Chestnutt, M., Prendergast, T., Stauffer, J.. (1999) Lung. In Tierney, L., McPhee, S., Papadakis, M.. *Current Diagnosis and Treatment* (38th Ed.) Norwalk, CT: Appleton and Lange.

Childhood Asthma Management Program (CAMP) Research Group. (2000). Long-term effects of budesonide or nedocromil in children with asthma. *New England Journal of Medicine;* 343(15): 1054–1063.

Christensen, C.C., Ryg, M., Refvem, O. K., & Skjonsberg, M. S. (2000). Development of severe hypoxaemia in chronic obstructive pulmonary disease patients at 2,438 m (8,000 ft) altitude. *Eur Resp J, 15,* 635–9.

Clark, D. J., Grove, A., Cargill, R. I., & Lipworth, B. J. (1996). Comparative adrenal suppression with inhaled budesonide and fluticasone propionate in adult asthmatics. *Thorax, 51,* 262–266.

Connolly, M. J., Crowley, J. J., Charan, N. B., Nielson, C. P., & Vestal, R. E. (1992). Reduced subjective awareness of bronchoconstriction provoked by methacholine in elderly asthmatic and normal subjects as measured on a simple awareness scale. *Thorax, 47,* 410–413.

Costello, J., Meltzer, S., & Bleecker, E. R. (1994). Summary: The pharmacology of leukotrienes in asthma. *Advances in Prostaglandin Thrombaxone Leukotrones Research, 22,* 263–268.

Coultas, D. B., Gong, H., Jr., Grad, R., Handler, A., McCurdy, S. A., Player, R., Rhoades, E. R., Samet, J. M., Thomas, A., & Westley, M. (1994). Respiratory diseases in minorities in the United States. *American Journal of Respiratory and Critical Care Medicine, 149*(3 Pt 2), S93–S131.

Cunha, B. A. (1996). Community-acquired pneumonia. Cost-effective antimicrobial therapy. *Postgraduate Medicine, 99,* 109–117.

Cunha, B. A., & Ortega, A. M. (1996). Atypical pneumonia. *Postgraduate Medicine, 99,* 123–132.

Davis, P. P., & Bayard, P. J. (1988). Relationships among airway reactivity, pupillary alpha-adrenergic and cholinergic responsiveness and age. *Journal of Applied Physiology, 65*(1), 200–204.

Dean, E., & Khoshoo, V. (1999). Reduced respiratory morbidity following RSV bronchiolitis in infants treated with ribovarin: A prospective study. *116*(4), S 251+.

Dean, N. C., Silver, M. P., Bateman, K. A. (2000). Frequency of subspeciaty primary care for elderly patients with community acquired pneumonia. *Chest, 117,* 393–397.

Dougherty, J., Bethany, D., Aboussouan, L.. (2003). Long-acting beta2 agonists for stable COPD. *Annals of Pharmacotherapy.* 37 (9); 1247–1255.

Drug Facts and Comparisons. (2003). Erwin Kastrup (Ed.). St. Louis, MO: Wolters Kluwer Co.

De Boer, W. I. (2002). Cytokines and therapy in COPD. *Chest,* 121(5): S209–S219.

DuBuske, L. M. (1994). Asthma: Diagnosis and management of nocturnal symptoms. *Comprehensive Therapy, 20*(11).

Durie, P. R., & Pencharz, P. B. (1992). Cystic fibrosis: Nutrition. *British Medical Bulletin, 48*(4), 823–846.

Elkus, R., & Popovich, J., Jr. (1992). Respiratory physiology in pregnancy. *Clinical Chest Medicine, 13*(4), 555–565.

Eller, J., Ede, A., Schaberg, T., et al. (1998). Infective exacerbations of chronic bronchitis: Relation between bacteriologic etiology and lung function. *Chest, 113:* 1542–1548.

Fahey T., Stocks N., Thomas T.. (1998). Quantitative systematic review of randomized controlled trials comparing antibiotic with placebo for acute cough in adults. *British Medical Journal* 316: 906–910.

Fein, A. M. (1994). Pneumonia in the elderly: Special diagnostic and therapeutic considerations. *Medical Clinics of North America, 78*(5), 1015–1034.

Fein, A. M. (1996). Treatment of communityacquired pneumonia: Clinical guidelines or clinical judgment? *Seminars in Respiratory and Critical Care Medicine, 17*(3), 237–241.

Ferguson, G. T., Enright P. L., Buist, A. S., et al. (2000). Office spirometry for the lung health assessment in adults. A consensus statement from the National Lung Health Education Program. *Chest, 117*(4), 1146–1161.

Fete, T. J., & Noyes, B. (1996). Common (but not always considered) viral infections of the lower respiratory tract. *Pediatric Annals, 25*(10), 577–584.

Figueroa, V., Carlos, M., Parks, E., et al. (2002). Abnormal lipid concentrations in cystic fibrosis. *Am J of Clin Nutrit, 75*(6), 1005–1012.

File, T. (1997). Management of community-acquired pneumonia. *Infectious Disease Practice, 21,* 9–12.

File, T., Tan, J., & Plouffe, J. (2001). Bacterial pneumonia: Community acquired and nosocomial in immunocompetent hosts. In R. M. Rakel & E. Bope (Eds.), *Current therapy* Philadelphia: W.B. Saunders.

File, T. M., Tan, J. S., & Plouffe, J. F. (1996). Community-acquired pneumonia. What's needed for accurate diagnosis. *Postgraduate Medicine, 99*(1), 95–107.

Finder, J. (1999). Understanding airway disease in infants. *Current Problems in Pediatrics.* Mar; 29(3): 65–91.

Fineland, M., & Dublin, T. D. (1939). Pneumococcal pneumonias complicating pregnancy and the puerperium. *JAMA, 112,* 1027–1032.

Forstner, G. G., & Durie, P. R. (1996). Cystic fibrosis. In W. A. Walker, P. R. Durie, J. R. Hamilton, et al. (Eds.), *Pediatric gastrointestinal disease* (2nd ed., pp. 1466–1487). St. Louis, MO: Mosby.

Fraser, D. (1997, November). Assessing the elderly for infections. *J Gerontological Nursing, 23*(11), 5–10.

Frederiksen, B., Lanng, S., Koch, C., & Hoiby, N. (1996). Improved survival in the Danish center-treated cystic fibrosis patients: Results of aggressive treatment. *Pediatric Pulmonology, 21,* 153–158.

Galgiani, J. N., Ampel, N. M., Catanzaro, A., et al. (2000). Practice guidelines for the treatment of coccidioimycosis. Infectious Disease Society of America. *Clinical Infectious Disease,* 30: 658–661.

Gales, M., & McClain, P. (1997). Coccidioidomycosis. A mycotic infection on the rise. *Clinical Reviews, 7,* 71–84.

Gizycki, M. J., Hattotuwa, K. J., Barnes, N., Jeffery, P. K. (2002). Effects of Fluticasone proprionate on inflammatory cells in COPD: an ultrastructural examination of endobronchial biopsy tissue. *Thorax.* 57:779–803.

Godden, D. J., Ross, S., Abdella, M., McMurray, D., Douglas, A., Oldman, D., Friend, J. A., Legge, J. S., & Douglas, J. G. (1994). Outcomes of wheeze in childhood: Symptoms and pulmonary function 25 years later. *American Journal of Respiratory Critical Care Medicine, 149*(1), 110–112.

Grant, C. C., Duggan, A. K., Santosham, M., & DeAngelis, C. (1996). Oral prednisone as a risk factor for infections in children with asthma. *Archives of Pediatric and Adolescent Medicine,* 58–63.

Green, M. (1997). Viral pneumonias. In E. Gillis & M. Kagan (Eds.), *Current pediatric therapy* (15th ed., pp. 637–638). Philadelphia: W. B. Saunders.

Groothius, J. R., Simoes, E. A., Hemming, V. G., & the Respiratory Syncytial Virus Immune Globulin Study Group. (1995). Respiratory syncytial virus (RSV) infection in preterm infants and the protective effects of RSV immune globulin (RSVIG). *Pediatrics, 95,* 463–467.

Guthrie, R. (2001). Community-acquired lower respiratory tract infection:etiology and treatment. *Chest,* 120(6): 2021–2035.

Hammerschlag, M. (1996). Chylamydia. In Behrman, et al. (Eds.), *Textbook of pediatrics* (15th ed., pp. 827–830). Philadelphia: W. B. Saunders.

Hanson, M. A., & Midthun, D. E. (1992). Outpatient care of COPD patients. *Postgraduate Medicine, 91,* 89–95.

Hayes, F. J., O'Brien, A., O'Brien, C., Fitzgerald, M. X., & McKennon, M. J. (1995). Diabetes mellitus in an adult population with cystic fibrosis. *Irish Medical Journal, 88*(3), 102–104.

Heath, J., & Mongia, R. (1998). Chronic bronchitis: Primary care management. *Am Fam Physician,*

Horsburgh, C., Feldman, S., Ridzon, R. 2000. Guidelines from the Infectious Diseases Society of America. Practice guidelines for the treatment of tuberculosis. *Clincal Infectious Disease,* 31:633–639.

Hunter, M., & King, D. (2001). COPD: Management of acute exacerbations and chronic stable disease. *American Family Physician, 64,* 603–612, 621–622.

Infectious Disease Society of America website: www.idsociety.org

Ingram Jr., R. H. (1994). Chronic bronchitis, emphysema, and airways obstruction. In K. J. Isselbacher, E. Braunwald, G. D. Wilson, J. Martin, A. S. Fauchi, & D. L. Casper (Eds.), *Harrison's principles of internal medicine* (pp. 1197–1206). New York: McGraw Hill.

Jarjour, N., Gelfand, E., McGill, K., & Busse, W. W. (1996). Alternative anti-inflammatory and immunomodulatory therapy. In J. Szefler, D.Y.M. Leung (Eds.), *Severe asthma: Pathogenesis and clinical management* (pp. 333–369). New York: Marcel Dekker.

Jarvis, B., Faulds, D. (1999). Inhaled fluticasone proprionate: A review of its therapeutic efficacy at dosages < or = 500 mcg/day in adults and adolescents with asthma. *Drugs, 57*(5), 769–803.

Joint Committee of the American College of Obstetrics and Gynecology (ACOG) and the American College of Allergy, Asthma and Immunology (ACAAI). Position Statement. 2002. The use of newer asthma and allergy medications during pregnancy. Annuals of Allergy, Asthma and Immunology. 84: 475–480.

Kaliner, M., & Lemanske, R. (1992). Rhinitis and asthma. *JAMA, 268*(20), 2807–2829.

Kalsiter, H. (2001). Treating children with asthma. *West J Med, 174,* 415–20.

Kamada, A. K., & Szefler, S. J. (1995). Glucocorticoids and growth in asthmatic children. *Pediatric Allergy and Immunology, 6,* 145–154.

Kimpen, J. L. (2001, June). Management of respiratory synctial virus infection. *Curr Opin Infect Dis., 14*(3), 323–328.

Klein, J. (1997). Pneumonias. In E. Gellis & M. Kagan (Eds.), *Current pediatric therapy* (15th ed., pp. 572–574). Philadelphia: W. B. Saunders.

Knutson, D., & Braun, C. (2002). Diagnosis and management of acute bronchtis. *Am Fam Physician, 65,* 2039–2044.

Krieger, B. (1996). Respiratory tract infections in the elderly. *Pulmonary Perspectives, 8,* 1–4.

Laitinen, A., & Laitinen, L. A. (1994). Airway morphology: Endothelium/basement membrane. *American Journal of Respiratory and Critical Care Medicine, 150,* S14–17.

Landau, L. I. (1996). Risks of developing asthma. *Pediatric Pulmonology, 22,* 314–318.

Landbo, C., Prescott, E., Lange, P., Vestbo., J., & Almdal, T. (1999). Prognostic value of nutritional status in chronic obstructive pulmonary disease. *American Journal of Respiratory Critical Care Medicine,* 160(6); 1856–1861.

Lanng, S., Thorsteinsson, B., Nerupo, J., & Koch, C. (1992). Influence of the development of diabetes mellitus on clinical status in patients with cystic fibrosis. *European Journal of Pediatrics, 151*(9), 684–687.

Leeper, K. (1996). Severe community acquired pneumonia. *Seminars in Respiratory Infections, 11*(2), 96–108.

Lemanske, R. F. (2001). Origins and treatment of airway inflammation in childhood asthma. *Pediatric Pulmonology Supplement, 21,* 17–25.

Levison, M. (1998). Pneumonia, including necrotizing pulmonary infections. In A. Fauci et al. (Eds.), *Harrison's principles of internal medicine* (14th ed.). New York: McGraw-Hill.

Li, J. T., & O'Connell, J. O. (1996). Clinical evaluation of asthma. *Annals of Allergy, Asthma & Immunology, 76,* 1–15.

Lim, W. S., MacFarlane, J. T., Colthorpe, C, L. (2001). Pneumonia and pregnancy. *Thorax,* 56: 398–405.

Lim, W. S., Lewis, S., MacFarlane, J. T. (2000). Severity prediction rules in community-acquired pneumonia: a validation study. *Thorax,* 55: 219–223.

Lipworth, B., Fowler, S., & Wilson, A. (2002). Asthma and Allergy Research Group, Department of Clinical Pharmacology and Therapeutics. University of Dundee, Ninewells Hospital and Medical School, Dundee, Scotland. Paper presented at the April 2002 Annual International Meeting of the American Academy of Asthma, Allergy and Immunology.

Long, S. (1997). Pertussis. In Gellis & Kagan (Eds.), *Current pediatric therapy* (15th ed., pp. 611–613). Philadelphia: W. B. Saunders.

Louden, M. (2001). Bronchodilator controversies. *EMed J, 2*(5), 10+.

Luskin, A. (1994). Asthma therapy: What really works. Highlights of the Americancademy of Family PHysicians 45th annual Scientific Assembly. *Audio Digest, 42,* 1–2.

MacDonald, A. (1996). Nutritional management of cystic fibrosis. *Archives of Disease in Childhood, 74,* 81–87.

MacKay, D.N. (1996). Treatment of acute bronchitis in adults without underlying lung disease. *Journal of General Internal Medicine, 11,* 557–562.

Madinger, N. E., Greenspoon, J. S., & Ellrodt, A. G. (1989). Pneumonia during pregnancy: Has modern technology improved maternal and fetal outcome. *American Journal of Obstetrics and Gynecology, 161,* 657–662.

Mandell, L. A. (1996). Community-acquired pneumonia. *New England Journal of Medicine, 334*(13), 861–864.

Mandell L., Bartlett J., Dowell S., File T., Musher D. & and Whitney C. (2003). Update of practice guidelines for the management of community-acquired pneumonia in immunocompetent adults. *Clinical Infectious Disease,* 37:1405–1433.

Mannino, D. (2002). COPD: Epidemiology, prevalence, morbidity and mortality and disease heterogeneity. *Chest, 121*(5), S121–127.

Marras, T. K., MacNee, W., Calverly, P.M.A. (2003). Management of COPD. *Thorax,* 58 (11): 1006 +.

Martinez, F. D., Wright, A. L., Taussig, L. M., Holberg, C. J., Halonem, M., Morgan, W. J., Group Health Medical Associates. (1995). Asthma and wheezing in the first six years of life. *New England Journal of Medicine, 332,* 133–138.

Marrie, T., Lau, J., Wheeler, S.L ., et al. (2000). A controlled trial of a critical pathway for treating community-acquired pneumonia. *Journal of the American Medical Association,* 283: 749–755.

McFadden, E. R., Jr. & Gilbert, I. A. (1994). Exercise-induced asthma. *New England Journal of Medicine, 330,* 1362–1367.

Meissner, C, Long, S. and the American Academy of Pediatric Committee on Infectious Diseases and the Committee on Fetus and Newborn. (2003). Palivizumab and respiratory syncytial virus immune globulin intravenous for the prevention of respiratory syncytial virus infection. *Pediatrics,* 112(6): 1442–1452.

Metlay, J. P., Fine, M. J. 2003. Testing strategies in the initial management of patients with community-acquired pneumonia. *Annals of Internal Medicine,* 138:109–118.

Milgrom, H., & Bender, B. (1995). Behavioral side effects of medications used to treat asthma and allergic rhinitis. *Pediatrics in Review, 16*(9), 333–335.

Mittl, R. L., Jr., Schwab, R. J., Duchin, J. S., et al. (1994). Radiographic resolution of communityacquired pneumonia. *American Journal of Respiratory and Critical Care Medicine, 149,* 630–635.

Morgan, M. D. L. (2003). Preventing hospital admission for COPD: role of physical activity. *Thorax,* 58; 95 +.

Moroney, C. (1996). Pharmacologic Update: Management of pneumonia in elderly people. *Journal of the American Academy of Nurse Practitioners, 6*(5), 237–241.

Mouton, C., Bazaldua, O., Pierce, B., Espino, D. (2001). Common infections in older adults. *American Family Physician,* 63:257–268.

Munn, M. B., Groome, J., Atterbury, J. L. et al. (1999). Pneumonia as a complication of pregnancy. *Journal of Maternal and Fetal Medicine,* 8: 151–154.

Musher, D. (1998). Pneumococcal infections. In A. Fauci et al., (Eds.), *Harrison's principles of internal medicine.* New York: McGraw-Hill.

Nathwani, D., MacClean, A., Conway, S. et al. (1998). Varicella infection in pregnancy and the newborn. A review prepared for the British Society for the study of infections. *Journal of Infections,* 36(Suppl 1): 59–71.

National Asthma Education and Prevention Program (NAEPP). (2002). Expert Panel Report 2: Update on Selected Topics 2002. Bethesda, MD: National Institutes of Health, National Health Blood Institute. Retrieved from: http://www.nhlbi.nih.gov/guidelines/asthma/asthsumm.htm 23 July 2002.

National Institute of Allergy and Infectious Diseases (NIAID) Conference on "Community-Acquired Pneumonia in Adult and Elderly Populations," June 3 and 4, 1998.

National Institutes of Health/National Heart, Lung and Blood Institute (NIH/NHLBI). (1993). Executive summary: Management of asthma during pregnancy. National Institute of Health/National Heart, Lung, and Blood Institute, NIH publication #93-3279A.

Newman, S. R., & Clarke, S. W. (1993). Bronchodilator delivery from gentlehaler, a new low-velocity pressurized aerosol inhaler. *Chest, 103*(5), 1442–1446.

Niederhauser, U. P. (1997). Prescribing for children: Issues in pediatric pharmacology. *Nurse Practitioner, 22*(3), 16–18.

Niederman, M. S. (2002a). Community-acquired pneumonia: Management controversies, Part 1: practical recommendations from the latest guidelines. *Journal of Respiratory Diseases, 23*(1), 10–18.

Niederman, M. S. (2002b). Community-acquired pneumonia: Management controversies, Part 2: Atypical pathogens and penicillin resistance take center stage. *Journal of Respiratory Diseases, 23*(3), 147–154.

Nolan, C. M., Goldberg, S. V., Baskin, S. E. (1999). Hepatotoxicity associated with INH preventive therapy. *Journal of the American Medical Association,* 281: 1014–1018.

Norman, D. C. (1999). Special infectious disease problems in geriatrics. *Clin Geriatrics,* 1 (Suppl), 3–5.

Okamoto, L. J., Noonan, M., DeBoisblanc, B. P., & Kellerman, D. J. (1996). Fluticasone propionate improves quality of life in patients with asthma requiring oral corticosteroids. *Annals of Allergy, Asthma, & Immunology, 76,* 455–461.

Oswald, H., Phelan, P. D., Lanigan, A., Hibbert, M., Carlin, J. B., Bowes, G., & Olinsky, A. (1997). Childhood asthma and lung function in mid-adult life. *Pediatric Pulmonology, 23,* 14–20.

Pauwels, R. A., Busit, A. S., Claverley, P. M., et al. (2001) Global strategy of the diagnosis, management and prevention of chronic obstructive pulmonary disease: NHLBI/WHO Global Initiative for Chronic Obstructive Lung Disease (GOLD) Workshop Summary. *Am J Resp Crit Care Med, 163,* 1256–1276. Website: goldcopd.com/workshop/index .html

PDR Generics (2nd ed.) (2002). Montvale, NJ: Medical Economics.

Pederson, S. (2000). *American Journal of Respiratory Critical Care Medicine, 161,* S182–185.

Pedersen, S. (1996). Inhalers and nebulizers: Which to choose and why. *Respiratory Medicine, 90,* 69–77.

Peloquin, C. A., & Berning, S. E. (1994). Infection caused by *Mycobacterium tuberculosis. Annals of Pharmacotherapy, 28,* 72–84.

Pennachio, D. (2001). CAP: Advice from the new guidelines: The guidelines for managing this ubiquitous and sometimes insidious disease have been updated. *Patient Care 35*(23), 36044.

Pirzada, O. M., & Taylor, C.J. (1999). Long-term macrolide antibiotics improve pulmonary function in cystic fibrosis. *Pediatric Pulmonology,* Suppl 19: 263+.

Powell, D. (1996). Mycoplasmal infections. In R. E. Behrman, R. M, Klegman & W. E. Nelson. (Eds.), *Textbook of pediatrics* (15th ed.; pp. 824–827). Philadelphia: W. B. Saunders.

Powers, S. W, Patton, S. R., & Byars, K. C., et al. (2002). Caloric intake and eating behaviors in infants and toddlers with cystic fibrosis. *Pediatrics, 109(5),* E75+.

Powers, S. W., & Patton, S. R. (2003). A comparison of nutrient intake between infants and toddlers with and without cystic fibrosis. Journal of the American Dietetic Association. Dec; 103(12): 1620–1625.

Prakash, U. (1996). Pulmonary diseases. In *Mayo International Medicine Board Review.* Rochester, MN: Mayo Foundation for Medicine.

Prober, C. (1996). Pneumonia. In Behrman et al. (Eds.), *Textbook of pediatrics* (15th ed. pp. 716–721). Philadelphia: W. B. Saunders.

Puchelle, E., de Bentzmann, S., & Zahm, J. M. (1995). Physical and functional properties of airway secretions in cystic fibrosis—Therapeutic approaches. *Respiration, 62*(suppl. 1), 2–12.

Ramsey, B. W., Farrell, P. M., P. Pancharz, & The Consensus Committee. (1992). Nutritional assessment and management in cystic fibrosis: A consensus report. *American Journal of Clinical Nutrition 55*(1), 108–116.

Reid, D. Withers, N. Francis, L. Wilson, J. Kotsimbos, T. (2002). Iron deficiency in cystic fibrosis: Relationship to lung disease severity and chronic Pseudomonas aeruginosa infection. *Chest, 121*(1), 48–55.

Rennard, S., Farmer, S. (2002). COPD in 2001: A major challenge for medicine, the pharmaceutical industry and society. *Chest, 121*(5), S 113–120.

Rigby, A. S., Pirzada, O. M., & Taylor, C. J., et al. (2000). Risk factors for liver disease in cystic fibrosis. *Am I Human Genetics, 67*(4), 213+.

Rigby, F., & Pastorek, J. G., II. (1996). Pneumonia during pregnancy. *Clinical Obstetrics and Gynecology, 39*(1), 107–119.

Rubin, R. H. (1996). Mycotic infections. *Scientific American,* June 274, 6–12.

Rubin, R. H., & O'Hanley, P. (1995). Infections due to gram-negative bacilli. *Scientific American* December 273, 24–27.

Rubin, B. (1999). Emerging therapies for cystic fibrosis lung disease. Chest. 115: 1120–1126.

Rubin, B., & Henke M.O. (2004). Immunomodulatory activity and effectiveness of macrolides in chronic airway disease. *Chest.* Feb; 125 (2Suppl): 70S–78S.

Saade, G. R. (1997). Human immunodeficiency virus (HIV)-related pulmonary complications in pregnancy. *Seminars in Perinatology,* 21:336–350.

Saage, M. S., Greybill, R. J., Larsen, R. A. et al. (2000). Practice guidelines for the management of cryptococcal disease. Infectious Disease Society of America. *Clinical Infectious Disease,* 30:710–718.

Sanchez, I., & Guiraldes, E. (1995). Drug management of noninfective complications of cystic fibrosis. *Drugs, 50*(4), 626–635.

Scharma, S. (2003). Pulmonary disease and pregnancy. Sept 25, emedicine.com

Schatz, M. (1999). Interrelationship between asthma and pregnancy: a literature review. *J Allergy Clin Immunol, 103*(2 pt 2), S330–336.

Schatz, M. (2001). The efficacy and safety of asthma medications during pregnancy. *Seminars in Perinatal Medicare, 25*(3), 145–152.

Schatz, M., Zeiger, R. S., Hoffman, C. P., & the Kaiser-Permanente Asthma and Pregnancy Study Group. (1990). Intrauterine growth is related to gestational pulmonary function in pregnant asthmatic women. *Chest, 98*(2), 389–392.

Schidlow, D. V., & Callahan, C. W. (1996). Pneumonia. *Pediatrics in Review, 17*(9), 300–309.

Schindler, M. (2002). Do bronchodilators have an effect on bronchiolitis? *Critical Care Medicine, 2* 111+.

Shulman, V., Alderman, E., Ewig, J. M. & Bye, M. R. (1996). Asthma in the pregnant adolescent: a review. *Journal of Adolescent Medicine,* 18: 168–176.

Schreiber, J. R., & Jacobs, M. R. (1995). Antibiotic-resistant pneumococci. *Antimicrobial Resistance in Pediatrics, 42*(3), 519–532.

Sethi, S. (1999). Etiology and management of infections in chronic obstructive pulmonary disease. *Clin Pulm Med, 6,* 327–332.

Sethi, S. (2002). Acute exacerbations of COPD: A "multipronged" approach to the use of antibiotics remains controversial. *J Resp Dis, 23*(4), 271–225.

Sin, D. D., McAlister, F. A., Man, S.F., Anthonisen, N. R. (2003). Contemporary management of COPD. *Journal of the American Medical Association,* Nov 5; 290(17): 2301–2312.

Spahn, J. D., & Kamada, A. K. (1995). Special considerations in the use of glucocorticoids in children. *Pediatrics in Review, 16*(7), 266–272.

Stockley, R. A. (2002). Neutrophils and pathogenesis of COPD. *Chest, 121*(5), 151+.

Streetman, D. D., Bhatt-Mehta, V. Johnson, C. E. (2001, July-August). Management of acute severe asthma in children. *Ann Pharmacothera, 37*(7-8), 1249–1260.

Streetman, D. D., Bhatt-Mehta, V., Johnson, E. (2002). Management of acute severe asthma in children. *Annals of Phamacotherapy,* July-August, 37(7–8): 1249–1260.

Thompson, A. (1997). Pneumonia. In R. Hoekelman, S. Friedman, et al. (Eds.), *Primary pediatric care* (pp. 133–145). St. Louis: Mosby-Year Book.

Toogood, J. H. (1993). Making better—and safer—use of inhaled steroids. *The Journal of Respiratory Diseases, 14*(2), 221–237.

VanSchayck, C. P., Loozen, J., Wagena, E. et al. (2002). Detecting patients at high risk of developing COPDH in general practice: Cross sectional case finding. *British Med J, 324*(7350), 1370–1373.

Vestbo, J., Sorenson, T., Lange, P. et al. (1999). Long-term effect of inhaled budesonide in mild and moderate COPD: a randomized controlled trial. *Lancet, 353,* 1819–1823.

Virrki, R., Rikalainem, T., Svedstrom, E., Mertsola, J., Ruskanem, O. (2002). Differentiation of bacterial and viral pneumonia in children. *Thorax,* 57(5): 438–441.

Wallings, A. (2001). Oral mucolytics provide benefits in chronic bronchitis. *Am Fam Physician, 64*(12), 2000.

Weinstein, A. G., Bender, B., Apter, A., Milgrom, H., Kobrynski, L., et al. (2002). *Achieving adherence to asthma therapy: AAAAI Quality of Care for Asthma Committee paper.* Milwaukee, WI: American Academy of Allergy Asthma and Immunology. Retrieved from: http://www.aaaai.org/members/asthma_cmte_paper.pdf 23 July 2002.

Wenzel, S. E., & Kamada, A. K. (1996). Zileuton: The first 5-lipoxygenase inhibitor for the treatment of asthma. *The Annals of Pharmacotherapy, 30,* 858–864.

West, S., Zeng, L., Lee, B. L, Kosorok, M., et al. (2002). Respiratory infections with pseudomonas aeruginsoa in children with cystic fibrosis: Early detection by serology and assessment of risk factors. *Journal of the American Medical Association, 287*(22),2958–68.

White, K. R., Munro, C. L., & Boyle, A. H. (1996). Nursing management of adults who have cystic fibrosis. *Medsurg Nursing, 5*(3), 163–167.

Wohl, M. E. B., & Majzoub, J. A. (2000). Asthma, steroids and growth. *New England Journal of Medicine, 343,* 1113+.

Wolthers, O. D. (1996). Long-, intermediate-, and short-term growth studies in asthmatic children treated with inhaled glucocorticosteroids. *European Respiratory Journal, 9*(4), 821–827.

Woolcock, A., Lundbeck, B., Ringdal, N., & L. A. Jacques. (1996). Comparison of addition of salmneterol to inhaled steroids with doubling of the dose of inhaled steroid. *American Journal of Respiratory Critical Care Medicine, 153,* 1481–1488.

Wouters, E., Creutzberg, E., & Schols, A. (2002). Systemic effects in COPD. *Chest, 121*(5), S 127–131.

Yang, E., & Rubin, B. K. (1995). "Childhood" viruses as a cause of pneumonia in adults. *Seminars in Respiratory Infections, 10*(4), 232–243.

Yang, K. D. (2000). Childhood asthma: Aspects of global environments genetics and management *23*(11), 641–661.

Yankaskas, J., Marshall, B., Sufian, B., Simon, R. & Rodman, D. (2004). CF adult care: consensus conference report. *Chest,* 125: 1S–39S.

Yu, N. C., & Maurer, J. R. (1996). Communityacquired pneumonia in high-risk populations. *Seminars in Respiratory and Critical Care Medicine, 17*(3), 255–257.

CHAPTER ❖ 23

EYE DISORDERS

Joanne K. Singleton ◆ Robert V. DiGregorio ◆ Victor Joe Yim

The eye is a sophisticated and sensitive organ. Eye disorders occur across the lifespan, with the most common disorders resulting from inflammation, infection, trauma, or increased intraocular pressure. The following common eye disorders seen in primary care will be reviewed in this chapter: corneal abrasion, disorders of the eyelid (hordeolum, chalazion, and blepharitis), conjunctivitis, glaucoma, and uveitis. Primary care providers should be able to diagnose and treat many of these conditions; however, several, once suspected, require an immediate ophthalmology consultation. For those conditions in which treatment is initiated and managed by an ophthalmologist, primary care providers must be fully aware of current management plans and expected outcomes.

CORNEAL ABRASION

The cornea is a transparent, avascular, biconvex structure of the eye that receives rich sensory innervation from the trigeminal, or fifth, cranial nerve. Major functions of the cornea include refraction of light and protection of the eye from injury and infection. The epithelium is the outermost layer of the five layers that comprise the cornea. Corneal abrasion is the result of localized loss of the epithelium. Common causes of corneal abrasion include direct trauma, foreign bodies, and contact lenses. Differentiation of traumatic corneal abrasion from that associated with contact lens wear is critical in the treatment and management of this condition.

The baseline history should include a thorough assessment of the injury: when it occurred, where it occurred, and especially what occurred. Common symptoms associated with corneal abrasion include pain, reduced visual acuity, lacrimation, photophobia, foreign body sensation, and blepharospasm (involuntary movement of the eyelids). Additionally, question patients about known drug allergies or sensitivities, past and current medical conditions, family history of glaucoma, head injury, hypermetropia (farsightedness), presbyopia (inability to focus on near objects), and current medications.

The following signs should be evaluated on physical examination: lid swelling, visual acuity measured by the Snellen chart, conjunctival injection, circumcorneal injection, anterior chamber depth, and fluorescein dye uptake by damaged corneal tissue. To evaluate the corneal defect, fluorescein dye 2% is topically applied to the affected eye, and the eye is examined using a Wood's lamp or a cobalt blue slit lamp. Contact lenses must be removed before applying the fluorescein dye. Damaged corneal epithelium tissue will take up the fluorescein, and fluorescein will react with the light, thereby outlining the affected area. Short-acting topical anesthetic drops may be required to facilitate the examination (Bertolini & Pelucio, 1995; Jampel, 1995; Knox & McIntee, 1995).

SPECIFIC CONSIDERATIONS FOR PHARMACOTHERAPY

When Drug Therapy Is Needed

Treatment should relieve pain, reduce the risk of or prevent bacterial infection, and promote healing. Corneal abrasions usually heal within 48 hours, whether left untreated or covered with an eye patch (Jampel, 1995). Pharmacotherapy, while not absolutely necessary, is often used for pain relief related to ciliary muscle spasm and the prevention of secondary infections (Jampel 1995; Knox & McIntee, 1995). Steroids should be avoided since their use is associated with enhanced bacterial replication and herpes simplex activation.

Short- and Long-Term Goals of Pharmacotherapy

The short-term goal of treating corneal abrasions is pain relief. The long-term goals of treating corneal abrasions are complete cure and prevention of infection. In the context of corneal abrasion therapy, these long-term goals should be attainable within 24 to 48 hours.

Nonpharmacologic Therapy

Controversy exists in the literature regarding the role of immobilizing the eyelids with a patch. Although commonly done, there is no definitive evidence that patching an eye results in faster healing. In the past it was believed that patching an eye for 24 to 48 hours provided greater comfort for the patient by immobilizing the eyelid so it would not rub against the abrasion. Recent studies, however, have found that eye patching did not improve healing rates or reduce pain in patients with corneal abrasion. Given the theoretical harm of loss of binocular vision and possible increased pain, many researchers caution the use of this practice (Flynn, Damico, & Smith, 1998). Recent controlled clinical trials have also demonstrated that eye patching does not appear to be beneficial in the treatment of traumatic corneal abrasion as compared with a course of topical antibiotic ointment (Le Sage, Verreault, & Rochette, 2001). *It must be noted that corneal abrasions associated with contact lens injuries should not be managed with an eye patch and must be treated with ophthalmic antibiotics* (Bertolini & Pelucio, 1995; Jampel, 1995; Knox & McIntee, 1995).

Time Frame for Initiating Pharmacotherapy

Since corneal abrasions are associated with a significant amount of pain, and infections can develop rapidly, treatment should be initiated as soon as possible. Corneal abrasions generally heal within 48 hours because the epithelium regenerates rapidly; thus, cycloplegic therapy should not be needed beyond 48 hours. Antibiotics are generally empirically utilized for approximately 1 week.

Pain relief due to cilliary spasm is generally achieved within 30 to 60 min after cycloplegic preparations are administered (*Ophthalmic Drug Facts,* 1996). However, patients may still have pain from exposed corneal nerve endings. General healing occurs within 48 hours.

Patient/Caregiver Information

Patients should be advised how to prevent future corneal abrasions; for example, if corneal abrasions are due to work-related trauma or a foreign body, use of protective eye wear should be encouraged. Contact lens wearers should be reminded to clean their lenses more frequently.

Further, patients should be advised not to wear contact lenses at night, to request disposable contacts when appropriate, and to clean lenses frequently.

OUTCOMES MANAGEMENT

Selecting Appropriate Agents

Topical steroids should be avoided. Homatropine hydrobromide 2–5% or cyclopentolate 0.5–2% are appropriate cycloplegic agents based on a 30-minutes onset of action and moderate duration of action (1–3 days). Homatropine is a more cost-effective agent than other cycloplegics. The usual dose of these agents is one or two drops of the solution prior to antibiotic instillation, and patching is used when indicated. Patients with a heavily pigmented iris may require higher doses. The lower-percentage solutions are reserved for pediatric use.

Choice of an antibiotic agent should be based on the type of abrasion, with antipseudomonal agents used exclusively for contact lens wearers and sulfacetamide for all others. Although gentamicin is the most inexpensive of the antipseudomonal agents, an increased resistance of *Pseudomonas aeruginosa* to gentamicin has made tobramycin or "fourth-generation" fluoroquinolones (moxifloxacin, gatifloxacin) preferred agents. Efficacy is established by the relief of pain, decreased inflammation, and absence of infection.

Monitoring for Toxicity

Prolonged use of cycloplegic products may produce irritation and edema in the eyelid. Systemic toxicity presents as anticholinergic poisoning with dryness of the mouth, blurred vision, tachycardia, fever, urinary retention, dysarthria, vasodilation, coma, and even death.

Followup Recommendations

Followup examinations for patients with corneal abrasions should be scheduled for 24 hours after the initial examination and treatment. Followup should include evaluation of common complications of corneal abrasion: recurrent erosion, corneal ulceration, and secondary iritis.

DISORDERS OF THE EYELID: HORDEOLUM, CHALAZION, AND BLEPHARITIS

Eyelids, accessory organs of the eye, are lined with elongated sebaceous glands called meibomian glands, the smaller sebaceous glands of Zeis at the edge of the lid, and the modified sweat glands of Moll at the border of the lids. Projecting from the margin of the eyelids are eyelashes that are lubricated by fluid from these glands.

A hordeolum, or the common stye—an acute inflammation of a hair follicle of the eyelash or a gland of the eyelid—forms when there is infection and blockage of the gland(s). The cause of infection is usually *Staphylococcus aureus*. A hordeolum resembling a pimple appears on the lid margin and may be internal with pointing onto the conjunctival surface of the lid. It is red, tender, and painful, and may be accompanied by moderate conjunctival injection (Crouch & Berger, 1995).

A chalazion results from a chronic inflammation of a meibomian gland. It is not usually preceded by acute inflammation and appears approximately 2 mm or more from the margin of the eyelid, with pointing of the lesion inside the lid (Diegel, 1986). Secondary infection may develop in surrounding tissue.

Blepharitis is an inflammation of the eyelid margins and associated structures. It is a chronic condition, usually bilateral, and is seen in all age groups, but especially in the elderly population. Although there are elaborate classification schemes for blepharitis, the two basic classifications are seborrheic and infectious, which may be found together. Patients often identify a history of hordeola or chalazia. Blepharitis may present with an associated conjunctivitis and tear deficiency, which is a risk factor for this condition. Factors that may contribute to acute phases of blepharitis and cause inflammation and irritation include: eye makeup, contact lens buildup, smoke, smog, and chemicals (Raskin, Speaker, & Laibson, 1992; Smith & Flowers, 1995; Wittpenn, 1995).

The usual organism found in blepharitis is staphylococcus, primarily *S. aureus* and secondarily *S. epidermidis*. Patients present with inflamed eyelids, moderate erythema, fibrinous scaling and crusts, and may have loss of lashes.

Eyelid inflammation in patients with seborrheic blepharitis is less prominent and is accompanied by greasy or oily scaling. There is a high incidence of other seborrheic dermatoses in these patients, i.e., rosacea, psoriasis, seborrhea, and dandruff (Wittpenn, 1995).

Patients who present with blepharitis often complain of itching, burning, and a chronic foreign body sensation. There is no cure for blepharitis since those affected by staphyloccus are most likely susceptible to the organism and suffer from reinfection; those with seborrheic blepharitis may have other underlying dermatologic pathologies.

The baseline history in patients with conditions of the eyelid should include identification of onset, symptoms, previous occurrences, and response to treatment, as well as known drug sensitivity. Common symptoms of hordeolum include pain, redness, and tenderness on palpation of the affected eyelid. In addition to the baseline history for hordeolum, the patient with chalazion should be asked about changes in visual acuity, a feeling of pressure on the affected eye, and tenderness or pain of the affected eyelid. In patients with blepharitis, the baseline history should also include presence of skin problems and exposure to eye makeup, contact lens buildup, smoke, chemicals, or smog.

On physical examination, evaluate the following signs for disorders of the eyelid: visual acuity, eyelid abnormalities, pointing of the lesion, abnormalities of the sclera and conjunctiva, and adenopathy, particularly in the preauricular area. In patients with blepharitis, use a magnifier to inspect the eyelids and assess erythema, scaling, and ulcers.

Diagnostic tests are not indicated for either a hordeolum or chalazion; in refractory cases of blepharitis a culture should be obtained.

SPECIFIC CONSIDERATIONS FOR PHARMACOTHERAPY

When Drug Therapy Is Needed

The initial treatments of hordeolum, chalazion, and blepharitis are primarily nondrug regimens. The aim of treatment for a hordeolum is to stimulate drainage of the gland and to eliminate the infectious bacteria. Patients need to be aware that there is currently no cure for blepharitis and that the goals of treatment are to control symptoms and prevent secondary complications.

Chalazia that are large or persist for several months may require treatment. Local or systemic treatment is generally not successful, and incision and curettage are recommended.

Antibiotic ointment is valuable in the treatment of blepharitis because it adheres to the eyelid margin; however, if more than small amounts are used, it can cause blurring of vision and therefore should be used at night. Antibiotic drops can be used during the daytime but may not be as effective as the ointment.

The drugs of choice are bacitracin and erythromycin. Gentamicin and tobramycin may also be used, although they may not be well tolerated in chronic treatment. In patients with coexisting conditions, additional treatment directed at the concomitant condition is necessary.

Topical antibiotics may be useful for refractory cases, and systemic antibiotics may be substituted if topical therapy fails. Topical antibiotics are more commonly used in the treatment of blepharitis, with therapy focused on the eradication of *S. aureus*.

Short- and Long-Term Goals of Pharmacotherapy

The short- and long-term goals of treating a hordeolum or chalazion are reversal of the blocked meibomian gland(s). Blepharitis is a disorder without a cure; the goals of therapy are geared toward a reduction in episode frequency. During the acute phase, direct the therapy at controlling the disease process. This first phase usually lasts 2 to 8 weeks. Over the long term, a reduction in episode frequency is achieved by determining the minimal amount of therapy necessary to maintain control.

Nonpharmacologic Therapy

Nonpharmacologic therapy centers on warm compresses applied to the affected area several times a day. The refractory chalazion can be removed surgically. Meticulous lid hygiene is essential for managing blepharitis. Lid hygiene should consist of warm eyelid scrubs with a cotton-tipped applicator, with either a 1:5 dilution of baby shampoo or a commercial eye scrub. Identification and removal of contributing factors, e.g., cosmetics, are essential to reducing the frequency of episodes.

Time Frame for Initiating Pharmacotherapy

Nonpharmacologic and pharmacologic therapy should begin as soon as possible. Therapy should be continued until the hordeolum or chalazion is relieved. Antibiotics are generally used for 5 to 7 days. Blepharitis treatment consists of two phases; the acute phase lasts from 2 to 8 weeks, and the maintenance phase lasts indefinitely.

Relief of these disorders varies. Chalazia resolve spontaneously after 3 to 4 months without therapy. If the hordeolum or chalazion persists, the patient should be referred to an ophthalmologist. Blepharitis may be controlled in as little as several days to 8 weeks; however, chronic therapy is needed to maintain the therapeutic goal (Dreyer, 1996; Raskin et al., 1992; Smith & Flowers, 1995).

Patient/Caregiver Information

Patients or their caregivers should apply the antibiotic ointment evenly over the margins of the eyelid. Ointment can cause blurring and loss of binocular vision; patients should be advised not to drive.

Patients who present with hordeola need to be instructed in eye hygiene. Makeup should not be worn until the stye has resolved, current eye makeup should be discarded, and the same eye makeup should not be used for long periods of time.

OUTCOMES MANAGEMENT

Selecting Appropriate Agents

Infection of the meibomian glands is usually caused by staphylococcus. The agent of choice for treating this infection is bacitracin. Alternative therapies have included aminoglycosides (gentamicin, tobramycin), vancomycin, and quinolones (ciprofloxacin, norfoxacin). The quinolones and the aminoglycosides have shown equal efficacy in several studies (Bloom, Leeming, Power, et al., 1994; Gwon, 1992; Miller, Vogel, Cook, & Wittreich, 1992). The quinolones typically are the most expensive of the available therapies. Thus, these agents are reserved for refractory cases or for patients who cannot tolerate aminoglycoside preparations. Systemic therapy, if warranted, is generally initiated by an ophthalmologist and can be accomplished cost effectively with oxacillin, amoxicillin, or occasionally tetracycline (contraindicated in pregnant women and young children).

Monitoring for Efficacy and Toxicity

Efficacy is primarily judged by the eradication of the hordeolum or chalazion. Efficacy in blepharitis therapy is observed when the apparent lid dermatitis has disappeared and reported symptoms have resolved. There is no need to monitor for toxicity.

Followup Recommendations

Since a hordeolum should resolve within 2 weeks of treatment, followup is usually not required. Chalazia that have not resolved after 3 to 4 months should be evaluated by an ophthalmologist for possible surgical excision. Sometimes a chronic chalazion may actually turn out to be a misdiagnosed carcinoma. Patients who present with chalazia and secondary infection should be treated and reevaluated in 2 weeks, whereas patients with small chalazia do not need followup care.

Chronic blepharitis should be followed closely until a maintenance phase is clearly established. Patients with mild cases of blepharitis can receive followup care at regularly scheduled appointments to evaluate effectiveness of maintenance treatment. In more severe cases, patients should be reevaluated in 10 to 14 days.

GLAUCOMA

The term *glaucoma* actually refers to a group of optic nerve disorders reflecting a variety of changes that alter the functional anatomy of the eye. This disease is associated with excessive intraocular pressure that will lead to the characteristic visual field loss and optic nerve atrophy. The two major types of glaucoma are open-angle and closed-angle. Both types can be primary, or inherited, or secondary, related to injury or underlying disease or precipitated by medications, diabetes mellitus, and acute or chronic use of steroids. Glaucoma is the second most common cause of blindness, and the most common among African-descended populations. Risk factors include; age, race, heredity, myopia, (Bensinger, 1994; Gelvin, 1994; Goldberg & Friedman, 2001; Long & Long, 1994; Rosenberg, 1995; Tucker, 1993). This section only discusses primary open-angle glaucoma, the most prevalent form of glaucoma.

Primary open-angle glaucoma—often called the "silent blinder"—is an inherited, bilateral disorder, usually seen after the age of 40, with the greatest incidence in those over 75. In primary open-angle glaucoma, there is a slow, gradual increase in intraocular pressure due to a low-grade outflow obstruction of the aqueous fluid from the anterior chamber. This causes a gradual loss in peripheral vision; if untreated, it will lead to a reduction of the central field of vision. In the early stages of the disease, midperipheral field vision may be affected; however, irreversible damage has occurred before the patient experiences visual changes. Medical management using drug therapy is usually initiated by an ophthalmologist and comanaged by the primary care provider (Bensinger 1994; Gelvin, 1994; Long & Long, 1994; Rosenberg, 1995; Tucker, 1993).

The baseline history should include identification of risk factors as well as loss of peripheral vision, in either one or both eyes, and onset. Medication history and known drug sensitivities must also be identified.

The physical examination should include measurement of intraocular pressure (the acceptable range is 10–21 mm Hg) a funduscopic examination to assess the disk for cupping, and gross measurement of visual fields by direct confrontation. Patients in whom open-angle glaucoma is suspected should be referred to an ophthalmologist for a complete examination (Bensinger, 1994; Long & Long, 1994; Uphold & Graham, 1994).

Current diagnostic tests used to screen for open-angle glaucoma include tonometry, ophthalmoscopy, perimetry (evaluation of visual fields) and corneal pachymetry and optic nerve imaging. Sensitivity and specificity of tonometry and ophthalmoscopy are poor for predicting open-angle glaucoma. Such a diagnosis is best made by perimetry, which has good sensitivity and specificity in identification of visual field damage in open-angle glaucoma. It is not an effective screening tool since it detects irreversible versible field loss rather than early disease (Tucker, 1993).

SPECIFIC CONSIDERATIONS FOR PHARMACOTHERAPY

When Drug Therapy Is Needed

The goal of therapy is to reduce the intraocular pressure to prevent further damage to the optic nerve and vision loss. Glaucoma is primarily medically managed, although surgical interventions are possible. Medical management centers on reducing ocular hypertension and minimizing drug-induced adverse reactions. The choice of a medication regimen is usually made by an ophthalmologist (Gelvin, 1994). It also should be noted that primary open-angle glaucoma can be aggravated or induced by corticosteroids, while other types of glaucoma can be aggravated or induced by corticosteroids as well as medications such as anticholinergics, benzodiazepines, phenothiazines, and tricyclic antidepressants (Abel, 1995). Patients with a history suggestive of glaucoma should have a thorough medication history taken for possible drug association.

Short- and Long-Term Goals of Pharmacotherapy

The short- and long-term goal in comanaging the glaucoma patient is to lower intraocular pressure and stave off resultant optic nerve atrophy and loss of vision.

Nonpharmacologic Therapy

Modern surgical techniques such as laser surgery and filtration surgery serve as alternatives to medical therapy in unresponsive patients. Recent studies have shown some benefit from iridectomy and iridotomy in the treatment of narrow angles and preventing primary angle closure glaucoma (Nolan, 2002).

Time Frame for Initiating Pharmacotherapy

Medical therapy should be initiated when the optic disk exhibits pathologic changes in addition to an increase in intraocular pressure. Glaucoma management is chronic, despite a relative lack of symptoms in the patient. See Drug Table 401.1.

Patient/Caregiver Information

Ocular hypertension is similar to cardiovascular hypertension in that it is a silent disease, with successful management dependent upon the patient's participation in her or his medication regimen. Patients and caregivers should receive extensive counseling regarding the importance of regular use of their prescribed medical therapy regardless of a disappearance of symptoms. See Table 23–1 for basic information both patients and caregivers can use to help administer eyedrops.

OUTCOMES MANAGEMENT

Selecting Appropriate Agents

Topical beta-adrenergic antagonists have long been the first line of treatment in chronic open-angle glaucoma. Timolol 0.5% has been the gold standard by which other glaucoma medications have been compared. Timolol and other beta blockers such as betaxolol decrease aqueous production and thus lower intraocular pressure. Patients with reactive airway disease, heart failure, or cardiac conduction blocks should be monitored closely because of the systemic absorption of these drugs. Patients must also be monitored for other serious side effects such as depression, impotence, and exercise intolerance.

TABLE 23–1. Patient and Caregiver Information for Administering Ophthalmic Solutions and Suspensions

1. Wash hands thoroughly prior to administration.
2. Tilt the patient's head backward or have the patient lie down.
3. Gently grasp the lower eyelid and pull the eyelid away from the eye, forming a pocket.
4. Without coming in contact with fingers or the eye itself, position the dropper over the eye and instill a drop.
5. Have the patient look down.
6. Release the eyelid and have the patient close the eye.
7. Using a fingertip, gently apply pressure to the inside corner of the eye for several minutes.
8. Do not rub the eye.
9. Do not rinse the dropper.
10. Do not use eyedrops if their color has changed.
11. Wait 3–5 min between medications when administering multiple eye preparations.

Source: Adapted from Ophthalmic Drug Facts (1996).

Pilocarpine eye drops of varying concentrations from 1 to 8% have long been used in the treatment of glaucoma. They allow increase aqueous outflow and can lower intraocular pressures very effectively. However, they too have serious side effects to consider, including retinal tears and detachments, browaches, and chronic pupillary miosis (constriction) with myopic shift. Carbonic anhydrase inhibitors are another class of medications available in both oral and drop form that lower intraocular pressure by direct inhibition of the carbonic anhydrase in the ciliary body, which reduces the production of aqueous humor in the eye.

Acetazolamide (Diamox) has long been the oral carbonic anhydrase inhibitor of choice; however, systemic side effects such as depression, impotence, renal stones, and metabolic abnormalities are possible side effects. More recently, carbonic anhydrase inhibitors in a drop form have been made available (dorzolamide (Trusopt^R^) and brinzolamide (Azopt^R^) in the hope of decreasing the risk of the systemic side effects.

More promising pressure-lowering medications have become available recently with fewer side effects, more pressure-lowering effect and lower frequency of dosing. A new class of glaucoma medication is the prostaglandin derivatives, which include latanoprost (Xalatan®), bimatoprost (Lumigan®), and travoprost (Travatan®). These medications decrease intraocular pressure in large part by increased uveoscleral outflow (drainage). Their most commonly seen side effects include conjunctival hyperemia, iris pigment color changes (lighter colored became darker), uveitis and cystoid macular edema, increased growth of eyelashes, and pigmentary changes of the eyelids. This class of medication has been shown to consistently lower intraocular pressure to a greater degree than the gold standard medication, timolol, and this difference was found to be statistically significant.

These new medications now offer patients with glaucoma lower intraocular pressures with less possibility of serious systematic side effects than older classes of medications such as the beta-adrenergic antagonists and carbonic anhydrase inhibitors. In fact, many glaucoma patients no longer need surgery because of the introduction of these newer agents (*FDA News,* 2001).

A final class of medications is the adrenergic agonists, which include dipivefrin, apraclonidine, and brimonidine. Brimonidine (Alphagan®), a relatively selective alpha-2 adrenergic agonist, has recently come into favor because of its strong pressure-lowering properties. It appears to lower intraocular pressure both by decreasing aqueous production and increasing uvealscleral outflow. It may also have a neuroprotective effect on the optic nerve and has been successfully combined with other glaucoma medications to further lower intraocular pressure. Common side effects include conjunctival hyperemia, headaches, ocular allergic reactions, and fatigue/drowsiness. Many of the above medications have been combined to have additive effects in lowering intraocular pressures.

Monitoring for Efficacy

Intraocular pressure monitoring and visual fields are evaluated on a regular basis after initiation of therapy.

Monitoring for Toxicity

In cases of acute overdosage with these preparations, the eye should be flushed with warm tap water or saline solution. Many of these products contain benzalkonium chloride as a preservative agent and should be avoided by soft contact lens wearers (Chapman, Cheeks, & Green, 1990).

Followup Recommendations

Followup care should be provided by a ophthalmologist. Followup should occur at 2-week intervals initially, followed by 3-month intervals once stabilization has occurred. Patients must continue therapy even after symptoms have resolved. Primary care providers comanage through their understanding of the antiglaucoma medications, of their potential for systemic effects, and of the high frequency with which patients either do not use their eye medications or do not administer them correctly.

CONJUNCTIVITIS

Conjunctivitis is an inflammation of the conjunctiva. The classification of conjunctivitis is primarily based on cause: allergic, bacterial, chemical, fungal, parasitic, and viral.

Ocular allergy is often the cause of allergic conjunctivitis. It is usually differentiated from infectious conjunctivitis based on seasonality, intense itching, and recurrence.

Bacterial conjunctivitis is seen worldwide and occurs in all age groups. Common bacterial pathogens include: *Staphylococcus aureus* (common in adults), *Streptococcus* species (common in children), *Haemophilus influenzae, Neisseria gonorrhoeae, Proteus* species, *Klebsiella,* and *Moraxella.* Contamination with the invading organism causes an acute inflammatory response that is most often self-limiting. However, in patients whose immune status is compromised, bacterial conjunctivitis can progress to a sight-threatening infection.

Gonococcal conjuntivitis may be seen in individuals who come in contact with infected genital secretions. Presenting as a copious purulent discharge that may result in corneal perforation, gonococcal conjuntivitis is considered an ophthalmologic emergency. Gonococcal ophthalmia neonatorum—gonococcal infection in the neonate—presents as a serosanguinous discharge, which rapidly changes to purulent exudate 24 to 48 hours after delivery. Instillation of silver nitrate drops or erythromycin ointment at birth has resulted in a significant decrease in this infection.

Viral conjunctivitis is usually caused by adenoviruses. The more benign condition, commonly seen in children, is pharyngoconjunctival fever, caused by adenovirus types 3 and 7. Adenovirus types 8 and 9 cause epidemic keratoconjunctivitis, which is highly contagious. Treatment for viral conjunctivitis caused by adenoviruses is aimed at relief of symptoms. Viral ocular infection can also occur with the herpes simplex and zoster viruses; when suspected, an immediate ophthalmologic consultation is required (Silverman, & Bessman, 2001).

Fungal conjunctivitis is rare. It is seen most often in patients who are immunosuppressed or who are receiving broad-spectrum antibiotic therapy or glucocorticoid therapy.

Chlamydia trachomatis is an obligate intracellular bacteria that is responsible for both trachoma, which is the leading cause of preventable blindness worldwide, and chlamydial inclusion conjunctivitis, which is associated with the sexually transmitted form of the disease. There are different serotypes of chlamydia that cause the different disease entities. Trachoma is an infectious disease common in third-world countries and associated with poor hygiene, inadequate sanitation, and the common housefly (which is thought to be the vector that spreads the disease). Trachoma is treated with topical and oral tetracycline or erythromycin. Chlamydial inclusion conjunctivitis is seen most commonly in association with the sexually transmitted form of the disease, but may also be spread via shared eye cosmetics and inadequately chlorinated swimming pools. Chlamydia strains have been isolated from a high percentage (30–60%) of men with sypmptomatic nongonoccal urethritis (Lietman, & Whitcher, 1999). The coexistence in women of chlamyadial conjunctivitis and positive cervical cultures is extremely high. Treatment includes 3 weeks of oral tetracycline, doxycycline, or erythromycin. A single dose of 1 gram of azithromycin may also be effective. Laboratory confirmed chlamydial conjunctivitis should prompt the practitioner to evaluate and treat for coinfection with other sexually transmitted diseases and treatment of partners.

Chemical conjunctivitis can be caused by any offending agent that comes in contact with the eye. The most common offending agents are chemicals found in eyedrops. Additional offending agents may include: eye makeup, household cleaning agents, and insect bites in the periorbital area.

Characteristics of conjunctivitis include loss of vision; itching, tearing, and diffuse conjunctival hyperemia will be present. Distinguishing features in bacterial conjunctivitis include mucopurulent discharge, with morning matting of the eyes, usually unilateral at onset but after a few days becoming bilateral; in viral conjunctivitis foreign body sensation, excessive tearing, clear to mucoid discharge, preauricular adenopathy, and corneal infiltrates or punctate staining may be present; and in allergic conjunctivitis excessive itching is present with a stringy discharge. Treatment is directed at the specific organism. Gram staining is the gold standard for determining the cause in bacterial conjunctivitis; however, it is reserved for cases that do not respond after 48 to 72 hours of treatment.

A baseline history should include onset of symptoms; contact with anyone with pinkeye; upper respiratory symptoms; type of discharge; matting of eyelids upon awaking; photophobia; history of allergies, *Chlamydia,* herpes simplex, or herpes zoster; and chemical irritants or insect bites in the area of the eye. Known drug sensitivities must also be identified.

On physical examination visual acuity should be measured, preauricular nodes should be evaluated, and a complete examination of the external structures of the eye should be performed. In addition, evaluate discharge and culture if purulent and perform a funduscopic examination. Patients with conjunctivitis who have changes in visual acuity, photophobia, and pain should be referred for ophthalmologic consultation.

Bacterial conjunctivitis should improve with treatment within several days; the viral version may not resolve for several weeks and is contagious, so patients must be advised not to rub their eyes and cross-contaminate the other eye or another person. Allergic conjunctivitis is relieved with treatment, and chemical conjunctivitis is relieved after identification and removal of the offending agent.

SPECIFIC CONSIDERATIONS FOR PHARMACOTHERAPY

When Drug Therapy Is Needed

Conjunctivitis is usually a self-limiting inflammatory disorder associated with multiple causes, including bacteria, viruses, allergens, chemicals, and mechanical irritants. It may be difficult to differentiate bacterial and viral conjunctivitis in clinical settings, so many health providers treat all presumed cases of infective conjunctivitis with a broad spectrum of antibiotics. Treatment with antibiotics, is associated with significantly better rates of clinical remission (Sheikh, Hurwitz, & Cave, 2002). Allergic conjunctivitis is differentiated by the presence of itching in addition to seasonal recurrence. The treatment of allergic conjunctivitis includes antihistamines, decongestants, mast-cell stabilizers, and cold compresses. If bacterial and allergic conjunctivitis are ruled out, viral conjunctivitis may be considered and treated with antiviral agents.

Short- and Long-Term Goals of Pharmacotherapy

The primary goal in managing conjunctivitis is achieving comfort for the patient, followed by cure.

Nonpharmacologic Therapy

Warm compresses and eye scrubs are considered as adjunctive therapies to antibiotics for bacterial conjunctivitis. Cold compresses and identification and eradication of causative allergens are beneficial for allergic conjunctivitis. Epidemic keratoconjunctivitis ("pink eye") should be treated with isolation precautions, good handwashing, and lubricating and nonsteroidal eye drops. Conjunctivitis secondary to chemical or foreign body exposure should be treated with copious amounts of water, saline, or eyewash solution.

Time Frame for Initiating Pharmacotherapy

Therapy should be initiated as soon as possible for patient comfort. Antibiotics are generally used for approximately 5 to 7 days. Antivirals are generally used for 14 to 21 days. Therapy for allergic conjunctivitis may be necessary for several months if the allergen cannot be eliminated.

Bacterial conjunctivitis usually resolves in 48 to 72 hours with treatment and in 2 weeks without treatment. Viral conjunctivitis responds to therapy in 2 to 3 weeks. Response to allergic conjunctivitis therapies should be seen within a few days. See Drug Tables 401.3, 401.4, 401.5.

Patient/Caregiver Information

Patients and caregivers should be advised that overuse of over-the-counter (OTC) sympathomimetic decongestants can lead to rebound vasodilation, worsening the conjunctivitis. Additionally, patients with certain types of glaucoma should be instructed not to use sympathomimetics. Patients and caregivers should be warned that viral conjunctivitis is highly contagious; handwashing must be used as a means to prevent spread of the infection to others, as well as not sharing bed linens. When ophthalmic ointments are used, patients should be advised not to drive because of loss of binocular vision.

OUTCOMES MANAGEMENT

Selecting Appropriate Agent

Antibiotic therapy is generally aimed at eradicating *Staphylococcus* and *Streptococcus* bacteria. Therapy may be initiated in a cost-effective manner with erythromycin or bacitracin ophthalmic ointments; however, many practitioners also use fortified aminoglycoside and cephalosporin preparations especially for corneal ulceration. These fortified antibiotics are not commercially available and must be compounded by a pharmacist familiar with sterile product preparation. Topical quinolones, such as ciprofloxacin and norfloxacin, have been shown to have comparable efficacy to the aminoglycosides and present a more costly alternative. Therapy should be guided by local resistance patterns and experience.

Neonatal conjunctivitis (ophthalmia neonatorum) occurs in the first month of life. Historically, this was an important cause of blindness prior to prophylactic regimens of silver nitrate and/or erythromycin ointment. The causative bacterium in this form of conjunctivitis is usually *N. gonorrhoea,* the consequence of maternal venereal disease. The U.S. Centers for Disease Control currently recommend topical erythromycin ointment at birth for prophylaxis.

The treatment of viral herpes conjunctivitis is aimed at inactivating the sight-threatening herpes simplex virus. Infections of adenovirus types 3 and 8 are not sight-threatening and are usually self-limiting. The treatment of the herpes simplex virus consists of either vidarabine 5% or idoxuridine 0.5% ointment five times a day, or trifluridine 1% solution nine times per day.

The most cost-effective therapy for allergic conjunctivitis is removal of the causative allergen. Unfortunately, this is not always possible. Symptoms may be managed by ophthalmic decongestants (e.g., Visine), oral and local (drops) antihistamines, decongestant-antihistamine combinations (Naphcon forte, Vasocon-A solution), mast-cell stablizers (Alomide®, Crolom®), topical NSAIDs (Acular®). The newest agents, H1 receptors and mast-cell stabilizer combinations (ketophen fumarate [Zaditor®], nedocromil [Alocril®], olopadatine [Patanol®] are recommended for use in adults and children with itching of the eyes due to allergic conjunctivitis. These agents should be chosen based on individual response. The newer agents, lodoxamide and levocabastine, have been noted to be at least as effective as cromolyn with less frequent administration necessary. A new ophthalmic solution Azelastine (Optivar®) has been approved by the FDA (May 2002), for treatment of allergic conjunctivitis. In the category of alternative medicine, eye drops made from Euphrasia rastkoviama can be used for various forms of conjunctivitis by general practitioners and ophthalmologists (Stoss, Michels, Beutke, & Gorter, 2002).

Monitoring for Efficacy

Efficacy can be seen with a reduction and overall elimination of symptoms.

Monitoring for Toxicity

There are many minor toxicities associated with the agents used for symptomatic treatment of conjunctivitis. These include rebound hyperemia with overuse (more than 48 hours) of the decongestant. Prolonged use of topical decongestants may also cause corneal edema. Antihistamines are associated with anticholinergic side effects, including dilated pupils, flushing, dry mouth, fever, ataxia, and hallucinations 30 to 120 minutes after administration. Ophthalmic cromolyn may be associated with a transient stinging or burning sensation.

Followup Recommendations

Bacterial conjunctivitis should be followed closely for response in 48 to 72 hours. If no response is seen, a Gram stain should be obtained to determine etiology. Patients should be reevaluated within 48 hours if there is no improvement. Severe cases, after response to treatment, should be followed up in 10 to 14 days; in mild cases no followup is necessary if symptoms resolve.

UVEITIS

Uveitis is inflammation in any part of the uveal tract, which includes the iris, ciliary body, and choroid. Adjacent ocular structures may also be involved. Uveitis is categorized as: *anterior uveitis,* which involves the iris (iritis) or both the iris and the ciliary body (iridocyclitis); *intermediate uveitis,* which affects the retinal vessels and the peripheral area of the retina and uveal tract; and *posterior uveitis,* which involves the posterior choroid (choroiditis), the retina (retinitis), or both (chorioretinitis). In *panuveitis,* inflammatory signs are both anteriorly and posteriorly distributed. Uveitis may be caused by infectious and noninfectious disorders, is associated with numerous systemic diseases, or may be idiopathic (McClusky, Fowler, & Lightman, 2000).

The most common conditions associated with anterior uveitis include sarcoidosis, ankylosing spondylitis, Reiter's syndrome, juvenile rheumatoid arthritis, inflammatory bowel disease, herpes simplex, tuberculosis, and trauma. Posterior uveitis is most commonly caused by toxoplasmosis and is also associated with syphilis, HIV/AIDS, tuberculosis, and cytomegalovirus. Posterior uveitis may be associated with sarcodosis and embolic retinitis (Gordon, 2001).

Uveitis may be acute or chronic. It may be asymptomatic or present with decreased visual acuity, pain, photophobia, tearing, small and irregular pupils, diffuse conjunctival hyperemia with ciliary flush, and complaint of blurred vision and floaters. Early diagnosis of chronic anterior uveitis is more likely to be made in patients who have associated systemic conditions and have had ongoing ophthalmic evaluations. *If uveitis is suspected, the patient should be immediately referred for an ophthalmology consultation.*

A baseline history must include the following: symptoms and their onset, circumstances surrounding their onset, occupational and environmental exposure, social and sexual history, and current illnesses and their symptoms.

On physical examination the following should be evaluated: visual acuity; pupil size, shape, and response to light; conjunctiva for flush or perilimbal injection; funduscopic examination; and consensual photophobia. A slit-lamp examination should be performed to confirm the presence of any inflammatory cells in the anterior chamber. If a systemic condition is present, additional physical assessment may be indicated.

SPECIFIC CONSIDERATIONS FOR PHARMACOTHERAPY

When Drug Therapy Is Needed

Therapy is aimed at symptom relief, reduction of inflammation, and restoring or preserving vision. Treatment is based on severity, as well as the general health of the patient. The need for therapy is usually determined upon referral to an ophthalmologist (DeGrezia, Robinson, 2001; McClusky et al., 2000; Shields, 2000).

Short- and Long-Term Goals of Pharmacotherapy

The initial management of uveitis is geared toward the reduction of symptoms and pain related to inflammation. Long-term goals of therapy are directed toward treatment of the underlying causative systemic disease, and prevention of complications such as permanent synechiae—adhesion of parts, especially the iris to the lens and cornea—and the preservation of vision (McClusky et al., 2000).

Time Frame for Initiating Pharmacotherapy

Therapy, if needed, should be initiated upon diagnosis. The duration of therapy is determined by the patient's response and resolution of underlying disease states. The time it will take for a therapeutic response depends on the underlying cause.

Patient/Caregiver Information

Patients who are experiencing photophobia should wear sunglasses.

OUTCOMES MANAGEMENT

Selecting Appropriate Agents

Treatment, when necessary, is usually initiated with a short-acting cycloplegic agent and a topical steroid. Topical steriods are contraindicated if the causal agent is infection. The choice of cycloplegic agent is made based on the severity of disease, with homatropine 5% for mild to moderate disease and atropine 1 to 4% for moderate to severe disease. Cycloplegic agents are avoided if the client has or is at risk for glaucoma. Cyclopentolate should be avoided since it may further aggravate the uveitis (Dreyer, 1996). The corticosteroid of choice is prednisolone acetate 1% ophthalmic suspension (Gordon, 2001). Systemic corticosteroids and immunosuppressants are reserved for unresponsive cases or for those cases in which the disease manifests systemically and visual acuity is affected. Prednisone is the oral corticosteroid of choice. Immunosuppressants used include cyclosporine, azathioprine, and mercaptopurine. NSAIDs are also used.

Monitoring for Efficacy

Relief of pain should be seen within 3 days of initiating corticosteroids along with resolution of photophobia and maintenance or improvement of visual acuity.

Monitoring for Toxicity

Corticosteroid use is associated with a multitude of systemic adverse effects including cataract formation, glaucoma, retinopathy, activation of herpes, depression, psychosis, mania, euphoria, headache, diabetes and glucose intolerance, growth suppression in children, Cushing's syndrome, abnormal hair growth, nausea, peptic ulcers, sodium retention and edema, hypokalemia, myopathies, osteoporosis, acne, and poor wound healing.

Followup Recommendations

Serious and sight-threatening uveitis should be followed by an ophthalmologist. Some sources advise that all uveitis should be seen first by an ophthalmologist, with comanagement by other providers for underlying causes and treatment.

REFERENCES

Abel, S. (1995). In L. Young & M. A. Koda-Kimble (Eds.), *Applied therapeutics: The clinical use of drugs* (6th ed.; pp. 49-1–49-23). Vancouver, WA: Applied Therapeutics.

Bensinger, R. (1994). Glaucoma: A general perspective. *Journal of the Florida Medical Association, 81* (4), 243–247.

Bertolini, J. (2001, April 30). Glaucoma, acute angle closure. *EmMedicine Journal, 2*(4). Retrieved March 3, 2002. http://www.emedicine.com/emerg/topics752.htm.

Bertolini, J., & Pelucio, M. (1995). The red eye. *Emergency Medicine Clinics of North America, 13*(3), 561–578.

Bloom, P. A., Leeming, J. P., Power, W., Laidlaw, D. A., Collum, L. M., & Easty, D. L. (1994). Topical ciprofloxacin in the treatment of blepharitis and blepharoconjunctivitis. *European Journal of Ophthalmology, 4*(1), 6–12.

Chapman, J., Cheeks, L., & Green, K. (1990). Interactions of benzalkonium chloride with soft and hard contact lenses. *Archives of Ophthalmology, 108*(2), 244–246.

Crouch, E., & Berger, A. (1995). Ophthalmology. In R. E. Rakel (Ed.), *Textbook of family practice* (pp. 1345–1379). Philadelphia: W. B. Saunders.

Diegel, J. T. (1986). Eyelid problems: Blepharitis, hordeola, and chalazia. *Postgraduate Medicine, 80*(2), 271–272.

DeGrezia, M., & Robinson, M. (2001). Opthalmic manifestations of HIV: An update. *Journal of the Association of Nurses in AIDS Care, 12*(3), 22–32.

Dreyer, A. (1996). In E. Herfindal & D. Gourley (Eds.), *Textbook of therapeutics: Drug and disease management* (6th ed.; pp. 437–450). Baltimore: Williams & Wilkins.

Drug and Therapy Perspectives. (2001) Range of topically active medications for treatment of glaucoma may reduce the need for surgery. *Adis International Limited.* 17 (10) 5–10. Retrieved 3/16/02 from www.medscape.com./viewarticle/4046499.

Dunn, J. P., & Nozik, R. A. (1994). Uveitis: Role of the physician in treating systemic causes. *Geriatrics, 49*(8), 27–32.

FDA News. (2001, March 16). FDA approves two new interocular pressure lowering drugs for the management of glaucoma. Department of Health and Human Services 101–08. Retrieved 3-16-02 from http://www.fda.gov/bbs/topics/NEWS/ 2001

Flynn, A., Damico, F., & Smith, G. (1998) Should we patch corneal abrasions? A meta-analysis. *Journal of Family Practice,* 47(4), 264–270. Retrieved 3/16/02 from http://205.3=232.111.21/bin/rdas.dlll.

Gelvin, J. (1994). Co-management of patients with glaucoma. *Optometry Clinics, 4*(2), 81–100.

Goldberg, I. (2001). Worldwide issues in glaucoma research. *American Academy of Opthalmology.* 2001 Annual Meeting. Retrieved May 11, 2002 from http://medscape.com/ viewartcle/420835.

Gordon III, K. (2001, May/June). Iritis and uveitis. *eMedicine Journal, 2* (7). Retrieved May 12, 2002 from http://www.emedicine.com/emerg/topic284.htm

Gwon, A. (1992). Ofloxacin vs tobramycin for the treatment of external ocular infection. *Archives of Ophthalmology, 110*(9), 1234–1237.

Jampel, H. (1995). Patching for corneal abrasions. *JAMA, 272*(19), 1504.

Knox, K., & McIntee, J. (1995). Nurse management of corneal abrasion. *British Journal of Nursing, 4*(8), 440–442, 459–460.

LeSage, N., Verreault, R., Rochette, L. (2001). Efficacy of eye patching for traumatic corneal abrasions: a controlled trial. *Annals of Emergency Medicine,* 38(2), 129–134.

Lietman, T., & Whitcher, J. P. (1999). Chlamydial conjunctivitis. *Opthalmology Clinics of North America, 12*(1), 21–32.

Long, K., & Long, R. (1994). Treating open-angle glaucoma. *Nurse Practitioner Forum, 5*(4), 205–206.

McClusky, P,. Fowler, H., & Lightman, S. (2000). Management of chronic uveitis. *British Medical Journal, 300,* 555–558.

Miller, I., Vogel, R., Cook, T., & Wittreich, J. (1992). Topically administered norfloxacin compared with topically administered gentamicin for the treatment of external ocular bacterial infections. *American Journal of Ophthalmology, 113*(6), 638–644.

Nolan, W. (2002). Irdectomy and iridotomy for treating narrow angles and preventing primary angle-closure glaucoma. *The Cochrane Review* (1). Retrieved March 2, 2002 form the Cochrane Library http://205.232.111.21/bin.rdas.dll.

Raskin, E., Speaker, M., & Laibson, P. (1992). Blepharitis. *Infectious Disease Clinics of North America, 6*(4), 777–787.

Rosenberg, L. (1995). Glaucoma: Early detection and therapy for prevention of vision loss. *American Family Physician, 52*(8), 2289–2298.

Sheikh, A., Hurwitz, B., & Cave, J. (2002). Antibiotics versus placebo for acute bacterial conjunctivitis. *The Cochrane Review* (1), Oxford: update software. Retrieved March 16, 2002 from the Cochrane Library http://205.232.111.21/bin.rdas/dll.

Shields, S. R. (2000). Managing eye disease in primary care, part 1-3. *Postgraduate Medicine,* 108 (5), 69–134.

Silverman, M. A., & Bessman, E. (2001). Conjunctivitis. *eMedicine, 5*(2). Retrieved March 30, 2002 from http://www.emedicine.com/ermerg/topic110.htm.

Smith, R., & Flowers, C., Jr. (1995). Chronic blepharitis: A review. *CLAO Journal, 21*(3), 200–206.

Stoss, M., Michels, C., Beutke, R., & Gorter, R.W. (2000) Prospectives cohort trial of euphrasia single-dose eye drops in conjunctivitis. *Journal of Alternative and Complementary Medicine,* 6 (6), 499–508.

Tucker, J. (1993). Screening for open-angle glaucoma. *American Family Physician, 48*(1), 75–80.

Uphold, C., & Graham, M. (1994). *Clinical guidelines in family practice.* Gainsville, FL: Barmarrae Books.

Wittpenn, J. (1995). EyeScrub: Simplifying the management of blepharitis. *Journal of Ophthalmic Nursing and Technology, 14*(1), 25–28.

CHAPTER ❖ **24**

EAR DISORDERS

Jeanette F. Kissinger ◆ Kathleen J. Sawin

Ear conditions are some of the most frequently occurring problems treated in primary care, especially among infants and children. This chapter reviews the treatment of selected ear conditions across the age span: acute otitis media, otitis media with effusion (serous otitis media), otitis externa, labrynthitis, and perforated tympanic membrane.

The Agency for Health Care Policy and Research (AHCPR) guidelines on otitis media (Stool et al., 1994), after a comprehensive meta-analysis of the literature, generated the following definitions of these selected types of otitis:

- *Acute otitis media* (AOM) is inflammation of the middle ear with signs or symptoms of middle ear infection.
- *Otitis media with effusion* (OME) is fluid in the middle ear without signs or symptoms of infection.
- *Persistent acute otitis media* (PAOM) is middle ear inflammation with signs of infection that do not resolve after initial treatment.
- *Otitis externa* (OE) is inflammation of the external auditory canal.
- *Perforated tympanic membrane* (PTM) is alteration of the integrity of the tympanic membrane caused by internal pressure or external trauma.

OTITIS MEDIA

Otitis media (inflammation of the middle ear) encompasses a number of clinical conditions with a variety of names. The National Center for Health Statistics and others (Schappert, 1992; Teele, Klein, Rosen, & The Greater Boston Media Study Groups, 1983) indicate that otitis media (OM) is the most frequent primary care illness diagnosed in infants and children younger than 15 years of age, accounting for 24.5 million visits in 1990 alone. Over 90% of children experience an episode of AOM before age 2. By the age of 3, approximately 80% of children have been diagnosed with otitis media, with 40% having had three or more infections (Richer & Lebel, 1997; Miser, 2001). In most developed countries, the leading cause of antibiotic use in children is the treatment of AOM (Johnson & Belman, 2001). In the United States and Australia, antibiotic use is 98%; in the Netherlands it is 31% (Glasziou, Del Mar, Hayem, & Sanders, 2000). In a study by Block, Hedrick, Kratzer, Nemeth, and Tack (2000), causative organisms for AOM were identified by tympanocentesis. Of the 134 pathogens isolated from a sample of 125 children aged 6 months through 12 years, 51.5% were *Streptococcus pneumonia,* 32.8% were *Haemophilus influenza,* beta-lactamase-positive in 18 of 44 strains; 11.2% were beta-lactamase–positive *Moraxella catarrhalis* and 4.5% were *Streptococcus pyogenes. S. pneumonia* is the most predominant pathogen causing AOM, estimated at 7 million cases annually in the United States (Pichichero, Reiner, Brook, Gooch, Yamauchi, Jenkins, & Sher, 2000a). Resistance of these bacteria to commonly used antibiotics is a growing concern (see discussion under Selecting Appropriate Agents below). The Union of Concerned Scientists (USC), in their support of HR3804 (Preservation of Antibiotics for Human Treatment Act of 2002), state that over half of all

U.S. antibiotic production is fed each year to healthy chickens, pigs, and cows. This greatly contributes to the problem of resistance (Mellon, Letter, USC, June 3, 2002). It is estimated that in 8–25% of cases of OM, viruses such as influenza A virus, respiratory syncytial virus, and coxsackievirus may be implicated (Johnson & Belman, 2001).

Certain populations seem to be at greater risk for otitis media. HIV-infected children with decreased T4 lymphocytes, in the first 3 years of life, have a threefold increase in risk for recurrent OM infection. Children under the age of 2 are more likely to have resistant organisms, as are those with recurrent (rAOM) or persistent AOM, which occurs in 20 to 30% of the pediatric population (Pichichero, 2000b). The clinical course of AOM over the past few decades has shown that serious complications such as mastoiditis have nearly disappeared. There are more recurrent middle ear infections and prolonged silent effusions instead (Joki-Erkkila, Pukander, & Laippala, 2000). Pichichero et al. (2000a) suggest that first-line therapy for prevention of rAOM should be removing risk factors that are modifiable. They suggest following the guidelines set forth by the Committee on Immunization Practice of the Centers for Disease Control and Prevention for influenza vaccine for those children whose rAOM is always worse during flu season. The pneumococcal conjugate vaccine should be given to children before year one and best before the second OM in order to prevent recurrent otitis media (Research Briefs, 2003).

SPECIFIC CONSIDERATIONS FOR PHARMACOTHERAPY

When Drug Therapy Is Needed

The recent guidelines developed by the American Academy of Pediatrics (AAP) and American Academy of Family Physicians (AAFP) in 2004 include the following:

> Observation without use of antibacterial agents in a child over 6 months with uncomplicated AOM is an option for selected children based on diagnostic certainty, age, illness severity, and assurance of follow-up. Observation is appropriate only when followup can be ensured and antibacterial agents started if systems persist or worsen.
>
> If the patient fails to respond to the initial management option within 48 to 72 hours, the clinician must reassess the patient to confirm AOM and exclude other causes of illness. If AOM is confirmed in the patient initially managed with observation, the clinician should begin antibacterial therapy. If the patient was initially managed with antibacterial agent(s), the clinician should change the antibacterial agent(s).

Several studies support the guidelines. Some data suggest that use of antibiotics for AOM in children provides only a small benefit. The Evidence Report on Management of Acute OM, conducted by the Agency for Healthcare Research and Quality (AHRQ) (2000), cites studies finding resolution of AOM, without antibiotic treatment, from 92.3% at 24 to 48 hours and 74% at 24 to 72 hours. The pooled estimate was 81.1% for resolution in 1 to 7 days. Glasziou et al.'s (2000) review of randomized trials of antibiotic versus placebo in children with AOM, a total of 2202 children, found no reduction in pain in 24 hours and only a 28% reduction in pain at 2 to 7 days. Approximately 80% of the children without antibiotic treatment had resolved the AOM spontaneously. They suggested that antibiotic use may provide a reduction of risk of mastoiditis in populations where it is more prevalent. Damoiseaux, van Balen, Hoes, Verheij, and de Milker (2000), from a study of 240 children aged 6 months to 2 years with AOM, found no differences in otoscopic and tympanometric outcomes between the amoxicillin and placebo group. They concluded that the small amount of antibiotic benefit did not justify prescribing antibiotics at the initial visit. In the algorithm for treatment of children 1 to 3 years of age with OME, antibiotic treatment is an option at initial diagnosis, at six weeks, and at a three-month followup. Observation and hearing evaluation are also an option. Decongestants and antihistamines are not supported in the treatment of this condition in any age population (Richer & LeBel, 1997, p. 2023; Stool et al., 1994). If OME persists after three months, especially with hearing loss, aggressive treatment is indicated (Stool et al., 1994; Terris, Magit, & Davidson, 1995). The guidelines recommend that healthcare providers need to inform patients fully as to the side effects and costs of antibiotic therapy as well as the benefits and harms of other options for care.

Not only are OTC cold remedies ineffective against AOM, but the use of intranasal sprays may increase the probability of AOM following an upper respiratory infection (Glasziou, Del Mar, Hayem, et al., 2002).

Short-Term and Long-Term Goals of Pharmacotherapy

The short-term goal of treatment for AOM is to resolve the infection in the middle ear and to restore normal, painless hearing. This is in contrast to OME treatment for which the short-term goal is to eliminate fluid in the middle ear and restore normal hearing. The short-term goal of treatment of OE is to resolve the local inflammation of the ear canal and prevent the extension of the inflammation to the pinna. AOM can be accompanied by OME, but OME can occur without AOM.

Long-term goals of treatment for AOM include prevention of recurrent episodes, intracranial complications (Munz, Farmer, Auger, O'Gorman, & Schloss, 1992), and hearing loss and the resulting speech, language, and cognitive developmental delays (Terris et al., 1995). The long-term goal of treating OME is principally the prevention of hearing loss and the resulting speech, language, and cognitive developmental delays (Terris et al., 1995). Although the causal relationship between sensorineural hearing loss and language is well established, a causal relationship between conductive hearing loss with OME and subsequent language and speech delays has not been established (Berman, 1995). The AHCPR panel did find a weak relationship between OME and abnormal speech and language development in children under 4 and a weak relationship between OME and expressive language, behavior, and development in children over 4. Golz, as reported in Clinical Capsules of Family Practice News (2003), studied 80 children (40 of each gender) aged 6.5 to 8 years old who had recurrent AOM and prolonged OME during the first five years of life. He found a significant deficit in reading ability when compared to a control group of healthy children, The lack of clarity regarding the role of OME in these delays contributes to the variability in treatment options. In each of the conditions of the middle ear, the goals of treatment are frequently achieved by antibiotic treatment. This discussion is aimed at the treatment of otherwise healthy patients with no craniofacial or neurologic abnormalities or sensory deficits. Another emerging, potentially preventive measure, that was the focus of a large randomized placebo-controlled trial, is the use of a bacterial nasal spray which replenishes alpha streptococci. It is thought that the a. Streptococci interfere with the common middle ear pathogens (Roos, Hakansson & Holm, 2001). See Table 24–1 for nonpharmacologic therapy and prevention for OME and OM.

TABLE 24–1. Nonpharmacologic Therapy and Prevention for OME and OM

Tympanostomy tubes	Change of day-care setting
Adenoidectomy	Breastfeeding until 6 months
Tonsillectomy	Avoiding supine bottle feeding
Equilibrating pressure techniques	Avoiding passive smoke

Source: AAP/AAFP (2004); Linder et al. (1997)

Time Frame for Initiating Pharmacotherapy

At the time of treatment AOM should be treated in the child under 6 months; children 6 months to 2 years with a certain diagnosis; or children over 6 months if severe illness. If AOM and non-severe illness is present, then observation is an option. If AOM treatment is initiated, a full course of antibiotics should be used. In both treated and observed children the families should be instructed to return for evaluation if the child is not substantially improved in 48–72 hours (AAP & AAFP, 2004). Follow-up of all cases of AOM needs to be scheduled in two or three weeks. The timing of OME treatment is complicated particularly in children and involves the possibility of antimicrobial treatment at one of several decision points (Stool et al., 1994). There is evidence that spontaneous resolution occurs for many children under age 3 with asymptomatic OME (Zeisel et al., 1995). (See Drug Table 102.)

ASSESSMENT AND HISTORY

A history of pain, fever, prior episodes of AOM and/or OME, upper respiratory infection (UR), hearing difficulties, speech delays, exposure to passive smoking, placement in a childcare center, and packs per year smoked by teenagers and adults are important aspects of the history of AOM. OME can be asymptomatic and highly prevalent in children under 2 in group daycare settings (Zeisel et al., 1995). The hallmark of AOM is acute inflamed tympanic membrane (TM) and middle ear infection. Changes in the landmarks and/or diminished landmarks secondary to a bulging TM may also be present. The clinician has to be alert to the possibility that a red TM when a child is actively crying may be a normal response and not an indicator of AOM. A pneumatic otoscope can be used to test the mobility of the TM, which is reduced when exudate or fluid collects behind it. However, pneumatic otoscope evaluation is not necessary when it is evident that the TM is inflamed and bulging. Forced movement of the TM would only cause unnecessary pain to the patient. A pneumatic evaluation requires that the examiner obtain a tight seal. In many adults and some children, using a ear speculum with a specifically designed cuff will aid in achieving an airtight seal.

Fluid behind the TM without signs of inflammation is the hallmark of OME. Bubbles or a fluid line may be seen, or the short process of the umbo can be prominent if the drum is retracted. Pneumatic otoscope evaluation is preferable to otoscope evaluation alone whenever OME is suspected (Belkengren & Sapala, 1995). A tympanogram, when available, can quantify the mobility of the TM and can be a valuable tool in accurately assessing response to treatment.

It is common for AOM to occur concomitantly with other infections such as viral URI, pharyngitis, sinusitis, and influenza. Ear pain may occur without AOM or OME from a source other than the ear. Complications from AOM may include meningitis, lateral sinus thrombosis, and chronic suppurative otitis media, as well as hearing loss and possible speech delay. Labrynthitis can be a complication of acute or chronic otitis media, and is often overlooked in children (Sun, Parnes, & Freeman, 1996).

Patient/Caregiver Information

Use of a pacifier by children under 2 years of age in daycare centers increases AOM risk 1.6 times, and for children 2 to 3 years old, the risk increases 2.9 times. One study by Niemela, Uhari, and Mottonen (1995) failed to show a strong association between AOM and breast-feeding, parental smoking, thumb sucking, use of a bottle, or social class. The panel of experts who developed the AHCPR guidelines found that while bottle-feeding and placement in childcare are associated with increased incidence of OME, removal from childcare facilities does not decrease incidence (Stevenson & Brooke, 1995; Stool et al., 1994).

The absorption of some newer broad-spectrum antibiotics that are prodrug esters, such as cefpodoxime proxetil (Vantin) or cefuroxime axetil (Ceftin), requires metabolism to become an active agent. Thus, their absorption is enhanced when given with food (Gerchufsky, 1995).

There is some evidence that children in daycare who have been given a flu shot have decreased incidence of AOM and OME during the flu season (Clements, Langdon, Bland, & Walter, 1995). If prednisone (a corticosteroid) is used for children, the tablets can be crushed and added to jelly to make the bitter taste more palatable (Berman, 1995). A common practice, meant to reduce ear pain, is to instill warm olive oil in the affected ear. In a comparative study, Hoberman, Paradise, Reynolds, and Urkin (1997) found that Auralgan provided greater pain relief within 30 minutes.

In a small but important study of nurse practitioner (NP) outcomes when treating OM, Matas, Brown, and Holman (1996) found the NP very effective. Parents reported 93% achieved completion of the medication regime. However, parents and providers can have different perceptions about information shared in a healthcare visit for AOM. Even when teaching is documented in the chart, parents may not hear or may not perceive getting important information about the care of their child. Healthcare providers need to develop multiple strategies to share critical information such as the rationale for completing the antibiotic course of treatment and the need for followup and behavioral changes helpful for prevention of future episodes of OM.

OUTCOMES MANAGEMENT

Selecting an Appropriate Agent

Antibiotics are the mainstay of therapy for the treatment of acute otitis media, although disagreement exists as to which agent(s) should be first-line. Selection of an agent to treat AOM requires consideration of factors such as the patient's age, OM history, drug hypersensitivity, prior antimicrobial response, and associated illness. Drug therapy should be active against the common middle ear pathogens (including *S. pneumoniae, H. influenzae,* and *M. catarrhalis*).

Amoxicillin is recommended by the AAP/AAFP guidelines as the drug of choice for most children. The dose should be 80–90 mg/kg/day (AAP & AAFP, 2004). The other antimicrobials are considered second-line for patients with persistent or recurrent AOM, for patients in other high-risk groups, or for special situations. There is no evidence for children free from AOM symptoms after the initial course of antibiotic treatment that further treatment results in faster resolution of effusion (Mandel, Casselbrant, Rockette, Bluestone, & Kurs-Lasky, 1995).

Of growing concern is the increase of resistant strains of *S. pneumoniae* and *H. influenzae* in Europe and in areas of the United States. This has led to treatment failures with such commonly used antimicrobials as TMP-SMX, beta-lactams, and macrolides. Clinicians should be aware of the resistance patterns in their communities and prescribe accordingly.

Many agents are effective against beta-lactamase–producing strains of *H. influenzae* and *M. catarrhalis.* See the in vitro spectrum of activity of antibiotics used in upper respiratory tract infections shown in Table 24–2.

Some older antibiotics that have poor activity against *H. influenzae* (erythromycin, penicillin, and first-generation cephalosporins) should not be used to treat AOM. Sulfonamides alone are not effective because of poor activity against pneumococcus and group A streptococcus. In penicillin-allergic patients, TMP-SMX or erythromycin-sulfisoxazole (EES-SSX) are reasonable choices. These drugs should be avoided in patients with known sulfonamide allergies.

Infants younger than 4 to 6 weeks of age are likely to be infected with *Staphylococcus aureus* and gram-nega-

TABLE 24–2. In Vitro Spectrum of Activity of Antibiotics used in Upper Respiratory Tract Infections

Antibiotic	Streptococcus pneumoniae	*Haemophilus influenzae* Beta-Lactamase Negative	*Haemophilus influenzae* Beta-Lactamase Positive	*Moraxella catarrhalis* Beta-Lactamase Negative	*Moraxella catarrhalis* Beta-Lactamase Positive	Group A Beta-Hemolytic Streptococci
Ampicillin or amoxicillin	+	+	−	+	−	+
Azithromycin	+	+	+	+	+	+
Ceftriaxone	+	+	+	+	+	+
Clarithromycin	+	+	+	+	+	+
Erythromycin	+	−	−	+	−	+
Erythromycin-sulfisoxazole	+	+	+	+	+	+
Trimethoprim-sulfamethoxazole	+	+	+	+	+	−
Amoxicillin-clavulanate	+	+	+	+	+	+
Cefaclor	+	+	±	+	+	+
Cefixime	+	+	+	+	+	+
Cefpodoxime proxetil	+	+	+	+	+	+
Cefprozil	+	+	+	+	+	+
Cefuroxime axetil	+	+	+	+	+	+
Loracarbef	+	+	+	+	+	+

+ = organism highly susceptible to antibiotic; ± = moderately susceptible to antibiotic; − = nonsusceptible to antibiotic.

Source: DiPiro et al. (1997)

tive enteric bacilli. These infants often need to be hospitalized for evaluation of systemic infection and generally require parenteral antibiotics for initial therapy (Canafax & Geibink, 1994). Infants younger than 6 months may be infected with *Chlamydia trachomatis* since it is a common cause of acute respiratory infections in that age group (Klein, 1995). The treatment of meningogenic labrynthitis complicating acute or chronic otitis media is most effectively achieved by cephalosporins. Of the cephalosporins, there is evidence that ceftazidime may be the optimum choice (Sun, Parnes, & Freeman, 1995, 1996).

Amoxicillin versus amoxicillin-clavulanate for first-line therapy. Many practitioners are tempted to start a patient on amoxicillin-clavulanate for first-line therapy since it is "broader-spectrum" than amoxicillin. This raises concern for a number of reasons. First, the amoxicillin-clavulanate is more expensive and likely to cause more adverse gastrointestinal effects than amoxicillin. Second, overuse of drugs like amoxicillin-clavulanate contributes to the growing problems of bacterial resistance. It is estimated that approximately 30% and 10% of cases of otitis media are due to *H. influenzae* and *M. catarrhalis,* respectively. If 30% of *H. influenza* and 90% of *M. catarrhalis* are beta-lactamase–producing, then 16% of cases of AOM are due to beta-lactamase–producing strains. It is clear that the incidence of resistance is not high enough to warrant abandonment of amoxicillin as first-line therapy (Klein, 1995). The caveat is that if a patient does not improve within 48 to 72 h, switching therapy from amoxicillin is reasonable. *Please note:* Some antibiotics may not be approved for use in certain age groups. Refer to Drug Table 102 for specific information.

Alternative initial therapies. Amoxicillin-clavulanate failure has been related to nontypable *H. influenzae,* history of previous episodes, gender (boys), and race (nonwhite) in a study of 99 children, mean age 21.4 months. This study found no relationship between compliance and drug failure (Patel et al., 1995). The use of broad-spectrum antibiotics as a first-line therapy should be deferred except for patients who have three or more previous episodes of AOM, who have polymicrobial infections (Patel et al., 1995), who are in conditions or situations that preclude sequential dosing for multiple days, who have not responded previously to amoxicillin, or who are considering air travel within the next three days. In addition, regional antimicrobial susceptibility may influence the clinician's decision (Canafax & Geibink, 1994). In these cases several options may be considered. Traditional dosing of a broader-spectrum antibiotic (i.e., Ceclor t.i.d. 10 to 14 days), use of a broader-spectrum antibiotic with less frequent dosing (i.e., Suprax given once daily for 10 days), or the use of nontraditional dosing of some agents has been shown to be safe and effective.

Recent studies of nontraditional dosing have supported the use of the following:

- A one-time intramuscular injection of ceftriaxone (50 mg/kg) in children 5 months to 5 years with uncomplicated AOM (Ceftriaxone and otitis, 2000).

- A 5-day treatment with cefpodoxime proxetil (8 mg/kg per day) for children 5 months to 12 years old (Cohen, 1995).
- A daily dose of azithromycin, 10 mg/kg per day for 3 days in children 6 months to 12 years (Daniel, 1993; Principi, 1995), faster resolution of symptoms was reported with azithromycin use in both studies. A single dose of azithromycin (30 mg/kg) is as effective as a 5 day regime (Dunne, 2003).
- A 5-day course of cefuroxime axetil in uncomplicated AOM (Adam, 2000).
- A 5-day course of cefdinir, 14 mg/kg/day divided b.i.d., in pediatric AOM was as clinically effective as a ten-day course of cefprozil 30 mg/kg/day divided b.i.d. (Block et al., 2000).

Cefpodoxime proxetil was found to be one of the most active compounds against *H. influenzae* and *S. pneumoniae.* Children who are very ill, who have recently been hospitalized, who have already had antibiotic treatment, who have had known exposure to resistant pneumococci, or who have an immunodeficiency are candidates for initial treatment with second-line agents. There is also some evidence that ibuprofen alters the disease pathogenesis of AOM. When given with an antimicrobial agent, the incidence of effusion and the degree of mucosal thickness at day 10 is less (Diven, Evans, Swarts, Burckart, & Doyle, 1995). For recurrent or refractory AOM, the Centers for Disease Control and Prevention recommend: (1) amoxicillin/clavulanate in combination with amoxicillin (80 to 90 mg/kg/day); (2) cefuroxime axetil (30 mg/kg/day); and (3) ceftriaxone (up to 3 injections for optimal clinical success) (Pichichero, 2000b).

In most cases OME resolves spontaneously within three months. The AHCPR guidelines discuss treatment of uncomplicated OME in children under 3 by the use of observation or antibiotic therapy, but recommend environmental risk factor control counseling for all. The use of antibiotics at the initial diagnosis only achieved 16% increased resolution of the OME. If the patient still has OME three months after diagnosis, by pneumatic otoscopy and tympanometry, the patient needs to be referred for hearing evaluation. The algorithm developed by AHCPR tracks each decision point and the considerations for antibiotics at several stages. Presence of speech and/or hearing problems in children may accelerate the treatment plan (Stool et al., 1994). An alternative interpretation of the meta-analysis of OME treatment suggests a third option for treatment: an antibiotic plus a corticosteroid. Limited data suggest this combination is significantly more effective than an antibiotic alone. However, if this option is used, it is critical to assess the exposure of the child to varicella. Children who have been exposed within the last month should not be treated with steroids due to risk of disseminated disease (Berman, 1995).

When the clinician determines that OME needs to be treated with antibiotics, the same parameters used to identify the drug of choice for AOM can generally be used to determine the drug of choice for OME. There is no evidence that antihistamines or decongestants are effective in treatment of OME in children (Stevenson & Brooke, 1995). However, they are frequently used in adults to control symptoms of URI. Their effect on prevention or treatment of OME is unknown.

Monitoring for Efficacy

A typical course of treatment for AOM is 10 to 14 days for children less than 2 years of age. Signs and symptoms should improve within 48 to 72 h. Common reasons for lack of improvement include noncompliance, adverse effects, short duration of therapy, or the presence of resistant organisms. These factors should be taken into account before switching to another agent. The guidelines indicate that if no improvement is seen within 48–72 h, switching to an agent with a broader spectrum of activity, such as ceclor or cefuroxime, is appropriate.

When there is still no improvement, some clinicians suggest a culture of the middle ear effusion by tympanocentesis to guide antimicrobial selection. Antimicrobial prophylaxis may be reasonable in patients who have a clearing of the middle ear effusion between episodes.

If there is recurrence within one month of the initial episode, the clinician can assume the same organisms caused the infection. However, resistance to initial therapy can also be assumed and a second-line antibiotic should be prescribed. However, if the recurrence occurs more than one month following the initial episode in a child free of symptoms, the same treatment can be repeated. If children have more than four episodes of AOM in six months or six episodes in twelve months, prophylaxis treatment should be considered (Richer & LeBel, 1997).

There is some evidence that recurrent infections can be prevented by daily use of either amoxicillin 20 mg/kg daily or sulfisoxazole 75 mg/kg per day for 3 to 6 months (Berman, 1995). Prophylaxis with azithromycin was found to equal amoxicillin in preventing recurrent AOM (De Diego et al., 2001). However, Goldstein and Sculerati (1994) found that only 46% of the patients they studied claimed compliance with this regimen. It would be important to monitor the status of children on this regimen for recurrent infections. Qualitative investigations may be helpful in understanding the experience of maintaining a preventive antimicrobial regimen in families and identifying the barriers to consistent achievement of prophylactic treatment.

Surgical treatment with placement of ear tubes is considered in patients who continue to have middle ear infections despite prophylactic treatment (Berman, 1995). In a study of 429 children less than 3 years of age, with persistent OME, Paradise, Dollaghan, Campbell et al. (2003) found the insertion of tympanostomy tubes did not improve cognitive, language, speech or psychosocial development. Most healthy children will outgrow OM by the age of 6 or 7 years.

Monitoring for Toxicity

Data support up to 30% incidence of diarrhea in children with antibiotic treatment of AOM. Skin care and fluid replacement strategies need to be reviewed (Mitchell, Van, Mason, Norris, & Pickering, 1996). In addition, spacing of medication evenly throughout the day may decrease the incidence of diarrhea.

Some antimicrobials may aggravate gastrointestinal symptoms that may already be present in an ill patient. These drugs include amoxicillin-clavulanate, EES-SSX, cefuroxime axetil, and cefixime. Side effects such as skin rash, diarrhea, and nonspecific gastrointestinal complaints are reported in as many as 20% of patients. These effects are thought to be due to an associated viral infection. General guidelines suggest that if the symptoms are severe or the rash urticarial, further use of the drug should be avoided.

Followup

A followup evaluation for AOM is recommend within one to two weeks of completing a course of therapy. In OM with effusion, followup will depend on the plan the provider has chosen.

OTITIS EXTERNA

The incidence of otitis externa (swimmer's ear) is higher in the summer months but overall incidence is unknown. This infection is usually bacterial, commonly caused by *Pseudomonas aeruginosa* and *S. aureus,* although occasionally fungus may be involved. When otitis externa (OE) is very localized, it is usually due to an infected hair follicle in the external canal. OE is termed malignant or necrotizing when it extends into the soft and bony tissues surrounding the ear canal. This condition has been classically seen in diabetic and immunosupressed patients.

SPECIFIC CONSIDERATIONS FOR PHARMACOTHERAPY

When Drug Therapy Is Needed

The identified organisms usually require topical antibiotic treatment or antifungal treatment. The short-term goal is resolution of pain, inflammation, and edema with the restoration of normal hearing. In recurrent OE, the goal is prevention of repeat episodes and prevention of extension to periauricular tissue.

Nonpharmacologic Therapy

Use of preventive ear plugs and swimming caps is common but of unknown value. There is no known nonpharmacologic treatment of the disease. If the condition is secondary to a furuncle, an adjunct treatment can be the application of heat.

Time Frame for Initiating Pharmacotherapy

Treatment should be initiated at the time of diagnosis. The medication should be continued for one week (Hoole, Pickard, Ouimette, Lohr, & Greenberg, 1995). If this is a recurrent infection, the medication should be continued for ten to fourteen days after cessation of symptoms. (See Drug Tables 102 and 402.)

Assessment Needed Prior to Therapy

Otitis externa is suggested by a history of pain on movement of the external ear and decreased unilateral hearing on the affected side; it is confirmed by visualization of the canal with an otoscope. Exudate, inflammation, or narrowing of the canal secondary to edema is usually present. Occasionally otorrhea is present. Pain can be reproduced by manipulation of the pinna and pressure on the tragus. If systemic symptoms such as fever, joint pain, paresis, or palsy are present, a complete neurologic exam is indicated.

Ask the patient if he or she was swimming. Even when swimming in waters that have passed environmental standards, OE still occurs. Persons with recurrent OE should take precautions. No controlled studies were found, but current clinical practice is to use two to three drops of a 1:1 solution of white vinegar and 70% ethyl alcohol in the ear canal before and after swimming (Hay,

Groothuis, Hayward, & Levin, 1995,). Swimming should be avoided during the acute phase. If on the otoscope examination the TM is clearly abnormal with no landmarks visualized and an apparent hole, or if a portion of the TM is missing, a diagnosis of perforated TM exists. If the TM looks somewhat abnormal and there is a question about a localized perforation in a child, a pneumatic otoscope can be used to clarify the diagnosis. A drum that moves, even slightly, cannot be perforated.

Assessment for malignant otitis externa includes a thorough history that may be characterized by persistent ear pain following treatment for OE in individuals with a compromised immune system. Increased drainage and/or odor or visible growth in the canal is frequently present. In addition, the clinician needs to assess the cranial nerves. Extensive cranial nerve paresis may be present (Boringa, Hoekstra, Roos, & Bertelsmann, 1995).

Patient/Caregiver Information

When the ear canal is very edematous, the insertion of a wick, on which the treatment solution is dropped, is effective in distributing the medication in the canal. The wick will spontaneously drop out of the canal when the edema resolves. The patient then drops the medication directly into the ear canal for the remainder of the treatment regime.

OUTCOMES MANAGEMENT

Selecting an Appropriate Agent

OE treatment is usually local and consists of Cortisporin otic solution four drops four times a day for adults and three drops four times a day for children. If perforation is suspected, Cortisporin otic suspension needs to be used. In addition, the canal needs to be kept dry and protected from the wind. There is no evidence to support the addition of oral antibiotics to the topical treatment in mild to moderate OE (Hannley, Denneny, & Holzer, 2000). If the TM perforation coexists with AOM, oral antibiotics need to be included in the plan.

Some alternative drugs have been found to be helpful: 2% acetic acid in propylene glycol (VoSol or VoSolH) has been found to be an effective alternative for uncomplicated OE (Mengel & Schwiebert, 1993). When OE is accompanied by a chronic suppurative OM, Supiyaphun, Tonsakulrungruang, Chochaipanichnon, Chongtateong, and Samart (1995) recommend the use of 0.3% ofloxacin otic solution for two weeks. Drugs recommended for malignant OE are the cephalosporins, penicillins, and aminoglycosides for a prolonged duration. Although initial assessment and treatment of malignant OE is appropriate for the primary care provider, referral to the appropriate specialist is recommended. Clinicians should use the Evidence Report/Technology Assessment (AHRQ, 2000) and its updates as their primary source regarding clinical guidelines, performance measures, and the most efficacious treatment of ear disorders.

Monitoring for Efficacy

If the OE does not respond to medication within 48 hours, a fungal organism needs to be considered. Nystatin otic solution is the choice if the clinician suspects a fungal causation. If symptoms are not resolved in seven days, referral to your collaborating physician is recommended. If normal hearing is not restored, referral to an ENT specialist is indicated.

Monitoring for Toxicity

Toxicity of topical treatment is unusual. If there is any increase in drainage/odor or urticaria, the drug should be discontinued. In cases of malignant OE, refer immediately to a specialist for consideration of a gallium scan and hospitalization for treatment (Boringa et al., 1995). Follow-up is generally not needed if symptoms resolve.

REFERENCES

Adam, D. (2000). Short-course antibiotic therapy for infections with a single causative pathogen. *Journal of International Medical Research, 28* Suppl. 1:13A-24A.

Agency for Healthcare Quality and Research. (2000). Management of acute otitis media. Summary, Evidence Report/Technology Assessment: Number 15, June. Rockville, MD *www.ahrq.gov/clinic/epcsums/otitisum.htm.*

American Academy of Pediatrics (AAP) and the American Academy of Family Physicians (AAFP). (2004). Clinical Practice Guidelines: Diagnosis and management of acute otitis media. Retrieved April 4, 2004 at: *http://www.aap.org/policy/aomfinal.pdf*

Belkengren, R, & Sapala, S. (1995). Pediatric management problems. *Pediatric Nursing, 21* (3), 304–305.

Berman, S. (1995). Otitis media in children. *New England Journal of Medicine, 332* (23), 1560–1565.

Block, S. L., Kratzer, J., Nemeth, M. A. & Tack, K. J. (2000). Five-day cefdinir course vs. ten-day cefprozil course for treatment of acute otitis media. *Pediatric Infectious Disease Journal, 19*(12 Suppl):S147–52.

Boringa, J. B., Hoekstra, O. S., Roos, J. W., & Bertelsmann, F. W. (1995). Multiple cranial nerve palsy after otitis externa: A case report. *Clinics of Neurology and Neurosurgery, 97* (4), 332–335.

Canafax, D. M., & Geibink, G. (1994). Antimicrobial treatment of otitis media. *Annals of Otology, Rhinology and Laryngology, 103,* 11–14.

Ceftriaxone and otitis in children: new indication. Only in special circumstances. (2000). *Prescrire International, 9*(48): 99–102.

Clements, D. A., Langdon, L., Bland, C., & Walter, E. (1995). Influenza A vaccine decreases the incidence of otitis media in 6 to 30 month old children in day care. *Archives of Pediatric Adolescent Medicine, 149,* 1113–1117.

Clinical Capsules. (2003). Otitis media and reading ability. *Family Practice News,* Dec. 15, 33 (24) 38.

Cohen, R. (1995). Clinical experience with cefpodoxime proxetil in acute otitis media. *Pediatric Infectious Disease Journal, 14* (4 Suppl.), S12–18.

Damoiseaux, R. A., van Balen, F. A., Hoes, A. W., Verheij, T. J. & de Melker, R. A. (2000). Primary care based randomised, double blind trial of amoxicillin versus placebo for acute otitis media in children aged under 2 years. *BMJ, 320* (7231):350–4.

Daniel, R. R. (1993). Comparison of azithromycin and co-amoxiclav in the treatment of otitis media in children. *Journal of Antimicrobial Chemotherapy, 31* (Suppl. E), 65–71.

De Diego, J. L., Prim, M. P., Alfonso, C., Sastre, N., Rabanal, L. & Gavilan, J. (2001). Comparison of amoxicillin and azithromycin in the prevention of recurrent acute otitis media. *International Journal of Pediatric Otorhinolaryngology, 58*(1):47–51.

Diven, W. F., Evans, R. W., Swarts, J. D., Burckart, G. J., & Doyle, W. J. (1995). Effect of ibuprofen treatment during experimental acute otitis media. *Auris Nasus, Larynx, 22* (2), 73–79.

Dunne, M.W. (2003). Efficacy of single-dose azithromycin in treatment of acute otitis media in children after a baseline tympanocentesis. *Antimicrobial Agents and Chemotherapy, 47*(8), 2663–2665.

Gerchufsky, M. (1995). Understanding upper respiratory tract infections. *Advance for Nurse Practitioners, 3* (3), 25–27.

Glasziou, P. P., Del Mar, C. B., Hayem, M. & Sanders, S. L. (2000). Antibiotics for acute otitis media in children. *Cochrane Database of Systematic Reviews,* (4):CD00219.

Glasziou, P. P., Del Mar, C. B., Hayem, M. & Sanders, S. L. (2002). Antibiotics for acute otitis media in children. *Cochrane Database of Systematic Reviews,* (3), Oxford: Update Software.

Goldstein, N. A., & Sculerati, N. (1994). Compliance with prophylactic antibiotics for otitis media in a New York city clinic. *International Journal of Pediatric Otorhinolaryngology, 28* (2–3), 129–140.

Hannley, M. T., Denneny, J. C. 3rd. & Holzer, S. S. (2000). Use of ototopical antibiotics in treating 3 common ear diseases. *Otolaryngology —Head & Neck Surgery, 122*(6):934–40.

Hay, W. H., Groothuis, J. R., Hayward, A. R., & Levin, M. J. (1995). *Current pediatric diagnosis and treatment.* Norwalk, CT: Appleton & Lange.

Hoberman, A., Paradise, J. L., Reynolds, E. A., & Urkin, J. (1997). Efficacy of Auralgan for treating ear pain in children with acute otitis media. *Archives of Pediatric Adolescent Medicine, 151*(7), 675–678.

Hoole, A. J., Pickard, C. G., Jr., Ouimette, R. M., Lohr, J. A., & Greenberg, R. A. (1995). *Patient care guidelines for nurse practitioners* (4th ed.). Philadelphia: J. B. Lippincott.

Johnson, C. E. & Belman, S. (2001). The role of antibacterial therapy of acute otitis media in promoting drug resistance. *Paediatric Drugs, 3*(9):639–47.

Joki-Erkkila, V. P., Pukander, J. & Laippala, P. (2000). Alteration of clinical picture and treatment of pediatric acute otitis media over the past two decades. *International Journal of Pediatric Otorhinolaryngology, 55*(3):197–201.

Klein, J. O. (1995). Otitis externa, otitis media, mastoiditis. In G. L. Mandel, J. E. Bennett, & R. Dolin (Eds.), *Bennett's principles and practice of infectious diseases* (4th ed., pp. 579–585). New York: Churchill Livingston.

Management of acute otitis media. Summary, Evidence Report/Technology Assessment: Number 15, June 2000. Agency for Healthcare Quality and Research, Rockville, MD. *http://www.ahrq.gov/clinic/epcsums/otitisum.htm.*

Mandel, E. M., Casselbrant, M. L., Rockette, H. E., Bluestone, C. D., & Kurs-Lasky, M. (1995). Efficacy of 20- versus 10-day antimicrobial treatment for acute otitis media. *Pediatrics, 96* (1 Pt. 1), 5–13.

Matas, K. E., Brown, N. C., & Holman, E. J. (1996). Measuring outcomes in nursing centers. *Nurse Practitioner, 21* (6), 116–125.

Mellon, M. (Letter, June 3, 2002). Warning: The chicken in this package has been fed large quantities of antibiotics. Union of Concerned Scientists. *www.ucsusa.org.*

Mengel, M. B., & Schwiebert, L. P. (1993). *Ambulatory medicine: The primary care of families* (pp. 119–125). Norwalk, CT: Appleton & Lange.

Miser, W. F. (2001). To treat or not to treat otitis media — That's just one of the questions. *Journal of the American Board of Family Practice, 14,* 474.

Mitchell, D. K., Van, R., Mason, E. H., Norris, D. M., & Pickering, L. K. (1996). Prospective study of toxigenic clostridium difficile in children given amoxicillin/clavulanate for otitis media. *The Pediatric Infectious Disease Journal, 15* (6), 514–519.

Munz, M., Farmer, J. P., Auger, L., O'Gorman, A. M., & Schloss, M. D. (1992). Otitis media and CNS complications. *Journal of Otolaryngology, 21* (3), 224–226.

Niemela, M., Uhari, M., & Mottonen, M. (1995). A pacifier increases the risk of recurrent acute otitis media in children in day care centers. *Pediatrics, 96* (5 Pt. 1), 884–888.

Paradise, J. L., Dollaghan, C. A., Campbell, T. F., Feldman, H. M., Bernard, B. S., Colborn, D. K., Rockette, H. E., Janosky, J. E., Pitcairn, D. L., Kurs-Lasky, M., Sabo, D. L. & Smith, C. G. (2003). Otitis media and tympanostomy tube insertion during the first three years of life: Developmental outcomes at the age of four years. *Pediatrics, 112,* 265–277.

Patel, J. A., Reisner, B., Vizirinia, N., Owen, M., Chonmaitree, T., & Howie, V. (1995). Bacteriologic failure of amoxicillin-clavulanate in treatment of acute otitis media caused by non-typeable *Haemophilus influenzae. Journal of Pediatrics, 126* (5 Pt. 1), 799–806.

Pichichero, M. E. (2000). Recurrent and persistent otitis media. *Pediatric Infectious Disease Journal, 19*(9):911–6.

Pichichero, M. E. (2000). Evaluating the need, timing and best choice of antibiotic therapy for acute otitis media and tonsillopharyngitis infections in children. *Pediatric Infectious Disease Journal, 19*(12 Suppl):S131–40.

Pichichero, M. E., Reiner, S. A., Brook, I., Gooch, WM 3rd., Yamauchi, T., Jenkins, S. G. & Sher, L. (2000). Controversies in the medical management of persistent and recurrent acute otitis media. Recommendations of a clinical advisory committee. *Annals of Otology, Rhinology & Laryngology—August Supplement,* 183:1–12.

Principi, N. (1995). Multicentre comparative study of the efficacy and safety of azithromycin compared with amoxicillin/clavulanic acid in the treatment of paediatric patients with otitis media. *European Journal of Clinical Microbiology and Infectious Diseases, 14* (8), 669–676.

Research Briefs. (2003). Pneumococcal jab not whole solution for otitis media. *The Lancet, 361* (2), 189–195.

Richer, M., & LeBel, M. (1997). Upper respiratory tract infections. In J. T. DiPiro, R. L. Talbert, G. C. Yee, G. R. Matzke, B. G. Wells, & L. M. Posey (Eds.), *Pharmacotherapy: A pathophysiologic approach* (3rd ed). Stamford, CT: Appleton & Lange.

Roos, K., Hakansson, E. G. & Holm, S. (2001). Effect of recolonisation with interfering a streptococci on recurrences of acute and secretory otitis media in children. Randomised placebo-controlled trial. *British Medical Journal, 322:* 336–342.

Ruben, R. J., Wallace, I. F., & Gravel, J. (1997). Long-term communication deficiencies in children with otitis media during their first year of life. *Acta Otolaryngologica (Stockholm) 117*(2), 206–207.

Schappert, S. M. (1992). *Office visits for otitis media: United States, 1975–90. Advance data from vital and health statistics of the Centers for Disease Control/National Center for Health Statistics,* (p. 214). Washington, DC: U.S. Department of Health and Human Services.

Stevenson, L., & Brooke, D. S. (1995). Managing otitis media with effusion in young children. *Journal of Pediatric Health Care, 9* (1), 36–39.

Stool, S. E., Berg, A. O., Berman, S., Carney, C. J., Cooley, J. R., Culpepper, L., Eavy, R. D., Feagans, L. V., Finitzo, T., Friedman, E. M., et al. (1994). *Otitis media with effusion in young children: Clinical practice guideline* (12), AHCPR publication no. 94-0622. Rockville, MD: Agency for Health Care Policy and Research, Public Health Service, U.S. Department of Health and Human Services.

Sun, A. H., Parnes, L. S., & Freeman, D. J. (1995). Pharmacokinetic profiles of ceftazidime in cochlear perilymph, cerebrospinal fluid and plasma: A high-performance liquid chromatographic study. *ORL Journal of Oto-rhino-laryngology and Related Specialties, 57* (5), 256–259.

Sun, A. H., Parnes, L. S., & Freeman, D. J. (1996). Comparative perilymph permeability of cephalosporins and its significance in the treatment and prevention of suppurative labyrinthitis. *Annals of Otology, Rhinology and Laryngology, 105* (1), 54–57.

Supiyaphun, P., Tonsakulrungruang, K., Chochaipanichnon, L., Chongtateong, A., & Samart, Y. (1995). The treatment of chronic suppurative otitis media and otitis externa with 0.3 percent ofloxacin otic solution: A clinico-microbiological study. *Journal of the Medical Association of Thailand, 78* (1), 18–21.

Teele, D. W., Klein, J. O., Chase, C., Menyuk, P., & Rosner, B. A. (1990). Otitis media in infancy and intellectual ability, school achievement, speech, and language at age 7 years. *Journal of Infectious Diseases, 162* (3), 685–694.

Teele, D. W., Klein, J. O., Rosen, B., & The Greater Boston Otitis Media Study Group. (1983). Middle ear disease and the practice of pediatrics. Burden during the first five years of life. *JAMA, 249* (8), 1026–1029.

Terris, M. H., Magit, A. E., & Davidson, T. M. (1995). Otitis media with effusion in infants and children. Primary care concerns addressed from an otolaryngologist's perspective. *Postgraduate Medicine, 97* (1), 137–138, 143–144, 147.

Zeisel, S. A., Robert, J. E., Gunn, E. B., Riggins, R., Evans, G. A., Roush, J., Burchinak, M. R., & Henderson, F. W. (1995). Prospective surveillance for otitis media with effusion among black infants in group child care. *Journal of Pediatrics, 127* (6), 875–880.

CHAPTER ❖ 25

GASTROINTESTINAL DISORDERS

Jeanette F. Kissinger ◆ Karen W. Jefferson ◆ Sharon A. Jung

This chapter covers the pharmacotherapy of selected common and uncommon gastrointestinal (GI) problems seen in primary care settings. Common symptoms such as nausea, vomiting, diarrhea, constipation, hemorrhoids, and flatus will be reviewed as well as the treatment and diagnosis of inflammatory bowel syndrome, peptic ulcer disease, gastroesophageal reflux, and hepatitis. Several new pharmacologic treatments have been introduced since the last edition of this book and will be included here.

NAUSEA AND VOMITING

Nausea and vomiting (N & V) are common but annoying problems experienced by virtually all patients and providers. Although seldom life-threatening conditions in the primary care setting, these symptoms can result in considerable concern, discomfort, and time lost from daily activities.

Nausea and vomiting may present as primary symptoms or they may be part of a complex clinical presentation. Symptoms may be self-induced, as in cases of bulimia or anorexia nervosa; caused by external stimuli such as acute infection, drug toxicity, food intake, and emotional stress; the result of metabolic conditions such as myocardial infarction, pregnancy, and diabetic ketoacidosis; or gastrointestinal disorders such as obstruction, peptic ulcer disease, or motility disorders.

SPECIFIC CONSIDERATIONS FOR PHARMACOTHERAPY

When Drug Therapy Is Needed

For many patients, N & V are self-limiting conditions that resolve without medical or drug therapy. When N & V are the predominant symptoms, the primary care provider's main concern is dehydration, especially with pediatric and geriatric patients. Nausea is entirely subjective and is commonly described as the sensation (or sensations) that immediately precede vomiting. Vomiting, in contrast, is a highly specific physical event that results in the rapid, forceful evacuation of gastric contents in retrograde fashion from the stomach up to and out of the mouth (Quigley, Hasler, & Parkman, 2001). Intervention will be directed toward (1) correction of any fluid, electrolyte, or nutritional deficiencies that may have resulted from the vomiting itself or the food aversion that may accompany these symptoms; (2) identification and elimination of the underlying cause of the symptoms where possible; and (3) the suppression or elimination of the symptoms themselves if the primary cause can be identified easily and promptly eliminated (Quigley, Hasler, & Parkman, 2001). For patients whose symptoms are caused by life-threatening illnesses such as bowel obstruction or myocardial infarction, immediate referral is indicated.

Short- and Long-Term Goals of Pharmacotherapy

Pharmacotherapy for N & V has two goals: to provide symptomatic relief for the patient and to maintain his or her hydration status.

Nonpharmacologic Therapy

Nonpharmacologic therapy consists of GI rest with gradual increases in bland foods. See also Table 25–1.

For morning sickness in the first trimester of pregnancy, avoidance of foods that provoke symptoms is the preferred treatment. Suggestions for relief include minimizing of odors, eating desired food (regardless of the time of day), and small morning feedings. Traditional recommendations are saltines and ginger ale; alternatively, potato chips and lemonade in the morning may allow women to eat regular meals for the remainder of the day (Erick, 1994). Vitamin B_6 (25 mg/day) PO is thought to be useful (Goroll, May, & Mulley, 1995).

In children with vomiting and/or diarrhea, volume depletion can occur rapidly. A solution of oral rehydration therapy (ORT) can be easily made in the home—see Table 25–2—or offer commercial ORT solutions, i.e., Pedialyte.

Time Frame for Initiating Pharmacotherapy

After ensuring that N & V are not indicative of an underlying condition needing immediate attention, it is reasonable to wait 24 hours to see if symptoms abate on their own. For motion sickness and travel-related prophylaxis, patients should be instructed to take medication 20 to 30 min before initiation of travel. Transdermal patches should be applied 2 to 3 hours prior to travel.

Metoclopramide PO should be started 15 to 30 min before specific migraine therapy and repeated in 4 to 6 hours (DiPiro & Bowden, 1997).

Chemotherapy-associated nausea and vomiting can be classified as acute, delayed, or anticipatory, depending upon the chemotherapeutic agent. Initiation of treatment should be based on the type of N & V as well as the agent used. Acute N & V usually occur within 1 to 4 hours after the start of chemotherapy and resolve within 24 hours. Delayed N & V may not begin for 24 hours and may last for several days (Morrow, Hickok, & Rosenthal, 1995). Some chemotherapeutic agents may have both an acute and a delayed phase (Morrow et al., 1995). Anticipatory N & V are associated with provoking stimuli, such as sight, smell, sound, and remembrance of past experiences.

TABLE 25–1. What the Patient Can Do to Treat Nausea and Vomiting

- No solids for 8 h.
- Clear liquids only (no milk) until 8–12 h have passed without vomiting. Start with 1 tbsp (15 cc) every 10 min. If vomiting does not occur, double the amount each hour. If vomiting does occur, allow stomach to rest 1–2 h and then start again. The key is to gradually increase the amount of fluid until taking 8 oz every hour.
  Older children and adults: Gatorade, Pedialyte, or Ricelyte may be combined with flavored gelatin to make them more palatable.
  Pedialyte, Ricelyte, or Kao Lectrolyte should be given to infants and small children since they tend to become dehydrated quickly. Resume breast/bottle feeding as soon as possible.
- Bland food after 8 h without vomiting:
  Saltines, bland soups (chicken noodle), rice, mashed potatoes
  Also acceptable is BRAT (bananas, rice, applesauce, toast)
- Resume normal diet as soon as possible

Source: Adapted from Uphold & Graham (1994) with permission.

TABLE 25–2. Homemade Oral Rehydration Therapy (ORT) Solution

1/2 or 1 tsp salt
1/2 tsp baking soda
4 tbsp sugar
1 L (or 4-1/3 cups) water

Mix or shake together all ingredients until the salt, baking soda, and sugar have dissolved in the water. Water should be kept at room temperature. Give frequent small sips to prevent dehydration and loss of electrolytes.

Source: Adapted from Sears & Sack (1995).

Assessment and History Taking

The determination of whether to initiate therapy should be based on a targeted medical history and physical examination. The history should include the following information:

- Timing of symptoms; relation to meals or other activities
- Self-treatments initiated and results
- Related signs/symptoms such as diarrhea and chest pain
- Current medications
- Presence of other medical problems, especially diabetes, renal disease, pregnancy, or peptic ulcer disease
- Recent history of travel (especially to areas with poor sanitation)
- Ingestion of foods commonly causing vomiting

The physical examination should include:

- Vital signs, including blood pressure and orthostatics
- Assessment of skin turgor and mucous membranes

- Abdominal examination to assess for distention, organ enlargement, visible peristalsis, abnormal bowel sounds, organ enlargement, and flank tenderness
- Screening neurological examination to assess for weakness

Consider the following diagnostic tests if symptoms are prolonged or especially severe:

- Serum chemistry (to check BUN/creatine; check glucose and anion gap, especially if the patient is diabetic)
- Liver function tests or AST and ALT (to rule out hepatitis)
- EKG (if myocardial infarction is suspected)
- Serum drug levels if an overdose is suspected (especially digitalis and theophylline)
- Pregnancy test if last menstrual period was more than 1 month ago
- X-ray to rule out obstruction (if symptoms present with acute abdominal pain)

Antiemetics have been implicated in contributing to or altering the course of Reye's syndrome and are not recommended for use in children. Their use should be limited to episodes of prolonged vomiting whose etiology is known.

Drug therapy should be minimized with pregnancy. No antiemetic is approved for use during pregnancy, although metoclopramide has been used without reports of fetal problems (Goroll et al., 1995).

Use of antiemetic drug therapy may make the diagnosis of acute abdomen more difficult. Therefore, it is important to rule out emergency conditions such as myocardial infarction, paralytic ileus, or bowel obstruction before starting antiemetics.

Patient/Caregiver Information

Primary emphasis should be on maintenance of hydration status, especially when diarrhea is also present. Giving very small sips of rehydration solution can assist. Instruct the patient and caregiver on Uphold and Graham's (1994) therapy regimen (Table 25–1). A reduction of personal and environmental activity and stimuli such as household smells and loud noises can serve as comfort measures. Teach patients to rinse their mouths after vomiting to minimize bad taste and corrosion of tooth enamel.

OUTCOMES MANAGEMENT

Selecting An Appropriate Agent

Motion Sickness. The differences in onset and duration of action of each drug should be kept in mind when selecting a drug for the prevention of motion sickness. Patients with mild to moderate motion sickness generally respond well to antihistamines such as dimenhydrinate (50–100 mg PO every 4–6 h, with a maximum dose of 400 mg a day), diphenhydramine (25–50 mg PO three to four times a day, up to 300 mg a day), and scopolamine. Scopolamine is more effective against motion sickness, with a faster onset of action but a relatively short duration compared to the antihistamines. By releasing drug constantly, at a rate of 0.5 mg every 72 h transdermal scopolamine (Transderm-Scop) provides an effective drug concentration over a prolonged period while minimizing the adverse effects. Scopolamine is also effective after nausea has started (Mitchelson, 1992).

Migraine Headaches and Pain. Migraines require treatment of the headache as well as therapy for the N & V. Metoclopramide increases the absorption or effectiveness of concurrent analgesic therapy and also acts as an antiemetic (Mitchelson, 1992). Phenothiazines such as prochlorperazine may be helpful in suppressing vomiting that is the result of migraines.

Chemotherapy-Associated Nausea and Vomiting.[1] When choosing an agent for patients receiving chemotherapy, there are many things to consider, including mechanism of action of the antiemetic agent, type of N & V to be treated, factors specific to the chemotherapy drug, as well as patient specific factors. The mechanism of chemotherapy-induced N & V is a complex interaction between neurotransmitters and receptors in the central and peripheral nervous systems (Hesketh, Van Belle, Aapro, et al., 2003). Dopamine type 2 and serotonin type 3 ($5HT_3$) receptors seem to be the most important. Other involved receptors include dopamine, opiate, histamine, acetylcholine, and neurokinin1 (Hesketh, Van Belle, Aapro, et al., 2003). Antiemetics are used to block the receptors and prevent the transmission of information used to induce N & V. Drug factors include emetogenicity of the chemotherapeutic agent, route of administration, rate of administration, other chemotherapy drugs given in combination, and number of consecutive days the treatment will be given. Certain chemotherapy drugs are more likely to cause N & V than others, and the antiemetic agents chosen should match that potential. Most

[1]ACKNOWLEDGMENT: Cynthia J. Simonson, RN, MS, CS, AOCN, ANP, Massey Cancer Center, Virginia Commonwealth University, Richmond, Virginia, is acknowledged with gratitude for her contribution to the section "Chemotherapy-Associated Nausea and Vomiting" in this chapter.

chemotherapy regimens are a combination of agents, and the antiemetics chosen should match the drug in the regimen with the most potential to cause N & V. If two drugs with moderate potential are given together, their combined potential should be considered, and a stronger antiemetic should be given. Consecutive days of treatment are additive and may require the addition of a stronger antiemetic. Patient specific factors include age of the patient—younger more susceptible than older; gender—female more susceptible than male; prior exposure to chemotherapy, especially if N & V were not well controlled; and prior history of alcohol abuse that decreases the risk of N & V (Schnell, 2003). All of these risk factors should be assessed and the antiemetic agents chosen should match their combined potential. See Table 502.3

The antiemetic activity of corticosteroids (dexamethasone or methylprednisolone) has been beneficial when they are employed as single agents in mild or moderate emetogenic chemotherapy, but they are less effective against highly emetogenic agents. Therefore, combination therapy with corticosteroids is a good choice when a single agent fails. (Gonzales & Adams, 2002).

Phenothiazines are helpful in mild to moderate emetogenic chemotherapy, but have limited efficacy against highly emetogenic agents. Therefore, they are generally used in combination with other agents or as alternative agents. The piperazine compounds (thiethylperazine, prochloperazine, and perphenazine) as a class have the greatest antiemetic activity and produce less sedation and hypotension; however, they have the highest incidence of extrapyramidal effects (Gonzalez & Adams, 2002).

The cannabinoids, dronabinol and nabilone, have been effective in patients refractory to other antiemetic therapy. Because of their high frequency of side effects and abuse potential, cannabinoids are not first-line antiemetics and should be used as alternative antiemetics or in combination therapy. Younger patients are more tolerant of cannabinoid-induced psychologic effects (Tramer, Carroll, & Campbell, et al., 2001).

Serotonin antagonists, such as ondansetron, dolasetron, and granisetron, have been very effective in the treatment and prevention of chemotherapy-associated N & V. They are considered first-line treatment for highly to moderately emetogenic chemotherapy (Gonzales & Adams, 2002).

Studies comparing the three serotonin antagonists have found them to be comparable. The combination with dexamethasone has been shown to increase the effectiveness of the serotonin antagonist in patients receiving highly emetogenic chemotherapy. Aprepitant, a new drug, is an oral neurokinin-1 antagonist. Adding aprepitant to the combination of a serotonin antagonists and dexamethasone has been shown to significantly enhance the efficacy of the regimen and has been shown to be effective through multiple cycles of highly emetogenic chemotherapy (De Witt, Herrstedt & Rapoport, 2003; Hesketh, Grunbery, Cralla et al, 2003).

These agents are very expensive. Therefore, these agents are considered the drug of choice only for patients who are receiving highly emetogenic chemotherapy, those unable to tolerate the adverse effects, or those refractory to other antiemetic therapy.

Benzodiazepines (lorazepam and midazolam) are agents with anxiolytic and amnestic properties; therefore, they are helpful in the prevention of anticipatory N & V associated with chemotherapy (Gonzales & Adams, 2002).

Mechanical Obstruction or Motility Disorders. Pro-kinetic agents are very effective in the treatment of mechanical obstruction or motility disorders. Cisapride, as well as metoclopramide, can stimulate the GI tract in patients with diabetic gastroparesis. However metoclopramide has been shown to decrease N & V more than cisapride (Agostinucci et al., 1986; Gralla, Itri, Pisko, et al., 1981; Tami & Waite, 1988).

Postoperative Vomiting. The incidence of postoperative N & V depends upon the anesthesia used, the age of the patient, and the concurrent medications used. Benzquinamide, phenothiazines, and butyrophenones are very helpful. Metoclopramide has not been shown to be effective, possibly because of its short duration of action compared to the duration of the anesthetic agent (Mitchelson, 1992).

Monitoring for Efficacy

Symptoms should improve within a short period of time, usually with one or two courses of medication. If symptoms do not resolve after maximum, frequent doses of antiemetic medication, the patient should be switched to a different agent with a different mechanism of action. N & V associated with an underlying process may require correction of the underlying cause before complete resolution of symptoms can occur. If the N & V are the result of a drug toxicity, symptoms should abate after the serum concentration of the offending drug starts to fall within the therapeutic range. If the symptoms continue despite a normal serum concentration, the drug should not be restarted. Select an alternative agent. Signs and symptoms of dehydration, electrolyte disturbances, and volume depletion should be monitored with frequent evaluation of mucous membranes and skin turgor. Fluid replacement should be initiated if necessary. Followup is not usually indicated after resolution of symptoms.

Migraine headache–associated emesis requires time for the underlying condition to abate. If the patient does not show improvement with metoclopramide or the patient cannot take the drug orally, prochlorperazine suppositories can be used.

N & V can occur following chemotherapy; other antiemetic agents should be added to the regimen if chemotherapy-associated N & V fail to respond adequately to the initial treatment. A patient's prior history with chemotherapy-associated N & V greatly affects the emetic control of subsequent therapy. Use of benzodiazepines may be beneficial to prevent subsequent anticipatory N & V. If good control is obtained with a particular regimen, maintain the regimen for successive therapy.

DIARRHEA

Diarrhea, or the abnormal frequency and liquidity of bowel movements, is another familiar condition in primary care practices. Virtually all diarrhea seen in an outpatient setting is due to infection, has an antibiotic association, is food- or drug-induced, or is the result of inflammatory bowel disease. Diarrhea can be classified as acute or chronic, depending on whether it persists for more than 3 weeks (McQuaid, 1997).

Most infectious diarrhea is acute. Chronic diarrhea can occur as a result of infections in several situations, such as:

1. Pathogens that can be parasites or bacteria.
2. Immunosuppressed individuals, such as those with HIV infection or on steroids or other immunosuppresants.
3. Some infections clear, but persons develop chronic symptoms, such as irritable bowel syndrome with diarrhea. Occasionally, ulcerative colitis develops after an acute infection (Lee & Surawicz, 2001).

Most patients have simple diarrhea manifested by watery stools, low-grade fever, mild malaise, abdominal cramps, and nausea (Nathwani & Wood, 1993). Although most episodes are short-term and self-limiting, serious effects such as dehydration, perforation, perianal skin breakdown, weight loss, and nutritional compromise can result if symptoms do not resolve and the condition becomes chronic. Approximately 5 to 10% of patients who seek medical care for diarrheal illness present with dysentery (Nathwani & Wood, 1993). In most studies, classic travelers diarrhea (TD) is defined as passage of greater than or equal to 3 unformed stools in a 24-hour period with one or more accompanying symptoms of entire disease, such as nausea, vomiting, abdominal cramps, fever, tenesmus or bloody stool (Rendi-Wagner & Kollaritsch, 2002).

SPECIFIC CONSIDERATIONS FOR PHARMACOTHERAPY

When Drug Therapy Is Needed

In general, diarrhea is self-limiting. Patients who are at special risk, however, such as small children, pregnant women, elderly patients, and patients with pre-existing illnesses, are at an increased risk of developing complicated and long-lasting disease. Other complications may include dehydration (particularly in children), reactive arthritis, postinfectious enterpathy, and campylobacter jejuni-associated Guillian-Barré syndrome (Rendi-Wagner & Kollaritsch, 2002). The most disastrous consequences of infectious diarrhea (dysentery) are related to dehydration and toxic megacolon, and are seen with *Clostridium difficile.* All patients with dysentery should receive antibiotic therapy (McQuaid, 1997). In travelers' diarrhea, symptoms are usually mild and short-lived, lasting 1 to 5 days—just enough to spoil a vacation.

Short- and Long-Term Goals of Pharmacotherapy

The short-term goal of treatment for diarrhea is prevention or reversal of fluid and electrolyte disturbances and any resultant metabolic complications. Long-term goals of treatment include prevention of recurrent episodes and prevention of antibiotic-resistant organisms.

Nonpharmacologic Therapy

Oral rehydration therapy in either homemade (see Table 25–2) or commercial forms, such as Pedialyte, should precede or accompany all other therapies. This is especially important in children and the elderly to prevent loss of fluids and electrolytes.

Persons who develop travelers' diarrhea should practice good food hygiene. This includes avoiding tap water and ice cubes, unreliable restaurants, raw seafood, uncooked foods, and unpeeled fruits. Bottled or boiled water should be used even for tooth brushing. Because contaminated food or beverages are the most important vehicle of transmission of all pathogens that cause TD, precautions regarding dietary habits (the rule of "boil it, cook it, peel it, or forget it!") remain the cornerstone of prevention (Rendi-Wagner & Kollaritsch, 2002; Virk, 2001).

Discontinue any antibiotics that are associated with the development of *Clostridium difficile* or change to another antibiotic with less incidence of causing this problem.

Regular dietary intake should be maintained. A BRAT diet (bananas, rice, applesauce, tea/toast) can assist in maintaining nutrition status and avoiding dehydration. In adults, dairy products should be avoided during the time of symptoms and for several days after resolution because lactose intolerance accompanies many cases of diarrhea (Richter, 1995). Children can continue to receive lactose-containing products (Brown, 1994).

Good perianal hygiene can avoid skin irritation and breakdown. After each loose stool, rinsing the perineum with warm water and patting the area dry with a cotton towel will minimize discomfort. Toilet paper should be avoided. Witch hazel pads (Tucks) are soothing. Apply hydrocortisone cream or an emollient such as petrolatum jelly to the perineum. Sitz baths for 10 minutes, two or three times a day, are a comfort measure.

Time Frame for Initiating Pharmacotherapy

Assurance of adequate hydration is the initial step in treatment. Consideration of whether antibiotics would be useful can be based on the epidemiological setting and the medical history. Empiric antibiotic treatment for diarrhea in otherwise healthy adults in industrialized countries is not recommended (Scott & Edelman, 1993).

Even though empirical use of antibiotics is not recommended, antibiotics are still commonly used, however, and include quinolones, TMP-SMX, doxycycline, and some nonabsorbable antibiotics (Seale, 2002).

Recent attention has been given to the use of probiotics for prevention of traveler's diarrhea. They are microorganisms that are nonpathogenic and reportedly are helpful in effectively aiding in the treatment of intestinal disturbances that include traveler's diarrhea. Rendi-Wagner and Kollaritsch (2002) relate that the principal concept of protection mediated by nonpathogenic bacteria remains appealing, but until now, no probiotic medication has been demonstrated to provide clinically relevant worldwide protection against TD; therefore, a general recommendation for the use of such preparations cannot be provided.

A number of studies have confirmed that bismuth subsalicylate (BBS) has a protective efficacy of up to 65%. Optimal protection rates were reported when the substance was administered as 2 tablets 4 times daily (2.1 g/day) for a maximum period of 3 weeks. It seems that the optimal antibacterial effect is provided by simultaneous ingestion of contaminated food and BSS (Rendi-Wagner & Kollaritsch, 2002).

The most commonly reported adverse reactions associated with BSS were transient blackening of tongue and stools, constipation, tinnitus, and nausea. It should be noted that BSS can deplete the absorption of doxycycline (Rendi-Wagner & Kollaritsch, 2002). In most European countries BSS preparations are not licensed. According to Rendi-Wagner and Kollaritsch (2002), most European countries do not use this product for traveler's diarrhea because of the large number of tablets required and the subsequent side effects.

The decision to initiate treatment for travelers' diarrhea will depend on the severity and duration of the diarrhea, and the past medical history of the traveler. Mild diarrhea is generally self-limiting and requires only symptomatic treatment. If the patient is dehydrated, rehydration should be initiated promptly and antidiarrheal agents initiated for relief of symptoms. If the diarrhea is severe or the patient high-risk (i.e., is immunocompromised or has gastrointestinal disease or low gastric acidity), antibacterial agents should be started.

The use of antidiarrheal drugs is not recommended for treatment of acute diarrhea in children. Additionally, for children and pregnant women neither quinolone-based prophylaxis nor treatment are approved (Rendi-Wagner & Kollaritsch, 2002).

See Drug Table 501.8.

Assessment and History Taking

To determine the kind or even desirability of therapy a targeted medical history and physical examination are needed. The history and examination should include the following:

- Timing of symptoms; relation to meals; acute or chronic condition
- Related signs and symptoms
- Current medications, especially antibiotics
- Presence of other medical problems, especially diabetes, renal disease, pregnancy, peptic ulcer disease, HIV infection
- Recent history of travel (especially to areas with poor sanitation)
- Ingestion of foods commonly causing diarrhea
- Self-treatments initiated and results

The physical examination should include assessment of:

- Vital signs, including BP for postural hypotension, temperature, weight
- Skin turgor, mucous membranes
- Abdomen to check for tenderness, distention, guarding, rebound, abnormal bowel sounds, organ enlargement or masses, visible peristalsis
- Rectal exam and fecal occult blood check (if positive, do CBC with differential to determine if infectious process or occult bleed)
- Screening neurologic examination to assess for weakness

Consider the following diagnostic tests if symptoms do not resolve within 3 days:

- Stool bacterial culture
- Stool examination for ova and parasites
- *Clostridium difficile* toxin assay (if recent history of antibiotics)
- CBC with differential (to rule out infectious process or if fecal occult blood test is positive)

Patient/Caregiver Information

The importance of thorough handwashing with soap and water after each episode of loose stool should be stressed. Hand lotions can minimize dryness, and towels used for hand drying should be changed daily.

Education about the importance of maintaining nutritional input should be provided. Many patients have misconceptions about the use of ORT agents and should be instructed that their use is to prevent dehydration, not to reduce the actual symptoms of diarrhea. Also, since food products like Gatorade or Jello do not contain the proper ratios of essential elements, they should not be used as a treatment for diarrhea. (See Table 25–1 for recommendations.)

OUTCOMES MANAGEMENT

Selecting an Appropriate Agent

Antibiotics are the mainstay of therapy for the treatment of diarrhea of infectious etiology. Selection of an agent requires consideration of the patient's allergy history, previous drug history, age, whether the patient is pregnant, the severity of the diarrhea, antibiotic resistance pattern in the community, and suspected pathogen.

The management of travelers' diarrhea can be divided into prophylaxis and treatment. The role of antibiotics in prophylaxis of traveler's diarrhea is controversial. Risks of adverse effects and fear of developing resistant strains of bacteria are the primary reasons for not recommending antibiotic prophylaxis to all (Seale, 2002). Antibiotic prophylaxis may be considered in people with (1) a previous history of travelers' diarrhea, (2) an underlying illness that would be worsened with the development of diarrhea, or (3) travel plans to an area with poor sanitation for less than 3 weeks. In the past 10 years four fluoroquinolones (norfloxacin, ciprofloxacin, ofloxacin, and levofloxacin) have attracted considerable attention as a result of their excellent safety profile and wide spectrum of coverage of enteropathogenic agents. It was shown that when taken daily in a single low dose—for instance, 400 mg of norfloxacin per day or 250 mg of ciprofloxacin per day—the protection against TD is up to 90%, providing that the enteropathogens present in the region of study are susceptible to the agent (Rendi-Wagner & Kollaritsch, 2002). Thus far, quinolones remain the drugs of choice when chemoprophylaxis is indicated; for instance, patients with severe baseline disease. However, side effects have been observed, such as skin rash, vaginal candidiasis, CNS reactions, phototoxicity, and gastrointestinal complaints. Very rarely, there have been severe events, including anaphylaxis (Rendi-Wagner & Kollaritsch, 2002). Antimicrobial therapy is recommended if symptoms worsen or continue for more than 24 h, for diarrhea associated with fever, for severe diarrhea, and for symptoms that recur when symptomatic therapy is discontinued. Seale, (2002) reports a study that added the use of an anti-motility drug: Two doses of TMP-SMX were compared with or without loperamide versus loperamide alone in a randomized controlled trial. The combination therapy was noted to be most efficacious in controlling symptoms. A dose-ranging study of rifaximin, a nonabsorbable antibiotic used for 5 days, when compared to TMP-SMX showed 11% clinical failure and with TMP-SMX a 29% clinical failure. A statistically nonsignificant benefit was noted with use of rifaximin, 200 mg 3 times a day. Efficacy of ciprofloxacin with and without loperamide was evaluated in a randomized controlled trial on 142 U.S. military personnel. Ciprofloxacin for 3 days with loperamide was better in decreasing the number of liquid stools (Dupont, Jiang, Ericsson, et al., 2001). If used, caution should be exercised in using opiate-based anti-motility drugs because they can cause sedation, nausea, and vomiting. Therefore, anti-motility drugs should not be used in patients with high fever or bloody stools, and they should be discontinued if symptoms persist for more than 48 hours. They can serve as an alternative agent in nondysenteric traveler's diarrhea. Antibacterial drug therapy should be active against the principal pathogens responsible for travelers' diarrhea. *Escherichia coli* is the most frequently isolated pathogen (30–70%) in all parts of the world, with *Shigella* species occurring 5 to 20% of the time (Nathwani & Wood, 1993). Salmonella, *Vibrio parahaemolyticus* and campylobacter species are less common (Nathwani & Wood, 1993). *Campylobacter* species are subject to seasonal variation, predominating in the winter months. *C. difficile* is the most frequent nosocomial pathogen of the gastrointestinal tract (Lee & Surawicz, 2001).

According to Dupont, Jiang, Ericsson, et al. (2001), ciprofloxacin was noted to have a clinical benefit in the treatment of travelers with diarrhea who were in Jamaica and Mexico. It was additionally noted that a Spanish study showed that campylobacter jejuni was isolated in 2.2% of symptomatic travelers in Africa, Latin America, and Asia. There was a high prevelance of resistance found to ampicillin and tetracycline (33% and 37%); resistance to ciprofloxacin was noted at 12.5%. The fluoroquinolone drugs (ciprofloxacin, norfloxacin, and ofloxacin) have similar efficacy; the choice should depend upon concurrent medications and cost. Doxycycline and the fluoroquinolones should not be given to pregnant women or children under the age of 12 years.

Up-to-date detailed information for travelers is available from the Centers for Disease Control's annual bulletin *Health Information for International Travel,* or the CDC phone line (401-332-4559).

The drug of choice for treatment of *Clostridium difficile* pseudomembranous colitis is metronidazole. Most cases are treated with metronidazole, 500 mg 4 times a day for 10 days, or vancomycin, 125 to 500 mg 4 times a day for 10 days (Lee & Surawicz, 2001). Metronidazole is as effective as vancomycin and much lower in cost. In addition, with the widespread use of vancomycin, resistance has developed to this antibiotic. Vancomycin can be considered as backup therapy if there is no response to metronidazole. Although antimotility drugs promote relief of diarrheal symptoms, they should be avoided in these patients.

Intestinal parasites such as *Giardia lamblia* microsporidia, *Entamoeba histolytica, Isospora belli,* and *Cryptosporidium parvum* are all frequent causes of waterborne diarrheal outbreaks in humans. Infections with these organisms are generally self-limiting except in children, the elderly, and immunocompromised patients. Stool cultures should be done to determine appropriate, organism-specific treatment. Empiric therapy is not recommended (Liu & Weller, 1996).

Immunocompromised patients will require more aggressive therapy. Approximately 50% of patients with HIV infection will have a diarrhea infection, although the etiology may be elusive. Evaluations to identify the causative organisms may include sigmoidoscopy and/or upper and lower endoscopy.

Cholera, a serious diarrheal disease in both children and adults caused by *Vibrio* species, requires aggressive rehydration. Two days of tetracycline have been effective in clearing the stool of vibrios (Islam, 1987). For tetracycline-resistant cholera, erythromycin and norfloxacin have been used successfully (Scott & Edelman, 1993); furazolidone is an alternative antibiotic for children.

Monitoring for Efficacy

For travelers' diarrhea, after the initiation of antimicrobial therapy, diarrhea should subside within 24 to 36 hours. Temperature should return to normal within 24 hours. For *Clostridium difficile* diarrhea, relapse is frequent despite the extreme sensitivity of the organism to antibiotic therapy. Relapses respond well to retreatment with vancomycin or metronidazole. Similarly, those who fail to respond to metronidazole may respond to vancomycin.

CONSTIPATION

Constipation is defined as the infrequent or difficult evacuation of feces. It results from delayed colonic transit time, usually the consequence of a sedentary lifestyle, inadequate intake of fluids and high-fiber foods, or the habitual ignoring of the urge to defecate. This common problem, which impacts all age groups, is one of the most frequent reasons for self-medication. Constipation affects as many as 26% of elderly men and 34% of elderly women and is a problem that has been related to diminished perception of quality of life (Schaefer & Cheskin, 1998).

SPECIFIC CONSIDERATIONS FOR PHARMACOTHERAPY

When Drug Therapy Is Needed

The normal frequency of bowel movements can vary greatly, and the usual pattern of the individual must be taken into account. For some, daily or even two to three times a day may be the norm, while others will have bowel movements only every 3 to 5 days. Individual differences may be the result of diet and/or exercise. A change in the patient's usual pattern may be reason for intervention. Although not common, metabolic and endocrine disturbances can be the reason for the constipation, and they must be ruled out.

Short- and Long-Term Goals of Pharmacotherapy

The establishment of normal bowel patterns, that is, the comfortable passage of formed stool on a regular basis, should be the goal of pharmacotherapy.

Nonpharmacologic Therapy

The primary prevention of constipation consists of adequate dietary intake of fluids and fibrous foods, moderate exercise, and recognition of the urge to defecate. Nonpharmacologic therapy consists of changing a sedentary lifestyle, increasing dietary fiber (bran cereal, whole grain breads, fruits, and vegetables), and maintaining an adequate fluid intake, usually a minimum of six to eight glasses of noncaffeinated beverages daily.

Time Frame for Initiating Pharmacotherapy

Conservative therapy for constipation can be initiated when a patient complains of feeling bloated or having difficulty moving his or her bowels.

See Drug Tables 501.9, 501.10.

Assessment and History Taking

A screening history and physical examination should determine that intestinal obstruction, drug-induced constipation, and metabolic and endocrine disorders are not the causes of the patient's constipation. The history should include the following:

- Patient's usual bowel habits (if alternating with diarrhea, consider irritable bowel syndrome)
- Recent dietary intake
- Activity level
- Other medications (including OTCs, such as iron, in addition to medications such as narcotic analgesics and/or opioids)
- Previous use of laxatives, enemas
- Other medical problems
- Signs of hypothyroidism
- Somatic complaints that might indicate depression
- History of current pregnancy, postpartum status, or recent abdominal surgery

The physical examination should include:

- Abdominal examination checking for bowel sounds, distention, tenderness, rebound
- Anal check for fissures, irritation, and hemorrhoids; rectal examination for hemorrhoids, fecal impaction, and occult blood

Diagnostic tests to consider to rule out obstruction and metabolic and endocrine disorders as causes of constipation include:

- Abdominal x-ray (if the constipation is of acute onset, accompanied by abdominal pain)
- Thyroid stimulating hormone (TSH) (if there are other signs of hypothyroidism)
- Serum chemistry (if diabetes, hypokalemia, or hypercalcemia is suspected)

If the patient also has nausea, vomiting, or abdominal pain with constipation, do not give laxatives.

Patient/Caregiver Information

For prevention and for initial therapy, a change in dietary habits to include foods high in fiber should be a priority for patients with constipation. The adequate intake of foods such as fruits, vegetables, and whole grain breads will result almost immediately in decreased GI transit time. Over the long term, such a diet is correlated with decreased colon cancer and diverticulosis.

Urge patients to avoid long-term or chronic use of laxatives and enemas. Although they are generally safe and well-tolerated drugs, the potential for dependence exists if laxatives are used regularly over long periods of time. Patients should work toward lifestyle changes including increased exercise, increased fluid intake, and increased dietary fiber.

OUTCOMES MANAGEMENT

Selecting an Appropriate Agent

Bulk-forming agents, such as wheat bran, absorb water and make soft, bulky stools without systemic side effects. They are taken by mixing with a full glass of water or juice and must not be chewed or swallowed dry. These agents are quite effective if taken on a regular basis. They can be purchased in bulk at health food stores or supermarkets and are inexpensive for daily use.

Psyllium preparations are more expensive but also effective with regular use. They may contain large amounts of dextrose and should be avoided by patients who have diabetes. These agents are excellent choices, as are stool softeners, for patients with hemorrhoids, for women who are pregnant, or for patients in whom Valsalva's maneuvers can be difficult or harmful, such as post-MI patients or patients who have had recent surgery.

Stool softeners or emollients work by allowing water in the intestine to enter the stool. They are used for prevention of constipation and are less useful in its treatment. Emollients are useful in patients who are pregnant and post-MI patients, in whom straining should be avoided.

Mineral oil or liquid petrolatum lubricates and softens the stool. Its long-term use should be avoided because of the potential for impairing the absorption of vitamins A and D. They should not be given to children under 6 years of age.

Enemas are used only in cases of fecal impaction and seldom indicated in the primary care setting. Stimulants increase GI peristalsis but can often also cause GI cramping.

Saline laxatives should be used with caution in patients with decreased ambulatory ability, because they may experience incontinence as the result of laxative use. These laxatives usually work within 2 to 6 hours and are indicated when fast, complete bowel evacuation is needed. Saline laxatives can result in considerable fluid loss, so they should not be used in the elderly or in patients with hypertension or cardiac conditions.

Nonpregnant patients showing no result from conservative therapy might find symptom relief with the use of cisapride 10 mg three to four times a day (Gardner, Beckwith, & Heyneman, 1995).

Monitoring for Efficacy

Moderate exercise, increasing noncaffeinated fluids to six to eight glasses daily, prune juice, bulk-forming agents, or stool softeners should show effects within 2 days. If there is no effect within 1 week, a more thorough workup is indicated.

INFLAMMATORY BOWEL DISEASE

The two inflammatory bowel diseases (IBDs)—Crohn's disease (CD) and ulcerative colitis (UC)—have similar symptoms but also important differences. UC is a mucosal disease and confined to the colon. In contrast, Crohn's disease affects any part of the gastrointestinal tract. UC causes a cascade of abdominal cramping, diarrhea, rectal bleeding, and weight loss. CD is characterized by chronic intestinal inflammation and periodic exacerbations with a variety of local and systematic manifestations (Ruymann & Richter, 1995). The chronic nature of the symptoms of IBD makes management a challenge; however, the majority of patients can be managed in a primary care setting, with referral to gastroenterologists necessary only for the most severe cases.

SPECIFIC CONSIDERATIONS FOR PHARMACOTHERAPY

When Drug Therapy Is Needed

Drug therapy acts at multiple sites, locally—depending on the location of the intestinal lesions—and systemically—to minimize inflammation. Drug therapy for UC and CD is indicated to enable patients to maintain as normal a lifestyle as possible, prevent nutritional deficiencies, and minimize the physiologic and social impact of the disease. Such treatment offers most patients relief from the symptoms of diarrhea, bleeding, abdominal cramps, flatulence, and pain. Drug therapy is the first line of defense against both diseases for patients with uncomplicated disease. Surgical intervention is reserved for patients with drug- or disease-related complications or for whom medical treatment has failed.

Short- and Long-Term Goals of Pharmacotherapy

The long-term goal of pharmacotherapy is to control mucosal inflammation and minimize the systemic impact of disease. Short-term goals are to induce and maintain remission of symptoms and to assist in the maintenance of an adequate nutritional status. However, clinical signs of remission are often difficult to interpret because they are so varied and subjective.

Nonpharmacologic Therapy

A positive therapeutic alliance between patient and provider is essential in the care of patients with long-term, frequently relapsing conditions such as IBD. Patients can experience a sense of trust and caring by working together with a provider to monitor the ups and downs of symptom exacerbation and medication efficacy and side effects common in IBD.

For all patients with cramping and diarrhea, an empiric trial of a milk-free diet will eliminate symptoms that may be due to lactose intolerance (DiPiro & Bowden, 1997). The constipation symptoms that may be a part of

IBD can be treated with bulk-type laxatives. However, fiber should be reduced when patients have active disease symptoms of cramping and diarrhea (Ruymann & Richter, 1995).

Nutritional support is important to prevent or minimize weight loss, or inadequate intake of vitamins and minerals. Multiple therapies are used to ensure an adequate nutritional status and minimize inflammation. In UC, therapy must make up for the increased nutritional loss as a result of diarrhea and the often decreased intake. Large doses of fish oil capsules (Max-EPA, Purepa) three times a day have been found to reduce the number of relapses or the need for steroids (Belluzzi, Brignola, Campieri, et al., 1996; Stenson, Cort, Rodgers, et al., 1992); however, some patients dislike the taste and resultant fishy breath.

In CD, bowel rest can be obtained with the preparations of an elemental diet such as Ensure, Sustacal, or Magnacal. In severe cases, total parenteral nutrition (TPN) for short periods of time may be indicated to improve symptoms, inflammation, and nutritional status (DiPiro & Bowden, 1997). Children and adolescents can alternate these nutritional therapies with steroids to allow them to obtain the nutrients needed for normal growth and development (DiPiro & Bowden, 1997). TPN should only be used for patients with severe malnutrition and/or intolerance to an elemental diet. Patients with steatorrhea should reduce their overall fat intake.

All patients with CD should take a multivitamin with minerals. Patients on long-term steroid therapy should supplement it with vitamin D and calcium supplements. Patients on sulfasalazine should supplement with folic acid (1 mg/day) (Ruymann & Richter, 1995). Patients who have had ileal resections should supplement with vitamins A, B_{12}, and D. Oral or parenteral iron supplements will be necessary if anemia is present.

Smoking, acetaminophen use, and increased sugar intake have been associated with increased symptoms of CD (Podolsky, 1991), so avoiding or minimizing use can be suggested to patients.

Nonsmoking has been positively correlated with the incidence of UC, and a role for nicotine has been suggested. Transdermal nicotine patches have been found to improve symptoms for some patients (Pullan, Rhodes, Ganesh, et al., 1994), although nicotine gum was less helpful (Lashner, Hanauer, & Silverstein, 1990).

The National Ileitis and Colitis Foundation can provide patient education and support; check for the availability of local chapters. Exploration of sources of stress and their relationship to symptom manifestation may be productive for some patients, along with support for individualized stress relief and relaxation activities.

Time Frame for Initiating Pharmacotherapy

Because of the relapsing nature of IBD, treatment depends on the patient's clinical picture. Pharmacotherapy should be instituted when symptoms occur. CD can present in an insidious manner; fever, weight loss, perianal disease, and fistulas indicate the need to start treatment. Sulfasalazine, aminosalicylic acid (5-ASA) preparations, or antibiotic therapy are used to treat mild CD. For disease of the colon, sulfasalazine is generally given for 4 to 8 weeks; if there is a positive response, therapy is continued for 4 to 6 months (Ruymann & Richter, 1995) and then stopped if the patient has no symptoms. Corticosteroid therapy is indicated for the short-term induction of remission in patients with moderate or severe symptoms. Immunosuppressive therapy can be used in CD patients who are dependent on corticosteroids or have persistent perianal disease or fistulas (Hanauer, 1996).

In patients with mild cases of UC, which are less associated with rectal bleeding, urgency, frequency, and rectal pain, treatment should be based on severity of symptoms and location of disease. Patients with mild to moderate disease can generally be treated with either oral or topical 5-ASA compounds or sulfasalazine. Patients with severe symptoms need close monitoring and may require hospitalization for treatment and observation of toxic megacolin. Costicosteroids are generally required to bring the acute disease under control. As in CD, immunosuppressive therapy is indicated for long-term treatment in patients with UC who are dependent on corticosteroids or do not respond to aminosalicylate corticosteroid therapy (Hanauer, 1996).

Patients with ulcerative proctitis should be differentiated from patients with more extensive disease. Ulcerative proctitis can generally be treated with topical compounds. Oral or topical therapy also can be used for disease of the distal colon or rectum.

With immunosuppressive drugs, therapy may take up to 6 months to show a positive effect. Aminosalicylates such as mesalamine can take several weeks to months to show effects (Shah & Peppercorn, 1995).

See Drug Tables 102.9, 102.10.

Assessment and History Taking

Since the laboratory workup that will give a definitive diagnosis is based on the patient's symptoms, a thorough history about the onset, timing, and nature of symptoms is essential. Ask about extracolonic disease manifestations, which can be seen in both UC and CD, such as blurred vision, headaches, eye pain, photophobia, mouth sores, and joint pain. Ask also about the associated signs and symptoms of active hepatitis, cholelithiasis, or kidney stones that are often seen in patients with IBD (Ruymann & Richter, 1995). History about family disease, recent travel, and/or antibiotic use is also helpful in ruling out other causes of symptoms.

In the physical examination, focus on the following areas:

- Vital signs, weight, body mass index
- Skin surfaces, especially of extremities and tibial surfaces of arms and legs for lesions of erythema nodosum
- Mouth, checking for lesions
- Thorough eye examination
- Thorough abdominal examination
- Rectal and perianal examination

To diagnose UC, flexible sigmoidoscopy without cleansing preparation is useful; if this gives only nonspecific findings, a stool culture and sensitivity and/or rectal biopsy may be more helpful (Ruymann & Richter, 1995). A barium enema or colonoscopy can assist in an uncertain diagnosis, but should not be performed during acute attacks since the risk of bowel perforation is increased.

In CD, a barium enema or air contrast barium enema can show the characteristic skip patterns of CD and provide a definitive diagnosis. In difficult to diagnose cases, sigmoidoscopy or colonoscopy also can be helpful. Radiologic tests should be minimized during pregnancy. A CBC, sedimentation rate, serum chemistry, and stool exam for occult blood can provide useful baseline information.

Patient/Caregiver Information

Sulfonamide drugs can result in hypersensitivity reactions of rash and fever or the dose-related side effects of nausea, vomiting, and headaches (Hirschfeld & Clearfield, 1995). Titrating the dose of the sulfasalazine can help to minimize headaches; taking these drugs with food will minimize other side effects (Hanauer & Baert, 1994). Sulfonamides also interfere with the bioavailability of digoxin so patients should be warned of signs and symptoms of inadequate digoxin dosing. Sulfa should not be taken at the same time as iron preparations (Ruymann & Richter, 1995).

Patients given metronidazole should be warned to avoid all alcohol and alcohol-containing products.

Patients should be told to contact their provider if they experience fever, increased diarrhea, rectal bleeding, or increased abdominal pain.

OUTCOMES MANAGEMENT

The primary end points of therapy should be the induction and remission of disease. In UC, the severity of disease can be assessed on the basis of clinical features using endoscopy and the criteria of Truelove and Witts (Hanauer, 1996). The Gastrointestinal Advisory Panel of the Food and Drug Administration has defined remission of UC as "absence of inflammatory symptoms (e.g., rectal bleeding) along with mucosal healing" (Hanauer, 1991). Assessing disease activity in patients with CD is more difficult because the clinical pattern and complications are more heterogeneous (Hanauer, 1996). The Crohn's Disease Activity Index has been used and consists of clinical variables and assessment of a patient's well-being. However, these end points are often difficult to define in IBD (Hodgson & Hazlan, 1991).

Maintenance therapy should be aimed at preventing recurrence of active disease.

Selecting an Appropriate Agent

Treatment options are determined by the location, the extent, and the severity of disease, and by the patient's response to current or past therapy.

Corticosteroids have been the most widely used and efficacious agents for the induction of remission of both moderate to severe active ulcerative colitis and Crohn's disease (Griffin & Miner, 1995). These agents are not useful as maintenance therapy for disease in remission or prophylaxis (Peppercorn, 1990; Shah & Peppercorn, 1995). The addition of corticosteroids to sulfasalazine for the treatment of patients with active Crohn's disease results in more rapid initial improvement, but not better overall results (Linn & Peppercorn, 1992). Therefore, corticosteroids are used primarily in severely ill patients or in patients who have failed with sulfasalazine or mesalamine. Once symptomatic improvement has been induced, steroids should be tapered to avoid their associated ill effects. The corticosteroid of choice should be one that is low in mineralocorticoid activity and high in antiinflammatory activity, such as prednisone or methylprednisolone.

Rectal administration of steroids has proven effective in patients with localized distal colitis, whereas oral corticosteroids are active against mild to moderate disease (Peppercorn, 1990). The use of topical rectal corticosteroids can minimize the adverse-effect profile as well as tenesmus and the urgent call to stool in patients with mild UC that is limited to the distal colon and rectum (Geier, Miner, Danielsson, Hellers, & Lyrenas, 1987). Foam preparations and suppositories are easier to administer than hydrocortisone enemas. However, even local administration can lead to Cushing's syndrome and adrenal suppression (Hanauer, Meyers, & Sachar, 1995; Mulder & Tygat, 1993). Newer oral and topical steroids with minimal side effects are currently used in Europe and expected to become available soon in the United States. In children, steroid therapy, using an alternating dose schedule, has minimized the effect on growth hormone. Since there may be better absorption of gluccocorticoid from intact than from inflammed mucosa, a lower dose can be used as healing occurs (Petitijean, Wendling, Tod, et al., 1992). In patients with severe UC, the absorption of oral corticosteroids may be decreased, requiring parenteral therapy. Corticotropin has been shown to be superior to hydrocortisone in patients naive to corticosteroid therapy; hydrocortisone is superior in patients previously treated with corticosteroids (Meyers, Sachar, Goldberg, & Janowitz, 1983).

The initial and subsequent dose of corticosteroid therapy should be individualized based upon the severity of symptoms and disease, and the corticosteroid used. Corticosteroid therapy should not be abruptly stopped, but gradually tapered as symptoms are controlled.

Sulfasalazine, a combination of 5-ASA and sulfapyridine, is effective for the initial treatment of UC and CD; it also is useful in preventing relapses. In CD this drug is only effective in patients with disease involving the colon or the ileum; it is not effective in patients with only small bowel disease (Malchow, 1984). Sulfasalazine will induce remission in up to 75% of patients with UC. Remission will be maintained in 70% of patients compared to 24% of those receiving placebo (Linn & Peppercorn, 1992). Since sulfasalazine is generally considered less effective than steroids, it is reserved for mild cases. It can also be combined with oral steroids for early treatment. Relapse rates appear to be dose-related, with higher doses resulting in lower frequencies of relapse (Griffin & Miner, 1995). For both UC and CD, a sulfasalazine dose of 500 mg qid PO can be initiated and increased rapidly to 4 g daily. As symptoms are relieved, decrease to the lowest dose necessary to control symptoms, usually 2 to 4 g/day (Ruymann & Richter, 1995). Doses greater than 4 g/day tend to increase side effects.

Despite its widespread acceptance, the usefulness of sulfasalazine has been limited by its adverse-effect profile (Peppercorn, 1990), which is a dose-related function of the sulfapyridine moiety (Hanauer, 1996; Geier et al., 1987). To counter this, the active component of sulfasalazine, 5-aminosalicylate, was isolated. Mesalamine, the generic name for 5-aminosalicylate, is hydrolyzed quickly in the stomach and well absorbed in the proximal small intestine. It does not reach disease sites in the distal colon and rectum. However, mesalamine can be administered via retention enemas or suppositories. Studies with patients with distal colitis have shown this form of administration to be more effective than placebos and as effective as sulfasalazine (Biddle & Miner, 1990; Campieri, DeFranchis, Bianchi Porro, et al., 1990). Because local contact is necessary for therapeutic efficacy, rectal administration of mesalamine should be used only in patients with disease confined to the distal colon (Hanauer, 1996). For long-term prophylaxis, oral forms of therapy are preferable to enemas or suppositories (Peppercorn, 1990).

In an attempt to increase the area of treatment, controlled-release (Pentasa) and delayed-release (Asacol) versions of mesalamine and a dimer of 5-aminosalicylic acid (olsalazine) have been developed for the treatment of disease in the small intestine and colon. In general, these oral aminosalicylates are therapeutically equivalent to sulfasalazine in the treatment of active disease or the maintenance of remission in mild or moderate UC. However, they may be better tolerated than sulfasalazine and can be used in patients unable to tolerate sulfasalazine (Linn & Peppercorn, 1992; "Olsalazine for Ulcerative Colitis," 1990). Pentasa has been shown to be useful as well in achieving and controlling remission in patients with active CD (Hanauer, 1993). Asacol also may prove useful in maintaining Crohn's disease in remission (Pallone et al, 1991). The recommended dose for Pentasa is 1.5 to 4 gs/day PO, in four divided doses; Asacol doses are 800 to 2400 mg/day PO, in three divided doses. For the maintenance of remission with olsalazine, the dose is 500 mg twice daily.

A switch to metronidazole 250 to 500 mg PO, three times a day, may be helpful for patients with mild to moderate CD who are unresponsive to sulfasalazine or olsalazine (Ruymann & Richter, 1995). Metronidazole 750 to 2000 mg PO per day is also effective for perianal complications in CD; treatment needs to be long-term (Ruymann & Richter, 1995). Many clinicians are using other antibiotics, especially ciprofloxacin in patients with CD who are intolerant or unresponsive to metronidazole (Hanauer & Baert, 1994; Peppercorn, 1993). Antibiotics, including metronidazole, have not been shown to be reliably effective in UC unless the patient has a concurrent infection with *Clostridium difficile.* Research findings do not support their use (Hanauer & Baert, 1994).

For CD patients who are refractory to aminosalicylates and/or steroids or who are steroid-dependent, the use of immunosuppressive therapies such as azathioprine (2.0–2.5 mg/kg per day PO) and 6-mercaptopurine (1–1.5 mg/kg per day PO) are indicated (Hanauer & Baert, 1994) and may allow tapering of the steroids (Ewe, Press, & Singe, 1993). Azathioprine has been shown to prolong remission in corticosteroid-dependent patients with UC (Hawthorne, Logan, & Gawkey, 1992). Caution is needed in the use of these agents because of their toxicity. The incidence of hematologic adverse effects is relatively low with initiating doses of 50 mg per day for both agents (Griffin & Miner, 1995). Parenteral methotrexate (25 mg intramuscularly or subcutaneously per week) has allowed significant reduction in steroid use in chronically active CD and UC (Geier & Miner, 1992; Hanauer & Baert, 1994). Other immunosupressive treatments include mycophenolate mofetil, tacrolimus, and cyclosporin.

Both steroids and sulfasalazine have been successfully used in pregnancy (Hanan, 1993). Steroids do not appear to have an effect on the fetus.

Monitoring for Efficacy

Patients requiring parenteral corticosteroid therapy should see symptomatic relief within 72 hours. Loftus, Loftus & Sandborn (2003) found 60% of patients symptom free in 5 days. They should then be changed to oral therapy. Remission should be achieved within 2 to 4 weeks; steroids should then be slowly tapered (Hanauer, 1996). If the disease recurs during the taper, the steroid dose should be increased for several days and a slower taper then started. Approximately 25% will not improve. They may successfully be treated with intravenous cyclosporin (Loftus, Loftus & Sandborn 2003).

Improvement shown by a decrease in pain and severity of diarrhea, with an increase in appetite and overall quality of life, should be seen with 4 to 6 weeks of maintenance therapy. Treatment should continue as the patient improves, even after resolution of symptoms (Hanauer & Baert, 1994).

Patients requiring immunosuppressive therapy (azathioprine, 6-mercaptopurine) may require 25-mg-per-day PO increases over the 50-mg initial doses to a maximum of 2 mg/kg per day (Hirschfeld & Clearfield, 1995). Therapeutic benefit from immunomodulators may require 3 to 6 months of therapy (Hanauer & Baert, 1994).

For patients placed on metronidazole, if there is no response within 4 to 8 weeks, the drug should be discontinued. If patients do respond to metronidazole, the drug can be continued for 3 to 4 months and then tapered (Peppercorn, 1990).

Monitoring for Toxicity

Sulfa drugs often cause nausea and headaches. Their allergic manifestations include hemolytic anemia, bone marrow suppression, and generalized hypersensitivity reactions that can be fatal (Hanauer, 1996). Sulfasalazine's effects are dose-related and can be minimized by administering less than 4 g per day. To minimize gastrointestinal effects, administer the drug with meals, initiate therapy at low doses, and titrate up slowly. If adverse effects occur, discontinue the drug until the effects abate and reinstitute at a lower dose. Patients should also be monitored for rash, fever, hematologic reactions, lupus-like syndrome, and hepatotoxicity.

Watery diarrhea is the most common adverse effect of olsalazine and can be avoided by starting with low doses and titrating up.

Anal irritation and pruritus have been associated with rectally administered mesalamine.

For patients on steroid therapy, be alert for cataracts, metabolic bone disease, and osteonecrosis. Monitor blood pressure and serum glucose levels.

Bone marrow suppression is dose-related when using immunomodulators. Monitor with a complete CBC with differential weekly for the first month and then monthly thereafter (Hirschfeld & Clearfield, 1995). The drug should be discontinued or dose decreased if the white blood cell count or platelets decrease. Because azathioprine and mercaptopurine have been associated with pancreatitis in 3 to 15% of patients, monitor amylase and lipase and be alert to patients' complaints of abdominal pain (Hanauer, 1996; Hanauer & Baert, 1994). Symptoms usually occur after several weeks of therapy.

Be alert for perforation or severe bleeding in all patients. Some patients may be refractory to treatment and need referral to gastroenterologists. Patients with UC who have high-grade dysplasia or suspected cancer or who are unresponsive to maximum treatment should be referred for surgery, which is curative. In CD, surgery is not curative but necessary when patients have an obstruction.

Followup Recommendations

Initial therapy may require a followup evaluation every 2 to 8 weeks. Maintenance therapy for at least 6 months to 1 year may be necessary for patients with UC, based on the severity of attacks, the response to treatment, and the history of relapse (Hanauer & Baert, 1994; Ruymann & Richter, 1995). At least annual followup with a primary care provider is indicated for patients with currently asymptomatic IBD.

PEPTIC ULCER DISEASE

Peptic ulcer disease (PUD) is a heterogeneous group of disorders involving the upper gastrointestinal tract. Duodenal and gastric ulcers are the most common types of peptic ulcer; however, ulcers of other areas of the gastrointestinal tract do occur. It is a disease that results from an imbalance between the body's aggressive forces and its defensive factors. PUD can be acute and short-lived or chronic and characterized by remission and recurrences. There are three etiologic groups into which PUD can be divided: (1) massive acid hypersecretion, for example, Zollinger-Ellison syndrome; (2) drug-induced, for example, from the intake of nonsteroidal antiinflammatory agents; or (3) infectious, from *Helicobacter pylori.*

A number of factors can predispose someone to PUD. The hypersecretion of gastric acid in individuals with increased parietal cell mass can lead to the development of ulcers. Through direct mucosal irritation and prostaglandin inhibition, drugs such as nonsteroidal antiinflammatory agents and aspirin can induce ulcer formation. The disruption of the architecture of the gastroduodenal mucosa from an inflammation associated with *H. pylori* can cause ulcers. Cigarette smoking, alcohol intake, and psychological stress have been implicated in ulcer formation. Age and family history may also play a role in the development of certain types of ulcers (Katz, 1991).

SPECIFIC CONSIDERATIONS FOR PHARMACOTHERAPY

When Drug Therapy Is Needed

The mortality of PUD has declined over the last decade. Less than 2% of patients with ulcers receiving therapy are expected to have a complication such as bleeding, perforation, or obstruction (Katz, 1991). However, PUD remains one of the most common GI diseases that results in loss of work and high medical costs. The natural history of PUD is associated with ulcer recurrence. It is widely accepted that *H. pylori* is a major etiologic factor leading to peptic ulcer disease, and about 6 to 20% of persons infected with *H. pylori* are later found to have the disease. The infection is found in 90 to 95% of patients with duodenal ulcers and 50 to 70% of patients with gastric ulcers (Knigge, 2001). Complications are reported to develop every year in 2.7% of patients without a history of bleeding or perforation and in 5% of those with previous complications.

Short- and Long-Term Goals of Pharmacotherapy

The short-term goal of treatment for PUD is resolution of pain or symptoms, promotion of ulcer healing, and prevention of complications. In Zollinger-Ellison syndrome, the goal of therapy is symptomatic pain relief and control of gastric acid secretion. The long-term goal of PUD treatment is the prevention of ulcer recurrence.

Nonpharmacologic Therapy

Patients should be counseled to avoid the following:

- Completely cease and avoid cigarette smoking
- Decrease caffeine-containing foods
- Avoid or limit corticosteroids and nonsteroidal antiinflammatory drugs
- Avoid foods that cause discomfort
- Abstain from foods late in the evening that will stimulate nocturnal acid secretion
- Develop a personal stress reduction program

Time Frame for Initiating Pharmacotherapy

Patients should be treated at the time of diagnosis to prevent the complications of bleeding or perforation. *H. pylori*–infected patients without symptoms need not be treated. Patients infected with *H. pylori* and with a gastric or duodenal ulcer should be treated with a full course of antibiotics along with an antisecretory agent (Berardi, 1997). For drug-induced ulcers, the offending drug should be discontinued and treatment with an antisecretory agent should be initiated. For patients who require continued NSAID therapy, enteric-coated formulations taken with meals may minimize recurrence but concurrent omeprazole (40 mg per day PO) administration may be necessary (Berardi, 1997; Goroll et al., 1995). In patients with Zollinger-Ellison syndrome, control of the excess amount of gastric acid output is important. Successful medical management can be achieved by titrating the 60-mg-per-day PO initial dose of omeprazole according to patient response (Berardi, 1997).

See Drug Tables 501.5, 501.6.

Assessment and History Taking

Assessment of the patient should include evaluation of pain—including the type, timing (i.e., episodic or continuous), and duration of pain, its association with meals, and what relieves the pain. The history should also include:

- Presence of related symptoms such as intermittent nausea, vomiting, belching
- Past medical history, including previous PUD occurrence, hyperparathyroidism, cirrhosis, pancreatitis, arthritis
- Medication history
- Smoking history
- Family history of ulcers

The physical examination should include:

- Abdominal examination, checking for rebound, tenderness, bowel sounds
- Rectal examination, checking for occult blood

Diagnostic tests should include:

- Radiologic and endoscopic tests
- Cultures and stains of endoscopically obtained specimens if *H. pylori* is suspected
- Acid-secreting tests for those unresponsive to therapy and/or if gastrinoma or other hypersecretory states are suspected

Laboratory tests should include:

- Hemoglobin, hematocrit
- BUN and creatinine
- Stool occult blood test

Patient/Caregiver Information

Patients should be counseled to:

- Avoid cigarette smoking
- Decrease caffeine-containing foods
- Minimize foods that cause symptoms
- Avoid corticorsteroids, aspirin, and nonsteroidal anti-inflammatory drugs
- Develop a personal stress management plan

OUTCOMES MANAGEMENT

Selecting an Appropriate Agent

Presently, H_2-receptor antagonists, sucralfate, omeprazole, antacids, and antibiotics are all indicated for the treatment of PUD. The therapeutic regimen should be chosen based upon etiology of the ulcer, comparative efficacies, adverse-effect profiles, pharmacokinetic properties, potential drug interactions, and cost.

H_2-receptor antagonists are indicated for the treatment of both duodenal and gastric ulcers. H_2-receptor antagonists have comparable healing rates of 70 to 95% after 4 to 8 weeks of therapy, respectively. Famotidine and nizatidine are the most potent and possess the longest duration of action; however, all the H_2-receptor antagonists can be administered once daily for the treatment of acute duodenal ulcers (Gitlin, McCullough, Smith, et al., 1987). All H_2-receptor antagonists are eliminated by a combination of hepatic metabolism, glomerular filtration, and renal tubular secretion. Renal excretion is the major route of elimination for famotidine and nizatidine; therefore, dosage adjustments are recommended for patients with moderate to severe renal insufficiency (creatinine clearance < 50 mL/min).

Sucralfate is a nonsystemic agent that has been approved only for the treatment of duodenal ulcers. This drug should not be used in a patient who may have a compliance problem because it must be administered four times a day. Sucralfate may be helpful for patients who have difficulty in swallowing because it is available as a suspension.

Antacids serve two roles in the treatment of PUD: pain relief and healing. Because one of the goals of PUD therapy is elimination of symptoms, antacids can be given on an "as needed" basis to provide pain relief. Antacids have a rapid onset of action (5–15 min); however, the duration of action is only 2 hours. Therefore, these agents are *not* recommended for patients who might have difficulty taking medications on a frequent and regular basis. Because of the adverse-effect profile and the multiple daily dosing, antacids are primarily used for symptomatic relief of pain or for patients unable to tolerate other therapies.

Omeprazole and lansoprazole are potent and highly specific inhibitors of gastric acid secretion. These agents are effective in the treatment of duodenal ulcers, Zollinger-Ellison syndrome, and *H. pylori*–associated ulcers. Because hypersecretion and resistance develop with the use of H_2-receptor antagonists, these drugs are the drugs of choice for the treatment of Zollinger-Ellison syndrome. They relieve symptoms and heal ulcers faster in PUD than H_2-receptor antagonists (2 to 4 versus 4 to 8 weeks). Because of the prolonged achlorhydria caused by these agents, they should be reserved for patients who have severe disease, a greater likelihood of complications, refractory PUD disease, or *H. pylori*– associated ulcers (Bardham, Naesdal, Bianchi, et al., 1991; Hixson, Kelley, Jones, et al., 1992).

Single agent therapy should not be used because of the unacceptably low eradication rates. In addition, dual therapy is no longer recommended because cure rates for all regimens are under 85%. Clinical trials have shown that multidrug regimens (triple therapy) are the most effective treatment, with eradication rates up to 96%. The regimen of choice is a PPI or ranitidine bismuth citrate (Tritec) plus two antibiotics for 14 days. These agents have superior efficacy to and are better tolerated than the standard bismuth-based triple therapy, consisting of bismuth subsalicylate, metronidazole (Flagyl, Protostat), and tetracycline hydrochloride (Knigge, 2001). Antimicrobial resistance among *H. pylori* isolates may limit the use of regimens containing metronidazole or clarithromycin (Biaxin). The background incidence of antibacterial resistance among *H. pylori* isolates in the United States is about 11% for metronidazole and 4% for clarithromycin. Standard bismuth triple therapy plus a PPI achieves eradication rates of more than 95% and can be used as a backup in patients in whom triple therapy has failed. However, documentation of these treatment failures in the literature is scarce (Knigge, 2001). In patients unable to tolerate metronidazole's side effects, clarithromycin 500 mg bid amoxicillin 1 gram bid, and a proton pump inhibitor for 14 days were equally efficacious and cost effective.

Monitoring for Efficacy

The treatment course is dependent upon the type of ulcer and its etiology. Duodenal ulcers should show improvement and healing within 4 to 8 weeks. Gastric ulcers generally require more time, up to 12 weeks of therapy. If the ulcer has not healed within the specified period of time, retreatment for an additional 4 weeks is indicated. Patients who do not heal with 3 to 4 months of therapy are considered refractory and should be evaluated for noncompliance or other causes for impaired healing (e.g., smoking, nonsteroidal drug use, alcohol use). Therapeutic options available for refractory ulcers include higher doses and more frequent dosing of H_2-receptor antagonists, or proton pump inhibitors. Omeprazole has been shown to work better than continued H_2-receptor antagonists for the treatment of refractory PUD (Bardham et al., 1991; Guerreiro, 1990).

H. pylori infection is one of the most common in the world. Its association with peptic ulcer disease and gastric MALT lymphoma is now undisputed, and numerous tests are available to detect the infection. PPI-based triple therapy is considered the gold standard of treatment. There is no vaccine to prevent *H. pylori,* but a number of investigators have begun to study the possibility of developing one (Knigge, 2001).

Patients with diagnosed drug-induced ulcers should see improvement rapidly when the causative agent is removed (Howden, Jones, Peace, Burget, & Hunt, 1988). H_2-receptor antagonists will heal small ulcers (< 0.5 cm) within 8 weeks; larger ulcers may require 12 weeks of therapy. Continued NSAID therapy may delay healing of small ulcers but does not appear to prevent healing. Misoprostol 200 μ g qid PO can prevent NSAID-associated ulcers in patients who require continuous NSAIDs.

The medical goal of therapy for Zollinger-Ellison syndrome is pain relief and control of gastric secretion, which can be achieved by titrating the drug dosage to a postdrug gastric acid secretion of less than 10 mEq/h PO for the last hour before the next dose of medication. If large once-daily dosing does not control acid secretion, administer the total daily dose in two divided doses for better gastric acid control (Frucht, Maton, & Jensen, 1991).

Monitoring for Toxicity

All H_2-receptor antagonists have a similar adverse-effect profile: All cause rashes, central nervous system alterations (e.g., confusion) and gastrointestinal disturbances. Famotidine has been associated with headaches and should be avoided in patients with a history of migraines. Because of its antiandrogenic effects, cimetidine has been associated with gynecomastia and impotence. Thrombocytopenia has been associated with the use of ranitidine and famotidine, and patients should be monitored for this periodically. With long-term use, proton pump inhibitors have been associated with hypergastrinemia, which may lead to carcinoid tumors of the stomach (Maton, 1991). With short-term therapy, omeprazole and lansoprazole are well tolerated despite gastrointestinal discomforts.

All antibiotics can cause gastrointestinal disturbances and rashes. Alcohol must be avoided in patients taking metronidazole.

Misoprostol is contraindicated in women of childbearing age unless contraceptive measures are utilized. The diarrhea associated with misoprostal is dose-related, but with reduced dosage the protection against drug-associated ulcers is impaired.

Followup Recommendations

Healing of the ulcer and/or eradication of *H. pylori* should be documented via endoscopy at least 4 weeks after completion of therapy for patients who are of high risk for complications or patients who are candidates for long-term maintenance therapy. For low-risk patients, documentation is optional because the recurrence of symptoms will identify those with reappearing ulcers or in whom infection has not been eradicated (Fennerty, 1995). Current literature supports the urea breath test for *H. pylori* post-treatment testing. The test is the most accurate method to document eradication of *H. pylori* following treatment. A positive breath test indicates active infection (Knigge, 2001). If positive, these patients should undergo endoscopy for visualization of ulcers and histological and culture testing.

Patients not responsive to antibiotic therapy can receive a second course of therapy. These patients should also have a fasting gastrin secretion test done to rule out Zollinger-Ellison syndrome. Consultation with a gastroenterologist should be considered to rule out gastric cancer, especially for patients over 50 (Berardi, 1997; Goroll et al., 1995; Katz, 1995).

GASTROESOPHAGEAL REFLUX

Gastroesophageal reflux disease (GERD) is a disorder in which the gastric contents are regurgitated into the esophagus, leading to irritation and injury to the esophageal mucosa. Heartburn, or pyrosis, is the primary symptom; however, symptoms such as cough and chest pain can also occur. Atypical symptoms include odynophagia, dysphagia, chest pain, cough and reactive airway disease (Kaynard & Flora, 2001). Gastroesophageal reflux events have been shown to occur by three mechanisms: (1) transient lower esophageal sphincter (LES) relaxation, (2) abdominal strain, and (3) a low resting LES pressure (Fennerty, Castell & Fendrick, 1996). GERD is likely the most common gastrointestinal disease seen in primary care (Kaynard & Flora, 2001). In the differential diagnoses, cardiac causes for any unexplained chest pain should be considered.

SPECIFIC CONSIDERATIONS FOR PHARMACOTHERAPY

When Drug Therapy Is Needed

Although lifestyle modification may alleviate the symptoms of mild disease, drug therapy is necessary for patients with more severe disease. The long-term exposure of the esophagus to refluxed material can result in serious complications, including hemorrhage, strictures, and ulceration (Katz, 1995).

Short- and Long-Term Goals of Pharmacotherapy

The initial goal of therapy is to eliminate the symptoms of retrosternal pain and diminish the frequency and duration of esophageal reflux. The long-term goal is to prevent relapse, recurrence, and esophageal injury.

Nonpharmacologic Therapy

Lifestyle modifications remain the cornerstone of initial therapy. These include the following:

- Dietary restrictions (e.g., avoid fatty foods and large meals, peppermint, onions, garlic, chocolate)
- Not eating for a least 3 hours before lying down; no bedtime snacks
- Sleeping with the head of the bed elevated to decrease nocturnal esophageal acid contact time
- Weight reduction
- No cigarette smoking

Time Frame for Initiating Pharmacotherapy

Lifestyle modifications alone remain limited, and pharmacotherapy for GERD is indicated when symptoms continue or are severe.

See Drug Tables 501.1, 501.5, 501.6.

Assessment and History Taking

The medical history should include specific questions about:

- Nature and frequency of pain and its relationship to sleep and meals
- Anorexia and recent weight loss
- Presence of symptoms of dysphagia, regurgitation, increased salivation, odynophagia, bleeding
- Dietary precipitants such as coffee, tomato or orange juice, spicy foods
- Use of anti-inflammatory drugs
- Smoking history
- Alcohol use
- Conditions such as pregnancy, scleroderma, achalasia

During the physical examination look for:

- Presence of cough, hoarseness, hiccups
- Presence of occult or frank blood in the stool

Laboratory tests that may be useful in the diagnosis of GERD include:

- 24-hour ambulatory esophageal pH study to quantitate and document reflux of gastric contents

- Barium swallow and/or an endoscopy may be the best initial test; the latter is the most sensitive test for detecting esophageal strictures
- Endoscopy is useful in assessing mucosal damage or documenting the presence of Barrett's epithelium, hiatal hernia, and/or strictures (Katz, 1995)

Patient/Caregiver Information

Patients should be counseled to:

- Avoid or stop smoking; consider use of nicotine gum or patches
- Lose weight if necessary
- Wear loose-fitting clothes to prevent abdominal or sternal pressure
- Avoid lying flat while watching television or sleeping
- Avoid foods that irritate the gastric mucosa (ie, spicy food) or foods that stimulate acid production (ie, alcohol)
- Avoid foods that lower the esophageal sphincter (ie, fatty meals, chocolate, peppermint)
- Avoid eating prior to going to bed
- Avoid bending over after eating
- Elevate head of bed with blocks

OUTCOMES MANAGEMENT

Selecting an Appropriate Agent

For patients with mild symptoms and nonerosive disease, therapy can include antacids, prokinetics, or H_2-receptor antagonists. The use of antacids is effective in relieving symptoms (DeVault & Castell, 1995). Because antacids have a short duration of action and do not heal esophagitis, they are recommended for use only with other therapies to provide symptomatic relief.

For patients with moderately severe symptoms and nonerosive or mildly erosive disease, prokinetics and H_2-receptor antagonists are usually efficacious. Response to an H_2-receptor antagonist depends upon dose, duration of therapy, and severity of the disease. Overall, 50 to 70% of symptomatic patients will respond with complete or partial resolution of symptoms when treated with H_2-receptor antagonists (Fennerty et al., 1996). The healing rates of esophagitis will vary depending upon the severity of the disease as well as the duration and dosage of the drug therapy. Studies have shown variable results (0–82%) in endoscopic healing of esophagitis with these agents (DeVault & Castell, 1995). For those with moderate symptoms and nonerosive disease, H_2 receptors can be administered in standard doses but on a more frequent basis (twice daily) (DiPiro & Bowden, 1997). For those with more severe disease or those who fail standard therapeutic doses, 1.5 to 2 times the standard doses should be utilized. Only twice-daily administration and high doses of H_2-receptor antagonists will suppress acid approximately to the levels attained by proton pump inhibitors. These results appear to depend upon the severity of the esophageal lesions and the dose given.

The role of prokinetic drugs (e.g., metoclopramide, cisapride) in the treatment of GERD is limited. Metoclopramide has shown minimal symptomatic improvement in promoting endoscopic healing, and because of the side-effect profile, its use is limited (Ramirez & Richter, 1993). The recommended regimen for metoclopramide orally is 10 mg taken 20 to 30 minutes prior to meals and at bedtime. In contrast, cisapride has been shown to be as effective as H_2-receptor antagonists, with comparable improvement of both symptoms and endoscopic healing in patients with GERD (DeMicco, Berenson, Wu, et al., 1992; Geldof, Hazelhoff, & Otten, 1993). A randomized trial involving patients with reflux esophagitis demonstrated that cisapride 20 mg qid PO provided better endoscopic healing (69%) than 10 mg qid PO (57%) (Faruqui, Sigmund, Smith, et al., 1992). However, because cisapride has no clinical advantage over H_2-receptor antagonists and is more expensive, it is not recommended as a sole agent for the treatment of GERD. A study comparing single-drug regimens (cisapride, ranitidine, and omeprazole) and two combined drug regimens (ranitidine plus cisapride and omeprazole plus cisapride) in patients with erosive reflux esophagitis found that omeprazole alone or in combination with cisapride was more effective than ranitidine alone or cisapride alone (Greenberger, 1997). Cisapride also may be beneficial in combination with an H_2-receptor antagonist in patients with delayed gastric emptying.

For patients with moderate to severe erosive esophagitis, a proton pump inhibitor omeprazole, lansoprazole, rabeprazole and esomeprazole is considered the drug of choice. These agents have a greater antisecretory effect and have been shown to be superior to the H_2-receptor antagonists. Omeprazole has been shown to heal approximately 60% of patients with esophagitis compared to 30% healing with H_2-receptor antagonist after 4 weeks (Bianchi Porro, Pau, Peracchia, et al., 1992; Havelund, Laursen, & Lauritsen, 1994). After 8 weeks of therapy, healing rates further increased to 35% and 80% for ranitidine and omeprazole, respectively. The higher healing rate for omeprazole was also accompanied by faster and more substantial symptom relief.

Patients with GERD without esophagitis or who have frequent recurrent symptoms should be placed on a maintenance program with an antisecretory agent or prokinetic agent if delayed gastric emptying is present. Other patients may have symptomatic relapses and failure of healing of esophagitis.

Proton pump inhibitors have been shown to be more effective than other therapies in controlling acid and in preventing recurrence of erosive esophagitis (Dent, Yeomans, Mackinoon, et al., 1994; Hallerback et al, 1994). Maintenance therapy with PPIs is often required after esophagitis is healed and symptoms are relieved. Attempts to reduce the dosage or switch to less effective medications usually result in recurrence (Kaynard & Flora, 2001).

Monitoring for Efficacy

Patients should see relief of symptoms such as heartburn within 4 weeks. If patients continue to have symptoms or there is incomplete healing of the esophagitis, consider increasing the dose and/or the frequency of the drug. For patients with resistant GERD who are already on a proton pump inhibitor and have gastroparesis, cisapride may be a helpful addition. Effective maintenance therapy depends on the severity of the disease and may require only lifestyle changes and antacids (Lieberman, 1987), or continuous maintenance therapy with acid-suppressing medications may be necessary (Howden, Castell, Cohen, et al., 1995). For many patients, esophagitis is a chronic relapsing disease, and the majority of patients will have a recurrence within 6 to 12 months after therapy is discontinued (Fennerty et al., 1996).

Monitoring for Toxicity

Cisapride has been associated with gastrointestinal upset and rhinitis. Therefore, patients with chronic sinusitis should be monitored for an exacerbation of this condition. H_2-receptor antagonists have a similar adverse-effect profile, which includes rash and gastrointestinal disturbances. Cimetidine is associated with impotence and gynecomastia, and famotidine has been associated with headaches. Thrombocytopenia can occur with all H_2-receptor antagonists but is more common with famotidine and ranitidine.

With long-term use, omeprazole has been associated with hypergastrinemia, which has the potential to lead to carcinoid tumors of the stomach. Therefore, patients placed on long-term proton pump inhibitors should be monitored for this.

Followup

Patients should be followed up within 4 weeks after diagnosis and initial treatment. Because this condition is associated with a high relapse and recurrence rate, patients should be followed closely.

EXCESSIVE FLATUS

Flatus, or the passage of intestinal gas through the anus, is a natural byproduct of digestion. Differing physiology and/or dietary intake, however, can result in excessive, noisy, or malodorous eruptions that can be embarrassing. Several over-the-counter preparations are available to minimize excessive flatus or bloating, none of which are considered highly effective.

SPECIFIC CONSIDERATIONS FOR PHARMACOTHERAPY

When Drug Therapy Is Needed

Based on personal criteria, patients generally decide when to initiate therapy. Generally, their immediate and longer term goals of elimination of all flatus are not able to be met; minimizing the number and/or intensity of events is a more realistic goal.

The most important nonpharmacologic therapy for flatus is simple dietary modification, which is generally indicated for all patients. To minimize swallowed air in the stomach, patients should eliminate carbonated beverages and gum chewing, avoid rapid eating or drinking, and ensure that dentures fit well. Alternatives to anticholinergic drugs should be found; these drugs cause dry mouth, which can also lead to aerophagia ("Simethicone for Gastrointestinal Gas," 1996).

See Drug Table 501.2.

Assessment and History Taking

Before therapy, patients should be evaluated for history or signs and symptoms of other GI disorders, such as diverticulosis, irritable bowel syndrome, or inflammatory bowel disease. Symptoms such as abdominal pain, alternating diarrhea and constipation, and passage of mucus or bloody stools should be considered together and not treated individually. Provider discretion should determine if a physical examination is indicated. Consider an abdominal examination checking for tenderness, rebound, and masses; a rectal exam to rule out impaction; and a stool guaiac test to check for occult blood.

Patients and caregivers should be reassured that their symptoms are not unusual. A daily chart of flatus events, noting specifics and timing of food ingestion and time and quantification of eruptions, can be helpful in determining which foods might be eliminated. Provide patients with education about the most common causes of flatus and appropriate dietary modification. Carbonated beverages, lactose-containing foods, beans, and certain vegetables such as cabbage, cauliflower, and broccoli are common causes of flatus.

SELECTING AN APPROPRIATE AGENT

Antibiotics are not recommended for the treatment of flatus. Although there was at one time hope that antibiotic manipulation of the intestinal flora could assist in the elimination of flatus, results have not proven successful (Danzl, 1992).

Simethicone, a combination of dimethylpolysiloxanes and silica gel, acts as an antifoaming agent. It causes gas bubbles to coalesce by lowering their surface tension. Although simethicone-containing products (Maalox Anti-Gas, Mylanta Gas Relief, Mylicon, etc.) are heavily advertised for treatment of flatus, well-controlled, double-blind studies in infants, postoperative patients, and healthy volunteers found no significant differences between subjects and controls ("Simethicone," 1996).

Alpha-galactosidase preparations (e.g., Beano) contain an enzyme intended to break down indigestible oligosaccharides found in high-fiber foods. Although minimal studies have been done with these products, they are considered generally safe and do provide relief for some patients (Ganiats, Norcross, Halverson, Burford, & Palinkas, 1994). The breakdown of the oligosaccharides produces galactose, so these products should be avoided in patients with galactosemia.

Anticholinergic agents decrease colonic contractions. These agents are not recommended because such contractions cannot be suppressed indefinitely; their resultant pressure must have an eventual outlet.

HEMORRHOIDS

Hemorrhoids are a common condition in the population over age 50 and in women of all ages who have been pregnant. They result from the pressure of large, firm stool, from partial blockage of the anal canal, and/or from increased venous pressure from conditions such as congestive heart failure or pregnancy. Hemorrhoids generally present with painless rectal bleeding, rectal itching, or anal discomfort.

SPECIFIC CONSIDERATIONS FOR PHARMACOTHERAPY

When Drug Therapy Is Needed

Patients can experience considerable pain, pressure and discomfort from symptomatic hemorrhoids. Therapeutic interventions can provide prompt relief for many patients.

Alleviation of the patient's discomfort, promotion of healing, and prevention of future attacks are the goals of therapy.

Nonpharmacologic Therapy

Local application of a cold pack can provide symptomatic relief. Finding a sitting position that avoids direct pressure on the symptomatic hemorrhoid is essential. This may be facilitated by the use of donut-shaped inflatable rings or soft foam pillows that distribute the pressure evenly. Warm sitz baths two or three times a day for 15 to 20 min are often soothing. A high-fiber diet and bulk-forming agents can result in soft, easily passed stools, minimizing local pressure on the anus. These should be continued after resolution of the acute problem as preventive measures against recurrence.

Time for Initiating Pharmacotherapy

Preventive therapy in the form of a high-fiber diet and bulk-forming agents can be suggested to all patients as a preventive measure. Localized therapy for hemorrhoids can be initiated at onset of acute symptoms.

See Drug Table 304.

Assessment and History Taking

The history of the patient with hemorrhoids should include questions about the nature, onset, and duration of symptoms; the usual nature of his or her bowel movements; and whether the patient has had a history of constipation or hemorrhoids in the past. Also determine if the patient is pregnant, has any systemic illnesses, has a history of anorectal surgery, or is taking any medications that might cause constipation or increased venous pressure. The physical examination should include a thorough inspection of the anal area and a digital rectal exam. Thrombosed or prolapsed hemorrhoids found on examination should be referred for surgical intervention. Anal fissures should receive antibiotic treatment and/or surgery.

Patient/Caregiver Information

Reduction of rectal pressure, constipation, and straining with defecation is the best long-term method for prevention of future hemorrhoids.

OUTCOMES MANAGEMENT

Selecting an Appropriate Agent

External creams or ointments are preferable to medicated suppositories inserted into the rectum with less local effect.

Most over-the-counter preparations contain topical anesthetics that provide relief from pain or pruritus. Benzocaine, one of the commonly used anesthetics, can give relief in several minutes but also produces local allergic reactions that can be worse than the original symptoms. Pramoxine is a less sensitizing anesthetic (Goroll et al., 1995). Astringents such as witch hazel provide inexpensive relief for some patients.

During pregnancy products such as Preparation H and Anusol Hc are acceptable (Remick, 1994). Topical steroids should be minimized because of the possibility of systemic absorption through the rectal mucosa.

Monitoring for Efficacy

If a patient complains of continued pain after all attempts at symptom relief, referral to a surgeon can be made for surgical treatment. Hemorrhoids that prolapse produce severe symptoms, reoccur repeatedly, or bleed heavily despite local treatments should also be referred to a surgeon for evaluation.

Monitoring for Toxicity

Patients should be warned that any increased symptoms after using the OTC or prescribed medications may be the result of local irritation and medication reaction. The medication should be discontinued and an alternative used that does not contain the offending product's main ingredient.

Followup

Patients should be encouraged to return for alternative medication within 1 week if the initial recommendations offered no relief. Surgical consultation may be necessary.

HEPATITIS

Hepatitis is an acute or chronic inflammation of the liver as a result of viral infection from one of five distinct viruses (A, B, C, D, and E) or chemical exposure, including alcohol.

SPECIFIC CONSIDERATIONS FOR PHARMACOTHERAPY

When Drug Therapy Is Needed

Pharmacotherapy in the primary care setting is limited to prophylactic immunizations for specific risk groups. Hepatitis A (HAV) viral-specific immunization is available for international travelers and children in daycare; immune globulin (IG) is indicated for household contacts of known cases of hepatitis A. Hepatitis B (HBV) vaccine, given in a series of three doses, is indicated for sexually active adults, healthcare workers, and the children of chronic carriers. An HBV prophylaxis regimen is suggested after percutaneous or mucous membrane exposure to known carriers of hepatitis B surface antigen (HBsAg). For more complete guidelines on immunization and postexposure prophylaxis against hepatitis A, B, and C, see the guidelines from the U.S. Preventive Services Task Force, Guide to Clinical Preventive Services (1996).

Short- and Long-Term Goals of Pharmacotherapy

The goals of pharmacotherapy are the prevention of infection in individuals who are exposed to any of the known hepatitis viruses.

Nonpharmacologic Therapy

Since hepatitis A and E are transmitted primarily by the fecal-oral route, meticulous attention to hygiene and handwashing after use of the toilet and changing diapers is indicated.

Condoms, either male or female, should be used with all sexual encounters to prevent spread of HBV. To prevent parenteral HBV spread, counsel patients to avoid injection drug use and not to share needles or drug apparatus. Universal precautions should be practiced by healthcare workers when in contact with blood and fluids. Family members of known HBV carriers should be educated about universal precautions.

Time Frame for Initiating Pharmacotherapy

Injections of HAV IG can be given immediately before travel exposures and last up to 3 months. For longer exposures, IG can be repeated every 4 to 6 months. IG should be given as soon as possible after exposure to household, sexual, and daycare center contacts; its use after 2 weeks is not effective. HAV vaccine is effective 14 to 21 days after IM administration (Benenson, 1995).

The hepatitis B vaccine series is recommended for all infants. Special attention should be given to vaccinating children from populations with high rates of hepatitis B infection, including Alaskan Natives, Pacific Islanders, and immigrants from countries with endemic HBV infection (Committee on Infectious Diseases, 1994). Immunization against HBV is also recommended for all adolescents. Emphasis should be on adolescents and adults who (Committee on Infectious Diseases, 1994):

1. Have sexually transmitted diseases
2. Have more than one sex partner
3. Are injecting drug users
4. Are homosexual men or bisexual men or women
5. Are sexual contacts of high-risk individuals
6. Work in contact with blood or body fluids

There are two timetables for administration of HBV vaccine: a three-dose schedule, which is initial, 1 to 2 months later, and 6 to 18 months later; or a four-dose schedule with the first dose at birth, followed at 1, 2, and 6 months of age (Benenson, 1995).

Hepatitis B immune globulin (HBIG) IM is indicated as soon as possible, but within 24 hours, after percutaneous or mucous membrane contact with blood that may contain HBsAg. An HBV vaccine series should be started at the same time in unimmunized persons. If the vaccine series cannot be started at the time of HBIG administration, a second dose of HBIG should be given 1 month after the first (Benenson, 1995). Sexual contacts of patients with acute HBV infection should also receive HBIG and initiation of an HBV vaccine series within 2 weeks of exposure.

See Drug Table 106.

Assessment and History Taking

The medical history should include specific questions about:

- Common presenting symptoms, including jaundice, fatigue, muscle pain, decreased appetite, nausea, vomiting, diarrhea, right upper quadrant abdominal pain, and low-grade fever
- Illnesses in household and sexual contacts
- Presence of darkened urine and white, chalky-colored stool
- History of recent travel
- Substance use, including alcohol and injection drugs
- Sexual partners and practices
- Work-related exposures
- Medication history, including OTCs

The physical examination should include:

- Skin examination to document the presence of jaundice on skin, sclerae, or mucous membranes
- Abdominal examination, checking for liver and spleen enlargement and/or tenderness

Laboratory tests should include (Uphold & Graham, 1994):

- CBC
- Liver function tests
- Prothrombin time
- Urinalysis
- Total and direct bilirubin
- Hepatitis screening panel, which will include HAV IgM antibody (IgM anti-HAV), HBV surface antigen (HBsAg), and HBV core antibody (anti-HBc)
- Additionally, the hepatitis screening panel should include screening for hepatitis C

Patient/Caregiver Information

Education should be provided about hand washing, condoms, and nonsharing of parenteral drug apparatus, as discussed above.

OUTCOMES MANAGEMENT

Selecting an Appropriate Agent

Two formulations of HBV vaccine are available: a plasma-derived version (Heptavax-B), which has been extensively tested and found safe, and a recombinant vaccine (Recombivax HB); both result in high rates of conversion. To avoid unnecessary prophylaxis in those already immune, prevaccination testing for anti-HBs may be done. There is no adverse effect in giving HBV vaccine to individuals with previous HBV infection. One milliliter (10 g of the recombinant vaccine or 20 μg of the plasma-derived vaccine) (or 0.5 mL in children less than 10 years old) intramuscular injections should be given in the deltoid region. Hemodialysis patients should receive higher doses because of less effective antibody response (Jacobs, 1997).

For postexposure prophylaxis of HBV, 0.06 mL/kg IM of HBIG should be given, with a second dose 1 month later (Benenson, 1995). For infants of mothers who are HBsAg positive, HBIG 0.5 mg intramuscularly is indicated within 12 hours of birth (U.S. Preventive Services Task Force, 1996).

Twinrix, a combination of Hepatitis A Inactivated and Hepatitis B (Recombinant) Vaccine, was recently approved for the prevention of hepatitis A and B in adults 18 years and older. The combination therapy of oral ribavirin with interferon alfa-2b, recombinant (Intron A) injection was approved for the treatment of chronic hepatitis C in patients with compensated liver disease who have relapsed after alpha interferon therapy or were previously untreated with alpha interferons. Patients with hepatitis should be referred to a specialist for examination and evaluation of various treatment options.

Human leukocyte alpha-interferon and adenine arabinoside (ara-A) have been shown to inhibit serum viral markers in patients with chronic HBV infection. Patients that are HBsAg carriers for over 1 year and symptomatic should be referred to a gastroenterologist for liver biopsy and possible treatment.

Monitoring for Efficacy

Testing for anti-HBs after vaccination should be done to ascertain that seroconversion has occurred. Revaceination with the same three-dose schedule is indicated for individuals who have no detectable antibody response. Protection against chronic HBV infection remains for at least 10 years even though anti-HBs become undetectable (Committee on Infectious Diseases, 1994).

Monitoring for Toxicity

As for all immunizations, pain at the injection site and occasional mild constitutional symptoms (Jacobs, 1997) may be experienced.

Followup

After an HBV vaccine series, immunity is maintained for an indeterminant time. Future recommendations for booster doses may be required to ensure immunity through adolescence and adulthood.

IRRITABLE BOWEL SYNDROME

Irritable bowel syndrome (IBS) presents as a combination of abdominal pain and altered bowel habits (either diarrhea or constipation) that is not explained by any detectable pathology. Symptoms are often aggravated by stress and begin in the second and third decades (McQuaid, 1997).

SPECIFIC CONSIDERATIONS FOR PHARMACOTHERAPY

When Drug Therapy Is Needed

Patients are frequently concerned about their condition and request drug therapy for relief of the distressing symptoms of IBS. However, drugs should be cautiously initiated since many patients are taking multiple medications prescribed from various attempts to alleviate symptoms. One suggestion is to initially stop all nonessential medications that may affect bowel habits and reintroduce them in a stepwise, selective manner (Goroll et al., 1995).

Short- and Long-Term Goals of Pharmacotherapy

The goal of pharmacotherapy is to work as an adjunct to diet and emotional support of the patient to minimize the disruptive symptoms of IBS.

Nonpharmacologic Therapy

A food/symptom diary can allow patients to see relationships among symptoms, food choices, and life events and assist in making dietary changes. However, a balance must be struck between avoidance of foods that provoke symptoms and becoming a slave to diets and food choices. Even if fruits and vegetables provoke symptoms, they should be eaten in small amounts. A trial of a lactose-free diet is indicated for all patients. The limiting of simple sugars, including sorbitol and fructose, has lessened symptoms in up to one-third of patients (Greenberger, 1995). These sugars are found in large amounts in colas, "sugar-free" gum, apples, cherries, and several special diet foods. Flatulence-producing foods such as beans, cabbage, and cauliflower can be minimized. Many patients are unable to tolerate caffeine (McQuaid, 1997). A high-fiber diet (20–30 g per day) and bulking agents can be useful in breaking the diarrhea-constipation pattern and should be recommended for most patients (McQuaid, 1997). Regular exercise and an increase in the intake of fluids, especially water and dilute juices, can often help minimize symptoms of constipation.

The development of a personal stress management plan and, if necessary, psychological counseling can be useful to many patients.

Time Frame for Initiating Pharmacotherapy

At the initial visit for IBS complaints, discontinue previous medications related to GI symptoms and initiate dietary changes as discussed above. Follow up with patient in 2 weeks. Drug therapy should be reserved for patients who do not respond to these conservative measures (McQuaid, 1997).

See Drug Tables 311.1, 501.3, 501.4, 501.8.

Assessment and History Taking

The goal of assessment is to rule out organic causes of the patient's symptoms before the initiation of drug therapy. The baseline history should elicit specific information on:

- Full constellation of GI symptoms, including pain, flatus, bloating, distension, diarrhea, and constipation and their pattern of occurrence; disappearance of symptoms is common with IBS (Uphold & Graham, 1994)
- Recent history of weight loss (a positive answer to this usually rules out IBS) (Uphold & Graham, 1994)
- Diet, specifically for foods with diarrheogenic potential, including nonabsorbable sugars such as sorbitol (Greenberger, 1995)
- Relationship of life stress to symptom occurrence

The physical examination should document weight loss and the presence of any masses, organ enlargement, tenderness, rigidity, or guarding of the abdomen. A rectal examination and fecal occult blood test should also be performed.

Routine laboratory tests should include CBC, sedimentation rate, thyroid function tests, and stool occult blood test. With predominant diarrhea symptoms, consider stool for ova and parasites, 24-hours stool collection, flexible sigmoidoscopy (in patients less than 40 years old), or barium enema/colonoscopy (in patients over age 40) (McQuaid, 1997).

Patient/Caregiver Information

Primary care providers should reassure patients about the functional nature of their symptoms and stress the ongoing nature of both the symptoms and the provider relationship.

OUTCOMES MANAGEMENT

Selecting an Appropriate Agent

Antispasmodic drugs such as dicyclomine 10 to 20 mg PO, three to four times a day; propantheline 15 mg PO, three times a day; and hyoscyamine 0.125 mg PO have anticholinergic effects that may be useful in relieving intermittent cramping pain. They are useful on a short-term or as-needed basis, or can be given 30 to 60 min before meals to relieve postprandial pain. They should not be used on a long-term basis (Goroll et al., 1995; McQuaid, 1997).

Antidiarrheal agents such as loperamide 2 mg PO, three to four times a day, or diphenoxylate with atropine 2.5 mg PO, four times a day, can be used prophylactically when diarrhea would be socially inconvenient. For patients in whom constipation is the main symptom even after dietary changes and bulking agents, cisapride 5 to 10 mg a day PO may be useful (McQuaid, 1997).

Patients with chronic, unremitting abdominal pain may benefit from antidepressants. The tricyclic amitriptyline 50–100 mg PO, once a day, is worth a trial because of its anticholinergic activity (Goroll et al., 1995).

Monitoring for Efficacy

The chronic nature of the disease should be stressed along with the waxing and waning of symptoms regardless of pharmacotherapy. Try dietary changes and a bulking agent for 2-week trial. Consultation with a gastroenterologist can be considered for patients in whom a reasonable trial of dietary changes, bulking agents, and dicyclomine are unsuccessful.

Monitoring for Toxicity

Chronic use of antispasmodics can make constipation and pain worse.

REFERENCES

Bardham, K., Naesdal, J., Bianchi, P., Petrillo, M., Lazzaroni, M., & Hinchliffe, R. (1991). Treatment of refractory peptic ulcer with omeprazole or continued H_2 receptor antagonists: A controlled clinical trial. *Gut, 32* (4), 435–438.

Belluzzi, A., Brignola, C., Campieri, M., Pera, A., Boschi, S., & Miglioli, M. (1996). Effect of an enteric-coated fish-oil preparation on relapses in Crohn's disease. *New England Journal of Medicine, 334* (24), 1557–1560.

Benenson, A. (Ed.). (1995). *Control of communicable diseases manual* (16th ed.). Washington, DC: American Public Health Association.

Berardi, R. (1997). Peptic ulcer disease and Zollinger-Ellison syndrome. In J. Dipiro, R. Talbert, G. Yee, G. Matzke, B. Wells, & L. Posey (Eds.), *Pharmacotherapy: A pathophysiologic approach* (3rd ed.). Stamford, CT: Appleton & Lange.

Bianchi Porro, O., Pace, F., Peracchia, A., Bonavina, L., Vigneri, S., & Scialabba, A. (1992). Short-term treatment of refractory reflux oesophagitis with different doses of omeprazole or ranitidine. *Journal of Clinical Gastroenterology, 15* (3), 192–198.

Biddle, W., & Miner, P. (1990). Long-term use of mesalamine enemas to induce remission in ulcerative colitis. *Gastroenterology, 99,* 113–118.

Brown, K. (1994). Dietary management of acute diarrheal disease: Contemporary scientific issues. *Journal of Nutrition, 124* (8 Suppl.), 1455S–1460S.

Campieri, M., DeFranchis, R., Bianchi Porro, G., et al. (1990). Mesalamine (5-ASA) suppositories in the treatment of ulcerative proctitis or distal proctosigmoiditis: A randomized controlled trial. *Scandanavian Journal of Gastroenterology, 25,* 663–668.

CDC. (1996/1997). *Health Information for International Travel.* Atlanta: DHHS.

Committee on Infectious Diseases, American Academy of Pediatrics. (1994). *1994 Red book.* Elk Grove Village, IL: AP.

Danzl, D. (1992). Flatology. *Journal of Emergency Medicine, 10,* 79–88.

DeMicco, M., Berenson, M., & Wu, W., et al. (1992). Oral cisapride in GERD: A double-blind, placebo-controlled multicenter dose-response trial [abstract]. *Gastroenterology, 102,* A59.

Dent, J., Yeomans, N., Mackinoon, M., Reed, W., Narielvala, F., & Hetzel, D. (1994). Omeprazole vs ranitidine for prevention of relapse in reflux oesophagitis: A controlled double-blind trial of their efficacy and safety. *Gut, 35*(5), 590–598.

DeVault, K., & Castell, D. (1995). Guidelines for the diagnosis and treatment of gastroesophageal reflux disease. *Archives of Internal Medicine, 155*(20), 2165–2173.

De Witt, R., Herrstedt, J., Rapoport, B., Carides, A., Carides, G., Elmer, M., Schmidt, C., Evans, J., Horgan, K. (2003). Addition of the oral NK_1 antagonist aprepitant to standard antiemetics provides protection against nausea and vomiting during multiple cycles of cisplatin-based chemotherapy. Journal of Clinical Oncology, 21(22), 4105–4111.

DiPiro, J., & Bowden, T. (1997). Inflammatory bowel disease. In J. Dipiro, R. Talbert, G. Yee, G. Matzke, B. Wells, & L. Posey (Eds.), *Pharmacotherapy: A pathophysiologic approach* (3rd ed.). Stamford, CT: Appleton & Lange.

DuPont, H. L., Jiang, Z. D., Ericsson, C. D., Adachi, J. A., Mathewson, J. J., DuPont, M. W., Palazzini, E., Riopel, L. M., Ashley, D., & Martinez-Sandoval, F. (2001). Rifaximin versus ciproflaxin for the treatment of traveler's diarrhea: a randomized, double-blind clinical trial. Clinical Infectious Diseases, 33(11), 1807–1816.

Erick, M. (1994). Battling morning (noon and night) sickness. *Journal of the American Dietetic Association, 94*(2), 147–148.

Ewe, K., Press, A., & Singe, C. (1993). Azathioprine combined with prednisolone or monotherapy with prednisolone in active Crohn's disease. *Gastroenterology, 105,* 367–372.

Faruqui, S., Sigmund, C., Smith, R., et al.. (1992). Cisapride in the treatment of GERD: A double-blind placebo-controlled multicenter dose-response trial. *Gastroenterology, 102*(4), A66.

Fennerty, B. (1995). "Cure" of *Helicobacter pylori. Archives of Internal Medicine, 155,* 1929–1931.

Fennerty, M., Castell, D., & Fendrick, M. (1996). The diagnosis and treatment of gastroesophageal reflux disease in a managed care environment. *Archives of Internal Medicine, 156,* 477–484.

Frucht, H., Maton, P., & Jensen, R. (1991). Use of omeprazole in patients with Zollinger-Ellison syndrome. *Digestive Diseases and Sciences, 36*(4), 394–404.

Ganiats, T., Norcross, W., Halverson, A., Burford, P., & Palinkas, L. (1994). Does Beano prevent gas? A double-blind crossover study of oral alpha-galactosidase to treat dietary oligosaccharide intolerance. *Journal of Family Practice, 39*(5), 441–445.

Gardner, V., Beckwith, J., & Heyneman, C. (1995). Cisapride for the treatment of chronic idiopathic constipation. *Annals of Pharmacotherapy, 29*(11), 1161–1163.

Geier, D., & Miner, P. (1992) New therapeutic agents in the treatment of irritable bowel syndrome. *American Journal of Medicine, 93,* 199–208.

Geier, D., Miner, P., Danielsson, A., Hellers, G. O., & Lyrenas, E. (1987). A controlled randomized trial of budesonide versus prednisolone retention enemas in active distal ulcerative colitis. *Scandanavian Journal of Gastroenterology, 22,* 987–992.

Geldof, H., Hazelhoff, B., & Otten, M. (1993). Two different dose regimens of cisapride in the treatment of reflux oesophagitis: A double-blind comparison with ranitidine. *Alimentary Pharmacology and Therapeutics, 7*(4), 409–415.

Gonzales, J. A., & Adams, C. S. (2002). Antiemetic agents in cancer chemotherapy. *Onocology Special Edition, 5,* 53–58.

Goroll, A., May, L., & Mulley, A. (1995). *Primary care medicine: Office evaluation and management of the adult patient.* Philadelphia: J. B. Lippincott.

Gralla, R., Itri, L., Pisko, S., Squillante, A., Kelsen, D., & Braun, D. (1981). Antiemetic efficacy of high-dose metoclopramide: Randomized trials with placebo and prochlorperazine in patients with chemotherapy-induced nausea and vomiting. *New England Journal of Medicine, 305*(16), 905–906.

Greenberger, N. (1997). Update in gastroenterology. *Annals of Internal Medicine, 126,* 221–225.

Griffin, M., & Miner, P. (1995). Conventional drug therapy in inflammatory bowel disease. *Gastroenterology Clinics of North America, 24*(3), 509–521.

Guerreiro, A. (1990). Omeprazole in the treatment of peptic ulcers resistant to H_2 receptor antagonists. *Alimentary Pharmacology and Therapeutics, 4*(3), 309–313.

Hallerback, B., Unge, P., Carling, L., Edwin, B., Glise, H., & Havu, N. (1994). Omeprazole and ranitidine in long-term treatment of reflux oesophagitis. *Gastroenterology, 107*(5), 1305–1311.

Hanan, I. (1993). Inflammatory bowel disease in the pregnant woman. *Comparative Therapeutics, 19,* 91–95.

Hanauer, S. (1991). Guidelines for the clinical evaluation of drugs for patients with inflammatory bowel disease. *Federal Register, 56,* 27.

Hanauer, S. (1993). Long-term management of Crohn's disease with mesalamine capsules (Pentasa). *American Journal of Gastroenterology, 881,* 343–351.

Hanauer, S. (1996). Inflammatory bowel disease. *New England Journal of Medicine, 334*(13), 841–847.

Hanauer, S., & Baert, F. (1994). Medical therapy of inflammatory bowel disease. *Medical Clinics of North America, 78*(6), 1413–1426.

Hanauer, S., Meyers, S., & Sachar, D. (1995). The pharmacology of anti-inflammatory drugs in inflammatory bowel disease. In J. Kirsner & R. Shorter (Eds.), *Inflammatory bowel disease* (4th ed.). Baltimore: Williams & Wilkins.

Havelund, T., Laursen, L., & Lauritsen, K. (1994). Efficacy of omeprazole in lower grades of gastrooesophageal reflux disease. *Scandanavian Journal of Gastroenterology, 201*(Suppl.), 69–73.

Hawthorne, A., Logan, R., & Gawkey, C. (1992). Randomized controlled trial of azathioprine withdrawal in ulcerative colitis. *British Medical Journal, 305,* 20–22.

Hesketh, P., Grunberg, S., Cralla, R., Warr, D., Roila, F., De Wit, R., Chawla, S., Carides, A., Ianus, J., Elmer, M., Evans, J., Beck, K., Reines, S., Horgan, K. (2003). The oral neurokinin-1 antagonist aprepitant for the prevention of chemotherapy-induced nausea and vomiting: a multinational, randomized, double-blind, placebo-controlled trial in patients receiving high-dose cisplatin – the Aprepitant Protocol 052 Study Group. Journal of Clinical Oncology, 21 (22), 4112–4119.

Hesketh, P., Van Belle, S., Aapro, M., Tattersall, F., Naylor, R., Hargreaves, R., Carides, A., Evans, J., Horgan, K. (2003). Differential involvement of neurotransmitters through the time course of cisplatin-induced emesis as revealed by therapy with specific receptor antagonists. European Journal of Cancer, 39 (8), 1074–1080.

Hirschfeld, S., & Clearfield, H. (1995). Pharmacologic therapy for inflammatory bowel disease. *American Family Physician, 51*(8), 1971–1975.

Hixson, L., Kelley, C., Jones, W., et al. (1992). Current trends in the pharmacotherapy for peptic ulcer disease. *Archives of Internal Medicine, 152,* 726–732.

Hodgson, H., & Hazlan M. (1991). Assessment of drug therapy in inflammatory bowel disease. *Alimentary Pharmacology and Therapeutics, 5,* 555–584.

Howden, C., Castell, D., Cohen, S., Freston, J., Orlando, R., & Robinson, M. (1995). The rationale for continuous maintenance treatment of reflux esophagitis. *Archives of Internal Medicine, 155*(14), 1465–1471.

Howden, C., Jones, D., Peace, K., Burget, D., & Hunt, R. (1988). The treatment of gastric ulcer with antisecretory drugs. *Digestive Diseases and Sciences, 33*(5), 619–624.

Islam, M. R. (1987). Single dose tetracycline in cholera. *Gut, 28*(8), 1029–1032.

Jacobs, R. (1997). General problems in infectious diseases. In L. Tierney, S. McPhee, & M. Papadakis (Eds.), *Current medical diagnosis and treatment* (36th ed.). Stamford, CT: Appleton & Lange.

Katz, J. (1991). The course of peptic ulcer disease. *Medical Clinics of North America, 75*(4), 831–841.

Katz, P. (1995). Disorders of the esophagus: Dysphagia, noncardiac chest pain and gastroesophageal reflux. In L. Barker, J. Burton, & P. Zieve (Eds.), *Principles of ambulatory medicine* (4th ed.). Baltimore: Williams & Wilkins.

Kaynard, A., & Flora, K. (2001). Gastroesophageal reflux disease: Control of symptoms, prevention of complications. *Postgraduate Medicine, 110*(3), 42–53.

Knigge, K. L. (2001) The role of *H. pylori* in gastrointestinal disease: A guide to identification and eradication. *Postgraduate Medicine, 110*(3), 71–82.

Lashner, B., Hanauer, S., & Silverstein, M. (1990). Testing nicotine gum for ulcerative colitis patients: Experience with single-patient trials. *Digestive Diseases and Sciences, 35,* 827–832.

Lee, S. D., & Surawicz, C. M. (2001). Infectious causes of chronic diarrhea. *Gastrointerology Clinics of North America, 30*(3), 679–91.

Lieberman, D. A. (1987). Medical therapy for chronic reflux esophagitis: Long-term follow-up. *Archives of Internal Medicine, 147*(10), 717–720.

Linn, F., & Peppercorn, M. (1992). Drug therapy for inflammatory bowel disease. *American Journal of Surgery, 164,* 85–89.

Liu, L., & Weller, P. (1996). Antiparasitic drugs. *New England Journal of Medicine, 334*(18), 1178–1184.

Loftus, C.Q., Loftus, E.V. Jr., & Sandborn, W.J. (2003). Cyclosporin for refractory ulcerative colitis. *Gut,* 52(2), 172–174.

Malchow, H. (1984). European cooperative Crohn's disease study: Results of drug treatment. *Gastroenterology, 86,* 249–254.

Maton, P. N. (1991). Omeprazole. *New England Journal of Medicine, 324*(14), 965–975.

McQuaid, K. (1997). Alimentary tract. In L. Tierny, S. McPhee, & M. Papadakis (Eds.), *Current medical diagnosis and treatment.* Stamford, CT: Appleton & Lange.

Meyers, S., Sachar, D., Goldberg, J., & Janowitz, H. (1983). Corticotropin versus hydrocortisone in the intravenous treatment of ulcerative colitis: A prospective, randomized, double-blind clinical trial. *Gastroenterology, 85,* 351–357.

Mitchelson, F. (1992). Pharmacological agents affecting emesis. *Drugs, 43*(4), 443–463.

Morrow, G., Hickok, J., & Rosenthal, S. (1995). Progress in reducing nausea and emesis. *Cancer, 76,* 343–357.

Mulder, C., & Tygat, G. (1993). Topical corticosteroids in inflammatory bowel disease. *Alimentary Pharmacology and Therapeutics, 7*(2), 125–130.

Nathwani, D., & Wood, M. (1993). The management of travellers' diarrhoea. *Journal of Antimicrobial Chemotherapy, 31*(5), 623–626.

Olsalazine for ulcerative colitis. (1990). *Medical Letter, 32,* 105–106.

Pallone, F., Prantera, C., Cottone, M., et al. (1991). Maintenance treatment of Crohn's disease with oral 5-ASA. *Gastroenterology, 100,* A237.

Peppercorn, M. (1990). Advances in drug therapy for inflammatory bowel disease. *Annals of Internal Medicine, 112,* 50–60.

Peppercorn, M. (1993). Is there a role for antibiotics as primary therapy in Crohn's? *Clinical Gastroenterology, 17,* 14.

Petitijean, O., Wendling, J., Tod, M., et al. (1992). Pharmacokinetics and absolute rectal bioavailability of hydrocortisone acetate in distal colitis. *Alimentary Pharmacology and Therapeutics, 6,* 351–357.

Podolsky, D. (1991). Inflammatory bowel disease. *New England Journal of Medicine, 325*(13), 928–937.

Pullan, R., Rhodes, J., Ganesh, S., Mani, V., Morris, J., Williams, G., Newcombe, R., Russell, M., et al. (1994). Transdermal nicotine for active ulcerative colitis. *New England Journal of Medicine, 330*(12), 811–815.

Quigley, E. M., Hassler, W. L., & Parkman, H. P. (2001). AGA technical review on nausea and vomiting. *Gastroenterology, 120*(1), 263–286.

Ramirez, B., & Richter, J. (1993). Review article: Promotility drugs and the treatment of gastroesophageal reflux disease. *Alimentary Pharmacology and Therapeutics, 7*(1), 5–20.

Remick, M. (1994). Promoting a healthy pregnancy. In E. Youngkin & M. Davis (Eds.), *Women's health: A primary care clinical guide.* Norwalk, CT: Appleton & Lange.

Rendi-Wagner, P. & Kollaritsch, H. (2002). Drug prophylaxis for travelers' diarrhea. Clinical Infectious Diseases, 34(5), 628–634.

Richter, J. (1995). Evaluation and management of diarrhea. In A. Goroll, L. May, & A. Mulley (Eds.), *Primary care medicine: Office evaluation and management of the adult patient.* Philadelphia: J. B. Lippincott.

Ruymann, F., & Richter, J. (1995). Management of inflammatory bowel disease. In A. Goroll, L. May, & A. Mulley (Eds.), *Primary care medicine.* Philadelphia: J. B. Lippincott.

Schaefer, D. C., & Cheskin, L. J. (1998). Constipation in the elderly. American Family Physician, 58(4), 907–915.

Scott, D., & Edelman, R. (1993). Treatment of gastrointestinal infections. *Baillieres Clinical Gastroenterology, 7*(2), 477–499.

Schnell, F. (2003). Chemotherapy-induced nausea and vomiting: the importance of acute antiemetic control. The Oncologist, 8 (2), 187–198.

Seale, J. P. (2002). Travel risks: update on traveler's diarrhea and other common problems. Consultant, 42(14), 1778–1785.

Sears, S., & Sack, D. (1995). Medical advice for the international traveler. In L. R. Barker, J. Burton, & P. Zieve (Eds.), *Principles of ambulatory medicine* (4th ed.). Baltimore: Williams & Wilkins.

Shah, S., & Peppercorn, M. (1995). Inflammatory bowel disease therapy: An update. *Comprehensive Therapy, 21*(6), 296–302.

Simethicone for gastrointestinal gas. (1996). *Medical Letter, 38* (977), 57–58.

Stenson, W., Cort, D., Rodgers, J., Rubakoff, R., DeSchryver-Keeskemeti, K., Gramlich, T., & Becken, W. (1992). Dietary supplementation with fish oil in ulcerative colitis. *Annals of Internal Medicine, 116*(8), 609–614.

Tami, J. A., & Waite, W. W. (1988). Metoclopramide suppository considerations. *Drug Intelligence in Clinical Pharmacology, 22*(3), 268–269.

Taylor, J., Zagari, M., & Murphy, K. (1997). Pharmacoeconomic comparison of treatments for the eradication of Helicobacter pylori. *Annals of Internal Medicine, 157,* 87–94.

Tramer, M. R. Carroll, D., Campbell, F. A., Reynolds, D. J. M., Moore, R. A., & McQuay, H. J. (2001). Cannabinoids for control of chemotherapy induced nausea and vomiting: Quantitative systematic review. *Britsh Medical Journal, 323*(16), 1–8.

Uphold, C., & Graham, M. (1994). *Clinical guidelines in family practice.* Gainesville, FL: Barmarrac Books.

U.S. Preventive Services Task Force. (1995). *Guide to clinical preventive services.* Baltimore: Williams & Wilkins.

Virk, A. (2001). Medical advice for international travelers. *Mayo Clinic Proceedings, 76*(8), 831–40.

CHAPTER ❖ 26

MUSCULOSKELETAL DISORDERS

Kathleen F. Jett ◆ Pamela B. Lester

Musculoskeletal disorders are common causes for persons to seek out the services of a healthcare clinician. Specific disorders range from inconveniences, such as sprains, to the cause of considerable disability (arthritis) and increased risk for death (fall related to osteoporosis).

The prevalence of arthritic and musculoskeletal conditions is likely to increase as the U.S. population shifts toward an aging high-risk society. In an era of managed care systems and cost containment, healthcare providers are challenged to support and maintain optimum functioning for individuals afflicted with musculoskeletal conditions by utilizing preventive measures and the most cost-effective treatment regimens. This chapter discusses the pharmacological and nonpharmacological management of the major arthritic and musculoskeletal conditions encountered in primary care.

RHEUMATOID ARTHRITIS

Rheumatoid arthritis (RA) affects 2.1 million people, or approximately 1% of the total population, with devastating effects of joint abnormality and disability within the first few years of the disease. Often initially presenting during the most productive years of work (between the 30s and 50s), the cost in individual person-hours due to lost work days averages 3.8 monthly with indirect costs of $281 (Newhall-Perry, Law, Ramos, et al., 2000).

The incidence (number of new cases occurring annually) of rheumatoid arthritis (RA) increases with age, with a peak incidence seen in persons aged 50 and older. By 2020, it is projected that arthritis will affect 59.4 million (18.2%) persons in the United States (CDC, 1996). RA is seen in women three times more often than in men (Ruoff, 2002). Rheumatoid arthritis is characterized by a fluctuating, symmetric, inflammatory polyarthropathy evidenced in pain and morning stiffness in affected joints and erosive synovitis. It may lead to extra-articular involvement and the destruction of the articular and periarticular structures. The pain accompanied by constant change in symptoms can have devastating effects on the individual and family, affecting physical, psychological, and spiritual health. In the presence of RA, joint destruction leads to bony deformities despite therapy. The changes result in disability, and in some cases, premature death (Mochan, 2001).

ETIOLOGY

The exact etiology of RA, a systemic autoimmune disorder, is unknown. However, it is known that RA is genetically linked, and the HLA-DRB chains appear to be markers for the disease. The destructive process of RA appears to begin with the activation of the T-cells, which results in proliferation of synovial cells, activation of pro-inflammatory cells from the bone marrow, and secretion of cytokines (including interleukin[IL]-1 and tumor necrosis factor a[TNF-a]) by macrophages and fibroblast-like synovial cells (Feldman & Maini, 1999). It is suggested that the disease-triggering agent is transmitted to the synovium via the bloodstream. The result is an activation and/or injury to the synovial microvascular endothelial cells. Continuous inflammation of the synovium gradually destroys collagen, narrowing the joint space and eventually damaging and destroying bone. In progressive RA, destruction to the cartilage accelerates when the fluid and inflammatory cells accumulate in the synovium to produce a pannus—a growth composed of thickened synovial tissue. The pannus produces more enzymes, which destroy nearby cartilage, aggravating the area and attracting more inflammatory white cells, macrophages, thereby perpetuating the inflammatory process. This process results in joint immobilization, muscle spasm and shortening, bone and cartilage destruction, ligamentous laxity, and altered tendon function; it can also harm other organs (Palmer, 1995). The disease course is characterized by remissions and exacerbations.

SPECIFIC CONSIDERATIONS FOR PHARMACOTHERAPY

Short-Term and Long-Term Goals of Therapy

Optimal management includes early diagnosis and a plan for the initiation of treatment options. The goals for the treatment of persons with RA are to alleviate pain, control symptoms, and to decrease the probability of the disability through the prevention or limitation of joint destruction and the preservation of joint function. In doing so, the quality of life for the person with RA may be maximized (Birnbaum, Barton, Greenberg, et al., 2000).

Assessment and History Taking

The typical history of the RA-afflicted individual is an insidious onset of peripheral joint pain and stiffness over a period of several weeks. In addition to morning stiffness, joint pain, and swelling, many patients experience constitutional symptoms of fatigue, malaise, or weight loss (Semble, 1995). Acute disabling polyarticular arthritis can occur, but disabling nonarticular presentation is rare. During the first month or two the extra-articular features, symmetrical inflammation, and the serologic findings may be absent. The differential diagnosis of RA includes osteoarthritis, gout, septic arthritis, and systemic lupus erythematosus (ACR, 2002).

A complete physical examination with particular attention to the musculoskeletal system is essential. RA can afflict any joint, with the wrist and hand, specifically the metacarpal phalangeal (MCP) and proximal interphalangeal (PIP) joints, most involved. The swan-neck deformity with ulnar deviation of MCP joints along with radial deviation of the wrist is a classic RA deformity. Other classic deformities are the boutonnière, with flexion of the PIP and hyperextension of the DIP joints of the fingers, and hammertoes, which occur with metatarsophalangeal joint subluxation (see Table 26-1).

Diagnostic Tests. No specific laboratory test, histologic, or radiographic finding diagnoses RA. The rheumatoid factor is found in 85% of patients, and its presence tends to correlate with increased disease severity and poorer

TABLE 26–1. Baseline Evaluation of Disease Activity and Damage in Patients with Rheumatoid Arthritis

Subjective
Degree of joint pain
Duration of morning stiffness
Duration of fatigue
Limitation of function
Physical examination
Actively inflamed joints (tender and swollen joint counts)
Mechanical joint problems: loss of motion, crepitus, instability, malalignment, and/or deformity
Extraarticular manifestations
Laboratory
Erythrocyte sedimentation rate/C-reactive protein level
Rheumatoid factor*
Complete blood cell count†
Electrolyte levels†
Creatinine level†
Hepatic enzyme levels (AST, ALT, and albumin)†
Urinalysis†
Synovial fluid analysis‡
Stool guaiac†
Other
Functional status or quality of life assessments using standardized questionnaires
Physician's global assessment of disease activity
Patient's global assessment of disease activity
Radiography
Radiographs of selected involved joints§

* Performed only at baseline to establish the diagnosis. If initially negative, may be repeated 6–12 months after disease onset.

† Performed at baseline, before starting medications, to assess organ dysfunction due to comorbid diseases. AST = aspartate aminotransferase; ALT = alanine aminotransferase.

‡ Performed at baseline, if necessary, to rule out other diseases. May be repeated during disease flares to rule out septic arthritis.

§ Helps to establish a baseline for monitoring disease progression and response to treatment.

Source: ACR (2002).

prognosis. An erythrocyte sedimentation rate (ESR) is used to document the inflammatory process. Synovial fluid leukocytosis (WBC > 2000/mm), histologic findings of chronic synovitis, and radiologic erosions may be seen after two years. A routine urinalysis and chemistry profile to determine kidney function should be performed prior to therapy. A uric acid level will help differentiate RA from gout. C-reactive protein, which is present in all individuals, is elevated in RA but is nonspecific (Abelson, Elkon, Pischel, et al., 2002).

Radiographic findings associated with RA include soft tissue swelling, osteoporosis, narrowed joint spaces, and marginal erosions. The finding of osteoporosis, marginal erosions, and reactive bone formation distinguishes RA from other arthritic conditions.

Extra-articular Manifestations. RA is a systemic disease, and individuals will need to be monitored for development of extra-articular signs and symptoms (Mochan, 2001). The rheumatoid nodule is the most common extraarticular sign, occurring in 40% of seropositive patients. The nodules form subcutaneously, in crops, over the bursae and along a tendon sheath and are more prevalent during the active phase. Although they can be found anywhere, including the viscera, they are commonly seen over the olecranon, the extensor surface of the forearm, and the Achilles tendon. Vasculitic lesions with splinter hemorrhages and necrotic areas on the fingertips and around the nails may be present. A disproportionate number of men are afflicted with severe extraarticular symptoms, e.g., vasculitis and Felty's syndrome (Mochan, 2001).

Baseline and periodic eye examinations are needed. Ocular involvement, including keratoconjunctivitis sicca, episcleritis, scleritis, and necrotizing scleritis (NS); marginal furrows; peripheral ulcerative keratitis (PUK); choroidal lesions; and retinal vasculitis, will afflict 25% of RA clients. The development of NS or PUK and vasculitis elsewhere in the body is a grim prognostic sign (Ruoff, 2002).

A baseline CBC is needed, since a common hematologic manifestation is a hypochromic-microcytic anemia with a low iron and low or normal iron-binding capacity. RA-associated anemic patients fail to respond vigorously to iron therapy with a brisk reticulocytosis. A significant confounder for gastrointestinal bleeding is that the ulcerogenic anti-inflammatory medications for treatment can produce a positive occult stool blood. Ferritin levels are not helpful in the differential diagnosis, and the clinician must restrict a detailed workup (bone marrow, x-ray, and endoscopy) to selected cases. Another hematologic manifestation is Felty's syndrome, which is a combination of RA, splenomegaly, leukopenia, and leg ulcers.

A baseline electrocardiogram is warranted to assess cardiac-associated extraarticular manifestations including involvement of the valves, pericardium, myocardium, and aorta. Inflammatory pericarditis and effusion usually develop during an acute exacerbation. Inflammatory lesions similar to the RA nodules can promote conduction defects, valvular dysfunction, embolic processes, and possibly myocardiopathy. Fifty percent of autopsied RA patients exhibited some cardiac pathology, as did 50% of RA cardiac asymptomatic patents undergoing echocardiography (Gabriel, Crowson, Luthra, et al., 1999).

Common neurologic manifestations include cervical spine–related myopathies with neck pain and associated bilateral sensory paresthesias of the hands. Entrapment neuropathies occur when a peripheral nerve passes through a compartment also occupied by a scarred synovium or tendon sheath. The severity of symptoms depends upon the degree of inflammation and the posture and stress on the joint. Nerves most frequently involved are the posterior interosseous nerve in the antecubital fossa, the femoral nerve anterior to the hip joint, the peroneal nerve adjacent to the fibular head, and the interdigital nerve at the metatarsal phalangeal (MTP) joint (Feldman & Maini, 1999).

Common respiratory associated involvement is manifested by inflammation of the cricoarytenoid joint. The symptoms are episodic laryngeal pain, dysphonia, and occasional pain with swallowing. Symptomatic pleuritis may occur when nodules develop on the lung parenchyma. Small effusions may be seen on chest x-ray. Along with the extraarticular manifestations, there is a general consensus that comorbid conditions (cardiovascular, pulmonary, and renal diseases) are increased in RA patients and RA itself may be a marker for increased risk for these problems (Goroll, Mag, & Mulley, 2000).

Time Frame for Initiating Pharmacotherapy

According to the American College of Rheumatology, optimum management requires an early diagnosis and timely institution of disease-modifying therapy prior to joint destruction (ACR, 2002). The optimal initiation strategy is currently under investigation. The response to currently available therapies varies between patients.

See Drug Tables 306, 307, and 319.

Patient/Caregiver Information

Patients receiving long-term corticosteroids should be advised to wear a medical alert bracelet. Any changes in vision must be reported immediately by patients taking hydroxychloroquine (HCQ). Sulfasalazine therapy results in discoloration of body fluids, namely urine and sweat, and may lead to permanent discoloration of contact lenses. Avoidance of alcohol is recommended during any course of drug therapy, but is especially important in patients receiving methotrexate (MTX). Women of child-bearing potential must be counseled on effective methods of contraception while receiving DMARD therapy. All drugs have unique effects on fetal development, and the benefits and risks of use should be individually evaluated.

Patient education remains the cornerstone of RA management. Patients and families need information about the disease course, therapeutic options, medication toxicity, and available community resources. Arthritis self-help and group support courses have been effective in increasing efficacy. The local chapter of the Arthritis Foundation can be an excellent resource for educational materials and information about support groups and classes.

OUTCOMES MANAGEMENT

Approach to Therapy

The new paradigm for treatment of RA is to obtain an early, definitive, accurate diagnosis. Then the plan is to begin early aggressive treatment that will maximize the response of the affected joints, sustain-long term effects, and change the course of disease progression—i.e., slow, stop, or perhaps reverse the disease. In the primary care setting, suspicions of a diagnosis of RA should be referred to a specialist (e.g., rheumatologist) for definitive diagnosis, the development of the treatment plan, and initiation of pharmacologic intervention. However, since this is a chronic disease with broad implications for the person's general health and well-being, monitoring of the progression of the disease and the response to the treatments is a cooperative effort of all involved with the person. The key to optimal outcomes is early and aggressive treatment in order to reduce joint destruction, thereby minimizing or delaying the permanent disability that often accompanies this disease. Treatment involves a combination of patient education, physical and occupational therapy, and, often, psychological support to assist with the lifestyle and image adjustments that may be necessary. Figure 26–1 provides an outline of the usual management of RA according to the 2002 update from the American College of Rheumatologists.

Pharmacologic therapies available for the treatment of RA include the nonsteroidal anti-inflammatory drugs (NSAIDs and COX-2s), glucocorticoids, and a class known as disease-modifying antirheumatic drugs or DMARDs.

See Table 26–2, Table 26–3 and Drug Tables 306, 307, and 319.

Current practice guidelines recommend starting DMARDs within three months of diagnosis in active disease to minimize joint erosion (ACR, 2002). NSAIDs and nonpharmocological therapies are also initiated at this time in order to alleviate pain and inflammation and maximize function. While the optimal initiation strategy of DMARDs is not yet known, a simplified plan is used whenever possible. All DMARDs have a slow onset of action and are associated with significant toxicity requiring frequent monitoring.

The newest biologicals have had a more rapid onset and a sustained response in clinical trials. Optimal treatment therapy would be a highly effective regime that provided symptom relief and inhibition of the disease progression, a safe, well-tolerated simple regime that requires minimal monitoring. Efficacy of the treatment regime would be sustained over time.

Nonsteroidal Anti-inflammatory Drugs. Nonsteroidal anti-inflammatory drugs are used for treatment and symptomatic relief of many musculoskeletal conditions. An overview of NSAIDs as a class is provided here, and each is discussed individually as it is applicable to each disease state. This drug class includes aspirin, nonacetylated salicylates, nonsalicylate NSAIDs, and selective 1 cyclooxygenase 2 inhibitors.

The exact mechanism of NSAIDs' anti-inflammatory and analgesic properties that are beneficial in musculoskeletal disorders remains unknown but may be related to the ability of NSAIDs to inhibit cyclooxygenase, decrease prostaglandin synthesis in inflamed tissue, and potentially interfere with other proinflammatory substances (Zuoff, 2002). Cyclooxygenase inhibition by NSAIDs leads to decreased prostaglandin synthesis. Prostaglandins play an important part in inflammation, gastrointestinal (GI) protection, and maintenance of renal perfusion. In addition, NSAIDs affect the activity of other inflammatory mediators such as bradykinins and leukotrienes and the production of oxygen radicals, influence cellular processes, and inhibit leukocyte migration and lymphocyte activation. The newer NSAIDs known as COX-2 inhibitors do not interfere with the gastro-protective effect

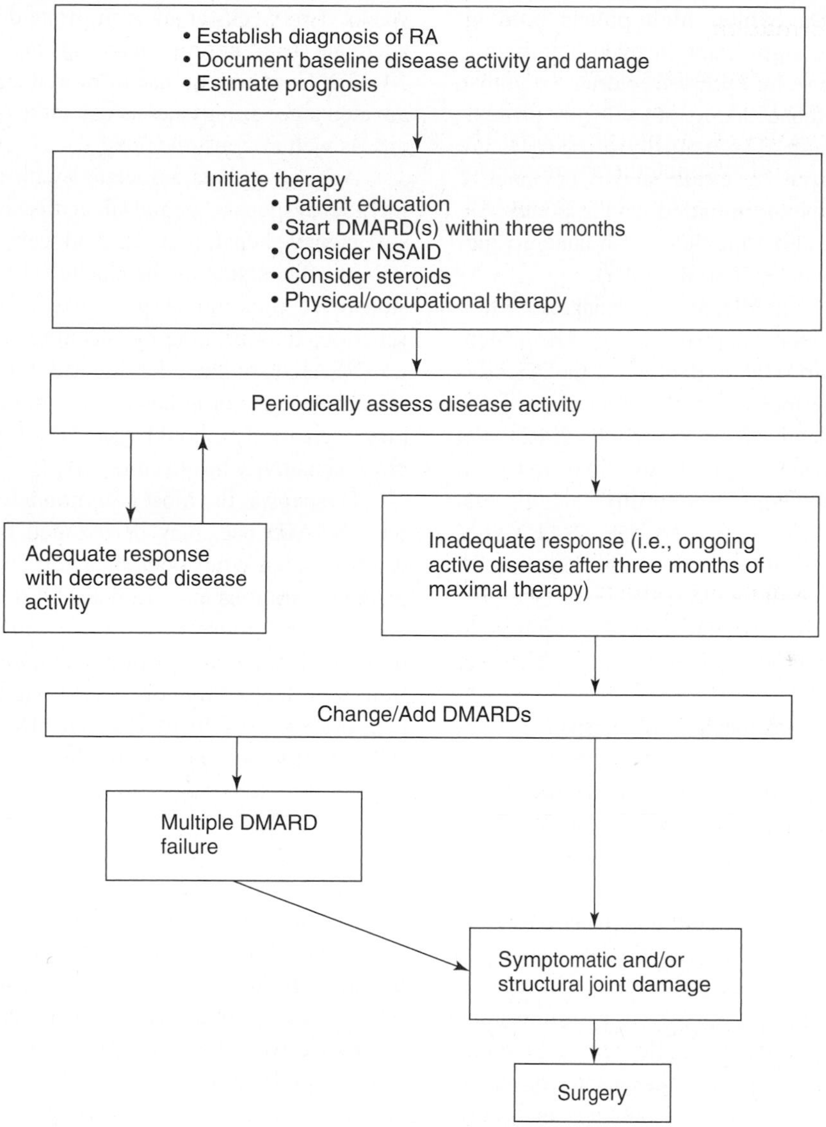

FIGURE 26–1. Outline of management of rheumatoid arthritis (Adapted from ACR, 2002)

of the cyclooxygenase-1 but rather act on cyclooxygenase-2. This newly described enzyme is associated with pro-inflammatory mediators only and does not appear to affect prostaglandin synthesis. This should result in fewer gastrointestinal side effects.

While there are a number of COX-1 NSAIDs approved for the use with RA, only COX-2s celecoxib and valdecoxib are approved for the use with RA. The much higher costs of the COX-2s limit their use on a long-term basis.

In RA, NSAIDs alleviate pain, reduce joint swelling, and maintain joint function. However, this class of drugs has not been shown to alter the disease course or slow the progression of joint destruction.

Pharmacokinetic parameters of the various NSAIDs are given in the NSAID Drug Table 306. Absorption of NSAIDs is rapid and complete. Coadministration with food interferes with the rate, but not the extent of, absorption. Theoretically, analgesia onset may be slightly delayed with food ingestion, but this may not be clinically significant. All NSAIDs exhibit high protein binding. This becomes clinically significant in hypoalbuminemic patients who cannot clear the excess free drug, i.e., those with renal failure and those taking other highly protein-bound drugs, e.g., dilantin. The majority of NSAIDs are metabolized by the liver to either active or inactive metabolites, which are then eliminated via the kidney. Aspirin and the nonacetylated salicylates also undergo metabolism in the gastric mucosa (ACR., 2002).

NSAIDs currently available in nonprescription strength include ibuprofen, naproxen, and ketoprofen. Although few direct comparative data exist, the NSAIDs appear to be equally effective in the treatment of the majority of muscoskeletal disorders (ACR, 2002). On an individual basis, however, great variability exists in both clinical response and tolerability among the various agents. Failure to respond to one NSAID does not indicate a failure of the entire class. Selection of an NSAID from a different or even the same chemical class and trials of many NSAIDs may be required to achieve an adequate clinical response (Simon & Smith, 1998).

Aspirin remains a reasonable and inexpensive RA treatment option, although higher doses may be necessary (3900–6500 mg/day). Blood levels can be monitored and a target level of 20 to 30 mg/dL correlates with an anti-inflammatory response. Levels higher than 30 mg/dL may produce significant toxicity.

Nonacetylated salicylates, including choline salicylate, choline magnesium trisalicylate, salsalate, and diflunisal are also effective. These agents are weak inhibitors of cyclooxygenase, which allows for fewer gastrointestinal side effects, less renal toxicity, and little to no antiplatelet effect. A potential disadvantage of these agents, however, is their relatively high cost. The usual maintenance dose for the nonacetylated salicylates is 3 to 4.5 g/day.

Nonsalicylate NSAIDs are reasonable alternatives to aspirin, equally efficacious, generally better tolerated, and do not require blood level monitoring. Selection of a particular NSAID product, whether aspirin, nonacetylated salicylate, or nonsalicylate NSAID, is based on trial and error and patient-specific response.

Consider cost when selecting an NSAID. Using a stepped-care approach, prescribe the least expensive NSAIDs initially and then progress to more expensive agents if necessary for substantial cost savings to patients and institutions without compromising adequate patient care.

The analgesic effect of NSAIDs occurs quickly, whereas anti-inflammatory actions may take 1 to 2 weeks. Two weeks at an appropriate dose is considered an adequate trial before changing the patient to another NSAID. Concomitant use of more than one NSAID is not advised since simultaneous use increases the risk for toxicity as well as consumer cost.

Adverse effects associated with the use of NSAIDs include dyspepsia, peptic ulcer disease (PUD), renal insufficiency, hepatotoxicity, and central nervous system (CNS) effects such as headache (HA), dizziness, confusion, or depression. Aspirin irreversibly affects platelet function, thus prolonging bleeding time. The nonsalicylate NSAIDs, on the other hand, exhibit reversible platelet effects once the drug has been removed. Patients with aspirin sensitivity should use NSAIDs with caution as cross-sensitivity has been reported.

Dyspepsia, the most common adverse effect reported with NSAID use, may be avoided by advising that the drug be taken with food. Buffered and enteric-coated aspirin preparations may decrease GI discomfort. Other less common, yet more severe GI complications include ulceration, bleeding, perforation, and gastric outlet obstruction. Risk factors for severe GI toxicity include advanced age, prior history of PUD or GI bleeding, cardiovascular (CV) disease, higher NSAID dosage, and concurrent corticosteroid use (ACR, 2002). Excess alcohol intake and smoking may also increase the risk of GI toxicity.

Renal toxicity may also occur as a result of NSAID use. All NSAIDs have the potential to cause reversible renal insufficiency, interstitial nephritis, and nephrotic syndrome. Although these complications are relatively uncommon, the elderly and patients with preexisting renal disease, congestive heart failure (CHF), cirrhosis, atherosclerosis, or any underlying condition affecting renal blood flow are at higher risk for developing NSAID-induced renal insufficiency (ACR, 2002). Patients taking diuretics may also be at risk. Monitoring renal function weekly for several weeks is indicated in high-risk patients following initiation of NSAID therapy (ACR, 2002).

NSAIDs may induce a transient elevation in liver enzymes. Routine laboratory monitoring is generally not indicated unless the patient has underlying liver disease (ACR, 2002).

Nonpharmacologic Therapy

A variety of nonpharmacologic treatment options exist, ranging from self-medication and self-help groups, yoga, water exercise and hydrotherapy, heat and paraffin baths, and referral to surgical intervention with joint replacement. Surgery is an option for patients with intractable pain or loss of function that ultimately interferes with activities of daily living. Many mechanical assistance devices are available to improve physical functioning. Treatment is multidisciplinary and may include podiatry and occupational, physical, and psychological therapies.

Glucocorticoids. This class of drugs effectively relieves symptoms associated with RA. Because of the toxicities associated with high doses and long-term use, continuous use is indicated only for life-threatening complications or refractory RA. Glucocorticoids in low doses (10 mg/day of prednisone or equivalent) are generally adequate to reduce joint swelling, relieve pain, and allow patients to resume activity (ACR, 2002). They are also used as interim therapy while waiting for DMARDs to take effect. Tapering or discontinuation should be initiated as early as possible, but this may be difficult in many RA patients.

Limited intra-articular injections are a safe and effective method to provide relief and improve function, especially in patients with a limited number of affected joints (ACR, 2002). The use of injections is limited to one or two joints and indicated only for those joints with significant inflammation. For each joint there is usually a three injection limit and may take months to show improved function. Commonly used medications include hyaluronan and sodium hyaluronate. The same joint should not be injected more than once within a 3-month period (ACR, 2002). If this schedule is not adequate to control joint symptoms, reevaluate the treatment regimen.

Potential adverse effects associated with low-dose glucocorticoids use include skin thinning, bruising, increased appetite, weight gain, fluid retention, acne, hypertension (HTN), hyperglycemia, atherosclerosis, gastric ulcers and associated bleeding, glaucoma, cataract formation, osteoporosis, avascular necrosis, impaired wound healing, increased susceptibility to infection, and development of a cushingoid appearance (ACR, 2002). Adequate patient counseling is important regarding adverse effects, duration of therapy, risks of long-term administration and difficulties with tapering, and the dangers of suddenly stopping glucocorticoid therapy.

DMARD. The use of the class of drugs known as DMARDs (disease modifying antirheumatic drugs) are the current mainstay of the long-term management of RA. They are the only drugs that are thought to actually slow joint destruction by inhibiting the inflammatory process of the disease. However, they may take 3–6 months to show affect and must be used with great caution to minimize the risk of side effects and to monitor early signs of toxicity. In general, only a highly skilled specialist, such as a rheumatologist, should initiate them. Long term monitoring is often done cooperatively between the primary care provider and the specialist. See Table 26–3. The most commonly used DMARD is methotrexate. Minocycline, cyclosporin and staphylococcal protein A immunoadsorption may be given as adjuncts to reduce the potential inflammation and infection associated with DMARD therapy (see Table 26–2).

Methotrexate. Methotrexate, a cytotoxic agent inhibiting dihydrofolate reductase, is the DMARD of choice for initial therapy by many rheumatologists. MTX is available both orally and parenterally for use as a single dose of 7.5 to 25 mg per week. Intramuscular (IM) injections of MTX are reserved for patients intolerant to oral MTX or in whom efficacy has decreased over time.

Toxicities associated with MTX include GI symptoms (common), pulmonary toxicity and hypersensitivity pneumonitis (uncommon), bone marrow suppression (uncommon), and hepatic fibrosis (rare) (ACR, 2002; Ruoff, 2002). Toxicity risks increase in patients with renal insufficiency, folate deficiency, concomitant use of antifolate drugs (e.g., Co-Trimoxazole), alcohol abuse, diabetes, and obesity (ACR, 2002). There is also the concern of increased risk of lymphomas with long-term use (Cohen, et al., 2002).

Lung toxicity may be increased in smokers and patients with underlying lung disease. Pulmonary hypersensitivity presenting as fever, cough, and dyspnea may lead to pulmonary fibrosis. This toxicity can occur at any time regardless of dose or duration of therapy (ACR, 2002; Bathon, Martin, Fleischmann, et al, 2000; Lipsky, van der Heijde, St. Clair, et al. 2000).

Hepatotoxicity may present as irreversible fibrosis or cirrhosis. Transient increases of LFTs commonly occur with MTX therapy, but correlate poorly with the development of hepatic fibrosis. An increase of LFTs to greater than three times the baseline level requires discontinuation of MTX. Risk factors for MTX-associated liver disease include age, duration of therapy, obesity, diabetes mellitus (DM), alcohol use, and a history of hepatitis B or C (Walker, Funch, Dryer, et al., 1993). Patients with known liver disease should avoid using MTX; however, if MTX must be used in this patient population, a pretreatment biopsy is recommended. Liver biopsy is also recommended in patients with persistent LFT abnormalities while receiving or following discontinuation of the drug (ACR, 2002; Williams, 1993). Routine liver biopsies are

TABLE 26–2. Recommended Monitoring Strategies for Treatment of Rheumatoid Arthritis

			Monitoring	
Drugs	***Toxicities Requiring Monitoring***[a]	***Baseline Evaluation***	***System review/examination***	***Laboratory***
Salicylates, nonsteroidal anti-inflammatory drugs	Gastrointestinal ulceration and bleeding	CBC, creatinine, AST, ALT	Dark/black stool, dyspepsia, nausea/vomiting, abdominal pain, edema, shortness of breath	CBC yearly, LFTs, creatinine testing may be required[b]
Hydroxychloroquine	Macular damage	None unless patient is over age 40 or has previous eye disease	Visual changes, funduscopic and visual fields every 6–12 months	
Sulfasalazine	Myelosuppression	CBC, and AST or ALT in patients at risk, G-6PD	Symptoms of myelosuppression,[c] photosensitivity, rash	CBC every 2–4 weeks for first 3 months, then every 3 months
Methotrexate	Myelosuppression, hepatic fibrosis, cirrhosis, pulmonary infiltrates or fibrosis	CBC, chest radiography within past year, hepatitis B and C serology in high-risk patients, AST or ALT, albumin, alkaline phosphatase, and creatinine	Symptoms of myelosuppression,[c] shortness of breath, cough, DOE, nausea/vomiting, lymph node swelling, jaundice, dark urine	CBC, platelet count, AST, albumin, creatinine every 4–8 weeks
Gold, intramuscular	Myelosuppression, proteinuria	CBC, platelet count, creatinine, urine dipstick for protein	Symptoms of myelosuppression,[c] edema, rash, oral ulcers, diarrhea	CBC, platelet count, urine dipstick every 1–2 weeks for first 20 weeks, then at the time of each (or every other) injection
Gold, oral	Myelosuppression, proteinuria	CBC, platelet count, urine dipstick for protein	Symptoms of myelosuppression,[c] edema, rash, diarrhea	CBC, platelet count, urine dipstick for protein every 4–12 weeks
D-penicillamine	Myelosuppression, proteinuria	CBC, platelet count, creatinine, urine dipstick for protein	Symptoms of myelosuppression,[c] edema, rash	CBC, urine dipstick for protein every 2 weeks until dosage stable, then every 1–3 months
Azathioprine	Myelosuppression, hepatotoxicity, lymphoproliferative disorders	CBC, platelet count, creatinine, AST or ALT	Symptoms of myelosuppression,[c]	CBC and platelet count every 1–2 weeks with changes in dosage, and every 1–3 months thereafter
Glucocorticoids (oral ≤10 mg of prednisone or equivalent)	Hypertension, hyperglycemia, osteoporosis hypertension, hyperglycemia, hyperlipidemia, cataracts, gastric irritations	BP, chemistry panel, bone densitometry in high-risk patients	BP at each visit, polyuria, polydipsia, edema, shortness of breath, visual changes, weight gain, fracture	Urinalysis for glucose yearly

Ethanercept	Abdominal pain, diarrhea	Evidence of infection or risk for infection	Acute or chronic infections, including T.B.	Monitor for injection site reaction, CBC
Anakinra	Aplastic anemia, lymphoma	Evidence of infection or malignancy	Injection site reaction, monitor carefully patients with asthma, avoid live vaccines	CBC
Leflunomide	Diarrhea, alopecia, rash, headache, theoretical risk of immuno-suppression pancytopenia	Hepatitis B and C in high risk persons, CBC, creatinine, LFTs.	Diarrhea, alopecia, rash, headache, inter-current liver, gallbladder and renal disease, pregnancy or delayed menses. Known teratogen, unexplained weight loss.	CBC, creatinine, monthly LFTs for the first 6 months and every 1–2 months thereafter.
Infliximab (only used with MTX)	None recognized	Evidence of infections or risk of infections	Acute or chronic infections	Monitor for infusion site reaction.
Minoclycline	Hyperpigmentation, dizziness, vaginal yeast infections	None	Hyperpigmentation, dizziness, vaginal yeast infections	None
Cyclosporin	Renal insufficiency, anemia, hypertension	CBC, creatinine, LFTs, uric acid, BP	Hypertrichosis, parathesias, nausea, gingival hyperplasia, edema, BP	Creatinine every 2 weeks until dosage is stable, then monthly; periodic CBC, LFTs and potassium.
Staphylococcal protein A immunoadsorption	Anemia, hypotension during procedure	CBC, creatinine, BP	Joint pain, fatigue, lightheadedness, infection at site, BP	CBC
Adalimumab	None recognized	CBC, SMAC21	Acute or chronic infections, including T.B. demyelinating disease	CBC SMAC-21

[a]Potential serious toxicities that may be detected by monitoring before they have become clinically apparent or harmful to the patient. This list mentions toxicities that occur frequently enough to justify monitoring. Patients with comorbidity, concurrent medications, and other specific risk factors may need further studies to monitor for specific toxicity.

[b]Package insert for diclotenac (Voltaren) recommends that AST and ALT be monitored within the first 8 weeks of treatment and periodically thereafter. Monitoring of serum creatinine should be performed weekly for at least 3 weeks in patients receiving concomitant angiotensin converting enzyme inhibitors or diuretics.

[c]Symptoms of myelosuppression include fever, symptoms of infection, easy bruisability, and bleeding.

CBC = complete blood cell count (hematocrit, hemoglobin, white blood cell count) including differential cell and platelet counts; ALT = alanine aminotransferase; AST = aspartate aminotransferase; LFTs = liver function tests; BP = blood pressure.

Source: Used with permission from American College of Rheumatology (2002).

TABLE 26–3. RA Drug Costs and Approximate Time to Benefit

Drug	Approximate Time to Benefit	Annual Cost (generic) in Dollars ($)
Hydroxychloroquine	2–6 months	1,056 (559)
Sulfasalazine	1–3 months	509–763 (205–308)
Methotrexate (MTX)	1–2 months	Oral 697–1859 (259–691) Injectable 419–806 (42–81)
MTX (SQ) plus infliximab	A few days–4 months	13,940–36,694
Azathioprine	2–3 months	579–1,737 (471–1,414)
D-penicillamine	3–6 months	865–2,595 (398–1,194)
Gold, oral	4–6 months	1,622
Gold, IM	3–6 months	198 (142)
Etanercept	A few days–12 weeks	15,436
Anakinra	4 weeks	Not available
Leflunomide	4–12 weeks	2,938

Annual drug costs for comparison purposes only. Based on 2001 Red Book and the usual maintenance dose. Values do not include costs of administration. (Adapted from ACR, 2002).

not cost-effective for patients receiving MTX with normal LFTs (Sandoval, Alarcon, & Morgan, 1995).

Myelosuppression, generally presenting as leukopenia, may also occur. Folate deficiency, renal insufficiency, and use of antifolate drugs increase the risk of cytopenias (ACR, 2002). Severe bone marrow suppression is uncommon with recommended doses.

Common toxicities include mucositis, mild alopecia, and GI symptoms such as anorexia, nausea, vomiting, dyspepsia, and diarrhea. These adverse effects may be precipitated by an underlying folate deficiency. Concurrent administration of folic acid 1 mg/day or as a single dose of 7 mg/week is recommended to prevent toxicity. Folinic acid, or leucovorin, may also be used, but it is more expensive than folate.

MTX is absolutely contraindicated in conception or pregnancy. MTX is teratogenic, as well as an abortifacient, and can lead to infertility in both men and women. Couples wishing to become pregnant should wait a minimum of three months or one ovulatory cycle following discontinuation of MTX therapy by men or women, respectively (ACR, 2002).

Concurrent administration of drugs affecting immune function should be avoided due to additive risks of bone marrow suppression. MTX concentrations may increase in patients with renal insufficiency also receiving NSAIDs, thus increasing the risk of toxicity (ACR, 2002).

Hydroxychloroquine. Hydroxychloroquine (HCQ), an antimalarial compound, is effective in treating mild to moderate RA, although it is used less commonly now with the new DMARDs available. It is one of the least toxic and least costly DMARDs to monitor (ACR, 2002). Initiated at a single daily dose of 400 mg, HCQ may then be decreased to 200 mg per day once efficacy has been established. Dosage adjustments are indicated in patients with decreased renal function. Retinal damage (rare) is the major toxicity associated with HCQ use and is preventable with appropriate monitoring (Table 26–2). Patients older than 70 years of age who have received a cumulative dose of more than 800 g are at the greatest risk of developing retinal toxicity (ACR, 2002). Other rare and less serious toxicities associated with HCQ include GI symptoms, myopathy, blurred vision, accommodation difficulty, abnormal skin pigmentation, and peripheral neuropathy.

Sulfasalazine. Sulfasalazine (SSZ), a drug consisting of sulfapyridine and 5-aminosalacylic acid (5-ASA), is a well-established treatment for inflammatory bowel disease. SSZ has various immunomodulatory and anti-inflammatory effects that may contribute to slowing the progression of joint damage (Bresnihan, 2001). Initial dosing in RA patients consists of 500 mg daily, increased by 500 mg weekly to a target dose of 2 to 3 g per day. SSZ has shown an efficacy equal to gold and penicillamine. It has been proven to be more efficacious and have a faster onset of action than HCQ and auranofin (Ruoff, 2002). The use of SSZ is contraindicated in persons allergic to sulfa. It can be used during pregnancy but is not advised during lactation (Bresnihan, 2001).

Common adverse effects include skin rash, photosensitivity, HA, and GI symptoms (ACR, 2002). Myelosuppression, unrelated to dose, generally manifests as leukopenia in 1 to 3% of patients during the first three to six months of therapy (ACR, 2002). Early detection by routine monitoring (Table 26–2) and drug discontinuation reverses the bone marrow suppression. Oligospermia may also occur and normalizes upon discontinuation of the drug. Administration of enteric-coated SSZ increases tolerability.

Azathioprine. Azathioprine (AZA), a purine analog, is initiated at 1.25 to 1.5 mg/kg per day and then increased to 2 to 2.5 mg/kg per day after three months if necessary. Dosage adjustments are necessary in patients with renal failure. Severe toxicity is uncommon with the low doses used in RA. The most common adverse effect of AZA is GI intolerance, which leads to discontinuation of the drug in ~10% of patients (ACR, 2002). Other adverse effects include reversible bone marrow suppression; rarely hepatitis and pancreatitis, and an increased risk of lymphoma with long-term use. Concomitant administration of allopurinol increases AZA concentrations and the risk of toxicity. If concurrent administration is necessary, decrease the AZA dose by 75%. Simultaneous use of angiotensin-converting enzyme inhibitors (ACEIs) or allopurinol in the presence of renal insufficiency increases the risk of AZA-associated bone marrow suppression (ACR, 2002).

Gold. The injectable gold products gold sodium thiomalate and aurothioglucose are administered intramuscularly starting with a test dose of 10 mg. If no adverse effects occur, a 25 mg dose is given the next week, followed by 50 mg administered weekly until a total cumulative dose of 1 g is reached, toxicity appears, or remission occurs. Once the patient improves, the dosing interval is increased to 2 weeks and then to 3 to 4 weeks as tolerated. Disease exacerbations may require reinstitution of weekly injections.

Stomatitis and rash occur commonly with gold therapy (ACR, 2002). Pruritis without rash may also occur. A nitritoid reaction consisting of flushing, weakness, nausea, and dizziness has been reported within 30 minutes of injecting gold thiomalate. Hematologic, renal, and pulmonary toxicities are serious enough to require frequent monitoring (Table 26–2), but occur rarely (ACR, 2002).

Oral gold, auranofin, is more convenient than the injectable form and causes fewer side effects, but is also less efficacious (Wood, 1994). Diarrhea resulting from auranofin therapy is generally dose-related and may necessitate discontinuation of the drug.

D-Penicillamine. A metabolite of penicillin, D-penicillamine is initiated at 250 mg given daily on an empty stomach. Doses may be increased 125 to 250 mg per day every 1 to 2 months to a maintenance dose of 750 mg per day.

Common, less severe side effects include pruritic rash, stomatitis, nausea, anorexia, and transient decreased or altered taste (ACR, 2002). Dysguesia is temporary and may resolve even if the drug is continued. More severe but rare toxicities include myelosuppression (especially leukopenia and thrombocytopenia), renal toxicities including proteinuria, renal failure, and nephrotic syndrome, and autoimmune syndromes such as myasthenia gravis, Goodpasture's syndrome, or a lupus-like illness. Titrating the dose decreases the incidence of thrombocytopenia (ACR, 2002). Bronchiolitis, cholestatic hepatitis, dermatomyositis, and polymyositis rarely have been reported. Two types of rash have been reported. A rash occurring early in therapy (<6 months) is generally mild and represents a reaction that will resolve when the drug is discontinued. D-Penicillamine may be restarted once the rash has resolved. A rash occurring late in therapy (<6 months) is usually more severe and requires permanent discontinuance of the drug (ACR, 2002).

New Therapies. New agents have been approved for use in conjunction with methotrexate (MTX) for persons who fail to achieve adequate benefit from MTX or one of the other DMARDs alone or who cannot tolerate the medications. The most effective new treatments are a class of biologics that include TNF-alpha antagonist therapies. There is a theoretical increased risk of lymphoproliferative disease.

Etanercept is a soluble receptor protein that binds to circulating TNF-alpha. It has been found to be effective whether used alone (25 mg. subcutaneously, twice weekly) or in combination with MTX. According to the package insert, more than 60% of patients treated with etanercept achieved an ACR 20 response, and 40% achieved an ACR 50 response (Weinblatt, Kremer, Bankhurst, et al., 1999).

Infliximab is a chimeric monoclonal antibody that binds circulating TNF-alpha. Combining infliximab with methotrexate reduces antibody production. The most common side effects are GI distress and fatigue. In one study TB was also associated with the use of infliximap (Kagen, 2004).

Leflunomide is a reversible inhibitor of de novo pyrimidine synthesis, with active metabolites that inhibit the rate-limiting step in pyrimidine synthesis and also inhibit IL-1 and TNF-alpha. Pyrimidine is required for mitogen-induced proliferation of T cells, and inhibition of pyrimidine synthesis is an important step in RA (Breedveld & Dyer, 2000; Strand, Cohen, Schift, et al., 1999; Weinblatt, Kremer, Coblyn, et al., 1999).

Anakinra is an exogenous recombinant IL-1 receptor antagonist that augments diminished levels of naturally occurring IL-1 Ra, as a counterbalance to the detrimental effects of the disease—heightened activity of IL-1 in bone resorption and erosion. Anakinra binds to IL-1 receptors, thus preventing receptor activation and joint cartilage. Anakinra is administered as a 100-mg self-administered daily subcutaneous injection using a specifically designed injector device provided by the manufacturer. Injection site reactions, especially during the first four weeks are the most common side effect. In clinical trials the reaction has caused discontinuation (Calabrese, 2002).

Adalimumab is a recombinant human IgG1 monoclonal antibody specific for human tumor necrosis factor

(TNF). It is supplied in single-use, 1 ml pre-filled glass syringes for subcutaneous injection every other week. There is a black box warning about the risk of infections especially in persons with latent tuberculosis. It is advised that patients should be tested for TB and treated as appropriate prior to the initiation of adalimumab therapy (CDC, 2002). Adalumimab may be combined with methotrexate or other DMARDs for greater efficacy of decreasing joint erosion in recalcitrant cases.

Monitoring for Efficacy

There has been a paradigm shift from the traditional value placed on laboratory tests and radiological findings to assess RA status and therapeutic response. Currently, more emphasis is placed on the patient's self-report of functional status. Patients should be assessed for relief of symptoms at two week intervals until stabilized.

The American College of Rheumatology recommends that a systematic rating be used for the response to treatment. At each visit the number of tender and swollen joints are assessed. In addition the physician's assessment of disease activity, the serum C-reactive protein concentration and the patient's assessment of pain, disease activity, and physical function are measured. A score of ACR 20 indicates a reduction of at least 20% in the number of affected joints as well as at least a 20% reduction in at least three of the other five parameters. Similar assessments for scores of ACR 50 or ACR 70 are also possible (ACR, 2002).

Psychosocial Factors. Arthritis patients frequently report disease activation with stressful events. Relationships between stress, the immune system, and other biological variables are being researched. The current RA management paradigm includes the assessment and monitoring of the psychosocial constructs of learned helplessness, self-efficacy, and mood affect. Useful tools include the Health Assessment Questionnaire (HAQ), the Arthritis Impact Measurement Scale (AIMES), the Modified Health Assessment Questionnaire (MHAQ), and the McMaster Toronto Arthritis Questionnaire (MACTAR). Additional tools that may be of benefit include the Beck Depression Inventory (BDI) and the Center for Epidemiological Studies Depression Index (CES-D). Optimal, ongoing management includes a comprehensive, coordinated, and multidisciplinary approach (Covic et al., 2000; Smarr, Parker, Kosciulek, et al. 2000; Strahl, Kleinknecht & Dinnel, 2000).

OSTEOARTHRITIS

Osteoarthritis (OA), also call degenerative joint disease (DJD), is the most common joint disease affecting the majority of persons over 65, often beginning often in the 40s. It is the leading cause of disability in both men and women. For persons under 45, OA is found most often in men, with a reversal for those over 45, when it is seen with increasing frequency in women (NIH, 2002).

At least 85% of all persons over 75 are thought to have x-ray evidence of the disease without symptoms. It is estimated that there are 43 million Americans affected with OA, with an annual economic burden estimated to be about $65 billion (Freeman, 2001). Compared with RA, OA with its increased prevalence has a 30-fold greater economic impact when work days lost, healthcare visits, diagnostic testing (arthroscopy), and joint replacement (arthroplasty) are considered (Brandt & Slemenda, 1993). Gabriel, Crowson, and O'Fallon (1995) analyzed the population-based Rochester Project data and found that persons with OA, adjusted for age and sex, incurred substantial incremental medical costs due to comorbid conditions and experienced significantly greater work disability than non-OA persons.

The knees, followed by the hips, are the joints most commonly affected due to their weight bearing roles. Also affected are fingers, thumbs, neck, and the lower back. In advanced stages, OA of the hands results in the orthopedic deformities of Bouchard and Heberden's nodes found in the proximal (PIP) and distal (DIP) interphalangeal joints respectively.

Besides age and gender, other risk factors associated with OA include obesity, mechanical stress, genetic disposition, previous inflammatory diseases. According to Felson (1995), data from the Framingham osteoarthritis study showed that for women, weight is the predominate risk factor for OA; for men, obesity is second to major knee injury as a preventable risk factor.

PATHOGENESIS

The exact cause of OA is not understood; however, biomechanical stress, biomechanical changes in the joints, and genetics all may play a part (ACR; 2000). The risk factors are cumulative. OA occurs when the surface layers of the cartilage in the joint breaks down. The articular surfaces of the joint rub together leading to pain and decreased function. Over time, osteophytes (bone spurs) may develop along the joint edges and particles may break off and float in the joint itself. OA may be idiopathic (primary) or the result of trauma or other disease in the joint (secondary). Although joint cartilage is the primary target, OA involves the articular cartilage, synovium, subchondral bone, ligaments, and neuromuscular system. Growth factors counteract this process in younger persons.

Genetic factors with autosomal dominant transmission in women and recessive inheritance in men are present with OA. The mother of a woman with DIP joint OA is twice as likely to have Heberden's nodes, and the patient's sister has a threefold chance compared with the mother and sister of a nonaffected woman (Brandt & Slemenda, 1993; Jimenez & Dharmavaram, 1994). Major trauma and repetitive use are strongly associated with OA. Human and animal studies show that damage to the anterior cruciate ligament or meniscus can result in knee OA. Occupations at risk for OA include jackhammer operators, cotton mill workers, coal miners, shipyard workers, and others who are subjected to repetitive stressful movement throughout the day. Farmers have a propensity for hip OA (Cooper, 1995). According to Lane's (1995) review of the literature, low-impact exercise activity does not increase the risk for OA. However, persons who participate in high impact sports or on a competitive level seem to be at greater risk. Longitudinal studies need to be conducted with a cohort of lifelong exercisers.

SPECIFIC CONSIDERATIONS FOR PHARMACOTHERAPY

When Drug Therapy Is Needed

The most common pharmacologic agents used in the treatment of osteoarthritis include NSAIDs, analgesics, and occasionally intraarticular corticosteroids. The hyaluronic acids hyaluronan and hylan G-F20 have been found effective for some persons with OA of the knee, especially those with severe pain. It should be noted that the majority of the research that has been done to test efficacy of modalities has been specific to OA of the knee (ACR, 2000). A number of experimental agents are also being currently evaluated.

Short- and Long-Term Goals of Pharmacotherapy

The primary goals of pharmacotherapy in the management of osteoarthritis is to minimize the painful symptoms associated with the underlying degenerative process, decrease inflammation if present, and to stop or slow joint damage. Controlling the pain allows the patient to maintain joint mobility, thereby maintaining or improving the patient's overall quality of life.

Nonpharmacologic Therapy

Nonpharmacologic therapies of some type are always used as adjuvant therapy with pharmacotherapeutics. Pain-relieving techniques include the use of heat (hydrotherapy or paraffin) and cold, acupuncture, and in severe cases, surgery. Techniques that may both relieve pain and protect the joint include cushioning the insoles of the shoes, low-impact exercise, weight loss, the use of walking aids and assistive devices, and minimizing repetitive movement or other stresses to the joint. Using a firm mattress may provide relief to the back, and modified cushions can provide support. Splints for limited periods of time may provide relief for overused joints. In the cases of knee and hip OA, weight loss and exercise may be the most important of these techniques. Physical therapy is important in both pain relief and in the return or maintenance of range of motion in the joints. (King & Halpern, 2002).

Yoga exercises have demonstrated benefits for pain relief and relaxation for all types of arthritis (Galas, 1996). The exercise is a gentle modality for decreasing joint stiffness and improving flexibility. The deep breathing and gentle stretching exercises are a mental, physical, and spiritual pathway to improved overall functioning.

In terms of surgery, replacement procedures are available for all extremity joints. However, the knee and hip joint replacements have demonstrated the best mobility and pain relief outcomes. Earlier surgical interventions are possible with advanced arthroscopic techniques. Other surgical procedures employed in the early stages include joint abrasion, wash out, and debridement (Edelson, Burks, & Bloebaum, 1995).

Assessment and History Taking

Joint pain associated with increased use stiffness with rest are the hallmark symptoms of OA. The pain is described as dull and aching and is relieved by rest in the initial stages. With later-stage disease, the pain occurs with rest and is frequently present at night. Localized joint stiffness is present after periods of rest for a short time during acute inflammatory flares. (Schumacher, Klippel, & Koopman, 1993).

Physical findings include pain on passive motion stiffness, locking, and crepitus. The patient with OA of the knee or hip usually presents with an antalgic gait favoring the affected joint (Hooker, 1996). Joint enlargement may be present because of increased synovial fluid or proliferative cartilage and bone changes. Joint tenderness may be elicited with acute synovitis. Joints commonly afflicted include the knee, hands, hip, foot, and spine. The elbow, shoulders, and toes are usually spared, and occupational or metabolic problems should be considered when these joints are involved (Moskowitz & Goldberg, 1993).

A common finding in OA of the hands is Heberden's nodes: spurs formed on the dorsolateral and medial aspects of the distal interphalangeal joints. These nodes usually develop slowly over months or years. They can, however, develop suddenly with an acute inflammatory process. Other common findings are: flexor and lateral deviations of the distal phalanx; Bouchard's nodes at the PIP joint; and the squared hand appearance, which results from involvement and tenderness of the first carpometacarpal joints. The trapezoid-scaphoid joint is frequently involved.

The Subcommittee of the American College of Rheumatology (ACR) has accepted specific criteria for the diagnosis of OA of the hand. For such a diagnosis to be made, the subcommittee suggests that the person have hand pain, aching, or stiffness and three of the four additional findings: (1) hard tissue enlargement of at least two of ten select joints, (2) hard tissue enlargement of the DIP joints, (3) swelling in less than three MCP joints, and (4) deformity of at least one of the ten select joints. For more details on diagnosis, see updates from the Arthritis Foundation (www.arthritis.org) or the ACR (www.rheumatology.org).

Persons affected with hip OA experience localized groin, anterior, or lateral thigh pain, and morning stiffness. Overuse of these joints precipitates pain. On physical examination they have pain and limited range of motion. With knee involvement, there is pain in and around the knee, which increases with weight bearing and improves with rest, along with the morning stiffness and the gel phenomenon. On physical examination, there is tenderness upon palpation, bony enlargement, crepitus, and diminished range of motion. The stiffness associated with OA typically lasts <30 min and resolves with movement of the joint. Inflammation is not commonly seen in OA, and its presence indicates a need for evaluation of other causes (ACR, 2000).

Diagnostic tests. An erythrocyte sedimentation rate that may be slightly elevated and CBC rules out acute infection. A rheumatoid factor may be considered when the primary affected site is the hands. Diagnostic radiographic findings of OA include joint space narrowing in mild cases and the presence of osteophytes with subchondral bony sclerosis (eburnation) in advanced cases (Hooker, 1996). Standing anterior-posterior knee x-rays are superior to plain knee views in detecting subtle joint space narrowing. Other x-ray findings in OA include cysts. Arthroscopy, CT, and MRI are helpful in the differential diagnosis of nonosteoarthritic lesions (Moskowitz & Goldberg, 1993). Joint aspiration may be performed when the signs of inflammation or joint effusion are present. Future tests may include immunoassay to detect molecular markers of cartilage matrix metabolism.

Patient/Caregiver Information

In addition to taking medications for the relief of pain, patients afflicted with osteoarthritis need to maintain an exercise and weight-monitoring program and learn to protect their joints from injury and stress. Many household and lifestyle modifications can improve mobility and well-being for the arthritis patient. Examples include using a large plastic bag or piece of lining fabric on upholstered car seats to make sliding into the car easier, asking for a table near the entrance of a restaurant to reduce walking, and asking the newspaper carrier to hang the paper in a plastic bag on the front doorknob.

OUTCOMES MANAGEMENT

Selecting an Appropriate Agent

Analgesics. Acetaminophen has long been considered first-line therapy in the treatment of osteoarthritis, either alone or in combination with other treatments or modalities (Felson, Lawrence, Hochberg, et al., 2002). Potential advantages of acetaminophen over NSAIDs include comparable efficacy with fewer adverse effects and lower overall cost. Clinical trials evaluating the efficacy of acetaminophen for the treatment of osteoarthritis of the knee have found that, at doses up to 4000 mg/day, acetaminophen is comparable to naproxen and to both analgesic and anti-inflammatory doses of ibuprofen (Bradley Brandt, Katz, et al., 1991; Williams, Ward, Egger, et al, 1993). For adequate control of symptoms, acetaminophen is typically dosed between 3000 and 4000 mg/day (Hochberg, Altman, Brandt, et al., 1995a; Moskowitz & Goldberg, 1993; Oddis, 1996). At therapeutic doses, acetaminophen is generally well tolerated. Potential adverse effects include rash, renal failure, and hepatotoxicity. Renal failure is typically associated with long-term use, and hepatotoxicty to excessive consumption of acetaminophen or use of acetaminophen in conjunction with regular alcohol intake. To minimize the risk of toxicity, a total daily dose of 4000 mg should not be exceeded and the patient should be advised to avoid alcohol consumption. Infrequently, not more than two or three alcohol-containing drinks should be consumed per day while taking acetaminophen.

Topical analgesics also can be used in the management of osteoarthritis either as sole therapy or in conjunction with systemic therapy. Commonly used agents include methysalicylate creams or capsaicin cream (Altman, Aven, Holmburg, et al., 1994; Deal, Schnitzer, Lipstein, et al., 1991). These agents are typically applied to the affected joint three or four times a day. Capsaicin cream reduces the pain associated with osteoarthritis by acting on substance P, a neurotransmitter that communicates painful stimuli from the peripheral to the central nervous system. Capsaicin depletes substance P at sensory nerve terminals and prevents its further synthesis and reaccumulation in the neuron. With the use of capsaicin cream, a local stinging or burning sensation is common; however, this sensation usually dissipates after several days of therapy (Altman et al., 1994; Deal et al., 1991). Symptomatic relief is usually experienced after approximately 1 to 2 weeks of therapy.

Opioid analgesics, especially those with codeine, are considered in the management of osteoarthritis in circumstances where no other treatments have been found to be adequate (ACR, 2000). Tramadol, a centrally acting synthetic opioid analgesic can be prescribed for persons for whom acetaminophen, NSAIDs, and COX-2 inhibitors have been either not effective or not tolerated. It is approximately equal to ibuprofen for OA of the knee. It can also be used as adjunctive therapy with NSAIDs. At the therapeutic doses of 200 to 400 mg/day in 3 to 4 divided doses, the side effects of nausea, constipation, or drowsiness are minimal. Seizures have occurred with persons with preexisting epilepsy or who are also taking medications that decrease the seizure threshold (Roth, 1998).

Nonsteroidal Anti-inflammatory Drugs. Despite their higher risk for adverse side effects, the nonselective NSAIDs and COX-2 specific inhibitors are the most commonly prescribed medications for the treatment of the pain associated with OA. They have been found to be more effective for moderate pain than acetaminophen (ACR, 2000).

In addition to aspirin and nonacetylated salicylates, there are a variety of NSAIDs and the newer COX-2 inhibitors available for the treatment of osteoarthritis. The choice between an NSAID and a COX-2 must be the result of the evaluation of risk, especially for that of a gastrointestinal bleed. Factors that increase risk include age over 65, concomitant use of corticosteroids, anticoagulants, and perhaps smoking and ETOH intake. Felson et al. (2002) describes a number of studies comparing the use of NSAIDs and COX-2 inhibitors for OA of the knee. Both COX-2 drugs currently available have been found superior to placebo and comparable to naproxen (celecoxib) and ibuprofen or diclofenac (refecoxib). For those persons at risk for bleeding, NSAIDs with gastroprotection may be an alternative to the costly COX-2s. Misoprostal 200 mg four times a day or the addition of omeprazole has been found to be comparable agents for gastroprotection (Hawkey, Karrasch, Szczpanski, et al., 1998). Refer to the rheumatoid arthritis section for a general discussion of these, including mechanism of action, pharmacokinetics, precautions, and adverse effects, and for a review of the anti-inflammatory options.

Joint Injections. The uses of both corticosteroidal and hyaluronic injections into the knee have been used to at least temporarily to treat severe pain of the knee. Steroids must always be used with caution and prolonged use can lead to an increase in the rate of deterioration of the joint. Hyaluronic acid is a substance that naturally occurs in the joint and is involved with lubrication and nutrition. While it is listed in the NIAMS/NIH website as a possible therapy, this treatment is controversial in the research literature. Studies that both support (Altman & Moskowitz, 1998) and refute the use of injections in the treatment of OA (Felson & McAlindon, 2002) can be found in the current literature.

Neutriceuticals. Eisenberg, Davis, Ettner, and colleagues (1998) found that as many as 26% of all persons who self-reported arthritis used complementary and alternative therapies. Among those used were glucosamine (1500 mg/day) and chondroitin. While these are widely used with positive anecdotal reports from patients, the research thus far has been inconclusive. They appear to be safe with minimal to no side effects and may prove to have some effect on disease process. However, studies can be found that both support and refute the claims of symptom relief (Houpt, McMillan, Wein, et al., 1999; McAlindon, LaValley, Gulin, & Felson, 2000; Rindone, Hiller, Collacott, et al., 2000; Chao & Vega, 2004; Schneiderman, 2001).

Monitoring Efficacy

Therapeutic drug efficacy is monitored by an improvement in the individual's range of motion, activity level and subjective report of pain. Along with the physical activity tolerance, the psychosocial dimension should improve.

Monitoring Toxicity

The Drug Tables on NSAIDs and analgesics (301, 306, 307, and 601.1) provide the potential toxicities, baseline evaluations, and frequency of monitoring for the therapeutic agents prescribed for OA.

Followup

Initially, the individual should be assessed at 2 to 3 week intervals until optimal pain relief is achieved and activity levels have improved. Clients should be encouraged to increase activity levels and maintain a weight reduction program during followup visits. Exploration of the psychological dimension is important during the followup visit.

OSTEOPOROSIS

Osteoporosis is the most common bone disease and is characterized by decreased bone mass and therefore strength. The most significant consequences of osteoporosis are nontraumatic bone fractures, estimated at 1.5 million annually (Chopra, 2002). While it affects white, non-Hispanic, postmenopausal women the most, it can affect all persons from all racial and age groups. Estimates from the 2000 Census suggest that 28 million people in the United States may be affected by low bone density. Eighteen million people are thought to have osteopenia (or bone thinning), and 10 million, osteoporosis; 80% in each group are women. It is further estimated that one out of two women over the age of 50 will experience an osteoporosis-related fracture at some time in her life (Khan, Tan, Briseno, & Heffron, 2002; NIH, 2000; NOF, 2002). If a woman sustains a fracture between the ages of 20 and 50, she is 74% more likely to sustain another (Wu, Mason, Horne, et al., 2002). Of those who sustain an osteoporosis-related fractures only about 30% will regain their pre-injury function and at one year, 20% will have died (NIAMS, 2000). The direct costs associated with osteoporotic fractures has reached $20 billion annually (Columbia, 2004).

CLASSIFICATION AND PATHOGENESIS

Low bone mass is classified as either osteopenia or osteoporosis and measured as a deviation of bone mineral density (BMD) from that of a young, normal, healthy white women. Most bone loss is the result of the normal changes with aging, particularly estrogen deficiency. Other causes of bone loss or insufficient bone density include nutritional deficiencies, several disease conditions including endocrine disorders and the use of a certain medications (Kessenich, 2000). The use of glucocorticoids for greater than two months is particularly noted as a causative factor for osteoporosis (Davidson & DeSimone, 2002).

The basic pathology of osteoporosis is that bone resorption exceeds bone formation. Bone remodeling is the process that constitutes a homeostatic balance between bone formation and resorption. Annually, adults replace 25% of their cancellous bone mass via activation of the bone remodeling units (Rungby, Hermann, & Mosekilde, 1995). This process involves osteoblasts (bone resorption) and osteoclasts (bone formation) (Khosla & Riggs, 1995; Silver & Einhorn, 1995). The process is controlled by a number of hormonal and physiologic process and cycles. Other factors that regulate this process include vitamin D, calcium, parathyroid hormone, calcitonin, growth hormone of the anterior pituitary, and estrogen. With the right nutrition, bone mass builds throughout childhood and the teens, reaching a peak in the twenty's. As a woman enters her third decade, her BMD begins to decline slowly until menopause. In the absence of estrogen replacement, the rate of decline increases rapidly, especially in the first three to five years after cessation of menses. By the time a woman reaches the age of 80, she may have lost 70% of her peak bone mass (NAMS, 2002).

According to the North American Menopause Society (2002), in addition to gender (female) and age, the major factors which increase one's risk for osteoporosis are genetics, lifestyle, and menopause-related estrogen deficiency. White non-Hispanic women are at the greatest risk for osteoporosis and associated fractures. African American women are at significantly less risk. Japanese women have lower peak BMD but have a lower rate of hip fracture (NIH, 2001). Children of women with osteoporosis and first-degree relatives have lower bone mass than expected (NAMS, 2002). Modifiable risk factors include nutritional deficiencies (especially calcium and vitamin D), low body weight, exercise and activity, smoking, and heavy alcohol consumption.

A number of medical conditions and drugs increase one's risk for osteoporosis. Among the conditions, disorders of absorption, hypogonadism, hyperthyroidism, and hyperparathyroidism are especially dangerous, as are the use of anticonvulsants, lithium, oral glucocorticoids, heparin, and cytotoxic agents (Khan et al., 2002; NIH, 2001; NAMS, 2002).

SPECIFIC CONSIDERATIONS FOR PHARMACOTHERAPY

Prevention of osteoporosis and subsequent fractures becomes the primary focus when caring for persons at risk for osteoporosis.

When Drug Therapy Is Needed

Both the North American Menopause Society and the National Institute of Health recommend that all postmenopausal women with any of the following indicators be considered for pharmacological management:

- a BMD T score of less than –2.5 of the hip or spine
- a BMD T score of –2.0 to –2.5 and one risk factor in addition to menopausal state
- any fracture that is considered to be osteoporosis related (with or without a BMD score)

While the recommendations for both the prevention and treatment of osteoporosis have been developed from the study of postmenopausal women, they are believed to be of use to men and younger women as well as indicated below (NIH, 2001).

Prescription medications, in combination with mineral supplementation and nonpharmacologic therapy, play an important role in the overall management of osteoporosis. Pharmacotherapy available for prevention and treatment of osteoporosis includes calcium, vitamin D, estrogen replacement, biphosphonates, salmon-calcitonin, and the newer parathyroid hormones.

Short- and Long-Term Goals of Pharmacotherapy

Goals of pharmacologic therapy are to optimize bone mass and preserve skeletal integrity, and ultimately, reduce the incidence of fractures and maintain normal physical function (Hodgson & Johnston, 1996).

Nonpharmacologic Therapy

Modification of controllable risk factors such as smoking cessation, reducing alcohol consumption, increasing exercise, and maintaining adequate nutritional intake of calcium and vitamin D remains the hallmark of both management and prevention. All must accompany any pharmacological treatment (NIH, 2001; Putukian, 1994).

There is agreement that weight-bearing exercise provides the highest level of osteogenic stimulation and that immobility leads to rapid bone loss (Taaffe, Robinson, Snow, & Marcus, 1997). However, less intense exercise, including walking, strengthening, and stretching, may have an even greater beneficial effect in the reduction of injuries associated with falls (NIH, 2001).

For persons with established osteoporosis, preventing fractures becomes paramount: one approach is to decrease one's fall risk. See Table 26–4 for suggestions to decrease the risk of falls and potential fractures (Galsworthy & Wilson, 1996). Eliminating the use of drugs that increase the risk for falls, such as sedatives, antihypertensives, and diuretics, is another important preventive measure.

Time Frame for Initiating Pharmacotherapy

Prevention of osteoporosis begins early in life by achieving and maintaining bone mass through adequate calcium balance. Initiation of estrogen therapy at the time of natural or surgical menopause (MP) provides the greatest preventive benefit, but is now questionable, due to associated risks.

See Drug Tables 605, 606.

Assessment and History Taking

All women seen in primary care should be regularly screened for both the presence of risk factors and for the diagnosis of osteoporosis. In this way, modifiable risks may be reduced and prompt treatment can be initiated to minimize bone loss and the risk for fracture and disability. The screening and assessment include a history determination of risk factors, including comorbid conditions,

TABLE 26–4. Minimizing the Opportunities for Falls

- Remove all throw rugs.
- Move electrical cords and wires out of the walking paths.
- Repair or replace unsteady or easily toppled furniture.
- Move commonly used items to low, easily reached shelves.
- Avoid the use of step stools or ladders.
- Keep all walking or standing surfaces dry and skid-resistant.
- Install securely mounted grab bars anywhere they may be helpful, e.g., kitchen, living room, porch, bathroom.
- Install or place telephones around the residence at strategic locations.
- Keep frequently used walking paths inside and outside of the home clear of clutter and well lighted at all times.

past injuries, diet, exercises, and menstrual and family history. Additional screening should include risk factors for falling. Physical exam includes dentition, weight, height and height history, palpation of the spine, range of motion of the joints, and muscle strength testing (Kessenich, 2000). A home safety inspection is ideal but not often possible.

Diagnostic tests. The measurement of bone mineral density (BMD) with dual-energy x-ray absorptiometry (DEXA) has become the gold standard for the both the diagnosis of osteoporosis and the evaluation of the effectiveness of treatment. The measurement results in a "T-Score," the number of standard deviations from that of a normal healthy young woman. The World Health Organization has established the diagnostic categories of osteopenia (1 to 2.5 standard deviations below normal) and osteoporosis (2.5 or greater deviations from normal). Other scans, such as the single-energy x-ray absorptiometry ultrasound, have also been used. Biochemical urine and serum markers of resorption and formation are available. However, they are very costly and are primarily used in research; clinical use is controversial. With further development they may be of greater use in the future (Kessenich, 2000).

Patient/Caregiver Information

Information should be given to the patient on how to prevent falls and decrease fractures (Table 26–4). Other preventive measures include wearing sturdy low-heeled shoes and maintaining adequate lighting throughout the house. An active exercise program is essential to maintain adequate bone mass. Calcium supplements should be taken on an empty stomach between meals. The exception is calcium carbonate, which is taken with food. Avoid foods, such as spinach, that decrease calcium absorption. Foods high in calcium include low-fat or skim milk (1 cup = 300 mg of calcium), swiss cheese (1 oz = 272 mg), canned sardines with bones (3 oz = 375 mg), low-fat fruit yogurt (1 cup = 300–400 mg), sesame seeds (3 tbsp, whole = 300 mg), and broccoli (1 stalk, cooked = 150 mg) (Galsworthy & Wilson, 1996).

OUTCOMES MANAGEMENT

Selecting an Appropriate Agent

Calcium and Vitamin D Supplementation. The recommended daily intake of calcium is given in Table 26–5. Dietary sources of calcium include dairy products, green vegetables, nuts, and some fish. Supplementation is recommended for men and women not meeting daily requirements through diet alone and those receiving the pharmacotherapy mentioned above (Hodgson & Johnston, 1996). Increasing age and ingestion of certain foods (e.g., oxalate-containing foods such as spinach) are associated with decreased calcium absorption. Vitamin D added to calcium supplementation enhances calcium bioavailability. This therapy is especially important in populations at risk for vitamin D deficiency such as those living in institutions or in regions with low levels of sunlight. (Hockwald, Harman-Boehm & Castel, 2004)

TABLE 26–5. Optimal Calcium Requirements Recommended by the National Institutes of Health Consensus Panel

Age Group	Optimal Daily Intake of Calcium, mg
Women	
25–50	1000
>50 (PMP) on estrogens	1000
>50 (PMP) not on estrogens	1500
>65 ± estrogens	1500
Men	
25–65	1000
>65	1500

Source: From National Institutes of Health (1994).

Numerous calcium and vitamin D products are available without a prescription. Table 26–6 lists the various salts and calcium content per product. Calcium carbonate is generally recommended because of high calcium content and low cost. Because over-the counter (OTC) calcium products are not regulated by the Food and Drug Administration (FDA), the use of brand name products is suggested to ensure adequate bioavailability. With the exception of calcium carbonate, which requires an acid environment for absorption, other calcium products should be taken between meals to increase bioavailability (Hodgson & Johnston, 1996; NIH, 2001). Absorption is greatest with single doses of 500 mg or less (NIH, 2001). Side effects occur infrequently, with constipation being the most common complaint. Hypercalciuria rarely occurs at recommended doses (Hodgson & Johnston, 1996).

TABLE 26–6. Calcium Supplementation Products

Calcium Salt	Elemental Calcium, %
Calcium carbonate	40
Calcium phosphate, tribasic	39
Calcium acetate	25
Calcium citrate	21
Calcium lactate	13
Calcium gluconate	9
Calcium glubionate	6.5

The greatest effects of calcium supplementation have been shown in elderly women five or more years following menopause. Increased bone mineral density and a decreased risk of vertebral and nonvertebral fractures have been demonstrated in this population (Hodgson & Johnston, 1996; NIH, 1994; Chapuy, Arlot, Duboeuf, et al., 1992). Calcium supplementation alone cannot counter the loss of bone mass during the early postmenopausal years, but is recommended as an adjunct to estrogen replacement therapy. Lifetime administration of calcium and vitamin D is recommended for optimal effect.

Vitamin D in recommended doses of 400 to 800 IU daily may be obtained from supplements, sunlight, vitamin D–fortified liquid dairy products, cod liver oil, and fatty fish (NIH, 2001). Calcitriol, a vitamin D analog, is currently not recommended for the treatment of osteoporosis.

Estrogen. Postmenopausal estrogen replacement (ERT) is the most effective therapy for both the prevention and treatment of osteoporosis. For the woman with an intact uterus, estrogen must be used in combination with progesterone (HRT) due to its link to endometrial hyperplasia. Estrogen, acting through receptors on the osteoclasts, inhibits bone reabsorption, thus decreasing bone turnover (Kanis, 1995). Multiple studies have demonstrated that ERT/HRT started at menopause initially increase BMD by 4–6% in the spine and 2–3% in the hip. After three years these increases are maintained as long as the therapy continues (NIAMS, 2002). Bone loss returns with the cessation of the ERT or HRT.

Common side effects associated with HRT may include premenstrual symptoms, such as bloating, irritability, bleeding or spotting, and the potentiation of migraine headaches. Contraindications include known or possible pregnancy, thromboembolitic disease and smoking.

Unfortunately we have learned from the Woman's Health Initiative that HRT increases the risk for coronary heart disease, strokes, pulmonary emboli and invasive breast cancers while it decreases the risk for colorectal cancers and hip fractures (Brucker & Youngkin, 2002). With this new information, HRT can no longer be considered a first line approach to osteoporosis, especially for use longer than five years. Fortunately the new drugs are available and may be substituted.

Bisphosphonates. This class of drugs inhibits osteoclast activity, decreases bone turnover, and alters bone metabolism to favor bone formation rather than resorption. They are indicated for the prevention and treatment of osteoporosis in both men and women. In clinical trials, bisphosphonates have been found to increase BMD in the spine and hip and decrease the risk of fracture by 30 to 50% (NIH, 2001). They have been the drug of choice for women who cannot or will not take ERT/HRT and in men and women who have steroid-induced osteoporosis (Davison & DeSimone, 2002).

All can cause gastric irritation and must be taken first thing in the morning on an empty stomach, with a full glass of water (not other fluids), and the person must remain upright for 30 minutes after dosing. They should not be prescribed for persons who cannot follow these instructions or have severe renal impairment. Concurrent administration of calcium and vitamin D are required.

Alendronate is now available in daily and weekly dosing for both prevention (5 mg/day or 35 mg/week) and treatment (10 mg/day or 70 mg/week). It has been shown to incrase BMD from 1 to 10% when used for two to seven years (Tonino, Meunier, Emkey, et al., 2000). Newer risedronate at doese of 5 mg/day also has been found to incraese BMD and decrease fractures, especially after three years of use (Harris Watts, Genent, et al., 1999).

SERMs. SERMs are selective estrogen receptor modulators, which provide the benefit of estrogen without the potential deleterious effects on the endometrium and the breast. Raloxifene (60 mg/daily) is the only SERM approved in the United States at this time, and it can be used for both the prevention and treatment of osteoporosis. Like estrogen it decreases bone turnover by inhibiting resorption. After two years, it has been found to increase BMD by 2.4% in both the spine and the hip (Delmas, Bjarnason, Mitlak, et al., 1997) and after three years reduced the risk for vertebral fracture by 35 to 50% (Ettinger, Black, Mitlack, et al., 1999). Other benefits appear to include a reduction in risk of invasive breast cancer after three to five years. It does however have possible side effects of DVTs and hot flashes. It cannot be used with persons that have prolonged periods of immobility.

Calcitonin. Salmon calcitonin therapy is indicated for men and women who cannot tolerate the other pharmacological modalities. It is recommended for women who are at least five years postmenopausal, and it may also be particularly helpful for those with associated back pain. Calcitonin is a peptide hormone that inhibits bone resorption but much less so then the other agents. While intramuscular injections are available, it is most often prescribed as an intranasal formulation (NAMS, 2002). Doses of 200 IU (one spray) daily, alternating nostrils, has been found to be the most effective. The only potential side effect of the nasal preparation is irritation of the mucosa. In a large, randomized study of 200 IU/day for five years, the vertebral fracture risk rate was decreased by 33%; however, no protective effect was found for the hip (Chestnut, Silverman, Andriano, et al., 2000). Calcitonin has the added benefit for providing pain relief for some persons with OA of the spine. Its mechanism in doing so is unknown.

Anabolics. After years of research a new and promising treatment has been added for both postmenopausal and glucocorticoid-induced osteoporosis.

Synthetic parathyroid hormone (PTH) has been found to stimulate bone formation and significantly increase bones mass and consequently reduce the risk for spinal fractures and to a lesser extent, non-spinal fractures in men and women. In animal studies some rats which received high doses of PTH developed osteosarcoma, but this has not yet been seen in humans (Crandall, 2002; NOF, 2004; Raggett & Partridge, 2004).

Side effects include dizziness, leg cramps, nausea, low energy and headaches and may indicate the rare event of the development of hypercalcemia. Due to this risk it should not be used in persons with Paget's or other bone metabolism disorders, children and young adults with open epiphyses, and in persons who have had or will have radiation of the bone. It is a pregnancy Category C. It has not been found to have any significant drug interactions.

Teriparatide (Forteo®) is the only approved product at this time. It is self-administered in daily subcutaneous injections of 20 mcg for 24 months and is available in 28-day supplies in disposable pen devices. For more information see www.forteo.com.

Combination Therapy. Research is also being conducted relating to the use of combination therapies, the role of statins, and the effectiveness of phytoestrogens and nitric oxide (NIAMS, 2002)

Monitoring for Efficacy

Measuring osteoporosis drug efficacy is a long-term process. Optimal efficacy is achieved by increasing bone mass, preventing fractures, and maintaining activity levels. DEXA Scans are used for monitoring the effectiveness of treatment.

Monitoring for Toxicity

Drugs used in the prevention and treatment of osteoporosis are generally well tolerated. Routine monitoring for adverse effects is important in maintaining patient compliance with long-term therapy.

Followup Recommendations

Appropriate followup is necessary following initiation of drug therapy. A return visit 4 to 6 weeks later is important for assessing compliance and adverse effects (Kleerekoper & Avioli, 1993). Once the patient is stable, annual followup is recommended. Women receiving hormone replacement therapy need to be instructed on monthly breast self-examination. Yearly gynecologic exams and mammography are also recommended. Bone mineral density studies are indicated for monitoring where appropriate, but should not be a routine monitoring parameter in asymptomatic prevention patients (Hodgson & Johnston, 1996). The elderly patient with comorbid conditions is often seen more frequently.

GOUT

Gout is a painful arthritic disease caused by the deposition of monosodium urate crystals in connective tissue, joint spaces, or both. It can result in swelling, redness, erythema, pain, and stiffness.

The deposition of calcium pyrophosphate dihydrate (CPPD), crystals results in a similar condition known as pseudogout, or chondrocalcinosis (AF, 2002).

EPIDEMIOLOGY

Middle-aged men in their fifth decade are most often afflicted, with postmenopausal women comprising the second highest-risk population. Gout is the most common cause of inflammatory arthritis in men over age 30 and is rarely seen in women prior to menopause. Gout accounts for about 5% of all arthritic conditions (NIAMS, 2002). Approximately 20% of younger gout-afflicted persons demonstrate a familial pattern (Beutler & Schumaker, 1994).

Acute gout may be precipitated by medications (see Table 26–7), minor trauma, acute illness, or excessive intake of alcohol or high purine foods. Persons with gout have a higher incidence of poorly controlled chronic diseases associated with renal insufficiency, such as hypertension and diabetes mellitus (Terkeltaub, 1993).

TABLE 26–7. Commonly Prescribed Drugs That Can Cause Gout

Alcohol (ethanol)
Diuretics
Nicotinic Acid
Levodopa
Aspirin (low doses)

More recently, researchers have noted an association between gout and heart disease. In both are commonly found insulin resistance and hyperlipidemia (Wortmann, 2002).

Older persons are more at risk for developing gout due to the increased number of medications they consume. They must be managed carefully since they usually have some degree of diminished renal functioning (Gonzalez, Miller, & Agudelo, 1994). The increased number of elderly women presenting with gout has been attributed to the almost 25% of Americans over aged 65 taking thiazide diuretics (Star & Hochberg, 1994; Terkeltaub, 1993).

PATHOGENESIS

Gout results when either the body increases the production or decreases the elimination of uric acid. This often results in hyperuricemia (> 7 mg/dL) (Pittman & Bross, 1999). Uric acid production in humans occurs from the ingestion of purine-containing foods and from the endogenous synthesis of nucleic acids. The kidney is the major route of uric acid excretion and under normal conditions accounts for 60% of the disposal. Insufficient renal excretion of uric acid is responsible for the majority (90%) of patients with primary hyperuricemia. Individuals whose kidneys underexcrete uric acid (the majority of gout patients) maintain inappropriately high serum urate concentrations (Pittman & Bross, 1999). The gut, through bacterial oxidation, is the major extrarenal disposal of urate. Compared with the kidney, the gut has a limited capability to deal with an increased urate load.

The exact mechanism that promotes spontaneous gouty inflammation remains elusive. Monosodium salt crystals may be found oversaturated joint tissues in the acute attack. The tophi, found later in the disease, are accumulations of crystals. However, the crystals can also be found in unaffected (asymptomatic) joints. An initial attack of gout most often affects the joint of the great toe, a condition known as podagra. It can also affect the instep, ankles, heels, knees, fingers, and elbows (Pittman & Bross, 1999).

SPECIFIC CONSIDERATIONS FOR PHARMACOTHERAPY

When Drug Therapy Is Needed

Once gout has been diagnosed, treatment is relatively straightforward and in the majority of cases can be handled on an outpatient basis. Agents available for the treatment of an acute attack of gouty arthritis include colchicine, NSAIDs, and corticosteroids (Van Doornum & Ryan, 2000). Agents used to manage symptomatic hyperuricemia include allopurinol and the uricosuric agents. Selection of an appropriate therapeutic regimen should be based on an assessment of efficacy versus toxicity through evaluation of patient-specific parameters. Asymptomatic hyperuricemia does not require treatment (Davis, 1999).

Short- and Long-Term Goals of Pharmacotherapy

The major short- and long-term goals of therapy include alleviation of pain associated with the acute attack as well as prevention of recurrent attacks and extraarticular manifestations of the disease (Meiner, 2001). Educate the patient regarding correctable factors, such as obesity, diet, use of thiazide diuretics, and alcohol consumption, as well as compliance with medications (Schesinger & Schumacher, 2001).

Nonpharmacologic Therapy

Gout attacks can be prevented by decreasing alcohol intake, and avoiding specific foods and medications that may have precipitated previous attacks. Dietary modifications with low-purine-containing foods have not demonstrated marked efficacy. The patient should maintain enough hydration to produce a urinary output of 2 L per day. This amount will aid urate excretion and decrease urate precipitation in the urinary tract.

Time Frame for Initiating Pharmacotherapy

In treating an acute attack of gouty arthritis, pharmacotherapy should be initiated at the first sign of symptoms. Delay in initiating palliative therapy typically results in a reduction of the medications' effectiveness. Any therapy that alters serum urate concentrations, such as allopurinol or the uricosurics, should not be initiated during an acute episode. If the patient is already on antihyperuricemic therapy, the dose should not be adjusted. Use or adjustment of these agents during an acute attack may cause exacerbation of symptoms or precipitation of a relapse due to changes in plasma urate concentrations (Emmerson, 1996; Star & Hochberg, 1993). If necessary, antihyperuricemic therapy should be initiated one to two weeks following the resolution of an acute attack.

See Drug Tables 306, 316, and 601.1.

Assessment and History Taking

There are four basic stages of gout: asymptomatic hyperuricemia, acute gouty arthritis, intercritical gout, and chronic tophaceous gout. It may be a misnomer to label asymptomatic hyperuricemia as gout since not all individuals who have hyperuricemia will develop gout. Acute gouty arthritis is characterized by an acute onset of intense pain usually in the first metatarsophalangeal joint, but the midfoot, ankles, knees, and wrists can be affected. The attack commonly occurs during the night. Classically, the joint is tender, swollen, warm, and erythematous. Chills and mild fever may accompany the pain. Early in the disease process, attacks tend to subside spontaneously in 3 to 10 days with or without treatment. Another attack may occur months or years later. Acute attacks may be precipitated by trauma, alcohol, drugs, surgical stress, and acute medical illness.

Gout can have an atypical subclinical presentation without the acute signs and symptoms. Acute gout should be suspected anytime a person has a sudden episode of joint pain, unilaterally or bilaterally, even if his or her symptoms do not meet the classic presentation.

Intercritical gout is the interval occurring between acute attacks. The patient is asymptomatic and exhibits no abnormal physical findings. Monosodium urate (MSU) crystals are present in 97% of synovial fluid aspirated from previously affected joints.

Chronic tophaceous gout develops gradually over a ten-year period. The synovium, subchondral bone, olecranon bursa, Achilles tendon, and subcutaneous tissue on the extensor forearm surfaces are the usual sites for tophi development (Pittman & Bross, 1999). Diagnostic aspiration may be necessary since tophi can be confused with rheumatoid or other nodules.

Individuals who overexcrete uric acid may present with an acute episode of flank pain as a consequence of urolithiasis. With long-standing untreated disease, patients may present initially with an acute urinary tract infection caused by stone formation and blockage.

Prior to the initiation of therapy, assessment of renal and hepatic function is recommended for the elderly patient.

Diagnostic Tests. Radiographs are useful to show soft tissue swelling and exclude septic joint changes, calcifications, and spur formations from other processes. A finding of calcified tophi may be difficult to differentiate. With chronic disease states, intra-articular or periarticular asymmetric round or oval bony erosions with sclerotic margins are seen (Kane & Sturrock, 2002).

The presence of MSU crystals in aspirated synovial fluid is considered the diagnostic marker for gout (Beutler & Schumaker, 1994; Star & Hochberg, 1994). Synovial fluid leukocyte cell counts are elevated from 20,000 to 100,000/mm and are predominately neutrophils (Tate, 1993). The serum uric acid level may not be elevated in some patients with acute gout and is considered to be of limited value since 30% of patients have normal levels during an acute attack (Joseph & McGrath, 1995; McCarty, 1994). However, serial measurements to follow treatment response are helpful. Additional tests may include a 24-hour urine uric acid measurement to assess renal stone risk, to detect underlying factors in the gout, and to determine the treatment. Urinary uric acid excretion greater than 750 to 1000 mg/day on a regular diet suggests uric acid overproduction. Aspirin, phenylbutazone, alcohol consumption, and contrast dye can affect uric acid excretion and should be withheld prior to testing (Tate, 1993).

Patient/Caregiver Information

Patients must avoid dehydration and large amounts of alcohol. They should be encouraged to drink enough fluids to maintain an urinary output of at least 2 L per day. Their fluid intake will need to be increased during hot dry weather. In order to obtain maximum pain relief, it is important to start pharmacotherapy at the first sign of an attack. Patients should contact their healthcare provider as soon as symptoms begin.

OUTCOMES MANAGEMENT

Selecting an Appropriate Agent for Acute Gout

Nonsteroidal Antiinflammatory Drugs. Nonsteroidal antiinflammatory drugs have been a mainstay in the treatment of acute gout and, unless contraindicated, are often the drugs of choice. NSAIDs should not be given to patients with active peptic ulcer disease or with a recent history of gastrointestinal bleeding (Star & Hochberg, 1993). Risk versus benefit must be carefully assessed before using NSAIDs in patients with other comorbid conditions, including renal dysfunction, congestive heart failure, uncontrolled hypertension, asthma, and inflammatory bowel disease (Pratt & Ball, 1993; Star & Hochberg, 1993). Use of NSAIDs in these patient populations can potentially lead to a worsening of their underlying disease state. Patients who appear to be at higher risk of developing gastrointestinal bleeding secondary to

NSAID use include the elderly, patients receiving high-dose therapy, those with a prior history of gastrointestinal bleeding, and patients receiving concomitant anticoagulation therapy (Polisson, 1996; Pratt & Ball, 1993). The COX-2 inhibitors are potentially safer NSAIDs for persons at risk for GI bleeding.

Colchicine. When an NSAID is not effective or is contraindicated, colchicine has been found to be highly effective for both the treatment of an acute attack and for the prevention of reoccurrences. Colchicine is an antimitotic agent that has been used for years in the treatment of gout. Although the mechanism by which colchicine exerts its effect has not been fully elucidated, it appears to inhibit the migration and phagocytosis by leukocytes. With phagocytosis decreased in the tissues, there is less lactic acid, which limits the deposition of the crystals in joint tissue and diminishes the inflammatory response. Colchicine also appears to decrease the release of chemotactic factors (Emmerson, 1996; Moreland & Ball, 1991).

In treating an acute attack, colchicine can be given either orally or intravenously. Unfortunately, the oral dose necessary for symptomatic relief almost inevitably leads to the development of gastrointestinal side effects, such as nausea, vomiting, diarrhea, and abdominal cramping (Agarwal, 1993).

To effectively abort an acute attack, the medication should be initiated in the first 12 to 36 hours. Delay in initiating therapy reduces the medication's effectiveness. The usual oral dosage is 1.2 mg initially, followed by 0.5 to 0.6 mg every 1 to 2 h until pain is relieved or until abdominal discomfort, nausea, vomiting, or diarrhea develops. A total dose of 7.8 mg should not be exceeded. In elderly patients and patients with renal or hepatic dysfunction, a decrease in dose is necessary (Boomershine, 2002; Emmerson, 1996; Pratt & Ball, 1993). Due to impaired elimination, these patients are more likely to develop cumulative toxicity to colchicine. A general guideline is to decrease the dose by approximately 50% in this patient population (Emmerson, 1996; Pratt & Ball, 1993).

Intravenous administration of colchicine is typically reserved for patients who are unable to take oral medications or for situations where gastrointestinal side effects must be avoided (Pittman & Bross, 1999). It can be given in 1 mg doses, not to exceed 4 mg in 24 hours. The use of intravenous colchicine has been associated with an increased risk of toxic side effects, including bone marrow suppression and renal or hepatic cell damage, and, therefore, is not routinely used in practice. Intravenous colchicine should not be used in patients with combined renal and hepatic dysfunction, a creatinine clearance of <10 mL/min, extrahepatic biliary obstruction, and immediate prior use of oral colchicine (Pratt & Ball, 1993). In order to prevent local tissue reaction or sclerosis, colchicine should be diluted with 20 mL of normal saline and delivered through an intravenous catheter over approximately 10 minutes. Colchicine is incompatible with dextrose and, therefore, should only be diluted with normal saline to prevent precipitation.

Common side effects associated with the use of NSAIDs include headache, dizziness, gastrointestinal complaints, and renal impairment (Brooks & Day, 1991; Furst, 1994; Simon, 1995). Administering the agents with food may decrease the incidence of gastrointestinal intolerance. See section on NSAID use earlier in this chapter. Indomethacin is one NSAID that has been used extensively over the years in the treatment of acute gout. A typical regimen of indomethacin is 50 mg 3 to 4 times a day for 1 to 2 days, reduced to 25 mg 2 times a day for 5 to 7 days. Common alternatives to indomethacin are naproxen sodium (825 mg × 1, then 275 mg q 8 hours until pain resolved) or sulindac (200 mg twice a day until pain resolved) (van Doornum & Ryan, 2000).

Corticosteroids. Corticosteroids have been shown to be beneficial in the treatment of acute gouty arthritis. In most cases, they are reserved for refractory cases or cases where the use of colchicine and NSAIDs is contraindicated (Davis, 1999). At the relatively low doses and short duration of therapy used in the treatment of gout, the corticosteroids are generally well tolerated. Potential side effects include fluid retention, hyperglycemia, and CNS effects.

Corticosteroids may be administered either orally, parenterally, or intraarticularly. Presence of a septic joint should be ruled out prior to the use of corticosteroids. In the treatment of acute gout, often involving multiple joints, oral doses of prednisone from 20 to 40 mg/day are recommended. This dose is administered for the first 3 to 5 days and then gradually tapered off over a 1- to 2-week period (Pratt & Ball, 1993; Star & Hochberg, 1993). For patients unable to take oral medications, particularly those in the hospital setting, an equivalent intravenous dose of methylprednisolone may be given. Intra-articular administration of corticosteroids is useful in cases involving one or two large joints. Triamcinolone acetonide at a dose of 10 to 40 mg, depending on the size of the joint, may be used for intraarticular injections (Pratt & Ball, 1993).

Prophylactic Treatment of Acute Gout. The ideal time to initiate pharmacological prophylactic therapy remains controversial. Some initiate prophylaxis after the first acute attack, others do not initiate it until the attacks have become frequent or there are signs of tophi or neuropathy (Pittman & Bross, 1999). Other factors to consider include potential toxicity, drug cost, patient compliance, and patient tolerance of acute attacks (Pratt & Ball, 1993). Nonpharmacologic intervention is often considered first-line therapy in preventing recurrent attacks. This consists of weight reduction, restriction of dietary purine and alcohol intake, and avoidance of drugs known to increase serum urate concentrations (low-dose salicylate, niacin, pyrazinamide, and thiazide and loop diuretics) (Fam, 1995). Compliance with these measures may circumvent the need for daily drug therapy.

Patients with recurrent attacks, despite compliance with nonpharmacologic intervention, are typically started on prophylactic drug therapy. Small daily doses of oral colchicine or NSAIDs are effective. One of these agents also should be started prior to initiating therapy with an antihyperuricemic agent to prevent precipitation of an attack. For prophylactic therapy, colchicine is usually dosed at 0.6 mg one to four times weekly. To minimize the chance of toxicity, the smallest effective dose should be used (Pratt & Ball, 1993). In patients with no other comorbid conditions affecting the elimination of colchicine, prophylactic doses are generally well tolerated. In patients with impaired renal function (creatinine clearance < 50 mL/min), reversible myopathy and neuropathy have been observed with long-term use (Kuncl, Duncan, & Watson 1987; Wallace, Singer, Duncan, et al., 1991). NSAIDs can also be used as prophylactic therapy, but their long-term use may be associated with a higher incidence of gastrointestinal adverse effects (Kot, Day, & Brooks, 1993). No consensus exists regarding the duration of prophylactic therapy; however, recommendations range from 6 months to 1 year of an attack-free interval following the normalization of serum urate concentrations (Emmerson, 1996; Kot et al., 1993).

Selecting an Appropriate Agent for Hyperuricemia

For patients with symptomatic hyperuricemia, the goal of treatment is to reduce and maintain the serum urate concentration below 6.0 mg/dL in order to prevent recurrent attacks and reverse the deposition of urate crystals in tissues (Pittman & Bross, 1999). There are currently two classes of drugs that can effectively lower serum urate concentrations: uricosuric agents and allopurinol. Selection of an agent is based on patient-specific parameters, including the overproduction or underexcretion of uric acid, renal function, and the presence of tophaceous gout. Uricosuric agents are preferred in cases of normal or underexcretion of uric acid, normal renal function, and nontophaceous gout (Pratt & Ball, 1993; Star & Hochberg, 1993). Allopurinol is the preferred agent in cases of overproduction of uric acid, renal impairment, and chronic tophaceous gout (Pratt & Ball, 1993; Star & Hochberg, 1993). The presence of both overproduction (high purine intake) and underexcretion (low clearance) of uric acid is fairly common. In this case, allopurinol may be the preferred agent because it is effective in handling both problems (Emmerson, 1996). To reduce the risk of precipitating an acute attack of gout, these agents should not be initiated until 1 to 2 weeks have passed following the resolution of an attack and a prophylactic agent (colchicine or NSAID) has been used for several days.

Probenecid and Sulfinpyrazone. Probenecid and sulfinpyrazone are two uricosuric agents that have long been used in the management of hyperuricemia in persons who are underexcretors of uric acid. The uricosuric agents act to lower serum urate concentrations by inhibiting the reabsorption of uric acid from the proximal tubule, thus increasing its excretion. These agents should be avoided in patients with excessive uric acid excretion, impaired renal function (creatinine clearance < 50–60 mL/min), inadequate urine flow (< 1 mL/min), and a history of renal calculi. The normal reduction of renal function in older persons generally limits their usefulness in this population (Pittman & Bross, 1999). Probenecid is initiated at a dose of 500 mg once daily and increased as needed to a maintenance dose of 1–2 g/day in divided doses to maintain serum urate concentrations < 6 mg/dL. Common adverse effects include gastrointestinal intolerance, rash, and nephrolithiasis. Formation of renal calculi may be minimized by starting with low-dose therapy and titrating slowly, maintaining high urine output, and alkalinizing the urine during initial therapy (Emmerson, 1996; Pratt & Ball, 1993; Star & Hochberg, 1993). The risk of developing renal calculi occurs each time therapy is restarted; therefore, compliance with uricosuric therapy must be emphasized. Due to its site of action, probenecid inhibits the excretion of a number of medications, thus enhancing their efficacy and/or toxicity. Some of these agents include penicillins, indomethacin, dapsone, acyclovir, and methotrexate. Concomitant use of salicylates may interfere with the uricosuric effect of probenecid (Davis, 1999).

Sufinpyrazone, a more potent uricosuric agent, is initiated at a dose of 100 mg/day and titrated as needed up to

800 mg/day given in divided doses. Potential adverse effects include gastrointestinal intolerance, nephrolithiasis, platelet dysfunction, and rarely bone marrow suppression. It must be used very cautiously in persons who are anticoagulated, have other bleeding, or have peptic ulcer disease.

Allopurinol. The xanthine oxidase inhibitor. Allopurinol decreases the production of uric acid through inhibition of the enzyme xanthine oxidase, which is responsible for the breakdown of purines to uric acid. In cases of renal insufficiency, allopurinol is preferred over the uricosurics. However, due to potential toxicity secondary to accumulation of the active metabolite, oxypurinol, the dose must be adjusted. Allopurinol is typically started at a dose of 100 mg/day and titrated up to a maintenance dose of 300 mg/day as needed to effectively lower serum urate concentrations (Kot et al., 1993). Smaller daily doses are recommended for patients with glomerular filtration rates < 50 mL/min (Vazquez-Mellado, Morales, Pacheco-Tona, & Burgos-Vargas, 2001). Depending on the degree of renal insufficiency, doses as low as 100 mg every other day or every third day may be necessary. As with the uricosurics, prophylactic therapy with colchicine or NSAIDs should be started prior to initiating allopurinol in order to minimize the risk of precipitating an acute attack of gout (Day, Birkett, Hicks, et al., 1994; Emmerson, 1996; Pratt & Ball, 1993; Star & Hochberg, 1993).

Common adverse effects associated with allopurinol use include gastrointestinal intolerance, hypersensitivity reactions, and skin rash. Fairly rare, yet serious adverse effects include toxic epidermal necrolysis, fever, leukopenia, vasculitis, interstitial nephritis, and hepatotoxicity. These effects tend to occur more commonly in patients receiving concomitant thiazide diuretic therapy and in those with renal insufficiency. Important drug interactions associated with allopurinol include increased serum concentrations of methotrexate, azathioprine, and theophylline secondary to inhibition of their metabolism.

Monitoring for Efficacy

Therapeutic drug efficacy is monitored by improvement in the patient's symptoms. Following prompt initiation of therapy for an acute attack, resolution of severe pain commonly occurs within several hours. Initially, the patient should be assessed in 1 week to verify that the acute attack has resolved. Residual pain is common; therefore, therapy is typically continued for 5 to 7 days. After the acute attack has resolved, the need for prophylactic therapy must be evaluated. Nonpharmacologic interventions should be emphasized.

Monitoring for Toxicity

Toxicity may occur with any of the agents used in the treatment and prevention of gouty arthritis. See the discussions of individual drugs for potential toxicities.

Followup Recommendations

Initially, the individual should be assessed at a 1- or 2-week interval to verify that the acute attack has resolved. If it is not the patient's first attack, the need for prophylactic therapy must be evaluated. Nonpharmacologic interventions also must be emphasized.

LOW BACK PAIN

Back pain represents one of the most common complaints for which healthcare is accessed. Marras (2000) reports that 80% of the general population experiences an episode of back pain during their lifetime between the age of 25 to 80. The chronicity of low back pain is estimated to be above 39%, according to Batt and Todd (2000). Chronicity is defined as persistent symptoms lasting over three months. Symptoms can be either be localized to the spine or may refer to the lower extremity. In most cases chronic back pain stems from repetitive injury or accumulation of microtrauma. Microtrauma usually occurs prior to the incident for which treatment is sought.

ETIOLOGY

Ninety percent of back pain in adults is attributed to a mechanical disorder, and the remaining 10% stems from one of more than 60 nonmechanical etiologies: rheumatologic, infectious (urinary tract, prostatitis, pelvic inflammatory disease, herpes zoster, epidural abscess), neoplastic, endocrine (diabetes), hematologic, referred from the abdomen (abdominal aortic aneurysm, perforated ulcer, pancreatitis, and endometriosis), and miscellaneous causes (Marras, 2000). Mechanical back pain is caused by overuse or strain, trauma, or spinal anatomic deformity. Common mechanical disorders associated with low back pain include muscle strain, osteoarthritis of the apophyseal joints, spinal stenosis, herniated disk with or without radiculopathy, or spondylolisthesis. Most back pain results from the pain-sensitive areas, including anterior and posterior ligaments, vertebral bodies, facet synovial lining, paraspinal muscles, sacroiliac joint, and neural tissue within the neural canal and foramen. The intervertebral disk is not sensitive to pain; therefore pain from a damaged disk must result from irritation or entrapment of pain-sensitive structures and tissue. Sprains in the lumbar and thoracic region are the result from sudden loading or torsional movements. They can result from direct or indirect trauma that forces the spinal segment(s) beyond their normal range of motion, as well as from compressive loading forces. The more common injury to the lumbar region is a sudden extension movement with rotation. The lumbar spine depends heavily on the surrounding musculature to increase its stability during mechanical loading.

The mechanism for muscular strains of the lower back is similar to those for sprains, elsewhere causing sudden contraction or stretching of the involved musculature. Sudden eccentric loading of an already contracting muscle is also a common cause of musculature strain. Strains can result from a single episode of muscle overload but also frequently from cumulative stress. Factors such as poor posture, muscular imbalance, poor conditioning, weak abdominal muscles, and inflexibility of the hamstrings, hip flexors, and/or back extensors can increase one's susceptibility to muscular low back strains (Marras, 2000).

SPECIFIC CONSIDERATIONS FOR PHARMACOTHERAPY

When Drug Therapy Is Needed

Conservative treatment of low back pain is most efficacious when a comprehensive program is initiated early, immediately after an injury. Although 80% of injuries resolve within 2 to 4 weeks, the microtrauma suffered in the injury increases susceptibility to further injury, and patient education is paramount to successful recovery. Multidisciplinary rehabilitation should focus on functional restoration, psychological factors, patient education, and pain management through appropriate medication, modalities, manual therapy, and others. Pharmacologic agents commonly used in the management of low back pain include acetaminophen, NSAIDs, and muscle relaxants. Other agents used to provide symptom control include opioid analgesics, corticosteroids, and antidepressants; however, the efficacy of these agents in the treatment of low back pain is debated.

Short- and Long-Term Goals of Pharmacotherapy

The primary short-term goal of pharmacotherapy is to provide symptom control to allow for activity tolerance until recovery occurs. Achieving this goal permits the patient to continue functioning normally both at work and home. Long-term management of back pain focuses primarily on nonpharmacologic therapy rather than prolonged drug therapy. Among other things, goals of long-term therapy include adequately educating the patient regarding low back problems and recommending activity modification. In the case of chronic back pain, clinicians and therapists should direct treatment to the physical and psychological issues related to chronicity.

Nonpharmacologic Therapy

Many therapeutic options with varying efficacy are utilized for relief of back pain. The management goal of back pain has shifted from a focus on the pain toward helping the patient improve activity tolerance. Limited physical activity for 2 days is recommended for patients without neurological deficits. Most patients will recover faster when they resume their normal activities.

A commonly utilized treatment modality is spinal manipulation. Short-term (1 month) spinal manipulation is recommended for patients with uncomplicated low back pain. Continuous long-term therapy has no proven benefit (Arnheim & Prentice, et al., 2000).

Physical therapy also is widely used for mechanical back pain. Typically, a 1- to 2-week physical therapy program in conjunction with pharmacological agents is effective. Some patients benefit from exercise and being taught improved body mechanics by the physical therapist.

Relaxation and stress management modalities, including yoga, meditation, imagery, and counseling, are employed with the patient afflicted with chronic back pain. Frequently, the patient's psychological status is a major factor contributing to the condition. Relationship conditions in marriage, at home, or at work may be intolerable for the patient, and stress management is an important aspect of treatment. For these patients, all stress, tensions, and frustrations are psychologically channeled to the back muscles. Traction, which was once widely used, has demonstrated no significant results other than keeping the patient passive and nonfunctional. Transcutaneous electrical nerve stimulation (TENS) is another treatment modality that has demonstrated equivocal efficacy in a few controlled studies (Arnheim, & Prentice, 2000). An ice pack (wrapped in a towel) placed on the back for 10 to 20 min every hour provides relief for some patients. For those who cannot tolerate the ice therapy, moist heat is very effective. The heat should be applied for 20 min five to six times a day. A moist hot towel applied to the back covered with plastic and a heating pad is very effective.

Most low back pain resolves within 4 weeks with conservative management. Only 1 to 2% of patients will require surgery. According to outcome studies, surgery has demonstrated no appreciable efficacy. Back pain prevention education programs by employers are a key element of management.

Time Frame for Initiating Pharmacotherapy

Once the diagnosis of back strain or musculoskeletal pain has been made, pharmacotherapy should be initiated immediately to encourage movement and minimize the complications associated with immobilization (Junge, et al., 2001).

See Drug Tables 301, 302, and 306.

Assessment and History Taking

The management plan for most back pain patients is derived from a detailed history and physical. Four basic questions should guide the workup of the patient with back pain:

1. What was the mechanism of injury?
2. Is there an underlying systemic problem such as cancer, abdominal aneurysm, or infection?
3. Is there a neuro-deficit present that warrants a consultation?
4. Is there a psychosocial component that may amplify or prolong the pain?

Plain x-rays are indicated for a few selected cases: pain sustained by a fall or forceful trauma, pain that does not improve with conservative therapy, possible metastatic cancer, older osteoporotic high-risk patients, patients over age 70, and patients using steroids (Batt & Todd, 2000). Patients with neurological signs and symptoms should receive an MRI. The history begins with a description of the circumstances associated with the onset of pain. This includes the type of work and usual position. Does the patient primarily sit or stand throughout the day? For possible litigation purposes, the exact location, conditions, wet or slippery floor, exact height of the fall, or force of the injury must be documented. Most work-related low back pain is due to mechanical strain (Marras, 2000). A previous history of back pain and its sequelae should be elicited. A detailed description of the pain is mandatory. Is the pain worse with activity or rest? Pain worse at night is usually indicative of disk disease. Is the pain localized or does it radiate? Be specific as to the radiation of the pain. Is it above or below the knee and which aspect of the leg? Neurological deficits should be ascertained by asking about the presence of extremity weakness or numbness and bowel or bladder deficits. Infectious processes can be detected by asking about fever, chills, dysuria, frequency, or vaginal discharge for females. Males over age 50 should be asked about prostate problems such as difficulty with stream and frequent voiding.

A history of coexisting predisposing factors should be elicited. For example, hypertension is a risk factor for an aortic aneurysm, and post-menopausal status poses a risk for vertebral fractures. Both conditions produce back pain. The psychological status of all patients should be assessed by inquiring about their life stressors and ability to cope (Frank, & Souza, 2001).

The physical examination begins by observing the patient ambulate to detect list or leg lag. Next, to rule out neurological deficits, the patient is asked to walk on his or her toes (S1) and heels (L4,5). The spine, paravertebral muscles, and costovertebral angles are palpated for tenderness. The patient should perform range of motion as tolerated. The patient's ability to squat and rise tests strength of the quadriceps and L4 innervation. Against resistance, dorsiflexion of the great toe tests L5. Testing for straight leg raising is performed with the patient sitting and lying. Pain below the knee at 70 degrees or less is indicative of L5 and/or S1 nerve root irritation. Pain that is relieved by plantar flexion of the ankle or external limb rotation suggests a herniated disk. A possible herniated disk diagnosis is further confirmed with the crossover strength leg raising (SLR) test. With this test, pain occurs when the elevated uninvolved leg produces similar pain distribution. Next, deep tendon reflexes and peripheral pulses are compared. Dorsiflexion and extension strength of the great toe is elicited to determine muscle weakness associated with neurological deficit. Hip range of motion and abdominal examination are performed with the patient supine. Pelvic and rectal examinations may be indicated by the history (Arnheim & Prentice, 2000).

Patient/Caregiver Information

Patients need to be instructed to refrain from operating moving vehicles or operating machines while taking narcotic analgesics and muscle relaxants. The patient should sleep on a firm mattress or place a board under the mattress to provide additional back support. A pillow under knees while laying on the back relieves pressure Laying on the side with a pillow between knees keeps the hips in anatomical position and relieved L_4 L_5 S_1 nerve pressure. When the back pain subsides, back stretching and abdominal strengthening exercises are preventive measures for subsequent episodes. In appropriate cases weight reduction is advisable. When lifting heavy objects, the patient should bend the knees and use the large quadriceps and hamstring muscles. Back rehabilitation classes that teach back exercises are very beneficial. Yoga is another modality that enhances back muscle stretching and mind/body relaxation. It is important to emphasize tension and stress management and reduction and the role they play in reducing back pain. Patients should always be instructed to seek care immediately for increased extremity numbness or weakness or decreased ability to void or move their bowels.

OUTCOMES MANAGEMENT

Selecting an Appropriate Agent

Analgesics. Acetaminophen, a primarily centrally acting analgesic with little to no anti-inflammatory activity, is considered a safe, effective, and low-cost agent for initial treatment of acute low back pain. Patients who experience inadequate pain relief with acetaminophen are often given a trial of NSAIDs. Use of an NSAID provides both analgesic and anti-inflammatory activity. As in the treatment of other musculoskeletal disorders, no one NSAID has been found to be superior to the others. There may, however, be great variability in efficacy among agents on an individual basis. Therefore, a patient may be given a trial of another NSAID, typically from a different class, if little to no pain relief is obtained after a 2-week period.

Short-term use of oral opioid analgesics provides another option for the treatment of severe, acute low back pain (AHCPR, 1994). The use of opioid analgesics should rarely extend beyond a 1- to 2-week period. Risk versus benefit must be assessed before initiating therapy with opioids because of potential CNS side effects and the potential for developing tolerance and physical dependence with this class of drugs. Commonly prescribed agents include codeine-containing products and synthetic opioids (e.g., hydrocodone, oxycodone). See the Drug Table 303 for further information on dosing and side effects.

Muscle Relaxants. Muscle relaxants are another class of agents commonly used in the treatment of various painful musculoskeletal conditions, including low back problems. These agents are targeted toward the relief of muscle spasm, which may or may not be associated with the pain. Based on findings in the literature, the efficacy of muscle relaxants remains somewhat inconclusive.

For treatment of low back problems, the centrally acting skeletal muscle relaxants are frequently prescribed. Rather than causing direct relaxation of skeletal muscle, these agents appear to act centrally through a sedative effect, which ultimately results in depression of neuronal activity (Guzman, Rosmin, et al., 2001). Commonly used skeletal muscle relaxants include carisoprodol, chlorzoxazone, cyclobenzaprine, metaxalone, methocarbamol, and orphenadrine citrate.

Although these agents may provide some symptomatic relief, their use is associated with a number of potential adverse effects. The side effect most commonly reported with these agents is drowsiness, which occurs in up to 30% of patients. Other reported CNS side effects include dizziness, headache, confusion, and agitation. Use of these agents in conjunction with alcohol or other CNS depressants may lead to cumulative toxicity.

Caution must be exercised with the use of chlorzoxazone. The FDA-approved labeling changes for chlorzoxazone warn of the rare idiosyncratic and unpredictable hepatotoxicity associated with its use. Early signs and symptoms of hepatotoxicity patients should be aware of include fever, rash, anorexia, nausea, vomiting, fatigue, right upper quadrant pain, dark urine, or jaundice (Nightingale, 1995). With long-term use, liver function tests should be monitored and if abnormality develops, the drug should be discontinued. Hepatotoxicity has also been associated with the use of metaxalone and all others in this class.

Both cyclobenzaprine, which is structurally similar to the tricyclic antidepressants, and orphenadrine, which is an analog of diphenhydramine, have anticholinergic properties. Use of these agents may be associated with the presence of dry mouth, blurred vision, urinary retention, and constipation. These agents should be avoided in patients with prostatic hypertrophy, angle-closure glaucoma, and underlying cardiac abnormalities. See Drug Table 314 for other commonly reported adverse effects and precautions.

In addition to adverse effects, concern exists over the potential for dependence and abuse of some of the centrally acting skeletal muscle relaxants secondary to their CNS effects. Dependence and withdrawal have been observed with the use of carisoprodol and cyclobenzaprine. To minimize the risk of dependence and abuse, ideally, these agents should be prescribed only for brief periods to provide acute symptomatic relief and discontinued gradually to avoid possible withdrawal symptoms. They typically can be limited to a 1- to 2-week course of therapy.

Other agents used with relaxant properties include diazepam (benzodiazepine), baclofen (antispasmodic), and dantrolene sodium (peripherally acting skeletal muscle relaxant). Diazepam appears to exert its muscle relaxant properties through augmentation of the inhibitory effect of the neurotransmitter gamma-aminobutyric acid (GABA) at spinal and supraspinal sites. Although diazepam has not shown superiority over centrally acting skeletal muscle relaxants in the treatment of muscle spasm and pain, it may provide some advantage in treating anxiety associated with painful conditions. The prolonged use of diazepam in the treatment of musculoskeletal disorders is limited because of its CNS depressant properties and its potential for dependence and abuse.

The antispasmodic agent baclofen, which is chemically related to GABA, elicits its effect through inhibition of the transmission of both monosynaptic and polysynaptic reflexes at the level of the spinal cord. This agent is indicated primarily for the relief of muscle spasticity associated with multiple sclerosis and spinal cord lesions. It is not indicated for the treatment of muscle spasms associated with rheumatic disorders. In patients with severe spasticity unresponsive to maximum oral therapy, baclofen may be administered by the intrathecal route. When initiating therapy with baclofen, it should be titrated up slowly to minimize the risk of side effects.

Dantrolene sodium appears to produce skeletal muscle relaxation through a direct peripheral effect rather than a central effect. This agent inhibits the release of calcium ions from the sarcoplasmic reticulum, ultimately leading to skeletal muscle relaxation. It is indicated for the treatment of muscle spasticity associated with upper motor disorders such as spinal cord injury, stroke, cerebral palsy, and multiple sclerosis. Like baclofen, it is not indicated for the relief of spasms associated with rheumatic disorders. Dantrolene use has been associated with hepatotoxicity caused by an idiosyncratic or hypersensitivity reaction to the medication. The risk for hepatotoxicity appears to be greatest for females over the age of 35 who are receiving other medications, in particular, estrogen therapy.

Corticosteroids. In the treatment of low back pain, there is no indication for the use of oral or intravenous corticosteroids (AHCPR, 1994). The use of corticosteroids for trigger point, facet joint, and epidural injections has been evaluated and they are widely used for temporary relief. Because of potential complications, use of these invasive measures is typically not recommended for the treatment of acute low back problems.

Monitoring for Efficacy

The typical course of treatment for acute low back problems is 1 to 2 weeks with up to 80% of patients symptomatically improving within this time period.

Monitoring for Toxicity

With many of the agents used in the management of low back pain, the most common and use-limiting side effects are CNS-related. These CNS effects include drowsiness, dizziness, headache, agitation, and confusion. Often, tolerance develops to these side effects; however, if they persist or are intolerable, the agent should be discontinued. The use of a number of centrally acting skeletal muscle relaxants has been associated with the development of hepatotoxicity. If one of these agents is used, the patient must be warned of early signs and symptoms of hepatotoxicity, and liver function tests should be monitored regularly. See Drug Tables 301, 302, 306 and 314 for specific agents associated with hepatotoxicity.

Followup Recommendations

The patient should be instructed to return for a followup visit immediately if bladder or bowel problems occur or if there is increased extremity numbness or weakness. Patients with acute injuries covered by workman's compensation are usually reevaluated within 1 week to determine the ability to resume full or partial work activities.

Prevention of back injury classes are recommended along with physical therapy evaluation for potential risk evaluation.

TENDINITIS, BURSITIS, SPRAINS, AND STRAINS

Persons experience muscle, tendon, or ligament strains or sprains as a result of trauma and overuse. During the past decade, reported workplace-associated overuse injuries have escalated, and the repetitive movement syndrome accounts for 30 to 50% of workplace injuries (Marras, 2000). In addition, the increased numbers of persons engaged in exercise activities (running and aerobic exercise) have produced a variety of musculoskeletal complaints. The most common problems are discussed below.

Stiff neck syndrome, which results when patients are subjected to strenuous positions (plumbers and others who must work in awkward positions). *Tension neck syndrome* is experienced by patients who sit at a desk and have poor posture (computer operators and accountants). These problems are not associated with an injury, but result from maintaining an incorrect posture for a prolonged time. The patient has neck pain and stiffness, often with a dull headache. The pain may spread to the upper thoracic regions, and the trapezius and levator muscles are tender with palpation. Radicular symptoms are usually absent, and if tingling sensations are present, consider other causes. *Occipital cephalalgia* results from restricted motion of the occipital-cervical joints. It commonly occurs from prolonged tucking of a telephone under the chin, from extended desk or computer work or from lying on a couch watching television with a pillow propping the head. These patients have intense unilateral pain, sometimes associated with migraine-like headaches (nausea and photosensitivity) and dizziness. The occipital muscular triangle is tender.

Tendinitis is an inflammation of a tendon sheath as a result of overuse or injury. Common areas afflicted include the elbow (epicondylitis), the shoulder (rotator cuff and adhesive capsulitis with frozen shoulder), the extensor tendon of the wrist and thumb, or the lower extremity (hamstring or Achilles tendon). Diabetics and arthritic patients are prone to developing tendinitis of the hands, and wrists (carpal tunnel syndrome) and shoulder (adhesive capsulitis). Patients experience pain with motion and occasionally paresthesia of the affected area. The affected area is usually tender, occasionally minimally swollen, but usually with no erythema.

Bursitis resulting from trauma, overuse, crystal-induced diseases (e.g., gout), connective tissue disease (e.g., rheumatoid arthritis), and infections (e.g., gonorrhea) commonly involves the elbow, shoulder, and the hip. Trochanteric bursitis of the hip, which is frequently underdiagnosed, is characterized by a chronic, intermittent aching pain in the lateral aspect of the hip. It results from inflammation of the four trochanter bursae and often secondarily from tendinous calcification (Arnheim & Prentice, 2000). The pain can be sharp and intense and increases with external rotation and abduction along with other hip movements. The pain can be reproduced by resisted abduction and external rotation. Patients will have localized tenderness over the greater trochanter and may have a positive Patrick's fabere test (Arnheim & Prentice, 2000).

Patients with bursitis of the shoulder complain of nocturnal diffuse shoulder pain in addition to specific abduction pain ranging from 70 to 110 degrees (painful arc). The pain is poorly localized to the deltoid area and may radiate down the arm. There should be no neurovascular compromise.

Musculoskeletal injuries with sprains and strains are among the most common complaints in primary care (Arnheim & Prentice, 2000; Buolinson 1997). When an injury is sustained, a specific inflammatory process initiates the symptoms of redness, swelling, heat, and pain. Ninety percent of ankle sprains involve the anterior or posterior talofibular ligament of the lateral malleolus. Injury to the medial malleolus is more likely to result in a fracture. There is usually a history of ankle inversion or eversion with or without a "pop." The presence of an audible sound indicates more serious injury, and the patient may be nauseated, lightheaded, and diaphoretic. With more serious injuries, the patient is unable to ambulate after the injury and there is immediate swelling and redness. With less serious injuries, swelling and pain may not occur until 8 to 12 hours after the injury. Neurovascular intactness and point tenderness, which are more specific for fracture, must be assessed. Ankle sprains are graded from I to III (Arnheim & Prentice, 2000). A grade I sprain is mild with minimal swelling and ecchymosis, no instability or functional disability, and full range of motion. A grade II sprain has moderate to severe pain, decreased range of motion, and swelling and ecchymosis with an incomplete ligament tear. A grade III sprain is more severe with a complete ligamentous tear and must be referred to an orthopedic surgeon for management. An x-ray can rule out fracture and is warranted for all high-risk injuries and for patients with severe pain or who are unable to ambulate.

NONPHARMACOLOGICAL TREATMENT

An effective simple treatment for tendinitis, bursitis, and ligamentous injuries is described by the acronym RICE (rest, ice, compression, and elevation). Put the affected area to rest to diminish swelling and inflammation. Compression can be attained with ace bangages. Elevation of the extremity by sling or simply propping the foot higher than the heart will aid in recovery. Persons with grade II and III ankle injuries will need crutches for 2 to 5 days. Most patients with grade I injuries can ambulate with an ace bandage. Cold therapy application, 15 to 30 min three to five times a day during the initial 24 to 72 h after an injury or work-induced syndrome reduces cellular metabolism and allows marginally viable cells to survive. Cold therapy is also applied to prevent reactive swelling after rehabilitative exercises (Arnheim & Prentice, 2000). During the subacute and chronic stages of the pain, when the swelling has subsided, moist heat application, 15 to 30 min three to five times a day, increases blood flow, promotes tissue healing, and loosens stiff joints and muscles. Moist heat may be applied, as suggested for back pain. A whirlpool bath is also an effective way to apply moist heat. Ultrasound transmits high-frequency acoustic energy deep heat waves to the injury and is used in the rehabilitative stage after the acute inflammation has subsided (Arnheim & Prentice, 2000). The use of a supportive device such as an elastic wrist band or carpal splint during the acute inflammatory phase of tendinitis is often therapeutic.

See Drug Table 306 for pharmacological treatment of these conditions.

REFERENCES

Rheumatoid Arthritis

Abelson, A., Elkon, K., Pischel, K., & Sigal, L. (2002). A common sense guide to rheumatologic tests. *Patient Care for Nurse Practitioners,* 6.

American College of Rheumatology (ACR) Ad Hoc Committee On Clinical Guidelines. (2002). Guidelines for management of rheumatoid arthritis. *Arthritis and Rheumatism, 46*(2), 328–346.

Bathon, J. M., Martin, R. W., Fleischmann, R. M., et al. (2000). A comparison of etanercept and methotrexate in patients with early rheumatoid arthritis. *New England Journal of Medicine, 343,* 1586–1593.

Birnbaum, H. G., Barton, M., Greenberg, P. E., Sisitsky, T., Auerbach, R., Wanke, L. A., & Buatti, M. C. (2000). Direct and indirect costs of rheumatoid arthritis to an employer. *Journal of Occupational Environmental Medicine, 42* (6), 588–596.

Breedveld, F. C., & Dayer, J. M. (2000). Leflunomide: Mode of action in the treatment of rheumatoid arthritis. *Annals of Rheumatic Disease, 59,* 841–849.

Bresnihan, B. (2001). Treating early rheumatoid arthritis in the younger patient. *Journal of Rheumatology, 28* (Suppl), 4–9.

Calabrese, L. H. (2002). Anakinra treatment of patients with rheumatoid arthritis. *Annals Pharmacotherapeutics, 36*(7), 1204–9.

CDC. (1996). Factors associated with prevelent self-reported arthritis and other rheumatic conditions—United States, 1989–1991. *MMWR, 45*(23), 487–491.

Center for Disease Control. (2000). Targeted tuberculin testing and treatment of latent tuberculosis infection. *MMWR, 49*(RR-6), 26–38.

Covic, T., Adamson, B., & Hough, M. (2000). The impact of passive coping on rheumatoid arthritis pain. *Rheumatology (Oxford), 39,* 1027–1030.

Feldman, M., & Maini, R. (1999). The role of cytokines in the pathogenesis of rheumatoid arthritis. *Rheumatology (Oxford), 38*(suppl 2), 3–7.

Gabriel, S. E., Crowson, C. S., Luthra, H. S., Wagner, J. L., & O'-Fallon, W. M. (1999). Modeling the lifetime costs of rheumatoid arthritis. *Journal of Rheumatology, 26*(6), 1269–1274.

Goroll, A. H., May, L. A., & Mulley, A.G. Jr. (Eds). (2000). *Primary care medicine: Office evaluation and management of the adult patient.* Philadelphia: Lippincott Williams & Wilkins.

Kagen, L. (2004, January). An update on the newer therapies for rheumatoid arthritis. *The Clinical Advisor,* 10–16.

Lipsky, P., van der Heijde, D., St. Clair, E., et al. (2000). Infliximab and methotrexate in the treatment of rheumatoid arthritis. Anti-tumor Necrosis Factor Trial in Rheumatoid Arthritis with Concomitant Therapy Study Group. *New England Journal of Medicine 343,* 1594–1602.

Mochan, E. (2001). Updata on rheumatoid arthritis: Tumor necrosis factor inhibition. *Consultant,* 1561–1563.

Newhall-Perry, K., Law, N. J., Ramos, B., et al. (2000). Direct and indirect costs associated with the onset of seropositive rheumatoid arthritis. *Journal of Rheumatology, 27,* 1156–1163.

Palmer, D. G. (1995). The anatomy of the rhematoid lesion. *British Medical Bulletin, 51*(2), 267–285.

Ruoff, G. (March, 2002). Rheumatoid arthritis: Emerging treatments. *Consultant,* 297–306.

Sandoval, D. M., Alarcon, G. S., & Morgan, S. L. (1995). Adverse events in methotrexate-treated rheumatoid arthritis patients. *British Journal of Rheumatology, 34*(Suppl 2), 49–56.

Semble, E. L. (1995). Rheumatoid arthritis: New approaches for its evaluation and management. *Archives of Physical Medicine and Rehabilitation, 76,* 190–201.

Simon, L. S., & Smith, T. J. (1998). NSAID mechanisms of action, efficacy, and relative safety. *Postgraduate Medical Special Report,* 12–16.

Smarr, K. L., Parker, J. C., Kosciulek, J. F., et al. (2000). Implications of depression in rheumatoid arthritis: Do sub-types really matter? *Arthritis Care Research, 13,* 23–32.

Strahl, C., Kleinknecht, R. A., & Dinnel, D. I. (2000). The role of pain, anxiety, coping and pain self-efficacy in rheumatoid arthritis patient functioning. *Behavior Research Therapy, 38,* 863–873.

Strand, V., Cohen, S., Schiff, M., et al. (1999). Treatment of active rheumatoid arthritis with leflunomide compared with placebo and methotrexate. *Archives of Internal Medicine, 159,* 2542–2550.

Walker, A. M., Funch, D., Dryer, N. A., et al. (1993). Determinants of serious liver disease among patients receiving low-dose methotrexate for rhematoid arthritis. *Arthritis and Rheumatism, 36,* 329–335.

Weinblatt, M. E., Kremer, J. M., Bankhurst, A. D., et al. (1999). A trial of etanercept, a recombinant tumor necrosis factor receptor: Fc fusion protein in patients with rheumatoid arthritis receiving methotrexate. *New England Journal of Medicine, 340,* 253–259.

Weinblatt, M. E., Kremer, J. M., Coblyn, J. S., et al. (1999). Pharmacokinetics, safety, and efficacy of combination treatment with methotrexate and leflunomide in patients with rheumatoid arthritis. *Arthritis Rheumatology, 42,* 1322–1328.

Williams, H. J. (1993). Rheumatoid arthritis: Treatment. In H. R. Schumacher, J. H. Klippel & W. J. Koopman (Eds.), *Primer on the rheumatic diseases* (10th ed.). Atlanta: Arthritis Foundation.

Wood, A. J. J. (1994). Second-line drug therapy for rheumatoid arthritis. *New England Journal of Medicine, 330,* 1368–1375.

www.hopkins-arthritis.somjhmi.edu: Excellent information about RA diagnosis, pathophysiology, and treatment options.

www.rheumatology.org: American College of Rheumatology website, which includes a search feature to find a local rheumatologist.

http://my.webmd.com/condition_center/rha: WebMD provides good general information about RA.

http://www.nih.gov/niams/healthinfo/juvarthr.htm.: Comprehensive information on juvenile RA.

Osteoarthritis

Altman, R. D., Aven, A., Holmburg, C. E., et al. (1994). Capsaicin cream 0.025% as monotherapy for osteoarthritis: A double-blind study. *Seminars in Arthritis and Rheumatism, 23*(6), 25–33.

Altman, R & Moskowitz, R. (1998). Intra-articular sodium hyaluronate (Hyalgan) in the treatment of patients with osteoarthritis of the knee: A randomized clinical trial. Hyalgan Study Group. *Journal of Rheumatology, 25,* 2203–12.

American College of Rheumatology (ACR). (2000). Subcommittee recommendations for the medical management of osteoarthritis of the hip and knees. *Arthritis and Rheumatology, 43*(9), 1905–1915.

Bradley, J. D., Brandt, K. D., Katz, B. P., et al. (1991). Comparison of an anti-inflammatory dose of ibuprofen, an analgesic dose of ibuprofen, and acetaminophen in the treatment of patients with osteoarthritis of the knee. *New England Journal of Medicine, 325*(2), 87–91.

Brandt, K. D., & Slemenda, E. W. (1993). Osteoarthritis, epidemiology, pathology, and pathogenesis. In H. R. Schumacher, Jr., J. H. Klippel, & W. J. Koopman (Eds.), *Primer on the rheumatic diseases* (10th ed.). Atlanta: Arthritis Foundation.

Chao, S. & Vega, C. (2004, January). Alternative approaches to relieving the pain of osteoarthritis. *The Clinical Advisor,* 21–26.

Cooper, C. (1995). Occupational activity and the risk of osteoarthritis. *Journal of Rheumatology, 22(1)*(Suppl. 43), 10–12.

Deal, C. L., Schnitzer, T. J., Lipstein, E., et al. (1991). Treatment of arthritis with topical capsaicin: A double-blind trial. *Clinical Therapeutics, 13*(3), 383–395.

Edelson, R., Burks, R. T., & Bloebaum, R. D. (1995). Short-term effects of knee washout for osteoarthritis. *American Journal of Sports Medicine, 23*(3), 345–349.

Eisenberg, D., Davis, R., Ettner, S. Appel, S., Wilkey, S., Van Rompay, M., & Kessler, R. (1998). Trends in alternative medicine use in the United States, 1990–1997: Results of a national follow-up study. *Journal of the American Medical Association, 280*(18), 1569–1574.

Felson, D., Lawrence, R., Hochberg, M., McAlindon, T., Dieppe, P., Minor, M., Blair, S., Berman, B., Fries, J., Weinberg, M., Long, K., Jacobs, J., & Goldberg, V. (2002). Osteoarthritis: New insights: Part 2 Treatment approaches. *Annals of Internal Medicine, 133*(9), 726–737.

Felson, D., & McAlidon, T. (2002). Osteoarthritis: New insights [letter]. *Annals of Internal Medicine, 136*(1), 88.

Freeman, S. (2001, September). Diagnosis and management of osteoarthritis. *American Journal for Nurse Practitioners,* 9–24.

Gabriel, S. E., Crowson, C. S., & O'Fallon, W. M. (1995). Costs of osteoarthritis: Estimates from a geographically defined population. *Journal of Rheumatology, 22*(Suppl. 43), 23–25.

Galas, J. (1996, May–June). Yoga all gain no pain. *Arthritis Today,* 30–32.

Hawkey, C., Karrasch, J., Szczpanski, L., Walker, D., Barkun, A. Swannell, A., & Yeomans, N. (1998). Omeprazole compared with misoprostol for ulcers associated with nonsteroidal anti-inflammatory drugs. *New England Journal of Medicine, 338*(11), 727–734.

Hochberg, M. C., Altman, R. D., Brandt, K. D., et al. (1995). Guidelines for the medical management of osteoarthritis (parts one and two). *Arthritis and Rheumatism, 38*(11), 1535–1546.

Hooker, R. S. (1996). Osteoarthritis of the hip and knee: Managing a common joint disease. *Clinician Reviews, 6,* 54–68.

Houpt, J., McMillan, R., Wein, C., & Paget-Dellio, S. (1999). Effect of glucosamine hydrochloride in the treatment of pain of osteoarthritis of the knee. *Journal of Rheumatology, 26,* 2423–2430.

Jimenez, S. A., & Dharmavaram, R. M. (1994). Genetic aspects of familial osteoarthritis. *Annals of Rheumatic Diseases, 53,* 789–797.

King, O. & Halpern, B. (2002). Osteoarthritis: A quick guide to exercise therapy for older patients. *Consultant, 42*(10), 1362–1368.

Lane, N. E. (1995). Exercise: A cause of osteoarthritis. *Journal of Rheumatology, 22*(1)(Suppl. 43), 3–6.

McAlindon, T., LaValley, M., Gulin, J., & Felson, D. (2000). Glucosamine and chondroitin for treatment of osteoarthritis: A systematic quality assessment and meta-analysis. *JAMA, 283*(11), 1469–1475.

Moskowitz, R. W., & Goldberg, V. M. (1993). Osteoarthritis: Clinical features and treatment. In H. R. Schumacher, Jr., J. H. Klippel, & W. J. Koopman (Eds.), *Primer on the rheumatic diseases* (10th ed.). Atlanta: Arthritis Foundation.

Oddis, C. V. (1996). New perspectives on osteoarthritis. *American Journal of Medicine, 100*(Suppl. 2A), 10S–15S.

Rindone, J., Hiller, D., Collacott, E., Nordhaugen, N., & Arriola, G. (2000). Randomized, controlled trial of glucosamine for treating osteoarthritis of the knee. *Western Journal of Medicine, 172,* 91–94.

Roth, S. (1998). Efficacy and safety of tramadol HCL in breakthrough musculoskeletal pain attributed to osteoarthritis. *Journal of Rheumatology, 25*(7), 1358–1363.

Schneiderman, H. (2001, December). Update on glucosamine treatment for osteoarthritis. *Consultant,* 1788–1789.

Schumacher, H. R., Jr., Klippel, J. H., & Koopman, W. J. (1993). *Primer on the rheumatic diseases* (10th ed.). Atlanta: Arthritis Foundation.

Williams, H. J., Ward, J. R., Egger, M. J., et al. (1993). Comparison of naproxen and acteaminophen in a two-year study of treatment of osteoarthritis of the knee. *Arthritis and Rheumatism, 36*(9), 1196–1206.

Osteoporosis

Brucker, M. & Youngkin, E. (2002). What's a woman to do?: Exploring HRT related questions raised by the Woman's Health Initiative. *Lifelines, 6*(5), 408–417.

Cauley, J. A., Seeley, D. G., Ensrud, K., et al. (1995). Estrogen replacement therapy and fractures in older women. *Annals of Internal Medicine, 122,* 9–16.

Chapuy, M. C., Arlot, M. E., Duboeuf, F., et al. (1992). Vitamin D3 and calcium to prevent hip fractures in elderly women. *New England Journal of Medicine, 27,* 1637–1642.

Chesnut, C., Silverman, S., Andriano, K., Genent, H., Gimona, A., Harris, S., Kiel, D., LeBoff, M., Maricic, M., Miller, P., Moniz, C., Peacock, M., Richardson, P., Watts, N., & Baylink, D. (2000). A randomized trial of nasal salmon calcitonin in postmenopausal women with established osteoporosis: The prevent recurrence of osteoporosis fractures study. PROOF study group. *American Journal of Medicine 109*(4), 267–76.

Chopra, A. (2002). Impact and pathogenesis of osteoporosis. *Annals of Long Term Care, 10*(3), 27–33.

Crandall, C. (2002). Parathyroid hormone for the treatment of osteoporosis. *Archives of Internal Medicine, 162*(20), 2297–2309.

Davidson, M., & DeSimone, M.E. (2002). Osteoporosis update: Targeting risks, managing wisely. *Clinical Reviews 12*(4), 76–82.

Delmas, P., Bjarnason, N., Mitlak, B., Ravoux, A., Shah, A., Huster, W., Craper, M., & Christiansen, C. (1997). Effects of raloxifene on bone mineral density, serum cholesterol concentrations and uterine endometrium in postmenopausal women. *New England Journal of Medicine, 337*(23), 1641–7.

Ettinger, B., Black, D., Mitlack, B., Knickerbocker, R., Nickelsen, T., Genent, H., Christainsen, C., Delmas, P., Zanchetta, J., Stakkestad, J., Gluer, C., Krueger, K., Cohn, F., Eckert, S., Ensrud, K., Aviolo, L., Lips, P., & Cummings, S. (1999). Reduction of vertebral fracture risk in postmenopausal women with osteoporosis treated with raloxifene: Results from a 3-year randomized clinical trial. *Journal of the American Medical Association, 282*(7), 637–45.

Folsom, A. R., Mink, P. J., Sellers, T. A., et al. (1995). Hormonal replacement therapy and morbidity and mortality in a prospective study of postmenopausal women. *American Journal of Public Health, 85,* 1128–1132.

Galsworthy, T. D., & Wilson, P. L. (1996). Osteoporosis: It steals more than bone. *American Journal of Nursing, 96*(6), 27–33.

Grady, D., Rubin, S. M., Petitti, D. B., et al. (1992). Hormone therapy to prevent disease and prolong life in postmenopausal women. *Annals of Internal Medicine, 117,* 1016–1037.

Harris, S., Watts, N., Genent, H., McKeever, C., Hangartner, T., Keller, M., Chesnut, C., Brown, J., Eriksen, E., Hoseyni, M., Axelrod, D., & Miller, P. (1999). Effects of risedronate treatment on vertebral and non-vertebral fractures in women with postmenopausal osteoporosis: A randomized controlled trial. *Journal of the American Medical Association, 282*(14), 1344–52.

Hockwald, O., Harman-Boehm, I. & Castel, H. (2004). Hypovitaminosis D among inpatients in a sunny county. *Israeli Medical Association Journal, 6*(2), 82–7.

Hodgson, S. F., & Johnston, C. C. (1996). AACE clinical practice guidelines for the prevention and treatment of postmenopausal osteoporosis. *Endocrine Practice, 2*(2), 155–169.

Kanis, J. A. (1995). Treatment of osteoporosis in elderly women. *American Journal of Medicine, 98* (Suppl. 2A), 2A-60S–2A-66S.

Kessenich, C. (2000, February). Osteoporosis in primary care: The role of biochemical markers and diagnostic imaging. *American Journal for Nurse Practitioners,* 24–29.

Khan, M., Briseno, K., Tan, C., & Heffron, W. (2002, April 15). Osteoporosis: What to tell patients about prevention and treatment. *Consultant,* 597–602.

Khosla, S., & Riggs, B. L. (1995). Treatment options for osteoporosis. *Mayo Clinic Proceedings, 70,* 978–982.

Kleerekoper, M., & Avioli, L. V. (1993). Evaluation and treatment of postmenopausal osteoporosis. In M. J. Favus (Ed.), *Primer on metabolic bone diseases.* New York: Raven Press.

National Institute of Arthritis and Musculoskeletal and Skin Conditions. (2000). Osteoporosis: Progress and promise. www.niams.nih.gov Accessed 3/23/02.

National Institute of Health. (1994). Consensus development panel on optimal calcium intake. *JAMA, 272*(24), 1942–1948.

National Institutes of Health. (2001). Osteoporosis prevention, diagnosis and therapy: Consensus statement. *JAMA, 285,* 785–795.

North American Menopause Society. (2002). Management of postmenopausal osteoporosis: Position statement of the North American Menopause Society. Menopause, 9(2), 84–101.

Columbia University College of Physicians & Surgeons. (2004). The state of the art in the management of osteoporosis. *Interdisciplinary Medicine, 5*(5), 1–66. Also available at www.nof.org/professionals Accessed 3/28/04.

National Osteoporosis Foundation. (2002). Medications to prevent and treat osteoporosis. www.nof.org accessed 3/26/04.

Putukian, M. (1994). The female triad: Eating disorders, amenorrhea, and osteoporosis. *Medical Clinics of North America, 78*(2), 345–356.

Raggett, Q. & Partridge, N. (2004). Parathyroid hormone: A double-edged sword for bone metabolism. *Trends in Endocrine Metabolism, 15*(2), 60–5.

Silver, J. J., & Einhorn, T. A. (1995). Osteoporosis and aging. *Clinical Orthopedics and Related Research, 316,* 10–20.

Taaffe, D., Robinson, T., Snow, C., & Marcus, R. (1997). High-impact exercises promotes bone gain in well-trained female athletes. *Journal of Bone and Mineral Research, 12,* 225–260.

Tonino, R., Meunier, P., Emkey, R., Rodriguez-Portales, J., Menkes, C., Wasnick, R., Bone, H., Santora, A., Wu, M., Desai, R., & Ross, P. (2000). Skeletal benefits of alendronate: 7-year treatment of postmenopausal osteoporetic women. Phase III Osteoporosis treatment study group. *Journal of Clinical Endocrinology Metabolism, 85*(9), 3109–15.

Wu, F., Mason, B., Horne, A., Ames, R., Clearwater, J., Liu, M., Evans, M., Gamble, G., & Reid, I. (2002). *Archives of Internal Medicine, 162*(1), 33–6.

Gout

Agarwal, A. K. (1993). Gout and pseudogout. *Primary Care, 20,* 839–855.

Arthritis Foundation (AF). (2002). Calcium pyrophosphate dihydrate crystal deposition disease (CPPD) (pseudogout). www.arthritis.org/research. Accessed 3/28/04.

Beutler, A., & Schumaker, R. (1994). Gout and pseudogout. *Postgraduate Medicine, 95*(2), 103–116.

Boomershine, K. (2002). Colchicine induced rhabdomyolysis. *Annals of Pharmacotherapeutics, 36*(5), 824–6.

Brooks, P. M., & Day, R. O. (1991). Nonsteroidal antiinflammatory drugs—Differences and similarities. *New England Journal of Medicine, 324*(24), 1716–1725.

Davis, J. (1999). A practical guide to gout: Current management of an old disease. *Postgraduate Medicine, 106*(4), 115–116, 119–123.

Emmerson, B. T. (1996). The management of gout. *New England Journal of Medicine, 334*(7), 445–451.

Fam, A. G. (1995). Should patients with interval gout be treated with urate lowering drugs? *Journal of Rheumatology, 22*(9), 1621–1623.

Furst, D. E. (1994). Are there differences among nonsteroidal antiinflammatory drugs? Comparing acetylated salicylates, nonacetylated salicylates, and nonacetylated nonsteroidal antiinflammatory drugs. *Arthritis and Rheumatism, 37,* 1–9.

Gonzalez, E., Miller, S. B., & Agudelo, C. A. (1994). Optimal management of gout in older patients. *Drugs and Aging, 4*(2), 128–134.

Joseph, J., & McGrath, H. (1995). Gout or pseudogout: How to differentiate crystal-induced arthropotis. *Geriatrics, 50*(4), 33–39.

Kane, D., & Sturrock, R. (2002). Diagnosis gouty arthritis. *Practitioner, 246*(1633), 260–2, 264–5.

Kot, T. V., Day, R. O., & Brooks, P. M. (1993). Preventing acute gout when starting allopurinol therapy: Colchicine or NSAIDs? *Medical Journal of Australia, 159*(2), 182–184.

Kuncl, R. W., Duncan, G., & Watson, D. (1987). Colchicine myopathy and neuropathy. *New England Journal of Medicine, 316*(25), 1562–1568.

McCarty, D. J. (1994). Gout without hyperuricemia. *JAMA, 271*(4), 302–303.

Meiner, S. (2001). Gouty arthritis: Not just a big toe problem. *Geriatric Nursing, 22*(3), 132–134.

Moreland, L. W., & Ball, G. V. (1991). Colchicine and gout. *Arthritis and Rheumatism, 34*(6), 782–786.

National Institute of Arthritis and Muscular and Skin Diseases (NIAMS). (2002). Questions and answers about gout. www.NIAMS.GOV/hi/TOPICS/qout Accessed 3/28/04.

Pittman, J., & Bross, M. (1999). Diagnosis and management of gout. *American Family Physician, 60*(9), 2504–2507.

Polisson, R. (1996). Nonsteroidal anti-inflammatory drugs: Practical and theoretical considerations in their selection. *American Journal of Medicine, 100* (Suppl. 2A), 31S–36S.

Pratt, P. W., & Ball, G. V. (1993). Gout—Treatment. In H. R. Schumacher, Jr., J. H. Klippel, & W. J. Koopman (Eds.), *Primer on the rheumatic diseases* (10th ed.; pp. 216–219). Atlanta: Arthritis Foundation.

Schlesinger, N., & Schumacher, H. (2001). Gout: Can management be improved? *Current Opinions in Rheumatology, 13*(3), 240–4.

Simon, L. S. (1995). Actions and toxicity of nonsteroidal anti-inflammatory drugs. *Current Opinion in Rheumatology, 7,* 159–166.

Star, V. L., & Hochberg, M. C. (1993). Prevention and management of gout. *Drugs, 45*(2), 212–222.

Star, V. L., & Hochberg, M. C. (1994). Gout: Steps to relieve acute symptoms, prevent further attacks. *Consultant, 34,* 1697–1706.

Tate, G. A. (1993). Gout: Clinical and laboratory features. In H. R. Schumacher, Jr., J. H. Klippel, & W. J. Koopman (Eds.), *Primer on the rheumatic diseases* (10th ed.). Atlanta: Arthritis Foundation.

Terkeltaub, R. (1993) Gout: Epidemiology, pathology, and pathogenesis in rheumatic diseases. In H. R. Schumacher, Jr., J. H. Klippel, & W. J. Koopman (Eds.), *Primer on the rheumatic diseases* (10th ed.). Atlanta: Arthritis Foundation.

van Doornum, S., & Ryan, P. (2000). Clinical manifestations of gout and their management. *Medical Journal of Australia, 172*(10), 193–7.

Vazquez-Mellado, J., Morales, E., Pacheco-Tena, C., & Burgos-Vargas, R. (2001). Relation between adverse events associated with allopurinol and renal function in patients with gout. *Annals of Rheumatic Diseases. 6*(10), 981–983.

Wallace, S. L., Singer, J. Z., Duncan, G. J., et al. (1991). Renal function predicts colchicine toxicity: Guidelines for the prophylactic use of colchicine for gout. *Journal of Rheumatology, 18,* 264–269.

Wortmann, R. (2002). Gout and hyperuricemia. *Current Opinions in Rheumatology, 14*(3), 281–6.

Low Back Pain

AHCPR. (1994). Acute low back problems in adults. *AHCPR Pub # 95-0642.* Rockville, MD: U.S. Department of Health and Human Services.

Arnheim, D., & Prentice, W. (2000). *Principles of athletic training* (10th ed.). Boston: McGraw-Hill.

Batt, M., & Todd, C. (2000). Five facts and five concepts of rehabilitation of mechanical low back pain. *British Journal of Sports Medicine, 34*(4), 261–313.

Brolinson, P. (1997). Practical approach to low back pain. *Sports Medicine in Primary Care, 3*(4), 30–36.

Frank, A. O., & Souza, L. H. (2001). Conservative management of low back pain. *International Journal of Critical Psychology, 55*(1), 21–30.

Guzman, J., Rosmin, E., et al. (2001). Multidisciplinary rehabilitation for chronic low back pain: Systematic review. *British Medical Journal, 23,* 1511–1520.

Mannion, A., Junge, A., et al. (2001). Active therapy for chronic low back pain (part 3). *Spine, 26*(8), 920–929.

Marras, W. S. (2000). Occupational low back disorder causation and control. *Ergonomics, 43*(7), 880–902.

Nightingale, S. L. (1995). Chlorzoxazone warning on hepatotoxicity is strengthened. *JAMA, 274*(24), 1903.

Tendinitis, Bursitis, Sprains, and Strains

Arnheim, D., & Prentice, W. (2000). *Principles of athletic training* (10th ed.). Boston: McGraw-Hill.

Brolinson, P. (1997). Practical approach to low back pain. *Sports Medicine in Primary Care, 3*(4), 30–36.

Marras, W. S. (2000). Occupational low back disorder causation and control. *Ergonomics, 43*(7), 880–902.

CHAPTER ❖ 27

DERMATOLOGIC DISORDERS

Candace M. Burns ◆ Glen E. Farr

Approximately 7% of patients treated in primary care settings have dermatological problems. Conditions are seen across the life cycle and those addressed in this chapter include: bacterial, fungal, viral, and yeast infections of the hair, skin, and nails; infestations, bites, and stings; dermatitis; acne; sunburn, minor burns, and recognition of possibly cancerous skin lesions; and psoriasis and pityriasis rosea.

Treatment is dependent upon accurate diagnosis. Thorough examination of the skin requires inspection and palpation of the entire body, nails, scalp, and hair in good light. The sequence of the appearance, onset, and duration of lesions—both primary and secondary changes—is very important. It is beyond the scope of this chapter to detail assessment of the skin and appendages.

BACTERIAL INFECTIONS

Bacterial infections usually develop in skin that has been damaged by chemical, mechanical, or thermal trauma, infection, or inflammation. The two most common organisms causing infection are *Staphylococcus aureus* and *Streptococcus pyogenes* (group A streptococcus) (Barker, Burton, & Zieve, 1999; Goroll, May, & Mulley, 2000; Hirschmann, 1996; Hall, 2000; Morris, 2003). In children, Haemophilus influenza is a frequent cause (Morris, 2003). Bacterial skin infections may be divided into *primary infections*—impetigo, ecthyma, folliculitis, furuncle, carbuncle, cellulitis, sweat gland infections—and *secondary infections*—cutaneous diseases with secondary infection, infected ulcers, infected eczematoid dermatitis. Systemic bacterial infections such as chancroid and gonorrhea are dealt with elsewhere in the text. Refer to Chapter 36.

PRIMARY INFECTIONS

Impetigo is a superficial but contagious skin infection usually caused by group A *S. pyogenes. S. aureus* causes about 10% of cases (Wells, Dipiro, Schwinghammer, & Hamilton, 2000). Although common in children, it may be seen at any age or among those living in close quarters. Lack of good hygiene is a predisposing factor, and it is common in hot, humid climates. There are two forms:

- *Nonbullous impetigo* lesions begin as small thin-walled vesicles or pustules on an erythematous base that rupture and discharge a honey-colored serous fluid that forms yellow-brown crusts when dried (Weston, Lane, & Morelli, 2002). Lesions are most commonly seen on the face, nares, and extremities. Impetigo develops in skin damaged by previous minor trauma such as cuts, abrasions, or insect bites. The involved areas may be pruritic, and regional lymph node enlargement may be present. A rare complication (<1% cases) of nonbullous impetigo is acute poststreptococcal glomerulonephritis. It occurs with selected strains of *S. pyogenes* (Dockery, 1997; Hirschmann, 1996).

- *Bullous impetigo* is less common. The characteristic lesions are thin-walled bullae usually less than 3 cm in diameter that rupture easily. The lesions may form on untraumatized skin, and the fluid may be amber, white, or yellow pus. Once the blister ruptures, the erythematous base dries to a shiny "varnish-like" crust (Dockery, 1997). The usual causative organism is *S. aureus*. Satellite lesions are caused by autoinoculation (Parker, 2001).

Ecthyma, another superficial bacterial infection, is deeper than impetigo and commonly seen in children, usually on the buttocks and thighs. It is commonly caused by beta-hemolytic streptococci. The primary lesion is characterized by a vesicle or vesicopustule arising on an erythematous base. The lesion enlarges to a diameter of 3 cm but proceeds to deep erosions in the epidermis covered by a thick, dry, dark, hard crust (Hall, 2000; Odom James, & Berger, 2000; Weston et al., 2002).

Folliculitis is a common bacterial infection of the hair follicle usually caused by coagulasepositive staphylococci. The infection may be superficial or deep. In the superficial form, the erythema and swelling are limited to the shallow portion of the hair follicle. The lesion is characterized by a red, elevated, slightly tender pustule. Hair comes from the center of the pustule (Parker, 2001). Deeper infections involving the entire hair follicle usually have a larger area of erythema and are quite painful. Pseudomonas folliculitis is a form of folliculitis that develops after exposure to a contaminated hot tub or other type of pool. The infection can occur several hours or days after the exposure and is most commonly seen on the legs, buttocks, and arms.

Cellulitis and *erysipelas* occur when the superficial streptococcal infection spreads to the deeper dermis and subcutaneous fat, cellulitis, and dermal lymphatics (Wells et al., 2000). Systemic symptoms of fever, tachycardia, confusion, regional lymphadenitis, and hypotension may also occur. Predisposing factors include edema, inflammation, tinea pedis, and skin permanently damaged by trauma, i.e., burns, radiation, or surgery. A number of bacteria can cause cellulites, such as group A streptococcus, *S. aureus,* and *H. influenzae* (Wells et al., 2000). Facial cellulitis in young children 6–36 months may develop from *influenzae,* which causes a bluish hue in the lesion (Weston et al., 2002). Periorbital cellulitis—infection of the tissues around the eye—is commonly seen as edema and pain and often accompanied by mild fever. Orbital cellulitis is generally due to a contagious sinus infection characterized by proptosis, restricted eye movement, pain with eye movement, and high fever (Eisenbaum, 1997). Cellulitis may also occur in normal skin. It is characterized by erythema and brawny edema that is tender with poorly defined borders. *Clostridium perfringens* and group A streptococcus cause the most aggressive spread of cellulitis of a wound that has been incised (Wells et al., 2000). Staphylococcal cellulitis spreads more slowly than streptococcal, which may spread within hours and lead to septicemia (Weston et al., 2002).

Furunculosis is an acute staphylococcal infection of the hair follicle in which the cellulitis has spread into adjacent dermis accompanied by a greater degree of pain and inflammation. The lesion is characterized by an inflamed, tender nodule with a pustular center through which the hair emerges. Furuncles can be anywhere on the body.

A *carbuncle* is an extensive infection of several adjoining hair follicles (furuncles) with several openings onto the surface of the skin. Carbuncles are more commonly seen in adults on the neck and back and are more common in patients with diabetes mellitus.

Sweat gland infection is quite rare; however, prickly heat, a sweat retention disease, frequently develops secondary infection (Hall, 2000; Odom et al., 2000).

SECONDARY INFECTIONS

Secondary bacterial infection of the skin is a complicating factor of another skin disease, including ulcers. Delay in treating the primary disease can predispose the patient to secondary infection. The presence of a secondary bacterial infection can also make correct diagnosis of the primary disease more challenging.

S. aureus, including methicillin-resistant *S. aureus* (MRSA); streptococci; enterococci; Enterobacteriaceae; and anaerobes are common organisms causing secondary infection of skin disorders, including diabetic foot ulcers. The increased prevalence of these infections is believed due to antimicrobial overuse and to long-term use of antimicrobials to suppress infections in those persons who are immunosuppressed. (Goldstein, Citron, & Nesbit, 1996; Wells et al., 2000).

SPECIFIC CONSIDERATIONS FOR PHARMACOTHERAPY

When Drug Therapy Is Needed

Bacterial skin infections should be treated as soon as possible to prevent spread and to contain the progression to a more serious condition. Cleanliness and correct treatment of superficial skin trauma may help prevent infections such as impetigo. The affected area should be cleansed regularly with antibacterial soaps and topical antiseptics, or antibiotics should be applied to cuts, bites, and abrasions.

Short- and Long-Term Goals of Pharmacotherapy

The goal of treatment is to prevent acute and long-term complications. Eradication of the offending organism and supportive therapy are of immediate concern while avoiding superinfection, systemic infection or other complications, scarring, or disability as well. Open ulcers colonized by bacteria share the treatment goal of resolving the infection and addressing the cause of the ulcer as well.

Nonpharmacologic Therapy

Primary prevention is an important part of overall treatment. Patients should be encouraged to improve their hygiene with more frequent bathing and use of a bactericidal soap to decrease pathogen spread—scrubbing and removal of crusts is not effective, however (Weston et al., 2002). Warm compresses may be applied to furuncles to promote drainage of the pus; large furuncles and carbuncles may require incision for drainage.

Clothing and bedding should be changed frequently and washed with hot, soapy water. The health history should include use of drugs that can cause lesions that mimic or cause pyodermas, such as iodides, bromides, testosterone, corticosteroids, and lithium (Dockery, 1997; Hall, 2000). Patients with chronic skin infections should be assessed to rule out diabetes mellitus or other predisposing systemic diseases and immunosuppression. Patients should also be instructed to avoid oily hair care products and tanning oils as appropriate. Furuncles, if fluctuant, require incision and drainage.

Time Frame for Initiating Pharmacotherapy

Treatment should be initiated as soon as the diagnosis is made. Instructing the patient/caregiver about interventions to prevent future infections is an important part of therapy. In cases in which the infection is contagious, the patient should use separate towels and washcloths, bedding, etc.

Overview of Drug Classes for Treatment

Since the normal skin flora is generally responsible for primary infections, antibiotics to treat coagulase-positive staphylococci or beta-hemolytic streptococci are the mainstays of therapy. They include the macrolide antibiotics (erythromycin, neomycin), penicillins, cephalosporins, and mupirocin. Secondary infection medications will need to be directed at those organisms found in primary infections, as well as organisms such as *Proteus, Pseudomonas,* and *Escherichia coli.*

See Drug Tables 102, 805.

Assessment and History Taking

Bacterial skin infections are generally characterized by pain at the site of infection, with significant individual variability. However, impetigo is often painless. Pruritis is generally present with impetigo, cellulitis, folliculitis, and erythrasma. Scratching may cause further trauma to the skin and lead to secondary infection. Chills, fever, and malaise may develop acutely and signify spread of the infection to deeper tissues or the bloodstream.

Cultures of the skin and biopsies have marginal value. However, Gram's stain and culture of pus or deeply necrotic material may be of value. Magnetic resonance imaging (MRI) or computerized tomographic (CT) scans are useful with severe cellulitis in diabetics and can distinguish preseptal from postseptal cellulitis. Bone scans and bone biopsies with culture may be indicated in selected cases of cellulitis to reveal concomitant osteomyelitis. Wood's lamp is useful in erythasma since the infected skin fluoresces coral red (Middleton, 1996).

Patient/Caregiver Information

Symptoms of common adverse drug reactions (ADRs) and drug toxicity, administration issues, and contraindications are listed in Drug Tables 102 and 805. Information should be taught to each patient and caregiver as appropriate and applicable. Information relative to significant food and drug interactions as discussed below should also be included in patient/caregiver education. Patients are generally placed on bed rest; getting up to use the bathroom is generally permitted. The importance of not scratching the affected areas must be stressed with the patient and caregiver. Also, it is important to teach the patient to take or use the medication(s) as indicated. The patient should be instructed to report progress or lack thereof to the primary care provider.

OUTCOMES MANAGEMENT

Selecting an Appropriate Agent

Impetigo and ecthyma. Superficial impetigo, if mild, can be treated with topical polysporin ointment, neosporin, or mupirocin. However, topicals can prolong the "carriage state" of the pathogen on the skin, so systemic antibiotics are best (Weston et al., 2002, p. 46). Moderate to severe impetigo and ecthyma require a 10-day course of a beta-lactamase–resistant drug such as dicloxacillin, cephalexin, cloxacillin, or erythromycin in addition to the topical therapy (Weston et al., 2002). Ecthyma lesions can produce scarring so should be treated more aggressively, even for mild cases.

Folliculitis. Following warm soaks to aid the extraction of the pustule and reduce the inflammation, folliculitis may be treated with topical anti-infective agents such as bacitracin, neomycin, or mupirocin. In superficial folliculitis, this is all that may be necessary. For more widespread or deeper lesions, oral antibiotics directed at *S. aureus* organisms are required (cloxacillin, dicloxacillin, cephalexin) (Weston et al., 2002).

Cellulitis. In addition to the application of cool wet compresses, oral antibiotic therapy is required for cellulitis. Penicillinase-resistant penicillins or cephalosporins are generally used. Dicloxacillin seems to be particularly beneficial. Acute illness requires hospitalization and prompt antibiotic treatment (Weston et al., 2002).

Furunculosis and carbuncles. Treatment with warm wet compresses will relieve the pain and assist in both relieving the pustule and in penetration of topical agents. Topical and systemic therapy is necessary and mimics that used for more widespread folliculitis. Incision and drainage is preferred for furunculosis and abcesses (Weston et al., 2002).

Monitoring for Efficacy

Resolution of the infection is the primary endpoint. If improvement or eradication is not seen in 1 week, cultures may be necessary.

Significant Food and Drug Interactions and Management

Food interactions relate to the oral antibiotics used for these conditions. Erythromycin absorption is quicker without food, but many patients do not tolerate the GI side effects of this drug. In that case, food may be taken without losing overall effectiveness. Dicloxacillin should be given on an empty stomach for maximal absorption.

Monitoring for Toxicity

Neosporin ointment may have a potential for causing a contact dermatitis if used long-term. The macrolide antibiotics (erythromycin) may cause GI intolerance as mentioned above.

Followup Recommendations

If after a week of treatment for impetigo, the lesions have not resolved, antibiotic resistance or poor compliance should be suspected. At this point, a new culture should be obtained from the base of the lesion below the crust. Antibiotic therapy should be adjusted accordingly. Ecthyma lesions are slower to heal, but can be evaluated at 1 week as well. If improvement is not seen at that point, cultures should be done.

FUNGAL AND YEAST INFECTIONS

Superficial fungal infections are common, infecting and surviving on dead keratin, i.e., the top layer of the skin (stratum corneum or keratin layer). Dermatophytes are responsible for the vast majority of skin, hair, and nail fungal infections. Lesions vary in appearance and should be verified for appropriate diagnosis and treatment.

DERMATOPHYTES

Superficial fungal infections of the stratum corneum of the epidermis affect various sites of the body. Therefore, fungal diseases of the skin are classified according to the location of the infection into the following clinical types: tinea of the feet (tinea pedis), tinea of the hands (tinea manus), tinea of the nails (onychomycosis), tinea of the groin (tinea cruris or "jock itch"), tinea of smooth skin (tinea corporis), tinea of the scalp (tinea capitis), and tinea of the beard and moustache (tinea barbae) (Skinner & Baselski, 1996).

Tinea pedis, or "athlete's foot," is common. Blisters occur between the toes and on the soles and sides of the feet. In chronic infections, the entire sole is dry and covered with a fine silvery white scale. The skin is pink, tender, and pruritic. Secondary bacterial infection, maceration, and fissures are common. The diagnosis of tinea pedis in the prepubertal child is uncommon; atopic or contact dermatitis is a more likely diagnosis in this age group (Hall, 2000; Morelli & Weston, 1997).

Primary prevention should be taught to all patients: Wear shower shoes or thongs in public or communal showers and locker rooms and footwear made of natural fibers (e.g., leather shoes, cotton or wool socks), avoid going barefoot, and change socks daily.

Acute vesicular tinea pedis is a highly inflammatory fungal infection of the foot. It is seen in individuals who wear occlusive shoes. This acute infection often develops after a chronic infection. Vesicles from a few to many form on the sole and dorsum of the foot. The vesicles may fuse into bullae or remain as collections of fluid under the thick scale on the sole of the foot. Secondary bacterial infection is common. All forms of *tinea pedis* are uncommon in children until after puberty (Weston et al., 2002).

Tinea of the hands is quite rare. Careful differential diagnosis—i.e., contact dermatitis, atopic eczema, psoriasis—is essential. The primary lesions appear as blisters on the palms and fingers at the edge of red areas with clear borders. It is frequently seen in association with tinea pedis.

Onychomycosis of the toenails is quite common and frequently accompanies tinea of the foot, whereas fungal infection of the fingernails is rather uncommon. The nail detaches distally and laterally with subsequent thickening and deformity. Yellowing of the nail indicates separation from the nail bed (Weston et al., 2002). Most cases of onychomycosis are caused by Trichophyton rubrum and Trichophyton mentagrophytes. Oral treatment is most effective (Moossavi & Scher, 2003). Secondary infection is common.

Tinea cruris is a common fungal infection of the groin area, mostly in men, and is seen on the crural fold, scrotum, penis, thighs, perianal area, and buttocks. The primary lesions appear bilaterally as fan-shaped, red, scaly patches with a sharp, slightly raised border. Small vesicles may be seen in the active border (Hall, 2000). Secondary bacterial infection may occur. It is especially common in the summer months as it thrives in warm, moist areas.

Tinea of the smooth skin—ringworm of the skin—is most commonly seen in children, can occur at any age, and is highly contagious. The primary lesions are round, oval, or semicircular scaly patches with slightly raised borders that are usually vesicular. Secondary infection can occur.

Tinea capitis can occur in two forms, noninflammatory and inflammatory. The noninflammatory type occurs most frequently in children aged 3 to 8, usually in the posterior scalp, causing gray, scaly round patches with broken hairs appearing as bald areas. Secondary bacterial infection is rare (Hall, 2000). The inflammatory type is characterized by pustular, scaly, round patches with broken hairs resulting in patchy baldness and frequently is seen in children and farmers. Secondary bacterial-like infection is common (Hall, 2000). Fungal culture is recommended in cases of suspected tinea capitis (Morelli & Weston, 1997). Healthcare providers should consult the local health department regarding guidelines for school attendance.

Tinea of the beard and moustache appears as follicular, pustular, or sharp-bordered ringworm-type lesions or deep, boggy inflammation masses (Hall, 2000). Secondary infection is common. *Tinea versicolor* causes scaling, oval patches that are white, red, or brown on the trunk, upper arms, and neck that may coalesce into larger, continuous areas (Parker, 2001).

CANDIDIASIS

Candidiasis (moniliasis) is a fungal infection caused by *Candida albicans,* resulting in lesions in the mouth, vagina, skin, nails, lungs, and gastrointestinal tract. Other types of *Candida* are *tropicalis* and *glabrata* (Roberts & Barbee, 2000). The organisms live in the normal flora of the mouth, vaginal tract, and gastrointestinal system. Pregnancy, oral contraceptives, antibiotic therapy, certain endocrinopathies (e.g., diabetes mellitus), and factors related to immunosuppression allow the yeast to become pathogenic (Habif, 1996). The specific appearance of the lesion varies with the location of the infection.

Oral candidiasis, or "thrush," is common in neonates, young children, and immunocompromised adults. It is characterized by discrete or confluent white patches on the buccal mucosa, tongue, gingiva, palate, and or oropharynx. Thrush develops in 5 to 10% of neonates, who usually acquired it during delivery (Ray, 1996). The first sign of AIDS is frequently oral candidiasis (Wells et al., 2000). AIDS patients and others who are immunocompromised—such as from chemotherapy—may have severe pain from esophageal infection (Roberts & Barbee, 2000). Prolonged wearing of dentures (especially all night long), poor dental hygiene, and factors associated with aging increase the risk of developing thrush in the older adult. Broad-spectrum antibiotics, systemic corticosteroids, and cytotoxic and/or radiation therapy are common predisposing factors (Hall, 2000; Ray, 1996).

Candida vulvovaginitis and *balanitis* are covered in Chapter 35.

Candida intertrigo commonly occurs on the surfaces of the gluteal, perineal, and inguinal folds; scrotum; axillae; inframammary regions; and pannus folds of the abdomen. Moisture, heat, and friction lead to maceration and erythema. Lesions are characterized by vesicopustules, bright erythema, and superficial erosions, surrounded by peripheral scaling; satellite pustules are usually seen (Ray, 1996). Diaper or perineal dermatitis is a variation of intertrigo that affects the perigenital, perianal, inner thighs, and buttocks (Roberts & Barbee,

2000). The warm, moist, occluded environment and the ammoniacal urine contribute to the process (Ray, 1996).

Candidal paronychia and *onychia* develop in individuals who have their hands in water or do other wet work for prolonged periods of time, e.g., dishwashers, bartenders, and food handlers. The infection develops in the nail plate and nail folds. The disease is characterized by swollen, erythematous, painful nail folds and mild serous or purulent discharge (Hall, 2000; Ray, 1996; Roberts & Barbee, 2000). Secondary infection may occur.

Congenital and *neonatal candidiases* are commonly seen in the newborn. Congenital candidiasis usually occurs within 12 h of birth and is characterized by a generalized erythema and vesiculopustules over the head, neck, hands, feet, and trunk. Oral thrush may develop with time. Neonatal candidiasis is acquired during birth, but lesions do not manifest until several days after delivery. Erythema, vesiculopustules, and erosive lesions resembling intertriginous candidiasis are diffuse and accentuated in the skin folds.

SPECIFIC CONSIDERATIONS FOR PHARMACOTHERAPY

When Drug Therapy Is Needed

Fungal and candidal infections can be disfiguring if left untreated and allowed to progress. Nail infections can be particularly difficult to resolve if the entire nail and bed are involved. Tinea versicolor will leave hypopigmented spots on the skin that will take sunlight or UV radiation to recolor. Additionally, these infections can be contagious, so quick resolution prevents spread of infection to others.

Short- and Long-Term Goals of Pharmacotherapy

Stopping the spread of infection, both on the patient and to others, and eradication of infectious agent should be high on the priority list. In the more difficult cases, such as onychomycosis, maintaining remission and managing outbreaks when they occur may be all that can be done.

Nonpharmacologic Therapy

Since fungal infections are contagious, patients should be taught to avoid sharing combs, headgear, and other personal items. Candidiasis thrives best in warm, moist environments, so the keys to prevention are to maintain good hygiene and ventilation and to keep the skin as dry as possible. Caregivers should remind patients to remove dentures at night and brush teeth daily; wear clean, cotton clothing or other fabrics that "breathe"; wear cotton underwear, socks, and cotton gloves inside rubber gloves when hands are wet for long periods of time; and change diapers frequently. Cornstarch powder should be avoided since it provides nutrients for *Candida* growth (Ray, 1996).

Time Frame for Initiating Pharmacotherapy

Treatment should be initiated as soon as possible after proper diagnosis.

Overview of Drug Classes for Treatment

Topical antifungal agents may be divided into (1) polyene antibiotics, such as nystatin, which is effective against *Candida* but not dermatophytes; (2) imidazoles, such as clotrimazole, sulconazole, and ketoconazole, which are fungistatic at low concentrations and fungicidal at high concentrations; and (3) allylamines, such as terbinafine, and butenafine, which are fungicidal. The latter two classes are effective against yeasts as well as dermatophytes. Selenium sulfide shampoos are also very effective in certain tinea infections, such as tinea versicolor.

Oral agents include nystatin for candidal infections, griseofulvin for tinea infections, and ketoconazole, fluconazole, and itraconazole for either of these or mixed infections.

See Drug Tables 102.10, 103.

Assessment and History Taking

Correct diagnosis is essential to proper treatment. Refer to the specific description of each type of lesion. Direct visualization under the microscope showing the branching hyphae in keratinized material is the most important test for correct diagnosis (Habif, 1996; Roberts & Barbee, 2000). Potassium hydroxide (KOH 5%) wet mount is one standard test for diagnosis, though hyphae may difficult to see at times (Habif, 1996; Roberts & Barbee, 2000). Chlorazol fungal stain, Swartz Lamkins fungal stain, or Parker's blue-black ink clearly stain hyphae, making them visible under the microscope (Habif, 1996). Fungal culture is necessary for fungal infections of the hair and nails (Habif, 1996). A sterile cotton swab moistened with sterile water or on an agar plate and rubbed vigorously over the lesion yields good results and is preferable for use with children (Cohn, 1992; Elewski & Weil, 1996; Habif, 1996).

Patient/Caregiver Information

Information about correct application of medications as described in the relevant drug tables should be taught to the patient and caregiver as appropriate. Refer above by disorder for patient education relative to prevention. Ketoconazole and itraconazole should not be taken within 2 h of use of antacids. Both medications should be taken with a full meal. Patients and caregivers should also be instructed about common adverse drug reactions (ADRs) and toxic effects.

OUTCOMES MANAGEMENT

Selecting an Appropriate Agent

Selecting an agent is based on location, causative organism (or likely causative organism if a KOH prep or culture evaluation is not done), and severity. Topical therapy is relatively ineffective for *tinea capitis.* Therefore, treatment includes selenium sulfide for 1 to several days to reduce spore shedding *and* oral griseofulvin to eradicate the fungus. Griseofulvin is only effective against dermatophytes. It also has slight antiinflammatory activity. Since the infection will require a few months of therapy with an oral agent, it is a good idea to confirm the diagnosis with a scraping or culture. After 6 weeks, KOH preparation cultures should be repeated. Treatment should continue for 2 weeks after cultures are negative.

Tinea corporis treatment consists of topical imidazole antifungals twice daily (clotrimazole, miconazole) or once daily (ketoconazole, sulconazole) for 4 to 6 weeks. The preparation should be placed thinly over the lesion and the surrounding skin about 1 cm out from the area. For more widespread infection, the treatment of choice is griseofulvin. Patients whose infection is resistant to treatment or who cannot tolerate griseofulvin can use oral ketoconazole, although side effects are higher (Parker, 2001). Note that miconazole is not effective against *Microsporum* and sulconazole is only effective against *Trichophyton.* Itraconazole is a systemic azole that is effective. Terbinafine (Lamisil) 250 mg per day is a newer fungicide that may be used for 2 weeks for systemic treatment of *tinea corporis* (Parker, 2001).

Tinea cruris and mild *tinea pedis* usually subside with a few days of topical imidazoles. *Tinea manus* may also respond well to topical imidazoles, but will require 6 to 8 weeks of therapy. Refractory tinea pedis or manus requires oral griseofulvin or ketoconazole.

Candidiasis may be treated with topical nystatin cream or an imidazole cream. Do not use the ointments. Topicals are applied two times a day until complete clearing is seen, generally in 2 to 3 weeks. In resistant cases, amphotericin B 3% lotion or cream four times daily, or oral ketoconazole (10–14 days) may be necessary. Other oral topicals are mystatin or clortrimazole (Roberts & Barbee, 2000). Topical drying powders (such as dry talc) may be helpful in preventing recurrences. Systemic therapy with ketoconazole, fluconazole, or itraconazole is used for immunocompromised individuals with difficult to treat candidiasis (Roberts & Barbee, 2000).

Paronychial Candida infections are best treated with liquid clotrimazole or cyclopirox since delivery to areas is difficult. Concurrent *Pseudomonas* infection is not uncommon and should be treated appropriately. *Onychomycosis* treatment is difficult (Weston et al., 2002). If no contraindications, itraconazole therapy, delivered orally one week a month for 3 to 5 months (called pulse therapy).

Tinea versicolor treatment should be initiated with topical selenium sulfide 2.5% lotion lathered and left on for 15 to 20 min every night for 2 weeks. Alternatively, some evidence exists that applying selenium sulfide to the body after an evening shower, sleeping overnight with the lotion on the body, and rinsing it off in the morning may resolve the infection. A reapplication 1 week later may be required in resistant cases. Alternative therapies include ketoconazole shampoo daily for 2 weeks, sodium thiosulfate applied daily for 2 weeks, zinc pyrithione 1% daily for 2 weeks, or imidazoles twice daily for 2 weeks. Sulfur soaps are effective prophylactically. Repigmentation of the hypopigmented spots is necessary to totally visualize the resolution. Ketoconazole orally, 200 to 400 mg depending on the extent, once and repeated in 1 week may be needed.

There are several other agents available for treatment of these conditions. Cyclopirox is as effective as imidazoles for all three types of fungi and is effective against all species of dermatophytes. It is applied twice daily. Other azoles that are helpful are econazole, miconazole, and clotrimazole (Parker, 2001). The allylamines (naftifine, terbinafine) may be alternative agents for candidiasis and tinea versicolor. Haloprogin, an older agent, is only effective for tineas. Tolnaftate, undecylenic acid, and Whitfield's ointment are over-the-counter alternatives.

Monitoring for Efficacy

Monitoring will require visual inspection, and repeating a KOH preparation and culture.

Significant Food and Drug Interactions and Management

Ketoconazole and itraconazole should not be taken within 2 h of antacids. Both should be taken with a full meal. Griseofulvin is better absorbed if given with milk or food, particularly fatty foods. This may also reduce side effects. Griseofulvin may also decrease the effectiveness of oral contraceptives, anticoagulants, and barbiturates. A disulfiram-like reaction may also occur if this drug is taken with alcohol. Ketoconazole should not be given with antacids since it needs an acid medium to be absorbed; ketoconazole can increase blood levels of both digoxin and cyclosporine, so proper monitoring is important.

Monitoring for Toxicity

Topical therapy is rarely a problem in terms of toxicity. In some instances irritation and stinging have been noted. If burning, erythema, or pruritis occur, switching to another agent may prove beneficial. Skin discoloration with amphotericin B can occur. Discontinuing the offending agent will resolve the problem.

The most common side effects of griseofulvin include diarrhea and headache. Both usually resolve after the initial week of therapy; however, persistence requires a dose reduction. Nausea, vomiting, urticaria, and photosensitivity occur occasionally. *Candidal* infections, and rarely leukopenia and proteinuria, may occur. Note that griseofulvin is teratogenic and impairs absorption of birth control pills. Young women who are sexually active need to be made fully aware of this and instructed to use two forms of birth control during treatment.

Ketoconazole may elevate liver function tests, so pretreatment and periodic analysis during treatment is necessary. All the oral antifungal agents may alter the pharmacokinetics of several other drugs, so care should be taken when concomitantly prescribing these agents.

Followup Recommendations

Depending on the circumstances and location and extent of involvement, followup can be once, at 6 to 8 weeks, or every few months.

ACNE

Acne vulgaris is a disease of the pilosebaceous unit of the skin. It is the most common skin disease in the United States, (Cayce, Careccia, Hancox et al., 2004; Roberts & Barbee, 2000). It affects 85% of the population between the ages of 12 and 25 years, frequently persisting or recurring in the third, fourth, and fifth decades (Whitmore, 1996). Eight percent of adults 25 to 34 years of age and 3% of 35- to 44-year-olds experience some form of acne (Bergfeld, 1995; Kaminer & Gilchrist, 1995; Thiboutot & Lookingbill, 1995). Acne is more severe and frequent in young males than young females, but between 20 and 50 years of age, the incidence is about the same (Roberts & Barbee, 2000). However, it is increasing among white women. Neonatal acne occurs in response to maternal androgen, first appears at 2 to 4 weeks of age, and lasts until 4 to 6 months (Weston et al., 2002). The disease can contribute to psychosocial problems such as clinical depression, anxiety, self-imposed isolation, low self-esteem, and negative body image (Whitmore, 1996). Neonatal acne that is more severe appears to be associated with later severe adolescent acne (Weston et al., 2002).

Acne vulgaris is a chronic disorder of the sebaceous glands, particularly those on the face, chest, and back, where the glands are the largest and most dense. Sebum from the glands reaches the surface by emptying into the hair follicle and flowing along the hair shaft; the two skin appendages form the pilosebaceous unit (Whitmore, 1996).

There are two primary types of acne lesions: noninflammatory and inflammatory. Noninflammatory acne lesions are further subdivided into closed comedones and open comedones. Inflammatory acne lesions are comprised of papules or pustules and nodules (Koda-Kimble, Young, Kradjan, & Guglielmo, 2002).

The initial acne lesion is the comedo, a plug formed by the impaction of the opening of the pilosebaceous duct by keratin debris and dried sebum. The closed comedones are also known as "whiteheads." The open comedones—"blackheads"—are due to oxidation of melanin and sebum in the plugs (Weston et al., 2002; Whitmore, 1996). Erythematous tender papules form when comedones become inflamed as the normal skin bacteria, *Propionibacterium acnes,* proliferate in response to increased sebum. Pustules form as the inflammation progresses and in severe cases become cystic due to abscess formation deep in the dermis. Scarring may occur from acne and is usually of the pitted type.

Four conditions must be present for acne to occur: (1) androgen-stimulated sebum production; (2) *P. acnes,* the anaerobic diphtheroid that constitutes most of the normal follicular flora and proliferates in response to increased sebum; (3) altered keratinization and desquamation of the cells lining the follicles; and (4) a host inflammatory response (Roberts & Barbee, 2000; Whitmore, 1996).

Neonatal acne may occur in the newborn shortly after birth or in infancy. Acneiform lesions generally occur on the nose and cheeks. The large sebaceous glands are stimulated by maternal androgens. The lesions generally clear without treatment.

When Drug Therapy Is Needed

Due to the external nature of this disorder, it can have profound psychological sequelae (Cayce, Careccia, Hancox et al., 2004). Further, if the more severe cases are left untreated, scarring and chronic infection can occur.

Short- and Long-Term Goals of Pharmacotherapy

The goals of treating acne are to reduce the acute inflammation and redness, minimize or prevent recurrences, and eliminate the potentially disfiguring consequences.

Nonpharmacologic Therapy

Patients should be instructed to gently wash the face with the fingertips two times a day using a mild soap (Koda-Kimble et al., 2002). Avoid oil-based skin care, makeup, and hair care products. Acne can result from friction from clothing (tight bras or other garments) and from equipment such as helmets, headbands, and baseball caps (Weston et al., 2002). Overly vigorous washing or scrubbing may lead to a more severe condition (Cayce, Careccia, Hancox et al., 2004).

Certain medications—hormonal contraceptives, ACTH, androgens, corticosteroids, lithium, iodides, phenytoin, anabolic steroids, isoniazid, and high doses of vitamin B_2 (riboflavin), B_6 (pyridoxine), and B_{12} (cyanocobalamin)—have been associated with acne (Weston et al., 2002; Whitmore, 1996).

Natural sun exposure and ultraviolet light therapy have not been found to affect the course of the disease. There is no evidence that particular foods are acnegenic. Therefore, food restrictions are not indicated.

Surgery to remove open comedones, closed comedones, and occasionally very small pustules is suggested by some. The instrument used (comedo extractor) has a flat surface with a central orifice. The contents of the lesion are expressed when firm even pressure is exerted around the lesion. The orifices of closed comedones may need to be enlarged by the use of vitamin A acid topically for 3 to 4 weeks to soften the closed comedones. Removal of closed comedones is important because they are the precursors of inflammatory lesions (Strauss, 1991). Weston et al. (2002) advise "there is no convincing evidence that dietary management, mild drying agents, abrasive scrubs, oral vitamin A, ultraviolet light, cryotherapy, or incision and drainage have any beneficial effects in the management of acne" (p. 22).

Time Frame for Initiating Pharmacotherapy

Treatment should be initiated as soon as acne develops.

Overview of Drug Classes for Treatment

Effective treatments include topical keratolytic agents topical antibiotics, systemic antibiotics, and oral retinoids (Wells et al., 2000; Weston et al., 2002). Topical keratolytic agents are considered the main therapies for acne, and the two types are (1) retinoids and (2) antibacterial plus keratolytic properties agents (Weston et al., 2002). Some benefit has been demonstrated by oral contraceptives for acne vulgaris. Antiandrogen topicals are being studied but have not proven very effective (Weston et al., 2002). Mild cases of comedonal acne may respond to a topical retinoid or benzoyl peroxide, whereas inflammatory lesions benefit from topical antibiotics. More severe inflammatory acne is treated with systemic antibiotics. Recalcitrant cases often require oral isotretinoin or hormonal therapies (Koda-Kimble et al., 2002).

See Drug Tables 102, 605, 801.

Assessment and History Taking

The type of acne, inflammatory or noninflammatory, and severity of the condition influence the treatment plan. The history should include duration, location of lesions, seasonal variation, aggravation by stress, any causes of friction, current treatment of the condition (topical, systemic) and treatment of other coexisting conditions, over-the-counter medication use, past treatment and outcomes, family history of skin disorders, drug and other allergies, general health, impact of the disease including psychosocial, and for women premenstrual exacerbation, menstrual history, pregnancy status and history, use of oral contraceptives, and use of cosmetics, moisturizers, and hair care products. The physical examination should include type and number of lesions, location, gradation, complications, and other associated findings (Habif, 1996; Hall, 2000).

Patient and Caregiver Information

The information regarding medication use, common ADRs, and toxic effects (refer to Drug Tables 102, 605, 801) should be taught to patients and caregivers as appropriate. Explain the mechanism of acne to the patient and caregiver. The treatment plan and a realistic time table also should be presented. Since acne often causes significant psychosocial effects, patients are often impatient and want immediate results. The treatment of acne and improvement of appearance generally takes several weeks. Patients and caregivers often require reassurance and emotional support.

OUTCOME MANAGEMENT

Selecting an Appropriate Agent

For the typical case of mild to moderate acne vulgaris, a clinician may begin by recommending exclusively topical therapy. Erythromycin or clindamycin may be applied either once or twice a day when the acne is predominately inflammatory. These antibiotics may be used alone or combined with tretinoin cream 0.025 to 0.05% applied sparingly at bedtime. Although more involved, the latter regimen treats both the comedonal and inflammatory phases of the disease. Alternatives include topical erythromycin or clindamycin in the morning and benzoyl peroxide 2.5 to 10% in a lotion base applied in the evening. The combination drug containing benzoyl peroxide and erythromycin (benzamycin) may be applied twice a day and gives very good clinical results.

Other agents may be substituted for erythromycin or clinidamycin when appropriate (ineffectiveness or adverse reactions). Tetracycline 0.25% is modestly effective. Meclocycline sulfosalicylate 1% cream is somewhat more effective than tetracycline and less staining.

More severe inflammatory acne may be treated using oral rather than topical antibiotics. Systemic agents useful in treating acne include estrogens, antiandrogens, tetracycline, erythromycin, minocycline, and clindamycin. Historically, the first choice of oral antibiotic has been one of the tetracyclines, such as tetracycline 250 mg four times a day, doxycycline 100 mg twice a day, or minocycline 50 mg or 100 mg once or twice a day depending upon the severity of the acne. Erythromycin is a good choice if the patient appears to be tetracycline-resistant. The dose is the same as for tetracycline. Tetracycline or erythromycin should be continued for 1 to 3 months until the lesions are suppressed (Weston et al., 2002). Generally, the patient will respond to therapy within 6 weeks. Clindamycin 150 mg daily may also be used. The combination gel of clindamycin and benzoyl peroxide offers a recently approved (2001) topical that has proven useful. Penicillins and cephalosporins are of little use in acne. The quinolones, such as ciprofloxacin, are effective in acne, but are quite costly and have not been demonstrated to be superior to less expensive antibiotics. Sulfanilamide drugs, such as Co-Trimoxazole, are often effective in acne that is resistant to tetracyclines or erythromycin. Tretinoin cream should be used concomitantly at bedtime. Resistance to the commonly used antibiotics for treating acnes is growing, according to a report from the 2001 Annual Meeting of the American Society for Microbiology. The recommendation was to restrict antibiotic use and test other regimens.

Patients with severe nodular acne or those who do not respond to topical and oral therapy may be considered for oral isotretinoin therapy. This drug can actually cure acne after a 20-week course, but has considerable precautions associated with it. Most notable is the danger to a fetus. Women of childbearing age should be made aware of the well-documented teratogenic effects of the retinoids and use dual methods of birth control during therapy (Sykes & Webster, 1994; Weston et al., 2002).

Isotretinoin is a known tertogen, so stringent methods of contraception are mandatory when this drug is used in women with childbearing potential. The 2002 FDA requirement of a new program to encourage the safe and appropriate use of this agent: SMART (System to Manage Accutane Related Teratogenicity). This program became effective in April 2002 and requires:

- All female patients will need two negative pregnancy tests before starting Accutane® and one negative test every month.
- All Accutane prescriptions will have to have a special *Accutane Qualification* sticker indicating to the pharmacist that the physician and patient are "qualified" for Accutane.
- Laboratory monitoring is required:
  - qualitative hCG (human chorionic gonadotropin) or urine pregnancy tests
  - lipid levels

In addition to the tetratogenic effects of isotretinoin, several side and adverse effects have been reported including:

- Cheilitis
- Musculoskeletal adverse effects, e.g., arthralgias
  - 2002 FDA requirement to list this in the warnings section of the package insert
  - ~30% of clients get low back pain

- Some concern that it may cause osteoporosis and increase the likelihood of bone fractures.
- Nose bleeds (epistaxis) and bleeding gums.
- Depression and suicide (In December 2000, there were reports of 66 suicides and 1373 other psychiatric adverse events associated with isotretinion.)

Roche has strengthened the labeling for Accutane to state that eligible patients "*must have severe disfiguring acne that is recalcitrant to standard therapies.*" This includes a "medication guide" and a consent form that must be distributed to the patient informing him or her of the serious risks of Accutane, including birth defects and mental changes.

- This includes that they have watched the videotape provided by Roche that gives information about contraceptive methods. Also, females must have obtained a negative result for the second urine pregnancy request, which is to be conducted on the second day of the next normal menstrual period of at least 11 days after the last unprotected act of sexual intercourse, whichever is later. Without the consent form, prescribers could be liable if a patient develops problems.

Adapalene, another topical retinoid, causes less hypopigmentation than tretinoin. Tazarotene is approved for both acne and psoriasis, but it is more irritating than tretinoin or adapalene, according to *The Medical* Letter, June 2002. Azelaic acid has anti-inflammatory, antibacterial, and comedolytic propertries.

Estrogens have been given to female patients with severe, recalcitrant, pustulocystic acne. Estrogens reduce sebum secretion and therefore may reduce the formation of acne. There may also be an indirect action on the sebaceous gland. Women for whom oral contraception is not contraindicated may be prescribed ethinyl estradiol at 30 to 35 μg. Several oral contraceptives are FDA approved for acne (Caufield, 2003; Cayce, Careccia, Hancox et al., 2004). EstrostepFe® and Ortho-Tricyclen® have been approved for moderate acne vulgaris in women 15 years or older. (Cayce, Careccia, Hancox, et al., 2004). The combination oral contraceptives are adjunct therapy to decrease production of sebum. A temporary flare of acne may occur during the initial cycles of therapy and upon discontinuation, and patients should be forewarned of this possibility. The antiandrogen spironolactone has been used for short-term control of acute acne at 100 mg daily with promising results. This potassium-sparing diuretic is most useful in women with hyperandrogenism secondary to polycystic ovarian syndrome (PCOS) and adrenal hyperactivity manifested by hirsuitism and acne.

Corticosteroids have been shown useful for men and women with androgen excess caused by a variety of endocrine disorders. Patients with resistant cystic acne should be tested for androgen excess. If apparent, therapies should be directed at lowering adrenal androgen production without totally suppressing the pituitary-adrenal axis. It is best to turn this form of treatment over to an endocrinologist for further workup and treatment.

Significant Food and Drug Interactions and Management

Caution is necessary when prescribing oral antibiotics to patients with acne. Erythromycin and the sulfa drugs can upset the stomach and although their absorption is more rapid on an empty stomach, food may minimize the irritation. Tetracycline, doxycycline, and minocycline should not be taken with dairy products or products (such as antacids) containing magnesium, aluminum, or calcium, all of which bind to the drug and reduce the extent of absorption. Tetracycline is best taken on an empty stomach. Minocycline is not affected by food.

Monitoring for Efficacy

Acne is a common self-limiting disease for which there are several effective therapeutic modalities. Concepts of therapy should be conveyed to the patient, and the importance of compliance should be emphasized. Achievement of clinical effectiveness by any given therapeutic regimen may require 6 to 8 weeks. Patients may also notice an exacerbation of acne after initiation of therapy. Inflammatory acne lesions may take approximately 4 weeks to surface; thereafter, new follicular plugging should be under control after 2 months of effective therapy. For topical agents, all acne-prone areas should be treated because the purpose of therapy is to prevent or minimize the formation of new lesions and to minimize the risk of scarring, a permanent endpoint for moderate to severe disease.

Monitoring for Toxicity

Many of the topical agents used contain alcohol, which may dry and irritate the skin, causing redness and inflammation. A similar outcome can be expected with the use of topical corticosteroids. Since inflammation promotes new skin growth and may actually aid in the healing process, remind the patient that it will pass. In most cases, reducing the number of applications per day will help. If irritation continues, discontinuing use may be necessary. Switching to a gel or cream-based topical agent should be considered. Maintaining adequate fluid intake may also be of benefit. Adolescents may need special support to continue treatment. Use of a moisturizer after medication application that does not promote comedones is essential, such as Moisturel®, Purpose® lotion, or Neutrogena® Moisture (Weston et al., 2002). Gel use every other day may be necessary.

Tetracycline antibiotics should not be prescribed to patients under 9 years old to avoid the risk of bone and tooth pigmentation. They are contraindicated in pregnancy. Long-term therapy with tetracyclines has been associated with the development of skin pigmentation and pigmented osteoma cutis (bluish or skin-colored, firm dermal lesions, typically on the face) (Walter & Macknet, 1991).

Sulfa drugs are known to cause hypersensitivity to the sun, and patients should be warned to use sunscreen. Rarely, blood dyscrasias have been noted, so a periodic CBC (every 6 months) would be appropriate.

Adverse effects with the use of oral isotretinoin and all other oral retinoids are particularly bothersome. The most common include generalized dryness of the skin and mucous membranes and hair loss. These all resolve after discontinuing the drug. Patients may experience myalgias and arthralgias. Abnormalities in laboratory parameters may also occur, such as elevation in triglycerides, cholesterol, and sometimes liver transaminases. But the greatest concern regarding oral retinoids is their extraordinary teratogenicity (Hall, 2000; Lammer, Chen, & Hoar, 1985; Stern, Rosa, & Baum, 1984).

VIRAL INFECTIONS

Common viral diseases of the skin include herpes simplex, warts (verrucae), varicella and herpes zoster, and exanthematous diseases (measles, German measles, roseola, and erythema infectiosum). Since these disorders are distinct, treatment varies for each disease. There is no specific antiviral drug yet available.

Primary care providers have a major responsibility to ensure that all individuals receive primary prevention for the common viral diseases for which there is an FDA-approved vaccine. Refer to Chapter 11 for specific guidelines about immunization administration.

HERPES SIMPLEX

The herpes simplex virus (HSV) is a member of the herpesvirus family that includes varicella (herpes zoster), cytomegalovirus, and Epstein-Barr virus (infectious mononucleosis). Herpes simplex viruses are divided into two major groups: type 1 (HSV-1) and type 2 (HSV-2). In general, HSV-1 causes diseases above the waist and HSV-2 causes diseases below the waist. However, either virus can infect any site on the skin or mucous membranes. Type 1 is generally the cause in infants and children with gingivostomatitis (Weston et al., 2002).

Herpes simplex viruses are transmitted through close personal contact via mucous membranes and broken epithelium. Primary infection in adults is usually through sexual contact. Primary infection in children is usually through close personal contact with infected adults or other children. In general, herpes simplex is characterized by recurring, localized painful vesicles that progress into erosions with crusts. The primary signs and symptoms vary with the location of the vesicles as follows (Hall, 2000; Sams & Lynch, 1996).

1. *Primary herpetic gingivostomatitis* is characterized by sore throat and fever. Painful vesicles and erosions occur on the tongue, palate, pharynx, gingivae, buccal mucosa, and lips. Incubation time from exposure ranges from 3 to 10 days, and it may persist for 2 to 6 weeks before resolving.
2. *Recurrent herpes labialis* occurs after the primary herpetic gingivostomatitis and is characterized by periodic localized vesicles on the vermilion border of the lip, commonly known as "fever blisters" or "cold sores." They usually resolve in 5 to 7 days. Recurrences may be triggered by trauma, sunburn, emotional stress, fatigue, menses, and upper respiratory infections.
3. *Herpetic whitlow* is herpes simplex infection of the fingers and hands. It is estimated that 2 to 5% of the normal adult population shed the virus in saliva, thus dental technicians, dentists, nurses, and physicians are at risk for acquiring the virus. Incubation time is 5 to 7 days. The primary infection is characterized by painful, deep, clustered vesicles; fever and regional lymphadenopathy may be present.
4. *Genital herpes* usually occurs within 5 to 10 days after sexual contact. Painful vesicles occur on the penis, vulva, or anus and rupture after a few days. Healing occurs usually within 2 weeks. Fever, headache, fatigue, and lymphadenopathy may accompany the vesicles. Patients may shed the virus prior to the eruption of lesions or development of symptoms.
5. *Neonatal herpes simplex* generally occurs in the presenting part of the newborn initially. Clusters of vesicles and bullae erode and crust. Mothers of the in-

fants may be asymptomatic of the disease, making anticipation difficult even in high-risk pregnancies. The incubation period is 2 to 4 weeks. Neonatal herpes simplex may be fatal due to rapid progression to systemic infection. Early diagnosis is essential for the infant to receive appropriate intravenous therapy with acyclovir.

WARTS

Warts (verrucae) are epithelial hyperplasia caused by the human papillomavirus (HPV); there are more than 150 subtypes identified to date (Goodheart, 2000). They can occur on any cutaneous or mucosal surface and have varying appearances depending upon the specific site and type of HPV. Human papillomavirus is transmitted by direct contact (Roberts & Barbee, 2000) or indirectly by contact with infected surfaces, e.g., shower floors or swimming pools. Incubation averages 3 months but ranges from 2 months to years with half of all warts spontaneously resolving within 2 years (Roberts & Barbee, 2000).

The contagiousness of warts varies with the type of wart, the amount of virus it contains, and host susceptibility. A subclinical stage exists during which transmission can occur. Genital warts are particularly contagious, with contact infectivity rates higher, as high as 85% for HPV types 6 and 11 (Roberts & Barbee, 2000).

Most warts occurring in immunologically normal individuals remain benign. However, several types of HPV predispose infected individuals to the development of squamous cell carcinoma and cutaneous carcinomas of renal transplant patients. A number of HPV types, including 16, 18, 31, 33, and 35 are significantly associated with cervical cancer. See Chapter 36 for additional information on genital HPV.

Children 6 to 12 years of age commonly develop warts. It is estimated that 65% of warts in children resolve spontaneously within 2 years (Jarratt & Dahl, 1991; Weston et al., 2002).

The characteristics of warts vary with location and specific type of HPV as follows:

1. *Common warts* (verrucae vulgaris) generally occur on the hands, distal forefingers, and distal nail areas (Goodheart, 2000). In children they often occur on the elbows and knees. Initially, they appear as translucent vesicles and progress to hyperkeratotic papules 0.25–1+ cm in diameter. The warts may demonstrate punctate hemorrhages or "black dots" representing thrombosed dermal capillaries (Goodheart, 2000; Roberts & Barber, 2000; Stone & Lynch, 1996).
2. *Flat warts* (verrucae planae) are flat, skin-colored papules usually a few millimeters in diameter and occurring most commonly on the face, neck, forearms, knees, and backs of the hands. They may be quite numerous. Shaving spreads them (Goodheart, 2000).
3. *Plantar warts* appear as circumscribed, thickened, slightly elevated papules with surface callus and thrombosed capillaries often visible. The entire heel or plantar surface of the foot may be covered with warts in severe infections. Confluent plaques called mosaic warts may also appear. Plantar warts may be confused with corns and calluses. A callus does not have tiny black dots representing hemorrhages, and a corn has a central nonbleeding core; warts demonstrate punctate bleeding points.
4. *Genital warts* (condylomata acuminata) most commonly occur as pale pink warts with numerous discrete narrow to wide projections on a broad base. The surface is smooth and moist and lacks hyperkeratosis. Warts may coalesce in the rectal or perianal area to form large, cauliflower-like masses. Another type of genital wart seen primarily in young, sexually active patients is multifocal, often with bilateral, red- or brown-pigmented, slightly raised, smooth papules (Habif, 1996). Lesions may occur in the external genitalia, perianal and pubic areas, intravaginally, and in the anal canal. Cervical lesions in women and anal lesions in men predispose to intraepithelial neoplasia. Genital warts in children should raise the question of sexual abuse although warts can be transmitted by the child or by a caregiver with warts on the hands.

VARICELLA

Varicella—chicken pox—is a highly contagious viral infection transmitted through airborne droplets or vesicular fluid. Patients are contagious from 2 days prior to onset of the rash until all lesions have crusted. The incubation period averages 2 weeks with a range of 9 to 21 days. The prodromal symptoms may be absent or consist of low-grade fever, chills, malaise, and headache.

The rash begins as crops of lesions on the trunk and spreads to the face and extremities (Weston et al., 2002). The severity of the disease varies greatly from mild to very severe. Lesions at different stages appear at the same time in any body area. Lesions begin as 2 to 4 mm red papules that gradually develop irregular borders (rose petal) as a thin-walled vesicle appears on the surface (dew drop). The lesions break within 8 to 12 h and crust. Pruritus accompanies the vesicular stage of the lesion.

Complications include secondary bacterial infection, encephalitis, acute cerebellar ataxia, Reye's syndrome, pneumonia, hepatitis (immunocompromised patients), and thrombocytopenia (Habif, 1996; Weston et al., 2002). Patients with defective, cell-mediated immunity or those on immunosuppressive drugs, especially systemic corticosteroids, generally experienced a prolonged course of the disease, more extensive eruption of lesions, and a greater incidence of complications (Habif, 1996). Pregnant women should be immediately referred to their obstetrical care provider for followup.

Varicella vaccine is available and approved for children and adults as primary prevention.

HERPES ZOSTER

Herpes zoster—shingles—is a common viral disease caused by latent varicella virus (Parker, 2001). It results from the reactivation of the virus and is seen in 10 to 20% of people in the United States (Elliott & Sams, 1996). It can occur at any age but is more common in adults over 50 years old, (Parker, 2001). When seen in children, it most often occurs in cases in which the mother had varicella during pregnancy, at which time the infant became infected and a latent infection was established (Elliott & Sams, 1996; Weston et al., 2002). Although not as contagious as the primary infection (varicella), it can cause varicella in unimmunized individuals.

The virus may spread to motor root ganglia and cause peripheral muscle weakness, leading to ophthalmoplegia or Bell's palsy. Involvement of sacral dermatomes can occasionally lead to urinary retention, frequency, and hematuria that generally resolve with time (Elliott & Sams, 1996). If the skin close to the eyes, is involved, ophthalmologic examination is indicated (Weston et al., 2002).

The primary lesion is characterized by painful, multiple groups of vesicles or crusted lesions usually unilateral along one or two dermatomes. The prodrome consists of fever, malaise, headache, and localized pain and paresthesia lasting 1 to 4 days. Resolution occurs in approximately 2 weeks.

Pain is the most common problem in herpes zoster. Postherpetic neuralgia, defined as pain lasting longer than 1 month, is seen in 10 to 15% of patients, and 50% of those who develop an outbreak after age 60 (Roberts & Barbee, 2000). It resolves within 2 months in 50% of patients and within 1 year in 75%, but it may persist for many years in a small percentage (Elliott & Sams, 1996; Hall, 2000).

VIRAL EXANTHEMS

Viral exanthems include maculopapular skin conditions such as rubeola (measles), roseola, rubella (German measles), and erythema infectiosum and other cutaneous eruptions that occur with acute viral syndromes (Weston et al., 2002). Herpes simplex also falls in this category. If the mucous membrane is affected, it is called an enanthem. Exanthems are common causes of generalized rashes, especially in children. Historically, exanthems were referred to by the order in which they were differentiated from other exanthems, i.e., measles "first," scarlet fever "second," rubella "third," erythema infectiosum "fifth." More than 50 agents are known to cause viral exanthems (Frieden, 1996). The common exanthems are described as follows:

1. *Rubeola* (measles) is caused by infection with a paramyxovirus. A vaccine is available for primary prevention immunization. There are three forms of measles: typical, modified, and atypical. The incubation period averages 9 to 14 days. Typically, measles is characterized by a prodrome of 3 to 5 days of high fever, upper respiratory tract congestion, conjunctivitis, and cough (Weston et al., 2002). A pathognomonic lesion appears during the prodrome consisting of Koplik's spots, small white or blue-gray dots on an erythematous, granular base located on the buccal mucosa. Enlargement of the preauricular lymph nodes is common. The dots begin to fade within 2 to 3 days after the onset of the exanthem.

   The measles exanthem typically begins on the forehead and behind the ears at the hairline and spreads to involve the total body. Lesions begin as discrete erythematous papules and then become confluent, lasting about 4 to 7 days. Fever may persist for several days in addition to adenopathy, pharyngitis, and splenomegaly. Complications include pneumonia, otitis media, laryngotracheobronchitis, myocarditis, and encephalitis (rare).

   Modified measles generally occurs in partially immune hosts such as infants less than 9 months of age, persons with partial immunization failure, and those with secondary infection (Frieden, 1996). The course of the disease is generally shorter and milder than typical measles. Death from measles in the United State, estimated to be 1 per 1000, is more likely in young infants, and immunocompromised and malnourished children (Weston et al., 2002).

Atypical measles is a characteristic syndrome that occurs in individuals previously immunized with killed virus vaccine (not used in the United States since 1967) and is now quite rare. The disease is more abrupt; pneumonia is common and may be life-threatening.

2. *Rubella* (German measles) is a common viral infection that is usually benign in children. However, if a pregnant women contracts the disease during the first trimester, it can cause birth defects in the fetus. The incubation period averages 17 days. The prodrome consists of fever and malaise. Before the rash erupts, only mild lymphadenopathy may be present (Weston et al., 2002). The rash appears on the face first and is similar to the measles rash but is usually less intense and of shorter duration, 2 to 3 days. Lymphadenopathy is common.
3. *Roseola* (exanthema subitum) is a common childhood rash. It is caused by the human herpesvirus 6 or herpesvirus 7 (Leach, Sumaya, & Brown, 1992). It most commonly occurs in children under 2 years of age (Weston et al., 2002). The incubation period is 5 to 15 days. The prodrome is a high fever of 3 days' duration, followed by the appearance of the rash. The lesions are characterized by maculopapules 2 to 5 mm in size with irregular configurations most commonly on the neck and trunk with a duration of 1 to 2 days. Pruritus is uncommon.
4. *Erythema infectiosum* (fifth disease) is caused by human parvovirus B19. It primarily affects children, but during epidemics may affect adults. The incubation period is 1 to 7 days. The prodrome may consist of headache, fever, malaise, nausea, and muscular aches. The rash begins on the cheeks as pink macules or papules that coalesce to form confluent erythematous patches resembling slapped cheeks (Weston et al., 2002). The rash on the body is measles-like with a duration of 6 to 10 days. Itching is usually present. The presence of petechiae or purpura in an acral distribution may occur (Frieden, 1996). Infection of pregnant women during the first trimester can result in hydrops fetalis or fetal death in up to 19% of the cases (Frieden, 1996). Sore throat, arthritis, and rash (the STAR complex) may be caused by parvovirus B19, as may rubella and several other viral diseases such as Eptsein-Barr (Weston et al., 2002).

SPECIFIC CONSIDERATIONS FOR PHARMACOTHERAPY

When Drug Therapy Is Needed

The need for drug therapy varies with the specific viral infection. Herpes, varicella, and measles viruses are highly contagious and require prompt attention to limit the spread of infection. Some warts, such as condylomata acuminata, are also contagious. In some instances, failure to adequately treat a topical viral infection can result in scarring.

Short- and Long-Term Goals of Pharmacotherapy

The goals of treatment of viral infections are to prevent secondary infection when applicable, minimize itching and discomfort, and address the social concerns, stigma, and altered body image that may occur with some of the diseases, e.g., genital infections or warts.

Nonpharmacologic Therapy

Herpes simplex. Primary gingivostomatitis is often accompanied by a painful mouth. Pain can be minimized with frequent mouthwashes of sodium bicarbonate in warm tap water or rinsing the mouth with a topical anesthetic such as viscous lidocaine. Systemic analgesics may be used if the infection is severe. If the infection is protracted and the individual is likely to become dehydrated, referral for hospitalization for rehydration and treatment with intravenous acyclovir may be indicated.

Herpetic lesions of the body and extremities can be treated with Burrow's compresses 20 min three times per day. Fever may be treated with acetaminophen unless contraindicated. Sunscreens (specifically formulated for the lips) can be applied to the lips to help prevent sun-induced herpes simplex.

Warts. There are several surgical procedures that may be used to remove common warts. However, care must be taken to avoid scarring that may be more painful and problematic than the wart itself. Surgical procedures include electrosurgery and liquid nitrogen applied to the wart with a cotton-tipped applicator. Freezing of plantar or palmar warts may cause painful hemorrhagic blisters.

Both techniques require specific training and equipment of the primary care provider.

Time Frame for Initiating Pharmacotherapy

Therapy should be initiated promptly with the earliest symptomatology after proper diagnosis has been made.

Overview of Drug Classes for Treatment

Warts may be treated with simple noninvasive methods, such as topical application of keratolytics, and/or soaking and filing. More extensive or resistant warts may require cryosurgery with liquid nitrogen, or laser surgery. Podophyllin is generally reserved for condylomata acuminata, and acyclovir for herpes.

For pain resolution, primarily with herpes zoster, topical capsaicin or oral tricyclic antidepressant medications are used.

See Drug Tables 106, 301, 306, 311.1.

Assessment and History Taking

Herpes simplex often follows a history of infection, trauma, stress, or sun exposure. Physical examination may reveal regional lymph nodes as swollen and tender. A Tzanck smear is positive for large multinucleated cells; immunofluorescence tests are positive (Berger, Goldstein, & Odom, 1997).

The pain of herpes zoster generally follows along a nerve, followed by painful grouped vesicular lesions. Upon physical examination, the lesions are usually unilateral although some lesions may occur outside the affected dermatome. Lesions are usually on the face and the trunk; regional lymph node swelling is inconsistent (Berger et al., 1997). Herpes zoster in children may not be painful and usually has a mild course (Weston et al., 2002).

Patient and Caregiver Information

Patients and caregivers should be instructed in nonpharmacologic interventions for care as previously described. The indication for use of the medications, ADRs, and toxic effects of the drug therapies (refer to Drug Tables 106, 301, 306, 311.1) should be taught as appropriate. Primary prevention through immunization should be encouraged when applicable.

Cloths or towels used for compresses by the patient may contain infectious viruses for several hours after use. Family members should be taught not to use these items before they are laundered in hot, soapy water.

OUTCOMES MANAGEMENT

Selecting an Appropriate Agent

Appropriate therapy for warts requires consideration of the patient's age and underlying health status as well as the number of warts and their location. According to a task force of the American Academy of Dermatology's Committee on Guidelines of Care (Drake, Ceilley, Cornelison, et al. 1995), acceptable indications for treatment of warts include (1) the patient's desire for therapy; (2) presence of such symptoms as pain, bleeding, itching, or burning; (3) lesions that are disabling or disfiguring; (4) large numbers of lesions or large-sized lesions; (5) a desire to prevent spread to unblemished skin; and (6) an immunocompromised state.

Treatment of common, flat, and plantar warts is typically daily self-application of topical 17% salicylic acid. If possible, the wart should be soaked for several minutes in warm water and then gently scraped with a file or pumice stone before applying the salicylic acid. The salicylic acid should be applied with a toothpick by micro drops (Weston et al., 2002) and left on overnight under occlusion. The next day the site should be washed and pared with an emery board. If the wart has not resolved after 6 weeks, the patient should be referred to a dermatologist for cryotherapy. Also available are transdermal patches, generally provided with securing tape and an emery board.

Salicylic acid 40% plaster is the product of choice for plantar warts. The process used is to trim the wart down, apply the plaster for 5 days, trim again, and repeat until resolution.

Several immunologic therapies exist for treatment of warts. Imiquimod cream may be applied as directed for 1 to 2 months to induce interferon production by keratinocytes (Weston et al., 2002). Oral cimetidine has been used for 3 months by some dermatologists to improve immunity to HPV while another therapy locally is applied. Injections of alpha interferon may be used twice weekly in adults only.

Retinoic acid, 0.025% or 0.05%, an antiproliferative agent, may be used for flat warts once or twice daily for 4 to 6 weeks (Weston et al., 2002).

Condylomata acuminata are successfully treated with a solution of podophyllin 25% in tincture of benzoin applied weekly. Care should be given to applying the mixture only to the affected surface since it can cause irritation of the surrounding tissue from its antimitotic action. The mixture is left on for 4 h and then washed off. Following a few applications, the mixture may be left on for up to 24 h except on the genitals. Resolution can occur after a few applications, or it may take as many as 25 applications. If podophyllin is ineffective, cryosurgery is the next line of therapy. Podophylum therapy should not be used for more than 4-6 weeks for genital warts. Podofilox, a purified podophyllotoxin, may be applied by the patient with a toothpick twice daily for 3 days, then none for 4 days, then another 3 days if warts are still present (Weston et al., 2002). Podophyllum may be neurotoxic in large doses.

Localized herpes simplex of the cutaneous tissues is treated with oral acyclovir, famciclovir, or valacyclovir (Weston et al., 2002). If the area infected is small, topical antiviral therapy may be used. With severe cases, intravenous infusions may be necessary, but this is beyond the scope of this book. For initial herpes simplex treatment, for example, acyclovir 200 mg 5 times daily for 10 days is necessary. Recurrent bouts will need only 5 days of therapy. The dose is doubled in immunocompromised patients and duration is 14 days. Ongoing prophylactic acyclovir therapy can be given at 400 mg twice daily for up to 12 months for those patients having six or more episodes yearly. See Chapter 36 for genital herpes therapy.

Varicella (chickenpox) is treated symptomatically with calamine lotion, acetaminophen, and acyclovir or another antiviral agent. Weston et al. (2002) advises that healthy children should not be treated with antivirals, but should receive symptomatic therapy such as soothing baths and oral antihistamines. Children at risk for complications should receive antiviral therapy. Never give salicylates to children for discomfort. The dose of acyclovir is 20 mg/kg per day for 5 days. A vaccine is available now that is given between the ages of 12 to 18 months. Whether protection lasts until adulthood is yet to be determined. Children with secondary bacterial infections should receive antistaphylococcal therapy (Weston et al., 2002). If the vaccine is given within 72 hours from exposure to varicella, the disease is prevented or less severe. Herpes zoster is symptomatically treated with Burow's Solution, compresses, analgesics, calamine lotion, hot soaks, and capsaicin cream. Prednisone 60 mg daily for 2 weeks may also be needed along with acyclovir 800 mg five times daily for 10 days. This should be started as soon as the diagnosis is made. Valacyclovir 1 g three times daily for 7 days is indicated for zoster in the immunocompetent patient. Famciclovir 500 mg three times daily for 7 days is also available. If more than 48 h have elapsed since the outbreak began, this therapy will only be marginally beneficial. The therapy reduces the development of new lesions, which may be beneficial in patients experiencing excruciating pain. Oral amitriptyline may help post herpetic pain (Parker, 2001).

Rubeola and rubella are treated with rest and acetaminophen for relief of discomfort. Vaccine is available and indicated in rubeola.

Pain may be managed by nonpharmacologic means (wet to damp dressings to reduce the dry, cracking nature of the lesions) and by pharmacologic means. Analgesics such as NSAIDs and acetaminophen help. Narcotics may be necessary. Topical capsaicin cream applied four times daily to the affected dermatome has been proven useful in diminishing the pain. Relief comes slowly, however, with days to weeks before full pain relief. Oral amitriptyline in doses of 12.5 to 150 mg per day also may decrease the discomfort of postherpetic neuralgia (Max, Schafer, Culnane, et al., 1988).

Monitoring for Efficacy

Elimination of the virus is not always possible when treating these disorders. They are notorious for their recurrence, with remission and less frequent occurrences being the goals. Absolute resolution does happen and should be the aim of therapy.

Significant Food and Drug Interactions and Management

Oral acyclovir may be taken without regard to meals. Information about specifics for food/drug interactions for any antiviral agent should be determined before prescribing.

Monitoring for Toxicity

Nausea and vomiting have been reported with patients taking acyclovir oral capsules. It is generally considered safe and effective with minimal side effects.

Topical application of salicylic acid can be irritating to surrounding unaffected tissue, causing some burning and irritation. Podophyllin causes stinging and burning as local wart necrosis occurs. Capsaicin, derived from peppers, causes discomfort in the initial 1 to 3 days as substance P is depleted.

Nonsteroidal antiinflammatory drugs should not be used in patients with renal failure and have several notable drug interactions. GI upset may also occur, so they should be taken with food.

Amitriptyline should be used with caution in elderly patients and those with cardiac abnormalities.

Followup Recommendations

Most warts may be followed at the patient's discretion. Because of the frequent application and potential toxicity of podophyllin, daily application and observation should be the norm for condylomata acuminata, unless the over-the-counter brand is used. It has a lower strength and is applied twice daily for a longer period of time. Patients may choose to follow this themselves.

Followup for herpes simplex and zoster infections is done with each outbreak. Herpes zoster may require closer supervision of disease progression. Herpes simplex requires significant patient education to avert the spread of infection.

INSECT INFESTATIONS, BITES, AND STINGS

This section addresses the treatment of common dermatologic disorders caused by infestations, namely scabies (mite infestation), pediculosis (lice infestation), and the bites and stings from commonly encountered arthropods.

SCABIES

Scabies is caused by an infestation with the female *Sarcoptes scabiei* mite. It is transmitted through close personal contact and affects all socioeconomic levels, both sexes, and individuals of all ages. The adult mite is approximately ⅓ mm in length and has a flattened, oval body with wrinkled, transverse corrugations and eight legs (two are brush-like) (Habif, 1996). The female mite attaches to the skin, digs a burrow (primary lesion), and lays approximately two or three eggs per day for the duration of her 1-month life. The eggs hatch within 3 to 4 days and mature within 14 days. Fecal pellets (scybala) are deposited along with the eggs and appear as dark, oval masses. Secondary lesions of excoriations of the burrows may be the only visible lesion. In severe, chronic infestations, secondary bacterial infection may develop in the form of impetigo, cellulitis, or furunculosis.

In adults the most common areas affected are the waist, pelvis, elbows, hands (especially finger webs), feet and ankles, penis and scrotum, buttocks, and axillae. Infants, young children, and the elderly may have lesions on the head and neck. Atypical (crusted or Norwegian) scabies may occur in patients who are immunocompromised [e.g., have human immunodeficiency virus (HIV)] or who are mentally retarded (Weston et al., 2002).

The initial phase of the disease is asymptomatic, with the pruritic rash developing in about 14 to 28 days. The primary symptom is intense itching, especially at night. The pathognomonic lesion is the burrow appearing as a pink-white linear or curved ridge with a tiny vesicle at one end. A skin scraping with an oil or potassium hydroxide mount reveals a mite, eggs, or fecal pellets.

Scabies may be overlooked in elderly patients in nursing homes. The inflammatory reaction may be muted although the patient itches intensely and may be misdiagnosed as "senile pruritus" (Orkin & Maibach, 1991).

In the elderly, it may manifest as a diffuse truncal infection (Walker & Johnston, 2003).

PEDICULOSIS

Infestations with lice have been documented for thousands of years. More deaths have occurred from diseases transmitted by lice than from any insect-borne disease other than the malaria mosquito (Orkin & Maibach, 1991).

The louse is a six-legged, wingless, dorsoventrally flattened, bloodsucking insect. There are three types: *Pediculus humanus corporis,* which infests the body and clothing, *P. humanus capitis,* which infests the head, and *Phthirus pubis,* which infests the pubic area and is considered a sexually transmitted disease (Hall, 2000; Orkin & Maibach, 1991; Weston et al., 2002). Pediculosis is most commonly seen in individuals with poor hygiene, and head lice are commonly seen in school children. The louse is 2 to 4 mm in length and transmitted by contact with infested clothing, bedding, and combs. Since lice bite the skin and live on the blood, they cannot live without human contact and die within 2 to 3 weeks. The oval eggs, or "nits," are deposited on hairs or fibers of clothing by the female louse. Eggs hatch within 30 days. The female louse lives for about 30 days and produces eggs every 2 weeks (Weston et al., 2002). Body lice are most commonly seen as linear excoriations on the trunk. Secondary infection often masks the primary lesions. Nits and lice can often be found in the seams of the infested clothing.

In head and pubic pediculosis, the nits are generally found attached to hairs; lice are rarely found. Erythema and scaling of the scalp may be present. Cervical lymphadenopathy (e.g., posterior) and febrile episodes are also common. *Pthirus pubis* on the eyelashes or hair of children should alert the primary care provider to the possibility of sexual abuse, but other modes of transmission do occur.

The bites of lice are relatively painless and often go unnoticed. The clinical signs and symptoms are caused by the patient's reaction to the saliva or anticoagulant injected into the dermis by the louse during feeding (bloodsucking). Individual sensitivity varies greatly. The sites of feeding may exhibit 2 to 3 mm erythematous macules or papules within hours to days of the bite. Others may develop an almost immediate reaction with flare and wheal formation (Hall, 2000; Orkin & Maibach, 1991).

ARTHROPOD BITES AND STINGS

Bites and stings from common arthropods such as mosquitos, fleas, ticks, hymenoptera (ants, bees, wasps), and spiders are common. Prior to treatment in the nonallergic individual, assessment will usually find local swelling, papule or wheal formation, pruritis, erythema, and mild discomfort. An allergic individual may experience a more severe local reaction or a systemic reaction of urticaria, hypotension, respiratory distress, angioedema, anaphylaxis, and death.

Two species of spiders have a venom strong enough to produce toxic reactions: the brown recluse spider (*Loxosceles reclusa*) and the black widow spider (*Latrodectus mactans*). The brown recluse spider commonly inhabits old buildings, storage sheds, wood piles, garages or basement storage areas, and occasionally closets. Therefore, the victim commonly reports being bitten while working around one of these areas or after donning boots, jackets, etc., that have been stored for a period of time. The venom of the brown recluse spider contains sphingomyelinase, which acts on the cell membranes resulting in dermonecrotic activity and a lipase that induces disseminated intravascular hemolysis (Dockery, 1997). The brown recluse spider bite generally has two types of responses, a localized cutaneous reaction and a systemic reaction marked by intravascular hemolysis, acute vasculitis, platelet thrombi, and leukocyte infiltrates (Dockery, 1997). The more severe reaction most frequently occurs in children and debilitated patients. A blue-gray halo develops around the site of the bite, and a cyanotic vesicle or bulla may appear. Pain may be severe. The necrotic tissue may extend deep into muscle. Within 12 to 24 h after the bite, the patient commonly reports fever, chills, nausea, vomiting, and urticaria. The patient may not have seen the spider; therefore, the history of activities when the bite occurred facilitates diagnosis.

In mild reactions, treatment is symptomatic with rest, ice compresses, pain control, and antibiotics to prevent secondary infection; warm compresses and exercise worsen the lesion. Tetanus toxoid may be indicated. Dapsone may be required in more severe cases, and referral of the patient to a hospital emergency room may be indicated. Surgical excision of the wound and skin grafting also may be required for severe reactions.

The black widow spider bite, although commonly believed to be a fatal bite, has a mortality of less than 1% (Dockery, 1997). The bite itself may not have been felt, and there may be minimal local reaction. The venom is a neurotoxin that produces symptoms of general toxemia 10 to 15 min after the bite, including muscle spasms and cramps, especially of the legs and abdomen; numbness that gradually spreads from the site of the bite to the entire torso; headache; sweating; increased salivation; nausea and vomiting; and a diffuse macular rash (Dockery, 1997). Syncope and coma may develop (Weston et al., 2002). The acute phase generally subsides within 48 h and gradually resolves in 2 to 4 days. The patient should be referred to an emergency room for treatment. An antivenom is available for bites in the very young, the debilitated, or for those with severe reactions. Mild reactions can be treated with cool compresses, analgesics for pain, and muscle relaxants.

Hymenoptera, ants, bees, wasps, and hornets commonly sting adults and children. The bite of the fire ant usually causes immediate pain that quickly subsides. The small red wheal becomes a vesicle over several hours. After 24 h, the vesicles become pustules that usually resolve in about 10 days. Multiple ant stings can cause severe allergic reactions requiring emergency treatment. Individuals with mild local reactions can be treated with cool compresses, antipruritic lotions, oral antihistamines, and thorough cleansing of the bites to prevent secondary infection.

The honeybee is the only stinging insect that leaves its barbed stinger and venom sac in the victim (Dockery, 1997). The venom of stinging insects contains histamines and vasoactive agents that are hemolytic and neurotoxic. The nonallergic patient generally reports moderate to severe pain at the time of the bite and a localized wheal, erythema, pruritis, and edema. Systemic reactions vary from mild to severe as previously described. Localized stings in nonallergic individuals are treated with cool compresses and mild analgesics for the pain. Antihistamines may be indicated in more severe localized reactions.

Prepackaged bee-sting kits including epinephrine 1;1000 in prefilled syringes and antihistamine tablets are available for allergic individuals. Patients should be instructed to carry them when participating in activities during which a sting might occur and in the use of the kit. Parents and caregivers should be taught how to care for allergic children and the elderly. The allergic individual also should be instructed to wear a medical alert tag or bracelet.

Tick bites are usually painless and self-limiting; however, ticks can carry organisms that cause serious disease, e.g., Lyme disease or Rocky Mountain spotted fever. Prevention of tick bites is important. Patients who camp in woods or hike in tall grasses are at risk. Therefore, remind them to wear long pants with the cuffs tucked into boots, long-sleeved shirts, turned-up collars, and hats with brims and to treat clothing with repellents.

SPECIFIC CONSIDERATIONS FOR PHARMACOTHERAPY

When Drug Therapy Is Needed

Treatment is required to eradicate the infestation of both scabies mites and lice. Patients should be questioned about itching in family members and close personal contacts, including classmates of school children. Selective treatment of asymptomatic family members at high risk for acquiring the infestations from a confirmed case may be appropriate, e.g., if the infested patient shares a bed with another individual. Sexual contacts should also be treated.

Most common bites and stings should be thoroughly washed with soap and water to cleanse the wound to prevent secondary infection. The area should be kept clean and itching avoided until the wound has healed.

Short- and Long-Term Goals of Pharmacotherapy

The goals of therapy are to eradicate the infestation, relieve the itching, treat secondary infection as needed, and educate the patient about the transmission of the disease to minimize the possibility of future infestations. Instruction in good personal hygiene should be conducted as appropriate. Individuals, especially school children, should be taught to avoid sharing combs, clothing, caps, etc., with others.

Patients should be instructed that the treatment destroys the insects and eggs, but the response to the sensitizing substances may last for several weeks; i.e., itching may persist for several weeks. If the rash persists and itching is intense, requiring treatment, topical corticosteroids and oral antihistamines may be necessary.

Patients must be cautioned not to overtreat themselves or family members, since these drugs can be toxic. Patients should be instructed NOT to repeat the treatment unless it is specifically prescribed by their health care provider.

Nonpharmacologic Therapy

Scabies. At the conclusion of therapy, all articles of clothing, bedding, and towels should be laundered with hot, soapy water and rinsed in hot water. Alternatives to this would be to dry-clean the clothes or place them in a sealed plastic bag for 30 days. Outerwear and furniture do not need to be cleaned because mites survive only a short time when deprived of the human host. Spraying upholstery with pyrethrin may help.

Pediculosis. Good hygiene, frequent bathing, use of clean clothing (including underclothing), and proper nutrition are important nonpharmacologic aspects of therapy. All clothing, bedding, towels, or other articles worn or used for 3 days before or during treatment must be machine-washed in hot water and dried in a hot dryer for at least 20 minutes. Items that cannot be washed should be dry cleaned, then hung outside for 2 days or sealed in a plastic bag for 10 days. Pressing woolens at home is also effective, but pay special attention to the seams of clothing. If items cannot be laundered or dry-cleaned, placing the items in plastic bags tightly sealed for at least 2 weeks will also kill the lice. Combs, brushes, barrettes, curlers, and other articles used in the hair must be soaked in an antiseptic solution, rubbing alcohol, or lice-killing shampoo for 1 to 2 hours, or boiled for 5 to 10 minutes.

Floors, furniture, play areas, etc., should be thoroughly vacuumed to remove hairs that contain nits with viable eggs.

Arthropod Bites and Stings. Cleansing of the wound with a mild soap and water should be done as soon as possible. The wound should be checked for the presence of a stinger, foreign body, or the insect itself (a tick), and it should be removed if needed. Local reactions are generally treated with ice compresses, topical antipruritics, oral antihistamines, and mild analgesics as needed. Scratching should be avoided to prevent secondary infection. For secondary infection, topical or oral antibiotics may be required. Systemic allergic reactions necessitate the use of epinephrine, antihistamines, and supportive care. Primary prevention should include use of appropriate repellents, barrier clothing, and avoidance of areas containing the arthropods.

Time Frame for Initiating Pharmacotherapy

Treatment should be instituted as soon as a diagnosis is made. Treatment for scabies should be preceded by a tepid bath or shower and drying with a towel.

Cutaneous manifestations of bites and stings often will be the only clinical expressions of an acute systemic allergic reaction. Therefore, individuals allergic to bites and stings should be instructed to carry a kit containing self-injecting epinephrine and oral antihistamines at all times when exposure might occur and taught how to use it. Allergic individuals should also be instructed to wear a medical alert tag or bracelet.

Overview of Drug Classes for Treatment

There are three major forms of medications for the treatment of scabies: lindane, crotamiton, and sulfur (see Drug Table 806). Sulfur is generally not used in adults because it is messy and odoriferous, and it stains clothing easily. It is good for infants and is used by applying a 10% ointment to the site for 24 h on three consecutive nights. Alternative medications for the treatment of scabies include permethrin, thiabendazole, and coal tar. Lindane and pyrethrins are commonly used for pediculosis infestations. The applications of the drugs when treating scabies and pediculosis are different, as noted below. Urticaria and redness may require topical corticosteroids, antihistamines, or antibiotics.

Insect bites and stings are generally benign, but in some patients can lead to serious consequences. Antihistamines are effective for mild cases. Corticosteroids may be necessary for more severe or prolonged cases.

See Drug Tables 102, 601, 705, 807.

Assessment and History Taking

Infestations, stings, and bites are characterized by a history of localized rash with pruritis. Specific signs and symptoms were described previously for each vector.

Patient and Caregiver Information

Specific patient and caregiver information is discussed in the section on nonpharmacologic treatment for each vector. The patient and caregiver should be taught the correct use of medications and encouraged to complete the course of drug therapy as prescribed. Patients and caregivers also should be taught about ADRs and the toxic effects of the drugs.

OUTCOMES MANAGEMENT

Selecting an Appropriate Agent

Scabies. Patients and family members should be treated with an overnight application of lindane or permethrin cream. The application should be from the neck down, left on for 8 to 14 h (generally overnight), and then washed off. Emphasize that all areas must be treated, especially between the fingers and toes, the groin, and the axilla. One fluid ounce (lindane) or 30 g (permethrin) should suffice. If there are scabetic lesions on the head and neck (usually seen only in children), they are also treated, but great care is needed to avoid the eyes, nose, and mouth. Permethrin and lindane are safe for children over 2 years of age. Alternatively, crotamiton is used and applied in the same fashion as lindane, but reapplied in 24 h. It is then left on for an additional 24 h. Permethrin 5% cream (Elimite) may be substituted for lindane in infants 2 months of age and older. Be sure the hands are covered with same type of clothing in infants and toddlers to prevent licking the scabicide (Weston et al., 2002).

Pediculosis. Treatment consists of the application of topical therapies such as pyrethrins or permethrin (over-the-counter), or lindane or malathion (prescription). The shampoo formulation should be used for hairy areas; the cream or lotion can be used elsewhere. The formulation should be left on for 5 min and then rinsed off. A repeat application 1 week later is necessary for lindane since it does not kill the nits. Since nits attach to the hair shaft, a fine-tooth comb should be used to remove them once they have been treated.

Secondary infection may be treated with topical mupirocin 2% ointment applied three times daily or with appropriate oral antibiotics.

Eyelash involvement is treated with petrolatum applied twice daily for 9 days followed by removal of any nits.

Ovide® lotion (0.5% malathion) was found to kill head lice most rapidly and effectively (Comparative efficacy, 2001). Combination 1% permethrin crème rinse and TMP/SMX is an effective alternative, but it is recommended to be saved for single therapy failures (Head lice infestation, 2001). Head lice therapies should be applied only after living nymphal or adult lice or apparently viable nits have been observed to avoid overdiagnosis and mismanagement (Overdiagnosis and consequent, 2000). Wet combing with malathion was found twice as effective as bug-busting in a UK study (Comparison of wet, 2000). Permethrin, pyrethrin, and malathion were found to be equally effective (Interventions for treating, 2000), but resistance to these products in the United States is increasing, and Meinking et al. (2002) found that Ovide is the only one that has not lost effectiveness. Of concern is the more serious infestations causing pyodermas and severe excoriations of the scalp, indicating a need for treatments that do not require nit removal for success, that have a strategy to prevent resistance, that are safe and effective, and that people will be willing to use (Meinking et al., 2002).

Arthropod bites and stings. Simple acute urticaria may be treated with an antihistamine such as diphenhydramine. In some cases, a short course of a glucocorticoid in a moderate dose may be necessary (e.g., prednisone 40 mg PO once daily for 4 days). For children, 2 mg/kg/d of prednisone for 5 days is recommended (Weston et al., 2002). A similar treatment can be used for angioedema unless it is associated with upper airway obstruction. Necrotic tissue may need to be removed surgically to prevent toxin spread (Weston et al., 2002).

Venom immunotherapy may be recommended as the treatment of choice for the prevention of recurrent systemic sting reactions. Treatment of this nature should be referred to the appropriate specialty practitioner.

Monitoring for Efficacy

Resolution of the infestation or diminishing of the erythema and urticaria is the primary endpoint to treating these conditions.

Significant Food and Drug Interactions and Management

Agents used for pediculosis and scabies are topical and have no food interactions. Corticosteroids should be taken with food.

Monitoring for Toxicity

Lindane is a neurotoxin and therefore should be avoided in infants, pregnant or lactating women, and persons with seizure disorders or numerous excoriations, which potentiate absorption.

Followup Recommendations

Patients may choose to monitor themselves without followup, but should be warned to return at the first sign of infection or continued symptoms.

DERMATITIS

Common dermatitis includes asteatotic dermatitis, atopic and contact dermatitis ("eczema"), and seborrheic dermatitis. Eczematous dermatitis is an inflammatory response of the skin to a wide variety of external and internal agents (Parker, 2001). The cause of the dermatitis often is unknown.

Eczematous dermatitis is classified according to general appearance, location, and presenting symptoms and acute, subacute, and chronic stages. The acute stage is characterized by vesicles, blisters, or bullae; erythema; and moderate to severe pruritis. The subacute stage is characterized by erythema, scaling, and fissuring with a scalded appearance, mild to moderate pruritus, and discomfort commonly described as "burning" in character. The chronic stage is characterized by lichenification (thickening and dryness giving a "washboard" appearance to the skin) with fissures and excoriations.

Asteatotic dermatitis is a common condition also known as chronic "winter itch" because it is frequently seen during the winter and in geographical areas of low humidity. It is characterized with dehydration, erythema, dry scaling, and fine superficial cracking of the skin. It results from a decrease in skin surface lipids (Dockery, 1997; Hall, 2000). Frequent bathing in hot water and use of deodorant soaps can aggravate the condition. Elderly individuals are most commonly affected.

Atopic dermatitis is a chronic inflammation of the skin. Patients often have associated allergic rhinitis and a family history of atopy is often reported (Barker et al., 1995; Dockery, 1997; Hall, 2000; Weston et al., 2002). Atopic dermatitis can be divided into subtypes based on the age of onset: infantile (2 months to 2 years), childhood (2 years through adolescence), and adult. Areas of involvement are typically those that the patient can scratch: infantile (cheeks, extensor arms, and legs), childhood (flexural arms, legs, neck, wrists, and ankles), and adolescent and adult (flexural surfaces, face, neck, upper chest, wrists, knees, hands, and feet) (Barker et al., 1995; Weston et al., 2002). Acute lesions are characterized by erythema, edema, papules, vesicles, erosions, crusts, and scale. Chronic lesions are characterized by lichenified plaques. Secondary bacterial infections may also occur.

Contact dermatitis may present as primary irritant contact dermatitis, allergic contact dermatitis, and photoallergic contact dermatitis. Lesions are seen in any of the stages from mild erythema or vesicles to large bullae with a significant amount of oozing. In primary irritant dermatitis, the patient is usually exposed to the irritant for a relatively short period of time and is not immunologically mediated. About 70 to 80% of all cases of contact dermatitis are of the irritant variety (Barker et al., 1995; Parker, 2001). Irritant contact dermatitis is characterized by a scalded, erythematous appearance of the skin with peeling of the most superficial epidermis. Common agents causing irritant dermatitis include agents with extremes of pH such as harsh soaps and cleansers. Diaper contact dermatitis is the most common form in pediatrics (Weston et al., 2002). Frequent handwashing is the most frequent cause of irritant contact dermatitis (Parker, 2001). Latex sensitivity poses a serious hazard for some individuals, and avoidance is the only answer.

Allergic contact dermatitis is caused by a delayed hypersensitive reaction (Parker, 2001). A common cause of allergic contact dermatitis is plant dermatitis caused by the *Rhus* genus, which includes poison ivy, oak, and sumac. It is the oleoresin oil within the plants that is the allergen. Sensitive individuals may continue to develop lesions for up to 3 weeks after exposure. Other common allergens include nickel compounds (costume jewelry), neomycin, benzocaine, fragrances and preservatives in cosmetics and personal hygiene products, paraphenylenediamines (shoe dyes), rubber products, ethylenediamines, and the chromates (Dockery, 1997). Repeated exposure to an antigen may cause widespread papulvesicular dermatitis, called an "id reaction" (Weston et al., 2002).

Occupational allergic contact dermatitis frequently occurs. It is estimated that 65% of all industrial diseases are dermatoses (Hall, 2000). Common allergens include potassium dichromate in cement, dyes, or textiles; epoxy resins in adhesives, finishing products, and casings for electrical devices; rosin in adhesive materials; thiuram, mercaptobenzothiazole, and carbamates in rubber products; glycerol monothioglycolate and paraphenylenediamine in hair wave and dye formulations; and acrylates in methylmethacrylate used in orthopedic surgery, dentistry, and nail sculpturing (Barker et al., 1995). A very detailed history is important for correct diagnosis, including questions regarding improvement when away from work or while on vacation.

Allergic contact dermatitis is unusual in children under the age of 3 years since this type of dermatitis occurs after a variable number of exposures with a sensitizer (Dockery, 1997). However, in children, the foot may be a site for allergic contact dermatitis to occur. Children frequently wear shoes for extended periods of time and the increased heat and perspiration can exacerbate an allergic contact dermatitis from shoe materials (Dockery, 1997). Differential diagnosis from tinea pedis is essential for initiation of correct therapy.

Photoallergic dermatitis may be seen with drugs such as chlorpromazine, promethazine, *p*-aminobenzoic acid, phenothiazines, tincture of benzoin, and povidone-iodine solutions.

Contact urticaria, although not strictly a dermatitis, is a contact reaction to latex that is very prevalent, especially in healthcare workers. Reactions vary from itching after wearing latex gloves to anaphylaxis.

Nummular eczema (discoid eczema) is characterized by coin-shaped papulovesicular lesions on the arms and legs and is of unknown etiology. Many factors may contribute, however, including dry skin, cold weather, wool clothing, irritating soap, and frequent bathing (Parker, 2001). It is most frequently seen in middle-aged and older adult men. Pruritis is mild to severe (Parker, 2001).

Seborrheic dermatitis is a common idiopathic dermatitis occurring in about 3 to 5% of the population (Barker et al., 1995). It is characterized by inflammatory hyperproliferation of the skin affecting areas of the body where sebaceous glands are plentiful (i.e., scalp, facial hair areas, presternal chest, axilla, umbilicus, inguinal folds, gluteal cleft, and perianal skin). The lesions appear as greasy, scaly, reddish, and yellow-brown patches. (Note: Dandruff is a similar but noninflammatory erythematous scaling of the skin in the seborrheic areas.) The etiology of seborrheic dermatitis is not known; however, it has been associated with the presence of *Pityrosporum ovale,* a yeast commonly present on the skin (Barker et al., 1995; Faergemann, Jones, Hettler, & Loria, 1996; Parker, 2001). Treatment with antifungal agents (e.g., terbinafine) has proven very successful. Infants frequently present with seborrheic dermatitis commonly called "cradle cap," which is characterized by greasy adherent scales on the vertex of the scalp. Secondary infection can occur.

SPECIFIC CONSIDERATIONS FOR PHARMACOTHERAPY

When Drug Therapy Is Needed

Treatment should be initiated as soon as the condition is diagnosed. However, drug therapy may not be indicated in asteatotic dermatitis. Rather, educate the patient about skin care and decreasing the number of baths or showers and encourage the use of topical emollients containing lanolin, glycerine, urea, and lactic acid or other alpha-hydroxy acids.

Short- and Long-Term Goals of Pharmacotherapy

Try to determine the causative nature of the dermatitis so the patient can avoid the antigen source. Education is important in preventing future occurrences. Caution the patient to remove the antigen as soon as possible after exposure and rinse with warm, soapy water. For example, for poison ivy, oak, or sumac, the area should be washed with soap within 15 minutes after exposure, so the sensitizing oil cannot be spread to other parts of the body (Koda-Kimble et al., 2002). Any clothing, shoes, or equipment should be washed, as will as under the fingernails. Ultimately, it is hoped that more severe reactions, more widespread coverage, and scarring can be avoided. Prevention of secondary infections, caused by excoriating the skin, is also important.

Nonpharmacologic Therapy

The source(s) of the irritant(s) should be determined in contact dermatitis and photodermatitis, and the patient should be instructed about interventions to avoid future exposure. When a medication is determined to be the causative factor, the medication should be discontinued under the supervision of a healthcare provider and alternative drug therapy initiated as appropriate. Patients should be instructed about their drug allergy and to wear a medical alert tag or bracelet.

Time Frame for Initiating Pharmacotherapy

Removing the causative agent and rinsing with warm soapy water in appropriate circumstances should be done immediately. Prevention of long-term complications should then be addressed.

Overview of Drug Classes for Treatment

Treatment of dermatitis reflects the inflammatory nature of the disorder. Management with low- to midstrength corticosteroids may be all that is necessary. For more severe dermatitis, higher-strength topical or oral corticosteroids are available. Treating pruritus with diphenhydramine or hydroxyzine and treating secondary infections with antibiotics also may be necessary.

See Drug Tables 601, 803, 807, 808.

Assessment and History Taking

A thorough health history, including a detailed occupational history, is essential to the effective treatment of dermatitis. Exposure(s) to the irritant(s) must be identified so that the patient and caregiver can be taught to avoid future exposure as much as possible. Elimination of the offending irritant is essential to optimal treatment. Assessment should include mechanism of response, number of exposures, nature of the substance, mode of onset, and distribution (Habif, 1996).

Patient and Caregiver Information

Once the offending irritants have been identified, patients and caregivers should be taught to avoid future exposure. If the offending agent is a medication, the healthcare provider who prescribed the medication should be notified immediately, the offending medication discontinued, and an alternative medication prescribed. Patients with drug allergies or other life-threatening allergies should wear a medical alert tag or bracelet to identify themselves as allergic.

The patient should be instructed to take oral corticosteroid medications with food to minimize stomach irritation.

OUTCOMES MANAGEMENT

Selecting an Appropriate Agent

Mild cases of contact dermatitis are usually treated with topical corticosteroids. Newer, more potent corticosteroids control both the symptoms and the spread of dermatitis. It is rarely necessary to use antipruritics. Adjunctive use of menthol and camphor lotions, cool soaks, and wet-to-dry soaks may be helpful in controlling pruritus (Millikan & Shrum, 1992). When the face is involved, only low-potency corticosteroids (like hydrocortisone 1% cream) should be used. For diaper-caused dermatitis, frequent changes, lubrication with a greasy ointment for protection of the skin after cleansing, and exposure to air are suggested (Weston et al., 2002). Use of steroid topical creams/ointments is not advised.

For more lichenified lesions that are not on the face, midpotency (e.g., triamcinolone, betamethasone valerate) to high-potency (e.g., fluocinonide, betamethasone) fluorinated steroids must be used. Use of systemic corticosteroids is generally reserved for patients who have a history of severe, widespread reactions or those in whom more than 30% of the body is involved. Patients with involvement of the hands, face, or genitals also are candidates for aggressive systemic corticosteorid therapy (Millikan & Shrum, 1992; Parker, 2001).

Some patients also require oral antibiotics for recurrent infection. Coverage should include *S. aureus*.

For patients unresponsive to therapy, other therapies, including phototherapy or photochemotherapy with UVB radiation or psoralen and UVA radiation, may be prescribed by a dermatologist.

Nummular dermatitis and asteatotic eczema are treated in a similar fashion to that described for contact dermatitis. Seborrheic dermatitis requires the addition of tar and antiyeast shampoos (e.g., selenium or ketoconazole) to the regimen. Since selenium sulfide shampoo is readily available in over-the-counter products, at a lower cost, recommend this first.

Monitoring for Efficacy

Relief of symptoms and resolution of the dermatitis are realistic goals for managing most of these patients. Temporary remission may be all that can be expected with seborrheic dermatitis.

Significant Food and Drug Interactions and Management

Most of the products used to treat dermatitis are topical, thus eliminating the food and drug interaction potential. Corticosteroids should be taken with food to minimize GI irritation.

Monitoring for Toxicity

All the topical corticosteroids can cause burning, itching, irritation, and erythema of the skin. The higher the potency, the higher is the likelihood of this occurring. The highest-potency corticosteroids can also cause skin atrophy and hypothalamic-pituitary-adrenocortical (HPA) axis suppression with long-term use.

Oral corticosteroids will cause HPA axis suppression with continued use at modest dosages. Patients who are at risk for complications of fluid retention caused by the mineralocorticoid effects of prednisone may benefit from the substitution of dexamethasone. This may be useful in older patients with cardiac problems and patients taking diuretics.

Diphenhydramine and hydroxyzine can cause drowsiness, but this side effect decreases with continued use. Patients driving or operating heavy equipment should be treated cautiously.

Followup Recommendations

Depending on severity, followup may be determined by the patient. In those patients requiring systemic therapy (corticosteroid or antibiotic), followup is in 1 week.

SUNBURN, SUNSCREENS, AND MINOR BURNS

Primary prevention of sunburn, the use of sunscreens, and the clinical management of minor burns will be described in this section. Sunburn—excessive exposure to ultraviolet radiation (UVR)—causes multiple health problems in addition to skin cancers. Skin cancer is the most common and also the most preventable cancer (American Cancer Society [ACS], 2002).* It is estimated that 50% of all people who live to age 65 will have at least one form of skin cancer.

There are approximately 1 million cases a year of highly curable basal cell or squamous cell cancers. It is projected that there will be 53,600 cases of the most serious skin cancer, melanoma, in 2002. It is estimated that 9600 deaths will be due to skin cancer, 7400 from malignant melanoma and the remainder from other skin cancers. About 90% of skin cancers can be prevented by protection from the sun's rays (ACS, 2002).

A relationship between ultraviolet B (UVB) exposure and the development of basal cell and squamous cell carcinoma has been documented. High-dose exposure to UVR generally increases the risk for development of malignant melanoma. Chronic exposure to ultraviolet A (UVA) and UVB increases the rate of skin aging and wrinkling. The cumulative effect of repeated sunburns in childhood is also a major risk factor for melanoma (ACS, 2002; Whiteman & Green, 1994).

Patients should be taught the long-term consequences of sun exposure (i.e., photoaging) and the benefits of regular sunscreen use and avoidance of sunburns. Appropriate use of sunscreens and reduction of the risk for skin cancer can be accomplished through aggressive patient teaching and counseling by the primary care provider.

Of the total solar radiation that reaches the earth, ultraviolet (UV) light accounts for about 3% and visible and infrared comprise the remainder. UV light is further divided into three subgroups: UVC, UVB, and UVA. UV radiation is measured as wavelengths of light in units of nanometers (nm).

UVC (200–290 nm) is considered potentially the most carcinogenic, but is almost completely absorbed by the ozone layer of the atmosphere. The UVB spectrum (290–320 nm) causes most sunburns. UVA (320–400 nm) can be up to 1000 times more intense than UVB, penetrates much deeper into the skin than any other UV wavelength, and can potentiate the carcinogenic effects of UVB (ACS, 2002; Farmer & Naylor, 1996). In addition, significant UV damage occurs prior to the development of perceptible UV-induced erythema (Farmer & Naylor,

*The American Cancer Society has a national toll-free number (1-800-ACS-2345) for obtaining general information as well as patient education materials about sun exposure, skin cancers, and skin examination guidelines for both the primary care provider and the patient.

1996). UVA contributes substantially to photoaging (wrinkling, drying) and may cause immunologic effects (ACS, 2002; Griffiths, 1992).

DNA damage is required before the tanning mechanisms are activated, specifically, pyrimidine dimer formation. DNA damage thus appears to be the trigger for the tanning response, meaning one cannot begin to tan until there is at least some damage. This suggests that there is no safe form or degree of tanning and that all UV radiation causes some skin damage (ACS, 2002; Eller, Yaar, & Gilchrist, 1994). Repeated miniexposures should not be overlooked since this type of incidental exposure accounts for 80% of the total exposure over a lifetime (Engle, 1995). In addition, the use of artificial tanning lamps and booths that use exposure to UVR should be avoided.

The ability to tan is largely determined genetically. Individuals with darker constitutive (i.e., non-sun-induced) pigmentation require different levels of UV protection. There are six skin types based on the relative amount of constitutive pigmentation. See Table 27–1 for a general guide to skin type.

The incidence of melanomas in light-complected individuals (skin types I–III) is several times greater than those with darker skin types (types IV–VI) even in similar geographic regions (Farmer & Naylor, 1996; Miller & Weinstock, 1994; Wentzell, 1996).

Regular sunscreen use has been shown to reduce the formation of precancerous actinic keratoses (AKs) by 36%. A dose-response–specific relationship has been found between the amount of sunscreen used and AK formation (Farmer & Naylor, 1996).

The development of benign nevi, one of the known risk factors for melanoma, is associated with personal sun exposure, especially multiple sunburns (Garbe, Buttner, & Weiss, 1994; Richard, Grob, & Gouvernet, 1993).

TABLE 27–1. A General Guide to Skin Type

Type I	• Low levels of constitutive pigmentation; very fair • Never tan; always burn • Redheads, light-complected blonds • Freckled; Celtic descent
Type II	• Slightly higher levels of constitutive pigmentation; fair • Always burn; able to tan small amounts after multiple sun exposures • Light-skinned individuals; blue-eyed • Slavic and Germanic descent
Type III	• Moderate levels of constitutive pigmentation • Infrequently burn; tan readily • Caucasians with brown/black hair (NOTE: Most white individuals fall into pigmentation types II and III.)
Type IV	• Moderate levels of constitutive pigmentation • Rarely burn; tan heavily with moderate sun exposure • Individuals of Asian, Native American, Mediterranean, and Latin American descent
Type V	• Dark constitutive pigmentation • Individuals become measurably darker with sun exposure • Light-complected African Americans, East Indian descent
Type VI	• Heaviest constitutive pigmentation • Dark-skinned African Americans

SPECIFIC CONSIDERATIONS FOR PHARMACOTHERAPY

When Drug Therapy Is Needed

The problem is summarized by this statement: "The skin never forgets an injury . . . . The eventual condition of the skin results from a summation of all the injuries it has received" (Farmer & Naylor, 1996). Prevention is the key to maintaining healthy skin throughout one's life.

Sunscreens act either physically or chemically. Physical sunscreens provide a mechanical barrier to sunlight; for example, zinc oxide paste and titanium dioxide scatter ultraviolet light. Clothing and beach umbrellas are also effective as physical sunscreens, but ultraviolet light may be reflected from sand and water to reach under a beach umbrella and cause burning.

Chemical sunscreens absorb a specific portion of the ultraviolet light spectrum. When the light is absorbed by the sunscreen, several changes may occur in the absorbing compound:

- Light energy is converted to heat.
- The sunscreen molecule may dissociate into atoms or radicals.
- The molecule may be excited to higher energy levels and its energy transferred through collision with another molecule, followed by a chemical reaction.
- The compound may become excited and lose its energy immediately by fluorescence or later by phosphorescence.

The literature shows disagreement on the value of sunscreen agent protection. However, there is evidence that these products provide some protection, depending on the degree of photosensitization. A photoallergic response is characterized by a delayed onset, occurs in sensitized skin, and recurs with subsequent exposures to ultraviolet light. Ultraviolet light above 320 nm can elicit a photoallergic response, so compounds that absorb energy throughout the ultraviolet region may be the most desirable for this purpose if they are used in adequate amounts. The following are sunscreen compounds known to have the propensity to cause a photoallergic response: barbiturates, chlorothiazide, chlorpromazine, demeclocycline, erythromycin, phenylsulfonylurea, promethazine, psoralens, quinidine, quinine, sulfas, and tetracycline.

Short- and Long-Term Goals of Pharmacotherapy

Sunscreen agents should be considered for protection against sunburn and premature aging of the skin. They also may reduce actinic or solar keratosis and some types of skin cancer. Treatment of first-degree burns is aimed at healing with minimal scarring, preventing infection, and minimizing pain and discomfort.

Nonpharmacologic Therapy

Requirements for protection from UVR are generally based on pigmentation skin type, presence of precancerous skin lesions, usual extent of UVR exposure, and history of skin cancer. It is important for the healthcare provider to obtain a thorough health history, including occupational and avocational/recreational history, as well as to conduct a thorough assessment of the skin in accordance with ACS guidelines (ACS, 2002).

For example, outdoor workers (e.g., construction workers, farmers, military personnel) and individuals whose recreation takes them out of doors (e.g., golfers, cyclists) require specific teaching and counseling relative to their extensive sun exposure. However, it is generally believed that most individuals should develop the positive health behavior of routinely using a sunscreen whenever they spend any time outside. Patients should be taught the following:

- Avoid sun exposure during the period when the UVR is most intense, i.e., from 10 A.M. to 4 P.M.
- UVA remains constant throughout the day.
- UVA is not blocked by glass; UVB is.
- UVR intensity increases by 4% for every 1000 ft of increase in elevation.
- Approximately 60 to 80% of UV radiation can penetrate a thin cloud.
- Snow reflects as much as 85% of the sun's rays.
- Shade and clouds do not provide adequate protection from UVR. Rays bounce from all directions off sand, water, patio floors, and snow. Approximately 70 to 80% of the UVR burning power penetrates clouds, and rays can even penetrate the surface of the water (ACS, 2002).

There are several ways to protect the skin from UVR, including clothing, physical sunscreens, and chemical sunscreens such as the ones with SPF values. Patients should be instructed to wear protective clothing that provides good physical coverage to high-exposure areas (e.g., hats with 2- to 3-in brims to shade the face, neck, and ears and long sleeves to cover the arms). A general guide is that if one can see light through the fabric, then UVR can penetrate it (ACS, 2002).

Physical sunscreens (e.g., zinc oxide and titanium dioxide) and chemical sunscreens (e.g., ones with SPF values) will be discussed in the drug therapy section. Table 27–2 summarizes recommendations for protection from sun exposure for adults.

A common misconception among many people is that after applying a SPF 15 sunscreen and staying out in the sun for 4 h, they can reapply the sunscreen and stay out in the sun another 4 h. At the end of 4 h, they have received their dose of sun for the day! They should go indoors or cover up so as not to receive *any* additional sun exposure. To increase exposure time, apply a sunscreen with a higher SPF initially. Several broad spectrum sunscreens, such as Photplex® and Shade UVA Guard,® block both UVA and UVB rays.

TABLE 27–2. UVR Protection Recommendations for Adults

Risk	Nonpharmacologic Therapy	Pharmacologic Therapy
High		
Skin types I–III; outdoors more than ½ day; history of precancerous lesions, skin cancer, recreational and occupational exposure; individuals wanting to decrease photoaging, photosensitivity disorders/drugs	Maximum protection; long-sleeve heavy cotton shirt, long pants, hat with wide brim; avoid sun from 10 A.M. to 4 P.M. when possible	SPF 30 sunscreen
Moderate		
Skin types III–IV; minimum occupational and recreational exposure	Hat and shirt to cover face, ears, and arms; avoid sun from 10 A.M. to 4 P.M. when possible	SPF 15 sunscreen
Minimum		
Skin types V and VI	Hat and shirt to cover face, ears, and arms; avoid sun from 10 A.M. to 4 P.M. when possible	SPF 8–15 sunscreen

Infants and children require special consideration. It is believed that people may receive up to 80% of their total life's exposure to UV light by the age of 18, and that by using sunscreens during that time, the number of skin pathologies can be reduced by up to 80% (American Academy of Pediatrics [AAP], 1995; ACS, 2002). The American Academy of Pediatrics (AAP) and the American Academy of Dermatology (AAD) (1995) cite the dangers of sunburn in infants and children. A baby's sensitive skin is thinner than adult skin, so a baby will burn more easily than an adult. In addition, sunburn can cause fever and dehydration in children. Sunburn in a child can be very dangerous, and severe sunburn in a child under 1 year of age is an emergency; parents should be instructed to notify their healthcare provider immediately (AAP, 1995). Do not use sunscreens on infants younger than 6 months (ACS, 2002). Infants under 6 months of age should be kept out of direct sunlight and placed in shade. In addition, the child's clothing should cover the total body; use long, lightweight pants, long-sleeved shirts, and hats with brims that shade the face and cover the ears. Clothing should be made of tightly woven fabrics that do not allow light to penetrate. Hold clothing up to a lamp or window and see how much light shines through: the less light, the better. Clothing made of cotton is both cool and protective. The bill of a hat should be facing forward to cover the child's face. Child-sized sunglasses with UV protection should be used to protect the child's eyes (AAP, 1995; Battan, Dart, & Rumack, 1997; Pion, 1996).

Burn Classification. Sunburn is usually a *first-degree* burn characterized by a delayed response to the UVR developing approximately 3 to 6 h after exposure and peaking within 12 to 24 h. The response is characterized by erythema, pruritus, tenderness, and pain, and may progress to edema, vesiculation, and even blistering. It involves the superficial layers of the epidermis. It blanches with pressure and shows little edema. A *second-degree* burn involves the epidermis and dermis. Generally, a distinction is made between superficial and deep second-degree burns based on the amount of dermis involved. Deep second-degree burns involve the entire papillary dermis with penetration to some or all of the reticular dermis. Second-degree burns are characterized by painful red blisters or broken epidermis with a weeping edematous surface. *Third-degree* burns involve all the layers of the epidermis and dermis with penetration into underlying fat and muscle. Third-degree burns are generally painless because the nerve tissue in the area has been destroyed.

All second-degree burns greater than 5 to 10% of the body, all third-degree burns, all burns associated with electrical current, and all burns of the ears, eyes, face, hands, feet, and perineum should be referred to a hospital prepared to handle burn patients. The remaining first-degree and second-degree burns less than 5% of the body should receive wound care and close followup. The goals of therapy are to decrease inflammation, prevent infection, relieve pain, and promote healing.

Nonpharmacologic treatment for first-degree burns includes application of cool, wet compresses of water, milk, or oatmeal to reduce discomfort and edema and mild analgesics for discomfort. Dressings or prophylactic antibiotics are not required. Infants and children should be referred to a physician or emergency room for initial treatment as previously described.

Second-degree burns require protection of the wound from potential infection. If the skin is intact, the burn should be washed with water and a mild antiseptic soap. Chemical burns should be flushed with running water for 15 to 30 min. A syringe or dental water device can be used to remove embedded debris. Management of blisters is somewhat controversial. Some believe blisters provide a protective barrier and should remain intact. Others suggest that the fluid beneath blisters is a medium for bacterial growth.

Silver sulfadiazine is the topical antibiotic of choice. (Refer to Drug Table 805.) Dressings are prepared by applying nonadherent gauze saturated in sterile saline to the burn and covering with a thick dressing to facilitate drainage. Followup is in 2 days to evaluate for infection. The patient should be instructed about the signs of infection and when to call the health care provider. Pain relief is accomplished with a nonsteroidal agent. Tetanus prophylaxis is indicated, and previously immunized patients should receive a booster as needed (Monafo, 1996; Peate, 1992).

Time Frame for Initiating Pharmacotherapy

The vast majority of individuals should be taught to use a sunscreen any time their skin is exposed to UVR because of the effects of miniexposures over time and long-term consequences of UV exposure. In addition, those individuals taking drugs with photosensitivity side effects and individuals with photosensitive disorders should be taught to use maximum UVR protection strategies.

Typically, burns managed in the outpatient setting are small, superficial thermal burns that do not effect areas of critical function (e.g., hands, joints) or of cosmetic concern (e.g., face). These wounds usually meet the criteria for first-degree or minor second-degree burns. Persons with larger or deeper burns, circumferential burns of an extremity, burns complicated by an underlying medical condition, or burns of the hands, joints, or face and infants and children with burns are best treated as inpatients (Clayton & Solem, 1995).

Overview of Drug Classes for Treatment

Initial outpatient management of burns includes pain control, cleansing of the wound, debridement of blisters or bullae, and application of a suitable dressing. An up-to-date tetanus immunization should be confirmed.

See Drug Table 805.

Assessment and History Taking

Assessment of the skin is an essential component of all patient visits. A thorough history of the patient's habits of sun exposure is important, including hobbies, occupations, and other activities that take the patient outdoors. This is essential to the accurate determination of overall sun exposure of the patient and prescription of appropriate sunscreens, including protective clothing. Sensitivity to sunscreen preparations should also be assessed.

The primary healthcare provider should perform a thorough physical examination of the patient's skin to detect any suspicious lesions that may be cancerous or precancerous. The patient may require referral to a dermatologist or oncologist as appropriate.

Accurate assessment of burns is essential to appropriate treatment. Referral to a hospital prepared to care for burn patients may be indicated as previously described.

Patient and Caregiver Information

Patients and caregivers should be taught the optimal methods of protecting their skin from harmful exposure to the sun during periods of outdoor activities. This includes correct selection and use of sunscreen preparations as well as the use of protective clothing and actual avoidance of sun exposure during the times of the day when the rays are most harmful. Special precautions for infants and children should also be taught to caregivers.

Patients with burns should be taught the correct way to care for the burn at home. Signs and symptoms of infection should also be taught to the patient and caregiver.

Patients and caregivers should be taught to examine their skin once a month in accordance with ACS guidelines. Literature is available from the ACS for use with patients.

OUTCOMES MANAGEMENT

Selecting an Appropriate Agent

Before recommending a sunscreen or suntan product, one should know the active ingredient and its maximum absorption, molar absorptivity, and concentration. Actual effectiveness in patients is difficult to determine precisely because individuals react in varying degrees to sunlight. The minimal erythemal dose (MED), the amount of sunlight needed for a minimum perceptible erythema (redness), is used to gauge the degree of sensitivity of both protected and unprotected skin to sunlight. The protection factor (PF), the ratio of the MED for protected skin to that for unprotected skin, is used to measure the relative effectiveness of sunscreens (the larger the PF value, the greater is the protection).

Individuals should be taught to select a sunscreen that provides the appropriate amount of protection for their skin type and the extent of UVR exposure. The goal of therapy is to prevent sunburn and minimize UVR exposure to reduce the extent of photoaging. Table 27–2 summarizes UVR photoprotection in adults.

Self-tanning products consist primarily of dihydroxyacetone (DHA). They are nontoxic and have a protein-staining effect in the stratum corneum of the skin. They may accentuate freckles and seborrheic keratoses, which may not be cosmetically desirable. Tanning accelerators are generally nontoxic and are a natural component of the skin in the normal melanogenic process. Tanning promoters (e.g., 5-methoxypsoralen) are not available over-the-counter in the United States and have been documented as highly phototoxic and carcinogenic. Tanning pills contain canthaxanthin and are toxic to both skin and eyes. They are not available over-the-counter in the United States.

Management of Minor Burns

Pain control. Most burn patients will experience intense pain because of the exposure of nerve endings that generally lie beneath the epidermal layer. Any manipulation of the wound, for instance during debridement, will further stimulate the pain response. Immediate cooling of the wound may lessen the severity, but rarely will diminish the pain to such a level that drugs are not necessary. Narcotics are almost always necessary and may be needed until the wound has healed over. Generally, the combinations of acetaminophen with codeine (e.g., Tylenol with Codeine No. 3) or acetaminophen with oxycodone (e.g., Percocet, Tylox) are the preferred choices, the latter being more potent. Aspirin products should be avoided since they have antiplatelet activity, which may impair the healing process.

Cleansing and wound protection. Most wounds are cleansed and dressed once daily. More frequent changes increase patient discomfort without improving the clinical rate of healing. Many protective and antibacterial products have been marketed for wound healing, but all have similar outcomes. Silver sulfadiazine is most commonly used. After cleaning the wound with mild soap and water, silver sulfadiazine is spread over it in a thin layer and a dressing is applied. A less expensive and equally effective alternative is bacitracin ointment. It is important to use a protective agent with antibacterial properties early in management. Microorganisms proliferate rapidly in burn wounds, especially in those severe enough to impair immune function. Topical antimicrobial agents increase the interval between injury and colonization and maintain low levels of wound flora.

Adjuvant therapies. As a wound heals, the skin dries and is prone to itching. Initially, it is best to use moisturizers without added ingredients since the skin is sensitive. Simple petroleum jelly (Vasoline) or lotions suffice. Other agents containing urea and fragrances may be used as the skin matures. If the itching is particularly bothersome and unrelieved by topical therapy, diphenhydramine (Benadryl) or hydroxyzine (Atarax, Vistaril) orally may be used. These do have a tendency to cause drowsiness, so the patient should be duly warned of the side effects.

Monitoring for Efficacy

Patients should be monitored for risk of excessive UVR exposure; correct use, sensitivity, and toxicity of sunscreens, and assessed for precancerous and cancerous lesions as previously described. Patients should be referred to a dermatologist for diagnosis and treatment for precancerous and cancerous lesions immediately. Patients also should be taught how to examine their skin monthly for changes in existing moles and appearance of new ones. The ACS has numerous patient education materials that can be used to assist in teaching patients about skin care and assessment.

Patients should be taught to apply sunscreens correctly. Sunscreens should be applied at least 30 to 60 min prior to sun exposure. This allows for penetration of the skin for maximum efficacy. They should be reapplied after sweating, swimming, or exercising. However, remind them that *reapplication does not extend the amount of time the individual can spend out in the sun.* Nine teaspoons of sunscreen are considered adequate to cover the average adult; ½ teaspoon each to the face, neck, arms, both shoulders, back, and torso, and 1 teaspoon to each of the legs and feet (ACS, 1998). The patient should be instructed to read the label of the sunscreen product carefully and follow the instructions and precautions.

Sunscreens for children should be selected by the caregiver rigorously. The sunscreen should screen out both UVA and UVB radiation. The SPF should be at least 15, and the sunscreen should be applied at least 30 min before going outside (AAP, 1995). The sunscreen should be water-resistant or waterproof. Waterproof sunscreens should be reapplied at least every 2 h. An adequate amount (refer to package directions) should be used and rubbed in well. Be sure to cover the baby's face, nose, ears, feet, and hands, and the backs of the knees. Zinc oxide, an effective sunblock, can be used as extra protection on the nose, cheeks, tops of the ears, and shoulders (AAP, 1995).

The sunscreen should be tested on the baby's wrist for any type of reaction before applying it all over; however avoid the eyes. If the child cries or complains that the sunscreen burns his or her eyes, a different brand of sunscreen may be tried or try a sunscreen stick or sunblock with titanium dioxide or zinc oxide. If a rash develops, the caregiver should be instructed to contact the healthcare provider (AAP, 1995).

Patients with first- or second-degree burns should be followed up within 2 days to evaluate for healing, pain control and infection. Thereafter, weekly office examinations help in the monitoring of healing rate and for early signs of infection. Wounds should heal within 2 to 3 weeks. If healing takes longer, concern over infection and the potential for scarring should guide the therapy.

Significant Food and Drug Interactions and Management

Since all of the agents used to treat burns and minimize the effect of UVR are topical, food and drug interactions are not a problem.

Monitoring for Toxicity

As previously described, sunscreens should be tested prior to application by using a small amount in the inner aspect of the arm and waiting 24 h to determine whether there is a reaction to the agent. Sunscreens should be removed with bathing or showering after UVR exposure, especially in children, to reduce the chance of absorption.

Followup Recommendations

Patients should be followed up at least yearly when the annual skin examination is conducted. Use of sunscreens, protective clothing, and monthly skin self-assessment can be evaluated at that time.

SKIN CANCER

Sun exposure increases the risk of skin cancers. It is beyond the scope of this book to address this topic thoroughly; however, assessing for neoplastic damage to the skin is important. Lesions that fail to heal, bleed and/or itch, and change in appearance, size, shape, or color should be examined by a dermatologist. Malignancies of the skin occur most often on sun-exposed areas of the skin and are more frequent in Caucasians. The main types include (Roberts & Barbee, 2000):

- *Basal cell carcinoma:* Slow growing pearly or shiny papules or nodules with a rolled border; may have crusting; color can be pink, red, brown, blue, or black; may be round or oval; may have indentation in the center (umbilication); usually asymptomatic; metastasis is rare; managed with excision, cryosurgery, or electrosurgery.
- *Squamous cell carcinoma:* Indurated plaques, papules, or nodules with keratotic scales, crusts, ulcerations that are thick; shape may be round, oval; may have umbilication; appear in months or years; managed with surgery or radiation.
- *Malignant melanoma:* Three-fourths of deaths from skin cancer are from this disease; incidence is increasing rapidly; may be macular, popular, or nodular and colors vary from black, gray, blue, brown to pink. *Cardinal signs* are: **A**symmetry; irregular **B**order; mottled or haphazard **C**oloring; **D**iameter greater than 6 cm; and **E**levation of surface. A genetic link has been identified in some families.

Skin cancer is preventable. The patient needs to be taught how to assess his or her own skin by the healthcare provider and urged to avoid severe sunburn.

PSORIASIS AND PITYRIASIS ROSEA

PSORIASIS

Psoriasis is a common, chronically recurring papulosquamous skin disease of multifactorial etiology (Naldi & Rzany, 2001). About 5 million Americans (1 to 2% of the population) have the disease (Naldi & Rzany, 2001; Stern, 1996; Zanolli, 1996). The annual costs of treating psoriasis exceed is believed to 1.6 billion. There is an equal sex incidence although females may be affected earlier in life than males (Camisa, 1995). Psoriasis occur more often in whites than in Asians or African Americans and only rarely in Native Americans (Abel & Morhenn, 1996; Naldi & Rzany, 2001). Most patients with psoriasis are treated in primary care settings; psoriasis is the third most common reason for patients to visit a dermatologist (Stern & Nelson, 1993).

Psoriasis is characterized by whitish, scaly patches of varying size most commonly seen on the elbows, knees, and scalp. However, there is wide variation in severity and distribution of the skin lesions and the disease is marked by exacerbations and remissions. Usually asymptomatic, about 20% of people with psoriasis complain of pruritus (Koda-Kimble et al., 2002).

Adults account for 84% of the office visits for psoriasis (Stern, 1996). Although lesions may occur just after birth, onset is most common in the second to fourth decades of life, with a mean age of onset of 27.8 years (Abel & Morhenn, 1996). If a child develops psoriasis, an affected family member is more likely to be found than if onset of the disease is as an adult (Weston et al., 2002).

The disease is influenced by environmental, immunological, and genetic factors. The exact modes of inheritance are unknown. Certain HLA antigens are more common among populations of psoriasis patients, so a gene linked to or related to HLA genes may be one predisposing factor (Roenigk, 1991; Weston et al., 2002). Kinetic cell studies have shown that in psoriasis the epidermal cells proliferate rapidly, completing a germinative cell cycle more rapidly than do the cells of normal skin. The normal epidermal turnover time is 28 to 56 days. In psoriasis, the epidermis renews itself in just 3 to 4 days. Psoriasis is not contagious and is often worse in the winter due to low indoor humidity and relative absence of sunlight.

There are four major subtypes of psoriasis based on the appearance of the lesions:

1. *Chronic plaque psoriasis* is the most common type. Patients exhibit one to many erythematous, clearly demarcated, oval plaques several centimeters in diameter. The plaques are covered by silvery-white scales.
2. *Guttate psoriasis* is the second most common type. It is characterized by an acute exanthum-like eruption with flat-topped scaly papules usually 1 mm to 1 cm in diameter over the entire body. It frequently follows an infection after 2 to 3 weeks, such as streptococcal pharyngitis or a viral upper respiratory infection, es-

pecially in children and young adults. (Parker 2001; Weston et al., 2002).

3. *Erythrodermic psoriasis* is infrequently seen. It is characterized by a generalized exfoliative erythroderma. It can be serious and life threatening (Parker, 2001).
4. *Pustular psoriasis* is also uncommon. It is characterized by a generalized scaly plaque. In addition, small, superficial nonfollicular pustules develop. The pustules generally resolve in a few days, but usually recur.

The two major clinical characteristics of psoriasis are:

1. The primary lesions are papules or maculopapules.
2. The majority of the lesions are covered with imbricated scale.

The scale is usually silver-white, silver-gray, or mother-of-pearl in color and occurs in thin mica-like layers. If the scale is removed, minute bleeding points are exposed (Auspitz's sign). Once the initial lesion forms, it continues to enlarge by peripheral extension and gradually becomes more indurated and slightly more elevated, becoming a plaque. A plaque may cover several centimeters and gradually join other plaques to cover large areas. Other common sites of involvement are the sacral and perianal areas, genitalia, and nails. The patient may experience a burning sensation and pruritus in acute exacerbations of the disease.

Physical trauma in the active phase results in development of linear patterns of psoriasis in the injured areas (Koebner's phenomenon) (Weston et al., 2002). Such isomorphic lesions also may be seen on the hands of factory workers in jobs requiring extensive use of the hands; they also occur in golf and tennis players.

More than 33% of psoriasis patients have nail involvement characterized by pitting of the nail plate, onycholysis (separation of the nail from the nail bed with resulting white color caused by air between the plate and the bed), and subungual hyperkeratosis (scale between the plate and the bed) (Naldi & Rzany, 2001; Weston et al., 2002). Secondary bacterial or fungal infections may result in black or green discoloration of the nail plate.

PITYRIASIS ROSEA

Pityriasis rosea is a common skin disease that occurs primarily on chest and trunk of young adults and is characterized by papulosquamous, oval, erythematous discrete lesions. It is mildly to moderately pruritic and occurs most often in the spring and fall. Face lesions are rare in white adults but are rather common in children and patients of African American descent (Sauer & Hall, 1996). Females ages 10 to 35 are most frequently affected (Gutierrez, 1999). A "herald patch" lesion 2 to 10 cm round to oval resembling a patch of "ringworm" may precede the general rash by 2 to 10 days. The lesions are salmon-colored in Caucasians and hyperpigmented in African Americans. The etiology is unknown, contagiousness is unknown, and recurrence is not usual (2%). However, there is some belief that the rash is viral in origin (Habif, 1996). The disease is benign and self-limited (Gutierrez, 1999).

SPECIFIC CONSIDERATIONS FOR PHARMACOTHERAPY

When Drug Therapy Is Needed

Although the exact causes of psoriasis and pityriasis rosea are unknown, treatment approaches are reliable and offer good control of the disorder. Since the disorders are visually apparent, emotional and psychological considerations warrant intervention in even the mildest of cases.

Short- and Long-Term Goals of Pharmacotherapy

Psoriasis is often a lifelong relapsing and remitting disease, so modes of therapy should be selected with long-term consequences in mind. The goal of therapy is to achieve complete clearing of lesions (partial clearing is acceptable at times), using regimens with minimal toxicity and maximum patient acceptability. Consideration should be given to the patient's ability to maintain an active home and work environment with little interference from this disorder.

Pityriasis rosea is generally self-limiting. Treatment of pruritis with oral antihistamines and topical corticosteroids may be appropriate when pruritis is present (Parker, 2001).

Nonpharmacologic Therapy

Factors that tend to exacerbate psoriasis include alcohol use, obesity, emotional upsets or stress, infection, trauma to the skin, and certain drugs (i.e., lithium, beta blockers, antimalarials, indomethacin). Patients should be instructed to eat a balanced diet to attain and maintain optimal weight and to avoid stress and fatigue. They should also be told that it can be controlled, it is completely epidermal, with underlying inflammation, and they should continue therapy until it is clear.

Natural sunlight is effective adjunctive therapy for psoriasis in many patients. Psoriasis often improves in the summer months. Some patients move to warm, sunny climates to maximize sun exposure year round.

Phototherapy in the form of artificial ultraviolet light exposure is a specialized treatment. Ultraviolet therapy (UVB) in increasing suberythema doses, once or twice a week, can be used after a daily thin application of a 2% tar salve, similar to the Goeckerman regimen (Abel & Morhenn, 1996; Roenigk, 1991; Hall, 2000). Weston et al. (2002) advise that artificial ultraviolet phototherapy is effective for children, and a mineral oil or petrolatum lubrication of the skin prior to therapy assists with a more uniform penetration of the affected area. Treatment with UVB three times a week for 18 to 24 weeks has been shown to be successful.

Psoralen plus ultraviolet A (PUVA) therapy uses a combination of oral psoralen and UVA for persistent or extensive psoriasis. It requires a special UVA light source, equipment, and specially trained personnel (Weston et al., 2002). Clearing of psoriasis is more likely to occur with higher doses of psoralen (Naldi & Rzany, 2001). PUVA therapy increases an individual's risk for nonmelanoma (but not melanoma) skin cancer. Therefore, patients should be followed indefinitely for the later development of skin cancer. There are numerous precautions when administering PUVA therapy. A detailed discussion of this therapy is beyond the scope of this chapter. UVB therapy is agreed upon as effective but has not been shown to be more effective than other therapies (Naldi & Rzany, 2001).

Erythrodermic and pustular psoriasis may be very difficult to treat, and such patients should be referred to a dermatologist as soon as possible for initial treatment (Whitmore, 1996).

Pityriasis rosea lesions have been found to resolve more quickly when exposed to direct sunlight or UVB administered in five consecutive treatments when used during the first week of the rash (Habif, 1996). Children and adolescents usually respond well to one UVL exposure (natural sunlight or sunlamp) (Weston et al., 2002).

Time Frame for Initiating Pharmacotherapy

Psoriasis is a lifelong disease and therefore will never be cured. To minimize the extent of skin involvement and to decrease the likelihood of progression beyond the epidermal layer, pharmacotherapy should be started at the earliest evidence of disease.

See Drug Table 802.

Assessment and History Taking

Patients should be assessed for return of the lesions, overall disability, and discomfort. The Psoriasis Area and Severity Index quantifies disability and discomfort. This disease is characterized by remissions and exacerbations and cannot be cured. However, there have been reported cases of spontaneous remission with no recurrence that have not been explained.

Arthritis has been reported to affect nearly one-third of psoriasis patients. Many view psoriasis and psoriatic arthritis as one disease affecting two organ systems. However, others believe the two are separate disorders. Regardless of etiology, the patient should be treated aggressively to minimize progression of the disease (Whitmore, 1996). Referral to a rheumatologist should be considered.

Patient/Caregiver Information

Although there is no cure for psoriasis, the disease can be managed. The overall goal of therapy is to achieve remission in which most or all of the lesions resolve. However, exacerbations and remissions are the typical course of the disease. There is also significant variability in the extent of the disease and the psychological and social response to the disease.

OUTCOMES MANAGEMENT

Selecting an Appropriate Agent

Selection of specific therapies depends upon the degree of body surface involvement and the clinical subtype of the disease. In many cases, combination therapy may be used to enhance the efficacy and to enable the use of lower doses, thereby decreasing the toxicity of each individual agent.

For chronic plaque psoriasis, mild emollients and keratolytics with low-potency topical corticosteroids are usually all that is necessary. Over-the-counter products available are plain white petrolatum or mineral oil, hydrocortisone 1%, coal tar ointments or shampoos (5%), zinc pyrithione shampoo, and salt water. If the plaque becomes more generalized, topical agents become less useful and can become quite expensive. Therefore, consideration must be given to oral psoralen therapy in combination with ultraviolet A radiation. This therapy is generally given three times weekly until the outbreak clears, and is repeated as necessary.

Topical corticosteroids may be necessary though they do not influence lesions (Weston et al., 2002). Products with triamcinolone 0.1% (ointment) or fluocinonide with 10% salicylic acid are particularly useful. However, tachyphylaxis can develop to these products.

Trigel, anthralin, and ketoconazole shampoo have been successful for scalp psoriasis, or ketoconazole 400 mg daily for 1 month may be tried.

Guttate psoriasis may be treated in the same fashion as described above and usually responds very well. Conversely, erythrodermic and pustular psoriasis may be very difficult to treat. Initial therapy includes bed rest, warm baths, and bland emollients, generally in combination with systemic therapy with etretinate, methotrexate, or cyclosporine. Systemic agents may be continued or the patient switched to PUVA therapy as tolerated once the disease is controlled. Many patients exhibit signs and symptoms of sepsis (vasodilation, increased cardiac output, fever, elevated white blood cell count with neutrophilia).

Methotrexate azathioprine and hydroxyurea should be reserved for severe recalcitrant psoriasis (Parker, 2001). Methotrexate has been used since the late 1950s with some success. There are currently 30,000 patients using it for psoriasis. It is contraindicated in liver disease. Oral administration is more convenient for the patient, but produces more nausea, and compliance may be an issue. Intramuscular administration is less convenient for the patient, but it minimizes these problems. The oral dose is 2.5 mg every 12 h for three doses; the intramuscular injection is given once as a 7.5 mg dose. The dose is increased as needed with the effective range being 7.5 to 25 mg. The average dose is 15 mg. After 1.5 to 2.0 g, a biopsy of the liver should be considered (Parker, 2001). Duration of therapy is dependent on cumulative dose and biopsy; a 3-year maximum is recommended.

Etretinate (ethyl ester of retinoic acid) and acitretin (metabolite of etretinate) are particularly effective in pustular psoriasis.

Calcipotriene (synthetic analog of vitamin D) is approved for plaque psoriasis and is equal in effectiveness to topical steroids, coal tars, and dithranol (Naldi & Rzany, 2001). It should not be used on the face and is applied twice daily for up to 8 weeks. A maximum of 300 g a week is suggested. Improvement is usually seen in 2 weeks. Only 10% of patients show complete clearing. It is better tolerated than anthralin but not as well tolerated as topical steroids.

Each patient should be assessed as an individual relative to disease severity, symptom, and level of physical, psychological, and social disability.

Monitoring for Efficacy

Psoriasis is a common hyperproliferative epidermal disorder for which several effective therapeutic modalities control rather than cure the condition. Recognition of the pathogenic factors associated with psoriasis, selection of an appropriate treatment regimen, and monitoring for adverse effects as well as disease progression often lead to a satisfactory outcome.

Achievement of clinical efficacy by any given therapeutic regimen requires days to weeks. Initial dramatic response may be achieved with some agents such as corticosteroids; however, sustained benefit with pharmacologically specific antipsoriatic therapy usually requires about 2 to 4 weeks for noticeable response.

Significant Food and Drug Interactions and Management

Oral corticosteroids and methotrexate may be taken with food if GI upset is noted. It is suggested that etretinate always be taken with food.

Drugs that may cause toxic levels of methotrexate include barbiturates, phenylbutazone, phenytoin, probenecid, salicylates, and sulfonamides. Severe bone marrow suppression can occur when methotrexate is combined with trimethoprim. It is ineffective with concomitant folic acid.

Monitoring for Toxicity

For most of the agents used to treat psoriasis, hypersensitivity and photosensitivity are the major concerns. If acute inflammation, rash, burning, and/or blistering lesions occur at the area of application, discontinue use. Calcipotriene is 6% systemically absorbed, so when used regularly over a large area patients may demonstrate signs of hypercalcemia or vitamin D toxicity.

The most important side effects of methotrexate are acute cytopenias and chronic hepatitis and cirrhosis. The most important side effect of etretinate is the induction of mutations in a developing fetus. Because it has been detected in tissue many years after dosing, it should never be used in women of childbearing potential. It can also lead to hepatotoxicity. Cyclosporine's side effects include hypertension, nephrotoxicity, paresthesias, hypertrichosis, hyperuricemia, and anergy.

Over a long period of time, PUVA therapy increases an individual's risk of nonmelanoma skin cancer. Therefore, patients should be followed indefinitely to evaluate for these occurrences.

Followup Recommendations

Followup is determined by the type of therapy and the recurrence of lesions. Patients should be monitored closely for efficacy of treatment and side effects and toxicity specific to the drug therapy prescribed (Abel & Morhenn, 1996; Barker et al., 1995). Vitamin and mineral deficiencies may occur because of the increased epidermal cell turnover rate of all the skin (Barker et al, 1995). Psoriasis that begins in childhood usually worsens in adulthood (Weston et al., 2002). Emotional support is needed by all patients.

REFERENCES

Abel, E., & Morhenn, V. (1996). Psoriasis. In D. Demis (Ed.), *Clinical dermatology.* Philadelphia: Lippincott-Raven.

American Academy of Pediatrics and the American Academy of Dermatology. (1995). *Fun in the sun: Keep your baby safe. Guidelines for parents.* Elk Grove, IL: AAP.

American Cancer Society. (2002). *Facts & Figures: Skin cancer.* Atlanta: Author.

Barker, L., Burton, J., & Zieve, P. (1999). *Principles of ambulatory medicine.* Baltimore: Williams & Wilkins.

Battan, F., Dart, R., & Rumack, B. (1997). Emergencies, injuries, and poisoning. In W. Hay, J. Groothius, A. Hayward, & M. Levin (Eds.), *Current pediatric diagnosis and treatment.* Stamford, CT: Appleton & Lange.

Berger, T., Goldstein, S., & Odom, R. (1997). Skin and appendages. In L. Tierney, S. McPhee, & M. Papadakis (Eds.), *Current medical diagnosis and treatment.* Stamford, CT: Appleton & Lange.

Bergfeld, W. (1995). The evaluation and management of acne: Economic considerations. *Journal of the American Academy of Dermatology, 32* (Suppl.), S52–S56.

Camisa, C. (1995). Treatment of severe psoriasis with systemic drugs. *Dermatology Nursing, 8*(2), 107–118.

Caufield, K. (2004). Controlling fertility. In E. Youngkin, & M. Davis (Eds.), *Women's health: A primary care clinical guide* (3rd ed.). Upper Saddle River, NJ: Prentice Hall.

Cayce, K., Careccia, R., Hancox, J., Feldman, S., & McMichael, A. (2004). ACNE: A clinical review for the primary care practitioner. *NPPR Continuing Medical Education.*

Clayton, M., & Solem, L. (1995). No ice, no butter. *Postgraduate Medicine, 97*(5), 151–165.

Cohn, M. (1992). Superficial fungal infections. *Postgraduate Medicine, 91*(2), 239–252.

Comparative efficacy of treatments for pediculaosis capititis infestations: Update 2000. (2001). *Archives of Dermatology, 137,* 287–292.

Comparison of wet combing with malathion for treatment of head lice in the UK: A pragmatic randomized controlled trial. (2000). *Lancet, 12,* 540–544.

Dockery, G. (1997). *Cutaneous disorders of the lower extremities.* Philadelphia: W. B. Saunders.

Drake, L., Ceilley, R., Cornelison, R., et al. (1995). Guidelines of care for warts: Human papillomavirus. *Journal of the American Academy of Dermatology, 32*(1), 98–103.

Eisenbaum, A. (1997). Eye. In W. Hay, J. Groothuis, A. Hayward, & M. Levin (Eds.), *Current pediatric diagnosis and treatment.* Stamford, CT: Appleton & Lange.

Elewski, B., & Weil, M. (1996). Dermatophytes and superficial fungi. In W. Sams & P. Lynch (Eds.), *Principles and practice of dermatology.* New York: Churchill Livingstone.

Eller, M., Yaar, M., & Gilchrist, B. (1994). DNA damage and melanogenesis. *Nature, 372,* 413–414.

Elliott, G., & Sams, W. (1996). Viral vesicular diseases. In W. Sams & P. Lynch (Eds.), *Principles and practice of dermatology.* New York: Churchill Livingstone.

Engle, J. (1995). Choosing sunscreen products. *American Druggist, 212*(2), 36.

Faergemann, J., Jones, T., Hettler, O., & Loria, Y. (1996). Pityrosporum ovale (*Malassezia furfur*) as the causative agent of seborrhoeic dermatitis: New treatment options. *British Journal of Dermatology, 134* (Suppl. 46), 12–15.

Farmer, K., & Naylor, M. (1996). Sunexposure, sunscreens, and skin cancer prevention: A year-round concern. *Annals of Pharmacotherapy, 30,* 662–673.

Frieden, I. (1996). Viral exanthems. In W. Sams & P. Lynch (Eds.), *Principles and practice of dermatology.* New York: Churchill Livingstone.

Garbe, C., Buttner, P., & Weiss, J. (1994). Associated factors in the prevalence of more than 50 common melanocytic nevi, atypical melanocytic nevi, and actini lentigines: Multicenter case-control study of the Central Malignant Registry of the German Dermatological Society. *Journal of Investigative Dermatology, 102,* 700–705.

Goldstein, E., Citron, D., & Nesbit, C. (1996). Diabetic foot infections: Bacteriology and activity of 10 oral antimicrobial agents against bacteria isolated from consecutive cases. *Diabetic Care, 19*(6), 638–641.

Goodheart, H. P. (2000). Superficial viral infections. Part 1: Diagnosis of nongenital warts (verrucae). *Women's Health in Primary Care, 3*(10), 729–732.

Goroll, J., May, L., & Mulley, A. (2000). *Primary care medicine.* Philadelphia: J. B. Lippincott.

Griffiths, C. (1992). The clinical identification and quantification of photodamage. *British Journal of Dermatology, 127* (Suppl. 41), 37–42.

Gutierrez, K. (1999). *Pharmacotherapeutics: Clinical decision-making in nursing.* Philadelphia: W.B. Saunders Co.

Habif, T. (1996). *Clinical dermatology.* St. Louis: Mosby–Year Book.

Hall, J. (2000). *Sauer's manual of skin diseases* (8th ed.). Philadelphia: Lippincott Williams & Wilkins.

Head lice infestation: Single drug versus combination therapy with one percent permethrin and trimethoprim/sulfamethoxazole. (2001). *Pediatrics, 107,* E30.

Interventions for treating head lice. (2000). *Cochrane Database Syst Rev.* CD001165.

Hirschmann, J. (1996). Bacterial infections of the skin. In W. Sams & P. Lynch (Eds.), *Principles and practice of dermatology.* New York: Churchill Livingstone.

Jarratt, M., & Dahl, M. (1991). Viral infections. In M. Orkin, H. Maibach, & M. Dahl (Eds.), *Dermatology.* Norwalk, CT: Appleton & Lange.

Kaminer, M., & Gilchrist, B. (1995). The many faces of acne. *Journal of the American Academy of Dermatology, 32* (Suppl.), S6–S14.

Koda-Kimble, M. A., Young, L. Y., Kradjan, W. A., & Guglielmo, B. J. (2002). *Handbook of applied therapeutics* (7th ed.). Philadelphia: Lippincott, Williams & Wilkins.

Lammer, E., Chen, D., & Hoar, R. (1985). Retinoic acid embryopathy. *New England Journal of Medicine, 313,* 837–841.

Leach, C., Sumaya, C., & Brown, N. (1992). Human herpesvirus-6: Clinical implications of a recently discovered ubiquitous agent. *Journal of Pediatrics, 121,* 173–181.

Max, M., Schafer, S., Culnane, M., et al. (1988). Amitriptyline, but not lorazepam, relieves post-herpetic neuralgia. *Neurology, 38,* 1427.

Meinking, T. L., Serrano, L., Hard, B., Entzel, P., Lemard, G., Rivera, E., Villar M. E. (2002). Comparative in vitro pediculicidal efficacy of treatments in a resistant head lice population in the United States. *Arch Dermatol, 138*(2):220–4.

Middleton, D. (1996). Cellulitis and other bacterial infections. In M. Mengel & L. Schwiebert (Eds.), *Ambulatory medicine in the primary care of families.* Stamford, CT: Appleton & Lange.

Miller, D., & Weinstock, M. (1994). Nonmelanoma skin cancer in the United States: Incidence. *Journal of the American Academy of Dermatology, 30*(5), 774–778.

Millikan, L., & Shrum, J. (1992). An update on common skin diseases. *Postgraduate Medicine, 91*(6), 103–104, 107–108.

Moossavi, M. & Scher, R. (2003 November) A hands-on guide to common nail disorders. *The Clinical Advisor,* 10–19.

Monafo, W. (1996). Initial management of burns. *New England Journal of Medicine, 335*(21), 1581–1585.

Morelli, J., & Weston, W. (1997). Skin: General principles and diagnosis. In W. Hay, J. Groothius, A. Hayward, & M. Levin (Eds.), *Current pediatric diagnosis and treatment.* Stamford, CT: Appleton & Lange.

Morris, Andrew. (2003) Cellulitis and erysipelas. In F. Godlee (Ed.), *Clinical Evidence.* London: BMJ Publishing Group.

Naldi, L., & Rzany, B. (2001). Chronic plaque psoriasis. *Clinical evidence, 6.*

Odom, R., James, W., & Berger, T. (2000). *Andrews' diseases of skin: Clinical dermatology* (9th ed.). Philadelphia: W.B. Saunders Co.

Orkin, M., & Maibach, H. (1991). Ectoparasitic diseases. In M. Orkin, H. Maibach, & M. Dahl (Eds.), *Dermatology.* Norwalk, CT: Appleton & Lange.

Overdiagnosis and consequent mismanagement of head louse infestations in North America. (2000). *Pediatr Infect Dis J, 19,* 689–693; discussion 694.

Parker, F. (2001). Skin diseases of general importance. *Cecil textbook of medicine,* W. B. Saunders. Retrieved 9/8/02 from http://www.merckmedicus.com

Peate, W. (1992). Outpatient management of burns. *American Family Physician, 45*(3), 1321–1330.

Ray, T. (1996). Candidiasis and other yeast infections. In W. Sams & P. Lynch (Eds.), *Principles and practice of dermatology.* New York: Churchill Livingstone.

Richard, M., Grob, J., & Gouvernet, J. (1993). Role of sun exposure on nevus. First study in age-sex phenotype-controlled population. *Archives of Dermatology, 129,* 1280–1285.

Roberts, M. J., & Barbee, K. (2000). Dermatologic health. In P.V. Meredith & N.M. Horan (Eds.), *Adult primary care.* Philadelphia: W. B. Saunders Co.

Roenigk, H. (1991). Papulosquamous diseases. In M. Orkin, H. Maibach, & M. Dahl (Eds.), *Dermatology.* Norwalk, CT: Appleton & Lange.

Sams, W., & Lynch, P. (1996). *Principles and practice of dermatology.* New York: Churchill Livingstone.

Sauer, G., & Hall, J. (1996). *Manual of skin diseases.* Philadelphia: J. B. Lippincott.

Skinner, R., & Baselski, V. (1996). Dermatophytes and superficial fungi. In W. Sams & P. Lynch (Eds.), *Principles and practice of dermatology.* New York: Churchill Livingstone.

Stern, R. (1996). Utilization of outpatient care for psoriasis. *Journal of the American Academy of Dermatology, 35,* 543–545.

Stern, R., & Nelson, C. (1993). The diminishing role of the dermatologist in the office-based care of cutaneous diseases. *Journal of the American Academy of Dermatology, 29,* 773–777.

Stern, R., Rosa, F., & Baum, C. (1984). Isotretinoin and pregnancy (Review). *Journal of the American Academy of Dermatology, 10,* 851–854.

Stone, M., & Lynch, P. (1996). Viral warts. In W. Sams & P. Lynch (Eds.), *Principles and practice of dermatology.* New York: Churchill Livingstone.

Strauss, J. (1991). Acne and rosacea. In M. Orkin, H. Maibach, & M. Dahl (Eds.), *Dermatology.* Norwalk, CT: Appleton & Lange.

Sykes, N., & Webster, G. (1994). Acne: A review of optimum treatment. *Drugs, 48*(1), 59–70.

Thiboutout, D., & Lookingbill, D. (1995). Acne: Acute or chronic disease? *Journal of the American Academy of Dermatology, 32* (Suppl.), S2–S5.

Walker, G, & Johnstone, J. (2003). Scabies. In F. Godlee (Ed.), *Clinical Evidence.* London: BMJ Publishing Group.

Walter, J., & Macknet, K. (1991). Pigmentation of osteoma cutis caused by tetracycline. *Archives of Dermatology, 110,* 113–114.

Wells, B.G., Dipiro, J.T., Schwinghammer, T.L., & Hamilton, C.W. (2000). *Pharmacotherapy handbook* (2nd ed.). Stamford, CT: Appleton & Lange.

Wentzell, J. (1996). Sunscreens: The ounce of prevention. *American Family Physician, 53*(5), 1713–1715.

Weston, W. L., Lane, A. T., & Morelli, J. G. (2002). *Color textbook of pediatric dermatology* (3rd ed). St. Louis, MO: Mosby.

Whiteman, D., & Green, A. (1994). Melanoma and sunburn. *Cancer Causes and Control, 5,* 564–572.

Whitmore, E. (1996). Common problems of the skin. In L. Barker, J. Burton, & P. Zieve (Eds.), *Principles of ambulatory medicine.* Baltimore: Williams & Wilkins.

Zanolli, M. (1996). Psoriasis and Reiter's disease. In W. Sams & P. Lynch (Eds.), *Principles and practice of dermatology.* New York: Churchill Livingstone.

CHAPTER ❖ 28

HEMATOLOGIC DISORDERS

Margaret A. Fitzgerald

This chapter focuses on the assessment and management of anemias—iron, folate, and vitamin B_{12} deficiencies—along with information on thrombus formation and the treatment of selected disorders of coagulation, encountered in primary care practice.

ERYTHROPOIESIS

Red blood cell (RBC) production (erythropoiesis) occurs in marrow located in the vertebrae, ribs, sternum, skull, sacrum, pelvis, and proximal epiphyses of long bones such as the femur and humerus. In the child, nearly all marrow is active in RBC production (Hoffbrand, Pettit & Moss, 2001a).

RBCs arise from undifferentiated stem cells containing DNA needed for mitosis and RNA needed for protein synthesis. Stem cells can be committed to developing into certain cell lines by the influence of growth factors, a group of glycoproteins that influence the differentiation of stem cells to their mature forms and regulate the number of these cells produced. Erythropoietin, a glycoprotein growth factor produced primarily by the kidney, influences the undifferentiated stem cell to form the RBC precursor (Hoffbrand, et al., 2001a).

For erythrocytes to form, a number of conditions must be present. The marrow must be intact and capable of cell production with adequate supplies of micronutrients critical to RBC production. These micronutrients include vitamins B_{12}, C, E, B_6, thiamin, riboflavin, pantothenic acid, and folic acid. Also, certain metals such as iron, manganese, and cobalt as well as amino acids must be present in the marrow (Hillman & Ault, 2002a, 2002b; Hoffbrand et al., 2001a).

In addition, factors influencing bone marrow stimulation, such as the erythropoietin mechanism, should be intact. The continued production of RBCs is in great part regulated by erythropoietin, a hormone primarily produced by the kidney (90%) and the liver (10%). Erythropoietin production is stimulated by the presence of low blood oxygen tension in the renal tissue. The kidney then interprets this as a situation consistent with anemia or other clinical conditions indicating the oxygen-carrying capability of the blood is diminished, such as hypoxia, poor cardiac output, or acute blood loss. As a result, erythropoietin excretion is increased and the number of stem cells committed to RBC formation increases. When adequate blood oxygen tension is detected, erythropoietin excretion is limited, thus promoting homeostasis (Hoffbrand et al., 2001a). Critical to erythropoietin production is the function of the kidney. In end-stage renal failure, kidney tissue damage severely limits erythropoietin production. As a result, anemia is a significant problem. This can be treated with recombinant erythropoietin (Duffy, 2000a). Also, adequate amounts of androgens and thyroxin—other hormones contributing to erythropoiesis—must be present (Hoffbrand et al., 2001a). Normal hematologic values are shown in Table 28–1.

TABLE 28–1. Normal Hematologic Values

	Female Adult	Male Adult	Neonatal	Infant	Childhood
Hemoglobin	12–15 g/dL	13–17 g/dL	14–24 g/dL	10–15 g/dL	11–16 g/dL
Hematocrit	36–45%	39–51%	48–70%	30–45%	32–42%
RBC count	4–5.3[a]	4.4–5.7[a]	4.8–7[a]	4.1–6.4[a]	4–5.3[a]
MCV	81–100 fL	81–100 fL	96–108 fL	82–91 fL	82–91 fL
MCHC	32–37%	32–37%	32–33%	32–36%	32–36%
RDW	11.5–14.5%	11.5–14.5%	11.5–14.5%	11.5–14.5%	11.5–14.5%
Reticulocyte count	0.5–2.5%	0.5–2.5%	0.5–2.5%	0.5–2.5%	0.5–2.5%

[a]measured in millions/mm^3.

MCV = mean cell volume; MCHC = mean corpuscle hemoglobin concentration; RDW = red cell distribution width.

Source: Desai (2004).

THE LIFE CYCLE OF THE RED BLOOD CELL

The length of time from development of the committed stem cell to circulating young RBC is about 1 week. These young forms, known as reticulocytes, mature in about 24 h in circulation. The normal RBC life span is 90–120 days. During that time, 85% will be engulfed by the macrocyte-macrophage system. In this system, the hemoglobin is broken down into its components. The iron is largely extracted for reuse and placed back in plasma circulation. The amino acids in the globin chains are conserved. The remaining 15% of RBCs undergo hemolysis in circulation (Hardy, 1996). The presence of chronic infection can shorten the life span of the RBC. In addition, conditions causing chronic inflammation, such as in rheumatoid arthritis, cancer, and liver disease, can truncate the RBC life span (Linker, 1996).

ANEMIA: DEFINITION AND CAUSES

Anemia is defined as a decrease in the level of hemoglobin (Desai, 2002). This results in decreased oxygen-carrying capability of the blood as well as a reduction in the reverse transport function of the RBC in carrying carbon dioxide and waste away from cells.

An important concept to bear in mind is that anemia is simply a sign of an underlying disease and only occurs when the hematologic reserves are exceeded. For example, in the healthy adult, the marrow reserve allows for new RBC production at two to three times normal in the face of acute blood loss. This can rise to six to eight times normal in the face of hemolysis (Hardy, 1996). Thus, anemia occurs in the presence of a clinical insult severe enough to disturb the normal homeostatic mechanisms and exceed reserves.

An anemia is usually classified by its underlying etiology. For example, the problem may be decreased RBC production related to a lack of a vital micronutrient, such as in iron, folate, or vitamin B_{12} deficiency. Reduced RBC production also can be seen in clinical situations when the RBC synthesis is reduced in the presence of chronic infection and/or inflammation. Bone marrow can be suppressed due to the use of certain drugs, such as large doses of alcohol. As normal RBC cell death occurs without the production of new RBC forms, anemia can occur (Linker, 1996).

The classification of anemia also includes those caused by premature RBC destruction, or hemolysis. Intrinsic factors precipitating hemolysis include certain inherited hemoglobinopathies such as sickle cell anemia and G6PD deficiency. Less common is hemolysis caused by extrinsic factors such as immune responses and thrombotic thrombocytopenia (Linker, 1996).

Anemia can also be caused by acute blood loss. Blood volume losses of up to 20% of the total blood volume are tolerated by a healthy individual; losses in excess of 1 liter usually produce symptoms because venospasm cannot compensate by redistributing circulating volume (Hillman & Ault, 2001c). More common in primary care is an anemia caused by chronic lower-volume blood loss, as from heavy menstrual flow or a small volume gastrointestinal bleed. This scenario may also lead to a combined anemia: The patient not only loses RBCs at a level exceeding replacement but also develops iron deficiency. Since the iron from the RBC wasted via blood loss cannot be recycled, a vital source of iron is forfeited (Hillman & Ault, 2002a).

As a result of the mechanisms causing anemia, remember that pharmacologic intervention to correct the presenting hematologic disorder is only part of the treatment plan. Correcting or modifying the underlying disease process is critical. When the diagnosis of anemia is established, the underlying cause can usually be identified by determining the following:

- *What is the cell size?* Is the RBC unusually small (microcytic)? Since hemoglobin is a major contributor to cell size, microcytosis is usually seen in anemia in which hemoglobin synthesis is impaired, such as iron deficiency anemia and the thalassemias. Is the RBC unusually large (macrocytic)? Macrocytosis is most commonly caused by impaired RNA and DNA synthesis in the young erythrocyte. Folic acid and vitamin B_{12} contribute significantly to this process. Thus, a lack of either or both of these micronutrients can cause a macrocytic anemia. Is the RBC of normal size (normocytic)? Generally, in these anemias there is no problem with RNA, DNA, or hemoglobin synthesis. Acute blood loss and chronic disease are two common reasons for normocytic, normochromic anemia (Zuckerman, 2000).
- *What is the RDW?* RDW is the degree of variation in RBC width. This also may be noted as anisocytosis on RBC morphology (Treseler, 1995). RDW measurement is elevated when red blood cells are of varying sizes, implying that cells were synthesized under varying conditions. For example, in an iron deficiency anemia, normal-sized cells produced prior to the iron depletion will continue to circulate until their 90- to 120-day life span ends. At the same time, the new, smaller, iron deficient cells containing less hemoglobin are produced. Therefore, there will be wide variation in cell size and an increase in RDW. Since minor variation in cell size is normal, RDW is only considered increased when it is above 15% (Desai, 2004).
- *What is the hemoglobin content (color) of the cell?* The hemoglobin content of the cell is reflected in the mean (average) corpuscle hemoglobin concentration (MCHC). It is reported as a percentage of the cell's volume. Since hemoglobin gives the RBC its characteristic red color, the suffix *-chromic* is used to describe the MCHC. Thus, when a cell has a normal MCHC, it is a normal color, or normochromic. When there is an impairment of hemoglobin synthesis, such as in iron deficiency anemia or thalassemia, the cells are pale, or hypochromic, and the MCHC is low. RBCs are seldom hyperchromic, or containing excessive amounts of hemoglobin (Desai, 2004).
- *What is the reticulocyte production index?* The body's normal response to anemia is to increase reticulocyte production in order to increase the hemoglobin level. Thus, an increase in the reticulocyte count, reticulocytosis, is an expected normal response to a drop in hemoglobin; if absent, suspect impaired marrow function or lack of erythropoietin stimulus (Hoffbrand et al., 2001).

CLINICAL PRESENTATION OF ANEMIA

The clinical presentation of anemia is highly variable as compensation is common because most anemias are gradual in onset. In addition, the oxyhemoglobin dissociation curve is moved to the right as the hemoglobin drops. As a result, the oxygen molecule is given up more freely by the RBC. Thus, symptoms of anemia seldom present unless the hemoglobin is below 10 g/dL (Hoffbrand & Pettit, 2001b).

Complaints of deep, sighing respiration with activity, often associated with a sensation of rapid, forceful heart rate, may be reported. This reflects the decreased oxygen-carrying capability of the blood and a corresponding compensatory mechanism. Fatigue and headache may also present. In the patient at risk or with coronary artery disease, angina may be reported. In the infant and younger child, the caregiver may report irritability and delay of large motor skills, primarily due to poor muscle tone (Lane, Armstrong, Ingrim, & Lance, 1995).

The physical examination usually contributes little to a diagnosis of anemia unless the anemia is severe. Pallor of the skin and mucous membranes is not reliable and usually only seen when anemia is severe (hemoglobin below 8 g/dL). In the elderly or patients with coronary artery disease, congestive heart failure signs (distended neck veins, rales, tachycardia, right upper quadrant abdominal tenderness, hepatomegaly) may be seen in severe anemia. An early systolic murmur may be heard, owing to the increase of blood flow over the heart valves. Neurologic findings such as paresthesia or difficulty with balance and, in extreme cases, confusion may be found in vitamin B_{12} deficiency anemia. Findings for specific anemias are found in their corresponding section in this chapter (Hoffbrand & Pettit, 2001b).

IRON DEFICIENCY ANEMIA

Iron deficiency is the most common reason for microcyclic anemia in adults and children (Hillman & Ault, 2002a). A number of factors contribute to the development of iron deficiency anemia (IDA). In the adult, diet is rarely a cause of iron deficiency. An estimated 8 years of poor iron intake in an adult would be needed to elicit IDA

(Hoffbrand & Pettit, 2002a). Rather, chronic blood loss, causing a wasting of the RBCs' recyclable iron, is the most common cause. In premenopausal women, blood loss from the reproductive tract is a significant contributor to IDA (Ries & Santi, 2001). The average woman loses 50 mL of blood monthly, increasing five- to sevenfold in the presence of heavy menstrual flow. In these women with menorrhagia, replacing wasted iron with diet alone would be unlikely, as 3 to 4 mg/day is needed (McLaren, 2002). Pharmacologic iron supplementation to avoid anemia probably is necessary.

Normal daily iron losses equal absorption, so iron balance is a tightly regulated system. Adult males and postmenopausal women require 1 mg iron per day. The woman during reproductive years requires 1.5–3 mg/day, in part because of the monthly loss of RBCs with the menses. Children have higher iron demands due to growth and increase in blood volume. In all these circumstances, iron requirements are achievable with a well-balanced diet.

Blood loss from the gastrointestinal tract is also a common cause of IDA in adults (Ries & Santi, 2001). This blood loss is usually low-volume and chronic, such as from aspirin or other NSAID use or peptic ulcer disease (Duffy, 2000b). One milliliter of packed red blood cells contains 1 mg of iron, so even daily losses of 2–3 mL of blood via the gastrointestinal tract can lead to iron deficiency.

The term infant is born with iron stores that will be exhausted by age 4 months if no dietary iron supplementation is given. Preterm infants will deplete their stores more rapidly since fetal iron storage is primarily an activity of the third trimester. Iron-enriched formula and/or breast milk used as the major caloric source in the first year of life assists in meeting the rapidly growing infant's iron needs and largely prevents the development of IDA in early childhood. However, early childhood is a period of high iron use. As a result, dietary iron deficiency is a significant cause of IDA in the child aged 6 to 24 months. In the child over 2, the most common cause of IDA is chronic blood loss (Hillman & Ault, 2002b).

SPECIAL CONSIDERATIONS FOR PHARMACOTHERAPY

When Drug Therapy Is Needed

The diagnosis of iron deficiency anemia must be established before initiating iron therapy. A number of other conditions, such as thalassemia trait and plumbism (lead poisoning), can mimic IDA. Misinterpretation of laboratory data can lead to the inappropriate treatment of a benign condition (thalassemia minor) or a potentially life-threatening disease (plumbism). The laboratory diagnosis of IDA is supported by the following findings:

- *Early disease:* Low normal hemoglobin, hematocrit, and total RBC count and normocytic, possibly hypochromic, RDW >15%.
- *Later disease:* Microcytic, hypochromic anemia with low RBC count and elevated RDW > 15%.
- *Low serum iron:* Reflects iron concentration in circulation. This level may be falsely elevated due to recent high iron intake.
- *Elevated total iron-binding capacity (TIBC):* An indirect measure of transferrin, a plasma protein that easily combines with iron. When more transferrin is available for binding, the TIBC rises, reflecting iron deficiency.
- *Iron saturation less than 15%:* Calculate by dividing the serum iron by the TIBC.
- *Low serum ferritin:* The body's major iron storage protein.
- *Absence of iron from bone marrow,* if aspiration is done.

In IDA, the order of the fall of the laboratory markers is as follows: Ferritin, marrow, serum iron, TIBC (rise), RDW (rise), hemoglobin, RBC indices. As a result, a drop in hemoglobin or RBC indices is a late rather than early marker of disease (Desai, 2004).

Prevention of IDA in Pregnancy. Fifteen to 25% of all pregnancies are complicated by anemia, with IDA accounting for 95%. During the first half of pregnancy, iron requirements are only slightly increased and likely can be met by diet. However, during the later half of pregnancy and the postpartum period, iron requirements for RBC replacement increase dramatically because of increased red cell mass, and rapid fetal growth, and anticipated blood loss at the time of the birth (Nuwayhid, Nguyen & Khalife, 1999).

Iron absorption by the duodenum doubles during pregnancy. In spite of this, iron needed by the woman in the second half of pregnancy is equivalent to 3.5 mg/day, likely exceeding what can be supplied by even the most prudent diet. Total pregnancy iron needs are about 1000 mg (500 mg for fetal use, 300 mg for maternal RBC use, and 200 mg to compensate for loss). As a result, prescription prenatal vitamins usually contain 60 mg of elemental iron as ferrous sulfate 300 mg.

Short- and Long-Term Goals of Pharmacotherapy

The short-term goal of pharmacotherapy is resolution of the iron deficiency–induced anemia and treatment of the underlying cause of the IDA. The long-term goal is restoration and maintenance of iron stores.

Nonpharmacologic Therapies

The rate of iron absorption from the duodenum and proximal jejunum increases significantly during times of great iron needs (pregnancy, childhood growth spurts) as well as disease states such as IDA (Hoffbrand et al., 2001c). Those with the greatest iron needs should receive nutritional counseling so as to minimize the risk of IDA development and make use of this natural adaptive process.

Iron is found in abundance in meat protein, the most available dietary iron source. Animal source iron is easily extracted for use. Plant sources of iron are much more tightly bound and thus less available (Ries & Santi, 2001).

Time Frame for Initiating Pharmacotherapy

Iron therapy should be initiated as soon as the IDA diagnosis is made. Usually iron therapy is continued for 2 to 3 months after hemoglobin correction to ensure that iron stores have been replenished.

See Table 28–2.

Assessment and History Taking

The primary assessment needed is the definitive diagnosis of IDA: the presence of a microcytic, hypochromic anemia with abnormal iron studies consistent with the diagnosis. There are no specific contraindications to treating IDA. However, the issue of iron's ability to interact with many medications (see Table 28–3) needs to be considered before its initiation. The condition causing IDA, such as chronic blood loss and poor diet, must also be treated.

TABLE 28–2. Iron Preparations

Form	% Elemental Iron	Recommended Dose Range
Ferrous fumarate	33	Adult: 200 mg bid–qid
Ferrous gluconate	11.6	Adult: 325–650 mg qid Child: 16mg/kg/day
Ferrous sulfate	20.0	Adult: 300 mg bid–qid Child: 10 mg/kg tid

Source: Ries and Santi (2001).

OUTCOMES MANAGEMENT

Selecting an Appropriate Agent

Supplemental or pharmacologic iron is available in a number of forms. Ferrous sulfate ($FeSO_4$) is the most commonly used and represents an inexpensive, effective treatment option. Each 325 mg tablet contains 65 mg of elemental iron, with an absorption rate of approximately 25%. Since the person with IDA can absorb a maximum of 50 to 100 mg of iron daily, a dose range of 200 to 400 mg of elemental iron is recommended (Ries & Santi, 2001). However, the duodenum remains relatively refractory to iron absorption for 6 h after a large dose is ingested. Therefore, for the multiple doses that fit within this recommendation (3 to 6 tablets), dosing would need to be on a rigid, round-the-clock schedule. The most commonly recommended regime for adults is ferrous sulfate 325 mg three times a day (Ries & Santi, 2001).

In children, 4 to 6 mg/kg per day of elemental iron in three divided doses daily is needed to correct IDA. Less severe IDA can be treated with 3 mg/kg per day. For the preterm infant receiving iron therapy as prophylaxis to compensate for low iron stores, the recommended dose is 0.5 to 2 mg/kg per day as a single dose. The most commonly used pediatric iron forms are ferrous sulfate elixir 220 mg/5 mL for toddlers and preschoolers and ferrous sulfate liquid 75 mg/0.6 mL for use in infants (Wynne, 2002).

Alternative oral iron forms include ferrous gluconate and ferrous fumarate, each containing a different amount of elemental iron per tablet. The prescriber must adjust the recommended number of tablets per day to ensure that the appropriate dose of elemental iron is being taken; see Table 28–2. Sustained-release and enteric-coated iron products should be avoided. These products are less likely to release iron in the proximal jejunum and duodenum, the area of best iron absorption (Ries & Santi, 2001). Iron deposited in the alkaline environment of the small intestine, common when sustained-release products are used, forms an insoluble complex and is not utilized (Wynne, 2002). In addition, the cost of sustained-release products usually is considerably higher.

Iron also is available in an injectable form as iron dextran. Indications for its use include intestinal diseases, such as sprue, that limit ability to absorb oral preparations, and for those receiving parenteral nutrition only. Resolution of IDA is not more rapid when using injectable iron, although stores may be replenished more rapidly.

TABLE 28–3. Drug Interactions with Oral Iron Therapy

Drug	Effect	Comment
Antiacids	Decreased iron absorption	Separate use by ≥ 2 h
Caffeine	Decreased iron absorption	Separate use by ≥ 2 h
Fluoroquinolones (ciprofloxacin, ofloxacin, levofloxacin, others)	Decreased fluoroquinolone effect	Avoid concurrent use if possible or separate doses by ≥ 6h
Levodopa	Decreased levodopa and iron effect	Separate medications by as much time as possible, increase levodopa dose as needed
Antihypertensives (ACE inhibitor, methyldopa)	Decreased antihypertensive effect	Separate medications by ≥ 2h, monitor BP Additional effect with IV iron—When ACE inhibitors given concurrently, increased risk of systemic reaction to iron (fever, arthralgia, hypotension); concurrent use should be avoided
Tetracycline	Decreased tetracycline and iron effect	Do not use concurrently or separate by ≥ 3–4h or use an enteric-coated iron product
Thyroid hormones	Decreased thyroxine effect	Take thyroid hormones ≥2 h before or 4 h after iron dose
Histamine-2 receptor antagonists	Decreased iron absorption	Minor interaction

Source: Tatro (2001).

Using injectable iron can cause an allergic reaction ranging from local inflammation to anaphylaxis. For that reason, a test dose of 0.5 mL IM (using the Z track technique to minimize the risk of tissue staining and/or irritation) should be administered or over 5 m if given IV. If no reaction is noted, the needed therapeutic dose is calculated by body weight or through the use of a formula to calculate the iron dose needed to correct the anemia. Caution must continue to be used with injectable iron therapy since allergic reactions have been noted in those who have previously received the product without difficulty (Hillman, & Ault, 2002a).

Patent/Caregiver Information

Drug interactions with iron are numerous and potentially serious (see Table 28–3). In general, the iron dose should be separated by at least 2 h from any other medication.

Optimally, ferrous sulfate should be taken on an empty stomach to enhance iron absorption. In addition, taking vitamin C 200 mg or more with the iron dose increases its absorption by at least 30% (Hillman, & Ault, 2002b). However, both these strategies significantly increase the risk of gastrointestinal upset.

Iron staining of the teeth may be seen when liquid preparations are used. In addition, children may find the taste objectionable. Mixing the medication with orange juice to mask its taste and having the child sip the mixture through a straw placed toward the back of the mouth may help with both problems. Since the staining is superficial, it will resolve after iron therapy is complete. Brushing the teeth after an iron dose may also minimize this problem.

Iron Therapy Side Effects

Gastrointestinal irritation, epigastric pain, nausea, and vomiting are reported by more than 10% of those who take iron (Lane et al., 1995). Although this can be largely eliminated by taking the drug with a meal, recognize that this will reduce iron absorption. Length of treatment may need to be extended as a result. Another strategy to reduce iron-induced GI upset is to initiate the therapy with a single dose once a day, and then add additional doses on a weekly basis until the desired dose is reached. Changing from one iron source to another, particularly to a form with a lower amount of elemental iron per tablet, can be helpful (Ries & Santi, 2001). Prescribing the needed dose in elixir form may help with gastrointestinal irritation because of its rapid dispersion.

Constipation is also reported in more than 10% of those on iron therapy. Adding extra fiber and liquid to the diet can often help. If constipation persists, lower the dose and extend the length of treatment so the patient can complete the needed therapeutic course (Hillman & Ault, 2002b).

Monitoring for Efficacy

Reticulocytosis begins quickly after initiation of iron therapy, with the reticulocyte count peaking 7 to 10 days into therapy. Hemoglobin rises at a rate of 2 g/dL every 3 weeks in response to iron therapy and will likely take 2 months to correct. As a result, the following laboratory tests may be used to evaluate the resolution of IDA: reticulocytes at 1 to 2 weeks to ensure marrow response to iron therapy, hemoglobin at 6 weeks to 2 months to ensure anemia recovery, and ferritin at 2 months after measure of normal hemoglobin (or 4 months after initiation of iron therapy) to ensure documentation of replenished iron stores (Hoffman et al., 2001b).

Monitoring for Toxicity

In children, iron overdose is common and potentially life-threatening. The most common source of this poisoning is maternal prenatal vitamins. In addition, ferrous sulfate tablets may resemble candy. Although the lethal level of poisoning has not been established, ingestion of elemental iron of 25 mg/kg will likely cause symptoms, of 50 mg/kg potentially serious reactions, and of 75 mg/kg severe signs and symptoms. In large doses, iron is corrosive to the gastric mucosa, allowing a large amount of systematic absorption. Virtually every body system is negatively affected by this toxic level of iron exposure.

When a child presents with a history consistent with iron overdose, a plain x-ray of the abdomen will reveal iron tablet fragments ingested within the past 2 hours. The film will not, however, reveal the multivitamins with low iron doses, nor, due to its rapid dispersion, iron elixir. Iron does not bind with activated charcoal nor can it be lavaged from the upper gastrointestinal system. Bowel decontamination with a polyethylene glycol solution given via nasogastric means may help remove undissolved tablets (Nolan, 1997).

Deferoxamine is a specific agent for the management of iron overdose, acting as a chelating agent. Its use is continued until iron levels are reduced (Hillman & Ault, 2002d). Supportive care for airway and circulatory maintenance is critical.

Followup Recommendations

Iron deficiency anemia occurs secondary to another condition, such as pregnancy, bleeding, or poor nutrition. Followup care for the person recovering from IDA should include care for the underlying condition.

MEGALOBLASTIC ANEMIAS CAUSED BY FOLATE OR VITAMIN B_{12} DEFICIENCIES

Folate (the reduced form of folic acid) and vitamin B_{12} are essential for DNA synthesis. When deficiencies of either of these micronutrients exist, DNA synthesis in the RBC is impaired, leading to distinctive changes in the RBC and bone marrow. The most clinically distinct change is the development of macrocytosis caused in part by the cell's high RNA:DNA ratio. This change is reflected in an increase in RBC mean cell volume (MCV). Since hemoglobin production is unaffected, cell color is maintained, yielding a normochromic cell, reflected in the measure of mean corpuscular hemoglobin concentration (MCHC) (Ries & Santi, 2001).

FOLATE DEFICIENCY ANEMIA

Through a complex reaction, folic acid is reduced to folate. Folate donates one carbon unit to oxidation at various levels, reactions vital to the proper DNA synthesis. Folic acid (pteroylglutamic acid) is a water-soluble B-complex vitamin found in abundance in peanuts, fruits, and vegetables. The standard diet contains approximately 50 to 500 µg/day as absorbable folate. During times of accelerated growth, such as childhood growth spurts and pregnancy and hemolytic anemia, the folic acid requirements increase from the baseline of 50 µg/day to 100–200 µg/day. Folate is absorbed throughout the gastrointestinal tract (Sancher, 2002).

The usual nonspecific findings in anemia may be present in folate deficiency. Diarrhea, sore tongue, and anorexia are common, with forgetfulness and irritability seen less often. Scleral icterus and splenomegaly may be seen. These findings also are seen in pernicious anemia (Sancher, 2002).

Special Consideration for the Woman Who Is Pregnant or Planning a Pregnancy

About 1% of all pregnancies are affected by folate deficiency, accounting for 10% of pregnancy-related anemias. Given that normal stores of folic acid last 3 to 4 months, the condition is usually diagnosed in the later part of pregnancy (50%) or in the postpartum period (50%) (Nuwayhid, Nguyen, & Khalife, 1999). Folic acid transfers readily through the placenta to the fetus, with fetal levels usually higher than maternal levels. Thus, there is evidence that pregnancy is a maternal folate-depleting event. Repeated or multiple pregnancies, in particular, cause depletion of the maternal RBC folate levels (Briggs, Freeman, & Yaffee, 2002).

Folic acid has been assigned pregnancy risk category A (Briggs, et al., 2002). Folate deficiency during pregnancy can be largely avoided through the consistent use of prescriptive prenatal vitamins, each tablet usually containing 0.8 to 1 mg of folic acid. Over-the-counter prenatal vitamins contain significantly less of this micronutrient, usually about 0.4 mg per tablet.

Supplementation should continue through lactation since approximately 0.5 mg of folic acid per day is transferred to breast milk (Hillman, 1996). Accumulation of the vitamin in human milk takes preference over maintaining maternal folate levels. The folic acid level is low in colostrum, with levels rising as true milk production is established. Refrigerating breast milk for short periods of time does not appear to alter its folic acid content, whereas protracted frozen storage (up to 3 months) causes a progressive drop in levels to below the recommended daily folate requirement for an infant (Briggs et al., 2002).

Maternal folic acid deficiency is likely a teratogenic state, particularly during neural tube formation. To reduce the rate of neural tube defects in their offspring, women planning a pregnancy should be advised take additional folic acid, 0.4 mg daily for 3 months, prior to conception. This recommendation should be extended to all women capable of conception. Over-the-counter multivitamin or diet supplementation with vitamin-fortified foods can easily supply the recommended folate dose. If the woman has a history of giving birth to a child with a neural tube defect, the folic acid dose should be increased to 4 mg daily 3 months preconception and continued at least through the first 12 weeks of pregnancy (Briggs et al., 2002).

If the pregnancy is unplanned or preconception counseling was not sought, initiating folic acid supplementation during the first 7 weeks of pregnancy appears to offer some neural tube protection (Briggs et al., 2002). This can be supplied by a prescription prenatal vitamin supplement. However, if the pregnant woman cannot tolerate the prenatal vitamin supplement because of nausea, a common condition, she likely will be able to take folic acid alone without difficulty.

Phenytoin (Dilantin) use in pregnancy presents a particularly difficult situation. As a result of pregnancy-related changes in drug metabolism and excretion, phenytoin doses usually need to be increased 30 to 50% above the prepregnancy dose in order to maintain seizure control. In addition, the pregnant woman requires folic acid supplementation to avoid developing anemia and to assist in neural tube formation in the fetus, thus potentially reducing phenytoin levels and negatively affecting seizure control. In this situation, monitoring free phenytoin levels is critical to the health of the mother and unborn child. In addition, the woman taking phenytoin should have serum and RBC folate levels measured preconception and during the period of organogenesis to ensure the best pregnancy outcome (Briggs et al., 2002).

Short- and Long-Term Goals of Pharmacotherapy

The short-term goal of pharmacotherapy is resolution of the folate deficiency–induced anemia and treatment of the underlying cause of the folate deficiency. The long-term goal is restoration and maintenance of folate stores.

Nonpharmacologic Therapies

Folic acid deficiency often can be avoided or, if present, treatment enhanced by a high folic acid diet. The most common causes of folic acid deficiency anemia are inadequate dietary intake, seen in the elderly, alcoholics, and the impoverished as well as those with a decreased ability to absorb folic acid, patients with malabsorption syndromes such as sprue and celiac disease. Also, children given folic acid–poor goat's milk in place of cow's milk may become folate-deficient. As it is heat-labile, up to 90% of folic acid can be destroyed through excessive cooking or food reheating (Hillman, 1996), leaving those who eat little fresh food at higher risk. In addition, unusually high folic acid utilization can be seen when cell division is high—during pregnancy, childhood growth spurts, hemolytic anemia, inflammation, and rheumatoid arthritis—leading to folic acid deficiency (Hoffbrand et al., 2001b). Thus diet counseling for these high risk groups is critical.

Time Frame for Initiating Pharmacotherapy

Intervention is initiated when the diagnosis is established. Folic acid supplementation should be continued until the anemia is resolved (1–2 months) and continued as long as the risk for its development exists.

Assessment and History Taking

Folic acid deficiency anemia takes some months to develop. In the absolute absence of dietary folic acid, the body stores are exhausted within a few months, with liver stores depleted in 4 to 6 weeks. At that time, the serum folate drops. In an additional 5 weeks, hypersegmented neutrophils develop, again reflecting the contribution of folic acid to cellular DNA synthesis. The RDW rises. In 17 weeks, reduced RBC folate levels and macrocytosis are noted, with megaloblastic bone marrow changes at week 19 and the appearance of anemia at week 20. These changes may take longer to occur when folic acid intake is decreased but not absent, or when it is available but demands are increased. (Hillman & Ault, 2002e)

When a megaloblastic anemia is found, screening needs to be performed for both folic acid and vitamin B_{12} deficiency by obtaining serum levels of both micronutrients. Since vitamin B_{12} deficiency can cause irreversible neurologic damage if not promptly treated, ruling out its presence is critical to safe practice.

Phenytoin can cause a macrocytic anemia reversible with folic acid supplementation. At the same time, folic acid supplementation in large doses causes increased metabolism of phenytoin, possibly reducing its therapeutic efficacy. As a result, phenytoin levels should be carefully monitored when folic acid supplementation is required (Tatro, 2001).

Patient and Caregiver Information

Informing the patient and/or caregiver about folic acid dietary supplementation is important in obtaining the anemia's resolution. Pharmacologic folic acid supplements require no specific advice on timing of dose.

Outcomes Management

Selecting an Appropriate Agent. Folic acid is supplied primarily in an inexpensive generic form. Recommended doses for folic acid replacement in the adult range from 0.5–1 mg/day to 5 mg/day (Hoffbrand et al., 2002e), with the usual dose being 1 mg/day (Linker, 1996). Folic acid is generally well tolerated, with doses of 50–100 recommended daily amounts (RDA) needed before toxic effects are noted. The underlying cause of the folate deficiency also must be treated.

Monitoring for Efficacy. Reticulocytosis occurs rapidly, with a peak at 7 to 10 days into folic acid therapy. The hematocrit rises by 4 to 5% per week and generally returns to normal in 1 month. Leukopenia and thrombocytopenia resolve within 2 to 3 days of therapy. A repeat hemogram in 1 to 2 months assists in the monitoring of therapeutic effect. Resolution of the related signs and symptoms generally follows the time frame needed for the resolution of the anemia (Hillman & Ault, 2002e).

Monitoring for Toxicity. Folic acid is a water-soluble vitamin that is easily excreted. As a result, even in overdose, toxicity is seldom seen.

Followup Recommendations. Folate deficiency anemia occurs secondary to another condition. Followup care for the person recovering from folate deficiency anemia should include care for the underlying condition.

VITAMIN B_{12} DEFICIENCY

Vitamin B_{12}, a member of the cobalamin family, is found in abundance in foods of animal origin and is essential to the development of the red blood cell. When vitamin B_{12} is ingested orally, it binds with intrinsic factor, a glycoprotein produced by the gastric parietal cells and transported systematically. Within the portal blood flow, the vitamin is attached to transcobalamin II (TC II), polypeptide synthesized in the liver and ileum. Intrinsic factor is not absorbed, and the new compound is transported to the bone marrow and other sites where it is available for use in red blood cell formation. Two additional glycoproteins, transcobalamin I (TC I) and III (TC III), combine with B_{12} and are used in the formation of granulocytes (Linker, 1996). In synergy with folic acid, vitamin B_{12} plays a role essential to RBC DNA synthesis. When deficiencies of either of these micronutrients exist, DNA synthesis in the RBC is impaired, leading to the distinct changes in the RBC and bone marrow (Ries & Santi, 2001). The most clinically distinctive change is the development of macrocytosis caused in part by the cell's high RNA:DNA ratio. This change is reflected in an increase in RBC MCV. Since hemoglobin production is unaffected (Ries & Santi, 2001), cell color is maintained, yielding a normochromic cell, reflected in the measure of MCHC.

The most common form of vitamin B_{12} deficiency is *pernicious anemia,* a disorder that causes atrophy of the stomach and is probably autoimmune in nature. With this atrophy, secretion of the intrinsic factor ceases and achlorhydria is present. Without intrinsic factor, a vital link of B_{12} delivery is lost. Rarely, vitamin B_{12} deficiency can be caused by a highly restricted vegan-type diet in which all animal products are omitted and no supplementation is taken (Linker, 1996).

Physical manifestations of vitamin B_{12} deficiency include those noted with other anemias. However, this anemia can be particularly severe, with presenting hematocrits as low as 10 to 15%, since the disease is slow in developing and compensation is common. Vitamin B_{12} deficiency can cause a characteristic group of neurologic problems, including peripheral neuropathy, difficulty with balance, and memory changes (Linker, 1996), as well as oral irritation and icterus (Hoffbrand et al., 2001d). Without treatment, these neurologic changes may become permanent. Since the disease is most common in elderly women, an older woman presenting with a sore tongue, fatigue, new-onset forgetfulness, and a gait disturbance should be tested for this disorder.

When Drug Therapy Is Needed

As the neurologic complications can be irreversible if left untreated, prompt recognition and treatment of pernicious anemia is essential. In addition, the degree of anemia is often severe, necessitating swift intervention to prevent cardiac decompensation.

Short- and Long-Terms Goals of Pharmacotherapy

The short-term goals of treatment include the reversal of neurologic signs and the reversal of anemia. Long-term goals include maintenance of a normal blood count and an intact neurologic status.

Nonpharmacologic Therapies

As mentioned, most individuals have ample dietary vitamin B_{12} and need no supplementation. However, those who do not ingest animal products should be advised either to supplement the diet with vitamin B_{12} orally or to use B_{12}-rich foods, such as brewer's yeast (Sancher, 2002).

Time Frame for Initiating Pharmacotherapy

Vitamin B_{12} therapy should be initiated when the diagnosis is made. Usually there is a brisk hematologic response, and the anemia is resolved within 2 months. Reversal of neurologic abnormalities is generally slower, but improvement is seen quickly.

Assessment and History Taking

As with folate deficiency anemia, vitamin B_{12} deficiency anemia is a macrocytic (elevated MCV) normochromic (normal MCHC) anemia. However, the degree of macrocytosis is generally marked (MCV 110–160 Pl), exceeding that seen in folate deficiency. Additional hematologic changes include the presence of hypersegmented neutrophils, often with leukopenia. The platelet count is often reduced as well (Linker, 1996).

Any person presenting with a macrocytic anemia should be assessed by history and physical examination for the neurologic changes seen in vitamin B_{12} deficiency. In addition, serum folate and B_{12} should be measured as part of the initial evaluation of macrocytic anemia to ensure that B_{12} and not folate deficiency is the problem. In vitamin B_{12} deficiency, the serum B_{12} will be low, whereas serum folate is elevated or normal. However, RBC folate is often low, reflecting the interaction of these micronutrients during RBC formation (Hoffbrand et al., 2001d).

If the serum B_{12} level is abnormally low, a Schilling's test is usually done. This is an indirect test of intrinsic factor deficiency, used to confirm the etiology of the vitamin B_{12} deficiency (Sancher, 2002).

Patient/Caregiver Information

The importance of treatment and appropriate followup must be stressed. With pernicious anemia, lifelong intervention is needed to avoid recurrence and relapse. The family of the patient can be instructed on giving the injection.

Outcomes Management

Selecting an Appropriate Agent. Vitamin B_{12}, usually supplied as cyanocobalamin or hydroxocobalamin, is available in generic form both orally, and parenterally, and in a gel nasal spray. Vitamin B_{12} injections may be given by the patient, family member, or healthcare provider's office or with the assistance of the visiting nurse. With all forms, strict adherence to recommended use schedule is critical to avoid hematologic relapse and neurologic sequelae.

The usual initial vitamin B_{12} dose is 100 µg IM or deep SC every day or every other day for 1 to 2 weeks for a total of at least 7 doses, then weekly for 1 month, then monthly for the rest of the lifespan (Sancher, 2002). Traditionally, doses as high as 1000 µg per injection have been used. However, a cyanocobalamin dose of more than 100 µg in a single injection exceeds the capability of available binding sites. Excess is excreted via the kidney and wasted. Concomitant administration of folic acid and iron may help with hematologic recovery (Hillman & Ault, 2002e). Orally, a higher dose of vitamin B_{12}, usually 1000 mcg/day, is needed. Vitamin B_{12} is also available in a nasal gel, usually used weekly at a dose of 500 mcg. These forms are usually appropriate for maintenance therapy after hematologic and neurologic recovery and vitamin B_{12} stores replenishment have been achieved.

When the etiology of the macrocytic anemia has not yet been established, a prudent course of action is to initially give parenteral vitamin B_{12} while giving folic acid 1 to 2 mg/daily. With this plan, no intervention time is lost. Once the appropriate diagnosis is established, the correct vitamin supplement is continued (Hoffbrand et al., 2002e).

Monitoring for Efficacy. The hematologic response is generally rapid once therapy is given. Reticulocytosis is brisk and peaks at 5 to 7 days. Hypokalemia, caused by serum to intracellular potassium shifts, is common if the anemia was particularly severe (Linker, 1996) and will be most likely seen with the peak of reticulocytosis. Monitoring serum potassium daily during the first week of therapy, especially in those on diuretic therapy, at other risk of hypokalemia, or on digoxin, is important. If hypokalemia occurs, oral potassium replacement at 40 mEq/d is usually sufficient. Concomitant oral iron therapy is indicated if there is iron deficiency or low iron stores. Full hematologic recovery usually takes about 2 to 3 months (Sancher, 2002).

Reversal of vitamin B_{12} deficiency signs and symptoms is generally rapid. A sense of improved well-being is usually reported within 24 h of the onset of treatment. Neurologic changes, if present under 6 months, reverse quickly. However, if these changes have been present for a protracted period, neurologic reversal is likely not possible (Linker, 1996).

Monitoring for Toxicity. Vitamin B_{12} is a water-soluble compound, with excess drug being easily eliminated by the kidney. As with most therapeutic vitamin replacements, it is well tolerated and has virtually no side effects other than localized irritation at the site of injection. On rare occasions, reaction may be seen in the person who has a cobalt allergy. An intradermal test dose may be given before initiating therapy.

Followup Recommendations. Recovery from pernicious anemia is usually rapid and without complications. However, if hematologic recovery is not achieved or is unusually slow, the presence of a second anemia should be investigated. Increasing the vitamin B_{12} dose is seldom needed. Patient followup is usually dictated by the presence of other health problems.

ANEMIA ASSOCIATED WITH RENAL FAILURE

Anemia occurs commonly in the person with select chronic health problems, such as acute and chronic inflammatory conditions (infection, arthritis), renal insufficiency, and hypothyroidism. In part, the anemia is caused by reduced erythropoietin response in the marrow, resulting in hypoproliferation of RBCs coupled with a shortened RBC lifespan. These anemias are second only to iron deficiency in occurrence (Hillman & Ault, 1995). Treatment of the underlying cause is usually sufficient in all but anemia associated with renal failure.

When the glomerular filtration rate falls below 30 to 40 mL/min, renal erythropoietin synthesis is reduced; a hypoproliferative normochromic, normocytic anemia develops, usually with hemoglobin ≥ 8 g/dL (Hillman & Ault, 2001f). Patient symptoms such as altered exercise capacity and sexual function that are often attributed to renal disease are often attenuated if hemoglobin is corrected to 11 to 12 g/dL with the use of recombinant human erythropoietin (epoetin alfa) (Sancher, 2002).

ERYTHROPOIETIN THERAPY

Recombinant human erythropoietin (epoetin alfa) is used in the treatment of anemias associated with ESRD, HIV, and cancer. The drug can be administered parenterally (SC or IV) up to 3 times per week with an expected rise in hematocrit of approximately 4% over two weeks. At the beginning of therapy, a CBC should be checked 2 to 3 times per week to ensure that hematocrit is not rising more rapidly because of the increased risk of seizure and hypertension. If hct rise is too rapid, or when hct goal is met, the epoetin alfa dose should be reduced. Iron therapy will also be needed if iron stores are marginal or deficient (Hillman & Ault, 2001f; Sancher, 2002).

Coexisting hematologic problems, such as micronutrient deficiencies, also must be treated. See Table 28–4 for specific information about epoetin alfa.

THROMBUS FORMATION AND ANTITHROMBOTIC THERAPY

Pathologic thrombus formation, leading to blood vessel occlusion, causes a variety of clinically significant conditions. With arterial thrombi, the tissue supplied by the vessel may become necrotic, such as in myocardial infarction. With venous thrombosis, the tissue drained by the affected vein usually becomes edematous and/or inflamed, such as in deep vein thrombophlebitis in the leg (Majerus, Broze, Miletich & Tollefsen, 1996). While a variety of medications are available to alter coagulation including antiplatelet drugs such as aspirin, dipyridamole, clopidogrel, and abciximab, as well as thrombolytics, this section focuses on the prevention and treatment of thrombosis with warfarin, unfractionated heparin (UFH) and low molecular weight heparin (LMWH, enoxaparin, dalteparin, ardeparin).

TABLE 28–4. Therapeutic Form of Erythropoietin

Drug	Dose Range	Pharmacology	ADR	Comment
Epoetin alfa	10–300 U/kg TIW IV/SC until hct≥ 36% or increased by 4% in a 2-week period; titrate therapeutic dose to maintain hct 33–36%	Same action as endogenous erythropoietin	HA, arthralgia, fatigue, GI symptoms, HTN especially w/rapid volume expansion	Due to increased requirements during expansion of RBC mass, give w/$FeSO_4$ 325 mg bid-tid unless evidence of excessive Fe stores Peak effect seen in 2-3 weeks into therapy. Check hct 2–3 times per week during first weeks of therapy

HEMATOLOGIC FACTORS INFLUENCING COAGULATION AND THROMBOLYSIS

Blood coagulation can be activated by a variety of pathways via the tissue factor (TF) pathway (formerly known as the extrinsic pathway) and the contact activation pathway (known as the intrinsic pathway). Expressed by injured endothelial cells, TF is the clinically most significant initiator of coagulation. TF binds to and activates Factor VII and the TF/VIIa complex, then activates Factor X and Factor IX to Xa and IXa respectively. In the presence of Factor XIIa, IXa can also convert Factor X to Xa. The contact activation pathway is activated when Factor XII comes in contact with a foreign surface. The resulting Factor XIIa then activates Factor XI, which in turn activates Factor IX. Factor IXa then activates Factor X. These pathways work together to provide maximum stimulation of Factor X that, in the presence of Factor V, activates prothrombin to thrombin; this is also known as the common pathway.

Equally important as blood coagulation is the blood's ability to avoid clot formation. In the larger arteries, clot risk is usually limited as aggregating platelets are dislodged by high velocity blood flow and thrombus formation is avoided. In smaller arteries and veins, blood flow is slower with platelet aggregation more likely to occur and clot risk higher. Working against thrombus formation, tissue factor pathway inhibitor (TFPI) binds to and inactivated the TF- VIIa- Xa complex. Antithrombin III inactivates circulating thrombin while proteins C and S are contributors to a complex process that down-regulates thrombin activity by preventing the activation of Factor V. If a clot does form, circulating plasminogen is incorporated into the thrombus; healthy endothelial cells adjacent to the vessel injury site release tissue plasminogen activator (t-PA) and activate plasminogen to plasmin, causing thrombolysis on the clot surface and minimizing thrombus size. At the same time, a number of factors, including plasminogen activator inhibitor (PAI-1), produced by the liver and endothelial cells, inhibit fibrin degradation by plasmin to limit thrombolysis (Hillman & Ault, 2001g).

SPECIFIC CONSIDERATIONS FOR PHARMACOTHERAPY

When Drug Therapy Is Needed

Drug therapy includes preventive measures as well as treatment for acute thrombotic conditions. Drug therapy is needed in clinical conditions that increase thrombosis risk and for intervention in thrombotic conditions. Heparin and warfarin reduce risk of thrombus formation and prevent extension of existing thrombus; neither drug has intrinsic thrombolytic activity. Anticoagulation therapy is typically contraindicated in clinical situations where the risk of hemorrhage is greater than the potential benefits of therapy, such as in substance abuse, dementia, or psychosis.

Short- and Long-Term Goals of Pharmacotherapy

The short- and long-term goals of anticoagulant therapy are to prevent or minimize the negative effects of thrombus formation. Since this is often associated with a potentially life-threatening condition, accurate assessment and swift, appropriate intervention are critical.

Time Frame for Initiating Therapy

Anticoagulant therapy should be initiated immediately upon the recognition of its need. Inappropriate delay may lead to unnecessary morbidity and mortality.

Assessment and History Taking

Accurate diagnosis of thrombosis or assessment of thromboembolic risk is crucial prior to initiating anticoagulant therapy. The type of diagnostic testing will vary according to the site of the thrombus.

Patient/Caregiver Information

In home heparin therapy, patient and caregiver information includes comprehensive education on the parenteral administration of drug, including the appropriate handling of injection equipment to avoid patient infection, injection technique, as well as stressing the importance of injection site rotation and avoiding rubbing or trauma to the injection site to minimize bruising and tissue injury. Information on appropriate used syringe disposal is critical.

As with any narrow therapeutic index medication, the patient and caregiver must be well aware of warfarin drug–drug and drug–food interactions (see Table 28– 5). For both warfarin and heparin users, wearing a medical alert bracelet is advisable as well as advising all healthcare providers about the use of these medications. Activities of daily living and grooming should be modified to minimize trauma risk; work site modification may also be in order. Since tobacco use enhances thrombus formation and may attenuate anticoagulation effectiveness, working with the patient for smoking cessation is a critical goal.

TABLE 28–5. Warfarin, Drug, and Food Interactions

Increased Anticoagulant Effect	Decreased Anticoagulant Effect	Variable Effects
Alcohol	Barbiturates	Phenytoin (both increased and decreased effect noted, as well as increase in phenytoin level)
Amiodarone	Carbamazepine	
Cimetidine	Chlordiazepoxide	
Clofibrate	Cholestyramine	
Cotrimoxazole	Griseofulvin	
Erythromycin	Nafcillin	
Fluconazole	Rifampin	
Isoniazid	Sucralfate	
Metronidazole	Dicloxacillin	
Miconazole	Azathioprine	
Omeprazole	Cyclosporine	
Phenylbutazone	Trazodone	
Piroxicam		
Propafenone		
Propranolol		
Acetaminophen (inconsistent)		
Ciprofloxacin		
Dextropropoxyphene		
Disulfiram		
Itraconazole		
Quinidine		
Tamoxifen		
Tetracycline		
Flu vaccine		

Source: Tatro (2001)

Patient and family should be advised to report any unusual bleeding promptly, such as blood in stools or urine, excessive menstrual bleeding, bruising, recurrent or excessive bleeding from the nose or gums, persistent oozing from superficial injuries, or bleeding from any lesion.

Warfarin therapy is contraindicated during pregnancy. Freely crossing the placenta, warfarin is a potent teratogen. A recognizable pattern of facial, skin, bone, and central nervous system deformity is found in up to 30% exposed fetuses. If anticoagulant therapy is needed during pregnancy, heparin, with a large molecule incapable of placental transfer, is the preferred agent (Hillman & Ault, 2002).

OUTCOMES MANAGEMENT

Selecting an Appropriate Agent

Heparin. Heparin is a naturally occurring carbohydrate found in mast cell secretory granulocytes. Unfractionated heparin (UFH) is a mixture of chain fragments with molecular weights varying from 3000 to 30,000 d, with an average of 15,000. UFH binds to and potentiates antithromboplastin III to help inactivate thrombin and inhibit factor X and Xa activity. Low molecular weight heparin (LMWH, molecular weight <9000 d) differs from UFH in that it contains smaller chain fragments that only inhibit factor X and Xa. It does not have appreciable antiplatelet effect or the ability to increase microvascular permeability. LMWH has pharmacokinetic advantages over UFH, including a lower binding affinity for endothelial cells and a number of plasma proteins, leading to a more predictable dose-dependent response and a longer half-life.

Warfarin. A vitamin K antagonist, warfarin is an oral drug that acts against coagulation Factors II, VII, IX, and X. Highly protein-bound, warfarin is a narrow therapeutic index (NTI) medication and is subject to numerous drug interactions. The mechanisms of the interactions range from displacement of warfarin from the protein-binding site to induction of hepatic enzymes, decreased drug metabolism, and others (Tatro, 2001) (see Table 28–5).

In the case of treating an acute thrombotic disease—for example, deep vein thrombophlebitis or pulmonary embolism—warfarin therapy is overlapped with heparin for 4 to 5 days until the INR is at goal. This is necessary to overlap heparin with oral warfarin because of the initial transient hypercoagulable state induced by warfarin; the length of this state is related to half-lives of protein C, protein S, and the vitamin K-dependent clotting Factors II, VII, IX, and X (see Tables 28–6, 28–7).

Long-term anticoagulation definitely is indicated for patients with recurrent venous thrombosis and/or persistent or irreversible risk factors. With IV UFH use, the goal is to achieve and maintain an elevated aPTT of at least 1.5 times control, and most commonly between 1.5 to 2.5 times control. With complex pharmacokinetics and a $T\frac{1}{2}$ = 60 to 90 minutes, aPTT should be checked after initial heparin bolus and continuous maintenance infusion. A typical initial heparin bolus dose is 80 μ/kg, while a constant maintenance infusion of 18 μ/kg is most often used (Schreiber, 2002).

Monitoring for Efficacy

To achieve the anticoagulant effect with warfarin, 3 to 4 days of therapy is needed. The dose may be initiated in the nonurgent situation as 5 mg (a common maintenance dose) or with a higher dose of 10 mg daily for 2 days, followed by a lower maintenance dose. The latter regimen affords greater anticoagulation effect in the first 48 h of intervention. Daily doses range from 1 to 15 mg (Hillman & Ault, 2002). If rapid anticoagulation is needed, heparin should be given initially and then discontinued after 5 days of warfarin therapy (Stauffer, 1996).

The prothrombin time (PT) is used as the measure of warfarin's efficacy. It is commonly measured in an International Normalized Ratio (INR). After the first warfarin dose, PT prolongation is seen in about 48 to 72 h. Daily PT measurement is generally done until the desired INR is reached, and then weekly to monthly testing continues throughout therapy (Treseler, 1995). Table 28–6 shows recommendations for different conditions and lengths of treatment with warfarin.

TABLE 28–6. Indications and Length of Warfarin Treatment

Condition	INR	Duration of Therapy
Acute venous thrombosis		
First episode	2–3	3–6 months
High risk of recurrence	2–3	Indefinitely
antiphospholipid syndrome	3–4	Lifelong
Prevention of systemic embolus		
Tissue heart valves	2–3	3 months
Valvular heart disease after thrombotic event	2–3	Indefinitely
Mechanical heart valve	2.5–3.5	Indefinitely
Acute myocardial infarction	2–3	As deemed by clinical presentation
Atrial fibrillation		
Chronic or intermittent	2–3	Lifelong
Cardioversion	2–3	3 weeks before and 4 weeks after conversion to sinus rhythm

Sources: Horton, J., & Bushwick, B. (1999).

Monitoring for Toxicity

As outlined in the patient/caregiver information section, any unusual bleeding should be considered potentially related to the anticoagulation therapy and promptly reported.

In IV UFH therapy, aPTT should be monitored every 6 hours while the patient is on IV heparin until the dose stabilizes. If aPTT is slightly outside of desired range, the infusion is increased or decreased (see Table 28–8). Protamine by IV infusion can by used to rapidly reverse, within 5 minutes, the effects of heparin, with 1 to 1.5 mg needed to neutralize 100 U heparin, Less protamine, protamine 0.5 to 0.75 mg will neutralize 100 U heparin over 30 to 60 minutes while a 0.25 to 0.375 mg produces the same effect over ≥ 2 hours (Schreiber, 2002).

Due to thrombocytopenia risk with UFH use, a platelet count also should be obtained. A modest, transient thrombocytopenia (> 75,000 but < 100,000) most often appears within 48 to 72 hours of initiation of heparin therapy and resolves within 4 days, even if therapy is continued. In heparin-induced thrombocytopenia (HAT), the platelet count is severely depressed (<75,000) and is usually noted within 5 to 10 days of heparin initiation. Risk of new clot development (white clot syndrome) is significant. With HAT, heparin in all forms, including line flushes, should be discontinued immediately. With >6 month's of heparin use, osteoporosis risk is possible. With LWMH use, aPTT monitoring is not needed and platelet effect is minimal (Lexi-Drugs, 2002).

Warfarin's efficacy is reduced if the INR is less than 2.0, and the risk of bleeding is increased when the INR exceeds 4.0. That said, the prescriber should conservatively approach intervention in mildly elevated INRs 4–9 or to mildly reduced INRs (<2), unless a very high risk of bleeding or thrombosis exists. A modest adjustment in warfarin therapy and/or more frequent INRs is usually the safest and most efficacious way to handle this common situation (see Table 28–7) (Bushwick, 1999). Vitamin K is typically used if significant bleeding accompanies prolonged INR, but this will not have effect on hemostasis for 24 h. If prolonged INR and enclosed space or severe bleeding occurs, fresh frozen plasma has a rapid effect on hemostasis (Schreiber, 2002).

TABLE 28–7. Warfarin: Initiation of Therapy and Long-term Management

Warfarin's full anticoagulation effect takes about 3 to 4 days of use to achieve. If immediate anticoagulation effect is needed, initiate heparin therapy while also starting warfarin 5 to 10 mg qd for 2 days then reduce to 5 mg qd. Check INR daily; when at goal, discontinue heparin.
If there is no need for immediate anticoagulation, warfarin should be initiated at 5 mg/d, anticipating therapeutic effect in about 4 days.
If INR is not within goal during warfarin therapy, check for adherence to recommended therapy prior to adjusting dose as well as use of medications or foods that may interfere with warfarin effect.

INR goal = 2 to 3	Action
At desired range	Repeat INR at interval determined by duration of therapeutic INR and underlying condition 4–6 weeks if stable condition and typically therapeutic INR At least weekly when underlying condition can impact coagulation state (malignancy, clotting disorder, use of medications that can influence warfarin effect)
INR < 2	Increase weekly dose by 5–20% Repeat INR 2–3 times/week until within desired range
INR 3 to 3.5	Decrease weekly dose by 5–15% Repeat INR 2–3 times/week until within desired range
INR 3.6 to 4	Consider withholding 1 dose, decrease weekly dose by 10–15% Repeat INR 2–3 times/week until within desired range
INR > 4 without complications and no indication for rapid reversal of anticoagulation effect	Consider withholding 1 dose, decrease weekly dose by 10–20% Repeat INR 2–3 times/week until within desired range
INR > 4 and need for rapid reversal of anticoagulant effect	Vitamin K 2.5–5 mg PO × 1–2 doses or 3 mg SC or slow IV
INR goal = 2.5 to 3.5	Action
At desired range	Repeat INR at interval determined by duration of therapeutic INR and underlying condition 4–6 weeks if stable condition and typically therapeutic INR At least weekly when underlying condition can impact coagulation state (malignancy, clotting disorder, use of medications that can influence warfarin effect)
INR < 2	Increase weekly dose by 10–20% Repeat INR 2–3 times/week until within desired range
INR 2 to 2.4	Increase weekly dose by 5–15% Repeat INR 2–3 times/week until within desired range
INR 3.5 to 4.6	Decrease weekly dose by 5–15% Repeat INR 2–3 times/week until within desired range
INR 4.7 to 5.2	Consider withholding 1 dose, decrease weekly dose by 10–20% Repeat INR 2–3 times/week until within desired range
INR > 5.2 without complications and no indication for rapid reversal of anticoagulation effect	Withhold 1–2 doses, decrease weekly dose by 10–20% Repeat INR 2–3 times/week until within desired range
INR > 5.2 and/ or need for rapid reversal of anticoagulant effect	Vitamin K 2.5 mg PO × 1–2 doses or 3mg SC or slow IV

Source: Horton & Bushwick (1999)

TABLE 28–8. Guidelines for Heparin Infusion Management

aPTT results	Action
< 1.5 times control	Increase infusion rate by 25%
1.5–2.5 times control	Usual desire range, continue with current infusion
2–3 times control	Decrease infusion rate by 25%
> 3 times control	Decrease infusion rate by 50%

REFERENCES

Briggs, G., Freeman, R., & Yaffee, S. (2002). *Drugs in pregnancy and lactation* (6th ed.). Baltimore: Williams & Wilkins.

DeGowin, R., & Brown, D. (2000). Lymphadenopathy. In DeGowin's *bedside diagnostics* (7th ed.) (pp. 488–994.) New York: McGraw Hill.

Desai, S., (2004). *Clinician's guide to laboratory medicine* (3rd. ed.). Hudson, OH: Lexi-Comp, Inc.

Duffy, T. (2000a). Normochromic, normocytic anemias. In J. Bennett, & F. Plum, *Cecil's textbook of medicine* (21st ed.) (pp. 853–855). Philadelphia: W. B. Saunders.

Duffy, T. (2000b). Microcytic and hypochromic anemias. In J. Bennett, & F. Plum, *Cecil's textbook of medicine* (21st ed.) (pp. 838–843). Philadelphia: W. B. Saunders.

Hardy, W. (1996). Common hematologic-oncologic problems. In R. Rubin, C. Vos, D. Derksen, A. Gately, & R. Quenzer, *Medicine: A primary care approach* (pp. 311–316). Philadelphia: W. B. Saunders.

Hillman, R. (1996). Hematopoietic agents. In J. Hardman, L. Limbird, P. Molinoff, & R. Ruddon, *Goodman & Gillman's The pharmacologic basis for disease* (9th ed.) (pp. 1311–1340). New York: McGraw-Hill.

Hillman, R., & Ault, K. (2002a). Iron deficiency anemia. In *Hematology in clinical practice* (3rd ed). (pp. 51–61) New York: McGraw-Hill.

Hillman, R., & Ault, K. (2002b). Microcytic anemias. In *Hematology in clinical practice* (3rd ed). (pp. 91–103) New York: McGraw-Hill.

Hillman, R., & Ault, K. (2002c). Blood loss anemias. In *Hematology in clinical practice* (3rd ed). (pp. 116–126) New York: McGraw-Hill.

Hillman, R., & Ault, K. (2002d). Hemachromatosis. In *Hematology in clinical practice* (3rd ed). (pp. 161–171) New York: McGraw-Hill

Hillman, R., & Ault, K. (2002e). Macrocyitc anemias. In *Hematology in clinical practice* (3rd ed). (pp. 91–103) New York: McGraw-Hill.

Hillman, R., & Ault, K. (2002f). Anemias associated with a reduced erytrhopoeitin response. In *Hematology in clinical practice* (3rd ed). (pp. 41–50) New York: McGraw-Hill.

Hillman, R., & Ault, K. (2002g). Normal hemostasis. In *Hematology in clinical practice* (3rd ed). (pp. 301–307) New York: McGraw-Hill.

Hoffbrand, A., Pettit, J., & Moss, P. (2001a). Blood cell formation. In *Essential hematology* (4th ed) (pp. 1–11) London: Blackwell Scientific.

Hoffbrand, A., Pettit, J. & Moss, P. (2001b). Hypochromic anaemia and iron overload. In *Essential hematology* (4th ed)(pp. 28–42) London: Blackwell Scientific.

Hoffbrand, A., Pettit, J. & Moss, P. (2001c). Erythropoiesis and general aspects of anaemia. In *Essential hematology* (4th ed)(pp. 12–27) London: Blackwell Scientific.

Hoffbrand, A., Pettit, J. & Moss, P. (2001d). Megaloblastic anaemias and other microcytic anaemias. In *Essential hematology* (4th ed)(pp. 43–56) London: Blackwell Scientific.

Hoffbrand, A., Pettit, J. & Moss, P. (2001e). Thrombosis and antithrombotic therapy. In *Essential hematology* (4th ed)(pp. 273–288) London: Blackwell Scientific.

Horton, J., & Bushwick, B. (1999). Warfarin therapy: Evolving strategies in anticoagulation. *American Family Physician, 59* (3) 635–647.

Majerus, P., Broze, B., Miletich, J., & Tollefsen, D. (1996). Anticoagulant, thrombolytic and antiplatelet drugs. In J. Hardman, L. Limbird, P. Molinoff, R. Ruddon, *Goodman & Gillman's The pharmacologic basis for disease* (9th ed.) (pp. 1341–1359). New York: McGraw-Hill.

McLaren, G. (2002). Iron deficiency. In Rankel, R., Bope, E., *Conn's Current Therapy* (pp. 355–359). Philadelphia: W. B. Saunders Company.

Nolan, R. (1997). Poisoning. In R. Hoekelman, S. Friedman, N. Nelson, H. Siedel, & M. Weiztman, *Primary pediatric care* (pp. 1738–1750). St. Louis: C. V. Mosby.

Nuwayhid, B., Nguyen, T., Khalife, S. (1999). Medical complications of pregnancy. In *Essentials of obstetrics and gynecology* (3rd ed) (pp 234–262). Philadelphia: W. B. Saunders.

Ries, C., & Santi, D. (2001). Agents used in anemias: Hematopoietic growth factors. In B. Katzung, *Basic and clinical pharmacology* (pp. 549–563). Norwalk, CT: Appleton & Lange/McGraw Hill.

Sancher, R. (2002). Pernicious anemia and other megaloblastic anemias. In R., Rankel. & E., Bope, *Conn's Current Therapy.* (pp. 366–368). Philadelphia: W. B. Saunders Company.

Schreiber (2002). Deep venous thrombosis and thrombophlebitis. In *eMedicine Journal* Vol. 3, No. 1., available at www.emedicine.com, accessed 6.6.02.

Tatro, D. (2001). *Drug interaction facts.* St. Louis: Facts and Comparisons.

Wynne, A. (2002). Anemia. In A., Wynne, T, Woo, & M., Milliard, *Pharmacotherapeutics for Nurse Practitioner Prescribers.* (pp. 811–824). Philadelphia: F. A. Davis Company.

Zuckerman, K., J. (2000). An approach to anemias. In J. Bennett, & F. Plum, *Cecil's textbook of medicine* (21st ed.) (pp. 840–847). Philadelphia: W. B. Saunders.

CHAPTER ❖ 29

NEUROLOGIC DISORDERS

Stephanie G. Metzger ◆ Janet C. Horton ◆
William R. Garnett ◆ Kathleen Sawin

Conditions affecting the nervous system remain one of the great frontiers in healthcare, with gains in basic neuroscience creating new pharmacologic interventions to improve the quality of life in what were once considered nontreatable conditions. The focus of this chapter is on the more common neurologic problems encountered in primary care, usually managed by the primary care provider in conjunction with a consulting neurologist.

The chapter focuses on the current common drugs utilized in specific conditions so the primary care provider is knowledgeable regarding their use, concurrent drug interactions, toxicities, and systemic changes that they may bring about.

TRAUMATIC BRAIN INJURY

Traumatic brain injury (TBI) is a health issue anywhere vehicles, sports, or violence is found. The average TBI incidence rate of combined hospitalization and mortality is 95 per 100,000 individuals. TBI was initially studied in terms of penetrating head wounds incurred during World War II. This was the beginning of correlation between focal injury and functional deficits. Mechanism of injury varies by age with motor vehicle collision being prevalent in the younger population and falls in older individuals. Populations at most risk for sustaining a TBI are males ages 15 to 24, children under 5, and adults over 75. Lower socioeconomic status also places an individual at risk for TBI. Nonaccidental brain injury is associated with child abuse and partner violence. Survival from TBI is based on the degree and extent of brain injury, which varies greatly based on cause. Overall, 22% of TBIs are fatal. Ninety-one percent of firearm-related TBIs result in death as compared to 11% of fall-related TBIs. Each year more than 230,000 individuals are hospitalized and survive a TBI. There are approximately 5.3 million individuals in the United States with a TBI-related disability (Guerrero, Thurman, & Sniezek, 2000; Thurman, Alverson, Dunn et al., 2000).

PATHOPHYSIOLOGY

TBI is divided into two distinct injuries. The primary brain injury is the direct result of the mechanical damage that occurs at the time of the injury. The secondary brain injury is the result of interrelated pathophysiologic processes caused by the trauma. The secondary brain injury may cause neuronal damage resulting from cerebral hypoxia, increased intercranial pressure, or decreased cerebral blood flow. Shearing and pressure-gradient forces that cause diffuse axonal injury, hypoxic-ischemic injury, and tissue hemorrhage cause major injury to the brain. Tissue hemorrhage is classified according to anatomical location: epidural, subdural, or intracerebral. Damage from the injury may not be visible on neuroimaging studies. Severe injuries associated with diffuse axonial injury often harm the brain stem and ascending reticular system, thus resulting in coma (Vanore, 2000). The outcome of TBI is often a degree of impairment in cognitive and/or functional abilities.

PROGNOSIS

Recovery from TBI is multifaceted and complicated by the fact that the individual often does not appear to be injured, especially in the case of mild TBI or postconcussive syndrome (Dikmen, Machamer, & Temlin, 2002). Difficulty with attention, memory, and multitask abilities are often seen for time intervals from weeks to months post-injury. These difficulties may result in personality changes, anger, aggression, or depression. It is important that any individual who has sustained even a mild TBI be evaluated by a neuropsychologist to assess need for cognitive retraining and compensation techniques as well as psychotherapy (Anderson, Parmenter, & Mok, 2002). Also present may be physical symptoms such as vertigo and headache. The headache may be migraines in nature and must be treated as such (Thornhill, Teasdale, Murray, et al., 2000).

Individuals who have sustained a moderate TBI experience recovery following the event up to years post-injury. The most rapid recovery is in the first 6 months, followed by the next 6 months. However, recovery does take place even years after the event (Goranson, Graves, & Allison, 2003). It was previously thought that children recovered more completely than adults due to the immature patterning of the brain. This has been shown to be incorrect through study of outcome data (Arciniegas & Silver, 2001).

A severe TBI is often associated with diffuse axonal injury as well as coma. These individuals require a critical care team to manage the secondary extracerebral complications of TBI. The brain controls not only the organs of the body but also the processes of autonomic and hormonal function. The precise complications that may be present are dependent upon both location and severity of the injury (Mosenthal, Lavery, Addis, et al., 2002).

A team of individuals trained in many fields—including nursing, medicine, psychology, occupational, physical and speech therapy, as well as social work and therapeutic recreation—are integral in the rehabilitation process. Their availability, coupled with the severity of the brain injury, will determine the cognitive and functional outcome the individual achieves. It is imperative that family be included in all aspects of care and that the practitioner realizes that there are many different definitions of family. The residual effects of TBI require pharmacotherapeutic treatment, healthcare services, and services related to the disabilities that may be resultant such as vocational/educational, socialization, and self-care abilities (Heinemann, Sokol, Garvin, & Bode, 2002).

SPECIFIC CONSIDERATIONS FOR PHARMACOTHERAPY

When Drug Therapy Is Needed

Pharmacological treatment in traumatic brain injury centers around treatment of sequelae of TBI such as headache, sleep disorders, and cognitive deficits. Table 29–1 lists common symptoms that may require pharmacological management.

Short- and Long-Term Goals of Pharmacotherapy

The goal of pharmacotherapy is to manage the physical, cognitive, and emotional changes occurring as a result of the injury. It is imperative that the treatment encompasses a thorough assessment of all variables and to realize that each sequelae may not have a corresponding pharmacotherapeutic treatment option. Short-term goals center around treatment of the sequelae with the lowest dosage used for the shortest duration of time. The long-term goal is to transition management of the sequelae to the primary care provider as well as the physiatrist.

Nonpharmacologic Therapy

The goal of nonpharmacological treatment of TBI is restoration of preinjury cognitive and functional ability. Cognitive impairments are almost ubiquitous following moderate to severe TBI. The most common cognitive deficits are grouped into the areas of attention and arousal, memory, sensory/perceptual function, language and communication, intellect, and executive function. Rehabilitation is the process of treatment with short- and long-term

TABLE 29–1. Common Deficits Seen in Brain Injury

Agitation	Fatigue
Anxiety	Headache (vascular or migraines)
Ataxia	Hearing loss/tinnitus
Cognitive dysfunction	Hemiparesis
Depression	Sleep disorders
Diplopia	Spasticity
Dysphagia	Tremor
Emotional lability	Visual changes

Source: Adapted from Horn & Zasler (1996).

goal setting to facilitate the individual's ability to reach his or her fullest potential. Potential must be explored from preinjury status and integrate physiologic and anatomic goals along with the goals of the individual and family, environmental considerations, and resources available (Montgomery, Oliver, Reisner & Fallat, 2002; Glenn, 2002).

Time Frame for Initiating Pharmacotherapy

In mild to moderate brain injury it is better to delay drug therapy for a number of weeks after injury. Cognitive impairments are the most common sequelae that are possibly amenable to pharmacological intervention (Glenn, 2002). However, the most common side effect of such intervention is sedation, which may be damaging to neurotransmitters and detrimental to the recovery process. This is especially crucial for individuals who have sustained a mild TBI resulting in postconcussive syndrome. Symptom management may necessitate the use of drugs that impede recovery from TBI. Table 29–2 lists examples of drugs that impede recovery. Individuals who have sustained a severe TBI often require many of these medications due to agitation as well as the need to provide ventilatory support and other life-enhancing interventions. If sedatives are necessary, short acting is preferred to long acting (Glenn, 2002).

Overview of Drug Classes for Treatment of Head Injury

Pharmacologic interventions may positively influence recovery. Some medications may benefit neurotransmitter systems and enhance cognitive recovery. The choice of medication options is based on the anatomic localization of the injury, injury size, and age of patient. Response varies between individuals as only 10 to 15% of neurotransmitters are identified. Interaction with brain receptor neuropeptides may influence brain plasticity and therefore enhance recovery (Glenn, 2002).

The drugs utilized in head injury are primarily from seven major groups: stimulants, dopaminergics, antipsychotics, antidepressants, anticonvulsants, and antianxiety agents including beta blockers. Many of the drugs are used for several different groups of symptoms. Drug utilization in this section is addressed by symptom: attention and arousal, psychosis, agitation and aggression, cognition, affective disorders (particularly depression), and seizures.

TABLE 29–2. Drugs that May Impede Recovery from Brain Injury

Benzodiazepines	Phenothiazines
Clonidine	Phenoxybenzamine
GABA	Phenytoin
Haloperidol	Prazosin
Phenobarbital	

Source: Adapted from Dombovy (1997).

Assessment

Pharmacologic intervention is a team approach in the critical care arena combining neurology and psychiatry with critical care specialists. The primary care provider will see individuals who present for followup if the injury was severe enough to warrant hospitalization. The primary care provider may also be consulted by individuals following a traumatic event for complaints of headaches, irritability, depression, difficulty thinking clearly, and inability to work. In many cases, these are individuals who were not hospitalized after the trauma; therefore, the provider may be unaware that the symptoms may be related to a TBI. Changes most commonly experienced by the individual and not noticed by others are related to changes in cognition as well as in personality and memory. Such changes may be subtle and a comprehensive history that may include neurobehavioral-rating scales is essential. Following a TBI, the individual may be unaware of these subtle changes. Assessment must include alcohol and drug assessments as well as a detailed medication assessment. Medications taken prior to injury will be reinstituted at lower levels in order to assess efficacy, especially psychotropic drugs. A dose schedule of one-third to one-half of the previous dose is usually necessary (Perini, Rago, Cicolini, et al., 2001). Often on the initial head CT scan, damage is absent, although magnetic resonance imaging (MRI) performed months after the event may show focal punctate densities.

Patient/Caregiver Information

Individuals who have sustained a TBI may have little to no insight into any changed behaviors or changes related to their cognitive abilities. TBI is therefore referred to as the silent disability because the individual may look unchanged even in the face of severe changes in behavior or cognition. Families may be both unaware and unprepared for this sequelae, especially related to the need for constant supervision. This sequelae can be especially difficult related to employment because the individual may appear to have cognitive abilities that are not present. Support groups and resources for education are essentials on an ongoing basis (Montgomery, Oliver, Reisner, & Fallat, 2002).

OUTCOMES MANAGEMENT

The goal of pharmacotherapeutic intervention is both short term and long-term symptom management. Sleep disturbance is a sequelae that affects outcome in all areas: attention and arousal, psychosis, agitation and aggression, affective disorders, cognition and posttraumatic seizures. Antidepressants are often useful for treatment in one or more of these areas. Common drugs that may be utilized are listed in Table 29–3 with dosages, side effects and other information provided in the drug reference tables. Treatments for ulcer prophylaxis and pain control are discussed in other chapters. Symptoms and medication use and monitoring are individually addressed below.

Attention and Arousal

Selecting an Appropriate Agent. General arousal is mediated by the reticular activating system, which projects to the entire cerebrum, midbrain, and lower brain, as well as the spinal cord. Damage to one or both cerebral hemispheres and/or the reticular activating system results in disorders of attention and arousal.

The arousal medications used in brain injury primarily act on the catecholaminergic system. The traditional stimulant, dextroamphetamine, blocks the reuptake of norepinephrine, and higher doses can block the reuptake

TABLE 29–3. Common Drugs Used in Brain Injury*

Generic (Trade) Name	Uses for Specific Behaviors in Head Injury
Drugs Used in Cognitive Function and Arousal[a]	
Dextroamphetamine (Dexadrin)	Cognitive function and arousal (stimulant)
Methylphenidate (Ritalin)	Cognitive function and arousal (stimulant)
Amantadine (Symmetrel)	Cognitive function and arousal (dopamine agonist), Parkinsonian symptoms
Bromocriptine (Parlodel)	Cognitive function and arousal (dopamine agonist)
L. Dopa/Carbidopa (Sinemet)	Cognitive function and arousal (dopamine agonist)
Trazadone (Desyrel)	Sleep and antidepressant
Drugs Used in Psychosis, Anxiety, and Aggression[b]	
Haloperidol (Haldol)	Anti-psychotic
Fluphenazine (Prolixin)	Anti-psychotic
Clozapine (Clozaril)	Anti-psychotic, anxiolytic
Buspirone (Buspar	Anxiety, especially post-aggressive syndrome
Propanolol (Inderal)	Anxiety, especially post-aggressive syndrome
Mania Therapeutic Drugs	
Lithium carbonate (Lithobid)	Mania/manic depression, aggressive behavior and agitation
Clonidine (Catapres)	Mania
Mania and Anti-Seizure Drugs	
Carbamazepine (Tegretol)	Mania, anti-seizure, aggression/agitation, lancinating neurogenic pain
Valproic acid (Depakene, Depakote)	Mania, mood lability, seizures, aggression/agitation, myoclonus
Other Anti-Seizure Medications[c]	
Clonazepam (Klonopin)	Anti-seizure (myoclonic)
Phenytoin (Dilantin)	Anti-seizure
Phenobarbital (Phenobarb)	Anti-seizure
Antidepressants[d]	
Fluoxetine (Prozac)	Antidepressant, mood lability, "emotional incontinence"
Sertraline (Zoloft)	Antidepressant
Paroxetine (Paxil)	Antidepressant, mood lability
Nortriptyline (Aventyl or Pamelor)	Antidepressant, mood lability
Desipramine (Norpramin)	Antidepressant

*Please refer to Drug Tables for further information on mechanism of action, dosages, toxicity, side effects, and interactions.
[a]As a group, can increase dopamine activity, paranoia, euphoria, agitation, irritability.
[b]Anti-psychotic drugs as a group can cause hypertension, sedation and confusion, Parkinsonian syndrome, acute dystomia. May impede neuronal brain recovery in subacute stage.
[c]As a group, can decrease cognition and cause depression.
[d]All antidepressants can increase seizure frequency. Continue this drug group six months after remission of symptoms. Some anticonvulsants increase therapeutic blood levels of the antidepressants.

of dopamine. In the presence of psychomotor retardation, antiparkinsonian drugs are utilized. Amantadine acts on the dopamine receptor both before and after the synapse and probably increases cholinergic and GABAnergic activity. Bromocriptine is both a dopamine receptor antagonist and agonist. In its midrange dose it primarily acts as an agonist.

The amphetamines methylphenidate and levodopa all improve arousal level. Antidepressants may also have a stimulating effect. Levodopa and bromocriptine have had successful use in patients with long-term loss of arousal. Cholinergic agonists have a detrimental effect in the acute stage of TBI, but are therapeutic in some persistent vegetative states.

Two drugs commonly used are methylphenidate (0.3 mg/kg bid) or dextroamphetamine (0.2 mg/kg bid). They tend to increase alertness and improve mood as well as task performance. These medications may require titration upward to 60 mg/day bid or tid with dosage increases every 5 to 7 days (Whyte, Vaccaro, & Grieb-Neff, & Hart, 2002).

The dopamine agonist Sinemet (L-dopa/carbidopa) is used to improve alertness and concentration; decrease fatigue, sialorrhea, and hypomania; and improve memory. The dosage used is 10/100 to 25/250 qid. Another dopamine agonist, bromocriptine, is used to treat cognitive initiation problems with a starting dose of 2.5 mg/day and treatment for at least 2 months. The drug is thought to help with increasing goal directed behaviors.

Another medication used in brain injury to improve impulsivity, emotional lability, and general arousal is amantadine at initial dosages of 50 mg b.i.d. to 400 mg/day, increasing the dose at 3-day to weekly intervals by 100 mg/day.

Monitoring for Efficacy and Toxicity. The major risk of the stimulant drugs is the increase in dopamine activity, leading to symptoms of overstimulation. The symptoms of overstimulation with dextroamphetamine and methylphenidate include paranoia, dysphoria, agitation, and irritability. Bromocriptine may cause sedation, nausea, psychosis, headaches, and delirium; amantadine may cause confusion, hallucinations, edema, and hypotension (Whyte et al., 2002). Side effects of confusion and lethargy are particularly troublesome in terms of TBI recovery (Anderson, Parmenter, & Mok, 2002). Careful titration both upward and downward of dextroamphetamine and methylphenidate is necessary to minimize side effect profiles. Because depression can arise with sudden withdrawal, slow titration off dextroamphetamine and methylphenidate is as important as slow titration at their initiation. Several recent studies cite little increased risk of seizures with methylphenidate, dextroamphetamine, and bromocriptine, but amantadine appears to lower the seizure threshold in some subjects.

Psychosis

Selecting an Appropriate Agent. Acute posttraumatic psychosis and anxiety following traumatic brain injury is common. Antipsychotic drugs are used only when other measures of environmental management are not appropriate or fail. These drugs as a group produce significant side effects at very small doses. Consequently, the recommended doses are often one-third to one-half of what might normally be prescribed in traditional psychosis. In addition, manufacturers may warn prescribers not to give these drugs to individuals who have sustained a TBI.

Antipsychotics are indicated when the behaviors resemble classic schizophrenia, such as hallucinations, paranoid or bizarre ideations, and loose associations. The drugs to avoid are those with a high anticholinergic effect, which can impair memory and new learning, as well as cause constipation, urinary retention, and blurred vision.

The drugs most commonly used are haloperidol, clozapine, lorazepam, buspirone, and propanolol. Their mechanisms of action, specific use, dosage, and interactions are listed in Drug Tables 205.5, 308.6, 309.2, 312.2, 312.3.

Monitoring for Efficacy and Toxicity. Although the risk is small, the use of neuroleptics may promote seizure activity. Other more common risk factors include the development of tardive dyskinesia and neuroleptic malignant syndrome. As a group, the drugs can cause hypertension, hypotension, sedation, confusion, parkinsonian syndrome, and acute dystonia. In the acute phase, the drugs may impede brain recovery.

Agitation and Aggression

Selecting an Appropriate Agent. In early brain injury, agitation is expected, and in the majority of patients this symptom subsides as recovery proceeds. The incidence of agitation following a severe brain injury varies between 11 and 50%, depending on the type of injury and the study involved. If aggression is present to the point of blocking medical intervention or the individual is at risk of self-harm, the benzodiazepines have been found to be helpful. If agitation causes a clinical emergency, haloperidol is the first-line treatment due to less sedative effects. In a minority of long-term patients, agitation and aggression remain. Another source of aggression and agitation is improper use of medications that aggravate this behavior. The most common offenders are haloperidol, lorazepam, and diazepam, which can lead directly to aggressive behaviors or indirectly as a rebound effect once the medication begins to wear off. Nonpharmacologic interventions include removing the source of frustration by controlling the environment, reducing the amount of stimulation, and setting a lower level of expected behavior. An aggressive approach to both environmental structure and medication use is helpful in the small number of patients in whom the behavior becomes chronic.

The traditional approach to this behavior in other diseases is the use of neuroleptics, but in brain injury these drugs appear to have little efficacy. Stimulant medications and tricyclic antidepressants produce a calming effect due to actions on inattention, distractibility, and cognition. Carbamazepine and valproate may be used for episodic dyscontrol variant aggression (Perino et al., 2001).

Benzodiazepines are used, but their efficacy in the long term is in doubt. In the short term they are very effective, particularly lorazepam. The beta blockers are more widely known for their use as antihypertensives. The drug propranolol is useful with unprovoked rage and aggression in chronic TBI. The suggested dose is quite high, so use of other drugs first is suggested because of the hypotensive effect.

Affective Disorders

Selecting an Appropriate Agent. The two common affective disorders in brain injury are mania and depression. The mania is often viewed in terms of agitation and aggression and treated as such. There is some thought that the depression seen in brain injury may be a straightforward chemical defect from the brain injury itself or a superimposed depression from the event of the brain injury. In any case, the depressive behaviors are similar, with psychomotor slowing, sparse speech, and changes in sleep and appetite. In brain injury the depression can be acute or delayed and is often dependent on the amount of insight an individual may have at different times regarding the brain injury.

The drugs of choice in treating depression in brain injury are the serotonin selective reuptake inhibitors (SSRIs), particularly sertraline and fluoxetine. These drugs have fewer anticholinergic side effects with a lower incidence of dyskinesias. In addition, lability of mood (excessive crying or laughing) is often treatable with SSRIs and other antidepressant medications such as amitriptyline (Elavil) and sertaline (Zoloft) (Fann, Uomoto, & Katon, 2001). Other drugs used to treat depression in head injury include the neuroleptics.

Cognition

Altered or decreased cognitive abilities following TBI are reported by survivors to be more disabling than residual functional deficits. Limited agents are effective for treatment, especially in the pediatric population (Cock, Fordham, Cockburn & Haggard, 2003). Cognitive impairment affects multiple areas of the brain but particularly the hippocampus, cerebral cortex, and cerebellum. The neurotransmitters involved include the ACh (acetylcholine) amino acid neurotransmitters such as gamma-aminobutyric acid (GABA), neuropeptides, and ACTH fragments, as well as opioids. The cholinergic agents show promise in treating cognitive deficits, but no studies currently exist to support their use in memory and learning disorders. The effective utilization of any of these drugs can change with time, as the brain changes in relationship to the injury; the drugs should all receive periodic weaning trials and decreased dosages as tolerated.

Posttraumatic Seizures

Selecting an Appropriate Agent. The incidence of seizures in traumatic brain injury is 4 to 7%. Penetrating injuries, depressed skull fractures, intracranial hemorrhage, prolonged duration of posttraumatic amnesia, and loss of consciousness all increase the risk of seizures (Asikainen, Kaste, & Sarna, 1999). Consequently, seizures are more frequent in individuals treated in a rehabilitation setting, and the incidence of seizures is higher the first 5 years postinjury. Focal seizures are more common than generalized seizures. Those with mild brain injuries have no greater seizure incidence than the general population. Additional predisposing factors to seizure development are alcoholism, epilepsy, and age. Children may have seizures immediately after injury but are not as predisposed to develop epilepsy as adults. If an individual has a seizure, early use of antiseizure medications is warranted to prevent increasing cerebral pressure or hypertension, but prolonged use of anti-seizure medications after the first 6 months may only increase the risk of further seizures.

The incidence of posttraumatic seizures following TBI is greater the more severe the brain injury. The risk of exacerbating secondary brain injury is greatest during the first 24 hours post-injury. High-risk injuries for developing posttraumatic seizures are those with dural penetration or intercranial hemorrhage (Asikainen, Kaste, & Sarna, 1999).

Periodic EEG monitoring will be used to determine if seizure medications can be discontinued. However, the absence of epileptiform activity does not guarantee that seizures will not reoccur once the medication has been withdrawn. The decision to withdraw medication will be made by the neurologist, but the primary care provider will follow the individual long term and monitor for signs and symptoms suggestive of seizure activity.

The antiseizure medications, particularly phenytoin, phenobarbital, and carbamazepine, can impair cognition and behavior at subtherapeutic and therapeutic levels. Conversely, in some patients, carbamazepine may improve mood, attention, information processing, and general functioning because this drug, as well as valproic acid, has mood-stabilizing properties. These two drugs are the drugs of choice with seizure activity in TBI (Cope, 1994, p. 586). In some cases aggressive or agitated behavior may be related to seizures or a postictal state and may thus respond to antiseizure medication.

Monitoring for Efficacy and Toxicity. See the seizure section of this chapter for a fuller discussion of efficacy and toxicity in antiseizure medications.

ATTENTION DEFICIT/HYPERACTIVITY DISORDER

BACKGROUND

Attention deficit hyperactivity disorder (ADHD) has burgeoned during the last decade. ADHD is now recognized as a disorder present in both children and adults. Increasing numbers of people of all ages are being evaluated and diagnosed with ADHD. The classic signs and symptoms of ADHD are impulsivity, defined as inadequate attention to internal stimuli; distractability, defined as inadequate attention to external stimuli; and hyperactivity, defined as physical interaction with outside stimuli. Adult ADHD may go unrecognized, although the individual may be experiencing difficulties across multiple dimensions such as in the home, at work, and in the community. Many negative consequences result from undiagnosed ADHD, including antisocial and criminal behavior; poor academic, vocational, or social functioning; and difficulties with substance abuse. The number of individuals being diagnosed with ADHD is increasing, as there is an increased awareness of the symptoms and treatment that improve success rates for this neglected but often treatable disorder (Faraone, Biederman, Spencer, et al., 2000).

CURRENT ISSUES IN ADHD

Diagnosis, treatment, and management of ADHD have evolved over the years. In 1980 the American Psychiatric Association recognized inattention as central to ADHD diagnosis, shifting emphasis from hyperactivity as the cardinal symptom. As diagnosis for ADHD without hyperactivity became established, a hybrid diagnosis of attention deficit hyperactivity disorder became classified based on a list of symptoms relating to inattention, impulsivity, and hyperactivity. This diagnosis was further refined in 1994 by the American Psychiatric Association in DSM-IV, which recognized and defined the predominance of inattention as a separate symptom from the hybrid diagnosis. DSM-IV recognizes three subtypes of ADHD: predominantly inattentive, predominantly hyperactive, and a combined type (American Psychiatric Association, 1994).

The American Academy of Pediatrics, the Academy of Child and Adolescent Psychiatry, as well as the Southern Medical Association, have published guidelines for assessment and evaluation of ADHD across the lifespan. Two clusters of ADHD symptoms are defined: symptoms of inattention and symptoms of hyperactivity-impulsivity. The individual must meet 6 of 9 criteria under one or both clusters to warrant further evaluation for ADHD. The symptoms must be inconsistent with the child's current developmental level; have been present and causing impairment for at least 6 months, with some symptoms occurring before the age of 7, and be present in two or more settings. Comorbidities may be present but the symptoms must not be attributable to other diagnoses (America, 2001; American Academy of Pediatrics, 2000; Bussing & Gary, 2001; Elliott, 2002).

According to DSM-IV, an estimated 3 to 5% of children in the United States have ADHD. The newly released diagnostic guidelines by the American Academy of Pediatrics estimated the incidence to be between 4 and 12% of all children. During childhood a disproportionate number of males are diagnosed with ADHD as compared to females. In the adult population, which has a 2 to 4% incidence of ADHD, the male to female ratio is 1:1. It is hypothesized that the lower incidence of ADHD in females in childhood is because inattention is the primary symptom manifested and ADHD may be missed or overlooked, with a subsequent delay in pharmacological treatment for females. Therefore, the ratio in childhood may be closer

TABLE 29–4. DSM IV Diagnosis and Criteria for ADHD

Approved Diagnosis

1. ADHD, predominately inattention (Criteria A1, B, C, D, E met)
2. ADHD, predominately hyperactive/impulsive (Criteria A2, B, C, D, E met)
3. ADHD, mixed (Criteria A1, A2, B, C, D, E met)
4. ADHD, not otherwise specified (prominent symptoms that do not meet criteria)
5. (In partial remission) a suffix used for individuals, especially adults and some adolescents whose present symptoms do not fully meet criteria

Criteria

For any ADHD related diagnosis, all of the following need to be present:

A. Six or more symptoms of inattention (A1) or hyperactivity/impulsivity (A2) (see below) present for 6 months to a degree that is maladaptive and inconsistent with developmental level

B. Symptoms that caused impairment present before age 7

C. Impairment from symptoms present in two or more settings (home, school, work)

D. Evidence of clinically significant impairment in social, academic, or occupational functioning

E. Symptoms do not occur only during course of pervasive developmental disorder or other psychotic disorder and are not better accounted for by another mental disease diagnosis

A1. Criteria for Inattention

a. Often fails to give close attention to details or makes careless mistakes in schoolwork or other activities.
b. Often has difficulty sustaining attention in tasks or play activities.
c. Often does not seem to listen when spoken to directly.
d. Often does not follow through with instructions and fails to finish schoolwork, chores, or duties in the workplace (not due to oppositional behavior or failure to understand instructions).
e. Often has difficulty organizing tasks and activities.
f. Often avoids, dislikes, or is reluctant to engage in tasks that require sustained mental effort (such as schoolwork or homework).
g. Often loses things necessary for tasks or activities (toys, school assignments, pencils, books, or tools).
h. Is often easily distracted by extraneous stimuli.
i. Is often forgetful in daily activities.

A2. Criteria for Hyperactivity/Impulsivity

Hyperactivity

a. Often fidgets with hands or feet or squirms in seat.
b. Often leaves seat in classroom or in other situations in which remaining seated is expected.
c. Often runs about or climbs excessively in situations in which it is inappropriate (in adolescents or adults may be limited to subjective feelings of restlessness).
d. Often has difficulty playing or engaging in leisure activities quietly.
e. If often "on the go" or often acts as if "driven by motor."
f. Often talks excessively.

Impulsivity

g. Often blurts out answers before questions have been completed.
h. Often has difficulty awaiting turn.
i. Often interrupts or intrudes on others (butts into conversations or games).

Source: APA (1994), pp. 83–85.

to 1:1 than the current estimates (Gaub & Carlson, 1997; USDHHS, 1999).

ADHD has a considered impact on familes as parents of children with ADHD experience higher levels of stress, self-blame, social isolation, depression, and marital discord (Kaye, 2002).

CURRENT ISSUES IN TREATMENT

ADHD is rooted in neurobiological and molecular genetics that may combine with environmental risk factors to cause ADHD. ADHD is a public health issue based on prevelance, impairment, treatment effectiveness and chronicity. ADHD is diagnosed in all countries studied, producing similar statistics. A genetic link is based on family studies, twin studies, and adoption studies. Specific genes implicated with ADHD are mutations in the thyroid and dopamine transporter genes as well as several other chromosome areas being researched. There is no single gene that causes ADHD. Numerous studies of individuals with ADHD have shown decreased blood to the prefrontal lobe as well as its pathways.

Individuals with ADHD share common characteristics referred to as symptoms of ADHD, yet there are unique characteristics and differences between each individual with ADHD. These differences must be addressed in order to provide successful clinical management. Considerations include but are not limited to age and intellectual ability, severity and urgency, treatment history, comorbidity, family factors such as psychopathology, willingness and ability to adhere to recommended treatment options and desire related to specific treatment options (Brown, 2000). It is imperative to discuss ADHD with patients and families using the facts related to the scientific basis of the disorder (Barr, Wigg, Bloom, et al., 2000; Crosbie & Schachar, 2001).

According to a national survey, evaluation and treatment for ADHD is often initiated by the primary care provider. This study documented that 72% of primary care providers will manage ADHD alone, while only 20% will manage ADHD with comorbidity (Chan, 2002). Referral to psychiatry is mandated if the diagnosis is at all suspect for a mental disorder or neurology if suspect of a neurological disorder such as seizures (Kaye, Montgomery, & Munson, 2003). Accurate diagnosis and treatment of attention deficit disorder in the primary care setting requires an accurate and thorough developmental history, recognition of cardinal features as well as a working knowledge of the neurobiology, psychopharmacology, and behavioral treatment of ADHD (Elliott, 2002).

It is essential to recognize and treat comorbid disorders before attempting to treat ADHD. Pharmacological treatments such as stimulants may exacerbate differential conditions. Treatment of anxiety or depression may add clarity to symptoms that may or may not be related to ADHD. Differential diagnosis and frequently occurring comorbidities include disorders of initiating and maintaining sleep, age appropriate high activity level, substance abuse, developmental disorders, epilepsy, disorders of the special senses such as vision or hearing, personality disorders, Tourette's or Asperger's syndrome, autism, obsessive compulsive disorder, mood disturbances and anxiety disorders, psychotic disorder, adjustment or oppositional disorder, learning and language deficits, chronic lead poisoning, anemia and thyroid dysfunction (Zametkin & Ernst, 1999).

Eight percent of females with ADHD and 14% of males with ADHD also have bipolar disorder. Depression is present in 35% of females with ADHD and 25% of males. Anxiety disorders are found in approximately half of all individuals with ADHD. Pharmacotherapeutic intervention for ADHD lowers the risk for substance abuse in adolescents (Brown, 2000).

SPECIFIC CONSIDERATIONS FOR PHARMACOTHERAPY

When Drug Therapy is Needed

Pharmacotherapeutic treatments should not be initiated prior to a comprehensive diagnostic evaluation. An interdisciplinary team including, but not limited to, primary care provider, neurologist/psychiatrist, psychologist, speech pathologist, occupational therapist, physical therapist, audiologist, and educator is the gold standard for evaluation. However, all disciplines may not be utilized, depending on information obtained in the history, as well as availability. If resources are limited and such a team cannot be readily established, pharmacotherapeutic treatment may be initiated but rigid followup must be ensured (Kaye, Montgomery, & Munson, 2002). Caution must be present to evaluate for comorbid conditions that may be complex and complicate treatment.

Short- and Long-term Goals of Pharmacotherapy

The aim of pharmacotherapy is to improve attention and control impulsivity and excessive motor behaviors that interfere with daily life and to treat concomitant anxiety and depression. Assessing problem behaviors prior to treatment and outlining targeted tasks is necessary to establish outcome measures specific to the individual. Examples of outcome measures include the amount of time a child can attend to specific school-related tasks, the ability to complete homework in a reasonable amount of time, the ability to play with schoolmates in appropriate ways, and sleeping with fewer interruptions. For the adult it may mean the ability to complete work assignments in shorter periods, better sleep patterns, and improved family and social relationships.

Nonpharmacologic Therapy

The key treatments in ADHD are control of the environment and education. Establishing a partnership with the adults who work with the person with ADHD is a primary goal. The team around the child with ADHD works together to provide consistent structure, counsel about specific detrimental and alternative behaviors, and control environmental stimulation to maximize success. This may require special placement within the educational system.

Education and counseling, individually or in groups and before and during pharmacological therapy, can be useful for children, teens, and adults with ADHD. Local support groups are helpful. Educational information should include a discussion of the biologic aspect (rather than character disorder) of the disease. Coping behaviors may help with organizational skills; avoiding fatigue may also improve skills. Open communication between family members tis helpful since the individual often lacks self-awareness (Fargason & Ford, 1994).

Time Frame for Initiating Pharmacotherapy

The first step in treatment is education of the individual and family related to ADHD. The most effective treatment for ADHD combines pharmacotherapeutic intervention with behavioral therapy. However, medication intervention alone is superior to behavioral intervention alone. Stimulants are the first line of treatment for ADHD, with antidepressants being added as needed (Rasmussen, Desantis, & Opler, 2001).

Overview of Drug Classes

Stimulants are the most effective treatment for the symptoms of ADHD, and about 70% of individuals improve with use, often seeing sudden and dramatic improvements in behavior. Antidepressants may also be useful for treatment of ADHD. Other classes include nonadrenergic specific reuptake inhibitors, monoamine oxidase inhibitors, selective seroronin reuptake inhibitors, alpha-2 nonadrenergic agonists, cholinergic agents, and antipsychotic agents. Antipsychotic agents may be mildly effective in improving behavioral symptoms in children but have a limited role in the treatment of adult ADHD (Wimmett & Laustsen, 2003).

Assessment Prior to Therapy

Accurate diagnosis and treatment of attention deficit disorder in the primary care setting requires an accurate and thorough history focusing on developmental history as well as a comprehensive physical examination. Diagnosis is aided by the use of questionnaires and symptom rating scales. The most frequently used questionnaire is the Conners, which has a version for parents, teachers and a self report version (Conners, 1998). Collateral reports from schools or employment agencies along with neuropsychological testing may be necessary prior to initiating therapy. Side effects related to nutritional status and cardiogenic side effects must be monitored. Genetic evaluation may be useful to limit the differential diagnosis list and provide information for future family planning.

Patient/Caregiver Information

Children treated with stimulants and antidepressants need parents and teachers to be knowledgeable about the primary and secondary effects of these medications. The two most common side effects of stimulant medications are lethargy and appetite suppression. Weight, height, and head circumference are monitored at each visit. In general, these drugs require tapering dosages prior to discontinuation in order to maintain treatment gains.

OUTCOMES MANAGEMENT

Selecting an Appropriate Agent

Stimulants available for use in individuals with ADHD include methylphenidate; D-amphetamine; D,L-amphetamine; and magnesium pemoline. These psychostimulants have onset of actions from 30 to 60 minutes and have a peak clinical effect of 1 to 2 hours post administration. They may be further subdivided by duration of action with short-acting methylphenidate lasting 2 to 5 hours, intermediate-acting D, L-amphetamine lasting 4 to 6 hours, and longer-acting sustained release preparations lasting 8 to 12 hours. Extensive literature documents the efficacy of methylphenidate treatment. It appears as if ADHD in preschoolers is more treatment refractory as compared to other age groups. The literature clearly documents behavioral improvement but also improved self-esteem and cognitive, social and family functioning in school age children. Based on this finding, the importance of treating individuals with ADHD beyond school or work hours is supported. Treatment for ADHD must include evening, weekends, and vacation time because ADHD is always presented. Both behavior and cognition are responsive to different doses of stimulants, and behavior and cognition improve in a dose-dependent fashion. Doses sufficient to improve behavior do not constrict attention or yield an over focusing phenomenon (Pelham, Arnoff, Midlam, et al., 1999).

Tricyclic antidepressants (TCAs) are useful in the treatment of ADHD because they modulate norepinepherine and serotonin. TCAs have advantages because their half-life is approximately 12 hours, and there are positive effects on sleep hygiene, mood, anxiety, and tics. Bupropion hydrochloride, a new generation antidepressant, has been shown to increase the ability to concentrate (Wilens, Spencer, Biederman, et al., 2001).

Monoamine oxidase inhibitors (MAOIs) have been shown to be effective in treatment of adult and pediatric ADHD. The potential for hypertensive crises in individuals using MAOIs limits the potential for use. Trials are underway using transdermal preparations, which carry a more favorable safety profile (Brown, 2000).

Selective serotonin reuptake inhibitors are not beneficial for treatment of cardinal symptoms of ADHD. Usefulness is demonstrated in individuals with a comorbidity of ADHD and depression (Brown, 2000).

Alpha-2 nonadrenergic agonists are used for their effect on behavior and possibly cognition. Use must be carefully monitored based on the possible cardiac effects when combining these agents with stimulants (Gutgesell, Atkins, Barst, et al., 1999; Wilens, Spencer, Swanson, et al., 1999).

Antipsychotics may have a mildly efficacious effect in children with ADHD. However, the long-term adverse effect of tardive dyskinesia limits usefulness. The primary care provider would not initiate this class of treatment.

Research has been promising in regards to a nonstimulant preparation atomoxetine for treatment of ADHD. Atomoxetine's effects are limited to norepinephrine, and it is not a controlled substance. This treatment has been shown to be effective in the pediatric population and may be a first-line treatment for adults (Michelson, Faries, Wernicke, et al., 2001).

Monitoring for Efficacy and Toxicity

Efficacy is monitored by behavioral control, social, and academic performance as well as nutritional status. The patient, family and school personnel need to be included in monitoring efficacy. Rating questionnaires are often helpful. Some centers will do a blind trial of medications—1 to 2 weeks on medicine and 1 to 2 weeks off medicine, with the child/family/school and sometimes even the clinician blinded to the treatment order. Comorbid conditions may be apparent or develop after initial diagnosis and continued assessment for emerging symptoms is critical.

Concerns related to long-term administration of stimulants on growth persist. A common side effect of stimulants is appetite suppression as stimulants are known to routinely produce anorexia, abdominal discomfort and weight loss. Appetite suppression is found in about 80% of individuals taking stimulant medication and can be managed by giving stimulants after meals and snacks. Appetite patterns are usually such that there is an average breakfast intake followed by a smaller intake at lunch and increasingly larger intake from the late afternoon to bedtime. Noticeable weight loss is present in approximately 10 to 15% of children (Mannuzza & Klein, 1999).

Stimulant effect on height is much less clear, with the inability to substantiate the claim that stimulants cause decreased height velocity. This issue has crucial significance related to the theory of providing a drug holiday to allow for catchup growth. This theory must take into consideration the possibility of a drug holiday causing exacerbation of symptoms (America, 2001).

Slight increases in pulse and blood pressure are occasionally observed, and the clinical significance of this is finding is unclear. Rarely, stimulant-associated toxic psychosis occurs with visual hallucinations. Premoline therapy has been associated with hypersensitivity reactions involving an increase in liver function tests after several months of treatment. Liver function should be monitored and families need to be instructed to monitor for the symptoms of hepatitis (Pliska, Browne, & Wynne, 2000).

Abuse potential related to stimulants is of concern. However, research has shown that the abused substance of choice for individuals with ADHD is marijuana, not stimulant medication. Treatment with stimulants substantially reduces the risk of substance abuse due to cognitive and behavioral improvements (Mannuzza & Klein, 1999).

ADHD is a major component of disability for individuals with Tourette's syndrome. Recent studies suggest that ADHD, Tourette's syndrome, and obsessive-compulsive disorder may have common mechanisms stemming from related anatomical sites (Lechman & Cohen, 1999). However, it is prudent to consider the risks and benefits of using stimulants in individuals with tics and ADHD. The risk of developing temporary tics is less than 1%.

TCAs have the potential for cardiotoxic risk in the pediatric population. It is imperative that a baseline EKG and interval EKGs be obtained. Likewise, overdose with TCAs are potentially lethal, and care must be taken regarding inaccessible storage (Gutgesell, Atkins, Barst, et al., 1999).

Followup Recommendations

No longer is ADHD a diagnosis treated with the use of stimulants until puberty when the condition was thought to remit. As many as 5% of the population may have ADHD and many of these individuals do not demonstrate hyperactivity. ADHD may be present throughout the life span for as many as half of the children diagnosed with ADHD and this discontinuation of treatment is individualized.

Although, the diagnostic criteria for ADHD state that at least some of the symptoms must have been present prior to the age of 7, ADHD is being increasingly diagnosed in adults. The follow-up pattern will be based on the age at diagnosis, medication prescribed, and behavioral therapy used.

Long-term surveillance of children should include data from school and parents using standardized instruments, when possible. Close monitoring for side effects when new medications are used or dosing is increased is imperative. Medications used to treat ADHD should be started low and be increased slowly (at weekly intervals in children and no more than every 3 days in adults).

Parents or adult patients should be counseled to contact the healthcare provider if side effects occur while the child/adult is on medication, especially if the medication is being titrated. Frequent return visits or close telephone contacts are useful when dosage is being adjusted. Children should be seen initially at 1-month intervals. After stabilization of medication, visits can be scheduled at 3- to 6-month intervals if the child is doing well and then yearly intervals maybe appropriate for stable adolescents. Adults should be followed at least yearly and more closely when medication changes are instituted. Due to the severity of the potential side effects, the fact that methylphenidate is a schedule 2 controlled medication and may need collaborative signatures in some states, and the co-morbid conditions often seen in this population, referral for initial management of children and adults as well as close collaboration with a physician for ongoing management is highly recommended.

STROKE

Cerebrovascular accident (CVA), or stroke, refers to a sudden loss of brain function resulting from a disruption of blood flow in one of three ways. Ischemic strokes, caused by occlusion of an artery account for 80 to 85% of cerebrovascular events. Hemorrhagic strokes, caused by a ruptured artery, account for 10 to 15% (American Heart Association, 2002). A small percentage are caused by other or unknown causes, including cerebral ischemia, artery dissection, coagulopathy, infection, and amyloid angiopathy. Stroke is the third leading cause of death and leading cause of neurologic disability in the United States. It is estimated that more than 700,000 strokes occur each year with more than 4.4 million people living with stroke and its concomitant disabilities (AHA, 2002). Although the mortality rate from stroke has improved steadily over time, decreasing 13% between 1989 and 1999 (AHA, 2002), the declines are not due to decreased incidence of stroke, but to improvement of diagnostic accuracy and advances in treatment of the acute phase of stroke.

The incidence of stroke doubles with every decade after age 55. Mortality ranges from 7.6% for ischemic and 37.5% for hemorrhagic events in the first 30 days post events (AHA, 2002). 22–30% of stroke individuals die within 1 year. The percentage is even higher among patients over the age of 65. More than 50% of stroke individuals die within 8 years. Although almost 50 to 70% of patients who suffer strokes regain full functional independence, as many as 15 to 30% are permanently disabled (AHA, 2002). The size and the location of the stroke lesion are key factors in specific neurological losses and recovery prognosis.

In acute stroke, disruption of circulation to the brain results in neural injury and death, generally within minutes. Pressure on adjacent tissue causes additional ischemic injury, which may be reversible if reperfusion is quickly obtained. Damage to surrounding neuronal tissue can recover spontaneously within hours to weeks following the actual event. The most common site of stroke is the middle cerebral artery (MCA) or one of its smaller tributaries. The MCA is the primary vascular source for the cerebral cortex, and damage to the MCA may result in loss of motor function, as well as loss of sensory function and language (aphasia) if the stroke affects the predominant left hemisphere.

The most common deficits following stroke are hemiparesis, sensory deficits, dysarthria, visual-perceptual deficits, cognitive deficits (particularly memory impairment), bladder control, and hemianopsia (Gresham, 1995). Symptoms vary in severity, depending on type, location, and duration of impaired blood flow to the brain.

The result of acute vascular changes can be a transient ischemic attack (TIA) with complete resolution of all neurologic changes within 24 h. A TIA is a short-lived approximately 5- to 20-min, neurological deficit with no permanent neurologic loss that can act as a warning sign for other neurologic changes.

Full recovery from a stroke can occur for up to a year and beyond, although most recovery occurs in the first 1 to 3 months. Recovery is due to spontaneous neurologic recovery as well as the patient's regaining skills through comprehensive rehabilitation. Recent studies have shown that physical rehabilitation undertaken 3 years following stroke can improve functional skill in dressing, bathing, and transfers, freeing the individual of the need for physical assistance (Margolis & Wityk, 1997).

The unmodifiable risk factors for stroke are age, gender, prior stroke, race, and family history. Despite recent advances in acute stroke management and improving stroke recovery, the best method to reduce the burden of stroke remains prevention. The most significant risk factors for stroke are hypertension, heart disease, diabetes, and cigarette smoking. Other risks include obesity, high blood cholesterol levels, prior history of stroke or TIA, illicit drug and alcohol use, and genetic conditions (Goldstein, Adams, Becker, et al., 2001).

The incidence of stroke doubles with every decade after 55 (Kannel, 1988). The incidence of stroke is greater among men; however, prevalence is greater in women, due in part to the fact that women live longer. Stroke-related fatality rates are also higher in women than men. The 1999 stroke mortality was 38.5% in men compared with 61.5% in women (AHA, 2002; Bousser, 1999). African Americans and Hispanic Americans have higher stroke incidence and mortality rates compared with whites (AHA, 2002). Frey, Jahnle, and Bulfinch (1998) found that differences in smoking history and heart disease accounted for part of the race/ethnicity stroke difference, with much of the risk in African Americans due to differences in hypertension, diabetes, and educational achievement. Individuals with a family history of stroke are at greater risk, while those with prior history of stroke have up to a tenfold increased risk for a subsequent stroke (American Stroke Association, 1999).

Although many risk factors cannot be modified, it is beneficial to recognize individuals at increased risk and modify any factors they can control. The modifiable risk factors are hypertension, diabetes, high cholesterol levels, coronary heart disease, smoking, illicit drug use, obesity, and heavy alcohol use (Goldstein et al., 2001; Gresham, 1995).

High blood pressure is the most significant modifiable risk factor for stroke. Blood pressure readings above 160/95 mm Hg have a ten- to twelve-fold risk of stroke compared to blood pressure in the 140/90 range Even borderline high blood pressure (140/90 to 154/94) is associated with a 50% increase in stroke risk (Kannel, 2000).

After hypertension, heart disease is the second most important risk factor for stroke. Cardiovascular conditions that increase the risk for stroke include endocarditis, valve replacement, atrial fibrillation, left ventricular hypertrophy, known cardiac thrombi, ventricular aneurysm, mitral regurgitation, mitral valve prolapse, coronary artery disease, and congestive heart failure. Having one stroke increases risk for a subsequent stroke up to tenfold (Kobayashi et al., 1997). Risk for recurrent stroke is greater in the first 6 months (European Stroke Prevention Study II, 1997; Wolf et al., 1999).

Diabetes carries a two- to threefold risk of stroke, which can be reduced by hypertension control, daily glucose control, and monitoring of glycohemoglobin levels (Margolis & Wityk, 1997). A total serum cholesterol level higher than 200 mg/dL is associated with increased stroke risk, apparently by accelerating cornary atheroscelerosis. If LDL is higher or HDL lower than recommended, risk is further increased (Koran-Morag, Tanne, et al., 2002). Several recent studies have shown that inflammatory response to plaque in the blood may be the most important contributing factor in stroke. Statin drugs (e.g., pravastatin, simvastatin, and atorvastatin) used to lower cholesterol may also serve to reduce blood levels of C-reactive protein (CRP), a protein associated with severe arterial inflammation, thus lowering the risk of stroke through several mechanisms. New guidelines regarding the role of inflammation in cardiovascular health are expected in the near future (Stein, Balis, Grundy et al., 2001; Hess, Dumcuk, Bass & Yatsu, 2000).

Cigarette smoking has long been established as a major risk factor for stroke. Smoking increases the risk of stroke by 50% in all gender and age groups: The risk is directly proportional to the number of cigarettes smoked. Smoking is associated with reduced blood vessel elasticity, increased blood levels of fibrinogen, increased platelet aggregability, decreased high-density lipoprotein (HDL) cholesterol levels, and increased hematocrit (AHA, 2002; Weinburger, 2002). Alcohol consumption at more than two drinks per day carries a 50% increased risk of cardiac arrhythmias, increased blood pressure, abnormal blood clotting mechanisms, and a higher risk of cerebral hemorrhage (Margolis & Wityk, 1997). Illicit drug abuse, particularly the use of amphetamines, "crack" cocaine, and heroin, has been associated with an increased risk of both ischemic and hemorrhagic stroke even in first-time users (Sloan, Kittner, Feeser, et al., 1998; Petitti, Sydney, Quesenberry et al., 1998). Obesity (identified as a body mass index [BMI] ≥ 30 kg/m^2), particularly abdominal obesity with a waist-hip ratio over 1, increases stroke risk. The role of obesity in stroke is related to its association with increased blood sugar, blood pressure, and blood lipid levels (Goldstein et al., 2001).

The relationship of oral contraceptives and hormone replacement therapy (HRT) to stroke risk is controversial. Much of the perceived risk associated with oral contraceptives is based in early studies with high-dose preparations. Studies of second-generation oral contraceptives containing lower doses of estrogens found a small increase in risk of stroke. The researchers concluded that the risk of unwanted pregnancy and sequelae posed the greater risk than stroke (Gillum, Mamidipudi, & Johnston, 2000). Results from the HERS II study of Hormone Replacement Therapy (HRT) (2002) found no evidence of overall benefit for cardiovascular health, and recommendations were made that HRT should not be used for the purpose of reducing risk for CHD events in postmenopausal women (Grady et al., 2002). In July 2002 the Women's Health Initiative trial discovered that the risks from long-term use of an estrogen-progestrone combination HRT is linked to higher rates of breast cancer and

CHD, causing them to stop the trial (Rossouw et al., 2002). Although the absolute relative risk attributed to estrogen plus progesterone was low, new recommendations are expected regarding the impact of hormone replacement therapy on CHD. Current data on HRT and stroke risk appears to be inconclusive; decisions on the use of HRT should be made in an individual risk-to-benefit basis (Fowler, 2001; Paganini-Hill, 2001).

Comorbid conditions of hypertension, heart disease, diabetes mellitus, obesity, and arthritis all predispose the individual with a stroke to a recurrent stroke and can compromise the ability to participate in rehabilitation as well as life in general. Good medical management of these comorbidities is essential to maintaining the quality of life.

SPECIFIC CONSIDERATIONS FOR PHARMACOTHERAPY

The aim of this section is threefold: First, a general overview of medications used to treat modifiable risk factors; second, a discussion of medications used in the treatment of acute TIA and stroke including antithrombolytic agents; and third, a general review of medications commonly used for the relief of symptoms following stroke.

When Drug Therapy Is Needed

Modifying risk factors to prevent new and further stroke is the first goal of drug intervention. The second goal is management of emergent events, including the use of antithrombotic therapy. The specific sequelae of the stroke, including but not limited to spasticity, mood disorders (particularly depression), alterations in bowel and bladder function, and attention deficits, amenable to drug therapy are covered below.

Short- and Long-Term Goals of Pharmacotherapy

The primary goal in managing a patient with stroke is to minimize functional and cognitive deficits associated with stroke. In embolic stroke, about 33% of patients may regain some or all of their previous function if treated within 3 h of stroke onset with a thrombolytic agent.

The long-term goals of pharmacotherapy are the prevention of stroke and of recurrent stroke through modification of known risk factors. There is a 5% incidence per year of stroke following TIA and having one stroke increases risk for a subsequent stroke up to tenfold (Kobayashi et al., 1997). The second long-term goal is appropriate use of pharmaceuticals for disability symptom relief.

Nonpharmacologic Therapy

Nonpharmacologic prevention of stroke therapy is similar to prevention directed toward coronary artery disease. Promotion of lifestyle modification is encouraged: Weight control, aerobic exercise for 30 minutes three times weekly, and appropriate stress management is recommended. Strongly encourage patients to stop smoking and limit alcohol intake. An in-depth history of substance abuse should be included as part of a complete health evaluation for all patients (Weinberger et al., 2002; Wolf et al., 1999).

Surgery may be used to prevent stroke, treat acute stroke, or to repair vascular damage or malformations in and around the brain. Individuals with a high degree of carotid stenosis (70–99% stenosis of any carotid vessel) show a better outcome with surgery because the risk of stroke without surgery is higher than the 5% risk with surgery (Gasecki & Hachinski, 1993). The key to a better outcome with carotid endarterectomy is a technically competent surgeon who performs the procedure frequently and has a low rate of complications.

Stroke occurs in 5 to 10% of individuals following coronary artery bypass surgery. The skill of the surgeon and his complication rate are factors in the outcome as well as close monitoring of oxygen levels.

Acute, post-stroke rehabilitation in specialized stroke care units has proven to be effective in reducing stroke mortality and increasing the number of patients making full functional recovery (Evans, 2001). Acute stroke teams have expertise in stroke etiology, brain areas involved, specific neurologic deficits, and complications that occur with stroke (Evans, 2001). The stroke team decreases mortality as well as maintenance of blood pressure, better treatment of hyperthermia, and control of hyperglycemia than traditional care. Hyperthermia with an increase in temperature of 2.7°F doubles the risk of poor outcome after stroke (Margolis & Wityk, 1997).

Following stroke, the services of a full rehabilitation team are useful, including speech pathologists, certified rehabilitation or neurologic nurses, physical therapists, occupational therapists, neuropsychologists, social workers and recreational therapists, as well as consulting neurologists and physiatrists. In most instances, physical therapy is the foundation of the rehabilitation process.

Time Frame for Initiating Pharmacotherapy

In general there are three treatment phases for stroke: preventive therapies, therapy immediately during or after a stroke event, and treatment of stroke sequelae. With the exception of a new acute stroke, the time frame for initiation of pharmacotherapy for stroke prevention and for symptom relief is within a day or week depending on the symptoms being addressed.

In a new acute stroke, time to pharmacologic intervention is crucial. The term "brain attack" advocated by many healthcare professionals emphasizes the emergency nature of the event. In the acute phase of stroke, rapid assessment and initiation of appropriate therapy is essential to minimize permanent damage to the brain and resulting neurological dysfunction (Weinberger, 2002). Within a 3-hour window, the patient must undergo a CT to locate or rule out a hemorrhage and to identify type of infarction. Emergency blood work is necessary to determine blood-clotting capabilities prior to treatment with thrombolytic agents. Emergency management includes stabilization and assessment of factors that may influence prognosis (such as dysphagia). Patients who present after the 3-hour window should be evaluated for etiology of stroke but are usually not eligible for acute therapy (Newman, 2002; Thomassen, Waje-Andreassen, & Maintz, 2001). Patients who have a stroke of known cardioembolic basis are at risk for recurrent stroke within 7 days of the initial event and should be placed on prophylactic anticoagulation (Weinberger, 2002).

Overview of Drug Classes for Treatment

Many drug groups are utilized in treating the modifiable risk factors in stroke: Antihypertensive agents, lipid-reducing agents, agents to treat obesity, and smoking cessation agents are all utilized.

In acute stroke, treatment is dependent on the diagnosis of ischemic stroke, the presence of ischemia, and the use of thrombolytic agents, as well as the necessity of treating concurrent hypertension accompanying the stroke and other forms of coronary artery disease.

In treating the sequelae of acute stroke, the drug classes include antispasmolytics, drugs to control incontinency, drugs for anxiety and depression, and pain relievers.

Assessment Needed Prior to Therapy

Assessment of stroke risk is recognizing the unmodifiable risk factors of age and sex and assessing those risk factors that can be modified. This assessment includes elevation of blood pressure, general hypertension, diabetes mellitus, obesity, use of oral contraceptives, cigarette smoking, cardiovascular disease (particularly atrial fibrillation, left ventricular hypertrophy, and carotid artery stenosis), and alcohol or drug abuse.

In acute stroke or TIA, rapid assessment of neurological status and life-threatening conditions is essential to minimize permanent damage and reduce complications. Measures must be taken to ensure adequate respiration and oxygenation and to identify and treat any causes of hypertension. Once the patient is stabilized, a full history, general physical examination, and full neurologic examination including overall mental status, cranial nerve status, motor strength, sensory changes, coordination, and communication should be completed. The second most important task after stabilizing the patient is to determine the etiology of the stroke. Because a clinical evaluation cannot discriminate between certain strokes and other nonstroke conditions, brain imaging with CT or MRI is essential to the diagnostic evaluation. Brain imaging differentiates stroke from nonstroke conditions, locates or rules out hemorrhage, and identifies location, size, and type of infarction (Newman, 2002). CT scans within hours to days of an ischemic stroke may not show new lesions. Additional tests to rule out other metabolic etiologies and provide important diagnostic information include electrocardiogram (EKG), full blood chemistries, complete blood count, clotting times, serum glucose, electrolytes, creatinine and blood urea nitrogen, urinalysis, and urine culture and sensitivity. (Margolis & Preziosi, 1996; Thomasson et al., 2001).

In assessing treatment after stroke, the pharmacologic agents utilized are for symptomatic relief. For the long-term treatment of stroke sequelae, see the sections covering spasticity, incontinency, pain relief, depression, and anxiety.

Patient/Caregiver Information

Individuals need to understand their role in stroke prevention through good control of modifiable risk factors and adherence with prescribed drug routines. At the same time patients and families need to realize that risk factors that cannot be altered—such as age, gender, race, and previous stroke—will benefit from stringent management of modifiable risk factors.

Despite high mortality rates and functional impairment due to stroke, many families and patients do not recognize the symptoms of stroke or recognize that seeking treatment is urgent (ESPS II, 1997). Although many factors influence delay in seeking treatment, inadequate knowledge of stroke and symptoms is most often identified as the primary reason (Yoon & Byes, 2002). Classic symptoms include hemiparesis (weakness affecting one side of the body), aphasia (impaired ability to understand speech or writing or to communicate), hemianopia (loss of vision in half of the visual field in one or both eyes), or an alteration in sensory perception. Teaching the public these signs and symptoms of stroke and that stroke is a medical emergency needs to be a priority of public health education.

If the onset of symptoms is within 3 h and a protocol for the use of thrombolytic agents is available at a local facility, then the individual and family need to be directed to that facility. Regardless of time frame, transfer to a facility with a stroke team in place may improve acute treatment, prevent complications, lessen the length of an acute hospital stay, and lessen stroke care costs.

Patient and caregiver information following a stroke includes specific guidelines for general and rehabilitation care, as well as measures needed to try and prevent further strokes. This includes information and treatment plans to modify further risk factors; the goals and pharmacologic treatment of spasticity, incontinency, cognitive impairments, speech, and dysphagia, and basic rehabilitation measures in daily as well as extended activities of daily living. In some cases caregivers need information regarding skilled care facilities, assisted living programs, home health services, financial issues, and healthcare proxies.

OUTCOMES MANAGEMENT

This section considers pharmacologic agents in three groups: the drugs used in the prevention of stroke, the drugs used in acute stroke, and the drugs used after a completed stroke.

Drugs Used in Stroke Prevention

The early prevention of stroke recurrence, immediately following stroke, is a vital component of stroke management. The objectives for stroke prevention are similar to those for cardiovascular disease and many of the same drugs are utilized. Antiplatelet and anticoagulant agents are a diverse class of drugs that have been successfully used for over 20 years in secondary stroke prevention. These agents include aspirin, the adenosine antagonists, ticlopidine and clopidogrel, and warfarin. Although nonsteroidal antiinflammatory agents (NSAIDs) have a transient effect on platelets, there is no long-term benefit, and their use in stroke prevention is limited.

Researchers continue to study drugs that will prevent stroke or stroke damage. Current studies on the use of dietary folate, vitamin E, certain ACE-inhibitors, and the thiazide diuretics as therapy for stroke prevention show promise, but to date no recommendations concerning their use have been endorsed. Observational data support the benefit of vitamin E supplementation for stroke prevention but results of controlled clinical trials are inconsistent (HOPE, 2000). Given the low costs and risk associated with supplements, healthcare practitioners may choose to recommend folate and vitamin E supplements pending further study regarding their role in stroke prevention (Pearce, Boosalis, & Yeager, 2000). Some of the promising drugs for use as neuroprotectants include choline precursors such as lecithin, citicoline, and CDP-choline, magnesium sulfate, and gavestinel. The effectiveness of these drugs is conditional on use within 1 hour of the onset of symptoms (Mitka, 2002). Increasing evidence suggests that statins play an important role in stroke reduction. The reduction in stroke with statin use may not be completely related to cholesterol reduction but may involve neuroprotectant and anti-inflammatory effects (Hess et al., 2000).

There is a growing interest in the concept of combination therapy for use in stroke prevention. This includes the use of clopidogrel or ticlopidine with aspirin, warfarin in combination with aspirin or dipyridamole (75 mg), and aspirin (325 mg). The combination of low-dose aspirin with extended release dipyridamole has been shown to be more effective than either drug alone for select patients. In the ESPS II (1997) the relative risk reduction for secondary stroke prevention was 37% with the use of a combination of extended-release dipyridamole and aspirin. The risk of major bleeding in the combination was no greater than that seen with aspirin alone. However, a 7.4% withdrawal from the trial was attributed to severe adverse events associated with DP (primarily headache and GI events).

Acetylsalicylic Acid (Aspirin). Aspirin (ASA) is the best studied and most widely used antiplatelet agent for primary and secondary stroke prevention. ASA results in a small but statistically significant reduction in mortality and disability when given within 48 hours after ischemic stroke. Aspirin therapy may be used safely in combination with low doses of subcutaneous heparin for deep venous thrombosis prophylaxis after stroke (Wolf et al., 1999). Aspirin inhibits platelet activation by inhibiting platelet cyclooxygenase and thromboxane production and reduces the risk of stroke by 25% (Chen et al., 2000). ASA is more effective in men than women. The optimal dose for either primary or secondary stroke prevention has been the subject of much study and debate. In 1998, the FDA recommended aspirin doses between 50 and 325 mg/d for secondary prevention of stroke, provided contraindications such as allergy and gastrointestinal bleeding are not present, and the patient has or will not be treated with thrombolytic agents (Hayden et al., 2002). There is a slight increase in the rate of hemorrhagic stroke in patients treated with aspirin, but on a risk-to-benefit assessment this is outweighed by the decrease in rate of ischemic strokes. Although the balance of benefits and risks are most favorable in patients at high risk of CHD, aspirin therapy is considered beneficial for a wide range of patients and should be considered for all patients at risk for recurrence (Chen et al., 2000). The chief side effect of ASA therapy is gastric irritation and consequent GI bleeding.

Ticlopidine and Clopidogrel. Ticlopidine (Ticlid) and Clopidogrel (Plavix) are thienopyridine derivative antiplatelet drugs that act by blocking the adenosine diphosphate pathways (ADP) receptor on platelets. Unlike aspirin, the effect takes 4 to 7 days to attain full platelet inhibition but can last up to 5 days after discontinuing therapy. The thienoyridines appear slightly more effective in preventing serious vascular events in high-risk patients (Graeme, Hankey, Sudlow, & Dunbabin, 2000; Hankey, Sudlow, & Dunbagin, 2000). In the TASS study (Grotta, Norris, Kamm, et al., 1992; Hass et al., 1989), patients receiving ticlopidine (500 mg/d) had a 21% decrease in all types of stroke at 3 years compared with those receiving aspirin (1300 mg/d). In the CAPRIE trial (CAPRIE, 1996), the largest study of clopidogrel to date, clopidogrel was more effective in prevention of strokes than aspirin. Compared with either aspirin or clopidogrel alone, the combination of aspirin 75 to 325 mg/d and clopidogrel, 75 mg/d resulted in an additional 20% reduction of vascular events in patients with CVD. The drug is utilized more in women, those failing ASA therapy, and with vertebrobasilar symptoms. Compared with ASA, thienopyridines have significantly less incidence of gastric upset and GI bleeding, but a significant increase in the incidence of skin rash and diarrhea. The risk of skin rash and diarrhea are greater for ticlopidine than for clopidrogel. Ticlopidine has several potentially dangerous side effects—e.g., neutropenia and thrombotic thrombocytopenic purpura—and should be reserved for patients with aspirin allergies. When patients are placed on ticlopidine, complete blood counts should be checked every 2 weeks for the first 3 months to detect thrombocytopenia. Clopidogrel appears to be safer than ticlopidine, making it a better, but more expensive, choice for patients who are aspirin intolerant (Graeme et al., 2000; Hankey et al., 2000).

Warfarin. Warfarin (Coumadin) is used in prevention of secondary stroke and significantly reduces risk of systemic embolism in patients in atrial fibrillation after minor stroke (Mohr et al., 2001). It acts by inhibiting clotting mechanisms in the liver. In the Chimowitz et al., (1995) study, warfarin was significantly better than ASA for stroke prevention in patients with symptomatic stenosis of a major intracerebral artery. In terms of stroke prevention, warfarin is more effective and less costly overall than ASA in patients with nonvalvular atrial fibrillation (Gage et al., 1995; Mohr et al., 2001). Therapy is started with an initial dose of 5 to 10 mg/d then individualized according to patient response as indicated by international normalized ratio (INR). The anticoagulation effect should be kept at a target INR of 2.5 but may vary in some conditions. The use of warfarin requires daily monitoring until the INR reaches the therapeutic range (2.0 to 4.0) and then less frequently once an individual is stabilized (Ansell et al., 2001; Mohr et al., 2001). Bleeding is the main complication of oral anticoagulant therapy. The risk of bleeding may be reduced dramatically by maintaining the INR range to 2.0 to 3.0 (Ansell et al., 2001). One of the primary factors limiting warfarin use is the challenges of closely monitoring the level of anticoagulation; thus, a cooperative patient and adequate laboratory facilities are required. Contraindications to its use may include heavy use of alcohol, history of GI bleeding, risk of falls, underlying hepatic or renal disease, use of antiplatelet agents, and thyrotoxicosis (Mohr et al., 2001).

Nimodipine. Nimodipine (Nimotop) is a calcium channel blocker used to reduce neurologic deficits following subarachnoid hemorrhage (SAH). Although the exact mechanism of action is unknown, it is thought to inhibit the uptake of calcium into damaged neurons and consequent neurocellular damage and cerebral vasoconstriction. The oral dose is 60 mg (two 30 mg capsules) every 4 hours for 21 consecutive days, preferably initiated within 96 hours of the hemorrhage. The chief side effect is hypotension, and in some cases this may necessitate discontinuing the drug. Other less common side effects include thrombocytopenia, rash, abdominal cramping, and elevated liver enzymes (AHFS, 1996).

Drugs Used in Acute Stroke Care

The primary goal of acute therapy is reperfusion of the occluded arterial territory and prevention of additional damage. Although there are few therapies that directly reduce damage to neural tissue, there is much that can be done to improve the outcome of stroke patients.

Thrombolytic Agents. Tissue plasminogen activator (t-PA) (alteplase, tenecteplase, and urokinesase) has been licensed in the United States since 1996 for use within 3 hours of onset of ischemic stroke. The findings of the National Institute of Neurological Disorders and Stroke (NINDS) rt-PA trial (1995), showed a highly significant increase in the number of patients making full neurological recovery from stroke (12% absolute risk reduction) with no increase in mortality. In contrast, streptokinase has not shown the same results (Donnan et al., 1996). Eligibility criteria for the use of intravenous tissue plasminogen activator is based on the NINDS trial protocol (see Table 29–5 for inclusion & exclusion criteria for thrombolysis in acute ischemic stroke). Therapy should be initiated as soon as possible to optimize benefits. The efficacy is time-based to within 3 hours of the acute stroke (Hacke et al., 1998; Fisher & Ratan, 2003). Bleeding is the major complication of thrombolytic therapy. Brain imaging to rule out hemorrhage, complete blood count (CBC), glucose levels, blood coagulation studies, and informed consent must be obtained prior to treatment with thrombolytic agents. If possible, hypertension must be controlled Use of ASA or Ticlid does not preclude the use of t-PA. Patients on warfarin or heparin should not be given t-PA for treatment of acute ischemic stroke. The inpatient hospital setting must have the ability to care for cerebral hemorrhage, which can occur following its use. Patients given t-PA should not receive other antithrombotic or antiplatelet drugs within 24 hours of therapy. Intravenous r-TPA is given in a dose of 0.9 mg/kg (maximum of 90 mg) 10% of the dose in a bolus and the remainder infused over 1 hour (DiPiro et al., 2002; Wolf et al., 1999).

TABLE 29–5. Inclusion and Exclusion Criteria for Intravenous tPA in Acute Ischemic Stroke

Criteria for Inclusion
Age 18 or older
Measurable stroke-related neurologic deficits not resolving
Time of symptom onset > 3 hours prior to beginning treatment
Criteria for Exclusion
Evidence of intracranial hemorrhage on noncontrast head CT
Rapidly improving stroke symptoms
High clinical suspicion of subarachnoid hemorrhage, known cerebral aneurysm or arteriovenous malformation
Recent internal bleeding (e.g., GI/GU bleed within 21 days)
Platelet count > 100,000/mm^3
Patient has received heparin within 48 hours
Recent use of anticoagulant (e.g., warfarin)
Intracranial surgery, major head trauma or previous stroke within 3 months
Major head surgery or serious trauma within 14 days
Arterial puncture at noncompressed site within 7 days
Lumbar puncture within 7 days
Witnessed seizure at stroke onset
Recent acute myocardial infarction
SBP > 185 mm Hg or DPB > 110 at time of treatment
Pregnancy

Sources: Hacke et al. (1998); Ninds (1995) Fisher, (2003).

Hypertension Management. In ischemic stroke, acute hypertension will usually resolve and begin to fall within hours of the event. The initial rise in systemic blood pressure is protective to ensure adequate blood flow to cerebral vessels. Stroke due to hemorrhage and initial hypertension in ischemia may, however, require aggressive treatment to prevent end-organ damage (heart, liver, and kidneys). If cerebral pressure autoregulation is impaired, an elevated blood pressure increases cerebral blood flow, which leads to increased intracranial pressure. The goal of reducing systemic hypertension is maintenance of cerebral perfusion to prevent further brain injury. If blood pressure is reduced too quickly or by drugs inducing cerebral vessel dilatation, the increase in cerebral edema causes cerebral blood vessel damage with vascular leakage and more cerebral edema. See Table 29–6 for guidelines for blood pressure management in stroke and hemorrhage.

Hypertension should be treated if the calculated mean blood pressure (sum of systolic blood pressure plus diastolic blood pressure times 2 and divided by 3) is over 130 mm Hg or systolic pressure is over 220 mm Hg. In such cases, the best parenteral drugs are those that are easily titrated, have a short duration of action, and minimal effect on cerebral blood vessels, such as labetalol or enalapril. Sodium nitroprusside may be indicated for the immediate reduction of blood pressure of patients in hy-

TABLE 29–6. Blood Pressure Management in Stroke and Hemorrhage

Neurological Condition	Hypertension Management
Acute stroke	Lower B/P slowly and gently Watch for signs of clinical deterioration in neurologic status
Ischemic stroke	Lower B/P only if repeated measurements are > 220 mm Hg systolic or > 120 mm Hg diastolic or there is evidence of end-organ failure or aortic dissection Lower B/P from 185–181/110–105 in patients with a history of HTN Lower B/P from 170–160/100–95 in patients with previously normal B/P
Intracerebral hemorrhage	Lower B/P from 185–180/110–105 in patients with a history of HTN Lower B/P from 170–160/100–95 in patients with previously normal B/P
Subarachnoid hemorrhage	Lower to prestroke levels

Sources: Adams, et al. (2003); Torbey & Bhardwai (2001).

pertensive crises. Concomitant longer-acting antihypertensive medication should be administered so that the duration of treatment with sodium nitroprusside can be minimized (Adams et al., 2003; Torbey & Bhardwai, 2001). For some individuals, treatment with oral agents such as captopril or nicardipine is adequate. Sublingual use of a calcium antagonist should be avoided due to rapid absorption and secondary precipitous drop in blood pressure (Adams et al., 2003). Labetalol (Trandate), an alpha and beta blocker, acts by decreasing systolic vascular resistance without reflex tachycardia by beta-adrenergic receptor blockage and improves cerebral perfusion pressure by a decrease in intracerebral pressure. The dose of labetalol is 0.05 mg/kg IV with response in 5 to 10 min. The dose can be repeated every 10 min or continuously infused at 0.5 to 2 mg/min. Enalapril (Vasotec) is an angiotensin-converting enzyme inhibitor that reduces the peripheral vascular resistance without provoking a reflex sympathetic stimulation thus retaining favorable end-organ perfusion (Kay et al., 1996). Once the desired B/P is reached, the infusion can be stopped and oral medications initiated.

In the office setting, if the individuals blood pressure is over 180/100 with a new stroke, hospital treatment is required. If blood pressure is mildly elevated, the oral agents used most frequently are captopril and nicardipine.

Management of Acute Myocardial Infarction. In acute stroke, there is a 12% incidence of acute MI that accompanies the stroke, as well as a higher rate of EKG changes, some of which are thought to be neuronal in origin. If EKG changes occur with stroke, patient survival is decreased by 50% in the first 3 years. Consequently, following stroke, appropriate ASA treatment at 325 mg per day in asymptomatic stroke survivors is recommended. If the individual has symptoms of cardiac disease, other treatment is recommended depending on their cardiac status (Hayden et al., 2002).

Congestive Heart Failure. Congestive heart failure can occur with stroke and requires appropriate acute treatment (see Chapter 20).

Seizure Management. Utilization of antiseizure medications will not prevent the onset of seizures. Seizures complicate 2% of strokes at onset: Half are generalized and half partial (focal). They are generally of no prognostic significance and do not require antiseizure medication. The risk is higher in patients with large MCA infarcts and ICH, each of which have a 10% risk of recurrent seizures or epilepsy. Most epilepsy development occurs in the first year following stroke.

Injury to the cortex carries a higher risk of seizure than injury to deeper cortical areas, both in infarction and hemorrhage, as does metabolic imbalance and multiple cerebral infarction. If recurrent seizures do occur, monotherapy with conventional anticonvulsant treatment may be initiated in some cases for recurrent events (see section on seizures for specifics of treatment options). Metabolic clearance for antiepileptic drugs does decline in the elderly, so frequently this group of patients needs less drug than a younger population. Weaning off seizure medications may be initiated at 1 year given a normal EEG and no recurrent seizures (Bladin, Alexandrov, Bellavance, et al., 2000).

Drug Use Following Stroke

Incontinence. Incontinence and bladder retention can occur after stroke. Medication use is delayed until specific diagnosis is made and behavioral therapies are initiated. The most common cause of initial incontinence in a previously hospitalized patient is a urinary tract infection. It is important to eliminate the cause before other therapy is initiated. If the patient remains persistently incontinent, assessing any previous history of incontinence and prostate disease is imperative, followed by a cystometrography study. If detrusor instability and hyperreflexia are found, specific medications are helpful as well as the utilization of incontinence devices.

Urinary Retention. Males with existing prostate disease can develop retention, which is most clearly indicated by a high postvoid residual (over 100 cc) if catheterized immediately. It is not uncommon for individuals with a mild stroke to present in the office setting with a large retentive bladder. Specifics for medication treatment are discussed in Chapter 34.

Spasticity. Spasticity following stroke includes a range of clinical problems including increased muscle tone, abnormal limb posture, excessive contraction of antagonist muscles, and hyperactive cutaneous and tendon reflexes. The prevalence of stroke-related disability is high, and spasticity may be a significant factor. Spacticity occurs within hours to up to 38 days after a stroke, first in the proximal muscles of the hip and shoulder, and then more distally. The presenting pattern is usually flexor then extensor synergy. The extensor synergy in the leg can help with gait. Spasticity can resolve with the return of voluntary muscle control. The specifics of treatment and pharmacotherapeutics are in Chapter 14. Management strategies include a multidisciplinary team approach utilizing a variety of rehabilitation techniques. Pharmacologic treatment can be difficult with this population because of the sedating properties of many of the drugs (ASA, 2002).

Upper Lower Extremity Pain. Reflex sympathetic dystrophy (RSD) or Complex Regional Pain Syndrome, is a clinical syndrome occurring in acute paralysis characterized by ipsilateral distal limb pain, swelling, erythema, contractures, and hyperalgia. It is commonly seen 1 to 5 months after stroke and is primarily diagnosed by a positive bone scan that shows an elevated nuclear uptake. An underlying predisposition has been suggested, but the pathogenesis is not completely understood; however, it may be related to reduced sympathetic outflow to the affected extremity. Many clinicians believe that RSD is best thought of as a "reaction pattern" to an injury or to activity restrictions following injury (Franklin, 1999). Secondary signs of RSD include osteoporosis, muscle atrophy, temperature changes, and vasomotor instability. Although physical therapy is the mainstay of treatment, pharmacologic interventions are needed to manage pain. Choice of agent is based on the type of pain. NSAIDs are commonly used to treat constant pain associated with inflammation; anti-depressants (e.g., amitriptyline, nortriptyline, trazodone) are often used for constant pain or spontaneous (paroxysmal) jabs and sleep disturbances; and anti-epileptics (e.g., carbamazepine, gabapentin) may relieve constant pain as well. Clonazepam (Klonopin) or Baclofen is used to treat muscle cramps (spasms and dystonia) (Karlsson, 1999; Kirkpatrick, 2000). Other interventions include cortiocosteroids, vasodilators, and alpha- or beta-adrenergic-blocking compounds. Several studies suggest that clonidine (Clonidine Patch) may decrease pain in RSD by inhibiting the sympathetic nervous system (Kirkpatrick, 2000). The use of opioids in RSD treatment remains controversial due to potential hazards associated with their use. Elevation of the extremity may be helpful. Injection of a local anesthetic, such as lidocaine, is sometimes used (Kirkpatrick, 2000).

Deep Vein Thrombus. Thromboembolism is rare in the first few weeks after stroke (around 1% in the first week, although higher if defined radiologically rather than clinically). Early mobilization, antiplatelet drugs, and rehydration all contribute to prevention, however, for acute stroke patients with restricted mobility the use of prophylactic low-dose heparin or low-molecular-weight heparin is recommended (Ansell et al., 2001). Heparin markedly reduces the incidence of DVT and pulmonary thromboembolism but is associated with higher risk of systemic hemorrhage. Low molecular weight heparin offers the major benefits of convenient dosing and possible outpatient treatment and less thrombocytopenia and recurrent venous thromboembolism than unfractionated heparin. Treatment with heparin (5000 units every 12 hours) or low molecular weight heparin (e.g., dalteparin 200 IU/kg/day in 1 or 2 doses) should be continued for at least 5 days. The treatment does not require laboratory followup. Oral anticoagulation (warfarin) should be overlapped with heparin therapy and should be continued for at least 3 months (Ansell et al., 2001).

Immobility or a stroke that limits ambulation to less than 30 ft per day requires prophylactic treatment with heparin; 5000 units every 12 h is recommended. Twenty percent of individuals on low-dose heparin still develop DVT, and 10% of these individuals will develop pulmonary emboli, which carry a 10% fatality rate (Potter, 1993).

Depression. Depression and related neuropsychiatric complications are common after stroke (about 50% incidence) but are often underdiagnosed and undertreated. The primary cause is a biological response to brain injury and a change in neurotransmitters, (Gainotti, Marra, Antonucci, & Paolucci, 2001).

Poststroke depression has negative effects on cognitive and functional recovery. Pharmacological intervention can dramatically improve function and quality of life. Standard depression scales and the DSM-IV criteria are used to determine the diagnosis. Regardless of etiology, depression should be treated. In stroke the serotonin reuptake inhibitors (SSRIs) (e.g., paroxetine [Paxil], fluoxetine [Prozac or Sarafem], or sertraline [Zoloft]), are a first-line drug choice, because they produce less lethargy and sedation than other antidepressants. In addition, sertraline (Zoloft) may have cognitive benefits as well. A second choice is tricyclic antidepressants. They require monitoring of cardiac conduction, heart rate, and blood pressure, particularly if left ventricle dysfunction is present.

Anxiety. A recent stroke review (Margolis & Wityk, 1997) showed an increase in general anxiety disorders of 25% following stroke. The symptoms were insomnia, excessive fatigue, and irritability. This group benefited by treatment with antidepressant rather than anxiolytic medications, which tended to be too sedating. The serotonin reuptake medications (SSRIs) were the recommended medications because of fewer side effects.

Dementia. Stroke can cause, contribute to, or coexist with dementia. In some elderly patients with mild dementias, the compensatory capacity of the brain may be overcome with the stroke. The prevalence of dementia in stroke is 26 to 52% if the individual is over 80 (Erkinjuntti, 2001). See the dementia section of this chapter regarding specifics of pharmacologic treatment.

Sexuality. Many changes can occur in sexual relationships and functioning after a stroke. The alterations can be related to physiologic and cognitive changes, use of medications, alterations in autonomic nervous system function, fear of another stroke, and diminished self-image. These changes need to be addressed by providers, and not ignored.

Drugs Not to Use in Stroke. In a retrospective analysis of the Sygen in Acute Stroke Study (Goldstein, 1995), a small but significant relationship between certain drug classes and a poor functional and motor outcome was noted. The drugs showing poorer outcome at 84 days after stroke were all given in the first month after stroke. The classes included benzodiazepines, phenytoin, phenobarbital, and dopamine. It is postulated that these drugs may inhibit stroke recovery by impairing the use of associated neurons at the site of the stroke, as well as inhibiting resolution of diaschisis.

Followup Recommendations

Followup in the office setting is based on the medication regimes of patients and their medical stability. Initially, several specialists may be involved because of cognitive or funcitonal issues. Care by these specialist may decrease with the patient's improvement. Event management may be by the primary care provider.

MULTIPLE SCLEROSIS

Multiple sclerosis (MS) is the most common neurologic diagnosis of young adults. Evidence suggests that this is an autoimmune condition, affecting 250,000 to 350,000 young adults younger than 40, with one peak in the mid-20s and another peak in the mid-40s. More women than men are affected with prevalence ranging from 1.1 to 2.8, and it is more common in Caucasians. The disease is more prevalent in North America and Northern Europe and migration after age 15 shows a prevalence to the country of origin (Donohoe, 1995).

The exact etiology is unknown. A proposed etiology is an autoimmune regulation abnormality. The actual mediator of myelin destruction has not been established but this activity has been attributed to the action of macrophages, killer T cells, lymphocytes, antibodies or a combination of these. Two genetic markers, HLA-DR2 on chromosome 6 and immunoglobulin GM on chromosome 14, are found more frequently in MS. There is a familial tendency, with identical twins showing a 26% chance of both twins having the disease if one develops it, and 2.5% in fraternal twins and first-degree relatives, a 5 to 15 times greater ratio than the general population. Although a viral infection is suspected, no active or latent virus has been located in brain or spinal cord tissue. There is a decreased risk of exacerbation in pregnancy, but there is an increased risk of exacerbation postpartum. The family's ability to carry out childcare should play a role in the decision of women to bear children (Donohoe, 1995).

The pathophysiology of MS is one of CNS demyelination of nerve fibers, sparing of axons, gliosis, and development of inflammatory cells. Plaques ranging from 1 mm to 4 cm are scattered throughout white matter and to some degree in grey matter. The areas usually showing early pathology are the optic nerves and chiasm and the areas surrounding the blood vessels in the cerebellum, cerebrum, and cervical spinal cord. Plaques that are actively forming create increased edema with a number of lymphs, macrophages, and plasma cells. The chronic lesions show astrocyte hyperplasia and a reduced number of oligodendrocytes that appear as scars. The disease is thought to be initiated by an immune response against a virus that cross-reacts with myelin or oligodendrocyte cells; the antigen that is produced is still unknown. The pathology of MS lesions is different in the early stages of the disease, during chronic MS, and during acute exacerbations.

One current hypothesis is that a defect in suppressor T-cell function lowers the threshold of T-cell activity. Cytokines (tumor necrosis factor and interleukin-2), interferon, and prostaglandins are present in MS and implicated in the regulation of the immune system and in autoimmune reactions. The use of MRI in judging the development of new plaques that may be clinically silent allows an objective measure of drug utilization and drug suppression of new plaque formation as a marker of drug efficacy (Donohoe, 1995).

The clinical manifestations of MS are in Table 29–7 and the diagnostic test studies are in Table 29–8. Symptoms may be classified as primary, secondary, and tertiary. Patients may appear in the office with an acute "attack" or exacerbation. They may present with complaints of visual changes, fatigue, heat intolerance, sensory disturbance, weakness and spasticity in the legs, bowel and bladder dysfunction, ataxic gait, paresthesias in the extremities, and sexual dysfunction. On clinical neurologic examination these patients show changes in ocular movement, changes in visual acuity, trigeminal neuralgia and optic neuritis, increased tone in the legs, a decrease in

TABLE 29–7. Clinical Signs and Symptoms of Multiple Sclerosis

Area of Dysfunction	Signs and Symptoms
Cranial nerves	Blurred central vision, faded color, blind spots (optic neuritis), diplopia, dysphagia, facial weakness, numbness, pain
Fatigue	Overwhelming weakness, not overcome by increased physical effort
Motor dysfunction	Weakness, paralysis, spasticity, abnormal gait
Cerebellar dysfunction	Dysarthria, tremor, incoordination, ataxia, vertigo
Cognitive dysfunction	Impaired short-term memory, difficulty learning new information, word-finding trouble, short attention span, decreased concentration, mood alterations (depression)
Sensory dysfunction	Paresthesia, decreased proprioception and temperature perception, Lhermitte's sign (electric shock sensation down spine into legs)
Bowel and bladder dysfunction	Fecal urgency, constipation, bladder urgency, incontinence
Sexual dysfunction	Women: decreased libido and orgasmic ability, decreased genital sensation Men: erectile, orgasmic, and ejaculation dysfunction

Source: Adapted from Donohoe (1995).

motor strength, bilateral clonus of knees and ankles, upgoing toes bilaterally, decreased appreciation of position, and decreased appreciation of vibration. A significant number of patients have cognitive impairment and emotional changes. Cognitively, in 50 to 60% there is difficulty with processing new information, difficulty recalling new information, and deficits in nonverbal problem solving. There may be deficits in sequencing and organizational skills, along with poor judgment, impulsivity, and inability to appreciate the consequences of an action. The Mini Mental Status Examination is helpful in assessing mental status. Emotional changes range from depression to a pseudobulbar affect that is often seen as euphoria, as well as significant amounts of fatigue, anxiety, and mental confusion.

The clinical course is marked by great variability and is unpredictable. The number and frequency of the acute "attacks" do not predict future disability. There are two major phases of disease: exacerbating-remitting and chronic-progressive. Patients in the first group average one attack per year, but after several years the disease usually becomes more chronic-progressive in 50% of individuals with MS. The attacks or exacerbations consist of new signs or worsening of old clinical signs or symptoms that last more than 24 h in the absence of fever or infection. Some individuals who present with chronic-progressive disease then change to an exacerbating-remitting disease pattern. Twenty percent present with chronic-progressive disease and are usually over 40 years of age.

TABLE 29–8. Diagnostic Tests and Results for Multiple Sclerosis

Test	Result
Magnetic resonance imaging	White matter lesions (plaques) of brain, brainstem, and spinal cord
CSF analysis (lumbar puncture)	Presence of oligoclonal bands and an increase in protein, lymphocytes, and IgG
Evoked potentials (visual, brainstem, somatosensory)	Prolonged impulse conduction
Urodynamic studies	Neurogenic bladder
Myelogram, skull and spine x-rays, CT scan	Rule out other neurologic disease

Source: Adapted from Donohoe (1995).

SPECIFIC CONSIDERATIONS FOR PHARMACOTHERAPY

When Drug Therapy Is Needed

As with other neurologic conditions, MS is managed with the assistance of a consulting neurologist who has in-depth training in the disease and its manifestations. Although not necessarily prescribing, the primary care provider needs an understanding of the drugs and their usual efficacy as well as side effects.

Short- and Long-Term Goals of Pharmacotherapy

The goals of therapy in MS are to decrease the severity, intensity, and duration of exacerbations, enhance recovery from exacerbations, prevent relapse and the onset of progressive disease, halt or reverse progressive disease, and provide symptomatic relief from the complications of MS (Bainbridge, Corboy, & Gidal, 2002).

Nonpharmacologic Therapy

The timing of therapy and specific goals are less clear in MS because of the unpredictability of the condition. Third-party payers are less familiar with the disease and somewhat reluctant to pay for therapy unless specific goals of treatment are established and met in an approved time frame. The goal of rehabilitation is to minimize functional loss despite the possibility of progressive neurologic impairments. This means the prevention of further hospitalization and preventing or delaying long-term care by adapting energy, skills, home modification, continuing employment, and cognitive rehabilitation (see the section on brain injury) as needed (Dombovy, 1997).

Symptomatic treatment areas include fatigue, spasticity, ataxia, pain, dysarthria, respiratory dysfunction, and bowel and bladder dysfunction. Learning energy conservation techniques from a physical and occupational therapist is helpful. Spasticity, muscle weakness, and ataxia often benefit from gait analysis and the use of assistive devices to ensure safety in ambulation, the necessity of wheelchair use, and proper transfer techniques. The key to reimbursement for these therapies is specificity in prescription with clear-cut goals. Pain in MS is often helped by relaxation techniques and electric stimulation. Dysarthria and respiratory dysfunction are often improved through the use of short-term speech therapy, as well as respiratory therapy to teach appropriate breathing techniques.

Bowel dysfunction is often related to constipation. It is the result of decreased exercise and consequent low motility as well as lesions or plaques on nerves that control normal bowel motility. The goal of therapy is regular bowel movements. Nonpharmacologic techniques include drinking 8 to 10 glasses of water per day (this can be problematic in bladder dysfunction). Other diet considerations include a high-bulk diet with fruits, vegetables, and whole grain cereals. Establishing a regular evacuation time is helpful, allowing 15 min of relaxation is necessary, and this may require 2 to 3 weeks to establish. Avoiding the use of a bedpan is helpful because the bowel is more active in an upright position. Exercising without causing extreme fatigue is helpful. Not having a bowel movement for 3 to 4 days and having very hard bowel movements or liquid bowel movements can result in further problems. Early intervention is helpful, so patients need to feel free to call the primary care provider with these kinds of problems. It is important to assess bowel function and use the nonpharmaceutical treatments as well as pharmaceutical treatments to maintain good bowel function.

Bladder dysfunction due to poor positioning and plaque formation on nerves and brain also is common. The bladder problems need followup with a urologist to obtain cystometric studies of bladder function. High residual urine is often a cause of urinary tract infections. If possible individuals with MS can be taught intermittent catheterization to maintain low residual urine. This may require catheterization up to 4 to 6 times a day, depending on the ability of the bladder to void and empty. Techniques to prevent urinary tract infection include the minimum intake of 2 to 3 qt of fluid per day, limiting caffeine to 2 cups per day, drinking cranberry juice, which inhibits bacteria from implantation on the bladder wall, and washing the genital area with warm water and soap twice a day. Bladder emptying may require more relaxation and time than usual in the face of dysfunction and more frequent emptying. Depending on the results of urine cystometric studies, some patients are taught to perform Credé's maneuver on their bladders. Patients need to know the symptoms of bladder infection to act appropriately and seek guidance. These symptoms include increased frequency, urgency to urinate, pain, burning with urination, and foul-smelling or cloudy urine. Because of the increased bacterial resistance to antibiotic treatment, urine cultures are necessary prior to starting treatment; prolonged prophylactic antibiotic use is not an appropriate alternative in this group of patients because it increases resistance to antibiotics.

Time Frame for Initiating Therapy

The time frame for therapy is dependent on the specifics of treatment. Treatment is undertaken either to slow the progress of the disease or to manage symptoms. In an acute exacerbation, it usually begins within a day of symptom relief or long-term prevention of new attacks. Symptomatic relief does not require such a strict time frame.

Overview of Drug Classes for Treatment

To prevent new plaque formation or acute exacerbations, patients are placed on immunomodulators; the ones currently approved by the FDA are both derivatives of interferon. The two commonly used are interferon beta-1a (Avonex) and interferon beta-1b (Betaseron). The two newest drugs in this category are glatiramer (Copaxone) and mitoxantrone (Novantrone). However the first is very expensive ($10,000/year) and the second, a cancer drug, was approved for MS in 2000 (Bryant, Clegg, & Milne, 2001; Coyle & Hartung, 2002). Further, the potential clinical benefits of mitroxamtrone appear to be only modest and the use of the drug carries a potential for serious toxicity (Goodin et al., 2003).

Anti-cholinergics remain the first-line treatment for bladder dysfunction, but alternative therapies are undergoing clinical trials. With a range of new pro-erectile oral medications available, interest has grown in treatment of multiple sclerosis-related erectile failure. Female sexual dysfunction is also now gaining some attention, with new classification criteria and methods for assessing and treating these patients. During an acute exacerbation, steroids are used to decrease inflammation and may be given orally (prednisone) or IV (methylprednisolone). The nitrogen mustard derivative cyclophosphamide (Cytoxan) and methotrexate are now also used (off label) to prevent acute inflammation. These oncology chemotherapy drugs have been shown to slow the rate of progression of MS in some people and are used when individuals do not respond to steroid use.

Symptomatically, treatment class is dependent on the symptom. The antispasm medications include baclofen, diazepam, and dantrolene. Options in the treatment of tremors include isoniazid, propranolol, and clonazepam. Bladder dysfunction may require oxybutynin and propantheline bromide. Bowel dysfunction may require bulk additives, stool softeners, and stimulants. Fatigue is treated with amantadine and pemoline, whereas mood alterations may require antidepressants, both SSRIs, and tricyclics.

Assessment Needed Prior to Drug Therapy

Once the diagnosis of MS is confirmed by a neurologist, appropriate followup by the primary provider is helpful in understanding the patient's baseline of disease so that any new acute exacerbation can be adequately evaluated and treated. A thorough neurologic examination is helpful to rate both baseline and function at exacerbation. Symptomatic treatment also will require regular visits to ascertain the effectiveness of drug treatment.

Patient and Caregiver Information

The unpredictability of the disease and its cycle of remission and exacerbation (and in some individuals, progressive nature) make information necessary and helpful. Patients need both physical and emotional support with the disease and assessment of family systems is helpful to ascertain the need for outside support (Rudick, 1993). In addition, healthcare proxies and at some point placing financial affairs in order is necessary. A recommended support source is the local Multiple Sclerosis Society as well as the regional neurologic clinic treating individuals with multiple sclerosis. Symptomatic intervention will require specific teaching as the medications are utilized.

OUTCOMES MANAGEMENT

This section focuses on the treatments to prevent the continued development of MS and those used in acute exacerbations, and briefly reviews the drugs used in symptomatic therapy.

Drugs Used to Prevent Exacerbations

Interferon Beta-1b (Betaseron). The interferons are from a large protein family, the cytokines, which "interfere" with viral infection on tissue culture. The drugs have antiviral, antiproliferative, and immunomodulatory activities. Interferons are naturally occurring agents in humans, primarily manufactured by white blood cells. The drugs appear to inhibit exacerbations in the first 2 years of therapy but have less benefit in years 3 through 5, although the rate of change over placebo is significant. The drugs' efficacy is judged by the number of new plaques seen on MRI. However, plaque formation does not always correlate with clinical signs and symptoms (Kelly, 1996).

Betaseron was released by the FDA in July 1993 for the treatment of relapsing MS. This immunomodulator is thought to act by augmenting suppressor cell function, increasing cytotoxicity of natural killer cells, and increasing macrophage activity. Interferon beta reduces the activity of interferon gamma, which decreases the inflammation produced in MS by its autoimmune response (Gidal et al., 1996).

The current dosage is 8 million units given subcutaneously every other day. Therapy is often begun at 4 million units and increased to 8 million after 1 to 2 weeks to diminish the initial side effects. The side effects are flu-like symptoms with fever, chills, and myalgias as well as injection site redness and swelling in almost all users. The drug can increase temperature, causing a loss of motor function in some MS patients, so it is better given at night. At times walking may be difficult, and patients may need temporary assistance in transfers and toileting due to adverse drug effects (Kelly, 1996). Clinical results suggest that the beneficial effects of Interferon Beta may be dose and frequency-dependent. Taken together, these findings indicate that treatment with IFN beta should be started as early as possible in the course of MS, and suggest that, in order to maximize patent benefit, the highest possible dose of IFN beta should be chosen (Grigoriadis, 2002). Nonsteroidal antiinflammatory agents or acetaminophen taken before and 24 h after administration are helpful, as is applying ice to the local injection site. Other adverse effects include shortness of breath, tachycardia, and depression, which requires close monitoring for suicide risk. Blood work before therapy includes baseline hemoglobin, complete blood counts, platelets, and liver function tests (RMSC, 1995).

Interferon Beta-1a (Avonex). This drug was released for general use in 1994. In early trials, patients taking interferon Beta-1a had a lower relapse rate and decreased disease progression compared to patients taking placebo. Also, there were fewer enhancing lesions in patients taking the active drug. More recently, this drug has been shown to slow brain atrophy and decrease cognitive decline. It is given by IM injection once weekly at 4 million units (30 μg) and can be given by the patient or a family member. It has similar side effects with flu-like symptoms, muscle aches, fever, chill, and weakness, and use of nonsteroidal antiinflammatory agents before and for 24 h after the injection is suggested, as well as ice application to the injection site. The drug may cause abortion and is not recommended for women trying to become pregnant; birth control must be practiced. It requires baseline hemoglobin, complete blood counts, platelet, and liver function tests; these are repeated after 1, 2, and 3 months on drug and then every 3 months. Its adverse effects can include exacerbation of seizures and heart disease, so some individuals may not be candidates for this treatment. Depression may also increase, requiring frequent monitoring and examination for suicide risk. The drug needs refrigeration, but not freezing, at home once reconstituted (RMSC, 1993).

Glatiramer Acetate (Copaxone). This drug was formerly known as copolymer-1 and is a synthetic polypeptide consisting of L-alanine, L-glutamic acid, L-lysine and L-tyrosine. It is thought to act by decreasing cell-mediated immune response against myelin basic protein. It contributes to the "bystander" suppression at the site of the MS lesions. It may also suppress T-cell activation. In relapsing-remitting MS, the drug showed a reduction in relapse rate over placebo in patients who are in early stages of the disease. The side effects include site reaction and systemic reactions of brief chest tightness and flushing (Gidal et al., 1996). It has few long-term side effects on initial testing. The drug is given daily at 20 mg subcutaneously (Johnson, 1996). Generally glatiramer acetate is effective (Boneschi et al., 2003) at relapse prevention and is well tolerated with mild pain and pruritus at the site of injection being the most commonly reported side effects. About 10% of patients will develop a transient reactions of chest tightness, flushing and dyspnea. Flu-like symptoms have also been reported. While this drug has been shown to slow the progression of MS, there have been no comparative trials with the interferons (Bainbridge, Corboy, & Gidal, 2002).

Mitoxantrone (Novantrone) has recently been approved by the FDA for reducing the neurologic disability and/or the frequency of clinical relapses in patients with secondary progressive MS, progressive-relapsing MS, or worsening progressive relapsing MS. It is administered in doses of 12 mg/m^2 every three months. The life time cumulative dose is 140 mg/m^2. An evaluation of left ventricular ejection fraction should be done when the cumulative dose reaches 100 mg/m^2. Other side effects associated with this drug are nausea, alopecia, menstrual disorder, amenorrhea, upper respiratory tract infection, urinary tract infection, and leucopenia (Bainbridge, Corboy, & Gidal, 2002). Some authors recommend caution with this drug, indicating that the potential clinical benefits of mitroxamtrone appear to be only modest and the use of the drug carries a potential for serious toxicity (Goodin et al., 2003).

Methotrexate. This chemotherapeutic agent slows the rate of progression in MS in some patients. It is thought to work by suppressing the immune system so it does not attack myelin. Patients with worsening disease who are not responsive to steroids can be given this drug. The oral dose is 7.5 mg per week usually taken as three tablets of 2.5 mg each in the morning with food. In the first 6 months side effects can include nausea, loss of appetite, mouth sores, mood alteration, dizziness, fatigue, hair loss, easy bruising, diarrhea, headaches, rash, and photosensitivity. It also requires blood monitoring before treatment; at 1 month, 2 months, and 3 months; and thereafter for decreases in red and white cell production, as well as altered liver and kidney function. The drug also can produce immunosuppressant diseases such as pneumonias, fungal infections, and herpes zoster (shingles). It can produce birth defects during and 6 months following treatment so birth control should be practiced. Folic acid 1 mg per day may reduce some of the side effects. Using aspirin or its derivatives and drinking alcoholic beverages is contraindicated. Use of nonsteroidal antiinflammatories should be under the direction of a primary care provider. Patients are advised to report dry cough over 2 days, mouth sores, signs of infection, and unusual bleeding (RMSC, 1995).

Cyclophosphamide (Cytoxan). Cyclophosphamide is another chemotherapeutic medication used in MS when the condition worsens and is unresponsive to steroid therapy. It is given IV in a clinic setting and dosing is based on height and weight. Usually the drug is given monthly for 6 months. The drug kills rapidly dividing cells (blood cells, hair cells, and mucous membrane cells). The side effects include nausea, vomiting, and loss of appetite at 6 to 8 h after the dose, diminishing over 1 to 2 days. Other side effects are hair loss, changes in taste, lowered blood cell counts with slow healing and increased bleeding times, bladder irritation, mouth sores, and facial tingling or burning during the injection. It also affects reproduction both during and for 4 months posttreatment, requiring the use of birth control. Patients and family need to call the provider if fever is greater than 100ºF and the patient has burning on urination, frequent or foul-smelling urine, sore throat, cough, swelling or redness at the injection site, and worsening of MS symptoms (RMSC, 1996).

Corticosteroids. Steroid use appears to reduce the intensity and duration of an exacerbation but does not change the overall loss of function. There is no consensus on dose, administration route, or duration of steroid therapy in MS. One protocol calls for methylprednisolone 1 g IV given each day for 3 to 5 days followed by oral prednisone at 60 mg and tapered over the next 11 to 18 days in patients with a substantial increase in their disability due to an exacerbation (Anderson & Goodkin, 1996).

Drugs Used in Symptomatic Treatment of MS

The primary care provider will spend the most time with MS patients in order to treat their symptoms and for counseling. Symptom management primarily centers around urinary tract infections, urinary incontinence, constipation, and spasticity. In a Dutch study, family counseling focused on disease explanation, emotional support, and coping strategies (Donker, Foets, & Spreeuwenberg, 1996). MS is costly, with patients over 65 on alpha blockers, anticholinergics, cholinergics, tricyclic antidepressants, anticonvulsants, antifatigue agents, antispasticity agents, and antibiotics for UTI in one Nova Scotia study. The average drug costs were 65% greater for MS patients than in comparable age groups (Sketris, Brown, Murray, Fisk, & McLean, 1996).

The symptoms reviewed here include spasticity, fatigue, tremors, bowel and bladder dysfunction, and mood dysfunctions.

Spasticity. Spasticity is an increase in resistance to movement. Range of motion exercises two to three times daily remain a mainstay of treatment. Spasticity can also be effective in allowing ambulation of a weakened extremity, and removal of the spasticity can impair gait. Excess spasm is debilitating and needs treatment. Treatment of spasticity is usually initiated for an ambulatory individual. The primary drug is oral baclofen given two to three times daily, increased by 5 mg every 3 days as tolerated. Many patients easily tolerate 60 to 80 mg per day. Telephone contact is helpful in establishing dosage parameters. The adverse effects increase with higher doses and include weakness, drowsiness, leg swelling, confusion, and sedation. Monitoring for liver function is necessary. The drug requires weaning since abrupt termination can lead to agitated behavior, paranoid ideation, and seizures. Supplemental doses of diazepam (Valium) 1 to 2 mg or clonidine 0.1 to 2 mg are often helpful and well tolerated.

Dantrolene sodium often is not effective in MS because it causes weakness and sedation, but it is used in nonambulatory patients (Marshall & Ragland, 1996). The dosage is 25 mg daily and is gradually increased to 100 mg four times daily. The adverse effects are diarrhea and toxic hepatitis.

Intrathecal baclofen administered through a subcutaneous pump has had good results in selected patients with intractable spasticity, allowing a fraction of the oral dose. This requires surgical implantation of an abdominal pump, with tubing placed into the spinal canal. The cost, locating the proper surgeon to carry out the procedure, and ongoing maintenance limit its usefulness. Even after pump removal lasting reduction of severe spasticity has been documented, and lower dosing is often achieved after months of therapy (Dressnandt & Conrad, 1996). Other drugs used for spasticity include diazepam, tizandine, tiagabine, and gabapentin (Bainbridge, Corboy & Gidal, 2002).

Fatigue. Over three-quarters of individuals with MS complain of excessive fatigue, which worsens during afternoon hours and with an increase in ambient temperature. It requires the patient to sit, lie down, and sleep. Training in energy conservation techniques is helpful. The drug of choice in excessive fatigue is amantadine hydrochloride in doses of 100 mg once or twice daily, and it is effective in about half the MS patient population. Pemoline 37.5 mg and fluoxetine hydrochloride 10 to 20 mg once or twice a day are also used. The adverse effects are anxiety and insomnia. Patients who respond do so within several days, and 1-week drug holidays every month are effective in diminishing drug tolerances. Other drugs used to treat the fatigue associated with MS are amantadine, antidepressants, modafanil, methylphenidate, dextroamphetamine (Bainbridge, Corboy, & Gidal, 2002).

Tremor or Ataxia. This is a most disabling symptom and one of the least responsive to treatment. The drug that seems to be effective is clonazepam 0.5 mg at bedtime and increasing slowly to 2 mg four times per day, given to an end-point of sedation or effective control of cerebellar tremor. Another recommended drug is primidone 125 to

250 mg daily in two to three doses. Oblative cerebellar surgery is done in some individuals with poor results (Rudick, 1993).

Bowel Dysfunction and Bladder Dysfunction. Over half of MS patients experience constipation, evacuation urgency, and incontinence. High fluid intake, bulk laxatives, and stool softeners with a regular evacuation time are helpful. In addition to the nonpharmacologic objectives outlined earlier, there are medications that can improve bladder function once a diagnosis is established. Detrusor spasticity will respond to anticholinergic agents, such as oxybutynin chloride at 2.5 to 5 mg two to three times daily or propantheline bromide at 15 mg orally three to four times each day. Dry mouth and constipation are common side effects. Bladder retention usually is best treated by intermittent catheterization but may also respond to terazosin hydrochloride 5 mg orally three to four times a day. Other drugs used to treat bowel or bladder dysfunction are propantheline, oxybutinin, dicyclomine DDAVP, self-catherization, imipramine or amitriptyline, prazosin, botulinum toxin type A (Bainbridge, Corboy, & Gidal, 2002).

Mood Alterations. The most common mood disorder present in individuals with MS is depression, but bipolar affective disease and anxiety disorders also occur more commonly in MS than the general population. The risk of suicide is higher in this population, requiring a routine review of suicide risk. One-third of the MS population will experience a major depression requiring treatment, usually in younger patients with less overall disability. The patients respond better to a combined regime of pharmacotherapy and psychotherapy. Medical treatment for depression in this group is often prolonged, requiring treatment for 18 months before successful medication withdrawal.

The current first-line drug of choice for depression in MS is the SSRI agent fluoxetine, at 10 to 20 mg per day each morning, because the side effects are less. The traditional tricyclic agent used is amitriptyline 25 mg at bedtime and increased by 25 mg each week to 75 to 100 mg daily. Adverse effects of tricyclics include dry mouth, urinary retention, and drowsiness (Scott, Allen, Price, et al., 1996). The anticholinergic properties of amitriptyline is helpful in individuals with bladder spasm.

MS patients can present with manic-depression as the first sign of the disease. These individual do respond well to lithium (Scott et al., 1996).

Other Symptoms in MS. Chronic pain and acute pain in extremities is reported and tricyclic antidepressants are used. Lumbar pain is often related to mechanical stress on the spine, spasticity, and weakness and may benefit from NSAIDs. Degenerative disc disease can also occur mechanically from the weakened back structure. Trigeminal neuralgias also occur in MS and may respond to carbamazepine 100 to 200 mg two to three times each day (Anderson & Goodkin, 1996).

Labile behavior with a persistent euphoria is not unknown in MS. The euphoria is thought to be the result of structural brain damage and dementia as well. The display of emotion without subjective content can be disabling. Some patients respond well to antidepressants to treat this condition.

Psychosis can also occur, probably due to temporal lobe and frontal lobe plaque formation. Lack of insight and persecutory delusions may ensue, as well as visual hallucinations. Followup with a psychiatrist familiar with MS may be helpful in treatment (Rodgers & Bland, 1996).

Followup Recommendations

In the office setting for individuals with stable disease, medical followup may be dependent on other disease states in the MS patient. For individuals with chronic remitting disease, 3-month followup visits may be necessary to keep abreast of symptom relief. Alternating visits with the consulting neurologist also may be helpful.

VERTIGO

Vertigo is usually described as a sensation of "spinning or rotating," and this sensation is often accompanied by nausea. Dizziness is described as a sensation of "light-headedness or imbalance." The two are difficult to separate and are often treated as one entity. More than 90 million Americans experience vertigo or dizziness at some point in their life (Smith, 2002). The prevalence of vertigo increases with age, causing many researchers to consider it a "geriatric syndrome" (Tinetti, Williams, & Gill, 2000).

Vertigo and dizziness are not disease entities but rather the symptoms of pathological or physiological processes. Spatial orientation is primarily an automatic function. Continual sensory monitoring evaluates the body's position in space with reference to the surrounding environment. The brain then integrates the feedback from this sensory monitoring and enables one to maintain balance, move around, and interact with other objects. When this process is disturbed or a compromised, the result is a sensation of spinning or vertigo. These disturbances may be of central (brainstem or cerebellum) or, more commonly, peripheral (inner ear or vestibular nerve) origin (See Table 29–9). The associated symptoms and signs help differentiate cardiovascular, neurologic, psychological, sensory, and medication-related etiologies of vertigo. The most frequently reported symptoms are dizziness, unsteadiness or imbalance when walking, sensations of spinning or turning, and nausea. Because the vestibular system interacts with many parts of the nervous system and with multiple organ systems, symptoms may also be experienced as problems with vision, hearing, muscles, thinking, and memory. Symptoms may be mild, lasting minutes, or severe, lasting days, weeks, or months.

Vertigo can effectively be relieved by pharmacological treatment, physical therapy, surgery, or psychotherapy according to the diagnosis. Treatment of the underlying disease usually eliminates the symptoms of vertigo and dizziness. In about 10% of all cases, no distinct cause is ever established (Ruckenstein, 2001). Although usually not life-threatening, vertigo can impose many limitations on an individual's ability to perform activities of daily living and, if prolonged, results in diminished quality of life.

Less than half of the patients who complain of dizziness actually have diseases of the vestibular system (Baloh, 1994). Infections, injuries, and lesions in the brain, inner ear, and related structures can create disturbances in the sense of balance. The history and physical examination are the most useful tools in determining the diagnosis. The length of attacks may provide the best diagnostic clues. Peripheral vertiginous disorders usually cause attacks of vertigo lasting a few seconds to minutes while those of central vertiginous disorders tend to last for days or weeks or may be unremitting.

TABLE 29–9. Etiologies of Vertigo

Central (Brain)
Anemia
Anxiety, Phobia, and Panic
Asthma, Pneumonia
Cardiac Arrhythmias, Congestive Heart Failure
CVA (Stroke)
Drugs affecting the CNS (esp. sedatives, anticonvulsants, loop diuretics)
Encephalitis
Migraine
Multiple Sclerosis, Parkinson's disease
Tumor: Acoustic Neuroma
Peripheral (Ear)
Autoimmune ear disease
Benign Paroxysmal Positional Vertigo
Degenerated Otoconia (cupololithiasis)
Drugs (aminogycosides, quinine, ASA)
Ear Trauma
Meniere's Disease
Otitis
Vestibular Neuronitis

Medications that act on the central nervous system can be the general cause of dizziness due to depression of the CNS and cerebellar dysfunction from tranquilizers, anticonvulsants, and alcohol use. Antihypertensives can elicit postural hypotension and subsequent dizziness if the blood pressure is too low to maintain adequate blood supply to the posterior cerebellar and cerebral blood vessels.

Vertigo from cardiovascular or respiratory etiology includes cerebrovascular accident (CVA), cardiac arrhythmias, hypotension, hypertension, congestive heart failure, anemia, pneumonia, and asthma. Vertigo can present as dizziness with or without accompanying symptoms. The dizziness is constant and not necessarily related to movement. It is most often seen in older adults.

Vertigo caused by CNS disturbances is usually accompanied by multiple neurologic deficits including cerebral ataxia and other cranial nerve abnormalities such as diplopia, dysarthria and nystagmus. If other nervous system deficits accompany the vertigo, the clinician is not just dealing with simple vertigo but a more complex problem. The presence of marked nystagmus with little vertigo is often a symptom of central disease. The CNS disturbance also can be of vascular origin with vertebrobasilar artery insufficiency. This type of dizziness can last minutes to hours and be positional and directly related to vasodilator use and arterial occlusive disease. It can also be a symptom of migraine headache. Demyelinative disorders (e.g., MS and Parkinson's disease) must be considered in prolonged vertigo episodes resistant to medical treatment. Vertigo is the initial complaint in 5% of patients with MS and is observed in up to 50% of patients with MS (Ruckenstein, 2001). Rarely, acoustic neuromas (a slow-growing tumor on the nerve from the inner ear to the brain) may interfere with the normal function of the vestibular system. Vertigo may be part of a group of symptoms in autoimmune diseases (i.e., Lyme disease, syphilis, systematic lupus erythematosus) when the disease process affects the CNS. Brain injury with concussion and whiplash injury to the cervical spine should be considered in all patients without discernable cause for symptoms.

Another etiology of vertigo is of psychological origin. Vertigo presents as a symptom of anxiety, phobias, or panic syndrome. In this condition, the dizziness is not episodic, but a constant condition with no remission during waking hours. Body movement can improve the dizziness, which is usually the opposite of vestibular dizziness, and the vertigo may appear only in certain situations such as a crowded room.

Peripheral vertigo (eighth cranial nerve or inner ear deficits) presents with associated nausea, tinnitus, and deafness but no central nervous system deficits. One cause is viral and bacterial infections (i.e., otitis media, acute sinusitis) with symptoms resolving as the illness runs its course. Another cause is ototoxicity brought on by medication use, particularly with aminoglycoside antibiotics. Even ceremun impaction can cause dizziness if the surrounding tissue begins to swell; removal of ceremun is all that is necessary to treat the vertigo.

Benign paroxysmal positional vertigo (BPPV) is the most common peripheral vestibular disorder. BPPV, which is diagnosed by the presence of peripheral nystagmus after taking a new head position, accompanied by severe vertigo and nausea with symptoms quickly fading, usually in seconds to minutes once the head is in a new position. BPPV is not accompanied by hearing loss, and caloric testing is normal. In many cases, BPPV is thought to be the result of clogging in the labyrinth processes, resulting in the inability of endolymph tissue to move freely. BPPV can also accompany head trauma.

If the vertigo is accompanied by tinnitus (ringing in the ears), fluctuating hearing loss, and aural fullness, the condition is Ménière's disease. In Ménière's disease an attack usually involves severe vertigo (spinning or whirling), imbalance, nausea, and vomiting. The average attack lasts 2 to 4 hours, and several attacks may occur within a short time. Physiologically there is swelling of the endolymph of the middle ear. It commonly occurs between 30 and 60 years of age. In 75% of the individuals with Ménière's disease only one ear is affected; in the other 25%, both ears are affected. In most cases, residual tinnitus and a progressive hearing loss occurs in the affected ear(s). It too can accompany brain injury (Knox & McPherson, 1997).

The duration of the vertigo is a clue to its etiology with BPPV lasting only seconds, vertebrobasilar insufficiency and migraine vertigo lasting minutes to hours, Ménière's disease vertigo lasting hours, and dizziness of days duration due to viral neurolabyrinthitis, vascular occlusion, and trauma.

The pharmacotherapy and other treatments discussed below are only specific to BPPV and Ménière's disease. Like other diseases in this section, referral to a neurologist or otolaryngologist may be necessary, with concurrent treatment.

SPECIFIC CONSIDERATIONS FOR PHARMACOTHERAPY

When Drug Therapy Is Needed

Medical management is aimed at prevention, symptom alleviation, and in some cases, cure. There are, as yet, no drugs known to absolutely cure vertigo without the possibility of serious side effects, the most common being permanent hearing loss.

Short- and Long-Term Goals of Pharmacotherapy

The aim is symptom relief in short- and long-term treatment of vertigo. Direct injection of medications into the inner ear often results in cure in the case of Ménière's disease.

Nonpharmacologic Therapy

Nonpharmacologic therapy is directed to two goals. The first is aimed at removing any clogs within the endolymph, and the second is to carry out vestibular retraining, desensitizing the individual to movement that causes the dizziness. In some cases of BPPV, otolithic debris is thought to be attached to the posterior canal, plugging the canal. Dislodging the plug through a repositioning maneuver can cure BPPV often in just one to three treatments, so that the clot falls into the utricular vestibule (Gans, 1996). Vestibular training with symptomatic medication use is more effective than drug use alone in BPPV (Fujino et al., 1996).

The two most common treatments of BPPV are the Semont maneuver (also called the liberatory maneuver) and the Epley maneuver (also called the canalith repositioning procedure). Both are very effective, with approximately an 80% cure rate. They are both intended to dislodge the debris out of the sensitive posterior canal of the ear to a less sensitive location. Both maneuvers take about 15 minutes to accomplish. The Semont maneuver involves rapidly moving the patient from lying on one side to the other. The Epley maneuver involves guided sequential movement of the head into four positions. The recurrence rate for BPPV after these maneuvers is about 5%, and in some instances a second treatment may be necessary. If exercises are unsuccessful in controlling symptoms, a surgical procedure called "canal plugging" may be recommended. Canal plugging stops the posterior canal's function without affecting the functions of the other parts of the ear. This procedure poses a small risk to hearing (Froehling, 2000; Nuovo, 2001).

Another treatment option includes vestibular rehabilitation or balance retraining exercises. In habitual training, the etiology of the vertigo may not be a clog in the endolymph canal. The goal is to help a person compensate for a loss or imbalance within the vestibular system. The habituation treatment involves excessive stimulation of the labyrinth canal and the use of balance activities to help maximize the use of the remaining vestibular function, sight, and sensation in the feet to maintain a sense of balance. Balance retraining therapy is of significant benefit for fall prevention especially in elderly patients (American Academy of Otolaryngology, 1998; Smith, 2002). Several studies show that physical therapy is more efficacious than the use of medications (Grizzi, 1995), showing a 63 to 70% improvement rating with therapy and only a 37% improvement with medications. Nonmedicinal treatment works even in vertigo of many years duration. Vestibular training shows better results in individuals with unilateral vestibular disease.

Avoidance of some drug classes is also effective for a minority of persons with vertigo. Eliminating caffeine, alcohol, and salt may relieve the frequency and severity of attacks. The initial treatment for Ménière's disease is a low-salt diet of 1 to 2 g of sodium per day, with or without the addition of a diuretic (Brookes & Knox, 1996). Eliminating tobacco use and reducing stress levels may also help to lessen the severity of the symptoms. Medications that help to control allergies, reduce fluid retention, or improve blood circulation in the inner ear may also help. In some cases a shunt, a tiny silicone tube, is inserted in the inner ear to drain off excess fluid. In cases of severe Ménière's disease, chemoablation or surgical ablation (labyrinthectomy when hearing is lost, vestibular nerve section when it is not) may be necessary in severe or refractory cases (NIOCD, 2001).

Time Frame for Initiating Pharmacotherapy

In terms of immediate symptomatic relief, the treatment should begin immediately. After an acute attack, maintenance or prophylaxis treatment is initiated in an attempt to prevent future attacks. As a last resort, in unremitting vertigo, it may be necessary to destroy the endolymph canals through injection of neurotoxins.

Overview of Drug Classes for Treatment

The drug classes used in vertigo include steroids as antiinflammatories, diuretics to reduce the amount of fluid within the inner ear, antiemetics for nausea, antidepressants for symptomatic relief, vestibular suppressants (including the calcium channel blocker nimodipine), and aminoglycosides to destroy the endolymph in severe cases of vertigo.

Assessment Needed Prior to Therapy

The initial workup begins with a brief general examination, including careful attention to the cardiovascular, lung, and abdominal systems, noting tachycardia, arrhythmias, shortness of breath, and abdominal swelling and bruits. Neurologic examination should include assessment of balance, gait, eye movements, and hearing. Potentially serious neurologic disease should be suspected in patients with focal neurologic signs, severe ataxia, nystagmus changing direction, vertical nystagmus, and abnormal eye movement. The examination includes the head, with attention to the ear canal and hearing, as well as eliciting specifics on subjective ringing of the ear. In addition to the cranial nerves, the examination needs to include cerebellar function and the presence of nystagmus. Checking for vertical and horizontal nystagmus, assessing the fatigue and latency of response in eye movements, and checking for positional nystagmus by having the patient go quickly from sitting to supine and turning the head, noting the presence of nystagmus, fatigue, and accompanying vertigo, should be done routinely. Potentially serious neurologic disease should be be suspected in patients with focal neurologic signs, severe ataxia, nystagmus changing direction, vertical nystagmus, and abnormal eye movement. A modified caloric test may be helpful in establishing the differentiation of central and peripheral nystagmus, but it is not necessary to establish the diagnosis.

In some instances, sudden or fluctuating hearing loss, vertigo, and ringing in the ears can be a presentation of otosyphilis and/or AIDS; testing for both diseases and a screening CBC may be warranted (Linstrom & Gleich, 1993). Another cause of vertigo can be vertebral artery insufficiency, which may warrant further ultrasound testing if the condition is suspected.

Patient/Caregiver Information

Once a diagnosis is established, thorough education about the various treatments is helpful, including vestibular and balance retraining through a physician specialist or physical therapist. Information on the action and side effects of medications for symptomatic relief is necessary. The patients and caregivers should understand that some cases of vertigo can improve over time, but in

Ménière's disease the condition is chronic and may require ongoing treatment.

OUTCOMES MANAGEMENT

Selecting an Appropriate Agent

Drug therapy in BPPV and Ménière's disease does not have high efficacy, with less than half of the patient population obtaining relief from medication. For both Ménière's disease and BPPV, using nonpharmaceutical therapeutics along with attempting symptom relief with medications can improve outcome. Traditionally, the first-line drug group is the vertigo suppressants with newer treatments including direct injection of steroids into the middle ear to reduce the inflammation. Steroid use does not cause the hearing loss that accompanies the use of the aminoglycosides.

The traditional first-line drug is meclizine hydrochloride (Antivert), classified as an antiemetic and used to treat the nausea accompanying vertigo. It is an antihistamine, suppressing labyrinth excitability and acting centrally to depress vestibulo-cerebellar pathways. It is long-acting, having a half-life of 6 h and single-dose effect of 8 to 24 h. It will depress the CNS, with resulting drowsiness among other side effects. For the control of vertigo, the usual dose is 25 to 100 mg per day in divided doses (ASHSP, 2002).

The calcium channel blocker nimodipine was successful in 50% of patients within a small sample in relieving vertigo in Ménière's disease. Calcium channel blockers are a common form of treatment in Europe and may act as vestibular suppressants because vestibular hair cells are rich in calcium channels. The drug may also act because of its general sedating properties (Rascol et al. 1995).

The neuroleptics (haloperidol, chlorpromazine) act by blocking dopaminergic receptors in the brainstem, reducing the neurovegetative symptoms paralleling vertigo. They act in 4 to 12 h given as oral agents or suppositories (Rascol et al. 1995).

Another drug group commonly used is the benzodiazepines, which potentates the inhibitory g-aminobutyric acid and inhibits vestibular responses. Diazepam 5 to 10 mg 2 to 3 times daily can be valuable in the acute period. The primary action is as a muscle relaxer and an antianxiety agent, allowing the patient to rest.

Current studies on the use of pentoxifylline, dimenhydrinate and cinnarizine combination therapy, and intratympanic dexamethasone for relief of vertigo and/or Meniere's disease show promise but to date no recommendations concerning their use has been endorsed. The histamine analogue betahistine has been the focus of recent studies. Betahistine with or without a diuretic may provide a means of providing maintenance medical treatment. Several controlled clinical trials have shown a significant improvement in vertigo, hearing loss, and tinnitus in the short term (Brookes, 1996). Although commonly used in Europe with mixed results, it is not recommended for use in the United States.

Low-dose methotrexate can be considered for patients when long-term treatment is required or when a steriod or cyclophosphamide is contraindicated. Results from a recent study shows oral methotrexate to be a safe and effective treatment for immune-mediated bilateral Meniere's disease, and provides good control of vertigo and stabilization of hearing in most patients (Kilpatrick, Sismanis, Spencer, & Wise, 2000). In low doses (7.5 to 25 mg/wk) few of the side effects associated with methotrexate as used in cancer chemotherapy have been reported. Many of these adverse reactions can be diminished by supplemental folic acid therapy (1 mg/day). Methotrexate is a teratogen so it should not be prescribed for pregnant or potential child-bearing women.

Other oral medications used in Ménière's disease include diuretics (furosemide, chlorothiazide) to reduce the inner ear endolymph swelling and antidepressants to inhibit CNS response to the sensation of dizziness.

Otolaryngologists also use direct injection of medications through the tympanic membrane into the inner ear to control unremitting vertigo. Some physicians, viewing Ménière's disease as an immune-mediated disease, advocate initial treatment with steroids to decrease endolymph swelling; this does not cause any hearing loss. Dexamethasone is injected directly into the inner ear through the round window and accompanied by IV injection of dexamethasone. The drug decreases and restores normal fluid balance (Shea & Gee, 1996).

Initially, direct injection of streptomycin was used, which did cure the vertigo but also left the patient with complete hearing loss to the treated ear. Indications for streptomycin are now limited, particularly with the current interest in intratympanic delivery of gentamicin for managing vertigo. Several studies showed a rate of control of vertigo of 90%, though a cochleotoxic effect is seen in 15 to 25% of cases. Modifications to the amount of drug strength and injection techniques have allowed better control for hearing loss and stabilization of the vertigo, with one third of the patients experiencing hearing loss as a result of the injections (Driscoll, Kasperbauer, Facer, et al., 1997; Hirsch & Kamerer, 1997; Seidman, 2002). There are other reported cases of gentamicin treatment in peripheral vestibular disorder other than Ménière's disease (Brantberg, Bergenius, & Tribukait, 1996). For many individuals, hearing loss is a small price to pay for return of function and relief from the disability of severe vertigo.

Monitoring for Efficacy

Although effective in some cases, the long-term use of meclizine with concurrent CNS depression must be kept in mind when attempting use of heavy machinery or driving, so the drug itself can cause a significant change in daily function. Meclizine use in children has not been studied.

Monitoring for Toxicity

Additive CNS depression can occur with meclizine when used with alcohol, barbiturates, or tranquilizers. The anticholinergic effects of the drug can cause increased symptoms of angle-closure glaucoma and prostatic hypertrophy. Like other antihistamines it can cause systemic dermatitis, CNS depression, changes in cardiac function, and interaction with other depressants.

Scopolamine has been used in the treatment of vertigo. There are cases of reported addiction to scopolamine in the literature, and the drug manufacturers warn of easy addiction (Luetje & Wooten, 1996). Indeed, this drug was off the market for several years. Extended use over weeks to months may lead to withdrawal symptoms of nausea, vomiting, headache, and dizziness, requiring treatment to allow for drug withdrawal. Primary addictive signs are the nausea, vomiting, and headache rather than the occurrence of dizziness. Some patients require hospitalization for symptom control for 72 h while the drug is cleared from their systems. The other adverse effects of scopolamine include dry mouth, drowsiness, blurred vision, dry eyes, dizziness, disorientation, restlessness, giddiness, hallucinations, and confusion. Skin rashes and contact dermatitis can also occur.

Followup Recommendations

The important treatment breakthrough for vertigo is the positional maneuvers that can cure benign positional vertigo. Finding a clinician who understands the condition and is skilled in the maneuvers can lead to cure. The association of BPPV and Ménière's disease requires followup on all patients with vertigo. In both conditions, vestibular rehabilitation can help the brain reorganize its visual, vestibular, and proprioceptive signals to allow full function once again. Newer dosing of intratympanic steroids or gentamicin at lower doses can give relief without further hearing loss in many patients with intractable vertigo and Ménière's disease.

DEMENTIA

Although commonly associated with a loss of memory, the term *dementia* refers to a loss in cognitive functioning and in thinking abilities. According to the American Psychiatric Association (APA, 1997), "the essential features of a dementia are multiple cognitive deficits that include memory impairment and at least one of the following: aphasia, apraxia, agnosia, or a disturbance in executive functioning (the ability to think abstractly and to plan, initiate, sequence, monitor, and stop complex behavior)." In the late stages of the disease, it can interfere with attention and consciousness. This disorder of memory, cognition, and personality gradually interferes with ability to perform in social or occupational situations. Dementia affects approximately 5 to 8% of persons age 65 and older, 15 to 20% of persons over age 75, and 25 to 50% of persons over age 85 (Brookmeyer, Gray, & Kawas, 1998). At any given time, well over 4 million Americans have some form of dementia that limits their capacity to live independently, creating an immense financial, social, and emotional burden on families and society in general (Kawas & Morrison, 1997). In most early to middle stages of dementia, the individual is alert and has the physical capacity to be independent but may be unable to process information and plan and carry out safe actions (Costa et al., 1996).

Most forms of dementia are progressive, creating a subtle, slow decline in function that does not become apparent until a specific event draws attention to the cognitive dysfunction. The diagnosis of dementia is made by history, patterns of cognitive losses, neurologic and physical examination, and laboratory and radiologic testing. It is important to exclude treatable secondary causes.

Dementia can be of primary or secondary origin. Examples of primary degenerative dementias are the dementias of Alzheimer's disease (AD), Parkinson's disease, Pick's disease, and Huntington's disease. Other irreversible causes of dementia include the vascular dementias, traumatic dementias, and cerebral infections. Until recently, there was little but symptomatic treatment available for the primary dementias. Reversible or secondary dementias can be of iatrogenic, vascular, infectious, metabolic, neurophysiologic, or psychological origin. They include such conditions as neurosyphilis, vitamin B_{12} deficiency, hypothyroidism, chronic drug ingestion, chronic subdural hematomas, brain tumors, and depression. The most common iatrogenic causes are medications, and the drug classes known to cause dementia are listed in Table 29–10. The secondary dementias are often improved or completely resolved by treating the underlying cause(s) (APA, 1997).

Regardless of etiology, individuals with dementia have many common symptoms, including changes in cognition, function, and behavior. The hallmark of many dementias is memory disorder, particularly immediate recall and declarative memory (i.e., Who is the president of the United States?). Word-finding difficulties are also a common cognitive complaint, as is sentence syntax in later stages. Losses in recognizing visual spatial relationships can also accompany dementias. These losses result in functional impairment in dealing with the basic activities of daily living and instrumental activities of daily living (banking, using the telephone, taking medications, meal planning, and shopping). Apathy is often present early in the disease process with patients exhibiting a noticeable lack of interest and reduced concern. Although personality symptoms are a late sign in Alzheimer's disease, other dementias can cause early personality changes, mood disturbances, delusions, hallucinations, and psychosis. The earliest symptom can be depression. The most difficult behavioral change is the occurrence of verbal and physical aggression, which can be progressive and pose serious stress on caregivers (Costa et al., 1996).

As with other neurologic conditions, determining the cause of cognitive functioning decline or loss is the key to therapeutic interventions. In addition, it is not uncommon for an individual to have more than one cause of dementia; for example, multi-infarct dementia can occur along with Alzheimer's disease (Hollister & Gruber, 1996).

The diagnosis of Alzheimer's disease requires a progressive loss in memory (either new recall or recalling previously learned functions), loss in one or more cognitive areas (aphasia, apraxia, agnosia, and decline in executive thinking), no disturbance in consciousness, onset between ages 40 and 90 (most often after age 65), and absence of any systemic disorder or brain disease accounting for other causes of the dementia (Costa et al. 1996: Woo & Lantz, 1995; Peterson et al., 2001). The pathology in Alzheimer's disease is the formation of neurofibrillary tangles and dendritic plaques in the cerebral cortex and hippocampal formation with a resultant loss in choline acetyltransferase in those areas (Woo & Lantz, 1995). Alzheimer's disease, which accounts for 50 to 75% of total dementia cases, affects women more than men, due in part to the longer lifespan of women.

TABLE 29–10. Drug Classes Known to Cause Dementia

Antiarrhythmic agents	Antiparkinsonian agents
Antibiotics	Antipsychotic (neuroleptic) agents
Anticholinergic agents	Corticosteroids
Anticonvulsants	Decongestants
Antidepressants	H_2 receptor agonists
Antiemetics	Hypnotics
Antifungal agents	Nonsteroidal anti-inflammatory drugs
Antihistamines	Narcotic analgesics
Antihypertensive agents	Radiocontrast media
Antimanic agents	Sedative/hypnotic agents
Antineoplastic agents	Skeletal muscle relaxants

SPECIFIC CONSIDERATIONS FOR PHARMACOTHERAPY

When Drug Therapy is Needed

In all dementias, both primary and secondary, there is a need for appropriate symptomatic relief. In the reversible or secondary dementias, drug therapy is directed at alleviating the primary problem and consequently the changes in cognitive functioning. In the primary, irreversible dementias there are now drugs that can slow down the disease progression in select individuals and may stabilize functional losses, allowing the individual to maintain a higher level of cognitive functioning for a longer duration of time. In addition to treatment of cognitive deficits, medical management of general health and associated noncognitive symptoms is essential. Visual and hearing deficits are common in older persons and may intensify symptoms of cognitive decline. Efforts should be made to ensure that corrections (e.g., glasses, hearing aids) are optimal, operating, and properly used (Cummings et al., 2002).

Short- and Long-Term Goals of Pharmacotherapy

The goal of treatment for patients with dementia should be directed at optimizing their physical and psychosocial functioning and providing support for their caregivers. Drug therapy in primary dementias, particularly in Alzheimer's disease, is directed to slowing the cognitive impairments present in individuals with mild to moderate AD. The second goal of drug therapy in all the dementias is relief of symptoms and, if possible, to use one medication for those with moderate to severe dementia.

Nonpharmacologic Therapy

Managing and treating patients with dementia is an involved process that requires frequent followup due to the progressive nature of the disease. Followup at 3- to 4-month intervals is helpful in reviewing the functional and behavioral limitations seen with progressive dementias for the patient as well as the primary caregivers. It is important for healthcare providers to be aware of symptoms associated with dementia to facilitate early intervention when cognitive changes occur (Cummings et al., 2002). The family and caregivers are often important sources of information. Healthcare providers should solicit and consider their input in treatment planning. This alone may encourage enough problem solving so individuals with progressive dementias can be maintained in a home setting for appropriate lengths of time.

Dementia is progressive and irreversible, but initiating pharmacologic therapy for cognitive decline and nonpharmacologic and pharmacologic treatments for the psychotic and behavioral sequelae of dementia can enhance quality of life. Nonpharmacologic symptom relief can incorporate a multitude of interventions, including reality orientation, behavioral intervention, occupational activities, environmental modification, validation therapy, reminiscence, and sensory stimulation. There is evidence that continuous reassessment of patient problems in dementia renders better quality of life and improved patient survival (Applegate & Burns, 1996). Specific interventions include elder day care for socialization, exercise, stimulation, medical followup, and physical therapy and to meet nutritional needs. Having a stable routine and environment with limited distractions and consistent behaviors is often a key to consistent behavior in the early to middle stages of dementia. All patients and families should be informed that even mild dementia increases the risk of accidents. Adequate supervision, ensuring safety regarding wandering, environmental modification to prevent falls, restrictions on driving, and the use of other dangerous equipment should be discussed early in the disease process. Other safety measures should include an evaluation of suicidal ideation and the potential for violence (APA, 1997).

Specific problem behaviors can be eliminated through good planning. For example, limiting fluids after 7 P.M. may eliminate evening incontinence, and daily walking and limiting daytime napping may be helpful in eliminating nocturnal behaviors. Ensuring respite care via specific healthcare workers and other family members may eliminate stress for the primary caregiver. Reexploring all local options in terms of day care, assisted care, and nursing home care should be attempted at periodic intervals. Last, healthcare proxies and living wills need addressing while individuals can still participate in these decisions.

Time Frame for Initiating Pharmacotherapy

The time frame for initiating symptom relief in dementias is symptom-dependent. Treatment is most effective when initiated early in the disease progression to slow the rate of cognitive decline and preserve physical and mental functioning. Individuals with severe vegetative signs of primary dementia do not respond well to drug therapy nor do individuals who show minimal impairments, such as in higher-order abstract reasoning, calculation deficits, and immediate recall.

Outcome measures for any therapy directed at cognitive stability, functional impairment, or behavioral instability should include retesting cognitive function by using the Mini-Mental Status Scale, a functional impairment measure such as the Functional Independence Measure, and behavioral assessments, as well as caregiver burden. Additional benefits of initiating therapy includes a decrease in behavior disturbances, which may delay nursing home placement and reduced demands on caregivers (Cummings, 2000). Caregiver burden is often the factor leading to nursing home placement.

Specific cholinesterase inhibitor therapy usually is initiated when an individual is diagnosed with mild to moderate Alzheimer's disease, usually defined as a score of 10 to 24 on the Mini-Mental Status Examination or a similar scale. This drug group is not effective in individuals with very mild or very severe Alzheimer's disease.

Overview of Drug Classes for Treatment

Treatment of the primary dementia may be considered as symptomatic, neuroprotective, and psychotropic. The drug classes used to treat the primary dementias include neurotransmitter inhibitors as primary therapy in AD as well as antidepressants, anxiolytics, nonsteroidal antiinflammatory drugs, antipsychotics, and sedatives for symptom relief in all the dementias. A thorough assessment of the patient, the family, and the home environment is essential to develop a comprehensive and appropriate treatment plan. The assessment should also identify the patient's decision-making capacity. The primary caregiver's needs and risks should also be assessed when developing a plan of a care for the patient (Cummings et al.,

2002). Incorporating the patient's and primary caregiver's input when developing the plan of care enhances chances of compliance with the treatment.

Assessment Needed Prior to Therapy

Individuals who present with memory changes, difficulty with abstract thinking, disorientation, and confusion require a full and careful history as well as laboratory and physical assessment before determining a diagnosis. The assessment should include the patient's medical problems, functional status, cognitive status, behavioral problems, and psychotic symptoms. Bolla, Filley, & Palmer (2000), described the classic symptoms of dementia as "the four "A"s: Amnesia (loss of memory initially for recent events and ultimately for remote events); Agnosia (total or partial loss of the perceptive faculty by which persons and things are recognized); Apraxia (inability to carry out a motor function in the absence of any motor weakness, such as having muscle power but being unable to dress oneself); and Aphasia (may include naming difficulties of familiar objects such as parts of clothing)." In the preliminary assessment, ascertaining behavioral and cognitive changes from both the patient and significant others is very helpful. Ask specific questions regarding falls and recent trauma, changes in the home environment, and information related to new and/or changes in medication to rule out head trauma, medication toxicity, or psychological stressors as the cause of behavioral change. Alzheimer's disease presents with an insidious onset, gradual progression, and absence of focal findings, remaining primarily a diagnosis of exclusion, a "definite" diagnosis can be made from pathologic evaluation only (Costa et al., 1996).

For a thorough and complete assessment of dementias and Alzheimer's disease see the AHCPR Guideline Number 19 on *Recognition and Initial Assessment of Alzheimer's Disease and Related Dementias* (Costa et al., 1996) or the *Alzheimer's Disease Assessment Scale* (Mohs, 1996). A physical examination of all systems is necessary as well as a valid mental status examination, such as the Mini-Mental Status Examination or other valid and reliable dementia screens, such as the Alzheimer's Disease Assessment Scale. (Cummings et al., 2002). Repeating the screening test over time is helpful in quantifying the effects of both pharmacologic and nonpharmacologic treatment. A full neuropsychologic evaluation can help characterize the type of dementia and help rule out depression as part of the etiology. A short group of four neuropsychologic tests have proven reliable in determining the diagnosis of Alzheimer's disease. In addition to the Mini-Mental Status Examination, they are the Blessed Information-Memory Concentration Test, the Blessed Orientation-Memory-Concentration Test, and the Short Test of Mental Status. All are available in AHCPR Guideline 19 (Costa et al., 1996).

The two common differential diagnoses to consider in assessing for dementia are delirium and depression. Acute delirium can indicate the development of an acute medical condition. It is marked by disturbances in consciousness, behavioral changes over hours to days (but not months), evidence of physical signs on focused examination, and alteration in cognition, which it shares with dementia. Although depression can coexist with dementia, it can also lead in itself to significant cognitive changes. In depression the individual gives a feeling of being down or irritated at all times with a decreased interest in most activities. There can also be significant weight gain or loss, with daily insomnia or hypersomnia.

If radiology examination is necessary for the diagnosis, it is usually a brain CT or MRI. The brain CT or MRI can determine white matter changes, presence of infarction or neoplasm, or hydrocephalus and determine demyelinating diseases. The location of brain atrophy can also give clues to etiology. The blood tests for persons presenting with possible dementia include CBC, serum B_{12} level, TSH, HIV, and VDRL serologies. If indicated, it may be necessary to obtain CSF testing to rule out meningitis or encephalitis. Even if a secondary cause of dementia is found, further assessment following treatment may be necessary to rule out a concomitant dementia.

The second most common cause of dementia after Alzheimer's disease is multiinfarct dementia. In this group the cognitive losses may be more focal. In order to prevent further disease, especially if large cerebral arterial vessels are involved, anticoagulation treatment may be started or carotid endarectomy used. Another possible reversibly cause of dementia is normal pressure hydrocephalus with the cognitive changes accompanied by incontinence and balance and gait changes. If the patient responds well to withdrawal of 50 cc of CSF (i.e., improvement in gait 1 and 24 h after the lumbar puncture), the patient may respond well to ventricular shunting (Chan & Hachinski, 1997). An electroencephalogram may be indicated if seizures are considered.

Another helpful guideline to consider in cases of dementia with an uncertain diagnosis is the use of neuropsychologic testing. Neuropsychological testing can serve several purposes: to give information to patients and their families on the specifics of cognitive deficits, assist in diagnosis, contribute to treatment recommendations, and provide a baseline measure for treatment and disease progression (Costa et al., 1996).

Patient/Caregiver Information

Once a diagnosis is established, there are several resources available for families. Primary care practitioners should encourage the use of local social service agencies and support organizations, including the Alzheimer's Association, for help and education in managing the day-to-day activities of dementia caregiving, legal and financial issues, respite care, and future care needs and options. A classic reference for families is *The 35-Hour Day* (Mace, 1981). See Table 29–11 for a list of organizations.

OUTCOMES MANAGEMENT

The pharmacologic treatments listed in this section are limited to the newer medications used to treat Alzheimer's disease and those for symptom treatment in all dementias.

Selecting an Appropriate Agent

Recently, drug agents have been developed to compensate for cerebral damage. The use of cholinesterase inhibitors to preserve the decreasing amount of acetylcholine found in the brains of individuals with Alzheimer's disease has been found to be useful (Gidal et al., 1996). Higher concentrations of acetylcholine may increase communication between nerve cells and temporarily improve the symptoms of the disease (Alzheimer's Association, 1996). More recently, it is postulated that cholinesterase inhibitors may be neuroprotective, slowing down or preventing formation of amyloid fragments (Schneider, 1996).

TABLE 29–11. Resources for Caregivers of Persons with Alzheimer's Disease

- Administration on Aging (Department of Health & Human Services)
  1-202-619-7501
  http://www.aoa.dhhs.gov
- Alzheimer's Disease Education & Referral Center
  1-301-495-3311 or 800-438-4380
  adear@alzheimers.org
- Alzheimer's Association
  1-800-272-3900
  www.alz.org
- Family Caregiver Resource Centers
  1-800-445-8106
  www.caregiver.org
- Elder Care Locator
  1-800-667-1116

Check local telephone directory for additional resources.

Cholinesterase inhibitors are the only medications approved by the U.S. Food and Drug Administration as treatment for AD. These agents have been shown to produce improvements in memory, social interaction, and cognition and delay decline in cognitive functioning in patients with mild to moderate AD (APA, 1997; Cummings, 2000). Beneficial response to a cholinesterase inhibitor can be determined by stabilization or delay in cognitive decline and improvement of behavioral problems based on evidence of behavioral or functional changes, caregivers' reports, or use of a mental status questionnaire (Cummings et al., 2002). Cholinesterase inhibitors should be reassessed on a regular basis and discontinued if the individual is unresponsive or noncompliant. The drug should be discontinued if, after 6 months, there is continued deterioration at pretreatment rate or if deterioration accelerates while on drug (Small et al., 1997). If patients do not respond to one agent in the class, they may respond to another. When switching from one agent to another, deterioration during withdrawal is common and requires careful monitoring.

Four cholinesterase inhibitors are currently available: tacrine, donepezil, rivastigmine, and galantamine. Tacrine (Cognex), the first inhibitor to show a significant improvement in cognitive function in patients with mild to moderate AD, was associated with significant adverse effects, including hepatotoxicity. Tacrine is rarely used since the introduction of several other cholinesterase inhibitors with similar efficacy profiles and low risk of adverse effects.

A second cholinesterase inhibitor, Aricept (donepezil hydrochloride), was FDA-approved in January 1997. This Drug is thought to be more stable, longer-acting, and provide higher concentrations of cholinergic transmitters in the central nervous system. This drug is not hepatotoxic. It is given to individuals with mild to moderate Alzheimer's disease initially at 5 mg per day, advancing to 10 mg per day in A.M. Side effects typically occur in the first few weeks of therapy and decline with continued drug use. The most common side effects are diarrhea, nausea, vomiting, insomnia, fatigue, and anorexia. The drug is taken with food. Some patients may experience an initial increase in agitation, which subsides after the first few weeks of therapy (Rogers et al., 1998). No stated interactions with other drugs are currently listed. Other drugs in this class include rivastigmine (Exelon), approved in 1999, and galantamine hydrobromide (Reminyl), approved in 2001, for the treatment of mild-to-moderate AD and age-related dementias.

Data on rivastigmine and galantamine demonstrated a significant benefit in patient cognition, behavior, and functioning, with adverse events consistent with the cholinergic actions of the drugs (Pearson, 2001; Rosler et al., 1999; Wilcock, Lilienfeld, & Gaens, 2000). In patients who used rivastigmine, the most common side effects included nausea, vomiting, anorexia, dyspepsia, and asthenia. These side effects were usually transient and mild to moderate in severity. Adverse reactions were usually less frequent later in the course of treatment. Adverse events might be reduced with more frequent, smaller doses of rivastigmine (Corey-Bloom, 1998; Rosler et al., 1999). Initial dose is 1.5 mg twice a day, titrated up to no more than 6 mg twice a day. Galantamine showed significant treatment effects at daily doses of 16 to 32 mg. Starting dosage is 8 mg/day, increasing to 16 mg/day after at least four weeks. The daily dose may be increase to 24 mg/day after an additional 4 weeks. Common side effects of the drug are gastrointestinal in nature, with a small percentage of patients experiencing nausea, vomiting, anorexia, diarrhea, and weight loss. Low dosage and a slow rate of titration (minimum 4 weeks) reduce the gastrointestinal symptoms (Wilcock, Lilienfeld & Gaens, 2000). As with any cholinergic agent, rivastigmine and galantamine increases the effect of other cholinergic agents and decreases effects of anticholinergic agents. Anticholinergic drugs or drugs with anticholinergic side effects (e.g., antihistamines, antispasmodics, tricyclic antidepressants, antipsychotics) may antagonize the effects of the cholinesterase inhibitors, thus reducing their effectiveness. Other drugs under consideration in this class include ENA 713 and metrifonate.

In October 2003, the FDA approved memantine (Namenda), a NMDA-receptor antagonist, as the first treatment for moderate to severe Alzheimer's disease. Unlike the cholinesterase inhibitors that temporarily boost levels of acetylcholine, memantine works by regulating the activity of glutamate, a chemical involved in information processing, storage, and retrieval. Preliminary data suggest that memantine may not be as effective in individuals with mild to moderate Alzheimer's disease. The dosage shown to be effective in clinical trials was 10 mg twice a day following a 4-week titration. The most common adverse affects in the trial studies were headache, dizziness, constipation and confusion (FDA, 2003). Memantine is expected to be available in the United States in early 2004.

Estrogen therapy is postulated to act as a neurotransmitter modifier by enhancing the action of cholinesterase transmission and through improved blood flow to the brain, which inhibits arteriosclerotic plaque buildup (Birge, 1996). The effect of receiving estrogen before, during, or just after menopause in the prevention or delay of Alzheimer's disease is not yet established (Mulnard, Cotman, Kawas, et al., 2000).

Another treatment under review is the use of agents to prevent or inhibit neuronal degeneration (Thal et al., 1996). Experimental treatments include giving neuronal growth factors (cholinergic neurotropin). There are several other experimental agents under study, including antioxidants, monoamine oxidase-B inhibitors, antiinflammatory agents, and calcium channel blockers (to prevent calcium influx, proposed to cause neuronal death due to release of intracellular enzymes). The support for the use of nonsteroidal antiinflammatory agents and estrogen is primarily through survey research. Preliminary results from studies of Vitamin E (2000 IU/d) show it has no effect on cognition or behavior but it does exhibit disease-modifying effects. Selegiline (10 mg/d) showed a modest reduction in the rate of decline of functions in patients with AD but is not recommended except for patients ineligible for, intolerant of, or unresponsive to cholinesterase inhibitors (Doody et al., 2000). Evidence to support the use of other antioxidants, prednisone, NSAIDs, or herbal medications such as ginkgo biloba is insufficient to recommend use as standard therapies. Immune therapy, although still in the experimental phase, is promising. In animal models, vaccination with amyloid [beta] prevented memory loss and reversed brain abnormalities. No clinical trials have yet been conducted (Wiebe & Nicolle, 2002). Last, it is postulated that genetic gene transfer may eliminate some forms of Alzheimer's disease.

The second goal of therapy is symptomatic treatment of the psychoses, mood disorders, and behavioral problems associated with dementia. In all symptomatic treatment, the smallest dose that alleviates the symptom should be used with frequent monitoring and periodic drug withdrawal to ascertain that the drug is actually effective in symptomatic relief.

Individuals with advanced dementias, particularly AD, may show signs of frank psychosis. The symptoms may include delusional episodes, agitation, hallucinations, hostility, and hyperactivity along with diminished independence in ADLs and loss of language skills. Using neuroleptics for symptom control is often attempted. However, if the patient is in a nursing home setting and subject to OBRA guidelines, a diagnosis of psychosis must be made prior to treatment. At this time there are no controlled studies on the efficacy of neuroleptics in the treatment of dementias. Many of the drugs may alleviate the symptoms but can lead to further cognitive decline, increased sedation, tardive dyskinesias, and Parkinsonian symptoms. In a review of several studies, trazodone at

150 mg per day had the least side effects (Sunderland, 1996). One drug frequently used is haloperidol at 1 to 2 mg per day, but side effects include imbalance, rigidity, and falls, which limit its effectiveness. For some, substituting clozapine is effective in reducing psychotic symptoms, but the mental status of the patient may decline. Risperidone (Risperdal) at 1 mg/day is effective in decreasing the symptoms of delusions, agitation, and vocalizations with fewer extrapyramidal symptoms (EPS) but also slightly decreases cognitive skills (Reynolds & Strayer, 2000). Olanzapine (Zyprexa) 2.5 mg (up to a maximum 10 mg) at bedtime is generally well tolerated. The reduction in psychotic symptoms may allow a patient to stay longer in the home setting.

Depression is common in individuals with dementia, occurring 50% of the time (Brookmeyer, Gray, & Kawas, 1998). Depressed mood may be improved by stimulation-oriented treatments or changes in the environment, but most patients with moderate or persistent depression benefit from treatment with antidepressant drugs. Although the tricyclic antidepressants may be used—e.g., nortriptyline, (Pamelor) 10 to 30 mg per day, despiramine (25 to 75 mg per day) and trazodone (75 to 200 mg per day), the first line treatment is the selective serotonin reuptake inhibitors (SSRIs), which tend to produce fewer side effects, particularly sedation (Chan & Hachinski, 1997; Cummings & Cole, 2002). The choice of agent—e.g., sertraline (Zoloft), 50 to 200 mg per day; paroxetine (Paxil), 20 to 50 mg per day; or fluoxetine (Prozac), 20 mg per day—is based on the side effect profile and characteristics of the individual patient. Agents with anticholinergic side effects (e.g., amitriptyline or impramine) should be avoided. Because of the risk of postural hypotension, monamine oxidase inhibitors (MAOIs) should be reserved for patients who do not respond to other treatments (APA, 1997; Cummings et al., 2002).

Agitation and psychosis are common in patients with dementia and often coexist. The agitation in dementia can actually be depression and more responsive to antidepressants than traditional medications prescribed for agitation. The use of psychotropic medications has been shown to be very effective, but dementia patients are often very susceptible to severe side effects and require close observation and frequent adjustments in dosage (APA, 1997). The medications used in agitation, particularly in Alzheimer's disease, are thioridazine (Melleril) at 10 to 20 mg per day (up to 80 mg) and haloperidol (Haldol) at 0.25 to 0.50 mg once or twice daily up to 3 to 5 mg per day. Haloperidol in particular can cause associated movement disorders and further cognitive losses; it requires careful use and frequent trials off the medication. Active delusions also may respond to haloperidol and melleril (Chan & Hachinski, 1997). Risperidone (0.25 to 3 mg per day) is less likely to cause extrapyramidal reactions but shares the same risks associated with high-potency agents. Clozapine also causes fewer extrapyramidal reactions but is associated with sedation, postural hypotension, elevated seizure risk, and risk of agranulocytosis, which requires routine blood monitoring.

Another common symptom in dementia is anxiety. The medication treatment includes lorazepam (Ativan) 0.5 to 1.0 mg per day, alprazolam (Xanax) at 0.25 to 0.5 mg up to bid and oxazepam (Serax) 10 mg up to bid (Chan & Hachinski, 1997). Anticonvulsants—e.g., carbamazepine and valproic acid—also have been shown to have anti-agitation effects. The SSRIs are less well studied but may be appropriate for nonpsychotic patients with mild anxiety or behavioral disorders (Cummings et al., 2002). Lithium and beta blockers are not recommended due to the potentially serious side effects.

Pharmacologic therapy is generally not recommended for nonaggressive behaviors such as wandering. Drugs should only be considered when all non-pharmacologic interventions have proven unsuccessful. If it becomes necessary, drug choices include antipsychotics, minor tranquilizers, and antidepressants (APA, 1997). Patients who wander should be registered in the Alzheimer's Association Safe Return Program and should be protected by appropriate use of safety latches and gates (APA, 1997; Cummings et al., 2002).

Insomnia can become the caregiver's burden. Preventing reversal of the sleep-wake cycle is important, and daily exercise is often helpful. Treatment can include warm milk at bedtime, trazodone (Desyrel) 20 to 50 mg per day; zolipidem (Ambien), 10 to 20 mg per day; or temazepam (Restoril), 7.5 mg to 15.0 mg all given at bedtime or 1 to 2 h before bedtime (ADA, 1997; Chan & Hachinski, 1997). Temazepam may induce daytime sedation due to its long half-life. Benzodiazepines and chloral hydrate are not recommended except for very brief use due to their risk of daytime sedation, rebound insomnia, and worsening of cognition and delirium. Diphenhydramine is not recommended due to its anticholinergic effects (APA, 1997).

Monitoring for Efficacy

Given the lack of reliable testing and the use of symptomatic treatment, appropriate cognitive and functional testing, levels of independence in ADLs, specific symptom relief, and caregiver burden are good vehicles for assessing drug efficacy (Cummings et al., 2001; Doody et al., 2000).

Monitoring for Toxicity

Although FDA approved, tacrine is no longer recommended as a first line treatment for AD due to its hepatotoxic side effects. For patients who take breaks in rivastigmine therapy for longer than 3 days, therapy should be resumed at the lowest daily dose (Rosler et al., 1999). Severe vomiting with esophageal rupture has been reported when reinitiation of therapy is resumed at high doses (AD Association, 2002).

Followup Recommendations

In very stable patients with dementia, followup is recommended every 3 to 4 months. In patients under symptomatic treatment, followup every 4 to 8 weeks may be necessary. Dementia is a dynamic, progressive disease and keeping abreast of new problems, eliminating drug therapy when symptoms subside, and providing support for the caregivers enhances the quality of life of the patient and the caregivers.

HEADACHE

Acute new-onset headache is a symptom, not a neurologic disorder. The National Headache Foundation reports that more than 45 million Americans experience chronic, recurring headaches, and 28 million experience migraines. In children and adolescents the percentage is approximately 20%. The types of headaches are tension, migraine, mixed tension and migraine, cluster, sinus, acute, hormonal, and chronic progressive headaches. Some individuals may suffer from more than one type of headache. The amount of physical dysfunction in activities of daily living produced by a headache is a classification parameter. In this country serious headaches have a huge economic and social impact due to lost work, lost income, difficulty with daily living activities, and social dysfunction. Although most individuals do not seek healthcare for their headaches, it is one of the most common presenting symptoms in primary care (de Lissovoy & Lazarus, 1994).

Diagnosis of headache is difficult due to its episodic nature, with occurrence and remission and the need to rely on the patient's description. Careful history and assessment are necessary in order to rule out serious underlying disease. It is imperative that this detailed assessment rule out tumors, intercranial bleeds, and other serious neurological problems before proceeding to treatment. Assessment of any severe onset headache needs to be aggressive, rule out these conditions, and consultation with physician is recommended. The treatment of common primary headaches will be discussed in this chapter as they are within the scope of most primary care providers. A classification of headaches is contained in Table 29–12. Migraine may be both underdiagnosed and undertreated even in the face of substantial disability because individuals are not able to recognize their headaches as migraine or adequately self-report symptoms. Migraine affects approximately 18% of women and 6% of men but is undiagnosed in 59% of women and 71% of men. Prevalence of migraine is inversely related to socioeconomic status as measured by income and or education (Lipton, 2002).

In the pediatric population migraine and tension headaches are the two most common types of recurrent headaches. Cluster headache is rare before puberty and most prominent in males. Sinus headache, posttraumatic headache, benign paroxysmal headache associated with fever, psychological factors, and substance exposure or withdrawal may also be causes of headache in the pediatric population. Cluster headaches are sometimes classified as a migraine variant. Chronic daily headaches can be of migraine or tension-type origin and are particularly common in analgesia overuse, resulting in a rebound headache response (Lipton & Stewart, 1997).

Neurology evaluation and or consultation with a headache clinic may be necessary if worsening headaches or daily headaches are present, headaches are unresponsive to pharamacotherapy, or a present as unilateral or with focal neurological symptoms.

The International Headache Society (IHS) established diagnostic criteria for adult headache in 1988. These criteria are listed in Table 29–12.

Migraine headaches are a chronic disease with episodic exacerbations marked by nausea, possible vomiting, photophobia, and phonophobia. An aura, a focal neurologic symptom, can precede migraine. Migraine may also have prodromes, changes in mood or behavior. Migraines as an episodic disorder produce changes in gastrointestinal and autonomic functions as well as cause headache.

The significant dysfunction of migraine headaches may lead the patient to the healthcare provider. One-third of individuals experiencing migraines require bedrest, and 50% account for 90% of the lost work time caused by migraines, leading to an economic cost in the billions of

TABLE 29–12. Diagnostic Criteria of Headaches

- Chronic daily headache
  1. Lasts 4–15 h per day, occurs daily or near daily (over 15 days per month), occurs over 180 days per year
  2. Transformed migraine (with or without analgesic overuse)
  3. Transformed tension-type headache (with or without analgesic overuse)
  4. New persistent daily headache
  5. Cervicogenic headache
     - Idiopathic
     - After neck trauma
  6. Post-head-trauma headache
     - With migrainous features
     - Without migrainous features
- Migraine headache
  1. Migraine without aura (history of five previous attacks)
     - Lasts 4–72 h untreated or unsuccessfully treated
     - Has at least two of the following:
       - Unilateral location
       - Pulsating quality
       - Moderate to severe intensity (inhibits/prohibits daily activities)
       - Aggravated by walking, stair climbing, or other physical activity
     - Has one of the following:
       - Nausea and/or vomiting
       - Photophobia or phonophobia
  2. Migraine with aura (history of two attacks)
     - Has three or more of the following:
       - One or more reversible aura symptoms of focal, cerebral, cortical, or brainstem dysfunction
       - One aura over 4 min or two or more auras in succession
       - Each aura limited to 60 min
       - Headache after aura or simultaneously with aura
- Tension headache
  1. Has two of the following:
     - Pressing or tightening quality
     - Mild to moderate intensity that does not prohibit activities
     - Not aggravated by physical exercise
  2. Has both of the following:
     - No nausea or vomiting, but anorexia can occur
     - Photophobia and/or phonophobia generally absent and do not occur together
- Cluster headache
  1. Severe unilateral, orbital, supraorbital, and/or temporal pain lasting over 15 min to 180 min (history of five previous attacks)
  2. Headache associated with one of the following:
     - Conjunctival injection
     - Lacrimination
     - Nasal congestion
     - Rhinorrhea
     - Forehead and facial sweating
     - Eyelid edema
     - Miosis
     - Ptosis
  3. Frequency is one every other day to eight a day
- Differential headaches
  - Neoplasm
  - Knife-blade
  - TMJ headache
  - Occipital neuralgia
  - Exertional headache
  - Paroxysmal hemicrania

For all of the types, the history and physical examination show no other organic causes of headache, and if another disorder is present it does not coincide with the headache.

Please consult The International Classification of Headache Disorders, 2nd edition, for operational headache classification criteria which are beyond the scope of this chapter. (Headache Classification Subcommittee of the International Headache Society. (2004). The International Classification of Headache Disorders, 2nd edition *Cephalalgia, 24*(Suppl), 1–150. This supplement can be retrieved from: http://216.25.100.131/ihscommon/guidelines/pdfs/ihc_II_main_no_print.pdf

Sources: Adapted from Solomon (1997), Mathew (1997), and Silberstein, Young, & Lipton (1997).

dollars per year. Migraines can occur in children, being described by children as young as 8 years old. In males the prevalence is constant at 6%, with a much higher percentage (17%) in females, peaking at 25% for women in their 40s and then declining. The decreased incidence of headaches in women does coincide with declining estrogen levels and approaching menopause, but women still experience more migraine than men even into their 80s.

A small percentage of women (6%) have migraine associated with the onset of menses (plus or minus 2 days) (MacGregor, 1997). Falling estrogen levels are postulated to be related to changes in neurotransmitters through one or more of four ways: a decrease in serum dopamine beta-hydroxylase, a dysfunction in opioid control of the hypothalamic-pituitary-adrenal axis, a decrease in magnesium levels, and a platelet dysfunction. In some women with migraines pregnancy abates the migraines, but 10% of pregnant women experience their first migraine with pregnancy (MacGregor, 1997). Migraine may also occur in the athlete secondary to prolonged exertion and effort with the mechanism being similar to spontaneous migraine. Headache is triggered in athletes by estrogen fluctuations and stress along with chemicals present in foods and behaviors such as limited dietary intake and decreased sleep (Lane, 2000).

There is a familial component to migraine headaches, particularly to the occurrence of familial hemiplegia accompanying the headache. There is some indication of an ion channel gene abnormality in some families. In addition, some individuals have emotional trigger features to their migraine headaches. The pathophysiology of migraine headaches does indicate a reduced cortical blood flow in migraines with or without aura. About 3% of the population with migraines may also experience seizures associated with their migraines. These seizures may be due to spreading changes in electrical or chemical potential brought on by the migraine headache (Welsh & Lewis, 1997). Migraine headaches have a documented association with psychiatric disorders, particularly depression and anxiety. It is not clear which is the antecedent to the other (Merikangas & Stevens, 1997).

Tension headaches are also commonly called stress headaches. These headaches are not severe, are usually bilateral, and are not exacerbated by increased physical activity. They are not marked by nausea and vomiting, photophobia, or phonophobia. The pericranial muscles are usually tense, and the headache is not brought on by systemic or organic disease.

Cluster headaches are marked by sharp, severe, unilateral pain lasting 15 to 180 min in the orbital, supraorbital, or temporal area. The attacks can be 1 to 8 a day and have a higher occurrence in heavy smokers. Accompanying autonomic signs include tearing, conjunctival redness, nasal congestion, facial sweating, and ptosis.

The majority of individuals who seek help do so because they are experiencing headaches daily. Although chronic tension headaches initially were described as the only form of daily headache, recent work tends to point to more than one type of headache becoming daily and chronic, either from a migrainous or tension type and often related to analgesic overuse. Headaches can evolve into daily events, often starting as occasional headaches while individuals are in their teens. About 20% of daily headache sufferers have a sudden onset possibly due to trauma, viral illness, septic meningitis, surgery, or other illness.

Individuals with chronic excessive analgesia use experience related rebound headaches characterized by daily headaches. The headache can vary in severity, location, and type with a low threshold of intellectual or physical activity bringing on the headache. Patients complain of many related symptoms: asthenia, nausea, restlessness, anxiety, irritability, decreased memory, decreased concentration, decreased attention, and depression. If using daily ergotamine medications, they can complain of cold extremities, tachycardia, paresthesias, decreased pulse, hypertension, light-headedness, extremity muscle pain, or leg weakness. Daily headaches often occur from 2 to 5 A.M. and with decreased REM sleep, and individuals awaken with a severe headache.

SPECIFIC CONSIDERATIONS FOR PHARMACOTHERAPY

When Drug Therapy Is Needed

Drug therapy in headaches is aimed at treating the headache at the time it occurs and aimed at prophylactic treatment to prevent headaches. The aim of drug use is to start with milder and then more potent analgesics as needed. The use of prophylactic medication is usually reserved for moderate to severe headaches and those occurring more than twice a week. Unfortunately, with analgesic and some prophylactic medications, there can be a rebound dependency effect with headache recurrence; thus frequent medication use can lead to more frequent headaches.

Short- and Long-Term Goals of Pharmacotherapy

The goals of medication use are the relief of headache and, in more severe, frequent headaches, the prevention of headache. A secondary goal in frequent headaches is prevention of drug dependency and more rebound headaches.

Nonpharmacologic Therapy

Regular patterns of sleep, exercise, and eating are helpful in preventing headaches, thereby reducing the need for medication as well as rebound headache. A regular sleep pattern is essential and behaviors need to be established to promote sleep. Headache sufferers, particularly those with migraine, often can identify trigger factors that should be avoided in preventing headaches. Some foods can trigger migraines, such as tyramine-containing food (red wine, aged cheese), monosodium glutamate, alcoholic beverages, and caffeine. Some individuals also find it helpful to avoid milk products, citrus products, and chocolate. Some medications can also cause headache, and stress management might be helpful in curbing frequent headaches. Stress management techniques include biofeedback, acupuncture, and behavioral counseling.

Alternative treatments such as biofeedback, acupuncture, healing touch, massage, vibratory medicine, use of flower essences, herbal and aroma therapy, and magnet therapy are used by individuals to treat headache. These nontraditional approaches must not be overlooked or ignored by providers.

Time Frame for Initiating Pharmacotherapy

With all headaches, the earlier the pharmacotherapy is initiated, the easier it is to treat the headache. In headache treatment it is imperative to take enough drug when the headache begins to abort it. The longer it takes to obtain relief (requiring more than one drug dose), the longer is the headache and its disability. In prophylactic headache relief, it is important that the medication be taken consistently. Prophylactic treatment is considered when two or more headaches per month produce disability lasting 3 or more days per month and when symptomatic medications are ineffective.

Overview of Drug Classes for Treatment

There are many drug classes used in the treatment of headache. The analgesic groups for mild to moderate headache include aspirin, acetaminophen, and NSAIDs (Naprosyn, Anaprox, ibuprofen, Voltaren); analgesic combinations including caffeine (Excedrin, Anacin) and butalbital (Fiorinal, Midrin); combination analgesics with narcotics (Fiorinal with Codeine, Tylenol with Codeine); and narcotics (Darvon, Darvocet, Dilaudid, Demerol, morphine). Acute migraine and cluster headaches are treated with serotonin agonists (ergotamine and dihydroergotamine, D.H.E., sumatriptan). Headache prophylaxis includes beta-adrenergic blocking agents (propranolol, timolol), ergot alkaloids (methysergide), NSAIDs, antidepressants, and valproic acid. The advent of pharmacotherapeutic agents in the triptan family is changing the approach to treatment of migraine because these agents are thought to reverse the mechanism of migraine therefore stopping pain and the associated symptoms. Recently, antiepileptic drugs (AEDs)—e.g., gabapentin, topiramate, and zonisamide—have been used for the prophylaxis of migraine headaches. Triptans may be administered in IM injection, nasally, and orally to abort an acute migraine. Some patients who have failed one triptan will respond to another.

Assessment Needed Prior to Therapy

A sudden onset of severe headache in a person with or without a history of severe headaches can be a medical emergency. Frequently, the person will call and say, "This is the worst headache of my life," and with or without focal symptoms this person should be seen by a healthcare provider within a short period of time to evaluate the possible etiology. Headaches that worsen over a period of weeks or months or headaches that occur three or more times a week may also justify emergent laboratory and radiology diagnostics to rule out other diseases.

A careful history during evaluation is necessary for headaches. This includes a careful description of the headache and if more than one type of headache occurs. For each type it is helpful to know its location, duration, temporality, warning symptoms, associated symptoms, alleviation or palliation of pain, medication use, and familial headache history. Asking the patient what she or he thinks causes the headaches is also helpful. Two types of headache may mean one is a rebound headache from prolonged, daily use of medication (which may or may not be for the headache itself), particularly if used prophylactically. Common medications known to cause headache include estrogens, vasodilators, and oral contraceptives.

If it is difficult for the patient to give this kind of specific information regarding the headache episodes, keeping a headache diary for 1 month may be helpful. For each headache ask the person to write out the warning signs, time the headache began and ended, type of pain, location, and intensity of pain on a 1 to 10 scale. Logging events prior to the headache (exercise, conflicts), foods eaten, hours of sleep, and treatment attempted is also helpful. Because headaches can be a symptom of other disease, a careful general examination and specific neurologic examination looking for focal symptoms is also necessary.

Patient/Caregiver Information

Individuals seeking headache relief need assistance in treatment for pain relief. They also need advice on headache etiology and headache prevention. These patients can be anxious and need reassurance that their chronic recurring headaches are usually benign. Making patients partners in headache relief enhances their success in treatment.

OUTCOMES MANAGEMENT

Selecting an Appropriate Agent

The order of medication use in mild to moderate headaches is analgesics; combination analgesic drugs with caffeine (potentiates the analgesic), butalbital, and/or narcotics; and NSAIDs (Silberstein, 1993). For moderate to severe headaches, ergot derivatives and sumatriptan are used, but not at the same time. D.H.E. is more effective in headache relief and associated autonomic symptoms and rebound headaches are less likely; there also is less nausea. To prevent migraine, beta blockers, ergot alkaloids, NSAIDs, antidepressants, and valproic acid are used.

Combination drugs are often used to enhance the analgesic action, reduce the total amount of medication, relieve anxiety, and for product convenience. Opiates can be used to prevent severe pain, and most individuals are careful with their use. Some individuals find other combinations and higher doses of medications other than opiates taken early in the headache as effective with less side effects (Sheftell, 1997). Recently, loading doses of intravenous valproic acid have been reported to quickly abort an acute migraine headache, obviating the need for opiate use and reducing the chance for drug dependency.

Monitoring for Efficacy

In acute migrainous headache the use of oral medications can be delayed due to decreased gastric motility. The side effects of many of these medications may also limit their effectiveness. Aspirin can potentiate nausea, and opioids can induce sedation. Ergot derivatives can lead to nausea, vomiting, and dependency (rebound headache). Rebound headache can occur with ergotamine with as little as 3 mg three times per week. Both ergot and sumatriptan are effective in relieving acute migraine (Mathew, 1997). However, sumatriptan, which causes less nausea, has a higher incidence of rebound headache (Drugs for migraines, 1995).

Monitoring for Toxicity

Children younger than 15 should not use aspirin for headache because of the risk of Reyes's syndrome, making acetaminophen preferable. Patients with a history of gastritis and ulcers or other bleeding disorders should also use acetaminophen. NSAIDs, used symptomatically and prophylactically, need careful monitoring because of occult gastric disease. Ergotamine can cause vascular occlusion and gangrene with overdosage (over 6 mg in 24 h or 10 mg per week), and the action is potentiated by beta-adrenergic blockers, dopamine, erythromycins or troleandomycin, liver disease, and fever (Drugs for migraines, 1995). D.H.E. is less toxic. Ergotamine and D.H.E. are contraindicated in renal failure, liver failure, pregnancy, coronary artery disease, peripheral vascular disease, hypertension, and sepsis. Recently, CYP3A4 inhibitors (ritonavir, nelfinavir, indinavir, erythromycin, clarithromycin, troleandomycin, ketoconazole, and itraconazole) have been reported to inhibit the metabolism of ergotamine tartrate and caffeine (Cafergot), resulting in life-threatening peripheral ischemia. Sumatriptan use is associated with chest pain and one report of myocardial infarction. Both sumatriptan and ergot derivatives are vasoconstrictive and can be additive. Their use needs to be sequentially separated by 24 h.

Followup Recommendations

Chronic headache sufferers need routine followup at 3- to 6-month intervals, primarily because of the frequent development of rebound headache. Warning signs of rebound headaches include increased medication tolerance and increased headaches. Limiting dosages to lower than the dosage producing the daily headache is useful, as is using different classes of medications to limit headaches. Educated, informed patients will often work with the provider to help themselves counter the effects of this disabling symptom and chronic disease. Referral to a headache clinic is appropriate if the individual does not respond to headache relief measures and the number of headaches is increasing.

PARKINSON'S DISEASE

The neuronal degenerative syndrome termed Parkinson's disease (PD) typically occurs when a loss of 40 to 80% of the dopaminergic cells occurs in the substantia nigra. This results in an imbalance between dopamine and acetylcholine with resulting difficulty in controlling skeletal muscle and autonomic nervous system activity. There is also a genetic component to the disease. The early treatment of PD involved the inhibition of acetylcholine. In the 1960s levodopa (L-dopa) was introduced as replacement therapy.

The majority of causes of PD are unknown but some causes are known, such as repeated trauma (pugilistic syndrome), carbon monoxide poisoning, heavy metal poisoning, illicit drug use, encephalitis, and medications that interfere with the dopamine function in the brain such as tranquilizers and antipsychotic medications (see Table 29–13). Theoretically, the release of radicals generated by oxidation reactions from dopamine metabolism may also play a role in the development of PD (Stern, 1997).

Patients with PD with good health management can now live 10 or more years with a relatively normal life and much longer with physical limitations (Silberstein, 1996).

The idiopathic, often insidious onset of PD is between ages 40 and 70 with a progressive course. The classic presentation is of a tremor at rest, first seen in the hands, face, and tongue and a stiffness (rigidity) marked by slowness or paucity of movement (bradykinesia). The early tremor is usually unilateral, unintentional, and slow

TABLE 29–13. Drugs That Can Cause Parkinsonism

Calcium channel blockers	Methyldopa
Captopril	Phenothiazines/butyrophenones
Chlorpromazine	Phenytoin
Diltiazem	Prochlorperanine
Haloperidol	Valproate
Lithium	Verapamil
Metaclopramide	Vincristine

with a pill-rolling motion seen in the hands. There is a loss of facial expression, decreased blinking, and gait changes marked by shuffling steps, little arm swing, and stooped posture.

Other signs include frequent falls, micrographia, hypophonia, excess salivation, and altered tendon reflexes (but downward toes). Concurrent symptoms can include depression, dysarthria, and fatigue. Numerous changes in the autonomic nervous system (impotence, increased salivation, orthostatic hypotension, paroxysmal sweating, seborrheic dermatitis, and urinary frequency) also occur.

Cognitive impairment is present in 15 to 30% of individuals who present with PD and is more prominent in individuals without tremor. Many other complain of difficulty with word-finding and thinking speed. Dementia is present in 15 to 35% of individuals who present with PD, often in those with little tremor. Consequently, cognitive testing is necessary for any individual who presents with PD symptoms. The dopaminergic medications used in treatment may also produce hallucinations or psychosis more readily in this population as well as toxic delirium (agitation, confusion, and worsening of the PD symptoms), necessitating lower doses of medications.

SPECIFIC CONSIDERATIONS FOR PHARMACOTHERAPY[1]

When Drug Therapy Is Needed

Because the cause is unknown and there is no cure, the primary treatment is symptomatic relief. Because of the probable role the release of oxygen free radicals plays in the development of the disease, early treatment is important. As the stiffness, tremor, slow movement, and gait difficulties worsen, dopaminergic drug treatment becomes necessary. In the late stages of the disease, the autonomic nervous system changes and possible occurrence of psychosis and dementia require symptomatic treatment (Stacy & Brownlee, 1996).

Short- and Long-Term Goals of Pharmacotherapy

The short-term goal of therapy is symptomatic control. The long-term goal is careful use of medications to prevent side effects and to some extent the necessity of adding further medications to control the side effects of the dopaminergic agents. Side effects of levodopa usually develop within 3 years of starting therapy.

[1]See additional note, page 623.

Nonpharmacologic Therapy

Complementary therapies such as meditation, biofeedback and therapeutic massage can help reduce tremor and rigidity. Tai Chi has been demonstrated to increase balance and decrease falls in the elderly without PD and may be helpful to those with PD. In addition, caffeine use has been associated with lower rates of PD (Ross et al, 2000). Use of botanicals (herbal) supplements and nutritional supplements should be discussed with a health care provider knowledgeable about movement disorders. Deep brain stimulation (DBS) was approved in 2000 by the FDA as a treatment for PD and has shown promise as a mechanism to allow patients to use lower doses of antiparkinson medications after the surgery (Imke, 2003). All these procedures continue to require antiparkinsonism medication. On an experimental basis, neural fetal tissue and adrenal medullary tissue are implanted in the striatum to alleviate the disease (Alexander, 1997).

Patient education allowing patient choice in medication treatment can produce better outcomes. Long-term decisions include employment, financial resources, caregiving decisions, health care proxies, and the use of self-help strategies.

Time Frame for Initiating Pharmacotherapy

Patients usually complain of the impairment related to movement slowness and imbalance more than the tremor, although the tremors can be socially embarrassing. A mild tremor not interfering with daily activities does not usually require treatment. Pharmacologic treatment of PD is usually initiated when daily functioning becomes impaired.

Overview of Drug Classes for Treatment

The drug classes used in PD include using the dopamine precursor levodopa to replace the lost dopamine. Levodopa and carbidopa levodopa/benserazide (Sinemet) are given together to prevent peripheral metabolism of levodopa allowing more of the drug to reach the brain. Levodopa may also be given with COMT (catechol-O-methyltransferase) inhibitors which inhibits the metabolism of levodopa in peripheral tissues and the brain allowing more drug to reach the site of activity. Dopamine agonists act directly on the receptor, bypassing the need for replenishment or release from neurons. Monoamine oxidase B (MAO-B) inhibitors are used to inhibit the catabolic breakdown of dopamine, and the MAO-B inhibitor selegiline is often used prior to major symptomatic control because of its possible effects as an antioxidant agent.

One class of anticholinergics, the antimuscarinics, block the effects of the unopposed acetylcholine activity and are used as second-line drugs to counteract tremor. Amantidine, classified as an antiviral medication, is used to increase the effects of dopamine levels at the nerve ending. The development of the second generation dopamine agonists, e.g. ropinirole (Requip) and pramipexole (Mirapex), that are better tolerated than the first generation drugs has led many clinicians to initiate therapy with these drugs. This has the advantage of delaying the use of levodopa which has been associated with a "wearing off" effect (PSG, 2002; Rascol, 2000). If psychotic symptoms induced through levodopa and MAO-B use cannot be controlled by limiting or withdrawing drugs, then antipsychotic agents may be utilized.

ADDITIONAL NOTE: PARKINSON'S DISEASE

Useful guidelines for the comprehensive treatment of Parkinson's disease, usually conducted in collaboration with a neurologist, can be found as a supplement in the journal *Neurology,* published in March 1998. These guidelines include algorithms for pharmacologic and nonpharmacologic treatment, including algorithms for exercise, support, nutrition, and problems associated with Parkinson's disease, such as dysautonomias, falls, motor complications, neuropsychiatric problems, and sleep disorders. In the pharmacologic treatment plan, algorithms are presented for no response, suboptimal peak response, "wearing off" response, unpredictable "on" and "off" response, and freezing (motor blocks) (Olanow & Koller, 1998).

Assessment Needed Prior to Therapy

The nature of this disease leads to easy misdiagnosis, and the treatment of the disease has become a neurologic subspecialty. The most common misdiagnosis by the primary care provider is essential familial tremor. This condition is five times as common as PD but less disabling with only 5% of patients seeking treatment. It is usually treated by primidone or propranolol. Drug-induced parkinsonism should be suspected when the symptom onset and progression are bilateral and the symptoms include abnormal movements of face and mouth. The currently used drug most commonly causing this complex of symptoms is metoclopramide (Reglan) (Imke, 2003). Some older BP drugs (resperpine and methyldopa) might also induce tremors confused for PD. Symptoms may cease after terminating the offending drug. However, long-term use may result in irreversible side effects. For the neurologist, misdiagnosis can also occur with patients actually having other conditions such as progressive supranuclear palsy, multiple system atrophy, corticobasal ganglionic degeneration, and vascular parkinsonism or for patients under age 50 with Wilson's disease.

Dementia is a common finding (approximately 20% on initial assessment) with the diagnosis of PD, and a screening mental status examination (Mini-Mental Status Examination) at initial assessment is often helpful. If the disease is accompanied by dementia, the differential diagnosis then includes Alzheimer's disease and Pick's disease. The current changes in drug therapy in PD are dynamic, and individuals with rapidly progressing disease may be best managed by a neurologist or special PD clinic aware of current treatment modalities.

Patient/Caregiver Information

There are local chapters of the national Parkinson's disease organization in almost all areas of the country. In addition to group support, current information on family and patient educational materials, nutritional guidance, and exercise can be offered. Patients who are educated about their disease and medications usually fare better and are able to manipulate their medications to allow maximum possible functioning. Functionally, great gains can be made to help with gait, balance, ADLs, and speech problems (dysphagia, hypophonia) through referral to physical, occupational, and speech therapists. Because PD is a chronic disease, counseling regarding occupation, caregiving decisions, and financial concerns needs addressing by appropriate therapists.

The four major organizations involved are the American Parkinson's Disease Association, Inc., the National Parkinson's Foundation, the Parkinson's Disease Foundation, and the United Parkinson's Foundation/International Tremor Foundation. They are helpful in addressing medical treatment, self-help strategies, and research advances.

OUTCOMES MANAGEMENT

Each of the major groups of drugs used in PD are presented below with its specific action, side effects, monitoring issues, toxicities, and follow-up recommendations. See Fig. 29–1 for an overview of medications used in Parkinson's disease. As patients become functionally disabled, symptomatic treatment is started. The drug choice is also based on the presence of cognitive disease, age, extent of disability, symptoms, and response to initial drug therapy (Silberstein, 1996). Dopamine agonists may

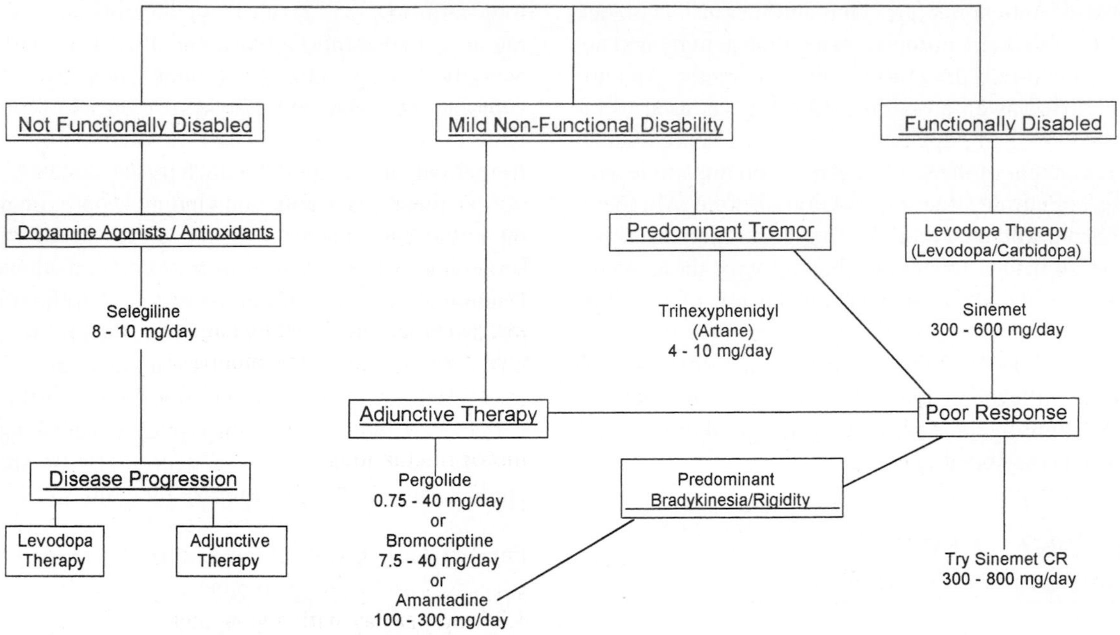

FIGURE 29–1. Medications used in Parkinson's disease.

be indicated either before or in conjunction with levodopa to allow the use of less levodopa. Over time and with disease progression, L-dopa almost universally develops side effects limiting its efficacy because of "on-off" phenomena. Depression, dementias, and psychosis are common problems in Parkinson's disease. A section outlining common drugs used for these problems in PD follows the discussion on antiparkinsonian medications.

NEUROPROTECTIVE AGENTS

After initial diagnosis and before there is any functional deficit interfering with daily life, early use of selegiline (Eldepryl, L-deprenyl), an MAO-B inhibitor dopamine agonist, is recommended. Selegiline may be neuroprotective by reducing free oxygen radical production through diminished oxidative metabolism of dopamine. It also has mild dopaminergic effects. Both effects allow delayed use of levodopa, necessary because of its long-term side effects of motor fluctuation and "on-off" phenomena (Ahlskig, 1996).

Selegiline is also used as an adjunct medication, primarily to reduce on the amount of dopa therapy and resulting motor fluctuations, usually allowing a 10 to 30% decrease in L-dopa therapy. Some patients do not tolerate both drugs well because of the combined dopaminergic effects with hallucinations and nausea, but a 5-year study showed good results with combined therapy (Myllyla, Sontaniemi, Hakulinen, Maki-Ikola, & Heinonen, 1997), in contrast to the earlier 2-year DATATOP study (Hely & Morris, 1996).

The usual dose is 5 to 10 mg per day. The drug should be taken early in the day since it has a mild amphetamine metabolite that may cause sleep disturbance and anxiety. The drug can also cause increased sedation when given with narcotics. Meperdine (Demerol) is contraindicated with patients on selegiline and this medicine should be discontinued 30 days before any hospitalization. If a patients is hospitalized on this medicication all personnel need to be vigilant to the risk of drug interactions causing pyscosis or malignant hypertension (Imke, 2003). Overdosing may be dangerous because of the MAO inhibition with a "cheese response" (or red wine or chocolate), producing hypertension, increased heart rate, headaches, and vomiting from absorption of tyramine. A new form of selegiline given transdermally, desmethylselegiline (DMS), is under development and showing fewer side effects than oral dosing.

Although the manufacturer of selegiline now warns against its use with SSRIs, commonly given in PD for depression, a new review of 2000 patients on combined selegiline and SSRI, found that the incidence of SSRI reaction with selegiline was 0.24% with no deaths (Richard et al., 1997). The reported reaction is one of seizures, anxiety, level of consciousness, or remotely, pseudopheochromocytoma.

Another side effect of the drug is its effect on the cardiovascular system. Patients with Parkinson's disease have changes in their cardiovascular systems, slowing of heart rate, and decreased autonomic vascular regulation with position change. Selegiline tends to exacerbate this condition in some individuals, especially under stressed conditions such as the tilt table, Valsalva's maneuver, and sudden standing with a delay in autonomic response of over 2 min from the stressor onset. These changes suggest an increased risk for orthostatic hypotension in selegiline users and a need to test BP lying, sitting, and standing during routine office visit followup. Many researchers caution providers about the use of this drug, as the long-term benefits vs. side effects are unknown.

DOPAMINE AGONISTS

The dopamine agonists directly stimulate specific subclasses of dopamine receptors. By reducing the turnover of dopamine, these drugs may reduce the toxic byproducts of dopamine metabolism, hydrogen peroxide and free radical accumulation. The second generation dopamine agonists, ropinirole and pramipexole, lack the ergoline chemical structure of the first generation dopamine agonists, e.g. bromocriptine and pergolide. The second generation dopamine agonists mimic the action of dopamine at post synaptic dopamine (D2) receptors and are more selective for these receptors than the first generation drugs. The second generation dopamine agonists may also have possible neuroprotective effects. In addition the second generation dopamine agonists have fewer and less sever side effects than the first generation drugs. They do not generate oxidative metabolites. These drugs may be used as initial therapy in Parkinson's Disease to delay the initiation of levodopa, as adjunctive therapy in patients who are uncontrolled on levodopa, and to reduce the dose of levodopa. The limitations of the second generation dopamine agonists are that they do not completely prevent the development of levodopa-related adverse events, do not treat all features of Parkinson's Disease such as freezing, postural instability, autonomic dysfunction, and dementia, and do not stop the disease progression. Side effects that have been associated with ropinirole and pramipexole include nausea, dizziness, somnolence, orthostatic hypotension, hallucinations, and dyskinesias (PSG, 2002). Drug Table 318 also lists other adjunctive medications not as commonly used as the ones described below. All of the dopamine agonists can cause nausea, vomiting, and orthostatic hypotension so slow titration is a key in treatment, and the drugs must be weaned slowly to prevent a rebound worsening of symptoms. Drugs specifically contraindicated when using dopaminergic agents in PD are neuroleptics, centrally active dopamine antagonist antiemetics (prochlorperazine, promethazine), and catecholamine-depleting agents such as reserpine. The dopamine agonists are also more expensive than Sinemet (carbidopa-levodopa), but their use may delay the onset of motor fluctuations, reducing levodopa requirements and decreasing the disability from motor fluctuations.

Bromocriptine (Parlodel) is an ergot alkaloid, with D2 receptor agonist activity. The drug is also used in conjunction with levodopa and by itself in the early stage of Parkinson's disease. In conjunction therapy the dose is 1.25 mg per day with a slow increase to 7.5 to 10 mg per day in three to four divided doses until adequate control is achieved. The dose may go as high as 30 mg per day. Its side effects include nausea, somnolence, orthostatic hypotension, back pain, confusion, and hallucinations.

Pergolide (Permax) also is an ergot preparation that is 10 times more potent than bromocriptine, stimulating the D2 receptors and having a partial effect on the D1 receptors. It is used early on as initial therapy and as adjunctive therapy in later Parkinson's disease with L-dopa. The early titrating dose is 0.125 mg per day, increased by 0.125 mg every 5 days to a total dose of 0.75 to 1.0 mg per day in three or four divided dosages. The usual dose in conjunction therapy is 0.05 mg daily, increased slowly to 0.2 to 0.6 mg per day until adequate control is achieved, or reachieved as the disease progresses. The drug's side effects are somnolence, nausea, orthostatic hypotension, confusion, back pain, and hallucinations.

More specific dopamine agonists are under development. Transcutaneous preparations are also being developed, and subcutaneous dopamine agonists (such as apomorphine which was approved in 2004) are useful in specific cases for advanced PD and severe unpredictable "off" periods (Stern, 1994).

Anticholinergics

Anticholinergics were the first drugs used to treat PD and primarily provide relief of severe tremor with less effect on bradykinesia, rigidity, and postural instability. These compounds block muscarinic receptors, thus restoring the balance between dopaminergic and cholinergic influence in the basal ganglia. Artane (trihexyphenidyl) is primarily used in disabling tremor in younger patients without many other disease symptoms. Its side effects include dry eyes, dry mouth, urinary retention, loss of concentration, and hallucinations. It is poorly tolerated in the elderly. The starting dose is 1 mg/day, increased by 1-mg increments to 5 to 12 mg per day in three or four divided doses, raising the dose every 3 to 5 days. The drug is usually effective for only 3 to 6 months. A less potent anticholinergic agent, procyclidine, can be tried if ttrihexyphenidyl has too many adverse effects.

Benztropine (Cogentin) is also used in the treatment of tremor, either alone or with other agents. The dosage is 0.5 to 6 mg per day, and it can also produce confusion, sleepiness, blurred vision, and dry mouth.

Amantadine

Amantadine (Symmetrel) is a known antiviral agent that enhances dopamine release, has antimuscarinic effects, and may increase dopamine synthesis and inhibit dopamine reuptake. The drug has a modest effect on bradykinesia and rigidity with less effect on tremor. The drug is also a mild psychostimulant. The drug's effect is time-limited, usually 3 to 6 months. Amantadine is usually well tolerated in doses of 100 to 300 mg per day given in two or three divided doses. The common adverse effects are dose-dependent ankle edema and livedo reticularis (a purple mottling of the skin), as well as anticholinergic side effects of confusion, sleepiness, blurred vision, and dry mouth. The medication is available in an elixir (50 mg/5 mL) for smaller dosing and use in severe dysphagia. The drug is cleared by the kidney and needs dosage reduction in impaired renal function.

Levodopa Therapy

Levodopa, combined with carbidopa (Sinemet) or benserazide (which inhibit the peripheral metabolism of levodopa) and/or entacapone (which is a COMT inhibitor in the peripheral tissue and the brain allowing more levodopa to reach the site of activity), are the cornerstone of PD therapy. Levodopa is an intermediate byproduct of tyrosine. Carbidopa, a peripheral amino acid decarboxylase inhibitor, eliminates many of the severe GI effects of levodopa. Levodopa is absorbed in the gut, peaking in 1 h and lasting 3 to 8 h. The progression of PD, with fewer dopaminergic neurons available to take up the levodopa, contributes to the erratic clinical response of levodopa in long-term treatment. The effect is simple and complex motor fluctuations marked by dyskinesias, end-of-dose deterioration (wearing-off effect), and random fluctuations (on-off effect).

Treatment with levodopa begins when the disability affects social or occupational function with as low a dose as needed. The drug may be started alone or in conjunction with dopamine agonists to enable low-dose levodopa for as long as possible. Over time and with disease progression, individuals may require more medication in order to continue their daily functioning. Two controlled-release levodopa preparations are also in use, Sinemet-CR and Madopar HBS (hydrodynamically balanced system). The bioavailability of the drugs is less than in Sinemet so the drug dosages are actually higher, despite fewer daily doses. In advanced disease, patients like better control of their dyskinesias and on-off and wearing-off phenomena and will use a combination of controlled-release and regular Sinemet.

The treatment goal is relieving functional disability. Initial treatment may begin with Sinemet 25/100 (25 mg carbidopa and 100 mg levodopa), one-half tablet once daily, increasing by one-half tablet every 3 to 5 days to one tablet three times daily. Sinemet usually starts working in 30 min. The last dose should be given in mid- to late afternoon as it is not needed during sleep and may cause vivid dreams or nightmares. If nausea occurs, the drug may be given with meals.

Sinemet-CR is prescribed as the first-line drug in levodopa therapy using 50/200, one-half tablet twice daily, titrating up to two full tablets daily. As the disease progresses, the dosing may go to tid. Treatment response to Sinemet-CR usually takes 1 h. Because the actual bioavailability of Sinemet-CR is less than plain Sinemet, the controlled release forms require higher doses. As the disease progresses, the dosage may be titrated to two to four tablets daily. Keeping a diary of dose response is helpful in establishing a better response to dosing. A dosage of 1000 mg per day with no response implies the diagnosis is other than Parkinson's disease.

Adding standard Sinemet, dopamine agonists, or other secondary drugs when symptom control is inadequate (Stern, 1997) may be necessary with disease progression. The early morning bradykinesia and later dyskinesia complications of levodopa therapy have many approaches. One approach is the use of a combination of regular and controlled-release Sinemet early in the morning and perhaps again at midafternoon to shorten the time of drug efficacy. Individuals over time may find only minutes of time that are free from the bradykinesia if on too little Sinemet. Conversely, they can experience dyskinesias if on the Sinemet for a number of years. Another treatment option is to add dopamine agonists and reduce the amount of Sinemet used. Still another approach is to dilute the Sinemet to a liquid form and take it every 2 to 3 h to ensure a drug steady state.

Keeping a very time-specific log of drug dosing and side effects is helpful in altering drug therapy to produce better function and "smooth" the transitions. If predominant tremor is an issue, anticholinergics are used in addition to Artane. The anticholinergics can cause hallucinations, and patients must be monitored carefully for behavioral changes. The fluctuations in drug effect may also be related to food intake. The levodopa/carbidopa competes with large amino acids for transportation across the blood-brain barrier. Thus, it is helpful to coordinate protein intake with medication use. Other side effects associated with levodopa involve the CNS (anxiety, nervousness, confusion, depression, nightmares, hallucinations, insomnia), the GI tract (abdominal cramps, constipation, peptic ulcer), and the cardiovascular system (orthostatic hypotension, irregular heart rate, hypertension), and motor abnormalities. Concern has been raised that levodopa may increase oxidative metabolites which may exacerbate the progression of Parkinson's Disease, but recent data does not support this.

DRUGS USED FOR DEPRESSION, DEMENTIA, AND PSYCHOSIS IN PARKINSON'S DISEASE

Depression

The classic symptoms of depression—psychomotor retardation, insomnia, poor concentration, and anorexia—are often overlooked in PD because the symptoms resemble the signs of PD. Approximately 40% of patients with PD will suffer from depression. The depression should be treated aggressively using tricyclics, serotoninergic uptake blockers (SSRIs), psychotherapy, and possible electroshock therapy.

A drug commonly used is amitriptyline (Elavil, Endep) with starting doses of 12.5 to 75 mg per day given at bedtime, which may be increased up to 100 to 300 mg per day. Its effects include improving mood, helping with sleep fragmentation, and possibly aiding in the control of tremor. Some patients have an early morning dystonia, or leg cramping, that is also helped by this drug. The side effects include early morning lethargy, dry mouth, hallucinations, and confusion, so starting with low doses and slow titration is often necessary.

The SSRIs are another choice in treating the depression because they cause fewer extrapyramidal side effects than tricyclic agents. Both fluoxetine and buspirone are in common use.

Dementia

Loss in cognitive function is common. The usual dementia medications to improve memory have traditionally shown a poor clinical response in this patient population.

Psychosis

Hallucinations both visual and auditory, are common in PD. Some patients may also become paranoid. Infrequent hallucinations not altering the patient's functioning are usually not treated. Recording hallucinations before drug treatment is necessary to ascertain if hallucinations are related to just the disease or the drug treatment as well. The drugs used in the treatment of PD, particularly anticholinergic and dopaminergic compounds, can also cause confusion, sleep disturbance, frightening nightmares, and hallucinations. If the hallucinations are drug-related, titrating down dosages and eliminating their use late in the day may be effective. If the reaction is severe enough, it may require hospitalization.

The antipsychotic medication clozapine (Clozaril) is the cited drug of choice in psychosis. It can be used with a starting dose of 12.5 to 50 mg h.s. to treat the insomnia, hallucinations, and psychosis from dopaminergic medications and occasionally helps with tremor. Patients who present with hallucinations that are not drug-induced alone may require doses of up to 200 mg per day. This drug does not have the severe extrapyramidal side effects associated with traditional neuroleptics. However, it can cause agranulocytosis in 1% of patients so monitoring of neutrophil count is necessary if a patient is on this drug.

Other medications used to treat psychosis include molindone starting at 2.5 and up to 20 mg per day. However, this drug may worsen the symptoms of PD. The possibility that estrogen may slow the progression of PD or impact the symptoms is currently under investigation. With new data on the lack of cardiac benefit and the risks of HRT, menopausal women with PD need to discuss the use of HRT with both their neurological and women's health providers (Lieberman, 2002). For discussion of the assessment and treatment of constipation due to neurogenic bowel and sexual function due to neurological conditions, including PD, see the chapter on individuals with disabilities (Chapter 11).

Followup Recommendations

Careful monitoring of Parkinson's disease symptoms and drug therapy every 3 to 6 months and even sooner if the disease is rapidly progressive is necessary. A daily log of symptoms and drug use is helpful for the clinician and patient to establish optimum drug utilization. If the disease is refractory to medication and presents in an atypical manner, referral to a neurologist specializing in Parkinson's disease is helpful.

SEIZURES

A seizure is a transient, finite paroxysmal abnormal neuronal discharge that interrupts brain function. Seizure types are manifested through clinical features as well as characteristic electrographic patterns. Epilepsy is a chronic condition of recurrent seizures. Seizures may have known correctable causes such as is the case with acute metabolic changes such as hypoglycemia or drug abuse and drug withdrawal. Seizures with an identified correctable cause are not labeled as epilepsy. Seizures may also be caused by an underlying condition such as Alzheimer's, stroke or traumatic brain injury (Lackner, 2002). As may as 30% of seizures are caused by CNS disorders or insults such as meningitis, trauma, tumors or exposure to toxins.

A febrile seizure is a type of seizure that occurs in relationship to a fever. Febrile seizures occur in 2% to 5% of all children and occur in infants and children between 6 months and 5 years of age. Children who experience an initial febrile seizure prior to 1 year of age have about a 50 percent chance of having another febrile seizure. By comparison children older than 1 year of age who experience an initial febrile have only a 30 percent chance of having a second febrile seizure. Children with a history of febrile seizures have a slightly higher risk of developing epilepsy by age 7 as compared to children who have not experienced a febrile seizure (AAP, 1999; Rosen, 2001).

Simple febrile seizures are defined as primary generalized seizures of less than 15 minutes duration and not recurring within a 24 hour period. Complex febrile seizures are defined as focal, prolonged, lasting more than 15 minutes, and may or may not occur in a flurry. Treatment following the first simple febrile seizure involves identifying the causes of the fever as well as initiating treatment with anti-pyretic agents such as acetaminophen and ibuprofen. Diagnostics may involve a lumbar puncture to diagnose meningitis. Febrile seizures usually do not require evaluation by EEG, blood studies, or neuroimaging. The key to treatment of febrile seizures is to initiate fever management as soon as a fever is present. Patients with benign febrile seizures do not need chronic anti-epileptic drug (AED) therapy. If the child has recurring febrile seizures, caregivers may give the child rectal diazepam (Rosen, 2001).

There are diverse etiologies of epilepsy as evidenced by various pathophysiologic alterations in the brains of individuals with epilepsy. For approximately half of the individuals with epilepsy there is no clear etiology and epilepsy is idiopathic. However, symptoms present at the onset of the seizure provide valuable information crucial to the diagnosis of the seizure type (Brodie & Kwan, 2002). Seizures are classified by the part of the brain affected or involved. Initiation of seizures may begin with alteration in sensory or emotional phenomena, consciousness, and motor activity. It is critical to differentiate between alterations related to epilepsy and other brief alterations in consciousness or abnormal movements. Syncope, drug abuse, transient ischemic attacks and pseudoseizures must be eliminated from the differential diagnosis. In the pediatric population behaviors such as breath holding, gastroesophageal reflux and head banging may be mistaken for epilepsy. Diagnosis of seizure type may be difficult and referral and collaboration with a neurologist is recommended.

There are two classification systems of epilepsy. The International Classification of Epileptic Seizures (ICES) was developed in 1964, and revised in 1981 by the International League Against Epilepsy. This classification system is based on three factors: clinical seizure symptoms, ictal (during the seizure) EEG findings and interictal (between seizures) EEG findings. The ICES classification system divides seizures into two categories of partial and generalized. Partial seizures initiate in one hemisphere of the brain and may be classified as simple, complex or partial seizures secondarily generalized. Generalized seizures that begin in both hemispheres of the brain without localization

The second classification system is the International Classification of the Epilepsies and Epileptic Syndromes (ICE) developed in 1985 and revised in 1989 by the Commission of Classification and Terminology of the International League Against Epilepsy. This classification divides epilepsy into partial and generalized seizures as well as according to epilepsies with known etiologies from those that are idiopathic. Further elaboration related to the classification systems are beyond the scope of this chapter (Dreifuss & Norldi, 2001).

Overall, epilepsy may also be characterized by clusters or grouping of symptoms. Classification of epileptic syndromes is based on the type or types of seizures as well as characteristic EEG patterns, symptoms, focus in the brain, precipitating factors as well as factors such as age, family history, cycling and severity or chronicity of the seizures. Seizure syndromes are useful in that they provide a means of communication about epilepsy as well as provide a format to evaluate treatment and formulate prognosis. If the predominant seizure type is partial or focal, the epilepsy is classified as location related. If the seizures are generalized, the classification is generalized. Seizure syndromes are further subdivided into primary or idiopathic, epilepsies and symptomatic or lesional epilepsies (Celano, 1998). Examples of common epileptic syndromes are: neonatal seizures, childhood absence epilepsy, Infantile spasms, benign focal epilepsy of childhood and juvenile myoclonic epilepsy.

SPECIFIC CONSIDERATION FOR PHARMACOTHERAPY

When Drug Therapy is Needed

Pharmacotherapeutic intervention for epilepsy is highly specific and the response of specific seizure types to antiepileptic drug (AED) intervention varies. Some pharmacotherapeutic interventions exacerbate seizures if used for the incorrect type of epilepsy. For example, carbamazepine exacerbates absence seizures. Therefore it is critical to diagnose seizure type prior to initiating pharmacotherapeutic treatment.

Monotherapy is desirable, but the goal of treatment is to be seizure-free with minimal side effects from medications. If necessary, several monotherapy options should be tried to eliminate the seizures. Each AED is titrated to clinical response, meaning the elimination of the seizures or intolerable side effects. The inability to stop the seizures or intolerable side effects after of monotherapy with 2 or 3 AEDs is a reasonable point to consider polytherapy. Seizures that are difficult to control are best managed by a neurologist rather than a primary care provider. A referral to a comprehensive epilepsy center is considered for seizures that are intractable to polytherapy with 2 or more agents or due to intolerable side effects (Garnett & Gloyd, 2001).

Short- and Long-Term Goals of Pharmacotherapy

Control of epilepsy is defined by the Centers for Disease Control (CDC) as no seizures and no side effects. Pellock, Dodson, and Bourgeois (2001) also include "the absence of stigma" to the definition of good control. Table 29–14 outlines the approach to anticonvulsant management.

Nonpharmacologic Treatment

Twenty percent of individuals with epilepsy do not achieve adequate seizure control through pharmacologic treatment. These individuals have drug resistant or intractable epilepsy. Intractable seizures in childhood may be treated with the ketogenic diet, usually in combination with AEDs. Surgery is an option for people who do not respond to drug therapy.

Surgical sectioning of the corpus callosum is based on the shared information between the hemispheres of the brain which is responsible for not only the spread but also the synchronization of seizure activity. Sectioning the anterior two-thirds of the corpus callosum preserves sharing of visual information and may decrease or eliminate seizures. If this is not effective, the remainder of the corpus callosum may be sectioned at a later time. The success rate is approximately 75%. This option is usually reserved for individuals experiencing drop attacks.

Vagus nerve stimulation (VNS) involves repeated electrical stimulation of regions of the brain such as the cerebellum and vagus nerve to produce remote inhibitory effects on the cerebral cortex. The VNS resembles a pacemaker and is implanted just below the left clavicle and the wire is inserted via an incision in the neck and is attached to the left vagus nerve.

Alternative treatment options are also used in the treatment of epilepsy. Pyridoxine (Vitamin B_6) may be

TABLE 29–14. Planning an Anticonvulsant Regimen

1. Select the proper drug for the seizure type.
2. Determine the initial dosage based on weight and potential toxicity or interactions.
3. Increase the dosage until the therapeutic effect is achieved or until limited by side effects or toxicity.
4. Monitor levels as indicated (total/free; metabolites).
5. Use the highest tolerated dosage and add a second drug if the therapeutic level is inadequate.
6. If possible, taper the first drug off.
7. NEVER stop an antiepileptic drug abruptly.

beneficial for pyridoxine-dependant seizures. Infantile spasms may respond to adrenocorticotropic hormone or corticosteroids. Individuals with seizures may use herbal remedies, vitamin supplements and acupuncture. There is no scientific evidence supporting these alternative therapies however, some individuals with epilepsy use such treatments and it is important that these treatments are discussed with the provider to make sure that there is no interaction or side effect from combination with traditional pharmacotherapeutic management.

Assessment Needed Prior to Therapy

Assessment for new onset seizures may be initiated by the primary care provider or a neurologist. An intensive history from patient and caregiver is obtained. This includes a thorough description of the event including activities before and precipitating factors and condition of the individual after the event. A past medical history and social history must also be obtained. Exposures to lead, toxins, medications, and illicit drugs and alcohol must be explored. A complete physical examination and neurologic exam is also necessary. Diagnostic tools may include an EEG, blood studies, urine studies and possibly neuroimaging to rule out structural lesions or brain abnormalities (Buelow, 2001).

Scientific evidence suggests that the variance in female hormones as well as reproductive state may influence seizure frequency and pattern. Approximately one-third of women with epilepsy experiencing a twofold or greater increase of seizure frequency. Variance is related to rapid progesterone withdrawal, menstruation or estrogen elevation prior to ovulation. Reproductive disorders and infertility occur more often in women with epilepsy as compared to women without epilepsy. AEDs that induce liver enzymes therefore decreasing the effectiveness of oral contraceptives include: carbamazepine, phenytoin, phenobarbital, primidone, oxcarbazepine and topiramate. AEDs that do not decrease oral contraceptive effectiveness are: gabapentin, levetiracetam, lamotrigine, tiagabine, valproate and zonisamide (Morrell, 2002).

Individuals over 60 make up the second largest group of individuals with epilepsy. They are surpassed only by children under the age of 3. The most common types of seizures in the older individual are tonic-clonic, simple or complex partial seizures. Absence seizures are rare in this population (Arroyo & Kramer, 2001, Leppik, 2001, McAuley & Anderson, 2002, Morell 1999, Yerby, 2001). Within the older population, pharmacotherapeutic intervention centers on a single non-sedating anticonvulsant. Renal and hepatic clearance often are decreased with age and therefore reduced dosages are necessary. Due to the decrease in protein binding for highly protein-bound drugs, free anticonvulsant levels must be monitored.

Patient/Caregiver Information

It is essential that patients and families be informed that epilepsy is a syndrome of symptoms, a chronic disorder consisting of abnormal firing of neurons. Epilepsy is NOT punishment, mental retardation or demonic possession. As many as 30 to 50 percent of individuals with epilepsy do not take their AEDs as prescribed which is a major cause of failure to respond to AEDs, as well as a trigger for status epilepticus. Strategies for improving adherence include, reinforcing adherence at each visit, obtaining patient's perceived barriers to medication usage, tailoring dosing to individual's schedule, and simplifying the dosage regimen to at most two times per day. Seizures result in the loss of the right to a driver's license with the return of the driver's license being dependant on seizure control. The laws regulating driving vary for each state. Storage of medications must be out of the reach of children and avoidant of extremes of temperature and humidity. Women of child bearing potential must be informed that AEDs may result in the loss of contraceptive protection and may change the clearance of AEDs. AEDs have the potential for teratogenicity and are also passed into breast milk (Gidal, Garnett, & Graves, 2002). Children and adolescents face stigma and negative attitudes that can impact self-esteem and decrease self-management and social competence (Raty, Wilde Larsson, & Soderfeldt, 2003). Addressing quality of life with epilepsy must be a part of any treatment plan (Austin & Santilli, 2001; Birgeck et al., 2002).

Patient education regarding first aid for each seizure type must be taught. In the case of tonic clonic seizures it is necessary to: ease person to floor and loosen constricting clothing, remove objects from the area that may be harmful, do not force anything hard between teeth, turn the person's head to the side, and if the seizure is still in progress after 5 minutes, make plans to transport the patient to the ER. For complex partial seizures first aid involves: no restraint of the individual unless absolutely necessary and make suggestions to guide the exhibited behavior if possible. There is no specific first aide for absence seizures except removing the individual from a place where they can be injured. Safety for individuals who have incompletely controlled seizures includes: no driving, swimming only in the presence of others who can swim and are trained as a lifeguard, avoiding glass shower stalls as well as caution with mechanical equipment and stoves.

OUTCOMES MANAGEMENT

General information about antiseizure medicines is followed by specific information on the most commonly used seizure medications.

Overview of Drug Classes: Selecting an Appropriate Agent

The individual or in the case of pediatrics the parents or caregivers are vital to the selection of medication. The individual is the one to report the side effects. Side effects are generally divided into four categories: dose related, idiosyncratic reactions, long term side effects and delayed effects (Asconape, 2002). If the AED has a known major side effect, patient education is essential in the monitoring process. It is helpful to provide written information regarding AED therapy. The Epilepsy Foundation website www.epilepsyfoundation.org is a valuable resource for such information.

AEDs are not initiated at standard starting dose and there is no uniform titration schedule. This is all tailored to patient response. The individual characteristics of each drug must be considered when initiating therapy. If an AED is metabolized by the liver, the dose should be modified by a neurologist. Likewise, Phenytoin is bound by formula or milk and must be given one hour prior or one hour after a feeding. If an individual can not tolerate a change in feeding schedule an alternate medication may need to be utilized (Pellock, Dodson, & Bourgeosis, 2001).

Monitoring for Efficacy

Adjustments of AED dosing may yield one of three scenarios. The increase may result in no seizures and no side effects or the seizures may continue but side effects increase or the seizures may continue and no side effects are present. AEDs have target ranges that serve as guidelines for medication titration (Fraught, 2001). Individual response may vary greatly within each range. Patients may require dosages above the range; however the percentage of patients experiencing side effects rapidly increases. In dosages below the range, the percentage of individual's not gaining benefit significantly increases (Kammerman & Wasserman, 2001).

Each AED has a half-life which represents the time at which the body would eliminate one half of the AEDs dose. If a medication is increased or decreased, it requires five half lives to establish the steady state. This must be considered when making dosing adjustments. Individuals must be informed of the time frame involved prior to experiencing any medication related change (Fisher & Patel, 2001).

Status epilepticus (SE) is a symptom of severe CNS malfunction and is defined as a seizure lasting more than 30 minutes or recurrent seizures lasting more that 30 min where the patient does not regain consciousness (Leszczyszyn & Pellock, 2001). There is both convulsive and nonconvulsive SE. Prolonged or uncontrollable SE has a poor prognosis. The neurologist is the primary health care provider for these individuals.

Monitoring for Toxicity

Therapeutic plasma levels, frequently used in the management of seizures and titration of AEDs, are not absolutes but rather guides. Medication adjustment is based on therapeutic ranges as a guide and medications are titrated to clinical response, not AED level. The patient is being treated, not the drug level. Plasma levels of AEDs are monitored but these results may be difficult to interpret as samples may be obtained during various times of the day. The gold standard is to measure plasma levels at the same time either before the first dose of the day is given or at the end of the day prior to the next dose. Plasma levels obtained at these times reflect trough levels of the AED. This is the lowest point at which the plasma level will be during any given day. If the individual is experiencing toxic side effect, it may be helpful to monitor the plasma level at the time the side effect occurs (Garnett, 1995).

Further, monitoring for side effects is critical. Gilliam and colleagues (2004) have found monitoring for side effects with a 19-items self-report instrument promising. Clinicians using the scale netted a 2.8-fold increase in AED modification and significant improvement of quality of life scores without increasing seizure frequency.

Overview of Commonly Used Antiepileptic Drugs

The antiepileptic drugs (AEDs) may be divided into first and second generation AEDs. The first generation AEDs are phenobarbital, phenytoin, ethosuximide, carbamazepine, valproic acid, and benzodiazepines which were the only available AEDs until the early 1990's. Because there was a recognized need for additional AEDs, the Antiepileptic Drug Development program, which was a cooperative alliance between the Epilepsy Branch of the NIH, the pharmaceutical manufacturers, and clinical investigators, was developed. Through this program numerous compounds were screened for AED activity and those with promise were brought to clinical trials resulting in eight new AEDs. These second generation drugs are felbamate, gabapentin, lamotrigine, topiramate, tiagabine, levetiracetam, oxcarbazepine, and zonisamide. This increases the opportunity to find the right drug or combination of drugs for a given patient but complicates the decision process because of the increased number of potential combinations. Also, there have been new delivery systems for the first generation AEDs.

Antiepileptic drugs (AEDs) should be chosen for the specific seizure type that the patient has. The first generation AEDs were primarily effective in simple and complex partial and generalized tonic clonic seizures. Valproic acid has been shown to be effective for other types of generalized seizures, e.g. absence and myoclonic. Ethosuximide is only effective for absence seizures. Absence seizures are unique pharmacologically. They respond to ethosuximide, valproic acid, lamotrigine and zonisamide but may be exacerbated by phenytoin or carbamazepine. The second generation AEDs were initially tested in patients with refractory partial seizures because animal models indicated they would be effective for this seizure type and this is the largest population with refractory seizures. Some of the second-generation AEDs, e.g., lamotrigine, topiramate, levetiracetam, and zonisamide, may be useful in patients with generalized seizures. For example, zonisamide and lamotrigine appear to be effective for myoclonic seizures.

There are very few direct comparative studies of the AEDs. The two Veteran's Cooperative trials comparing the first generation AEDs are landmark trials. In the first VA cooperative study, phenobarbital, phenytoin, primidone, and carbamazepine were compared in a prospective, double-blind, randomized trial. This study demonstrated that more patients could be maintained on either phenytoin or carbamazepine than phenobarbital or primidone. Base on tolerance, carbamazepine was considered the drug of first choice especially for partial seizures. In the second VA Cooperative Trial, carbamazepine was compared to valproic acid in a design similar to the first study. Using outcome that combined efficacy and tolerance, this study demonstrated that there was no difference between the two drugs for patients with generalized seizures but that carbamazepine was superior to valproic acid for patients with partial seizures. Many clinicians consider carbamazepine to be the initial drug for patients with partial seizures. In some epilepsy centers, clinicians are initiating therapy with the second generation AEDs although most of them are approved only for adjunctive use.

The selection of an AED for a particular patient will depend on seizure type, dosage form available, potential for drug interactions, adverse drug reactions (ADRs), gender and age.

Seizure Type. The AED selected must be appropriate for the type of seizure the patient has. Most AEDs, with the exception of ethosuximide, are effective for partial seizures. However, not all AEDs are effective for generalized seizures. Only ethosuximide, valproic acid, lamotrigine, and zonisamide are effective for absence seizures. Valproic acid, lamotrigine, and zonisamide have been shown to be effective for juvenile myoclonic epilepsy. Carbamazepine and phenytoin may exacerbate absence seizures.

Dosage Forms Available. The choice of an AED may be affected by the dosage form available. For example, a very young or old patient make not be able to swallow an oral solid. There an AED may be chosen because it is available as a liquid, a "sprinkle" that can be mixed with food, a dispersible tablet, or can be extemporaneously made into a liquid. Of course, if the patient cannot take anything by mouth, an intravenous or intramuscular form is essential.

Potential for Drug Interactions. Drug interactions are common with the AEDs. While this does not contra-indicate their use, it does increase the monitoring that is required. An AED may be selected because it is known not to interact with other drugs or other AEDs that it might be used with.

Adverse Drug Reactions. All of the AEDs are associated with some adverse reactions. One of the treatment goals is to have no seizures with no or a minimal incidence of side effects. Therefore, an AED may be selected because it has a lower potential for side effects rather than because it is believed to have superior efficacy.

Gender. Women with epilepsy have special needs that include cosmetic changes associated with AEDs, contraception, infertility, complications of pregnancy, catamenial seizures, and an increase in seizures associated with hormonal replacement therapy. Some of the cosmetic changes associated with AEDs that may be of special concern to women are weight gain with valproic acid, weight loss associated with felbamate, topiramate, and zonisamide; alopecia and change in hair color associated with valproic acid; and gingival hyperplasia, excessive hair growth, and acne associated with phenytoin. Carbamazepine, oxcarbazepine, phenobarbital, phenytoin, and topiramate have been associated with a decreased efficacy of oral contraceptives. With these AEDs a higher estrogen/progestin OC is advised. The patient may also be advised to use a second method of contraception. Epilepsy and AEDs have also been associated with infertility. This may result from reproductive and endocrine disorders, polycystic ovarian disease, social stigma, or concern about teratogenicity. Hormonal, metabolic, psychological, pharmacokinetic and physiologic changes during pregnancy may increase the incidence of seizures. The pregnant female should be seizure free and the AED therapy should be continued during the pregnancy. Seizures per se can cause tetratogenicity. The dose of the AEDs may need to be increased during the third trimester and reduced immediately post-partum. Women with epilepsy do have more complications during pregnancy that include vaginal bleeding, hyperemesis gravidarium, pre-eclampsia, abruptio placentae, premature labor, and weaker uterine contractions. To minimize the complications of pregnancy women with epilepsy should receive preconception counseling. At this time, the AED with the least potential for tetratogenicity should be selected. Phenytoin is associated with about a 4 to 6% incidence of birth defects. Valproic acid and carbamazepine are associated with a 1% incidence of spina bifida. The second generation AEDs appear to be less teratogenic. However, the numbers of women who have taken the second generation AEDs during pregnancy is low. Women who can become pregnant need to be on a multivitamin with 0.4 to 1.0 mg of folic acid. Women who plan to become pregnant should be under medical supervision and after a assessment to rule out vitamin B deficiency, should begin 4–5 mg of folic acid supplementation daily per prescription before conception. This supplementation should not be in a multivitamin format. (Wilson et al., 2003). She should receive vitamin K_1 10 mg/day during the last month of pregnancy. Also, the AED levels should be carefully monitored during the third trimester because the clearance seems to increase until immediately after delivery. While there have been complications in the offspring of women with epilepsy, they should be reminded that about 95% of women with epilepsy deliver a healthy baby. Women with epilepsy who are taking AEDs during pregnancy should be registered with the North American Antiepileptic Drug Pregnancy Registry by calling 888-233-2334. It has been reported since 1885 that some women will have an increase in seizures during menses. This increase in seizure frequency is called catamenial epilepsy and is defined as all or most of a woman's seizures occur during a 7 day period, form 3 days before through the early phase of the cycle. Catamenial epilepsy has been treated with progesterone, clomiphen, and acetazolamide. Finally, older women requiring hormonal replacement therapy (HRT) have been reported to experience an increase in seizures (AAN, 1998; Morrell, 1999, 2002).

Age. The very young and the very old present unique treatment options. It may be difficult to recognize seizure activity in very young patients. Also, their pharmacokinetics are not the same as adults. Therefore, the dose must be individualized. It is important to remember that the onset of new seizures has a bimodal distribution with the highest peaks occurring in the very young and in patients over age 65 years. Partial seizures are the most common seizure type in the older patients. However, auras are less frequent or are more non-specific. Automatisms are less frequent and the postictal confusion may be prolonged. Finally, the seizure may be mis-diagnosed as altered mental status, confusion, memory disturbance, or a TIA. The elderly are more likely to have more severe consequences of seizures because of injuries occurring during falls. The elderly have altered pharmacokinetics and are taking more drugs making drug interactions more likely (Arroyo & Kramer, 2001).

First Generation Antiepileptic Drugs (Faught, 2001, Garnett, 1995, Garnett & Gloyd, 2001, Gidal 2002)

Phenobarbital/Primidone. This is the oldest AED still in common use. Phenobarbital elevates seizure threshold by decreasing postsynaptic excitation, possibly by stimulating postsynaptic GABA-ergic inhibitory processes. This drug is available in a variety of dosage forms including a parenteral form, a solution, and a tablet. The drug displays linear pharmacokinetics meaning that the increase in serum concentration is proportional to the increase in dose. Phenobarbital has a very long half life (36 to 96 hours). This means that the drug can be dosed once a day. However, it will take up to three weeks to achieve a new steady state after a change in dose. Therefore, dosage adjustments should be made very gradually. The drug is effective for partial and generalized seizures. However, the use of phenobarbital is limited by the incidence of side effects. In children, phenobarbital causes paradoxical hyperactivity. In adults, phenobarbital impairs cognition and causes CNS depression. It has been associated with an increase in falls in the elderly. Phenobarbital is a ubiquitous inducer of the cytochrome P-450 system and is associated with numerous drug interactions.

Primidone (Mysoline) is metabolized to phenobarbital and to phenylethylmalonamide. Because primidone has intrinsic antiepileptic activity, it may be effective in a few patients who have failed phenobarbital. The half-life of primidone is shorter than phenobarbital and consequently must be given more frequently. However, because it is metabolized to phenobarbital, it rarely should be added to phenobarbital. Also, steady state will be reached with primidone before it is reached with phenobarbital. Therefore, dosing adjustments should be made on the time to reach steady state with phenobarbital. The potential for ADRs and drug interactions with primidone is similar to phenobarbital.

Phenytoin. Phenytoin (Dilantin) was introduced in 1938 and remains the most frequently prescribed AED. Phenytoin inhibits seizure activity primarily by blocking sodium activated voltage channels. It may have some effect on calcium channels and on serotonin. It has been used mainly for partial and tonic-clonic generalized seizures.

It is a drug with complicated pharmacokinetics which makes dosing difficult. The amount of drug absorbed is affected by dose. The absorption of doses greater than 400 mg may saturate necessitating an increased dosing interval. Phenytoin is metabolized in the liver primarily by CYP2C9 but CYP2C19 is also involved. The first metabolite is further metabolized to a glucoronide which is excreted in the urine. Phenytoin displays Michaelis-Menton pharmacokinetics which means that the body's ability to metabolize phenytoin saturates. This happens at doses used clinically with the result being that in some patients a small change in dose will result in a significantly larger increase in serum concentrations. Unfortunately, there is no good clinical method for predicting which patient and at what dose a patient will saturate the metabolism. Consequently, dosage adjustments should be made very carefully. A clinical guideline for dosing is to increase the dose by 100 mg/day if the phenytoin concentration is less than 7 mcg/ml, to increase the dose by 50 mg/day if the phenytoin concentration is between 7 and 12 mcg/ml, and to increase the dose by 30 mg/day if the phenytoin concentration is greater than 12 mcg/ml. Although the half life of phenytoin is usually assumed to be 24 hours, the Michaelis-Menton pharmacokinetics means that the half-life of phenytoin is dependant on the concentration. The half-life is longer when the serum concentrations are higher. However, dosage adjustment of phenytoin should not be made more rapidly than every seven days. Phenytoin is highly protein bound (>90%). Since it is the unbound fraction that diffuses across the blood brain barrier to exert the pharmacologic activity, changes in the free fraction will alter the response. For example, patients with low albumin, chronic renal failure, a very young or advanced age, and other highly protein bound drugs will have an increase in the free or unbound drug. In these patients monitoring the total serum concentration of phenytoin may be misleading. Phenytoin is extensively metabolized in the liver and its metabolism can be induced and inhibited by other drugs. Also, phenytoin is an enzyme inducer and increases the metabolism of other drugs metabolized by cytochrome P-450. There have been numerous ADRs reported with phenytoin. Some such as nystagmus, ataxia, lethargy, and cognitive impairment are concentration related. Others such as gingival hyperplasia, anemia, hirsutism, and osteomalacia are idiosyncratic.

Phenytoin is available in a variety of dosage forms including a parenteral formulation, a chewable tablet, a suspension, and oral capsules. Fosphenytoin (Cerebrex) is a diphosphate ester of phenytoin and is much more water soluble. Therefore, fosphenytoin can be given by IV infusion faster with less thrombosis and vascular irritation. The suspension does need to be shaken but remains in suspension sufficiently for accurate dosing. An appropriate calibrated measuring device should be used to measure phenytoin suspension. Recently, a controlled release formulation of phenytoin (Phenytek) was approved. This allows for once a day dosing but has been limited by being available only as a 200 mg or 300 mg capsule.

Ethosuximide. Ethosuximide (Zarontin) is the most frequently used of the succimide AEDs. It inhibits NADPH-linked aldehyde reductase necessary for the formation of gamma-hydroxybutyrate which has been associated with the induction of absence seizures. It is effective uniquely for absence seizures. The use of ethosuximide for seizure types other than absence should be questioned. This drug is available as a capsule and an oral solution.

The drug is well absorbed and is extensively metabolized to inactive metabolites. The half-life of ethosuximide is 30 to 60 hours suggesting that once a day dosing is appropriate. However, the incidence of gastrointestinal side effects increases with once a day dosing and the drug is usually given twice a day. Other side effects associated with ethosuximide include drowsiness, CNS depression, and hiccups. Drug interactions with ethosuximide are rare. The availability of a capsule and syrup provides flexibility in dosing patients who have trouble swallowing an oral solid dosage form.

Carbamazepine. Carbamazepine (Tegretol, Tegretol-XR, Carbatrol) was originally developed for trigeminal neuralgia. Carbamazepine blocks seizure activity primarily by inhibition of voltage gated sodium channels. It may also have some effect on serotonin. The two VA Cooperative Studies indicated that carbamazepine is the initial drug of choice for patients with partial seizures and that it is also effective for patients with generalized tonic-clonic seizures.

The absorption of carbamazepine from immediate release tablets is slow and erratic. Because absorption is dissolution rate dependant, bioavailability may be decreased at higher doses. Carbamazepine binds primarily to alpha-glycoprotein and is not displaced by drugs binding to albumin. Carbamazepine is metabolized primarily by CYP3A4. Carbamazepine has a half-life that becomes shorter with continued dosing because of auto-induction. The half-life of carbamazepine in drug naive individuals is approximately 36 hours. However, carbamazepine induces its own metabolism and with continued dosing the half-life may be 8 to 10 hours. If the patient is taking enzyme inducing drugs the half-life may be even shorter. Carbamazepine has an active metabolite that contributes to its efficacy and to its toxicity. Some drugs, e.g. valproic acid and felbamate, will cause an increase in the concentration of the active metabolite without increasing the concentration of the parent drug. Carbamazepine is an enzyme inducer and its metabolism can be induced and inhibited. The most common side effects of carbamazepine include CNS depression, skin rash, hyponatremia, and leukopenia. The CNS side effects have been correlated with peak concentrations with immediate release tablets and may be decreased by the use of extended release formulations. Leukopenia is common with carbamazepine but does not necessarily mean that the patient has bone marrow suppression. It is common for patients to have a low white blood cell count, especially a neutropenia, while on carbamazepine. However, it appears that carbamazepine alters the storage of neutrophils but does not inhibit their mobilization or function. Patients with low WBC on carbamazepine are not immuno-suppressed and do not have an increase in infections or autoimmune disorders. While bone marrow suppression has been reported with carbamazepine, it is very rare.

Carbamazepine is available as a chewable tablet, suspension, immediate release tablet, controlled release tablet, and a sustained release capsule. Concern has been voiced about variability in the bioavailability of the generic immediate release tablets. The suspension is absorbed more rapidly than the immediate release tablet necessitating more frequent dosing to avoid higher peaks and lower troughs. The extended release formulations (Tegretol-XR and Carbatrol) offer the advantage of twice a day dosing. This is an aid to adherence and may decrease peak related side effects. The controlled release tablet (Tegretol-XR) should not be crushed and patients should be informed that the shell or casing of the dosage form will be excreted in the feces. The sustained release dosage form (Carbatrol) is a capsule which can be opened and the contents mixed with food. This would be an alternative to patients who cannot swallow an oral solid. It has also been well tolerated in adults for as long as 36 months (Hogan, Garnett, Thadani, and the Carbatrol Study Group, 2003). The controlled release tablet (Tegretol-XR) and the sustained release dosage form (Carbatrol) are not generic dosage forms of carbamazepine. They are unique delivery systems. In a short-term study in volunteers, the sustained release dosage form (Carbatrol) provided more reliable absorption although the two dosage forms were bioequivalent.

Valproic Acid. Valproic acid (Depakene, Depakote, Depakote-ER) increases GABA by inhibiting its degradation. It also blocks the sodium voltage gated channel, the T-calcium channel, and possibly the potassium channel. It is a broad spectrum AED and has been used to treat partial seizures and a variety of generalized seizures. Valproic acid is available as a syrup, a gelatin capsule, a delayed release tablet, a "sprinkle," an extended release tablet, and an IV formulation.

The absorption of valproic is dependent on the dosage form. Absorption from the syrup and gelatine capsule is faster than from the delayed release (Depakote) or extended release (Depakote-Sprinkles, Depakote-ER) formulations. Valproic acid is highly (>90%) protein bound. At concentrations less than 90 mcg/ml the percent free, or the unbound fraction, is around 10%. However, at concentrations greater than 90 mcg/ml, the binding saturates and the percent free increases at a disproportionate rate to the increase in dose. This can make the monitoring of total serum drug levels misleading. Valproic acid is extensively metabolized by the liver and its metabolism may be induced or inhibited. Valproic may inhibit the metabolism of other drugs.

The most common side effects of valproic acid include gastrointestinal distress, tremor, alopecia, weight gain, thrombocytopenia, and elevated liver function tests.

Depakote, which has an enteric coating that does not dissolve in the acidic mileau of the stomach, was developed to avoid contact of valproic acid with the GI mucosa. The fine tremor associated with valproic acid appears to be dose related. Although alopecia occurs, the hair does return and some patient like the new texture better. Weight gain may be a limiting side effect. Interestingly, alopecia and weight gain were not associated with the development of the extended release formulation (Depakote-ER) formulation of valproic acid. Other rare side effects of valproic acid include an association with ovarian cysts, pancreatitis, and hepatotoxicity. The hepatotoxicity appears to occur primarily in patients less than two years of age who may also have an inborn error of metabolism and/or multiple other drugs.

Benzodiazepines. Lorazepam (Ativan) given intravenously has replaced diazepam (Valium) in many hospital for the treatment of continuous seizures because it has a longer duration of anticonvulsant activity. However, diazepam is absorbed better rectally and there is a rectal enema of diazepam (Diastat) that can be used by caregivers when the patient has prolonged seizure activity. The formulation is approved for acute repetitive seizures but data suggest that rectal diazepam is also effective for status epilepticus and febrile seizures.

Second Generation Antiepileptic Drugs (Faught, 2001, Garnett, 1995, Garnett & Gloyd, 2001, Gidal 2002)

Felbamate. Felbamate (Felbatol) was the first of the second generation AEDs. It also was the first AED to be associated with CNS stimulation rather than sedation. It blocks the glycine receptor on the NMDA complex which prevents the release of glutamate. Although this drug was very effective in patients with refractory seizures, its use has been limited because of its association with aplastic anemia and acute hepatic failure. The onset of these severe adverse reactions was between 68 and 354 days after beginning therapy. The incidence of aplastic anemia was estimated at 1 in 3000 patient exposures and the incidence of hepatitis was estimated at 1 in 10,000 patient exposures. A history of cytopenia, AED allergy or significant toxicity, viral infection, and/or immunologic problems may predispose patients to aplastic anemia. While felbamate is still available and is still used in the treatment of refractory epilepsy, it is a drug that should be initiated by an epileptologist. Felbamate is available as a tablet and an oral suspension.

Gabapentin. Gabapentin (Neurontin) was designed to be a GABA agonist but it does not react at either GABA receptor. It does increase GABA be increasing its production or decreasing its rate of synthesis. Gabapentin may modulate specific ion channels and decrease the levels of glutamate, a neurotransmitter involved in seizure and pain propagation. Gabapentin is available as capsules and tablets of varying strengths and as an oral solution.

Gabapentin is unique in that it binds to a L-amino acid carrier protein in the gut. This binding is saturable resulting in decreased bioavailability of gabapentin at higher doses. Gabapentin is not metabolized by liver enzymes and is not protein bound. This means that gabapentin has a very low potential for pharmacokinetic drug interactions. Since the drug is excreted unchanged in the urine, the dose and/or dosing interval should be decreased in patients with significant renal impairment. A replacement dose should be given after hemodialysis.

Gabapentin is generally well tolerated with CNS depression, e.g. fatigue, somnolence, dizziness, and ataxia being the most frequently reported side effects. The incidence of these side effects appears to be lower than with traditional AEDs. Other reported side effects include weight gain, edema, and behavioral abnormalities. The dose of gabapentin can usually be titrated rapidly.

Gabapentin is primarily useful in patients with partial seizures who have failed initial treatment. It should be noted that many clinicians will increase the dose of gabapentin beyond the upper limit of 3600 mg/day which is listed in the package insert. Doses as high as 10 Gm/day have been reported. Gabapentin does not appear to be useful in patients with generalized seizures but is effective in patients with neuropathic pain and some psychiatric disorders including bipolar affective disorder.

Lamotrigine. Lamotrigine (Lamictal) blocks neuronal sodium and calcium channel and also blocks the release of excitatory neurotransmitters such as glutamate and aspartate. Lamotrigine was originally approved for use in patients with refractory partial seizures. However, it has been used as monotherapy for patients with partial and generalized seizures. Lamotrigine is an alternative AED for patients who have absence or juvenile myoclonic seizures. It is also useful in the Lennox-Gastaut syndrome. Lamotrigine is available as a chewable/dispersible tablet and immediate release tablets of varying strengths.

The absorption of lamotrigine is rapid and unaffected by food. Lamotrigine is extensively metabolized in the liver and its metabolism can be induced, e.g. phenytoin, carbamazepine, phenobarbital, and inhibited, e.g. valproic acid. Lamotrigine does not stimulate or inhibit the metabolism of other drugs that are metabolized by the cytochrome P-450 system and is not highly protein bound resulting in a low potential for pharmacokinetic drug interactions. Lamotrigine is reported to have a pharmacodynamic interaction with carbamazepine. While lamotrigine does not affect the concentration of the parent carbamazepine or the pharmacologically active metabolite, there is an increase in CNS side effects when lamotrigine is added to the drug regimen of a patient taking carbamazepine. It has recently been reported that when oral contraceptives were given to a patient who had previously been well controlled on lamotrigine that break through seizures occurred.

Lamotrigine is generally well tolerated with CNS depression, e.g. diplopia, drowsiness, ataxia, and headache being the most frequently reported side effects. However, the most serious side effect associated with lamotrigine is skin rash. This rash is typically described as being an erythematous and morbiliform rash. It typically develops three or four weeks after the initiation of therapy and is usually mild to moderate in severity. However, some patients will develop a more serious rash such as a Stevens-Johnson reaction. The incidence of rash is associated with a high initial dose, a rapid dosage titration, and concurrent use of valproic acid. Therefore, the dose of lamotrigine should be initiated at a very low dose and gradually titrated upward.

Topiramate. Topiramate (Topamax) was initially approved for adjunctive therapy in patients with refractory partial seizures. However, topiramate has multiple mechanisms of action and is useful in primary generalized seizures. It is effective in the treatment of Lennox-Gastaut syndrome. Topiramate has also been used for conditions other than epilepsy, e.g. migraine headache. Topiramate is available as a "sprinkle" capsule and as an immediate release tablet.

Approximately 50% of an administered dose of topiramate is metabolized by the liver and the rest is excreted unchanged in the liver. The metabolism of topiramate may be induced or inhibited. Topiramate is not highly bound to plasma proteins but it is highly bound to erythrocytes leading to some non-linearity in the correlation of administered dose versus achieved concentration. In vitro studies have demonstrated that topiramate inhibits CYP2C19. Clinically this translates into an interaction with phenytoin. Some patients on phenytoin will experience an increase in phenytoin concentrations when topiramate is added to their drug regimen. It has been suggested that patients who are most likely to experience this interaction are at the point where they saturate their ability to metabolize phenytoin. Slight increases in the concentrations of digoxin and valproic acid have been reported with topiramate. Women taking oral contraceptives are warned to report any spotting or break through bleeding while taking topiramate.

The most common side effects associated with topiramate involved CNS depression, e.g. ataxia, fatigue, somnolence, dizziness, attentional deficits confusion, and "thinking abnormally." However, in some patients topiramate has been associated with significant depressed cognitive functioning including word finding skills. These more severe expressions of CNS depression are associated with large initial doses, rapid dosage titration, and large maintenance doses. Therefore, the dose of topiramate should be initiated at doses of 25 to 50 mg per day and dosage increases should not be greater than 25 to 50 mg every week. Doses greater than 600 mg/day have not been associated with increased efficacy. Other side effects associated with topiramate are nephrolithiasis, paresthesia, mood alterations, anorexia, and weight loss.

Tiagabine. Tiagabine (Gabatril) is a potent and specific inhibitor of GABA uptake into glial and other neuronal elements. Thus, tiagabine enhances the action of GABA by decreasing its removal from the synaptic space. Tiagabine is second-line therapy of patients with refractory partial seizures who have failed traditional therapy. It does not appear to have any activity against generalized seizures. Tiagabine is available as an immediate release tablet in varying strengths.

Tiagabine is well absorbed and is highly protein bound. It is metabolized in the liver by CYP3A4. Enzyme inducers, e.g. phenytoin and carbamazepine have been reported to increase the clearance of tiagabine. Also, valproic acid may increase the free fraction or percent unbound of tiagabine. The half-life and the free fraction may be increased in patients with significant liver disease. Tiagabine does not alter the binding of other highly protein bound drugs such as warfarin, phenytoin, and valproic acid.

The most commonly reported side effects with tiagabine are dizziness, asthenia, nervousness, tremor, diarrhea, and depression. The CNS side effects may be reduced by taking the drug with food which decreases the rate but not extent of absorption. Also, a slow dosage titration is required. It appears that a daily dose of at least 30 mg of tiagabine is needed for efficacy. Doses up to 56 mg/day have been used.

Levetiracetam. The mechanism of action of levetiracetam (Keppra) is unknown. It does not appear to work by any of the known mechanisms of other AEDs. Also, it is not effective in the traditional animal models used to screen for drugs with antiepileptic potential. However, it does inhibit burst activity and has been shown to be effective in patients with refractory partial seizures. Thus, the mechanism of action of levetiracetam appears to be novel. Levetiracetam is available as an immediate release formulation and a solution.

Levetiracetam is rapidly absorbed and has minimal protein binding. Approximately two-thirds of levetiracetam is excreted unchanged in the urine with the rest being metabolized by liver pathways that do not involve the cytochrome P-450 system. Therefore, levetiracetam has a very low potential for drug-drug interactions but the dose and/or dosing interval should be decreased in patients with impaired renal function.

Levetiracetam is generally well tolerated. The most frequently reported side effects are sedation, fatigue and coordination difficulties. Interestingly, there was an increase in upper respiratory tract infections associated with the use of levetiracetam in Phase III clinical trails. There was also a slight decrease in white blood cell counts. However, the patients were not immuno compromised. Some behavioral side effects have also been reported.

The initial dose that is recommended for levetiracetam is 500 mg orally twice a day. Some patients respond at the initial dose. The initial dose should be titrated slowly to decrease the incidence of CNS side effects.

Oxcarbazepine. Oxcarbazepine (Trileptal) is structurally related to carbamazepine and is a prodrug. Oxcarbazepine does not have direct pharmacologic activity but is metabolized to a monohydrate derivative (MHD) that is pharmacologically active. The mechanism of action of oxcarbazepine is the same as carbamazepine. Like carbamazepine, oxcarbazepine is indicated for partial and primary generalized convulsive seizures. Also, like carbamazepine, it has been used for trigeminal neuralgia and neuropathic pain. Oxcarbazepine is available as an immediate release tablet and as an oral suspension.

Oxcarbazepine is well absorbed and is metabolized to a MHD which is further metabolized by a glucuronide conjugation pathway with some intact drug being excreted unchanged in the urine. Autoinduction has not been reported with oxcarbazepine. Oxcarbazepine has been reported to decrease the bioavailability of oral contraceptives, to inhibit CYP2C19 causing a 40% increase in the concentration of phenytoin, to induce the UGT isozymes causing a decrease in the concentration of lamotrigine. The MHD does not appear to induce or inhibit other drugs but its metabolism can be affected by other drugs.

The side effects associated with oxcarbazepine are similar to those associated with carbamazepine. While it has been reported that oxcarbazepine is better tolerated than carbamazepine, it should be noted that oxcarbazepine has only been compared to immediate release carbamazepine and has not been compared to a controlled release carbamazepine formulation which has less peak to trough fluctuations. Hyponatremia, defined as a serum sodium < 125 mol/L occurs in up to 25% of patients taking oxcarbazepine. This rate is higher than the rate of hyponatremia associated with carbamazepine. While many of these patients have been asymptomatic, the serum sodium should be monitored in patients taking oxcarbazepine. Approximately 25% to 30% of patients experiencing a rash with carbamazepine will also experience a rash on oxcarbazepine. Oxcarbazepine is more expensive than carbamazepine or any of the other second generation AEDs.

Zonisamide. Zonisamide (Zonegran) has multiple mechanisms of action and clinical experience indicates that this is a broad spectrum AED. In addition to being effective for patients with partial seizures, zonisamide is also effective a variety of generalized seizure types including tonic-clonic convulsive seizures, absence seizures, and juvenile myoclonic seizures. Zonisamide is available as a capsule. However, the capsule can be opened and mixed with food and a solution can be made extemporaneously.

Zonisamide is well absorbed and is not highly protein bound. It is metabolized by CYP3A4 and n-acetylation with about 30% of the drug being excreted unchanged in the urine. Zonisamide does not induce or inhibit the metabolism of other AEDs. However, its metabolism may be induced and inhibited. Zonisamide has a very long half, e.g. 63 to 69 hours. This would allow once a day dosing. With once a day dosing the fluctuation in serum concentrations is about 28% and with twice a day dosing the fluctuation is about 14%. However, once a day dosing may improve adherence in some patients. Because of the long half life, the recommendation for dosing adjustments is every two weeks.

The most common side effects associated with zonisamide are somnolence, dizziness, anorexia, headache, nausea, agitation and irritability. These side effects were more common with a rapid dosage increase. Zonisamide is a sulfonamide and patients with a true allergy to sulfonamides may a hypersensitivity reaction to zonisamide. Other side effects reported with zonisamide include nephrolithiasis, weight loss, a reversible decline in renal function, and oligohydrosis.

Time Frame for Initiating Pharmacotherapy

A first seizure is usually not treated with antiseizure drugs unless there is clear evidence of pathology. No drugs currently in use can prevent the development of epilepsy, and a diagnosis of epilepsy is not proven until the presentation of another seizure. The course of action following the first seizure is a diagnostic workup. If a focus for the seizure is found on MRI or EEG, then treatment may be initiated since the likelihood of a seizure recurrence is high.

In febrile children, a generalized seizure of less than 15 min with normal neurologic status and a normal lumbar puncture is usually not treated with medication. A focal onset and seizure lasting over 15 min is treated acutely and further evaluated with EEG, brain imaging, and cerebral spinal fluid examination and, if warranted, treatment is begun. An afebrile child with normal neurologic status and a normal EEG is usually followed with no medical treatment. If the afebrile child has abnormal neurologic signs, with abnormalities on EEG and brain imaging, the child is usually treated. Persons with abnormal EEGs showing generalized discharges or focal spikes are usually treated with medications. An exception is rolandic epilepsy in childhood.

REFERENCES

Traumatic Brain Injury

Anderson, M., Parmenter, T., & Mok, M. (2002). The relationship between neurobehavioral problems of severe traumatic brain injury (TBI), family functioning and the psychological well-being of the spouse/caregiver: path model analysis. *Brain Injury, 16,* 743–757.

Anderson, S. & Bergedalen, A. (2002). Cognitive coorelates of apathy in traumatic brain injury. *Neuropsychiatry Neuropsychological Behavioral Neurology, 15,* 184–191.

Arciniegas, D. B. & Silver, J. M. (2001). Regarding the search for a unified definition of mild traumatic brain injury. *Brain Injury, 15,* 649–652.

Asikainen, I., Kaste, M., & Sarna, S. (1999). Early and Late Posttraumatic Seizures in Traumatic Brain Injury Rehabilitation Patients: Brain Injury Factors Causing Late Seizures and Influence of Seizures on Long-Term Outcome. *Epilepsia, 10,* 581–589.

Cock, J., Fordham, C., Cockburn, J. & Haggard, P. (2003). Who knows best? Awareness of divided attention difficulty in a neurological rehabilitation setting. *Brain Injury, 17*(7), 561–574.

Depalma, J. A. (2001). Measuring quality of life of patients of traumatic brain injury. *Critical Care Nursing Quarterly, 23,* 42–51.

Dikmen, S., Machamer, J., & Temkin, N. (2001). Mild head injury: facts and artifacts. *Journal of Clinical & Experimental Neuropsychology, 23,* 729–738.

Dombovy, M. L. (1997). Mechanisms of recovery following neurological injury and the role of rehabilitation. *Continuum: Lifelong Learning in Neurology, 3.*

Glenn, M. B. (2002). A differential diagnostic approach to the pharmacological treatment of cognitive, behavioral, and affective disorders after traumatic brain injury. *Journal of Head Trauma Rehabilitation, 17,* 273–283.

Goranson, T. E., Graves, R. E., Allison, D., & LaFreniere, R. (2003). Community reintegration following multidisciplinary rehabilitation for traumatic brain injury. *Brain Injury 17*(9), 759–774.

Guerrero, J., Thurman D. J., & Sniezek, J. E. (2000). Emergency department visits association with traumatic brain injury: United States, 1995–1996. *Brain Injury, 14,* 181–186.

Heinemann, A. W., Sokol, K., Garvin, L., & Bode, R. K. (2002). Measuring unmet needs and services among persons with traumatic brain injury. *Archives of Physical Medicine & Rehabilitation, 83,* 1052–1059.

Horn, L. J., & Zasler, N. D. (1996). Medical rehabilitation of traumatic brain injury. Philadelphia: Hanley and Belfus.

Headache Classification Committee of the International Headache Society. (1988). Classification and diagnostic criteria for headache disorders, cranial neurakgias and face pain. *Cephalagia, 8,* 1–96.

Meythaler, J. M., Brunner, R. C., Johnson, A., & Novack, T. A. (2002). Amantadine to improve neurorecovery in traumatic brain injury-associated diffuse axonal injury: a pilot double-blind randomized trial. *Journal of Head Trauma Rehabilitation, 17,* 300–313.

Montgomery, V., Oliver, R., Reisner, A., & Fallat, M. E. (2002). The effect of severe traumatic brain injury on the family. *Journal of Trauma-Injury Infection & Critical Care, 52,* 1121–1124.

Mosenthal, A. C., Lavery, R. F., Addis, M., Kaul, S., Ross, S., Marburger, R., Deitch, E. A., & Livingston, D. H. (2002). Isolated traumatic brain injury: age is an independent predictor of mortality and early outcome. *Journal of Trauma-Injury Infection & Critical Care, 52,* 907–911.

Perino, C., Rago, R., Cicolini, A., Torta, R., & Monaco, F. (2001). Mood and behavioural disorders following traumatic brain injury: clinical evaluation and pharmacological management. *Brain Injury, 15,* 139–148.

Saper, J. R., Lake, A. E., & Tepper, S. J. (2001). Nefazodone for chronic daily headache prophylaxis: an open-label study. *Headache, 41,* 465–474.

Thornhill, S., Teasdale, G. M., Murray, G. D., McEwen, J., Roy, C. W., & Penny, K. I. (2000). Disability in young people and adults one year after head injury: prospective cohort study. *BMJ, 320,* 1631–1635.

Thurman, D. J., Alverson, C. A., Dunn, K. A., Guerrero, J., & Sniezek, J. E. (1999). Traumatic brain injury in the United States: a public health perspective. *Journal of Head Trauma Rehabilitation, 14,* 602–615.

Vanore, M. L. (2000). Care of the pediatric patient with brain injury in an adult intensive care unit. *Critical Care Nursing Quarterly, 23,* 38–48.

Whyte, J., Vaccaro, M., Grieb-Neff, P., & Hart, T. (2002). Psychostimulant use in the rehabilitation of individuals with traumatic brain injury. *Journal of Head Trauma Rehabilitation, 17,* 284–299.

Attention Deficit Hyperactivity Disorder

American Psychiatric Association. (1994). Diagnostic and Statistical Manual of Mental Disorders (DSM-IV). Washington, DC: American Psychiatric Association.

American Academy of Pediatrics Subcommittee on Attention-Deficit/Hyperactivity Disorder and Committee on Quality Improvement. (2001). Clinical practice guideline: treatment of the school-aged child with attention-deficit/hyperactivity disorder. *Pediatrics, 108,* 1033–1044.

Arnold, L. E. (2001). Alternative treatments for adults with attention-deficit hyperactivity disorder (ADHD). *Annals of the New York Academy of Sciences, 931,* 310–341.

Barr, C. L., Wigg, K. G., Bloom, S., Schachar, R., Tannock, R., Roberts, W., Malone, M., & Kennedy, J. L. (2000). Further evidence from haplotype analysis for linkage of the dopamine D4 receptor gene and attention-deficit hyperactivity disorder. *American Journal of Medical Genetics, 96,* 262–267.

Blondis, T. A., & Roizen, N. J. (1996). Management of attention-deficit disorders and hyperactivity. In A. J. Capute & J. A. Pasquale, Developmental Disabilities in Infancy and Childhood (2nd ed.). Baltimore: Paul H. Brookes, pp. 437–449.

Brown, T. (Ed.). (2000). *Attention Deficit Disorders and Co morbidities in Children, Adolescents and Adults.* Washington, DC: APA Press.

Brue, A. W. & Oakland, T. D. (2002). Alternative treatments for attention-deficit/hyperactivity disorder: does evidence support their use? *Alternative Therapies in Health & Medicine, 8,* 68–70.

Bussing, R. & Gary, F. A. (2001). Practice guidelines and parental ADHD treatment evaluations: friends or foes? *Harvard Review of Psychiatry, 9,* 223–233.

Conners, C. K. (1998). Rating scales in attention-deficit/hyperactivity disorder: use in assessment and treatment monitoring. *Journal of Clinical Psychiatry, 59 Suppl 7,* 24–30.

Crosbie, J. & Schachar, R. (2001). Deficient inhibition as a marker for familial ADHD. *American Journal of Psychiatry, 158,* 1884–1890.

Elliott, H. (2002). Attention deficit hyperactivity disorder in adults: a guide for the primary care physician. *Southern Medical Journal, 95,* 736–742.

Faraone S. V., Biederman, J. (1998) Neurobiology of attention-deficit hyperactivity disorder. *Biological Psychiatry, 44* (10):951–8.

Faraone, S. V., Biederman, J., Spencer, T., Wilens, T., Seidman, L. J., Mick, E., & Doyle, A. E. (2000). Attention-deficit/hyperactivity disorder in adults: an overview. *Biological Psychiatry, 48,* 9–20.

Hunt, R.D., Arnsten, A. F., & Asbell, M. D. (1995). An open trial of guanfacine in the treatment of attention-deficit hyperactivity disorder. *Journal of the American Academy of Child & Adolescent Psychiatry, 34,* 50–54.

Gaub, M. & Carlson, C. L. (1997). Gender differences in ADHD: a meta-analysis and critical review. [erratum appears in J Am Acad Child Adolesc Psychiatry 1997 Dec; 36(12):1783.]. *Journal of the American Academy of Child & Adolescent Psychiatry, 36,* 1036–1045.

Gutgesell, H., Atkins, D., Barst, R., Buck, M., Franklin, W., Humes, R., Ringel, R., Shaddy, R., & Taubert, K. A. (1999). AHA Scientific Statement: cardiovascular monitoring of children and adolescents receiving psychotropic drugs. *Journal of the American Academy of Child & Adolescent Psychiatry, 38,* 1047–1050.

Kaye, D. L., Montgomery, M. E., Munson, S. W. (2002). *Child and Adolescent Mental Health:* Lippincott Williams & Wilkins Publishers.

Leckman, J., & Cohen, D. (1999). *Tourette's Syndrome: Ties, Obsessions, Compulsions.* Wiley and Song.

Mannuzza, S., & Klein, R. G. (1999). Adolescent and adult outcomes in attention deficit/hyperactivity disorder. In: H. C. Quay & A. E. Hogan (Eds), *Handbook of Disruptive Behavior Disorders* (pp. 279–294). New York, NY: Klumer Academic/Plenum Publishers.

Michelson, D., Faries, D., Wernicke, J., Kelsey, D., Kendrick, K., Sallee, F. R., Spencer, T., & Atomoxetine, A. D. H. D. (2001). Atomoxetine in the treatment of children and adolescents with attention-deficit/hyperactivity disorder: a randomized, placebo-controlled, dose-response study. *Pediatrics, 108,* E83.

Pelham, W. E., Aronoff, H. R., Midlam, J. K., Shapiro, C. J., Gnagy, E. M., Chronis, A. M., Onyango, A. N., Forehand, G., Nguyen, A., & Waxmonsky, J. (1999). A comparison of ritalin and adderall: efficacy and time-course in children with attention-deficit/hyperactivity disorder. *Pediatrics, 103,* E43.

Pliszka, S. R., Browne, R. G., Olvera, R. L., & Wynne, S. K. (2000). A double-blind, placebo-controlled study of Adderall and methylphenidate in the treatment of attention-deficit/hyperactivity disorder. *Journal of the American Academy of Child & Adolescent Psychiatry, 39,* 619–626.

Ramirez, P. M., Desantis, D., & Opler, L. A. (2001). EEG biofeedback treatment of ADD. A viable alternative to traditional medical intervention?. *Annals of the New York Academy of Sciences, 931,* 342–358.

Rasmussen, P. & Gillberg, C. (2000). Natural outcome of ADHD with developmental coordination disorder at age 22 years: a controlled, longitudinal, community-based study. *Journal of the American Academy of Child & Adolescent Psychiatry, 39,* 1424–1431.

Wilens, T. E., Spencer, T. J., Biederman, J., Girard, K., Doyle, R., Prince, J., Polisner, D., Solhkhah, R., Comeau, S., Monuteaux, M. C., & Parekh, A. (2001). A controlled clinical trial of bupropion for attention deficit hyperactivity disorder in adults. *American Journal of Psychiatry, 158,* 282–288.

Wilens, T. E., Spencer, T. J., Swanson, J. M., Connor, D. F., & Cantwell, D. (1999). Combining methylphenidate and clonidine: a clinically sound medication option. *Journal of the American Academy of Child & Adolescent Psychiatry, 38,* 614–9discussion.

Wimett, L. & Laustsen, G. (2003). Drug News: First new ADHD treatment in 30 years. *Nurse Practitioner, 28*(12), 50–53.

Zametkin, A. J. & Ernst, M. (1999). Problems in the management of attention-deficit-hyperactivity disorder. *N Engl J Med.* 7;340(1):40–6.

Volkow N. D., Wang G. J., Fowler J. S., Logan J., Gatley S. J., Gifford A., Hitzemann R., Ding Y. S., Pappas N. (1999). Prediction of reinforcing responses to psychostimulants in humans by brain dopamine D2 receptor levels. *Am J Psychiatry 157*(10), 1708–10.

U.S. Department of Health and Human Services (1999). *Mental Health, a Report of the Surgeon General.* Rockville Maryland: Department of Health and Human Services. Retrieved March 2004 at: http://www.mentalhealth.samhsa.gov/features/surgeongeneralreport/home.asp.

Stroke

Adams, H. P., Brott, T. G., & Adams, R. J. (2003). Guidelines for the Early Management of Patients With Acute Ischemic Stroke: A Statement for Healthcare Professionals From a Special Writing Group of the Stroke Council, American Heart Association. Available [On-line] http://www.americanheart.org/presenter.jhtml?identifier=1227. Accessed June 2004.

American Heart Association (2002). *Heart and Stroke Statistical Update.* Dallas, Tex: American Heart Association.

American Hospital Formulary Service. (1996). Drug Information. Gerald K. McEvoy, Ed. American Society of Health System Pharmacists.

American Stroke Association (1999). *Heart and stroke: A–Z guide.* Available [On-line] http://www.strokeassociation.org. Accessed June 2004.

Ansell, J., Hirsh, J., Dalen, J. Bussey, H., Anderson, D., Poller, L., Jacobson, A., Deykin, D., & Matchar, D. (2001). Managing oral anticoagulant therapy. In: Sixth ACCP Consensus Conference on Antithrombotic Therapy. American College of Chest Physicians. *Chest, 119*(1 suppl), 300S–320S.

Bladin, C. F., Alexandrov, A. V., Bellavance, A., et al. (2000). Seizures after stroke: a prospective multicenter study. *Archives of Neurology, 57,* 617–622.

Bousser, M. G. (1999). Stroke in women: the 1997 Paul Dudley White International Lecture. *Circulation, 99,* 463–467.

CAPRIE Steering Committee (1996). A randomised, blinded trial of clopidogrel versus aspirin in patients at risk of ischaemic events (CAPRIE). *Lancet, 348,* 1329–1339.

Chen Z. M., Sandercock P., Pan H. C., et al. (2000). Indications for early aspirin use in acute ischemic stroke: a combined analysis of 40,000 randomized patients from the Chinese acute stroke trial and the international stroke trial. On behalf of the CAST and IST collaborative groups. *Stroke, 31,* 1240–1249.

Chimowitz, M. I., Kokkinos, J., Strong, J., Brown, M. B., Levine, S. R., Silliman, S., et al. (1995). The warfarin-aspirin symptomatic intracranial disease study. *Neurology, 45,* 1488–1493.

Donnan, G. A., Davis, S. M., Chambers, B. R., Gates, P. C., Hankey, G. J., McNeil, J. J., Rosen, D., Stewart-Wayne, E. G., & Tuck, R. R. (1996). The Australian streptokinase (AKS) trial study group. *JAMA, 276,* 961–966.

Erkinjuntti, T. (2001). Vascualr dementia. Program and abstracts from the 17th World Congress of Neurology; June 17–22, 2001. London, UK. *Journal of Neurology Science, 187(suppl 1),* S117. Abstract 16.06.

European Stroke Prevention Study (ESPS) II: Efficacy and safety data. (1997). *Journal of Neurological Science, 151,* Supplement SL-S77.

Evans, A., Perez, I., Harraf, F., Melbourne, A., Steadman, J., Donalson, N. & Karlra, L. (2001). Can differences in management processes explain different outcomes between stroke unit and stroke team care? *The Lancet, 358(9293),* 1586.

Fisher, M. for Stroke Therapy Academic Industry Round table (2003). Recommendations for advancing development of Acute Stroke therapies. Stroke Therapy Academic Industry Round table 3. *Stroke 34,* 1539–1546.

Fisher, M. & Ratan R. (2003). New perspectives on developing acute stroke therapy. *Annals of Neurology* 53, 10–20.

Fowler, S. (2001). Hormone Replacement and Stroke. *Journal of Neuroscience Nursing, 33(3),* 173.

Franklin, G. (1999). *Complex regional pain syndrome (CRPS).* Washington. State Department of Labor and Industries, Olympia, WA.

Frey J. L., Jahnke H. K., & Bulfinch E. W. (1998). Differences in stroke between white, Hispanic, and Native American patients: the Barrow Neurological Institute stroke database. *Stroke, 29,* 29–33.

Gage, B. F., Cardinalli, A. B., Albers, G. W., & Owens, D. K. (1995). Cost-effectiveness of warfarin and aspirin for prophylaxis of stroke in patients with nonvalvular atrial fibrillation. *Journal of the American Medical Association, 274,* 1839–1845.

Gainotti, G., Antonucci, G., Marra C., & Paolucci, S. (2001). Relation between depression after stroke, antidepressant therapy, and functional recovery. *Journal of Neurology, Neurosurgery and Psychiatry, 71(2),* 258.

Gasecki, A. P., & Hachinski, V. C. (1993). Stroke recurrence and prevention. In R. W. Teasell (Ed.), Long-term consequences of stroke. Physical medicine and rehabilitation. *State of the Art Reviews, 7,* 43–54.

Gillum, L. A., Mamidipudi, S. K., & Johnston, S. C. (2000) Ischemic Stroke Risk With Oral Contraceptives A Meta-analysis. *The Journal of the American Medical Association, 284(1),* 72.

Goldstein, L. B., Adams, R., Becker, K., et al (2001). Primary Prevention of Ischemic Stroke. *Circulation, (103),* 163–182.

Goldstein, L. B., & Sygen in Acute Stroke Study Investigators. (1995). Common drugs may influence motor recovery after stroke. *Neurology, 45,* 865–871.

Grady, D., Herrington, D., Bittner, V., Blumental, R. et al. (2002). Cardiovascular disease outcomes during 6.8 years of hormone therapy; Heart and estrogen/progestin replacement study follow-up (HERS II). *The Journal of the American Medical Association, 288(1),* 49–58.

Graeme J. Hankey, G. J., Cathie L. M. Sudlow, C. L. M., & Dunbabin, D. (2000). Thienopyridines or Aspirin to Prevent Stroke and Other Serious Vascular Events in Patients at High Risk of Vascular Disease? A Systematic Review of the Evidence From Randomized Trials. NINDS [National Institute of Neurological Disorders and Stroke]-sponsored research study. *JAMA, The Journal of the American Medical Association, 283,* 1145–1150.

Gresham, G. E. (Ed.) and the Post-Stroke Rehabilitation Guideline Panel. (1995). *Post-stroke rehabilitation.* Clinical Practice Guideline No. 16, AHCPR Publication No. 95-0662. Rockville, MD: U.S. Department of Health and Human Services.

Grotta, J. C., Norris, J. W., Kamm, B., & the TASS Baseline and Angiographic Data Subgroup (1992). Prevention of stroke with ticlopidine: Who benefits most? *Neurology, 42,* 111–115.

Hacke W, Kaste M, Fieschi C, et al. (1998). Randomised double-blind placebo-controlled trial of thrombolytic therapy with intravenous alteplase in acute ischaemic stroke (ECASS II). Second European-Australasian acute stroke study Investigators. *Lancet, 352,* 1245–51.

Hankey, G. J., Sudlow, C. L. M., & Dunbabin, D. W. (2002). Thienopyridine derivatives (ticlopidine, clopidogrel) versus aspirin for preventing stroke and other serious vascular events in high vascular risk patients (Cochrane Review). *Stroke, 31,* 1779–1784.

Hayden, M., Pigonone, M., Phillips, C., & Mulrow, C. (2002). Aspirin for the primary prevention of cardiovascular events: A summary of the evidence for the U. S. Preventive Services Task Force. *Annals of Internal Medicine, 136,* 161–172.

Heart Outcomes Prevention Evaluation (HOPE) Study Investigators (2000). Vitamin E supplementation and cardiovascular events in high-risk patients: The HOPE Study results. *New England Journal of Medicine, 342,* 154–60.

Hess, D. C., Dumchuk, A. M., Brass, L. M., & Yatsu, F. M. (2000). HMG-CoA reductase inhibitors (statins): A promising approach to stroke prevention. *Neurology, 55(7),* 790–796.

Kannel, W. B. (2000). Vital Epidemiologic clues in heart failure. *Journal of Clinical Epidemiology, 53,* 229–235 (Abstract).

Kannel W. B. (1988). Contributions of the Framingham Study to the conquest of coronary artery disease. *American Journal of Cardiology,* 62, 1109–1112.

Karlsson, A. K. (1999). Autonomic dysreflexia. Spinal Cord, 37, 383–391.

Kay, R., Wong, K. S., Ling, Y., Chan, Y. W., Tsoi, T. H., Ahuja, A. T., & Kenton, E. J. (1996). Diagnosis and treatment of concomitant hypertension and stroke. *Journal of the American Medical Association, 88,* 364–368.

Kirkpatrick, A. F. (2000) *Reflex Sympathetic Dystrophy/Complex Regional Pain Syndrome (RSD/CRPS).* Reflex Sympathetic Dystrophy Syndrome Association of America (RSDSA) Available [online] at www.rsd.org. Accessed August 2002.

Kobayashi, S., Okada, K., Koide, H., et al. (1997) Subcortical silent brain infarction as a risk factor for clinical stroke. *Stroke, 32,* 280–299.

Koren-Morag, N., Tanne, D., Graff, E. & Goldbourt, U. (2002). Low- and high-density lipoprotein cholesterol and ischemic cerebrovascular disease: the Bezafibrate Infarction Prevention registry. *Archives of Internal Medicine, 162(9),* 993–100.

Margolis, S., & Preziosi, T. J. (1996). *Stroke.* Baltimore: The Johns Hopkins Medical Institutions.

Margolis, S., & Wityk, R. J. (1997). *Stroke.* Baltimore: The Johns Hopkins Medical Institutions.

Mitka, M. (2002). News about neuroprotectants for the treatment of stroke. *JAMA, The Journal of the American Medical Association, 287(10),* 1253–1260.

Mohr, J. P., et al. (2001). A comparison of warfarin and aspirin for the prevention of recurrent ischemic stroke. *New England Journal of Medicine, 345,* 1444–1451.

National Institute of Neurological Disorders and Stroke rt-PA Stroke Study Group. (1995). Tissue plasminogen activator for acute ischemic stroke. *New England Journal of Medicine, 333*(24), 1581–1587.

Newman, J. (2002). Diagnosis and treatment of stroke. *Radiologic Technology, 73(4),* 305(34).

O'Connell, J. E., & Gray, C. S. (1996). Atrial fibrillation and stroke prevention in the community. *Age and Aging, 25,* 307–308.

Paganini-Hill, A. (2001). Hormone replacement therapy and stroke: Risk, protection or no effect? *Maturitas, 38(3),* 243–261.

Pearce, K. A., Boosalis, M. G., & Yeager, B. (2000). Update on Vitamin Supplements for the Prevention of Coronary Disease and Stroke. *American Family Physician, 62,* 1359–1366.

Petitti, D. B., Sidney, S., Quesenberry, C., et al. (1998). Stroke and cocaine or amphetamine use. *Epidemiology, 9,* 596–600.

Rossouw, J. E., Anderson, G. L., Prentice, R. L., et al (2002). Risk and Benefits of Estrogen plus progestin in healthy post-menopausal women; Principle results from the Women's Health Initiative Randomized Controlled Trial. *JAMA, The Journal of the American Medical Association, 288(3),* 321–333.

Sloan M. A., Kittner, S. J., Feeser, B.R., et al. (1998) Illicit drug-associated ischemic stroke in the Baltimore-Washington Young Stroke Study. *Neurology, 50,* 688–1693.

Stein, D., Balis, D., Grundy, S., Adams-Huet, B., & Devaraj, S. (2001) Statins reduce levels of protein linked to inflammation, heart attack and stroke. *Circulation: Journal of the American Heart Association.* Available [On-line] http://www.americanheart.org/presenter.jhtml?identifier=12064. Accessed August 2002.

Stroke. (2002). In Dipro, J. T., Talbert, R. T., Yee, G. C., Matzke, G. R., Wells, B. G., & Posey, L. M. (Eds.), *Pharmocotherapy: A pathophysiological approach, fifth edition.* (pp. 384–388), New York, NY: McGraw-Hill.

Stroke Unit Trialists' Collaboration. (1997) Collaborative systematic review of the randomised trials of organised inpatient (stroke unit) care after stroke. British Medical Journal, 314, 1151–1159.

Thomassen, L., Waje-Andreassen, U. & Maintz, C. (2001). Acute stroke: the first 6 hours. *Journal of Neurology, Neurosurgery and Psychiatry, 71(3),* 424.

Torbey M. T., Bhardwai, A. (2001). Blood pressure management in critically ill neurologic patients. *Journal of Critical Illness 16(4),* 179–182.

Weinberger, J. (2002) Stroke and TIA: Prevention and management of cerebrovascular events in primary care. *Geriatrics, 57(1),* 38.

Wolf, P. A., Clagett, G. P., Easton, J. D, Goldstein et al., (1999). Statement on the Physicians Health Study Report, AHA Scientific Statement: Preventing Ischemic Stroke in Patients With Prior Stroke and Transient Ischemic Attack, #710178. *Stroke, 30,* 1991–1994.

Yoon, S. S. & Byles, J. (2002). Perceptions of stroke in the general public and patients with stroke: A qualitative study. *British Medical Journal, 324(7345),* 1065–1069.

Multiple Sclerosis

Anderson, P., & Goodkin, D. E. (1996). Current pharmacologic treatment of multiple sclerosis symptoms. *Western Journal of Medicine, 165,* 313–317.

Bainbridge, J. L., Corboy, J. R. & Gidal, B. E.M. (2002). Multiple Sclerosis in *Pharmacotherapy: A Pathophysiologic Approach.* Eds DiPiro Joseph T, Talbert Robert L, Yee Gary C, et al., McGraw-Hill, New York, page 1019–1030.

Boneschi, F. M., Rovaris, M., Johnson, K. P., Miller, A., Wolinsky, J. S., Ladkani, D., Shifroni, G., Comi, G., & Fillippi, M. (2003). Effects of glatiramer acetate on relapse rate and accumulated disability in multiple sclerosis: meta-analysis of three double-blind, randomized, placebo-controlled clinical trials. Multiple Sclerosis 9(4), 349–355.

Bryant J., Clegg A., Milne, R. (2001). Systematic review of immunomodulatory drugs for the treatment of people with multiple sclerosis: Is there good quality evidence on effectiveness and cost? *Journal of Neurology, Neurosurgery & Psychiatry. 70*(5):574–9.

Coyle, P. K & Hartung, H. P (2002). Use of interferon beta in multiple sclerosis: rationale for early treatment and evidence for dose- and frequency-dependent effects on clinical response. *Multiple Sclerosis, 8*(1):2–9

DasGupta, R. & Fowler, C. J. (2002). Sexual and urological dysfunction in multiple sclerosis: better understanding and improved therapies. *Current Opinion in Neurology; 15*(3): 271–8.

Dombovy, M. L. (1997). Neuro-rehabilitation. *Continuum: Lifelong Learning in Neurology, 3*(2), 130–132.

Donker, G. A., Foets, M., & Spreeuwenberg, P. (1996). Multiple sclerosis: Management in Dutch general practice. *Family Practice, 13*(5), 439–444.

Donohoe, K. M. (1995). Autoimmune disorders. In E. Barker (Ed.), *Neuroscience nursing* (pp. 559–585). St. Louis: C. V. Mosby.

Dressnandt, J., & Conrad, B. (1996). Lasting reduction of severe spasticity after ending chronic treatment with intrathecal baclofen. *Journal of Neurology, Neurosurgery and Psychiatry, 60,* 168–173.

Gidal, B. E., Wagner, M. L., Privetera, M. D., Dalmady-Isreal, C., Crismon, M. L., Fagan, S. C., & Graves, N. M. (1996). Current developments in neurology, part I: Advances in the pharmacotherapy of headache, epilepsy, and multiple sclerosis. *Annals of Pharmacotherapy, 30,* 1272–1276.

Goodin, D. S., Arnason, B. G., Coyle, P. K. Frohman, E. M., Paty, D. W. (2003). The use of mitoxantrone (Novantrone) for the treatment of multiple sclerosis: report of the Therapeutics and Technology Assessment Subcommittee of the

American Academy of Neurology. *Neurology, 25:61*(10). 1332–8.

Grigoriadis, N. (2002). Interferon beta treatment in relapsing-remitting multiple sclerosis. A review. *Clinical Neurology & Neurosurgery, 104*(3):251–8.

Jacobs, L. D., Cookfair, D. L., Rudick, R. A., Herndon, R. M., Richert, J. R., Salazar, A. M., et al. (1996). Intramuscular interferon beta-1a for disease progression in relapsing multiple sclerosis. *Annals of Neurology, 39,* 285–294.

Johnson, K. P. (1996). A review of the clinical efficacy profile of copolymer 1: New U.S. phase III trial data. *Journal of Neurology, 243* (Suppl. 1), S3–S7.

Kelly, C. L. (1996). The role of interferons in the treatment of multiple sclerosis. *Journal of Neuroscience Nursing, 24,* 114–120.

Marshall, L. L., & Ragland, D. (1996). Therapeutic management of multiple sclerosis. *Pharmacist,* 41–55.

NeuroCommunications Research Laboratories and Department of Neuroscience at the Institute for Biomedical Engineering and Rehabilitations Services of Touro College. (1996). Estrogen's impact on cognitive functions in multiple sclerosis. *International Journal of Neuroscience, 86,* 23–31.

Rochester Multiple Sclerosis Clinic Patient Information Sheet. (1993). *Beta interferon (Betaseron)* Strong Memorial Hospital, Rochester, NY.

Rochester Multiple Sclerosis Clinic Patient Information Sheet. (1995). *Methotrexate as a treatment for multiple sclerosis.* Strong Memorial Hospital, Rochester, NY.

Rochester Multiple Sclerosis Clinic Patient Information Sheet. (1996). *Cytaxan.* Strong Memorial Hospital, Rochester, NY.

Rodgers, J., & Bland, R. (1996). Psychiatric manifestations of multiple sclerosis: A review. *Canadian Journal of Psychiatry, 41,* 441–445.

Rudick, R. A. (1993). Multiple sclerosis. In R. T. Johnson & J. W. Griffin (Eds.), *Current therapy in neurologic disease* (pp. 158–163). St. Louis: C. V. Mosby.

Sandyk, R. (1996). Estrogen's impact on cognitive functions in multiple sclerosis. *International Journal of Neuroscience, 86,* 23–31.

Scott, T. F., Allen, D., Price, T. R. P., McConnell, H., & Lang, D. (1996). Characterization of major depression in symptoms in multiple sclerosis patients. *Journal of Neuropsychiatry and Clinical Neurosciences, 8,* 318–323.

Sketris, I. S., Brown, M., Murray, T. J., Fisk, J. D., & McLean, K. (1996). Drug therapy in multiple sclerosis: A study of Nova Scotia senior citizens. *Clinical Therapeutics, 18*(2), 303–318.

Swain, S. E. (1996). Multiple sclerosis primary health care implications. *Nurse Practitioner, 21,* 40–54.

Vertigo

American Hospital Formulatory Service (1996). Drug Information. Bethesda, Maryland. American Society of Health Systems Pharmacists.

Baloh, R. W. (1994). Approach to the dizzy patient. *Baillieres Clinical Neurology, 3*(3), 453–465.

Brantberg, K., Bergenius, J., & Tribukait, A. (1996). Gentamicin treatment in peripheral vestibular disorders other than Meniere's disease. *ORL, 58,* 277–279.

Brookes, G. B. (1996). The pharmacological treatment of Ménière's disease. *Clinical Otolaryngology, 21,* 3–11.

Driscoll, C., Kasperbauer, J. L., Facer, G. W., Harner, S. G., & Beatty, C. W. (1997). Low-dose intratympanic gentamicin and the treatment of Meniere's disease: Preliminary results. *Laryngoscope, 107,* 83–89.

Froehling, D. A. (2000). The Canalith Repositioning Procedure for the Treatment of Benign Paroxysmal Positional Vertigo: A Randomized ControlledTrial. *JAMA, The Journal of the American Medical Association, 284(10),* 1222.

Fujino, A., Tokumasu, K., Okamoto, M., Naganuma, H., Hoshino, I., Arai, M., & Yoneda, S. (1996). Vestibular training for acute unilateral vestibular disturbances: Its efficacy in comparison with antivertigo drug. *Acta Oto-laryngologica* (Suppl. 524), 21–26.

Gans, R. E. (1996). *Vestibular rehabilitation: Protocols and programs.* San Diego: Singular Publishing Group.

Grizzi, M. (1995). The efficacy of vestibular rehabilitation for patients with head trauma. *Journal of Head Injury Trauma, 10*(6), 60–77.

Hain, T. C. (1997). Vertigo and dysequilibrium. In R. T. Johnson & J. W. Griffin (Eds.), *Current therapy in neurologic disease* (pp. 8–13). St. Louis: C. V. Mosby.

Hirsch, B. E., & Kamerer, D. B. (1997). Intratympanic gentamicin therapy for Meniere's disease. *American Journal of Otology, 18,* 44–51.

Kilpatrick, J. K., Sismanis, A., Spencer, R. F., & Wise, C. M. (2000). Low-dose oral methotrexate management of patients with bilateral Meniere's disease. *Ear, Nose and Throat Journal, 79(2),* 82.

Linstrom, C. J., & Gleich, L. L. (1993). Otosyphilis: Diagnostic and therapeutic update. *Journal of Otolaryngology, 22*(6), 401–408.

Luetje, C. M., & Wooten, J. (1996, April). Clinical manifestations of transdermal scopolamine addiction. *Ear, Nose and Throat Journal,* 210–214.

National Institute on Deafness and Other Communication Disorders of The National Institutes of Health. (1998) *NIDCD Publication: Because You Asked about Meniere's Disease.* Last updated Nov. 2001. Available (Online) http://www.nih.gov/nidcd/health/pubs hb/meniere.htm. Accessed July 2002.

Nuovo, J. (2001) Treatment for Benign Paroxysmal Positional Vertigo. *American Family Physician, 63(2),* 357.

Rascol, O., Hain, T. C., Brefel, C., Benazet, M., Clanet, M., & Mostastruc, J-L. (1995). Antivertigo medications and drug-induced vertigo: A pharmacological review. *Drugs, 50*(5), 777–791.

Ruckenstein M. J. (2001). Managing dizziness and vertigo in older women. *Womens Health Primary Care, 4,* 241–250.

Seidman, M. (2002). Continuous gentamicin therapy using an IntraEAR microcatheter for Menoiere's disease: A retrospective study. *Otolaryngology—Head and Neck Surgery, 126,* 244–256.

Shea, J. J., Jr., & Gee, X. (1996). Dexamethasone perfusion of the labyrinth plus intravenous dexamethasone for Meniere's disease. *Otolaryngolic Clinics of North America, 29*(2), 358–368, April.

Smith, M. W. (2002). *Vestibular disorders.* Vestibular Disorders Association (VEDA) Available [online] http://www. vestibular.org. Accessed June 2004.

Tinetti, M. E., Williams, C. S., & Gill, T. M. (2000) Dizziness among older adults: a possible geriatric syndrome. *Annals of Internal Medicine, 132,* 337–344.

Dementia

Alzheimer's Association (2002). *Guidelines for Alzheimer's disease management.* Available [online] http://www.alz.org/resources /topicindex/diagnosis.asp. Accessed June 2004.

American Psychiatric Association. (1997). Practice guideline for the treatment of patients with Alzheimer's disease and other dementias of late life. *American Journal of Psychiatry, 154*(5 Suppl.), 1–33.

American Psychiatric Association (1997). Practice Guideline for the Treatment of Patients With Alzheimer's Disease and Other Dementias of Late Life: II. Disease Definition, Natural History, And Epidemiology. APA Steering Committee on Practice Guidelines. Available (online) http://www.psych .org/psych_pract/treatg/pg/pg_dementia_2.cfm. Accessed January 2004.

Applegate, W. B., & Burns, R. (1996). Geriatric medicine. *Journal of the American Medical Association, 275*(23), 1892–1893.

Birge, S. J. (1996). Is there a role for estrogen replacement therapy in the prevention and treatment of dementia? *Journal of the American Geriatric Society, 44,* 865–870.

Bolla, L. R., Filley, C. M., Palmer, R. M. (2000). Dementia DDx: Office diagnosis of the four major types of dementia. *Geriatrics, 55,* 34–46.

Brookmeyer, R., Gray, S., & Kawas. C. (1998). Projections of Alzheimer's disease in the United States and the public health impact of delaying disease onset. *Am J Public Health. 8(88),* 1337–1342.

Chan, R. K. T., & Hachinski, V. C. (1997). The other dementias. In *Current therapy in neurologic disease* (pp. 311–314). St. Louis: C. V. Mosby.

Corey-Bloom, J., Anand, R., Veach, J. et al. (1998). A randomized trial evaluating the efficacy and safety of ENA 713 (rivastigmine tartrate), a new acetylcholinesterase inhibitor, in patients with mild to moderately severe Alzheimer's disease. *Int J Geriatr Psychopharmacology, 1,* 55–65.

Costa, P. T., Williams, T. F., Albert, M. S., Butters, N. M., Folstein, M. F., Gilman, S., et al. (1996). *Recognition and initial assessment of Alzheimer's disease and related dementias.* Clinical Practice Guideline No. 19. AHCPR No. 97-0702. Rockville, MD: U.S. Department of Health Care Policy Research.

Cummings, J. L. (2000). Cholinesterase inhibitors: a new class of psychotropic agents. *American Journal of Psychiatry, 157,* 4–15.

Cummings, J. L., Frank, J. C., Cherry, D. Kohatsu, N., L., Kemp., B., Hewitt, L., & Mittman, B. (2002). Guidelines for managing Alzheimer disease. Part I. Assessment. *American Family Physician, 65,* 2263–2272.

Cummings, J. L., Frank, J. C., Cherry, D. Kohatsu, N., L., Kemp., B., Hewitt, L., & Mittman, B. (2002). Guidelines for managing Alzheimer disease. Part II. Treatment. *American Family Physician, 65(11),* 2525–2234.

Doody, R. S., Stevens, J. C., Beck, C. et al. (2001). Practice parameter: management of dementia (an evidence-based review). *Neurology, 56,* 1154–1166.

Federal Drug Administration's (FDA) Peripheral and Central Nervous System Drugs Advisory Committee (2003). FDA Approves Memantine (Namenda) for Alzheimer's Disease. *FDA News P03-82.* Last updated 10-16-2003. Available (Online) http://www.fda.gov/bbs/topics/NEWS/2003/NEW00961 .html. Accessed January 2004.

Federal Drug Administration's (FDA) (2003). Approval labeling text N21-487 Namenda TM (memantine hydrochloride). Last updated 10-20-2003. Available (Online) http://www. fda.gov/ cder/foi/label/2003/021487lbl.pdf. Accessed January 2004.

Gidal, B. E., Crismon, M. L., Wagner, M. L., Fagan, S. C., Privitera, M. D., Dalmady-Isreal, C., & Graves, N. M. (1996). Current developments in neurology, Part II: Alzheimer's disease, Parkinson's disease and stroke. *Annals of Pharmacotherapy, 30,* 1446–1451.

Hollister, L., & Gruber, N. (1996). Drug treatment of Alzheimer's disease. Effects on caregiver burden and patient quality of life. *Drugs and Aging, 8*(1), 47–56.

Kawas, C., & Morrison, A. (1997). Alzheimer's disease and other dementias. In *Current therapy in neurologic disease* (pp. 303–311). St. Louis: C. V. Mosby.

Mace, N. L. (1981). *The 35-hour day.* Baltimore: Johns Hopkins University Press.

Mohs, R. C. (1996). The Alzheimer's Disease Assessment Scale. *International Psychogeriatrics, 8*(2), 195–203.

Mulnard R. A., Cotman C. W., Kawas C., et al. (2001). Estrogen replacement therapy for treatment of mild to moderate

Alzheimer disease. *JAMA, The Journal of the American Medical Association, 283,* 1007–1015.

Patterson C. J., Gauthier S., Bergman H., Birks J., Flicker L. (2001). Selegiline for Alzheimer's disease. *Cochrane Database Syst Rev, 2,* CD000442.

Pearson V. E. (2001). Galantamine: a new Alzheimer drug with a past life. *Annals of Pharmacotherapy, 35(11),* 1406–13.

Petersen, R. C., Stevens, J. C., Ganguli, M., Tangalos, E. G., Cummings, J. L., DeKosky, S. T. (2001). Practice parameter: Early detection of dementia: Mild cognitive impairment (an evidence-based review). Report of the Quality Standards Subcommittee of the American Academy of Neurology. *Neurology, 56,* 1133–1142.

Reynolds, P. R. & Strayer, S. M. (2000). Neuroleptics for Behavioral Symptoms of Dementia. *Journal of Family Practice, 49(1),* 78.

Rogers, S. L., Farlow, M. R., Doody, R. S., et al. (1998). A 24-week, double-blind, placebo-controlled trial of donepezil in patients with Alzheimer's disease. *Neurology, 50,* 136–145.

Rösler, M., Anand, R., Cicin-Sain, A., Gauthier, S., Agid, Y., Dal-Bianco, P., Stähelin, H. B., Hartman, R., Gharabawi, M. (1999). Efficacy and safety of rivastigmine in patients with Alzheimer's disease: international randomised controlled trial. *British Medical Journal, 318,* 633–640.

Schneider, L. S. (1996). New therapeutic approaches to Alzheimer's disease. *Journal of Clinical Psychiatry, 57* (Suppl. 14), 30–36.

Small, G., Rabins, P., Barry, P., Buckholtz, N., et al. (1997). Diagnosis and treatment of AD and related disorders: Consensus statement of the American Association for Geriatric Psychology, Alzheimer's Association, and American Geriatrics Society. *The Journal of the American Medical Association 278 (16),* 1363–1371.

Sunderland, T. (1996). Treatment of the elderly suffering from psychosis and dementia. *Journal of Clinical Psychiatry, 57* (Suppl. 9), 53–56.

Thal, L. J., Schwartz, G., Sano, M., Weiner, M., Knopman, D., Harrell, L., Bodenheimer, S., Rossor, M., Philpot, M., Schor, J., & Goldberg, A. for the Psysostigmine Study Group. (1996). A multicenter double-blind study of controlled-release physostigmine for the treatment of symptoms secondary to Alzheimer's disease. *Neurology, 47,* 1389–1395.

Wiebe, S. & Nicolle, M. W. (2002). Recent developments in neurology. (Clinical Review). *British Medical Journal, 324(7338),* 656–661.

Wilcock G. K., Lilienfeld S., Gaens E. (2000). Efficacy and safety of galantamine in patients with mild to moderate Alzheimer's disease: multicentre randomised controlled trial. Galantamine International-1 Study Group. *British Medical Journal,* 321(7274), 1445–9.

Headache

Annequin, D., Tourniaire, B., & Massiou, H. (2000). Migraine and headache in childhood and adolescence. *Pediatric Clinics of North America, 47,* 617–631.

Evans, R. W. & Lipton, R. B. (2001). Topics in migraine management: a survey of headache specialists highlights some controversies. *Neurologic Clinics, 19,* 1–21.

Lipton, R. B., Diamond, S., Reed, M., Diamond, M. L., & Stewart, W. F. (2001). Migraine diagnosis and treatment: results from the American Migraine Study II. *Headache, 41,* 638–645.

Lipton, R. B., Stewart, W. F., & Liberman, J. N. (2002). Self-awareness of migraine: interpreting the labels that headache sufferers apply to their headaches. *Neurology, 58,* S21–S26.

Lipton, R. B., Stewart, W. F., Diamond, S., Diamond, M. L., & Reed, M. (2001). Prevalence and burden of migraine in the United States: data from the American Migraine Study II. *Headache, 41,* 646–657.

Olesen J., Goadsby P. (2000) Synthesis of migraine mechanisms. In Olesen J., Tfelt-Hansen P., Welch K. (eds) The Headaches, 2 ed. Philadelphia: Lippincott Williams & Wilkins.

Saper, J. R., Lake, A. E., & Tepper, S. J. (2001). Nefazodone for chronic daily headache prophylaxis: an open-label study. *Headache, 41,* 465–474.

Sheftell, F., O'Quinn, S., Watson, C., Pait, D., & Winter, P. (2000). Low migraine headache recurrence with naratriptan: clinical parameters related to recurrence. *Headache, 40,* 103–110.

Silberstein, S. D. (2002). Highlights from the 44th Annual Scientific Meeting of the American Headache Society June 21–23, 2002, Seattle, Washington. *Medscape Neurology & Neurosugery,* 4.

Silberstein S. (2000). Practice Parameter—Evidence-based guidelines for migraine headache (an evidence-based review): Report of the Quality Standards Subcommittee of the American Academy of Neurology for the United States Headache Consortium. *Neurology* 55:754–762.

Tfelt-Hansen, P. (2000) Prioritizing acute pharmacotherapy of migraine. In Olesen. J, Tfelt-Hansen. P, Welch. K, (eds). The Headaches, 2 ed. New York: Lippincott Williams & Wilkins.

Tfelt-Hansen, P., De, V., & Saxena, P. R. (2000). Triptans in migraine: a comparative review of pharmacology, pharmacokinetics and efficacy. *Drugs, 60,* 1259–1287.

Winner, P., Rothner, A. D., Saper, J., Nett, R., Asgharnejad, M., Laurenza, A., Austin, R., & Peykamian, M. (2000). A randomized, double-blind, placebo-controlled study of sumatriptan nasal spray in the treatment of acute migraine in adolescents. *Pediatrics, 106,* 989–997.

Parkinson's Disease

Ahlskig, J. E. (1996). Treatment of early Parkinson's disease: Are complicated strategies justified? *Mayo Clinic Proceedings, 71,* 659–670.

Alexander, G. E. (1997). Parkinson's disease. In R. T. Johnson & J. W. Griffin (Eds.), *Current therapy in neurologic disease* (pp. 268–274). St. Louis: C. V. Mosby.

Hely, M. A., & Morris, J. G. L. (1996). Controversies in the treatment of Parkinson's disease. *Current Opinion in Neurology, 9,* 308–313.

Imke, S. (2003). Parkinson's disease, more than meets the eye. *Advance for Nurse Practitioners, 11,* 42–54.

Important web cites www.parkinson.org (National Parkinson Foundation) www.apdaparkinson.com American Parkinson Disease Association.

Lieberman, A. (2002). The dopamine agonists Mirapex and Requip slow the rate of progression of PD. *Parkinson Report, 13*(3), 7–15.

Myllyla, V. V., Sotaniemi, D. A., Hakulinen, P., Maki-Ikola, O., & Heinonen, E. H. (1997). Selegiline as the primary treatment of Parkinson's disease—A long-term double-blind study. *Acta Neurologica Scandinovica, 95,* 211–218.

Olanow, C. W., & Koller, W. C. (1998). An algorithm for the management of Parkinson's disease: treatment guidelines. *Neurology, 50* (suppl 3), s1–s57.

Parkinson Study Group-PSG. (2002). Dopamine transporter imaging to assess the effects of Pramipexole versus Levodopa on the progression of Parkinson disease. *Journal of American Medical Association, 287,* 1653–1661.

Rascol, O., Brooks, D. J., Korczyn, A. D., De Deyn, P. P., Clarke, C. E., Lang, A. E. for The 056 Study Group. (2000). A five-year study of the incidence of dyskinesia in patients with early parkinson's disease who were treated with Ropinirole or Levodopa. *New England Journal of Medicine, 342,* 1481–1491.

Richard, I. H., Kurlan, M. D., Tanner, C., Factor, S., Hubble, J., Suchowerski, M. D., Waters, C., & the Parkinson Study Group. (1997). Serotonin syndrome and the combined use of deprenyl and an antidepressant in Parkinson's disease. *Neurology, 48,* 1070–1077.

Ross, G. W., Abbott, R. D., Petrovitch, H., Morens, D. M., Grandinetti, A, Tung, K. H., Tanner, C. M., Masaki, K. H., Blanchette, P. L., Curb, J. D., Popper, J. S., White, L. R. (2000). Association of coffee and caffeine intake with the risk of Parkinson disease. *Journal of American Medical Association,* 2674–2679.

Silberstein, P. M. (1996). Moderate Parkinson's disease. Strategies for maximizing treatment. *Postgraduate Medicine, 96*(1), 52–68.

Stacy, M., & Brownlee, H. J. (1996). Treatment options for early Parkinson's disease. *American Family Physician,* 1281–1287.

Stern, M. B. (1994). Movement disorders. In R. T. Johnson & J. W. Griffin (Eds.), *Current therapy in neurological disease* (pp. 242–246). St. Louis: C. V. Mosby.

Stern, M. B. (1997). Contemporary approaches to the pharmacotherapeutic management of Parkinson's disease: An overview. *Neurology, 49* (Suppl. 1), 82–89.

Seizures

American Academy of Pediatrics (AAP) (1999). Practice parameter: long-term treatment of the child with simple febrile seizures. *Pediatrics, 103* (6), 1307–1309.

Arroyo, S. & Kramer, G. (2001). Treating epilepsy in the elderly: safety considerations. Drug Safety, 24 (13), 991–1015.

Austin, J. K. & Santilli, N. (2001). Quality of life in children with epilepsy. Classification of Epilepsies in Childhood. In Pellock, J. M. Dodson, W. E. Bourgeois B. F. (Ed) *Pediatric Epilepsy: diagnosis and therapy.* 2nd ed. New York: Demos., 601–612.

Asconape, J. J. (2002). Some common issues in the use of antiepileptic drugs. *Seminars in Neurology, 22* (1), 27–39.

Birbeck, G. L. Hays, R. D., Cui, X., & Vickrey, B. G. (2002). Seizure reduction and quality of life improvements in people with epilepsy. Epilepsia 43(5), 535–8.

Brodie, M. J. & Kwan, P. (2002). Staged approach to epilepsy management. Neurology, 58, (8 Suppl 5), S2–8.

Buelow, J. M. (2001). Epilepsy management issue and techniques. *Journal of Neuroscience Nursing, 33* (5), 260–9.

Celano, R. T. (1998). Diagnosing pediatric epilepsy: an update for the primary care clinician. *Nurse Practitioner, 23*(3), 69–96.

Dreifuss, F. E. & Nordli, D. R. (2001). Classification of Epilepsies in Childhood. In Pellock J. M. Dodson, W. E., Bourgeois, B. F. (Ed) *Pediatric Epilepsy: diagnosis and therapy.* 2nd ed. New York: Demos. 69–80

Fisher, J. H. & Patel, T., (2001). Guide to antiepileptic agents. *CNS News Special Edition,* December, 101–107.

Faught, E. (2001). Pharmacokinetic considerations in prescribing antiepileptic drugs. *Epilepsia, 43, Suppl* (4) 19–23.

Garnett William R. "Antiepileptics" in *Therapeutic Drug Monitoring,* edited by Gerald E. Schumacher Appleton & Lange, Norwalk, Connecticut, 1995, 345–395.

Garnett, W. R. & Gloyd, J. C. (2001). Dosage form considerations in the treatment of pediatric epilepsy. In Pellock, J. M., Dodson, W. E., Bourgeois, B. F. (Ed) *Pediatric epilepsy: diagnosis and therapy.* 2nd ed. New York: Demos. 329–342.

Gidal, B. E., Garnett, W. R., & Graves, N. (2002). In DiPiro, J. T., Talbert, R. L, Yee G. C. et al. *Epilepsy, in Pharmacotherapy: A Pathophysiologic Approach,* 5th edition, editors DiPiro J. T., McGraw Hill, New York, pages 1031–1059.

Gilliam, F. G., Fessler, A. J., Baker, G., Vahle, V., Carter, J. & Attarian, H. (2004). Systematic screening allows reduction of adverse antiepileptic drug effects: a randomized trail. *Neurology, 62*(1), 23–27.

Hogan, R. E., Garnett, W. R. Thadani, V. M. and the Carbatrol Study Group. Tolerability and effects on quality of life of twice-daily extended release carbamazepine in adults with seizure disorders: an open 12- to 36-month continuation study. *Clinical Therapeutics, 25*(10), 2586–2596.

Kammerman, S. & Wasserman, L. Seizure disorders: Part 2 Treatment. Western Journal of Medicine, 175(3), 184–8.

Lackner, T. E. (2002). Strategies for optimizing antiepileptic drug therapy in elderly people. Pharmacotherapy. 22(3), 329–64.

Leppik, I. E. (2001). Epilepsy in the elderly. Current Neurology Neuroscience Reports. 1(4), 396–402.

Leszczyszyn, D. J. & Pellock, J. M. (2001). Status epilepticus. In Pellock, J. M., Dodson, W. E., Bourgeois, B. F. (Ed) *Pediatric epilepsy: diagnosis and therapy.* 2nd ed. New York: Demos. 275–300

McAuley, J. W. & Anderson, G. D. (2002). Treatment of epilepsy in women of reproductive age: Pharmacokinetic considerations. *Clinical Pharmacokinetics. 41*(8), 559–79.

Morrell, M. J. (2002). Epilepsy in women. *American Family Physician, 66*(8), 1489–92.

Morrell, M. J. (1999). Epilepsy in women: the science of why it is special. *Neurology, 53*(4 Suppl 1):S42–8.

Pellock, J. M. Dodson, W. E., Bourgeois B. F. (Ed) *Pediatric Epilepsy: diagnosis and therapy.* 2nd ed. New York: Demos.

Raty, L. K., Wilde Larsson, B. M., & Soderfeldt, B. A. (2003). Health-related quality of life in youth: a comparison between adolescents and young aduls with uncomplicated epilepsy and healthy controls. *Journal of Adolescent Health, 33*(4), 252–8.

Rosen, N. P. (2001). Febrile seizures. In Pellock, J. M., Dodson, W. E., Bourgeois, B. F. (Ed) *Pediatric epilepsy: diagnosis and therapy.* 2nd ed. New York: Demos. 357–372.

Yerby, M. S. (2001). Teratogenicity of anticonvulsant medication. In Pellock, J. M., Dodson, W. E., Bourgeois, B. F. (Ed) *Pediatric epilepsy: diagnosis and therapy.* 2nd ed. New York: Demos. 357–372.

Wilson, R. D., Davies, G., Desilets, V. Reid, G. J., Summers, A. Wyatt, P., Young, M. et al, Genetics Committee and Executive Council of the Society of Obsteritrics and Gynaecologists of Canada. The use of folic acid for the prevention of neuroal tube defects and other congenital anomalies. *Journal of Obstetrics and Gynaecology of Canda, 25*(11), 959–973.

CHAPTER ❖ 30

ENDOCRINE DISORDERS: THYROID AND ADRENAL CONDITIONS

Michael S. Monaghan ◆ Jeanette F. Kissinger ◆ Jeanne Archer

The endocrine system helps the body respond to changes from stressors like temperature, injury, electrolyte imbalances, changes in osmolality, or shock (Kirsten, 2000). Its purpose is to maintain a steady internal state in response to stimuli. Two components of the endocrine system, the thyroid gland and the adrenal gland, are discussed in this chapter as well as the conditions that may arise from disorders associated with these glands.

THYROID CONDITIONS

Metabolically, the thyroid gland and thyroid hormones influence virtually all cellular function. Normal growth and development depend on appropriate production of thyroid hormones. Conditions affecting the thyroid are common, occurring in approximately 10% of the general population (Shagam, 2001). Women are more frequently affected, at a three to four times greater rate. Further, the prevalence of thyroid conditions increases significantly with age. The first part of this chapter addresses the two major divisions of thyroid conditions: hypothyroidism and hyperthyroidism. Thyroid conditions as they pertain to children, pregnancy, and the elderly are then discussed, followed by drug-induced changes in thyroid function.

NORMAL THYROID FUNCTION

Thyroid hormones, thyroxine (T_4) and triodothyronine (T_3), are iodinated complexes synthesized and stored in the thyroid. T_3 is more physiologically active, having a biological half-life of approximately 1.5 days. T_4 is the major hormone circulating in blood, but is less physiologically active. T_4 has a longer biological half-life, up to 1 week (Shagam, 2001). T_4, though active, serves mainly as a reserve for T_3. T_4 can be converted to T_3 peripherally when increased thyroid hormone activity is required. Less than 20% of circulating T_3 is secreted by the thyroid; the majority is peripherally converted from T_4 (Reasner & Talbert, 2002).

Production and release of thyroid hormones are minutely regulated by the hypothalamic-pituitary-thyroid axis; see Figure 30–1. Changes in concentration of circulating T_3 and T_4 produce positive or negative stimuli to the hormonal regulation of the thyroid gland. Thyrotropin-releasing hormone (TRH) is released by the hypothalamus when concentrations of T_3 and T_4 drop below normal. TRH then stimulates the release of thyrotropin, also known as thyroid-stimulating hormone (TSH), which stimulates thyroid synthesis and release of T_3 and T_4. When adequate concentrations of circulating T_3 and T_4 are achieved, negative feedback stops further TSH release (Figure 30–1) (Shagam, 2001). Again, the majority of circulating T_3 is generated through peripheral conversion. Peripheral conversion of T_4 to T_3 is stimulated by cold temperatures. Peripheral conversion is inhibited by acute illness, chronic illness, starvation, and some medications, see Table 30–1 (Fitzgerald, 2002; Lazarus & Obuobie, 2000; Ram-schak-Schwarzer, et al., 2000). Together, the negative feedback process and peripheral conversion allow acute regulation of thyroid hormone synthesis and activity.

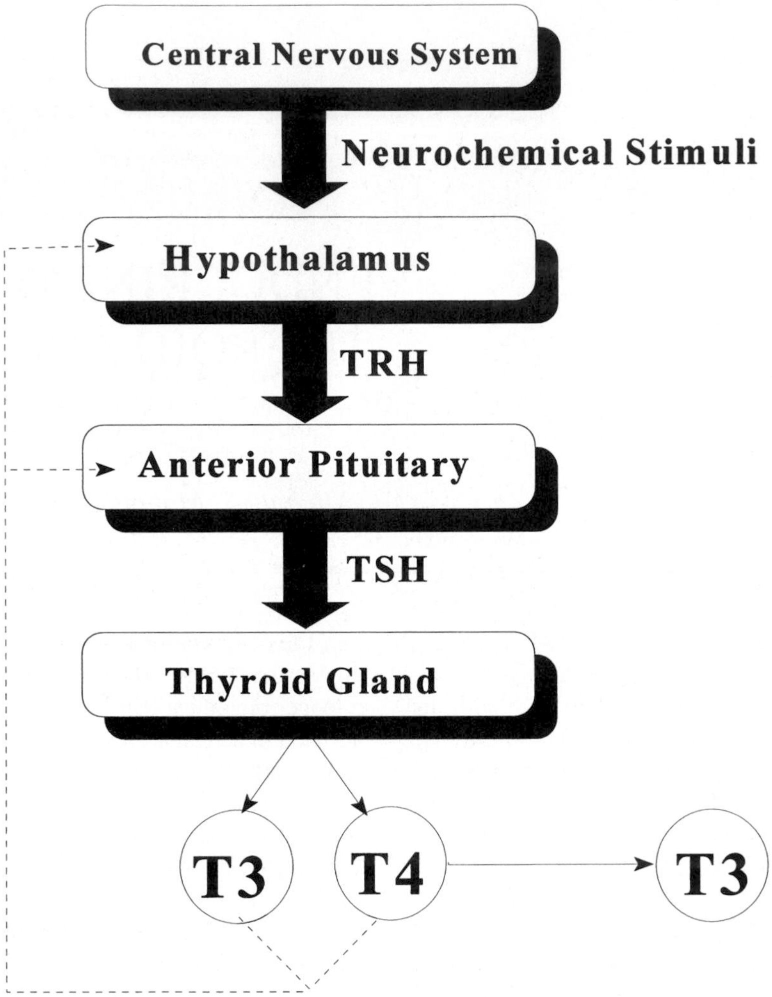

FIGURE 30–1. Hypothalamic-pituitary-thyroid axis illustrating the positive (heavy black arrows) and negative feedback (dashed arrows) stimuli that affect the hormonal regulators thyrotropin-releasing hormone (TRH) and thyrotropin (i.e., thyroid-stimulating hormone, TSH).

THYROID FUNCTION TESTS

Thyroid function tests (TFTs) are used to evaluate thyroid function and as a screening mechanism for the detection of thyroid conditions. Table 30–2 lists the common TFTs, their normal ranges, and findings in hypo- and hyperthyroidism. The initial laboratory test for evaluating thyroid conditions is the sensitive TSH assay (American College of Physicians, 1998; Bryer-Ash, 2001). The result from this measurement may then be used to determine which, if any, additional tests should be performed. One possible algorithm for use of TFTs in evaluating thyroid conditions is given in Figure 30–2. Once an abnormality in TSH is detected, a review of the patient's medications may provide the explanation. A number of medications can affect thyroid function, both clinically and subclinically. A drug-induced cause for the abnormal TSH measurement must be ruled out before further diagnostic investigation is pursued. [Refer back to Table 30–1 for common medications known to adversely affect thyroid function.]

Thyroid conditions may be classified as clinical or subclinical, based on presenting signs and symptoms in conjunction with TFT results (Madeddu, Spanu, Falchi, & Nuvoli, 1999). A patient with clinical or overt disease presents with signs and symptoms typically associated with hypo- or hyperthyroidism. Generally, *subclinical* im-

TABLE 30–1. Adverse Effects of Drugs on Thyroid Function.

Thyroid Function Affected	Drug	Comments
TSH response to TRH	Phenytoin	Decreases TSH response to TRH by up to 50%. Mechanism: enhancing cellular uptake and metabolism of T_4.
	High-dose salicylates NSAIDs?	Doses of about 4.0 gm suppress TSH response. Mechanism: dispacement of thyroid hormones from thyroid binding globulin (TBG). May occur with some nonsteroidal antiinflammatory drugs (NSAIDs).
	Levodopa	Chronic therapy suppresses TSH response. Mechanism: dispacement of thyroid hormones from TBG.
	Glucocorticoids	Impair basal and TRH-stimulated TSH concentrations.
	Dopamine blockers (i.e., neuroleptics)	Increase basal TSH and enhance TSH response to TRH.
	Theophylline	Increase TSH response through β-adrenergic stimulation of the hypothalamus.
Euthyroid hypothyroxinemia (clinically insignificant)	Phenytoin	Therapeutic doses decrease total T_4 (TT_4) by increasing metabolism of T_4. High doses can also impair binding of T_4 and T_3 to TBG.
	Carbamazepine	Decrease TT_4 by increasing metabolism of T_4.
	High-dose salicylates	Inhibit binding of T_4 and T_3 by TBG and prealbumin.
Euthyroid hyperthyroxinemia (clinically insignificant)	Cholecystographic agents (i.e., gallbladder dyes)	Inhibit peripheral conversion of T_4 to T_3.
	Other radiographic contrast media Propranolol, nadolol	Inhibit peripheral conversion of T_4 to T_3.
	Amiodarone	Inhibit peripheral conversion of T_4 to T_3.
	Estrogen preparations	Cause an increase in TBG values.
Hypothyroidism	Amiodarone	Release of iodine as drug is metabolized. Clinically significant in up to 10% of patients.
	Lithium	Blocks iodine uptake by the thyroid and release of thyroid hormones. Clinically significant in about 2% of patients.
Hyperthyroidism	Amiodarone	Released iodine can induce thyrotoxicosis. Clinically significant in about 3% of patients on long-term therapy.

Sources: Fitzgerald (2002); Lazarus & Obuobie (2000); Ramschak-Schwarzer et al. (2000).

plies an asymptomatic or presymptomatic status based on the measurements of TFTs. For example, a symptomatic patient with a high TSH and a low T_4 is classified as having clinical or overt hypothyroidism. A symptomatic patient with a low TSH and a high T_4 is classified as having overt hyperthyroidism. An asymptomatic patient with a high TSH and a normal T_4 has subclinical hypothyroidism. An asymptomatic patient with a low TSH and a normal T_4 has subclinical hyperthyroidism. Again, medications may produce TFT abnormalities in asymptomatic patients (Table 30–1). TFTs in patients on phenytoin or high-dose salicylates show a normal TSH and a low T_4. In patients on amiodarone or estrogen preparations, TFTs show a normal TSH and a high T_4.

TABLE 30–2. Laboratory Tests Used in the Evaluation of Thyroid Function.

Test	Normal Range*	Comments
Thyrotropin (thyroid stimulating hormone, i.e., TSH)	0.5–5.5 mU/L	Elevated in primary hypothyroidism (may be > 10); low or normal in pituitary/hypothalamic-related disease; low or undetectable in hyperthyroidism.
Total (free and bound) thyroxine (TT_4)	5.0–11.0 μg/dL	Elevated in hyperthyroidism; low in hypothyroidism.
Free thyroxine (FT_4)	0.6–2.1 ng/dL	Elevated in hyperthyroidism; low in hypothyroidism.
Total (free and bound) triiodothyronine (TT_3)	88–160 ng/dL	Useful in detecting mild hyperthyroidism; less so for mild hypothyroidism.
Triiodothyronine resin uptake (RT_3 U)	26–35%	Estimates the number of unoccupied binding sites (inverse relationship, i.e., a high RT_3 U indicates few unoccupied binding sites). Elevated in hyperthyroidism; low in hypothyroidism and thyroxine-binding globulin (TBG) excess.
Free thyroxine index (FT_4 I)	1.3–3.9 μg/dL	Calculated as the product of RT_3 U × T_4. Aids in interpreting abnormal T_4 levels due to elevation or depression of thyroid binding globulin levels (e.g., if total T_4 levels are elevated due to increase TBG, RT_3 U will be depressed, indicating a high amount of binding sites and the FT_4 I will be normal).

* Normal values may vary based on the laboratory.

Adapted from Hershman, Ladenson, & Paulshock, (1992).

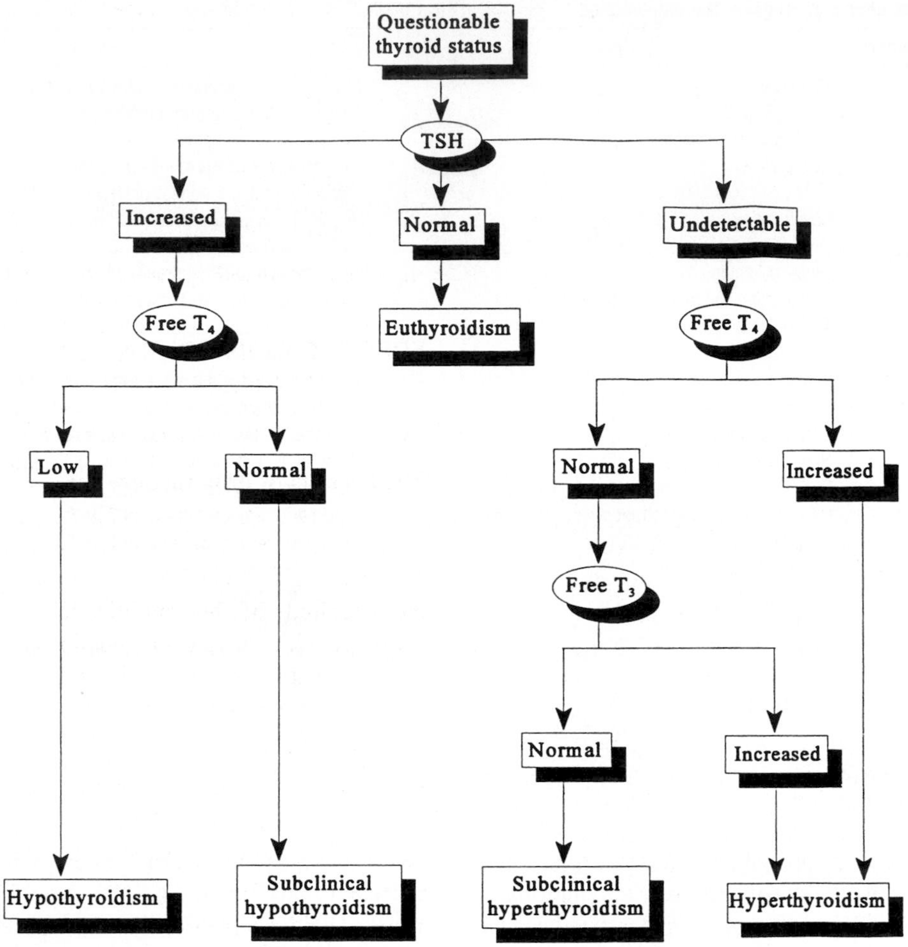

FIGURE 30–2. An algorithm for the evaluation of thyroid conditions using laboratory data, including measurements of serum thyrotropin (i.e., thyroid stimulating hormone, TSH), free T_4, and free T_3. *Source: Caldwell, Kellett, Gow, et al. (1985); Bryer-Ash (2001).*

HYPOTHYROIDISM

Hypothyroidism refers to the clinical syndrome caused by undersecretion of thyroid hormone from the gland (Herfindal & Gourley, 2000). Hypothyroidism may be classified as primary or secondary, based on the etiology. Primary hypothyroidism, by far the more common of the two, is caused by thyroid gland dysfunction. Secondary hypothyroidism, a relatively rare occurrence, is caused by failure of the hypothalamic-pituitary-thyroid axis due to pituitary or hypothalamic disease. Patients with secondary hypothyroidism generally present with other endocrine abnormalities such as adrenal insufficiency or hypogonadism. Table 30–3 lists major causes of hypothyroidism.

Symptoms of hypothyroidism may be nonspecific and vary among patients depending on gender, age, duration and severity of disease, and rapidity of onset of the deficiency ("AACE Clinical Practice Guidelines," 1995). Table 30–4 lists common signs and symptoms of hypothyroidism.

HYPERTHYROIDISM

Hyperthyroidism refers to the clinical syndrome produced by the body's exposure to the excessive action of thyroid hormone ("AACE Clinical Practice Guidelines," 1995). Common causes of hyperthyroidism are listed in Table 30–5. Graves' disease is the most common cause of

TABLE 30–3. Major Causes of Primary and Secondary Hypothyroidism

Classification	Mechanism	Etiology
Primary		
	Thyroid destruction	Chronic inflammation (i.e., Hashimoto's thyroiditis)
		Surgical thyroid gland removal
		Radioiodine thyroid gland ablation
		External irradiation
	Thyroid deficiency	Iodine deficiency—lack of hormonal substrate
		Iodine excess—interference with hormone release
		Drug-induced (i.e., amiodarone, lithium)
Secondary		
	Deficiency of TSH	Pituitary disease
	Deficiency of TRH	Hypothalamic disease

hyperthyroidism. Like Hashimoto's thyroiditis, it is an autoimmune disorder thought to be inherited secondary to familial clustering.

Symptoms of hyperthyroidism are caused by the action of supraphysiologic thyroid hormone and vary among patients depending on age, duration of disease, and the magnitude of circulating hormonal excess ("AACE Clinical Practice Guidelines," 1995). Elderly patients often present without classic signs and symptoms of hyperthyroidism, but almost always present with some cardiac manifestation (eg, congestive heart failure, atrial fibrillation, and angina). Table 30–6 lists common signs and symptoms of hyperthyroidism.

TABLE 30–4. Common Signs and Symptoms of Hypothyroidism

Signs	Symptoms
Thin brittle nails	Weakness, tiredness, lethargy, fatigue*
Thickened, doughy skin**	Cold intolerance*
Pallor	Headache
Puffy, mask-like face**	Loss of taste and/or smell
Yellowing of skin**	Deafness
Thinning of outer eyebrows**	Hoarseness
Edematous eyelids**	Absence of sweating
Thickening of tongue**	Weight gain*
Peripheral edema	Muscle cramps
Decreased deep tendon reflexes	Slow speech
Cardiomegaly**	Angina
Pleural/peritoneal/pericardial effusions	Constipation*
Bradycardia	Menorrhagia and/or galactorrhea
Hypertension	
Goiter	
Anemic from heavy menses	

Sources: Herfindal & Gourley (2000); Young & Koda-Kimble (1995).
*Classic symptoms.
** Signs of myxedema

TABLE 30–5. Major Causes of Hyperthyroidism

- Graves' disease
- Toxic adenoma
- Toxic multinodular goiter
- Painful subacute thyroiditis
- Silent thyroiditis
- Iodine-induced hyperthyroidism
- Excessive pituitary TSH or trophoblastic disease
- Excessive therapy with thyroid hormone

Sources: Franklyn (1997), Reasner & Talbert (2002), Lazarus & Obuobie (2000).

SPECIFIC CONSIDERATIONS FOR PHARMACOTHERAPY

When Drug Therapy Is Needed

The benefits of drug therapy must always outweigh risks before therapy is instituted. The need for drug therapy is based on the answers to two questions: (1) Is the patient experiencing signs and symptoms of disease? (2) What is the magnitude of abnormalities in TFTs? Once a diagnosis of clinical disease or subclinical disease is reached (refer to Figure 30–2), the decision to institute drug therapy must be individualized.

Hypothyroidism. In children with hypothyroidism, growth and mental development depend on adequate hormonal therapy (Koch & Sarlis, 2001). Since the function of virtually all organ systems depends on the euthyroid state, prompt treatment of clinical hypothyroidism is necessary. Treatment of subclinical hypothyroidism, common in the elderly, is more controversial. Poor left ventricular function and an increase in serum cholesterol are associated with thyroid dysfunction. Subclinical hypothyroidism may be associated with thyroid dysfunction. Subclinical hypothyroidism may be associated with coronary heart disease in both men and women (Bryer-Ash, 2001). Although irrefutable benefit has yet to be demonstrated,

TABLE 30–6. Common Signs and Symptoms of Hyperthyroidism

Signs	Symptoms
Thinning of hair	Heat intolerance
Proptosis, lid lag, lid retraction, periorbital edema	Weight loss common (or weight gain due to increased appetite)
Diffusely enlarged goiter	Increased sweating
Thyroid bruits, thrills	Palpitations
Flushed, moist skin	Pedal edema
Palmar erythema	Diarrhea
Increased deep tendon reflexes	Light menses or amenorrhea
Pretibial myxedema	Weakness, fatigue
Wide pulse pressure	Tremor, nervousness, irritability, insomnia

Source: Adapted from Young & Koda-Kimble (1995) with permission.

most endocrinologists treat subclinical hypothyroidism ("AACE Clinical Practice Guidelines," 1995). An individualized approach to the introduction of drug therapy must be taken. For example, thyroid replacement may aggravate preexisting myocardial ischemia in the elderly, and some cardiac intervention (e.g., coronary artery bypass graft) may be necessary prior to initiating replacement therapy to ensure benefit from drug therapy. Hypothyroidism in pregnancy is associated with gestational hypertension, premature labor, and low-birth-weight infants. Therapy can decrease neonatal morbidity.

Hyperthyroidism. Again, to maximize organ function, treatment of clinical hyperthyroidism is necessary. Hyperthyroidism can produce cardiomegaly and heart failure in newborns, as well as interfering with normal growth during adolescence (Mestman, 1999). In the elderly, untreated hyperthyroidism is associated with heart failure and atrial fibrillation. Hyperthyroidism, too, complicates pregnancy. Inadequately treated hyperthyroidism increases the risk of first-trimester spontaneous abortion, still births, and neonatal mortality (Mestman, 1999).

In summary, drug therapy for hyperthyroidism must be individualized. The selection of adjuvant therapy (e.g., beta-adrenergic blocking drugs) in an elderly person with heart failure secondary to hyperthyroidism must be done with great care so as to not worsen cardiac output. During pregnancy, some treatment modalities are absolutely contraindicated (e.g., radioiodine) secondary to fetal risks (Mestman, 1999).

Short- and Long-Term Goals for Pharmacotherapy

Hypothyroidism. The short-term goal for the treatment of hypothyroidism is to relieve signs and symptoms experienced by the patient. Long-term goals are to restore TSH concentration to within the normal range and reverse biochemical abnormalities (i.e., lipid abnormalities) of hypothyroidism.

Hyperthyroidism. Goals of therapy for hyperthyroidism are to minimize symptoms, eliminate excess circulating thyroid hormone, and prevent long-term sequelae caused by hyperthyroidism (Reasner & Talbert, 2002).

Time Frame for Initiating Pharmacotherapy

Hypothyroidism. For clinical hypothyroidism, pharmacotherapy is initiated at the time of diagnosis. Whether replacement therapy should be initiated at the time of detecting subclinical hypothyroidism is less certain. In a patient with an elevated TSH and a normal T_4, progression from subclinical to overt hypothyroidism occurs at a rate of at least 1 to 3% per year (Shrier & Burman et al, 2002). Therefore, some clinicians recommend repeating TFTs in 6 months and annually thereafter. Replacement therapy is begun only if there is a clear trend in the TFTs toward clinical hypothyroidism.

Hyperthyroidism. For clinical hyperthyroidism, pharmacotherapy is initiated at the time of diagnosis. For subclinical hyperthyroidism caused by toxic goiter, toxic adenoma, or toxic multinodular goiter, therapy is generally initiated at diagnosis. Subclinical hyperthyroidism caused by glucocorticoid use, severe illness, and pituitary dysfunction does not require standard therapeutic intervention ("AACE Clinical Practice Guidelines," 1995). See Drug Table 607.

Assessment and History Taking

A complete history and physical examination should be aimed at uncovering the signs and symptoms relevant to thyroid disease, listed in Tables 30–3 through 30–6. Baseline TFTs are necessary prior to drug therapy since these measurements will be used to determine the adequacy of treatment. Both pregnancy and certain medications can affect normal, expected TFT values. During pregnancy, circulating estrogen increases. Estrogen stimulates a 2.5-fold increase in thyroxine-binding globulin (TBG). This increased TBG results in increased total serum T_4 and T_3 concentrations, but no change in serum free T_4. Also, because of the increased binding, T_3 resin uptake will be decreased. Generally, the TSH will remain within the reference range (Glinoer, 1999). These changes must be taken into consideration when deciding when and if drug therapy is introduced and during the assessment of treatment.

Patient/Caregiver Information

Examples of patient information for drug treatment of hypo- and hyperthyroidism are given in Tables 30–7 and 30–8, respectively.

OUTCOMES MANAGEMENT

Selecting an Appropriate Agent

Hypothyroidism. Although several thyroid replacement agents are available, the American Association of Clinical Endocrinologists advocates the use of a high-quality brand preparation of levothyroxine ("AACE Clinical

TABLE 30–7. Example of Patient Information for the Treatment of Hypothyroidism Caused by Hashimoto's Thyroiditis

Levothyroxine

- Levothyroxine is a thyroid medicine belonging to the group of medications called hormones. It is used when the thyroid gland does not produce enough hormone.
- When you get this medicine refilled, make sure your pharmacist uses the same manufacturer's brand each time. This will help the medicine work best for you.
- Use this medicine only as directed. Do not use more or less of it, and do not take it more often than ordered. If you take a different amount than prescribed for you, you may experience symptoms of overactive or underactive thyroid. Take the medicine at the same time each day to make sure it always has the same effect.
- You may have to take this medicine for the rest of your life. It is very important that you do not stop taking this medicine without first checking with your healthcare professional.
- If you miss a dose of this medicine, take it as soon as possible. However, if it is almost time for your next dose, skip the missed dose and go back to your regular dosing schedule. Do not double doses.
- Make sure all healthcare professionals you see know you are taking this medicine. Also, make sure they are aware of other medicines you now take. If you start taking a new medicine, make sure you state that you take levothyroxine.
- It is very important that your healthcare professional check your progress at regular visits, to make sure this medicine is working properly. Any dose changes you may need are based on these visits.
- Report any problems such as chest pain, fast or irregular heartbeats, or shortness of breath.
- This medicine usually takes several weeks to have a noticeable effect on your condition. If you do not improve in about 3 weeks, check with your healthcare professional.

Source: United States Pharmacopeial Convention (2000).

TABLE 30–8. Example of Patient Information for the Treatment of Hyperthyroidism Caused by Graves' Disease

Methimazole

- Methimazole is used when the thyroid gland makes too much thyroid hormone. It works by slowing down your body's production of thyroid hormone.
- Use this medicine only as directed. Do not use more or less of it and do not use it for a longer time than prescribed. If you do, you increase the chances of side effects.
- This medicine works best when there is a constant amount in the blood. To help keep the amount constant, do not miss any doses. Also, if you are taking more than one dose a day, it is best to take the doses at evenly spaced times day and night.
- Usually you have to take this medicine for 6 months to a year. It is very important that you do not stop taking this medicine without first checking with your healthcare professional.
- If you miss a dose of this medicine, take it as soon as possible. If it is almost time for your next dose, take both doses together. Then go back to your regular dosing schedule.
- If you wish to become pregnant or become pregnant while taking this medicine, notify your healthcare professional.
- Make sure all healthcare professionals you see know you are taking this medicine. Also, make sure they are aware of other medicines you now take. If you start taking a new medicine, make sure you state that you take methimazole.
- It is very important that your healthcare professional check your progress at regular visits, to make sure this medicine is working properly and to check for unwanted effects.
- Check with your healthcare professional immediately if you develop a rash, cough, fever, or chills that do not go away within a week.
- This medicine usually takes several weeks to have a noticeable effect on your condition. If you do not improve in a month, check with your healthcare professional.

Source: United States Pharmacopeial Convention (2000).

Practice Guidelines," 1995). Three trade name products are now available (Synthroid, Unithroid, Levoxyl) and can be considered equivalent. Levothyroxine possesses consistent activity while having a long half-life. Desiccated products are available, but their potency is based on iodine content rather than hormone activity, and therefore they provide less predictable activity. Other products listed in Drug Table 607.3, liothyronine, liotrix, and thyroglobulin, offer no advantage over levothyroxine and should not be used to initiate therapy ("AACE Clinical Practice Guidelines," 1995). Generic levothyroxine brands may be used, but therapy should be initiated with one brand and that brand used to control and maintain thyroid replacement therapy. Available brands are not bioequivalent; the use of a single brand will prevent under- or overtreatment.

The initial dose (range 12.5–100 μg) for adults is based on the age, weight, and cardiac status of the patient, as well as the duration and severity of hypothyroidism ("AACE Clinical Practice Guidelines," 1995). Also, the duration and speed with which replacement therapy is attempted will be patient-specific. An appropriate initial dose of levothyroxine for most patients is 50 g/day for 1 month, which is then increased to 100 μg/day. The appropriate maintenance dose also will vary, but the mean replacement dose of levothyroxine is 1.6 g/kg per day ("AACE Clinical Practice Guidelines," 1995). The following examples illustrate initial and maintenance dosing. In young adults with no risk factors limiting rapid replacement (e.g., advanced age, cardiac disease, longstanding hypothyroidism), a conservative maintenance dose of 100 μg/day may be initiated. For elderly patients or those with a history of heart disease, the starting dose is 25 μg/day, which is then increased by 12.5 μg to 25 μg/day each month until the appropriate maintenance dose is achieved. This slower increase prevents aggravation of preexisting ischemic heart disease (Reasner & Talbert, 2000). Also, maintenance dosing in the elderly is generally less than 1.6 μg/kg per day, with adequate maintenance doses of 50 μg/day not uncommon in those over 60 years of age.

Levothyroxine tablets are also the agent of choice for the treatment of pediatric hypothyroidism. Tablets may be crushed and added to bottle contents for treatment of infants. The suggested replacement dose for pediatric patients, like adults, varies according to age and presence of risk factors (Kirsten, 2000). These risk factors are preexisting cardiac disease or extreme sensitivity to the effects of levothyroxine. Normal TFT values vary in early life and may be difficult to interpret without experience (American Academy of Pediatrics [AAP] & American Thyroid Association [ATA], 1993). Therefore, diagnosis and treatment of congenital hypothyroidism may require referral to a specialist.

During pregnancy, women will require an approximate 45% increase in levothyroxine dosing over their usual maintenance dose. Maintenance dosing returns to prepregnancy requirements after delivery.

Minimal amounts of levothyroxine are excreted into breast milk. No dosage adjustments are necessary secondary to breastfeeding. Further, any amounts reaching the breast milk are insufficient to treat neonatal hypothyroidism.

Hyperthyroidism. Three treatment modalities exist for the management of hyperthyroidism caused by Graves' disease: radioiodine, surgery, and antithyroid drugs (Franklyn, 1997; Reasner & Talbert, 2000). Radioiodine is currently the therapy of choice. Surgery is used when radioiodine or antithyroid agents are not optimal for patient-specific reasons. The antithyroid agents methimazole and propylthiouracil (PTU) are utilized to induce a remission. These agents are easy to use, have somewhat predictable therapeutic effects, and are inexpensive. They inhibit binding of iodine and inhibit coupling of reactions during thyroid hormone formation. PTU, unlike methimazole, also inhibits peripheral conversion of T_4 to T_3. This additional mechanism makes PTU useful in the treatment of severe hyperthyroidism (i.e., thyroid storm), when lowering serum T_3 aids in treatment.

Other differences between the two agents exist. Methimazole possesses a longer half-life, permitting once-daily dosing and potentially increasing compliance. PTU has a shorter half-life and must be dosed three times daily. PTU does not cross the placenta well and is the drug of choice for hyperthyroidism in pregnancy and breastfeeding. These agents are given until TFTs are within the normal range (ie, euthyroid) or a remission occurs. The ideal duration of therapy is not well defined; the length of therapy is usually 6 months to 2 years. A reasonable treatment course should be up to 18 months to maximize the chance of inducing a remission. Once the patient is euthyroid, the dose is decreased to the lowest possible dose that will maintain normal TFT values. For those experiencing severe hyperthyroidism, for children, and for patients who are pregnant or breast-feeding, PTU is the agent of choice (Reasner & Talbert, 2000). The effectiveness of both agents depends on patient compliance ("AACE Clinical Practice Guidelines," 1995). If the patient has a history of noncompliance, methimazole may be the preferred agent since the longer half-life permits once-daily dosing, particularly during maintenance therapy.

Iodine products (see Drug Table 607.2) are used as short-term adjuvant therapy in the treatment of hyperthyroidism. These products acutely block thyroid hormone release, inhibit thyroid hormone biosynthesis (i.e., Wolff-Chaikoff paradoxical effect), and decrease the vascularity of the gland (Reasner & Talbert, 2000). Therefore, they are most useful as adjuvants to surgery or emergent radiation administration since they are capable of producing a short-term (7–14 day) euthyroid state and decreasing gland vascularity.

Both radioiodine and antithyroid agents take several weeks to produce symptomatic relief. Because many of the symptoms caused by hyperthyroidism mimic excess beta-adrenergic activity (e.g., palpitations, tremor, sweating, heat intolerance), beta-adrenergic blocking drugs (beta blockers) may be used to control these symptoms until the gland-modifying agent takes action. Propranolol and nadolol are the agents of choice since they can block peripheral conversion of T_4 to T_3 as well as beta-receptor-mediated effects of catecholamines (see Table 30–1). Doses are titrated to a pulse less than 100 beats/min. Propranolol, the drug of choice for thyroid-induced atrial fibrillation, is initiated at dosages of 20 mg four times daily and titrated to pulse; very large doses may be required.

Monitoring for Efficacy

Hypothyroidism. Two to three weeks after the initiation of therapy, subjective benefit is experienced. But other signs and symptoms (e.g., weight gain, increased pulse, hoarseness, skin changes) may take months to correct.

Approximately 3 months after the initiation of therapy, TFTs [i.e., TSH and free T_4 (FT_4)] should be obtained. These measurements will then be used to make adjustments in replacement therapy. Also, after any dosage adjustment, TFT measurements should not be obtained for at least 6 weeks. This is because of the long half-life of levothyroxine and the length of time necessary to reach a steady state.

In pregnancy, as previously stated, elevated estrogen stimulates an increase in TBG, altering total T_4 (TT_4)

values but not FT_4. Therefore, the adequacy of replacement therapy in pregnancy also should be based on TSH and FT_4 laboratory values (Reasner & Talbert, 2000). Laboratory measurements should be made at 8 weeks' and 6 months' gestation. The goal of therapy is to normalize TSH values while maintaining FT_4 at the upper limits of normal.

Hyperthyroidism. Several weeks after the initiation of therapy, most patients experience subjective benefit (Reasner & Talbert, 2000). Beta blockers may be added to provide immediate symptomatic relief. If symptomatic improvement does not occur within this time frame, consider increasing the dose of the antithyroid agent.

Dosage adjustments are based on TFTs (i.e., TSH and TT_4). With appropriate dosing, TSH will increase to within the normal range and TT_4 will decrease to within the normal range. Laboratory assessment should occur monthly until a euthyroid state is achieved.

Monitoring for Toxicity

Hypothyroidism. With excessive thyroid replacement, symptoms of hyperthyroidism will occur. These symptoms—weight loss, increased sweating and palpitations—are similar to those listed in Table 30–6. Explain this to patients so they will contact a health care professional if these symptoms occur. Generally, laboratory assessment is not performed at less than 6-week intervals, again because of the long half-life of levothyroxine.

Hyperthyroidism. Adverse effects associated with the antithyroid agents are skin reactions, leukopenia, and rarely, agranulocytosis (Fitzgerald, 2002). Agranulocytosis is the most serious adverse effect and generally occurs within the first 3 months of therapy. Patients should be instructed to report the development of a rash, cough, fever, or chill that does not resolve within a week (see Table 30–8).

To determine if antithyroid agents are affecting leukocytes, a baseline white blood cell count (WBC) should be performed prior to the initiation of therapy. Frequent monitoring of the WBC does not predict who will develop agranulocytosis (Fitzgerald, 2002). Therefore, WBC should only be performed if the patient complains of flu-like symptoms and during TFT assessment.

Followup Recommendations

Hypothyroidism. Once a patient is euthyroid (as determined by TSH concentrations), a 6-month laboratory assessment should be performed. Patients should then be assessed, using TFTs, annually. At the time of laboratory assessments, an appropriate interim history (assessing symptoms of under- or overtreatment) and physical examination also should be performed ("AACE Clinical Practice Guidelines," 1995).

Hyperthyroidism. After treatment (e.g., surgery) patients should be seen at 4- to 6-week intervals until euthyroid (as determined by TSH concentrations). Once patient is euthyroid, a 6-month laboratory assessment should be performed. Patients should then be assessed using TFTs annually. At the time of laboratory assessments, an appropriate interim history (assessing symptoms of under- or overtreatment) and physical examination also should be performed ("AACE Clinical Practice Guidelines," 1995).

ADRENAL CONDITIONS

Adrenal conditions are rarely encountered by general clinicians, particularly compared to thyroid conditions. The adrenal glands rest above the kidneys and are composed of the adrenal medulla and the adrenal cortex. The adrenal medulla comprises 10% of the gland and secretes catecholamines. The hormones produced by the adrenal medulla are not essential for life. The adrenal cortex makes up the majority of the gland and secretes three classes of steroid hormones: the glucocorticoids, the mineralocorticoids, and the androgens. The glucocorticoids and mineralocorticoids are necessary for subsistence; in fact, life is not possible without adrenocortical function. Glucocorticoids regulate carbohydrate and protein metabolism. Mineralocorticoids regulate sodium, potassium, and fluid balance. A lack or overabundance of either steroid class produces disease. Androgens contribute to the pubertal growth of body hair, particularly the pubic and axillary hair of women. Excess androgen production can result in hirsutism and virilization. This section of the chapter addresses the two major divisions of adrenocortical disorders: hypofunction (e.g., adrenal insufficiency, or Addison's disease, and hypoaldosteronism) and hyperfunction (e.g., Cushing's syndrome, aldosteronism, and hirsutism). Where appropriate, adrenal conditions as they pertain to children and pregnancy are discussed.

NORMAL ADRENAL CORTEX FUNCTION

The major role of the adrenal cortex is the production of glucocorticoid and mineralocorticoid hormones. The major physiologic glucocorticoid synthesized and secreted is cortisol. Cortisol influences numerous processes in the body including the regulation of intermediary metabolism (i.e., glucose and lipid metabolism), inflammatory and immunologic responses, cardiac and hemodynamic function, calcium homeostasis, and normal growth and development. Normal cortisol secretion follows a diurnal pattern, with burst production occurring in response to stress, such as illness or trauma (Zafar & Wisgerhof, 1999). Therefore, normal cortisol production is necessary for the appropriate reaction to stress. The major physiologic mineralocorticoid is aldosterone. Aldosterone mainly affects the kidney's ability to regulate fluid and electrolyte balance (NIH, 1998). Aldosterone increases sodium reabsorption and potassium secretion. Water passively follows sodium movement; therefore, aldosterone affects extracellular fluid volume. Aldosterone also causes hydrogen ion secretion, thus affecting acid-base status.

Cortisol production and secretion are regulated by the hypothalamic-pituitary-adrenal axis (Figure 30–3). Changes in concentration of cortisol produce positive or negative stimuli to the hormonal regulation of the adrenal cortex. Corticotropin-releasing hormone (CRH) is released by the hypothalamus when increased concentrations of cortisol are required. CRH then stimulates the release of corticotropin [i.e., adrenocorticotropic hormone (ACTH)], which stimulates the adrenal cortex to release cortisol. When adequate concentrations of circulating cortisol are achieved, negative feedback stops further production and release of cortisol by the adrenal cortex (Figure 30–3).

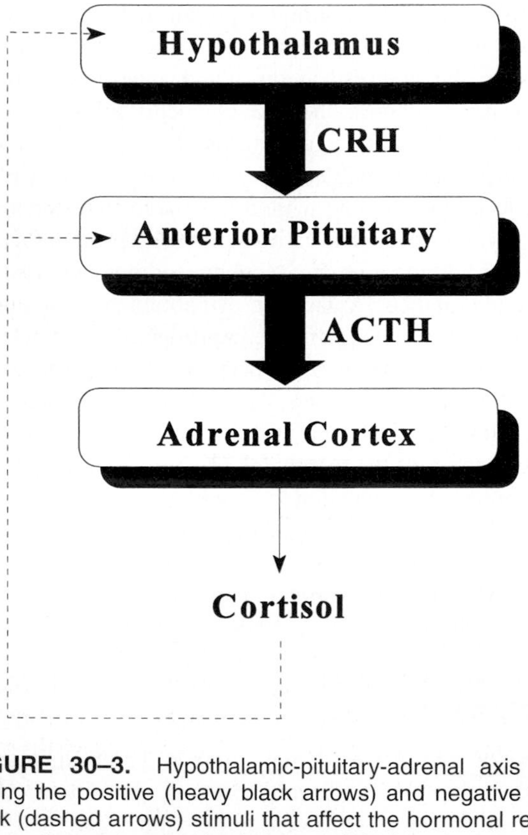

FIGURE 30–3. Hypothalamic-pituitary-adrenal axis illustrating the positive (heavy black arrows) and negative feedback (dashed arrows) stimuli that affect the hormonal regulators corticotropin-releasing hormone (CRH) and corticotropin (i.e., adrenocorticotropic hormone, ACTH).

Aldosterone production and secretion are governed mainly by the renin-angiotensin system (NIH, 1998). Four predominant factors influence aldosterone release: changes in renal tubular sodium chloride concentration, renal perfusion pressure, angiotensin II, and serum potassium concentration. When sodium chloride concentration falls, when intravascular volume is low, or when blood pressure falls, renin is released from the juxtaglomerular cells of the afferent renal arteriole. Renin stimulates angiotensin II production and release. Angiotensin II is a potent stimulator of aldosterone release. The presence of angiotensin II also blocks further renin release, thus providing feedback to inhibit the system. High serum potassium concentrations can also stimulate aldosterone release, whereas decreases in serum potassium inhibit aldosterone release.

ADRENOCORTICAL HYPOFUNCTION: ADRENAL INSUFFICIENCY

Adrenal insufficiency, by definition, is characterized by inadequate production of cortisol, aldosterone, or both. Adrenal insufficiency may be classified as primary or secondary, based on the etiology. Primary adrenal insufficiency, or Addison's disease, is caused by the destruction of the adrenal cortex (NIH, 2000). Primary adrenal insufficiency is associated with deficiencies in both cortisol and aldosterone. Secondary adrenal insufficiency stems from a hypothalamic-pituitary defect resulting in insufficient ACTH. Aldosterone production is usually adequate in secondary adrenal insufficiency. The differentiation between a primary and secondary etiology can be made through laboratory evaluation; see Figure 30–4. Table 30–9 lists major causes of primary and secondary adrenal insufficiency (Laureti, Aubourg, Calcinaro et al., 1998; Orth, 2001).

Symptoms common to both primary and secondary adrenal insufficiency are weakness, easy fatiguability, and weight loss. Table 30–10 lists common signs and

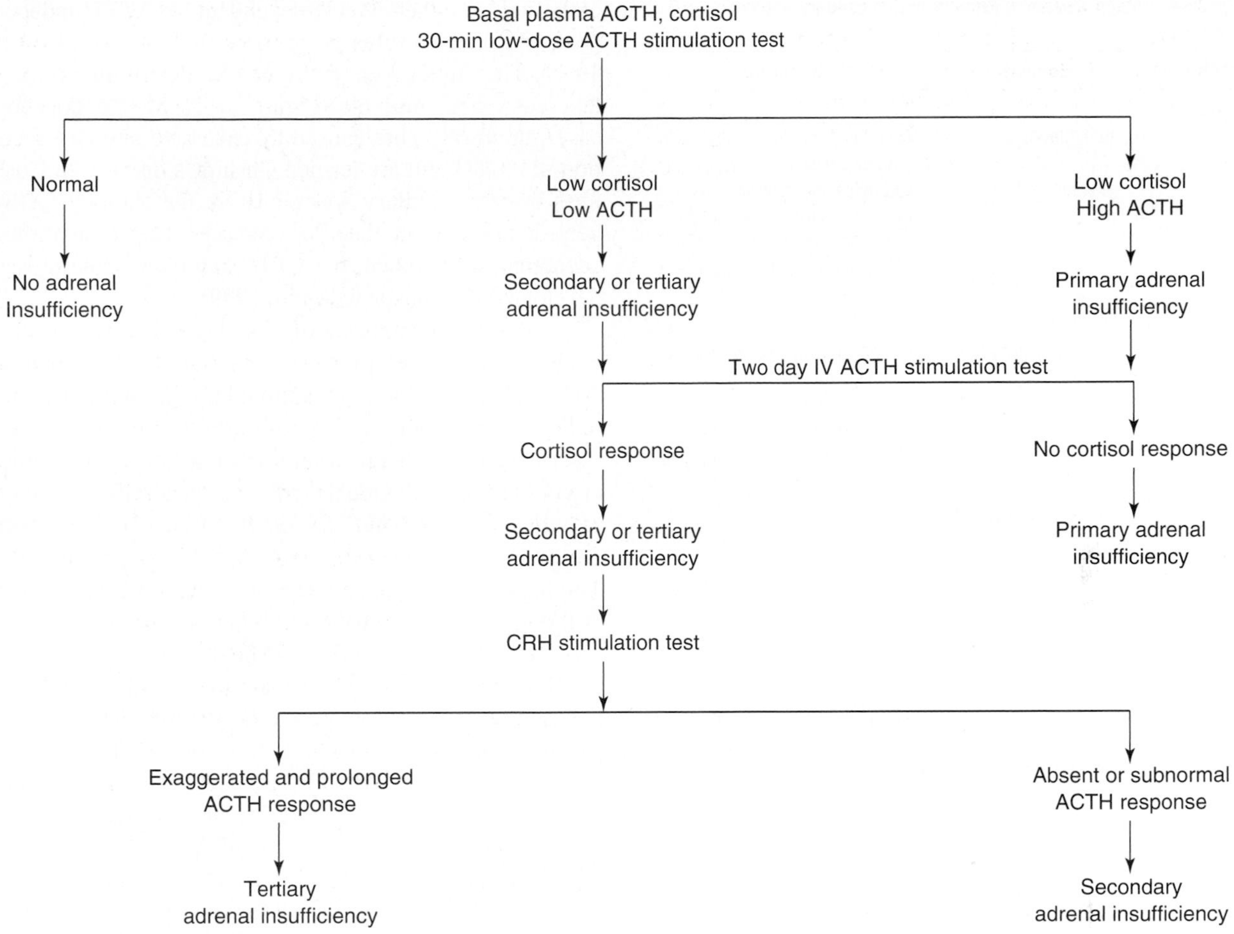

FIGURE 30–4. Diagnostic approach to suspected adrenal insufficiency. *Source: Orth (2002).*

symptoms of primary adrenal insufficiency (Kovacs, 2001, Lam, & Pater, Laureti et al., 1998; Orth, 2001). In comparison, patients with secondary adrenal insufficiency tend to have less hyperpigmentation and retain aldosterone activity, and therefore do not present with severe dehydration and electrolyte abnormalities. The clinical presentation of adrenal insufficiency depends on the rate and degree of loss of adrenocortical function. With acute stress, patients may present with addisonian crisis, a life-threatening emergency. Resembling shock patients, they present with severe dehydration and hypotension. Chronic adrenal insufficiency is associated with an insidious onset, and the symptoms at presentation are nonspecific.

ADRENOCORTICAL HYPOFUNCTION: HYPOALDOSTERONISM

Hypoaldosteronism is rare. This disorder can occur with Addison's disease or as the sole adrenocortical defect (NIH, 1998). When it is the sole defect, hypoaldosteronism is usually caused by hyporeninemic hypoaldosteronism, a defect in the secretion of renin. Hyporeninemic hypoaldosteronism generally occurs concurrently with renal disease, but also may occur in patients with normal renal function who have malignancies (Chung, Tanaka, & Fujita, 1996). Patients present with low serum sodium and high serum potassium concentrations.

TABLE 30–9. Major Causes of Primary and Secondary Adrenal Insufficiency

Classification	Etiology	Comments
Primary		
	Autoimmune	Accounts for approximately 80% of all cases
	Infections	Examples: tuberculosis—accounts for approximately 15–20% of all cases; fungal infections (i.e., histoplasmosis); HIV
	Adrenal hemorrhage	
	Metastatic disease	Examples: lung, gastric, breast, malignant melanoma
	Drugs	Two mechanisms: decreased steroid synthesis (i.e., ketoconazole) and increased clearance (i.e., rifampin)
	Severe Inflammatory disease	
Secondary		
	Glucocorticoid use	Major cause: synthetic steroids suppress adrenocortic otropic hormone (ACTH) release
	Pituitary disease	
	Hypothalamic disease	

Sources: Laureti et al., (1998), Orth (2001), Perry et al. (2002).

ADRENOCORTICAL HYPERFUNCTION: CUSHING'S SYNDROME

Cushing's syndrome is caused by chronic exposure to supraphysiologic glucocorticoids. The syndrome is most commonly due to excessive administration of exogenous glucocorticoids or may occur endogenously (Gums & Terpening, 2002). Major endogenous causes of Cushing's syndrome, classified as either ACTH-dependent or ACTH-independent, and their prevalence are listed in Table 30–11 (Orth, 1995). The etiology generally can be determined through laboratory evaluation (see Figure 30–5). Most endogenous cases, up to 68%, are caused by excessive pituitary secretion of ACTH and are termed Cushing's disease. In Cushing's disease, pituitary adenomas are the etiology for hypersecretion in more than 90% of cases. The cause of these adenomas is unknown, but CRH may play a role in their development (Johnson & Amin, 1999).

Signs and symptoms of Cushing's disease, listed in Table 30–12, develop over years (Gums & Terpening, 2002). Their development is thought to be caused by catabolic or antianabolic effects of cortisol. Two of the more common ones, facial rounding and fat accumulation around the supraclavicular areas, are generally referred to as *moon face* and *buffalo hump.* Striae are most commonly on the lower trunk and are red to purple in color. The hypertension seen in approximately 70% of patients is thought to be due to a combination of glucocorticoid and mineralocorticoid effects (Marsh & Kim, 1999).

Presentation in children may differ, with growth failure as the most common presenting abnormality. Iatrogenic Cushing's syndrome in children secondary to intranasal steroids has been reported by Perry, Findlay, and Donaldson (2002). They suggest that inquiry as to use of nasal steroids should be routine when children present with unexplained growth failure. Other signs and symptoms common in adults (see Table 30–12) are also present. Although Cushing's disease in adults is more common in women (at a ratio of 8:1), in children there is no female predominance.

Because of the adverse effects of cortisol on the reproductive state, pregnancy is rare in women with Cushing's disease (Fitzgerald, 2002).

TABLE 30–10. Common Signs and Symptoms of Primary Adrenal Insufficiency (Addison's Disease) and Percent Occurrence of Each

Sign or Symptom	Percentage
Weakness and fatigue	74–100
Weight loss	56–100
Hyperpigmentation	92–96
Hyponatremia	88–96
Hypotension	59–88
Hyperkalemia	52–64
Gastrointestinal symptoms	56
Postural dizziness	12

Sources: Kovacs et al., (2001), Laureti et al. (1998), Orth (2001).

TABLE 30–11. Causes of Cushing's Syndrome and their Prevalence, Classified as Corticotropin (i.e., Andrenocorticotropic Hormone, ACTH)-Dependent and ACTH-Independent

Classification	Etiology	Percentage of Patients
ACTH-dependent		
	Cushing's disease	68
	Ectopic ACTH syndrome	12
	Ectopic CRH syndrome	<1
ACTH-independent		
	Adrenal adenoma	10
	Adrenal carcinoma	8
	Micronodular hyperplasia	1
	Macronodular hyperplasia	<1

Source: Adapted from Orth (1995) with permission.

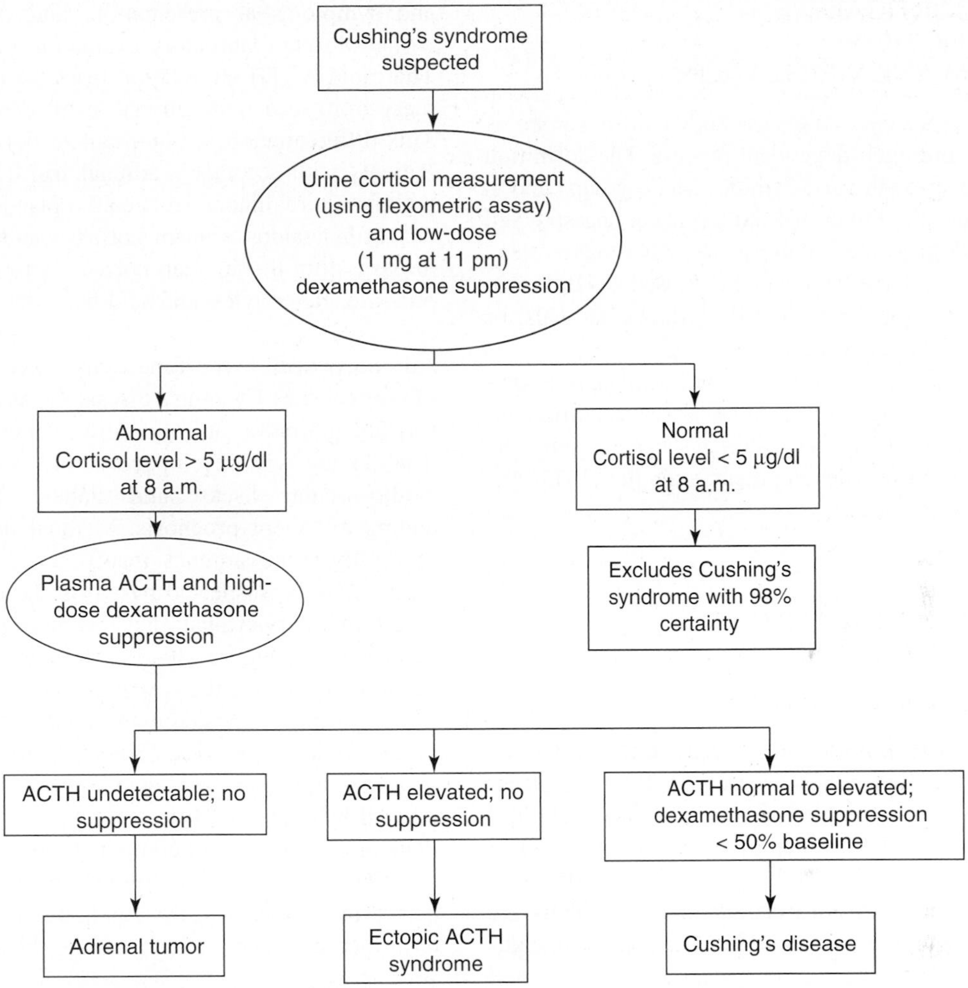

FIGURE 30–5. An algorithm for the evaluation of suspected Cushing's syndrome utilizing laboratory measurements, including serum corticotropin (i.e., adrenocorticotropic hormone, ACTH). *Sources: Fitzgerald (2002), Gums & Terpening (2002).*

TABLE 30–12. Common Signs and Symptoms of Cushing's Disease In Decending Order of Occurrence

Sign or Symptom
Central obesity
Facial rounding
Hirsutism
Deficits in cognitive function
Menstrual complications
Hypertension
Muscular weakness, muscle wasting
Back pain
Striae, thin skin
Acne
Psychiatric changes

Sources: Fitzgerald (2002); Forget, Lacroix, & Cohen (2002).

ADRENOCORTICAL HYPERFUNCTION: ALDOSTERONISM

Primary aldosteronism, caused by an increased production of aldosterone, is a rare disorder characterized by sodium retention, suppression of renin activity, hypokalemia, and hypertension (Sergev & Wisgerhof, 1999). The usual pathogenesis is an aldosterone-producing adrenocortical adenoma or bilateral adrenocortical hyperplasia (Sergev & Wisgerhof, 1999). Patients are commonly identified by detection of hypertension on a routine physical examination.

ADRENOCORTICAL HYPERFUNCTION: HIRSUTISM AND VIRILIZATION

Hirsutism, the presence of excess body hair in women, is primarily an androgen-dependent process. The definition of excess hair growth varies among ethnic groups and is more common in women of Mediterranean ancestry and least common in women of Japanese or North American Indian ancestry. Hirsutism can be caused by drugs or pathologic conditions involving the ovaries, adrenals, or skin (Plouffe, 2000); see Table 30–13.

Virilization, the masculinization of women, is associated with androgen-secreting tumors. The condition includes hirsutism, temporal balding, deepening of the voice, pectoral muscle development, and clitoral enlargement (Fitzgerald, 2002).

SPECIFIC CONSIDERATIONS FOR PHARMACOTHERAPY

When Drug Therapy Is Needed

Adrenocortical Hypofunction. Appropriate production of adrenocortical hormones is essential. Before replacement therapy was available, most patients died within 2 years of diagnosis. Drug therapy to replace insufficient cortisol and aldosterone production (i.e., Addison's disease) is essential to restore quality of life. Patients are suspected of having adrenal insufficiency based on signs and symptoms at presentation, and diagnosis is confirmed through laboratory evaluation (see Figure 30–4). The rapid ACTH stimulation test also distinguishes primary from secondary adrenal insufficiency (NIH, 1998). This differentiation is important to define drug therapy. Patients with secondary adrenal insufficiency generally do not require mineralocorticoid replacement.

In hypoaldosteronism not associated with Addison's disease, drug therapy can correct abnormalities in blood pressure, electrolytes, and acid-base status.

Adrenocortical Hyperfunction. Excessive production of cortisol (i.e., Cushing's disease) is associated with significant morbidity and mortality. Patients without medical therapy will develop comorbid conditions such as cardiovascular disease and diabetes mellitus, further adding to a poor prognosis. Medical therapies decrease morbidity. Like adrenal insufficiency, Cushing's syndrome may be suspected based on the clinical presentation. Laboratory evaluation is then used to confirm the diagnosis (see Figure 30–5). Delineating the etiology defines the medical therapy of choice.

In primary aldosteronism, medical therapy depends on the etiology (Gums & Terpening, 2002). Drug therapy is used only in primary aldosteronism caused by bilateral adrenal hyperplasia. Differentiating the etiologies can be done through the use of computed tomography (CT).

Therapy for women with hirsutism or virilization depends on the extent of the condition and etiology. Short-term measures may include waxing, bleaching, electroly-

TABLE 30–13. Common Causes of Hirsutism

Causes	Clinical Clues
Idiopathic or familial	Pubertal onset, regular menses; no dectectable hyperandrogenism
Ovarian	
Polycystic ovary syndrome/stein leventhal syndrome	Pubertal onset, irregular menses, family history
Androgen-producing ovarian neoplasms (uncommon [0.8%])	Explosive course, virilization, abdominal or pelvic pain
Insulin resistance syndromes	Diabetes, acanthosis nigricans, skin tags
Adrenal	
Nonclassic 21-hydroxylase deficiency	Family history, Ashkenazic Jews; 50% have mineralocorticoid deficiency
Androgen-producing adrenal neoplasms (carcinoma [rare])	Explosive course, virilization, abdominal or flank pain
Cushing's syndrome	Hypertension, muscle weakness, easy bruisability
Hyperprolactinemia	Headaches, seizures, weight gain, visual field cut, extraocular muscle disturbances, gynecomastia, fatigue, cold intolerance, constipation, muscle cramps, spinal cord lesions, herpes zoster, chest wall trauma, breast disease
Medications	
Anabolic steroids	Virilization
Phenytoin, minoxidil, cyclosporine, glucocorticoids	Growth of fine, nonpigmented hair in androgen-independent areas

Sources: Fitzgerald (2002); Plouffe (2000); Taylor, Pillay, & Setrakian (2000).

sis, or shaving, whereas longer-term solutions like weight loss may help to decrease hair growth. Women with dark hair and light skin pigmentation may benefit from laser therapy for facial hirsutism (Fitzgerald, 2002). In more severe cases, drug treatments can include oral contraceptives and antiandrogen drugs such as spironolactone, 50–100 mg bid on days 5.25 of the menstrual cycle, flutamide, 250 mg daily, or finasteride, 5 mg daily. Second- or third-line treatment includes GnRH analogs given in combination with estrogen-progestin therapy (Fitzgerald, 2002).

Short- and Long-Term Goals for Pharmacotherapy

Adrenocortical Hypofunction. The short-term goal for the treatment of adrenal insufficiency and hypoaldosteronism is to relieve patient signs and symptoms (including laboratory abnormalities) using the lowest effective dosing regimen that mimics normal physiologic adrenocortical function. The long-term goal is to improve quality of life (Orth, 2001).

Adrenocortical Hyperfunction. Goals for the treatment of Cushing's disease and aldosteronism are to alleviate symptoms, cure the hypercortisolism or aldosteronism, eliminate any tumor that threatens the patient's health, and minimize the risk of secondary endocrine deficiency and long-term dependence on medications (Orth, 2001).

Goals for the treatment of hirsutism/virilization may include cosmetic or medical treatment. The decision to utilize medical treatment may depend on the severity and degree of distress to the patient.

Time Frame for Initiating Pharmacotherapy

For all adrenocortical disorders, medical intervention is begun at the time of diagnosis. In acutely ill patients with suspected adrenal insufficiency (i.e., addisonian crisis), drug therapy is begun before laboratory confirmation of the suspected diagnosis is received because of patient acuity. Drug treatment may be lifelong, particularly in adrenal insufficiency. Patients who have an adrenal insufficiency should carry documentation so they can be given glucocorticoid therapy in an emergency (Zafar & Wisgerhof, 1999).

See Drug Table 601.

Assessment and History Taking

Adrenocortical Hypofunction. Laboratory data are *less* useful in monitoring the adequacy of adrenocortical replacement therapy than in monitoring thyroid conditions (Orth, 2001). Regardless, a number of laboratory tests are recommended for the diagnosis and treatment of adrenocortical hypofunction. The tests are serum concentrations of ACTH, cortisol, aldosterone, and electrolytes. Blood pressure is used to assess treatment of aldosterone disorders and therefore should be measured prior to the initiation of drug therapy. A baseline patient weight is also helpful.

Adrenocortical Hyperfunction. Prior to initiating therapy for adrenocortical hyperfunction, serum concentrations of ACTH, cortisol, aldosterone, and electrolytes should be obtained. Also, a urinary cortisol concentration should be measured. Baseline measurements of blood pressure and patient weight are necessary. Urine electrolyte levels are useful if primary aldosteronism is suspected.

Patient/Caregiver Information

Examples of patient information for drug treatment of Addison's disease and Cushing's syndrome are given in Tables 30–14 and 30–15, respectively. See also the discussion of patient education for adrenocortical hypofunction in the next section for additional information.

TABLE 30–14. Example of Patient Information for the Treatment of Addison's Disease

Hydrocortisone

- Your body naturally produces cortisone-like hormones that are necessary to maintain good health. Hydrocortisone is like those hormones. Because your body is not producing enough, you must take this medicine to make up the difference.
- Use this medicine only as directed. Do not use more or less of it and do not use it for a longer time than prescribed. If you do, you increase the chances of side effects. Take the medicine at the same time each day to make sure it always has the same effect.
- Take this medicine with food to help prevent stomach upset.
- You may have to take this medicine for the rest of your life. It is very important that you do not stop taking this medicine without first checking with your healthcare professional.
- If you take several doses of this medicine a day and you miss a dose, take it as soon as possible. If it is almost time for your next dose, take both doses together. Then go back to your regular dosing schedule.
- It is very important that your healthcare professional check your progress at regular visits to make sure this medicine is working properly. Any dose changes you may need are based on these visits.
- You should carry a medical identification card stating you have Addison's disease and you are taking this medicine.

Source: United States Pharmacopeial Convention (2000).

TABLE 30–15. Example of Patient Information for the Treatment of Cushing's Syndrome

Ketoconazole

- Even though this medicine is usually for the treatment of serious fungus infections, that is not why you are taking it. Your body naturally produces cortisone-like hormones that are necessary to maintain good health. Because you have Cushing's disease, your body makes too much cortisone. This medicine reduces the body's production of cortisone and helps treat Cushing's disease.
- Use this medicine only as directed. Do not use more or less of it, and do not take it more often than ordered. If you take a different amount than prescribed for you or you take it longer than prescribed, you increase the chances of side effects. Take the medicine at the same time each day to make sure it always has the same effect.
- If you miss a dose of this medicine, take it as soon as possible. However, if it is almost time for your next dose, skip the missed dose and go back to your regular dosing schedule. Do not double doses.
- Make sure all healthcare professionals you see know you are taking this medicine. Also, make sure they are aware of other medicines you now take. If you start taking a new medicine, make sure you state that you take ketoconazole.
- Liver problems are more likely to occur if you drink alcoholic beverages while you take this medicine. Therefore, you should not drink alcoholic beverages or use alcohol-containing products while you are taking this medicine.
- Talk with your healthcare professional before you take any over-the-counter stomach medicines such as antacids.
- This medicine may cause your eyes to become more sensitive to light than they are normally. Wearing sunglasses and avoiding too much exposure to bright light should help.
- Check with your healthcare professional immediately if you develop a rash, cough, fever, or chills that do not go away within a week. Also, check with your doctor if your urine becomes dark or your stools become lighter than normal.
- This medicine usually takes several weeks to have a noticeable effect on your condition. If you do not improve in a month, check with your healthcare professional.

Source: United States Pharmacopecial Convention (2002).

TABLE 30–16. Suggested Protocols for the Treatment of Acute and Chronic Adrenal Insufficiency

Acute Crisis

- Immediate correction of dehydration, sodium depletion, hypotension, and hypoglycemia with intravenous 5% dextrose and normal saline solution.
- Parenteral hydrocortisone 100 mg intravenous bolus followed by 100 mg every 8 h for 24–48 h.
- When the patient improves, convert hydrocortisone to 50 mg orally every 8 h for another 24–48 h.
- Taper oral hydrocortisone to a maintenance dose, usually 30–50 mg/day in divided doses.
- Consider Empire Antibiotics.

Chronic Therapy

- Hydrocortisone 15–20 mg orally every morning (by 8 A.M., approximately) and 5–10 mg orally between 4 and 6 P.M.
- Fludrocortisone 0.05–0.2 mg orally every morning.
- Increase hydrocortisone dose for trauma, surgery, infection or stress.

Sources: Fitzgerald (2002), Orth (2001).

OUTCOMES MANAGEMENT

Selecting an Appropriate Agent

Adrenocortical Hypofunction. Treatment of adrenal insufficiency differs depending on the onset of symptoms. In acute adrenal insufficiency, a patient is exposed to a major stressor (i.e., surgery, trauma) that requires an increased cortisol response. Because of adrenal insufficiency, the patient cannot adequately respond and a life-threatening condition ensues. Again, treatment is begun before laboratory confirmation is received. One potential protocol for the treatment of acute adrenal insufficiency is listed in Table 30–16. Because of the severity of illness, hospitalization is required with intravenous glucocorticoids. The underlying stressor must be identified and corrected to prevent future complications.

Treatment of chronic adrenal insufficiency differs slightly based on classification of the condition as primary or secondary. Primary therapy requires both glucocorticoid and mineralocorticoid replacement, whereas secondary usually requires only glucocorticoid replacement. Table 30–16 includes one potential treatment regimen. A goal of drug therapy is to mimic normal physiologic adrenal secretion. Without disease, endogenous cortisol secretion follows a diurnal rhythm, with 75% of the daily production occurring between 4 and 10 A.M. and another peak occurring in late afternoon or early evening. Dosing regimens should be designed taking this diurnal rhythm into account. Therefore, the total daily dose must be given in two to three divided doses. A suggested daily glucocorticoid replacement is the equivalent of hydrocortisone 12 to 15 mg/m^2, given two-thirds in the morning and one-third in the afternoon or evening. All regimens must be individualized based on the lowest effective dose possible. Some patients may subjectively improve using a three-times-a-day dosing regimen, hence improving their quality of life (Fitzgerald, 2002).

Patient education is extremely important. Patients must understand drug therapy is lifelong. Patients should understand the normal action of cortisol and how production increases in response to stress caused by illness, trauma, etc. They must then be able to adjust their glucocorticoid replacement therapy in response to personal need, similar to the way a person with diabetes increases insulin dosing in response to illness (i.e., sick-day management). A guideline is to double their usual dose for illness associated with vomiting and/or diarrhea not requiring medical attention. When a patient cannot use oral hydrocortisone then it must be administered IM. Patients must be aware of the adverse effects associated with therapy and how to recognize them (e.g., weight gain, edema). Also, patients must know what to do about missed doses (refer back to Table 30–14).

In the treatment of hypoaldosteronism, fludrocortisone alone is used in the same manner as listed in Table 30–16. Dosing is individualized based on response.

Adrenocortical Hyperfunction. Medical treatment of Cushing's syndrome is based on the etiology of hypercortisolism (NIH, 1998). Although the causes of Cushing's syndrome, as shown in Table 30–11, are many, surgery is the therapy of choice. Drug therapy plays only a palliative or adjunctive role. A number of medications have been used for these purposes. When drug therapy is used, the goal of therapy is to lower the mean serum cortisol concentration throughout the day into the range of 150 to 300 nmol/L (NIH, 1998). Four classes of agents are available: steroidogenic blocking drugs, adrenolytic drugs, neuromodulators, and steroid receptor antagonists.

The steroidogenic agents are metyrapone, aminoglutethimide, and ketoconazole. These agents inhibit the adrenal enzymes necessary for the production of cortisol. Currently, ketoconazole appears to be the most effective. It lowers cortisol production promptly with clinical and metabolic effects disappearing within 4 to 6 weeks (Zafar & Wisgerhof, 1999). Further, it has been recommended as the initial agent of choice for most patients. Effective dosages range from 800 to 1200 mg/day divided in two doses. Overall, few patients experience adverse effects. The major adverse effect seen is hepatotoxicity, which occurs in about 12% of patients.

The adrenolytic agent mitotane inhibits biosynthesis of adrenal steroids and destroys adrenocortical cells (Zafar & Wisgerhof, 1999). Side effects include anorexia, nausea, diarrhea, somnolence, pruritis, hypercholesterolemia, and hypouricemia. The recommended dose is 6 to 12 g/day in divided doses.

Neuromodulators used in Cushing's syndrome are bromocriptine, cyproheptadine, and valproate sodium. These agents are thought to decrease ACTH release through their effect on neurotransmitters. Limited success is seen with these agents.

One of the major causes of Cushing's syndrome is Cushing's disease. Again, Cushing's disease is typically caused by a pituitary adenoma. The therapy of choice for Cushing's disease is transsphenoidal adenomectomy (TSA). It is curative in approximately 80% to 85% of cases. Postsurgically, patients require daily glucocorticoid replacement therapy (same as in Table 30–16) for 6 to 12 months, until the hypothalamic-pituitary-adrenal axis recovers. In children, the therapy of choice has been pituitary irradiation with success rates up to 80%. However, newer reports suggest TSA is as effective as irradiation with fewer side effects. Therefore, TSA may be the preferred mode of therapy in children (NIH, 1998).

If TSA fails, pituitary irradiation is suggested. A lag time of 3 to 12 months occurs before hypercortisolism is controlled. Therefore, adjunctive drug therapy is used to control hypercortisolism during this time. In the authors' opinion, ketoconazole will probably become the agent of choice.

Ectopic ACTH syndrome is caused by non-pituitary tumors that secrete ACTH. The therapy of choice is surgical resection, but localization of the tumor with a cure is successful in only about 10% of cases. Therefore, 90% of cases require drug therapy. Again, ketoconazole will probably become the drug of choice. Serum and urinary cortisol concentrations can be measured and used to adjust drug therapy.

In patients with ACTH-independent disease caused by an adrenal adenoma, adrenal carcinoma, or adrenal hyperplasia, surgical resection or removal of the gland is the therapy of choice. If both adrenals are removed, lifelong replacement therapy is indicated (see Table 30–16). With unilateral adrenalectomy, contralateral gland atrophy is common and glucocorticoid replacement therapy is required up to 12 months. Adrenal carcinomas may not be completely resected and require palliative therapy. The drug of choice, at present, is mitotane.

Because so few pregnancies have occurred in women with Cushing's syndrome, no definitive recommendations regarding treatment can be made (Lo, Lo, & Lam, 2002).

As in the case of Cushing's syndrome, medical management of primary aldosteronism depends on the etiology. When the cause is an adrenocortical adenoma, surgical resection is the therapy of choice. When bilateral adrenocortical hyperplasia is the cause, drug therapy is indicated. The therapy of choice is spironolactone. In this particular indication, spironolactone appears to inhibit adrenal gland synthesis of aldosterone (Fitzgerald, 2002). The effective dosage range is 200 to 400 mg/day. It may take 4 to 8 weeks to see the full effect of therapy. Therefore, dosage adjustments usually are not performed until this time. Blood pressure is the primary monitoring parameter used to assess the appropriateness of therapy. In most patients, the drug is well tolerated.

Monitoring for Efficacy

Unlike hypothyroidism, no one test is available to appropriately assess adrenal insufficiency replacement therapy (Orth, 2001). Most clinicians assess the adequacy of therapy clinically. Patients without sufficient replacement retain or develop signs and symptoms of adrenal insufficiency. Patients with excessive replacement develop signs and symptoms of Cushing's syndrome. Thus, subjective improvement and questions regarding symptoms of disease are important markers in assessing drug therapy. Objectively, patient weight, blood pressure, signs of disease, and serum electrolytes are monitored and used to adjust replacement therapy. Most clinicians do not include measurements of serum cortisol and ACTH.

Symptoms usually subside within days from the initiation of therapy. Strength and hyperpigmentation generally take longer to improve (weeks vs. days) (Fitzgerald, 2002). Hyperpigmentation will ameliorate with appropriate replacement, and a lack of improvement may be used to assess the adequacy of therapy.

Adverse drug effects are monitored as well. Symptoms such as dyspepsia, edema, hypertension, hypokalemia, insomnia, and glucose intolerance all indicate an excess of glucocorticoid and/or mineralocorticoid therapy.

In hypoaldosteronism, dosage adjustments are based on serum electrolytes, particularly potassium, and blood pressure response.

REFERENCES

AACE clinical practice guidelines for the evaluation and treatment of hyperthyroidism and hypothyroidism. (1995). *Endocrine Practice, 1,* 54–62.

American Academy of Pediatrics & American Thyroid Association. (1993). Newborn screening for congenital hypothyroidism: Recommended guidelines. *Pediatrics, 91,* 1203–1209.

American College of Physicians. (1998). Clinical guideline, part 1. Screening for thyroid disease. *Annals of Internal Medicine, 129,* 141–143.

Bryer-Ash, M. (2001). Evaluation of the patient with a suspected thyroid disorder. *Obstetrics and Gynecology Clinics of North America, 28*(2), 421–38.

Caldwell, G., Kellett, H. A., Gow, S. M., Sweeting, V. M., Kellett, H. A., Becket, G. J., Seth, J., & Toft, A. D. (1985). A new strategy for thyroid function testing. *Lancet, 1,* 1117–1119.

Chung, U., Tanaka, Y., & Fujita, T. (1996). Association of interleukin-6 and hypoaldosteronism in patients with cancer. *New England Journal of Medicine, 334,* 473.

Fitzgerald, P. A. (2002). Endocrinology. In L. M. Tierney, Jr., S. J. McPhee, & M. A. Papadakis (Eds.), *Current medical diagnosis and treatment* (pp. 1121–1201). New York: Lange/McGraw-Hill.

Forget, H., Lacroix, A., & Cohen, H. (2002). Persistent cognitive impairment following surgical treatment of Cushing's syndrome. *Psychoneuroendocrinology, 27*(3), 367–383.

Franklyn, J. A. (1997). Management guidelines for hyperthyroidism. *Bailliere's Clinical Endocrinology and Metabolism, 11,* 561–571.

Glinoer, D. (1999). What happens to the normal thyroid during pregnancy? *Thyroid, 9*(7), 631–635.

Gums, J. G., & Terpening, C. M. (2002). Adrenal disorders. In J. T. DiPiro, R. L. Talbert, G. C. Yee, G. R. Matzke, B. G. Wells, & L. M. Posey (Eds.), *Pharmacotherapy: A pathophysiologic approach* (5th ed.; pp. 1379–1393). New York: McGraw-Hill.

Herfindal, E. T., & Gourley, D. R. (2000). *Textbook of therapeutics: Drug and disease management* (7th ed.). Philadelphia: Lippincott Williams & Wilkins.

Hershman, J. M., Ladenson, P. W. & Pawshock, B. Z. (1992). A savvy approach to thyroid testing. *Patient Care, 26*(3): 134–151.

Johnson, T. L., & Amin, M. B. (1999). Pathology of the adrenal glands. In J. C. Cerny (Ed.), *Medical and surgical management of adrenal diseases.* New York: Williams and Wilkins.

Kirsten, D. (2000). The thyroid gland: physiology and pathophysiology. *Neonatal Network, 19*(8), 11–26.

Koch, C. A., & Sarlis, N. J. (2001). The spectrum of thyroid diseases in childhood and its evolution during transition to adulthood: Natural history, diagnosis, differential diagnosis and management. *Journal of Endocrinological Investigation 24*(9), 659–675.

Kovacs, K. A., Lam, Y. M., & Pater, J. L. (2001). Bilateral massive adrenal hemorrhage. Assessment of putative risk factors by the case-control method. *Medicine, 80* 45.

Laureti, S., Aubourg, P., Calcinaro, F., et al. (1998). Etiological diagnosis of primary adrenal insufficiency using an original flowchart of immune and biochemical markers. *Journal of Clinical Endocrinology and Metabolism, 83,* 3163.

Lazarus, J. H., & Obuobie, K. (2000). Thyroid disorders-an update. *Postgraduate Medical Journal, 76,* 529–536.

Lo, C. Y., Lo, C. M., & Lam, K. Y. (2002). Cushing's syndrome secondary to adrenal adenoma during pregnancy. *Surgical Endoscopy, 16*(1), 219–220.

Madeddu, G., Spanu, A., Falchi, A., & Nuvoli, S. (1999). Clinical and laboratory assessment of subclinical thyroid disease. *Rays, 24*(2), 229–242.

Marsh, H. M., & Kim, J. G. (1999). Anesthesia for adrenal surgery. In J.C. Cerny (Ed.), *Medical and surgical management of adrenal diseases.* New York: Williams and Wilkins.

Mestman, J. (1999). Diagnosis and management of maternal and fetal thyroid disorders. *Current Opinion in Obstetric's and Gynecology 11*(2) 167–175.

National Institutes of Health. (1998). Adrenal conditions. Office of Health Reports. www.niddk.nih.gov. Accessed September 20, 2002.

National Institutes of Health. (2000). *Managing adrenal insufficiency.* Baltimore: Patient Information Pubs.

Orth, D. N. (1995). Cushing's syndrome. *New England Journal of Medicine, 332,* 791–803.

Orth, D. N. (2001). Causes of primary adrenal insufficiency. In B.D. Rose, (Ed.), Wellesley, MA: UpToDate, www. uptodate.com. Accessed September 17, 2002.

Perry, R.J., Findlay, C.A., & Donaldson, M.D. (2002). *Archives of Disease in Childhood, 87*(1), 45–48.

Plouffe, L. Jr. (2000). Disorders of excessive hair growth in the adolescent. *Obstetrics and Gynecology Clinics of North America, 27*(1), 79–99.

Ramschak-Schwarzer, S., Radkohl, W., Stiegler, C., Dimai, H. P., & Leb, G. (2000). Interaction between psychotropic drugs and thyroid hormone metabolism—An overview. *Acta Med Austriaca, 27,* 8–10.

Reasner, C. A., & Talbert, R. L. (2002). Thyroid disorders. In J. T. DiPiro, R. L. Talbert, G. C. Yee, G. R. Matzke, B. G. Wells, & L. M. Posey (Eds.), *Pharmacotherapy: A pathophysiologic approach* (5th ed.; pp. 1359–1378). New York: McGraw-Hill.

Sergev, O., & Wisgerhof, M. (1999). Primary aldosteronism. In J.C. Cerny (Ed.), *Medical and surgical management of adrenal diseases.* New York: Williams and Wilkins.

Shagam, J.Y. (2001). Thyroid disease: An overview. *Radiologic Technology, 73*(1), 25–40.

Shrier, D. K., & Burman K. D. (2002). Subclinical hyperthyroidism: Controversies in management. *American Family, 65,* 431–438.

Taylor, H.C., Pillay, I., & Setrakian, S. (2000). Diffuse stromal Leydig cell hyperplasia: A unique cause of postmenopausal hyperandrogenism and virilization. *Mayo Clinic Proceedings, 75*(3), 288–292.

United States Pharmacopeial Convention. (2000). Advice for the Patient USP DI Vol. II (20th ed.). Micromedex, Inc., Englewood CO: The United States Pharmacopeial Convention, Inc.

Young, L. Y., & Koda-Kimble, M. A. (Eds.). (1995). *Applied therapeutics: The clinical use of drugs* (6th ed.). Vancouver, WA: Applied Therapeutics.

Zafar, M. S., & Wisgerhof, M. (1999). Cushing's syndrome. In J. C. Cerny (Ed.), *Medical and surgical management of adrenal diseases.* New York: Lippincott Williams & Wilkins.

CHAPTER ❖ 31

ENDOCRINE DISORDERS: DIABETES MELLITUS

Martha J. Price ◆ *Daniel J. Kent*

The treatment of diabetes mellitus has been dramatically influenced in the past 25 years by improved diagnosis and classification of the disease, first by the National Diabetes Data Group in 1979, and most recently by an expert committee's review of the current state of the diabetes diagnostic and classification evidence (American Diabetes Association, 2004). Both classification efforts have helped to track and synthesize the most relevant information to better understand diabetes' etiology, pathophysiology and progression. The pharmaceutical market, too, has kept pace with these changes, and the projected treatment for the 21st century suggests that therapies, as we now know them, will give way to new and combined agents, including preventive therapies.

CHARACTERISTICS OF DIABETES MELLITUS

Diabetes mellitus is a metabolic syndrome characterized by hyperglycemia from an absolute or relative lack of the pancreatic hormone, insulin. Insulin is an essential hormone that allows glucose, the body's principal energy source, to enter insulin-dependent tissue—skeletal muscle, liver, fat cells. Elevated blood glucose and associated symptoms, such as polydipsia (increased thirst) and polyuria (increased urinary frequency) are diagnostic markers. More specifically, using the aforementioned American Diabetes Association (2004) criteria, a casual plasma glucose $>$200 mg/dl accompanied by symptoms of diabetes or a fasting plasma glucose of $>$126 mg/dl supports the diagnosis of diabetes mellitus. Unless hyperglycemia is unequivocal, FPG should be repeated on 2 separate occasions. Normal fasting glycemia range is 70 to 110 mg/dL. Weight loss and fluid and electrolyte imbalance may also accompany the onset, particularly in type 1 diabetes which is caused by pancreatic beta cell destruction. Type 2, the most common type of diabetes, may present more subtly over a period of years with symptoms of fatigue, blurred vision, and persistent infections, such as vaginal candidiasis. Classification of diabetes types, as accepted by the World Health Organization (1985) include type 1 diabetes, type 2 diabetes, secondary diabetes, gestational diabetes, and impaired glucose tolerance (IGT). In the short term, very elevated hyperglycemia may pose a threat to stable fluid and electrolyte balance. Long-term complications of diabetes result in chronic macrovascular, microvascular and neurologic changes, increasing the risk of disability and death from myocardial infarction, stroke, and end organ damage to eyes, kidneys, extremities, and autonomic functioning, such as gastrointestinal and sexual disorders.

Diabetes is genetically determined, and onset is influenced by environmental factors. Those factors are particularly best known in type 2 diabetes where obesity and sedentary lifestyles pose greatest risk. Persons of Hispanic, Native American, and African American ethnicity and those with a known family history of diabetes would do well to adjust diet and activity to prevent or delay diabetes onset (Diabetes Prevention Program Research Group, 2002).

THE TWO MOST COMMON TYPES OF DIABETES

Type 1 Diabetes

In type 1 diabetes the pathophysiology lies in the autoimmune destruction of the pancreatic beta cells, thus insulin replacement is the critical component of treatment. Hyperglycemia associated with this type of diabetes is often accompanied by elevated triglycerides, insulin resistance during very elevated hyperglycemia (over 250 mg/dl), production of ketones, alteration of counterregulatory hormone production, and weight loss. Failure to treat adequately with insulin results in catabolism, ketoacidosis, and death. If treatment is sufficient to prevent ketoacidosis, but not adequate to control continuous hyperglycemia, the risk of microvascular disease resulting in nephropathy, retinopathy, and neuropathy is increased. The Diabetes Control and Complications Trial (DCCT) (Diabetes Control and Complications Trial Research Group, 1993) and the United Kingdom Prospective Diabetes Study (UKPDS) conclusively demonstrated that diabetics who achieve and maintain near-normal glycemia can prevent or markedly slow such microvascular complications.

The current pharmacological goal of treating type 1 diabetes is to 1) replace insulin; 2) achieve a balance of insulin, food, and activity compatible with the individual's growth and development; and 3) achieve an average range of fasting blood glucose between 70 to 110 mg/dl. In addition to available insulin treatment, newer therapies are emerging that include insulin analogs, potential alteration and/or reduction in the rate or onset of pancreatic beta cell destruction, and altering metabolism via rate of carbohydrate absorption.

Type 2 Diabetes

Hyperglycemia is also the hallmark of *type 2 diabetes mellitus,* however, the etiology of this form of diabetes differs markedly from type 1. Its etiology includes a progression of events that includes alteration in beta cell production of insulin, resistance to insulin uptake at the target cells (skeletal muscle, liver, fat), and increased hepatic secretion of glycogen (DeFronzo, 1988). When insulin cannot link up with the insulin receptors along the target cell rim, glucose is prevented from entering the cell. It is not uncommon for relatively high doses of exogenous insulin to be required to overcome this insulin resistance. In contrast, smaller amounts of exogenous insulin are needed to suppress hepatic release of glycogen stores.

Type 2 diabetes is more likely to have associated obesity and hypertension, and the major mortality risks are from cardiovascular events—myocardial infarction and stroke. The common blood lipid pattern in this type of diabetes is very similar to those at risk for CVD—elevated total cholesterol and LDL-cholesterol, and lower HDL-cholesterol.

Not all people with type 2 are overweight (about 20% are not overweight), and this may actually be another variation in the genetic expression of diabetes as a disease. These individuals are more likely to exhaust their endogenous insulin supply, fail sulfonylurea therapy, and need insulin therapy to prevent severe hyperglycemia.

Children and Adolescents

The discussion of medications in this chapter applies to individuals of all ages. However, as diabetes in children and adolescents is a complex disease requiring multifaceted care, close followup by a pediatric diabetes treatment team is recommended. Type 1 diabetes in children is managed with a combination of insulin by injection or pump, meal planning, and blood glucose self-monitoring. Type 2 diabetes in children and adolescents is increasing exponentially and is an emerging public health problem. Presentation of type 2 in children and adolescents may be similar to older individuals. Parents report that short- and long-term complications, the complexity of day-to-day management, the challenges of transferring responsibility for diabetes self-management to their youth are their major concerns. The primary care provider should find the discussion of these issues in this chapter useful in understanding and participating in treatment and followup of type 1 and type 2 diabetes.

DIABETES AND PHARMACOLOGICAL AIMS

To understand the rationale of pharmacologic approaches for diabetes treatment, it is important to first understand what occurs when diabetes is *not* present. In the non-diabetes state, insulin and accompanying counterregulatory hormones—glucagon, growth hormone, glucocorticoids, and epinephrine—exist in a continuous rising and falling balance to keep blood glucose contained within a narrow range (fasting of 70–110 mg/dl; 4-6 mmol/l); casual plasma glucose $<$200 mg/dl (11.1 mmol/l). When this balance is upset because of lack of insulin or inability to use endogenous insulin, the treatment must be targeted to the areas of deficiency and/or defect.

Any attempt to artificially reproduce what the body would normally do if diabetes were not present brings with it the potential for untoward side effects of treatment. Diabetes therapies that directly reduce hyperglycemia also pose the risk of hypoglycemia. Hypoglycemic danger exists because insulin and oral hypoglycemic agents must be offered as *open-loop therapy, meaning that there is no automatic feedback loop for controlled release of counterregulatory hormones to keep blood glucose within a physiologic normal and safe range.* The body will be unable to respond with an automatic reduction in the agent's action if blood glucose begins to fall below normal (i.e., 70 mg/dl). Keeping the balance between a sufficient metabolically stable blood glucose level and avoiding hyperglycemia or hypoglycemia requires near constant vigilance and self-management. For this reason, food is an essential factor in the treatment of diabetes management. Sufficient calories and nutrients to sustain normal weight and activity will be required, and appropriate timing of both has to be coordinated with hypoglycemic drugs. Activity and exercise are also critical cornerstones of treatment, because diabetes mellitus, as a disease of metabolism, will effect how the body is able to access quick energy and store/release energy for activity needs. For these reasons, pharmacotherapeutics for diabetes will necessarily require concurrent attention to food and activity patterns as essential components of any treatment equation.

As more information becomes available about the pathophysiology of diabetes, the question for clinicians will be necessarily expanded from "*how can blood glucose control be achieved?*" to "*how will this particular therapy affect the processes and outcomes of the disease known as diabetes?*" This perspective is so important that it is suggested that the clinician view ALL pharmacological therapies with the questions posed in Table 31–1 in mind.

TABLE 31–1. Questions to ask when Selecting Antidiabetes Therapy

1. How will this agent affect blood glucose? (Does it exert a direct effect on lowering glucose and is severe hypoglycemia a possible side effect?)
2. How will this agent affect blood lipids?
3. How will this agent affect end-organs most frequently affected by diabetes?
4. How will this agent affect body weight?
5. How will this agent affect hepatic glucose production?
6. How will this agent affect counterregulatory hormones?
7. Will this agent likely be altered by over-the-counter, self-prescribed therapies?
8. What is the science base to support use of this agent within specific age ranges?
9. What food, activity, and monitoring conditions must be met for this agent to be safely administered? Can the patient or family meet these conditions?
10. Even if the agent is the drug of choice, is it the drug of choice for THIS patient given the pharmaco-dynamics and associated self-management requirements and costs?
11. What information is available regarding outcomes of long-term use of this agent?

SETTING GLYCEMIC GOALS

In addition to targeting therapies to reduce the organ damage of diabetes, whether microvascular or macrovascular, it is important to set safe, therapeutic targets for blood glucose. Setting glycemic goals needs to be considered within what is safest, in the short term, and most beneficial, in the long term, for the individual patient. Current science should guide this decision. The Diabetes Control and Complications Trial (DCCT) and the United Kingdom Prospective Diabetes Study (UKPDS) results indicate that the glycemic level is positively correlated to degree of rate of microvascular damage. That is, when glycemia levels are persistently above normal (HbA1c >7%), the rate of damage to eyes, kidneys, and nerves rises exponentially (Diabetes Control and Complications Trial Research Group, 1993). Those DCCT data also show that even modest reductions in HbA1c can reduce the rate of eye, kidney, and nerve damage. With glycated hemoglobins (HbA1c assay) nearing normal values (4–6%) the rate of end-organ damage is reduced substantially; *however,* the *risk of hypoglycemia* increases. Achieving consistence euglycemia may be contraindicated for some patients whose quality of life and safety (i.e., risk of hypoglycemia) would be adversely affected.

While the DCCT and UKPDS studies verify the protective effect that good glycemic control has on microvascular damage from diabetes, the science is accumulating about glycemic control's effect on macrovascular disease, i.e., risk of heart attack and stroke (UKPDS, 1995). Therefore, an essential focus of treatment for diabetes must continue to give concentrated attention to reducing cardiovascular risks—diet and exercise; no smoking or tobacco use; controlling hypertension; daily use of aspirin when possible to prevent CVD events; and appropriate use of ACE inhibitors and statins. (H.O.P.E. Study, 2000; H.P.S., 2002). Overall treatment is targeted to support maintenance of desired body weight, control of blood lipids, and reduction of hyperglycemia. These recommended risk reductions are often difficult to treat because they require, for the most part, lifestyle or major behavioral change.

Type 1 therapy should be aimed at insulin replacement via regimens that afford the best glycemic control given the patient's capacity and willingness to attend to multiple self-management behaviors and problem-solving techniques.

The treatment for Type 2 is targeted to supporting endogenous insulin production and utilization, a reduction in insulin resistance, and suppression of hepatic glucose release during nocturnal fasting (sleep). As the disease progresses with further reduction in insulin production, exogenous insulin may need to be added to oral therapies.

Thus, type 2 diabetes may actually require a combination of several therapies to achieve desired physiologic balance. A stepped approach to type 2 treatment is aimed towards improved glycemic control and reduction of cardiovascular risks. Diet and exercise remain important cornerstones to therapy for type 2 diabetes, and should be encouraged to the best that the patient can manage.

Consistent, ideal blood glucose levels (70–110 mg/dl for fasting blood glucose; a random blood glucose of 70–126 mg/dl) corresponds to a glycated hemoglobin (HbA1c) of approximately 6 to 7% or less. However, factors such as age, cognitive skills, accompanying co-morbidities, and psychosocial characteristics all need to be taken into consideration, when setting glycemia goals.

THE IMPORTANT ROLE OF SELF-MANAGEMENT IN EFFECTIVE DIABETES THERAPY

Whether the treatment plan is limited to diet and exercise or includes one or more pharmacotherapeutic agents, self-management is an essential ongoing activity for successful outcomes. Self-management will depend upon diabetes acuity, end organ damage, and perceived treatment goals. The actual activities prescribed for self-management will depend upon the age, cognitive and psychomotor skills, psychosocial resources and the value that the patient and/or his or her family place on treatment and self-management.

Obviously, there is no "easy" age at which to be diagnosed with diabetes. Each developmental stage presents its own demands and challenges. The child, adolescent or young adult in whom type 1 diabetes is most common, requires a treatment schedule that most mimics the insulin production and glucose utilization in the nondiabetic person. Without proper treatment, growth and development can be adversely affected. Yet near euglycemia targets place the type 1 patient at risk for hypoglycemia.

In the child under age 13, the treatment goals should target promotion of healthy growth and development while avoiding severe hyperglycemia and diabetic ketoacidosis and severe hypoglycemia. The older child will need to learn diabetes management skills that avoid acute complications and sustain the best possible glycemic control.

A tighter glycemic control regimen requires multiple decisions to be made during the course of the day regarding types and amounts of food, as well as types and amounts of insulin. These decisions must be made on a variety of data: blood glucose test results, physical signs and symptoms, and knowledge of which factors can or have affected blood glucose levels. Couple these treatment demands with the child's need to develop his or her own self-identity and social self, and the challenges for patients and their families come into sharper focus.

Questions abound about when to give the child responsibility and how much. Most of the family literature regarding diabetes has been focused on type 1 diabetes and the special challenges of the child and family with diabetes. The available evidence clearly shows that children who are provided with loving parental guidance, as well as caring and patient teaching per their own readiness, can succeed in learning to take on self-management (Giordano, Petrila, Banion, and Neuenkirchen, 1992; Hentinen & Kyngäs, 1996; Grey, Cameron & Thurber, 1991). Families will need accurate and supportive information from their healthcare provider. It will not be sufficient for the provider to know and prescribe the various diabetes pharmacotherapeutics; therapeutics he or she will also be required to skillfully guide and support the patient and family in the application of therapy and determine the readiness of the child to assume responsibility for tasks and decision making. This includes being aware of the support resources available to patients and families in the care setting, community, or region.

OTHER IMPORTANT PHARMACOTHERAPEUTICS FOR DIABETES MANAGEMENT

Although the remainder of this chapter is dedicated to discussion of those agents that specifically lower blood glucose, the reader is referred to Chapter 20 for information on the agents used to control cardiovascular disease and lipoprotein management as well as discussion of ACE-inhibitors as the drug of choice to reduce the progression and/or onset of diabetes renal disease. Diabetes pharmacotherapeutics are changing rapidly. Development and availability of new glucose-lowering agents will likely increase the complexity of designing effective diabetes treatment regimens. At the same time, diet and exercise remain powerful tools in the treatment of type 2 diabetes and should not be minimized or replaced entirely with drug therapy.

SPECIFIC CONSIDERATIONS FOR PHARMACOTHERAPY

NONPHARMACOLOGIC THERAPY

Because diabetes mellitus is a metabolic disease, nutrition and exercise remain the most essential part of diabetes management. In type 2 diabetes, weight management and exercise are the initial focus because insulin resistance can be dramatically improved with minimal weight loss (10% of body weight), and drug therapy is reserved for those requiring additional glycemic management (Franz, 1994). Even though type 1 diabetes will require insulin replacement, that replacement regimen will require coordination with meal planning, meal patterns, and adjusting insulin to match activity level and food intake. Establishing individual caloric needs necessary to maintain desired body weight is best achieved by balancing carbohydrate, fat, and protein intake. The American Diabetes Association recommends dietary intake of these nutrients to be individualized to the particular patient. However, the following can be used as a guide to plan nutrition therapy: carbohydrate intake of 50 to 60% with a fiber content of 20 to 30 gm daily, fat comprising less than 30% (10% saturated) of calories, and protein 10 to 20% of the total daily calorie content. Goals of therapy remain the same—euglycemia, optimal lipid management, weight management, and maintenance of self-management behaviors (Franz, 2002). Even before or along with a dietary referral, the primary care provider can easily reinforce good nutrition principles of quality or balance in healthy, low-fat food choices (the Food Guide Pyramid is an easy place to start), in appropriate quantities or serving sizes, and, if on glucose-lowering drugs, being consistent in the timing of meals and amounts of carbohydrates (Powers, 1996). The general benefits of exercise apply to all humans, including those with diabetes, and the primary care provider can promote participation in consistent, planned physical exercise (American Diabetes Association, 2004).

WHEN DRUG THERAPY IS NEEDED

Type 1 diabetes must be treated by replacing insulin. The ideal insulin replacement regimen would be to try to approximate the normal, physiological pattern of insulin release and glucose utilization. For the older adult with type 1 diabetes, this regimen may necessarily be modified to prioritize safety and quality of life. In type 1 diabetes, nutrition and exercise are important adjuncts to successful insulin therapy.

In type 2, dietary management and exercise are the cornerstones of treatment. About 80% of those with type 2 diabetes are likely to require weight reduction and effort at maintaining a desirable body weight. Evidence is now available to support primary use of ACE-inhibitors (HOPE, 2000) and lipid-lowering agents (HPS, 2002).

Diet and exercise alone may not be sufficient therapy for someone with type 2 diabetes, and if target glycemic goals are not attained by these requisite steps, then adding (not displacing diet and exercise) drug therapy must be considered. Generally, monotherapy is tried first, but combinations are becoming more common. Each step of therapy needs to be given sufficient trial and careful followup to see if glycemic targets (HbA1c and FPG goals) can be attained. This means careful attention to diet, exercise, and blood glucose monitoring and glycated hemoglobin data. The choice of therapy is matched to the specific pathophysiology defect, and in the case of type 2 is usually targeted at decreasing insulin resistance and improving endogenous insulin production. Thus, begin with monotherapy of metformin (UKPDS, 1995). Then, if goals are not achieved after a full 3-month trial, or are not sustained, a combination therapy is the next step. More specifics are given below by drug agent. Monitor each step as carefully as any scientific experiment. Keep as many glucose influencing factors as constant and controlled for as long as possible. The art of this treatment approach cannot be underestimated. To find a therapeutic regimen for each patient requires a full partnership between the patient and healthcare providers.

SHORT-TERM AND LONG-TERM GOALS OF PHARMACOTHERAPY

Setting specific glycemic goals using intermediate and longer-term markers of success are critical for patient motivation and accomplishment of desired health outcomes. Short-term markers include monitoring for improvement in blood pressure; blood lipids: cholesterol, low-density lipoproteins (LDLs), high-density lipoproteins (HDLs), and triglycerides; body weight reduction; and a trend toward the targeted hemoglobin A1c. The patient should be encouraged to participate in daily self-blood glucose monitoring frequently enough to discern whether treatment is effective. For type 2 patients on either monotherapy or two oral agents, a fasting and pre-evening meal glucose testing schedule may be sufficient. The patient who wants to achieve and maintain normal glycemic control will require blood tests and decision making throughout the day, including post prandial testing. Longer-term goals will focus on overall weight management, evidence of lipid control, and reduction of microvascular and macrovascular complications.

There is currently a controversy over the importance of post-prandial glycemic control. While evidence clearly supports overall glycemic control (i.e., HbAlc under 7%) to reduce microvascular and macrovascular damage from diabetes, the data are not available (except in pregnant women with diabetes) to show that post-prandial control makes a therapeutic difference in outcomes. If post-prandial normoglycemia is the goal, there are now pharmacotherapies available to make this possible, but each agent adds cost and patient self-management burden.

TIME FRAME FOR INITIATING AND MODIFYING PHARMACOTHERAPY

For those with type 1 diabetes, insulin therapy is initiated at the time of diagnosis. Primary care team support should target not only finding the most effective insulin dose, but also helping the patient incorporate this therapy into daily living. The challenge with this therapy is most often learning how to achieve pattern management. Pattern management is both collecting and using information from blood glucose test results along with the type of and timing of meals and the influence of varying levels of activity or exercise. When glycemic management is modified, it is useful to apply and monitor the changes for at least 1 to 2 weeks. Overall glycemic changes can be evaluated by laboratory data of a glycated hemoglobin as often as every 2 to 3 months. The major guide is whether the treatment approach is bringing about glycemic shifts towards the preferred targeted range.

In type 2 diabetes, initiating drug therapy depends first on an individual's ability to successfully use nutrition and exercise. A reasonable trial period, during which concerted effort is applied, is 2 to 3 months. If the target glycemic goal has not been reached by then, it is reasonable to consider adding oral drug therapy to the continued diet and exercise program. As with type 1, the glycemic targets will guide the therapeutic approach and determine over time if changes are needed.

ASSESSMENT AND HISTORY TAKING

The same principles of general health screening apply to persons with diabetes. However, careful monitoring for end-organ damage secondary to DM is essential. The American Diabetes Association publishes information on clinical practice recommendations for those providers who may encounter patients with diabetes (American Diabetes Association, 2004). General assessment for type 1 and type 2 diabetes should include review of current cardiovascular risks (smoking status, blood pressure, weight, exercise, and nutrition habits), routine retinal screening, evaluation of the presence of microalbuminuria, foot ulcer risk, as well as establishing a glycemic management plan appropriate to the individual patient's targeted treatment goals.

Laboratory evaluation should include glycated hemoglobin, fasting lipid profile, serum creatinine, urinalysis, albumin/creatinine ratio for microalbuminuria, thyroid function tests if indicated, and electrocardiogram in adults.

The frequency of visits thereafter need to be determined by treatment goals and the requisite monitoring to assess treatment effectiveness. At the very least an annual examination would be wise to repeat evaluation of cardiovascular risk factors and assessment of eyes, kidneys, feet, and glycemic control. In addition, an evaluation of the patient's self-management skills and behaviors as pertain to the treatment plan and patient's goals needs to occur. This can be done by careful review of the presence and frequency of hyper- and hypoglycemia symptoms, the blood glucose test results record, current medication regimen and how administered, and review of typical day's meals, work, and exercise times.

Encourage the patient to self-manage and self-monitor to help determine the effectiveness of a specific treatment approach. The questions in Table 31-2 can help both the patient and the healthcare provider determine treatment self-management requirements and effectiveness. For example, if insulin is prescribed, the patient has to know how to prepare and administer an injection, how to store insulin, how and when to test blood glucose, what and when to eat, and how to detect and treat mild or se-

TABLE 31–2. Questions to Help the Patient Evaluate the Effectiveness of Anti-Diabetes Therapies

1. How will this agent affect my blood glucose? (Does it exert a *direct effect* on lowering glucose and is severe hypoglycemia a possible side effect?)
2. How often do I need to test my blood glucose? What can/should I do with the information?
3. What are the short-term effects (including side effects) of the agent?
4. What are the long-term side effects of the agent?
5. How will this agent affect me in preventing or slowing diabetes complications?
6. How will this agent affect my weight?
7. How will this agent affect my cholesterol and lipid levels?
8. How will this agent affect hepatic glucose production?
9. How will this agent affect counterregulatory hormones?
10. Will this agent likely be changed by over-the-counter, self-prescribed therapies?
11. Is this the best agent for someone of my age, physical condition, and living situation?
12. Do I have to be careful about when and what I eat because of this agent?
13. Do I have to watch how exercise affects this agent? How can I prevent my blood glucose from going too high or too low because of exercise effects?
14. Does my family or live-in partner need to be taught how to treat a reaction to this agent? What if there is no one to do this for me?
15. How will I know if this treatment is not working? When or how often should I be in touch with the provider?

vere hypoglycemia. It may also be helpful for the patient to understand what insulin is intended to accomplish in terms of successful treatment. For example, the intention of therapy with insulin for a type 1 diabetic who makes no endogenous insulin is quite different from the prescription for a type 2 diabetic of a single bedtime dose of intermediate acting insulin to suppress nocturnal hepatic glucose release.

Although there are many literature resources for patients with diabetes mellitus, none are likely to be effective unless the healthcare provider or team can integrate the information into the specific patient's overall management plan. The American Diabetes Association (1660 Duke Street, Alexandria, VA 22314) has many kinds of educational materials—pamphlets, tapes, video, and low-literacy reading material—to assist patients and professionals in learning about and managing diabetes. Because much of the information is generalized, the healthcare team can assist with interpretation to make it most meaningful for the individual. The pharmaceutical industry also can help with developing disease management programs, setting up specific delivery approaches, and providing specific diabetes product aids. These products range from specific drug agents to durable goods, such as insulin delivery devices, including pens, air-jet injectors, glucose measuring monitors, test monitoring strips, and visual (large-type, Braille) devices.

OUTCOMES MANAGEMENT

SELECTING AN APPROPRIATE AGENT

Because hyperglycemia depends on the specific pathology, it is important to try to match the pharmacological agent with the targeted defect. In type 1 diabetes this choice is always insulin replacement. In type 2 diabetes, the disease can express in varying degrees of insulin resistance, compensated insulin production by the pancreatic beta cell, and hepatic glucose secretion. Individuals with type 2 diabetes and obesity generally have greater insulin resistance and require agents to improve this problem. Also, these individuals may benefit from bedtime doses of an intermediate acting insulin to suppress the release of hepatic glucose. Daytime use of metformin and/or sulfonylurea or insulin sensitizer are continued along with the bedtime NPH insulin. Continuing oral meds accomplishes support at different points in the pathophysiology chain and helps to control glycemia during the day and over meal times; however, if daytime blood glucose values begin to rise on this combination therapy, then it is appropriate to consider starting a daytime insulin regimen and discontinuing the sulfonylurea. Those type 2 diabetics who are non-obese are more likely to progress from oral agent therapy alone to daytime insulin supplements. The important caveat is that all diabetes changes over time and requires monitoring to assess its progress and effect on overall systemic health. Thus, therapies need to be evaluated and modified over time to achieve optimal glycemic control.

A stepped approach to targeting glycemic control in type 2 diabetes can be considered as long as appropriate judgment is applied to the patient situation and accounts for severity of hyperglycemic or hypoglycemic symptoms. Using a stepped approach is best done by first setting hemoglobin A1c and pre-meal targets. Later, if warranted, post-prandial targets can be set.

The following stepped sequence is a proposed guide as used by these authors and is based on consideration of available best scientific evidence. This is not intended to be a rigid recipe for drug therapy in type 2 diabetes management. As more diabetes agents and suggested combinations for use become available, the reader is encouraged to keep in mind not only the specific action of each agent, but also that specific agents may be needed at certain points in the disease progression. For example, insulin production in the type 2 patient will diminish over time and no longer be responsive to sulfonylureas or insulin secretogogues.

***Step 1** would be a prescription for a 6 week to 3 month trial of diet and activity.* Type 2 patients who present at diagnosis with mild symptoms and blood glucoses averaging under 250 mg/dl may be first treated with a concerted effort in diet and exercise for a period of 6 weeks to 3 months (Franz, 1994). Sources may vary in suggested length of time for trialing this step, but the reader is encouraged to choose a short time frame for evaluation follow-up in order to stay ahead of any needed adjustments.

If significant effort to diet and exercise do not achieve blood glucose targets, or if the patient is unable or unwilling to make or sustain such changes, then medications will be needed to achieve glucose control.

If the presentation is that of consistently higher blood glucose (well over 250 or 300 mg/dl), and with serious symptoms of fatigue, polydipsia, and polyuria, consideration should be given to aggressive, initial treatment with insulin, as well as dietary modification, to bring blood glucose levels to a more euglycemic state. Once accomplished, it may then be possible to start a short trial at step 2.

Step 2 would be to add a single oral agent, a biguanide (metformin) or sulfonylurea. Metformin is the preferred choice of the authors (DeFronzo, et al., 1995), and, if day time blood glucose levels remain or begin to be higher than the set target, a sulfonylurea might be added. A sulfonylurea choice needs to be based on some clinical judgment regarding how recent the diagnosis has been and whether or not it is likely that type 2 patient will be able to respond to stimulated insulin production.

***Step 3** is to* add late evening/bedtime NPH insulin to bring the fasting blood glucose into target (most often under 130 mg/ml). Some clinicians might add an insulin sensitizer in the form of a thiazolidinedione (TZD) at this point, but there remains a lack of clarity about the best point of inclusion of these agents. Because of their potential for serious side effects, and because there are data to support the value of adding evening NPH while continuing the daytime use of metformin, the authors' *Step 3* is to add bedtime NPH. (The authors use an initial dose of 12 units if patient weighs less than 200 lbs. and 20 units if patient weighs more than 200 lbs.) Dosing for NPH may need to increase weekly to achieve a fasting blood glucose (bg) target that has been set for the specific patient.

Step 4 is needed when daytime blood glucose levels (pre-meal) consistently exceed target. At this point, diet, exercise, metformin and evening NPH insulin are continued, and a daytime insulin regimen selected. There are multiple choices, such as a fast acting analog before all or select meals; or twice daily NPH; or twice daily Ultralente. If the patient has been on sulfonylureas up to this point, it is worth stopping this agent while continuing to evaluate the blood glucose patterns, but to continue with the metformin.

Variations or modifications in the suggested step-wise approach might be necessary for tight post prandial glycemic control (i.e., 2 hour post-meal average of <140 mg/dl). Agents that can help with this aim are the alpha glucosidase inhibitors, the short-acting insulin anlogs, or the insulin secretogues (meglitamines or phenylalnines).

One additional caveat to consider is that giving the maximum dose of an agent is not always warranted. The decision to increase dosage should be accompanied by careful evaluation of whether the increase improves overall glycemic control and diabetes health. If not, then the therapy is both ineffective and expensive, and another treatment approach should to be considered.

Alpha-Glucosidase Inhibitors

Alpha-glucosidase inhibitors are one of several classes of drugs that work to slow or delay the absorption of carbohydrates prior to their digestion to glucose and other monosaccharides. They exert their action on the brush border intestinal cells by binding to pancreatic amylase and alpha glucosidase to prevent hydrolysis of complex carbohydrates. An alpha-glucosidase inhibitor competes with carbohydrates for binding these enzymes in the small intestine, and the result is the slowing of the absorption of the monosaccharides from the gut. These agents are intended to reduce the post-prandial hyperglycemia. That is characteristically seen in patients with diabetes (Gavin et al., 1998).

The first of its class to become available in the U.S. is acarbose (Precose). Systemic absorption of this drug is less than 1%. The second agent is miglitol (Glyset), and, unlike acarbose, it is absorbed from the gut and is excreted via the kidneys (Sels et al., 1994). The FDA has approved use of these drugs in type 2 diabetes. Their action decreases the peak post-prandial rise in serum glucose by delaying and more evenly distributing the absorption of glucose. This gradual delay in absorption then allows a sluggish endogenous insulin response to a meal (as in type 2 diabetes) to "catch up" to and better manage the glucose load of the meal. Of course, this assumes that the dietary carbohydrate burden is controlled by appropriate type and amounts of carbohydrates, i.e., that the meal contains complex carbohydrates of prescribed proportions. Absorption of monosaccharides, or sucrose will be delayed by acarbose, so oral treatment of hypoglycemia must be accomplished with dextrose (commercially prepared glucose tablets) (Bayer Corporation, 1995).

Acarbose and miglitol induce action in the intestinal tract in the brush border cells starting proximal and continuing distally to the ascending colon. This action has been responsible for the most significant side effects and has led to dose-dependent flatulence, abdominal cramping, distention, belching, and diarrhea. These effects are due in part to the fermentation of the unabsorbed carbohydrates as they travel through the colon (Baliga & Fonseca, 1997; Conniff, 1995c). As more of the border cells are induced, the side effects tend to diminish with time; however, approximately 11% of patients will seek relief from this major side effect.

Before treating the uncomfortable side effects of abdominal bloating and flatulence, the practitioner needs to be aware that some products for flatulence relief also contain alpha glucosidase (an example is "Beano") and interfere with the therapeutic action of acarbose or miglitol and therefore are contraindicated in combination. Antacids and bismuth are appropriate alternatives for treating abdominal side effects. Patients with chronic abdominal and intestinal diseases should avoid the use of acarbose due to its action on intestinal border cells.

Side effects may be minimized by dosing to acclimatize acarbose within the colon. The starting dose for both acarbose and miglitol should begin at 25mg per day, then dosing up slowly to three times daily. These should be taken at the beginning of the meal for maximal effect. At 4- to 6-week intervals, the dose can be increased very slowly in 25 mg increments, depending on post-prandial blood glucose levels and patient tolerance (May, 1995). The maximal dose for acarbose is 50 mg three times daily for patients weighing less than 60 kg, and 100 mg three times daily if the person weighs more than 60 kg. The usual maintenance dose for miglitol is 50 mg three times a day. Some patients may require 100 mg three times daily for maximal benefit (Bischoff, 1995). Clinical response to these agents is defined as consistent 2-hour post-prandial glucose lowering. This effect is experienced by 35 to 50% of type 2 patients with diabetes. Acarbose is indicated in treatment for:

- Type 2: Primary treatment for mild to moderate postprandial hyperglycemia
- Type 2: Adjunct therapy for those on sulfonylureas, biguanides, and/ or insulin
- Type 1: *Not yet FDA approved for this group:* Potential adjunct therapy with insulin for controlling postprandial glucose excursions, However, risk for hypoglycemia may increase.

The effectiveness of acarbose to reduce post-prandial glucose serum concentrations and glycosylated hemoglobin has been demonstrated in patients managed by diet alone, diet plus metformin, diet plus sulfonylurea, and diet plus insulin therapy (Chaisson, 1994). Insulin-treated type 2 patients taking acarbose have been able to reduce insulin intake by 20%. Study subjects have experienced at least an additional 0.4% reduction in glycosylated hemoglobin levels while continuing to focus on diet and exercise (Coniff, 1995a). Combination tolbutamide plus acarbose has shown greater reduction in serum glucose concentrations than either will alone (Baliga & Fonseca, 1997; Conniff, 1995a), and so suggests that acarbose has better overall glycemic effect when combined with another hypoglycemic agent.

Lipid management may actually be improved slightly with acarbose, with enhancements seen in total cholesterol levels and the HDL-cholesterol ratio. It is likely that lipid reduction is a consequence of a reduction in hyperinsulinemia while on acarbose (Leonhardt, 1994).

Potentially significant elevations in hepatic transaminase levels may occur while on acarbose and should be monitored regularly. Transaminase levels usually return to normal once acarbose has been discontinued (Baliga & Fonseca, 1997; Conniff, 1995).

Caution is necessary when selecting an alpha-glucosidase inhibitor because of potential systemic absorption. If the agent is absorbed from the small intestine, it is prudent to exclude patients whose serum creatinine is >2.0 mg/dL. And, although the agents do not directly cause hypoglycemia when used as a monotherapy, there is a risk of hypoglycemia when they are used in combination with sulfonylureas or insulins (Johnson & Taylor, 1996). Treatment of hypoglycemia must be modified to use dextrose, NOT sucrose (table sugar) products, because the alpha-glucosidase inhibitor will inhibit conversion of sucrose to glucose (Bayer Corporation, 1995). Mild hypoglycemia would be best treated with dextrose tablets, which are commercially available as glucose tablets. More severe hypoglycemia will require either an injection (subcutaneous or intramuscular), glucagon or intravenous dextrose solution.

Biguanides

Compounds synthesized from the amino acid *guanidine* have been available in European markets for over 40 years. Of these, two have been removed (phenformin and butformin) because of the incidence of lactic acidosis. Metformin, however, is one biguanide with minimal propensity towards lactic acidosis, except in persons whose renal and cardiac function have been compromised. Metformin became available in the U.S. market in 1995.

Metformin acts in at least two ways to lower plasma glucose. Without altering insulin secretion or releasing or depleting insulin stores, metformin has been shown to increase muscle and adipose cell receptor sensitivity to glucose, thereby making glucose uptake more efficient. However, its primary action is thought to be suppression of hepatic glucose production and increased utilization of glucose by muscles, In a study reported by Riddle, et al. (1996), low dose metformin (500 mg) at bedtime was sufficient to suppress hepatic glucose release, while higher doses (1 to 2 grams) during the day were required to handle prandial glucose. Some patients best tolerate metformin with food, and the drug will still be of benefit if taken with a meal schedule rather than at bedtime. Because metformin can reduce glucose absorption from the gastrointestinal tract, some individuals may experience transient anorexia and weight loss. This weight loss is usually a modest 3 to 5 kilograms (Calle-Pascual, 1995; Dunn, 1995).

Advantages of metformin are that it provides little risk of hypoglycemia in either patients with or without diabetes. The incidence of hypoglycemia is greater when metformin is combined with a sulfonylurea or insulin than when it is used separately (Baliga & Fonseca, 1997; DeFronzo, 1995). Metformin has also been shown to improve the lipid profiles by decreasing LDL-cholesterol, triglycerides, and increasing HDL-cholesterol.

The addition of metformin to diet alone, or with a sulfonylurea or with insulin, has been successful in controlling blood glucose in those with type 2 diabetes (Hermann, 1994; UKPDS, 1995).

Metformin is appropriate for patients who have type 2 diabetes, whose serum creatinine is less than 1.4 or whose creatinine clearance is better than 50 ml/min. The (Cockcroft-Gault) formula for creatinine clearance is: and in whom diet and exercise alone have not achieved desired blood glucose levels. There is an advantage to using metformin with those eligible patients who are obese or would benefit from modest weight reduction (Chong, 1995).

$$\frac{(140 - \text{age [yrs]}) \times \text{Ideal body weight (kg)}}{72 \times \text{serum creatinine (mg/dl)}}$$
$$= \text{creatinine clearance for adult males}$$

$$\frac{(140 - \text{age [yrs]}) \times \text{Ideal body weight (kg)} \times 0.8}{72 \times \text{serum creatinine (mg/dl)}}$$
$$= \text{creatinine clearance for adult females}$$

The limiting side effects of metformin are predominantly those associated with gastrointestinal disturbances. These disturbances are prevalent in 10 to 35% of the patients and consist of bloating, nausea, abdominal cramping, diarrhea, and flatulence. These effects are controlled by slowly initiating therapy, starting with the lowest dose tolerated, usually 250 or 500 mg daily, then increasing the dosage every 1 to 3 weeks until the maximum effective dose is reached. Maximum daily dose is 2.5 grams, usually divided into 2 to 3 doses per day (Dunn, 1995). This slow-dosing approach often circumvents gastrointestinal side effects and enables patients to achieve full dose ranges with the benefit of optimal glycemic control.

Glycemic targets and benefits of metformin therapy are realized within 3 to 6 months once the patient is cycled to an optimal dose. During this time it is prudent to have the patient self-monitoring and recording blood glucose levels. This is especially important for those who are combining metformin therapy with that of a sulfonylurea or insulin regimen. When used in combination, metformin is more likely to improve the body's sensitivity to insulin and thereby lower blood glucose. Hypoglycemia may occur, and the dose of sulfonylurea and/or insulin may need to be reduced, or sometimes even stopped.

Metformin is the least likely of the biguanides to precipitate lactic acidosis. Even though lactic acidosis is rare, it has a high mortality rate and the use of concomitant drugs that can alter systems function (i.e., kidney, liver, cardiac) have the potential for complicating therapy (Lalau, 1995). Patients who are at risk for kidney, liver, cardiovascular, and electrolyte imbalances are at risk for lactic acidosis, and metformin is not appropriate therapy for these individuals. Metformin is not the drug of choice in the conditions just listed, nor should it be a part of therapy for frail, older adults, or patients in whom their creatinine clearance is less than 50 ml/min.

Because metformin excretion is through tubular secretion in the kidneys, lactic acidosis is more likely in those patients whose renal function has been diminished. The possibility of lactic acidosis may also be increased when contrast dyes for radiological procedures are required for those diabetic patients on metformin. In that circumstance, the practitioner needs to be alert to the potential for short-term decreased kidney function and lactic acidosis. Therefore, it is recommended that metformin be discontinued 24 to 48 hours prior to diagnostic or surgical procedures, and for at least six hours after the procedure or until hydration has been restored or assured. Similar situations apply also to hospitalizations or procedures where changes in renal function are likely to occur. This problem can be avoided by frequent monitoring of renal function and appropriate selection of patients for metformin therapy who are not expected to have major shifts in fluids, electrolytes, and kidney, cardiac, or respiratory function (Lalau, 1995).

Metformin is effective in reducing blood glucose for patients with type 2 diabetes who have failed diet and exercise alone. Comparison studies have shown that metformin is more likely to be effective in patients who are 120% or higher in their recommended body weight. It is more likely to provide the best glycemic control when used in combination with sulfonylurea (Baliga & Fonseca, 1997; DeFronzo, 1995; UKPDS, 1995). At least 80–90% of patients experience a decrease in fasting plasma glucose and overall HbA1c reduction by 58 mg/dL and 1.8%, respectively (DeFronzo, 1995).

Insulin

Insulin is a hormone that is made and secreted by the pancreas. It is essential for metabolism of nutrients—particularly carbohydrates. At present, insulin can only be replaced by injecting commercially prepared insulins. Available insulin preparations are biogenetically engineered using yeast or *E. coli* bacteria. This recombinant DNA technology has replaced insulins prepared from animals sources (beef and pork). Not only are these sources purified to less than 10 ppm of extraneous materials, but they are also molecularly the same as human insulin. All insulin preparations contain protein components and none are antigenic, although biogenetically engineered human source insulin may be somewhat less immunogenic than animal source insulin.

Originally insulin was derived from the extraction of animal pancreas—either pork, beef, or beef-pork combinations. In the early 1980s, so-called human insulin became available through semi-synthetic recombinant DNA technology. Most animal source insulins have been replaced with the human insulin product.

Most recently biomolecular alterations in the insulin protein structure have permitted development of insulin analogs. At present there are three very rapid acting analogs and one very long acting analog. The analogs do not have accompanying data regarding long-term use, and in the instance of glargine (trade name Lantus), there are only comparative data to NPH insulin. However, at the time of this chapter update, a new rapid acting analog, glulisine insulin (trade name, Apidra, from Aventis Corp.) has just received FDA approval (April 2004). Detimir, an intermediate/long-acting analog from Novo Nordisk, is currently pending final FDA approval.

Insulin preparations are also available by varying unit-dose concentrations, the most common of which is U-100, which means that 1 cc will equal 100 units of insulin. For special use situations, Regular insulin is also available in a concentration of U-500. (*Note:* Regular insulin will be denoted with a capital "R" to avoid confusion of the term "regular.") For convenience, insulin is available in fixed ratios of either 70/30 or 50/50, meaning that the solution contains 70% of an intermediate-acting insulin and 30% of a shorter-acting insulin, or, as in the 50/50 ratio, equal parts of each. In addition, a 75/25 ratio (Lispro protamine & Lispro) and a 70/30 (Aspart & Aspart protamine) have recently been made available as combination long-and rapid-acting analogs. Fixed dose mixed insulins have frequently been a source of insulin injection errors and require particular attentin to the analog vs. non-analog origins.

Insulin Actions. Insulin preparations can be further categorized by duration of action: ultra short acting insulin analogs, short-acting insulins, intermediate-acting insulins, and long-acting insulins. By adding either protamine or zinc to pure insulin, the action of insulin can be prolonged, and administration regimens can be prescribed that more nearly mimic the body's physiological secretion of insulin. Basicially, there are two physiologic insulin secretion patterns that insulin regimens try to duplicate: 1) a continuous basal level that provides continuous 24 hour insulin availability to match metabolic glucose requirements, and 2) bolus-released insulin in direct response to meal or glucose intake (see Figure 31–1). This physiological pattern also serves the purpose of stimulating glucose utilization and storage of glucose, fat and protein.

In type 1 diabetes, when insulin is no longer produced by the pancreas, the goal of insulin regimens is to provide both components of action-basal and meal-stimulated glucose utilization. For this reason, patients usually require a combination of insulins that can provide this physiological pattern.

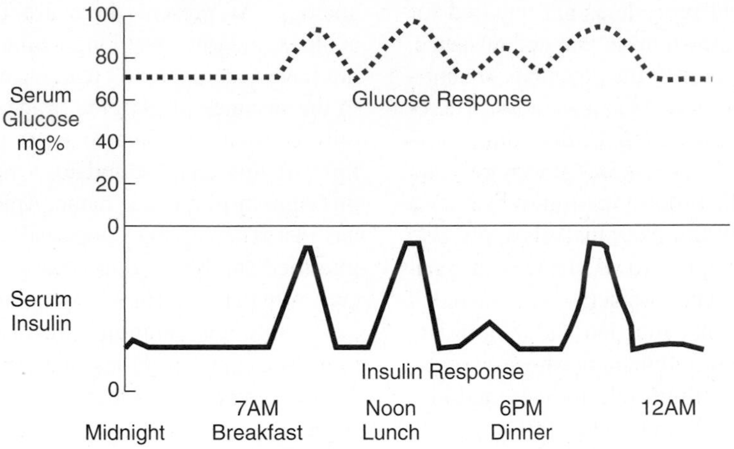

FIGURE 31–1. Physiologic insulin secretion in response to a meal or glucose intake.

In type 2 diabetes, it is common for hepatic glucose release to occur during the hours of sleep due to insufficient insulin production. To suppress or reduce this secretion of hepatic glycogen, an intermediate or longer acting exogenous insulin can be used. This helps to bring fasting glucose averages into or closer to target, and then oral agents in combination may be sufficient to control glycemic levels during the daytime or waking hours. However, because type 2 diabetes does not present in an homogenous pattern, some type 2 patients may require a combination of insulins and a regimen more similar to those advocated for type 1 patients in order to control blood glucose throughout the day and night.

Short-acting insulin (Regular) and ultra-short-acting insulins (lispro, trade name, Humalog; aspart, trade name Novolog; and glulisine, trade name, Apidra) (see Figure 31–2) are clear, colorless and all but Apidra (no available data on route administration other than subcutaneous) can be administered by an intravenous, intramuscular, or subcutaneous route. The available ultra-short-acting insulins are analogs designed for very fast absorption (5 to 15 minutes), while the short-acting Regular is absorbed and

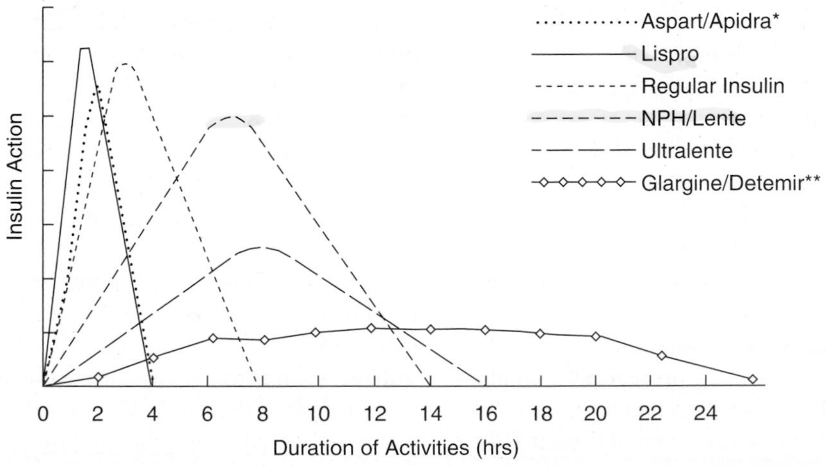

*Insufficient data to graph any significant differences between insulin glulisine and aspart or lispro (trade name vapidra)

FIGURE 31–2. Insulin pharmacokinetic action.

starts action within 30 to 60 minutes after administered. The ultra-short-action provides improved insulin availability for mealtime coverage.

For daily use, all injections of insulin are most commonly self-administered into the subcutaneous tissue, and for this reason there is a lag time between absorption and action. Regular insulin should be given 30 to 60 minutes prior to meals to maximize onset to peak of action. Analog ultra-short-acting insulins, because their molecular structure allows for very quick subcutaneous absorption, can be given just 5 to 15 minutes prior to meals (Anderson et al., 1995; Howey et al., 1995), providing patients with the flexibility to more accurately match insulin requirements to the quantity and types of carbohydrate in the meal. Lispro's quick onset and action can also reduce the post-prandial blood glucose rise.

Aspart insulin has slightly less rapid onset than lispro, but more rapid than Regular insulin; however, it lasts slightly longer than lispro.

Intermediate-acting insulins are used to provide the basal level insulin release and are administered as a single or twice-a-day injections. Twice-a-day injections of intermediate acting insulin are given about 10 to 12 hours apart, in the morning and either with the evening meal or at bedtime, depending on existing or targeted glucose patterns. Administering the intermediate evening dose at the evening meal may predispose the patient to nocturnal hypoglycemia about 2 or 3 A.M. If that occurs, the first step is to move the administration of the intermediate insulin to later in the evening, for example at 10 P.M.

Intermediate insulins, when combined with a regime of short-acting or ultra-short-acting insulin, offer patients more flexibility in meal planning and closer physiological insulin patterns with potentially better glucose control. Certain insulins mix well and are stable for extended periods of time. For example, NPH and Regular can be mixed and used up to 7 to 14 days (Peters, 1986), while Lente and Regular are stable for just 5 minutes before the Regular insulin bonds to the Lente and loses its rapid action (Heine, 1984). Lispro has similar mixing compatabilities and actions as Regular insulin.

Theoretically, the onset of action of intermediate insulin is 1 to 2 hours with peak action occurring in 6 to 8 hours and lasting 10 to 14 hours (as seen in Figure 31–2). When NPH and/or Lente insulins are mixed with Regular insulin, the rapid action of the Regular may be blunted, and instead of two action peaks, the action is sustained as one intermediate action peak. Patients experiencing otherwise inexplicable glucose variation may want to try separating these two insulins as separate injections to see if glycemic excursions become more manageable.

Glargine, a long-acting insulin analog, is absorbed slowly and action onset is gradual. This steady, slow absorption is reported to provide a long-lasting (up to 24 hours or more) and peakless effect (Ratner, et al. 2000). As a note of interest, the authors' clinical experience has found that most patients do better with the total daily basal insulin dose divided in half—that is, one half the dose given in the morning and the other half given 12 hours later in the evening. Some patients report a distinct, but small peak effect about 2 to 3 hours following administration.

Insulin mixtures take on particular kinetic profiles depending on the type of insulins and the ratios used in the mixture. Do not expect that the onset and length of action will be identical to the expected actions of the insulins in the mixture if they were given separately. An example is an NPH and Regular mixture of 70/30 will have one peak that occurs later than Regular alone, and earlier than NPH alone. The peak is also likely to be more intense.

Insulin dosing. For adults with type 1 diabetes who present with normal body weight, without infection, concurrent disease, or illness, the recommended beginning dose is 0.6 to 0.75 units per kg per day (American Diabetes Association, 1994b). To meet growth and hormonal changes, higher dosages for children (0.6–0.9 units/kg per day) and adolescents (up to 1.5 units/kg per day) may be needed. Patients who also have hyperglycemia and some degree of ketoacidosis may require higher doses of insulin (1.0–1.5 units/kg per day) until the hyperglycemia and accompanying insulin resistance improves. During times of illness or stress, insulin dosages as high as 2.5 units/kg/day may be required to compensate for inadequate blood glucose control, and must be changed as the patient's condition changes.

When taken along with Regular insulin, Aspart, or Lispro insulin, the dosage of intermediate insulin is approximately 60% of the total daily insulin requirement. This is often given as two-thirds in the morning and one-third of the total in the evening. Intermediate-acting and long acting insulin doses should be adjusted no more frequently than every 5 to 7 days, preferably with adequate supportive and guiding blood glucose data to provide sufficient pattern discernment of insulin requirements at various points throughout the day.

In type 1 diabetes, the person who is newly diagnosed may find that he or she enters a remission of sorts, referred to as the "honeymoon" period. Insulin dosage may be dramatically reduced, with requirements being as little as 0.1 to 0.3 units per kg per day (American Diabetes Association, 1994b). During this phase, it is recommended that the patient be continued on a low dose of insulin.

Women who have diabetes and become pregnant will require careful and, usually increased, insulin dose adjustment. Those who plan to become pregnant should try to achieve excellent preconception glucose control to secure the best possible outcome of the pregnancy. This level of control prior to conception is best achieved via multiple insulin injections per day, as well as 4 to 6 blood glucose tests per day. Consultation with a diabetologist and diabetes educator can help design an effective, individualized approach.

Patients with type 2 diabetes, on oral agents, usually begin insulin therapy with a small bedtime dose of intermediate insulin. A common starting dose for adults is 12 to 16 units of intermediate insulin, if blood glucose average is under 200 and weight is under 200. Those with weight over 200 and blood glucose average over 200 may have greater insulin resistance and require a starting dose of 20 to 30 units of NPH. The aim is to suppress hepatic glucose release during the night, and this suppression requires less insulin than that required to control prandial glucose loads. To assess the effectiveness of this regimen and the dose, the patient can be asked to test and average a week's worth of fasting blood glucose values. The bedtime insulin dose can be adjusted according to whether the average fasting test value is within the targeted fasting blood glucose range. Doses of 40 units or more will require reevaluation of therapy, as larger boluses of insulin may be unpredictably absorbed. If the fasting blood glucose is at target, but daytime targets cannot be achieved with sulfonylureas and/or metformin and/or acarbose, then the practitioner may need to consider adding daytime administration of insulin as well.

Type 2 patients using insulin as the principal therapy for blood glucose control may need high doses, even at or greater than 100 units per day. This will be determined by the degree of obesity and associated insulin resistance (American Diabetes Association, 1994c).

The need for self-management of insulin therapy with continual blood glucose monitoring cannot be overemphasized, and recommendations for target blood glucose testing should be individualized to meet the patient's need for insulin, meals, exercise, and glycemic homeostasis. For target blood glucose levels see Table 31–3. These targets may require adjustment for safety and feasibility for the patient.

TABLE 31–3. Optimal Blood Glucose Levels

Time	Level, mg/dL
Pre-prandial (30–60 min before meal)	70–120
1 h post-prandial	100–180
2 h post-prandial	80–120
3 A.M.	70–120

Insulin regimens. There are many dosage regimens for designing optimal insulin therapy. Depending on the type of diabetes and severity of insulin impairment, regimens may range from a single injection per day to 4 to 5 injections per day.

The simplest regimen is one injection per day. This may be given as a single pre-breakfast injection, or, as in the case of type 2 diabetes with elevated fasting blood glucose values, a single bedtime dose of intermediate acting insulin. Seldom is a single injection of insulin per day sufficient for glycemic management of type 1 diabetes.

If two injections of insulin are required per day, they may consist of only intermediate or longest acting insulin. However, a common insulin regimen of two injections per day is that of a "split-mixed" regimen. The morning regime contains intermediate- or long-acting insulin, with a bolus of Regular insulin, aspart or lispro. If Regular insulin is used, it should be injected 30 to 60 minutes prior to meal time for maximal results. The evidence supports mixing these two insulins together, however, if a patient is experiencing fluctuating blood glucose levels while keeping food (amounts of carbohydrate and timing) consistent, the patient can try using two separate injections: the intermediate- or long-acting in the thigh or buttock, and the Regular, aspart or lispro insulin administered in the abdomen. Also, if the ratio of Regular to intermediate or longer-acting insulin is greater than 1:2, and/or glucose variation is inexplicable, separate injections may be beneficial in achieving predictable absorption and desired duration.

The use of multiple insulin administrations per day (three or more) is often referred to as "intensive insulin therapy." Table 31–4 outlines three regimens that may be used.

Intensive regimens of multiple administrations of insulin require that the patient be testing his or her blood glucose at least four times a day and be able to make decisions about adjusting the dose of the shorter-acting insulins based on individual activity and eating patterns. These intensive regimens can help achieve near euglycemia, but they are not for everyone. Because of the concurrent blood glucose testing and insulin adjustments necessary, the patient also requires ongoing support and guidance from a knowledgeable, confident provider. An

TABLE 31–4. Three Models for Intensive Insulin Therapy

Method	Insulin Regime	Types of Insulins Used	Number of Injections
Model 1	Insulin dosage dependent on blood glucose	Regular insulin (or) Lispro (or) Aspart	Three Injections daily before meals
Model 2	Two-thirds of daily dose of intermediate insulin in the morning along with a bolus of fast-acting insulin Fast-acting insulin before dinner One-third of daily dose of intermediate insulin at consistent bedtime hour	NPH or Lente, and Regular insulin (or) Lispro (or) Aspart	Three injections daily • Intermediate + Regular before breakfast • Regular before dinner • Intermediate at bedtime
Model 3	Ultralente along with fast-acting insulin before breakfast Fast-acting insulin dose before lunch Ultralente along with fast-acting insulin dose with evening meal	Ultralente, (or) Glargine and Regular insulin, (or) Lispro, (or) Aspart.	Three injections daily; cannot mix Glargine or Ultralente with Regular or lispro or aspart.

individualized "sliding scale," or algorithm, for adjusting the dose of the shorter-acting insulins is needed, and patients must learn to use it. See the example of an adjustment guide for regulating Regular, Lispro, or Aspart in Table 31–5.

If the multiple injections do not achieve the targeted blood glucose goals, consider other methods of insulin delivery, such as an insulin pump. This equipment is expensive to obtain and maintain, requiring access to health personnel well versed in its use. For select patients, it may help to achieve near normal glycemic control.

Storing insulin. All unopened insulin should be stored in the refrigerator and kept from freezing. Patients should keep the bottle currently being used at room temperature away from exposure to heat and sunlight. Injectable medicine kept at room temperature causes less pain. Vials of insulin, once opened, can be used until the expiration date. The exception is Lispro insulin. This insulin analog should be used within 28 days once opened, even if refrigerated. Check the expiration date stamped on the vial. If traveling, patients should always keep insulin with them at a constant temperature. Because it is a protein, insulin is similar to egg whites (also protein) and can be easily affected by very hot or very cold temperatures. The insulated thermal packs or thermos bottles can be used to transport insulin while traveling. Remind the insulin-using patients to carry a letter from their healthcare provider when traveling abroad, in case care is needed at the arrival destination and to avoid problems with transporting syringes and insulin through customs.

TABLE 31–5. Sample of an Algorithm/Sliding Scale for Adjusting Short or Ultra-Short-Acting Insulins

Approach A: A guide can be set for dosing solely based on blood glucose values before the meal. Such a guide would look like the following example:
- If BG is less than 80 mg/dL, eat right away and take $^1/_2$ of the dose if BG were between 81–140 units.
- If BG is 81–140, take 4 units of short or ultra-short-acting insulin.
- Take an additional unit for every 40 mg/dL above 140 mg/dL, up to a maximum of 10 units.

Approach B: An ideal guide for dose adjustment of short or ultra-short-acting insulin before meals is based on both pre-meal BG and the amount of Carbohydrate (in grams) that will be consumed at that meal. This guide would look like the following example:
- If BG is less than 80 mg/dL, eat right away and then take ½ of the dose if BG were between 81–140.
- If BG is 81–140, take 1 unit for every 15 grams of carbohydrate in the meal to be eaten.
- Take an additional unit for every 40 mg/dL above 140 mg/dL, up to a maximum of 10 units.

Note: Approach A may be a simpler way to make adjustments and can also be used as the guide until a patient learns carbohydrate counting. Approach B requires that both provider and patient collaborate until the best insulin to carbohydrate ratio (this example used 1:15) is determined.

Insulin injection preparation. Visual inspection of each vial should be performed prior to withdrawing an insulin dose. Prior to the advent of insulin analogs, it was easy to tell which insulins were long- or short-acting. The long-acting insulins were cloudy because they were basically Regular insulin with either protamine or zinc added. Today, both short- and long-acting insulin analogs are clear, and it is incumbent upon the provider and the patient to devise visual cues to keep these insulins separate and easily identifiable. All insulins should look uniform in appearance and have no visible clumping or flocculation (floating pieces). Insulins that are normally cloudy (NPH, ULtralente, combinations of NPH + Regular) should be gently rolled or gently shaken to be certain the suspension is uniform before drawing it up in the syringe. After inspection and prior to withdrawing a dose of suspension (intermediate, long-acting) insulin from a vial, the vial should be gently rolled between the palms, not shaken.

Administration of insulin. Commercially available insulin needles are of such a fine gauge and short length that the injection can be made by inserting the insulin needle at a 90-degree angle into the adipose tissue of the abdomen, arms, thigh, or buttocks. A very lean person may find it necessary to pinch the skin and insert the needle into the adipose at a 30-degree angle. It is not necessary to prepare clean skin with alcohol or any other cleansing lotion or fluid. Insert entire length of needle, then deliver the contents of syringe quickly. Aspiration is not necessary. Do not inject into scar tissue and avoid the one inch area around the navel.

Other factors that will influence onset, peak, and duration of action include whether administration is into dermis/adipose/muscle, smoking; current blood glucose level; insulin sensitivity; metabolic state; and insulin antibodies. These multiple factors can best be controlled by consistent administration in both selected sites and by keeping food and exercise consistent.

To accommodate delivery convenience, many patients administer through a device known as an *insulin pen.* This product consists of insulin cartridges (as opposed to the usual vials), the pen device, and disposable needles. In most instances, the cartridges cost more than the ordinary vial insulin, but busy, on-the-go people may prefer this option. Other convenient—and more costly—products include air-jet injectors instead of the standard insulin syringe. Continuous subcutaneous insulin infusions (insulin pumps, CSII) are expensive in terms of cost for the technology (approximately $4,000+) and require further education and followup. However, they allow some individuals to achieve a more near-normal insulin delivery when the other intensive, multiple injection regimens have been unsuccessful.

Side effects of insulin. Adverse reactions from insulins are essentially those associated with hypoglycemia, especially in patients with type 1 diabetes who are active and intent on achieving near-euglycemia (The DCCT Research Group, 1993). A severe hypoglycemic reaction can result in coma, seizure, and the need for intravenous glucose or glucagon. Hypoglycemia can be strictly defined as blood glucose <50 mg/dl, and patients with clinical symptoms of hypoglycemia—tachycardia, palpitations, shakiness, sweating, dizziness, hunger—can reverse the symptoms with 10 to 15 gm of quick acting carbohydrate (see Table 31–6). Evaluate blood glucose in 15 minutes and 1 hour to assess response.

Hypoglycemia can be caused by three main factors, or a combination of all three: 1) too much insulin, 2) delay of food intake, 3) increase in activity or exercise. Alcohol consumption without concurrent carbohydrate intake may also predispose to hypoglycemia. Query patients to determine if they have recently started a new bottle of insulin, changed injection technique or major sites, experienced hormonal changes or symptoms of gastroparesis (delay in stomach emptying and reduction in intestinal peristalsis).

Patients intent on maintaining euglycemia will experience an increase in episodes of hypoglycemia. Unrealistic glycemic goals can endanger patients, so negotiate healthy patterns of control with them. Family, friends, school and work associates should be instructed on appropriate treatment for hypoglycemia and shown how to administer glucagon injection in the event the patient becomes unconscious.

Hypoglycemia-unawareness can occur in patients who have had type 1 for many years, and in those patients who have employed a regimen of very tight glucose regulation (Edleman, 1997). For those with long duration of the disease, it can become increasingly difficult to recognize and self-treat hypoglycemic symptoms. Monitoring and a readily available glucose source is essential for these individuals, as is re-negotiating blood glucose targets to a safer range. Those experiencing hypoglycemia due to tight glycemic control regimens may be able to improve symptom detection by meticulously avoiding hypoglycemia and allowing the blood glucose to run in the mid to high 100s mg/dL for several days (Edleman, 1997).

Nocturnal hypoglycemia that occurs in the early morning hours (around 3 or 4 A.M.) is more common in

TABLE 31–6. Suggested Fast-Acting Carbohydrates to Treat Hypoglycemia

Symptomatic Mild Hypoglycemia (shaky, sweating nervous, unable to swallow)
Goal: Administer 10–15 gm glucose:
2–3 glucose tablets
1/2 tube of glucose gel
4 oz of orange juice
1 small tube of cake icing
4 oz of regular (sweetened) soda
4–6 Lifesavers
Repeat dose every 15 minutes until bg is above 70 mg/dL.
Unresponsive Severe Hypoglycemia
Glucagon (kit)—1 dose injected subcutaneously (or) 50% dextrose and water administered intravenously

those patients who are trying to achieve near-euglycemia and/or in those who take intermediate-acting insulin with the evening meal. Patients may not awaken during these episodes, but may recall nightmares or awaken with a headache. Have the patient monitor the 3 A.M. blood glucose and adjust the regimen. For example, moving the intermediate-acting insulin to a bedtime hour (and being consistent in this administration), may avoid the middle of the night peak that occurs from evening meal intermediate-acting insulin.

Other side effects of insulin may occur through immunological effects. Lipoatrophy and lipohypertrophy can occur with repeated injections to the same puncture site. Injection rotation within the site area will help to prevent these changes to the adipose tissue, and subsequent variation in absorption. With glargine insulin some stinging can occur due to the relatively low pH of the analog. Stinging can be reduced if injected more slowly and at room temperature. Because glargine is clear and less stable when mixed with other insulins, it is not recommended to mix glargine with any other insulin.

Situations requiring immediate insulin therapy. Two metabolic situations increase insulin requirements, and both are often precipitated by illness or infection. *Diabetic ketoacidosis (DKA)* is most common in type 1 diabetes. Illness, trauma, or infection can create a need for more energy and more insulin. Because of the absolute absence of insulin, type 1 patients are more likely to begin experiencing a breakdown of fat into fatty acids when their insulin and energy requirements are in higher demand. These acid by-products, along with the release of counterregulatory hormones (further elevating hyperglycemia) create a metabolic state of ketoacidosis. The result is major fluid and electrolyte shift, and the treatment is immediate replacement of insulin and appropriate fluids.

In type 2 diabetes, since some insulin production capability remains, fat breakdown does not occur. This condition is called *non-ketosis, hyperglycemic, hyperosmosis (NKHH)*. Hyperglycemia is severe in NKHH, and, so too, are the fluid and electrolyte shifts. The comparative difference is that ketosis is not present, the sustained hyperglycemia may be significantly high (over 500 mg/dl), and osmolality is greater than 320 mOsm. Treatment calls for insulin replacement, along with fluid and electrolyte administration. Both conditions are life-threatening.

Illness is the common precipitator of both of these metabolic conditions, so it is essential that the patient with diabetes be aware of this potential when ill and take steps to prevent symptoms from progressing.

Meglitinides

One of several newer classes of drugs making their way through clinical trials are the meglitinides. Prandin™ is the agent that is currently available. Currently available with the generic name of repaglinide, it is the first of the meglitinide class.

Repaglinide works in a fashion similar to the sulfonylurea agents in that it stimulates insulin secretion from pancreatic beta cells (Owens et al., 2000). A partially restored early insulin response when foods are consumed appears to be the primary value of this drug. Repaglinide offers an alternative to patients who are allergic to sulfonylureas. However, it is not likely to offer further therapeutic effect when the patient has already exhausted sulfonylurea treatment. A possible therapeutic advantage, and yet to be more clearly understood, is that repaglinide action is diminished when glucose levels drop to near hypoglycemia. Also, unlike sulfonylureas that tend to have time-limited effectiveness of 2 to 5 years, repaglinide's ability to switch off during conditions of hypoglycemia may also promote resensitization and preservation of the beta cells. This action would, theoretically, offer more years of effective oral therapy for glycemic control. Long-term clinical studies have not been completed to support this theory.

Repaglinide has pharmacokinetic properties that require the drug be given just prior to meals 2 to 4 times daily (Owens, 2000). If a meal is missed or added, then so is the drug. This requires a rather intensive adherence schedule and may be difficult for some patients who have had problems structuring meals or remembering to take their medications. The most common adverse effects from repaglinide include influenza symptoms, respiratory infections, and rhinitis.

Weight gain on average was 3.3% in those treated with the agent. One potential advantage is that this drug has a kidney-sparing effect and may be used by patients with altered renal function. Because the drug is metabolized in the liver, frequent monitoring of liver function may be necessary.

In very short and limited clinical trials, the reported clinical benefits from this new oral hypoglycemic agent are improvements in glycemic control, ranging from 0.5 to 0.8% drop in HbA1c's. In patients on oral combination therapy the glycemic response appears to be slightly less. The dosing range is 0.5 to 4 mg given as 0.5 mg, 1 mg, or

2 mg tablets with each meal, and the maximum total daily dose is 16 mg. The starting dose is 0.5 mg with each meal.

Phenylalanines

This newest class of hypoglycemic drugs is derived from D-phenylalanine that uniquely resembles a sulfonylurea agent. The only agent available currently in this class is nateglinide (Starlix). Like sulfonylureas, the phenylalanine class binds to sulfonylurea receptors on the beta cell, thereby blocking the ATP-potassium channel that permit insulin release. The binding to the receptors is quickly reversed and less prolonged than sulfonylureas (Hanefeld et al., 2000). This action provides an explanation for the rapid rise and fall in insulin levels seen with each dose, which theoretically matches the endogenous insulin release seen in people without diabetes.

In the recent post-marketing phase IV trials, nateglinide was shown to have the benefit of less nausea and GI symptoms compared to biguanides or alpha-glucosidase inhibitors. And there are no special administration requirements besides taking each dose 1 hour before eating. Nateglinide is taken 30 to 60 minutes prior to a meal at a dose of 120 mg three times a day.

Hypoglycemia is potentially less common, since insulin levels more closely resemble the usual insulin response to meals. For those patients with concerns about maintaining a strict diet or who wish to avoid weight gain, nateglinide on average causes weight gains of 2 to 4 kg (Horton, 2000). While the side effects may be fewer or better tolerated, the effectiveness in reducing overall HbA1c and maintaining an improved glycemic response is less well documented. Clinical trials have shown that there is no clinical benefit from the use of nateglinide when sulfonylureas have been used and ultimately fail due to beta cell exhaustion. For individuals with irregular meal and eating habits, nateglinide may be beneficial in matching food, exercise, and daily activities with effectively treating post-prandial hyperglycemia. This is due to the short binding response at the receptor level that also may prevent hypoglycemia.

Sulfonylurea Drugs

The class of sulfonylurea drugs has expanded to 3 generations, with generations 1 and 2 showing unique differences in their kinetic and dynamic actions. Sulfonylureas are commonly referred to as oral hypoglycemic agents (OHAs). The first generation of these agents included tolbutamide (Orinase), chlorpropamide (Diabinese), tolazamide (Tolinase), and acetohexamide (Dymdor), and some of these are still in use today. The second generation agents are glyburide (DiaBeta, Glynase PresTab, Micronase), glipizide (Glucotrol, Glucotrol XL); the third-generation agent is glimepiride (Amaryl).

The mechanism of action of sulfonylureas is complex and still not completely understood. Study evidence shows that pharmacological actions can be seen both within the pancreas, where there is an increase in insulin release, and at the cellular receptor level, where an increase in the sensitivity and binding of insulin can be measured. A combination of these mechanisms probably produces the intended hypoglycemic effect (American Diabetes Association, 1996).

The major utility of the sulfonylurea class has been their ability to more efficiently and effectively increase circulating insulin levels to bring about reduced blood glucose levels. About 20% of patients will experience no therapeutic response to these agents, a condition called "primary failure." Another portion of users will initially respond with increased beta cell stimulation and resultant increased insulin secretion; however, over time (5–7 years) this effect may diminish, insulin levels fall and secondary failure will occur. The former is known as primary failure, in which the sulfonylureas immediately fail to produce any change in glycemic control. The latter, "secondary failure," is the term applied to that category of patients for whom sulfonylureas worked for a time.

While in the past the sulfonylurea drugs have been one of the first oral durgs for intial therapy, they are losing favor to more potent agents such as metformin, with or without insulin.

The therapeutic decision for what agent would be the best choice for a particular patient will necessarily stem from the kinetic profile of the drug, the patient's metabolic condition, and the therapeutic goal. This means it is best to consider the drug's metabolism and excretion, along with the duration of activity and the patient's blood glucose control targets. For example, tolbutamide, with its short half life, may be most appropriate for patients in whom hypoglycemia is to be avoided if possible. This group includes those who frequently experience hypoglycemia that are renally compromised or elderly (Lebovitz, 1991). Acetohexamide and tolazamide have intermediate duration of activity but contain active metabolites that can accumulate in those patients with renal failure and who are elderly. (American Diabetes Association, 1996; The DCCT Research Group, 1993). Chlorpropamide has the longest duration of action with active metabolites. Chlorpropamide is the least expensive OHA product available, yet its long action combined with the potential for hyponatremia, can complicate therapy in the elderly and renal-compromised patient (Shorr, 1997).

Of the second- and third-generation sulfonylurea agents, glimepiride, is similar in kinetics and therapeutic action to glyburide. Generally, the onset of action for the second generation agents is 1 to 4 hours and is best given 30 minutes to an hour prior to the breakfast and/or dinner meal. The duration of action for glyburide is 24 hours while glipizide's approaches 10 to 24 hours. When the patient reaches greater than 50% of the maximum daily dose, it may become necessary to split the daily dose. Once the total daily dose reaches 15 mg of glyburide or 30 mg of glipizide, the efficacy of blood glucose reduction decreases with increased dosing (Cefalu, 1996; Stenman et al., 1993). When the patient has reached maximum benefit from the sulfonylureas, additional blood glucose reduction can be achieved by adding agents from other glucose lowering classes, such as metformin and/or acarbose. Glyburide has shown to be more effective over the 24-hour period in reducing blood glucose and longer term glucose control, while glipizide has been more effective in reducing postprandial glucose levels, but circulating insulin levels tend to be elevated. High circulating levels of insulin may be associated with advancing atherosclerosis (Lebovitz, 1991). However, both medications have a similar effect on the HbA1c.

Patients who fail on monotherapy of oral hypoglycemic agents have been shown to do better on combination oral and insulin therapy in reducing long-term glucose levels. Specifically, the BIDS regimen (*b*edtime *i*ntermediate insulin and *d*aytime *s*ulfonylurea) has been demonstrated to be effective in those type 2 patients who have persistently elevated fasting blood glucose levels (Groop et al., 1992; Pugh et al., 1992; Riddle, 1990).

The side effects of sulfonylurea drugs are not extensive. The most common side effect (and therapeutic effect) that all sulfonylurea agents share is *hypoglycemia.* Depending on the duration of activity of the specific agent and the age and morbidity status of the patient, hypoglycemia can usually be easily treated with ingestion of simple carbohydrates, such as juice, hard candy, honey, or syrup. However, in the longer acting agents or those with active metabolites, the hypoglycemia may be significantly and seriously prolonged. The elderly tend to be more susceptible to it because of declining renal and liver function. This is true for even those agents with weak metabolites, such as glyburide. Elderly patients (>70 yrs) most likely to be at risk are those with poor nutritional status, fragile states of health, chronic diseases where fluid shifts occur and any compromised renal and hepatic function. Any of those conditions will warrant OHAs that are shorter acting and less likely to evoke a prolonged hypoglycemic reaction. In fact, a single dose of long-acting glargine may be the preferred agent for glucose control in those susceptible individuals.

Hypoglycemia can be a very serious complication with significantly poor outcomes, and treatment should include aggressive glucose replacement for as long as 24 to 48 hours with intravenous therapy. To avoid hypoglycemia for patients receiving OHAs, consider using the agent with the shortest duration of action, appropriate to existing renal and hepatic function, avoiding drug interactions, and thoroughly reviewing the patients potential for changes in fluid and nutrition status or shifts (Shorr, 1997).

Renal function can be an important consideration when starting a patient on an oral hypoglycemic agent. Most sulfonylureas have some diuresis action. However, acetohexamide and tolazamide have more than most, and all can cause fluid retention. Electrolyte imbalance can occur more frequently with the first generation agents, with hyponatremia being at greatest risk with chlorpropamide use. Cholestatic jaundice is particularly a problem with chlorpropamide; however, the other agents have this potential too, and it is recommended that patients be switched to insulin or an alternative non-sulfonylurea agent if this should occur.

Less common, but equally significant are hematological reactions such as thrombocytopenia, leukopenia, hemolytic anemia; maculopapular rashes; pulmonary reactions; and decrease in thyroid function (Hermann, 1994). Drug interactions can be an important cause of poor glycemic control and can change metabolism, elimination, and actions of the sulfonylurea agents. In general, the second- and third-generations of sulfonylurea agents will have less potential for interactions that produce significant glycemic changes.

The sulfonylurea drugs have been effective in reducing blood glucose in patients who have some inherent circulating and stored insulin. Of patients who use OHAs, 60 to 70% will have an initial response to therapy. Glycemic control will generally continue for two or more years; failures after this period of time occur 5 to 20% of the time. Excluding patient compliance problems, failure usually requires increasing the dose or frequency, switching to alternative agents; or adding an agent from a different class of OHAs. The success rate of oral combination therapy is time- and disease progression-dependent and may necessitate insulin therapy (Hermann, 1994; Lebovitz, 1991). Insulin therapy may be used during periods of stress, illness, or major life changes until stabilization of blood glucose is established and oral therapy can be reinstated. Changes in drug management should not preclude appropriate emphasis on dietary and exercise management and should complement lifestyle changes.

Thiazolidinediones

Thiazolidinediones (TZDs) act to lower blood glucose by reducing insulin resistance and improving insulin sensitivity in muscle and adipose tissue (Whitcomb, Saltiel, & Lockwood, 1996). Interestingly, the TZDs were first developed in Japan and designed to reduce triglyceride levels but were found to have a positive affect for improving HbA1c (Peters, 2001). While troglitazone (trade name Rezulin) was removed from the market in March 2000 because of significant liver toxicity, rosiglitazone (trade name Actos) and pioglitazone (trade name Avandia) remain available (Lebovitz, 2002), with more soon to be released. TZDs also cause some suppression of hepatic glucose output, but to a lesser degree than the biguanides. They are currently approved for use in type 2, *not type 1,* diabetes management as monotherapy or in combination therapy.

Currently, TZDs are approved for and found to be more effective when combined with sulfonylureas than when given as monotherapy (Boyle et al., 2002). On average, HbA1c's can be expected to drop by 1.8% when used in this combination, as compared to 0.7% when used alone. Results of glycemic improvement when insulin and a TZD are used in combination are slightly less than that seen with combination with sulfonylureas.

The thiazolidinedione class of antidiabetic agents by themselves do not contribute to hypoglycemia, such as may occur with either insulin or sulfonylurea therapy. TZDs cause significant weight gain and/or non-weight related edema in some, but not all, patients. However, for those where weight gain or edema do occur the undesired outcomes can be significant, especially for patients with cardiovascular co-morbidity. The incidence of edema or peripheral edema is 5.9% (Einhorn et al., 2000). Some TZD have a positive effect on triglycerides, high-density lipoproteins (HDL) levels, and low-density lipoproteins (LDLs). The lipid profile may be the most distinct difference between pioglitazone and rosiglitazone. While HDL and LDL generally improve by 5 to 18% with either agent triglycerides improve most prominently with pioglitazone on average 5 to 10% with not statistically significant differences for rosiglitazone and triglycerides (Einhorn et al., 2000, Peters, 2001).

Early reports show that these agents are generally well tolerated and that primary side effects from the TZDs are fluid retention, minor abdominal cramping, nausea, and upper respiratory infections. Edema should be carefully monitored with reported ranges 3–5% for monotherapy and 15% for those on combination therapy (Nesto, 2003). This can be especially serious for those patients with underlying COPD or CHF (Peters, 2001). Adverse effects may be minimized by careful selection of patients for TZD. Those who have predisposing congestive heart failure (Delea, 2003) or hepatic impairment are not appropriate candidates for TZD. Liver function tests (LFTs) should be done prior to starting therapy, then every other month for the first year. The drug should be discontinued if LFT show significant abnormal elevations (generally 1.5 to 3 times the upper limit of normal).

While early indications of glycemic improvement have been documented with the thiazolidinedione class of drugs the progression of long term macrovascular complication measures have not been reported. Several large long term trials (*PROACTIVE: PRO*spective pioglit*A*zones *C*linical *T*rial *I*n macro*V*asular *E*vents, *CHICAGO:* A study evaluating *C*arotid Intima-media T*HIC*kness (CIMT) in *A*therosclerosis using pio*G*litaz*O*ne, *PERISCOPE: P*ioglitazone *E*ffect on *R*egression of *I*ntravascular *S*onographic *C*ornary *O*bstruction *P*rospective *E*valuation) are currently under way to determine the full benefits of using this class of drugs.

To initiate monotherapy or combination therapy, the following guidelines are provided:

Monotherapy.

- Pioglitazone is initiated at 15 mg daily, but ultimately the most effective dose with the greatest reduction in A1c usually begins with dosages of 30 mg daily or more. (Nesto, 2003)
- Rosiglitazone 4 mg daily to start and will not likely show additional improvement with higher doses. (Nesto, 2003)
- Average improvement in HbA1c with 4 mg is about 0.8% within 12 weeks. If only minimal glycemic improvement is noted, an adjustment to 8 mg may bring a further reduction.

Combination therapy.

- Combination therapy with metformin (daily dose of metformin at 2000 mg/day) can be initiated with a pioglitazone dose of 15 mg. This has been shown to reduce HbA1c approximately 1% when added to therapy, with slightly greater reduction when the dose is boosted to 30 to 45 mg daily.

- When added to sulfonylurea therapy, pioglitazone has reduced A1c by 0.9% and 1.3% with doses of 15 mg and 30 mg, respectively. If pioglitazone is added to insulin, A1c fell an average of 0.7% with 15 mg.
- Changes in HbA1c with rosiglitazone in combination therapy with sulfonylureas, metformin, and insulin have been found to be similar to pioglitazone.
- When combined with insulin, the TZD's have been shown to reduce overall insulin dose requirements by 10 to 25%. This effect should be communicated to patients so that they can carefully monitor their own blood glucose and work with their healthcare providers to adjust insulin doses safely and therapeutically.

In 15% of patients, insulin therapy can be discontinued. An FDA warning was issued in 2001 regarding use of rosiglitazone (Avandia) and insulin and the subsequent onset of congestive heart failure (CHF) and cardiovascular events in patients with previously unknown cardiovascular disease (CVD). The warning cautions for monotherapy with this TZD (not to combine rosiglitazone [Avandia] and insulin) in those patients with known CVD, and careful monitoring in otherwise healthy patients for signs of CHF (HHS, 2001). This caution does not at present extend to other glucose-lowering agents in this class.

Drug Combinations

Drugs that can cause hyperglycemia or complicate treatment for hyperglycemia are not necessarily contraindicated in patients with diabetes, but they may require more attention for monitoring glucose levels and appropriate adjustment of the patient's drug regimen. The drugs that contribute to hyperglycemia and hypoglycemia are shown in Tables 31–7 and 31–8, respectively.

TABLE 31–7. Drugs Causing Hyperglycemia

Acetazolamide	Indapamide
Alpha blockers	L-Asparaginase
Beta blockers	Niacin-nicotinic acid
Butmetanide	Nicotine
Caffeine	Nonsteroidal anti-inflammatory drugs
Calcium channel blockers	Oral contraceptives
Cyclophosphamide	Pentamidine
Diazoxide	Phenobarbital
Epinephrine (sympathomimetics)	Phenytoin
Fish oils	Sugar-containing drug products
Furosemide	Thiazide diuretics
Hormones (glucagon, estrogens, thyroid, steroids)	

TABLE 31–8. Drugs Potentiating Hypoglycemia

Alcohol	Insulin
Alpha glucosidase inhibitors	MAO inhibitors
Anabolic steroids	Phenylbutazone
Beta blockers	Salicylates
Biguanides	Sulfinpyrazone
Clofibrate	Sulfonylureas
Fenfluramine	Tetracycline
Guanethidine	Thiazolidinedones

REFERENCES

Ahern, J. A., & Grey, M. (1996). New developments in treating children with IDDM. *Journal of Pediatric Health Care, 10*(4), 161–166.

American Diabetes Association. (1994a). *Maximizing the role of nutrition in diabetes management.* Alexandria, VA: Author.

American Diabetes Association (1994b). *Medical management of insulin-dependent (Type 1) diabetes (2nd Ed.).* Alexandria, VA: American Diabetes Association Clinical Education Series.

American Diabetes Association (1994c). *Medical management of non-insulin-dependent (Type II) diabetes* (3rd ed.). Alexandria, VA: American Diabetes Association Clinical Education Series.

American Diabetes Association. (1996). Consensus Statement: The pharmacologic treatment of hyperglycemia in NIDDM. *Diabetes Care, 19*(Suppl. 1), S 54–61.

American Diabetes Association. (2004). Clinical Practice Recommendations 2004. *Diabetes Care, 27*(1) (Suppl. 1).

American Diabetes Association Position Statement. (1995). Standards of medical care for patients with diabetes mellitus. *Diabetes Care, 12*(12), 365–368.

Anderson, J. H., et al. (1995). Insulin lispro compared to regular insulin in a crossover study involving 1,037 patients with type I diabetes. *Diabetes, 44*(Suppl 1), Abstract No. 228A.

Bailey, C. J., Path, M. R. C., & Turner, R. C. (1996). Drug therapy: Metformin. *New England Journal of Medicine, 334*(9) 574–579.

Baliga, B. S., & Fonseca, V. A. (1997). Recent advances in the treatment of type II diabetes mellitus. *American Family Physician,* pp. 817–824

Bayer Corporation, Pharmaceutical Division (1995). Precose package insert.

Bischoff, H. (1995). The mechanism of alpha-glucosidase inhibition in the management of diabetes. *Clin. Invest. Med, 18,* 303–311.

Boyle, P. et al. (2002). Effects of Pioglitazone and rosiglitazone on blood lipid levels and glycemic control in patients with Type

2 diabetes mellitus: a retrospective review of randomly selected medical records. *Clin. Thera.* 2002. Mar; 24(3): 378–96.

Delea, C. (2003) use of thiazolidindiones and risk of heart failure in people with type 2 diabetes. *Diabetes Care,* 26: 2983.

Calle-Pascual, A. L. (1995). Comparison between acarbose, metformin, and insulin treatment in type II diabetic patients with secondary failure to sulfonylurea treatment. *Diabetes Et Metabolism, 21*(4), 256–260

Cefalu, W.T. (1996). Treatment of type II diabetes. *Postgraduate Medicine, 99*(3), 109–119.

Chaisson, J. L. (1994). The efficacy of acarbose in the treatment of patients with non-insulin-dependent diabetes mellitus. *Annals of Internal Medicine. 121,* 928–935.

Chong, P. K. (1995). Energy expenditure in type II diabetic patients on metformin and sulfonylurea therapy. *Diabetic Medicine, 2*(5), 401–408.

Conniff, R. F. (1995a). A double-blind placebo-controlled trial evaluating the safety and efficacy of acarbose for the treatment of patients with insulin-requiring type II diabetes. *Diabetes Care, 18*(7), 928–932.

Conniff, R. F. (1995b). Multicenter, placebo-controlled trial comparing acarbose with placebo, tolbutamide, and tolbutamide plus-acarbose in non-insulin-dependent diabetes mellitus. *American Journal of Medicine, 98,* 443–451.

Conniff, R. F. (1995c). Reduction of glycosylated hemoglobin and postprandial hyperglycemia by acarbose in patients with NIDDM. *Diabetes Care, 18*(6), 817–824.

Decode Study (1999). Glucose tolerance and mortality: comparison of WHO and American Diabetes Assoc. Diagnostic Criteria. Lancet. 1999; 354: 617–21

DeFronzo, R. A. (1988). The triumvirate: B-cell, muscle, liver. A collusion responsible for NIDDM. *Diabetes. 37,* 867–887.

DeFronzo, R. A. (1995). Efficacy of metformin in patients with non-insulin-dependent diabetes mellitus: The multicenter metformin study group. *New England Journal of Medicine, 333*(9), 541–549.

Diabetes Prevention Program (2002 February 7), *New England Journal of Medicine,*

The Diabetes Control and Complications Trial Research Group. (1993). The effect of intensive treatment of diabetes on the development and progression of long-term complications in insulin-dependent diabetes mellitus. *New England Journal of Medicine, 329,* 977–986.

Dunn, C. J. (1995). Metformin: A review of its pharmacological properties and therapeutic use in non-insulin-dependent diabetes mellitus. *Drugs, 49*(5), 721–749.

Edleman, S. (1997). *Diabetes Interview* : Beware of hypoglycemia unawareness. Issue #61. (Available from *Diabetes Interview, 3715 Balboa Street, San Francisco, CA 98121.)*

Einhorn D. et al. (2000). Pioglitazone in combination with Metformin in treatment of type 2 diabetes mellitus; A Randomized placebo controlled trial. Clin Thera. 22:12; 1395–1409.

Franz, M. (Ed). (1994). *Maximizing the role of nutrition in diabetes management.* Alexandria, VA: American Diabetes Association.

Franz, M. J., (2002). Evidenced based nutrition principles and recommendations for treatment and prevention of diabetes and related complications Diabetes Care 25: 148–198.

Ganda, O. P. (1996). Rational therapy: Non-insulin-dependent diabetes mellitus. *ICPR.*

Gavin III, J. R., Reasner, C. A., Weart, C. W., & Labso, L. (1998). Oral antidiabetic drugs: One size does not fit all. *Patient Care, 32*(3), 40–68.

Ghazzi, M. N., Perez, J.E., & Antonucci, T. (1997). Cardiac and glycemic benefits of troglitazone treatment in NIDDM. *Diabetes, 46,* 433–439.

Giordano, B. P., Petrila, A., Banion, C. R., & Neuenkirchen, G. (1992). The challenge of transferring responsibility for diabetes management from parent to child. *The Journal of Pediatric Health Care. 6*(5), 235–239.

Goo, A. K. Y., Carson, D. S., & Bjelajac, A. (1996). Metformin: A new treatment option for NIDDM. *The Journal of Family Practice. 42*(6), 612–618.

Grey, M., Cameron, M. E., & Thurber (1991). Coping and adaptation in children with diabetes. *Nursing Research, 1*(40), 144–149.

Groop, L. C. et al. (1992). Morning or bedtime NPH insulin combined with sulfonylurea in treatment of NIDDM. *Diabetes Care, 15*(7), 831–834.

The Heart Outcomes Prevention Evaluation Study. (2000). Effects of an angiotension converting enzyme inhibitor, Ramapril, on cardiovascular risks in high-risk patients. *The New England Journal of Medicine,* Vol 342 (no. 3), 145–153.

Heart Protection Study. (2002). MRC/BHF Heart protection study of cholesterol lowering with simvastatin in 20,536 high risk individuals. *The Lancet.* Vol 360, July 6, 7–22.

Heine, R. J. (1984). Absorption kinetics and action of mixtures of short and intermediate-acting insulins. *Diabetologia, 27,* 558–562.

Hentinen, M., & Kyngäs, H. (1996). Diabetic adolescents' compliance with health regimens and associated factors. *International Journal of Nursing Studies, 33*(3), 325–337.

Hermann, L. S. (1994). Therapeutic comparison of metformin and sulfonylurea, alone and in various combinations: A double-blinded controlled study. *Diabetes Care, 17*(10), 1100–1109.

Hanefeld, M. et al. (2000). Rapid- and Short-Acting mealtime insulin secretion with nateglinide controls both prandial and mealtime glycemia. *Diabetes Care, 23,* 202–207.

HHS (2001). *FDA Drug Warning.* NDA-21-017, July 2001.

Horton, E. (2000). Nateglinide alone and in combination with metformin improves glycemic control by reducing mealtime glucose levels in Type 2 diabetes *Diabetes Care, 23,* 1660–1665.

Howey, D. C., et al. (1994). A rapidly absorbed analogue of human insulin. *Diabetes, 43*(3), 396–402.

Howey, D. C., et al. (1995). Effect of injection time on postprandial glycemia. *Clinical Pharmacology Therapy, 58,* 459–469.

Johnson, A. B., & Taylor, R. (1996). Does suppression of postprandial blood glucose excursions by the alpha-glucosidase inhibitor miglitol improve insulin sensitivity in diet-treated type II diabetic patients? *Diabetes Care, 19*(6), 559–563.

Krolewski, A. J. et al. (1995). Glycosylated hemoglobin and the risk of microalbuminuria in patients with insulin-dependent diabetes mellitus. *New England Journal of Medicine, 332,* 1251–1255.

Lalau, J. D. (1995). Role of metformin accumulation in metformin-associated lactic acidosis. *Diabetes Care, 18*(6), 779–784.

Lebovitz, H.E. et al. (2002). Evaluation of Liver function in Type 2 diabetic patients during clinical trials: Evidence that rosiglitazone does not cause hepatic dysfunction *Diabetes Care, 25*(5), 815–821.

Lebovitz, H. (1991). *Therapy for diabetes mellitus and related disorders.* Alexandria, VA: American Diabetes Association.

Lee, T. et al. (1994). Incidence of renal failure in NIDDM. *Diabetes. 43* , 572.

Leonhardt, W. (1994). Efficacy of alpha-glucosidase inhibitors in lipids in NIDDM subjects with moderate hyperlipidaemia. *European Journal of Clinical Investigation, 24*(Suppl. 3), 45–49.

May, C. (1995). Efficacy and tolerability of stepwise increasing the dosage of acarbose in patients with non-insulin-dependent diabetes, treated with sulfonylureas. *Diabetes Und Stoffwechsel, 4,* 3–8.

National Diabetes Data Group. (1979). Classification and diagnosis of diabetes mellitus and other categories of glucose intolerance. *Diabetes, 28,* 1039–1057.

NCEP. (1993). Expert Panel on Detection, Evaluations, and Treatment of High Blood Cholesterol in Adults: Summary of the second report of the national cholesterol education program (NCEP) expert panel on detection, evaluation, and treatment of high blood cholesterol in adults. *Journal of the American Medical Association, 269,* 3015–3023.

Nesto, RW; Beel, D. (2003). Thiazolidinedrone use, fluid retention and congestive heart failure: A consumer statement from the American Heart Association & American Diabetic Association *Circulation* 108: 2941.

Olefsky, J. (Personal communication to diabetes professional community of National Diabetes Education Initiative Faculty, November 12, 1997.)

Owens D. R. et al. (2000). Increased prandial insulin secretion after administration of a single preprandial oral dose of repaglinide in patients with type 2 diabetes. *Diabetes Care, 23,* 518–523.

Peters, A. L. (1986). Effect of storage on action of NPH and regular insulin mixtures. *Diabetes Care, 14,* 180–183.

Peters, A. (2001). Using Thiazolidinedrones Rosiglitazone and Pioglitazones in clinical practice. *Am. J. Managed Care, 7,* 3; 587–595.

Powers, M. (1996). *Handbook of diabetes medical nutrition therapy.* Gaithersburg, MD: Aspen Publishers.

Pugh, J. A., et al. (1992). Is combination sulfonylurea and insulin therapy useful in NIDDM patients? *Diabetes Care, 15* (8), 953–959.

Ratner R., et al (2000). Less hypoglycemia with Insulin Glargine in intensive Insulin Therapy for type I diabetes. Diabetes Care 23; 5: 639–643.

Riddle, M. C. (1990) Evening insulin strategy. *Diabetes Care, 13,* 676–686.

Riddle, M. C., McDaniel, P. A., Mitchell, M. C., Ahmann, A. J., & Karl, D. M. (1996). Lowdose metformin added to sulfonylurea: Comparison of two regimens. Scientific presentation at 56th Annual Meeting & Scientific Sessions of ADA, June 1996, San Francisco, CA.

Sambol, N. C. (1995). Kidney function and age are both predictors of pharmacokinetics of metformin. *Journal of Clinical Pharmacology, 35*(11), 1094–1102.

Sels, J. P., et al. (1994). Effect of miglitol (BAY m-1099) on fasting blood glucose in type 2 diabetes mellitus. *Netherlands Journal of Medicine, 44*(6): 198–201.

Shorr, RF. (1997, August). Incidence and risk factors for serious hypoglycemia in older persons using insulin or sulfonylureas *Arch Int. Med, 157,* 1681–1686.

Stenman, S., et al. (1993). What is the benefit of increasing the sulfonylurea dose? *Annals of Internal Medicine, 118*(3), 169–172.

United Kingdom Prospective Diabetes Study (UKPDS). (1995). Relative efficacy of randomly allocated diet, sufonylurea, insulin, or metformin in patients with newly diagnosed non-insulindependent diabetes followed for 3 years. *British Medical Journal, 310*(69–72), 83–88.

Vignati, L. et al. (1995). Treatment of 722 patients with type II diabetes with insulin lispro in a 6 month crossover study. *Diabetes, 44*(Suppl 1), Abstract No. 229A.

Whitcomb, R. W., Saltiel, A. R., & Lockwood, D. H. (1996). New therapies for NIDDM: Thiazolidinediones. In LeRoith, D., Taylor, S.I., Olefsky, J. M. (eds.), *Diabetes mellitus: A fundamental & clinical text.* Philadelphia, PA: Lippincott-Raven, pp. 661–668.

White, J. R. (1996). The pharmacologic management of patients with type II diabetes mellitus in the era of new oral agents and insulin analogs. *Diabetes Spectrum, 9,* 227–234.

World Health Organization (1985). *Diabetes mellitus: Report of a WHO study group.* Geneva, Switzerland: World Health Organization (Tech. Rep. Service., No. 727).

CHAPTER ❖ 32

OBESITY

Jeanette F. Kissinger ◆ Ellis Quinn Youngkin

Obesity is one of the greatest health and social problems plaguing the United States today. Sixty-one percent of U.S. adults aged 20 to 74 years are overweight or obese—(National Heart, Lung, 2002). In contrast, the National Population Health Survey of Canada in 1996/1997 reported 46% of Canadians being overweight or obese (Gilmore, 1999). Of the estimated 97 million U.S. adults overweight or obese, 34% have a body mass index (BMI) of 25.0 to 29.9, classifying them as overweight, and 27% (50 million) are obese with a BMI greater or equal to 30.0. Adolescents and prepubertal children overweight are 14% and 13%, respectively (National Center for Health Statistics [NCHS], 1999). The number of children who are overweight, Black, and Hispanic has more than doubled in the last 12 years (Tanner, 2001). C. Everett Koop, former surgeon general of the United States, refers to the problem as an epidemic (Fraser, 1997). It is reported as the second leading cause of preventable death behind cigarette smoking with 58 million afflicted and contributing to 300,000 deaths annually (Davis & Feller, 1997). The economic cost in 1995 attributed to obesity was $99.2 billion. Of this, $51.6 billion were direct medical costs for treatment of diseases related to obesity (National Institutes of Health [NIH], 1998). By the year 2000, the cost had risen to $117 billion (Kuritzky, 2002).

DEFINITIONS AND PREVALENCE OF OBESITY

In the early 90s obesity was defined by the National Institutes of Health as an excess of body fat resulting in impairment of health. The more accepted definition then for adult obesity was being 20% over ideal weight ("The Triumph of Obesity," 1997, "Weight Management," 1996). Since the late 1990s, the body mass index (BMI) has been shown to be clinically useful to define overweight and obesity; this measurement describes relative weight for height and is significantly correlated with total body fat content. An adult with a BMI of less than 18.5 is considered underweight; a normal range is 18.5 to 24.9, over weight is 25.0 to 29.9, obesity is 30.0 to 39.9, and extreme obesity is a BMI over 40. An adult with a BMI of 30 would be approximately 30 pounds over his or her "normal" or "desired" weight of 196 lbs (see Figure 32–1). There continues to be a larger percentage of women overweight than men; the prevalence of being overweight is much higher in non-Hispanic Black women (66.0%), in Mexican American women (65.9%), and in Mexican American men (63.9%) (NCHS, 1999; NIH, 1998). Since 1998, waist circumference has been recognized as the most useful marker for disease risk related to obesity (Kuritzky, 2002; NIH, 1998).

In children, obesity is defined with more difficulty because reference data on morbidity and mortality used for defining the problem in adults are less clear in children. In the past, the use of triceps skinfold thickness and weight for height, age, and sex in defining obesity for children, saying that if the triceps skinfold thickness is greater than or equal to the 85th percentile, and the weight for height, age, and sex is greater than or equal to the 85th percentile, the child is obese. The National Health and Nutrition Examination Survey (HANES) that is periodically conducted on children ages 6 to 11 years and adolescents aged 12 to 17 years, uses as the definitions for overweight and obesity a BMI at or above gen-

Weight (lb)	Height (ft, in) 4'10"	4'11"	5'0"	5'1"	5'2"	5'3"	5'4"	5'5"	5'6"	5'7"	5'8"	5'9"	5'10"	5'11"	6'0"	6'1"
130	27	26	25	25	24	23	22	22	21	20	20	20	19	18	18	17
135	28	27	26	25	25	24	23	22	22	21	20	20	19	19	18	18
140	29	28	27	27	26	25	24	23	23	22	21	21	20	20	19	19
145	30	29	28	27	27	26	25	24	23	23	22	21	21	20	20	19
150	31	30	29	28	27	27	26	25	24	24	23	22	22	21	20	20
155	32	31	30	29	28	28	27	26	25	24	24	23	22	22	21	20
160	34	32	31	30	29	28	28	27	26	25	24	24	23	22	22	21
165	35	33	32	31	30	29	28	28	27	26	25	24	24	23	22	22
170	36	34	33	32	31	30	29	28	28	27	26	25	24	24	23	22
175	37	35	34	33	32	31	30	29	28	27	27	26	25	24	24	23
180	38	36	35	34	33	32	31	30	29	28	27	27	26	25	25	24
185	39	37	36	35	34	33	32	31	30	29	28	27	27	26	25	24
190	40	38	37	36	35	34	33	32	31	30	29	28	27	27	26	25
195	41	39	38	37	36	35	34	32	32	31	30	29	28	27	27	26
200	42	40	39	38	37	36	34	33	32	31	30	30	29	28	27	26
205	43	41	40	39	38	36	35	34	33	32	31	30	29	29	28	27
210	44	43	41	40	38	37	36	35	34	33	32	31	30	29	29	28
215	45	44	42	41	39	38	37	36	35	34	33	32	31	30	29	28
220	46	45	43	42	40	39	38	37	36	35	34	33	32	31	30	29
225	47	46	44	43	41	40	39	38	36	35	34	33	32	31	31	30
230	48	47	45	44	42	41	40	38	37	36	35	34	33	32	31	30
235	49	48	46	44	43	42	40	39	38	37	36	35	34	33	32	31
240	50	49	47	45	44	43	41	40	39	38	37	36	35	34	33	32
245	51	50	48	46	45	43	42	41	40	38	37	36	35	34	33	32
250	52	51	49	47	46	44	43	42	40	39	38	37	36	35	34	33
255	53	52	50	48	47	45	44	43	41	40	39	38	37	36	35	34
260	54	53	51	49	48	46	45	43	42	41	40	38	37	36	35	34
265	55	54	52	50	49	47	46	44	43	42	40	39	38	37	36	35
270	56	55	53	51	49	48	46	45	44	42	41	40	39	38	37	36
275	57	56	54	52	50	49	47	46	44	43	42	41	40	38	37	36
280	58	57	55	53	51	50	48	47	45	44	43	41	40	39	38	37
285	59	58	56	54	52	51	49	48	46	45	43	42	41	40	39	38
290	60	59	57	55	53	51	50	48	47	46	44	43	42	41	39	38
295	61	60	58	56	54	52	51	49	48	46	45	44	42	41	40	39
300	62	61	59	57	55	53	52	50	49	47	46	44	43	42	41	40

FIGURE 32–1. Body mass index (BMI) self-assessment chart. An adult with a BMI over 25 is considered obese.

der- and age- specific 85th percentile for overweight and 95th percentile for obesity. With 13% and 14% prevalence respectively, the danger is that more than 80% of these children and adolescents will become overweight and obese adults (NIH, 1998).

The number of overweight and obese individuals in this country has climbed steadily in the last 20 years (McLellan, 2002; "Update," MMWR, 1997; "Weight Management," 1996). According to surveys, 33 to 40% of adult women and 20 to 24% of adult men are seeking to lose weight at any one time. Many more are trying to maintain their current weight. More Hispanic men are trying to lose weight than any other group of men. Mokdad, Bowman, Ford, and colleagues (2001), in a study of 184,450 adults from all 50 states, found that of those trying to lose weight, only 42.8% of the obese and 15.6% of those overweight had been counseled by their healthcare providers to lose weight.

A Tufts University report mapped obesity levels in the 33 largest U.S. metropolitan areas ("Mapping U.S. Obesity," 1997). New York had the largest percentage of obese residents (38%); Denver had the lowest (22%). The report blamed overconsumption secondary to the many restaurants and corner food vendors in New York; however, this would not explain the second highest ranking city's rate—34% for Norfolk, Virginia. Cities with higher percentages of obese individuals were found to have the following in common: higher unemployment rates, a higher number of food stores per person, larger African American populations, lower per capita income, and higher annual precipitation.

RISKS OF OBESITY

Multiple studies have verified that obesity puts the individual at risk for a number of serious physical conditions, as well as for psychosocial disadvantages. Reports of evidence from clinical studies and surveys (Carek, Sherer, and Carson, 1997; Gilmore, 1999; National Heart, Lung, 2002; NIH, 1998; Shintani, Ogawa & Nakao, 2002; "Update," 1997) state that being overweight or obese substantially raises the risk for morbidity and mortality associated with hypertension, hyperlipidemia, coronary heart disease, heart failure, stroke, diabetes mellitus, gallbladder disease, sleep apnea, and respiratory disease, asthma, endometrial, breast, prostate, and colon cancers, thyroid disorders, gout, back problems, and osteoarthrtis. Men who are at 150 to 300% of ideal body weight (extreme obesity) die at 12 times the rate of nonobese men (Isselbacher, Braunwald, Wilson, et al., 1995).

People who are obese are 50% more likely to have serum cholesterol levels of at least 250 mg/dL, as well as other lipid abnormalities. Hypertension is much more common in obese individuals, as is coronary heart disease (CHD) (National Cholesterol Education Program [NCEP], 2001). There is a five times greater incidence of non-insulin-dependent diabetes mellitus (type II) in individuals who are moderately obese, and this rises to ten times greater with severe obesity (Carek et al., 1997 NIH, 1998). A 15-year followup study of middle-aged men and women in Finland found that mortality from CHD and body mass index (BMI) were positively associated, and smoking further increased the risk ratio (Jousilahti, Tuomilehto, Vartianinen, et al, 1996). Obesity was said to be an independent risk factor for CHD mortality among men and a contributing factor among women.

The risk of morbidity such as stroke, ischemia, heart disease, and diabetes mellitus, is three to four times greater in people with a BMI greater than 28 than it is in the population generally (Rosenbaum, Leibel, & Hirsch, 1997). A study reported by the National Heart, Lung, and Blood Institute (NHLBI) (2002) found that an increased strong and independent risk of heart failure occurs with an excess in body weight, and the risk increases steadily as weight increases. For each value of 1 increment in BMI, the risk of heart failure increased 5% for men and 7% for women. Obese men had a 90% increase in risk; obese women's risk doubled. According to one study, BMI increased until age 50 in men, then plateaued (Lamon-Fava, Wilson, & Schaefer, 1996). BMI increased in women up to the 70s. Based on BMI, 72% of men and 42% of women had BMIs higher than 25, the traditional cutoff point for overweight (see Figure. 32–1). Reduced HDL cholesterol levels and hypertension were found to be the more strongly associated risk factors associated with higher BMI for both sexes. For women, elevated triglyceride levels, small LDL particles, and diabetes mellitus also were strongly associated with higher BMI. The "apple" figure (a central distribution of body fat) is a significant risk factor as opposed to a waist:hip ratio (WHR) that shows a more peripheral fat distribution ("pear shape") (Rosenbaum, et al., 1997). Both men and women increase their WHRs as they age. An increased health risk is associated with a WHR of 0.95 or more for men and 0.80 or more for women (Cerulli, Lomaestro, & Malone, 1998). The recommendation from the Clinical Guidelines on the Identification, Evaluation, and

Treatment of Overweight and Obesity in Adults (NIH, 1998) is to use the waist circumference cutoffs in conjunction with the BMI to identify the increased disease risk. The waist circumference (WC) is a better indicator of abdominal fat than the WHR. The WC can provide a useful estimate of increased abdominal fat, and thus an increased risk for associated disease, even when there is no change in BMI. To obtain an accurate WC, the subject should be standing. The tape measure should be parallel to the floor around the waist at the uppermost lateral point of the iliac crests. The tape should be snug, but not compress the skin. The measurement reading is taken at a normal minimal respiration. Cutoff points for WC in men are > 102 cm (> 40 in), and in women > 88 cm (> 35 in).

Troiano, Frongillo, Sobal, and Levitsky (1996) estimated the relationship between BMI and all-cause mortality in a meta-analysis. They concluded that a comparable increased mortality existed at both moderately low BMI levels and at extreme overweight levels for white men, which was related to smoking or existing disease. According to Dr. Koop, a study out of Harvard by Mason found that even mild to moderate overweight was associated with an increased risk of premature death (Fraser, 1997). One British study found that fatter or overweight children had higher blood pressure levels and higher cholesterol concentrations than normal-weight children, and advised reducing obesity in children as one appropriate action to prevent CHD in adulthood (Rona, Qureshi, & Chinn, 1996).

Death rates from colorectal cancer and prostatic cancer were reported to be higher in overweight men; death rates from endometrial, cervical, ovarian, breast, and gallbladder cancers were higher in obese women. Rates of renal disease and pregnancy complications, as well as those conditions mentioned previously, also are reported to be higher in overweight people (NIH, 1998).

Studies confirm that maternal obesity is associated with congenital malformation risks, especially neural tube defects (Prentice & Goldberg, 1996). This factor is an independent risk factor of other possible covariant confounders such as folate intake, smoking, socioeconomic status, maternal age, or maternal education. Some suggest that overweight or obese status influences folate to lose its protective influence in pregnancy.

Besides the physical risks, obesity causes serious social stigmata, with the obese person often being blamed for his or her own illness, labeled as lacking willpower, gluttonous, and lazy. Often, people who are normal weight are repulsed by obese individuals, leading to anger and withdrawal by the obese person. Consequently, depression and social isolation are common. Obese people have a lesser chance for employment and advancement; discrimination in college acceptance; less financial aid from parents and/or grants; fewer rental availabilities; and fever opportunities for marriage. Most of the research has been done on Caucasians. It is believed that other racial and ethnic groups are not as harsh in evaluating obese persons (NIH, 1998).

Children who are obese have particularly serious sequelae psychologically and socially. In one study of adolescent overweight girls, after 7 years, they were less likely to be married, had lower household incomes, and higher poverty rates regardless of aptitude scores or socioeconomic status at the beginning of the study (Gortmaker, Must, Perrin, et al., 1993). Conflicting data exist regarding the later adult morbidity effects of obesity in childhood. According to Rosenbaum and colleagues (1997), an increased risk of later morbidity is associated with childhood obesity, even if the person is not obese as an adult. A recent, large Australian cohort study found health risks as adults to be more common in those who were underweight as children than those who had excess weight as children (Wright, Parker, Lamont, & Craft, 2001). Hospitalizations of overweight and obese children have tripled in the last twenty years for increasing rates of diseases caused by obesity, such as diabetes and sleep apnea, according to a CDC study led by William Dietz (Neergaard, 2002).

The emphasis in developed countries on being attractive and thin is so great that huge amounts of money are spent by Americans annually to try to become or stay thinner, or for products associated with conditions caused by being overweight. The market, media ads, and mail orders have exploded with new products to help get slim . . . trim, and lose "cellulite." Their emphasis is not on decreasing the risk of obesity-related disease. In 1996, Gorsky et al. estimated a $70 billion cost of obesity-related disease. As addressed earlier in this chapter, the cost has already exceeded $117 billion. To reduce these escalating healthcare costs related to obesity, a strategy for prevention of excess weight, maintenance of normal weight, and reduction of overweight and obesity needs to include behavioral, nutritional, and activity modification with pharmacotherapy as a possible adjunct.

CAUSES OF OBESITY

As a chronic condition, obesity is rooted in many areas: inherited traits, lifestyle, and environment. Behavior is unlikely to be the only cause of obesity based on responses of lean and obese people to experimental perturbation of body weight (Rosenbaum, et al., 1997). Recidivism occurs almost inevitably in lean and obese people who lose weight. There is a great diversity of opinion over the relative importance of factors related to obesity. The average adult consumes and burns approximately one million calories a year, yet weight remains rather constant due to the compensatory mechanism of the body (hunger and hypothalamic satiety centers) to control and maintain its usual weight. The concept that obesity is the result of caloric intake exceeding the caloric need of the body is an oversimplification (James, Guo, & Liu, 2001; Ripoll, 2001). Because of differences in age, race, gender, activity level, metabolic rate, and habits like smoking and/or drinking, overeating in some people leads to obesity but in others to no weight change. The NIH, in their evidence report (1998), stated that several studies have shown that some people gain weight or lose weight more easily/quickly than other people. In support of this, other studies have shown that some obese people eat no more calories than thinner people. Contributing to the problem of obesity may likely be the overconsumption of foods high in fat than simply overeating in general. However, it is evident that even low fat intake with high caloric intake of carbohydrates contributes to weight gain. In addition, sedentary lifestyle is a major contributor to obesity, and Americans lead very inactive lives. Another influencing factor is the level of leptin. A deficiency of this protein results in excessive eating. Leptin's normal function is to influence the hypothalamus to decrease the production of neuropeptide Y (NPY). NPY stimulates the intake of food (Harrell, Bomar, McMurray, Bradley, and Deng, 2001; Ripoll, 2001; Shintani et al., 2002). Obesity that is mild to moderate is usually seen beginning in later life and can be attributed to a combination of genetic predisposition, diet high in fat and calories, infrequent exercise, and inadequate stress management (Cerulli et al., 1998).

These behavioral problems also are seen with children, as more data link the patterns of physical activity, hours watching television and videos, intake of saturated fats, and body fatness. The patterns for later life, including risk factors, are begun in childhood as the result of family behavioral patterns. Our sociocultural traditions promote overeating and the preference for high caloric foods. Food marketing in supermarkets, mass media, and restaurants is highly sophisticated and, together with the large portions served in restaurants and fast food places, promotes high caloric consumption (NIH, 1998). Only recently has the restaurant industry started to modify their selections in response to the nationwide focus on low carbohydrate intake and the glycemic index. A recent study found that certain behaviors of mothers interfere with the children's ability to self-regulate energy intake of food (Spruijt-Metz, Lindquist, Birch, et al., 2002). If the mother restricted what the children ate, they were more likely to be overweight. If the mother pressured the children to eat, the children tended to have lower total fat mass. Approximately one quarter of people suffering from severe obesity are said to have a binge-eating disorder (Andersen, 1996). These individuals graze or binge without purging.

Recent studies on the genetic influence on obesity suggest that 25 to 40% of individual differences in BMI may depend on genetic factors. This was the finding when a population of subjects with a wide range of BMIs had data on their siblings, parents, and spouses analyzed. However, in identical twin studies, where the twins were reared apart from each other, the genetic influence reaches 70% (NIH, 1998). Obese parents are more likely to have obese children, although many more factors influence the outcome. When both parents are obese, the child's chance of being obese is 80 to 90%; it is 40% with one obese parent, and 7 to 10% with no obese parents (Andersen, 1996). Women in the Nurses' Health Study who were overweight were more likely to have mothers who were in the heaviest of nine weight groups ("Birth Weight," 1996). First-degree relatives of overweight persons, in comparison to the general population, have the relative risk (RR) of 2 in becoming overweight themselves; a RR of 3 to 4 if the relative is moderately obese, and 5 if the relative is severely obese. Mendelian disorder studies with obesity seem to suggest there are several genes that have the capacity to increase the likelihood of becoming obese. It is thought that the regulation of energy balance is controlled by the hormone leptin involving both reward pathways and the pleasurable aspect of eating (Harold and Williams, 2003). The rodent gene for leptin and its receptor have been cloned, but their relationship to human obesity has not been established. One human study describes subjects with a leptin mutation. From all of this research, it suggests that in humans, the susceptibility genotypes for obesity may result from variations of several genes (NIH, 1998; Shintani et al., 2002).

In utero, overnutrition or undernutrition may influence the development and capabilities of the hypothalamic centers' control of food. There is some speculation that overnutrition in the third trimester and postnatal periods may influence adipose tissue cellularity, promoting obesity. Research from the Nurse's Health Study "Birth

Weight," found that women who weighed more than 10 lb at birth were 62% more likely to become obese in midlife than those who weighed under 8.5 lb ("Birth Weight," 1996).

Some conditions occasionally cause a secondary obesity. These include endocrine disease (hypothyroidism, Cushing's syndrome, hypogonadism, insulinoma), hypothalamic hyperphagia (Prader-Willi syndrome seen in children), genetic alterations (beta$_3$-adrenergic receptor coding gene mutation), neurologic disorders, and some drugs, such as prednisone (Andersen, 1996; Carek et al., 1997).

The reader is referred to the review of the regulation of energy storage, intake, and expenditure, neurophysiology of feeding, metabolic effects of weight perturbation as well as futile cycles, chemical mediators of energy homeostasis, and genetic factors in Rosenbaum and colleagues (1997). The discussion of these areas is beyond the scope of this chapter.

SPECIFIC CONSIDERATIONS FOR PHARMACOTHERAPY

WHEN DRUG THERAPY IS NEEDED

Pharmacotherapy may be needed as an adjunct to behavioral modification therapy. The literature, however, overwhelmingly supports behavioral, dietary, and activity modification therapies as the primary means toward long-lasting weight loss. Since these behavioral modifications are difficult for many people to begin or to maintain, and despite the fact that behavior therapy has proven to be a better way to maintain weight loss than pharmacotherapy, drug therapy may be indicated (Carek et al., 1997; Davis & Turner, 2001). Drug therapy has been shown to lead to a faster beginning weight loss, thus this method as an adjunct to behavioral therapies is commonly accepted for initial cotherapy by many practitioners. However, providers must remember that "the history of weight-reduction efforts as aided by drug treatments is not a bright or happy one," as will be discussed later in this chapter (Davis & Feller, 1997, p. 114). Children and adolescents are most successfully treated with realistic goals, a diet balanced in low-fat and high-fiber foods, moderate caloric reduction of 20 to 25%, increased physical activity, strong parental support, and behavioral therapy. (Davis & Turner, 2001; Williams, Campanaro, Squillace & Bollella, 1997). Drug therapy in these age groups is not advised.

SHORT- AND LONG-TERM GOALS OF PHARMACOTHERAPY

Of great importance is helping the obese person set realistic short-term goals, not impossible goals based on societal thinness standards (Rosenbaum et al., 1997). Pharmacotherapy, as a short-term therapy, is aimed at helping the individual get off to a faster start with weight loss, as well as promoting a more positive initial emotional response to therapy. The slower response to behavioral therapies that is the rule with behavioral, diet, and activity modifications may lead people to lose interest and motivation. When reducing morbidity and mortality risks are the long-term aims of weight loss, the use of drug therapy may be necessary.

If the weight level is mildly to moderately elevated and the patient has no serious complications, or worsening of complications, some providers feel any cycling of weight gain and loss is worse in promoting cardiovascular disease than remaining at a stable though somewhat increased weight (Andersen, 1996). Also, although anoretic drugs have some limited benefits, regaining of lost weight occurs rapidly once they are discontinued without continued maintenance of primary behavioral modification therapies concerning diet and exercise (Carek et al., 1997; Davis & Turner, 2001).

NONPHARMACOLOGIC THERAPY

Behavioral, diet, and exercise therapies are the mainstays of weight-loss and maintenance programs today. When drug therapy is used, it should be used in conjunction with these where possible, and monitoring should occur around the combination of therapy.

Behavioral Modifications

The initiation of any weight-loss program must begin with a mental and emotional dedication by the patient to change his or her behavior. Such alterations include lifestyle, dietary habits, and activity levels, but most of all, they include a mental framework that encourages and enhances continuing with the modifications. Behavioral changes are said to progress through stages, whatever the health adaptation or cessation behavior (Pender, 1997). The transtheoretical model, developed by Prochaska and DiClemente, is applicable to modifying one's life and behavior. The aims of behavioral programs are to find and alter the prior habits to eating, describe and improve the style of eating, and provide rewards for improved eating behavior (Bray, 2002). A summit meeting on obesity held in June 2004, sponsored by *Time* magazine and ABC News, focused on lifestyle changes including initiatives to restrict the availability of non0nutritional foods in schools. An interactive web site, www.smallstep.gov, sponsored by U.S. Health and Human Services encourages Americans to make small activity and dietary changes.

Dietary Modification

This is the most preferred therapy (Bray, 1993; Davis & Turner, 2001; NIH, 1998). Numbers of diet plans are touted to produce weight loss, with everything from decreased caloric intake to low fat intake as the primary factors for loss. A huge, multibillion dollar market exists for such diet plans and for food products to enhance weight loss. This chapter does not review dietary behavioral therapy or diet plans. The reader is referred to appropriate references for this information. However, suffice it to say that reducing total calories is the most important element of any diet (Bray, 2002). Eating a diet that is lower in calories than daily activity requires, low in fat (especially saturated fat), high in vegetables and fruits adequate in complex carbohydrates, and adequate in vitamins and mineral requirements and provides protein from low-fat dairy products, vegetable sources, or fish and chicken (no more than 5–6 oz a day) is considered a healthy nutritional plan. Low-fat diets are associated with short-term weight loss, which can be maintained if the diet is continued (Rosenbaum et al., 1997). The heart-healthy step 1 diet recommended by the National Cholesterol Education Program (2001) lists 30% of caloric intake from fat (with only 8–10% from saturated fat), 55% from carbohydrates, and 15% from protein. Diet therapy involves not only modification of intake of foods, but changes in all the contextual elements surrounding eating, such as environment and emotional states that are more conducive to con-trolling intake. It also must take into account the sociocultural influences that will have to change after years of habituation and familial influence. No other activity of daily living in the lives of individuals is so ensconced with who one is as an individual. Changing the habits related to eating is no small or easy task for anyone.

Physical Activity

Energy expenditure must be increased along with dietary modifications to attain the most success in weight loss. Without the congruence of these two methods, the needed calorie deficit cannot be achieved (Carek et al., 1997; NIH, 1998). Diet and exercise combined are able to decrease the number of people with glucose impairment who progress to frank diabetes mellitus by 58% (Bray, 2002). Again, this chapter does not cover the myriad of exercise and fitness therapies suggested as successful for weight loss and improved physical form. The lay literature promotes many programs, among the most popular, the low carbohydrate diets. The reader is urged to seek readings in appropriate references in planning and counseling individuals about weight loss and fitness. Needless to say, a thorough history and physical examination are indicated prior to the initiation of any concerted fitness regimen to make sure the person is not at risk for illness or injury related to such activities. Any exercise program must be geared to the individual's abilities and interests to be maintained, and should be monitored by the provider for safety. Walking, cycling slowly, cleaning the house, dancing, raking leaves, and gardening are among the lower energy-expending activities that are generally safer for older individuals. For those who are safely able, running, fast cycling, skating, skiing, and rowing offer higher energy expenditure, but require better physical fitness to begin with. Exercise that is of high intensity followed by low intensity (intermittent) leads to more weight and fat loss than exercise that is the same low to moderate intensity even though both continuous and intermittent expend the same number of calories (Davis & Turner, 2001; NIH, 1998; Rosenbaum et al., 1997). Again, developing a safe exercise plan requires assessment and incorporation of all facets of the person's life.

Surgical Therapy

The reader is referred to appropriate references for surgical therapy information. Procedures that reduce the absorptive surface to GI contents are safer today (Bray, 2002). Several new procedures in the last five years offer hope to those with a BMI greater than 35, lower than the BMI of 40 (severe obesity). An even lower BMI than 35 may qualify someone for surgery if major risk factors co-exist.

TIME FRAME FOR INITIATING PHARMACOTHERAPY

When to initiate drug therapy for obesity depends on the individual patient. The provider can offer such therapy after an initial evaluation to rule out contraindications, but the patient must be ready emotionally to try it. If the patient has tried and relapsed using nonpharmacologic therapies, she or he may be more ready to try a drug regimen to assist with weight loss. Also, if the patient has complications of obesity, such as hypertension, CHD, or arthritis pain, these diseases become strong motivators to begin a plan comprised of behavioral change, as well as dietary, exercise, and drug therapy. The sooner an obese person can begin a safe weight-loss plan, the better the chances are of decreasing risks of serious consequences.

Drug therapy is contraindicated in children and pregnant or lactating women. Nonpharmacologic combination therapy plans are advised for children and adolescents. Nonprescribed and unsupervised dieting in pregnancy and lactation may be dangerous to the fetus.

How long it takes to achieve the goals with drug therapy depends on the individual. Some people will need a "boost" for a few months or more, whereas others will need longer support. There is evidence that some drug therapies do promote and maintain long-term weight loss, but they have to be taken long-term (Carek et al. 1997).

See Drug Table 1002.

ASSESSMENT PRIOR TO THERAPY

Baseline History, Physical Examination, and Diagnostic Test Data

Anyone who is being evaluated for obesity needs a complete history and physical examination. Pulmonary and cardiac status need to be determined as well as a lipid profile. Causes of secondary obesity, such as thyroid disease, as well as complications of obesity itself need to be ruled out; thus, an extensive history and physical examination are indicated. Treatments will hinge on the these findings.

A diagnosis of obesity is based on comparison of the patient's weight to standard tables for height and frame (see Table 32–1), waist circumference (see Table 32–2), or by calculation of body mass index (BMI). An adult with a BMI over 25 is considered overweight. A BMI self-assessment chart is provided in Figure 32–1. A gross calculation of obesity can be made by calculating percentage of ideal body weight. The actual body weight is divided by ideal body weight, and the product is multiplied by 100. The ideal result is 100; over 120 is considered obese.

For children, see the previously discussed measurements of triceps skinfolds and growth above the 85th percentile. For adults, skinfold measurements of the triceps and subscapular sites with skin calipers (anthropometry) can provide more precise measures. When these are coupled with BMI, an accurate diagnosis can be made (see Table 32–3 for skinfold measures). Three skinfold measurements are taken at each site (triceps and subscapular), and the median values are summed. Marked deviations above or below the 50th percentile for young adults indicates abnormality. The normal for young men is 21 or 9.45% of body fat; normal for young women is 30 or 22.8% of body fat. Pender (1997) states that the "gold standard" for indirect body fat estimates is hydrostatic weighing, but this requires complex equipment and time and often causes anxiety to the patient.

TABLE 32–1. Weight Table According to Height And Frame

Height		Weight in Pounds (Frame)		
Feet	*Inches*	*Small*	*Medium*	*Large*
Adult Man				
5	2	128–134	131–141	138–150
5	3	130–136	133–143	140–153
5	4	132–138	135–145	142–156
5	5	134–140	137–148	144–160
5	6	136–142	139–151	146–164
5	7	138–145	142–154	149–168
5	8	140–148	145–157	152–172
5	9	142–151	148–160	155–176
5	10	144–154	151–163	158–180
5	11	146–157	154–166	161–184
6	0	149–160	157–170	164–188
6	1	152–164	160–174	168–192
6	2	155–168	164–178	172–197
6	3	158–172	167–182	176–202
6	4	162–175	171–187	181–207
Adult Woman				
4	10	102–111	109–121	118–131
4	11	103–113	111–123	120–134
5	0	104–115	113–126	122–137
5	1	106–118	115–129	125–140
5	2	108–121	118–132	128–143
5	3	111–124	121–135	131–147
5	4	114–127	124–138	134–151
5	5	117–130	127–141	137–155
5	6	120–133	130–144	140–159
5	7	123–136	133–147	143–163
5	8	126–139	136–150	146–167
5	9	129–142	139–153	149–170
5	10	132–145	142–156	152–173
5	11	135–148	145–159	155–176
6	0	138–151	148–162	158–179

Source: From Pender (1997, p. 122).

Concomitant Disease States and Contraindications

As mentioned previously, secondary obesity may be caused by a number of diseases. The management of these diseases is not covered in this chapter. Readers are referred to appropriate chapters in this book or other references for this information. Conditions contraindicating the use of the drugs for treating obesity are provided in

TABLE 32–2. **Classification of Overweight and Obesity by BMI, Waist Circumference and Associated Disease Risk***

	BMI	Obesity Class	Disease Risk* Relative to Normal Weight and Waist Circumference: *Men ≤102 cm (≤40 in) Women ≤88 cm (≤35 in)*	*>102 cm (>40 in) > 88 cm (>35 in)*
Underweight	<18.5			
Normal†	18.5–24.9			
Overweight	25.0–29.9		Increased	High
Obesity	30.0–34.9	I	High	Very high
	35.0–39.9	II	Very high	Very high
Extreme obesity	>40	III	Extremely high	Extremely high

* Disease risk for type 2 diabetes, hypertension, and CVD.

†Increased waist circumference can be a marker for increased risk even in persons of normal weight.

Source: (NIH, 1998).

Drug Table 1002 or in the subsequent sections dealing specifically with drug therapy for obesity.

PATIENT/CAREGIVER INFORMATION

All the literature agrees that pharmacotherapy for weight loss must be accompanied by an exercise regimen and a reduction in caloric intake. This requires, for most, a change in lifestyle. If the patient is committed to change, then the healthcare provider can work out a plan for the individual based on BMI, usual daily activity, and what the patient is willing to do for physical activity (energy expenditure). This will determine the amount of energy intake in calories that is needed to meet nutritional requirements but with sufficient deficit (300 to 500 calories per day) to provide for weight loss (Davis & Turner, 2001).

The patient should know that the medication will give him or her a "fast start" on losing weight, but will not continuously maintain weight loss. That will depend on the lifestyle changes made by the patient. If a patient is not losing weight while on medication, reassess readiness for change. He or she may benefit from learning strategies to *prevent weight gain.*

TABLE 32–3. **Triceps Skinfold Thickness Indicating Obesity (mm)**

Age (yr)	Males	Females
5	≥12	≥15
10	≥13	≥17
15	≥15	≥20
20	≥16	≥28
25	≥20	≥29
30 and above	≥23	≥30

Source: From Pender (1997, p. 122).

Patients should know when and how to take their medications (see Drug Table 1002). They should be told the possible side effects and how to counteract them when possible. A common irritating side effect is dry mouth and/or thirst. Tell them to chew sugarless gum or suck on sugarless lemon drops and increase fluid intake.

Patients taking serotonergic agents should be warned not to abruptly stop the medication, as this could cause depression.

OUTCOMES MANAGEMENT

SELECTING AN APPROPRIATE AGENT

The major classes of anorectic drugs approved by the FDA to treat obesity are noradrenergic (sympathomimetic) agents, norepireprhine-serotonin reputake inhibitor (noradrenergic/serotonergic) agent, serotonergic agents, and pancreatic (GI) lipase inhibitor (Bray, 2002; Wells, DiPiro, Schwinghammer, & Hamilton, 2000). Long-term use of anorectic agents with people who have no contraindications may be more advantageous than short-term therapy, which often results in regain of weight after therapy is discontinued (Wells et al, 2000).

Noradrenergic Agents

These agents act by activating central beta and/or dopaminergic receptors in the hypothalamus (Carek et al., 1997). Many are related chemically to the prototype agent amphetamine. Because amphetamine has such a high potential for abuse, its chemical structure has been modified to reduce stimulant effects, and the resulting newer agents are safer. Agents such as amphetamine, dexamphetamine, and phendimetrazine are now illegal for obesity treatment, and are controlled Schedule II substances. Abuse of the newer agents is rare if they are used according to the manufacturers' recommendations.

Leaders in the field of obesity treatment believe that true tolerance to a noradrenergic agent does not develop; however, patients reach a point in weight loss where they plateau, usually about 6 months after beginning therapy (Bray, 2001; Carek et al., 1997). They then must continue taking the drug even to maintain that weight, and no more weight is lost. This occurs, most likely, in response to the body's compensatory action of decreasing the metabolic rate as it senses the weight loss.

Specific noradrenergic agents (see the Monitoring for Toxicity section that follows for the typical noradrenergic side effects seen with these drugs; all are taken by mouth) are the following:

- *Diethylpropion* (Tenuate) is a Schedule IV prescription medication. The typical daily dose is 25 mg tid; the extended-release dose is 75 mg qd. It causes side effects more rarely than other drugs in this class (Carek et al., 1997) and may be used in patients with mild to moderate ATN (Wells et al., 2000)
- *Mazindol* (Mazanor, Sanorex) is a Schedule IV prescription medication. The typical daily dose is 1 mg tid or 1-3 mg qd. This drug enhances insulin secretion and may have hypolipidemic action that is independent of weight loss. Mazindol has been effective for short-term use; its stimulant activity is less than phentermine (Wells et al., 2000)
- *Phentermine* (Fastin or Ionamin) is a Schedule IV prescription medication. The typical daily dose is 30 mg in the morning or 8 mg before meals (Wells et al., 2000). It has less abuse potential than amphetamine and less stimulant activity. Works equally well if given alternate months or continuously (Carek et al., 1997; Nandigama, Newton—Vinson, & Edmondson, 2002).
- *Phendimetrazine tartrate* (Bontril, Plegine, PreM-2) is a Schedule III prescription medication. The typical dose is 35 mg bid or tid; the extended-release dose is 105 mg once qd. This drug increases free fatty acids and/or glycerol (Carek et al., 1997).
- *Benzphetamine* (Didrex) is a Schedule III prescription medication. The typical dose is 50 mg qd to tid (Carek et al., 1997).

According to Wells et al. (2000), there is a high abuse potential with benzphetamine and routine use is not recommended.

Noradrenergic/Serotonergic Agents

Monoamine reuptake inhibitor. A drug with anti-obesity activity, sibutramine (Meridia), was approved by the FDA for long-term use (Bray, 2001; Davis & Feller, 1997; Niff, 1998). It has little or no monoamine oxidase effect but has a broad monoamine reuptake inhibitor action, interfering with reuptake of 5-HT, dopamine, and norepinephrine. It enhances the ability to regulate hunger. Because of its effect on elevating heart rate and blood pressure, it is not recommended for anyone who has poorly controlled or uncontrolled hypertension, a history of coronary artery disease, congestive heart failure, stroke, arrhythmia or is over the age of 60. It is recommended only for those whose BMI is 30, or 27 with other risk factors. The drug was approved by the FDA over the objection of its scientific advisors. The FDA, recommends that all persons taking the drug have their blood pressure and heart rate checked before initiating therapy and have reevaluations of same at regular intervals (Weighing in, 1998; NP Therapeutics, 1998; Diet drug, 1998). The drug was recently reintroduced for use in Italy with strict limitations because of the adverse effects (Lorenzi, 2002). It is thought that it may be particularly helpful with obese type II diabetics. Side effects, said to be mild, include dry mouth, headache, constipation, and insomnia (Davis & Feller, 1997). This drug is, available in 5, 10, and 15 mg capsules.

Serotonergic Agents

Since August 1997, serious adverse effects resulting from the treatment of some obese individuals with two popular serotonergic agents have been verified, leading to banning of dexfenfluramine (Redux) and fenfluramine (Pondimin) by states and voluntary withdrawal from the market of both drugs by Wyeth-Ayerst, the manufacturer. Patients taking either drug were advised by the FDA to discontinue the drug immediately ("Redux and Pondimin," 1997). A Mayo Clinic cardiologist, Dr. Heidi M. Connolly, and colleagues found that 24 women who had taken the popular combination of drugs, known as fen-phen (fenfluramine and phentermine), for an average of 12 months had developed fibrous thickening of one or more cardiac valves, preventing complete closure of the valve and resulting in regurgitation (Connolly, Crary, McGoon, et al., 1997). Valves on both sides of the heart were involved, and eight women had developed new pulmonary hypertension. Upon histopathological examination, the leaflets and chordal structures had plaque-like encasement. So serious were the findings that *The New England Journal of Medi-*

cine allowed an early release of this study. The women in the study had no previous histories of heart disease and were young; the average age was 44 years. An advisory issued by the FDA warned the public and professionals of the results of this study and of 9 similar cases ("Off-label drug use," 1997). By September 1997, Florida had banned use of the drugs for 90 days, and other states followed suit. As of October 1997, more than 45 additional cases had been reported to the FDA, leading the manufacturer to withdraw the drugs from the market. Phentermine was not implicated in the complications (Napier, 1997).

Interestingly, both fenfluramine (a seroto-nergic agent) and phentermine (an adrenergic agent) were approved by the FDA years before problems arose with fenfluramine, simply because the two were not prescribed together; when used alone, neither was particularly hailed, thus both were prescribed at low rates (Davis & Feller, 1997). Phentermine, when used alone, is limited as an effective weight loss agent because of intolerance to its stimulatory activity (Cerulli et al., 1998).

The introduction of dexfenfluramine in 1996 with an accompanying flurry of publicity not only increased its use but fenfluramine's as well. As research showed that fen-phen actually helped obese persons lose weight more effectively than nutritional alterations alone, the prescribing of the two drugs "became a veritable medical craze" (Davis & Feller, 1997, p. 177). Not soon enough did the realization come that significant complications resulted in some people from use.

Serotonergic agents are structurally very similar to noradrenergic agents, but they work by a different mechanism (Carek et al., 1997). A racemic mixture of dexfenfluramine and levofenfluramine, fenfluramine was a highly selective serotonin agonist. It enhanced serotonin release into nerve synapses and inhibited its reuptake. Dexfenfluramine was the active form and was found to be effective in half the dose of fenfluramine (Voelkel, Clarke, & Higenbotham, 1997).

With the loss of these drugs for treating obesity, weight-loss clinics, providers, and consumers looked to fluoxetine (Prozac) to replace the "fen," and "phen-pro" was born (Davis & Feller, 1997). Although fluoxetine is believed to be an anorectic agent, it is not approved by the FDA for this purpose. In fact, Eli Lilly & Co., the manufacturer, does not endorse its use with phentermine for weight loss, a combination many have turned to as a replacement for fen-phen. Much research is needed before such a combination can be endorsed as safe or effective.

What is known about fluoxetine is that weight loss occurs in nonobese individuals as well as those who are obese or overweight (Carek et al., 1997). Weight loss is promoted for at least 5 to 6 months in people being treated for depression (Rosenbaum, et al., 1997). After 16 to 20 weeks of using 10 to 20 mg qd of fluoxetine, some patients regain weight (Carek et al., 1997). Fluoxetine is approved for depression, bulimia, and obsessive-compulsive disorder. It raises basal body temperature and may increase energy expenditure as well as inhibit serotonin reuptake. Mean weight loss between control and treatment groups in a 1-year double-blind, randomized study of white women was not significantly different with fluoxetine 60 mg daily and placebo, although a clinically significant amount of weight was lost by the fluoxetine group (Goldstein, Rampey, Enas, et al., 1994). The treatment group reported adverse effects significantly more often; controls reported "allergic reactions" significantly more often. Side effects of the drug therapy were asthenia, diarrhea, sweating, insomnia, somnolence, bronchitis, nervousness, nausea and vomiting, tremor, and thirst. Less than half of the patients in both groups completed the study. Of those who did, the treatment group had significantly greater mean weight loss after 7 consecutive months than the placebo group, but maintenance of weight control beyond this point was not successful. Fluoxetine was used in a study with obese patients who had type II diabetes, and were receiving insulin. Those receiving fluoxetine lost significantly more weight than the placebo group, and their daily insulin dosage significantly decreased on active treatment. Both groups had similar adverse effects, but the sample was small (Gray, Fujioka, Deuise & Bray, 1992). Goldstein, Hamilton, Masica, and Beardsley (1997) found that fluoxetine used to treat older patients with major depression was not associated with statistically significant weight loss. Fluoxetine has been found effective and safe for up to 16 weeks when used to treat patients diagnosed with bulimia nervosa (Goldstein, Wilson, Thompson, Potvin, & Rampey, 1995).

Sertraline (Zoloft) has a similar effect on appetite as fluoxetine, but paroxetine does not (Davis & Feller, 1997). Once again, the lack of data on the use of fluoxetine (and other similar drugs) with phentermine must lead providers to consider that a similar synergistic effect as with fen-phen may occur with phen-pro, and caution is urged.

Pancreatic (GI) lipase inhibitor. Orlistat (Xenical) acts by inhibiting pancreatic and gastric lipase, thus reducing the amount of fat from the diet absorbed by the GI tract (Bray, 2002). It is approved for long-term use in the United States by the FDA. Taken with each meal, orlistat is considered a minor adjunct to diet ("Orlistat: A second look," 2002). Two-year clinical trials showed that a mean weight loss occurred at the end of a year of up to 10% when the prescribed diet had 30% fat (Bray, 2002). Orlistat also causes a decreased absorption of fat-soluble vitamins. This results in soft stools and oily leakages. Concerns focus on whether the decreased fat absorption will cause patients to take in more fat, offsetting any benefit (Carek et al., 1997). Side effects of orlistat create a defecation urgency and frequency that may be very bothersome (Davis & Feller, 1997). Abdominal pain may be present. The problems are reported to decrease in the second year of use. Of concern is that fat-soluble vitamins A, D, E, K, and beta-carotene are not absorbed well when this drug is used, so multivitamin supplements should be taken at least 3 hours prior to taking the drug (Davis & Feller, 1997; Nitt, 1998). The best use of this drug requires dietary counseling to be effective (May, 2002).

Herbal Weight Loss Products and Concerns

By October 1997, in the wake of the fen-phen demise, Nutri/System was suggesting that two herbal products, St. John's wort (active ingredient is Hypericum) and ephedra, were the answer to an obese person's dilemma to lose weight (see Chapter 9 for more on these herbs) (Hendren, 1997). The herbal combination was touted to be a safe replacement; however, no studies on the effectiveness or safety of these two herbs in combination were reported "(Update '97," 1997). The largest U.S. manufacturers of St. John's wort sell it as a nutritional supplement and are barred from making health-related claims by federal law. However, ads, stepping close to the line of allowable, have trumpeted the "garden" as a safe way to lose weight in selling the herb.

In the herbal plan, 250 mg of Hypericum in a capsule and 334 mg of ephedra extract in another capsule were given (Davis & Feller, 1997). The second capsule also may have had additional herbs and substances in it supposed to increase fat metabolism, such as chromium, potassium, and magnesium phosphates. The combination was supposed to have an anorexic effect (ephedra) and suppress compulsive eating urges by raising dopamine levels in the brain (Hypericum) (Davis & Feller, 1997).

In fact, ephedra, also called ma huang, epitonin, Sida cordifolia, or ephedrine has been associated with several deaths and many adverse health reports (Wells et al., 2000). Of additional importance for the consumer to know is the Federal Trade Commission's requirement that product labels for Herbal Ecstacy, an ephedra-containing herbal product, contain health warnings ("FTC requires warning," 1997). The FDA cited 800 injuries and at least 17 deaths associated with ephedra. By November 1997, the FDA warned consumers that the combination of ephedra and St. John's wort could cause hypertension, insomnia, seizures, heart attacks, and stroke. Regulations that would limit the amount of ephedrine per dose and ban advertising recommending use of ephedra products for more than 7 days were proposed by the FDA (Jellin et al., 2002, 2000). The FDA warned companies that by advertising dietary supplements as weight loss products, they were violating federal law (Neergaard, 1997). Tyler (1998) attributed 22 deaths to ephedra. He stated that the June 1997 FDA recommended limitation on ephedra use of no more than 8 mg of ephedra alkaloids in a 6-hour period, or 24 mg per day, for no longer than 7 days made ephedra useless as a diet aid. His advice was, that an emphatic "no" be given to the question, "Should I take ephedra?" Based on documented adverse reactions and serious risks with ephedra, it has been banned from U.S. markets since March 2004.

Davis and Feller (1997) issued special cautions to diabetics and hypertensives against taking the herbal combination. Some diabetics may be taking chromium already to enhance insulin action, and adding more may be excessive. They also cite the dangers of ephedra. Chromium was not shown in a double-blind, placebo-controlled study to be effective (Wells et al., 2000). For the hypertensive, ephedra may interfere with the action of prescribed medications, putting the patient at risk.

Because so many people have turned to herbal alternatives to help with weight problems, Dr. Tyler, now deceased, dean emeritus of the Purdue University School of Pharmacy and Pharmacal Sciences, and distinguished professor emeritus of pharmacognosy, devoted an entire article in *Prevention* magazine to help the public have a better understanding of safety issues related to this topic (Tyler, 1998). In addition to discussing ephedra and St. John's wort, he discussed the following herbs being used for weight loss and the pros and cons of each:

- *Hydroxycitric acid (HCA):* Obtained from the brindall berry (Garcinia cambogia), HCA seems to decrease appetite in animals and subsequent food intake. However, no rigorous human studies have been done. Tyler stated that this product may work but recommended that many questions need to be answered by research before use, including substance activity and level after HCA is converted into a supplement; absorption efficiency; weight recidivism after stopping the herb; side effects; and length of time one can take the herb safely.

- *Diuretic and laxative herbs:* Listed were parsley, juniper, and dandelion leaves as diuretic herbs, and aloe, rhubarb root, buckthorn, cascara, and senna as laxative herbs. Many products have these herbs in them, so reading labels is important. Tyler warned that only water is lost with these herbs, thus weight is regained immediately upon stopping them. Using the laxative herbs indefinitely leads to dependence. They may cause diarrhea and severe abdominal cramping. Of greatest concern is potassium loss with low levels causing cardiac irregularities and possible heart failure (Tyler, 1998). Tyler reports the deaths of 4 women from these herbs in teas touted as teas for dieting. The use of these products to lose weight was discouraged.

One group of supplements that Tyler said might be helpful are dietary fiber products, although these are not approved or advertised as weight loss products (Tyler, 1998). He listed oat or barley bran, psyllium, or glucomanna capsules as ways to increase fiber, which might decrease hunger and cholesterol, colon cancer risk, and constipation. He cited a study where dieters either took a fiber supplement or not. The weight loss was nearly twice as great in the supplement group, who reported being less hungry. Tyler advised using small amounts to start (to decrease flatulence and diarrhea). Also, with psyllium and glucomannan capsules, patients need to be urged to drink additional fluids to be sure the product does not remain in the throat/esophagus, swell, and obstruct.

Investigational Agents

The following compound agents are being studied as possible weight-loss drugs (Bray, 2002, p. 1019):

- *Bupropion:* An antidepressant approved by the FDA, bupropion appears to lead to weight loss.
- *Topiramate:* A sulfamate, topiramate is used as adjunctive therapy for seizures. Studies have shown that patients who are being treated with it for epilepsy have lost weight.
- *Ciliary neurotrophic factor (CNTF):* Weight loss has been found with the use of this drug. It is currently being studied for this purpose.
- *Leptin:* A peptide mainly manufactured in adipose tissue, a deficiency of leptin is associated with immense obesity. It has been found that in obese people there is a high resistance to the effects of leptin; thus, greatly limiting its theraputic effectiveness (Batterham, R.L.; Cohen, M.A.; Ellis, S.M.; Le Roux, C.W.; Withers, D.J.; Frost, G.S.; Ghatei, M.A.; Bloom, S.R., 2003).

The following are a few of the molecules being studied for weight loss possibilities (Bray, 2002, p. 1019; Davis & Feller, 1997):

- *Glucagonlike peptide-1:* GI cells process this molecule from enteroglucagon molecules. It has been found to cause a decrease in food intake in people of all weights.
- *Ghrelin:* This molecule is produced in the stomach primarily. It is associated with increased food intake, so an antagonist is thought to have possibilities for weight loss.
- *Pentapeptide enterostatin:* Produced in the intestine, this molecule is associated with reduced fat intake.
- *Neuropeptide Y antagonist:* A very powerful molecule that stimulates food intake and decreases thermogenesis. Antagonists are being studied for either the Y-1 or Y-2 receptor.
- *Melanocortin-4 receptor:* When this receptor is lost in mice, they become obese. Antagonists to this receptor, thought to be signaled by the alpha-melanocyte-stimulating hormone, are being studied.

A very promising hormone, PYY3-36, has been identified by researchers in Oregon and Australia (Maugh, 2002). This hormone, a peptide, is produced in the intestines naturally, and its role is to promote cessation of eating once fullness is obtained. Batterham et al (2003) found that unlike leptin, PYY3.36 was effective in obese subjects as well as lean subjects. Obese subjects were found to be deficient in PYY3.36 which probably contributes to the pathogenesis of obesity. Studies are continuing to identify foods that stimulate greater release of the hormone or to produce an oral form of the hormone.

MONITORING FOR EFFICACY

The patient should be weighed every 1 to 2 weeks at first, then monthly as appropriate (Wells et al., 2002). Weight, waist circumference, body mass index, medical history, blood pressure, and acceptability and tolerance of the therapy should be assessed at each visit. Ideal body weight should be determined, and the patient should be monitored closely so that he or she does not fall below this weight. If the patient is averaging a weight loss of 1 to 2 lb per week, reinforce the positive behaviors including accurate medication taking. Reassess medication-taking behavior, diet, physical activity, and readiness to change. If still no weight loss, discontinue the drug (Nitt, 1998).

Evaluate the effect of weight loss on energy level, hypertension and risk factors (hyperlipidemia, hyperglycemia, etc.). Even when patients are not able to attain ideal body weight, a reduction of 5 to 10% of weight often produces clinically relevant benefits (Davis & Faulds, 1996).

MONITORING FOR TOXICITY AND FOLLOWUP

Noradrenergic Agents

Side effects of these agents include insomnia, headache, irritability, nervousness, dry mouth, sweating, nausea, elevations in heart rate and blood pressure, palpitations, and constipation (Carek et al., 1997). Diethylpropion, Phentermine, and mazindol can interfere with sleep (Carek et al., 1997). None of these agents should be given with a monoamine oxidase inhibitor due to the potential for interaction. Physical and/or psychologic dependence is rare if noradrenergic agents are administered according to the manufacturer's advice. Norandrenergic and serotonergic agents, separately or when used in combination, can cause primary pulmonary hypertension (Wells et al., 2000).

Serotonergic Agents

Side effects are similar to but usually more mild than the corresponding noradrenergic effects. They include sweating, nausea, vomiting, insomnia, diarrhea, somnolence, bronchitis, polyuria, asthenia, nervousness, tremor, and thirst. None of the serotonergic agents should be abruptly discontinued. Such cessation may result in depression. Fluoxentine's abrupt cessation may result additionally in muscle aches and paresthesias. Use of more than one SSRI simultaneously should be avoided as this may cause serotonin syndrome (Wells et al., 2000). Severe consequences are possible with this syndrome—seizures, renal failure, hypotension, DIC, dyspnea, hypertension, and even death.

Sibutramine. Those being treated with this drug must be monitored for more serious problems, such as hypertension, cardiac arrhythmias, and GI problems (Bray, 2002; Lorenzi, 2002). As mentioned earlier, sibutramine should not be given to people who are elderly, with stroke, congestive heart failure, myocardial infarction, or glaucoma or those taking MAOIs. Do not give with other SSRIs.

Orlistat. Use of this drug can cause transient diarrhea, increased flatus, anal leakage, anal urgency from the increased fecal fat being lost (Bray, 2002). If fat-soluble vitamins are not absorbed and, no supplements provided (2 hours later or earlier), deficiencies could result. Some statins' effects may be increased. Warfarin and cyclosporine levels must be monitored closely.

REFERENCES

Andersen, A. E. (1996). Eating and weight disorders. In J. D. Stobo, D. B. Hellmann, P. W. Ladenson, B. G. Petty, & T. A. Traill (Eds.), *The principles and practices of medicine.* Stamford, CT: Appleton & Lange.

Batterham, R. L., Cohen, M. A., Ellis, S. M., Le Roux, C. W., Withers, D. J., Frost, G. S., Ghatei, M. A, & Bloom, S. R. (2003, September 4). Inhibition of food intake in obese subjects by peptide YY3–36. *The New England Journal of Medicine, 349*(10), 941–8.

Birth weight, hypertension, and obesity. (1996). *Harvard Women's Health Watch, IV*(4), 7.

Bray, G. A. (1993). Use and abuse of appetite-suppressant drugs in the treatment of obesity. *Annals of Internal Medicine, 119*(7 Pt. 2), 707–713.

Bray, G. A. (2001). Drug treatment of obesity. Reviews in *Endocrine & Metabolic Disorders, 2*(4), 403–418.

Bray, G. A. (2002, July). Obesity: Is there effective treatment? *Consultant,* 1014–1020.

Carek, P. J., Sherer, J. T., & Carson, D. S. (1997). Management of obesity: Medical treatment options. *American Family Physician, 55*(2), 551– 558.

Cerulli, J., Lomaestro, B. M., & Malone, M. (1998, January). Update on the pharmacotherapy of obesity. *The Annals of Pharmacotherapy, 32,* 88–102.

Connolly, H. M., Crary, J. L., McGoon, M. D., Hensrud, D. D., Edwards, B. S., Edwards, W. D., & Schaff, H. V. (1997). Valvular heart disease associated with fenfluramine-phentermine. *New England Journal of Medicine, 337*(9), 581–588.

Davis, R., & Faulds, D. (1996). Dexfenfluramine: An updated review of its therapeutic use in the management of obesity. *Drugs, 52*(5), 696–724.

Davis, R. B., & Turner, L. W. (2001). A review of current weight management: Research and recommendations. *Journal of the American Academy of Nurse Practitioners, 13*(1), 15–19.

Davis, W. M., & Feller, D. R. (1997, December 8). Advances and retreats in the pharmacotherapy of obesity. *Drug Topics,* 114–121.

Diet drug to hit the shelves. (1998, February 13). *Sun-Sentinel,* 11A.

Fraser, L. (1997, March). C. Everett Koop, *1994 Report Shape up America. Reader's Digest,* 177–184.

FTC requires warning labels for Herbal Ecstacy. (1997, October 18). *Sun-Sentinel,* 12A.

Gilmore, J. (1999). Body mass index and health. *Health Reports, 11*(1), 31–34.

Goldstein, D. J., Hamilton, S. H., Masica, D. N., & Beasley, C. M., Jr. (1997). Fluoxetine in medially stable, depressed geriatric patients: Effects on weight. *Journal of Clinical Psychopharmacology, 17*(5), 365–369.

Goldstein, D. J., Rampey, A. H., Jr., Enas, G. G., Potvin, J. H., Fludzinski, L.A., and Levine, L.R., . . . (1994). Fluoxetine: A randomized clinical trial in the treatment of obesity. *International Journal of Obesity and Related Metabolic Disorders, 18,* 129–135.

Goldstein, D. J., Wilson, M. G., Thompson, V. L., Potvin, J. H., & Rampey, A. H. (1995). Long-term fluoxetine treatment of bulimia nervosa. *British Journal of Psychiatry, 166*(5), 660–666.

Gortmaker, S. L., Must, A., Perrin, J. M., et al. (1993). Social and economic consequences of overweight in adolescence and young adulthood. *New England Journal of Medicine, 329*(14), 1008–1012.

Gray, D. S., Fujioka, K., Devine, W., & Bray, G. A.. (1992). A randomized double-blind clinical trial of fluoxetine in obese diabetics. *International Journal of Obesity and Related Metabolic Disorders, 16* Suppl 4, 567–572.

Harrell, J. S., Bomar, P., McMurray, R., Bradley, C., & Deng, S. (2001). Leptin and obesity in mother-child pairs. *Biological Research for Nursing, 3*(2), 55–64.

Harrold, J. A., & Williams, G. (2003, October). The cannabinoid system: a role in both the homeostatic and hedonic control of eating? *The British Journal of nutrition, 90*(4), 729–34.

Hendren, J. (1997, October 18). Herb's popularity soars after ban on two diet drugs. *Sun-Sentinel,* 10A.

Isselbacher, K. J., Braunwald, E., Wilson, J. D., Martin, J. B., et al. (1995). *Harrison's principles of internal medicine,* New York: McGraw-Hill.

James, G. A., Guo, W., & Liu, Y. (2001). Imaging in vivo brain-hormone interaction in the control of eating and obesity. *Diabetes Technology & Therapeutics, 3*(4), 617–622.

Jellin, J. M., Batz, F., Hitchens, K., et al. (2002). *Pharmacist's Letter/Prescriber's Letter Natural Medicines Comprehensive Database.* (4th Ed.). Stockton, CA: Therapeutic Research Facility.

Jellin, J. M., Gregory, P., Batz, F., Hitchens, K., et al. (2000). *Pharmacist's Letter/Prescriber's Letter Natural Medicines Comprehensive Database.* (3rd Ed.). Stockton, CA: Therapeutic Research Facility.

Jousilahti, P., Tuomilehto, J., Vartianinen, E., Pekkanene, J., & Puska, P. (1996). Body weight, cardiovascular risk factors, and coronary mortality: 15-year followup of middle-aged men and women in eastern Finland. *Circulation, 93*(7), 1372–1379.

Kuritzky, L. (2002, July). Long-term management of obesity: Focusing on comorbid risk factors. *Clinical Spectrum,* 4–9.

Lamon-Fava, S., Wilson, P. W., & Schaefer, E. J. (1996). Impact of body mass index on coronary heart disease risk factors in men and women. The Framingham Offspring Study. *Arteriosclerosis, Thrombosis, and Vascular Biology, 16*(12), 1509– 1515.

Lorenzi, R. (2002). Sibutramine to re-enter the Italian market with specific caveats. *Reuters Medical News.* Retrieved 9/4/02 from http://www.medscape.com.

Mapping U.S. obesity. (1997). *Tufts University Health & Nutrition Letter, 15*(3), 1.

Maugh, T. H., II. (2002, August 18). Hormone reduces appetite, study says. *Sun-Sentinel,* 1A, 7A.

McLellan, F. (2002). Obesity rising to alarming levels around the world. *Lancet, 359*(9315), 1412.

Mokdad, A. H., Bowman, B. A., Ford, E. S., Vinicor, F., Marks, J. S., & Koplan, J. P. (2001). The continuing epidemics of obesity and diabetes in the United States. *The Journal of the American Medical Association, 286*(10), 1195–1200.

Nandigama, R. K., Newton-Vinson, P., & Edmondson, D.E. (2002). Phentermine inhibition of recombinant human liver monoamine oxidases A and B. *Biochemical Pharmacology, 63*(5) 865–869.

Napier, K. (December 1997). Special report. No more diet pills—What now? *Prevention,* 39–40.

National Center for Health Statistics (NCHS). (1999). *National Health and Nutrition Examination Survey* (NHANES). Fast stats a to z USDHHS. Internet posting: http://www.cdc.gov/nchs/fastats/overwt.htm, accessed September 7, 2002.

National Cholesterol Education Program: Third report of the expert panel on detection, evaluation, and treatment of high blood cholesterol in adults (Adult treatment panel III). (2001). National Heart, Lung, and Blood Institute, Bethesda, MD. NIH Publication No. 01-3305. U. S. Department of Health and Human Services.

National Heart, Lung, and Blood Institute Press Release. (July 31, 2002). NHLBIA's Framingham heart study finds strong link between overweight/obesity and risk for heart failure. *NHLBI Communications Office.* Retrieved NHLBINetwork @prospectassoci.com July 31, 2002.

National Institutes of Health, National Heart, Lung, and Blood Institute. (1998). Clinical guidelines on the identification, evaluation, and treatment of overweight and obesity in adults: The evidence report. U. S. Department of Health and Human Services, Public Health Service, NIH, NHLBI.

Neergaard, L. (1997, November 7). FDA targets herbal fen-phen. *Sun-Sentinel,* 8A.

Neergaard, L. (2002, May 2). Obesity-related illnesses increasing in children. *Sun-Sentinel,* 9A.

NP Therapeutics. (1998). *The Nurse Practitioner, 23*(1), 94–95.

Off-label drug use. (1997, October). *Harvard Women's Health Watch, V*(2), 2–3.

Orlistat: A second look. At best, a minor adjunct to dietary measures. (2002). *Prescrire International, 11*(57), 10–12.

Overweight, obesity threatens U.S. health gains. (2002). *FDA Consumer, 36*(2), 8.

Pender, N. J. (1997). *Health promotion in nursing practice* (3rd ed.). Stamford, CT: Appleton & Lange.

Prentice, A., & Goldberg, G. (1996). Maternal obesity increases congenital malformations. *Nutrition Reviews, 54*(5), 146–150.

Redux and Pondimin withdrawn from market. (1997, October). *Nurses Drug News, 1*(11), 1.

Ripoll, I. (2001, September 20). *Obesity and the dismetabolic syndrome.* Paper presented at Virginia Nurse Practitioner Program, Richmond, Virginia.

Rona, R. J., Qureshi, S., & Chinn, S. (1996). Factors related to total cholesterol and blood pressure in British 9 year olds. *Journal of Epidemiology and Community Health, 50*(5), 512–518.

Rosenbaum, M., Leibel, R. L., & Hirsch, J. (1997). Obesity. *The New England Journal of Medicine, 337*(6), 396–407.

Shintani, M., Ogawa, Y., & Nakao, K. (2002). Obesity induced by abnormality in leptin receptor and melanocortin-4 receptor. *Nippon Rinsho—Japanese Journal of Clinical Medicine, 60*(2), 404–409.

Spruijt-Metz, D., Lindquist, C.H., Birch, L.L., et al. (2002). Relation between mothers' child-feeding practices and children's Eadiposity. *American Journal Clinical Nutrition, 75,* 581–586.

Tanner, L. (2001, December 12). Number of overweight children rising quickly. *Sun-Sentinel,* 4A.

The triumph of obesity. (1997). In Women and obesity: A preventable disease. *Women's Health Digest, 1*(4), 263.

Troiano, R. P., Frongillo, E. A., Jr., Sobal, J., & Levitsky, D. A. (1996). The relationship between body weight and mortality: A quantitative analysis of combined information from existing studies. *International Journal of Obesity and Related Metabolic Disorders, 20*(1), 63–75.

Tyler, V. E. (1998, January). Question: Since prescription diet pills are not on the market any more, I'd like to try some of the herbal weight loss products. Do they work? *Prevention,* 81–85.

Update: Prevalence of overweight among children, adolescents, and adults—United States, 1988–1994. (1997). *MMWR, Morbidity and Mortality Weekly Report, 46*(9), 198–202.

Update 97: Weight-loss products: "Herbal" doesn't necessarily mean safe. (1997, December). *Mayo Clinic Health Letter, 15*(12), 4.

Voelkel, N. F., Clarke, W. R., & Higenbottam, T. (1997). Obesity, dexfenfluramine, and pulmonary hypertension. *American Journal of Respiratory and Critical Care Medicine, 155,* 786–788.

Weighing in on Meridia. (1998, February). *Harvard Women's Health Watch, 5*(6), 7.

Weight management: Making the leap to a healthy life. (1996). The Fitness Partner Connection. Reprinted from *International Food Information Council & Food Insight*(1992, July/August), 1–3.

Wells, B.G., DiPiro, J. T., Schwinghammer, T. L., & Hamilton, C.W. (2000). *Pharmacotherapy handbook*(2nd ed.). Stamford, CT: Appleton & Lange.

Williams, C. L., Campanaro, L. A., Squillace, M., & Bollella, M. (1997). Management of childhood obesity in pediatric practice. *The Annals of the New York Academy of Science, 817,* 225–240.

Wright, C. M., Parker, L., Lamont, D., & Craft, A. W. (2001). Implications of childhood obesity for adult health: Findings from Thousand Families Cohort Study. *BMJ, 323,* 1280–1284.

CHAPTER ❖ **33**

MENTAL HEALTH DISORDERS

B. J. Landis ◆ Charles C. Marsh

Most individuals experiencing psychological distress go to their primary care providers rather than to mental health specialists, and over half of mentally ill patients in the United States receive their psychiatric care exclusively in primary care settings (Afinson & Bona, 2001). This trend is likely to continue since the growing managed care systems limit patient access to specialists such as psychiatrists. However, treatment of mental illness has changed dramatically over the past 20 years. Many mental disorders have been linked to specific neurochemical imbalances that are amenable to pharmacologic intervention. Currently, pharmaceutical efforts are focused on developing more effective psychoactive drugs using new knowledge about neurotransmitters and receptors in the central nervous system. Mental health conditions covered in this chapter are the most common ones managed in primary care settings and include disorders of mood, anxiety disorders, insomnia, eating disorders, and substance abuse.

DISORDERS OF MOOD

These disorders have a disturbance in mood as the predominant feature (American Psychiatric Association [APA], 1994). Depression, a very prevalent condition seen in primary care, is associated with significant morbidity and mortality, lost productivity, diminished quality of life, and increased healthcare costs. Almost 18 million Americans are affected with depression each year, and the total estimated monetary costs of this illness exceeded $44 billion in 1990 (AHRQ, 2002). Likewise, anxiety disorders significantly diminish one's quality of life, and their financial cost to society is estimated to be greater than $40 billion per year (Krystal, D'Souza, Sanacora, et al., 2001). Despite the high prevalence of mood disorders, they are often underdiagnosed and consequently undertreated in primary care settings, the place that patients most likely first seek help.

MAJOR DEPRESSIVE DISORDER AND DYSTHYMIA

Clinical depression is a syndrome (a constellation of signs and symptoms) that is not a normal reaction to life's difficulties. Depression should not be confused with a sad mood that normally accompanies specific life experiences such as losses or disappointments. Also, a sad mood is only one of the many manifestations of depression, which may include apathy, anxiety, and irritability. These conditions tend to occur in families. Depressive disorders involve disturbances in emotional, cognitive, behavioral, and somatic regulation (DGP, 1993a). Suicide is the most serious consequence of depressive disorders, occurring at 30 times the rate of nondepressed individuals. (Kando, Wells, & Hayes, 1999).

Major depressive disorder (MDD) consists of a discrete major depressive episode that can be distinguished from the patient's usual level of functioning and is classified into several subgroups (psychotic, melancholic, atypical, seasonal, and postpartum). The subtypes are not all-inclusive but may be useful in selecting treatment regimens.

MDD is a primary disease not associated with nonmood psychiatric conditions (such as eating disorders, panic attacks, or obsessive-compulsive disorder), substance abuse, or medical conditions. Major depression is an acute and sometimes severe episode of depression with unrelenting symptoms persisting for at least 2 weeks; it is not secondary to a medical illness, substance abuse, or other psychological disorders even though it may coexist with these conditions. It may be a chronic disorder that needs long-term followup attention and treatment (APA, 1994; DGP, 1993a).

Melancholic depression is more common among older persons and is manifested by psychomotor retardation or agitation, anhedonia (inability to experience pleasure), worse depression in the morning, and early morning awakening.

Atypical depression is usually associated with younger age of onset and includes two broad categories of symptoms: (1) *vegetative*—marked overeating, oversleeping, and hypersensitivity to personal rejection; and (2) *anxious*—difficulty falling asleep, phobias, and sympathetic arousal along with marked anxiety.

Seasonal depression (seasonal affective disorder) is a well-documented mild to moderate chronic depressive disorder that recurs seasonally, most often during winter. It is more common in females and often presents with significant hypersomnia, lethargy, and weight gain. In addition to antidepressants, limited light therapy may be useful. The therapeutic response may be quick (4–7 days) or delayed up to 2 weeks.

Postpartum depression commonly occurs within 4 weeks to 1 year after childbirth and is more symptomatic than "postpartum blues," which occur briefly within 1 to 5 days after delivery. It is characterized by irritability, depression, insomnia, inability to cope, and tearfulness; however suicide ideation is infrequent. Eight to twenty percent of postpartum women develop this disorder (Bower & Katz, 2002).

Psychotic depression is characterized by hallucinations and delusions that are congruent with the patient's depressed mood. This psychotic variant is best managed in psychiatric settings.

Dysthymic disorder is characterized by a chronic, mild, insidious depressed mood with marked impairment of social functioning lasting 2 years or more. This disorder often exists with comorbid medical conditions such as a cerebrovascular accident, multiple sclerosis, AIDS, hypothyroidism, and cardiac transplantation. Many patients with dysthymia go on to develop a major depression (termed "double depression") that is difficult to treat. Dysthymia is usually manifested by sadness in adults and by either sadness or irritability in children and adolescents (DGP, 1993a; DePaulo, 1999; Moore & Bona, 2001).

Depression commonly presents with symptoms of sleep and appetite disturbances, anhedonia, fatigue, decreased libido, diminished ability to concentrate, indecisiveness, feelings of worthlessness or hopelessness, suicidal ideation, and psychomotor agitation or retardation. Almost 90% of depressed patients also experience anxiety symptoms.

Children and adolescents may also suffer from depression. Depressed adolescents are at high risk for suicide or substance abuse, particularly if the depression is untreated. Although the diagnostic criteria for depression are the same for any age group, young patients may present differently. Given the severity of psychosocial and academic consequences of depression in this population, a multidisciplinary treatment approach is recommended. Unexplained pain and changes in school performance, mood, social aggressiveness, or athletic activities are often presenting symptoms. Also, youngsters who are withdrawn, angry, impulsive, or self-destructive should be evaluated for depression. Nursing home residents and elders with concomitant physical illnesses are also at risk for depressive disorders. Depression can mimic dementia, but usually psychological distress is present only in the depressed patient. Depression in older adults should be treated as aggressively as for any medical illness (DGP, 1993a; Moore & Bona, 2001).

Specific Considerations for Pharmacotherapy

When Drug Therapy Is Needed. The foundation of treatment for MDD is an antidepressant agent to bring relief from the core symptoms. Most sources advocate using both pharmacotherapy and psychotherapy with frequent followup care by the primary clinician.

Basic principles for understanding and treating depression include the following:

1. Accurate diagnosis should rule out underlying physiologic causes.
2. Pharmacotherapy is only part of the treatment plan, which should include collaborative decision making with the patient and family and short-term psychotherapy.
3. No "magic bullet" exists.

4. Every drug has its side effects, and antidepressant choice depends on the drug's side-effect profile.
5. *Do not undertreat.*

Once the decision has been made to use an antidepressant drug, it is vital to use the proper dosage and duration of treatment. Factors to consider in drug selection include: age, family history, pattern of depression, suicidal potential, appetite, sleep habits, and coexistent diseases or other drugs being taken.

The treatment of depression occurs in three phases and gives direction for monitoring therapeutic outcomes: *acute, continuation,* and *maintenance* (APA, 2000). Acute phase goals are to eliminate symptoms of depression and restore psychosocial and occupational function. If treatment results in little or no symptom relief by 6 weeks or only partial relief by 12 weeks, the diagnosis and treatment plan should be reassessed. Substance abuse or underlying medical or psychiatric conditions may become apparent. The continuation phase is the middle stage in which the initially effective drug dosage is sustained. The treatment goal during the maintenance phase is to prevent recurrence of the depression. Some patients will require maintenance medication indefinitely. If depression responds to treatment, some sources recommend continuing the drug for at least 6 months and slowly tapering off over a 4-week period. Should symptoms recur, the effective dose should be returned to its prior level and maintained for another 3 to 6 months. Reports indicate that patients do well when psychotherapy is continued during the maintenance phase. A therapeutic alliance with the patient and family and primary provider is important over the long term to lessen the likelihood of recurrence. Three or more depressive episodes greatly increase the chance of another, and these patients are good candidates for long-term maintenance phase therapy. Using a lower dose of the effective antidepressant during maintenance phase is not recommended. It is best to maintain the medication at the effective dose (DePaulo, 1999; Howland & Thase, 2002).

Depression is commonly associated with nonmood psychiatric disorders such as substance abuse and eating disorders. If present, these nonmood disorders should be treated first; if depression continues, then the depression is treated. Depression often coexists with anxiety; adequate treatment of the primary depression will alleviate secondary anxiety symptoms.

A number of current theories offer explanations for the complex etiology of depression. Some of these theories are shown in Table 33–1. The biogenic amine theory of depression explains its cause as a deficiency of brain neurotransmitters—primarily norepinephrine, serotonin, and dopamine. Emerging neurobiology of depression suggests dysregulation in multiple interconnecting neuromodulating systems (Krystal et al., 2001). Antidepressants intensify neurotransmitter action by blocking reuptake inactivation into presynaptic nerve endings (e.g., tricyclic antidepressants, selective serotonin reuptake inhibitors) or by preventing transmitter degradation (e.g., monoamine oxidase inhibitors). Down-regulation of norepinephrine and serotonin receptors occurs with persistent use of antidepressants, which would explain the delayed onset of the drug. Pharmacotherapy is the cornerstone of treatment for depression whether there is an identifiable psychological cause or stressor. (Kando et al., 1999, Krystal et al., 2001).

TABLE 33–1. Theoretical Basis of Depression

Theory	Pathophysiology
Biogenic amine	Inadequate monoamine neuro-transmission produces depression, primarily from norepinephrine.
Receptor sensitivity	Downregulation of norepinephrine and serotonin receptors follows chronic administration of antidepressants.
Dysregulation	Failure of homeostatic regulation of the neurotransmitter system produces depression.
Permissive hypothesis	Decreased serotonin levels permit expression of affective state; decreased norpinepherine causes depression; elevated norepinepherine causes mania.
Role of dopamine	Elevation of dopamine neurotransmission in the nucleus accumbens may be common pathway for mechanism of antidepressant action.

Adapted from Kando, Wells, & Hayes (1999).

Short- and Long-Term Goals of Pharmacotherapy. Treatment goals include relieving signs and symptoms of depression, restoring psychosocial and occupational function, and avoiding relapse or recurrence of depression (DGP, 1993b; Howland & Thase, 2002). Current recommendations are to maintain effective drug therapy for up to 1 year at the same dosage level needed to achieve resolution of symptoms. Continuation therapy for at least 4 months after the acute episode is necessary to consolidate drug response and prevent relapse. Some experts consider depression a chronic condition and recommend lifetime maintenance of drug therapy in selected patients. Most experts recommend psychotherapy with pharmacotherapy whenever practical. Any treatment program should include support, advice, reassurance, and hope as well as monitoring drug side effects and adjusting dosage for patients receiving medication.

Nonpharmacologic Treatment. All phases of treatment (acute, continuation, and maintenance) are carried out in the context of *clinical management,* which includes education and discussion with patients and their families about the nature of depression, its course, and relative costs and benefits of treatment options. The focus is on resolution of obstacles to treatment adherence, monitoring and management of treatment side effects, and outcome assessment. The primary provider is in a unique position to coordinate the care of a multidisciplinary treatment team and facilitate a therapeutic alliance among health professionals, patients, and their families (DGP, 1993b).

Psychotherapy is combined with medication for patients with partial responses to either treatment alone and for those with a chronic history of depressive disorder. Referral to a psychologist or mental health specialist is necessary for these interventions. Supportive therapy focuses on management and resolution of current difficulties and life decisions using the patient's strengths and available resources. It includes supervision of more severe, complex, or chronic cases as well as active listening, education, reassurance, encouragement, and guidance. Short-term cognitive behavioral and interpersonal therapy, as well as social skills training (12–24 weeks), have demonstrated effectiveness in treating major depression. Postpartum depression responds to interpersonal therapy. Light therapy is a first-line treatment for well-documented seasonal affective disorder.

Hospitalization may be needed if psychosis is present, suicidal risk is significant, social support is inadequate, or a serious general medical condition exists. Electroconvulsive therapy (ECT) is a proven effective and rapid treatment for severely symptomatic patients who have failed to respond to medication trials or who are rapidly deteriorating. These patients are usually hospitalized and referral to a psychiatrist is required (APA, 2000; DGP, 1993b; DePaulo, 1999).

Time Frame for Initiating Pharmacotherapy. Patients should be treated promptly after diagnosis to relieve symptoms, improve functional impairment, and decrease suicide risk. The sooner antidepressant medication is started, the sooner patients will be afforded relief. Because all antidepressants may take up to 4 to 6 weeks to exert their effect and since short-term side effects may be common, patient support and encouragement to adhere to initial drug treatment recommendations are critical.

Overview of Drug Classes for Treatment

- *Selective serotonin reuptake inhibitors* (SSRIs) exert selective effects on serotonin and are the first-line antidepressant agents in the primary care setting because of their proven efficacy, favorable adverse-effect profile, long-term tolerance, once-daily dosing, and wide therapeutic index. These agents also may be used as secondary choices for patients who do not respond well to a trial with tricyclic antidepressants (Friedman & Kocsis, 1996; Howland & Thase, 2002). A warning was issued by the FDA on March 22, 2004, that SSRIs may be associated with worsening depression and suicide in some people (Shogren, 2004).
- *Tricyclic antidepressants* (TCAs) have been used to treat depression in the United States for over 30 years and their efficacy has been well documented. TCAs inhibit reuptake of norepinephrine and/or serotonin; secondary amines primarily increase norepinephrine availability in the CNS. Tertiary amines have a greater effect on serotonin levels. All TCAs are equally effective antidepressant agents with major differences in degree of anticholinergic, sedative, and orthostatic side effects. Importantly, their narrow therapeutic index and potential for overdose may be life-threatening. (Howland & Thase, 2002; Moore & Bona, 2001).
- *Monoamine oxidase inhibitors* (MAOIs) block monoamine oxidase from inactivating amine neurotransmitters, norepinephrine, dopamine, and serotonin in presynaptic neurons. MAOIs are potent antianxiety and antidepressant agents and may be very useful when anxiety is present with depression. However, the clinical utility of these drugs in primary care is limited by their adverse effects and drug-drug and drug-food interactions. Generally, a MAOI drug regimen is managed by a psychiatrist.
- *Other antidepressants: Bupropion* is an antidepressant similar to SSRIs in its energizing effects. It is free of the cardiovascular and anticholinergic side effects of TCAs at both therapeutic doses and in the setting of overdose. Its mode of action is unclear, although it appears to modulate effects of dopamine and norepinepherine. Bupropion has little or no effect on monoamine oxidase or the neurotransmitters serotonin and norepinephrine and, thus, is considered to be an antidepressant that affects different neural systems. For this reason, bupropion may be particularly useful in depressed patients who do not respond to or cannot tolerate SSRIs. Moreover, bupropion has no effect on sexual function and has gained utility in depressed patients treated with SSRIs who develop sexual dysfunction (impotence and delayed ejaculation in males and anorgasmia in females). Initial evidence indicates that bupropion may be especially useful in

bipolar depressed patients because it may have less of a proclivity to induce hypomania in such patients.

Trazodone and *nefazodone** are antidepressants that have in common triazolopyridine chemical structures. These drugs may be listed in some tables as tetracyclic antidepressants. Both of these agents tend to be sedative and orthostatic in their chemical effects. Trazodone is much more likely to cause these adverse effects than its more recently approved "cousin," nefazodone. However, nefazodone has the neurochemical properties of SSRIs, as well as some postsynaptic serotonergic effects. Given this profile, nefazodone can be used in patients who do not respond to SSRIs. *Venlafaxine* is another newer antidepressant that has a distinct neurochemical action among atypical agents. Termed a serotonergic noradrenergic reuptake inhibitor (SNRI), venlafaxine offers patients yet another alternative treatment to TCAs and may be used for the primary treatment of depression. Unlike some of the newer agents, venlafaxine has been shown to be effective even in severe depression compared to placebo and the SSRI fluoxetine. *Mirtazapine* is a novel, tetracyclic agent that has multiple effects on serotonin and antagonizes alpha$_2$ presynaptic receptors, with a net effect of increasing both norepinephrine and serotonin. It has few sexual side effects but has significant weight gain and sedating properties (APA, 2000; DePaulo, 1999; Howland & Thase, 2001).

Assessment and History Taking. A detailed personal and family history is essential to selecting an appropriate treatment regimen. A depressed patient may present with a variety of somatic complaints such as insomnia, headache, musculoskeletal pain, GI disturbance, and vague abdominal pain.

Anxiety, insomnia, and substance abuse are often superimposed on the depression. Men are more likely to present with physical complaints, whereas women are more apt to report feelings of sadness. Cultural differences should be considered in assessing presenting symptomatology of depression. Depression is a potentially fatal disease given the propensity for suicide, and this risk needs to be carefully assessed. Approximately 60% of suicides can be attributed to major depression. Many experts maintain that the risk of attempted suicide is greatest as the patient begins to respond to treatment and has the psychic energy to act upon suicidal thoughts. Thus, a history of prior suicide attempts, suicidal ideation, sense of hopelessness, physical illness, or substance abuse places the patient at high risk, requiring psychiatric referral for treatment. It is a myth that talking to a depressed patient about suicide may prompt the individual to act upon such self-destructive ideation. Rather, clinicians should routinely inquire about thoughts of suicide. If such thoughts are present, differentiate between fleeting thoughts of wishing life were over and recurrent suicidal ideation with a well-thought-out plan for self-injury. Seriously suicidal patients should always be referred immediately to a psychiatrist, and hospitalization is frequently required.

Determine if the depression is associated with a medical disease and take a drug inventory to assess for an adverse drug response. Endocrine disorders (e.g., diabetes mellitus, Cushing's disease), CNS disorders (e.g., Alzheimer's disease), CV disorders (e.g., CHF, CVA), and other diseases (e.g., cancer, malnutrition, lupus, AIDS) may be the underlying cause of depression. Antihypertensives and cardiovascular drugs (e.g., clonidine, digitalis, guanethidine, hydralazine, prazosin, propanolol), sedative-hypnotic drugs (e.g., alcohol, barbiturates, benzodiazepines), anti-inflammatory and analgesic drugs (e.g., indomethacin, opiates, phenylbutazone), steroids (e.g., corticosteroids, estrogen withdrawal, oral contraceptives), and miscellaneous other drugs (e.g., antineoplastics, antiparkinsonian agents, neuroleptics) may be associated with depression and should be reevaluated (Blazer, Grossberg, & Pollock, 1998; DGP, 1993a; Eisendrath & Lichtmacher, 2000).

A physical examination, CBC, chemistry panel, and thyroid function studies (T_3, T_4, TSH) are useful to rule out organic etiologies and guide selection of an antidepressant. A baseline EKG can detect cardiac conduction abnormalities prior to prescribing TCAs. Depression in the elderly may be difficult to distinguish from Alzheimer's disease and other dementia because their cognitive symptoms overlap. However, when depression is present without dementia, patients experience psychological distress and are aware of their cognitive deficits. Depression superimposed on chronic dementia may be responsible for agitation, insomnia, and apathy that frequently results in hospitalization. Controlling these behaviors may be the key to keeping patients home and out of the hospital.

See Drug Table 311.

Patient/Caregiver Information. A caring family able to provide social and environmental support during treatment can be a real asset to recovery from any illness, including depression. Patients and families need to learn at the outset of treatment about the nature of depression and that treatment can be effective for most patients. Education and counseling needs to deal with issues of side ef-

*See Addendum on p. 748.

fects and nonadherence. The primary clinician can instill a sense of hope. Inform patients and their families about target signs and symptoms that they can use to assess the therapeutic drug response (Friedman & Kocsis, 1996).

The patient and family need to understand that medications should be taken regularly, that they may take several weeks to work, and that there may be side effects that usually resolve with time. Avoid using OTC medications or herbal remedies that may interact with the antidepressant. Reassure them that antidepressants are not addictive but they need to be taken as prescribed. Patient and caregiver need information about special dietary restrictions when MAOIs are prescribed; see, for example, Table 33–2. Caffeine intake should be limited because it tends to increase nervousness in patients taking TCAs and MAOIs and can precipitate cardiac arrhythmias or hypertension in patients taking MAOIs. Table 33–3 contains patient, family, and health professional resources for managing depressive disorders.

Outcomes Management

In assessing treatment outcomes remember that the major reasons for a poor response to antidepressant drug treatment are inadequate therapy, insufficient dosage, or inadequate duration of treatment.

Selecting an Appropriate Agent. Selecting an antidepressant agent is based on the patient's age, general health status, clinical presentation, and past response to medication. Additional considerations include the drug's side-effect profile, potential drug interactions, and cost. If a patient has previously responded to a particular antidepressant, the same agent should be used again, unless it is contraindicated because of a newly diagnosed medical condition. Clinicians should be alert to increased depression, agitation, violent behavior, and suicidal behavior, in light of the recent FDA warning about SSRIs (Shogren, 2004).

Some experts consider the key issues in selecting an antidepressant to be the side-effect profile of the drug and any comorbidities of the patient. The patient's target symptoms should be matched with the drug's side-effect profile to maximize potentially beneficial side effects and minimize the unwanted ones. For example, if symptoms include agitation and insomnia, choose a sedating antidepressant (amitriptyline, nortriptyline, doxepin, nefazodone, or mirtazapine). If symptoms include anhedonia, anergia, and psychomotor retardation, choose an activating antidepressant (desipramine, sertraline, or bupropion). No studies substantiate that such a selection leads to a better drug response; however, it should enhance compliance by decreasing unwanted side effects and making the patient more comfortable (DGP, 1993; Kuzel, 1996; Moore & Bona, 2001). The main differences among

TABLE 33–2. Dietary Information for Patients Taking MAO Inhibitors

Prohibited Foods	
Aged cheeses[a]	Meats: canned, aged or processed
Anchovies	Monosodium glutamate
Avocado, ripe	Pods or board beans (fava beans)[a]
Beer	Raisins
Fermented foods	Sardines
Figs, canned	Sauerkraut
Herring[a]	Snails
Licorice	Soy sauce
Liver (chicken or beef >2 days old)	Yeast products[a]
Marmite (meat extract)	
Limited Intake Permitted	
American cheese: up to 2 oz daily	Sour cream: up to 2 oz daily
Chocolate: up to 2 oz daily	Wine (especially Chianti and sherry) and spirits: 3 oz of white wine or a single cocktail
Coffee: up to 2 oz daily: decaffeinated is unrestricted	
Cottage cheese: up to 2 oz daily	Yogurt: up to 2 oz daily

[a]High tyramine content.

Adapted from Wells, Mandos, & Hayes (1997).

TABLE 33–3. Resources for Managing Mood Disorders

National Alliance for the Mentally Ill (NAMI)
Colonial Place Three
2107 Wilson Blvd, Suite 300
Arlington, VA 22201
NAMI Helpline: 1-800-950-6364
www.nami.org/

National Mental Health Association (NMHA)
NMHA Information Center
1021 Prince Street
Alexandra, VA 23314-2971
Office: 703-684-7722
Information: 1-800-969-NMHA
www.nmha.org/

HCPR Clearinghouse
2101 E. Jefferson Street
Suite 501
Rockville, MD 20852
301-594-1364
www.ahcpr.gov/

National Depressive and Manic Depressive Association (NDMDA)
730 N. Franklin Street, Suite 501
Chicago, IL 60610
1-800-826-3632
312-642-0049
www.ndmda.org/

National Foundation for Depressive Illness, Inc.
P.O. Box 2267
New York, NY 10116
1-800-239-1265
www.depression.org/

these antidepressant agents are their differing side-effect profiles—muscarinic, histaminergic, and alpha-adrenergic responses. Remember too that starting dosages for elderly patients should be approximately half the usual adult dose. Maximum tolerated doses within the therapeutic blood level guidelines should be used for 4 to 6 weeks at therapeutic serum levels before concluding that they are not effective for an individual patient (Miller & Keitner, 1996).

Selective Serotonin Reuptake Inhibitors. Fluoxetine,[†] sertraline, paroxetine, citalopram, and escitalopram are effective antidepressants and are first-line agents in primary care treatment of major depression. Fluoxetine is more likely to cause agitation and anxiety, whereas paroxetine causes dry mouth and sedation. Start fluoxetine at 10 to 20 mg and sertraline at 50 mg once daily in the morning. Sertraline is equally effective as imipramine for treating dysthymia; however, 51% of imipramine-treated patients dropped out of a recent study because of adverse side effects compared with only 25% of the sertraline-treated patients (Friedman & Kocsis, 1996; Jessen, 1996; Kuzel, 1996). In double-blind trials, paroxetine was about as effective as imipramine in treating major depression. However, like all SSRIs, paroxetine inhibits activity of cytochrome P-450 isoenzymes and thus interacts with other drugs such as phenytoin, digoxin, and warfarin. Begin paroxetine at 20 mg in the morning. Start citalopram at 20 mg daily and titrate up to 40 mg/day after one week if necessary. Begin escitalopram at 10 mg daily and titrate up to 20 mg/day after one week if needed for a therapeutic response. The new delayed-preparation preparation, fluoxetine weekly, takes advantage of the drug's long half-life and is administered on a weekly basis to patients who have responded well to daily doses. This dosing might be particularly useful during the *maintenance phase* of MDD treatment. For women experiencing premenstrual dysphoric disorder (PDD), fluoxetine weekly can be used for the two weeks prior to menses each month.

Venlafaxine (Effexor) and fluvoxamine (Luvox) are two additional SSRIs. An extended-release form of venlafaxine is available (Effexor XR) for once-daily dosing. Dosing starts at 75 mg/d; it may be increased up to 225 mg/d by 75 mg/4 d increments. QT interval effects may occur in patients with heart problems.

Fluoxetine, paroxetine, and sertraline are first-line agents for treating postpartum depression and are considered safe for breastfeeding mothers (Bower & Katz, 2002; Kulin, Pastuszak, & Sage, 1998; Wisser, Gelenberg, & Leonard, 1999). SSRIs should not be used during pregnancy because recent studies warn that women taking fluoxetine, sertraline, or citalopram during their pregnancies delivered infants with brain injuries.

Basically, the SSRIs have comparable efficacy, but subtle patterns of difference have been noted among the various agents. In general, SSRIs tend to be "energizing"; thus, they may be a good choice for patients presenting with lethargy and loss of energy. However, they can cause agitation, restlessness, and insomnia, particularly if the patient presents with anxiety. Their advantage over TCAs are absence of weight gain, anticholinergic effects, and CV safety. Because SSRIs lack the CV toxicity of the TCAs, they present less danger from drug overdose. Some clinicians have found that SSRIs have better response rates with women, patients who are overweight, and those whose symptoms include overeating, oversleeping, or profound lethargy.

Coadministration with an MAOI is hazardous, and the interaction can produce excitement, rigidity, diaphoresis, and hyperthermia. There should be a 2-week "washout" before starting an MAOI after using an SSRI. A washout period of at least 5 weeks is recommended for fluoxetine because of its very long half-life. SSRIs inhibit cytochrome P-450 and may increase serum levels of benzodiazepines, anticonvulsants, antiarrhythmics, sulfonylureas, and warfarin (Preskorn, 1996). For the pediatric population requiring pharmacotherapy, SSRIs are the initial antidepressant of choice. Fluoxetine has FDA approval for use in children as young as 7 years of age.

SSRIs are especially effective in treating elderly patients because they do not contribute to constipation, orthostatic hypotension, and potential cardiotoxicity as do the TCAs. Fluoxetine has a long half-life and would not be first choice for elderly patients because of increased risk of adverse effects. As noted above, the potential for causing drug interactions in the elderly, who take more medications in general, should be assessed.

The most frequently reported SSRI side effects are insomnia, nausea, headache, dizziness, agitation, and assorted sexual dysfunctions. Side effects are usually worse at the beginning of treatment, so if doses are kept low for the first 2 to 3 weeks, these can be minimized. Titrating dosages gradually can often keep these effects tolerable for the patient. Start with half the normal dose for the first week, especially with elderly patients. Benzodiazepines (e.g., clonazepam) may be prescribed along with an SSRI to decrease anxiety and insomnia and can be tapered off as side effects are better tolerated. If sexual dysfunction threatens medication adherence, try lowering the

---

[†]An expert panel report on fluoxetine frm the National Toxicology Program is available at http://cerhr.niehs.nih.gov.

dose or instituting drug holidays over the two or three weekends a month (Eisendrath & Lichtmacher, 2000; Moore & Bona, 2001; Rens, 2002).

Tricyclic Antidepressants. Amitriptyline and doxepin have the greatest anticholinergic effects, are very sedating, and may be a good choice when the patient has psychomotor agitation and insomnia with the depression. Begin the medication at 50 mg taken at bedtime to minimize problems with side effects. Protriptyline is the least sedating TCA and is started at 10 mg at bedtime. Desipramine has an "energizing" effect and is a good choice for depression with psychomotor retardation and pronounced fatigue, but it may cause insomnia if taken too late in the day. Imipramine is the least costly with moderate sedative and anticholinergic activity.

TCAs are not recommended as first-line treatment for youth because of their lack of efficacy and potential side effects. Generally, only imipramine and clomipramine are recommended for children over 6 years of age. In children, adolescents, and young adults TCAs may produce tachycardia and mild hypertension. Therefore, a pretreatment EKG in young depressed patients should be performed. Generally, avoid TCAs and MAOIs in elderly patients because of their undesirable side effects. Be sure to treat depression in the elderly as aggressively as any other illness (Blazer et al., 1998; Moore & Bona, 2001; Worthington & Rausch, 2000). Elderly patients and men with prostatic hypertrophy do best with a nonsedating TCA that has relatively mild anticholinergic effects such as nortriptyline or desipramine; these agents cause the least amount of postural hypotension.

TCAs may produce lethal cardiovascular toxicity if overdosed because of the quinidine-like effect of these agents that causes prolonged interventricular cardiac conduction complicated by severe anticholinergic and alpha-adrenergic blocking effects. *Because a TCA overdose may be lethal, no more than 1 week's supply (1 g) should be prescribed at a time to a depressed patient who could potentially use the drug to carry out a suicide plan.*

The most common side effects of TCAs are anticholinergic effects, orthostatic hypotension, sedation, sexual dysfunction, and weight gain. TCAs are contraindicated in patients with prostatic hypertrophy, narrow-angle glaucoma, and certain cardiac arrhythmias.

Other Antidepressants. Bupropion has a relatively short half-life and should be dosed three times a day. The minimally effective dose is from 225 to 300 mg/day. Begin with 100 mg bid and increase to 100 mg tid after 3 days. Early experience with bupropion revealed a somewhat greater potential for causing drug-induced seizures, especially in patients who have an existing seizure disorder or who are prone to experience seizures (e.g., patients ingesting alcohol or benzodiazepines on a chronic basis, patients with recent head injury, and patients with other neurological disorders). Bupropion should not be prescribed for patients with eating disorders because of a high seizure incidence at higher doses in that patient population. Drug-induced seizures from bupropion are dose-related as well as correlated with high peak plasma level concentrations achieved soon after a dose is administered. Therefore, no more than 150 mg should be taken at one time. Warn patients not to "double-up" for missed doses of bupropion but continue taking individual doses as prescribed. A sustained-release preparation has recently obtained FDA approval and now circumvents many of the dosing peculiarities of the agent. Bupropion SR is available in 100, 150, and 300 mg tablets. It has fewer sexual side effects than the SSRIs or TCAs. Bupropion probably should be avoided in depressed patients with psychotic features or in individuals with schizophrenia-like disorders because the dopaminergic effects of the agent may give rise to an increase in psychotic symptomatology. (Eisendrath & Lichtmacher, 2000).

Trazodone's sedative effects are prominent, and many patients cannot tolerate the doses of 200 to 400 mg/day needed for its antidepressant effect. For this reason, it now is primarily used as a hypnotic agent for insomnia in doses of 50 to 75 mg at bedtime. This sedative feature of trazodone has led to its concurrent use with other, more activating antidepressants, such as SSRIs, desipramine, and bupropion. Priapism (sustained, painful erection in males sometimes requiring surgical detumescence and resulting in permanent impotency) is a rare adverse effect of trazodone that occurs in approximately 1 in 6000 males treated with the drug (Wells et al, 1997). Men receiving trazodone should be counseled to stop the drug immediately if changes in erectile function are noticed and notify their clinician. Given its rarity, priaprism is not a reason to avoid its use in males. However, patient education is necessary.

Nefazodone's sedative effects, although not as prominent as those seen with trazodone, are useful in depressed patients who also have symptoms of anxiety.* Begin with 100 mg bid and increase in increments of 100 mg/day each week up to the recommended dose. In older individuals, nefazodone's starting dose is 50 mg bid. Progressive increases in dosage up to an average of approximately 300 to 400 mg/day are recommended for younger patients. Some patients will have difficulty tolerating its sedative and orthostatic effects and will complain of sleepiness, lightheadedness, and/or dizziness. The side effects of the agent can often be made more tolerable by gradual dose increases. Priapism seems not to be a problem in men taking nefazodone, and sleep studies of nocturnal penile tumescence in normal volunteers serving as their control taking trazodone, nefazodone, or placebo at spaced time periods showed significant differences for trazodone compared to placebo, but no difference from placebo compared to nefazodone.

Nefazodone* is metabolized by the cytochrome P-450 isoenzyme system and inhibits the metabolism of other drugs. Therefore, nefazodone is contraindicated in patients taking the nonsedating antihistamines terfenadine and estimazole. Additionally, patients taking alprazolam or triazolam should have the dose of these benzodiazepines (BZDs) reduced by 50% if nefazodone is coadministered.

Venlafaxine has a short half-life and should be dosed twice daily. A starting dose of 25 mg bid or tid is recommended although some patients may experience early-onset side effects. Initial nausea and vomiting occasionally can be problematic, and slower introduction of the drug is necessary. It is better tolerated when the dose is gradually increased. Venlafaxine also can cause increased diastolic blood pressure, and blood pressure should be monitored, especially in hypertensive patients. It does not cause significant hypotension or sedation. Although venlafaxine is metabolized by the cytochrome P-450 enzyme system, it has a low potential for drug interactions and may be preferred in depressed patients taking multiple medications for other medical conditions that are metabolized by the liver. Modulation of serotonin levels effects impulsivity, sexual behavior, appetite, and aggression. Norepinepherine systems modulate vigilance, socialization, energy, and overall motivation while both serotonin & norepinepherine modulate anxiety, irritability, mood, emotion, & cognitive function. Based on these distinguishable profiles, a dual action agent, such as venlafaxin, may provide the broadest spectrum of therapeutic effect across the full range of depressive symptoms (Gutman & Nemerhoff, 2002; Kando et al., 1999).

Mirtazapine's most common side effects are dry mouth, weight gain, somnolence, asthenia, and constipation. Because of its relatively sedative pharmacology, it may be preferentially used in depressed patients with significant anxiety and/or insomnia. The recommended starting dose for mirtazapine is 15 mg at bedtime. After a few days, patients can be moved up to 30 mg/day. Some patients may require the maximal approved dose of 45 mg/day. Hepatic impairment of mild to moderate severity may cause up to a 33% decrease in hepatic clearance of mirtazapine and downward dosage adjustment is probably necessary if the patient has liver disease (Howland & Thase, 2002).

MAOIs are usually prescribed by a psychiatrist; however, the primary care provider may monitor the treatment regimen. Common adverse effects include tachycardia, sedation, insomnia, agitation, and sexual dysfunction (Jessen, 1996). MAOIs should not be administered with a TCA because of the potential for sudden, intense CNS and atropine-like effects.

If switching between SSRIs and MAOIs, allow a "washout" period because of the potential for serious interaction. When changing from a TCA to an MAOI, allow a drug-free interval of 1 week. When moving from fluoxetine to an MAOI, a drug-free interval of 5 weeks is recommended; when changing from sertraline or paroxetine, a 2-week interval is sufficient. When switching from an MAOI to an SSRI, a 2-week interval is recommended.

MAOIs are not recommended for patients under 16 years of age and contraindicated for patients over 60 years of age. The prevalence of CV disease in the elderly significantly increases the risk associated with MAOI therapy in this group of patients. Excessive hypotension from MAOI overdose and severe hypertension from drug or food interactions increase the risk with the elderly (Eisendrath & Lichtmacher, 2000).

Monitoring for Efficacy. Measuring treatment outcomes includes evaluation of target symptom relief and restoration of function. Symptom evaluation may be done through the clinical interview alone or in combination with a symptom-rating scale completed by the patient, such as the General Health Questionnaire (GHQ), Beck Depression Inventory (BDI), or Hamilton Depression Scale (HAM-D). A rating scale allows both practitioner and patient to assess treatment response, determine if medication dosage should be adjusted, and clarify if and when alternative treatments are needed (DGP, 1993b; Moore & Bona, 2001).

Monitor drug response and provide clinical management every 1 to 2 weeks. Patients with more severe symptoms should be seen weekly for the first 6 to 8 weeks of the acute phase of treatment. Weekly psychotherapy sessions are useful. The clinician should be available by phone particularly during this phase of treatment. During the continuation phase of treatment, monitor for symptom resolution at least every 4 weeks. The goal here is to prevent relapse; this phase lasts about 9 to 12 months. Dur-

Serotonin syndrome

ing the maintenance phase, the goal of treatment is to prevent recurrence. If depression responds to treatment, some sources recommend continuing the drug for at least 6 months and always tapering off over a 4-week period. Should symptoms recur, return the dose to its prior level and maintain for another 3 to 6 months (DGP, 1993b).

If treatment results in little or no symptom relief by 6 weeks or only partial relief by 12 weeks, reassess the diagnosis and treatment plan. Substance abuse or underlying medical or psychiatric conditions may become apparent. Monitor adherence, check blood levels, raise the dose, or change the medication. Medication underdosing is a common cause of poor treatment response. Refractory depression that is not responsive to first-line treatment probably requires referral. Monitor for symptom resolution at least every 4 weeks during this phase.

A specific length of time for a monotherapy drug trial has not been established, but some response should be noted after 3 to 4 weeks and the patient should have substantial symptom relief after 6 to 8 weeks of treatment. If there is little or no response to antidepressant therapy after 4 weeks at the full recommended dose, the drug trial should be considered a failure. If the patient has not responded at all or has only minimal symptomatic response to the medication, two steps are recommended: (1) reassess the adequacy of the diagnosis and (2) reassess the adequacy of treatment (DGP, 1993b). The main reasons for failed drug therapy are inadequate dosing and insufficient length of treatment (APA, 2000).

In general, monotherapy is preferred over a combination of drugs. Thus, switching medications is usually preferred over augmentation as an initial strategy. If the decision is to discontinue a medication, TCAs need to be tapered off over 2 to 4 weeks because patients may undergo gastrointestinal side effects caused by cholinergic rebound; MAOIs, bupropion, trazodone, nefazodone, venlafaxine, and mirtazapine do not require tapering. The shorter-acting SSRIs paroxetine and sertraline should be tapered off, whereas the longer-acting fluoxetine warrants no gradual reduction. After weaning off the medication, monitor the patient for 6 to 12 months for recurrence of symptoms. Inadequate treatment responses make chronic depression more likely and subsequent treatment more difficult.

Monitoring for Toxicity. Obtain a chemistry panel for liver and renal function when clinically indicated. Drug treatment regimens for patients with hepatic or renal impairment should be initiated by a psychiatrist or mental health specialist and managed collaboratively with the primary care provider.

SSRI toxicity may produce seizures, nausea, vomiting, excessive agitation, and restlessness. All SSRIs currently in use have been implicated in adverse drug interactions involving cytochrome P-450 enzymes. Most of these relate to elevated plasma levels of TCAs; fluoxetine is the most frequent offender. For this reason, SSRIs and TCAs should probably not be given concurrently unless the clinician is prepared to carefully monitor TCA plasma levels. Collaborative management with a psychiatrist or mental health specialist would be prudent. Fluoxetine has a longer half-life than other SSRIs and after withdrawing the drug, any TCA should be introduced at low dose (10 to 25 mg) and increased very slowly according to patient tolerance. Cimetidine and ketoconazole are strong cytochrome P-450 enzyme inhibitors and may interact with psychotropic drugs. Ranitidine could be substituted for cimetidine and fluconazole for ketoconazole because they are less likely to interact with psychotropic agents. Likewise, the antihistamines astemizole and terfenadine should not be taken with SSRIs. Sertraline and venlafaxine have the fewest interactions with other drugs (Moore & Bona, 2000).

Serotonin syndrome (SS) is an occasionally fatal disorder characterized by rigidity, hyperthermia, autonomic instability, myoclonus, and confusion. Using OTC sympathomimetics, such as cold remedies or diet pills, can precipitate SS in patients taking SSRIs. For mild cases of SS, an oral benzodiazepine may be sufficient; however, a plan for emergency treatment should be in place if symptoms continue. Referral to a psychiatrist or mental health specialist for management is recommended (Brown, Skop, & Mareth, 1996; Eisendrath & Lichtmacher, 2000).

TCAs can cause cardiac arrhythmias in toxic doses, and in patients with conduction disorders (bundle-branch disease), pose a serious risk for heart block even in normal therapeutic concentrations. Side effects include anticholinergic phenomena (dry mouth, constipation, blurred vision) and alpha blocking effects (sedation, orthostatic hypotension). They may lower the seizure threshold and can induce arrhythmias by increasing the heart rate and slowing cardiac conduction. High doses may produce severe postural hypotension, dizziness, tachycardia, palpitations, arrhythmias, and seizures. Amoxapine has caused extrapyramidal side effects.

Plasma TCA levels >1000 ng/mL indicate a major overdose and will generally cause EKG abnormalities; a prolonged corrected Q-T interval ($Q\text{-}T_c$) over 0.44 ms should cause concern. However, any elevated plasma level in conjunction with signs of toxicity should be regarded as potentially lethal. Nortriptyline has the most clearly defined therapeutic window for clinical response (50 to 150 ng/mL). Life-threatening CV symptoms include tachycardia and impaired conduction leading to AV block. At toxic levels, the EKG shows a prolonged QRS interval (Miller & Keitner, 1996).

Bupropion increases the risk of seizures in all patients at doses exceeding 450 mg/day or 150 mg/dose. Venlafaxine may increase diastolic blood pressure when used in high doses.

Mixed and indirect-acting sympathomimetics interact with MAOIs to produce a serious and potentially life-threatening hypertensive crisis. These sympathomimetics cause epinephrine to be abruptly released, which results in increased blood pressure. Patients need to be warned that many OTC preparations, particularly those for colds and weight loss (e.g., pseudoephedrine), can interact with the MAOI, producing a serious hypertensive crisis. Taking meperidine or dextromethorphan with an MAOI may lead to delirium, hyperpyrexia, convulsions, coma, and even death. A low tyramine diet also is required to avoid potential interactions. Refer again to Table 33–2. A hypertensive crisis presents with occipital headache, nausea, palpitations, tachycardia/bradycardia, and chest pain. Patients experiencing these symptoms should understand that this is an emergency situation and seek treatment promptly (Howland & Thase, 2002; Kando et al., 1999).

Followup Recommendations. Support, reassurance, and hope are essential to effective management and followup care for depression in primary care settings. Collaborative decision making with the patient, family, and clinician generally improves adherence to treatment and provides better outcomes.

Establishing a working relationship with a psychiatrist and other mental health specialists can be helpful for patient consultation or referral. Prompt consultation or referral is needed in the following situations: uncertain diagnosis; severe, recurrent episodes; coexisting complex medical problems; poor adherence; partial response to initial treatment; suicidal ideation; need for hospitalization; or at the patient's request (DGP, 1993b).

BIPOLAR DISORDER

Bipolar disorder, formally known as manic-depressive illness, is a cyclic disorder with alternating episodes of depression and mania. *Bipolar I* (manic-depressive) is characterized by a least one manic episode and one major depressive episode. *Bipolar II* is characterized by at least one major depressive episode accompanied by one hypomanic episode.

Bipolar disorder, affecting approximately 3% of the adult population the United States, is chronic, with recurrent symptoms and relapses over the course of a lifetime and causes substantial psychosocial morbidity. Onset of the disorder usually begins in early adulthood (20 to 29 years of age) when the patient exhibits periods of abnormal mood swings that can be euphoric, depressed, or a combination of both. Although rare in preadolescent children, the second most common age range of onset is 15 to 19 years. It presents as silly, excited, hyperactive, irritable, withdrawn, angry, paranoid, or explosive behavior with mood lability among adolescent patient populations. Bipolar disorder differs from unipolar disorders in several ways: It occurs more commonly in families, presents with a more acute onset, and patients have more episodes over a lifetime than patients with unipolar depressive disorders (APA, 2000; Keck, McElroy, & Arnold, 2001).

Patients with bipolar disorder present with target symptoms that include: (1) mood disturbances (irritable, expansive, euphoric, manipulative, labile with depression), (2) hyperactivity (sleep disturbances, rapid speech, flight of ideas, distractibility), (3) delusional symptoms (sexual, persecutory, religious, grandiose, threatening), and (4) schizophreniform reactions (tangential associations, ideas of reference, catatonia, hallucinations). These symptoms are present almost daily for more than 1 week. The target symptoms are important for monitoring effects of drug therapy during the course of treatment.

A *classic manic episode* with euphoric mood is a distinct period of abnormally and persistently elevated, expansive, or irritable mood that lasts at least a week. Mania is characterized in three stages: The initial stage is characterized by increased psychomotor activity and overconfidence; the intermediate stage is evidenced by greater psychomotor activity and delusional thoughts; and the final stage is evidenced by frenzied psychomotor activity, hallucinations, and disorientation. Not all patients progress from one stage to another, and often, the time between stages is short and difficult to recognize. Generally, these patients require hospitalization.

Patients may present with a *mixed episode* of bipolar disorder in which symptoms of both mania and depression occur almost daily for a least a week (Keck, McElroy, & Arnold, 2001). Other patients may switch from a manic to a depressive mood quickly. This "rapid cycling" occurs four or more times a year and is difficult to distinguish from a mixed episode.

Specific Considerations for Pharmacotherapy

When Drug Therapy Is Needed. Although major depression is frequently treated by primary care providers, bipolar disorder generally requires psychiatric referral for initial management of a manic episode. However, the treatment regimen may be monitored over time by the primary care provider. It is clinically important to distinguish between bipolar and unipolar mood disorders when selecting pharmacotherapeutic agents because antidepressants may precipitate mania in patients with bipolar disorder. Also, mania can be druginduced from stimulants or adrenergic drugs, such as amphetamines, cocaine, levodopa, ephedrine, tricyclic antidepressants, and monoamine oxidase inhibitors, as well as by high doses of corticosteroids. (Howland & Thase, 2002).

Treatment for bipolar disorder has three phases: (1) the acute phase involves treatment of the manic episode to afford the patient behavioral control; (2) the continuation phase further stabilizes the patient over time; and (3) the maintenance phase has the goal of preventing recurrence. Primary care clinicians will generally be concerned with management of the continuation and maintenance phases of treatment (Howland & Thase, 2002; Schiffer, 2000).

Bipolar disorder is a complex mood disorder because it appears to have multiple determinants and the clinical presentation differs significantly among individual patients. Several theories have been proposed to explain the underlying pathophysiology of the disorder and suggest the mechanism of various therapies. Some of these current theories are shown in Table 33–4.

Short- and Long-Term Goals of Pharmacotherapy. Treatment goals are to decrease the frequency, severity, and psychosocial consequences of recurring episodes and to improve functioning between episodes. Initial treatment of a manic episode focuses on prompt symptom relief and behavioral control. Long-term goals focus on preventing recurrence of either manic or depressive episodes. Most patients remain on a mood stabilizer indefinitely (Schiffer, 2000).

Nonpharmacologic Treatment. Psychotherapy can help patients learn how to manage their depression, fatigue, or obsessive ruminations and structure their daily activities to reduce mood lability during maintenance treatment. Psychotherapeutic modalities are most useful after mood episodes are stabilized. To reduce the incidence of relapse, patients can diminish psychosocial stress by carefully monitoring their sleep/wake/activity patterns. Fam-

TABLE 33–4. Theoretical Basis of Bipolar Disorder

Theory	Pathophysiology
Genetic Factors	There is a high genetic risk for first-degree biological relatives of individuals with bipolar I disorder. Current research is focusing on chromosomal abnormalities.
Neurotransmitter	1. There is a functional deficit of monoamine neurotransmitters (norepinepherine, serotonin) in the CNS, producing mood disorders. An excess results in mania and a deficit results in depression. 2. Dysregulation between neurotransmitter systems (norepinephrine, serotonin) produces a cyclic disturbance in mood rhythms. Excessive catecholamine activity may contribute to manic episodes; deficits in dopamine may contribute to the disorder. 3. Deficiency of gamma-aminobutyric acid, a major inhibitory CNS neurotransmitter, causes excessive stimulation that produces mania.
Sensitization	Initial psychosocial or physical stressors trigger a bipolar episode, but later episodes occur spontaneously due to increased sensitization and kindling of the CNS.
Neuroendocrine	Disruption in the hypothalamic-pituitary-thyroid axis contributes to mood disorders. Thyroid hormones may play a part in rapid-cycling bipolar episodes.
Membrane and Cation	Abnormal calcium and sodium homeostasis may cause mood fluctuations seen in bipolar disorder. The calcium secondary messenger system may be involved in the pathology. Several antimanic drugs (lithium, calcium channel blockers, and phenothiazine) have calcium antagonistic effects.
Secondary Messenger System	When neurotransmitters bind to postsynaptic receptors, a series of intracellular events occur that are mediated by chemical systems known as "secondary messengers." Studies related to these multiple interconnecting neuromodulatory systems have promise for new pharmacologic interventions.
Biologic Rhythms	Decentralization of circadian or seasonal rhythms may cause variations in mood and system patterns. Circadian rhythms may cause diurnal variations in mood, sleep disturbances, and seasonal recurrences of bipolar episodes. Depression appears to be most prevalent during spring and mania most prevalent during summer.

Adapted from Fankhauser & Benefield (1999).

ily therapy is particularly useful for women, and all patients benefit from supportive therapy, which focuses on management and resolution of life difficulties using the patient's strengths and resources. It can significantly reduce nonadherence to medication regimens so prevalent among bipolar patients. Support groups are a beneficial and cost-effective strategy to decrease denial, increase adherence to pharmacologic treatment, and reduce the need for hospitalizations. Some self-help and advocacy groups are organized under the National Depressive and Manic-Depressive Association. Referral to a psychologist or mental health professional is necessary for specialized interventions.

Hospitalization is usually necessary during the acute phase of a manic episode to control symptoms. Electroconvulsive therapy may be useful in severe mania or depression that does not respond to drug therapy. Patients are usually hospitalized and referral to a psychiatrist is required (APA, 1994b; Schiffer, 2000).

Time Frame for Initiating Pharmacotherapy. The key to managing bipolar illness is not aborting an acute episode but preventing recurrent manic and depressive episodes over time and diminishing the severity of those that do occur. However, treatment needs to be instituted promptly after diagnosis to relieve symptoms and manage manic behavior. A more rapid response can be obtained when drug treatment is begun in the early stage of mania (Keck, 2001).

Overview of Drug Classes for Treatment

Mood-Stabilizing Agents. These drugs are used in all phases of treatment of bipolar disorder. Lithium is the drug of choice for mania, but other agents (valproate, carbamazepine) have proven effective in managing manic episodes. Lithium, first reported to have antimanic effects in 1949, has been used for acute and preventive treatment of bipolar disorder in the United States since the mid-1960s. Lithium salts are chemically similar to sodium and alter reuptake of norepinephrine, serotonin, and dopamine. Lithium controls depressive as well as manic symptoms and is the initial drug of choice for treating bipolar disorder. It is an agent with a narrow therapeutic range, and patients frequently become toxic on the drug (Schiffer, 2000).

Anticonvulsants. Carbamazepine and valprorate, anticonvulsant medications, are effective alternatives to lithium for treatment of bipolar disorder. These agents are used primarily for treating acute mania in patients who respond poorly or are unable to tolerate lithium. Carbamazepine appears to increase norepinephrine and dopamine and enhance action of gamma-aminobutyric acid (GABA). It initially held much promise in controlling bipolar disorders; however, further study has shown it not to be as useful as lithium for many patients. Carbamazepine is a potent enzyme inducer of other drugs and also induces its own metabolism, making it difficult to regulate a therapeutic dosage. The agent does have some utility in rapid-cycling patients. (Howland & Thase, 2002).

Although carbamazepine has a longer history of research as an antimanic drug, most experts prefer to use valproate (available as valproic acid or divalproex sodium), either in conjunction with or as a substitute for lithium. The symptoms of mania and hypomania best treated by valproate are those of the "primary manic syndrome": increased activity, expansive mood, and decreased sleep. The agent appears to increase the action of GABA, which inhibits neurotransmitter stimulation. Two new anticonvulsants, lamotrigine and gabapentin, show some efficacy in treating intractable affective disorders. Case reports suggest a possible adjunctive role in treatment of refractory bipolar disorder (Eisendrath & Lichtmacher, 2000; Schiffer, 2000).

Other Agents. Antipsychotics and benzodiazepines (BZDs) are often required to augment treatment of an acute manic episode. These agents have a more rapid onset than lithium and allow faster symptom control. Clozapine and risperidone have been used with mood stabilizers because they cause less extrapyramidal side effects. When mania is controlled, these agents are gradually discontinued. Patients treated with antipsychotics require hospitalization. The BZDs (eg, clonazepam, lorazepam) are an alternative to antipsychotics and have minimal adverse effects with rapid sedation. BZDs are gradually tapered and discontinued when the manic episode is under control with the mood stabilizer (Eisendrath & Lichtmacher, 2000; Fankhauser & Benefield, 1999).

Antidepressants (e.g., MAOIs, bupropion) are often combined with a mood stabilizer during an acute depressive episode. MAOIs and bupropion are preferred agents; TCAs seem to initiate mania that is difficult to control. All antidepressants can precipitate a manic episode in patients with underlying bipolar disorder if they are not receiving a mood stabilizer (Schiffer, 2000). Please see Chapter 29 for information on anticonvulsants (valproic acid and carbamazepine) in the treatment of epilepsy.

Assessment and History Taking. A careful history and physical examination are essential to identify bipolar disorder. A positive family history of mood disorder is an important risk factor. The best predictor of mania is having a first-degree relative with bipolar I disorder. Talk with the family if possible because bipolar patients are usually unreliable reporters. Assess current medications and discontinue any precipitating drug such as a TCA, an MAOI, amphetamine, anticholinergic, antihypertensive, cocaine, ephedrine, glucocorticosteroid, hallucinogen, or levodopa. Consider exposure to illegal drugs such as cocaine, amphetamines, or hallucinogens particularly in younger patients. More than 60% of patients with a history of mania also have a history of substance abuse. Keep in mind that obsessive-compulsive, panic, and eating disorders frequently accompany bipolarity.

The baseline laboratory workup prior to starting lithium should include a CBC with differential, BUN, creatinine, electrolytes, thyroid function studies (TSH, T_3, T_4), and a pregnancy test for women of childbearing age. An EKG is recommended for patients with preexisting cardiac disease and those over age 40. In addition to the baseline workup, liver function studies are needed prior to prescribing carbamazepine or valproate (APA, 2000; Schiffer, 2000).

See Drug Tables 205.6, 308, 309, 311, 312, 313.

Patient/Caregiver Information. Psychoeducational programs for patients and their families are very important. Group sessions to discuss concerns about bipolar illness and drug treatment can help patients and their families adjust to this chronic condition. Denial and nonadherence are common among bipolar patients, so they need instructions repeated many times and written information is essential. Patients need to know how to recognize signs and symptoms of emerging mania or depression and when to seek prompt treatment. Keeping a diary of target symptoms is a useful way to identify mood changes.

Special instructions for lithium treatment include: (1) Take lithium with meals to reduce nausea; (2) take the medication at about the same time each day to maintain serum levels; and (3) drink at least 8 glasses of fluid per day and avoid dehydration. Patients and their families need to know signs of lithium toxicity and to stop the drug at the first hint of sickness: diarrhea, vomiting, or a fever that could lead to dehydration. Have them stop the lithium for at least 24 h after the illness. Remind patients that the frequent use of NSAIDs may increase lithium levels and suggest aspirin or acetaminophen because these agents have minimal effect on serum levels and can be used with lithium. Sulindac is another good choice for an antiinflammatory agent because it does not decrease renal clearance of lithium. Diuretics should be used cautiously: Regular use of thiazide diuretics can increase lithium levels while xanthines (coffee, theophylline, aminophylline) can decrease lithium levels. Refer to Table 33–3 for patient, family, and health professional resources.

Outcomes Management

Selecting an Appropriate Agent. The initial treatment plan for an acute manic episode should be determined by a psychiatrist or mental health specialist and usually requires referral and hospitalization. Neuroleptic drugs or BZDs are often required with a mood stabilizer to control the manic behavior until the antimanic agent (lithium, valproic acid, carbamazepine) begins to take effect in 1 to 2 weeks. Antipsychotics such as haloperidol and fluphenazine combined with lithium may produce neurotoxic syndromes and require careful monitoring. Clozapine and risperidone are less likely to cause extrapyramidal side effects than other antipsychotic agents when combined with lithium. However, use of antipsychotics is usually limited to psychotic patients who are under the care of a psychiatrist.

When bipolar depression occurs during maintenance treatment, add an antidepressant such as bupropion, desipramine, nortriptyline, fluoxetine, or sertraline cautiously and after consultation. Initial reports suggested that bupropion was less likely to induce mania, but further study is needed. Generally, use the lowest effective dose for the shortest length of time (Schiffer, 2000).

Mood-Stabilizing Agents. Traditionally, lithium carbonate is the primary pharmacologic choice for treatment and prophylaxis of bipolar disorder, but many patients in the manic phase do not respond to lithium or are intolerant of it. The drug is available in the United States as lithium carbonate in regular and extended-release tablets or capsules and lithium citrate in a syrup. The drug is contraindicated in patients with significant renal or CV disease and severe debilitation or dehydration. It should be used cautiously in patients with cardiac disease, decreased sodium intake (e.g., low-sodium diets for hypertension) or increased sodium loss, and those on NSAIDs. For an acute manic episode, start lithium at 600 mg three times a day or 900 mg twice a day for the extended-release form.

Side effects of lithium include gastrointestinal distress, weight gain, tremors, polyuria, and fatigue. These symptoms usually can be managed by adjusting the dosages, and they gradually subside in the first few months of treatment; however, up to half of patients discontinue taking maintenance lithium therapy because of persistent unacceptable side effects (Fankhauser & Benefield, 1999; Schiffer 2000).

Lithium is teratogenic and contraindicated in pregnancy and during breastfeeding. There is no information about its safety for children under 12 years of age. Lithium should be used cautiously with elderly patients; the dosage needs to be reduced to account for decreased renal function, and fluid intake must be carefully monitored to avoid dehydration. Individual drug dosage should be determined by a mental health specialist and monitored collaboratively with the primary care provider.

Valproic acid is a good alternative for patients who do not respond to lithium or cannot tolerate its side effects. It has potent antimanic properties and minimal to moderate antidepressant properties. In controlled trials, valproic acid was found to be as effective as lithium. The drug is available in the United States as valproate, divalproex, and valproic acid. Valproate is rapidly converted to valproic acid in the stomach, whereas divalproex is converted more slowly in the small intestine. Valproate has few serious side effects other than a dose-related thrombocytopenia and rise in liver function tests that may require discontinuing the drug. Patients at risk for serious hepatitis are those with preexisting liver disease and those currently receiving enzyme-inducing anticonvulsants. Valproic acid is metabolized by the P-450 system but is not an enzyme inducer.

Nausea, vomiting, and diarrhea are common side effects during early therapy, but usually resolve and rarely require discontinuation of the drug. It has a short half-life and requires multiple daily dosing. For an acute manic episode start valproic acid at 250 mg three times a day. It is contraindicated in patients with hepatic disease or abnormal liver studies. Divalproex is a form of valproate that is better tolerated and causes fewer gastrointestinal side effects.

Carbamazepine, a TCA compound similar to imipramine, is the most well-documented alternative to lithium and is used for patients who do not respond adequately to lithium and neuroleptics. It can be added to antidepressants, neuroleptics, or lithium in partial responders, but has been effective as a single agent. Unlike the TCAs, carbamazepine produces a better antidepressant response in patients with bipolar disorder than in those with unipolar depression. Carbamazepine appears to be effective in controlling both manic and depressive episodes.

For an acute manic episode, start at 200 mg twice a day and increase by 200 mg every 3 to 5 days up to 1200 mg/day four times a day. Give medication with meals to minimize gastrointestinal upset. Side effects include drowsiness, dizziness, unsteadiness, nausea, and diplopia. It is contraindicated in patients with a history of bone marrow depression or abnormal blood studies.

Other Agents. If the patient presents with a depressive episode, remember that all antidepressants have the potential to precipitate a manic episode in susceptible patients and may increase the risk of rapid cycling in bipolar patients. This risk is reduced if the patient is already taking a mood stabilizer such as lithium. Bupropion or an SSRI (paroxetine or sertraline) may be a better choice than a TCA if an antidepressant is added to the lithium. If the patient is already taking lithium prophylaxis and becomes manic, raise the dosage to prior therapeutic treatment levels in collaboration with the mental health specialist. (Eisendrath & Lichtmacher, 2000; Fankhauser & Benefield, 1999).

Monitoring for Efficacy. For manic episodes, a BZD or antipsychotic agent may be required initially for prompt symptom relief and behavior control. Mania symptoms begin to resolve in 1 to 2 weeks after beginning lithium. Changes in the target symptoms (abnormal mood, hyperactivity, delusions, and schizophreniform reactions) are used to monitor response to drug therapy. Generally, the acute phase of mania is managed by a psychiatrist or mental health specialist; once control is achieved, the primary clinician can monitor mental status every 2 weeks, then once a month, then 2 to 4 times per year. Lithium levels take 4 to 5 days to stabilize after adjusting the dosage, so there is no need to monitor levels more frequently. Serum levels should be drawn 12 h following the last dose of lithium.

Patients who respond only partially to lithium may benefit from adding either divalproex or carbamazepine to the treatment regimen. Unlike unipolar depression, antidepressants for bipolar depressive episodes are usually discontinued 1 to 2 months after symptoms are relieved (Eisendrath & Lichtmacher, 2000).

Monitoring for Toxicity. Lithium has a narrow therapeutic window, making it difficult to use; serum levels are necessary. Severe lithium toxicity can result in permanent neurologic damage or even death. Draw blood for drug levels as close as possible to 12 h after the last lithium dose. It is important to standardize timing to correctly interpret lab values. Monitoring serum lithium level assesses for toxicity and adherence to drug therapy. Lithium toxicity is manifested as follows: mild toxicity (serum level 1.0–1.5 mEq/L)—impaired concentration, lethargy, irritability, weakness, tremor, and nausea; moderate toxicity (serum level 1.6–2.5 mEq/L)—disorientation, confusion, drowsiness, restlessness, coarse tremor, muscle fasciculations, and vomiting; and severe toxicity (serum level >2.5 mEq/L)—impaired consciousness, delirium, extrapyramidal symptoms, convulsions, and coma.

During maintenance therapy with lithium, schedule weekly appointments until the patient is stable and then monthly for at least a year. Measure drug levels at each visit (draw blood sample 12 h after last dose). Check serum creatinine once or twice a year to assess renal function. If creatinine levels rise, consider a switch from lithium to divalproex or carbamazepine. This medication change should be done in collaboration with the mental health specialist. Monitor the patient more frequently to determine the response to any medication change. Some clinicians recommend assessing thyroid function periodically either by clinical findings or TSH assay because lithium can induce hypothyroidism and a nontoxic goiter. If hypothyroidism occurs and lithium is necessary, a thyroid supplement can be used (Schiffer, 2000).

Polyuria is a commonly reported side effect in maintenance therapy, and the patient should be encouraged to drink 8 to 12 glasses of fluids, preferably fruit juices containing electrolytes to avoid dehydration and possible lithium toxicity. If lithium carbonate causes persistent GI distress, consider switching to lithium citrate syrup. Assess for possible dehydration because this can cause the body to conserve water, sodium, and lithium and increase the risk of toxicity.

Evidence suggests that most patients on maintenance therapy do not exhibit withdrawal or rebound symptoms if the drug is discontinued abruptly. Nevertheless, some clinicians prefer to gradually taper off lithium if it is to be stopped. Although there are conflicting reports about irreversible renal damage due to long-term lithium therapy, there is clear benefit from the medication for patients who have a significant number of manic episodes. Although nephrosis has been rarely reported, the most significant renal effect induced by lithium is a disability of urine concentration. Urine specific gravity should be monitored annually.

Valproic acid may produce profound CNS depression and possible coma. Hepatic dysfunction is most likely to occur during the first 6 months of therapy. Liver function studies are essential before beginning treatment with valproic acid, followed by once-monthly liver panels for 3 months and less frequent panels thereafter. Early signs of carbamazepine toxicity are neuromuscular disturbances, such as double vision, muscular restlessness, twitching, and involuntary movements. Large overdoses may cause coma or convulsions. Monitor liver enzymes for potential toxicity every 3 months after stabilization during the continuation phase of treatment. Another frequent toxicity of carbamazepine is neutropenia. Although usually transient, occasionally patients may experience a severe neutropenia. A CBC with differentials should be monitored routinely (once every 2 weeks initially, then once a month, and then 3 to 4 times per year). If decreases in granulocyte counts are seen, patients should be followed more carefully. In general, the discontinuation of carbamazepine is not necessary unless the absolute granulocyte count approaches 1000 or below. (Eisendrath & Lichtmacher, 2000).

Followup Recommendations. Encourage patients to establish a regular schedule for sleeping, eating, exercising, and socializing, which promotes maintenance of stable moods. During followup visits, nurture the therapeutic alliance with the patient and family, monitor the patient's mood and behavior, continue patient and family education, and promote adherence to the maintenance regimen.

Treatment adherence is a major issue for patients with bipolar disorder. It is not unusual to hear patients complain that they feel less creative and productive when taking a mood stabilizer. To some extent, bipolar patients may enjoy their "high" episodes when they can perform at a more creative level. Whenever possible, the family should be involved in the patient's monitoring of the disorder. Often, patients themselves will not notice the onset of manic symptoms—such as increased talkativeness, "telephonitis," poor judgment in spending money, or increases in sexual activity—until these behaviors have taken their toll. Change in sleep patterns may herald development of a manic episode. Family members, once educated about the signs and symptoms of the disorder, can help control evolving decompensation, aid in early medical intervention, and prevent the need for hospitalization (Schiffer, 2000).

ANXIETY DISORDERS

Although everyone experiences feelings of apprehension and uneasiness when facing a stressful situation, the fears of individuals with an anxiety disorder are abnormally intense and irrational and significantly interfere with their lives. Anxiety and depression are often comorbid conditions. Anxiety disorders are frequently encountered in primary care settings with an estimated lifetime prevalence rate of 25% of the U.S. population. Characteristically a disorder of young adults, they affect women twice as often as men. As a complicating factor, 30 to 50% of patients with anxiety disorders are also clinically depressed. Substance abuse is frequently a complication of anxiety disorders because of patients' attempts at self-medication. Patients with untreated anxiety disorders are high utilizers of healthcare facilities for nonpsychiatric reasons and often have extensive workups for possible medical conditions (APA, 1994a, Kirkwood, 1999; Wu, 2002).

Anxiety is a distressing experience manifested in one's affective, cognitive, behavioral, and somatic domains. The affective component is characterized by fear and feelings of dread and terror that are cognitively countered with attempts to make sense of the distress. Various behaviors reflect the anxiety state or evolve into avoidance behavior in response to the stress. Somatic complaints resulting primarily from autonomic nervous system hyperactivity include systemic, cardiopulmonary, gastrointestinal, urinary, and neurologic symptoms. Generalized anxiety disorder, panic disorder, social phobia, obsessive-compulsive disorder, and post-traumatic stress disorder are the most common forms of anxiety seen in primary care settings (Worthington & Rauch, 2000).

Generalized anxiety disorder (GAD) is characterized by uncontrollable, chronic worry accompanied by insomnia, irritability, trembling, muscle tension, clammy hands, dry mouth, and palpitations. Unrealistic and excessive worry over physical conditions or circumstances persist for at least 6 months. The disorder is manifested in children by concern about their performance at school or in sporting events. GAD exhibits a chronic, prolonged course with a lifetime prevalence of 5%. It is often associated with drug and alcohol abuse, either as the underlying cause or as the patient's attempt to self-medicate the uncomfortable feelings. GAD includes both psychological (worry, tension), and somatic (tachycardia, palpitations, tremor, gastrointestinal upset) symptoms (APA, 1994a; Hidalgo & Davidson, 2001).

Panic disorder is a series of discrete periods of intense fear or terror that are accompanied by somatic or cognitive symptoms lasting less than 30 min. The attacks have a sudden onset, build to a peak rapidly, and are often accompanied by a sense of imminent danger or impending doom accompanied by an urge to escape. The lifetime prevalence of the disorder is 3.5% (APA, 1994). Onset usually occurs during adolescence or young adulthood. The patient experiences extreme apprehension, fear, terror, fear of death, and a desire to flee. Anticipatory anxiety and phobias usually follow one or more panic attacks. Agoraphobia (fear of being in places or situations from which escape might be difficult or embarrassing) often develops secondarily to the panic attacks. Patients begin to avoid situations that may precipitate panic attacks, which leads to restricted social interaction and occupational impairment (APA, 1998; Bradwejn & Koszycki, 2002).

Social phobia is characterized by extreme, persistent fear of social or performance situations. *Performance anxiety* is a discrete social phobia that can impair one's occupational or academic accomplishments. These individuals fear scrutiny, doing something embarrassing, or receiving a negative evaluation. Social phobia in children presents with crying, tantrums, clinging to familiar persons, and inhibited social interaction to the point of mutism. Young children may appear excessively timid in unfamiliar social situations, refuse to participate in group plans, and typically remain on the periphery of social activities. These children fail to achieve an expected level of functioning. When the onset is in adolescence, there may be a decline in social and academic achievement. Social phobia is a chronic and disabling condition with significant psychosocial, occupational, or academic morbidity. The lifetime prevalence rate of the disorder is 13% (APA, 1994a; Raj & Sheehan, 2001).

Obsessive-compulsive disorder (OCD) is characterized by recurrent obsessions that cause marked anxiety and/or compulsions to neutralize the anxiety. Thoughts and images occur repeatedly, causing increased anxiety, which, in turn, fosters compulsive ritualistic behavior. The obsessions and compulsions are time-consuming and significantly interfere with the patient's normal daily activities. OCD has a lifetime prevalence of 2.5% for adults and 1% for children. Obsessional themes usually focus on contamination by germs, toxic materials, or dirt; orderliness; sexual thoughts and impulses; religion; doubts; and aggressive thoughts of harming self or others. Patients with OCD are aware that their thoughts and behaviors are aberrant, but are powerless to respond rationally. The mean age of onset is 17 to 20 years of age. In children, OCD presents with symptoms similar to those in adults. These children experience a gradual decline in their school work because they are unable to concentrate. Almost 20% of patients have a positive family history of the disorder. Most patients have a chronic waxing and waning course with exacerbations that may be related to stress. About 15% of OCD patients show progressive occupational and social dysfunction (APA, 1994a; Swerdlow, 2001; Wells & Hayes, 1999).

Post-traumatic stress disorder (PTSD) can occur when the patient has suffered or witnessed an event or events that involved actual or threatened death or serious injury to the self or others that is persistently reexperienced. Combat experiences, natural disasters, assault, and rape as well as emotional or physical abuse are typical traumatic events leading to the disorder. The patient has symptoms of avoidance, numbing, and increased arousal that endures for more than 4 weeks. PTSD often presents with depression, anxiety, or substance abuse symptoms. Children have nightmares about monsters or threats to self, or relieve the trauma through repetitive play. PTSD was previously recognized as "combat fatigue" or "shell shock." PTSD is considered acute if symptoms last less than 3 months and chronic if they last 3 months or longer. It is a serious disorder with significant associated psychiatric morbidity, functional impairment, and disability. The prevalence rates of PTSD from community-based studies range from 1 to 14%, whereas prevalence rates among at-risk populations (e.g., combat veterans) range from 3 to 58% (APA, 1994a; Roca, 1999).

SPECIFIC CONSIDERATIONS FOR PHARMACOTHERAPY

When Drug Therapy Is Needed

Treatment of anxiety disorders occurs in two phases: stabilization and management. Pharmacotherapeutic agents are most needed during the stabilization phase to help the patient become more comfortable and to resume normal daily activities. Anxiolytics facilitate psychotherapy, which is the foundation of treatment in the management phase. During this phase, the patient learns to control fears and deal with residual phobias, cognitions, and psychosocial problems. The need for drug therapy may decrease during the management phase of treatment (Carter, Holloway, & Schwenk, 1994).

Generalized Anxiety Disorder. BZDs are the most frequently prescribed anxiolytic agents and are the drugs of choice for short-term or intermittent treatment of GAD. When long-term treatment is required, a non-BZD anxiolytic such as buspirone or venlafaxin can be used. Drugs with secondary anxiolytic properties such as antihistamines, beta blockers, and antipsychotics are also prescribed for GAD (Kirkwood & Hayes, 1997; Valente, 1996).

Panic Disorder. Although BZDs have been widely used for years to treat panic disorder, their side effects and dependence were problematic. Currently, SSRIs are recommended as standard first-line agents followed by TCAs. Paroxetine and sertraline are FDA approved for treatment of panic disorder (Bradwejn & Koszycki, 2002).

Social Phobia. SSRIs and BZDs are used in treating social phobia. Most of the SSRIs appear to be effective and paroxetine has received FDA approval for this disorder. TCAs and buspirone are not effective for managing social phobia (Zamorski & Ward, 2000). Clonazepam and alprazolam are effective BZDs in treating the disorder; the MAOI phenelzine also has documented efficacy for generalized social phobia. Alprazolam may be used for occasional performance anxiety on an "as needed" basis. Although beta blockers are ineffective for treating generalized social phobia, they are quite effective for performance anxiety. A beta blocker given prior to the feared performance can eliminate the troublesome physical manifestations of anxiety, such as palpitations and tremor.

Obsessive-Compulsive Disorder. SSRIs are the mainstay of OCD symptom relief. Higher doses than for depression are required. Initial trials with the dualacting agent, venlafaxin, appear to be effective and further study is continuing (Korn, 2000; Raj & Sheehan, 2001; Wells & Hayes, 1999).

Post-Traumatic Stress Disorder. Prompt treatment following the precipitating traumatic event is necessary to prevent PTSD anxiety from becoming chronic and disabling. Personality changes may occur if the disorder becomes chronic. Selection of a pharmacotherapeutic agent focuses on the target symptoms to be treated, such as depression, anxiety, or panic. Antidepressants (TCAs, MAOIs, SSRIs), BZDs (clonazepam), and buspirone are often used for PTSD but the SSRIs are most effective. Paroxetine and sertraline have been FDA approved for treatment of PTSD. Clonidine is used to minimize the physiologic hyperreactivity associated with PTSD. Long-term treatment is best managed by a mental health specialist using individual, group, and family psychotherapy. (Kirkwood, 1999; Raj & Sheehan, 2001, Wu, 2002).

The underlying pathophysiology of anxiety disorders is unknown, but current evidence suggests it is a biologic illness with genetic factors. Anxiety is likely the result of multiple interactions among the central nervous system (CNS) neurotransmitters—norepinephrine, serotonin, and GABA—on which the anxiolytic drugs act. Both excitatory and inhibitory neurotransmitters function together to regulate CNS activity. Norepinephrine is an excitatory neurotransmitter; serotonin and GABA are inhibitory. The majority of norepinephrine in the brain is located in the locus coeruleus (LC). When this area is stimulated, it activates the sympathetic nervous system, causing the characteristic somatic complaints accompanying the anxiety. When the GABA receptor is activated, it reduces the influx of chloride into the neuron, causing hyperpolarization that makes the neuron more difficult to fire when stimulated. BZDs enhance the actions of GABA, resulting in an anxiolytic effect. There are multiple subtypes of serotonin, which is located in the pons and midbrain. BZDs, antidepressants, and $alpha_2$ antagonists inhibit LC firing, decrease noradrenergic activity, and reduce symptoms of anxiety (Olson, 1995).

Anxiolytics increase the action of the inhibitory neurotransmitter GABA and are most needed initially during the stabilization phase of treatment. GAD tends to be chronic and may require continued drug therapy during the management phase of treatment. Although psychotherapy and behavioral therapy are the mainstays for treating panic disorder and social phobias, anxiety is a prominent feature and amenable to pharmacotherapeutic intervention. The underlying cause for OCD is poorly understood, but it is thought to be caused in part by abnormal serotonin neurotransmission, particularly in the orbital gyri of the frontal lobes. Various types of psychotropics have been used to treat OCD although none have controlled symptoms completely. Thus, cognitive behavioral therapy and pharmacotherapeutic agents have achieved the best treatment outcomes. Likewise, treatment for PTSD requires pharmacotherapy, behavior therapy, and psychotherapy. Pharmacotherapeutic agents provide relief from recurring nightmares and reduce psychological and physical distress. These agents make the patient more comfortable and enhance response to psychotherapy modalities. SSRIs are effective in reducing intrusive "flashbacks" and anxiety related to the initial traumatic event. The TCA clomipramine has been used as well as the BZDs alprazolam and clonazepam (Swerdlow, 2001; Wu, 2002).

Short- and Long-Term Goals of Pharmacotherapy

Short-term treatment goals are to relieve symptoms, minimize anxiety with anxiolytics, and prepare the patient for psychotherapy. These goals are accomplished during the stabilization phase of treatment. Long-term goals are to have the patient gain control of symptoms and restore psychosocial and occupational function. Psychotherapeutic and nonpharmacologic treatments during the management stage minimize the likelihood of relapse following drug discontinuation.

Nonpharmacologic Treatments

Psychotherapy is the major treatment modality for anxiety disorders, either individually or in group settings. However, response to psychotherapy may be significantly enhanced if the anxiety is minimized with appropriate medication.

Supportive therapy should be offered by the primary care provider and includes empathic listening, education, reassurance, encouragement, and guidance, forming the basis for a therapeutic alliance between patient and clinician. Insight-oriented therapy helps the patient to understand the association between circumstances, emotions, and symptoms, which helps reduce the response to anxiety. Behavioral therapies are effective psychotherapeutics in reconditioning or modifying behaviors. These include: relaxation techniques, such as progressive muscle relaxation to help increase tolerance of anxiety symptoms, especially in GAD, and reconditioning, whereby gradual exposure and desensitization to the feared situation is made, useful in treating social phobia. Cognitive therapy stresses reframing the interpretation of stressful events and is used for OCD, phobias, and panic disorder. Hyperventilation control is beneficial when patients produce physical symptoms such as dizziness, shortness of breath, tingling, tachycardia, and feelings of suffocation. Assertiveness training is particularly useful for patients with social phobia who fear negative evaluation. Structured problem solving empowers patients to become more effective in their social functioning. This intervention is useful in treating all anxiety disorders. Social skills training helps social phobic patients who need additional competence for social interaction. Although pharmacotherapeutic agents are useful in robustly treating panic disorder, they do not treat the agoraphobia or phobic avoidances that develop as a result of panic attacks nearly as well as nonpharmacologic interventions (Hidalgo & Davidson, 2001; Swerdlow, 2001; Worthington & Rauch, 2000; Wu, 2002).

Time Frame for Initiating Pharmacotherapy

Pharmacotherapy is initiated at the time of diagnosis during the stabilization phase to reduce anxiety and help the patient gain control of symptoms.

Overview of Drug Classes for Treatment

Benzodiazepines. BZDs were first used in the United States during the 1960s for treatment of anxiety. They have no antipsychotic or analgesic action; however, they are powerful anxiolytics. Although serotonin, norepinephrine, and dopamine may be to some extent involved with BZDs, they primarily exert their antianxiety effects by potentiating the inhibitory action of GABA. Unlike other

BZDs, lorazepam and oxazepam are metabolized solely by conjugation and thus are not affected by hepatic microsomal oxidation or liver disease. Other BZDs (e.g., diazepam) are metabolized in the liver to an active metabolite with a very long half-life.

Chronic use of BZDs can cause a withdrawal syndrome upon abrupt discontinuation. If high doses of short-acting BZDs are suddenly stopped, the withdrawal symptoms include increased anxiety, restlessness, and irritability. Therefore, these shorter-acting BZDs (lorazepam, oxazepam, alprazolam) should be discontinued gradually. BZDs with longer half-lives (diazepam, chlorazepate, chlordiazepoxide) are more slowly eliminated from the body and less likely to cause severe withdrawal symptoms (Kirkwood, 1999).

Azapirones. Buspirone is the only azapirone currently available in the United States. Its anxiolytic action is not known, but it does not interact with the GABA complex. Buspirone acts as a partial agonist on serotonin ($5HT_{1a}$) receptors and as both an agonist and antagonist on dopamine receptors. This mode of action results in decreasing anxiety without the sedative effects of other antianxiety agents. Unlike BZDs, buspirone has no muscle-relaxant, anticonvulsant, or sedative effects. Moreover, it has no abuse potential and may be taken for an extended period of time without bringing about dependency or withdrawal upon discontinuation. These characteristics make buspirone an attractive anxiolytic, particularly since substance abuse is frequently seen as a comorbid condition in anxiety disorders.

Antidepressants. TCAs that are generally sedative in their pharmacology (e.g., doxepin, amitriptyline) may be used as anxiolytics. Because of the sedative, orthostatic, and anticholinergic effects of these agents, tolerability may be a problem, especially in the elderly. Moreover, since GAD and clinical depression can coexist, special attention should be paid to the potential danger of a TCA overdose in depressed patients with suicidal ideation. Imipramine has been extensively studied in treating panic attacks. SSRIs were first introduced into the United States in 1988 for treatment of depression. Select SSRIs have been FDA approved for treating GAD, PD, social phobia, OCD, and PTSD. Extended-release venlafaxin, an antidepressant, has been FDA-approved for treatment of GAD (Gorman, 2000). MAOIs are potent antianxiety agents as well as antidepressants but are generally reserved for patients unresponsive to first-line drugs or who have medical problems that preclude using them. Because MAOIs have significant side effects and drug and food interactions, they may be difficult to monitor in a primary care setting.

Other Agents. Antihistamines such as hydroxyzine and diphenhydramine can be useful in treating anxiety largely because of their sedative effects. Such agents are not substances of abuse and may be preferentially used for patients in whom anxiety is intermittent and the clinician is concerned about prescribing a BZD because of their abuse potential and "street value." Beta blockers (propanolol, atenolol) that blunt the physiologic response to anxiety are used for occasional performance anxiety and in some cases of panic disorder. Antihypertensives (clonidine) are used as an adjunctive medication to reduce hyperarousal symptoms of PTSD (Bradwejn & Koszycki, 2002; Hidalgo & Davidson, 2001; Wu, 2002).

See Drug Tables 309.1, 309.2, 311.1, 311.4.

Assessment and History Taking

Most physiologic body systems are affected by anxiety (GI, GU, respiratory, CV), producing complaints of headache, fatigue, tremor, and general malaise. Consequently, patients present with a variety of unexplained physical symptoms such as dizziness, choking, chest pain, palpitations, trembling, paresthesias. An underlying medical problem may coexist with an anxiety disorder and must be appropriately recognized and treated. With numerous possible medical causes of anxiety, assessment should be focused on any medical conditions currently being treated.

The health history should center on the onset, quality, intensity, and duration of anxiety symptoms and what has been done to control them. A detailed history of present illness and family history are useful in predicting the patient's drug response. Anxiety may mask another psychiatric syndrome such as depression or psychosis. Any underlying medical or psychiatric disorder should be treated first. Obtain a history of current or past drug use (amphetamines, theophyllin, beta agonists, marijuana, OTC decongestants). CNS stimulants and depressants such as nicotine, caffeine, and OTC drugs containing stimulants can induce anxiety. Up to 20% of panic disorder patients self-medicate with alcohol and have a coexisting drinking problem. All drinking should stop prior to using BZDs.

Laboratory studies may include an EKG, chemistry panel for hypoglycemia and electrolytes, CBC, and a thyroid profile if clinically indicated. A routine urine drug screen may be needed if substance abuse is suspected. A thorough physical examination is required.

Patient/Caregiver Information

Patients need to understand that treatment of anxiety disorders is similar to that of any other complex, chronic health problem. Panic disorder and social phobia are fairly common conditions amenable to treatment. Reassure patients that they are not going to die during a panic attack, they are not losing their minds, and they can gain control of the disorder. Overcoming OCD is difficult and requires close collaboration with clinicians. Treatment success is directly related to patient motivation. Progress does not proceed in a straight line, but tends to fluctuate over time. PTSD treatment response is relatively slow and may take up to 8 weeks or more to see beneficial effects. Good social and community support minimizes the likelihood of substance abuse during treatment. Remind patients that medication adherence is very important and troublesome side effects that occur with initial treatment usually decrease over time. The primary provider should be available by phone particularly during the stabilization phase of treatment.

Often, simply educating patients about the nature of the disorder with reassurance that it can be treated is therapeutic. Also, advise patients to stop drinking caffeinated beverages and avoid excessive alcohol intake, and encourage patients who smoke to quit. Inform patients about relaxing techniques, such as deep breathing and progressive relaxation; imagery that focuses on a safe, pleasant mental picture; and positive self-talk to replace automatic negative thoughts. A regular exercise program (e.g., walking) can relieve tension and enable patients to get sufficient sleep. Provide printed information and instructions on relaxation strategies and advise patients about appropriate community resources (Valente, 1996). Table 33–5 contains patient, family, and health professional information for managing anxiety disorders.

Again, treatment with MAOIs requires rather strict dietary and other drug restrictions. Refer to Table 33–2. Additional specific information is included in sections that follow.

OUTCOMES MANAGEMENT

Selecting an Appropriate Agent

Benzodiazepines, azapirones, and sedating antidepressants are used for treating anxiety. Generally BZDs and TCAs are available in generic form and less expensive than newer agents. Cost should be a consideration in selecting an appropriate drug.

TABLE 33–5. Resources for Managing Anxiety Disorders

American Psychiatric Association 1400 K Street, N.W. Washington, DC 20005 202-682-6000 www.psych.org
Anxiety Disorders Association of America, Inc. 11900 Parklawn Drive, Suite 100 Rockville, MD 20852-02624 301-231-9350 www.adaa.org
International Society for Traumatic Stress Studies 60 Revere Drive, Suite 500 Northbrook, IL 60062 847-480-9028 www.istss.org
National Center for PTSD VA Medical Center (116D) White River Junction, VT 05009 802-296-5132 www.dartmouth.edu/dms/ptsd
National Anxiety Foundation www.lexington-on-line.com/naf.html National Institute of Mental Health Public Inquiries 6001 Executive Blvd., Room 8184 MSC Bethesda, MD 20892-9663 301-443-4513 www.nimh.nih.gov
American Psychological Association www.apa.org/psychnet
National Mental Health Consumers' Self-Help Clearinghouse www.mhselfhelp.org/
National Center for PTSD—Veterans Affairs www.ncptsd.org

Benzodiazepines. Diazepam is the oldest, most widely used of the BZDs. It has a rapid onset, is long acting, and is effective for situational anxiety, but it has a high abuse potential in some patients, particularly those with a history of alcohol abuse. Alprazolam, the only BZD that is FDA-approved for treatment of panic disorder, has a rapid onset (20 min), peaks in 1 to 3 h without sedation, and wears off in about 6 h. It is useful for treating infrequent, predictable panic attacks. Begin alprazolam at 0.5 mg tid and increase by 1 mg/day every 3 to 4 days up to 10 mg if needed. Because depression usually accompanies panic disorder, therapy often begins with alprazolam in conjunction with an antidepressant (SSRI or TCA). The BZD is tapered off after 10 to 14 days as the antidepressant begins to take effect. During an acute exacerbation of panic attack or GAD, consider a short course of lorazepam 1 mg tid for 5 days either as a monotherapy or as adjuvant therapy to a TCA or SSRI being used as maintenance treatment.

Patients with performance anxiety who have an occasional public speaking engagement can benefit from pharmacotherapy an hour or two prior to the stressful event. A short-acting BZD, such as oxazepam (10–15 mg) or alprazolam (0.25–0.5 mg), about 1 h before the speech may be all that is needed. Because of the potential for CNS depression and memory impairment, the patient should be familiar with the effects of the drug before using it for a planned presentation. Chronic medication use may be necessary for patients whose phobias have had a significant psychosocial impact or if feared situations are frequently encountered and unscheduled. Low-dose clonazepam (0.5 mg tid) is a good choice to manage frequent or unpredictable attacks. Its onset occurs in about 60 min and lasts 8 to 12 h. When used for phobias, lorazepam (1 mg tid) provides a response within 2 weeks. Often patients are able to reduce their dose gradually over time, and some are able to stop the medication altogether after 6 months.

If a BZD is selected, give an adequate dose to relieve symptoms; with careful patient selection and monitoring of compliance, dosage, and core symptoms, BZDs can be prescribed without fear of addiction. Dependency becomes a problem when BZDs are used more than three times per week or with daily use for more than 3 weeks. Moreover, patients with a history of substance abuse or unstable personalities are not good candidates for BZDs. The most common side effects are drowsiness, sedation, and psychomotor impairment. BZDs are effective in both generalized and discrete phobias such as performance anxiety; however, cognitive and psychomotor performance may be negatively affected. The tendency for abuse must be considered because of the high comorbidity of alcoholism with anxiety disorders. A 3- to 4-week course of BZD therapy is a safe choice to reduce risk of drug dependency.

Diazepam, alprazolam, and lorazepam are contraindicated in patients with narrow-angle glaucoma because of their anticholinergic side effects. BZDs must be used cautiously in patients with hepatic dysfunction and those who are elderly or debilitated. The elderly are much more sensitive to the side effects of BZDs and require lower doses. Elders are at risk for falls if BZDs with a long half-life such as diazepam are prescribed. Alprazolam (0.25 mg bid or tid), lorazepam (1–2 mg bid) or oxazepam (10 mg tid) are better choices for elderly patients and those with liver dysfunction. Hip fracture resulting from BZD-induced falls is an important concern. Safety and efficacy of BZD use in children under 18 years have not been established (Hidalgo & Davidson, 2001; Kirkwood, 1999; Wells & Hayes, 1999).

Azapirones. Buspirone is the drug of choice for GAD treatment because it has no abuse potential, can be used long-term, and is particularly beneficial when irritability and hostility are present. Unlike other anxiolytic agents, buspirone should be taken on a regular, daily basis to exert its therapeutic effects, not periodically on an "as-needed" basis. Like many other psychotropic drugs (e.g., lithium, antidepressants), response to buspirone may not be seen until after 4 to 6 weeks of treatment. Adequate doses are necessary for efficacy to be seen: Start it at approximately 7.5 mg bid and increase the dose up to 30 mg or more. Buspirone will not prevent withdrawal symptoms from BZDs; if a BZD is given initially, it should be tapered while buspirone is being increased. The subjective effects of buspirone are very different from BZDs, and it is not uncommon for patients who have taken BZDs to be disappointed in its effects and complain that it is not effective. Nevertheless, buspirone is effective when taken for an adequate length of time (4–6 weeks). The most commonly encountered side effects are nausea, headache, and dizziness, experienced early in the course of buspirone therapy and usually resolved with continued treatment. Patients should be encouraged to continue taking the medication if at all possible so that its anxiolytic effects can be evaluated. Safety and efficacy of buspirone use in children under 18 years have not been established.

Antidepressants. TCAs, SSRIs, and MAOIs are effective drugs for treating core symptoms of anxiety disorders. Generally, the TCAs, imipramine or doxepin, are used for managing panic disorder, especially if the patient has not responded to a trial of SSRIs. Begin imipramine or doxepin 100 mg daily and increase up to 300 mg/day, in divided doses, if necessary. Clomipramine was first marketed in 1990 for treating OCD. However, its success has been limited by adverse side effects and increased incidences of seizures and male sexual dysfunction. Start clomipramine at 25 mg daily and increase gradually as tolerated to 100 mg daily in divided doses within 2 weeks to a maximum total daily dose of 250 mg. Give clomipramine with meals to minimize gastrointestinal upset.

For elderly patients, start clomipramine at 25 mg daily, and increase as tolerated. Because it is very sedating, a bedtime dose with a snack may be safer for elders. For children over age 10, start at 25 mg daily, and increase to maximum total daily dose of either 200 mg or 3 mg/kg of body weight, whichever is less (Valente, 1996).

TCAs help decrease depressive and panic symptoms, nightmares, intrusive daytime thoughts, and flashbacks but have little effect on avoidance symptoms in patients with PTSD. Imipramine and amitriptyline have established efficacy for PTSD treatment. Response to TCAs is delayed for 4 to 6 weeks, so a BZD can be used during stabilization to bring prompt relief from anxiety. Later, taper off the BZD as the TCA becomes effective. Doses higher than recommended increase seizure risk. The most common side effects of TCAs include anticholinergic effects, orthostatic hypotension, sedation, sexual dysfunction, and weight gain. TCAs are useful for patients unable to take BZDs or who have only partial response to buspirone. The more sedating TCAs (e.g., doxepin, amitriptyline) may be used for their anxiolytic effects to treat GAD. Additionally, imipramine and trazodone are effective after 8 weeks of treatment. Because of their sedative, orthostatic, and anticholinergic effects, tolerability may be a problem, especially in the elderly. Moreover, since GAD and clinical depression can coexist, special attention should be paid to the danger of TCA overdose in depressed patients with suicidal ideation. Venlaflaxin extended release has been approved for treatment of GAD and would be a good initial choice.

SSRIs have a favorable side-effect profile making fluoxetine, sertraline, and paroxetine preferred agents in the treatment of panic disorder. Doses used should be similar to those used to treat depression. Occasional use of a BZD may be helpful early on in treatment to decrease anticipatory anxiety while the antipanic effects of the SSRI begin to be experienced (usually after 4–6 weeks of daily use). Fluoxetine, paroxetine, sertraline, and fluvoxamine have been approved for treating OCD and the new SSRI citalopram is being used successfully for anxiety disorders. Higher doses than used for antidepressants are frequently needed (e.g., fluoxetine 10 to 80 mg/day rather than 20 mg for depression). They relieve symptoms without the histaminic, cholinergic, and alpha-adrenergic effects seen with the TCAs. Fluoxetine is slightly energizing, and the usual dose is 60 to 80 mg/day. Sertraline can be started at 25 mg/d and increased to 200 mg/d. Citalopram is started at 10 mg/d and increased up to 60 mg/d. Fluvoxamine is slightly calming; it has a short half-life, no proconvulsive effects, and is not associated with abuse. The initial dose of fluvoxamine is 50 mg h.s., increased 50 mg/day every 4 to 7 days up to 300 mg daily. Doses greater than 300 mg should be given in divided doses bid. Safe use of fluvoxetine for children and adolescents has not been established. Although not approved for PTSD treatment, fluoxetine helps decrease the patient's withdrawal behavior and numbing symptoms. Several studies have shown fluoxetine particularly effective in social phobia. Nausea, insomnia, anxiety, and sexual dysfunction are common SSRI side effects. If an SSRI is not effective, imipramine may be used.

The MAOI agents phenelzine and tranylcypromine have been effective in treating social phobias in the short term, but improvement is not maintained when the medication is withdrawn. Phenelzine is effective in alleviating PTSD symptoms. However, its side effects and dietary and alcohol restrictions often preclude its use with this population of patients (Roca, 1999; Wu, 2002).

Other Agents. Beta blockers are effective in suppressing somatic and autonomic symptoms of anxiety, but do not alter the psychic symptoms. They blunt the peripheral catecholamine-mediated response of anxiety and thus are useful on an as-needed basis for "stage fright" or performance anxiety. Atenolol is effective for treating performance anxiety when given about 1 h prior to the feared performance. Although not approved for treatment of panic disorder, propranolol 10 to 40 mg is helpful on an as-needed basis to alleviate autonomic symptoms of anxiety. Fluoxetine has been found to be effective in treating social phobia. Antihypertensives such as clonidine (an alpha agonist) have been used as adjunct agents for treating hyperarousal symptoms of PTSD. Hydroxyzine, an antihistamine, is useful in decreasing anxiety at 50 to 100 mg q 6 hours as needed.

As a general rule, avoid prescribing any drug to a pregnant woman, particularly during the first trimester. The most teratogenic psychotropics are lithium and the anticonvulsants. If medication is required during a pregnancy, the patient should be referred to a specialist for management. Virtually all psychoactive drugs are excreted in breast milk, and mothers taking these medications should not breastfeed their infants.

Monitoring for Efficacy

Patients and their families need an objective method of rating the severity of their symptoms so that improvement can be measured. Identify the core symptoms that are expected to improve and set treatment goals. Monitor anxiety symptoms and note the degree of dysfunction in social, occupational, and interpersonal activities.

The stabilization phase of treatment may require up to 12 weeks to see maximum benefits from medications, and frequent contact with the patient is necessary to offer support during this time. It is important to monitor target symptoms and sufficiently alleviate anxiety to facilitate progress in psychotherapeutic interventions. BZDs relieve symptoms of anxiety promptly, whereas the antidepressants may take up to 12 weeks of treatment before maximum benefit is achieved; buspirone takes 4 to 6 weeks to become effective (Kirkwood, 1999).

Monitoring for Toxicity

Benzodiazepines. BZDs interact with all CNS depressants to produce additive effects. Although they have an extremely high margin of safety, even low doses of other CNS depressants such as alcohol dramatically increase the risk of toxicity. Coadministration with other sedative drugs (e.g., antihistamines, TCAs, alcohol) should be avoided. Caution patients to be careful driving or operating dangerous machinery, especially when a BZD and another sedative agent are just beginning to be taken concurrently.

Azapirones. Buspirone causes relatively few drug interactions and is generally well tolerated. Adverse effects include dizziness, drowsiness, dry mouth, headaches, fatigue, insomnia, and muscle spasms.

Antidepressants. TCAs can cause cardiac arrhythmias in toxic doses, and in patients with conduction disorders (bundle-branch disease) they pose a serious risk for heart block even in normal therapeutic concentrations. Side effects include anticholinergic phenomena (dry mouth, constipation, blurred vision) and alpha-blocking effects (sedation, orthostatic hypotension). They may lower the seizure threshold and can induce arrhythmias by increasing heart rate and slowing cardiac conduction. High doses may produce severe postural hypotension, dizziness, tachycardia, palpitations, arrhythmias, and seizures. Plasma TCA levels > 1000 ng/mL indicate a major overdose; however, any elevated plasma level in conjunction with signs of toxicity should be regarded as potentially lethal. Life-threatening CV symptoms include tachycardia and impaired conduction leading to AV block. An EKG shows a prolonged QRS interval in the presence of a toxic serum level.

SSRI toxicity may produce seizures, nausea, vomiting, excessive agitation, and restlessness. All SSRIs currently in use have been implicated in adverse drug interactions involving cytochrome P-450 isoenzymes. Serotonin syndrome is an occasionally fatal disorder characterized by symptoms such as mental status changes, seizures, myoclonus, and blood dyscrasias. Ingesting OTC sympathomimetics such as cold remedies or diet pills can precipitate the serotonin syndrome in patients taking SSRIs. For mild cases of serotonin syndrome, an oral benzodiazepine may be sufficient; however, a plan for emergency treatment should be in place if symptoms continue. Refer the patient to a psychiatrist or mental health specialist for management (Brown et al., 1996).

Followup Recommendations

If a BZD is used, the patient should be followed closely so as to avoid daily use of these potentially addictive agents. Try setting up a "contract" with the patient when the BZD is first prescribed, wherein the patient agrees not to use the drug more than 3 days a week.

Once an acute episode of GAD is controlled, patients should be encouraged to rely on nonpharmacologic aids to control anxiety on a long-term basis. Encourage continued exercise and relaxation techniques. Once patients with panic disorder are successfully treated, it is wise to follow up over time to ensure that medication adherence is maintained. Monitoring for concomitant alcohol use should be routine. Most importantly, patients should be encouraged to venture into previously feared situations. Panic disorder patients and their families should be advised to seek help early if panic attacks begin to reemerge to avoid a convoluted pattern of phobic avoidance. Most patients with OCD require prolonged followup to ensure continued benefit from drug therapy. Patients should be encouraged to seek psychotherapy from an individual familiar with the disorder.

EATING DISORDERS

Disturbed eating behaviors are prevalent in Western societies because of a perceived link between beauty and thinness. Teenage and young adult women are most often affected (about 1.2 million in the United States); athletes, dancers, and models are at particular risk. The prevalence of anorexia nervosa among female adolescents and young adults is about 1.0%, whereas the prevalence for bulimia nervosa in the same population is about 3% (APA, 1994). Eating disorders carry significant morbidity and a mortality rate that may be as high as 20% (Zerbe, 1996). Recognizing early signs of an eating disorder is essential if primary care providers are to intervene with preventive measures before a full-blown episode develops. Opportunities for recognition come during annual physical examinations for school, college, sports, or camp as well as family planning services.

Anorexia nervosa is characterized by refusal to maintain a minimally normal body weight. These patients are obsessed with food and fearful of becoming obese even when thin and losing weight. A distorted body image, coupled with a rigorous need to control some part of their life, drives their constant desire to lose weight. Obsessive-compulsive features both related and unrelated to food are prominent in anorexia. Weight loss is accomplished through fasting, dieting, excessive exercise (restrictive type), or purging with self-induced vomiting and misuse of laxatives, enemas, or diuretics after an eating binge (binge-purge type). Induced vomiting and laxative use are common purging methods. These patients commonly have an emaciated appearance and tend to withdraw from social activities. Females are usually amenorrheic. Over 90% of the patients are female with a mean age at onset of 17 years. This disorder is rarely seen in women over 40 years of age (APA, 1994).

Bulimia nervosa is characterized by uncontrolled, repeated episodes of binge eating followed by inappropriate compensatory behaviors such as self-induced vomiting, laxative abuse, diuretics, fasting, or excessive exercise to prevent weight gain. There are two subtypes of bulimia: *purging type* (self-induced vomiting, laxatives, enemas) and *nonpurging type* (fasting, excessive exercise following a binge). Bingeing is triggered by dysphoric mood, stress, or hunger following a period of fasting. Individuals with bulimia usually are within a normal weight range, but may have frequent weight swings. They tend to be very sociable and outgoing. These patients often have depressive symptoms and are at increased risk for bulimia if they have a positive family history of an eating disorder. Bulimia usually begins in late adolescence or early adulthood (APA, 1994a).

Although not a diagnostic category, *compulsive overeating* covers a wide variety of overconsumption of food driven by emotions. Some authorities consider it a nonpurging form of bulimia. In many instances of compulsive overeating, the pattern is not to binge but to "graze" or overconsume food throughout the day. Compulsive overeating is likely a major cause of obesity in the United States. Patients may benefit from psychotherapy to resolve underlying psychosocial problems. A sensible eating plan, appropriate exercise program, and self-help group participation (e.g., Overeaters Anonymous) offer the best strategies to control this behavior (Powers & Santana, 2002).

SPECIFIC CONSIDERATIONS FOR PHARMACOTHERAPY

When Drug Therapy is Needed

No pharmacologic agent has been found to remedy eating disorders, and psychotherapy remains the major therapeutic approach to treatment. Nutritional, cognitive, behavioral, and pharmacologic therapies should be integrated and coordinated with a mental health specialist, dietitian, gastroenterologist, and dentist as required.

Anorexia nervosa is a complex and often chronic disorder demanding a comprehensive treatment plan that coordinates medical management with individual and family psychotherapy. Medications should not be used routinely or as primary treatment for anorexia. Because of the potentially grave complications of anorexia, these patients should be initially referred to a specialist for a treatment regimen and then monitored collaboratively by the primary care provider. Cyproheptadine, metoclopramide, and selected antidepressants may be used to treat target symptoms. Bulimia nervosa treatment strategies include nutritional and rehabilitation counseling, psychotherapy, family interventions, and pharmacotherapy. Anticonvulsants (e.g., carbamazepine), antidepressants (TCAs, SSRIs, MAOIs), and other agents (e.g., cypropheptadine, BZDs) may be necessary (Zerbe, 1996). If depression coexists, as it often does with compulsive overeating, consider an SSRI, which tends to decrease depression and suppresses appetite.

The pathogenesis of eating disorders is unknown, but it likely involves an array of physiologic, emotional, sociologic, genetic, and family factors. Central nervous system neurotransmitter abnormalities have been suggested as the physiologic pathogenesis of eating disorders and are amenable to drug intervention. Alterations in serotonin metabolism appear to affect central neurotransmitter activity related to eating behaviors. Serotonin-mediated eating activity is located primarily in the medial hypothalamus. Stimulation of serotonin receptors in the paraventricular and ventromedial nuclei decreases carbohydrate intake, enhances satiety, and terminates eating. However, stimulation of presynaptic serotonin receptors initiates eating, probably by inhibiting the release of serotonin. When there is decreased food intake, norepinephrine is released in the paraventricular nucleus, which inhibits satiety. Simultaneously, norepinephrine is inhibited in the lateral hypothalamus. Dopamine has been associated with self-stimulation behavior in other disorders and may be related to the eating binges observed in bulimia (Marken & Sommi, 1999).

Short- and Long-Term Goals of Pharmacotherapy

The primary treatment goal for anorexia is to restore normal body weight (correct serious nutritional, fluid, and electrolyte imbalances, stop weight loss, and improve overall nutritional status) followed by establishment of healthy eating behaviors (Lipscomb & Agostini, 1995). Bulimia often presents with symptoms of major depression or bipolar disorder, and these patients should be started on appropriate medication. Long-term goals are directed at preventing relapse. Pharmacotherapeutic and psychotherapeutic interventions are directed at treating underlying psychological problems and changing disturbed eating behaviors (Smith, 2000).

Nonpharmacologic Treatment

Psychological and developmental issues, particularly regarding the role of family, are significant etiologic issues in eating disorders and are important considerations when selecting nonpharmacologic treatment strategies (APA, 1993). Although bulimic patients rarely require hospitalization, it may be necessary for the anorexic patient to restore weight and correct fluid and electrolyte imbalances. Criteria for referral and hospitalization include:

1. Weight loss greater than 40% of ideal weight or greater than 30% in 3 months
2. Rapid progression of weight loss
3. Cardiac arrhythmias
4. Persistent hypokalemia
5. Inadequate cerebral perfusion manifested by syncope, dizziness, and listlessness
6. Severe depression with suicide risk

All anorexic and bulimic patients require psychotherapy to reverse their abnormal eating patterns and distorted body image.

When the patient is not at medical risk, nonpharmacologic interventions are begun that include a refeeding regimen that begins with small increases in food intake. Add 200 calories to the diet every 2 to 3 days over several weeks. Anorectic patients need 3400 calories daily to begin gaining weight, but achieving this level of food intake will occur slowly. Supportive therapy, provided by the primary care clinician includes guidance on nutrition and exercise. Develop a therapeutic alliance with the patient, family, and treatment team. Cognitive behavioral therapy teaches the patient to identify irrational thoughts related to food, eating, and self-image. Behavior therapy helps the patient alter overt actions. Interpersonal psychotherapy helps the patient resolve role issues, social isolation, and prolonged grief reactions. Initially, treatment focuses on patient education about the disorder and, subsequently, on resolving interpersonal difficulties. Family therapy may be necessary, particularly if the patient is young, to change unhealthy family dynamics that could perpetuate the disorder. Psychotherapy may be individual or group-based and often includes the patient's family. Day treatment hospital programs, offered as an outpatient service, are less expensive than inpatient hospitalization yet give structured therapeutic care. The patient spends a half-day in a treatment program that includes one or two meals along with professionally supervised group therapy meetings (Krahn, 2002; Powers & Santana, 2002; Rigotti, 2000; Smith, 2000).

Time Frame for Initiating Pharmacotherapy

Early intervention with counseling and medication is essential to achieving good treatment outcomes. The first treatment priority for patients with eating disorders is to correct any medical complication from severe malnutrition or harsh purging. Initiate appropriate pharmacotherapy promptly for underlying mood disorders or anxiety coexisting with the eating disorder.

Overview of Drug Classes for Treatment

A range of pharmacotherapies for anorexia nervosa has been studied, and no pharmacologic agent has proven effective in promoting weight restoration. Treatment of anorexia requires a long-term, comprehensive, multidisciplinary approach that integrates medical management, individual psychotherapy, and family therapy (Smith, 2000).

Antidepressants. These drugs are used to improve depression and promote weight gain and have had some success in treating eating disorders. Studies show that the TCA clomipramine increases hunger and energy levels and maintains stable weight in anorexic patients. Imipramine and desipramine decrease the bingeing, vomiting, and depressive symptoms in bulimia. Although TCAs, MAOIs, and SSRIs have been efficacious in treating bulimia, only fluoxetine has FDA approval for use in eating disorders. The antidepressants have been effective in reducing binge eating and purging behaviors in bulimia.

The fluoxetine dose used for treating bulimia is higher than for depression (up to 60 mg/d). Fluoxetine has been beneficial in decreasing relapse rate in weight-restored anorexic patients, but is not effective against depression when the patient is underweight. It is thought that the patient's diet is deficient in carbohydrates, resulting in tryptophan depletion, and antidepressants are not effective in tryptophan-depleted states (Powers & Santana, 2002). The antidepressant bupropion is contraindicated in treatment of bulimia because of possible seizure induction.

Other Agents. Cyproheptadine, an antihistamine and serotonin antagonist, has had variable success in improving appetite and decreasing depression in some anorexic patients. It has fewer side effects than antidepressants and, although not always effective, it is a useful adjunctive treatment. Metoclopramide given before meals increases the rate of gastric emptying and relieves the gastrointestinal distress that often accompanies anorexia. Low-dose BZDs such as alprazolam given before meals reduces anxiety related to eating in both anorexics and bulimics. Lithium has been used for bipolar bulimics, but adverse side effects and toxicity risks from purging and laxative abuse limit its use (Krahn, 2002; Marken & Sommi, 1999; Zerbe, 1996).

See Drug Tables 308, 311, 313, 502.2, 705.

Assessment and History Taking

Anorexic patients often appear wasted and cachectic, making them easy to identify; bulimics are less immediately identifiable. Screening instruments may be helpful for detecting patients with eating disorders in a population at risk. However, two specific questions can be a quick predictor for detecting bulimia:

- Do you ever eat in secret?
- Are you generally satisfied with your eating patterns?

If the patient answers "yes" to the first and "no" to the second, explore further (Rock & Zerbe, 1995).

Initially, determine the degree of malnutrition, dehydration, and electrolyte disturbance, and determine if hospitalization and consultation or referral is needed. Explore the patient's attitude toward desired weight, weight loss, and eating habits; a 24 h diet recall is a useful tool for obtaining some of this information. Ask about bingeing, vomiting, laxatives, diuretics, diet pills, and daily exercise. Note symptoms of malnutrition and dehydration such as fatigue, skin changes, thirst, syncope, muscle cramps, and palpitations. Patients often present with complaints of amenorrhea, constipation, cold intolerance, lethargy, and heartburn.

Attention to family and psychosocial history may reveal a genetic link and/or a dysfunctional family that contributes to the eating disorder. Major life changes such as beginning college or a new job may trigger a bingeing episode. Low self-esteem or mood and anxiety disorders also affect eating behaviors. Look for indications of physical or sexual abuse because recent studies suggest a link with eating disorders (Zerbe, 1996).

The physical examination should assess for emaciation, severe hypotension, brittle hair, bradycardia, hypothermia, and very dry skin. There may be painless hypertrophy of the salivary glands, particularly the parotids. If the patient is inducing vomiting, dental enamel erosion may be noted as well as calluses on the dorsum of the hand from contact with teeth to induce vomiting. Broken blood vessels may be seen in the conjunctiva. Bulimics can induce vomiting with "tools" such as toothbrushes or spoons. Lanugo, fine downy hair, may be on the face and arms of the anorexic patient. A careful examination is required to rule out medical causes for weight loss and malnutrition such as malignancy, chronic infection, intestinal disorders, and endocrinopathies.

Laboratory studies should include a CBC, serum electrolytes, BUN, serum creatinine, urinalysis, and EKG. A thyroid profile is indicated because many symptoms mimic thyroid disorders. If the patient abuses laxatives, serum calcium and magnesium should be measured. Patients who have been underweight and amenorrheic for longer than 12 months may need a bone densitometry to assess for osteoporosis.

Patient/Caregiver Information

Educate the patient and family about eating disorders and particularly the dangers of insufficient protein and caloric intake, mental function impairment, lowered resistance to infection, heart arrhythmias, organ damage, and gastric or esophageal rupture. Inform the patient and family about community resources that can offer psychosocial support. Table 33–6 contains patient, family, and health professional resources for eating disorders.

OUTCOMES MANAGEMENT

Selecting an Appropriate Agent

Anorexia Nervosa. Individual, target symptoms of the anorexic patient guide selection of the appropriate pharmacologic agent. However, many anorexic patients do not respond to any medication.

Cyproheptadine, an antihistamine/serotonin antagonist, is used to stimulate appetite and decrease depression

TABLE 33–6. Eating Disorder Resources

American Anorexia/Bulimia Association Inc. 165 W. 46th Street, Suite 1108 New York, NY 10036 212-575-6200
National Association of Anorexia Nervosa and Associated Disorders Box 7 Highland Park, IL 60035 Hotline: 847-831-3438 www.anad.org/
Eating Disorder Awareness & Prevention Inc. 603 Stewart Street, Suite 803 Seattle, WA 98101 1-800-931-2237 www.edap.org

in patients that do not exhibit bulimic symptoms (purging). It has few adverse effects and has been found effective in severe anorexia. Give cyproheptadine 8 mg qid. Metoclopramide increases the rate of gastric emptying, which reduces the abdominal discomfort frequently seen in anorexic patients. Give 10 mg qid. 30 min before meals. A short course of alprazolam 0.25 mg may be given before meals to reduce severe anxiety when it limits eating. Long-term use should be avoided because of abuse potential.

Antidepressants are used with varying success to decrease depression and promote weight gain. Generally, these agents are used only if depression continues after the target weight has been reached. Cardiac abnormalities may result from starvation or chronic purging behaviors, and a baseline EKG is essential to rule out potential impairment. Desipramine is a good first choice TCA because it has a preferred low anticholinergic profile and is better tolerated in this group of patients. It is "energizing" and may be useful in countering fatigue symptoms. Start desipramine at 25 mg in the morning and slowly titrate up to 150 mg/day given in divided doses. An alternative choice is clomipramine 100 mg at bedtime; it increases hunger and energy levels and aids in maintaining a stable weight. The SSRI fluoxetine reduces obsessions and depression, maintains target body weight, and restores normal eating behavior. The effective dosage for anorexia is higher than for treating depression and ranges from 20 to 60 mg/day. Begin fluoxetine at low doses (10 mg in the morning) and slowly titrate up to a therapeutic level. Give medication in divided doses in the morning and at noon. The cost for fluoxetine may limit its use for some patients. Bupropion has been linked with increased seizure risk in patients with eating disorders and should be avoided in these patients (Marken & Sommi, 1999).

Bulimia Nervosa. Antidepressants reduce binge eating, vomiting, and depression as well as improve eating habits of bulimics. However, the adverse side effects of antidepressants limit their usefulness because bulimic patients have an increased sensitivity to them. The TCAs imipramine and desipramine and the MAOI phenelzine have been effective in treating bulimia. The SSRI fluoxetine reduces vomiting, bingeing, depression, carbohydrate craving, and pathologic eating habits. It is well tolerated in bulimic patients. Trazodone has fewer anticholinergic side effects than the TCAs but has limited controlled data reported. Desipramine and fluoxetine have a lower incidence of adverse side effects than the other agents and are good first-line drug choices. Dosages are the same for treating depression. Begin with a low dose and titrate up slowly to minimize initial side effects. Phenelzine should be used cautiously in bulimic patients because of its strict dietary requirements and potential for hypertensive crisis. A baseline EKG to rule out cardiac abnormalities is necessary prior to beginning an antidepressant. A personal or family history of seizures, cerebrovascular disease, and alcohol withdrawal puts a patient at risk for seizures when taking antidepressants.

Anticonvulsants are reserved for a subgroup of bulimic patients who also have symptoms of bipolar affective disorder and would benefit from mood stabilization. Dosages for carbamazepine and valproic acid are similar to those to treat seizure disorders, and prescribing information can be found in those sections.

A short course of alprazolam 0.25 mg tid before meals can be used to reduce severe anxiety associated with eating. Avoid long-term use because of the potential for abuse (Marken & Sommi, 1999).

Monitoring for Efficacy

Anorexia Nervosa. Measure treatment outcomes by evaluating resolution of target symptoms. The aims of treatment are to restore healthy weight and healthy eating patterns, correct dysfunctional thoughts and behavior, improve family support, and prevent relapse. Patients should be monitored every week until weight is stabilized, and there should be a 1 to 2 lb gain per week until the target weight is achieved. Check electrolyte balance and cardiac rhythm. Provide supportive therapy and help the patient and family assess treatment progress. During clinic visits, inquire about eating patterns, and review the patient's diet diary, feelings about eating, and any purging behavior. Regular menses should resume when the target weight is achieved.

Antidepressants should be tried for up to 8 weeks. If there is no improvement in mood, another antidepressant should be tried. If the medication is effective, it may be continued at the same dosage for up to 6 months. When TCAs are discontinued, they should be tapered off over a 2-week period to reduce anticholinergic rebound. No tapering is need for fluoxetine.

Bulimia Nervosa. Evaluate antidepressant effectiveness about 1 month after reaching therapeutic levels. Continue use for up to 12 months after the initial episode. Relapse following discontinuation of medication is prevalent, and long-term maintenance therapy should be considered (Marken & Sommi, 1999; Powers & Santana, 2002).

Monitoring for Toxicity

Careful monitoring of TCA and SSRI antidepressant side effects is essential because anorexic and bulimic patients are particularly sensitive to their anticholinergic and cardiovascular side effects. Antidepressant medication toxicity is discussed in the section on depression and dysthymia above. Information on carbamazepine and valproic acid toxicity can be found in the section on bipolar disorder.

Cyproheptadine may cause anticholinergic side effects as well as drowsiness and should not be administered concurrently with MAOIs. Metoclopramide may produce dizziness and drowsiness and a hypertensive crisis may occur if it is given together with an MAOI.

Followup Recommendations

Treatment of eating disorders is usually a long-term and complex undertaking that is best managed with the primary care provider working with a multidisciplinary team.

INSOMNIA

Approximately 70 million Americans suffer from sleep disorders, and for almost 60% of them they are chronic. They spend an estimated $100 billion/year on treating insomnia and related sleep disorders. In 1993, the National Center on Sleep Disorders Research (NCSDR) was created to address this growing public health problem. In addition to supporting research, the NCSDR launched a major effort to educate both the public and primary care providers about sleep disorders. (Hahn, 1996; Weilberg, 2000).

Insomnia is defined as a persistent difficulty initiating or maintaining sleep or experiencing sleep that is nonrestorative (APA, 1994). It implies fatigue, mood disturbance, or impaired performance. Basically, insomnia results from underlying physiologic or psychological processes. The disorder affects patients of all ages, especially the elderly because sleep patterns normally change with age. Problems are associated with sleep initiation (difficulty falling asleep), sleep maintenance (difficulty remaining asleep), or terminal sleep (difficulty with early morning awakening). The disorder may be considered as *primary* (idiopathic) or *secondary* (related to an underlying cause). About 10% of insomnia cases are due to a primary sleep disorder in which patients have objectively verified difficulty falling asleep or maintaining sleep in the absence of any identifiable underlying pathology. Transient insomnias related to acute situational factors such as stress are very common and affect about 85% of Americans at sometime in their lives. Primary insomnia results from endogenous abnormalities in the normal 24 h wake-sleep cycle that may occur with rotating shift work or as "jet lag" from travel. Some patients have a conditional insomnia in which they associate bedtime with frustration, anxiety, and a variety of sleep-preventing behaviors. These patients typically sleep well away from their own bedroom, such as when on vacation or lying on the living room sofa. Primary insomnia is rare in childhood or adolescence and typically begins in young adulthood or middle age (APA, 1994).

Secondary insomnia may be caused by multiple factors, such as drugs, alcohol, and caffeine use; psychiatric factors; or medical and neurologic illnesses. Stimulant drugs—amphetamines, cocaine, sympathomimetics, caffeine, and nicotine—may induce insomnia. Alcohol is a frequent cause for insomnia seen in primary care settings. Although alcohol induces sedation, the sleep is shallow, short, and not restorative. Activating antidepressants (SSRIs, phenelzine, bupropion) and phenylpropanolamine found in many OTC products can interrupt sleep. Caffeine intake may be an unsuspecting contributing factor. Common medications such as anticonvulsants, methylxanthines, antiarrhythmics, lipid-soluble beta blockers, and decongestants may interfere with sleep.

Up to half of all patients with chronic insomnia have underlying psychiatric disorders. Patients with depression have difficulty with falling asleep or early morning waking. Patients with agitated depression have diminished total sleep time and complain of overall exhaustion. During manic phases of bipolar disorder, patients have diminished total sleep time but do not feel tired. Patients with dysthymia may complain of feeling tired and irritable, of being unable to get enough sleep, and of never feeling rested. Patients with anxiety, particularly obsessive-compulsive disorder, often have great difficulty falling asleep because they lie in bed and ruminate. Those with post-traumatic stress syndrome fear going to sleep because of recurring, frightening nightmares, and sleep disturbances always accompany the psychoses. Medical problems such as chronic pain and cardiopulmonary dysfunction may cause orthopnea or paroxysmal nocturnal dyspnea, resulting in secondary insomnia. Urinary frequency associated with urinary tract infection or prostatism will prevent the patient from sleeping through the night. Patients with sleep apnea, a potentially serious breathing-related disorder, often present with a complaint of daytime sleepiness. *Sleep apnea* is caused by repeated periods of airway collapse followed by disruption of sleep. Most of these patients are unaware of how disrupted their sleep really is, but spouses report very loud snoring that interrupts their own sleep. Sleep apnea most often occurs in men over age 30, with a heavy upper body and a short, thick neck (APA, 1994; Eddy & Walbroehl, 1999; Weilburg, 2000).

SPECIFIC CONSIDERATIONS FOR PHARMACOTHERAPY

When Drug Therapy Is Needed

Management is determined by the underlying cause and duration of the insomnia. Treatment combines general measures to improve sleep, psychotherapeutic strategies, and pharmacotherapeutic agents. The treatment plan should be individualized based on underlying physiologic, psychological, or situational processes. General measures include treatment of any identified causes, patient education, and stress management techniques. Consider discontinuing all unnecessary medication and adjusting any unusually high drug dosages. Hypnotics are prescribed adjunctively for short-term or intermittent insomnia; however, medication should be used carefully to avoid precipitating excessive drug use and habituation. Anxiolytics and hypnotics should be avoided in the patient with sleep apnea.

The normal sleep-wake cycle is regulated by neuronal complexes located in the brainstem, basal forebrain, and hypothalamus with projections entering the cortex and thalamus. The reticular activating system maintains wakefulness; norepinephrine and acetylcholine in the cortex, and histamine and neuropeptides in the hypothalamus regulate neuronal activity during wakefulness. Sleep is promoted when the reticular activating system decelerates and serotonin neurotransmission in the raphe nuclei reduces sensory input, which inhibits motor activity. Norepinephrine is involved with dreaming, whereas serotonin is active during nondreaming periods. During sleep, the brain is extremely active and produces a pattern of stages that cycle throughout the night. The sleep pattern is altered with age, resulting in decreased overall sleep time.

Hypnotics, drugs that facilitate or produce sleep, are used to treat short-term or intermittent insomnia. Anxiolytics such as BZDs can be used as hypnotics because they act on the GABA and BZD receptors that decrease neuronal firing. The non-BZD agent zolpidem selectively binds to BZD receptor sites to induce sleep. Other agents such as antihistamines produce drowsiness that facilitates sleep (Jermain, 1999).

Short- and Long-Term Goals of Pharmacotherapy

Basically, insomnia is a symptom and should be treated following these management principles: (1) Any underlying medical or psychiatric disorder must be treated, (2) use nonpharmacologic treatment modalities, and (3) restrict use of hypnotics to transient or short-term insomnia only. Short-term insomnia is best managed by good sleep hygiene and other nonpharmacologic therapies. Patients with long-term or chronic insomnia will benefit from referral to a specialty sleep disorder clinic for evaluation and management.

Nonpharmacologic Treatment

Insomnia is a multidimensional problem requiring individualized treatment and nonpharmacologic behavioral interventions. The first-line insomnia treatment in the primary care setting is supportive therapy. Sleep hygiene measures center on environmental factors and behaviors that promote sleep. Stimulus control measures reinforce use of the bedroom only for sleeping or sexual activity, not for sleep-incompatible behaviors such as reading, eating, or watching television. Sleep restriction stresses no daytime napping. Relaxation techniques, such as progressive relaxation, guided imagery, and biofeedback, can help. Chronic insomnia responds well to psychotherapy and behavioral techniques. A sleep diary, found to correlate closely with polysomnography, is particularly useful in treating insomnia. Simply keeping the diary can improve one's sleep habits. Reviewing the patient's sleep diary and suggesting alterations may be all that is necessary to correct the problem. Sleep hygiene is an important treatment strategy and suggested measures are shown in Table 33–7. Stimulus control measures and sleep restriction are reported to be the most effective treatment modalities for chronic insomnia.

TABLE 33–7. Sleep Hygiene Measures

1. Have regular hours for going to bed and waking up each day.
2. Don't take naps during the day.
3. Get regular exercise early in the day.
4. Avoid heavy evening meals. However, if hungry at bedtime, have a *light* snack.
5. Plan quiet evening activities.
6. Use bedroom only for sleeping or sexual activity.
7. Environment should be quiet, dark, and have a moderate temperature.
8. Avoid caffeine—coffee, tea, and colas—during evening.
9. Avoid alcohol, particularly in the evening.
10. Avoid chronic tobacco use.
11. Avoid excessive liquids in the evening.

Adapted from Hartman (1995).

Referral to a psychologist or mental health specialist may be necessary for specialized psychological techniques, including cognitive restructuring, which encourages the patient to consider alternative, more rational beliefs about sleep and insomnia. In addition, psychotherapeutic interventions focus on assisting the patient to resolve conflicts and develop effective coping strategies.

Obstructive sleep apnea may respond to using plastic nasal strips placed across the bridge of the nose to keep the nasal passages open during sleep. Since obesity promotes the development of sleep apnea, weight management may be an important preventive intervention.

Time Frame for Initiating Pharmacotherapy

Lack of sleep can impair work performance, reflex response, cognitive abilities, and one's sense of well-being. Patients with insomnia have undoubtedly tried various sleep-producing techniques, home remedies, and OTC sleep preparations before presenting to a clinic. However, pharmacologic agents generally are used only after nonpharmacologic interventions have failed. Sleep disturbances seem to be an important early indicator of psychiatric illness, allowing primary care providers the opportunity to diminish morbidity associated with new or recurrent mood disorders by prompt intervention or referral to mental health specialists (Doghramji, 2002).

Overview of Drug Classes for Treatment

Benzodiazepine hypnotics have sleep-producing effects similar to barbiturate hypnotics, but they are much safer to use and have become the drugs of choice for treatment of insomnia. They promote the onset of sleep, reduce awakenings, and increase total sleep time. Nevertheless, BZDs tend to alter the sleep stages and shorten restorative sleep. These agents are associated with development of tolerance and rebound insomnia after long-term continuous use.

Two nonbarbiturate, nonbenzodiazepine hypnotics, zolpidem and zaleplon, have been approved for short-term use in treating insomnia. They are chemically unrelated to BZDs but are as effective in inducing sleep and increasing sleep quality. They bind selectively to type 1 BZD receptors. However, these new agents are much more expensive to use than BZDs.

Antidepressants such as amitriptyline, trazodone, and doxepin are prescribed for their hypnotic effects for patients who complain of nonrestorative sleep and should not receive BZDs.

Other agents may be used to avoid prescribing BZDs for insomnia. Some clinicians begin treatment with an OTC sleep preparation containing an antihistamine such as diphenhydramine or doxylamine. Melatonin is a hormone synthesized in the pineal gland that regulates sleep, mood, and ovarian cycles. Several small studies have linked melatonin supplements with improved sleep in elderly patients, but long-term studies have not been completed. Some reports suggest it is beneficial for "jet lag" and mild insomnia (Doghramji, 2002; Hahn, 1996; Jermain, 1999).

Assessment and History Taking

A careful history is the most important part of assessment to differentiate between primary and secondary insomnia. Get a full description of the problem and have the patient keep a sleep diary for 2 weeks. Interview the patient's bed partner, especially if sleep apnea is suspected. During the interview, ask about specific symptoms, onset, duration, and exacerbating/alleviating factors; daytime symptoms; past treatment; past medical and psychiatric history; and sleep hygiene patterns. Rule out underlying medical or psychiatric conditions, drug/alcohol abuse, medication use, occupational situations, and travel patterns that may contribute to the insomnia. A complete physical examination is needed to rule out an underlying physiologic cause. Laboratory studies are rarely necessary and included only if clinically indicated. Continuous daytime sleepiness and fatigue suggests sleep apnea. It is important to recognize the possibility of sleep apnea because prescribing sedatives may increase the danger of respiratory difficulties in these patients. The bed partner or family members usually report that the patient snores loudly. Sleep apnea is ordinarily diagnosed with polysomnography in a specialized sleep laboratory.

See Drug Table 310.

Patient/Caregiver Information

Education related to sleep in general and to insomnia in particular is an important part of overall management. Explain how to keep a sleep diary: recording time in bed, estimated sleep time, any awakening, time of morning arousal, estimated sleep quality, any unusual events, and associated symptoms. Record information in the diary first thing each morning. The sleep diary is usually kept for 2 weeks prior to evaluation by the clinician and patient.

Correct any misconception that alcohol can improve sleep. Although alcohol may cause one to fall asleep more rapidly, sleep becomes restless in 2 to 4 h with frequent awakening and is not restorative. If patients are taking BZDs, remind them not to use these drugs for insomnia because of the high abuse potential, greater tolerance, and rebound insomnia when discontinued (Eddy & Walbroehl, 1999; Hahn, 1996).

OUTCOMES MANAGEMENT

Selecting an Appropriate Agent

Benzodiazepine Hypnotics. Triazolam, temazepam, estazolam, quazepam, and flurazepam are used for managing short-term insomnia. Triazolam has the shortest duration of action (2 h half-life) and patients report less daytime sedation following its use. It is lipophilic, rapidly absorbed, and produces intense sedation in about 1 hour after administration. Begin with 0.125 mg h.s. Temazepam (15 mg h.s.) and estazolam (1 mg h.s.) are intermediate-acting BZD hypnotics used for patients who have difficulty remaining asleep. Temazepam and triazolam are most often used to induce sleep. Flurazepam (15 mg h.s.) and quazepam (7.5 mg h.s.) are long-acting agents because they form active metabolites with long half-lives. Flurazepam reduces both sleep-induction time and number of awakenings. All the BZD hypnotics, except temazepam, are metabolized in the liver and are affected by drugs that inhibit the cytochrome P-450 enzyme system (e.g., erythromycin, nefazodone*). Thus, temazepam may be a better choice for elderly patients and those with impaired liver function. BZDs are not prescribed to patients with a positive current or past history of drug abuse, and they generally are prescribed only for a short-term course of treatment.

Always use the lowest effective dose for the shortest length of time. Tolerance can develop when BZDs are used daily for over 4 weeks, so these drugs are best taken short-term or intermittently. Withdrawal may result in rebound insomnia, particularly with the short-acting agent triazolam. To avoid rebound insomnia following long-term use (greater than 6 months), gradually taper the dose to discontinuation. Elderly patients have an increased sensitivity to all the BZDs. Because there is an association between falls and hip fractures and the use of long-acting BZDs, flurazepam and quazepam should be avoided in this group of patients. BZDs should not be prescribed for patients with suspected sleep apnea or during pregnancy.

Nonbenzodiazepine Hypnotics. Zolpidem and zaleplon, two newer hypnotics, selectively act on the BZD type 1 receptors with minimal effect on sleep stages, consequently promoting a more natural sleep. They have little anxiolytic, muscle relaxant, or anticonvulsant effect. Although the potential for abusing zolpidem and zaleplon is minimized by the high incidence of nausea and vomiting at higher doses, their abuse and tolerance potential are unclear. They have a rapid onset and are useful for initiating and maintaining sleep. Begin with 10 mg h.s. for healthy adults; this can be increased up to 20 mg per night as necessary. For the elderly and those with liver impairment, use 5 mg h.s. The ultra-short half-life of zaleplon makes it the least likely to cause daytime sleepiness. Duration of its effect is limited to 4 h. Zolpidem has a longer half-life and would be a better choice for patients having difficulty remaining asleep during the night.

Antidepressants. These drugs are effective alternatives for patients who complain of nonrestorative sleep but should not take BZDs. Some clinicians prescribe a sedating antidepressant such as trazodone 50 mg h.s. to avoid using a BZD hypnotic. Trazodone is particularly effective for treating insomnia secondary to fluoxetine or bupropion therapy. Anticholinergic side effects may limit use of the tricyclic antidepressants such as amitriptyline, particularly in elderly patients.

Other Agents. OTC sleep preparations that contain diphenhydramine and doxylamine are readily available to patients. However, they alter sleep architecture and may cause confusion in the elderly. Melatonin, also available OTC, may be most beneficial for treating circadian pattern changes (e.g., "jet lag" or shift changes) in adults. Melatonin replacement therapy appears to be effective in treating insomnia in melatonin-deficient elderly patients. The usual dose is 1 to 3 mg taken about 2 h before desired bedtime for at least 7 days. Lack of research on its long-term effects may limit recommending its use. Table 33–8 contains a list of antianxiety agents often used in treating insomnia (Doghramji, 2002; Eddy & Walbroehl, 1999; Hahn, 1996).

TABLE 33–8. Agents Used in Treatment of Insomnia

Generic Name	Brand Name	Indications	Usual Dose Range (mg/day)[a]
BZD Hypnotics			
Alprazolam	Xanax	Anxiety-depression	0.75–4
	Generics	Panic disorder	1.5–10
Chlordiazepoxide	Librium	Anxiety	25–200
	Generics	Alcohol withdrawal	
Diazepam	Valium	Anxiety	2–40
	Generics	Alcohol withdrawal	
Lorazepam	Ativan	Anxiety	0.5–10
	Generics		
Chlorazepate	Tranxene	Anxiety	7.5–90
	Generics	Seizure disorders	
Oxazepam	Serax	Anxiety-depression	10–15
	Generics	Alcohol withdrawal	
Non-BZD Hypnotics			
Zolpidem	Ambien	Insomnia	5–10
Zaleplon	Sonata	Insomnia	5–10
Antihistamines			
Hydroxyzine	Vistaril	Anxiety, pruritis	50–400
	Atarax		
Diphenhydramine	Benadryl	Allergy	25–200
	Generics		
Antidepressants			
Amitriptyline	Elavil Generics	Depression	50–100
Doxepin	Sinequan	Depression	50–150
	Generics	Anxiety	
Trazodone	Desyrel	Depression	50–150
Dietary Supplement			
Melatonin	Melatonin	Circadian schedule changes	0.5–3000

Monitoring for Efficacy

Because insomnia is basically a subjective complaint, the patient's self-report is the most important determinant of improvement. If symptoms recur after a short-term drug course (2 weeks) for primary insomnia or if the patient is unresponsive to nonpharmacologic interventions, refer him or her to a specialist for management. Patients with chronic, long-term insomnia are best evaluated and treated by specialists at a sleep disorder clinic.

Monitoring for Toxicity

For antidepressants, refer to the section on major depression and dysthymia above. For antihistamines, refer to Drug Table 705. For BZD hypnotics, refer to the section on anxiety disorders above. Among the non-benzodiazepine hypnotics, zolpidem and zoleplon can produce headache, agitation, daytime drowsiness, and gastrointestinal upset. To date, use of melatonin remains controversial and little is known about its long-term effects and potential toxicity (Doghramji, 2002; Jermain, 1999; Eddy & Walbroehl, 1999).

Followup Recommendations

Patients should be evaluated after a week of treatment to assess drug effectiveness, any adverse effects, and adherence to nonpharmacologic interventions. The sleep diary should be evaluated after 2 weeks. Should a BZD be used for short-term treatment, followup is essential to monitor for appropriate use. Remind patients not to drink alcohol when taking BZDs. Provide printed information and counseling on precautions when using medications for sleep.

SUBSTANCE ABUSE

Substance abuse is the harmful use of alcohol, tobacco, or other drugs knowing they cause psychosocial problems or are physically damaging. It is a leading cause of premature but preventable illness, disability, and death in the United States (Department of Health and Human Services [DHHS], 1998). The abuse of alcohol and nicotine, the most widely used legal psychoactive drugs in the United States today, is discussed in this section. Alcohol abuse alone costs society almost twice as much as all other drugs combined, for a total of about $86 billion annually. Adults as well as older children and adolescents are at risk. The potential for fetal alcohol syndrome makes alcohol abuse of particular concern among women of childbearing age (Bjornson, Fiore, & Logan-Morrison, 1996).

Although tobacco use is the delivery system for the drug, nicotine, it is not thought of as substance abuse in the same way as other substances. However, any use of tobacco causes significant harm even when used in moderation. Tobacco dependence is a doubly serious problem not only because of health risks involved in its use but also because nicotine is an addictive psychoactive drug. *Smoking is the leading cause of preventable death in the United States today, with 430,000 tobacco-related deaths annually.* Exposure of nonsmokers to environmental tobacco smoke also poses a substantial health risk to these individuals. Infants and children exposed to environmental smoke have increased rates of chronic middle ear effusions, pneumonia, and other respiratory illnesses. Smoking cessation involves more than changing a habit because of the powerful addictive nature of nicotine. Counseling regarding the dangers of alcohol abuse and tobacco use should be included as a routine part of well-child care, and all complete health exams for adults should incorporate an in-depth history of alcohol and tobacco use. Given the significant morbidity and mortality associated with alcohol and nicotine abuse, prevention should be the first-line intervention strategy in all primary care settings (USDHHS, 1998).

ALCOHOL ABUSE

Alcohol abuse is a frequently encountered problem in primary care. Many individuals have suffered some adverse event in their lives from alcohol use and are able to modify their drinking behavior so that dependence and abuse do not become a problem (APA, 1994a). However, the psychiatric complications that may result from alcohol abuse and dependence are many, ranging from delirium to drug-induced mood and anxiety disorders. Additionally, individuals with mood or anxiety disorders may use alcohol as an attempt at self-treatment, only to complicate further the course of their underlying disorder. Prevention of alcohol abuse is the most important intervention strategy for primary care settings (USDHHS, 1998). Ideally, primary care providers should try to screen for and treat an alcohol problem in its early phases routinely, before it becomes an addiction and more difficult to manage. As needed, treatment programs should be recommended. Generally, outpatient alcohol treatment programs combine pharmacotherapeutic and psychotherapeutic treatment modalities. Inpatient care is costly and reserved for patients with severe, acute withdrawal syndrome; those who have failed previous treatment programs; or those who have a poor social environment (Prater, Miller, & Zylstra, 1999).

Specific Considerations for Pharmacotherapy

When Drug Therapy Is Needed. Because all the repercussions of alcohol use and abuse are well beyond the scope of this section, the management of outpatient alcohol withdrawal will be the focus. This disorder may require acute treatment and, left unattended, could result in serious medical (mostly neurologic) consequences such as seizures. Early detection and prompt intervention are essential for successful treatment outcomes.

Individuals who chronically abuse alcohol in large quantities expose themselves to the possibility of acute withdrawal upon abrupt cessation of drinking. The withdrawal syndrome is characterized by autonomic hyperactivity such as sweating, tachycardia, hand tremor, agitation, anxiety, and grand mal seizures (APA, 1994). Such symptoms are the result of unmasking a hyperactive autonomic state that develops because of the chronic consumption of alcohol and its sedating effects. Thus, treatment of alcohol withdrawal consists of replacing alcohol with another sedative agent (such as a benzodiazepine) with a longer half-life, from which the patient can then be gradually withdrawn without such severe neurological sequelae. Further, because alcoholics may ignore the need for adequate nutrition, the body usually becomes deficient in the B vitamins. Treatment of alcohol withdrawal syndrome requires patient monitoring, keeping an environment with minimal stimulation, and providing food, noncaffeinated fluids, rest, and reassurance.

Short- and Long-Term Goals of Pharmacotherapy. The short-term goal of alcohol withdrawal is to prevent or minimize occurrence of withdrawal symptoms and related psychiatric and nutritional problems. Long-term goals include maximizing the patient's motivation for abstinence from alcohol and preventing relapse by assisting the individual to rebuild a substance-free lifestyle. It is increasingly recognized that achieving motivation for abstinence is a critical first step in achieving long-term treatment goals. Pharmacologic agents are used in alcohol abuse treatment to decrease the urge to drink, blunt withdrawal symptoms, and to treat underlying psychological problems. Treating any coexisting mood or anxiety disorder will assist the patient in maintaining life-style changes and preventing relapse (Galanter, 1999; Hanna, 2000).

Nonpharmacologic Treatment. Over the years many nonpharmacologic treatment programs for alcoholism have evolved. Any successful program stresses both the importance of continued sobriety and basic lifestyle changes. Dealing with marital and other family issues, enhancing self-esteem, enriching job functioning and financial management, addressing relevant spiritual issues, and dealing with the possibility of homelessness are special issues for those in alcohol treatment programs. The primary care provider can offer supportive therapy, encouraging the patient to seek psychotherapeutic modalities such as cognitive-behavioral techniques, coping skills training, and relapse prevention. Psychotherapy is usually delivered in a group therapy setting. Self-help groups such as Alcoholics Anonymous (AA) are very successful because its members know all the tricks of the disease and the value of surrender and serenity. There are over 750,000 local chapters of AA in the United States. A treatment program that is negotiated with the individual patient and family, together with a multidisciplinary team approach, has the best chance of success. (Galanter, 1999). Table 33–9 contains patient, family, and health professional resources for managing alcohol abuse.

Time Frame for Initiating Pharmacotherapy. Outpatient drug treatment for alcohol withdrawal can be achieved successfully and is less emergent if the patient's degree of withdrawal is relatively mild to moderate. The time frame for initiating drug treatment for alcohol withdrawal may vary, depending upon the severity of symptoms. Immediate treatment is necessary and should be carried out on an inpatient basis if there is a history of severe alcohol withdrawal symptoms or recent head trauma. Fever of over 101°F, delirium or hallucinations, significant malnutrition, or serious medical complications of alcohol use also would warrant hospitalization for withdrawal management. Alcohol withdrawal symptoms occur after a period of abstinence or during a reduction in the amount of alcohol intake. The primary care provider should be cognizant of the fact that a withdrawal syndrome may occur inadvertently from a sometimes brief concurrent illness or during the course of a medical illness or trauma. Therefore, it is important to be aware of the possibility of alcohol withdrawal even though abuse may not have been previously recognized.

TABLE 33–9. Resources for Managing Alcohol Abuse

Alcoholics Anonymous (AA)
Grand Central Station
PO Box 459
New York, NY 10163
www.alcoholics-anoynmous.org/
Check local newspapers and phone book for information on local AA chapters.

American Academy of Pediatrics
www.aap.org/
Check website for drug and alcohol information for children.

PREVLINE
Prevention Online
DHHS
www.health.org/

National Institute on Alcohol Abuse and Alcoholism (NIAAA)
6000 Executive Blvd—Willco Building
Bethesda, MD 20892-7003
www.niaa.nih.gov/

National Institute on Drug Abuse (NIDA)
www.nida.nih.gov/

Overview of Drug Classes for Treatment. Pharmacotherapeutics are used for alcohol withdrawal to blunt withdrawal symptoms, reduce the urge to drink, and treat underlying psychiatric problems that may be contributing to the alcohol abuse. Benzodiazepines have a central role in alcohol withdrawal treatment. These agents suppress signs and symptoms of uncomplicated alcohol withdrawal, seizures, and delirium. Long-acting BZDs such as chlordiazepoxide and diazepam are more effective in preventing withdrawal seizures and ensuring a smoother withdrawal than short-acting BZDs. However, the short-acting agents such as lorazepam and oxazepam are less likely to cause sedation in the elderly, and they are not metabolized by the liver, making them preferred for patients with hepatic dysfunction.

Adrenergic agents like clonidine and atenolol are sometimes used to treat the autonomic hyperactivity seen during alcohol withdrawal. These are not sufficient for monotherapy because they do not control withdrawal seizures or hallucinations. Anticonvulsants, such as phenytoin, valproic acid, and carbamazepine, are very effective in treating a comorbid seizure disorder. They cannot be used to treat acute alcohol withdrawal because they do not prevent withdrawal seizures. Patients with a history of seizures are not good candidates for outpatient withdrawal and should be referred to a mental health specialist for management.

Nutritional supplements help restore nutritional deficiencies and facilitate the withdrawal process. These generally include multivitamins and thiamine supplements. Recently, the opiate antagonist naltrexone has been approved as an adjunctive treatment to lessen the craving for alcohol. Opioid dependence should be ruled out before its use. Disulfiram may be used as a short-term aversive therapy. It uncouples the oxidation of ethanol, resulting in temporary accumulation of acetaldehyde, a toxic compound producing unpleasant and potentially dangerous symptoms. Aversion therapy with disulfiram requires a patient who seeks total abstinence, requests the drug, has no underlying cardiovascular disease, and is willing to follow up with monthly evaluations (Crabtree & Polles, 1997; Hanna, 2000; Prater et al., 1999).

Assessment and History Taking. Obtain a thorough history of previous alcohol use and have this information confirmed by family members, if possible. A complete health assessment can determine if the patient is an appropriate candidate for outpatient withdrawal. Vital signs should be measured to monitor for autonomic hyperactivity. Observe for symptoms of mild withdrawal, including insomnia, irritability, anxiety, headache, GI distress, mild hypertension, and tremulousness.

Laboratory studies should include a chemistry panel, liver panel, and CBC. Plasma albumin, serum folate, and vitamin B_{12} level will aid in evaluating nutritional status. Consultation and collaboration with a specialist is recommended for outpatient withdrawal management.

The CAGE questionnaire, a brief screening instrument for alcohol abuse, is easily administered in a primary care setting (Mayfield, McLeod, & Hall, 1974). CAGE questions ask the patient about attempts to *c*ut down on drinking, being *a*nnoyed by criticism of drinking, feeling *g*uilty about drinking, and having an *e*ye-opener drink in the mornings for a hangover. Positive responses to two of the questions suggest possible alcohol abuse and further evaluation is indicated (USDHHS, 1998).

See Drug Tables 205.5, 308.2, 308.3, 309.1, 312, 313.

Patient/Caregiver Information. Whenever significant alcohol abuse or dependency is suspected, address the issue directly with the patient. Explaining the difference between appropriate alcohol use and abuse is an important step. Refer the patient to various community resources, such as an alcohol treatment program or Alcoholics Anonymous.

A supportive family who can provide close supervision is essential for outpatient management of alcohol withdrawal. Refer to Table 33–9 for resources. In addition, family members dealing with a problem alcoholic can get excellent support from their local Alanon, Alateen, and Adult Children of Alcoholics (ACOA) meetings.

Outcomes Management

Selecting an Appropriate Agent

Benzodiazepines. BZDs have been the most frequently used agents to treat alcohol withdrawal symptoms of autonomic hyperactivity such as tremors, anxiety, sweating, tachycardia, and hypertension. Tremulousness is the earliest appearing symptom and can be seen 6 to 12 h after the patient's last drink. Chlordiazepoxide, a long-acting BZD, is a good choice; diazepam is a reasonable substitute. Begin withdrawal by tapering chlordiazepoxide starting with 50 mg tid for 1 day, 50 mg bid for 1 day, 25 mg tid for 1 day, 25 mg bid for 1 day, 25 mg daily for 1 day, and then discontinue. Tapering of the BZD can be accomplished over a 5- to 7-day period of time depending on symptom manifestations. Tapering an acute dose over a 2-week period may be indicated (Janicak et al., 1993). The longer-acting BZDs may be erratically absorbed from the gastrointestinal tract if the patient is experiencing nausea and vomiting, and an intramuscular BZD may be required. In such cases, lorazepam intramuscularly is the preferred agent for injection because chlordiazepoxide and diazepam are poorly absorbed from the muscle. However, patients requiring parenteral medications for withdrawal treatment should be referred for inpatient care.

If liver function tests suggest possible hepatic complications, intermediate-acting BZDs, which do not depend on the liver for their metabolism, would be prudent. Examples of such agents are oxazepam and lorazepam, which are good choices for treating elderly patients in alcohol withdrawal. Begin BZD withdrawal by tapering over a 5- to 7-day period. Start with lorazepam 2 mg tid for 2 days, 2 mg bid for 2 days, 2 mg daily for 1 day, and then discontinue (Crabtree & Polles, 1997).

Antipsychotic agents may be needed for severe delirium and hallucinosis; low doses of haloperidol (1–10 mg/day) aid in the control of these symptoms. However, should the patient exhibit such symptoms of a severe withdrawal syndrome, he or she should be immediately referred to a specialist for inpatient care.

Adrenergic Agents. Beta-adrenergic blockers such as propanolol or atenolol may be administered to treat the autonomic hyperactivity seen in alcohol withdrawal.

Nutritional Supplements. Thiamine 100 mg/day for 3 days should be taken. A multivitamin preparation is given to restore possible deficiencies due to poor nutrition. Often, a prenatal multivitamin preparation is recommended because of its folic acid content.

Other Agents. Drugs to decrease alcohol consumption include naltrexone given 50 mg daily for up to 12 weeks to reduce cravings. The patient may request disulfiram to use as aversion therapy to deter drinking. Its important to remember that drug therapy should be only one part of a comprehensive, multidisciplinary alcohol treatment program (Baker, 2002; Hanna, 2000).

Monitoring for Efficacy

Benzodiazepines. The goal of BZD therapy is not to sedate patients but to treat for withdrawal. They should still be able to participate in other, nondrug therapeutic interventions.

Adrenergic Agents. When beta-adrenergic blockers are used to treat withdrawal symptoms, blood glucose should be monitored, especially in the first 36 h after drinking since the patient's poor nutritional status may result in hypoglycemia, which in turn could lower the seizure threshold.

Nutritional Supplements. Supplements such as a prenatal multivitamin may be continued indefinitely to augment adequate dietary intake. A 24 h diet recall or 3-day diet diary may be useful to monitor nutritional status.

Other Agents. If naltrexone is prescribed, a daily dose of 50 mg orally is usually given. A weekly dose of 350 mg may be given in three divided doses, e.g., 100 mg on Monday and Wednesday and 150 mg on Friday. Naltrexone is started after detoxification to avoid unintentional precipitation of withdrawal. Do not administer naltrexone to polysubstance abusers since it can induce opiate withdrawal in heroin or other chronic opiate users. It is only adjunctive therapy for alcoholism.

On occasion, disulfiram (250–500 mg/day for 3 days as a loading dose and maintained on 125–200 mg/day) may be useful to prevent relapse following withdrawal. It should be used only by well-motivated patients who are physically healthy. Patients must be warned of the reactions that will occur if alcohol is ingested while taking disulfiram: headaches, nausea, vomiting, and facial flushing. For these reasons, many primary care providers obtain written consent before starting a disulfiram regimen.

Monitoring for Toxicity. Benzodiazepine toxicity may be monitored by checking for oversedation. Patients undergoing alcohol withdrawal, who are asleep most of the day, provide evidence that more than adequate doses are being administered.

Beta-adrenergic blockers may be monitored by a family member watching for bradycardia, level of alertness, mobility, and difficulty breathing (if emphysema or asthma is present). A blood glucose level may be obtained after the first 2 days of use, or earlier if indicated. Beta blockers can have adverse effects on comorbid conditions such as diabetes, chronic obstructive pulmonary disease (COPD), and cardiomyopathies. Alpha-adrenergic agonists may be monitored by following the patient's blood pressure during clinic visits.

The most commonly reported side effect of naltrexone is gastrointestinal disturbances. It is potentially hepatotoxic, so serum transaminases should be measured before initiating therapy and periodically throughout. The hepatotoxicity seems to be readily reversible on discontinuing the drug. Serious disulfiram reactions can include chest pain, shock, and respiratory depression (Doering, 1999).

Followup Recommendations. Once alcohol withdrawal is controlled, patients and families both need to be counseled about obtaining help from a rehabilitation program for the patient and from support groups for family members, of which there are usually many in the community.

NICOTINE ABUSE

Tobacco use is the single greatest cause of preventable illness and death in the United States today. Smoking is a known cause of heart and lung disease, cancer, and stroke in this country. It is a dangerous activity because of significant health risks associated with smoking, the addictive nature of nicotine, and the hazard to others in a smoking environment. Exposure to second-hand smoke is a potential health hazard to infants and young children. Since passive smoking can aggravate symptoms of asthma and allergies and decrease pulmonary function, exposed children have higher rates of lower respiratory tract infections, middle ear infections, and lung cancer. Primary healthcare providers can play a key role in helping smokers stop smoking and preventing others from starting (USDHHS, 1998).

Specific Considerations for Pharmacotherapy

The three stages of smoking cessation are: (1) preparing to quit, (2) initial cessation, and (3) maintenance of cessation. Pharmacotherapy is used when the patient stops smoking. Nicotine replacement therapy (NRT) along with cognitive-behavioral interventions has proven to be the most successful program in maintaining smoking cessation.

When Drug Therapy Is Needed. The nicotine found in tobacco causes the release of epinephrine and norepinephrine, producing a pleasurable feeling to smokers. Tolerance develops quickly, and users must increase their intake to obtain the desired effect. A typical one-pack-per-day smoker absorbs 20 to 60 mg of nicotine a day. Tobacco (nicotine) withdrawal syndrome begins within 24 h after smoking cessation. Common symptoms of withdrawal include craving for tobacco, anxiety, headaches, gastrointestinal upset, mood changes, irritability, difficulty concentrating, changes in appetite, and craving for sweets. Pharmacotherapy is used to relieve these symptoms so the patient can focus on changing the behavioral dependency during the smoking cessation program. Bupropion, a newer antidepressant, is the first nonnicotine pharmacotherapeutic agent effective in smoking cessation. It is safe and may be used jointly with NRT. Other antidepressants and anxiolytics are potentially useful, but only nortriptylene has consistent empirical evidence of smoking cessation efficacy (MMWR, 2000).

Short- and Long-Term Goals of Pharmacotherapy. The short-term goal of pharmacotherapy is to relieve symptoms of nicotine withdrawal so that patients can concentrate on behavioral change. The major long-term goal is to prevent risks of relapse by continued encouragement and discussion of strategies to maintain abstinence from smoking.

Nonpharmacologic Treatment. Prevention is the first-line intervention strategy for all primary healthcare providers. It is particularly important for children and teenage patient populations because about 95% of adult smokers began smoking before age 20. Providers can use the National Cancer Institute's smoking prevention/cessation counseling principles:

- Anticipate a smoking risk.
- Ask about smoke exposure.
- Advise all smoking patients to quit.
- Assist smokers in quitting.
- Arrange for followup care.

Antismoking strategies should begin in early preteen years with constant reinforcement and efforts to promote nonsmoking as the norm. Establish a smoke-free clinic environment and make educational materials related to the dangers of smoking and benefits of quitting available. Successful smoking cessation programs must include nonpharmacologic treatment along with pharmacotherapy. When smokers are preparing to quit, increase their motivation by discussing the risks and benefits of smoking cessation related to their physical, psychological, and social status. The healthcare professional's advice to stop smoking is a powerful motivator for some patients. During *every* clinic visit, providers should advise smokers to quit, offer brief smoking cessation counseling, give educational materials, prescribe NRT when appropriate, and refer to a stop-smoking program when the patient is ready to quit.

Supportive therapy from the primary provider is important to the patient during a smoking cessation program. Personalizing reasons to quit improves the patient's motivation to begin a treatment program and maintain cessation. Supporting the patient's belief that he or she *can* stop smoking is key to beginning the change process of a smoking cessation program. These interventions can be intensive or brief advice to quit smoking (MMWR, 2000; USDHHS, 1998).

Time Frame for Initiating Pharmacotherapy. Pharmacotherapy is begun on the day the patient stops smoking. NRT should be coupled with cognitive-behavioral interventions with self-help manuals, audiotapes, referral to a structured program, group therapy, and followup counseling. NRT alone will not change smoking behaviors; it only mitigates nicotine withdrawal symptoms.

Overview of Drug Classes for Treatment. Nicotine withdrawal symptoms can be relieved by maintaining some exposure to nicotine other than by smoking. Chewing gum, transdermal patches, nasal sprays, and inhalers are available delivery methods for NRT. Other agents used for withdrawal symptoms include antidepressants (bupropion amd nortriptylene) and clonidine, a centrally acting adrenergic blocking agent. Bupropion is the first nonnicotine-containing agent FDA approved for smoking cessation. It relieves the symptoms of nicotine withdrawal (Prochazka, 2000).

Assessment and History Taking. Ask every child and adult about tobacco use. Obtain a history of smoking in the patient's home and work environments. Determine if the patient has tried to quit previously and how successful the effort was. Assess for any coexisting psychiatric disorders that may contribute to continuation of smoking.

Assess cardiovascular and circulatory status to rule out any contraindications to NRT, such as recent MI, worsening angina, arrhythmias, active peptic ulcer, or pregnancy. Women who are pregnant or nursing infants should not use NRT. Discuss any physical findings that may be associated with tobacco use, which tends to "personalize" the need for smoking cessation and reinforce a commitment to quit.

See Drug Table 1003.

Patient/Caregiver Information. Provide educational materials on the dangers of smoking, benefits of quitting, and community resources to help people stop smoking. Talk about nicotine addiction and smoking cessation program availability. Although nicotine gum and the patch became OTC products in 1996, patients still need a behavioral treatment program for the best smoking cessation outcomes. The nicotine nasal spray requires a prescription. Instruct patients not to smoke during NRT (gum, patch, or nasal spray) or use other nicotine products. Remind patients to wash their hands after applying nicotine patches or handling the nasal spray. Table 33–10 contains patient, family, and health professional resources for smoking cessation.

Outcomes Management

Selecting an Appropriate Agent. Patients who smoke more than one pack per day or smoke their first cigarette of the day within 30 min of waking are most likely to be addicted to nicotine and will benefit most from NRT. With nicotine chewing gum, the nicotine is absorbed through the oral mucosa while avoiding harmful effects of smoking. The gum comes in 2 and 4 mg strengths. Instruct the patient to pick a target date to quit smoking. After that date, chew the gum whenever there is an urge to smoke. Advise the patient to chew the gum slowly, just enough for a slight tingling taste, "park it" between the cheek and teeth for proper absorption, and chew for about 30 min. Up to 12 pieces of gum may be chewed at the beginning of withdrawal, but not more than 30 pieces of 2 mg gum should be used in 24 h. Common side effects of nicotine gum include mouth irritation, dizziness, nausea, headache, and excess salivation. Some patients have problems with the gum adhering to dental work. Remind patients to avoid coffee, tea, or colas immediately before or after using the gum to enhance nicotine absorption.

TABLE 33–10. Resources for Managing Smoking Cessation

American Academy of Family Physicians
111400 Tomahawk Creek Parkway
Leawood, KS 66211-2671
913-906-6000
www.aafp.org/

American Cancer Society
1-800-ACS-2345
www.cancer.org/

American College of Obstetricians and Gynecologists
409 12 St. SW
PO Box 96920
Washington, DC 20090-6920
www.acog.org/

National Cancer Institute
www.nci.nih.gov

National Heart, Lung, and Blood Institute (NHLBI)
www.nhlbi.nih.gov/

Nicotine Anonymous World Services
www.nicotine-anonymous.org/

Check local newspapers and the phone directory for smoking cessation programs sponsored by local chapters of the American Cancer Society, American Heart Association, or local health agencies.

The transdermal patch, available OTC, provides a means of maintaining a steadier level of nicotine replacement during the smoking cessation program. The patch is used with patients who are willing to set a stop date, have significant nicotine addiction (smoke more than one pack per day or have had withdrawal symptoms), are willing to refrain from smoking while using the patch, and will participate in a structured behavioral program. Patches may be used for 24 h a day or for 16 h a day and removed at bedtime. Instruct patients to apply the patch to a nonhairy area of the skin on the trunk or the upper, outer area of the arm. Rotate the sites to avoid skin irritation. The patch can be worn in the shower or while swimming; however, perspiration can loosen the patch.

Begin with a 21-mg/day patch (strongest) for 4 to 6 weeks, gradually taper down to a 14 mg/day patch for 2 to 4 weeks, and finally go to a 7 mg/day patch (lowest) for 2 to 4 weeks. If the patient weighs less than 100 lb, begin with a 14 mg/day patch. The most common side effect of the nicotine patch is skin irritation, so patients with psoriasis or atopic dermatitis should consider another NRT delivery system. Use cautiously in patients with severe renal impairment or insulin-dependent diabetes mellitus because nicotine increases release of catecholamines. Patients who complain of insomnia may do better with a 16-mg/day patch that is removed at bedtime. Headache, nausea, vertigo, and dyspepsia have been reported with using the patch (Nicotrol, 1997).

Nicotine nasal spray delivers nicotine to the nasal mucosa and provides a rapid response to nicotine craving. Patients should not smoke while using the nasal spray or use other nicotine-containing products. One dose of the spray delivers 1 mg of nicotine in two sprays (one spray in each nostril). Patients start on one or two doses per hour, increasing up to 40 mg (80 sprays) as needed to control withdrawal symptoms. Common side effects include nasal and throat irritation, watering eyes, sneezing, and cough. Usually, patients adjust to these symptoms during the first week of treatment. Nicotine nasal spray is contraindicated in pregnant or nursing smokers and is not recommended for patients with asthma or allergic rhinitis. Benefits of using NRT for patients with cardiovascular and peripheral vascular diseases must be weighed against the risks of continued smoking. Nicotine nasal spray should not be used for longer than 6 months.

Generally, NRT is contraindicated for patients with a history of recent MI, increasing angina, severe arrhythmias, pregnancy, or lactation. Safe use in children under 18 has not been determined (Nicotrol NS, 1997). For heavy smokers who are pregnant, fewer uterine contractions may occur with the lower nicotine levels in replacement therapy than if the woman continues to smoke. (Brideau, 1997; MMWR, 2000; Montalto, 2000).

Bupropion hydrochloride (Zyban) is an FDA-approved medication to aid smoking cessation that has shown minimal side effects. Used in combination with NRT, bupropion showed high long-term smoking cessation rates (Hurt, Sacks, Glover, et al., 1997; Prochazka, 2000). It is not recommended in pregnancy or lactation.

Monitoring for Efficacy. Phone or write patients within 7 days of the initial visit to remind them of their quit date. Schedule a clinic visit within 1 to 2 weeks after the patient's stop date. Assess smoking cessation progress to provide support and help prevent relapse. Remind the patient that relapse is common, and if it should happen, to try again immediately. The nicotine gum dose should be tapered after about 3 months and used for not more than 6 months. Although the patch may be used for up to 16 weeks, a 3-step, 10-week program is recommended and detailed instructions accompany the product. The nasal spray may be continued for up to 6 months (USDHHS, 1998).

Monitoring for Toxicity. Signs and symptoms of nicotine toxicity include pallor, nausea, salivation, vomiting, abdominal pain, diarrhea, vision disturbances, dizziness, and mental confusion. Nausea, heartburn, and palpitations are the most often reported side effects of NRT. Assess for adverse reactions at each clinic visit or phone contact.

Followup Recommendations. Regular followup with patients is critical to their smoking cessation success. Providers should use every clinic encounter to encourage the smoker to quit, to support smoking cessation efforts, and to refer to appropriate community resources.

NEFAZODONE ADDENDUM

As this book was goin to press, serzone (nefazodone) was removed from the U.S. market on June 14, 2004. The manufacturer, Bristol-Myers-Squibb, denies that safety concerns are the cause for the withdrawal; however, a strong liver toxicity warning was plaxed on the label in 2002, and risk of severe injury must be strongly considered with this drug's use (Neergaard, 2004).

REFERENCES

Afinson, T. J. & Bona, J. R. (2001). A health services perspective on delivery of psychiatric services in primary care including internal medicine. *Medical Clinics of North America,* 85(3), 597–616.

AHCPR. (2001). *Treatment of Depression: Newer Pharmacotherapies.* Publication No. 99-E014, accessed hstat.nlm.nih.gov.

AHRQ. (2000). *Improving quality of care for people with depression: Translating research into practice.* Fact Sheet. AHRQ Publication No. 00-P020. Rockville, MD: Author.

American Psychiatric Association (APA). (2000). *Practice guideline for major depressive disorder in adults.* Washington, DC: American Psychiatric Press, Inc.

American Psychiatric Association (APA). (1994a). *Diagnostic and Statistical Manual of Mental Disorders* (4th ed.). Washington, DC: American Psychiatric Press, Inc.

American Psychiatric Association (APA). (1994b). Practice guideline for the treatment of patients with bipolar disorder. *Am J Psychiatry* 151:12 (suppl) 1–29.

Baker, R. (2002). Alcoholism. In R. E. Rakel, & E. T. Bope, *Conn's Current Therapy 2002,* (54th ed.) W. B. Saunders, 1113–117.

Bjornson, W. M., Fiore, M. C., & Logan-Morrison, B. A. (1996). The growing problem of smoking in women. *Patient Care 30*(13): 143–165.

Blazer, D. B., Grossberg, G. T., & Pollock, B. G. (1998 May). Managing depression in the elderly. *Patient Care for the Nurse Practitioner,* 11–12.

Bowers, W. A. & Katz, V .I. (2002). Postpartum depression. In S. G. Gabbe, J. R. Niekbyl, & J. L. Simpson (Eds.), *Obstertics: Normal and problem pregnancies* (4th ed.). New York: Churchill Livingston, pp. 716–710.

Bradwejn, J. & Koszycki, D. (2002). Panic disorder. In R. E. Rakel & E. T. Bope (Eds.), *Latest Approved Methods of Treatment for the Practicing Physician* (54th ed.), 1144–1146.

Brideau, D. J. Jr. (1997). Using nicotine replacement therapies. *Patient Care,* 31, 31–44.

Brown, T. M., Skop, B. P. & Mareth, T. R. (1996). Pathophysiology and management of the serotonin syndrome. *Ann Pharmacotherapy* 30:527–533.

Crabtree, B. L. & Polles, A. (1997). Substance-related disorders. In DiPalma, J. R., DiGregorio, G. J., Barbieri, E. J., & Ferko, A. P. (Eds.). *Basic Pharmacology in Medicine* (4th ed) West Chester, PA: Medical Surveillance, Inc.

DePaulo, J. R. (1999). Affective disorders. In L. R. Barker, J. R. Burton, & P. D. Zieve (Eds.), *Ambulatory Medicine* (5th ed.). 167–182.

Department of Health and Human Services (DHHS). (1996). Quick reference guide for clinicians. Smoking cessation: Information for specialists. *Journal of American Academy of Nurse Practitioners, 8*(7), 317–322.

Department of Health and Human Services (DHHS). (1998). *Clinician's handbook of preventive services* (2nd ed.). Washington, DC: U.S. Government Printing Office.

Depression Guideline Panel. (1993a). Clinical practice guideline number 5. *Depression in primary care: Volume 1. Detection and diagnosis* (AHCPR Publication No. 93-0550). Washington, DC: U.S. Government Printing Office.

Depression Guideline Panel. (1993b). Clinical practice guideline number 5. *Depression in primary care: Volume 2. Treatment of major depression* (AHCPR Publication No. 93-0551). Washington, DC: U.S. Government Printing Office.

Doering, P. L. (1999). Substance-related disorders: Alcohol, nicotine, and caffeine. In J. T. DiPiro, R. L. Talbert, G. C. Yee, G. R. Matzke, B. G. Wells, & L. M. Posey (Eds.), *Pharmacotherapy: A Pathophysiologic Approach* (4th ed.). 30–35.

Doghramji, K. (2002). Insomnia. In Rakel, R. E. & Bope, E. T. (Eds.), *Conn's Current Therapy 2002* (54th ed). Philadelphia: W. B. Saunders.

Eddy, M. & Walbroehl, G. S. (1999). Practical therapeutics: Insomnia. *American Family Physician,* 59(7), 1911–1916, 1918.

Eisendrath, S. J. & Lichtmacher, J. E. (2000). Psychiatric disorders. In Tierney, L. M, McPhee, S. J., & Papadakis, M. A. (Eds). *Current Medical Diagnosis & Treatment.* pp. 1046–1053.

Fankhauser, M. P. & Benefield, W. H. (1997). Bipolar diorders. In DiPiro, J. T., Talbert, R. L., Yee, G. C., Matzke, G. R., Wells, B. G., & Posey, L. M. (Eds.). *Pharmacotherapy: A Pathophysiologic Approach.* (3rd ed.). Stamford, CT: Appleton & Lange, pp. 1419–1441.

Friedman, R. A. & Kocsis, J. H. (1996). Pharmacotherapy for chronic depression. *Psychiatr Clin North Am* 19(1):121–132.

Galanter, D. (1999). Alcohol. In M. Galanter & H. D. Kleber (Eds.), *Testbook of Substance Abuse Treatment* (2nd ed.). 151–164.

Gorman, J. M. (2000). Generalized anxiety disorder. *Clinical Comerstone* 3(3):37–46.

Gutman, D. & Nemeroff, C. B. (2002). The neurobiology of depression: Unmet needs. Accessed at www.medscape.com.

Hahn, M. S. (1996). In search of Mr. Sandman. ADVANCE for Nurse Practitioners (May) 36–42.

Hanna, E. Z. (1995). Approach to the patient with alcohol abuse. In Goroll, A. H., May, L. A., & Mulley, A. G. (Eds.). *Primary care medicine: Office evaluation and management of the adult patient* (3rd ed). Philadelphia: J.B. Lippincott.

Hartman, P. M. (1995). Drug treatment of insomnia: Indications and newer agents. *Am Fam Physician* 51:191–194.

Hidalgo, R. B. & Davidson, J. R. (2001). Generalized anxiety disorder: An important clinical concern. *Medical Clinics of North America,* 85(3), 691–710.

Howland, R. H. & Thase, M. E. (2002). Mood disorders. In *Conn's Current Therapy 2002,* 54th ed. pp. 1133–1139.

Hurt, R. D., Sacks, D. P., Glover, B. D. et al. (1997). A comparison of sustained release bupropion and placebo for smoking cessation. *The New England Journal of Medicine, 337,* 1195–1202.

Jermain, J. M. (1999). Sleep disorders. In J. G. DiPiro, r. L. Talbert, G. C. Yee, G. R. Matzke, B. G. Wells, & L. M. Powey (Eds). *Pharmacotherapy: A Pathophysiologic Approach* (4th ed.) New York: McGraw Hill, pp. 1056–1064.

Jessen, L. M. (1996). Depression. *Pharmacist,* 57–70.

Kahn, D. A. (1995). New strategies in bi-polar disorder part II: Treatment. *Journal of Practical Psychiatry Behavioral Health* 1:148–157.

Kando, J. C., Well, B. G., & Hayes, P. E. (1999). Depressive disorders. In J. T. DiPiro, R. L. Talbert, G. C. Yee, G. R. Matzke, B. G. Wells, & L. M. Posey (Eds.), *Pharmacotherapy: A Pathophysiologic Approach* (4th ed.). New York: McGraw Hill, pp. 1141–1160.

Keck, P. D., McElroy, S. L., & Arnold, L. M. (2001). Advances in the pathophysiology and treatment of psychiatric disorders: Implications for internal medicine. In *Medical Clinics of North America,* 85(3), pp. 645–661.

Kirkwood, C. K. (1999). Anxiety disorders. In DiPiro, J. T., Talbert, R. L., Yee, G. C., Matzke, G. R., Wells, B. G., & Posey, L. M. (Eds.). *Pharmacotherapy: A Pathophysiologic Approach* (4th ed.). Stamford, CT: Appleton & Lange.

Korn, M. L. (2000). Understanding and treating obsessive-compulsive disorder. *J Am Board Fam Practice* (13(4), 251–260.

Krahn, D. D. (2002). Bulimia nervosa. In Rakel, R. E. & Bope, E. T. (Eds.), Conn's Current Therapy 2002 (54th ed.). Philadelphia: W.B. Saunders.

Krystal, J. H., D'Sousa, D. C., Sanacora, G. et al. (2001). Current perspectives on the pathophysiology of schizophrenia, depression, and anxiety disorder. *Medical Clinics of North America,* 85(3), 559–577.

Kulin, N. A., Pastuszak, M. S., & Sage, S. R. (1998). Pregnancy outcome following maternal uise of the new selective serotonin reuptake inhibitors. *Journal of the American Medical Association,* 179(8), 609–610.

Kuzel, R. (1996). Management of depression. *Postgraduate Medicine, 99*(9), 64–67.

Marken, P. & Sommi, R. (1999). Eating disorders. In J. T. DiPiro, R. L. Talbert, G. C. Yee, G. R. Matzke, B. G. Wells, & L. M. Posey (Eds.), *Pharmacotherapy: A pathophysiologic approach* (4th ed.). Stamford, CT: Appleton & Lange, pp. 1056–1064.

Mayfield, D., McLeod, G., & Hall, P. (1974). The CAGE questionnaire: Validation of a new alcoholism screening instrument. *Am J Psychiat 131*(10):1121–1123.

Miller, I. & Keitner, G. (1996). Combined medication and psychotherapy. *Psychiatric Clinics of North America, 19*(1), 151–171.

MMWR. (2000). Reducing tobacco use: A report of the surgeon general. *MMWR,* 16(RR-16).

Montalto, N. J. (2000). Primary prevention and cessation of tobacco use. *Clinics of Family Practice,* 2(2), 423–448.

Moore, J. D. & Bona, J. R. (2001). Depression and dysthymia. *The Medical Clinical of North America,* 85(3),

Neergaard, L. (2004, May 20). Serzone pulled from market. *Sun-Sentinel,* 14A.

Nicotrol: Nicotine transdermal system. (1997). In *Physicians' desk reference* (51st ed.). Montvale, NJ: Medical Economics.

Nicotrol NS. (1997). In Physicians' desk reference (51st ed.). Montvale, NJ: *Medical Economics.*

Olson, J. (1995). Clinical pharmacology made ridiculously simple. Miami: MedMaster, Inc.

Powers, P. S. & Santana, C. A. (2002). Eating disorders: A guide for the primary care physician. *Primary Care: Clinics in Office Practice,* 29(1), 81–98.

Prater, C. D., Miller, K. E., & Zylstra, R. G. (1999). Outpatient detoxification of the addicted or alcoholic patient. *American Family Physician,* 60(4), 1175–1183.

Preskorn, S. H. (1996). Reducing the risk of drug-drug interactions: A goal of rational drug development. *J Clin Psychiatry 57* (suppl 1):3–6.

Prochazka, A. V. (2000). New developments in smoking cessation, *Chest,* 117(4), 1693–1755.

Raj, B. A. & Sheehan, D. V. (2001). Social anxiety disorder. *Medical Clinics of North America,* 85(3), 711–133.

Rens, V. I. (2002). Psychiatric disorders. In *Harrison's Online.* McGraw-Hill Companies. Accessmedicine.com.

Rigotti, N. A. (2000). Approach to eating disorders. In Goroll, A. H., May, L. A., & Mulley, A. G. (Eds.). Primary care medicine: *Office Evaluation and Management of the Adult Patient* (3rd ed). Philadelphia: J. B. Lippincott.

Roca, R. P. (1999). Anxiety. In L. R. Barker, J. R. Burton, & P. D. Zieve (Eds.), *Ambulatory Medicine* (5th ed.). pp. 148–163.

Rock, C. L. & Zerbe, K. J. (1995). Keeping eating disorders at bay. *Patient Care,* 29(18), 78–104.

Schwartz, R. H. (1996). Let's help young smokers quit. *Patient Care* 30(3):45–51.

Schiffer, R. B. (2000). Psychiatric disorders in medical practice. In L. Goldman & J. C. Bennett (Eds.), *Cecil Textbook of Medicine* (21st ed.). Philadelphia: W.B. Saunders.

Shogren, E. (2004, March 23). FDA orders suicide risk label. *Sun-Sentinel,* 1A, 8A.

Smith, D. (2000). The eating disorders. In Goldman, L. & Bennett, J. C. (Eds.). *Cecil Textbook of Medicine* (21st ed.). Philadelphia: W.B. Saunders.

Swerdlow, N. R. (2001). Obsessive-compulsive disorder and tic syndromes. *Medical Clinics of North America,* 85(3), 735–755.

Valente, S. (1996). Diagnosis and treatment of panic disorder and generalized anxiety in primary care. *Nurse Practitioner, 21*(8), 26–45.

Weilburg, J. B. (2000). Approach to the patient with isomnia. In Goroll, A. H. & Mulley, A. G. (Eds.), *Primary care medicine* (4th ed.). Philadelphia: Lippincott Williams & Wilkins.

Wells, B. G. & Hayes, D. E. (1999). Obsessive-compulsive disorder. In J. T. DiPiro, R. L. Talbert, G. C. Yee, G. R. Matzke, B. G. Wells, & L. M. Posey (Eds.), *Pharmacotherapy: A Pathophysiologic Approach* (4th ed.). 1197–1207.

Wells, B. G., Mandos, L. A., & Hayes, D. E. (1997). Depressive disorders. In J. T. DiPiro, R. L. Talbert, G. C. Yee, G. R. Matzke, B. G. Wells, & L. M. Posey (Eds.). *Pharmacotherapy: A Pathophysiologic Approach* (3rd ed.). Stamford, CT: Appleton & Lange.

Wisser, K. L., Gelenberg, A. J., Leonard, H. et al. (1999). Pharmacologic treatment of depression during pregnancy. *Journal of the American Medical Association,* 282: 1264–1269.

Worthington, J. J. & Rausch, S. L. (2000). Approach to the patient with depression. In A. H. Goroll & A. G. Mulley (Eds.). *Primary Care Medicine: Office Evaluation and Management of the Adult Patient* (4th ed.). pp. 1157–1159.

CHAPTER ❖ 34

URINARY TRACT DISORDERS AND MALE SEXUAL DYSFUNCTION

Linda D. Scott ◆ David H. Nelson

Urinary tract infections (UTIs) are some of the most frequently treated health problems in primary care. Infections of the upper and lower urinary tracts account for 8 million visits to healthcare providers, contribute to more than 1 million hospital admissions, and cost approximately $1 billion annually. Statistical data in the literature rarely differentiate between lower and upper UTIs. UTI syndromes range from uncomplicated to complex, relate to an inflammatory response, and describe an anatomical site of infection (Gupta, Hooton, & Stamm, 2001; Miller & Hemphill, 2001; Romanzi, 2002). Definitions of UTIs are listed in Table 34–1. This chapter addresses the treatment of selected urinary tract infections across the life span and covers lower UTIs; upper UTIs; stress urinary incontinence; and male urinary tract disorders, such as epididymitis, urethritis, prostatitis, benign prostatic hyperplasia (BPH), and male sexual dysfunction. It also presupposes that the treatment is for healthy patients who do not have renal complications or neurologic or urologic abnormalities.

LOWER URINARY TRACT INFECTIONS

Cystitis and *urethritis* (inflammation of the bladder and urethra) are characterized by dysuria, frequency, urgency, hesitancy, back pain, nocturia, and suprapubic heaviness or pain (Miller & Hemphill, 2001; Romanzi, 2002; Santen & Altieri, 2001). The most common pathogen of community-acquired UTIs is the gram-negative bacillus *Escherichia coli* (80%), followed by the gram-positive coccus *Staphylococcus saprophyticus* (5–15%), and less frequently, *Klebsiella pneumoniae, Proteus mirabilis, Pseudomonas aeruginosa,* and *Enterococcus faecalis* (Gupta, Hooton, & Stamm, 2001; McLaughlin & Carson, 2004; Miller & Hemphill, 2001; Romanzi, 2002).

The prevalence of UTIs relates to age and gender. In newborns and infants up to age 1, the prevalence of bacteriuria is 1%, more common in males, and relates to structural or functional abnormalities. UTIs in males after age 1 is rare, with incidence increasing after age 50 and relating to prostatic obstruction (McLaughlin & Carson, 2004; Miller & Hemphill, 2001; Romanzi, 2002; Santen & Altieri, 2001).

The incidence of UTIs after age 1 year is most common in females (1–5%) and dramatically increases by 1–4% after puberty. Risk factors for UTIs include family history of UTIs, increasing age, sexually transmitted diseases (STD), frequency of sexual intercourse, use of diaphragm and spermicide, delayed coital micturation, pregnancy, and history of recent UTIs. Symptomatic cystitis in females is commonly associated with chlamydia, *Neisseria gonorrhoeae,* herpes simplex infections, fungal infections, or mycobacterial (tuberculosis is the most common) infections. It is estimated that 40% of all females experience discomforts of UTIs in their lifetimes, accounting for 5 to 15% of annual visits to healthcare

TABLE 34–1. Definitions of Upper and Lower Urinary Tract Infections

Term	Definition
Lower Urinary Tract	
Uncomplicated cystitis	Infection in a healthy individual by a common pathogen. Presents with symptoms of dysuria, urgency, frequency, abdominal pain or fullness, afebrile with no systemic illness.
Asymptomatic cystitis	Infection with significant bacteria ($>10^5$ CFU/ml of urine) and the absence of symptoms.
Symptomatic cystitis	Complaints of dysuria, urgency, frequency, abdominal pain, or fullness in the presence of significant bacteria.
Recurrent	Infection occuring after documented resolution of previous infection and causation of different organism
Unresolved	Infection within 2 to 3 weeks after previous infection by the same organism. May be associated with pyelonephritis, stone, anatomical abnormality, acquired resistance, or inadequate coverage of second organism or nonadherence.
Complicated cystitis	Infection associated with structural, neurologic, or congenital abnormalities or distortion of urinary tract. Associated conditions include diabetes, pregnancy, age >65 years, UTI in prior 6 weeks, urinary symptoms >7 days, use of a diaphragm, and symptoms of upper UTI.
Upper Urinary Tract	
Uncomplicated pyelonephritis	Infection in a healthy individual by a common pathogen. Varies from mild to severe state and characterized by systemic symptoms of acute onset of fever (101° F or 38.5°C), headache, frank shaking chills, CVA tenderness, and nausea or vomiting or both.
Complicated pyelonephritis	Infection by common pathogen and associated with structural, neurologic, or congenital abnormalities that interfere with normal urinary flow. Associated with diabetes, pregnancy, age >65 years, UTIs in prior 6 weeks, stones, prostatic hypertrophy, and in dwelling catheter. Acute onset of systemic symptoms of fever (>101°F or 38.5°C), frank shaking chills, moderate to severe CVA tenderness, abdominal pains, nausea, vomiting, malaise, headache, dehydration, and possible hematuria. Varies from mild to severe state.

providers, with 20% of these experiencing recurrent UTIs. Risk factors for males are advancing age or homosexuality. Morbidity, time lost at work, cost of medical care, and psychological and emotional stress are experienced with urinary discomfort (Chancellor & Yoshimura, 2004; McLaughlin & Carson, 2004; Miller & Hemphill, 2001; Romanzi, 2002; Santen & Altieri, 2001).

UTI, specifically asymptomatic bacteriuria, is the most common complication of pregnancy. It occurs in 10% of normal pregnancies and is comparable to the prevalence in sexually active nonpregnant females of reproductive age. UTI places the pregnant female at risk for adverse outcomes, such as preterm labor, low birth weight infants, intrauterine growth retardation, and pyelonephritis (50% incidence), and chronic renal disease. Socioeconomic status, sickle cell trait, diabetes mellitus, and multiparity are factors that relate to increased prevalence, with a twofold increase during pregnancy (Delzell & LeFevre, 2000; MacLean, 2001; Miller & Hemphill, 2001; Romanzi, 2002).

The overall incidence of asymptomatic cystitis increases substantially after the age of 65 years and is approximately equal for both genders. The rate of incidence further increases for institutionalized and hospitalized elders. This relates to prostatic hypertrophy, poor bladder emptying with prolapse in females, absence of estrogen effects, fecal incontinence, neuromuscular diseases, and increased urinary instrumentation or catheterization (Miller & Hemphill, 2001; Romanzi, 2002; Santen & Altieri, 2001).

SPECIFIC CONSIDERATIONS FOR PHARMACOTHERAPY

When Drug Therapy Is Needed

Cystitis needs to be treated with antibiotics when the patient presents with symptoms and/or the disease is confirmed with diagnostic testing. Prompt diagnosis is essential because the incidence of disease varies according to age and gender; may be symptomatic or asymptomatic; and has the potential for renal scarring or serious damage to the urinary system (MacLean, 2001; McCue, 2000; Miller & Hemphill, 2001; Santen & Altieri, 2001). The key to diagnosis is confirmation of significant numbers of pathogens in an appropriate urine specimen. The type and extent of laboratory examination depends on the clinical situation (Gupta, Hooton, & Stamm, 2001; McCue, 2000; Miller & Hemphill, 2001). Healthcare providers need to educate patients fully about side effects and costs of antibiotic therapy as well as the benefits and harms of other options of care.

Short- and Long-Term Goals of Pharmacotherapy

The short-term goals of treatment for uncomplicated and complicated cystitis are to resolve the infection, restore normal physiological function of the urinary tract, and prevent future recurrence of infection. The long-term goals of treatment for uncomplicated cystitis are to prevent recurrent episodes of infection and renal complications. The long-term goals of treatment for complicated cystitis are to correct any physiological abnormality when possible and prevent reinfection or renal complications.

In each condition of the lower urinary tract, treatment goals are achieved primarily by antibiotic therapy and patient education.

Time Frame for Initiating Pharmacotherapy

Treatment for cystitis should be initiated when the patient presents with complaints or by laboratory confirmation of diagnosis to prevent the serious sequelae discussed. A course of antibiotics is the required therapy to eliminate causative bacteria. Significant improvement of symptoms is expected in 24 to 48 h (Gupta, Hooton, & Stamm, 2001; McLaughlin & Carson, 2004; Miller & Hemphill, 2001).

See Drug Tables 102.1–102.7, 102.10, 903.

Assessment and History Taking

Refer to Tables 34–2 and 34–3.

Patient/Caregiver Information

Educating the patient concerning signs and symptoms of the disease, drug therapy, and prevention measures is critical for positive outcomes. Refer to Table 34–4.

OUTCOMES MANAGEMENT

Selecting an Appropriate Agent

Patient factors of age, gender, presence or absence of symptoms, pregnancy, drug or environmental hypersensitivities, adherence to therapy regimen, and recent antibiotic therapy must be considered in selecting an appropri-

TABLE 34–3. Diagnostic Tests for Urinary Tract Infections

Urine Collection
- Midstream clean-catch voided specimens (preferably first morning specimen or wait 2 hours after last voiding)
- Single-time catherization if unable to obtain clean midstream specimen

Urinalysis
- Dipstick
  Positive leukocyte esterase test indicates pyuria
  Positive nitrite denotes presence of gram-negative bacteria only
  Positive blood indicates infection
- Microscopic analysis
  Significant pyuria = WBCs 10^2 CFU/mL
  Complete Gram's stain to identify if positive or negative plus shape and pattern
  Presence of hematuria or RBCs
  Sterile pyuria suggests presence of STDs or urethritis
- Urine culture and sensitivity
  Determine organism for type of cystitis
  Obtain with all children, all men, initial prenatal visits, and females with renal abnormalities, immunocompromise, diabetes mellitus, prolonged symptoms, three or more UTIs in past year, or pyelonephritis
  Significant hematuria is $\leq 10^2$ CFU/mL of urine
  Determine bacteria and antibiotic sensitivity

Tests for STDs
Wet mount for vaginal or urethral secretions
Neisseria gonorrhoeae culture
Chlamydia test

CBC with Differential for Systemic Symptoms

Consider Erythrocyte Sedimentation Rate

Rule out Pregnancy When Indicated

For Complicated Cystitis or Complicated Pyelonephritis
Refer for renal ultrasound, intravenous pyelogram (IVP), renal scan, renal biopsy, cystoscopy, voiding cystourethrogram

TABLE 34–2. Baseline Data: History and Physical Examination for Urinary Tract Infections

History
Onset and duration of symptoms and voiding patterns
Sequence of dysuria in voiding pattern
Past medical history (drugs, allergies, chronic diseases, previous genitourinary problems and treatment)
Sexual (LMP, length of menopausal state, sexual behaviors, frequency of coitus, risk for STDs)
Contraception

Physical Examination
Vital signs: note elevation of temperature and hydration status
Complete abdominal examination: note suprapubic tenderness
Costovertebral tenderness (CVA)
Females: Inspect perineum; complete pelvic, speculum, and rectal examinations if symptoms indicate or confusion in diagnosis
Males: inspect and palpate external genitalia; prostate, and rectal examination
Children: observe general appearance for pallor, diaphoresis, listlessness, signs of sepsis, and dehydration
Elders: usually asymptomatic and present with altered mental status, change in eating habits, or gastrointestinal symptoms

TABLE 34–4. Patient/Caregiver Information for Urinary Tract Infections

Drink adequate amounts of fluid, 2–4 L daily
Avoid excessive intake of carbonated beverages, coffee, tea, or alcohol
Ensure nutrition is adequate
Establish frequent, regular urinary elimination patterns
Avoid retention of urine or delay of elimination
Practice good perineal hygiene by wiping perineal area front to back
Wash hands before and after urination
Shower or bathe daily, taking particular attention to cleansing perineal area
Know the signs and symptoms of infection and how important it is to seek healthcare immediately

ate drug and regimen to treat UTIs. Drug features of cost, safety, urinary excretion, effects on bowel and vaginal flora, local sensitivity, and resistance patterns are important considerations (Gupta, Hooton, & Stamm, 2001; Le & Miller, 2001; Miller & Hemphill, 2001). Refer to Table 34–5 for antibiotic recommendations for the following lower and upper UTIs.

Symptomatic Uncomplicated Cystitis. The diagnosis is based on symptoms, and a pretreatment urine culture is not required. Single-dose therapy of trimethoprin-sulfamethoxazole (TMP-SMX) or fluoroquinolones (FQLNs) is not as effective and is associated with a higher failure rate than the 3-day course. Three-day courses are as effective as the traditional 7-to 10-day therapies and have fewer side effects (McLaughlin & Carson, 2004; Miller & Hemphill, 2001; Naber, 2001; Romanzi, 2002).

Asymptomatic Uncomplicated Cystitis. Therapy recommendations depend on the patient's age, presence of pregnancy, and urine culture ($\geq 10^2$ CFU/mL) (Delzell & LeFevre, 2000; MacLean 2001; McCue, 2000; Miller & Hemphill, 2001; Romanzi, 2002; Santen & Altieri, 2001). For therapy recommendations for children, pregnant females, and elders, refer to "Special Situations" in Table 34–5.

Recurrent. Differentiation between reinfection and relapse is critical for appropriate drug selection. Reinfection is viewed as a new UTI; however, serial reinfections require a review of the patient's health habits and risk factors. Changes in risk factors such as changing from a diaphragm to birth control pills or daily application of estrogen vaginal cream in postmenopausal females to decrease colonization of *E. coli,* and education about preventive measures may reduce the frequency of reinfection (Gupta, Hooton, Roberts, & Stamm, 2001; Hooton, 2001; Miller & Hemphill, 2001; Romanzi, 2002).

Unresolved. Relapse or treatment failure requires resolution of the source of infection and potentially a change of drugs. Further diagnostic evaluation is needed to rule out prostatitis, stones, occult upper UTI, or a resistant organism. Urine cultures guide antibiotic selection (Gupta, Hooton, Roberts, & Stamm, 2001; Hooton, 2001; Miller & Hemphill, 2001; Romanzi, 2002).

Complicated Cystitis. The choice of antibiotics is guided by the pretreatment urine culture (Gupta, Hooton, & Stamm, 2001; Hooton, 2001; Miller & Hemphill, 2001; Romanzi, 2002).

Symptomatic Relief. The patient needs to be aware that phenazopyridine changes the color of urine and other body fluids. Do not use antispasmodics, such as hyoscyamine, unless the patient's symptoms are severe, because they exert strong systemic anticholinergic effects (Gupta, Hooton, & Stamm, 2001; Hooton, 2001; Miller & Hemphill, 2001; Romanzi, 2002).

Special Situations. *Pregnant patients* with bacteriuria or pyuria must be treated aggressively, including close monitoring. Pretreatment urine cultures guide therapy. Amoxicillin and cephalexin are safe, but *E. coli* resistance is an ever-increasing problem (29% in 1992 to 38% in 1996) (Romanzi, 2002). Nitrofurantoin is safe, especially effective against *E. coli,* an excellent choice in beta-lactam allergy, and most often the best choice during pregnancy. FLQNs and tetracyclines are contraindicated in pregnancy because of potential harm on fetal bone development. Sulfas are avoided in late pregnancy because of risk of inducing kernicterus (Delzell & LeFevre, 2000; MacLean, 2001; Miller & Hemphill, 2001; Romanzi, 2002).

Drug selection for *children* and *elders* is guided by pretreatment urine cultures as necessary (McCue, 2000; Miller & Hemphill, 2001; Romanzi, 2002; Santen & Altieri, 2001).

Monitoring for Efficacy

Symptomatic Uncomplicated Cystitis. Symptom resolution within 24 to 48 hours is considered sufficient monitoring of outcomes. Persistence of symptoms or continued bacteriuria requires a urine culture before resuming therapy for 7 to 10 days. All patients with positive pretreatment cultures must have a posttreatment urine culture in 1 to 2 weeks on completion of therapy to verify sterilization of the urine (Delzell & LeFevre, 2000; McLaughlin & Carson 2004, Miller & Hemphill, 2001; Romanzi, 2002).

Asymptomatic Uncomplicated Cystitis. A posttreatment urine analysis (UA) or dipstick assessment of asymptomatic UTIs is recommended. Continued bacteriuria requires a urine culture before resuming therapy for 7 to 10 days. All patients with positive pretreatment urine

TABLE 34–5. Empiric Antibiotic Recommendations for Upper and Lower Urinary Tract Infections

Diagnosis	Antibiotic	Regimen	Preference
	Lower Urinary Tract: Cystitis		
Uncomplicated			
Asymptomatic **OR** symptomatic	TMP-SMX	Give for 3 days[a]	1st
	FLQN	Give for 3 days[a]	Alt[b]
Recurrent (single event)	Same as asymptomatic or symptomatic		
Recurrent (serial: associated with coitus)	TMP-SMX	Single dose postcoital[a]	1st
	FLQN	Single dose postcoital[a]	Alt[b]
Recurrent (serial: genetic risk)	TMP-SMX	For 3 days with onset of symptoms	1st
	FLQN	For 3 days with onset of symptoms	Alt[b]
Unresolved	Follow culture and sensitivity results	Treat for 14+ days	
Complicated	TMP-SMX	Give for 7–14 days[a]	1st
	FLQN	Give for 7–14 days[a]	Alt[b]
Symptomatic relief	Phenazopyridine	100–200 mg PO tid for maximum 3 days	
	Special Situations		
Pregnancy	Amoxicillin	500 mg PO tid for 14 days	1st
	Cephalexin	500 mg PO qid for 14 days	Alt
	Nitrofurantoin	50 mg PO qid for 14 days	Alt
	Nitrofurantoin SR	100 mg PO bid for 14 days	Alt
	Third-generation cephalosporin	Give for 14 days[a]	2nd
Children			
<6 weeks	Hospitalization		
>6 weeks	TMP-SMX	Give for 7–10 days[a]	1st
	Amoxicillin-clavulanate	Give for 7–10 days[a]	Alt
	Third-generation cephalosporin	Give for 7–10 days[a]	2nd
Elders			
Symptomatic	Same as for any adult		
Asymptomatic	No treatment indicated		
	Upper Urinary Tract: Pyelonephritis		
Uncomplicated			
(Mild to moderate symptoms)			
Gram-negative bacilli	FLQN	Give for 14 days[a]	1st
Gram-positive cocci	Amoxicillin	500 mg PO tid for 14 days	1st
	Amoxicillin-clavulanate	500 mg PO tid for 14 days	Alt
(Moderate to severe symptoms)	Hospitalization		
Complicated			
(Mild to moderate symptoms)	Same as uncomplicated		
(Moderate to severe symptoms)	Hospitalization		
	Special Situations		
Pregnancy	Hospitalization		
Children	Hospitalization		
Elders	Hospitalization		

[a]See drug table for specific doses for various agents or ages.
[b]First choice in areas of high resistance patterns of *E. coli* to TMP-SMX (>20%). Alt = alternative; FLQN = fluoroquinolone; TMP-SMX = trimethoprim-sulfamethoxazole

cultures must have a posttreatment urine culture 1 to 2 weeks after completion of therapy to verify sterilization of the urine (Delzell & LeFevre, 2000; McLaughlen & Canon, 2004; Miller & Hemphill, 2001; Romanzi, 2002).

Recurrent. Patients with infrequent reinfections need to be monitored as if they have separately occurring symptomatic or asymptomatic infections. Patients on chronic prophylaxis or selfdirected therapy require periodic urine cultures during and on completion of 6 to 12 months of therapy. If symptoms redevelop after discontinuation of prophylaxis, initiate a full course of therapy and follow with continuous prophylaxis (Gupta, Hooton, Roberts, & Stamm, 2001; Hooton, 2001; Miller & Hemphill, 2001; Romanzi, 2002).

Unresolved. Monitor patients with relapse infections periodically with urine cultures. Efficacy of therapy is achieved with symptom resolution. If relapse infections continue, refer the patient for comprehensive urological evaluation (McLaughlen & Carson, 2004; Miller & Hemphill, 200; Romanzi, 2002).

Complicated Cystitis. A urine culture in 1 to 2 weeks posttherapy is essential to demonstrate cure. A positive urine culture requires resolution of treatable risk factors and is followed by 2 weeks or more of antibiotic therapy. Urine culture results guide drug selection (Gupta, Hooton, Roberts, & Stamm, 2001; Hooton, 2001).

Special Situations. *Pregnant patients* with a positive urine culture must be screened for reinfection or relapse through the remainder of the pregnancy and at the 6-week postpartum examination. Serial reinfections or relapses require chronic prophylaxis with ampicillin 250 mg twice daily, nitrofurantoin 100 mg once daily, or cephalexin 250 mg twice daily. A comprehensive postpartum urological evaluation is essential (Delzell & LeFevre, 2000; MacLean, 2001; Miller & Hemphill, 2001; Romanzi, 2002).

Children with any treatment failure require a comprehensive urological diagnostic evaluation. Ureteral reflux in combination with infection may lead to permanent renal damage (Santen & Altieri, 2001).

Monitoring for Toxicity

Refer to the Drug Tables 102.1–102.7, 102.10, 903.

Followup Recommendations

Patient followup should be scheduled in 10 to 14 days if symptoms persist. Resolution of symptomatic and asymptomatic cystitis requires no followup. Reinfected cystitis and all patients with complicated cystitis require posttreatment urine cultures and correction of identified abnormalities on completion of antibiotic therapy or within 14 days. All pregnant patients require repeat urine cultures every 2 weeks until delivery and at postpartum examination (Delzell & LeFevre, 2000; Gupta, Hooton, Roberts, & Stamm, 2001; Miller & Hemphill, 2001; Romanzi, 2002).

UPPER URINARY TRACT INFECTIONS

PYELONEPHRITIS

Pyelonephritis (inflammation of the renal parenchyma and collecting system) varies from mild to severe states and is characterized by systemic symptoms and lower urinary tract symptoms. Differentiation of pyelonephritis from cystitis is not always possible. Clinical presentation, laboratory findings, and pathologic findings assist the clinician in determining a definitive diagnosis of pyelonephritis (Delzell & LeFevre, 2000; Gupta, Hooton, Roberts, & Stamm, 2001; Gupta, Hooton, & Stamm, 2001; Miller & Hemphill, 2001; Romanzi, 2002; Santen & Altieri, 2001; Talan, Stamm, Wooten, et al. 2000).

Pyelonephritis occurs when organisms ascend from the lower to upper urinary tract or arrive via the blood or lymphatic systems. The most common pathogen of pyelonephritis is the gram-negative bacillus *E. coli* (80–90%), with unique subgroups of specific virulence. Gram-positive *S. saprophyticus* accounts for 5 to 10% of cases and *K. pneumoniae, P. mirabilis, P. aeruginosa,* or *E. faecalis* present less frequently (Delzell & LeFevre, 2000; Gupta, Hooton, & Stamm, 2001; Miller & Hemphill, 2001; Romanzi, 2002; Santen & Altieri, 2001; Talan et al., 2000).

The prevalence of pyelonephritis relates to age and gender. In newborns and infants up to age 1, the prevalence of bacteriuria is 1 to 5%, and it is more prevalent in febrile infants (5%), more common in males, and connected with structural or functional abnormalities. Pyelonephritis in the ages of 1 to 3 years is more common in females and dramatically increases by 1 to 4% after puberty (Santen & Altieri, 2001). It is estimated that 250,000 episodes occur annually in adult women with as many as 100,000 hospitalizations (Talan et al., 2000). Pyelonephritis is five to ten times more common in women with diabetes mellitus than women without diabetes (Romanzi, 2002). Risk factors for pyelonephritis include frequency of sexual intercourse, use of diaphragms and spermicide, delayed coital micturation, pregnancy, history of recent UTIs, and history of structural abnormalities (Delzell & LeFevre, 2000; Gupta, Hooton, & Stamm, 2001; Miller & Hemphill, 2001; Romanzi, 2002; Santen & Altieri, 2001; Talan et al., 2000).

Pyelonephritis is the most common nonobstetric cause of hospitalization in pregnancies with an occurrence rate of 1 to 2%; up to 23% of these women will have recurrences in the same pregnancy (Delzell & LeFevre, 2000). Untreated or unidentified asymptomatic cystitis progresses to pyelonephritis in 20 to 40% of all pregnant females. Pyelonephritis places the pregnant female at risk for adverse outcomes, such as preterm labor, septicemia, intrauterine growth retardation, anemia, altered renal function, and chronic renal disease. The prevalence of pyelonephritis directly relates to normal physiological changes of pregnancy and needs to be monitored through routine prenatal screenings (Delzell & LeFevre,

2000; Gupta, Hooton, & Stamm, 2001; Miller & Hemphill, 2001; Romanzi, 2002; Talan et al., 2000).

The overall incidence of pyelonephritis increases after the age of 65 years and is approximately equal for both genders. The rate of incidence further increases for institutionalized and hospitalized elders. This relates to prostatic hypertrophy, poor bladder emptying with prolapse in females, absence of estrogen effects, fecal incontinence, neuromuscular diseases, and increased urinary instrumentation or catheterization (Gupta, Hooton, & Stamm, 2001; Miller & Hemphill, 2001; Romanzi, 2002).

SPECIFIC CONSIDERATIONS FOR PHARMACOTHERAPY

When Drug Therapy is Needed

Pyelonephritis is treated with antibiotics when the patient presents with symptoms or the disease is confirmed by diagnostic findings. One key to diagnosis is confirmation of significant numbers of pathogens in the urine. Prompt diagnosis and treatment are essential because the incidence varies according to age and gender, the degree of systemic illness may advance rapidly, and the potential for renal scarring leads to chronic hypertension or end-stage renal disease. The type and extent of laboratory and radiological examinations depend on the clinical presentation and patient history (Delzell & LeFevre, 2000; Miller & Hemphill 2001; Romanzi, 2002; Santen & Altieri, 2001). Healthcare providers need to educate patients to side effects and costs of antibiotic therapy as well as benefits and harms of other options of care.

Short- and Long-Term Goals of Pharmacotherapy

The short-term goals of treatment for uncomplicated and complicated pyelonephritis are to resolve the infection, restore normal physiological function of the urinary tract, and prevent further recurrence of infection. The long-term goals for uncomplicated pyelonephritis are to prevent recurrence of infection and renal complications. The long-term goals for complicated pyelonephritis are to correct the physiological abnormality when possible and prevent reinfection or renal complications. In each of the conditions of the upper urinary tract, the treatment goals are achieved primarily by antibiotic therapy and patient education.

Nonpharmacologic Therapy

Patient education of prevention measures is located in Table 34–4.

Time Frame for Initiating Pharmacotherapy

Pyelonephritis requires immediate treatment when patients present with complaints or laboratory confirmation of diagnosis to prevent the serious sequelae discussed. The clinician needs to determine the patient's degree of systemic illness (bacteremia) because that guides the treatment regimen of outpatient or inpatient care and the choice of oral or parenteral antibiotic therapy. The clinician should consider hospitalization of those patients who are pregnant, vomiting, dehydrating, and have a history of chronic disease or of nonadherence to therapies (Delzell & LeFevre, 2000; Miller & Hemphill 2001; Romanzi, 2002; Santen & Altieri, 2001).

See Drug Table 102.

Assessment and History Taking

Refer to Tables 34–2 and 34–3.

Patient/Caregiver Information

Education of the patient concerning signs and symptoms of the disease, drug therapy, and prevention measures is critical for positive outcomes. Refer to Table 34–4.

OUTCOMES MANAGEMENT

Selecting an Appropriate Agent

Consider age, gender, pregnancy, drug or environmental hypersensitivities, concurrent diseases, recent antibiotic therapy, recent institutionalization, adherence to therapy regimen, and presence, absence, or severity of symptoms when selecting appropriate drugs and regimen to treat pyelonephritis. Cost, safety, urinary excretion, effects on bowel and vaginal flora, local sensitivity, resistance patterns, and efficacy are important drug features. Laboratory findings guide antibiotic selection (Delzell & LeFevre, 2000; Le & Miller, 2001; Miller & Hemphill, 2001; Romanzi, 2002; Santen & Altieri, 2001).

Empiric therapy is based on the Gram's stain results and directed toward specific bacteria groups. The degree of systemic disease determines whether oral or parenteral therapy is required. Patients with nausea and vomiting, who are acutely ill, under 5 years old, over 65 years, immunosuppressed, diabetic, or pregnant must be hospitalized for parenteral therapy (Delzell & LeFevre, 2000; Le & Miller, 2001; Miller & Hemphill, 2001; Santen & Altieri, 2001).

Costs of failure to treat pyelonephritis promptly and aggressively often outweigh any potential drug costs. Pretreatment urine cultures allow for effective and economical antibiotic selection. With decreases in the patient's symptoms, a change from parenteral to oral therapy contributes to cost savings. Most oral FLQNs provide almost identical serum levels compared to parenteral and are an early option for oral therapy (Miller & Hemphill, 2001; Naber, 2001).

Uncomplicated and Complicated Pyelonephritis. Refer to Table 34–5. Patents with complicated pyelonephritis are generally hospitalized for parenteral therapy and resolution of the obstruction, stone, or complicating factor (Delzell & LeFevre, 2000; Gupta, Hooton, & Stamm, 2001; Miller & Hemphill, 2001; Romanzi, 2002; Santen & Altieri, 2001).

Special Situations. Pregnant patients with pyelonephritis require hospitalization for parenteral therapy (Delzell & LeFevre, 2000; MacLean, 200; Romanzi, 2002). In *males,* pyelonephritis is considered a complicated infection unless the urologic diagnostic evaluation proves otherwise (Miller & Hemphill, 2001; Romanzi, 2002). *Elders* tend to have more bacteremia than other age groups; therefore, a blood culture is prudent before initiating therapy (McCue, 2000; Gupta, Hooton, & Stamm, 2001; Miller & Hemphill, 2001; Romanzi, 2002). For *children* and for all groups, refer to Table 34–5.

Monitoring for Efficacy

Uncomplicated Pyelonephritis. Assess all patients' clinical responses to drug therapy within 12 to 72 hours. Utilize followup urine culture results to modify antibiotic therapy as needed. Resolution of clinical symptoms and a sterile urine culture within 2 weeks indicate that further therapy is not needed. A final urine culture is performed 2 months after therapy completion. If the patient's symptoms persist, assess for antibiotic resistance and perform diagnostic evaluation to rule out complicated pyelonephritis or abscess (Delzell & LeFevre, 2000; Miller & Hemphill, 2001; Romanzi, 2002).

Complicated Pyelonephritis. Continue medical management and utilize urine culture results for modification of antibiotic therapy. Resolution of clinical symptoms and a sterile urine culture 2 weeks after completion of drug therapy indicate that further drug therapy is not needed. The clinician needs to monitor for complications or obstruction until a final urine culture is obtained 2 months after therapy completion. If symptoms persist, expand the diagnostic evaluation, assess for a drug-resistant organism strain, and consider surgical intervention. If urine cultures indicate *S. aureus,* determine if it is a real pathogen or urine sample contaminant. This organism presents in renal tissue by blood rather than ascending the urinary tract and requires that an abscess be ruled out (Delzell & LeFevre, 2000; Gupta, Hooton, & Stamm, 2001; Miller & Hemphill, 2001; Romanzi, 2002; Santen & Altieri, 2001).

Special Situations. For *pregnant patients,* a urine culture is essential on completion of drug therapy and every 2 weeks until delivery. Those with serial relapse or reinfection cystitis and recurrent episodes of pyelonephritis need extensive diagnostic evaluation during pregnancy and up to 3 months postpartum (Delzell & LeFevre, 2000; MacLean, 2001; Miller & Hemphill, 2001; Romanzi, 2002).

Close monitoring of children is critical because the risk for recurrence of pyelonephritis is 40 to 50% in infants and 30% in older children and relates to an anatomical abnormality. Obtain urine cultures every 3 months after the infection is resolved and monitor febrile episodes. Educate parents on prevention measures, potential complications (such as renal scarring, end-stage renal disease, and hypertension), need for comprehensive evaluation by urologist, and the need to seek healthcare when signs and symptoms of pyelonephritis present (Santen & Altieri, 2001).

Assess *elders'* response to drug therapy within 12 h and then as recommended for all adults. Treatment response may be affected by multiply resistant or nosocomial organisms, such as *P. aerguinosa* or *E. faecalis.* Increased rates of hospitalization, institutional care, or catheter use by elders enhances the opportunity for treatment failure from these organisms (McCue, 2000; Romanzi, 2002).

Monitoring for Toxicity

Elders, diabetics, and patients with chronic disease or severe renal infections require blood urea nitrogen and serum creatinine tests to monitor renal function. Aminoglycoside doses are adjusted according to renal function as they are ototoxic and nephrotoxic. Moderate aminoglycoside serum levels in pyelonephritis without systemic involvement are appropriate and avoid toxicity. Systemic infections require higher levels of therapy and mandate the monitoring of blood levels. Depending on renal clearance, aminoglycoside dosing intervals range from 8 to 48 h (Le & Miller, 2001; Miller & Hemphill, 2001).

Followup Recommendations

Uncomplicated Pyelonephritis. An initial assessment of patients' symptoms is essential within 12 to 24 h by phone or office visit. Significant improvement of symptoms should occur in 12 to 48 h. A second assessment of the patient's symptoms needs to be scheduled in the office within 2 to 3 days. If symptoms persist or worsen in 24 to 48 h, the patient needs to be hospitalized for parenteral antibiotic therapy and diagnostic evaluation to determine etiology of complicated pyelonephritis. All patients with pyelonephritis require posttreatment urine cultures within 2 weeks of therapy completion and 2 months later (Delzell & LeFevre, 2000; Miller & Hemphill, 2001; Romanzi, 2002).

Complicated Pyelonephritis. After hospitalization, posttreatment urine cultures are required within 2 weeks of therapy completion and 2 months later. The urine culture guides further drug therapy to alleviate the infection. Further diagnostic evaluation to determine etiology and referral for correction of the problem is essential if this was not achieved during the hospital stay. Sufficient monitoring of complicated pyelonephritis may require 6 to 12 months to prevent reinfection or renal complications (Delzell & LeFevre, 2000; Miller & Hemphill, 2001; Romanzi, 2002). Refer to "Special Situations" for specific followup of pregnant patients, children, and elders.

STRESS URINARY INCONTINENCE

Stress urinary incontinence (SUI) is defined as the involuntary loss of urine during activities that increase abdominal pressure, such as coughing, sneezing, laughing, or other physical activities. Pathophysiologic changes of SUI in females relate to increased intraabdominal pressure from neuromuscular changes and hypermobility of the bladder base and urethra associated with poor pelvic support or intrinsic urethral sphincter failure or weakness. In males, pathophysiologic changes relate to overflow from an underactive or acontractile detrusor and are associated with prostate gland problems, urethral stricture, neurologic problems, or idiopathic detrusor failure. SUI from intrinsic sphincter deficiency (ISD) is characterized by continuous leakage at rest or with minimal exertion, such as postural changes (Beheshti & Fonteyn, 1998; Delancey & Ashton-Miller, 2004; Holroyd-Leduc & Straus, 2004; Thakar & Stanton, 2000; U.S. Department of Health and Human Services [USDHHS], 1996).

Risk factors for SUI include medications, smoking, fecal impaction, habitual straining during defecation, low fluid intake, high-impact physical activities, obesity, estrogen depletion, pelvic muscle weakness, pelvic floor trauma, vaginal infections, parity, pregnancy, vaginal delivery, episiotomy, and history of childhood sexual abuse. Urinary incontinence affects approximately 13 million Americans or 10 to 35% of adults and 50% of the 1.5 million nursing home residents. Females have twice the prevalence of incontinence. Approximately 26% of females between the ages of 30 and 59 years experience SUI or a combination of SUI and urge incontinence. Approximately 5 to 10% of all community-dwelling individuals older than 60 years have urinary incontinence (UI). It is estimated that 53% of all homebound elders are incontinent. UI is the second leading cause of institutionalization of elders. Direct costs of caring for persons of all ages with UI are more than $15 billion annually (Beheshti & Fonteyn, 1998; Delancey & Ashton-Miller, 2004; Holroyd-Leduc & Straus, 2004; Thakar & Stanton, 2000; USDHHS, 1996).

Patients underreport UI because of embarrassment, stress related to odor and appearance, and the belief that UI is normal, especially in females. Most affected individuals do not seek help for incontinence and may be reluctant to admit to their UI. Patients need to be asked if they are accidentally leaking urine, since 70% of UI is curable, but correct diagnosis is essential (Beheshti & Fonteyn, 1998; Holroyd-Leduc & Straus, 2004; Palmer, 2004; Thakar & Stanton, 2000; USDHHS, 1996).

SPECIFIC CONSIDERATIONS FOR PHARMACOTHERAPY

When Drug Therapy Is Needed

Therapy for SUI is primarily behavioral and pelvic floor exercise techniques, as they are the least invasive and have fewer potential side effects (Palmer 2004; USDHHS, 1996). Approximately 12 to 16% of patients are cured of stress and urge incontinence, and 54 to 75% of patients report improvement of symptoms with the use of behavioral techniques (Beheshti & Fonteyn, 1998; Thakar & Stanton, 2000; USDHHS, 1996).

Although no specific drug therapy for SUI exists (Newman, 2004), some drugs impact bladder contractility or urethral resistance. Alpha-adrenergic agonists increase striated or smooth muscle tone to increase urethral resistance. Tricyclic agents decrease bladder contractility and increase urethral resistance. Estrogen per vagina may help with urge in continence. An investigational SNRI, duloxetin, may prevent SUI by external urethral sphincter contractions (Newman, 2004).

The elimination, dosage adjustment, or schedule change of drugs that precipitate or contribute to SUI is considered a therapeutic action. All patients need a comprehensive assessment of their over-the-counter herbal or prescribed medications. Drugs that affect UI include anticholinergic agents, diuretics, caffeine, alcohol, antidepressants, psychotropics, sedatives, hypnotics, narcotics, antipsychotics, antispasmodics, antiparkinsonian agents, and phenothiazines and alpha-adrenergic blocking (Blaivas, Romanzi, & Heritz, 1998; Gray, 2004; Newman, 2004; USDHHS, 1996).

Short- and Long-Term Goals of Pharmacotherapy

The short-term goals of treatment for SUI are to decrease incontinent symptoms or episodes, improve management of SUI, and prevent complications. The long-term goals of treatment of SUI are to eliminate incontinent symptoms or episodes and prevent complications. The goals of treatment are best accomplished by behavioral techniques first, then drug therapy if needed.

Nonpharmacologic Therapy

Refer to "Patient/Caregiver Information" for additional information. Behavioral techniques and/or mechanical to surgical interventions require education and positive reinforcement. They consist of the following

- Pelvic floor exercises (PFEs) or Kegel exercises
- Voiding records (Bladder diary)
- Dietary modifications
- Fluid intake modification
- Eliminating constipation; regular bowel
- Smoking cessation
- Weight reduction
- Using incontinence pads or garments
- Biofeedback
- Physical, social, and environmental devices to facilitate toileting
- Penile clamps or external catheters or condoms
- Pessaries or vaginal cones for pelvic support
- Neuromodulation (electrical stimulation)
- Use of catheters (intermittent, indwelling, or suprapubic)
- Periurethral bulking agent injections
- Surgery such as pubovaginal sling and netro-pubic colpo-suspension Newman, 2004; Palmer, 2004; (Beheshti & Fonteyn, 1998; Buback, 2001; Holroyd-Leduc & Straus, 2004; Thakar & Stanton, 2000; US-DHHS, 1996).

Time Frame for Initiating Pharmacotherapy

SUI should be treated at the time of diagnosis to prevent increased symptomatology, patient embarrassment and discomfort, and complications. The degree of symptomatology, patient preference, and the clinician's judgment determine when drug therapy is initiated.

See Drug Tables 311.1, 501.10, 605, 703.

Assessment and History Taking

Refer to Tables 34–6 and 34–7.

Patient/Caregiver Information

Refer to Table 34–8.

OUTCOMES MANAGEMENT

Selecting an Appropriate Agent

Pharmacotherapy plays a minor role in the treatment of SUI. Many references do not even address the issue of drug therapy in SUI. Treatment success or failure with behavioral therapy, history of hypertension, history of cardiovascular disease, gender, and menstrual age are factors to consider in selecting drug therapy (Blaivas, Romanzi, & Heritz, 1998; Holroyd-Leduc & Straus, 2004; USDHHS, 1996).

Refer to Table 34–9. Alpha-adrenergic agonists are used to increase bladder sphincter tone, but are of questionable benefit. Topical estrogen in postmenopausal females may help to restore mucosal vascularity and tone. Oral estrogen is not recommended (Newman, 2004) Du-

TABLE 34–6. Baseline Data: History and Physical Examination for Stress Urinary Incontinence

History

Onset of SUI, duration, and characteristics, such as stress, dribble, or urge
Patient's most bothersome symptom(s)
Urinary habits, such as frequency, timing, and volume of voiding; continent and incontinent episodes
Precipitating factors, such as cough, sneeze, laugh, "on way to bathroom," high-impact exercise, surgery, trauma, recent pregnancy, onset of illness, or new medications
Current management of SUI, including protective devices and use of pads or briefs
Previous treatment for SUI and its effect; patient expectations of treatment
Presence of UTI symptoms, such as dysuria, nocturia, hesitancy, sensation of incomplete bladder emptying, hematuria, or vaginitis
Bowel habits, frequency, consistency of stool, and changes in bowel habits
Alterations of sexual function related to SUI
Amount of daily fluid intake and use of any diuretic fluids or irritants, such as caffeine
Complete past medical and surgical history
Review all patient medications
History of genitourinary and neurological systems
  In females, comprehensive obstetrical history, such as episiotomy, length of labor, baby's birth weight, and complications
  In males, postvoid dribbling, urgency, and problems with prostate
Assess patient for SUI risk factors
Determine any physical, social, and environmental barriers, such as disability, access to bathroom, work restrictions, or living arrangements
Assess a voiding record or diary for frequency of voiding, time of day, and precipitating events; may be initial assessment measure and evaluation measure to determine effectiveness of treatment

Physical Examination

Abdominal examination to detect masses, suprapubic tenderness or fullness, diastasis rectus, and estimation of postvoiding residual (PVR) urine
  In males, perform genital examination to detect abnormalities of the foreskin, glans, penis, and perineal skin; assess the consistency and contour of the prostate
  In females, perform a pelvic examination to assess perineal skin, urethra, pelvic prolapse (cystocele, vaginal vault prolapse, uterine prolapse), pelvic mass, perivaginal muscle tone, atrophic vaginitis, and to estimate PVR urine by abdominal palpation and percussion
Rectal examination to assess perineal sensation, resting and active sphincter tone, rectal mass, fecal impaction, and estimation of PVR
Neurologic examination and observe mobility

loxetine is expected to be FDA approved soon for SUI treatment (Newman, 2004).

Monitoring for Efficacy

Monitoring guidelines for drug efficacy in SUI therapy lack clarity because efficacy relates to subjective expectations and multiple effects of combined therapies. A paucity of empirical longitudinal studies provides few monitoring guidelines. Monitoring of drug efficacy is based on the pharmacological properties of selected drugs, sufficient time frames, such as weeks to months for optimum drug effects, and the reduction of incontinent episodes (Blaivas, Romanzi, & Heritz, 1998; USDHHS, 1996).

TABLE 34–7. Diagnostic Tests for Stress Urinary Incontinence

Postvoiding residual (PVR) urine: Catheterized specimen after patient voids; PVR <50 mL is adequate bladder emptying; PVR >200 mL is inadequate emptying.
Provocative stress testing: Have client relax, then cough vigorously; observe for urine loss from urethra.
Perineal pad test: Objective measurement of volume of urine loss.
Urinalysis: Detect contributing conditions, such as hematuria, pyuria, bacteriuria, gylcosuria, and proteinuria (dipstick acceptable for screening; microscopic analysis helpful).
Urine culture: If bacteria present in urinalysis.
Bedside cystometrogram (bladder capacity): Volume of first sensation of bladder fullness and presence or absence of uninhibited detrusor contractions. Have patient void in privacy to empty a comfortably full bladder. Catheterize for postvoiding residual volume (14 French straight catheter). Fill bladder using a 50-mL syringe (without piston or bulb) with 25 to 50 mL of room temperature sterile water; hold syringe 15 cm above pubic symphysis. Have patient void with first sensation; maximum capacity assumed when patient cannot hold anymore. Upward movement of column fluid indicates presence of involuntary bladder contractions. Involuntary contractions or severe urgency at low bladder volumes, $<250-300$ mL, suggests detrusor instability, especially if consistent with patient symptoms.
Suspected urinary obstruction, retention, or noncompliant bladder: Blood urea nitrogen, creatinine, calcium levels.
Uroflowmetry and other urine cytology: If patient has recent onset of irritative voiding or hematuria.

TABLE 34–8. Patient/Caregiver Information for Stress Urinary Incontinence

- Behavioral techniques
  - Habit training or scheduled voiding
  - Timed voiding
  - Bladder training
  - Prompted voiding
  - Relaxation techniques
  - Voiding or bladder record
- Importance of daily pelvic floor exercises (PFEs) or Kegel exercises to reduce SUI
- Dietary modifications to include a decrease or elimination of alcohol, sweetener substitutes, and caffeine
- Fluid intake modification by decreasing or increasing volume (individual needs and related health problems); recommend 48 to 64 oz per day to stimulate bladder's stretch receptors and dilute urine
- Eliminate constipation with high-fiber foods and daily exercise, such as walking
- Importance of smoking cessation
- Develop a weight reduction plan
- Proper use of absorbent pads or garments and meticulous skin care
- Strategies to overcome physical, social, and environmental barriers to facilitate toileting, such as accessible toileting facilities, adequate lighting in bathroom, grab bars in the bathroom, elevated toilet seats, and walkers or mobility aids
- In males, purpose and appropriate use of penile clamps or external catheters
- In females, purpose and proper use of vaginal cones, pessaries, electrical stimulation, and vaginal hormone therapies
- Signs and symptoms of UTI and to seek health care if these occur
- Purpose, dosage, and side effects of drugs
- Teach health promotion and prevention measures
  - PFEs for all females in schools and clinics
  - Weight reduction
  - Birth control methods
  - Consistent bladder and bowel habits
  - Proper lifting techniques to avoid abdominal strain
  - Postcoital voiding to prevent UTI

Monitoring for Toxicity

In using alpha-adrenergic agonists, monitor for adverse effects of hypertension, tachycardia, anorexia, insomnia, agitation, headache, sweating, and respiratory difficulty. Avoid the use of estrogen in women with thromboembolic disease, abnormal bleeding, pregnancy, or known or suspected breast or uterine cancer. (Blaivas, Romanzi, & Heritz, 1998; USDHHS, 1996) A progestogen is advised with estrogen if the uterus is present. Any bleeding should be explained. Imipramine use requires monitoring (see Drug Table 311.1).

TABLE 34–9. Pharmacotherapy for Stress Urinary Incontinence

Drug	Regimen
Alpha-adrenergic agonist	
Pseudoephedrine	15–30 mg PO tid
Hormones (postmenopausal women)	
Conjugated estrogen cream	1–2 g vaginally, periurethrally qd
Tricyclic antidepressant	
Imipramine HCl*	75 mg PO daily

*No long term studies support use.

Followup Recommendations

All patients require regular monitoring of behavioral therapy, PFEs, and drug efficacy. The degree of symptomatology, patient characteristics and adherence, and potential drug adverse reactions determine monitoring frequency. Positive reinforcement of the patient's efforts is critical to continuation and success of therapy (Blaivas, Romanzi, & Heritz, 1998; Newman, 2004; Palmer, 2004; USDHHS, 1996).

MALE URINARY AND RELATED PROBLEMS

EPIDIDYMITIS

Epididymitis (inflammation of the epididymis) is the most common acute scrotal pain in postpubertal males and accounts for more than 600,000 annual visits to healthcare providers in the United States. Pathogens reach the epididymis through the lumen of the vas deferens from infected urine, the posterior urethra, or seminal vesicles; underlying structural disorders are rare. Epididymitis is most commonly sexually transmitted and accompanied by asymptomatic urethritis, prostatitis, or cystitis in postpubertal boys and males under 35 years. *Neisseria gonorrhoeae* and more commonly *Chlamydia trachomatis* are the causative pathogens in 75% of all cases. In homosexual males, specifically the insertive partner, *E. coli* is the causative pathogen (Centers for Disease Control and Prevention, 2002; Cole & Vogler, 2004; DuFour, 2001; Luzzi & O'Brien, 2001; Marcozzi & Suner, 2001; *Morbidity and Mortality Weekly Report,* 2002 Woodward, Schwabs, & Sesterhenn, 2003).

Nonsexually transmitted epididymitis is generally seen in males older than 35 years or those who have recently experienced urinary tract surgery or instrumentation. It is commonly associated with UTI caused by gram-negative enteric organisms (Cole & Vogler, 2004; DuFour, 2001; Luzzi & O'Brien, 2001; Marcozzi & Suner, 2001; *Morbidity and Mortality Weekly Report,* 2002; Woodward, Schwabs, & Sesterhenn, 2003). An underlying urinary abnormality or anomaly is often present in infants and children, such as a pathological connection between the urinary tract, genital duct system, or bowel that results in contamination of the epididymis with coliform bacteria (Luzzi & O'Brien, 2001).

Epididymitis is characterized by gradual onset of pain, unilateral testicular pain and tenderness, fever, dysuria, urinary frequency, urgency, urethral discharge, and scrotum edema as the disease progresses. Nausea and vomiting are usually absent. Uncommon complications include testicular necrosis, testicular atrophy, and infertility. Common complications among immunocompromised patients include testicular cancer, tuberculosis epididymitis, and fungal epididymitis. Differentiation between epididymitis and testicular torsion must be made since the latter presents with sudden onset of severe pain and requires emergency treatment (Cole & Vogler, 2004; DuFour, 2001; Luzzi & O'Brien, 2001; Marcozzi & Suner, 2001; *Morbidity and Mortality Weekly Report,* 2002; Schubert, 2000; Woodward, Schwabs, & Sesterhenn, 2003).

A comprehensive analysis of the literature generates the following definitions (Cole & Vogler, 2004; DuFour, 2001; Luzzi & O'Brien, 2001; Marcozzi & Suner, 2001; *Morbidity and Mortality Weekly Report,* 2002; Schubert, 2000; Woodward, Schwabs, & Sesterhenn, 2003; Zdrodouska-Stefenow et al., 2000).

- *Sexually transmitted epididymitis* is an infection of the epididymis in a healthy individual by a sexually transmitted organism and associated with urethritis.
- *Nonsexually transmitted epididymitis* is an infection of the epididymis in a healthy individual by a common pathogen and associated with gram-negative enteric organisms

SPECIFIC CONSIDERATIONS FOR PHARMACOTHERAPY

When Drug Therapy Is Needed

Epididymitis is treated with antibiotics when the patient presents with symptoms. Prompt diagnosis and treatment are essential because of varying degree of illness, potential spread of sexually transmitted diseases, and potential urinary and renal complications. Bed rest and comfort measures are essential to provide relief of symptoms. Patients with severe symptomatology or who appear septic need to be hospitalized immediately for parenteral therapy (Cole & Vogler, 2004; DuFour, 2001; Luzzi & O'Brien, 2001; *Morbidity and Mortality Weekly Report,* 2002).

Short- and Long-Term Goals of Pharmacotherapy

The short-term goals of treatment for sexually transmitted epididymitis are to resolve the infection, restore normal physiological function, and prevent the spread and recurrence of infection. For nonsexually transmitted epididymitis, they are to resolve the infection, restore normal physiological function, and prevent further recurrence of infection. The long-term goals of treatment for both types of epididymitis are to prevent recurrence of infection and potential renal complications. In each of the conditions of epididymitis, the goals of treatment are achieved primarily by antibiotic therapy and patient education.

Time Frame for Initiating Pharmacotherapy

Epididymitis requires prompt diagnosis and treatment when patients present with clinical symptoms to prevent the serious sequelae discussed. Empiric treatment is indicated before culture results are available. Treatment failures require further evaluation, and culture results guide drug selection. Differential diagnosis to rule out testicular torsion and abscesses is critical for positive patient outcomes (DuFour, 2001; Luzzi & O'Brien, 2001; *Morbidity and Mortality Weekly Report,* 2002; Schubert, 2000).

See Drug Tables 102.3–102.6, 102.10, 102.11, 306.

Assessment and History Taking

Refer to Tables 34–10 and 34–11.

TABLE 34–10. Baseline Data: History and Physical Examination for Epididymitis

History
Onset, duration, and course of symptoms of scrotal pain, dysuria, urinary frequency, urgency, and urethral discharge (color, amount, and consistency)
Associated diseases, such as fever, nausea, vomiting, and diagnosed urinary tract infections and structural or neurologic abnormalities
History of new sexual partners and complaints, if any, of dysuria, urinary frequency, or genitourinary discharges
Physical Examination
Vital signs; note any temperature elevation
Inspect scrotum for erythema, edema, and torsion; usually indurated, enlarged, and tender if epididymitis present
Testicular tenderness, position, size, and consistency; testes are generally normal
Elicit Prehn's sign (passive elevation of testicles) as it relieves pain
Suprapubic tenderness and CVA tenderness
Rectal examination to elicit prostatic tenderness and urethral discharge

TABLE 34–11. Diagnostic Tests for Epididymitis

Urinalysis
- Pyuria in 20–95% cases

Urine culture and sensitivity and Gram's stain smear of uncentrifuged urine for gram-negative bacteria
Postpubertal males with STD
- Gram's stain of urethral discharge or intraurethral swab for *N. gonorrhoeae* and nongonococcal urethritis (≥5 polymorphonuclear leukocytes per oil immersion field)

Urethral discharge or intraurethral swab for chlamydia
Gonococcal culture of urethral discharge
CBC for elevation in leukocytes
Color Doppler ultrasound for hypervascularity and rule out testicle torsion
Older males
- Culture of expressed prostatic secretions (EPS) unless acute prostatitis suspected
- Assess for an obstruction of the bladder outlet, such as an intravenous pyelography, doppler ultrasound, scrotal ultrasound, or radionuclide scrotal imaging

Patient/Caregiver Information

Refer to Table 34–12.

OUTCOMES MANAGEMENT

Selecting an Appropriate Agent

Patient factors of age, sexual activity, sexual preference, drug or environmental allergies, concurrent diseases, degree of symptomatology, and adherence to therapy regimen guide antibiotic therapy selection. Empiric therapy is based on a patient's symptomatology and diagnostic findings. Treatment of males with HIV infection and epididymitis is the same as those without HIV (Cole & Vogler, 2004; DuFour, 2001; Luzzi & O'Brien, 2001; *Morbidity and Mortality Weekly Report,* 2002).

Sexually Transmitted Epididymitis. Empiric therapy for patients with sexually transmitted epididymitis is directed at *C. trachomatis* and *N. gonorrhoeae.* See Table 34–13. The patient's sex partner(s), for the 30 days prior to diagnosis, needs diagnostic evaluation and treatment (Cole & Vogler, 2004; DuFour, 2001; Luzzi & O'Brien, 2001; *Morbidity and Mortality Weekly Report,* 2002). See Chapter 36 for treatment of STDs.

TABLE 34–12. Patient/Caregiver Information for Epididymitis

Condom use during sexual intercourse to prevent risk of exposure to STDs
Bed rest with scrotal elevation and ice packs for pain
Scrotal support as needed
Warm sitz baths three times daily for relief of symptoms
Patients with STD epididymitis need to refer sex partners for evaluation and treatment
Avoid sexual intercourse until both patient and partner(s) have completed therapy and are without symptoms
Educate about signs and symptoms of septicemia or potential complications and the importance of seeking healthcare immediately

TABLE 34–13. Empiric Drug Therapy for Epididymitis

Drug	Regimen	Preference
Sexually Transmitted		
	Age: 17–35 years (Include sexual partners)	
Ceftriaxone	250 mg IM once	1st
Plus		
Doxycycline	100 mg PO bid for 10 days	1st
Allergic or intolerant to cephalosporins or tetracyclines		
Ofloxacin	300 mg PO bid for 10 days	Alt
Levofloxacin	500 mg PO bid for 10 days	Alt
Nonsexually Transmitted		
	Age: >35 years	
FLQN	Give for 10–14 days[a]	1st
Ofloxacin	300 mg PO bid for 10 days	1st
Levofloxacin	500 mg PO bid for 10 days	Alt
Third-generation cephalosporin	Give for 10–14 days[a]	Alt
Ampicillin with sulbactam	Give for 10–14 days[a]	Alt

[a]See drug table for specific doses for various agents
Alt = alternative

Nonsexually Transmitted Epididymitis. Empiric therapy for nonsexually transmitted epididymitis is directed at enterobacteriaceae common in UTIs. Selection of oral or parenteral therapy is based on the severity of patient symptomatology (Cole & Vogler, 2004; DuFour, 2001; Luzzi & O'Brien, 2001; *Morbidity and Mortality Weekly Report,* 2002). Refer to Table 34–13 also.

Drugs for comfort measures in epididymitis include nonsteroidal anti-inflammatory drugs (NSAIDs), such as ibuprofen and naproxen. Opiates, such as hydrocodone and oxycodone in combination with acetaminophen or aspirin are for patients with severe symptomatology (DuFour, 2001; Luzzi & O'Brien, 2001; *Morbidity and Mortality Weekly Report,* 2002).

Monitoring for Efficacy

Drug efficacy is determined by resolution of patient symptoms. Failure of symptoms to improve within 72 h requires reassessment of the patient (DuFour, 2001; Luzzi & O'Brien, 2001; *Morbidity and Mortality Weekly Report,* 2002).

Monitoring for Toxicity

Tetracyclines and FLQNs in males <17 years may cause abnormalities in cartilage and bone development.

Followup Recommendations

Prepubertal boys and older males with bacteriuria require posttreatment cultures on completion of therapy. Delayed or further diagnostic evaluation for urological abnormalities needs to be completed. In postpubertal and <35-year-old males, no followup or test of cure is needed if symptoms resolve. Failure of symptoms to improve within 72 h requires reassessment of the patient's symptoms, diagnosis, and therapy. Males with tenderness and swelling that persist after completion of therapy need evaluation for testicular cancer and tuberculosis or fungal epididymitis. These diseases are common among patients who are immunocompromised (Cole & Vogler, 2004; DuFour, 2001; Luzzi & O'Brien, 2001; *Morbidity and Mortality Weekly Report,* 2002).

URETHRITIS IN MALES

Urethritis (inflammation of the urethra) in males is known as nongonococcal or gonococcal urethritis (GU). Nongonococcal urethritis (NGU) is the most common STD syndrome and accounts for 4 to 6 million healthcare visits in the United States per year. The two major causative agents of NGU are *C. trachomatis* (35–45%) and *Ureaplasma urealyticum* (15–25%). Trichomonas vaginalis, herpes simplex, and the newly recognized genital *M. genitalium* account for the remaining cases. *N. gonorrhoeae* is the causative agent of GU; however, the patient may be coinfected with *C. trachomatis* (CDCP, 2002; Shahmanesh, 2001; Steele, 2000).

Urethritis may be symptomatic or asymptomatic, with the latter being common. Urethritis is characterized by a mucoid or purulent discharge (yellow, white, or cloudy), dysuria, and urethral itching or tingling. Diagnosis of NGU is based on the presence of a urethral discharge and laboratory confirmation of leukocytes on a Gram's stain smear. GU is diagnosed by the presence of a urethral discharge and confirmation of gram-negative diplococci in a urethral secretion or an intraurethral swab (CDCP, 2002; Shahmanesh, 2001; Steele, 2000).

Approximately 600,000 males develop recurrent or persistent urethritis annually because of lack of compliance with a therapeutic regimen or reinfection by untreated sex partner(s). Males with persistent or recurrent urethritis need to be retreated along with sex partners. Untreated urethritis may lead to severe complications, such as epididymitis, Reiter's syndrome, or infertility. The female sex partners of males with urethritis are at risk for mucopurulent cervicitis, chlamydial infections, pelvic inflammatory disease, ectopic pregnancy, and tubal infertility. The presence of STDs may facilitate transmission of the HIV virus. Early recognition and prompt, effective treatment may contribute significantly to decreasing potential complications and reducing heterosexual transmission of HIV (CDCP, 2002; Shahmanesh, 2001; Steele, 200).

A comprehensive analysis of the literature generates the following definitions:

- *Nongonococcal urethritis* is an inflammation of the urethra not caused by gonococcal infection and diagnosed by ≥5 polymorphonuclear leukocytes per oil immersion field on a smear of an intraurethral swab specimen.
- *Gonococcal urethritis* is an inflammation of the urethra caused by gonococci and diagnosed by the presence of intracellular gram-negative diplococci from an intraurethral swab.

SPECIFIC CONSIDERATIONS FOR PHARMACOTHERAPY

When Drug Therapy Is Needed

NGU and GU are treated with antibiotics when the patient presents with symptoms and diagnostic tests confirm identification of etiological organisms. Prompt diagnosis and treatment are essential to prevent serious renal, reproductive, and systemic complications. Therapy for a specific disease or infections is reportable to state health departments. Treatment compliance and partner notification are generally better with a specific diagnosis. If diagnostic tools are not available, the clinician should treat the patient for both types of infections; however, clinicians need to avoid the cost of treating two diseases (CDCP, 2002; Steele, 2000).

Short- and Long-Term Goals of Pharmacotherapy

The short-term goals for treatment of NGU and GU are to identify the causative agent, resolve the infection, restore normal physiological function, and prevent the spread and recurrence of the infection. The long-term goals are to prevent recurrence of infection and prevent potential complications. Both conditions respond to antibiotic therapy and patient education.

Time Frame for Initiating Pharmacotherapy

Treatment of urethritis should be initiated when the patient presents with complaints and by laboratory confirmation of causative organisms to prevent the serious sequelae discussed.

See Drug Table 102.

Assessment and History Taking

Refer to Tables 34–14 and 34–15.

Patient/Caregiver Information

Education of the patient about the signs and symptoms of the disease, drug therapy, and prevention measures is critical for positive outcomes. Refer to Table 34–16.

OUTCOMES MANAGEMENT

Selecting an Appropriate Agent

Empiric therapy is based on laboratory results. In the absence of a definitive diagnosis, therapy for NGU and GU must be initiated. Lack of patient compliance with the prescribed therapeutic regimen is a barrier in the effective treatment of STDs. Monitored single doses enhance compliance as in the case of doxycycline and azithromycin; however, dosages of azithromycin cost five to six times more than the cost of a week's supply of doxycycline. Evaluation and treatment of the patient's sex partner(s) are critical to prevent the spread of the disease or reinfection (CDCP, 2002; Steele, 2000). See Table 34–17.

Sex partners are treated with the same therapies except in the presence of pregnancy. Azithromycin and erythromycin are the choices for pregnant clients (CDCP, 2002; Steele, 2000).

TABLE 34–14. Baseline Data: History and Physical Examination for Urethritis

History

- History of onset and duration of symptoms, such as presence and color of urethral discharge, presence of dysuria, and urethral itching along with associated symptoms of fever, chills, nausea, vomiting, diarrhea, constipation, abdominal and back pain, and hematuria
- Sexual history, such as age of first intercourse, number of sexual partners, specifically within the last 30–60 days, frequency of sexual coitus, sexual behaviors (anal and vaginal coitus), and use of barrier methods
- Past history of STDs, including characteristics, frequency, duration, and effectiveness of treatments
- Past medical history including drug and environmental allergies; chronic diseases such as diabetes mellitus, multiple sclerosis, and cancer; and previous genitourinary problems and treatment

Physical Examination

- Vital signs, particularly noting temperature elevation
- Inspect and palpate external genitalia
- Examine urethra for mucopurulent discharge

TABLE 34–15. Diagnostic Tests for Urethritis

- Gram's stain of an intraurethral swab specimen
  - NGU confirmed with ≥5 polymorphonuclear leukocytes per oil immersion field
  - GU confirmed by the presence of intracellular gram-negative diplococci
- Asymptomatic males
  - First 10–20 mL of urine to screen for GU or NGU with leukocyte estrase test (LET); positive LET indicates *T. vaginalis* and must be confirmed with an urethral swab specimen Gram's stain
- *Neisseria gonorrhoea* cultures (GC) and chlamydia test
- Blood tests for syphilis and HIV
- Presence of systemic symptoms, order CBC with differential and consider erythrocyte sedimentation rate

Monitoring for Efficacy

Symptom resolution within 48 to 72 h is considered sufficient for monitoring of outcomes. Persistence or recurrence of symptoms requires further diagnostic evaluation (CDCP, 2002).

Monitoring for Toxicity

Tetracyclines and FLQNs in pregnant patients or patients in the puberty stage may cause abnormalities in cartilage and bone development. Metronidazole is contraindicated in the first trimester of pregnancy (CDCP, 2002).

Followup Recommendations

Persistence or recurrence of symptoms requires diagnostic evaluation. Assess the patient's compliance with the selected therapeutic regimen and for possible reinfection by untreated sex partner(s). Treatment failure or reinfection of NGU or GU requires the same therapeutic regimen after laboratory confirmation of the specific organ-

TABLE 34–16. Patient/Caregiver Information for Urethritis

- Condom usage during sexual intercourse to prevent the risk of exposure of STDs to self and partner(s)
- Refer sex partner(s) for evaluation and treatment
- Avoid sexual intercourse until the patient and partner(s) have completed therapy and are without symptoms
- Know about signs and symptoms of reinfection, septicemia, or potential complications and the importance of seeking health care immediately

TABLE 34–17. Empiric Drug Therapy for Urethritis

Drug	Regimen	Preference
Nongonococcal Urethritis (NGU)		
Azithromycin	1 g PO once	1st
OR		
Doxycycline	100 mg PO bid for 7 days	1st
Erythromycin base	500 mg PO qid for 7 days	Alt
Erythromycin ethylsuccinate	800 mg PO qid for 7 days	Alt
Ofloxacin	300 mg PO bid for 7 days	Alt
Levofloxacin	500 mg PO qd for 7 days	Alt
Gonococcal Urethritis (GU)		
Ceftriaxone	125 mg IM once	1st
OR		
Cefixime	400 mg PO once	1st
Ciprofloxacin[a]	500 mg PO once	Alt
Ofloxacin[a]	400 mg PO once	Alt
Levofloxacin[a]	500 mg PO once	Alt
If chlamydial infection is not ruled out, add NGU therapy.		

[a]Fluoroquinolone resistance reported in Pacific region, Asia, Hawaii, and California.
Alt = alternative

ism. Evaluate the patient for *T. vaginalis* with a microscopic wet mount from an intraurethral swab. If the wet mount is positive for *T. vaginalis,* treat the patient and sex partner(s) with a single, oral dose of metronidazole 2 gm or 500 mg bid for 5 days. A negative wet mount indicates that a change to an alternative drug is needed, such as from doxycycline to azithromycin (CDCP, 2002).

PROSTATITIS

Prostatitis (inflammation of the prostate gland) is one of the most common urologic diseases in adult males, accounts for 25% of office visits for genitourinary complaints, and occurs in 25 to 50% of all males at some time. The National Institutes of Health use an updated classification system for prostatitis (Table 34–18) that promotes more focused research. It may result from (1) an ascending uretheral infection, (2) reflux of infected urine, (3) direct extension or lymphatic spread of a rectal infection, or (4) hematogenous spread. In clinical practice, prostatitis is a general term to describe any unexplained symptoms that may occur of the prostate gland (Chow, 2001a; Collins, MacDonald, & Wilt, 2000; Lummus & Thompson, 2001; Nickel, 2003).

In bacterial prostatitis, gram-negative enteric organisms are the causative pathogens, similar in type and prevalence to those in UTI. *Escherichia coli* occurs in 75% of diagnosed cases and is followed by *P. mirabilis, K. pneumoniae,* and species of *Enterobacter, Pseudomonas,* and *Serratia.* There is some evidence, though controversial, that gram-positive organisms may play a role in chronic bacterial prostatitis (CBP). These gram-positive organisms include *S. epidermidis, S. aureus,* and diphtheroids. Over the last decade, sexually transmitted diseases have been associated with prostatitis and UTI in

TABLE 34–18. Definitions of Prostatitis

Term	Definition
Acute bacterial prostatitis (APB)	An uncommon, aggressive prostatitis that presents with a urinary tract infection and easily diagnosed by history and physical exam. An asystemic disease characterized by acute onset of fever, chills, dysuria, frequency, retention, urgency, nocturia, low back and perineal pain, generalized malaise, arthralgia, myalgia, and suprapubic discomfort. Prostatic massage contraindicated because of risk for precipitation of bacteremia. Urine culture identifies offending organism (usually *E. coli*). It resolves with antibiotic therapy and rarely reoccurs. Complications are bacteremia or frank sepsis, urinary outflow obstruction, or abscess formation.
Chronic bacterial prostatitis (CBP)	More common in older males and difficult to diagnose as the clinical presentation is less clear. The hallmark feature of CBP is a history of recurrent UTIs by the same pathogen. CBP is characterized by dysuria, urgency, frequency, nocturia, dribbling, hesitancy, loss of stream volume and force, pain in various sites (low back, perineal, suprapubic, scrotal, or penile), hematuria, and hematospermia or painful ejaculation for longer than 3 months. CBP symptoms wax and wane. Diagnosis is confirmed by the presence of 10 to 15 WBCs per high-power filed in a urine specimen, serial segmented cultures of urine, and pre- and post-massage test with inflammatory cells. Chronic pain and sexual dysfunction are potential complications.
Chronic pelvic pain syndrome (CPPS)	Most common type of prostatitis that affects males of all ages, five times as common as CBP, and a symptom complex of pelvic pain. It presents with symptoms similar to CBP of greater than 3 months duration. Clinical exam is normal with sterile urine and prostatic cultures. The subtypes are inflammatory or noninflammatory and based on the presence of leukocytes in EPS and prostatic urine. Etiology is unknown and treatment is ineffective with poor response to antibiotics. The condition is frustrating for the client and provider. Complications are associated with stress and sexual dysfunction.
Asymptomatic inflammatory prostatitis (AIP)	Defined as the presence of inflammatory cells in prostatic fluid, urine, or other tissue without clinical symptoms. It is generally discovered during routine testing for semen or biopsy specimens. The etiology, pathogenesis, and natural history are not clearly defined. Treatment is controversial and based on comorbid diseases.

males. These pathogens include *N. gonorrhoeae, T. vaginalis, C. trachomatis, Gardnerella vaginalis,* and *U. urealyticum* with *Chlamydia* being the most common. The clinician needs to consider the possibility of mixed infections that involve two or more pathogens (Chow, 2001a; Collins, MacDonald, & Wilt, 2000; Lummus & Thompson, 2001; Nickel, 2003).

SPECIFIC CONSIDERATIONS FOR PHARMACOTHERAPY

When Drug Therapy Is Needed

Bacterial prostatitis is treated with antibiotics when the patient presents with symptoms and diagnostic tests confirm identification of etiologic organisms. Prompt diagnosis and treatment are essential because of varying degrees of systemic illness and potential sequelae that may lead to prostatic edema, urinary retention, renal parenchymal infection, or bacteremia; chronic infections may produce prostatic stones. Diagnosis of acute bacterial prostatitis (ABP) requires immediate treatment with antibiotics with therapy duration of 4 to 6 weeks. Hospitalization and parenteral antibiotic therapy should be considered in the presence of comorbid illnesses, such as immunosuppression, liver disease, renal disease, cardiac disease, or diabetes. Symptomatic relief is achieved with analgesics (Chow, 2001a; Collins, MacDonald, & Wilt, 2000; Lummus & Thompson, 2001).

CBP is less life-threatening, requires long-term antibiotic therapy of months, and generally results from a relapsing subacute illness that is diagnosed by a positive culture. Many antibiotics fail to achieve the high concentrations that are needed to penetrate the prostatic fluid for an adequate cure rate. CBP is often frustrating to the patient, with continuation of symptoms and frequency leading to nonadherence to the prescribed therapy regime. Symptomatic control is achieved by the use of alpha-1 blocking agents and analgesics as necessary (Chow, 2001a; Collins, MacDonald, & Wilt, 2000; Lummus & Thompson, 2001).

CPPS requires an individualized approach because the etiological organism is unclear. It is proposed that either the offending organism is not identifiable by traditional means or the organism's characteristics, such as slime or bacterial biofilm, prohibit isolation or treatment However, the pain and inflammatory process are present. In noninfectious CPPS, increased intraprostatic pressure and voiding dysfunction lead to reflux of urine, retention of prostatic fluid, and chronic pain related to bladder or ureteral spasms (Lummus & Thompson, 2001). Current therapy consists of antibiotics to eradicate potential STD organisms and measures to control symptoms. Patients need reassurance that CPPS is self-limiting and not a life-threatening situation. The symptom complex and chronicity of the problem requires a referral to a urologist for diagnostic tests to rule out carcinoma of the bladder or other potential complications and determine the most appropriate treatment modality. AIP is diagnosed by a urologist while conducting diagnostic tests. Treatment and followup for AIP is controversial, not clearly defined, and focuses on comorbid diseases, such as prostate cancer or benign prostatic hypertrophy (Chow, 2001a; Collins, MacDonald, & Wilt, 2000; Lummus & Thompson, 2001).

Healthcare providers need to educate patients fully to side effects and costs of antibiotic therapy as well as to the benefits and risks of other options of care.

Short- and Long-Term Goals of Pharmacotherapy

The short-term goals for ABP and CBP are to resolve the infection, restore normal physiological functioning, and prevent the spread and recurrence of the infection. The long-term goals are to prevent recurrence of infection and potential complications. The short-term goals for CPPS and AIP are to control symptoms if present and refer patients for a comprehensive diagnostic evaluation to determine the etiology of illness. The long-term goals are to implement the prescribed therapeutic regimen, provide individualized comfort measures, and prevent potential renal complications.

Time Frame for Initiating Pharmacotherapy

Bacterial prostatitis requires prompt diagnosis and treatment. Treatment of ABP is based on clinical presentation, and therapy is adjusted according to urine culture results. Expressed prostatic secretion (EPS) is not always obtainable because massage of the prostate can cause bacteremia. The patient's degree of systemic illness guides the treatment regimen of outpatient or inpatient care and the choice of oral or parenteral antibiotic therapy. In CPS and CPPS, treatment is based on serial segmented urine cultures (Chow, 2001a; Collins, MacDonald, & Wilt, 2000; Lummus & Thompson, 2001).

See Drug Tables 102.4, 102.7, 102.10, 102.11, 306, 502.1.

Assessment and History Taking

Refer to Tables 34–19 and 34–20.

Patient/Caregiver Information

Education of the patient about the signs and symptoms of the disease, drug therapy, and prevention measures is critical for positive outcomes (Chow, 2001a; Collins, MacDonald, & Wilt, 2000; Lummus & Thompson, 2001). See Table 34–21.

OUTCOMES MANAGEMENT

Selecting an Appropriate Agent

Empiric therapy is based on the patient's symptomatology, laboratory findings, and presumptive diagnosis of ABP, CBP, or CPPS. Table 34–22 lists specific drug therapies. Effective antibiotic therapy in bacterial prostatitis is often difficult to attain because of poor prostatic tissue penetration by some agents commonly used in the treatment of UTI. Other agents penetrate the prostatic tissue, but are inactive against gram-negative rods. TMP-SMX and FLQN achieve reasonable tissue penetration. Treatment success in ABP is common because inflamed prostate tissue has increased permeability to drugs (Bundrick et al., 2003; Chow, 2001a; Collins, MacDonald, & Wilt, 2000; Lummus & Thompson, 2001).

TABLE 34–19. Baseline Data: History and Physical Examination for Prostatitis

History

Onset and course of illness and associated symptoms, such as urethral discharge, urethral meatal itching, fever, perineal pain, hematuria, hesitancy, decreased stream, painful ejaculation, incontinence, back pain, and weight loss
History of previous urinary tract infections and STDs with successes and failures of treatment
Sexual partner has symptoms of dysuria or STDs
Any new sexual partners
National Institutes of Health Chronic Prostatitis Symptom Index (NIH-CPSI) (self-administered index for impact of CBP or CPPS on daily life)

Physical Examination

General appearance for signs of systemic illness
Vital signs; note for elevation of temperature and hydration status
Complete abdominal examination; note bladder distention and suprapubic pain
External genitalia and scrotum for edema
Prostatic evaluation:
- ABP: *Do NOT palpate the prostate.* Prostate is extremely tender, warm, swollen, irregular, and partially or totally firm, soggy, or boggy
- CBP and CPPS: Carefully palpate prostate for size and shape; it usually feels normal, but may be irregular and mildly tender

TABLE 34–20. Diagnostic Tests for Prostatitis

Serial segmented cultures of urine and expressed prostatic secretion (EPS)
- Urine collection (two glass)
  - In uncircumcised male, instruct patient to tape foreskin back, cleanse meatus with soap and water, and then dry.
  - In circumcised male, instruct patient to cleanse meatus with soap and water, then dry.
- Patient collects first 5–10 mL of urine voided; label first bladder voiding as VB^1
- Clinician massages prostate from each lateral lobe to midline, about six to seven times on each side; milks urethra to produce secretion; collects secretions on swab, slide, or in cup; and labels as EPS.
- If unable to obtain all specimens on command, interpretation of results may be confusing.
- Microscopic examination of all specimens
  - Presence of >10 WBCs per high-power field in EPS indicates some type of prostatitis; Macrophages with oval fat bodies confirm this diagnosis

Culture all specimens
- Bacterial growth in VB^1 and VB^2 indicates cystitis
  - A 10-fold increase of bacteria in EPS and VB^2 indicates APB or CBP
  - >10 WBC in VB^2 indicates CPPS, inflammatory
  - Testing for antibody levels of IgA and IgG in common pathogenic bacteria in EPS and VB^2 may diagnose CBP. Elevation of antibody levels indicates bacterial prostatis
- CBC
- In CBP, consider transrectal ultrasound for prostate calculi.
- Older males, consider urine cytologies to rule out bladder malignancy.

Treatment failure in CBP is common and indicates the need for long-term, low-dose suppressive therapy. Cure rates are 50–90% for FLQNs and 32–71% for TMP-SMX. Carbenicillin indanyl sodium is effective, with cure rates of 60–74%; however, it is expensive and usually reserved for treatment failure with FLQNs.

Prostatic calculi preclude a cure, and evaluation for surgical removal of prostatic stones is recommended (Bundrick et al., 2003; Chow, 2001a; Collins, MacDonald, & Wilt, 2000; Lummus & Thompson, 2001).

Treatment of CPPS is controversial and mirrors treatment for CBP; cure is uncommon. Response rates vary

TABLE 34–21. Patient/Caregiver Information for Prostatitis

Bed rest as needed for symptom relief
Warm sitz baths three to four times daily
Adequate hydration (2–4 L daily)
Avoid irritants, such as alcohol, coffee, or tea
High-fiber diet for adequate bowel elimination to decrease abdominal pressure
Avoid spicy foods (decreases spasms)
Avoid urethral instrumentation
Use relaxation techniques daily
Educate about signs and symptoms of infection and importance of seeking health care immediately

TABLE 34–22. Empiric Therapy for Prostatitis

Drug	Regimen	Preference
Acute Bacterial Prostatitis (ABP)		
Outpatient Antibiotics		
FLQN	PO for 4 weeks minimum	1st
TMP-SMX	PO for 4 weeks minimum	Alt
Inpatient Antibiotics		
FLQN	IV then PO for 4 weeks minimum	1st
Cephalosporin	IV until able to switch to appropriate oral	Alt
Second-Third generation	Total 4 weeks therapy	
Aminoglycoside	IV until able to switch to appropriate oral	Alt
	Total 4 weeks therapy	
Symptomatic Relief		
NSAIDs	PO prn	1st
Opiates	PO prn	Alt
Chronic Bacterial Prostatitis (CBP)		
Antibiotics		
FLQN	PO for 3–4 months	1st
TMP-SMX	PO for 3–4 months	Alt
Symptomatic Relief		
Alpha-1 blockers	PO q d prn	1st
NSAIDs	PO prn	Alt
Opiates	PO prn	2nd
Chronic Pelvic Pain Syndrome (CPPS)		
Antibiotics		
FLQN	PO for 3–4 months	1st
TMP-SMX	PO for 3–4 months	Alt
Symptomatic Relief		
Alpha-1 blockers	PO q d prn	1st
NSAIDs	PO prn	Alt
Opiates	PO prn	2nd
Muscle relaxants (noninflammatory CPPS)		
Diazepam, baclofen	PO prn	3rd

Alt = alternative; FLQN = fluoroquinolone; NSAID = nonsteroidal anti-inflammatory drug

with 40% demonstrating some degree of improvement. Antibiotics, NSAIDs, sitz baths, muscle relaxants, and alpha-blocking agents are the empiric therapy. Alpha-blocking agents, such as Terazosin either with or without antibiotics, have demonstrated clinical improvement in up to 80% of patients. There is a strong association between depression and CPPS and antidepressant therapy may be considered (Leummus & Thompson, 2001).

Monitoring for Efficacy

Acute and Chronic Bacterial Prostatitis. Failure of symptoms to improve within 48 to 72 h requires reassessment of the patient. A referral to a urologist is indicated in treatment failure (Chow, 2001a; Lummus & Thompson, 2001).

Chronic Bacterial Prostatitis and CPPS. Treatment failure is common in both. If initially effective, long-term, low-dose suppressive therapy with antibiotics may be needed. In CBP, prostatic calculi preclude a cure and evaluation for removal of prostatic stones is recommended. In CPPS, a subset of patients may be infected with *Chlamydia trachomatis* or *Ureaplasma urealyticum* with a negative culture. A trial of doxycycline for 6 weeks is recommended (Chow, 2001a; Lummus & Thompson, 2001).

Monitoring for Toxicity

Refer to Drug Tables.

Followup Recommendations

Acute and Chronic Bacterial Prostatitis. Posttreatment urine and EPS cultures are required within two weeks of therapy completion (Chow, 2001a; Lummus & Thompson, 2001).

Chronic Pelvic Pain Syndrome. Monitor effects of doxycyline if prescribed. Refer to an urologist for comprehensive evaluation (Chow, 2001a; Lummus & Thompson, 2001).

BENIGN PROSTATIC HYPERPLASIA

Benign prostatic hyperplasia (BPH) or "prostatism" is a symptom complex defined as benign adenomatous hyperplasia of the periurethral prostate gland's stromal and glandular elements. The etiology of BPH is unclear; however, contributing factors include: (1) increased age, (2) increased 5-alpha-dihydrotestosterone (DHT), (3) increased estrogen, and (4) stimulation of alpha-adrenergic nerve endings that interfere with the opening of the bladder neck internal sphincter (Akduman & Crawford, 2001; Chow, 2001b; Irani, et al., 2003; Kim, Benson, Stern, & Gerber, 2002).

BPH is rare in males <40 years old and common in males >50 years (50%). Approximately 90% of males older than 80 years have microscopic evidence of BPH. It is estimated that approximately 35% of all males in the United States will require treatment for relief of symptoms of BPH during their lifetime. Approximately 400,000 transurethral resections are performed annually, and this procedure is rated the second most common procedure after cataract extraction in males over 65 years. The associated expense is estimated at $5 billion per year (Akduman & Crawford, 2001; Chow, 2001b; Irani et al., 2003; Kim et al., 2002).

BPH is characterized by obstructive or irritative symptoms or a combination of both in varying degrees with gradual worsening of symptoms. The enlarged prostate compresses the urethra to reduce or obstruct urinary flow, which results in obstructive symptoms of weak or decreased force of urinary stream, urinary hesitancy, postvoid or terminal dribbling, intermittency, abdominal straining to urinate, and incomplete bladder emptying. Irritative symptoms result from uninhibited smooth muscle contractions and detrusor instability and include nocturia, urinary frequency, urinary urgency, dysuria, and incontinence. BPH is the most common cause of hematuria. These symptoms frequently increase during periods of stress, exposure to cold, or use of sympathomimetic agents (Akduman & Crawford, 2001; Chow, 2001b; Irani et al., 2003).

Males seek healthcare for BPH because of worry, embarrassment, and progressive symptoms that affect their quality of life (Lowe, 2002; O'Leary, 2002). Complications of BPH may vary from recurrent UTIs, UTIs with possible sepsis, acute urinary retention, and uremia. Postoperative complications from transurethral prostate resection include morbidity, retrograde ejaculation, impotence, urinary incontinence, repeat surgeries, and lack of satisfactory long-term outcomes. Differential diagnosis is critical to rule out prostatic cancer, vesical neck obstruction, hyperreflexia from inflammatory or infectious conditions, and impaired detrusor contractility related to neurogenic, myogenic, or psychogenic factors (Akduman & Crawford, 2001; Chow, 2001b; Irani et al., 2003).

SPECIFIC CONSIDERATIONS FOR PHARMACOTHERAPY

When Drug Therapy Is Needed

Therapeutic regimens of BPH are in transition. The clinician needs to consider the degree of symptomatology, patient preference, pharmacologic agents, and surgical therapies in determining the best therapeutic regimen for each patient. The purpose of therapy in BPH is to decrease urological symptoms and to improve the rate of urinary flow. Urologists' primary therapy preference remains transurethral prostate resection (Akduman & Crawford, 2001; Chow, 2001b; Kirhy et al., 2004).

The degree of symptomatology is measurable by the American Urological Association (AUA) Symptom Index (USDHHS, 1996). It is a reliable, subjective tool for initial assessment of the patient's symptoms and periodic determination of disease progression or treatment effectiveness. The AUA Symptom Index is a self-administered seven-item questionnaire that rates the severity of symptoms on a scale from 0 (*not at all*) to 5 (*almost always*); items are summed to obtain a total score (Chow, 2001b).

Males with minimal to moderate symptoms or an AUA Symptom Index score of ≤7 may safely be followed by the strategy of watchful waiting and stand to gain little from any treatment, including surgery. Males with moderate to severe symptoms or an AUA Symptom Index score ≥8 may be offered the various treatment alternatives (including watchful waiting) or be scheduled for additional tests. Tests include flow rate recording, residual urine measurement, and pressure flow urodynamic studies to confirm the presence of BPH, rule out other causes of the patient's symptoms, and assist in determining the proper time for therapeutic interventions. Patients with refractory urinary retention, recurrent UTIs, recurrent gross hematuria, and bladder or renal insufficiency clearly related to BPH are candidates for surgery and should be referred to a urologist for a comprehensive evaluation (Akduman & Crawford, 2001; Chow, 2001b; Kirhy et al., 2004).

Patient preference is influenced by the degree of symptomatology, personal living circumstances, cost concerns, knowledge of therapeutic options, and probability of expected symptom improvement. Patient education includes the benefits and risks of watchful waiting and alternate therapies, such as behavioral techniques, drug therapy, balloon dilation, or surgery (Akduman & Crawford, 2001; Chow, 2001b; Lowe, 2002; O'Leary, 2002).

Sexual dysfunction and BPH coexist in aging men, and pharmacological agents can also impact negatively on sexual function. It is important to dialogue with aging patients about sexual concerns or use the Brief Sexual Function Inventory (BSFI), a self-administered 11-item questionnaire that assesses erection, ejaculation, problem assessment, and overall sexual satisfaction. The BSFI is available in multiple languages and validated in numerous cultures (O'Leary, 2002).

Ideal candidates for pharmacologic therapy are males with moderate symptoms, those unfit for surgery, or those who desire to avoid surgery.

Short- and Long-Term Goals of Pharmacotherapy

The short-term goals of therapy for BPH are to decrease the patient's symptoms and increase urinary flow. The long-term goals are to decrease the patient's symptoms, halt progress of the disease, increase urinary flow, and prevent complications of the disease to improve the patient's quality of life. The goals of treatment are achieved by watchful waiting, drug therapy, or surgery.

Time Frame for Initiating Pharmacotherapy

BPH should be treated at the time of diagnosis to prevent worsening of urinary symptoms and potential complications. The clinician's treatment decision should be based on the degree of symptomatology, patient preference, etiology of the disease process, and pharmacological agents (Akduman & Crawford, 2001; Chow, 2001b).

See Drug Tables 205.3, 602.2, 1001.

Assessment and History Taking

Refer to Table 34–23 and 34–24.

Patient/Caregiver Information

Education of the patient about signs and symptoms of the disease, drug therapy, and palliative measures is critical for positive outcomes (Akduman & Crawford, 2001; Chow, 2001b). Refer to Table 34–25.

OUTCOMES MANAGEMENT

Selecting an Appropriate Agent

Pharmacologic agents target two avenues of actions: (1) reduction of smooth muscle tone by alpha-1 blockade and (2) reduction of prostate size by hormonal manipulation.

TABLE 34–23. Baseline Data: History and Physical Examination for Benign Prostatic Hyperplasia

History
Onset and duration of symptoms
Initial assessment with the American Urological Association (AUA) Symptom Index: patient rates symptoms experienced over the past month, such as sensation of not emptying bladder after urination, occurrence of the need to urinate within 2 hours of last urination, episodes of having to start and stop during urination, difficulty postponing urination, weak urinary stream, occurrence of needing to push and strain to urinate, and the number of times got up from bed to urinate during the night
History of pain or discomfort, hematuria, recent onset of back or bone pain, anorexia, and weight loss
Patient records symptoms in a daily diary for a period of 1 week
Medical history, specifically about genitourinary problems and surgeries, such as urethral trauma, gonococcal urethritis, or urethral instrumentation; diabetes mellitus; and neurologic diseases that may cause a neurologic bladder dysfunction
Medication history: ask if cold or sinus medications aggravate their symptoms; use of drugs, such as anticholinergics that impair bladder contractility and sympathomimetics that increase outflow resistance
Physical Examination
Abdominal examination to detect a distended bladder from retention, renal tenderness, or a mass
Digital rectal examination (DRE) to estimate the size of the prostate, detect nodules or induration indicative of prostate cancer, and evaluate anal sphincter tone
Observe patient voiding or ask him to time urination to determine size and force of urinary stream (a male normally empties bladder of 300 mL of urine in 12–15 s)
Neurologic examination to detect neurogenic disease, such as multiple sclerosis

TABLE 34–24. Diagnostic Tests for Benign Prostatic Hyperplasia

Urinalysis to rule out UTI and hematuria
Creatinine to assess renal function (renal insufficiency increases risk for postoperative complications)
Prostate serum antigen (PSA) is optional; serum values of PSA increase in direct proportion to the volume of BPH; thus PSA levels may be as high as 10 μg/L without being indicative of prostate cancer; digital rectal examination (DRE) and PSA are the best strategy for detecting prostate cancer
Moderate to severe symptoms, consider urinary flow rate, postvoid residual urine, pressure flow urodynamic studies, and urethrocystoscopy

TABLE 34–26. Empiric Therapy for Benign Prostatic Hyperplasia

Drug	Regimen
Alpha-1 Blockers	
Terazosin[a]	1–10 mg PO qhs
Doxazosin[a]	1–8 mg PO qhs
Tamulosin[b]	0.4 mg PO qhs
Hormonal	
Finasteride	5 mg PO qd

[a]Start at lowest dose; advance to maximum tolerated dose in 1–2 week steps.
[b]Tapering up of dose not necessary. Occasionally, 0.8 mg dose may be needed.

Alpha-1 selective receptor blockers, such as terazosin, doxazosin, and tamulosin relax smooth muscle tone in prostatic tissue to produce immediate and significant improvement in urinary flow and irritative symptoms of BPH (Refer to Table 34–26). Dizziness, postural hypotension, and asthenia are common adverse effects of terazoxin and doxazosin, requiring a tapering up of their dose gradually until an effective dose is achieved. Tamulosin is selective for alpha-1 receptors found in prostatic tissue versus vascular tissue and is far less prone to trigger hypotension. Tapering up of the dose is not required (Akduman & Crawford, 2001; Chow, 2001b; Kirby et al., 2004).

For patients with a moderately elevated blood pressure, terazosin and doxazosin are good economical choices. For patients with persistent hypotension or low baseline blood pressure, tamulosin is considered a better agent. Finasteride is a 5-alpha-reductase inhibitor that blocks the conversion of testosterone to DHT. DHT promotes the hyperplasia of BHP and its reduction enhances gradual shrinkage of the gland. Finasteride has few side effects, lowers the serum concentration of prostate-specific antigen (PSA), and maintains a low toxicity profile. Sexual potency and functioning are maintained because finasteride spares testosterone levels while lowering DHT. In direct comparative studies, alpha-1 blockers provide quicker, more reliable relief than finasteride and work well on larger prostates (>40 cc) (Akduman & Crawford, 2001; Chow, 2001b; Kirby et al., 2004).

TABLE 34–25. Patient/Caregiver Information for Benign Prostatic Hyperplasia

- Limit fluid intake after dinner
- Avoid decongestants
- Void frequently
- Avoid sudden diuresis, which often occurs after drinking caffeine or alcohol
- Perform prostatic massage after intercourse
- Avoid certain medications, such as anticholinergics, tranquilizers, and antidepressants
- Educate how to assess for signs and symptoms of retention and obstruction and to seek health care if problems exist

Monitoring for Efficacy

Reassessment of the patient's symptoms using the AUA Symptom Index is essential after 6 months of *hormonal therapy,* along with peak uroflow diagnostic evaluation. The expectation is a decrease in the AUA Symptom Index Score from the initial assessment or scores from periodic monitoring. Reports show a mean score improvement of 2.7 points and peak flow improvement of 1.6 mL/s. For treatment failures consider alpha blockade therapy, watchful waiting, or surgical intervention (Chow, 2001b).

Reassessment of the patient's symptoms using the AUA Symptom Index is essential after obtaining optimal tolerated dosages of *$alpha_1$-selective blockers.* The expectation is a decrease in the AUA Symptom Index Score from the initial assessment or scores from periodic monitoring. Reports show a mean index score improvement of 4.5 points. For treatment failures consider hormonal therapy, watchful waiting, or surgical intervention (Chow, 2001b).

Monitoring for Toxicity

Finasteride has significant adverse effects on a developing fetus. Patients need to avoid fathering children while on the medication and avoid exposing pregnant patients to semen fluid as it can produce fetal abnormalities. Monitor for symptoms of postural hypotension and dizziness with doxazosin and terazosin. Advance the dose only as allowed (Akduman & Crawford, 2001; Chow, 2001b).

Followup Recommendations

All BPH patients need periodic assessments to monitor for progression of disease. Time frames for assessment depend on mode of therapy, such as watchful waiting or drug therapy. Assessments include the determination of changes in symptomatology and diagnostic evaluation, such as urinalysis, uroflow, and renal function. Comparison of AUA Symptom Index scores clearly delineates symptom relief and delay of disease progression. Elderly males need an annual monitoring of PSA and a digital rectal examination (DRE) to check for the development of prostate cancer. Patients undergoing surgery or balloon dilation are followed by a urologist (Akduman & Crawford, 2001; Chow, 2001b).

ERECTILE DYSFUNCTION

Erectile dysfunction (ED) is defined as the inability to attain or maintain an erection sufficient to allow sexual performance. An erection is a hemodynamic process mediated by neurogenic, endothelial, endocrine, and cortical (psychological) influences. Impairment of any element of the erectile apparatus or changes of its control leads to ED. It is estimated that 50% of ED is organic in nature (Astbury-Ward, 2000; Jensen & Burnett, 2002; Ralph & McNicholas, 2000; Rosen & Kostis, 2003).

Approximately 30 million males are affected in some degree by ED in the United States. Approximately 1% of males are affected by the age of 30; 40% by the age of 40, and 67% by the age of 70. Etiological factors of ED are diverse and may be hormonal, psychological, vasculogenic, or neurogenic (Table 34–27). The most common causes of ED are advancing age, diabetes mellitus (25 to 75% prevalence), cardiovascular disease, medications, and chronic health conditions. A current study suggests that ED is one of the first signs of cardiovascular disease as the narrow vessels of the penis are more sensitive to atheroscleortic blockage than the larger vessels of the heart. Health providers need to screen for ED to enhance the diagnosis of serious underlying medical conditions (Astbury-Ward, 2000; Jensen & Burnett, 2002; Ralph & McNicholas, 2000; Rosen & Kostis, 2003).

Males are reluctant to seek healthcare for ED because of embarrassment, low self-esteem, myths regarding the aging process, and uncertainty in how to discuss concerns. The denial of problems with ED or the omission of assessment for ED by healthcare providers leads to decreasing quality of life and lack of compliance with prescribed medication regimens. Patients at risk for ED need to be firmly and professionally asked if a problem with intimacy exists. The discussion, identification, and treatment of ED is more acceptable by patients and healthcare providers with the lifting of taboos, changes in societal attitudes, greater knowledge of human sexuality, accessibility of an oral medication (Viagara), and the media's coverage of Viagara since the late 1990s (Astbury-Ward, 2000; Eardley, 2001; Jensen & Burnett, 2002; Ralph & McNicholas, 2000).

TABLE 34–27. Etiological Factors of Erectile Dysfunction

Age	Fear of failure or anxiety
Alcohol abuse	Hypertension
Atherosclerosis	Neurogenic diseases
Associated medications	Alzheimer's disease
Analgesics	Diabetic neuropathy
Antiandrogens	Multiple sclerosis
Anticholingerics	Parkinson's disease
Antidepressants	Pelvic injury
Antihypertensives	Spinal cord injury
Antipsychotics	Stroke
Dopamine antagonists	Penile and uretheral lesions
H_2 blockers	Perineal trauma
Hormones	Peripheral vascular disease
Psychotropic drugs	Peyronie's disease
Thiazide diuretics	Prolonged bicycling
Tranquilizers	Prostatic disease
Cardiovascular disease	Benign prostatic hyperplasia
Cigarette smoking	Cancer
Chronic renal failure	Prostatitis
Diabetes mellitus	Vesiculoprostatitis
Depression	Psychological disorders
Endocrine disorders	Radical pelvic surgery
Adrenal disorders	Stress disorders/conflicts
Hyperthyroidism	
Hypothyroidism	
Pituitary tumor	
Hypogonadism	
Hyperprolactinemia	

SPECIFIC CONSIDERATIONS FOR PHARMACOTHERAPY

When Drug Therapy Is Needed

Therapeutic regimens of ED are in transition. Consider the degree of symptomatology, patient preferences, pharmacological agents, ease of administration, invasiveness of procedures, reversibility, cost, legal regulatory, approval, availability, mechanism of action, and surgical therapies in determining the therapeutic regimen for each patient. The aim is to decrease the symptoms of ED and improve the quality of life without interfering with prescribed health regimens of other health conditions. It is essential to eliminate, when possible, all iatrogenic causes of ED. Effective therapy may be the simple adjustment of current medication, such as diuretics, hypertensives, or psychotropic agents by reducing dosage or switching to an angiotensin-converting enzyme inhibitor, calcium channel blockers, or cardiac-selective beta blocking agent. First-line therapy includes oral erectrogenic agents, sexual education, and counseling, followed by intracavernosal injection therapy, vacuum-assisted devices, and penile implants (Astbury-Ward, 2000; Crowe & Streetman, 2004; Eardley, 2001; Jensen & Burnett, 2002; Leungwattanakij, Flynn, & Hellstrom, 2001; Padma-Nathan & Giuliano, 2001; Ralph & McNicholas, 2000; Roen & Kostis, 2003).

The degree of symptomatology relies on the patient's and the sexual partner's perceptions and is subjectively defined. Patient preference is influenced by the degree of symptomatology, personal relationships, cost concerns, knowledge of therapeutic options, and probability of expected symptom improvement. Patient education includes the benefits and risks of all therapies (Jensen & Burnett, 2002).

Short- and Long-Term Goals of Pharmacotherapy

The short-term goals of therapy for ED are to decrease the patient's symptoms and maintain compliance with any prescribed drug regimen for other health conditions. The long-term goals are to decrease the patent's symptoms, halt progress of disease, maintain compliance with any prescribed drug regimen for other health conditions, and prevent complications of diseases to improve the patient's quality of life.

Time Frame for Initiating Pharmacotherapy

ED is treated at the time of diagnosis to prevent further symptoms and potential complications. The clinician's treatment decision is based on degree of symptomatology, patient preference, the etiology of the disease process, and pharmacologic agents (Jensen & Burnett, 2002; Leungwattanakij, Flynn, & Hellstrom, 2001; Padma-Nathan & Giuliano, 2001).

Assessment and History Taking

Refer to Tables 34–28 and 34–29.

Patient/Caregiver Information

Education of the patient about signs and symptoms of the disease, drug therapy, human sexuality, need of counseling, and prevention measures is critical for positive outcomes and include the following (Astbury-Ward, 2000; Jensen & Burnett, 2002; Ralph & McNicholas, 2000).

TABLE 34–28. Baseline Data: History and Physical Examination for Erectile Dysfunction

History

Onset and duration of symptoms

Sexual history, such as age of first intercourse, number of sexual partners, frequency of sexual coitus, sexual behaviors (anal and vaginal coitus), sexual libido, and use of barrier methods

Sexual function, such as erectile function (consistent problem or situational), achieve orgasm, difficulties with ejaculation, intercourse satisfaction, overall sexual satisfaction, previous therapies for ED. Use the (1) Brief Sexual Function Inventory (BSFI), a self-administered 11–item questionnaire; (2) International Index of Erectile Function (IIEF) self-administered 15–item questionnaire; or (3) specific, direct questions that assesses erection, ejaculation, problems, and overall sexual satisfaction.

History of pain or discomfort, hematuria, recent onset of back or bone pain, anorexia, and weight loss

Frequency of early morning erections (sudden onset and preservation of erections on awakening or masturbation are characteristic of psychogenic disease whereas gradual onset and progressive loss of duration and strength of morning erections suggest organic disease)

Complete medical history, specifically about genitourinary problems and surgeries, such as urethral trauma, urethral instrumentation, or pelvic fracture, diabetes mellitus, neurologic diseases, and cardiovascular diseases

Complete medication history; any changes in ED while on medications

Physical Examination

Vital signs; note if any postural fall in blood pressure

General appearance for loss of secondary sexual characteristics

Skin examination for spider angiomata, palmar erythema, excessive dryness, hyperpigmentation, and other dermatological signs of endocrinopathy

Flaccid penis examination for tumor, inflammation, discharge, and phimosis of the foreskin

Erect penis examination for degree of chordee to erectile weakness

Testicular examination for size, masses, nodules, and tenderness

Elicit bulbocavernosus reflex (absence indicates neurological impairment)

Digital rectal examination (DRE) to estimate the size of the prostate and detect nodules, masses, or tenderness, and evaluate anal sphincter tone

Aorta and femoral arteries for rate, bruits, and other signs of occlusive disease, especially with history of claudication

Neurologic examination to detect neurogenic disease, such as multiple sclerosis that relates to etiology of ED

Pain sensation in genitalia and perianal areas

TABLE 34–29. Diagnostic Test for Erectile Function

Serum glucose; if elevated, do Glucose Tolerance Test to rule out diabetes mellitus
Fasting lipid profile
TSH
Serum total testosterone
Prolactin level if low testosterone present
LH and FSH
Prostate-specific antigen (PSA)
Urinalysis
If indicated: CBC, liver enzymes
Nocturnal penile tumescence or "postage stamp" test to assess the intactness of erectile apparatus (most sensitive test available). Instruct patient to wrap a ring of postage stamps snugly around a flaccid penis at bedtime and moisten overlapping stamps to seal the ring. Positive test is confirmed with breakage along the perforations in the morning.
Home monitoring of erections with Rigiscan for strength and number of erections
Other tests by urologist, such as Doppler ultrasonography, color flow tests, intracavernosal injection, or sacral reflex latency time

- Smoking cessation
- Positive lifestyle measures, i.e. exercise, proper nutrition, ideal body weight, limited use of alcohol, relaxation techniques
- Annual physical examination and screenings, i.e., vital signs, weight, lipid profile, glucose levels, etc.
- Etiology and progression of disease
- Use of coping mechanisms to reduce stress
- The purpose, dosage, and side effects of drugs
- Appropriate technique of self-administered injection prior to coitus or the use of vacuum-assisted devices
- Signs and symptoms of complications and importance of seeking health care

OUTCOMES MANAGEMENT

Selecting an Appropriate Agent

The key to therapy is having a complete history to be able to determine the etiology of ED. Discontinuing drugs or substituting alternative drugs is appropriate if ED is the result of a drug side effect. Antihypertensive drugs, such as thiazide diuretics, methyldopa, clonidine, and beta blockers, cause ED and loss of libido. Angiotensin-converting enzyme (ACE) inhibitors, calcium channel blockers, selective cardiac beta blockers, and peripheral $alpha_1$ blockers, such as prazocin and terazocin, are less likely to affect ED (Crowe & Streetman, 2004; Astbury-Ward, 2000; Jensen & Burnett, 2002; Padma-Nathan, 2003; Ralph & McNicholas, 2000; Rose & Kostis 2003).

Sildenafil, tadalafil, and vardenafil are selective inhibitors of cGMP-specific phophodiesterase type 5 (PDE5) that increase levels of cGMP in penile tissue to enhance the patient's response to nitric oxide released during sexual stimulation. Oral agents are preferred because of ease of administration and relatively low adverse effect profile. The three medications are contraindicated in patients using organic nitrates or nitric oxide donors, such as nitroglycerine, isosorbide mononitrate, isosorbide dinitrate, or nitroprusside. Vardenafil is contraindicated in patients taking alpha-blockers. Tadalafil is contraindicated on alpha-blockers except for tamulosin 0.4 mg once daily. Sildenafil in doses greater than 25 mg should not be taken within four hours of an alpha-blocker. Coadministration of strong inhibitors or inducers of CYP3A4 isoenzyme decrease or increase respectively hepatic clearance of the drugs. Sildenafil, tadalafil, and vardenafil vary in potency, onset of action, selectivity for other isoforms of phosphodiesterase, and half-life. The clinical significance of these differences have not been demonstrated by clinical use and head to head trials (Crowe & Streetman, 2004; Jensen & Burnett 2002; Padma-Nathan, 2003; Rose & Kostis 2003).

Other pharmacotherapeutic options for ED include intraurethral suppositories and intravavernosal injections. These methods require a referral and management by an urologist and are generally reserved for patients who failed oral or cannot tolerate oral therapy. Alprostadil (PGE1) is a small suppository that is inserted into the urethra with a plastic applicator and is contraindicated in pregnancy and female partners who frequently experience vaginitis (10%). Administration requires some degree of dexterity with the onset of actions of 10 to 30 minutes. Intracavernosal injections are the most effective method for treating ED; however, longitudinal studies show high dropout rates and lack of satisfaction due to adverse effects. Alprostadil, phentolamine, and papaverine are the drugs used in intracavernosal injections. Both options require a trial administration in the urologist's office for observation of efficacy, duration of erection, dosage adjustment to prevent priapism, and education on the proper technique for administration. A trial of oral yohimbine seeks to avoid the use of injections; however, it is ineffective and not recommended (Jensen & Burnett, 2002; Leungwattanakij, Flynn, & Hellstrom, 2001; Padma-Nathan & Guiliano, 2001)

Monitoring for Efficacy

Effects of drug therapy changes for ED range from a few days to several weeks. Frequent monitoring of blood pressure is essential when antihypertensive drugs are modified. The reduction of dosages for antipsychotics or the use of different antidepressants requires monitoring of therapeutic effects. Monitor the patient for overall sexual function and satisfaction as it is the hallmark of efficacy. Monitoring is achieved by using (1) Brief Sexual Function Inventory (BSFI), a self-administered 11–item questionnaire, (2) International Index of Erectile Function (IIEF) self-administered 15–item questionnaire, (3) Global Efficacy Question (GEQ), the healthcare provider asks if treatment has improved erections, or (4) specific, direct open-ended questions to the patient that assess sexual function, such as erectile function, achieve orgasm, ejaculation function, intercourse satisfaction, and overall sexual satisfaction (Astbury-Ward, 2000; Jensen & Burnett, 2002; Ralph & McNicholas, 2000).

Monitoring for Toxicity

A prolonged erection or priapism is the most important toxic effect to monitor. Erections lasting longer than 4 h require immediate physician intervention (Jensen & Burnett, 2002; Leungwattanakij, Flynn, & Hellstrom, 2001; Padma-Nathan & Giuliano, 2001).

Followup Recommendations

Dose adjustments of hypertensive, antidepressant, antipsychotic, or other drug therapies require followup recommendations for the respective treatment regimen. Patients using intracavernous injection therapy are evaluated every month for dosage adjustment, correct injection technique, and side effects.

Assess patients for physiological changes and adverse drug interactions. Regularly remind the partners of patients on intraurethral therapy that the drugs are contraindicated during pregnancy (Jensen & Burnett, 2002; Leungwattanakij, Flynn, & Hellstrom, 2001; Padma-Nathan & Giuliano, 2001).

REFERENCES

Akduman, B., & Crawford, E. D. (2001). Terazosin, doxazosin, and prazosin: Current clinical experience. *Urology, 58*(Suppl. 6A), 49–54.

Anonymous. (2000). Routine use of antibiotics and alpha-blockers to treat chronic prostatitis is not supported by evidence. *Research Activities, 243,* 6–7.

Astbury-Ward, E. (2000). The erectile dysfunction revolution. *Nursing Standard, 15*(11), 34–40.

Beheshti, P., & Fonteyn, M. (1998). Role of the advanced practice nurse in continence care in the home. *American Association of Critical Care Nurses, 9,* 389–395.

Blaivas, J. G., Romanzi, L. J. & Heritz, D. M. (1998). Incontinence. In P. C. Walsh, A. B. Retick, E. Darracott-Vaughn, A. J. Wein (Eds.), *Campbell's Urology* (7th ed., pp. 1007–1043). Philadelphia: W.B. Saunders.

Buback, D. (2001). The use of neuromodulation for treatment of urinary incontinence. *AORN, 73*(1), 175–178, 181–182, 184–187, 189–196.

Bundrick, W., Heron, S. P., Ray, P., Schiff, W. M., Tennenberg, A. M., Wiseinger, B. A., Wright, P. A., Wu, S. C., Zadeikis, N., & Kahn, J. B. (2003). Levofloxacin versus ciprofloxacin in the treatment of chronic bacterial prostatitis: A randomized double-blind multicenter study. *Urology, 62,* 537–541.

Centers for Disease Control and Prevention. (2002). Sexually transmitted diseases and treatment guidelines. *Morbidity and Mortality Weekly Report, 51*(RR-6), 1–84.

Chancellor, M. B., & Yoshimura, N. (2004). Treatment of interstitial cystitis. *Urology, 63* (Suppl. 1), 85–92.

Chow, R. D. (2001a). Prostatitis: Work-up and treatment of men with telltale symptoms. *Geriatrics, 56*(4), 32–36.

Chow, R. D. (2001b). Benign prostatic hyperplasia: Patient evaluation and relief of obstructive symptoms. *Geriatrics, 56*(4), 32–36.

Cole, F. L., & Vogler, R. (2004). The acute, nontraumatic scrotum: Assessment, diagnosis, and management. *Journal of American Nurse Practitioner, 16,* 50–56.

Collins, M. M., MacDonald, R., & Wilt, T. J. (2000). Diagnosis and treatment of chronic abacterial prostatitis: A systematic review. *Annals of Internal Medicine, 133,* 367–381.

Crowe, S. M., & Streetman, D. S. (2004). Vardenafil treatment for erectile dysfunction. *The Annals of Pharmacotherapy, 38,* 77–85.

Delancey, J. O., & Ashton-Miller, J. A. (2004). Pathophysiology of adult urinary incontinence. *Gastroenterology, 126,* (1 Suppl. 1), S23–S32.

Dezell, J. E., & Lefevre, M. L. (2000). Urinary tract infections during pregnancy. *American Family Physician, 61,* 713–720.

DuFour, J. L. ((2001). Assessing and treating epididymitis. *Nurse Practitioner, 26*(3), 23–24.

Eardley, I. (2001, November). *Erectile dysfunction: Breaking the silence.* Paper presented at the meeting of the 20th International Bayer Pharm Press Seminar, Mexico City, Mexico.

Gupta, K., Hooton, T. M., Roberts, P. L., & Stamm, W. E. (2001). Patient-initiated treatment of uncomplicated recurrent urinary tract infections in young women. *Annals of Internal Medicine, 135,* 9–16.

Gupta, K., Hooton, T. M., & Stamm, W. E. (2001). Increasing antimicrobial resistance and the management of uncomplicated community-acquired urinary tract infections. *Annals of Internal Medicine, 135,* 41–50.

Holroyd-Leduc, J. M., & Straus, S. E. (2004). Management of urinary incontinence in women: Scientific review. *Journal of the American Medical Association, 291,* 986–995.

Hooton, T. H. (2001). Recurrent urinary tract infection in women. *International Journal of Antimicrobial Agents, 17,* 259–268.

Irani, J., Brown, C. T., van der Meulen, J., & Emberton, M. (2003). A review of guidelines on benign prostatic hyperplasia and lower urinary tract symptoms: Are all guidelines the same? *British Journal of Urology, 92,* 937–942.

Jensen, P. K., & Burnett, J. D. (2002). Erectile dysfunction: Primary care treatment is appropriate and essential. *Advance for Nurse Practitioners, 10*(4), 45–52.

Kim, H. L., Benson, D. A., Stern, S. D., & Gerber, G. S. (2002). Practice trends in the management of prostate disease by family practice physicians and general internists: An Internet-based survey. *Urology, 59,* 266–271.

Kirby, R. S., Quinn, S., Mallen, S., & Jensen, D. (2004). Doxazosin controlled release vs tamsulosin in the management of benign prostatic hyperplasia: An efficacy analysis. *International Journal of Clinical Practice, 58,* 6–10.

Le, T. P., & Miller, L. G. (2001). Empirical therapy for uncomplicated urinary tract infections in an era of increasing antimicrobial resistance: A decision and cost analysis. *Clinicals of Infectious Diseases, 33,* 615–621.

Leungwattanakij, S., Flynn, V., & Hellstrom, W. J. G. (2001). Intracavernosal injection and intraurethral therapy for erectile dysfunction. *Urological Clinics of North America, 28,* 343–354.

Lowe, F. C. (2002). Goals for benign prostatic hyperplasia therapy. *Urology, 59*(Suppl. 2A), 1–2.

Lummus, W. E, & Thompson, I. (2001). Prostatitis. *Emergency Medical Clinics of North America, 19,* 691–707.

Luzzi, G. A., & O'Brien, T. S. (2001). Acute epididymitis. *BJU International 87,* 747–755.

MacLean, A. B. (2001). Urinary tract infection in pregnancy. *International Journal of Antimicrobial Agents, 17,* 273–277.

Marcozzi, D., & Suner, S. (2001). The nontraumatic acute scrotum. *Genitourinary Emergencies, 19,* 547–568.

McCue, J. D. (2000). Complicated UTI: Effective treatment in the long-term care setting. *Geriatrics, 55*(9), 48–61.

McLaughlin, S. P., & Carson, C. C. (2004). Urinary tract infections in women. *Medical Clinics of North America, 88,* 417–429.

Miller, O., & Hemphill, R. R. (2001). Urinary tract infection and pyelnephritis. *Emergency Medical Clinics of North America, 19,* 655–674.

Morbidity and Mortality Weekly Report. (2002). Evaluation of sexually transmitted diseases control practices for male patients with urethritis at a large group practice affiliated with a managed care organization: Massachusetts, 1995–1997. Retrieved April 5, 2002, from http://www.cdc.gov/mmwr/preview/mmwrhtml/mm50222a2.htm

Naber, K. G. (2001). Which fluoroquinolones are suitable for the treatment of urinary tract infections? *International Journal of Antimicrobial Agents, 17,* 331–341.

Newman, D. K. (2004, May). Stress urinary incontinence: Therapeutic strategies for managing stress urinary incontinence in women. *American Journal for Nurse Practitioners,* Special Supplement, 23–32.

Nickel, J. C. (2003). Classification and diagnosis of prostatitis: A gold standard? *Andrologia, 35,* 160–167.

O'Leary, M. P. (2002). Quality of life and α-blocker therapy: An important consideration for both the patient and the physician. *Urology, 58*(Suppl. 2A), 7–11.

Padma-Nathan, H. (2003). Efficacy and tolerability of Tadalafil, a novel phosphodiesterase 5 inhibitor, in treatment of erectile dysfunction. *American Journal of Cardiology, 9* (Suppl.), 19M–25M.

Padma-Nathan, H., & Giuliano, F. (2001). Oral drug therapy for erectile dysfuction. *Urological Clinics of North America, 28,* 321–334.

Palmer, M. H. (2004, May) Stress urinary incontinence: Prevalence, etilogy, & risk factors in women at 3 life stages. *American Journal for Nurse Practitioners,* Special Supplement, 5–14.

Ralph, D., & McNicholas, T. (2000). UK management guidelines for erectile dysfunction, *British Medical Journal, 321,* 499–503.

Romanzi, L. J. (2002). *Lower urinary tract infections and the primary care clinician: Gender-specific issues in assessment and treatment.* Littleton, CO: Medical Education Resources.

Rosen, R.C., & Kostis, J. B. (2003). Overview of p-5 Inhibition in erectile dysfunction. *American Journal of Cardiology,* 92(Suppl.), 9M–18M.

Santen, S. A., & Altieri, M. F. (2001). Pediatric urinary tract infection. *Emergency Medical Clinics of North America, 19,* 675–690.

Schubert, H. (2000). Emergency case: Acute testicular pain. *Canadian Family Physician, 46,* 1289–1290.

Shahmanesh, M. (2001). Why common things are common: The tale of non-gonococcal urethritis. *Sexually Transmitted Infections, 77,* 139–140.

Steele, R. W. (2000). Prevention and management of sexually transmitted diseases in adolescents. *Adolescent Medicine, 11,* 315–326.

Talan, D. A., Stamm, W. E., Hooton, T. M., Moran, G. J., Burke, T., Iravani, A., Reuning-Scherer, J., & Church, D. A. (2000). Comparison of ciprofloxacin (7 days) and trimethoprim-sulfamethoxazole (14 days) for acute uncomplicated pyleonephritis in women. *Journal of the American Medical Association, 283,* 1583–1590.

Thakar, R., & Stanton, S. (2000). Management of urinary incontinence in women. *British Medical Journal, 321,* 1326–1331.

U.S. Department of Health and Human Services. (1996). *Managing acute and chronic urinary incontinence* (AHCPR Publication No. 96-0686). Rockville, MD: Author.

Woodward, P. J., Schwab, C. M., & Sesterhenn, I. A. (2003). From the archives of the AFIP: Extratesticular scrotal masses, radiologic-pathlogic correlation. *Radiographics, 23,* 215–240

Zdrodows-Stefanow, B., Ostaszewska, I., Darewicz, B., Darewicz, J., Badyda, J., Pucito, K., Bulhak, V., & Szczurewski, M. (2000). Role of *chlamydia trachomatis* in epididymitis. Part 1: Direct and serologic diagnosis. *Medical Science Monitor, 6,* 1113–1118.

CHAPTER ❖ 3[illegible]

GYNECOLOGIC DISORDERS AND FEMALE SEXUAL DYSFUNCTION

Linda O. Morphis ◆ M. Sharm Steadman

This chapter focuses on gynecological problems often seen in primary care. Vulvar conditions, including folliculitis, vulvar dermatitis, vulvodynia, vulvar vestibulitis, and lichen sclerosus are discussed. Amenorrhea, dysfunctional uterine bleeding, premenstrual syndrome, dysmenorrhea, endometriosis, adenomyosis, and sexual dysfunction are also covered.

VULVAR CONDITIONS

In addition to vulvar tissue being under hormonal influence, the warm, moist environment makes it susceptible to many irritative and infectious conditions. To compound this susceptibility, the tissue is exposed to vaginal secretions, urine, and feces as well as nonabsorbent synthetic fibers and irritating products such as soaps, sprays, powders, daily use of peripads (scented ones are particularly irritating), and colored, scented toilet paper. It is little wonder that vulvar conditions are a common reason for visits to the practitioner (Breslin & Lucas, 2003).

Although some vulvar conditions may be difficult to diagnose and treat, careful assessment and management can relieve much discomfort and distress. Of paramount importance is the need to rule out serious conditions, realizing that premalignant and malignant vulvar lesions can, and do, occur. Consultation and referral are always warranted for any suspicious lesions.

FOLLICULITIS

Folliculitis is an infection of the hair follicles, usually caused by *Staphylococcus* (Markusen & Barclay, 2003; Shellow, 2000). *Pseudomonas aeruginosa* has been identified as the offending organism in the development of folliculitis following hot-tub sessions, with pustules appearing within 1 to 4 days. Superficial trauma from chemical and mechanical factors, such as shaving pubic hair, plays a role in the etiology (Curry, 2000). A nonbacterial type of folliculitis can be caused by the use of oils, cosmetics, cocoa butter, or coconut oil. Tight jeans or other restrictive clothing causes decreased air circulation, friction, and increased perspiration in the pubic or genital area, leading to folliculitis. *Candida albicans* can cause a yeast folliculitis (Curry, 2000; Stulberg, Penrod, & Blatny, 2002).

Specific Considerations for Pharmacotherapy

When Drug Therapy is Needed. Drug therapy will be needed to treat the infection if self-care, nonpharmacotherapy-measures fail to clear the folliculitis.

Short- and Long-Term Goals of Pharmacotherapy. The short-term goal is to treat infection and to relieve symptoms; the long-term goal is to prevent recurrence and complications.

Nonpharmacologic Therapy. Warm, moist compresses to the vulvar area, using water or saline, or warm sitz followed by patting dry with a clean towel and then thoroughly drying the area with a warm hair dryer setting to minimize discomfort. The prevention of predisposing causes is essential. Water in hot tubs and whirlpools must be properly treated. Other nonpharmacologic therapies include the elimination of irritating products; the use of an antibacterial soap only while infection is present and then changing to a nonalkaline, unscented, uncolored, pH-balanced soap; the use of a new or clean razor blade if shaving is continued; careful drying after bath or shower with a hair dryer on the warm setting; wearing all-cotton underwear; and leaving underwear off as frequently as possible, particularly at night.

Time Frame for Initiating Pharmacotherapy. Depending on severity, nonpharmacologic treatment guidelines alone may be initiated when the patient presents for care, with the understanding that if symptom relief does not occur within 3 days, pharmacotherapy should be begun. If presenting symptoms warrant, pharmacological treatment should begin with initial patient contact, with expected symptom relief within several days to 1 week.

See Drug Tables 103, 805.

Assessment and History Taking. On history, the patient will present with complaints of "bumps" in the area, mildly pruritic to nonpruritic. Questions related to shaving and use of irritating products, as well as presence of vaginal discharge should be included in history taking. Pelvic examination will show small superficial pustules at the base of the hair follicle, and mild erythema may be noted. Folliculitis lesions from *Pseudomonas* may be vesicular or pustular. Diagnostic tests for folliculitis are not indicated, as diagnosis is made by examining the area. Tests to rule out sexually transmitted infections, however, should be performed as indicated.

Patient/Caregiver Information. Patients should be instructed in the nonpharmacologic and pharmacologic application of treatment. Inform the patient if any diagnostic test is pending, and when she should return for followup.

Outcomes Management

Selecting an Appropriate Agent. Bactroban (mupirocin 2%) topical antibiotic ointment applied sparingly bid or tid is the treatment agent of choice for folliculitis (Shellow, 2000). Although this agent may be more costly than others, its effectiveness in the majority of cases justifies use. Unless pruritis is pronounced, oral antihistamines generally are not given. Yeast folliculitis requires treatment with an antifungal cream. Since underlying tissues are not affected in folliculitis, systemic antibiotics generally are not given unless constitutional or chronic symptoms are present. Phenoxymethyl penicillin is sufficient for streptococcal infection, Azithromycin is a good alternative. Dicloxacillin or cephalexin may be given for resistant staphlococcal species (Shellow, 2000).

Monitoring for Efficacy. See "Time Frame for Initiating Pharmacotherapy" above.

Monitoring for Toxicity. Toxicity to mupirocin is rare. Neomycin is a known contact sensitizer, with sensitization developing with long-term use in denuded areas (Sober, 1995). See Drug Table 102 for antibiotic information.

Followup Recommendations. Followup should be in 1 week to assess clearing of infection and adherence to guidelines for prevention. This could be by phone or office visit.

VULVAR DERMATITIS

This vulvar condition is generally irritative but noninfectious in nature. It is a contact dermatitis, can be acute or chronic, and results from contact with allergens or chemicals, use of the previously noted irritants, as well as tight, restrictive clothing (Markusen & Barclay, 2003). Pruritis is very common and often severe, with risk of secondary infection from scratching.

Specific Considerations for Pharmacotherapy

When Drug Therapy is Needed. Discomfort and pruritis from vulvar dermatitis produces both physiological and psychological distress, warranting drug therapy.

Short- and Long-term Goals of Pharmacotherapy. The short-term goal of pharmacotherapy is the re-lief of pruritis and irritation as quickly as possible, while the long-term goal is to prevent recurrence.

Nonpharmacologic Therapy. Nonpharmacologic therapy includes cool to tepid sitz baths or compresses to the vulvar area, patting rather than rubbing dry, and careful drying using the warm hair dryer setting. This drying regimen, plus use of a mild, nonirritating soap, wearing all-cotton underwear, leaving underwear off as frequently as possible, and avoiding tight, restrictive clothing and irritating substances, will greatly reduce the risk of recurrence.

Time Frame for Initiating Pharmacotherapy. Because of patient discomfort, treatment should be initiated with patient contact, and improvement in symptoms should be expected within 24 h after application of the topical agent.

See Drug Table 800.

Assessment and History Taking. History taking should include specific questions related to use of irritants, as well as the presence of any chronic conditions, including liver disease. The woman will complain of itching, burning, and stinging of the affected area.

The vulva will be erythematous on exam. Mild edema, increased temperature scaling, and linear excoriations from scratching may also be present. A wet mount should be done to rule out infections such as *Candida,* and a culture for herpes simplex virus (HSV) also should be done if questionable lesions are present.

Patient/Caregiver Information. Information should include instructions on how to use warm compresses and sitz baths. Avoidance of irritants is very important, and written information listing those products to avoid would be helpful. Patients should be told how to apply topical corticosteroids with emphasis placed on importance of short-term use. If oral corticosteroid therapy is indicated, appropriate information regarding side effects, interactions, and expected tapering regimen should be stressed (see Drug Table 601).

Outcomes Management

Selecting an Appropriate Agent. Appropriate topical corticosteroids include low-potency prescriptive preparations such as Aristocort or 0.5–1% OTC topical hydrocortisone, applied sparingly bid for 3 to 5 days (Lichtman & Duran, 1995). Oral antihistamines such as Atarax or Benadryl may also be used, particularly at bedtime if sleep is being disrupted. All these agents are fairly economical. For more severe acute problems, prednisone PO for 4 to 5 days with tapering over a 5 to 10-day period can be used (Curry, 2000). One commonly used regimen is 60 mg for 4 days, 40 mg for 5 days, and 20 mg for 5 days. It is important to use a therapeutic dose early in therapy.

Monitoring for Efficacy. Efficacy of treatment should be assessed in approximately 3 days. All symptoms, in mild cases, should be cleared in that time and physical examination should be negative. More severe cases may require a longer period to evidence healing.

Monitoring for Toxicity. Local adverse reactions are reported infrequently with topical steroids when used short-term, but may include burning, irritation, dryness, and contact dermatitis. Skin atrophy, striae, and hypopigmentation especially are associated with long-term use, and therefore should be avoided. Short-term use of oral corticosteroids should not cause toxicity (see Drug Table 601, for possible negative effects from long-term use).

Followup Recommendations. Stress the importance of continuing to avoid chemical or allergen irritants, nylon underwear, and tight-fitting garments. Lack of response to therapy requires referral to a specialist.

VULVODYNIA

Vulvodynia refers to chronic vulvar discomfort that may involve complaints of constant burning, stinging, irritation, and a feeling of rawness. The symptoms are not necessarily associated with sexual activity (Markusen & Barclay, 2003). Although women have presented to healthcare providers with these symptoms and complaints for decades, in 1982 the International Society for the Study of Vulvar Disease at long last defined vulvodynia as a distinct clinical entity.

What seems to have confounded the defining of this condition, as well as the diagnosis and treatment, is the fact that it is virtually without visible evidence of vulvar pathology or abnormality, other than an occasional subtle redness. Sensitivity to touch will be noted on examination, but no proportional causative etiology will be detected initially.

Numerous disorders that result in chronic vulvar discomfort may be associated with vulvodynia. Discussion of two of these—vulvar vestibulitis and lichen sclerosus—follows.

VULVAR VESTIBULITIS

Vulvar vestibulitis is a chronic syndrome characterized by exquisite tenderness of the minor vestibular glands, which exhibit marked erythema. Pain is elicited with attempted penetration, or by even touching the vaginal vestibule (Johnson, Johnson, Murray, & Apgar, 2000). The exact etiology is unknown, although many factors, including recurrent fungal, bacterial, and viral agents, have been indicated (Johnson, Johnson, Murray, & Apgar, 2000). It is most often seen in young adult women, and whether HPV is involved in the etiology is controversial (Markusen & Barclay, 2003). Other suggested causes include elevated urinary levels of calcium oxalate, allergic reactions and chronic dermatitis, hormonal changes, and psychological responses.

Specific Considerations for Pharmacotherapy

When Drug Therapy Is Needed. The psychological and physical pain of vulvar vestibulitis over months and even years can be tremendous. Activities of day-to-day life, work, and relationships are disrupted.

Short- and Long-Term Goals of Pharmacotherapy. Short-term and long-term pharmacologic goals are to relieve pain and discomfort and to restore a semblance of normalcy to daily life, work, and relationships.

Nonpharmacologic Therapy. Previously discussed nonpharmacologic therapies are included here. Needless to say, avoidance of irritants should be strictly observed, as they may not only aggravate the condition but also will add to discomfort. Additional nonpharmacologic therapies may include vaginal lubricants and a low oxalate diet along with the ingestion of calcium citrate tablets (Solomons, Melmed, & Heitler, 1991). Biofeedback could be investigated as a treatment modality. In addition, psychosocial support is extremely important, and consideration should be given to the formation of a support group for these women. Sexual counseling with emphasis on sexual gratification by means other than intercourse may be needed, as well as possible referral to a certified sex therapist for more intensive care. Severe vulvar vestibulitis that is unresponsive to conservative behavioral-based interventions may require surgery as a last resort. This involves a crescent-shaped. posterior vestibular excision followed by vaginal advancement (Botte, 2003).

Time Frame for Initiating Pharmacotherapy. Pharmacologic intervention should be initiated with patient contact. Achievement of goals is extremely variable, and may not occur at all.

See Drug Tables 311, 809.

Assessment and History Taking. Women often present with a history of postcoital vulvar burning localized to the posterior fourchette. The painful burning may eventually become so constant and severe that intercourse, as well as insertion of tampons, is impossible. The history will also include discomfort with sitting, biking, snug-fitting clothing, or anything that touches or rubs the vulva. As with other vulvar problems, questions concerning past infections, especially *Candida,* HPV, and HSV should be asked. Ruling out the use of irritative products, douching, overbathing, and scrubbing also is very important.

With physical examination, redness may be seen around the vestibule, especially where the Skene's and Bartholin's ducts open (Kaufman, 1995). Staining with acetic acid will promote strong acetowhitening, and although some sources feel HPV is not currently considered a causative factor (Markusen & Barclay, 2003), others differ. In 1988, Turner and Marinoff reported an association between HPV and vulvar vestibulitis. Umpierre et al. (1991) further identified HPV in tissue specimens of a sample of women with the condition. Diagnostic tests to rule out other infectious processes should be done as needed. Colposcopy can be very helpful in identifying areas of inflammation, and the use of a moist cotton-tipped applicator in finding a pattern of localized point tenderness with touch is most diagnostic of vulvar vestibulitis. Any suspicious area should, of course, be biopsied.

Patient/Caregiver Information. Women should be educated as much as possible concerning the known etiology of vulvar vestibulitis, emphasizing that it is a recognized physical entity. Encourage them to follow the recommended interventions, both pharmacologic and nonpharmacologic, and to avoid self-treatment until evaluation has been completed. If an antidepressant is prescribed, care should be taken to assure the patient that the prescription is not being given because the condition is "just in her head," but because of the antidepressant's effect on nerve endings and usefulness in treating chronic pain (Jones & Lehr, 1994). Ask her to keep a diary with notes about specific foods, activities, or events that seem to trigger discomfort, as well as any interventions that offer relief. Women should be informed of the possible long-term duration of this condition, as well as the possibility of spontaneous regression in 6 months to 1 year (Curry, 2000). Any available information concerning support groups should be given and the woman encouraged to attend.

Outcomes Management

Selecting an Appropriate Agent. Since the psychological impact of vulvar vestibulitis cannot be overlooked, use of antidepressants is often a treatment choice (McKay, 1993; Markusen & Barclay, 2003). Amitriptyline (Elavil) is often given with an initial dosage of 10 mg/day. This is increased by 10 mg/week until the desired effect of pain reduction is achieved, or a maximum of 50 mg/day has been reached.

For management of pain, 2 to 5% lidocaine in an emollient base may be carefully applied in the specific area daily and before intercourse (Markusen & Barclay, 2003).

The therapeutic success of intralesional injection of interferon is reported as 50% or higher. One million units of recombinant interferon alfa-2 is injected submucosally at a different location of the vestibule. The injections are three times per week for 4 weeks (a total of 12 injections) in a clockwise pattern, until the entire vestibule has been injected (Kaufman, 1995; Secor & Fertitta, 1992). This treatment is quite expensive. Although some studies have shown patient improvement, more research needs to be done to prove its efficacy. It is recommended that interferon be used only with consultation (Markusen & Barclay, 2003).

Monitoring for Efficacy. Women should be seen weekly if an antidepressant is ordered and if interferon injections are being given. Efficacy is determined by patient response, with the antidepressants being adjusted as previously noted, and interferon injections being given weekly. Since intercourse is not thought to have an effect on the prognosis of vulvar vestibulitis (Jones & Lehr, 1994), it need not be avoided during these treatments, and patient response can thus be monitored via degree of dyspareunia. Topical anesthetics may also be monitored in this way.

Monitoring for Toxicity. With amitriptyline, monitor for drowsiness, anticholinergic effects, and CNS overstimulation. Some women may experience galactorrhea with higher dosages (Weil, 1996); however, this response does not necessarily indicate toxicity.

Adverse reactions to interferon include flu-like symptoms. CBCs and liver function tests should be obtained to monitor for blood dyscrasias and hepatic problems (Weil, 1996), and although no set schedule seems to be available for these tests, it is prudent to obtain these tests at least every 4 weeks, and perhaps more frequently.

Topical lidocaine should be used with extreme caution since it may be a sensitizing agent in some patients if used over the entire vulva (Jones & Lehr, 1994).

Followup Recommendations. Followup appointments should be made weekly after initial contact, and treatment evaluated. Treatment outcomes are variable, and partial vulvectomy or vestibulectomy may be suggested to women with severe, long-term symptoms that fail to respond. This surgical intervention should be considered as a last resort, after all nonsurgical therapies have been ineffective.

LICHEN SCLEROSUS

This condition is one of the vulvar dystrophies, also called vulvar dermatoses. Lesions are white circumscribed or diffuse, atrophic or hypertrophic (Markusen & Barclay, 2003). All are pruitic and affect perimenopausal and menopausal women. Malignancy risk is under 5%.

Specific Considerations for Pharmacotherapy

When Drug Therapy Is Needed. Intervention with drug therapy is indicated, since the discomfort resulting from severe, chronic pruritis can be debilitating.

Short- and Long-Term Goals of Pharmacotherapy. The primary short-term goal is to relieve pruritis and its concomitant rubbing, scratching, and inflammation. The long-term goal is to build up the atrophic epithelium, and to prevent recurrence.

Nonpharmacologic Therapy. Nonpharmacologic treatments are those noted previously, with strict attention paid to avoidance of irritants and hot baths. Leaving underwear off entirely is the best option; however, this may cause undue discomfort in some women. Encourage the patient to at least leave underwear off at night and to wear loose-fitting, all-cotton, boxer-type underwear during the day.

Time Frame for Initiating Pharmacotherapy. Treatment is initiated upon patient contact for care, after diagnosis has been confirmed.

See Drug Tables 705, 807, 810.

Assessment and History Taking. Intense pruritis is the presenting complaint of women with lichen sclerosus, usually of long-term duration (Curry, 2000). Questions focused on previously prescribed treatments and self-treatment should be asked, as well as questions about the use of common irritants and chronic rubbing of clothes. Physical examination findings include a pattern of whitish, wrinkled, atrophic, parchmentlike skin. Affected areas may include the vulva, clitoral hood, perineal area, skinfold areas next to the thighs, buttocks, and a keyhole area around the anus (Kaufman, 1995). Excoriations and fissures may be present, and the introitus may be constricted. Topography is lost as the vulvar structures atrophy and contract and the labia minora blends with the labia majora. Intense pruritis leading to chronic scratching and rubbing results in lichenification, epithelial atrophy, and hyperkeratosis. Tentative diagnosis may be made from history and physical examination, but colposcopy with biopsy is necessary to confirm the diagnosis and to rule out dysplasia. Biopsy must always be done with any suspicious lesion of the vulva (Curry, 2000).

Patient/Caregiver Information. The patient should be educated about the strict avoidance of irritants, medication use, and the etiology and chronic nature of this condition. She should be given support and encouragement, since beneficial effects depend largely on compliance with recommendations.

Outcomes Management

Selecting an Appropriate Agent. With the stated goals in mind, a combination of high-potency topical steroidal cream, oral antihistamines, and testosterone cream is used. The high-potency steroid cream or ointment is applied twice daily for 4 weeks, then once every day for 8 weeks. Maintenance is 2 to 3 times a week with clobestasol propionate 0.05% or another topical steroid of a lesser dose (Markusen & Barclay, 2003). Clobestasol is most commonly used for treatment; the ointment may not burn as much as the cream. Beneficial effects should be noticed by the patient within 24 h. Two percent testosterone propionate ointment, which must be prepared by a pharmacist, may be prescribed to thicken the epithelium. The testosterone propionate in petrolatum is applied 2 to 3 times daily for 6 to 12 weeks, then twice weekly indefinitely until the lesion resolves. Testosterone side effects of virilization and metabolic changes may become problematic and require stopping use (Markusen & Barclay, 2003).

Monitoring for Efficacy. Subjective findings of decreased pruritis hopefully will be noted by the patient at the first followup visit, and as the weeks progress with adherence to pharmacologic and nonpharmacologic regimens, objective observations of decreased lichenification and atrophy should become evident. Testosterone propionate cream may be gradually decreased after epithelium is restored.

Monitoring for Toxicity. As previously noted, long-term use of topical corticosteroids in the vulvar area is not recommended; therefore, care must be taken to ensure proper use of this medication. The development of hirsutism, acne, and excessively oily skin may occur as androgenic side effects from testosterone. A serum testosterone level may be obtained if these problems are noted. They are annoying rather than posing an actual toxic effect, however, and should diminish if the treatment is discontinued.

Followup Recommendations. Followup should be scheduled 1 to 2 weeks after the initial visit, and then monthly. With improvement of the condition, thought should be given to placing the patient on oral hormone replacement therapy if no contraindications exist. Estratest, with its combination of estrogen and testosterone, might be considered, thereby providing the benefits of estrogen (including alleviation of atrophic vaginitis) and continuing effects of testosterone to maintain epithelial thickness.

MENSTRUAL DISORDERS

Much time, energy, thought, and money are given by women to the concerns of menstruation. Menses that are too frequent, too infrequent or absent, too scant, too heavy, too painful, or too bloating send women to pharmacies and healthcare providers every day. This section discusses four common menstrual problems: amenorrhea, dysfunctional uterine bleeding, premenstrual syndrome, and dysmenorrhea.

AMENORRHEA

Amenorrhea is the absence of menses. It may be primary or secondary and either a physiologic function or caused by a pathologic condition. *Primary amenorrhea* is the absence of menarche by age 14 with the lack of secondary sex characteristics, or by age 16 regardless of the development of secondary sex characteristics (Gordon & Speroff, 2002; Letterie, 2004). Women with these presenting characteristics warrant thorough evaluation by a specialist, and this condition is beyond the scope of this chapter.

Secondary amenorrhea is the cessation of menses for at least 3 (some sources say 6) months in a woman who has previously had regular monthly menstrual cycles. Secondary amenorrhea is a frequent cause of concern for many women. Although secondary amenorrhea can be a sign of a serious problem such as a pituitary tumor, pregnancy and menopause are frequent causes of missed menses. The condition also may occur because of suppression of the hypothalamus, which can result from physical and emotional stress, strenuous exercise, use of hormonal therapy, and sudden weight loss or gain. Other causes include polycystic ovary syndrome (PCOS), intrauterine scarring (Asherman's syndrome), and hypothyroidism (Gordon & Speroff, 2002; Hatcher et al., 1998; Letterie, 2004).

Specific Considerations for Pharmacotherapy

When Drug Therapy Is Needed. Amenorrhea is generally associated with reduced estrogen levels, and estrogen is closely associated with bone density. Prolonged amenorrhea with reduced estrogen can result in bone loss and subsequent higher risk of fractures (Conviser & Fitzgibbon, 1997). Fertility is associated with regular ovulation and menses, and the lack of these two normal functions may indicate decreased fertility in women hoping to conceive. In addition, women with amenorrhea caused by anovulation are at risk for endometrial hyperplasia from unopposed estrogen. For these, as well as other psychological and physiological reasons, drug therapy is needed.

Short- and Long-Term Goals of Pharmacotherapy. Pharmacotherapy goals are to restore cyclic ovulation and menses in premenopausal women, to prevent problems associated with estrogen and progesterone deficit, and to eliminate the risk of endometrial hyperplasia.

Nonpharmacologic Therapy. If the absence of menses is determined to be due to nonpathologic hypothalamic suppression, lifestyle changes may correct the problem. Learning to manage stress, reducing intensity of exercise, and gaining weight are therapy options. If a serious eating disorder is diagnosed, referral to a specialist is essential as this can be a life-threatening condition.

Time Frame for Initiating Pharmacotherapy. Treatment should begin as soon as the cause of amenorrhea is established.

See Drug Tables 603, 605, 607.

Assessment and History Taking. Assessment through a complete history and physical examination is essential to rule out pathology prior to therapy. Careful history taking alone can often reveal the cause of missed menses; oral contraceptives, hormonal injections, and implants for contraception can all affect regularity of menstrual flow. It also is very important to ask questions concerning frequency and intensity of exercise, eating habits, significant changes in body weight, and stressful lifestyle events. The questions all relate to hypothalamic suppression. A history of headaches, nipple discharge (galactorrhea), and changes in vision could suggest a pituitary adenoma. Presence of hot flashes, night sweats, and vaginal dryness in a younger woman could indicate premature ovarian failure, and in an older woman, the common symptoms of approaching menopause.

Height, weight, and vital signs should be taken. A complete physical examination with pelvic and Pap smears is needed. If, by general appearance and history, an eating disorder is suspected, the percentage of body fat should be measured. Note any hirsutism. If present, androgen-producing tumors must be ruled out with testosterone and dehydroepiandrosterone sulfate levels. Additionally, polycystic ovarian syndrome (PCOS) may be the cause of amenorrhea evidenced by chronic anovulation and hyperandrogenemia (Gordon & Neinstein, 2002; Gordon & Speroff, 2002). A luteinizing hormone/follicle-stimulating hormone (LH/FSH) ratio greater than 3:1 (high LH and low to normal FSH) accompanied by low elevations of androgens indicates PCOS or some other problem exists (Gordon & Speroff, 2002). The ovaries are usually enlarged but may be normal in size (Gordon & Neinstein, 2002). The thyroid gland should be palpated for enlargement and/or nodules. Hypothyroidism can stimulate an increased prolactin level. A sensitive urine pregnancy test should be done on all women to rule out pregnancy, as this is a very frequent cause of amenorrhea. After pregnancy is ruled out, diagnostic tests, at a minimum, should include thyroid-stimulating hormone (TSH) and serum prolactin levels. FSH levels may also be obtained to rule out premature ovarian failure or menopause. A second FSH level should be drawn 2 weeks after the initial level as a midcycle FSH level may be elevated normally and mimic menopause. Polycystic ovary syndrome is believed to be linked with insulin resistance, and in some women hirsutism and/or obesity are present, thus additional diagnostic testing for elevated androgens, diabetes, and lipids are needed (Gordon & Neinstein, 2002; Gordon & Speroff, 2002).

Patient/Caregiver Information. Information should be given concerning physical examination findings and laboratory results. The etiology of amenorrhea should be reviewed, as well as the health risks associated with amenorrhea. If contraception is not currently being used and the pregnancy test is negative, the woman should be counseled on contraceptive techniques if pregnancy is unwanted. All pharmacologic and nonpharmacologic treatments should be discussed in detail, as well as the need for any followup testing, evaluation, and referral. Women placed on oral contraceptives should be told that amenorrhea will likely return if the medication is stopped (Hatcher et al., 1998).

Outcomes Management

Selecting an Appropriate Agent

- Pregnancy must first be excluded.
- If TSH is elevated, treat for hypothyroidism.
- If the serum prolactin level is elevated (greater than 100 ng/mL), a CT scan or MRI should be ordered to evaluate the sella turcica for pituitary adenoma. If the scan is abnormal, refer the patient for further evaluation and possible treatment with bromocriptine (Parlodel), a dopamine agonist (Gordon & Speroff, 2002). If the scan is normal, hypothalamic suppression is responsible for the amenorrhea, and it should be treated with estrogen and progestin. Combined oral contraceptives are an appropriate choice, particularly if the woman desires birth control. Conjugated

estrogen and medroxyprogesterone acetate (MPA) prescribed as for postmenopausal hormone treatment may be appropriate for premature failure but should not be initiated to rpevent CVD (Letterie, 2004).

- If FSH is high, menopause (ovarian failure) is the cause of amenorrhea. Further evaluation of the younger woman less than 45 by an endocrinologist may be warranted. Treatment to replace the loss of hormones, whether premature or expected, may be indicated (Hatcher, 2004; Letterie, 2004).
- If TSH and serum prolactin levels are normal, administer a progestin challenge test. This consists of giving inexpensive MPA 10 mg PO daily for 5 days, progesterone in oil 200 mg IM, or 300 mg oral micronized progesterone (Gordon & Speroff, 2002). If withdrawal bleeding occurs in 2 to 7 days after completion of medication, the diagnosis of anovulation is established. Assuming no contraindications, low-dose oral contraceptives are a good option for anovulatory patients. MPA 10 mg daily for 10 days each month is also an acceptable treatment (Gordon & Speroff, 2002).
- If withdrawal bleeding does not occur with the progestin challenge, the patient may be hypoestrogenic and the endometrium should be "primed" for 21 days with conjugated estrogens 1.25 mg PO daily, followed by MPA 10 mg daily for 5 days (Gordon & Speroff, 2002; Goroll & Mulley, 2000), or conjugated estrogens 2.5 mg daily for 21 days, with the addition of MPA 10 mg daily on days 12 to 21, the last 10 days (Skrypzak, 1995). If withdrawal bleeding occurs, then hypothalamic-pituitary dysfunction is indicated. Further assessment should be directed toward understanding why there was insufficient endogenous estrogen available (Skrypzak, 1995). An FSH level should be drawn if one has not previously been obtained. If this level is low or normal, order a CT scan or MRI evaluation of the sella turcica and proceed as previously discussed. High FSH levels again indicate ovarian failure with menopause and should be thus managed. If withdrawal bleeding still does not occur, referral should be made to evaluate for end-organ (uterine) problems, such as Asherman's syndrome.
- If physical findings, the LH/FSH ratio, increased estrone, increased androgen levels, reduced SHBG levels, and reduced glucose response indicate PCOS, low-dose oral contraceptives are used if the woman does not desire fertility (Gordon & Speroff, 2002). Metformin is being used to improve peripheral insulin sensitivity with PCOS, though non-obese women have a better response (Gordon & Speroff, 2002). Decreases in weight of obese women help effectiveness. Androgenic effects are opposed by the estrogen; testosterone clearance is increased by the progestogen; and testosterone levels should decrease in about 3 months, with an actual decrease in the ovaries' size in 6 months by ultrasound. About 60–80% of women have an abnormal LH/FSH ratio (Gordon and Speroff, 2002). Women who desire fertility will need ovarian stimulation. Consultation with or referral to a specialist is advised.

Monitoring for Efficacy. Patient monitoring depends on the cause of amenorrhea and the treatment chosen. If hormonal therapy is used, patients should be seen in approximately 3 months to assess regulation of menses. It is recommended that the therapy be stopped after 6 months to assess spontaneous resumption of menses (Dambro, 1995).

Monitoring for Toxicity. If oral contraceptives have been prescribed, patients should be seen in 3 months for a blood pressure check and to assess for any side effects. See Chapter 18 on contraceptives for further discussion. Likewise, in Chapter 19 on hormone replacement therapy monitoring is discussed for those women who have been given exogenous estrogen and progestin.

Followup Recommendations. Followup should be as noted in monitoring for efficacy. Further workup for anovulatory women usually is not indicated unless the woman desires pregnancy. Women with chronic anovulation are at increased risk for endometrial carcinoma due to unopposed estrogen. Women with PCOS are at increased risk for cardiovascular disease, diabetes, and hypertension. Careful monitoring is indicated (Gordon & Speroff, 2002).

DYSFUNCTIONAL UTERINE BLEEDING

Dysfunctional uterine bleeding (DUB) is the abnormal, unpredictable bleeding of endometrial origin with no demonstrable organic pathology (Gordon & Speroff, 2002). Ninety percent of all DUB is caused by anovulation (Dambro, 1995). It occurs with conditions associated with anovulatory cycles, such as hypothyroidism, polycystic ovarian syndrome, and some of the other conditions previously discussed with amenorrhea. Since ovulation has not occurred, progesterone is not available to stabilize the endometrium. The endometrium, therefore, attains an abnormal height and is fragile, leading to spontaneous bleeding. As the endometrium from one site is shed, new sites break down in an asynchronous manner. There is no rhythmic vasoconstriction or orderly collapse to induce stasis and clotting. DUB is most commonly see in menarche, as regular ovulation is being established, and during perimenopause, as ovarian function is declining. However, it can occur at any time during a woman's reproductive years.

Specific Considerations for Pharmacotherapy

When Drug Therapy Is Needed. Unpredictable menstrual bleeding is, at the very least, physically and emotionally disconcerting. Risks of unopposed estrogen have previously been discussed, notably endometrial hyperplasia. Anemia can result if bleeding is heavy and prolonged. Drug therapy is also needed for those women who are anovulatory and desire pregnancy.

Short- and Long-Term Goals of Pharmacotherapy. Goals of therapy are to control bleeding and promote cyclic flow, prevent recurrences of irregular bleeding, prevent endometrial hyperplasia, and preserve fertility.

Nonpharmacologic Therapy. For women whose bleeding cannot be controlled with hormonal therapy, surgical measures may be necessary. Options include dilatation and curettage (D&C), endometrial ablation by laser destruction, and, as a last resort, hysterectomy (Griswold, 2004).

Time Frame for Initiating Pharmacotherapy. Therapy should be instituted after pregnancy and pathology have been ruled out and a diagnosis made.

See Drug Tables 306, 603, 605.

Assessment and History Taking. A complete history and physical examination are needed. Menstrual history, contraceptive history, problems with infertility, fibroid tumors, obesity, hirsutism, and lifestyle changes are all important areas to explore, as are any possible systemic diseases that could cause bleeding. A sensitive urine test to rule out pregnancy should be done on every woman with irregular bleeding. If bleeding has been prolonged, a hemoglobin and hematocrit should be obtained. Other laboratory tests should be considered to rule out a thyroid disorder or coagulopathy. If the woman has symptoms of menopause, an FSH would be in order. Bleeding in a postmenopausal woman must always be investigated. An endometrial biopsy will rule out pathology. Other causes of bleeding, such as cervical cancer or infection, should also be ruled out. If history and examination suggest polycystic ovarian syndrome, laboratory testing as discussed previously with amenorrhea is indicated (Gordon & Speroff, 2002; Goroll & Mulley, 2000).

Patient/Caregiver Information. A thorough, easy-to-understand explanation of the etiology, diagnostic procedures, and treatment plan should be given. Techniques to manage stress may be discussed as well as good nutrition, including ways to increase iron in the diet.

Outcomes Management

Selecting an Appropriate Agent. To stop abnormal bleeding that is nonpathologic, MPA 5 to 10 mg daily for 10 days can be given orally, or 100 mg of progesterone can be given in a single intramuscular injection. (Gordon & Speroff, 2002; Goroll & Mulley, 2000). This is frequently referred to as a medical D&C (Goroll & Mulley, 2000). To prevent bleeding from again occurring because of withdrawal after the MPA, low-dose combination oral contraceptives may be started once treatment is completed and bleeding has stopped. Oral contraceptives may be continued for several months, after which time menses may regulate. If prevention of pregnancy is desired, oral contraceptives should be continued. An advantage of this approach is the improvement of the hyperandrogenism that accompanies some cases of anovulatory bleeding, primarily polycystic ovarian syndrome.

If contraception is not needed, oral MPA 5 to 10 mg may be taken every month on the first or last 10 to 12 days to ensure cyclic endometrial shedding (Gordon & Speroff, 2002), thereby protecting against cellular changes and the risk of endometrial cancer associated with long-term unopposed estrogen stimulation.

Prostaglandin synthetase inhibitors (PGSIs) and nonsteroidal antiinflammatory drugs (NSAIDs) are nonhormonal agents that may be helpful in decreasing flow. These include mefenamic acid (Ponstel) 500 mg PO tid for 3 days, or naproxen (Naprosyn) 500 mg PO stat, then 250 mg PO tid for 5 days (Griswold, 2004). Ibuprofen is also included and is quite inexpensive. NSAIDs have been shown to decrease the endometrial blood flow by their antiprostaglandin effect. Alone, they may reduce blood loss by 30%.

Monitoring for Efficacy. With progestin therapy, bleeding should stop within 24 to 48 hours, and a heavy withdrawal bleed can be expected several days to 1 week after completing the MPA. A telephone call should be made in that time to assess efficacy. If this therapy does not stop acute bleeding, referral for a surgical D&C is indicated (Goroll & Mulley, 2000).

Ovulation can spontaneously resume when cyclic MPA is given; therefore, the treatment should be stopped for a month or two to evaluate for the return of regular cycles. Barrier contraception is indicated during this time if pregnancy is not desired. If this therapy is used, periodic visits, possibly every 6 months, should be scheduled.

Monitoring for Toxicity. The side effects most often associated with progestin therapy include weight gain, fatigue, depression, and acne (Hatcher et al., 1999). Also see Chapters 18 and 26 on oral contraceptives and NSAIDs use with musculoskeletal problems for side effects, as well as Drug Tables 306 and 603.

Followup Recommendations. Patients should be seen in 3 months if started on oral contraceptives. The importance of annual Pap smears should be emphasized. Patients should be encouraged to keep a menstrual calendar and to return should irregular bleeding, as well as no bleeding, occur. If conception is desired, referral should be made to a reproductive specialist.

PREMENSTRUAL SYNDROME

Premenstrual syndrome (PMS) is the cyclical recurrence of distressing physical, affective, and behavioral changes that can result in the deterioration of interpersonal relationships and personal health. These symptoms tend to peak premenstrually and disappear after the beginning of menses. In addition, perimenopausal symptoms have been found to reduce work efficiency, increase absenteeism, and have an impact on family and personal relationships (Barnhart, Freeman, & Sondheimer, 1995).

Approximately 75% of women in the general population complain of some minor premenstrual symptoms. However, depending on the criteria and population studied, only 20 to 50% of women experience moderate symptoms that prompt them to seek medical treatment. (Sagraves, 2001). Three to 5% of women have such severe symptoms that their level of functioning is significantly affected (APA, 2000). Although cultural variations exist according to cross-cultural studies, African American and Caucasian women in the United States report equal frequencies of various premenstrual symptoms, with frequency of symptom reported peaking in the 25 to 34-year-old group. Epidemiologic studies of PMS have not confirmed an unequivocal correlation between PMS symptoms and age, socioeconomic status, parity, diet or physical activity, menstrual characteristics, or personality (Rubinow, 1992).

Symptoms

Although the most commonly reported perimenstrual symptoms may be complaints of physical discomfort (bloating, cramping), the reports of mood changes or negative affect symptoms are often the most distressing. Although symptoms are multiple and diverse, they are often grouped into categories such as somatic (mastalgia, bloating, headache, pelvic pain, fatigue), mood (irritability, depression, mood swings), cognitive (poor concentration, confusion), and behavioral (social withdrawal, impulsiveness, appetite changes); see Table 35–1. With more than 100 reported symptoms attributed to the menstrual cycle, delineation of symptoms into symptom clusters may allow for an organized symptom-based approach to women's perimenstrual complaints.

Although most clinicians and researchers generally agree that PMS is not a psychiatric disorder, a subset of PMS with more severe behavioral symptoms, Premenstrual Dysphoric Disorder (PMDD), is included in the appendix of the *Diagnostic and Statistical Manual for Psychiatric Disorders* (DSM-IV). Characteristics of PMDD include depression, anxiety, lability of mood, and irritability that are comparable to a major depressive episode (APA, 2000). Diagnostic criteria are seen in Table 35–2.

Etiology

Although many theories have been proposed for the cause of premenstrual symptoms, none of the proposed etiological theories have been substantiated. Biologic theories have included hypotheses on neurotransmitter dysfunc-

TABLE 35–1. Symptom Clusters of Perimenstrual Complaints

Physical/Somatic	Affective/Behavioral	Cognitive	Fluid Retention
Headache	Depression	Mood lability	Breast tenderness/swelling
Abdominal cramps	Irritability	Difficulty concentrating	Weight gain
Generalized muscle aches/pain	Tension	Memory impairment	Abdominal bloating
Back pain	Anxiety	Confusion	Peripheral edema
Fatigue	Altered libido	Social avoidance	
Insomnia	Tearfulness or crying easily		
Dizziness/vertigo	Cravings for sweet or salty foods		

TABLE 35–2. Diagnostic Criteria for Premenstrual Dysphoric Disorder (PMDD)

1. Must have five or more of the following symptoms, including at least one of the first four:
   - Depressed mood, feelings of hopelessness, or self-deprecating thoughts
   - Marked anxiety or tension; feeling "keyed up" or "on edge"
   - Significant mood lability
   - Persistent anger or irritability; increased interpersonal conflicts
   - Decreased interest in usual activities
   - Lethargy, easy fatigability, or marked lack of energy
   - Changes in appetite; overeating or food cravings
   - Hypersomnia or insomnia
   - Subjective sense of difficulty in concentration
   - Physical symptoms such as breast tenderness, headache, joint or muscle pain, bloating, or weight gain
2. Symptoms occur during the last week of the luteal phase and remit within a few days after onset of menses.
3. Symptoms must seriously interfere with work or with usual social activities or relationships with others.
4. Symptoms not merely an exacerbation of another disorder (e.g., depressive, panic, dysthymic, or personality disorders).
5. Symptoms must be confirmed by prospective daily self-ratings during at least two symptomatic menstrual cycles.

Source: Adapted from APA (2000)

tion, prostaglandin excess, estrogen/progesterone imbalance, vitamin deficiencies, and psychogenic factors (Servino & Moline, 1995). However, no significant differences in serum concentrations of estradiol, progesterone, FSH, or LH have been found in women with PMS compared to controls (Sagraves et al., 2001).

Changes in prolactin concentrations have also not been found to be significantly different in women with or without PMS (Fankhauser, 1999). Alterations in gonadotropin-releasing hormone (GnRH) activity may play a key role in explaining some of the hormonal theories of PMS. Changes in GnRH and ovarian hormone production have been implicated in both the development or elimination of symptoms associated with PMS. GnRH must be released in the appropriate amounts and at the right pulse rate to stimulate gonadotropin secretion and to cause ovulation. Release of GnRH is regulated by positive and negative feedback from norepinephrine, dopamine, serotonin, ovarian hormones, and endogenous opiates. GnRH release is mediated by norepinephrine and serotonin, and its pulsating pattern is modified by endorphins, estrogen, and progesterone. Changes in any of these neurotransmitters may alter GnRH release, which eventually will down-regulate LH and FSH release and prevent ovulation. Suppression of ovulation results in the reduction of the cyclical changes in moods and physical symptoms associated with PMS (Fankhauser, 1999).

Serotonin deficiency has also been proposed as a theory for the development of PMS. Depressed serotonergic activity has been associated with depressed mood, irritability, anxiety, impulsivity, aggressiveness, and increased appetite (Rapkin, 1992). Lower serotonin levels during the luteal phase of the menstrual cycle have been found in women with PMS compared to normal controls (Rapkin, 1992). These findings may explain the similarities in mood and behaviors associated with PMDD and depression.

The pathophysiology of PMS/PMDD has yet to be clearly defined, but the currently accepted hypothesis asserts that normal hormone fluctuations of the menstrual cycle induce changes in the activity of various neurotransmitters, including serotonin and gamma-aminobutyric acid (GABA), in genetically susceptible women (Grady-Weliky, 2003; Sagraves et al., 2001).

Specific Considerations for Pharmacologic Therapy

When Drug Therapy Is Needed. Since a specific etiology for PMS has not been identified, a variety of pharmacological therapies have been tried.

Pharmacologic interventions have been initiated in an effort to correct the theoretical endocrine or neurochemical imbalances that have been proposed as the causative factors for PMS. Various forms of progesterone have been prescribed based on the progesterone deficiency theory; oral contraceptives have been prescribed based on the need for ovarian suppression; aldosterone inhibitors have been used for excess aldosterone secretion and its role in premenstrual fluid retention; and prostaglandin inhibitors have been tried for imbalances in circulating prostaglandins. The most effective therapy has been the use of selective serotonin reuptake inhibitors (SSRIs) because of the presumed role that an imbalance in the levels of the neurotransmitter serotonin may play in PMS.

Current pharmacologic therapy should be directed at the relief or prevention of symptoms to enable women to continue functioning with minimal interference with their activities of daily living. Symptomatic relief can be achieved with analgesics such as aspirin, acetaminophen or the NSAIDs, diuretics, anxiolytics, and antidepressants. GnRH agonists is a treatment used in extreme cases (Faukhauser, 1999).

A combination of treatments may be more effective than monotherapy if a woman is experiencing both incapacitating physical and behavioral symptoms. Drug therapy in combination with nonpharmacological interventions such as exercise, relaxation techniques, and dietary changes appears to hold the most promise in alleviating perimenstrual symptoms. Combination therapy may allow for lower doses of drugs, shorter duration of therapy, and less potential for adverse effects.

Short- and Long-Term Goals of Pharmacotherapy. The initial goal of therapy should be to understand the patient's perimenstrual experience and help her define and manage her symptoms and their related problems. Self-awareness of symptom severity and symptom patterns are the first steps of treatment. For some women, self-monitoring alone may be enough to assist them in making necessary changes in their relationships, stress load, and dietary and exercise routines. Only women with the most extreme manifestations of PMS are likely to require pharmacologic therapy. Initial symptom management should include multiple nonpharmacologic treatments. The woman should be included in the selection process as this promotes empowerment and a sense of self-control. An individualized treatment plan should be established initially and updated regularly until PMS severity is reduced and stabilized. The long-term goal of therapy is development of a treatment plan involving nonpharmacologic and pharmacologic agents and behavioral changes that lead to control of perimenstrual symptom severity and occurrence. This plan would allow the woman to continue her usual lifestyle without disruption.

Nonpharmacologic Therapy. Clinical experience indicates that patient education and support, stress reduction, a healthy diet, regular aerobic exercise, and vitamin supplements assist in relieving some of the symptoms associated with PMS and help a woman to feel more in control of her symptoms (Griswold, 2004). Many women will see a marked reduction in perimenopausal symptoms with these interventions, and only women with more severe symptoms may require additional drug therapy (Fankhauser, 1999).

Acknowledging that the symptoms experienced by patients are real can be therapeutic. Information regarding PMS and the functioning of a normal menstrual cycle needs to be provided. A prospective calendar of menstrual symptoms should be kept for 2 to 3 months to enhance patient awareness and assist in planning and implementing an individualized treatment plan. The patients should be encouraged to identify personal and professional stresses that contribute to PMS and develop coping strategies or adjust their lifestyle to modify or remove these stresses from their lives. Patients may benefit from referral to a psychologist, counselor, or support group to assist them in stress management techniques (Griswold, 2004). Lifestyle changes are recommended for all women with a diagnosis of PMS. Regular aerobic exercise, dietary changes, and modification of sleep habits may be the only treatment necessary for mild PMS.

The American College of Obstetricians and Gynecologists released guidelines for the management of PMS. These guidelines employ a stepped approach that combines pharmacologic and nonpharmacologic options based on severity of symptoms (ACOG, 2000). Guidelines are summarized in Table 35–3.

Although there is no evidence that nutritional deficiencies cause PMS, poor diet may exacerbate symptoms. Dietary changes that have been shown to reduce perimenstrual symptoms include reduction of sodium intake, increased intake of foods high in complex carbohydrates and low in protein, and reduction or elimination of caffeine, especially during the two weeks prior to menses (ACOG, 2000). Some authors recommend a diet that consists of 60% complex carbohydrates, 20% protein, and 20% fat (preferably high in omega-3 fatty acids). Cravings may be controlled by eating at more frequent intervals rather than increasing caloric intake (Brown, Freeman, & Ling, 1998).

Dietary supplementation with various vitamins and minerals has been tried for the relief of PMS symptoms, but actual clinical data to support their claims are limited.

Vitamin B6 (pyridoxine) has been traditionally been used to reduce mastalgia and improve mood, but a recent meta-analysis of clinical trials was unable to definitively show any overall benefit of pyridoxine in women with PMS (Wyatt, Dimmock, Jones, & O'Brien, 1999). However, limited evidence suggests that 50 to 100 mg of B6 daily may be helpful. Higher doses of pyridoxine ($>$ 100 mg/day) have been associated with development of peripheral neuropathy.

Use of vitamin E (alpha tocopherol) for treating PMS symptoms evolved from its use in treatment of fibrocystic breast disease. High-dose vitamin E (400 IU) has been shown to reduce mood symptoms and food cravings but has had minimal effects on physical symptoms, including breast tenderness. Lower doses of vita-

TABLE 35–3. ACOG Recommendations for Treatment of Premenstrual Disorders

Step One	Supportive therapy, complex carbohydrate diet, aerobic exercise, nutritional supplements (Calcium, magnesium, vitamin E), spironolactone
Step Two	SSRIs (fluoxetine or sertraline preferred); if no response, consider anxiolytic for specific symptoms
Step Three	Hormonal ovulation suppression (BCPs or GnRH agonists)

min E have provided no symptom relief (London, Bradley, & Chiamor, 1991).

The benefit of calcium supplementation in relieving PMS symptoms has been demonstrated by a number of clinical trials. Women who received 1200 mg of calcium carbonate per day noted a decrease in negative affect, water retention, food cravings, and pain. Overall, 84% of women in calcium group experienced a > 50% improvement in symptoms compared to 52% of women who received a placebo (Thys-Jacobs, Starkey, Bernstein, et al., 1998).

Trials of magnesium supplementation (200 to 360 mg/day) have produced varying degrees of improvement in mood and physical symptoms such as fluid retention (Facchinetti, Borela, Sances, et al., 1991; Walker, De Souza, Vickers, et al., 1998). The inconsistent findings may be related to dosage or the degree of magnesium depletion in study subjects.

Numerous herbal and natural dietary supplements have been marketed for relief of PMS symptoms. Most of these products have limited clinical data to support their claims. Evening primrose oil, which contains gamma-linolenic acid and essential fatty acids, has been promoted as relieving breast pain. A systematic review of clinical trials indicated inconsistent benefit in reduction of breast symptoms and limited to no effect on mood or other physical symptoms (Blommers et al., 2002; Budeiri, Liwan Po, & Dornan, 1996; Douglas, 2002; Fellin et al., 2002). Diets high in fish oil, which contains omega-3 fatty acids, may impair prostaglandin production and result in a reduction of menstrual pain and cramping (Harel, Biro, Kottenhahn, & Rosenthal, 1996). In one study, St John's wort has been shown to significantly improve mood and decrease breast tenderness and swelling (Stevinson, 2000). Studies with chaste-tree berry (vitex agnus castus) support its role in reducing the physical symptoms of PMS (Loch, Selle, & Boblitz, 2000). Other nonpharmacologic therapies that have been promoted for relief of PMS symptoms include phototherapy, acupuncture, transcutaneous electrical nerve stimulation (TENS), and spinal manipulation (Sagraves et al., 2001). See Chapter 10 for additional information on herbal therapies.

Time Frame for Initiating Therapy. Self-awareness of symptom severity and symptom patterns is the first step to treatment. For some women, self-monitoring alone may be enough to assist them in making appropriate lifestyle changes. Monitoring stress in relationships and work and the individual's reaction to these stressors is also an important first step. A trial of nonpharmacologic interventions is recommended prior to changing to or adding drug therapy. Pharmacologic interventions should be targeted either at symptom relief or at correcting a presumed endocrine or neurotransmitter imbalance. Drug therapy can be initiated at any time based on the clinical assessment and patient preferences.

See Drug Tables 208, 301, 304, 306, 307, 309, 310, 311, 603, 605, 608, 705.

Assessment and History Taking. Before initiating either nonpharmacologic or pharmacologic treatment for PMS, it is necessary to obtain a thorough description of the patient's symptoms and their severity, as well as the effect that these symptoms have had on her ability to function. The initial evaluation should include an assessment of the patient's menstrual, obstetric, and gynecologic history, family history of PMS or other affective disorders, and a complete drug history. It is important to explore the impact that her symptoms have had on her relationships, professional activities, and family life.

Information gathered from the PMS history provides general information about the woman's symptom experience, but retrospective symptom severity reports are likely to overestimate severity and do not provide data about symptom patterns. A prospective menstrual or PMS calendar kept for a minimum of two menstrual cycles is useful for women to describe their unique symptoms and symptom clusters and help to visualize symptom severity patterns. Several validated PMS self-rating scales are available to help identify symptoms and quantify their severity (Thys-Jacob, Alvir, Fratarcangelo, 1995).

The diagnosis of PMS requires that symptoms appear or increase in severity during the luteal phase and disappear or return to baseline shortly after the onset of menses. The National Institute of Mental Health (NIMH) has recommended that the diagnosis of PMS be made only if the symptom severity scores change by at least 30% during the luteal phase.

A general physical examination is recommended to help rule out other causes for the symptoms that the woman is experiencing. Other gynecologic disorders, endocrine abnormalities, and psychiatric illnesses need to be ruled out as either the cause or as concomitant conditions exacerbating the woman's symptoms.

There are no specific laboratory tests that can confirm the diagnosis of PMS, but there are several tests that should be considered to rule out other causes. TSH, CBC, prolactin levels and FSH, urinalysis, and cultures for STDs may help establish the presence of another diagnosis. Routine measurements of serum estrogen and progesterone levels are not recommended.

Patient/Caregiver Information. Women with PMS are usually relieved to learn that they have a recognized medical condition, that they are not crazy, and that there are effective treatments available to treat their symptoms. Education and support, along with self-monitoring of daily health and perimenstrual symptoms, are all the treatment some patients will need. Family members and coworkers also need to receive information on the condition to increase their awareness of the role that relationships play in symptom management. Many women find they can control their symptoms without pharmacologic intervention just by making changes in diet, exercise habits, and lifestyle. If pharmacologic therapy is indicated, the woman should receive complete information on how the drug works, potential adverse effects, and when to anticipate a therapeutic response. In addition, some women may benefit from participating in a self-help group where they can share problems and learn more effective strategies for self-management of PMS symptoms.

Outcomes Management

Selecting an Appropriate Agent. Pharmacologic interventions for PMS have been based on a number of theories that suggest that the symptoms of PMS are caused by imbalances or deficiencies of certain endogenously produced substances, including progesterone, estrogen, aldosterone, prostaglandins, and serotonin (Fankhauser, 1999). The medical literature indicates a growing support for the role of serotonin imbalance in PMS and a lack of evidence confirming the role of progesterone deficiency as a causal mechanism (Dimmock, Wyatt, Jones, et al., 2000; Wyatt, Dimmock, Jones, Obhrai, & O'Brien, 2001).

Selection of an appropriate agent for treatment of PMS may be accomplished by taking a symptom-focused approach, especially for the physical symptoms. Many of the mild physical symptoms associated with PMS (cramps, headache, and fluid retention) can be managed with nonprescription products, such as aspirin, acetaminophen, and nonprescription strength ibuprofen and naproxen.

NSAIDs may be effective in relieving breast and joint pain, abdominal cramps, and menstrual headaches but provide no relief from emotional or behavioral symptoms. Ibuprofen (Motrin) 200 to 400 mg every 4 to 6 h, or naproxen sodium (Anaprox) 550 mg followed by 275 mg every 6 to 8 h, should be begun at least 7 days prior to menses for maximum effectiveness (see Drug Table 306).

If menstrual headaches are not relieved by NSAIDs, other drugs such as beta blockers (see Drug Table 205) or tricyclic antidepressants (see Drug Table 311) may be given prophylactically to abort the occurrence of the headaches. Low-dose estradiol (see Drug Table 605), administered orally or by transdermal patch, may be helpful in decreasing the symptoms of a menstrual migraine if started within 3 days before menses and continued for 7 days through menstruation.

Increased breast tenderness and swelling unrelieved by diuretics, decreased caffeine intake, and Vitamin E may be relieved by bromocriptine, which suppresses prolactin secretion. Doses of 1.25–2.5 mg twice daily taken from ovulation until the start of menses have been shown to reduce breast engorgement and mastalgia. Severe symptoms may require treatment with danazol. Because of its significant antiestrogen effects, danazol 50 to 100 mg bid should be reserved for short-term use in refractory patients (Fankhauser, 1999).

Insomnia and complaints of restless sleep can be treated with nonprescription antihistamines such as diphenhydramine 25 to 50 mg at bedtime. Melatonin, kava and valerian, dietary supplements, may also help decrease sleep latency (see Ch. 10). Alternative treatments include low doses of sedative antidepressants such as trazodone, taken 1 to 2 h before bedtime. Chronic use of benzodiazepines as sedative hypnotics is not recommended because of the potential for physical dependence and rebound insomnia after discontinuation.

Diuretics (see Drug Table 208), such as the aldosterone inhibitor spironolactone (Aldactone) 25 to 50 mg bid, qid, have been used to treat the premenstrual fluid retention that may occur. Fluid retention or bloating generally responds well to nonpharmacologic measures such as decreased intake of high-sodium–containing foods and increased water intake. Diuretics, if used, should be taken only during the week prior to menses (ACOG, 2000).

If an etiology-based approach is taken to the treatment of PMS, data seem to suggest that drugs that effect serotonin and/or hormone activity are important to consider when selecting an agent. If serotonin dysregulation is considered an etiology for PMS, selective serotonin reuptake inhibitors (SSRIs) should be strongly considered for first-line therapy.

Although SSRIs primarily improve behavioral symptoms, some studies have also noted improvement in physical symptoms of PMDD (Dimmock et al., 2000). Data from placebo-controlled trials indicate that fluoxetine (Prozac), sertraline (Zoloft), and paroxetine (Paxil) are all effective in the management of PMS (Ericksson, Hedberg, Andersch, et al, 1995 Yonkers, Halbreich, Freeman, et al., 1997; Steiner Steinberg, Stewart, et al, 1995). In addition, nortriptyline, nefazodone, clomipramine (Anafranil), and fluvoxamine also have been shown to be effective based on limited clinical studies (Fankhauser, 1999). Response to SSRI therapy occurs rapidly, even with intermittent therapy, suggesting a mechanism of action that is different from that seen in the treatment of depression.

Since the SSRIs are similar in efficacy, the choice of agent should be based on patient symptoms, side-effect profile, and cost. An activating drug, such as fluoxetine, may be a good initial choice for the woman who is depressed with low energy; if the woman is experiencing significant problems with insomnia, irritability, or anxiety, sertraline or paroxetine may be a better initial choice. If one agent does not work or is not tolerated, try another SSRI before declaring treatment a failure and switching to another class of drugs. Allow sufficient time for a trial of a drug.

Currently, only fluoxetine, sertraline (Zoloft), and paroxetine (Paxil CR) have FDA-approved indications for PMDD (Grady-Weliky, 2003). Fluoxetine is approved for this indication under the brand name Sarafem, not Prozac, to reduce some of the perceived stigma by patients of having to take an antidepressant.

If cost is an issue, prescribe a higher-dose pill and have the patient cut it in half. For example, the 100-mg sertraline (Zoloft) tablet costs the same as the 50-mg tablet. Generic fluoxetine is now available at a significant cost savings compared to the brand name SSRIs.

Therapy should be initiated at half the recommended dose for depression. If tolerated, increase the dose after 1 to 2 weeks. Clinical trials have studied both full menstrual cycle dosing starting on day 1; others have limited treatment to the luteal phase only (last 14 days before menses) (Sagraves, et al., 2001). Another option is to use half the dosage for the first 2 to 3 weeks of the menstrual cycle and increase the dosage during the time when the woman becomes more symptomatic.

If an SSRI is ineffective, alprazolam (Xanax) is another option (see Drug Table 309). It is well tolerated and shown to be effective for PMS when taken only during the luteal phase (Freeman, Rickels, Sondheimer, & Polansky, 1995). Initiate therapy with 0.25 mg tid, and increase to a total of 1 to 1.25 mg/day. Use should be limited to only the luteal phase (some women may require only 4 to 5 days of therapy), and the dose should be tapered at the start of menses to avoid withdrawal symptoms. If alprazolam is contraindicated or ineffective, buspirone (BuSpar) 10 mg tid taken during the entire menstrual cycle is an effective alternative (Rickels, Freeman, & Sondheimer, 1989).

Regardless of the lack of evidence confirming progesterone deficiency as a causal mechanism for PMS, progesterone is still prescribed by many practitioners and anecdotal reports suggest dramatic responses in some women. However, numerous randomized placebo-controlled clinical trials have shown that neither natural progesterone (in suppositories or micronized oral preparations) nor synthetic progestins are more effective than placebo for PMS (Wyatt et al., 2001). Progesterone therapy for treatment of PMS is not FDA-approved, and the patient should be so informed (see Drug Table 605).

For women who experience symptoms that begin at ovulation or who have significant perimenstrual pain, suppression of ovarian function with low-dose oral contraceptives (see Drug Table 603) may decrease the severity of physical symptoms (Fankhauser, 1999). Monophasic pills are preferred because of fewer mood changes.

The newer oral contraceptive Yasmin contains estradiol and drospirenone, a progestin that has antimeralocorticoid activity similar to sprironalactone. In addition to inhibiting ovulation, it may reduce water retention, negative affective symptoms, and increased appetite (Brown, Ling, & Wan, 2002).

GnRH agonists may be indicated in women who continue to be symptomatic and do not respond to other hormonal regimens (see Drug Table 608). GnRH agonists relieve symptoms of PMS by producing a chemical oophorectomy. Available products include goserelin acetate (Zoladex), leuprolide acetate (Lupron Depot), and intranasal nafarelin acetate (Synarel). These agents induce a "pseudomenopause" and increase the risk of osteoporosis so their use should be reserved for severe cases only. GnRH agonists may be given for longer periods of time if the patient is given oral contraceptives concurrently as "addback" therapy (Surrey, 1999).

Many other pharmacological therapies have been tried for PMS (e.g., clonidine, lithium, valproic acid, carbamazepine, verapamil), but few controlled studies are available to confirm either their efficacy or safety. Additional controlled clinical studies are needed before these alternative therapies become a part of standard practice (Sagraves et al., 2001).

Monitoring for Efficacy. Determining efficacy or therapeutic failure with any of the pharmacologic treatments prescribed for the symptoms of PMS requires use for at least two menstrual cycles. Doses of SSRIs may be increased after 1 week of treatment if therapy was initiated with half the dose used for depression. After establishing a therapeutic response, doses may be reduced for the first

2 to 3 weeks of each menstrual cycle. An alternative would be to take just the SSRI during the luteal phase of the cycle. Assessment of the efficacy of NSAIDs and diuretics should be based on the patient's perception of the relief of physical symptoms.

Followup should be scheduled for 3 months for assessment of drug efficacy and lifestyle modifications. The patient should continue to keep her menstrual symptom calendar to provide objective documentation of treatment efficacy or failure.

Monitoring for Toxicity. Each of the therapies has its own unique side effects. Activating SSRIs, such as fluoxetine, may cause insomnia, irritability, and agitation, which may require a change to a less activating agent, such as sertraline or paroxetine. Loss of libido and anorgasmia have been reported with long-term use of some of the SSRIs (Woodram & Brown, 1998). A change to another agent or a drug holiday may restore sexual function. Benzodiazepines should be avoided in women with a history of alcohol or drug abuse. Abrupt discontinuation may produce withdrawal symptoms.

Oral contraceptives are generally well tolerated. However, depressive symptoms may be exacerbated in about one third of women. GnRH agonists may cause menopausal symptoms such as hot flushes, genitourinary changes, and mood changes and increase the risk of osteoporosis. These agents should be avoided in women who have a past or current history of depression. Treatment should be limited to 6 consecutive months to avoid adverse effects.

Overuse of NSAIDs may result in gastrointestinal irritation and bleeding, fluid retention, elevations in blood pressure, and renal insufficiency.

Chapter 19 on menopausal therapies and Chapter 18 on oral contraceptives contain more extensive discussions of the adverse effects associated with progesterone and estradiol. The Drug Tables also contain a more in-depth coverage of dosages, adverse effects, and drug interactions for all drugs discussed in this chapter.

DYSMENORRHEA

Dysmenorrhea is the most frequently encountered gynecological disorder (Silberstein, 2003). In the United States over half of women of childbearing age experience some degree of painful menstruation. Approximately 10% of these women have dysmenorrhea severe enough to incapacitate them for 1 to 3 days each month, resulting in increased absenteeism and economic loss (Coco, 1999). Dysmenorrhea is the leading cause of absenteeism for adolescent females and is reported to be one of the most frequent reasons for young females to seek medical advice.

Dysmenorrhea is classified as either primary or secondary. *Primary dysmenorrhea* occurs in the absence of pelvic pathology, whereas *secondary dysmenorrhea* occurs as the result of some other underlying gynecological condition, such as endometriosis, cervical stenosis, pelvic inflammatory disease (PID), or congenital malformations. Secondary dysmenorrhea should be considered when there is a history of recurrent PID, irregular menstrual cycles, menorrhagia, IUD use, or infertility (Coco, 1999).

Primary dysmenorrhea usually presents within the first 6 to 12 months after menarche, when ovulatory cycles are established. The pain typically begins 1 to 2 h before the onset of menstrual flow and lasts several hours up to 1 to 2 days, usually diminishing with onset of menstrual bleeding. The pain is characteristically a dull, crampy ache located in the suprapubic area with radiation to the lower back and anterior thighs. The pain often is accompanied by nausea, vomiting, diarrhea, headache, dizziness, and fatigue. The severity of primary dysmenorrhea is associated with the duration of menstrual flow, cigarette smoking, and early menarche (Harlow & Park, 1996).

The pathophysiology of primary dysmenorrhea is related to an increased production and release of prostaglandins ($PGF_{2\alpha}$ and PGE_2) in the endometrial lining, resulting in increased uterine contractions, vasospasm, and cramping (Silberstein, 2003).

Secondary dysmenorrhea usually occurs either with the first menses or after age 25. The pain often begins earlier and lasts longer than with primary dysmenorrhea. The characteristics of the pain vary depending on the etiology of the secondary dysmenorrhea.

Specific Considerations for Pharmacotherapy

When Drug Therapy is Needed. The pain and systemic symptoms associated with primary dysmenorrhea are thought to be prostaglandin-mediated so that the logical first-line treatment should involve prostaglandin inhibition with one of the NSAIDs or selective COX-2 inhibitors. Another therapeutic option would be one of the low-dose combination oral contraceptives. This option could be considered as primary therapy if the woman also needs a method of birth control (Sagraves et al., 2001). Cyclooxygenase-2 (COX-2) inhibitors, though use is limited because of cost, are FDA approved for dysmenorrhea (Silberstein, 2003).

By suppressing prostaglandin synthesis, NSAIDs decrease the concentration of $PGF_{2\alpha}$ in the endometrium, resulting in a decrease in uterine contractility, and systemic symptoms, nausea and diarrhea. Oral contraceptives suppress ovulation, which results in lower levels of prostaglandins in the endometrium and menstrual blood loss (Sagraves et al., 2001).

Treatment of secondary dysmenorrhea should be based on the etiology of the dysmenorrhea.

Short- and Long-Term Goals of Pharmacotherapy. The short-term goal of therapy should be to relieve the pain of dysmenorrhea and other associated symptoms. An NSAID with a quick onset of effect, such as ibuprofen (Motrin, others), diclofenac potassium (Cataflam), or naproxen sodium (Anaprox, Aleve), provides the most rapid alleviation of symptoms. Diuretics may help relieve some of the symptoms of bloating and water retention.

The long-term goals should be to prescribe either an NSAID or oral contraceptives to prevent or diminish future episodes of dysmenorrhea. NSAIDs are more effective when they are started prior to or at the onset of menses.

Time Frame for Initiating Therapy. If the woman is symptomatic at the time of the office visit, drug therapy with an NSAID should be started immediately to relieve symptoms. If the woman is not currently experiencing dysmenorrhea, she should be given a prescription to be used with the onset of her next menstrual period. Oral contraceptives may be initiated either on the first day of menses or on the first Sunday after the onset of menstrual bleeding. They will not provide acute relief of symptoms.

See Drug Tables 208, 306, 307, 603.

Assessment and History Taking. A complete menstrual history, sexual history, and description of symptoms should be taken prior to diagnosis or treatment. Physical findings are usually normal with primary dysmenorrhea and a pelvic examination may not be necessary in a nonsexually active adolescent with a typical presentation. Causes of secondary dysmenorrhea should be initially evaluated with a pelvic examination, Pap smear, pregnancy test, and cultures for STDs. Tests to identify specific pelvic pathology may include a pelvic ultrasound and exploratory laparoscopy.

Patient/Caregiver Information. Patients should be given information on the menstrual cycle and the causes of dysmenorrhea. Women with primary dysmenorrhea should be reassured that their symptoms are not caused by some other gynecological condition. Women with secondary dysmenorrhea may benefit from stress reduction and relaxation techniques or referral to a support group. Patient education should be provided on the medications prescribed including when they should be taken, when to expect pain relief, and potential side effects. See Tables 35–4 and 35–5.

Outcomes Management

Selecting an Appropriate Agent. The initial choice of therapy for primary dysmenorrhea should be one of the NSAIDs, which decrease both endometrial and menstrual fluid prostaglandin concentrations. NSAID selection should be based on overall effectiveness, onset of symptom relief, side effects, and cost as well having an FDA-approved indication for primary dysmenorrhea.

Certain classes of NSAIDs appear to be more effective than others in relieving the symptoms of dysmenorrhea. These include the indole acetic acids, propionic acids, salicylic acids, and fenamates (refer to Drug Tables 306, 307 for specific products). Mefenamic acid (Ponstel) may have a theoretical advantage over other NSAIDs because it appears to antagonize the action of formed prostaglandins at the receptor sites, in addition to inhibiting their production (Sagraves et al., 2001). However, its clinical use is limited by a high incidence of GI side effects and cost.

NSAIDs with the FDA-approved indication for primary dysmenorrhea include ibuprofen, diclofenac potassium (Cataflam), ketoprofen (Orudis), naproxen and naproxen sodium (Aleve, Anaprox), meclofenamate sodium (Meclofen), and mefenamic acid (Ponstel). All of these have a rapid onset of effect within 30 min to an hour after administration.

All of the approved agents are effective if used as soon as the pain begins or at the onset of menses. The medication should be continued for the first 2–3 days of menstrual flow. Ibuprofen is usually the drug of choice because it is inexpensive, available in several strengths, and can be purchased without a prescription.

If a clinical response is not seen with a particular agent, the subsequent doses should be increased or a

TABLE 35–4. What Patients Need to Know to Prevent or Treat Dysmenorrhea

Education regarding normal menstrual cycle and causes of dysmenorrhea
Aerobic exercise should be continued, as possible
Advise cessation of cigarette smoking
Use heating pads or hot water bottles
Limit sodium and caffeine intake
Increase dietary intake of omega-3 fatty acids
TENS (transcutaneous nerve stimulation)
Use relaxation techniques and stress therapy
Contact support groups

TABLE 35–5. ACOG Recommendations for Treatment of Premenstrual Disorders

Step One	Supportive therapy, complex carbohydrate diet, aerobic exer cise, nutritional supplements (calcium, magnesium, vitamin E), spironolactone
Step Two	SSRIs (fluoxetine or sertraline preferred); if no response, consider anxiolytic for specific symptoms
Step Three	Hormonal ovulation suppression (BCPs or GnRH agonists)

change made to an alternative agent (Sagraves et al., 2001). Alternative agents could include COX-2 selective inhibitors, such as celecoxib (Celebrex), rofecoxib (Vioxx), and valdecoxib (Bextra), in women who cannot tolerate the GI side effects of NSAIDs.

If a woman also desires a method of contraception, a combination oral contraceptive may be the initial drug of choice. They are effective in controlling symptoms of dysmenorrhea in more than 90% of women. If symptoms are relieved but still present after a trial of 3 to 4 months, an NSAID may be added to the regimen.

There are numerous nonprescription products that are marketed for the relief or prevention of dysmenorrhea symptoms. Most of these products contain various combinations of aspirin, acetaminophen, ibuprofen, caffeine, and "natural" diuretics. The effectiveness of any of these expensive products is limited to, at most, a mild analgesic effect unless they contain ibuprofen.

Monitoring for Efficacy. An appropriate NSAID should provide some symptomatic relief within 30 min to 1 h after ingestion. If pain relief does not occur, repeat and double the next dose. With the next menstrual cycle, start with the increased dose. If relief of symptoms does not occur, switch to another NSAID. A trial of 3 to 6 months should be adequate to determine the effectiveness of therapy. Therapy should be taken on a continuous basis through the first 48 to 72 h of menstrual flow rather than on an as-needed basis (Sagraves et al., 2001).

Oral contraceptives should be taken for three to four menstrual cycles to determine their clinical effectiveness. An NSAID may be added at that time if symptoms are improved but still occurring.

Monitoring for Toxicity. Adverse effects associated with NSAID use for primary dysmenorrhea should be uncommon except for gastrointestinal irritation, because of their limited, intermittent use. GI side effects can be reduced if NSAIDs are taken with food or an antacid, or change to a COX-2 inhibitor. Other side effects that might occur include dizziness, visual disturbances, rash, tinnitus, fluid retention, and increased risk of bleeding. (Refer to Drug Table 306 for a more inclusive list of side effects and contraindications) Potential side effects and contraindications with oral contraceptives would be the same as those experienced when prescribed as a method of birth control (see Drug Table 603).

ENDOMETRIOSIS AND ADENOMYOSIS

Endometriosis and adenomyosis are discussed together in this section as they have several similar characteristics. They both involve the growth of endometrial glands and stroma outside the uterine cavity; retrograde menstruation or spread through other pathways, such as the lymphatics, are the likely causes in endometriosis; a genetic tendency is associated with endometriosis; and they both cause painful, heavy menses; and the treatment is generally the same for both conditions (Gordon & Speroff, 2002).

The most common sites of endometrial implants outside the uterine cavity are the ovaries, broad ligament, posterior cul-de-sac, bladder serosa, fallopian tubes, and large bowel. The degree of disease does not always correlate with the severity of symptoms. With adenomyosis, endometrial tissue grows into the myometrium, or uterine wall (Forrest, 2004; Memarzadeh, Muse, & Fox, 2003).

SPECIFIC CONSIDERATIONS FOR PHARMACOTHERAPY

When Drug Therapy Is Needed

Severe, or even moderate, dysmenorrhea can be life-disrupting. For this reason alone, drug therapy is needed, since dysmenorrhea is a very common symptom of endometriosis and adenomyosis. Infertility, with all its emotional trauma, is associated frequently with endometriosis and occasionally with adenomyosis. Pharmacotherapy may be needed in the management and resolution of this stressful problem.

Short- and Long-Term Goals of Pharmacotherapy

Pharmacotherapy goals are to halt stimulation of the endometrial implants, decrease severity of symptoms, and preserve fertility if the woman so desires.

Nonpharmacologic Therapy

Herbal teas (such as that made from vitex berries, wild yam rhizome, and cramp bark), hot water bottles, and massage may help alleviate pelvic discomfort. Yoga, exercises to relieve pelvic congestion, warm tub baths, and biofeedback also may be useful.

In severe cases, surgical intervention may be necessary. Laparoscopic cautery or laser surgery is used for endometrial implants. Total hysterectomy and bilateral salpingo-oophorectomy may be done if all other medical and conservative surgical therapies have failed.

Time Frame for Initiating Pharmacotherapy

Therapy should be initiated after a diagnosis has been made; however, medications are frequently given to alleviate dysmenorrhea before a definitive diagnosis by laparoscopy is made.

See Drug Tables 306, 603, 605, 608.

Assessment and History Taking

A complete history and physical examination, with careful pelvic and rectovaginal assessment, is needed. A menstrual history, reproductive history, and sexual history should be obtained. Questions should be asked concerning dyspareunia, dysmenorrhea, STDs, PID, and infertility (Memarzadeh, Muse, & Fox, 2003).

On pelvic examination, tender uterosacral ligaments or tender nodules in the posterior cul-de-sac may be palpated with endometriosis. The uterus may become fixed and retroverted as the disease advances (Gordon & Speroff, 2002). In adenomyosis, the uterus is globular and diffusely enlarged as much as two to three times normal size. It may have a fine granular or nodular surface. In both endometriosis and adenomyosis, the uterus may be tender with compression (Star, 1995).

Although no specific laboratory tests are available for the assessment of endometriosis and adenomyosis, cultures should be taken to rule out gonorrhea and chlamydia, and a pregnancy test and Pap smear should be done. The CA-125 level may be elevated with endometriosis, but this is neither specific nor sensitive enough to help with diagnosis (Adamson, 1990). Definitive diagnosis of endometriosis is made by laparoscopy. The diagnosis of adenomyosis is frequently made incidentally by the pathologist after hysterectomy or on autopsy (Star, 1995).

Patient/Caregiver Information

Theories of etiology, diagnostic procedures, treatment options, and side effects should be discussed with the patient. Although various medical therapies may be effective, the definitive treatment of chronic pelvic pain associated with endometriosis and adenomyosis is total abdominal hysterectomy with bilateral salpingo-oophorectomy (Gordon & Speroff, 2002; Lu & Ory, 1995), and patients should be made aware of this. If pregnancy is desired, referral should be made to a competent fertility specialist.

OUTCOMES MANAGEMENT

Selecting an Appropriate Agent

If endometriosis or adenomyosis is suspected, the patient may be treated symptomatically as described in the section on dysmenorrhea. NSAIDs can offer symptomatic relief. Since endometriosis cannot be definitively diagnosed without a laparoscopy, referral to a gynecologist is needed not only for diagnosis but also for initial management and treatment. Continued management should be in consultation with the gynecologist.

Oral contraceptives may be given continuously to prevent ovulation and to provide relief from pelvic pain, dysmenorrhea, and dyspareunia (Gordon & Speroff, 2002). OCs have been found to be more effective in relieving menstrual pain and equal to GnRH analogues in other pain relief (Barton, 2001). Almost any combination oral contraceptive has been used with comparable success in promoting symptom relief (Lu & Ory, 1995).

Danazol, an androgen derivative that inhibits endometrial growth is one effective treatment modality (Gordon & Speroff, 2002). Although in the past danazol was given orally in two dosages of 400 mg/day, evidence shows that lower dosages of 400 mg/day can be used for less severe disease (Lu & Ory, 1995). Danazol is an appropriate treatment of endometriosis, but its side effects have decreased patient acceptance of this therapy. Lower doses, under 800 mg/d, may be less effective (Gordon & Speroff, 2002).

Progestin therapy has been shown to be as effective as danazol in the promoting the regression of endometriosis (Gordon & Speroff, 2002). The progestin most commonly used is medroxyprogesterone acetate (MPA) with the oral dosage being 10 to 30 mg/day for 6 months. It may also be given as an IM preparation (Depo-Provera) 100 mg every 2 weeks for four doses, followed by 200 mg/month for 4 months (Lu & Ory, 1995). With the lower cost of progestin therapy compared to danazol, the comparable effectiveness, and the potential for less serious side effects, it is frequently recommended over danazol.

Another class of drugs used to cause a regression in endometrial implants is the GnRH agonists. They are as effective as danazol or progestins (Gordon & Speroff, 2002). These agents decrease the secretion of FSH and LH. Within 6 weeks the circulating levels of ovarian hormones subsequently become so low, the treatment is sometimes called a *medical oophorectomy.* The following medications may be used (Koda-Kimble et al., 2002; Surrey, 1999). GnRH agonists may cause a loss of bone mineral density, so usually are stopped after 6 months (Memarzadeh, Muse, & Fox, 2003).

- Nafarelin (Synarel) intranasal spray, one spray (200 μg/spray) twice daily, administering the spray in a different nostril in the morning and in the evening. This should be continued for 6 months.
- Leuprolide acetate (Lupron or Lupron Depot) 0.5 to 1.0 mg/day SC or 3.75 to 7.5 mg/month IM, respectively.
- Goserelin acetate implant (Zoladex) 3.75 mg SC every 4 weeks for 6 months.

Monitoring for Efficacy

For oral contraceptives, monitoring for efficacy and side effects is the same as for women placed on cyclic oral contraceptive therapy. However, if breakthrough bleeding occurs, the tablet dosage may be increased to two per day, or additional conjugated estrogens, 1.25 mg/day for 2 weeks (Lu & Ory, 1995) or 2.5 mg/day for 1 week (Forrest, 2004).

If danazol therapy is being used, the patient should be seen in 6 weeks and if no improvement has occurred within that time, the dosage may be increased to 600 to 800 mg/day. Therapy usually is continued for 6 months, and up to 90% of patients will have alleviation of pelvic pain (Gordon & Speroff, 2002). A shorter treatment time also may be effective (Lu & Ory, 1995). Women should be seen every 1 to 2 months while receiving this therapy.

Efficacy for progestin therapy has been previously noted. As with danazol, women should be seen monthly or bimonthly and efficacy assessed.

Serum estradiol levels may be monitored when using GnRH. With nafarelin nasal spray, if the patient continues to have menses after 2 months of treatment, the dosage may be increased to 800 μg (Dambro, 1995).

Monitoring for Toxicity

Side effects of danazol include those typically associated with androgenic agents, as well as those associated with low estrogenic states, oily skin, acne, weight gain, emotional lability, vaginal dryness, and hot flashes are the most common. Less frequent may be hirsutism, decreased breast size, and deepening of the voice. The drug also may cause a mild elevation of liver function tests, a decrease in high-density lipoprotein levels, and an increase in low-density lipoprotein levels. Although these side effects usually are reversible when danazol is discontinued, there have been reported cases of permanent voice changes. It would be prudent to obtain LFTs and fractionated cholesterol levels prior to beginning therapy and every 6 months, and to avoid using this treatment in patients who have a history of hyperlipidemia.

Side effects of MPA have previously been discussed. Breakthrough bleeding with MPA is managed the same as with breakthrough bleeding with oral contraceptives, using conjugated estrogens. Untoward effects of estrogen should be monitored (see Chapter 18).

The primary concern with the GnRH agonists is osteoporosis secondary to low estrogen. Their use, therefore, is limited to 6 months. Although the loss of trabecular bone is measurable, it also is reversible (Whitehouse, Adams, Bancroft, Vaughan-Williams, & Elstein, 1990). Hypoestrogenic effects such as atrophic vaginitis, hot flashes, and others previously noted are certainly present with GnRH therapy.

Followup Recommendations

Since medical therapy is seen as suppressive rather than curative and recurrence of symptoms is common once the therapy has been discontinued, close follow-up is recommended and is dependent on the chosen therapy. Referral to, or consultation with, appropriate specialists should occur as indicated.

SEXUAL DYSFUNCTION

Sexual dysfunctions are currently classified into four major categories, according to the *Diagnostic and Statistical Manual of Mental Disorders* (DSM-IV-TR). These categories are (1) sexual desire disorders, including hypoactive sexual desire and sexual aversion disorder; (2) sexual arousal disorders, including female sexual arousal disorder and erectile disorder; (3) orgasmic disorders, including female and male orgasmic disorder, and premature ejaculation; and (4) sexual pain disorders, including dyspareunia and vaginismus (APA, 2000). Sexual dysfunction should be categorized as lifelong or acquired, general or situational, and affecting one or both partners (Rosen & Lieblum, 1995).

Hypoactive sexual desire (HSD) is a "deficiency or absence of sexual fantasies and desire for sexual activity and the disturbance must cause marked distress and interpersonal difficulty" (APA, 2000). The term is used when the etiology for low libido has not been determined. Other organic causes or other psychiatric disorders that may affect sexual desire such as depression need to be ruled out. HSD may be broken down into (1) primary HSD: total lack of sexual desire throughout a woman's life; (2) secondary HSD: loss of previous desire, such as after childbirth; or (3) situational HSD: lack of desire in particular situations but not in others. Common etiologies for HSD include sexual trauma (sexual abuse, incest, or assault) and high amounts of hostility and/or resentment in relationships. Physical causes include depression, high stress levels, medications, and low testosterone levels (Ayres, 1995).

Female orgasmic disorder is diagnosed by a "persistent or recurrent delay in, or absence of, orgasm following a normal sexual excitement phase. The diagnosis should be based on the clinician's judgment that the woman's orgasmic capacity is less than would be reasonable for her age, sexual experience and the adequacy of sexual stimulation she receives" (APA, 2000). Female orgasmic disorder (or anorgasmia) can be categorized as (1) primary anorgasmia: never experienced orgasm by any means including masturbation; (2) secondary anorgasmia: no longer experiences orgasms as a result of physical illness, relationship problems, medications, or stress; (3) situational anorgasmia: achieves orgasm only in certain situations; and (4) coital anorgasmia: can achieve orgasm by manual or oral stimulation but not from intercourse alone (Ayres, 1995).

Dyspareunia is a "recurrent or persistent genital pain in either a male or a female, which causes marked distress or interpersonal difficulty" (APA, 2000). Although one of the most common causes, it is not caused exclusively by lack of lubrication due to insufficient arousal. Lack of lubrication may also be caused by estrogen deficiency, infection, or medications.

Vaginismus is a "recurrent or persistent involuntary spasm of the musculature of the outer third of the vagina that interferes with sexual intercourse" (APA, 2000). Involuntary contraction of the vaginal muscles is often a physical manifestation of psychological or interpersonal factors. Contributing factors may include sexual trauma or abuse, negative family and religious psychosexual messages, and sexual fears and phobia (Rosen & Leiblum, 1995). Pain associated with PID or endometriosis, or fear of cancer, pregnancy, HIV infection, or other STDs also may be associated with vaginismus (Ayres, 1995).

SPECIFIC CONSIDERATIONS FOR PHARMACOTHERAPY

When Drug Therapy Is Needed

Unless the sexual dysfunction is secondary to a medical condition that requires a specific drug for management, such as depression, diabetes, or menopause, pharmacologic interventions should not be considered first-line therapy. They can be adjunctive therapy to nonpharmacologic interventions such as stress management, individual counseling, or couples therapy.

Anxiolytics and/or antidepressants can help in certain cases of sexual dysfunction related to fear, previous sexual abuse, relationship problems, or preoccupation with other life stressors. Depending on the age of the woman, dyspareunia may be related to hormone deficiency and can be relieved with the use of vaginal lubricants and oral or vaginal estrogen replacement.

The addition of oral or topical testosterone may diminish the loss of libido experienced by perimenopausal women. Anorgasmia may be related to medications that the woman may be taking for another medical indication, such as contraception or depression, which may require a change to an alternative agent with less effect on sexual functioning (Woodram and Brown, 1998). Antibiotics may be necessary to treat genitourinary infections that may be causing pain or changes in lubrication that may interfere with sexual pleasure (Ayres, 1995).

Short- and Long-Term Goals of Pharmacotherapy

The short-term goal of pharmacotherapy is to treat any medical condition that is causing pain or discomfort and interfering with normal sexual functioning. This could involve the use of antibiotics to treat genitourinary infections, use of vaginal lubricants, or use of vaginal estrogen creams. If the sexual dysfunction is related to stress or anxiety, short-term benzodiazepines could be prescribed along with behavior modification techniques.

Long-term goals involve appropriate treatment of medical conditions that have an association with sexual dysfunction, such as diabetes and depression. Efforts should be made to optimize management with appropriate drugs for those disease processes. Perimenopausal women should also be evaluated for signs and symptoms of estrogen deficiency that could be relieved with hormone replacement therapy.

Patients who present with a new onset of complaints of problems with sexual function or desire should always be questioned about their use of prescribed medications or substances of abuse. Common medications that can affect the various phases of sexual functioning include antihypertensives, antidepressants, antihistamines, neuroleptics, and histamine H_2 receptor antagonists. Excessive use of alcohol, cocaine, and narcotics may also interfere with the normal phases of sexual arousal (APA, 2000).

Nonpharmacologic Therapy

Counseling is the primary nonpharmacologic therapy for sexual problems. This may take the form of instruction on stress management techniques, counseling for the woman and her partner, or intensive individual psychotherapy.

Of the various approaches, the classic PLISSIT model (Annon, 1976), with its varying levels of intervention, is one of the most widely used. Increased knowledge and skill are required of the practitioner as the levels of intervention are progressively more complex. The four levels are permission, limited information, specific suggestions, and intensive therapy. The following is a brief description of each level:

1. *Permission:* This level is the least complex and provides the patient with the reassurance that she is normal and has professional permission to continue with whatever she is doing, provided the activity is not harmful or detrimental to herself or her partner.
2. *Limited information:* Factual information that addresses the patient's problem or concern is given at this level, with the hope of changing attitude and/or behavior. An example of this could be providing to someone information on how stress affects libido if she is concerned about diminished sex drive during a time of upheaval and change.
3. *Specific suggestions:* Recommendations for behavior change are given here. Suggestions may range from recommending a vaginal lubricant to specific positional changes to increase clitoral contact during intercourse. The nature of the sexual difficulty treated here is limited in scope. For instance, sexual dysfunction that arises from long-term sexual abuse cannot be appropriately addressed at this level.
4. *Intensive therapy:* This is the most complex level. It is used when sexual problems have not been resolved with the first three levels of intervention. Practitioners must have advanced training and skills to intervene at this level; therefore, referral to a sex therapist generally is made at this point.

Time Frame for Initiating Pharmacotherapy

Antidepressants and anxiolytics should only be initiated after nonpharmacologic interventions, such as stress management, counseling, and education about the normal sexual response cycle, have either been ineffective or refused by the patient. Treatment for genitourinary infections or hormone deficiency should be initiated as soon as the diagnosis is made.

Antibiotics should be given for the recommended number of days based on the causative organism and site of infection. Hormone replacement therapy must be taken continuously for symptomatic relief as well as for the long-term benefits of osteoporosis prevention. Anxiolytics and antidepressants are intended for short-term use. An adequate trial to determine the benefit of antidepressants would be 4 to 6 weeks. If effective, the antidepressant should be continued for 6 months.

See Drug Tables 102, 309, 311, 605.

Assessment and History Taking

Women who complain of any sexual dysfunction, no matter what the subsequent diagnosis, should be asked to complete a thorough history, including current health history, past medical and surgical history, and family history. This provides valuable information as to psychological contributors and rules out any organic cause for the dysfunction. The presence of physical symptoms should be explored; acute and chronic illnesses and current medications should be identified. Sexual habits and techniques should be discussed as well as any history of sexual assault and abuse. Lifestyle stressors, job/career stressors, financial stressors, and family and social support systems need to be identified as well as recent changes in the relationship that may contribute to the current problem. Since specific and intimate details are required, this interview must be handled in a respectful, professional manner, and the woman must feel comfortable and be assured that the information she supplies is totally confidential. She should be given a complete and thorough physical examination with careful attention to the thyroid gland. Pelvic examination should note any hooding (or covering) of the clitoris, which can result in decreased sensation, evidence of atrophy, and presence of discomfort at any time during the examination. Laboratory tests may include CBC, thyroid function tests, and any hormone studies deemed necessary.

Patient/Caregiver Information

The patient should receive education about the different phases of the normal sexual response cycle and what physiological or psychological factors can affect them. In some instances, reassure patients that what they are experiencing is considered normal (Anderson & Cyranowski, 1995). The woman needs to become aware of specific situations, individuals, and/or relationships that may be contributing to her dysfunction. Recommend stress management techniques and improving coping skills. Participation in support groups should also be encouraged depending on the patient's comfort level. If the dysfunction is the result of a medical condition that is not well controlled, the importance of compliance with a prescribed therapeutic regimen should be strongly reinforced. If drug therapy is prescribed as part of the management of the sexual dysfunction, the patient needs to understand how the drug needs to taken and any special instructions, potential adverse effects, and drug interactions.

OUTCOMES MANAGEMENT

Selecting an Appropriate Agent

Selecting an appropriate pharmacologic agent and its duration depends on the etiology of the sexual dysfunction. The patient's medication list should be reviewed for optimal therapy of concomitant medical conditions and drugs that possibly may exacerbate sexual dysfunction. See Table 35–6.

Decreased or inhibited sexual desire can often be treated with a short-acting benzodiazepine, such as alprazolam, or one of the SSRIs if the symptoms are stress- or depression-related. If the loss of libido is related to the use of an SSRI, change therapy to another antidepressant with a lower incidence of inhibition of libido and orgasm, such as buproprion (Wellbutrin), nefazadone (Serzone), or venlafaxine (Effexor XR)* (Croft, Settle, Houser, et al., 1999; Gregorian, Golden, Bakce, et al., 2002; Rajucci & Culhane, 2003). Other options for treatment include decreasing the dose of the SSRI to smallest effective dose or adding another drug to treat the sexual dysfunction such as cyproheptadine, yohimbine, or gingko biloba (Frye & Berger, 1998).

TABLE 35–6. Selected Drugs that May Decrease Libido or Prevent Orgasm

Antihypertensives
Thiazides
Methyldopa(Aldomet)
Clonidine (Catapres)
Beta blockers
Tricyclic antidepressants
Selective serotonin reuptake inhibitors
Fluoxetine (Prozac)
Sertraline (Zoloft)
Paroxetune (Paxil)
Citalopram(Calexa)
Phenothiazines
Narcotic analgesics

Additional agents may also cause erectile dysfunction.

If the woman is taking oral contraceptives, switching to an alternative product that contains a more androgenic progestin, such as Lo Ovral, Ovral, or Loestrin 1.5/30, may have a positive effect on libido. With perimenopausal women, the addition of either oral or vaginal estrogen supplements may be helpful. If the woman is already receiving estrogen replacement, supplementation with testosterone may be beneficial.A transdermal testosterone patch for women is being tested in 2004 by Procter and Gamble for release in 2005. Another, Tostella, will be available soon. Testosterone can be given as methyltestosterone 1.25 to 5 mg PO daily, Depo-Testosterone 50 mg IM every 4 weeks, or in the conjugated estrogen 0.625 mg/methyltestosterone 1.25 mg combination product (Estratest).

If the woman is experiencing anorgasmia, the first-line therapy would involve discontinuing any medication that may decrease libido or interfere with the ability to achieve orgasm. Vaginal atrophy may require the use of vaginal lubricants or hormone replacement therapy. Sildenafil (Viagra), vardenafil (Levitra), and tadalafil (Cialis) have been studied for their benefit in women with female sexual dysfunction. Outcomes have been inconsistent and pursuit of an FDA indication for women has been discontinued for sildenafil (Berman, Berman, Toler, et al., 2003; Data on file, Pfizer, 2004; Data on file, Lilly ICOS LLC).

*On June 3, 2004, Wyeth issued a warming that venlafaxine HCL may worsen depression and/or suicidality.

Dyspareunia may be caused by inadequate lubrication, vaginal atrophy, or vaginal infections. Vaginal lubricants such as Lubrin or Astroglide may need to be used prior to intercourse. Vaginal estrogen creams, such as Premarin or Ogen, provide symptomatic relief of vaginal atrophy secondary to estrogen deficiency. The creams need to be used on a daily basis until symptoms begin to subside. They then may be continued on an intermittent basis, usually twice a week. Vaginal infections, urinary tract infections, and pelvic inflammatory disease need to be treated with appropriate antibiotics.

Symptoms of vaginismus can sometimes be relieved with vaginal lubricants and hormone replacement therapy, but the intense constriction of the vaginal muscles may require analgesics for the pain and discomfort. In addition to counseling, benzodiazepines may assist in relieving some of the underlying anxiety that may exist.

Clinical efficacy is based on the relief of signs and symptoms since there are no laboratory tests to follow and the physical examination is usually normal. The exceptions would be if there was an infection or evidence of vaginal atrophy present. Length of treatment will vary based on the underlying problem and the patient's response. The schedule for followup will depend on the etiology of the sexual dysfunction.

Monitoring for Toxicity

The majority of the agents that are prescribed are well tolerated. However, it is important to assess whether the woman is pregnant before initiating therapy since all of the drugs that may be prescribed have a potential effect on pregnancy outcome. The exception is the vaginal lubricants, which have virtually no adverse effects. Chapters 18 and 19 on contraception and menopause contain a more extensive discussion of the adverse effects associated with the hormonal interventions. The benzodiazepines, antidepressants, and antibiotics are covered in depth in other chapters. The Drug Tables contain detailed coverage of drug dosages, adverse effects, and drug interactions for all the drugs discussed in this chapter.

REFERENCES

Adamson, G. D. (1990). Diagnosis and clinical presentation of endometriosis. *American Journal of Obstetrics and Gynecology, 162,* 568.

American College of Obstetricians and Gynecologists (ACOG). (2000). Clinical management guidelines for premenstrual syndrome. *ACOG Practice Bulletin, 15,* 1–8.

American Psychiatric Association (APA). (2000). *Diagnostic and statistical manual of mental disorders* (4th ed, text revision.). Washington, DC: Author.

Anderson, B. L., & Cyranowski, S. (1995). Women's sexuality: Behaviors, response and individual differences. *Journal of Consulting and Clinical Psychology, 63*(6), 891–906.

Annon, J. S. (1976). The PLISSIT Model: A proposed conceptual scheme for the behavioral treatment of sexual problems. *Journal of Sex Education and Therapy, 2,* 1.

Ayres, T. (1995). Sexual dysfunction. In W. L. Star, L. L. Lommel, & M. T. Shannon (Eds.), *Women's primary health care: Protocols for practice.* Washington, DC: American Nurses Association.

Barnhart, K. T., Freeman, E. W., & Sondheimer, S. J. (1995). A clinician's guide to the premenstrual syndrome. *Medical Clinics of North America, 79*(6), 1457–1472.

Barton, S. (Ed.). (2001). *Clinical evidence. Issue 6.* London, UK: BMJ Publishing.

Berman J. R., Berman L. A., Toler S. et al. (2003). Safety and efficacy of sildenafil citrate for the treatment of female sexual arousal disorder: a double-blind, placebo controlled study. *Journal of Urology,* 170:2333–8.

Blommers, J., de Lange-De Klerk, E., Juik, D., Bezemer, P., & Meijer, S. (2002). Evening primrose oil and fish oil for sever chronic mastalgia: A randomized, double-blind, controlled trial. *American Journal of Obstetrics Gynecology, 1875*), 1389–1394.

Botte, M. E. (2003). Dyspareunia. In T. M. Buttaro, J. Tybulski, P. P Bailey, & J. Sandberg-Cook (eds.), *Primary Care: A Collaborative Practice* (2nd ed.). St. Louis: Mosby

Breslin, E.T., & Lucas, V.A. (2003). *Women's health nursing: Toward evidence-based practice.* Philadelphia, PA: Saunders.

Brown, C. S., Freeman, E. W., & Ling, F. W. (1998). An update on the treatment of premenstrual syndrome. *Am J Man Care, 4,* 115–124.

Brown, C. S., Ling, F. W., & Wan, J. (2002). A new monophasic oral contraceptive containing drospirenone: Effect on premenstrual symptoms. *Journal of Reproductive Medicine, 47,* 14–22.

Budieri, D., Li Wan Po, A., & Dornan, J. C. (1996). Is evening primrose oil of value in the treatment of premenstrual syndrome? *Controlled Clinical Trials, 17,* 60–68.

Coco, A. S. (1999). Primary dysmenorrhea. *Am Fam Phys, 60,* 489–96.

Conviser, J. H., & Fitzgibbon, M. L. (1997). Eating disorders. In K. Allen & J. Phillips (Eds.), *Women's health across the lifespan.* Philadelphia: Lippincott.

Croft, H., Settle, E., Houser, T., et al. (1999). A placebo-controlled comparison of the antidepressant efficacy and effects on sexual functioning of sustained-release bupropion and sertraliine. *Clinical Therapeutics, 21* (4), 643–658.

Curry, S. L. (2000). Other disorders of the vulva, vagina, and uterus. In V. Seltzer & W. Pearse (Eds.), *Women's primary health care office practice and procedures* (2nd ed.). New York: McGraw-Hill.

Curry, S. L., & Barclay, D. L. (1994). Benign disorders of the vulva and vagina. In A. DeCherney & M. Pernall (Eds.), *Current obstetric and gynecologic diagnosis and treatment.* Norwalk, CT: Appleton & Lange.

Dambro, M. (1995). *The 5 minute clinical consult.* Baltimore: Williams & Wilkins.

Data on file, Lilly ICOS LLC.

Data on file. Pfizer Inc 2004.

Dimmock, P. W., Wyatt, K. M., Jones, P. W., et al (2000). Efficacy of selective serotonin-reuptake inhibitors in premenstrual syndrome: A systematic review. *Lancet, 356,* 1131–1136.

Douglas, S. (2002). Premenstrual syndrome. Evidence-based treatment in family practice. *Canadian Family Physician, 48,* 1789–1797.

Eriksson, E., Hedberg, M. A., Andersch, B., et al. (1995). The serotonin reuptake inhibitor paroxetine is superior to the noradrenaline reuptake inhibitor maprotiline in the treatment of premenstrual syndrome. *Neuropsychopharmacology, 12,* 167–176.

Facchinetti, F., Borela, P., Sances, G., et al. (1991). Oral magnesium successfully relieves premenstrual mood changes. *Obstetrics and Gynecology, 78,* 177–181.

Fankhauser, M. P. (1999). Menstrual-related disorders. In T. J. DiPiro, R. L. Talbert, G. C. Yee, G. R. Matzke, B. G. Wells, & L. M. Posey (Eds.), *Pharmacotherapy: A pathophysiologic approach* (4th ed.). Stamford, CT: Appleton & Lange.

Forrest, D. E. (2004). Common gynecologic pelvic disorders. In E. Youngkin & M. Davis (Eds.), *Women's health: A primary care clinical guide* (3rd ed.). Upper Saddle River, NJ: Prentice Hall.

Freeman, E. W., Rickels, K., Sondheimer, S., & Polansky, M. (1995). A double-blind trial of oral progesterone, alprazolam, and placebo in treatment of severe premenstrual syndrome. *Journal American Medical Association, 274,* 51–57.

Frye, C. B., & Berger, J. E. (1998). Treatment of sexual dysfunction induced by selective serotonin-reuptake inhibitors. *American Journal Health-System Pharmacology, 55,* 1167–1169.

Gordon, C., & Neinstein, L. (2002). Amenorrhea. In L. Neinstein, *Adolescent health care* (4th ed.). Philadelphia: Lippincott Williams & Wilkins.

Gordon, J. D., & Speroff, L. (2002). *Handbook for clinical endocrinology and infertility.* Philadelphia: Lippincott Williams & Wilkins.

Goroll, A. H., & Mulley, A. G. (2000). *Primary care medicine* (4th ed.). Philadelphia: Lippincott.

Grady-Weliky T. A. (2003). Premenstrual dysphoric disorder. *New England Journal of Medicine;* 348(5):433–438.

Gregorian, R. S., Golden, K. A., Bahce, A., Goodman, C., Kwong, W. J., and Khan, Z. M. (2002). Antidepressant-induced sexual dysfunction. *Annals of Pharmacotherapy;* 36:1577–89.

Griswold, D. (2004). Menstruation and related problems and concerns. In E. Youngkin & M. Davis (Eds.), *Women's health: A primary care clinical guide* (3rd ed.). Upper Saddle River, NJ: Prentice Hall.

Harel, Z., Biro, F. M., Kottenhahn, R. K., & Rosenthal, S. L. (1996). Supplementation with omega-3 polyunsaturated fatty acids in the management of dysmenorrhea in adolescents. *American Journal of Obstetrics and Gynecology, 174,* 1335–1338.

Hatcher, R. A., Trussell, J., Stewart, F., Stewart, G. K., Kowal, D., Guest, F., Cates, W., Jr., & Policar, M. S. (1999). *Contraceptive technology* (17th ed.). New York: Irvington.

International Society for the Study of Vulva Disease. (1991). Issue Committee report on vulvodynia, vulva vestibulitus, and vestibular papillomatosis. *Journal of Reproductive Medicine, 36,* 413.

Jellin, J.M., Gregory, P.J., Batz, F., Hitchens, K., et al. (2002). *Pharmacist's Letter/Prescriber's Letter Natural Medicines Comprehensive Database* (4th ed.). Stockton, CA: Therapeutic Research Faculty.

Johnson, B. J., Johnson, C. A., Murray, J. L., & Apgar, B. S. (2000). *Women's health care handbook* (2nd ed.). Philadelphia: Hanley & Belful.

Jones, K. D., & Lehr, S. T. (1994). Vulvodynia diagnostic techniques and treatment modalities. *Nurse Practitioner, 19*(4), 34.

Kaufman, R. H. (1995). Disease of the vulva and vagina. In D. Lemcke, J. Pattison, L. Marshall, & D. Cowley (Eds.), *Primary care of women.* Norwalk, CT: Appleton & Lange.

Koda-Kimble, M. A., Young, L., Kradjan, W., & Guglielmo, B. (2002). *Handbook of applied therapeutics* (9th ed.). Philadelphia: Lippincott Williams & Wilkins.

Letterie, G. S. (2004). Disorders of menstruation: From amennorrhea to menorrhagia. In Lemcke, D., Pattison, J., Marshall, L., & Cowley, D. (Eds.), *Current care of women: Diagnosis and treatment.* New York: McGraw-Hill.

Lichtman, R., & Duran, P. (1995). The vulva and vagina. In R. Lichtman & S. Papera (Eds.), *Gynecology: Well-woman care.* Norwalk, CT: Appleton & Lange.

Loch, E-G., Selle, H., & Boblitz, N. (2000). Treatment of premenstrual syndrome with a vital pharmaceutical formulation containing Vitex agnus castus. *Journal of Womens Health Gender Based Medicine, 9,* 315–320.

London, R. S., Bradley, L., & Chiamor, N. (1991). Effect of nutritional supplement on premenstrual symptomatology in women with premenstrual syndrome: A longitudinal study. *Journal of the American College of Nutrition, 10,* 494–499.

Lu, P. Y., & Ory, S. J. (1995). Endometriosis current management. *Mayo Clinic Proceedings, 70,* 453.

Markusen, T. E., & Barclay, D. L. (2003). Benign disorders of the New York: McGraw-vulva & vagina. In A. DeCherney & L. Nathan (eds.), Current Obstetric & Gynecologic Diagnosis & Treatment. New York: McGraw-Hill.

McKay, M. (1993). Dysesthetic (essential) vulvodynia: Treatment with amitriptyline. *Journal of Reproductive Medicine, 38*(1), 9.

Memarzadeh, S., Broder, M., Wexler, A., & Derroll, M. (2003). Endometriosis. In DeCherney, A. and Nathan, L. (eds.). *Current obstetrics & gynecologic diagnosis and treatment.* N.Y.: McGraw-Hill.

Nurnberg, H. G., Hensley, P. L., Lauriello, J., et al. (1999). Sildenafil for women patients with antidepressant-induced sexual dysfunction. *Psychiatric Services, 50,* 1076–1078.

Ragucci, K. R., and Culhane, N. S. (2003). Treatment of female sexual dysfunction. *Annals of Pharmacotherapy;* 37:46–55.

Rapkin, A. J. (1992). The role of serotonin in premenstrual syndrome. *Clinics in Obstetrics and Gynecology, 35,* 629–636.

Rickels, K., Freeman, E. W., & Sondheimer, S. (1989). Buspirone in treatment of premenstrual syndrome. *Lancet, 1,* 777.

Rosen, R. C., & Leiblum, S. R. (1995). Treatment of sexual disorders in the 1990s: An integrated approach. *Journal of Consulting and Clinical Psychology, 63*(6), 877–890.

Rubinow, D. (1992). The premenstrual syndrome: New views. *Journal of the American Medical Association, 268,* 1908.

Sagraves, R., Parent-Stevens, L., & Hardman, J. (2001). Gynecological disorders. In M. A. Koda-Kimble & L. Y. Young (Eds.), *Applied therapeutics: The clinical use of drugs* (7th ed.). Philadelphia: Lippincott Williams & Wilkins.

Secor, R. M., & Fertitta, L. (1992). Vulva vesiculitis syndrome. *Nurse Practitioner Forum, 3*(3), 161.

Sensing, E. C. & Bailey, P. P. (2003). Vulvar and Vaginal Disorders. In T. M. Buttaro, J. Tybulski, P. P. Bailey, & J. Sandberg-Cook (eds.), *Primary care: A colaborative practice* (2nd ed.). St. Louis: Mosby.

Skrypzak, B. (1995). Approach to abnormal vaginal bleeding. In D. Lemcke, J. Pattison, L. Marshall, & D. Coley (Eds.), *Primary care of women.* Norwalk, CT: Appleton & Lange.

Shellow, W. V. R. (2000). Approach to bacterial skin infections. In A. Goroll, L. May, & A. Mulley (Eds.), *Primary care medicine.* Philadelphia: Lippincott.

Sober, A. J. (1995). Dermatologic problems. In Goroll, A., May, L., & Mulley, A. (Eds), *Primary care medicine.* Philadelphia: Lippincott.

Solomons, C. C., Melmed, M. H., & Heitler, S. M. (1991). Calcium citrate for vulva vestibulitis. *Journal of Reproductive Medicine, 36,* 879.

Star, W. (1995). Pelvic masses. In W. Star, L. Lommel, & M. Shannon (Eds.), *Women's primary health care: Protocols for practice.* Washington, DC: American Nurses Association.

Steiner, M., Steinberg, S., Stewart, D., Carter, D., Berger, C., Reid, R., Grover, D., & Streiner, D. (1995). Fluoxetine in the treatment of premenstrual dysphoria. *New England Journal of Medicine, 332,* 1529–1534.

Stevinson, C. & Ernst, E. (2000). A pilot study of *Hypericum perforatum* for the treatment of premenstrual syndrome. *British Journal of Gynecology,* 107(7), 870–876.

Stulberg, D., Penrod, M., & Blatny, R. (2002). Common bacterial skin infections. American Family Physicians, 66(1), 119–124.

Surrey, E. S. (1999). Add-back therapy and gonadotropin-releasing hormone agonsits in the treatment of patients with endometriosis: can a consensus be reached? *Fertility and Sterility, 71,* 420–424.

Thys-Jacobs, S., Alvir, J. A. J., & Fratarcangelo, P. (1995). Comparative analysis of three PMS assessment instruments: The identification of premenstrual syndrome with core symptoms. *Psychopharmacology Bulletin, 31,* 389–396.

Thys-Jacobs, S., Starkey, P., Bernstein, et al. (1998). Calcium carbonate and the premenstrual syndrome: Effects on premenstrual and menstrual symptoms. *American Journal of Obstetrics and Gynecology, 179,* 444–452.

Umpierre, S. A., et al. (1991). Human papilloma virus DNA in tissue biopsy specimens of vulva vestibulitis patients treated with interferon. *Obstetrics and Gynecology, 78,* 693.

Walker, A. F., De Souza, M. C., Vickers, M. F., et al. (1998). Magnesium supplementation alleviates premenstrual symptoms of fluid retention. *Journal of Womens Health and Gender Based Medicine, 7,* 1157–1165.

Weil, E. K. (Ed.). (1996). *Nurse practitioner's prescribing reference.* New York: Prescribing Reference.

Whitehouse, R. W., Adams, J. E., Bancroft, K., Vaughan-Williams, C. A., & Elstein, M. (1990). The effects of nafarelin and danazol on vertebral trabecular bone mass in patients with endometriosis. *Clinical Endocrinology, 33,* 365.

Woodram, S., & Brown, C. S. (1998). Selective serotonergic reuptake inhibitor (SSRI)-induced sexual dysfunction. *Ann Pharmacotherapy, 32,* 1209–1215.

Wyatt, K. M., Dimmock, P. W., Jones, P. W., Obhrai, M., & O'Brien, S. (2001). Efficacy of progesterone and progestogens in management of premenstrual syndrome: Systemic review. *British Medical Journal, 323,* 1–8.

Wyatt, K. M., Dimmock, P. W., Jones, P. W., & O'Brien, S. (1999). Efficacy of vitamin B-6 in the treatment of premenstrual syndrome: systematic review. *British Medicial Journal, 318,* 1375–1381.

Yonkers, K. A., Halbreich, U., Freeman, E., et al. (1997). Symptomatic improvement of premenstrual dysphoric disorder with sertraline treatment: A randomized controlled trial. *Journal of the American Medical Association, 278,* 983–988.

CHAPTER ❖ 36

SEXUALLY TRANSMITTED INFECTIONS, VAGINITIS, AND PELVIC INFLAMMATORY DISEASE

Adrianne K. Tillmanns ◆ Susan Rawlins

Sexually transmitted infections (STI) continue to be a widespread problem in the United States with 15 million people becoming newly infected each year and more than 65 million people living with an incurable STI (Cates, 1999). This chapter is an overview of the common sexually transmitted infections (STIs), pelvic inflammatory disease (PID), infestations, and vaginitis. An important viral pathogen, the human immunodeficiency virus (HIV) is covered in Chapter 37 of this book. From the clinician's perspective, comprehensive management of patients with sexually transmitted infections is challenging. The clinician must be engaged in continuous reeducation to stay abreast of new developments such as emerging antibiotic resistance patterns, improved diagnostic tests, and new drugs and treatment regimens. In addition to being proficient at diagnosis and treatment, the clinician needs to be effective at preventing the spread of these infections, by educating and hopefully influencing change in the sexual behaviors that place patients at risk for acquiring or transmitting STIs.

The treatment regimens provided in this chapter closely follow the recommendations of the Centers for Disease Control and Prevention 2002 Guidelines for Treatment of Sexually Transmitted Diseases (STDs) (CDC, 2002a). However, additional current resources are used to supplement the CDC guidelines.

SYPHILIS

Syphilis is an acute and chronic infection caused by the anaerobic spirochete *Treponema pallidum*. This bacterial infection is noted for distinct stages, beginning with localized genital ulcers, progressing through multiple systemic manifestations, and eventually cardiovascular and neurological disease, blindness, and death if not treated. An untreated, infected mother can transmit the infection to her fetus. Syphilis cases had been declining in the United States since they peaked in 1990. In 1998, the low rates of infection coupled with the concentration of cases in a relatively small geographic area prompted the CDC to launch the National Plan to Eliminate Syphilis in the United States (CDC, 1999). The five strategies of the syphilis elimination plan are (1) to increase surveillance, (2) strengthen community involvement and partnerships, (3) rapidly respond to outbreaks, (4) improve and increase health promotion, and (5) expand clinical and laboratory services (CDC, 1999). Since the inception of this plan, progress has been made toward the goal. In 2000, there were 5,979 reported cases of primary and secondary syphilis in the United States, the lowest rate ever recorded since reporting began in 1941 and a 30% drop since 1997, the year before the national plan was initiated (CDC, 2000a). In the same time period, congenital syphilis rates dropped 51% and rates for primary and secondary syphilis among African Americans decreased by 41% (CDC, 2000b). While progress was made, certain groups have been identified as being at high risk for syphilis infection. These are (1) drug users, especially of crack cocaine; (2) those with a history of STD infections; (3) those who exchange drugs or money for sex; (4) those having multiple sex partners; and (5) those with non-heterosexual sexual preference (Bachmann, Lewis, Allen, et al., 2000; Hwang, Ross, Zack, et al., 2000; Lopez-Zetina, Ford, Weber, et al., 2000; & Nuttbrock, Rosenblum, Magura, et al., 2000). However, in 2003, more than 7000 cases were reported (Incidence, 2004). There have been increases reported in men who have sex with men (CDC, 2002b). One recent case report documents female-to-female transmission of syphilis (Campos-Outcalt & Hurwitz, 2002). Syphilis maybe transmitted orally (STDs that are, 2003).

SPECIFIC CONSIDERATIONS FOR PHARMACOTHERAPY

When Drug Therapy Is Needed

Syphilis requires prompt identification and treatment to prevent the transmission of infection to others, including infants, and the progression of disease. Efforts should be made to treat infected women before conception, because fetal infection has been documented with all stages of early syphilis infection (Hollier, Harstad, Sanchez, et al., 2001). The risk of neonatal syphilis after adequate treatment for maternal syphilis is increased with high maternal VDRL titers at treatment or delivery, early stage of maternal syphilis, short interval from treatment to delivery, and preterm delivery (Sheffield, Sanchez, Morris, et al., 2002). In adults, untreated syphilis can progress to destroy tissue and function in the heart, brain, skin, and bone. Although rare, one case report describes neurosyphilis presenting as acute psychosis in a 30-year-old pregnant and previously healthy woman (Kohler, Pickholtz, & Ballas, 2000).

Short- and Long-Term Goals of Pharmacotherapy

For all sexually transmitted infections, the short-term goals are to alleviate the acute symptoms and prevent the adverse health consequences of untreated infection, including PID, infertility, ectopic pregnancy, cancer, and death. Screening at-risk populations identifies infected, asymptomatic individuals and permits treatment before complications occur.

An additional important goal is to prevent the transmission of the infection to other individuals, including fetal and neonatal infection. A long-term goal is pre-exposure immunization of individuals at risk of acquiring vaccine-preventable infections. Finally, once the initial infection is treated, the long-term goal is to prevent the acquisition of new sexually transmitted infections.

Nonpharmacologic Therapy

Pharmacologic therapy is required to cure or relieve symptoms of most sexually transmitted infections. Because many STIs can result in lifelong, incurable infections, prevention is the only option. Prevention is the cornerstone of nonpharmacologic therapy. The two most reliable behaviors to prevent the acquisition of STIs are practicing sexual abstinence or being in a long-term, mutually monogamous relationship with an uninfected partner. Male latex condoms effectively prevent or reduce the risk of transmission of infections, especially those spread by fluids from mucosal surfaces (gonorrhea, chlamydia, trichomonas, etc.). Male condoms are less effective at preventing the transmission of infections that involve skin-to-skin transmission (HPV, HSV, syphilis, etc.) (CDC, 2002a). Nonlatex condoms are available for those with latex allergy. If the male partner cannot or will not correctly use a male condom, women have the option of using the female condom (Reality™). Although studies documenting the efficacy of the female condom in preventing the transmission of infections are lacking, if used consistently, it should substantially reduce the risk of transmission (CDC, 2002a). Dental dams are advised for oral sex.

STI prevention interventions can be directed toward individuals at risk or the social structures that support risky behaviors (Cohen & Scribner, 2001). Clinicians have the opportunity and responsibility to deliver prevention messages at each encounter with clients seeking healthcare. A recent study found that less than 50% of new or experienced OB/GYN physicians assessed condom use, number of sexual partners, or sexual partner risk profile during a general medical examination (Haley, Maheux, Rivard, & Gervais, 2002). Prevention messages to individuals are most effective if tailored to identified risks and describe specific behaviors that if employed will prevent infection (CDC, 2002a). Jaworski and Carey (2001) reported that female college students who received a one-session intervention teaching information, motivation, and behavioral skills had greater reductions in the number of sexual partners than the control group. Another successful prevention intervention involved lay health advisors who were trusted members of high-risk communities. These advisors distributed information and taught skills for reducing STD in their social networks and had documented improvements in STD prevention behaviors in their neighborhoods (Thomas, Eng, Earp, & Ellis, 2001). Structural interventions target conditions that are outside the control of the individual, such as access to condoms and clean needles, media messages that glamorize high-risk behaviors, and social support such as youth supervision (Cohen & Scribner, 2001).

Partner notification and disease reporting are important components of non-pharmacologic disease control. Partner notification, identifying sexual contacts of an infected individual and facilitating treatment, has been a major component of STD control for decades. Kohl, Farley, Ewell, & Scioneaux (1999) demonstrated the continued usefulness of partner notification for syphilis control, but also identified a need for additional strategies. Incorporating partner notification in the larger context of a social network-based approach can help identify core groups of high transmitters and may be useful in reducing the incidence of syphilis (Rothenberg, Kimbrough, Lewis-Hardy, et al., 2000). Every state requires the reporting of syphilis, gonorrhea, chlamydia, and AIDS. Reporting requirements for other STDs and HIV vary by state and clinicians should become familiar with local reporting requirements.

Time Frame for Initiating Pharmacotherapy

For all STIs, therapy should be initiated as soon as the diagnosis is confirmed. There is no need to delay treatment. Treatment delays provide a greater opportunity for transmission of the infection to sexual contacts and development of complications from disease progression.

Pharmacologic management should not be limited to the index patient, but extended to the sex partner(s) as soon as possible. Sexual partners of individuals with primary, secondary, or early latent syphilis who have been exposed within 90 days preceding diagnosis should be presumptively treated. Sexual partners exposed more than 90 days prior to the diagnosis should be evaluated and treated as clinically indicated. Sexual partners of individuals with latent syphilis should be evaluated and treated based on the results of laboratory and exam findings. A more thorough discussion of partner evaluation and treatment can be found in the 2002 CDC STD treatment guidelines (CDC, 2002a). Pregnant women must be screened and treated early to decrease congenital syphils (Gunter, 2003).

See Drug Tables 102.6, 102.11.

Assessment and History Taking

The physical signs and symptoms of syphilis have been described for hundreds of years and appear to have changed little over time. Syphilis has three symptomatic stages: primary syphilis, secondary syphilis, and tertiary syphilis. In addition, syphilis is noted for long periods of latency (latent syphilis) where serologic tests remain positive, but there are no signs or symptoms present (Garnett, Aral, Hoyle, Cates, & Anderson, 1997)

Primary Syphilis. After an incubation period of about 10 to 90 days, a painless chancre appears at the site of inoculation. Depending on the number of penetrating spirochetes, there may be more than one chancre. Common sites of penetrance are the fourchette, cervix, anus, labia, and nipples. The ulcer is usually round, painless, and red and has well-defined raised edges surrounding a granular base. The chancre is extremely infectious, but after about 3 to 8 weeks it heals spontaneously (Garnett et al., 1997).

Secondary Syphilis. If untreated, the disease disseminates and symptoms of secondary syphilis appear 2 to 6 weeks after manifestation of primary syphilis. Unique to secondary syphilis is the occurrence of a maculopapular rash on the palms of hands and soles of feet. This mucocutaneous eruption may also occur throughout the body or remain localized to a particular area. Along with the dermatological manifestations, a low-grade fever, headache, malaise, pharyngitis, anorexia, and arthralgia are also commonly observed. Whether therapy is initiated or not, the rash resolves after about 4 to 10 weeks. Unless treatment is received, the rash could spontaneously reappear anytime within 4 years; therefore, these individuals are still considered infectious (Garnett et al., 1997; Lukehart & Holmes, 1998). A recent study confirmed the most common manifestations of secondary syphilis as skin rash, lymphadenopathy, persistent chancre, mucus patches, condyloma lata, and split papules (Kumar, Gupta, & Muralidhar, 2001).

Latent Syphilis. Latent syphilis is defined as a positive serologic test for syphilis in the absence of clinical manifestations. Latent syphilis is considered early latent when the syphilis infection has been present for less than one year. Early latent syphilis is confirmed with any of the following documented within the past year: (1) seroconversion; (2) symptoms of primary or secondary syphilis; (3) or a sex partner with primary, secondary, or early latent syphilis. All other cases of latent syphilis are considered either late latent or syphilis of unknown duration. Individuals in the latent stage are hosts to the syphilis organism but are not able to transmit the infection to others (CDC, 2002a).

Tertiary Syphilis and Neuro-Syphilis. A small proportion (20 to 30%) of individuals with latent syphilis progress to tertiary syphilis. Tertiary syphilis can involve any organ system or tissue in the body, including cardiac or gummatous lesions. The central nervous system can be affected during any stage of syphilis and can present in a variety of ways, including but not limited to cognitive dysfunction, motor and sensory deficits, ophthalmic or auditory abnormalities, or signs of meningitis (CDC, 2002a; Garnett et al., 1997). The diagnosis and management of tertiary syphilis and neurosyphilis should be by experts in the field and is beyond the scope of this chapter.

Diagnosis

T. pallidum cannot be cultured in vitro; therefore, direct examination of the organism under darkfield microscopy or the use of serologic tests is necessary for laboratory diagnosis. Darkfield microscopy can be used to diagnose primary and secondary syphilis. This method is fairly sensitive and specific for *T. pallidum* because it involves the organisms from chancres, cutaneous external lesions, or mucous patches, which are examined under darkfield microscopy for motile treponemes. However, it requires the specimens to be examined immediately. The direct fluorescent antibody test, *T. pallidum* (DFA-TP), is another alternative that will also give immediate results. Its advantages over darkfield microscopy are that it does not require immediate examination of the specimen and it has higher specificity. (Larsen, Steine & Rudolph 1995; Lukehart, 1998).

Serological testing is divided into *nontreponemal* and *treponemal* tests. Nontreponemal tests measure antilipid antibodies that are specific for the treponeme cell surface. Commonly used nontreponemal tests include the Venereal Disease Research Laboratory (VDRL) test and rapid plasma reagin (RPR) test. False positives may occur (Gunter, 2003). The frequency of reactive nontreponemal tests depends on the stage of the infection with a reported 76% reactive in primary syphilis, 100% in secondary syphilis, 95% in early latent syphilis, and 70% in late latent syphilis. Reactivity is first detected 1 to 3 weeks after the primary chancre (Larsen, Steiner, & Rudolph, 1995). These tests are used for screening and to assess response to therapy. A fourfold decrease in titer (1:32 decreasing to 1:8) within 6 months of treatment indicates appropriate response to therapy. Conversely, a fourfold increase in titer in a previously treated individual indicates reinfection, treatment failure, or inadequate treatment (CDC, 2002a).

Treponemal tests are more sensitive for all stages of syphilis and are used to confirm positive nontreponemal tests. Examples of treponemal tests include the fluorescent treponemal antibody absorption (FTA-ABS) test, and *T. pallidum* particle agglutination (TP-PA). Because treponemal tests remain reactive for life, they are not useful to assess response to therapy. The false-positive rates for treponemal tests are 1 to 2% in the healthy population (Larsen et al., 1995).

OUTCOMES MANAGEMENT

Selecting an Appropriate Agent

Pharmacologic intervention should be initiated as soon as the diagnosis is confirmed to prevent the transmission of infection to others and to prevent potential progression to tertiary syphilis. Despite the development of many new antibiotics, the treatment of choice for the past 50 years has been parenteral penicillin G. In recent years, clinical trials and clinical experience continue to demonstrate and reconfirm the efficacy of penicillin for the treatment of this disease (CDC, 2002a). Treatment recommendations from the CDC are presented in Table 36–1.

The usual treatment of primary, secondary, and early latent syphilis in the non-penicillin allergic patient is a single intramuscular (IM) injection of benzathine penicillin G 2.4 million units. Similarly, the treatment of late latent syphilis is also with benzathine penicillin G 2.4 million units, but given once a week for 3 consecutive weeks. Only neurosyphilis requires treatment with intravenous penicillin G in order to achieve adequate drug levels in the cerebrospinal fluid (CSF) (CDC, 2002a).

Although not considered the gold standard, alternative antibiotics have been used for patients allergic to penicillin. Currently, the CDC recommends doxycycline 100 mg bid., or tetracycline 500 mg qid for 2 weeks to treat syphilis of less than 1 year in duration. (CDC, 2002a). For syphilis greater than 1 year in duration, doxycycline or tetracycline is another good option, and the treatment course is for 4 weeks (CDC, 2002a). Although most experts recommend the same treatment strategies for pregnant women or HIV-infected individuals as non-pregnant and HIV-negative individuals, other experts recommend more intensive therapies. A detailed description of these intensive recommendations can be found in the 2002 CDC treatment guidelines. Penicillin is the drug of choice for treating syphilis in pregnancy because it is the only drug known to reliably cure the infected fetus as well

TABLE 36–1. 2002 CDC Treatment Guidelines

Stage/Type of Syphilis	Recommended Regimen
Primary, secondary, or early latent	Benzathine penicillin G 2.4 million units IM in a single dose
Late latent, unknown duration, or tertiary	Benzathine penicillin G 2.4 million units IM once a week for 3 successive weeks (7.2 million units total)
Neurosyphilis	Aqueous crystalline penicillin G 18 – 24 million units per day, given as 3–4 million units IV every 4 hours or continuous infusion for 10 – 14 days or Procaine penicillin 2.4 million units IM once daily PLUS Probenecid 500 mg orally four times a day, both for 10 – 14 days.
Nonpregnant Penicillin-Allergic patients	
Primary, secondary, or early latent	Doxycycline 100 mg PO two times daily for 14 days or Tetracycline 500 mg PO four times daily for 14 days
Late latent, unknown duration	Doxycycline 100 mg PO two times daily for 28 days or Tetracycline 500 mg PO four times daily for 28 days
Neurosyphilis	Ceftriaxone 2 grams daily either IM or IV for 10 to 14 days.

as the mother. Pregnant women with a history of penicillin allergy should have skin testing with both major and minor determinants. Those women who are skin-test negative can receive conventional penicillin therapy. Those women who are skin-test positive should be desensitized before treatment with penicillin (CDC, 2002a).

Monitoring for Efficacy

Although the failure rate with penicillin is very low, it still can occur. Treatment failure or reinfection should be suspected if symptoms persist, recur, or if nontreponemal titers show a fourfold increase. These individuals should be retreated with the late latent regimen, unless neurosyphilis is diagnosed. Evaluation for HIV infection is also recommended (CDC, 2002a).

Monitoring for Toxicity

Patients should be informed of the possibility of developing the Jarisch-Herxheimer reaction. The Jarisch-Herxheimer reaction is not an allergic response to penicillin, but can result in myalgias, chills, headache, and rash. This reaction can usually be controlled with antipyretics. This reaction occurs commonly with primary and secondary syphilis and less frequently in latent syphilis (CDC, 2002a; Lukehart & Holmes, 1998). The Jarisch-Herxheimer reaction also complicates treatment of syphilis in pregnancy. In pregnancy the reaction is often accompanied by uterine contractions, decreased fetal activity, and occasionally by fetal distress. With a severely affected fetus, preterm labor, delivery, or fetal death may occur (Klein, Cox, Mitchell, & Wendel, 1990). This risk should not delay or deter treatment in pregnancy (CDC, 2002a).

Followup Recommendations

Followup evaluations including serology should be done at 6 and 12 months for primary and secondary syphilis and at 6, 12, and 24 months for latent syphilis (CDC, 2002a).

GONORRHEA

Gonorrhea is a sexually transmitted disease caused by the gram-negative diplococcus *Neisseria gonorrhoeae.* In the United States, approximately 600,000 new cases of gonorrhea are reported by the CDC each year (CDC, 2002a). The highest prevalence of gonococcal infection is in individuals 15 to 24 years of age. Of this group, the majority are women of lower socioeconomic classification, minority race, and unmarried status, living in inner city housing, and who became sexually active at an early age (Fox & Knapp, 1999). Gonorrhea can produce a spectrum of symptoms. The well-known male symptoms of dysuria and urethral discharge cause the patient to seek medical treatment. The symptoms of gonorrhea can be less obvious in women than in men, and in both men and women less recognizable symptoms can present. This can lead to a missed diagnosis by the clinician or a delay or failure to seek medical treatment by the patient. Complications such as pelvic inflammatory disease (PID), ectopic pregnancy, and infertility secondary to tubal scarring can result from unrecognized, untreated gonorrhea (CDC, 2002a; Fox & Knapp, 1999).

SPECIFIC CONSIDERATIONS FOR PHARMACOTHERAPY

When Drug Therapy is Needed

Pelvic inflammatory disease, infertility from tubal scarring, and ectopic pregnancy are several complications related to gonorrhea. Gonococcal infection during pregnancy can lead to spontaneous abortion, premature rupture of the amniotic membranes, chorioamnionitis, disseminated gonococcal disease, and arthritis. Ophthalmia neonatorum, a conjunctivitis caused by *N. gonorrhoeae* that can lead to blindness, is caused by transmission of the organism to infants during delivery. The goals of therapy and the time for initiating therapy are the same as those for syphilis.

See Drug Tables 102.1–5, 102.11.

Assessment and History Taking

In women, the cervix is the common site of infection with extension to involve the urethra in greater than 70% of culture-positive cases. Clinical signs and symptoms associated with cervical infection(s) in females are vaginal discharge, cervical discharge, and cervical mucopus or positive swab test result (Deceunick, Asamoah-Adu, Khonde, et al., 2000). Asymptomatic infection is common and reported as cervix 50%, rectum 85%, and pharynx > 90% (Bignell, 2001).

In the male population the primary site of infection is the urethra, characterized by burning and uretheral discharge. Rectal involvement may cause perianal pain and/or anal discharge. Asymptomatic infections have been reported as urethera <10%, rectum >85%, and pharynx >90%. Therefore, the rectum and posterior pharynx should be cultured (Bignell, 2001; Jephcott, 1997).

Pharyngeal infection occurs in approximately 5% of cases. There is a general consensus that oral pharyngeal infections occur more frequently in homosexual males than females and heterosexual males (Barlow, 1997).

Diagnosis of cervical gonococcal infection can be confirmed via Gram stains, endocervical cultures, or immunoassays (Macsween, Ridgway, & Geoffrey, 1998; Morse, 2001). The endocervical culture is the cornerstone of diagnosis. Culture methods have greater sensitivity and nearly 100% specificity and antibiotic sensitivity information. Although it is the gold standard, culture diagnosis of gonorrhea requires technical expertise, is expensive, and requires 24 to 48 hours for a full report (Jephcott, 1997).

Unlike endocervical cultures, Gram's stains provide immediate information for complete evaluation of the infection and generally are used in clinical practice. Under a microscope, *N. gonorrhoeae* appears as a gramnegative intracellular diplococcus ("Gonorrhea," 1994).

Immunoassays are other diagnostic alternatives to the aforementioned methods. Gonozyme is an enzyme-linked immunosorbent assay (ELISA) that is commercially available (Jephcott, 1997). Its advantages are quick results with minimal technical requirements. Although its specificity and sensitivity are high, they appear to be higher in females than males (Jephcott, 1997). Gonozyme should not be used for extragenital specimens or to assess treatment outcomes because of high crossreactivity with bacterial antigens at those sites; gonococcal antigens still persist despite cure (Jephcott, 1997). Other immunoassays include nucleic acid hybridization, polymerase chain reaction (PCR), and the ligase chain reaction technique. These assays appear to have better sensitivity and specificity compared with more traditional methods; however, technical skill for retrieving specimens and absence of antibiotic sensitivity information must be addressed before the value of these methods can be determined (Jephcott, 1997). The greatest benefit of the nucleic acid amplification tests may be the ability to screen for chlamydia or gonorrhea infection in non-traditional settings using urine or self-administered vaginal swabs.

Patients with gonorrhea are often coinfected with other STIs, particularly *C. trachomatis.* The CDC (2002a) recommends that patients receiving treatment for gonococcal infections be concurrently treated for chlamydia. This requires the addition of an antichlamydial antibiotic.

Because many strains of gonorrhea are sensitive to doxycycline and azythromycin, cotreatment for chlamydia in gonorrhea positive patients may delay the onset of antibiotic resistant gonorrhea.

OUTCOMES MANAGEMENT

Selecting an Appropriate Agent

The development of antibiotic resistance by *N. gonorrhoeae* has limited the usefulness of certain antibiotics, particularly penicillin and tetracycline. Emergence of strains resistant to the quinolone antibiotics also has been reported (Fox & Knapp, 1999). The occurence rate in the United States is currently less than 0.5% except in special populations including men who have sex with men (MSM), women whose male partners have sex with men, or infections acquired in Asia, the Pacific coast of the U.S., England and Wales. In these special populations quinolone resistance exceeds 5% which is the traditional level at which therapeutic regimens are changed. With the increasing emergence of quinolone resistance around the world and in MSM in the U.S., detailed sexual histories and travel histories are necessary for appropriate antibiotic selection (CDC, 2004a). Much has been written on the incidence and mechanism of antibiotic resistance in *N. gonorrhoeae* (CDC, 2004a; Fox & Knapp, 1999; Knapp, Wongba, & Limpakarnjanarat, 1997).

For uncomplicated gonococcal infections, the CDC (2002a) recommends the regimens outlined in Table 36–2. Cure rates achieved with any of these regimens for anal and genital infection are greater than 95%. For pharyngeal infection, ceftriaxone or ciprofloxacin is recommended. Cure rates with these drugs are greater than 90% (CDC, 2002a). For MSM, women whose male partner has sex with men, or infections acquired in areas with high rates of resistance, fluoroquinolones are not longer recommended as first-line therapy (CDC, 2004a).

Currently, there have not been any reports of gonococcal strains resistant to ceftriaxone. Ceftriaxone 125 mg provides sustained bactericidal concentrations in the blood with the same efficacy as higher doses; therefore, higher doses are not necessary (Fox & Knapp, 1999). Drawbacks to ceftriaxone are higher cost, pain at injection site (some practitioners suggest using a 1% lidocaine solution as a diluent to minimize the pain), and lack of commercially available dosage forms of less than 250 mg (CDC, 2002a).

Oral cefixime is a less invasive alternative to ceftriaxone but does not provide the sustained bactericidal concentration in the blood. Therefore, its use should be limited to uncomplicated genital and anal infection (CDC, 2002a) This drug has not been available in the U.S. since 2002. In February 2004, the Food and Drug Administration approved Lupin, Ltd. (Baltimore, Maryland) to manufacture and market cefixime, as yet, the 400-mg tablets

TABLE 36–2. 2002 CDC Treatment Recommendations for Gonorrhea

Infection	Recommended Regimen	Alternative Regimen
Uncomplicated gonococcal infection of the cervix, urethra, and rectum	Cefixime 400 mg orally single dose or Ceftriaxone 125 mg IM single dose or *Ciprofloxacin 500 mg orally single dose or *Levofloxacin 250 mg orally single dose or *Ofloxacin 400 mg orally single dose plus If *C. Trachomatis* infection not ruled out Azithromycin 1 g orally single dose or Doxycycline 100 mg orally BID for 7 days	Spectinomycin 2 g IM single dose or Cefotaxime 500 mg IM single dose or Ceftizoxime 500 mg IM single dose or Cefoxitin 2 g IM with probenecid 1 g orally or *Gatifloxacin 400 mg orally single dose or *Norfloxacin 800 mg orally single dose or *Lomefloxacin 400 mg orally single dose
Uncomplicated gonococcal infection of the pharynx	Ceftriaxone 125 mg IM single dose or *Ciprofloxacin 500 mg orally single dose plus If C. *Trachomatis* infection of other sites not ruled out Azithromycin 1 g orally single dose or Doxycycline 100 mg orally BID for 7 days	See CDC 2002a guidelines for alternatives
Gonococcal meningitis and endocarditis	Ceftriaxone 1–2 g IV q12h; meningitis: for 10–14 days; endocarditis: for at least 4 weeks; consultation with expert recommended	
Pregnancy	Cefrtriaxone 125 mg IM single dose or Cefixime 400 mg PO single dose	Spectinomycin 2 g IM single dose (for cephalosporin allergy) plus *C. trachomatis* therapy (see Chlamydia therapy)
Disseminated gonoccocal infection (DGI)	Cefriaxone 1 g IM or IV q 24 h	(see CDC 2002a for alternative initial regimens)

*Fluoroquinolones are not recommended as first line agents in MSM, women partners of MSM, or infections acquired in Asia, Pacific coast of the US, England, or Wales.

Adapted from CDC, 2002a.

to treat gonorrhea are not available; but the suspension (100 mg/5 mL) is available (CDC, 2004b).

The quinolones (ciprofloxacin, ofloxacin, and levofloxacin) have favorable pharmacokinetic properties. Each of the above quinalones is effective against most strains of *N. gonorrhoea* in the United States (except as noted above). Like ciprofloxacin, ofloxacin and levofloxacin are effective for anal and genital gonorrhea, but not as effective for pharyngeal infection (CDC, 2002,a).

Patients allergic to penicillin should be treated with a quinolone. Patients who are allergic to both penicillins and quinolones can be treated with spectinomycin 2 g IM (CDC, 2002a).

Pregnant women should receive cephalosporins for treatment of gonorrhea because quinolones are contraindicated during pregnancy. Quinolones should also be avoided in nursing mothers and in patients younger than 17 years of age. If there is an allergy to the cephalosporin or quinolones, spectinomycin 2 g IM is an effective alternative (CDC, 2002a).

All of the above regimens should include a drug regimen effective against possible coinfection with *C. trachomatis,* such as doxycycline 100 mg PO, twice daily for 7 days, or, azithromycin PO, given as a single dose (CDC, 2002a). *Clinicians should be aware that tetracycline and doxycycline are contraindicated in pregnancy.*

Azithromycin, given as a single oral dose of 2 grams (double the usual dose for treating *C. trachomatis*), has been demonstrated to be an effective treatment for gonorrhea (Anonymous, 2000; CDC, 2002a). However, this higher dose is not recommended due to the increased cost and higher incidence of GI intolerance when compared to the four regimens recommended by the CDC (CDC, 2002a).

Monitoring for Efficacy

Test-of-cure cultures are not required if CDC recommended therapies are used and symptoms resolve. However, if a non-recommended regimen is used or symptoms persist after treatment, test-of-cure should be considered. Where antibiotic sensitivity testing is available monitoring for the emergence of quinolone resistance in the heterosexual population is encouraged (Bignell, 2001; CDC, 2002a; CDC, 2004a). It has been suggested that test-of-cure cultures may be useful for patients with oral pharyngeal involvement (Barlow, 1997).

Monitoring for Toxicity

Ceftriaxone can cause pain at the injection site. Toxicities caused by a single 125-mg dose of ceftriaxone are rare. All of the recommended oral medications (ciprofloxacin, ofloxacin, levofloxacin, cefixime) may cause diarrhea and nausea in some patients.

CHLAMYDIA

Chlamydia has been recognized as the most commonly reported sexually transmitted bacterial infection in the United States. In the year 2000, the Centers for Disease Control and Prevention (CDC) estimated that greater than 700,000 chlamydial infections had been reported. Of the reported chlamydial cases, females were reported four times higher than males. The lower rates in men probably are attributed to the increased number of females who are screened for the disease. Chlamydia and its consequences can be very costly. The CDC estimates that for each dollar spent on screening and treatment, $12 is saved in treating secondary complications from untreated chlamydia (CDC, 2001a). Untreated chlamydial infections include complications, such as urethritis, cervicitis, pelvic inflammatory disease, chronic pelvic pain, infertility, and potentially fatal tubal pregnancy (Steinhandler, Peipert, Herber, et al., 2002). Differentiation of infection caused by *C. trachomatis* from infection caused by *N. gonorrhoeae* cannot be accomplished reliably based on signs and symptoms. Simultaneous infection with both *C. trachomatis* and *N. gonorrhoeae* is common among certain patient groups; therefore, treatment regimens for *N. gonorrhoeae* utilize a drug regimen with activity against both organisms (CDC, 2002a).

Individuals at high risk for chlamydial infection are young, sexually active adolescent women ranging in age from 15 to 24. Demographic characteristics commonly associated with the infection include nonwhite race, age < 25 years, unmarried, new or multiple sex partners, lack of condom use, history of other sexually transmitted infections, douching, mucopurulent cervical discharge, purulent vaginal discharge, cervical edema, ectopy, and friability (Steinhandler et al., 2002). A recent study found that the rate in teen men is near that of teen women (Incidence, 2004).

SPECIFIC CONSIDERATIONS FOR PHARMACOTHERAPY

When Drug Therapy Is Needed

In women, the sequelae of chlamydia are quite severe and include PID, ectopic pregnancy, and infertility (CDC, 2002a). Complications, such as urethral infection or swollen and tender testicles, can result from untreated chlamydial infections in men (CDC, 2001b). Pregnant women who are infected with *C. trachomatis* may transmit the disease to infants during birth (CDC, 2002a). There is also an increased risk of these infants developing neonatal conjunctivitis and pneumonia. If exposed, women with chlamydia have an increased risk of acquiring Human Immunodeficiency Virus (HIV) (CDC, 2001b).

See Drug Tables 102.4, 102.5, 102.11.

Assessment and History Taking

Approximately 70 to 80% of women who are infected with *C. trachomatis* are without symptoms. The presence of a green or yellow mucous cervical discharge along with polymorphonuclear leukocytes (PMNs) on an oil immersion field or wet mount, is associated with chlamydial infection (Steinhandler et al., 2002; Weinstock, Dean, Bolen, 1994). Many practitioners will treat these women without testing because these symptoms are highly predictive and a laboratory workup can be quite expensive.

Approximately 25 to 50% of men infected with *C. trachomatis* are without symptoms. Urethral infection with *C. trachomatis* can cause dysuria and mucopurulent discharge, or it can be completely asymptomatic. Generally, urethral infection with *C. trachomatis* causes less severe symptoms and is more often asymptomatic than urethral infections caused by *N. gonorrhoeae* (CDC, 2001b).

A portion of assessing the patient is affirming a positive test result for chlamydia, initiating treatment, and finally having a proper followup with a potential repeat screen. In order to begin these steps, it is important to consider if positive and negative test results truly indicate chlamydial infection and to evaluate the positive versus the negative predictive value of the test. Second, consider if a negative test-of-cure result truly indicates eradication of infection, thus evaluating the efficacy of the treatment.

It has been well documented that cell culture has been the test by which all others have been measured. Although culture is effective, it is important to note that barriers exist, such as being difficult to standardize, technically demanding, and expensive to perform. Manufacturers have recognized these barriers and have developed nonculture tests in which live organisms are not required and testing can be automated. Laboratory-based tests include culture, nucleic acid amplified test (NAAT), nucleic acid hybridization and transformation tests, enzyme immunoassay (EIA), and direct fluorescent antibody tests (DFA) (CDC, 2002c). Table 36–3 compares these techniques.

Cell culture methods have disadvantages, such as standardization incongruence, the need for increased incubation of 48 to 72 hours, transport requirements, increased cost. They are also laborious to carry out. Cell culture can be advantageous when the evidence is used in legal investigations. Additionally, cell culture is the only isolate that can be used for antimicrobial susceptibility testing (CDC, 2002c).

Nucleic acid amplified tests, as their name implies, are designed to amplify nucleic acid sequences specific to the organism being identified. NAATs do not require live organisms in order to complete the test. Examples of commercial tests available on the market are polymerase chain reaction (PCR) and ligase chain reaction (LCR). Specimens may be obtained from endocervical swabs in women, urethral swabs from men, and urine from both women and men. Oropharyngeal specimens and rectal specimens are not recommended when using the NAAT method. The advantage of NAATs is that screening using a urine sample can be less invasive than using cervical or

TABLE 36–3. Sensitivity and Specificity of Various Diagnostic Tests for *C. Trachomatis*

Test†	Sensitivity*	Specificity*	Positive Predictive Value*	Negative Predictive Value*	Test-for-Cure*
LCR on urine specimen	77.3–100	99.4–100	94.5–100	96.9–100	10 Positive at day 10; 0 at >day 21
PCR on Urine specimen	88.9–100	100	100	97.4–100	5–14 Positive at day 14; 0 at day> 21
DFA, EIA on cervical or urethral specimens	>70	97–99	>90	85–99	19 Positive at day 4; 0 at day 10
Culture on cervical or urethral specimens	70–90	100	100	93	27 Positive at day 2; 0 at day 5

*All values are given as percentages. Sensitivity indicates the probability of a positive test result given presence of disease; specificity, the probability of a negative test result given absence of disease; positive predictive value, the probability of disease given a negative test result; and test-for-cure, the number of days after start of treatment until test results are negative

† LCR indicates ligase chain reaction; PCR, polymerase chain reaction; DFA, direct fluorescent antibody; and EIA enzyme immunoassay.

Adapted from Reust, C., (2000).

urethral swabs. Potential false-negative results can occur, which can be a disadvantage (CDC, 2002c).

Enzyme immunoassay tests are reliable in detecting *C. trachomatis* infections. Advantages of EIAs are that specimens can be transported and stored without refrigeration, and processing is according to the labeling instructions of each manufacturer. There is an increased chance for a false-positive result due to cross-reaction, a disadvantage. The manufacturers developed assays with blocking agents to verify positive test results. Last, EIA agents should not be tested using rectal specimens due to the increased chance of fecal bacterial cross-reactivity (CDC, 2002c).

Direct fluorescent antibody (DFA) tests employ endocervical samples placed on a slide, dried, fixative applied, and processed ≤ 7 days after being obtained. The downside to this type of testing is that the clinician checking smears must be competent in fluorescent microscopy as well as proficient in identifying classic columnar cells. This test is time-consuming and labor intensive (CDC, 2002c).

There are a variety of tests available with varying specificity and sensitivity. Fortunately, advances in testing methods allow for a wide range of screening to be preformed in nontraditional settings such as schools, jails and detention centers, and street HIV or STI outreach programs. NAATs and culture using endocervical swabs are similar in sensitivity; however, urine specimens when applied to NAATs have slightly lower sensitivity. All other tests are similar in performance specificity. It is important to note at this time that there are no tests currently approved by the FDA that utilize vaginal specimens and NAATs as a primary method of detection. However, research continues to look promising in this area. Non-NAATs definitely have inferior sensitivity when using vaginal or urine specimens and are therefore not recommended (CDC, 2002c).

The CDC (2002c) continues to recommend annual screening for chlamydia in all sexually active adolescents, as well as for females 20 to 25 years old. Additionally, screening is recommended for all females who are sexually active with risk factors such as new sex partner, multiple sex partners, or any other appropriate risk factor that may indicate the need for more frequent screening.

OUTCOMES MANAGEMENT

Selecting an Appropriate Agent

Doxycycline has been widely used for the treatment of *C. trachomatis*. It is inexpensive and is generally well tolerated. Azithromycin has the advantage of being administered as a single oral dose, thus eliminating the potential for poor compliance. However, the cost to health care organizations for azithromycin is considerably higher than for doxycycline. Despite the high cost of purchasing this medication, Haddix, Hillis, and Kassler (1995) have demonstrated azithromycin to be cost-effective compared with doxycycline. Treatment recommendations from the CDC are presented in Table 36–4.

Alternative drug regimens have a limited role in the treatment of *C. trachomatis* because of the superiority of doxycycline and azithromycin in most clinical situations. Ofloxacin is equally effective, but it is more expensive than doxycycline. Like doxycycline, ofloxacin is contraindicated in pregnancy and nursing mothers and in patients younger than 17 years of age (CDC, 2002a). Erythromycin has been recommended as an alternative medication in the pregnant patient. Erythromycin base and erythromycin ethylsuccinate can cause GI intolerance and require qid dosing, which may result in poor patient compliance (CDC, 2002a).

Very high success rates are obtained with successful completion of either of the two recommended antibiotic treatment regimens (CDC, 2002a). If the 7-day doxycycline regimen is utilized, patients should be advised to avoid sexual contact until the treatment regimen is completed (CDC, 2002a).

The recommended antibiotic regimens are doxycycline 100 mg PO, bid for 7 days, or azithromycin 1 g PO, as a single dose. These treatments are both highly effec-

TABLE 36–4. 2002 CDC Treatment Recommendations for Chlamydia

Infection or Status	Recommended Regimen ORAL	Alternative Regimen ORAL
Adolescents/Adults	Doxycycline 100 mg twice a day for 7 days **or** Azithromycin 1 g single dose	Erythromycin base 500 mg four times a day for 7 days **or** Ofloxacin 300 mg twice a day for 7 days **or** Erythromycin ethylsuccinate 800 mg four times a day for 7 days **or** Levofloxacin 500 mg once a day for 7 days
Pregnancy	Erythromycin base 500 mg four times a day for 7 days **or** Amoxicillin 500 mg three times a day for 7 days	Erythromycin base 250 mg four times a day for 14 days **or** Erythromycin ethylsuccinate 800 mg four times a day for 7 days **or** Erythromycin ethylsuccinate 400 mg four times a day for 14 days or Azithromycin 1 g PO single dose

Adapted from CDC (2002a).

tive in eliminating the organism, and are cost-effective as well. In pregnant patients, doxycycline and ofloxacin are contraindicated. Some clinicians do use azithromycin in pregnant women, although safety and efficacy in pregnant patients has not been well established.

A single 1 g dose of azithromycin has been shown to be as effective as a 7-day course of doxycycline 100 mg bid. In addition, azithromycin has good tissue concentrations and very high intracellular levels even up to 4 days after administration (Weinstock et al., 1994). Although more expensive than doxycycline, azithromycin may be preferable for patients for whom medication compliance is an issue.

Monitoring for Efficacy

When the patient is treated with either doxycycline or azithromycin, retesting or test-of-cure cultures are not needed unless symptoms persist or reinfection is suspected. However, if erythromycin is used, a test of cure may be considered 3 weeks after the completion of therapy (CDC, 2002a).

Monitoring for Toxicity

Either doxycycline or azithromycin is capable of causing nausea and/or vomiting. Both agents generally are well tolerated.

HERPES GENITALIS

Herpes simplex virus (HSV) is a double-stranded DNA surrounded by a glycoprotein envelope (Yeung-Yue, Brentjens, Lee, & Tyring, 2002). Herpes simplex virus type 1 (HSV-1) and herpes simplex virus type 2 (HSV-2) are responsible for oral and genital infections, respectively (Yeung-Yue et al., 2002); the focus of this chapter will be on HSV-2.

In 1999, an estimated 500,000 people were seen for genital herpes infection (Gilson & Mindel, 2001). Genital herpes cases declined 17% in the 1990s, with the greatest declines in men and teens (Incidence, 2004). Herpes simplex type 2 is responsible for most cases of recurrent genital herpes (CDC, 2002a). The virus is transmitted by direct physical contact with the infected individual (kissing, sexual relations, or delivery of an infant through an infected vagina) (Yeung, Yue et al., 2002). Women are more likely than men to have HSV. The women who are at increased risk are those who are in the lower socioeconomic groups (less access to health insurance and clinics), have multiple sexual partners, do not use barrier contraception, practice vaginal douching, have sex at an early age, have high-risk partners, as well as use alcohol and drug (Swanson, 1999). Upon successful entry into the host, the virus invades the sensory nerve terminals up to the sensory sacral ganglia that innervate the skin and mucosa of the site of entry. The virus will either cause the clinical symptoms or it will remain dormant until "triggered" to reactivate (Yeung-Yue et al., 2002).

SPECIFIC CONSIDERATIONS FOR PHARMACOTHERAPY

When Drug Therapy Is Needed

Drug therapy helps reduce the duration of symptoms and infectivity. Drug therapy options include short courses of antiviral therapy for initial and recurrent episodes, or long-term suppressive antiviral therapy. Treatment depends on the severity and frequency of recurrence (Drake, Taylor, Brown, & Pillay, 2000). In addition, valcyclovir has been shown to reduce the risk of heterosexual transmission of genital herpes to susceptible partners with healthy immune systems when used as suppressive therapy in combination with safer sex practices (FDA, 2003).

The safety of acyclovir and valacyclovir in pregnant women has not been established. Currently, a registry is set up to monitor pregnant women receiving acyclovir or valacyclovir. Women who are prescribed either of these agents should be reported to this registry; telephone (800) 722-9292, ext 38465. Recent analysis of the database does not indicate an increased risk of major birth defects with the use of acyclovir. However, this analysis is still preliminary (CDC, 2002a).

Current CDC guidelines suggest treating the first clinical episode of genital herpes with oral acyclovir. For life-threatening maternal HSV infection, intravenous acyclovir is preferred.

See Drug Table 106.

Assessment and History Taking

Most individuals with primary genital herpes (no previous antibodies to HSV-1 or HSV-2) have no symptoms, but are extremely infectious through viral shedding (Yeung-Yue, et al., 2002). Approximately 37% of patients present with symptoms initially. Systemic symptoms may present as blisters and sores, local tingling and discomfort, dysthesia or neuralgic pain in the buttocks or legs, and malaise with fever (Drake et al., 2000).

Recurrent genital herpes is most common after a primary infection. Factors such as menses, trauma to the area, emotional stress, or altered immune status are known to trigger these recurrences. Fortunately, symptoms of recurrent disease are generally milder; few have systemic symptoms. The clinical presentation may include atypical rashes, fissuring, excoriation and discomfort of the anogenital area, cervical lesions, urinary symptoms, and extragenital lesions (Drake et al., 2000).

Diagnosis is based primarily on clinical manifestations that are confirmed by one of several tests. The Tzanck smear will provide immediate diagnosis. Viral culture is the gold standard for diagnosis and has the greatest specificity for differentiating between the HSV types. However, viral culture is time-consuming, and the sensitivity declines with recurrent disease when compared to primary disease. The Tzanack smear provides a diagnosis of herpes virus, but the finding is nonspecific and cannot differentiate between infection of HSV-1, HSV-2, or varicella zoster virus. EIAs, immunofluorescence, and antigen detection methods are also nonspecific. Polymerase chain reaction (PCR) is as specific as viral culture and more rapid; however, PCR is very costly. Currently there are two FDA approved type-specific HSV assays, POCkit™ HSV-2 (Diagnology) and HerpeSelect™ -2 ELISA IgG (Focus Technology, Inc.). Serologic testing can be beneficial in pregnant females to avoid viral infection to the neonate as well in individuals at high risk for transmission or acquisition of human immunodeficiency virus (HIV) (CDC, 2002a, Yeung-Yue et al., 2002).

OUTCOMES MANAGEMENT

Selecting an Appropriate Agent

Current therapy for genital herpes does not provide a cure. Instead, therapy helps reduce or suppress symptoms, viral shedding, and recurrent episodes. The main treatment modalities available for herpetic infections include acyclovir, valcyclovir, and famciclovir. Acyclovir has low bioavailability following oral administration. Valcyclovir and famciclovir both have increased oral bioavailability. Topical therapy offers minimal clinical benefit and is not recommended (CDC, 2002a, Yeung-Yue et al., 2002). Bathing in saline may provide some comfort. Valacyclovir is the prodrug of acyclovir; that is, it will be converted to acyclovir. Acyclovir has a bioavailability of only 15%, whereas valacyclovir has a bioavailability of 54% (Alrabiah & Sacks, 1996). Famciclovir is metabolized to penciclovir, an acyclic, guanosine analog that inhibits HSV DNA synthesis (Alrabiah & Sacks, 1996). Few studies have directly compared valacyclovir or famciclovir with acyclovir. However, results of clinical trials suggest that these two agents are comparable to acyclovir (CDC, 2002a).

First Clinical Episode of Genital HSV. Management of the first episode of genital HSV includes medication and extensive counseling. Either acyclovir, valacyclovir, or famciclovir could be used for treatment, and the duration of therapy is usually for 7 to 10 days or until healing is complete. Please refer to Table 36–5 for dosing guidelines (CDC, 2002a).

Patients should be counseled extensively on the natural history of the disease, recurrent episodes, asymptomatic viral shedding and sexual transmission. Patients should also be advised to notify their partners, abstain from sexual activity when the lesions or prodromal symptoms are present, and the risk of transmission during asymptomatic periods. In addition, the risk of neonatal transmission should be discussed with both partners

TABLE 36–5. 2002 CDC Treatment Guidelines for Genital Herpes Simplex Virus

Infection or Status	Recommended Regimen
First clinical episode of genital herpes	Acyclovir 400 mg orally three times a day for 7–10 days or Acyclovir 200 mg orally five times a day for 7–10 days or Famciclovir 250 mg orally three times a day for 7–10 days or Valcyclovir 1 g orally twice a day for 7–10 days
Episodic recurrent infection	Acyclovir 400 mg orally three times a day for 5 days or Acyclovir 200 mg orally five times a day for 5 days or Acyclovir 800 mg orally twice a day for 5 days or Famciclovir 125 mg orally twice a day for 5 days or Valacyclovir 500 mg orally twice a day for 3–5 days or Valacyclovir 1 g orally once daily for 5 days
Daily suppressive therapy	Acyclovir 400 mg orally twice a day or Famciclovir 250 mg orally twice a day or Valacyclovir 250 mg orally twice a day or Valciclovir 500 mg orally once a day or Valacyclovir 1 g orally once a day

Adapted from CDC (2002a).

(CDC, 2002a). Valacyclovir once daily reduces partner risk (Corey, Wald, et al., 2004).

Recurrent Episode of Genital HSV. After the first clinical episode, most patients will have recurrent events. Initiating therapy during the prodrome or within 1 day after the formation of lesions, helps alleviate symptoms. The recommended regimens for episodic recurrent infection is described in Table 36–5 (CDC, 2002a).

Some patients may have frequent recurrences (i.e., greater than six episodes per year). These patients may benefit from daily suppressive therapy, which has been shown to reduce genital herpes recurrences by >75%. Chronic suppression with valacyclovir has been shown to decrease transmission to uninfected heterosexual partners when combined with safer sex practices (FDA, 2003). Transmission to an uninfected partner is still possible during suppressive therapy. The use of acyclovir for suppressive therapy for as long as 6 years was shown to be safe and effective. The safety and efficacy profile for famciclovir and valacyclovir have been documented for 1 year. After 1 year of suppressive therapy, clinicians and patients should reevaluate whether therapy should be continued. Table 36–5 list the regimens and their doses for suppressive therapy (CDC, 2002a).

Severe Disease. Intravenous acyclovir 5 to 10 mg/kg q8h for 2 to 7 days or until clinical symptoms improve is recommended for severe genital HSV (CDC, 2002a).

Monitoring for Toxicity

Acyclovir is fairly well tolerated with gastrointestinal side effects being the most common problems.

LYMPHOGRANULOMA VENEREUM

Lymphogranuloma venereum (LGV) is a sexually transmitted infection caused by serovars L1, L2, or L3 of *Chlamydia trachomatis* (CDC, 2002a). LGV is rare in the United States, with only 42 cases reported in 2000 (CDC, 2001a), but is endemic in many tropical areas such as India, Africa, South East Asia, and some Caribbean islands (Anonymous, 1999). LGV is a chronic, systemic disease with a clinical course classically divided into three stages. These three stages are primary, secondary and tertiary or anorectogenital stage. A recent review of LGV is presented by Mabey and Peeling (2002).

SPECIFIC CONSIDERATIONS FOR PHARMACOTHERAPY

Short- and Long-Term Goals of Pharmacotherapy

The goals of pharmacotherapy are the same as those for syphilis.

Time Frame for Initiating Pharmacotherapy

As with other STIs, treatment should be initiated immediately once diagnosis is confirmed to prevent progression to the more severe secondary and tertiary stages.

See Drug Tables 102.5, 102.9, 102.11.

Assessment and History Taking

Lymphogranuloma venereum is an infection of the lymphatic tissue with extension of the inflammatory process to surrounding tissues. After an incubation period of 3 to 30 days, the primary stage is manifested by a painless papule, pustule, or shallow erosion on the coronal sulcus of males or the cervix, posterior vaginal wall, fourchette, or vulva of women. The initial lesion is transient and often goes unnoticed (Anonymous, 1999).

Secondary LGV follows the primary lesion within 10 to 30 days. In heterosexual men, secondary LGV most often causes unilateral, inflammed, swollen, and painful inguinal lymph glands. Bubo formation occasionally occurs, and ulceration and chronic fistula formation are possible. If both the femoral and inguinal lymph nodes are involved, they may be separated by the inguinal ligament forming the pathognumonic "groove sign." While classic, this "groove sign" occurs in only 15 to 20% of cases. The vast majority of individuals recover from this stage of LGV without sequelae (Anonymous, 1999; CDC, 2002a).

Persistent infection and spread of the disease leads to the chronic inflammation and progressive tissue destruction of tertiary LGV. Women and homosexually active men have involvement of the retroperitoneal, perirectal or perianal lymphatic tissues with resulting proctitis, fistulas, strictures, and chronic granulomas with disfiguring of the vulva (Anonymous, 1999). After thirty years without a published case report of LGV presenting as a rectovaginal fistula, there have been two more recent reports of rectal complications of LGV. In the first report, one otherwise healthy pregnant woman presented with rectal stricture (Papagrigoriadis & Rennie, 1998), and in the other report a healthy woman presented with rectal fistula due to LGV (Lynch, Felder, Schwandt, & Shashy, 1999).

Diagnosis

Diagnosis can be made when an individual has the typical clinical presentation and high (>1:64) or rising complement fixation titers and other causes of genital ulcers and inguinal lymphadenopathy have been ruled out (CDC, 2002a). Other tests that have been used to diagnose LGV include culture of material from LVG lesions, direct immunofluorescence of material from LGV lesions, enzyme immunoassay, detection of nucleic acid by amplification techniques, or alternative serology testing such as microimmunofluorescence (Anonymous, 1999).

OUTCOMES MANAGEMENT

Selecting an Appropriate Agent

As with other chlamydial infections, the agent of choice is doxycycline 100 mg twice a day for 21 days. Alternative agents for those who cannot take doxycycline are erythromycin 500 mg four times a day for 21 days. Although clinical studies on it use are lacking, some specialists recommend azithromycin 1 g orally once a week for 3 weeks as an effective treatment. The recommended treatment for pregnant or lactating women is erythromycin at the above recommended dose, and although safety and efficacy studies are lacking, azythromycin may be an appropriate therapeutic option (CDC, 2002a).

Monitoring for Efficacy

As with other STIs, monitor for resolution of symptoms.

Monitoring for Toxicity

The tetracyclines and macolides usually cause gastrointestinal symptoms, but most abate with time.

Followup Recommendation

Followup is recommended until signs and symptoms resolve, usually in 3 to 6 weeks (CDC, 2002a). Surgical repair of lesions, including reconstructive genital surgery, may be required for destructive lesions of advanced disease (Anonymous, 1999).

GRANULOMA INGUINALE

Granuloma inguinale, or donovanosis, is caused by the gram-negative rod *Calymmatobacterium granulomatis*. Although it is a very rare disease in developed countries, such as the United States and the United Kingdom, it is more common in tropical or semitropical countries (O'Farrell, 2001). Donovanosis is not a highly contagious disease and appears to require repeated exposure for complete infectivity. Whether sexual transmission is the only mode of infection is controversial because nonsexual transmission, such as repeated trauma of the infected site, has also been demonstrated. It is a genital disease that leads to painless, irregular, and granulomatous ulcers that can be quite disfiguring (O'Farrell, 2001).

SPECIFIC CONSIDERATIONS FOR PHARMACOTHERAPY

When Drug Therapy Is Needed

Drug treatment halts progression of the disease and allows for reepithelialization of ulcers (CDC, 2002a). Donovanosis lesions may be noticed on the cervix and can extend toward the pelvis. Lesions easily bleed with contact, have a "beefy red appearance" from increased vascularity, and can erode to form granulomatous ulcers (CDC, 2002a, p. 17; O'Farrell, 2001). Regional lymphadenopathy is absent (CDC, 2002a). If an ulcer progresses, lymphatic obstruction may occur. Dissemination can cause osteomyelitis of the cervix. Donovanosis may be more aggressive during pregnancy (O'Farrell, 2001).

See Drug Table 102.

Assessment and History Taking

Donovanosis as described above involves the cervix, but the majority of cases have lesions involving the external genitalia, with some involvement of the inguinal and anal regions. Lesions have been reported on the upper arms, chest, legs, mouth, jaw, and bones (tibia). Disseminated disease has also been reported to the abdominal cavity, bowel, spleen, liver, lung, uterus, and ovaries (O'Farrell, 2001).

Aside from the clinical presentation, the diagnosis is confirmed by a Wright's or Giemsa stain that reveals Donovan bodies, the infecting organisms (O'Farrell, 2001; Schaffer, 2003). The method is similar to a Gram stain, except that multiple swabs are taken in order to detect other co-infecting organisms (CDC, 2002a; O'Farrell, 2001). Donovanosis also can be identified using PCR techniques (O'Farrell, 2001). Other methods include serum complement–fixing antibodies or a positive skin test to intradermal Donovan antigen.

Differential diagnoses include carcinoma, secondary syphilis, chancroid, and amebiasis (Schaffer, 2004). Gonorrhea or syphilis are possible concurrent infections that should be part of the diagnostic evaluation (Hart, 1990).

OUTCOMES MANAGEMENT

Selecting an Appropriate Agent

Several available treatment options are available for donovanosis. The majority of therapies are long courses of antibiotics until lesions have completely re-epithelialized. The CDC (2002) recommends either doxycycline 100 mg orally twice daily or trimethoprim-sulfamethoxazole one double-strength (800 mg/160 mg) tablet orally twice daily for at least three weeks (CDC, 2002a; O'Farrell, 2001). Other regimens are available, such as ciprofloxacin 750 mg orally twice daily or erythromycin base 500 mg orally four times daily each to be administered for a minimum of three weeks (CDC, 2002a). Azithromycin has achieved healing using 500 mg daily for 7 days or 1 g orally once per week for at least 3 weeks (CDC, 2002a; O'Farrell, 2001). Gentamicin (1 mg/kg IV q8 h) can be added to any of the above regimens if lesions do not respond within the first few days of therapy (CDC, 2002a).

During pregnancy practitioners should use caution; doxycycline and ciprofloxacin are contraindicated in pregnancy. Sulfonamides also hold a relative contraindication. Erythromycin is recommended in the pregnant and lactating individuals and aminoglycoside may be needed as well. Azithromycin may be efficient in treating pregnant females; however, published studies are not available (CDC, 2002a).

Monitoring for Efficacy

Lesions should become less friable and less vascular within a few days. Optimal duration of therapy can vary, but should increase for larger ulcers. Many clinicians insist to continue therapy until re-epithelialization is complete (O'Farrell, 2001).

Monitoring for Toxicity

The most common side effects with these agents are gastrointestinal in nature and should resolve with continued therapy. If gentamicin is part of the treatment regimen, monitor for renal toxicity.

Followup Recommendations

Again treatment should continue until tissue has re-epithelialized and all signs and symptoms have resolved (CDC, 2002a; O'Farrell, 2001).

HUMAN PAPILLOMAVIRUS

Human papillomavirus (HPV) is the etiologic agent of two diseases that primarily infects the squamous epithelium of the lower anogenital tract of both males and females. The two diseases are condylomas (raised warts) and flat warts (subclinical disease and precancerous lesions) (Cox, Buck, Kinney, & Rubin, 2001). In addition, HPV virus can remain latent with no visible signs or symptoms in infected skin. HPV is the most common viral STI, with about 40 genital types (Munoz, Bosch, deSanjose, et al., 2003). Of these 40, 18 are high-risk for cervical cancer. 320,000 cervical cancers occurring annually implicate HPV as the primary etiology both molecularly and epidemiologically (Cox, et al., 2001). The most common nongenital and genital HPV types causing skin warts are type 1 (plantar warts) and type 3 (flat warts) (Cox, et al., 2001). The most common HPV types causing anogenital lesions are 6, 11, 16, 18, and 31, with types 6 and 11 causing benign genital warts (CDC, 2002a). Invasive carcinoma of the external genitalia is rare with types 6 and 11. The most common HPV types causing external genital squamous intraepithelial neoplasia and cervical dysplasia and malignancy are 16, 18, 31, 33, and 35 (CDC, 2002a). These types are also associated with anal and vaginal cancer. Other cancers are associated with HPV types, including laryngeal, conjunctival, and nasal with 6 and 11; oral cancer with 3, 6, 11, 16, 18, and 57; and sublingual cancer with 16 (CDC, 2002a; Cox et al., 2001). Women can be infected with multiple types simultaneously (CDC, 2002a).

HPV infection can be completely asymptomatic and undetectable to the patient, or there can be mild symptoms such as itching, local pain, and friability of the lesion. The goal of treatment is the removal of symptomatic visible warts. Wart removal does not eradicate HPV infection, and recurrence is likely. Similarly, there is no evidence that wart removal by any of the currently used modalities effectively reduces infectivity. Sex partners of patients with HPV infection are very likely to be infected. Treated patients and their partners should be counseled that the patient continues to be infective even though the warts have been removed.

SPECIFIC CONSIDERATIONS FOR PHARMACOTHERAPY

When Drug Therapy Is Needed

Topical drug therapies aimed at removal of symptomatic warts are among the local therapies available. There are no effective systemic drug therapies for HPV available. Local removal of warts does not eliminate HPV infection, and it is unclear if it decreases infectivity. "Debulking" of anogenital warts is thought by some experts to reduce the likelihood of transmission of the disease. The development of cervical dysplasia associated with HPV types 16, 18, 31, 33, and 35 is probably not affected by wart removal.

Short- and Long-Term Goals of Pharmacotherapy

Refer to the syphilis section for general guidelines for all STIs, including the time frame for initiating pharmacotherapy. Since pharmacotherapy does not lead to eradication of HPV, treatment goals are to reduce symptoms, if present, and prevent the transmission of the organism to new partners.

Nonpharmacologic Therapy

Both nonpharmacologic and pharmacologic therapies are used for "debulking" or wart removal. Currently used nonpharmacologic therapies include:

- Cryotherapy with liquid nitrogen or a cryoprobe
- Electrocoagulation
- Laser ablation
- Surgical excision

There are some advantages and disadvantages of each of these, depending upon the clinical situation and available resources.

For most exophytic genital and anal warts, cryotherapy with liquid nitrogen or a cryoprobe is the preferred treatment. Cryotherapy is widely available, simple for the provider to administer to the patient, and relatively inexpensive. Cryotherapy has no systemic toxicities and usually does not produce scarring.

Electrocoagulation requires local anesthesia (lidocaine), which is usually painful to administer. Large amounts of wart can be removed quickly. Scarring is common.

Laser ablation requires expensive equipment, general or local anesthesia, and a practitioner skilled in the technique. Precise control of the depth of tissue penetration can be accomplished with this modality. Laser ablation is probably the method of choice for treating flat cervical warts (Ferenczy, 1985).

See Drug Table 809.

Assessment and History Taking

There are a number of skin growths that can occur in the anogenital region that may be similar in appearance to HPV infection. These include moles, skin tags, molluscum contagiosum, and condylomata lata keratoses. Differentiation can be difficult and may require consultation with an expert. DNA hybridization tests are useful for identifying the HPV type, but this test is not recommended for screening purposes. Patients can be simultaneously infected with multiple HPV types.

OUTCOMES MANAGEMENT

Selecting an Appropriate Agent

The choice of therapy will depend on several factors, including individual provider experience; available treatment modalities and resources; the potential for treatment toxicity; the size, number, and anatomic location of the warts; and patient preference and convenience (CDC, 2002a). Warts that are easily visible and anatomically accessible to the patient may be treated with a patient-applied topical therapy, if desired. Patient-applied therapies require the provider to instruct the patient on which specific wart(s) to treat and ensure that the patient understands how to properly apply the medication. Other warts must be treated with provider-administered therapies. Lesions on moist surfaces and in intertriginous areas generally should be treated with a topical agent (CDC, 2002a). Drier area warts respond least to cryotherapy. Wart size, number, site, patient preference, cost, convenience, and adverse effects are factors influencing choice of therapy.

Podophyllin resin is a popular topical therapy for genital warts, but it is less effective than cryotherapy (Bashi, 1985). Podophyllin is most effective in mucosal areas, but has diminished effectiveness in dry, highly keratinized areas. Podophyllin should not be used for cervical warts. Podophyllin can cause significant local irritation, especially to the eyes and mucous membranes. Systemic absorption of podophyllin can cause a variety of unwanted toxicities including bone marrow suppression and severe gastrointestinal disturbances. Because of the potential for toxicity, the CDC recommends that no more than 0.5 mL be applied per session, and that no more than 10 cm^2 of wart be treated. Removing the drug by thorough washing 1 to 4 h after application is also suggested. Treatment sessions should be at least 7 to 10 days apart. Patient self-administration is not recommended, for obvious reasons. The CDC (2002a). advises that the safe use of podophyllin resin in pregnancy has not been established.

Imiquimod (Aldara) is available as a 5% cream. It is given as a patient-applied therapy. Patients should be instructed to apply imiquimod cream to the wart with a finger, at bedtime, three times a week for up to 16 weeks (CDC, 2002a). The treated area should be washed with soap and water 6 to 10 h following application. Mild to moderate skin reactions (erythema, erosion, excoriation/flaking, and edema) are common (Drugdex® Drug Evaluations, 2002). More frequent application is associated with an increase in adverse reactions. Like other topically applied drugs, imiquimod is more effective on mucosal surfaces and intertriginous areas and is less effective when applied to dry, highly keratinized skin.

As with other topical therapies for HPV, patients should be advised that the organism persists in their body despite the clearance of lesions. Patients should avoid sexual contact while on imiquimod therapy. Patients should be advised that imiquimod may weaken condoms and diaphragms and that concurrent use of imiquimod and condoms or diaphragms is not recommended. The safety of imiquimod in pregnancy is unknown (CDC, 2002a).

Podofilox (Condylox) is a topical antimitotic agent available in a 0.5% solution or gel. This agent, like imiquimod, is designed for patient self-application. Podofilox is indicated for the treatment of external genital or perianal warts, but is not approved for treatment of warts on mucous membranes (Drugdex Drug Evaluations, 2002). The patient should be instructed to apply podofilox solution or gel with a cotton-tipped applicator to specifically identified warts, twice daily, in the morning and in the evening, for 3 days. The minimum amount of drug necessary to cover the lesion should be applied. In areas where the treated wart comes in contact with opposing skin, the opposing skin should be held apart until the applied medication dries. For podofilox 0.5% gel, the patient may apply the drug with a finger, if desired. When using podofilox solution, application must be with a cotton-tipped applicator (supplied with the product). The patient should be instructed to discard the cotton-tipped applicator and wash hands after applying the medication. After the drug has been applied for 3 consecutive days, the drug should be withheld for the next 4 consecutive days. The 1-week cycle can be repeated up to 4 times. If the response to therapy after 4 weeks is incomplete, consider an alternative therapy. Like podophyllin, the amount of treated wart should be limited to no more than 10 cm^2, and no more than 0.5 mL of the drug should be applied in a 24-h period. The CDC (CDC, 2002a). advises that the safety of podofilox during pregnancy is unknown.

Trichloroacetic acid (TCA) and bichloroacetic acid (BCA) are strong acids that require careful application by the provider. The acid is carefully applied to the wart and allowed to dry, with great care taken to use a minimal amount so as not to get the product on surrounding tissue. The application can be reapplied every 1 to 3 weeks, if necessary. The acid liquid is thin and flows easily, like water. Wherever the acid has contacted tissue, a white frosty-appearing crust will form. In the case of a spill or overapplication, unreacted acid can be neutralized with sodium bicarbonate powder or talc. This must be done very quickly, or the acid will spread, coagulating the skin proteins that the acid comes in contact with. Alternatively, the affected area can be flushed with water, utilizing soap to neutralize the acid. Powdered sodium bicarbonate or talc may also be used to treat painful reactions to the acid treatment.

Intralesional injections of interferons have been used with some success (Friedman-Kien, Eron, Conant, et al., 1988; Kirby, Kiviat, Beckman, et al., 1988). Interferons are expensive, have systemic side effects, and are not any more effective than therapies that are less expensive and less potentially toxic. The CDC (2002a) does not recommend intralesional interferon for routine use. 5-fluorouracil (5-FU) has good efficacy (Rosemberg, Greenberg, & Reid, 1987), but it is very irritating (Krebs, 1987) and potentially toxic. A vaccine against HPV 16 showed very positive results (Koutsky et al., 2002), and other HPV vaccines are being tested (Galloway, 2003).

PELVIC INFLAMMATORY DISEASE

Pelvic inflammatory disease (PID) is an infection of the female genital tract characterized by pelvic or lower abdominal pain, often following the onset or cessation of menses. PID encompasses a spectrum of symptoms caused by a variety of circumstances. The causative microorganisms are predominantly sexually transmitted but may include other microorganisms, particularly normal vaginal flora. PID is the major medical and economic consequence of sexually transmitted infections in women of reproductive age (Washington, Arno, & Brooks, 1986). PID can be caused by trauma, surgery, or ascending infection. PID may be undetected or asymptomatic, or there may be severe symptomatology requiring hospitalization. A variety of sequelae may result from PID, especially impaired reproductive health. Some practitioners use the term PID interchangeably with acute salpingitis.

SPECIFIC CONSIDERATIONS FOR PHARMACOTHERAPY

When Drug Therapy Is Needed

PID is a systemic infection that may be associated with severe acute symptoms. As with other systemic infections, there is the possibility of bacteremia with septic shock, peritonitis, or abscess formation. Appropriate antibiotic therapy is essential to eradicate the organism, relieve acute symptoms, prevent the development of sequelae, and prevent the transmission of the disease to others. Less severe cases can be managed on an outpatient basis but also require appropriate antibiotic therapy.

Short- and Long-Term Goals of Pharmacotherapy

See the syphilis section for general goals. Avoiding or minimizing the impairment of the patient's reproductive health is an important goal.

Time Frame for Initiating Pharmacotherapy

See the syphilis section for general guidelines. Severe cases of pelvic inflammatory disease may require hospitalization and prompt initiation of parenteral antibiotics. See the CDC 2002 guidelines for hospitalization criteria.

See Drug Tables 102.1–5, 102.11.

Assessment and History Taking

The clinical diagnosis of PID is difficult because of the broad range and variable intensity of the symptoms. At one extreme, the patient with acute PID may present with minimal or unimpressive symptoms. At the other extreme, the patient may present with septic shock. Many patients have mild to moderate symptoms that are nonspecific for PID or may mimic other conditions.

The following three findings must be present to make a diagnosis of PID (CDC, 2002a). These three findings are referred to as the "minimum" criteria by the CDC:

- Lower abdominal tenderness
- Adnexal tenderness
- Cervical motion tenderness

The following findings may be present and can be used to increase the specificity of the diagnosis (CDC, 2002a):

- Documented *N. gonorrhea* or *C. trachomatis* infection
- Oral temperature > 38.3° C or 101°F
- Abnormal cervical or vaginal discharge
- Elevated erythrocyte sedimentation rate
- Elevated C-reactive protein
- Laboratory documentation of cervical infection with *N. gonorrhoeae* or *C. trachomatis*
- Presence of white blood cells (WBCs) on saline microscopy

The CDC has also listed the following "definitive" criteria for diagnosing PID:

- Histopathologic evidence of endometritis on endometrial biopsy
- Radiologic abnormalities (thickened fluid-filled tubes with or without free pelvic fluid or tuboovarian complex) on transvaginal sonography or other radiologic tests
- Laparoscopic abnormalities consistent with PID

Clinicians should culture for *C. trachomatis* and *N. gonorrhoeae;* however, the abundance of normal flora in the lower genital tract, as well as potential differences in the flora of the upper versus the lower genital tract can complicate the use of cultures for diagnosis. Any confirmed cases of *C. trachomatis* or *N. gonorrhoeae* will require treatment of sex partners. As is the case with most suspected or confirmed sexually transmitted diseases, the clinician would be prudent to test for HIV. Finally, the CDC recommends a low threshold of diagnosis because of the difficulty of diagnosis, and awareness of the potential for reproductive health impairment with even mild cases of PID.

OUTCOMES MANAGEMENT

Selecting an Appropriate Agent

A variety of organisms are capable of causing PID. Frequently encountered organisms include *N. gonorrhoeae, C. trachomatis*, gram-negative facultative bacteria, anaerobes, and streptococci. Since no single antibiotic has a spectrum of activity that can cover all of the most likely causative organisms of PID, empiric therapy is broad-spectrum and is achieved with a combination of antibiotics. The most popular antibiotic combinations for treating PID are listed in Table 36–6. Note that all of the listed regimens have gonococcal, anaerobic, gram-negative, and chlamydial coverage.

A diagnosis of PID is not synonymous with hospitalization in many cases. Parenteral antibiotic therapy can be

TABLE 36–6. 2002 CDC Treatment Guidelines for Pelvic Inflammatory Disease

Recommended Regimen	Alternative Regimen
Parenteral	
Regimen A	
Cefotetan 2 g IV every 12 h	Ofloxacin 400 mg IV every 12 h
or	or
Cefoxitin 2 g IV every 6 h	Levofloxacin 500 mg IV once daily
plus	With or without
Doxycycline 100 mg IV or orally q 12 h	Metronidazole 500 mg IV every 8 h
	or
	Ampicillin/sulbactam 3 g IV every 6 h
	plus
	Doxycycline 100 mg IV or orally q 12 h
Regimen B	
Clindamycin 900 mg IV every 8 h	
plus	
Gentamicin 2 mg/kg loading dose followed by maintenance dose 1.5 mg/kg every 8 h (IV or IM) (single daily dosing of gentamicin may be substituted for q 8 h dosing)	
Oral	
Regimen A	
Ofloxacin 400 mg orally twice a day for 14 days	
or	
Levofloxacin 500 mg orally once daily for 14 days	
With or without	
Metronidazole 500 mg orally b.i.d. for 14 days	
Regimen B	
Ceftriaxone 250 mg IM single dose	See CDC 2002 Treatment guide lines for alternative treatments.
or	
Cefoxitin 2 g IM + probenecid 1 g orally single dose	
Doxycycline 100 mg orally twice. for 14 days	
With or without	
Metronidazole 500 mg orally twice a day for 14 days.	

Adapted from CDC (2002a).

given in either an inpatient or an outpatient setting. The clinician should consider the severity of the illness, availability of resources and therapies, costs, patient compliance and acceptance, and antibiotic resistance patterns when considering hospitalization versus outpatient treatment and multidose continuous parenteral therapy versus oral or single-dose parenteral therapy. Some clinicians believe that all adolescent patients should be hospitalized for treatment because of the potential for poor compliance with oral antibiotic therapy, likelihood of engaging in risky sexual behaviors prior to completion of therapy, and potential for not returning for followup (Ivey, 1997).

The reader is referred to Table 36–6 for a listing of the antibiotic regimens recommended by the CDC. Other antibiotic regimens may work equally as well but have not been studied as extensively as the ones listed in the table. Note that even in the inpatient setting, the preferred route of administration of doxycycline is oral because of the potential for pain on infusion. Azithromycin has been shown to be highly effective against *C. trachomatis* in lower genital tract infections and has the advantage of single-dose oral therapy. Some clinicians endorse the use of azithromycin for compliance reasons, but because of the expense, it may not be cost-effective (Haddix et al, 1995); azithromycin is not endorsed by the CDC in the 2002 guidelines for the treatment of PID because of a lack of data on the use of azithromycin in treating upper genital tract infections.

The choice of antibiotic regimen to use in the treatment of PID is not straightforward. The reader is referred to the discussion in the treatment section for PID of the 2002 CDC guidelines (CDC, 2002a). The choice of antibiotic regimen should be guided by clinical experience and local antibiotic resistance patterns.

Monitoring for Efficacy

The patient should respond to therapy and improve clinically, as described by the CDC, within 72 h, whether oral or parenteral therapy is utilized. The CDC 2002 STD guidelines describe clinical improvement as defervescence, reduction in direct or rebound abdominal tenderness and reduction in uterine, adnexal, and cervical motion tenderness. Patients who are on oral therapy and do not improve within 72 h should be reevaluated and placed on parenteral therapy. Patients who are on parenteral therapy and do not improve within 72 h should be reevaluated and considered for surgical intervention.

Monitoring for Toxicity

If the patient receives parenteral regimen B (see Table 36–6), then the clinician may want to monitor gentamicin levels if this therapy is continued for more than 2 to 3 days, or if the patient has a condition that could complicate aminoglycoside dosing, such as renal impairment.

Followup Recommendations

Rescreening for *C. trachomatis* and *N. gonorrhoeae* 4 to 6 weeks after completion of therapy has been recommended by some experts (CDC, 2002a). Followup to prevent or detect reinfection is important. PID is a disease primarily of young women. The clinician needs to be sensitive to the living situation and circumstances of the patient in order to maximize followup and secondary prevention efforts.

INFESTATIONS

Scabies and pediculosis pubis are sexually transmitted insect infestations primarily seen in young adults, but they may be transmitted by nonsexual skin-to-skin contact and to a lesser degree by fomites (Venna, Fleischer, & Feldman, 2001). The distinctive symptoms and clinical findings usually lead to correct diagnosis with little delay.

Scabies infestation by the human itch mite *Sarcoptes scabiei* usually causes intense pruritis, which tends to be worse at night and after bathing in hot water (Venna et al., 2001). The itching occurs first on the webs and sides of the fingers, wrists, and elbows, and eventually spreads to other parts of the body.

Pediculosis pubis, often called "crabs," is an infestation of pubic hair with the louse *Phthirus pubis*, a member of the same family as the head louse and the body louse (Venna et al., 2001). The intense pubic itching and the sensation of insects crawling over the skin is characteristic of the infestation. Clinical diagnosis can be made by any of the following: nits or lice in the hair, intense pubic itching, and maculae cerulae near the lower abdomen or thigh area (Scott, 2001).

SPECIFIC CONSIDERATIONS FOR PHARMACOTHERAPY

When Drug Therapy Is Needed

Neither the itch mite nor the pubic louse is known to transmit any other type of disease (Venna et al., 2001). Both infestations cause intense itching and discomfort for the patient, and the scratching that accompanies the itching breaks the skin barrier, which can become secondarily infected.

Short- and Long-Term Goals of Pharmacotherapy

Short-term goals are to kill the insects on the patient, treat associated problems such as itching and secondary skin infection, treat personal contacts, and eradicate the mite from the physical environment (Venna et al., 2001). The long-term goal is to teach the patient safer intimacy practices to decrease the likelihood of future infections and the risk for other STIs.

Time Frame for Initiating Pharmacotherapy

Treatment should be initiated as soon as the diagnosis is confirmed.

See Drug Table 806.

Assessment and History Taking

The diagnosis is aided by a history of itching in household contacts and/or sexual partners. The physical examination and simple laboratory findings confirm the diagnosis.

Scabies should be considered in any patient who presents with itching. Using bright light and magnification, a thorough examination for the classic burrow or small, erythematous papules with surrounding erythema should be made (Venna et al., 2001). Once a suspicious lesion is found, a drop of mineral oil is placed on the skin and the lesion vigorously scraped. The material is placed on a slide, covered with a cover slip, and examined under low-power light microscopy. Diagnostic findings include the mite, eggs, egg cases, or fecal pellets (Venna et al., 2001).

Pubic lice can be identified with careful examination of the pubic hair or other sites where itching is present using bright light and magnification. Diagnostic findings include the louse itself or nits (egg casings) on the hair shafts.

Scabies and pubic lice often coexist with other STIs. A thorough search for other infections discussed in this chapter should be made (CDC, 2002a).

Patient/Caregiver Information

To help prevent absorption of toxic levels through the skin, patients should not bathe before using lindane; if a bath is taken, the skin should be dry and cool before application. If applying lindane to more than one person the caregiver should wear rubber gloves (Drugdex Drug Evaluations, 2002). Lindane should not be used by pregnant or nursing women or children younger than 2 years of age (CDC, 2002a; Gunter, 2003).

When applying any of the topical medications, special attention should be paid to the nails and cuticles and intertriginous areas to ensure adequate penetration of the medication. A clean toothbrush may aid in applying medication to nail and cuticle areas. The toothbrush must be thrown away after use (Drugdex Drug Evaluations, 2002). In addition, the medication should be applied to all crusts and scabs.

The itching that accompanies parasitic insect infestations is the result of the immune response to the insect. Once the insect is killed, the itching subsides gradually over a period of 2 to 4 weeks (Venna et al., 2001). Continued itching does not indicate treatment failure, and retreatment should only be instituted with healthcare provider approval. Unnecessary retreatment with lindane can lead to severe toxicity such as seizures or less serious problems such as contact dermatitis. Because symptoms can take up to 1 month to become apparent after infestation with scabies, all household and sexual partners should be treated whether symptomatic or not. Only sexual partners of people with pubic lice need to be treated.

Fomites play a minor role in transmission of scabies and pubic lice, and fumigation of the entire house is not necessary. Even so, patients should be instructed to decontaminate their environment by machine laundering in hot water or machine drying on hot cycles all bed linens, sleeping bags, clothes, and personal articles like bath towels (CDC, 2002a).

OUTCOMES MANAGEMENT

Selecting an Appropriate Agent

For scabies, the recommended treatment is permethrin cream (5%) applied to all areas of the body from the neck to the soles of the feet and washed off after 8–14 h (Brown, Becher, & Brady, 1995; CDC, 2002a). Permethrin is more expensive than lindane but is equally effective and has no known systemic side effects (Drugdex Drug Evaluations, 2002; Venna et al., 2001). Alternative regimens include:

1. Lindane (1%): 1 oz of lotion or 30 g of cream. Apply to all areas of the body from the neck to the soles of the feet and wash off after 8 h.
2. Sulfur (6%) precipitated in ointment: Apply to all areas of the body each night for three nights. Wash off all medication before applying the next dose and 24 h after the last dose.
3. Ivermectin 200 μg/kg in one single oral dose repeated in two weeks. Ivermectin has been useful in difficult cases; however, comparative studies to current therapy are not available (CDC, 2002a; Venna et al., 2001).

In addition to treatment for the infestation, patients may require a medication to control itching such as diphenhydramine 25 to 50 mg by mouth every 6 h or topical hydrocortisone.

For pubic lice, the CDC-recommended treatment (CDC, 2002a):

1. Permethrin 1% cream rinse applied to the affected area and washed off after 10 min.
2. Lindane 1% shampoo applied to the affected area and thoroughly washed off after 4 min.
3. Pyrethrins with piperonyl butoxide applied to affected area and washed off after 10 min.

For pubic lice infestation of the eyelashes, the only recommended treatment is occlusive ophthalmic ointment to the eyelid margins twice a day for 10 days. The other regimens should not be used near the eyes (CDC, 2002a).

Lindane should not be used by pregnant or lactating women, by children less than 2 years of age, or by people with extensive dermatitis. In addition, lindane should not be used by people with seizure disorders (CDC, 2002a; Venna et al., 2001).

Monitoring for Efficacy

The itching from scabies should decrease gradually over 2 to 4 weeks. If symptoms persist unchanged or if live mites are seen, patients can be retreated with an alternative regimen in 1 week (CDC, 2002a). Patients with crusted scabies may require multiple applications of medication over several weeks or a combination of oral and topical treatments (Meinking, Taplin, Herminda, Pardo, & Kerdel, 1995).

For pubic lice, followup is required only if symptoms do not resolve. If lice continue to be present or nits are present at the skin-hair junction, patients should be retreated (CDC, 2002a).

The most common causes of treatment failure for infestation include incorrect use of medication, failure to treat all infected body sites, or exposure to an untreated sexual partner (Venna et al., 2001).

Monitoring for Toxicity

Lindane is a moderately toxic insecticide with seizures being the most common neurologic adverse event. Most lindane toxicity comes from inappropriate use of the drug, leading to increased absorption in adults or when used in the pediatric or geriatric populations (Fischer, 1994). Symptoms of lindane toxicity include nausea, vomiting, respiratory, failure, aplastic anemia, and, rarely, death (Faber, 1996). Patients should report any adverse events to the healthcare provider. Adverse events related to other recommended treatments are limited to local burning or stinging (Venna et al., 2001).

Followup Recommendations

Patients may experience feelings of continued infestation even after successful therapy and need emotional support to completely resolve the psychological impact of infestation. If these issues are not addressed, patients may overuse medications and experience toxic reactions.

VAGINITIS

Vaginitis is one of the most prevalent problems of women in primary care and gynecologic practice settings and may be the result of either a sexually transmitted pathogen or an alteration in the normal vaginal flora. The healthy vaginal milieu is a delicate ecosystem with colonies of multiple organisms existing in dynamic balance. A variety of common activities such as douching, coitus, and hormonal fluctuations can disrupt this balance and result in vaginitis. Vulvovaginal candidiasis, bacterial vaginosis, and trichomonas vaginitis are the specific conditions that will be addressed. The diagnosis and treatment of atrophic vaginitis are discussed in Chapter 19. There are noninfectious causes of vaginal discharge such as vaginal or cervical cancer or discharge from a retained vaginal foreign body that are not addressed in this chapter, but they should be considered in the differential diagnosis of any vaginal discharge, especially one that does not respond to standard therapy.

VULVOVAGINAL CANDIDIASIS

Vulvovaginal candidiasis (VVC) is a common fungal vaginal infection of reproductive-aged women. Most cases are the result of overgrowth of *Candida albicans*, but the incidence of non-*albicans* infections is increasing. VVC is estimated to affect 20% of women annually (Geiger, Foxman, & Gillespie, 1996). In addition, 75% of women will experience at least one episode of VVC during their lifetime, with 40 to 45% of women experiencing two or more symptomatic episodes (CDC, 2002a). Hypoestrogenic, postmenopausal women seldom experience symptomatic VVC until started on estrogen replacement.

Women typically present with acute onset of pruritus and discharge. The vulva may be erythematous, edematous, and contain satellite lesions. Other symptoms, such as burning upon urination, are common (Haefner, 1999).

Several studies have identified a variety of risk factors for VVC. These include receptive oral sex, high-dose estrogen oral contraceptive use, spermacide use, sex during menses, pregnancy, diabetes, steroid use, systemic antibiotic use, and African American ethnicity (Geiger & Foxman, 1996; Geiger et al., 1996; Hellberg, Zdolsek, Nilsson, & Mardh, 1995; Hillier & Arko, 1996).

Recurrent VVC (four or more episodes per year) occurs in <5% of women (CDC, 2002a). Recurrent VVC is more often associated with infection with non-*albicans* species such as *C. glabrata* or *C. tropicalis* than are initial acute infections (Spinillo, Capuzzo, Egbe, Nicola, & Piazzi, 1995; Spinillo, Capuzzo, Gulminetti, et al., 1997).

Specific Considerations for Pharmacotherapy

When Drug Therapy is Needed. Although not life-threatening, the symptoms of VVC are distressing and disruptive to affected women. Prompt treatment is indicated to restore a healthy vaginal environment and improve the quality of life.

Short- and Long-Term Goals of Pharmacotherapy. The short- and long-term goals of therapy for all types of vaginitis are very similar. The short-term goal for therapy is to resolve signs and symptoms of infection. Long-term goals are to restore the vaginal ecology and manage risk factors to prevent recurrent infection.

Nonpharmacologic Therapy. Although not known to be effective for treatment of acute symptomatic VVC, nonpharmacologic therapy is a mainstay in prevention of recurrent episodes. The following measures should be kept in mind:

1. The daily ingestion of yogurt enriched with live *Lactobacillus acidophilus* bacteria has been associated with preventing the recurrence of yeast vaginitis (Elmer, Surawicz, & McFarland, 1996; Shalev, Battino, Weiner, Colodner, & Keness, 1996) and bacterial vaginosis.
2. Cotton underwear absorbs the normal vaginal secretions and allows air circulation to prevent continual moisture on the vulva.
3. Women with recurrent VVC should be encouraged to avoid occlusive clothing such as panty hose and tight jeans that prevent air flow and contribute to alterations of the vaginal environment, including overgrowth of yeast organisms.
4. Women should be encouraged to avoid douching. Douching alters the normal vaginal environment and encourages the overgrowth of a variety of organisms, increasing the incidence of yeast vaginitis, bacterial vaginosis, and pelvic inflammatory disease.

Time Frame for Initiating Pharmacotherapy. Therapy should be initiated as soon as the diagnosis is confirmed. There is no benefit from delay. A variety of therapeutic schedules are available to treat VVC including topical and systemic medications. If symptoms resolve, followup evaluation is not required.

See Drug Tables 103, 805.

Assessment and History Taking. Assessment for vaginal symptoms is usually straightforward and leads to a definitive diagnosis. The assessment includes a targeted history, physical examination, and simple office laboratory studies. Ideally, women should not be menstruating and should avoid intravaginal medications and sexual intercourse for 2 to 3 days before an examination for vaginitis (Secor, 1997).

The targeted history identifies events that may have altered the delicate balance of organisms that normally colonize the vagina. Factors reported to affect the vaginal ecosystem are broad-spectrum antibiotics, exogenous estrogen (menopausal replacements or high-dose oral contraceptives), contraceptives such as spermacides and latex devices, douches, vaginal medications, sexual intercourse, stress, and a change of sexual partners (ACOG, 1996). Other factors that may predispose patients to vulvovaginal candidiasis include uncontrolled diabetes mellitus, steroid use, and compromised immune status (chronic systemic illness such as lupus, HIV, or AIDS) (ACOG, 1996; Haefner, 1999). It is important to determine if the patient has initiated self-treatment for the presenting symptoms. Ferris, Dekle, and Litaker (1996) noted that only a minority of women were able to correctly diagnose VVC from signs and symptoms. Use of nonprescription antifungals may mask the signs and symptoms of other causes of vaginitis and may select for resistant yeast organisms (ACOG, 1996; Haefner, 1999). As with any skin surface, the vulvar and vaginal epithelia are susceptible to allergic and chemical irritation. Accordingly, the history should include a search for common chemical sources of irritation such as perfumed and medicated soaps and shampoos, laundry detergents, bath oils, perfumed or dyed toilet paper, and chemicals in swimming pools and hot tubs (ACOG, 1996).

The clinical exam and microscopy are most useful for diagnosis (Anderson et al., 2004). A careful inspection of the external genitalia, noting any erythema or pallor, edema, excoriation, or lesion such as blisters, fissures, or warts is needed. The femoral and inguinal lymph nodes are palpated and the presence of vaginal discharge at the introitus should be noted. If the woman reports external symptoms and no obvious abnormalities are noted, it is helpful to ask the woman to point to the area causing discomfort.

Next the clinician inserts the speculum, being careful to not traumatize the cervix. The color, amount, and consistency of the vaginal discharge as well as any cervical ectopy, friability, or mucus in the os are noted. The appearance of the vaginal walls and cervix should be noted. There are no controlled studies documenting the best method for collecting and preparing wet-mount slides of vaginal specimens for microscopic examination. Gant and Cunningham (1993) suggest that specimens for microscopic examination and pH determination of the vaginal discharge be collected from the lateral vaginal walls close to the cervix (between the speculum blades) with a cotton swab. Secor (1997) suggests a wooden or plastic spatula to avoid fiber artifacts. The posterior vaginal pool should be avoided since this contains discharge of cervical rather than vaginal origin. The specimen is then placed in a small test tube (e.g., a 5-cc red-top tube) with ½-in of fresh normal saline. The solution should be opaque with suspended cells and exudate. The pH of the discharge is best determined with narrow-range (4–5.5) pH paper (Haefner, 1999; Hillier & Arko, 1996). A strip of the paper may be held with ring forceps and placed against the lateral vaginal wall, or placed on the anterior lip of the withdrawn speculum. The history or physical findings may indicate a need for cervical cultures for gonorrhea and chlamydia or a Pap smear. Although not commonly needed in the workup of vaginal discharge, a colposcopy and biopsy may be indicated if cervical or vaginal lesions are found. The speculum is removed and a bimanual examination performed checking for evidence of upper-level involvement such as uterine, adnexal, or cervical motion tenderness.

Laboratory studies to identify the etiology of a vaginal discharge include ascertaining the pH, as described earlier, as well as microscopic evaluation. Vaginal cultures are rarely necessary except in recurrent infection or those recalcitrant to standard therapy. A saline wet-prep slide is examined for "clue" cells (epithelial cells stippled with bacteria), motile protozoa, white blood cells, epithelial cells, red blood cells, lactobacilli, and background bacteria.

A 10% potassium hydroxide (KOH) slide is examined to identify yeast organisms (CDC, 2002a). The KOH slide provides higher sensitivity for identifying yeast organisms than the saline slide.

The examination findings that indicate yeast vaginitis include erythema of the vulva and vagina with possible excoriations or discrete fine pustules. The vagina often has a thick curd-like discharge that adheres to the vaginal wall. Vaginal pH is most often normal. Under microscopy, *C. albicans* and *tropicalis* are dimorphic organisms and can be found as both hyphae and buds. In contrast, *C. glabrata* and other non-*C. albicans* species are monomorphic and exist only in bud form (Secor, 1997). The differentiation of *Candida* species is difficult without culture and is not necessary for treatment of simple yeast vaginitis.

Patient/Caregiver Information. Patients should be counseled to complete the full course of therapy even if symptoms resolve sooner. Many intravaginal medications contain mineral oil and may weaken latex condoms and diaphragms if used concurrently with or within 72 h of using oil-based intravaginal products (Haefner, 1999). Clinicians should take care to prescribe a non-oil-based product for women using latex condoms or diaphragms. The other option is for the woman to use nonlatex contraceptive devices.

Women should be discouraged from self-diagnosis and treatment with nonprescription antifungals. The use of nonprescription antifungals may have contributed to the increase in non-*albicans* species causing VVC. These non-*albicans* species are less sensitive to the nonprescription antifungals as well as the oral agent fluconazole (Tobin, 1995).

Only the topical azoles can be used safely after the first trimester (CDC, 2002a). Pregnant women should be counseled to insert only a small portion of the applicator very gently into the vagina to avoid trauma to the cervix. It is probably unwise for women with premature cervical dilatation to use vaginal applicators.

Outcomes Management

Selecting an Appropriate Agent. Faro, Apuzzio, Bohannon, et al. (1997) recommend topical azoles as a first-line treatment for VVC because of the high mycological and clinical cure rates, minimal systemic effects, and low side-effect profile. Sobel, Brooker, Stein, et al. (1995) found similar efficacy rates for oral fluconazole and topical clotrimazole. When compared to the oral preparations, the topical azoles are thought to provide quicker relief of symptoms. The oral agents, although more convenient for some women, have a greater risk of side effects and drug interactions (O-Prasertsawat & Bourlert, 1995). In addition, several non-*albicans* organisms are resistant to oral agents.

The topical agents are available in doses for a variety of treatment schedules from 1- to 7-day intravaginal therapy. For mild, short-duration, or first-episode VVC the short-course treatments of any product will usually result in high cure rates. It would seem prudent to select a topical agent with broad-spectrum activity to discourage the selection for non-*albicans* treatment failures. For more severe symptomatology (extensive inflammation, severe excoriation, etc.), for symptoms of long duration, or after multiple episodes of self-treatment, the longer course of therapy is recommended (Faro et al., 1997). Terconazole (a topical antifungal in 3- or 7-day dose regimens) appears to have the broadest spectrum of antifungal activity (Tobin, 1995), although clinical cure rates are comparable with all topical and oral agents.

Fluconazole 150 mg in a single dose is the only oral medication that is FDA-approved for the treatment of symptomatic VVC (Desai & Johnson, 1996). Ketoconazole, although not FDA-approved, has been used to treat chronic, recurrent symptomatic VVC.

Monitoring for Efficacy. A typical course of therapy for acute VVC is one oral dose of fluconazole or a 3 to 7 day course of terconazole. Signs and symptoms should start to improve within 2 days and be resolved within 4 to 6 days with oral therapy. Signs and symptoms should start to resolve within 1 to 1½ days and be resolved within 4 to 6 days with topical therapy (Slavin, Benrubi, Parker, Griffin, & Magee, 1992). Continuing symptoms are commonly related to incomplete treatment adherence or a mixed infection that was missed at diagnosis and, rarely, to resistance.

If short-course treatment does not resolve symptoms, consideration should be given to the 7-day topical treatment. The clinician should consider a mixed etiology for the vaginitis and reevaluate for other pathogens if the 7-day treatment does not relieve symptoms. Treatment failure and recurrent infections should be evaluated with yeast cultures.

Although rarely indicated now that broad-spectrum topical antifungals are available, gentian violet solution painted on the cervix, vagina, and vulva provides almost immediate symptomatic relief. The deep purple solution stains fabrics, and the woman should be counseled to protect her clothing.

Chronic recurrent VVC is a therapeutic challenge and is best managed by an expert. Women with chronic recurrent infections have often endured repeated symptomatic episodes with the accompanying workup and treatment, only to become symptomatic again. Treatment must be in the context of a partnership of the woman and clinician to determine the regime that balances the woman's needs and desires with the best options for cure or long-term remission. Treatment of the asymptomatic male partner is controversial, since it has not been shown to significantly reduce the recurrence rate in women. Chronic recurrent VVC requires long-term topical or oral treatment until symptoms resolve followed by either intermittent or long-term continuous maintenance. Patients with resistant yeast infection may require therapy with vaginal boric acid inserts. A dose of 600 mg twice daily for a duration of 14 days has been reported as successful by Sobel and Chaim (1997) and others (Bingham, 1999).

Monitoring for Toxicity. Toxicity is rare with topical therapy. The most common side effects are vaginal burning or itching (Haefner, 1999).

The oral agent fluconazole has been associated with a variety of side effects such as GI symptoms and adverse events including drug interactions, liver function abnormalities, congenital anomalies (Lee, Feinberg, Abraham, & Murphy, 1992; Nisson, 2002; Schaffer, 2004), and, rarely, angioedema (Abbot, Hughes, Patel, & Kinghorn, 1991) and anaphylaxis (Neuhaus, Pavic, & Pletscher, 1991). Significant drug interactions with oral fluconazole include serious arrhythmias when coadministered with nonsedating antihistamines. In addition, elevated serum levels of cyclosporine, anticoagulants, anticonvulsants, oral hypoglycemic agents, and theophylline can occur when these drugs are coadministered with oral antifungal agents (Faro et al., 1997). More research is required to document whether these interactions are a problem with single-dose oral azoles.

Followup Recommendations. If symptoms resolve with treatment, no followup is required. Women who remain symptomatic after a full 7-day course of a broad-spectrum antifungal should be reexamined for mixed infection and vaginal cultures should be performed.

BACTERIAL VAGINOSIS

Abnormal vaginal discharge is most often caused by bacterial vaginosis (BV) is the most common cause of abnormal vaginal discharge. BV develops when the normal balance of organisms in the vagina changes with loss of the normally predominant H_2O_2-producing lactobacilli and exuberant growth of a variety of strict and facultative anaerobes, including *Bacteroides, Peptococcus, Mobiluncus, Gardnerella, Streptococcus,* and *Mycoplasma* (Eschenbach, 1993, Hawes, Hillier, Benedetti, et al., 1996). The factors that cause this shift in vaginal flora are unknown. There are no established risk factors for BV, but it is more common in women who have multiple sex partners and is rare in women who have never been sexually active (CDC, 2002a). Bacterial vaginosis does not cause an inflammatory response, but surface changes in the epithelia result in the exposure of the cervix to immunologic shifts. Such shifts cause increases in inflammatory cytokines like interlukin 1β and decrease natural protectant molecules like secretory leukocyte protease inhibitors (Hillier, Soper, & Sobel, 2002). One study (Rein, Shih, Miller, & Guerrant, 1996) suggested that the lack of leukocytes in the vaginal discharge of women with BV was the result of destruction of these cells rather than the absence of a primary inflammatory response.

The most common presenting symptom of women with BV is a copious vaginal discharge, possibly with a foul odor that is more noticeable after coitus. A large portion of affected women (up to 50%) are asymptomatic (CDC, 2002a).

Specific Considerations for Pharmacotherapy

When drug therapy is needed. It was once accepted that asymptomatic women should not be treated (CDC, 2002a), but studies have identified significant morbidity associated with untreated BV (Morales, Schorr, & Albritton, 1994; Newton, Piper, & Peairs, 1997). Untreated BV has been associated with pelvic inflammatory disease, cervicitis, postoperative infection, abnormal cytology in the nonpregnant woman, and with preterm labor and low birth weight when untreated during pregnancy (Hillier, Nugent, Eschenbach, et al, 1995; Hillier, Kiviat, Hawes, 1996; Platz-Christensen, Sundstrom, & Larsson, 1994; Sweet, 1995). There is growing consensus that at the very least, routine screening and treatment would benefit women undergoing gynecologic surgery, elective abortion, or other invasive procedures and possibly those with abnormal Pap results. During pregnancy, screening and treatment are appropriate for all symptomatic women and should be considered for those women considered at high risk for preterm delivery either by history or physical findings (CDC, 2002a). Three of four studies have reported a reduced incidence of preterm delivery with systemic treatment of women with BV (CDC, 2002a). Until the risks and benefits of treating low-risk and asymptomatic pregnant women are known, this group deserves special caution.

Short- and Long-Term Goals of Pharmacotherapy. As with VVC, the short-term goal is to resolve symptoms and restore the vaginal ecosystem. There are no proven strategies for preventing recurrence, so the long-term goal should be to maintain the normal vaginal flora and a balanced vaginal ecosystem.

Nonpharmacologic Therapy. Nonpharmacologic therapy for BV is the same as for VVC. It is focused on restoring and maintaining a healthy vaginal ecosystem.

Time Frame for Initiating Therapy. Therapy should be initiated as soon as the diagnosis is confirmed in symptomatic women. A variety of therapeutic schedules are available to treat BV, including topical and systemic medications. If symptoms resolve, followup evaluation is not required.

See Drug Table 101.

Assessment and History Taking. The assessment for vaginal discharge is the same as for VVC. The laboratory findings that are diagnostic for BV include finding at least three of the following:

1. "Clue" cells on wet prep or gram stain
2. Fishy (amine) odor of vaginal discharge before or after addition of 10% KOH (positive "whiff" test)
3. pH of vaginal discharge > 4.5
4. A thin, adherent, white, homogenous vaginal discharge (CDC, 2002a)

The wet prep usually demonstrates few lactobacilli, few WBCs, and a large number of background bacteria. Cultures are not recommended because the bacteria responsible for BV are normal inhabitants of the vagina and can be cultured from at least 50% of normal women (CDC, 2002a). Other tests are available for diagnosis such as the FemExam® test card and Pip Activity TestCard™ (CDC, 2002a).

Patient/Caregiver Information. In addition to the general caregiver guidelines discussed for VVC, the woman with BV requires the following information. With oral administration of metronidazole, the most common side effects are mild nausea, dry mouth, a metallic taste, or mild headache (Hillier et al., 2002; Tracy: Webster, 1995). Patients can minimize these side effects by taking the medication in divided doses with food. Patients should be warned that metronidazole can cause abdominal distress, vomiting, flushing, or headache if alcohol is consumed during or for 24 h after completion of therapy. Although serum levels are much lower with intravaginal administration than with oral dosing, sensitive individuals could experience the same disulfiram-like reactions when intravaginal metronidazole is used concomitantly with alcohol. Patients should be advised to discontinue the medication and call their healthcare provider if numbness, tingling, or weakness develops in any extremity or if any other abnormal neurologic symptoms occur. Anyone taking antibacterial agents, including oral and intravaginal clindamycin, should be counseled to report diarrhea, especially bloody diarrhea.

Metronidazole is secreted in breastmilk. To minimize effects on the newborn, breastfeeding should be discontinued for 24 h after maternal ingestion of a single 2-g dose (Haefner, 1999). Expressed milk should be discarded.

Outcomes Management

Selecting an appropriate agent. Bacterial vaginosis can be effectively treated with oral or topical agents (Ferris, Litaker, Woodward, Mathis, & Hendrich, 1995). The selection should be guided by patient preference, clinician experience, and cost considerations. CDC (2002a) guidelines recommend metronidazole 500 mg po bid for 7 days. Other recommended treatment regimens for nonpregnant women include metronidazole gel 0.75%, 5 mg intravaginal applicatorful once daily for 5 days, or clindamycin cream 2% intravaginal applicatorful once daily for 7 days at bedtime (CDC, 2002a). Alternative treatments include metronidazole 2 g orally once, clindamycin 300 mg orally bid for 7 days, or clindamycin ovules 100 g intravaginally once daily at bedtime for 3 days (CDC, 2002a). The nonoral routes are associated with lower systemic side effects but significantly higher costs (Mikamo, Kawazoe, Izumi, et al., 1997).

The CDC (2002a) advises that "All symptomatic pregnant women should be tested and treated" for BV due to the dangers associated with this infection in pregnancy (p. 44). There is growing consensus but not complete agreement that to decrease the risk of preterm birth, screening and treatment of BV in high-risk women should be conducted at the first prenatal visit. Appropriate treatment regimens for high-risk pregnant women include metronidazole 250 mg tid for 7 days, metronidazole 2 g in a single dose, or clindamycin 300 mg bid for 7 days. If they are symptomatic with BV, pregnant women at low risk for preterm delivery should be treated with one of the above therapies or metronidazole gel 0.75%, one applicator bid for 5 days (CDC, 2002a). Because of reports from two randomized clinical trials of increased rates of preterm birth after treatment with clindamycin vaginal cream, the CDC does not recommend its use in pregnancy (CDC, 2002a).

Monitoring for Efficacy. Women who become asymptomatic during treatment need no further evaluation. For women who remain symptomatic or have symptoms return very shortly after completing treatment, one of the alternative treatment regimens should be used. For women with recurrent BV, Winceslaus and Calver (1996) achieved cure rates equal to current drug therapy and with no side effects using a single vaginal washout with 3% hydrogen peroxide. The hydrogen peroxide was retained in the vagina for 3 min before being drained. Some women may prefer this inexpensive treatment to repeated doses of costly intravaginal drugs or the side effects associated with repeated courses of oral medication.

Monitoring for Toxicity. Metronidazole has a low side-effect profile in the doses used to treat BV. The most consistent findings include mild nausea and diarrhea and a metallic taste in the mouth. More serious side effects can occur with higher doses or prolonged therapy, including neutropenia, paresthesias and peripheral neuropathies, confusion, hallucinations, and seizures (Kasten, 1999; Simms-Cendan, 1996). Corey, Doebbeling, DeJong, and Britigan (1991) reported metronidazole-induced pancreatitis in three patients treated for bacterial vaginosis. All signs and symptoms of pancreatitis resolved promptly after discontinuation of metronidazole. If administered concomitantly, metronidazole has been shown to increase the serum levels of warfarin, phenytoin, and lithium. In addition, phenobarbital, cimetidine, prednisone, phenazone, and rifampin have been shown to increase the metabolic clearance of metronidazole and may decrease its effectiveness Patients suspected of recurrent BV infections should be tested for *Candida*. The mechanism for patients developing a superinfection of *Candida* is unknown. It is important to treat the yeast infection with an appropriate antifungal until antimicrobial therapy is discontinued (Sobel, 2001).

Followup Recommendations. Bacterial vaginosis is a common condition with frequent recurrences in susceptible women. Treatment of male partners has not been shown to improve the woman's response to therapy or decrease recurrence rates. At this time, treatment of male partners is not recommended (CDC, 2002a).

TRICHOMONAS VAGINITIS

Trichomonas vaginalis is a protozoan parasite that can infect the urogenital tract in women and men. Worldwide, trichomonas vaginitis (TV) is thought to be the most common nonviral, nonbacterial sexually transmitted infection (Zhang, 1996). In symptomatic women, *T. vaginalis* infection is characterized by a copious, frothy, vaginal discharge and vulvar irritation. In addition to vaginal infection, trichomonads have been found in the urethra, Skene's glands, and Bartholin's gland. Women often become symptomatic during or shortly after menses when the pH of the vagina is raised by menstrual blood. This produces a favorable environment for trichomonad proliferation (Goode, Grauer, & Gums, 1994). In men, *T. vaginalis* can cause urethral discharge, but symptoms are often mild, if present at all (CDC, 2002a; Kreiger, 1995). The vast majority of cases of trichomonas infection are sexually transmitted, but the organism can survive for several hours on wet towels, bathing suits, toilet seats, and other fomites. *Trichomonas vaginalis* often coexists with other sexually transmitted pathogens; therefore, infected women should be screened for other sexually transmitted infections (Reynolds & Wilson, 1996).

Specific Considerations for Pharmacotherapy

When Drug Therapy Is Needed. Although most men are asymptomatic, trichomonas vaginitis causes acute symptoms in most women and treatment should be instituted to provide relief and prevent transmission to sexual partners. In addition to acute local symptoms and discomfort, trichomonas vaginitis during pregnancy has been associated with preterm rupture of membranes and preterm delivery (CDC, 2002a). Women coinfected with *Trichomonas* and *Chlamydia* have an increased risk of developing pelvic inflammatory disease when compared to women infected with *Chlamydia* alone (Paisarntantiwong, Brockman, Clarke, et al. 1995). Treating TV prevents the transmission to new sexual partners.

Short- and Long-Term Goals of Pharmacotherapy. Short-term goals are to eliminate the organism from the genital tract, resolve the symptoms of infection, and prevent the transmission to sexual partners. Long-term goals are to prevent adverse events in pregnancy and prevent recurrence through education on the use of barrier contraception and safer sex practices.

Time Frame for Initiating Pharmacotherapy. As with all STIs, pharmacotherapy should be instituted as soon as the diagnosis is confirmed. Treatment should be arranged for all sexual partners of the infected woman.

Assessment and History Taking. The basic history, physical examination, and office laboratory studies for all types of vaginitis, including TV, are the same as those for VVC.

Specific examination findings consistent with TV infection include any or all of the following: diffuse vulvar erythema; copious, sometimes frothy, vaginal discharge; inflamed vagina and cervix; and punctate hemorrhages (strawberry spots). Because the clinical features of TV are nonspecific, diagnosis relies upon the combination of clinical findings and laboratory results. Vaginal pH is almost always > 5.0 and many times approaches 6.0. A positive "whiff" test is often present. The wet prep reveals many WBCs and motile, flagellated protozoa. The presence of trichomonads on a Pap smear result is neither sensitive nor specific for infection, and treatment of asymptomatic women based on Pap findings alone could result in unnecessary treatment of up to 30% of cases (Weinberger & Harger, 1993).

Patient/Caregiver Information. TV is a sexually transmitted infection in almost all cases. Infected individuals should be counseled to inform all sex partners of the need for treatment regardless of the presence of symptoms. They should abstain from intercourse or have their male partners use condoms until all medication has been completed and all partners are asymptomatic. In addition, health promotion teaching should stress the importance of barrier contraception and safer sex practices at all times to reduce the risk of reinfection with TV or of acquiring other sexually transmitted infections.

Outcomes Management

Selecting an Appropriate Agent. Metronidazole is the only recommended treatment for TV in the United States. The recommended treatment for pregnant women after the first trimester, nonpregnant women, and all male sexual partners whether symptomatic or not is 2 g orally, given as a single dose. Alternatively, metronidazole can be given as 500 mg orally, twice daily for 7 days (CDC, 2002a). Sexual partners also should be treated, and patients should abstain from sex until each partner is cured (CDC, 2002a).

Because trichomonads infect the urethra, Skene's glands, and Bartholins's gland as well as the vagina, intravaginal metronidazole gel is not effective for treating TV (Tidwell, Lushbaugh, Laughlin, Cleary, & Finley, 1994). During the first trimester of pregnancy, symptomatic relief but not reliable mycologic cure can sometimes be obtained by using clotrimazole vaginal suppositories, 100 mg at bedtime for 6 to 8 days (Knodel & Kraynak, 1997, p. 2216). A study in nonpregnant women demonstrated similar results using two 100-mg clotrimazole vaginal tablets once a day for 7 days (duBouchet, Spence, Rein, Danzig, & McCormack, 1997).

Monitoring for Efficacy. Resolution of symptoms indicates effective therapy, and no further followup is needed. Even organisms with diminished susceptibility to metronidazole usually respond to higher doses (CDC, 2002a; Pearlman, Yashar, Ernst, & Solomon, 1996). If treatment failure occurs and symptoms remain, and reinfection is excluded, the diagnosis should be reconfirmed and the patient retreated with metronidazole 500 mg bid for 7 days. Patients who have had treatment failures may respond to a single 2-g dose of metronidazole for 3 to 5 days. Houang, Ahmet, and Lawrence (1997) reported successful treatment of four patients with culture-positive symptomatic resistant trichomonas vaginitis with a combination of oral metronidazole (200–400 mg tid), and 1% zinc sulfate douche followed by metronidazole vaginal suppositories (500 mg) bid. This regime included prophylactic douching and suppositories after menses for several months. The lower dose of oral medication resulted in fewer side effects than the standard therapy. Any patient in whom reinfection has been excluded, who fails to respond to standard therapy, or who is allergic to metronidazole should be managed in consultation with an expert (CDC, 2002a).

Monitoring for Toxicity. Metronidazole side effects and toxicity are the same as those discussed for BV.

Followup Recommendations. Trichomonas vaginitis is a sexually transmitted infection in almost all cases. Because most men are asymptomatic and there is a high transmission rate of infection between partners, all sexual partners of women with trichomonas vaginitis should be treated. *Trichomonas* often coexists with other sexually transmitted pathogens, and infected individuals should be screened for other conditions (Reynolds & Wilson, 1996).

SUMMARY

The diagnosis and treatment of vaginitis in women is usually straightforward and involves correlating the findings from history, physical examination, and simple laboratory studies. It is also evident that environmental factors as well as pathogens affect the vaginal milieu and that a clear understanding of normal vaginal flora has not been definitively established. In an observational study of the composition of the vaginal flora of healthy women over time, only 4 women out of the 26 in the study had "normal" vaginal microbiology throughout the study period (Priestly, Jones, Dhar, & Goodwin, 1997). A variety of conditions including candidiasis, BV, and *Ureaplasma urealyticum* were found intermittently throughout the study, and symptoms correlated poorly with microbiological findings. More research is required to define the "normal" vaginal environment, establish clear guidelines for screening pregnant and nonpregnant asymptomatic women, and determine the most appropriate treatment for the variety of conditions that affect the reproductive tract of women. Readers are urged to maintain currency as CDC guidelines are revised.

REFERENCES

Abbott, M., Hughes, D. L., Patel, R., & Kinghorn, G. R. (1991). Angioedema after fluconazole. *Lancet,338* (8767), 633.

Alrabiah, F. A., & Sacks, S. L. (1996). New antiherpesvirus agents: Their targets and therapeutic potential. *Drugs, 52*(1), 17–32.

American College of Obstetricians and Gynecologists (ACOG). (1996). *Vaginitis*. ACOG Technical Bulletin no. 226. Washington, DC: Author.

Anderson, M., Klink, K., & Cohrssen, A. (2004) Evaluation of vaginal complaints. Journal American Medical Association, 291(1), 1368–1379.

Anonymous. (2000). From the Centers for Disease Control and Prevention. Fluoroquinolone resistance in *Neisseria gonorrhea*, Hawaii, 1999, and decreased susceptibility to azithromycin in *N. gonorrhea*, Missouri, 1999. *JAMA, 284*(15), 1917–1919.

Anonymous. (1999). National guideline for the management of lymphogranuloma venereum. Clinical Effectiveness Group (Association of Genitourinary Medicine and the Medical Society for the Study of Venereal Diseases). *Sexually Transmitted Infections, 75*(Suppl 1), S40–2.

Bachmann, L., Lewis, I., Allen, R., Schwebke, J., Leviton, L.C., Siegal, H., & Hook, E. (2000). Risk and prevalence of treatable sexually transmitted diseases at a Birmingham substance abuse treatment facility. *American Journal of Public Health, 90*(10), 1615–1618.

Barlow, D. (1997). The diagnosis of oropharyngeal gonorrhea. *Genitourinary Medicine*, 73(1), 16–17.

Bashi, S. A. (1985). Cryotherapy versus podophyllin in the treatment of genital warts. *International Journal of Dermatology, 24*, 535–536.

Bignell, C.J. (2001). European guideline for the management of gonorrhea. *International Journal of STD & AIDS, 12*(3), 27–29.

Bingham, J. S. (1999). What to do with the patient with recurrent vulvovaginal candidiasis. *Sexually Transmitted Infections*, 75(4), 225–227.

Brown, S., Becher, J., & Brady, W. (1995). Treatment of ectoparasitic infections: Review of the English-language literature, 1982–1992. *Clinical Infectious Diseases, 20*(Suppl. 1), S104–S109.

Campos-Outcalt, D., & Hurwitz, S. (2002). Female-to-female transmission of syphilis: A case report. *Sexually Transmitted Diseases, 29*(2), 119–120.

Cates, W. Jr. (1999). Estimates of the incidence and prevalence of sexually transmitted diseases in the United States. American Social Health Association Panel. *Sexually Transmitted Diseases, 26*(4 Suppl), S2–7

Centers for Disease Control and Prevention (CDC) Division of STD Prevention. (1999). *The national plan to eliminate syphilis from the United States.* Atlanta: U.S. Department of Health and Human Services.

Centers for Disease Control and Prevention (CDC) Division of STD Prevention. (2000a). *Sexually transmitted disease surveillance, 1999.* Atlanta: U.S. Department of Health and Human Services.

Centers for Disease Control and Prevention (CDC). (2000b). *Tracking the hidden epidemics: 2000 Trends in STDs in the United States.* http://www.cdc.gov/nchstp/od/news/RevBrochure1pdfSyphilis.htm Accessed October 10, 2002.

Centers for Disease Control and Prevention (CDC). (2001a). *Sexually transmitted disease surveillance, 2000.* Atlanta, GA: U.S. Department of Health and Human Services, Centers for Disease Control and Prevention. Available at hHttp://www.cdc.gov/std/stats. Accessed October 10, 2002.

Centers for Disease Control and Prevention (CDC). (2001b). *Sexually transmitted disease facts—Chlamydia in the U.S., April 2001.* Available at http://www.cdc.gov/std Accessed 2002 October 10, 2002.

Centers for Disease Control and Prevention (CDC). (2002a). *Sexually transmitted diseases treatment guidelines. MMWR, 51*(RR-6), 1–82.

Centers for Disease Control and Prevention (CDC). (2002b). *Primary and secondary syphilis among men who have sex with men — New York City, 2001. MMWR, 51*(38), 853–856.

Centers for Disease Control and Prevention (CDC). (2002c). Screening tests to detect chlamydia trachomatis and *Neisseria gonorrhea* infections—2002. *MMWR, 51*(Recommendations and Reports 15), 1–27. Available at http://www.cdc.gov.mmwr Accessed October 18, 2002.

Centers for Disease Control and Prevention (CDC). (2004a). *Increases in Fluoroquinolone-Resistant Neisseria gonorrhoeae Among Men Who Have Sex with Men—United States, 2003, and Revised Recommendations for Gonorrhea Treatment, 2004.* MMWR, 53(16) 335–338.

Centers for Disease Control and Prevention (CDC). (2004b). Oral Alternatives to Cefixime for the Treatment of Uncomplicated *Neisseria Gonorrhoeae* Urogenital Infections. http://www.cdc.gov/std/treatment/Cefixime.htm Accessed 5/04/04.

Cohen, D., & Scribner R. (2001). An STD/HIV prevention intervention framework. *AIDS Patient Care & STDs, 14*(1), 37–45.

Corey, L., Wald, A., Patel, R., et al. (2004). Once-daily valacyclovir to reduce the risk of transmission of genital herpes. *New England Journal of Medicine, 350*(1), 11–20.

Corey, W. A., Doebbeling, B. N., DeJong, K. J., & Britigan, B. E. (1991). Metronidazole-induced pancreatitis. *Reviews of Infectious Diseases, 13*, 1213–1215.

Cox, T., Buck, H., Kinney, W., & Rubin, M. M. (2001). *Clinical proceedings, human papillomavirus (HPV) and cervical cancer*. Association of Reproductive Health Professionals (ARHP), 1–32.

Deceunick, G., Asamoah-Adu, C., Khonde, N., Pepin, J., Frost, E. H., Deslandes, S., Asamoah-Adu, A., Bekoe, V., & Alary, M. (2000). Improvement of clinical algorithms for the diagnosis of *Neisseria gonorrhea* and *Chlamydia trachomatis* by the use of gram-stained smears among female sex workers in Accra, Ghana. *Sexually Transmitted Diseases, 27*(7), 401–410.

Desai, P. C., & Johnson, B. A. (1996). Oral fluconazole for vaginal candidiasis. *American Family Physician, 54*(4), 1337–1340, 1345–1346.

Drake, S., Taylor, S., Brown, D., & Pillay, D. (2000). Improving the care of patients with genital herpes. *British Medical Journal, 321*(7261), 619–623.

duBouchet, L., Spence, M. R., Rein, M. F., Danzig, M. R., & McCormack, W. M. (1997). Multicenter comparison of clotrimazole vaginal tablets, oral metronidazole, and vaginal suppositories containing sulfanilamide, aminacrine hydrochloride, and allantoin in the treatment of symptomatic trichomoniasis. *Sexually Transmitted Diseases, 24*(3), 156–160.

Drugdex® Drug Evaluations: entanercept [online]. Drugdex® editorial staff, eds. Englewood: Micromedex®; expires 2002 September.

Elmer, G. W., Surawicz, C. M., & McFarland, L. V. (1996). Biotherapeutic agents: A neglected modality for the treatment and prevention of selected intestinal and vaginal infections. *JAMA, 275*(11), 870–876.

Eschenbach, D. A. (1993). History and review of bacterial vaginosis. *American Journal of Obstetrics and Gynecology, 169*(2S), 441–445.

Faber, F.M. (1996). The diagnosis and treatment of scabies and pubic lice. Primary Care Update for Ob/Gyns. 3(1),20–24.

Faro, S., Apuzzio, J., Bohannon, N., Elliott, K., Martens, M. G., Mou, S. M., Phillips-Smith, L. E., Soper, D. E., Strayer, A., & Young, R. L. (1997). Treatment considerations in vulvovaginal candidiasis. *Female Patient, 22*, 21–38.

Federal Drug Administration (2003). FDA Updates Labeling of Valtrex. FDA Talk Paper. http://www.fda/gov/bbs/topics/ ANSWERS/2003/ANS01250.html Accessed 05/04/2004.

Ferenczy, A. (1985). Comparison of 5-fluorouracil and CO_2 laser for treatment of vaginal condylomas. *Obstetrics and Gynecology, 64*, 773–778.

Ferris, D. G., Dekle, C., & Litaker, M. S. (1996). Women's use of over-the-counter antifungal medications for gynecologic symptoms. *Journal of Family Practice, 42*(6), 595–600.

Ferris, D. G., Litaker, M. S., Woodward, L., Mathis, D., & Hendrich, J. (1995). Treatment of bacterial vaginosis: A comparison of oral metronidazole, metronidazole vaginal gel, and clindamycin vaginal cream. *Journal of Family Practice, 41*(5), 443–449.

Fischer, T. F. (1994). Lindane toxicity in a 24-year-old woman. *Annals of Emergency Medicine, 24*(5), 972–974.

Friedman-Kien, A. E., Eron, L. J., Conant, M., Growdon, W., Bradiak, H., Bradstreet, P. W., Fedorczyk, D., Trout, J. R., & Plasse, T. F. (1988). Natural interferon-α for treatment of chondylomata acuminata. *JAMA, 259*(4), 533–538.

Fox, K. K., & Knapp J. S. (1999). Antimicrobial resistance in *Neisseria gonorrhea. Current Opinion in Urology, 9*(1), 65–70.

Galloway, D. (2003). Papillomavirus vaccines in clinical trials. *Lancet Infectious Diseases, 3*(8), 469–475.

Gant, N. F., & Cunningham, F. G. (Eds.). (1993). *Basic gynecology and obstetrics* (pp. 43–53). Norwalk, CT: Appleton & Lange.

Garnett, G., Aral, S., Hoyle, D., Cates, W., &. Anderson, R. (1997). The natural history of syphilis. Implications for the transmission dynamics and control of infection. *Sexually Transmitted Diseases, 24*(4), 185–200.

Geiger, A. M., & Foxman, B. (1996). Risk factors for vulvovaginal candidiasis: A case-control study among university students. *Epidemiology, 7*(2), 182–187.

Geiger, A. M., Foxman, B., & Gillespie, B. W. (1996). The epidemiology of vulvovaginal candidiasis among university students. *American Journal of Public Health, 85*(8, Pt. 1), 1146–1148.

Gilson, R. J. C., & Mindel, A. (2001). Sexually transmitted infections. *British Medical Journal*, 322(7295), 1160–1164.

Gonorrhea and chlamydial infections. (1994). *International Journal of Gynaecology and Obstetrics, 45*, 169–174.

Goode, M. A., Grauer, K., & Gums, J. G. (1994). Infectious vaginitis: Selecting therapy and preventing recurrence. *Postgraduate Medical Journal, 96*(6), 85–98.

Gunter, J. (2003). *2003 Sexually transmitted infection update.* New York, NY: McMahon Publishing Group.

Haddix, A. C., Hillis, S. D., & Kassler, W. J. (1995). The cost effectiveness of azithromycin for *Chlamydia trachomatis* infections in women. *Sexually Transmitted Diseases, 22*(5), 274–280.

Haefner, H. K. (1999). Current evaluation and management of vulvovaginitis. *Clinical Obstetrics & Gynecology, 42*(2), 184–195.

Haley, N., Maheux, B., Rivard, M., & Gervais, A. (2002). Unsafe sex, substance abuse, and domestic violence: How do recently trained obstetricians-gynecologists fare at lifestyle risk assessment and counseling on STD prevention? *Preventive Medicine, 34*(6), 632–637.

Hart, G. (1990). Donovanosis. In K.K. Holmes, P. A. Mardh, P. F. Sparling, P. J. Wiesner, W. Cates, S. M. Lemon, & W. E. Stamm (Eds.), *Sexually transmitted diseases* (2nd ed., pp. 273–277). New York: McGraw-Hill.

Hawes, S. E., Hillier, S. L., Benedetti, J., Stevens, C. E., Koutsky, L. A., Wolner-Hanssen, P., & Holmes, K. K. (1996). Hydrogen peroxide-producing lactobacilli and acquisition of vaginal infections. *Journal of Infectious Diseases, 174*(5), 1058–1063.

Hellberg, D., Zdolsek, B., Nilsson, S., & Mardh, P. A. (1995). Sexual behavior of women with repeated episodes of vulvovaginal candidiasis. *European Journal of Epidemiology, 11*(5), 575–579.

Hillier, S. L., & Arko, R. J. (1996). Vaginal infections. In S. A. Morse, A. A. Moreland, & K. K. Holmes (Eds.), *Atlas of sexually transmitted disease and AIDS* (2nd ed.; pp. 149–164). Baltimore, MD: Mosby-Wolfe.

Hillier, S. L., Kiviat, N. B., Hawes, S. E., Hasselquist, M. B., Hanssen, P. W., Eschenbach, D. A., & Holmes, K. K. (1996). Gynecology: Role of bacterial vaginosis-associated microorganisms in endometritis. *American Journal of Obstetrics and Gynecology, 175*(2), 435–441.

Hillier, S. L., Nugent, R. P., Eschenbach, D. A., Krohn, M. A., Gibbs, R. S., Martin, D. H., Cotch, M. F., Edelman, R., Pastorek, J. G., II, Rao, A. V., McNellis, D., Regan, J. A., Carey, J. C., Klebanoff, M. A., & the Vaginal Infections and Prematurity Study Group. (1995). Association between bacterial vaginosis and preterm delivery of a low-birth-weight infant. *New England Journal of Medicine, 333*(26), 1737–1742.

Hillier, S. L., Soper, D. E., & Sobel, J. D. (2002). Vaginal ecosystem: Current views. Bacterial Vaginosis: Balancing the approach to treatment. *Ob. Gyn. News*, Supplement, 1–11.

Hollier, L., Harstad, T., Sanchez, P., Twickler, D., & Wendel, G., (2001). Fetal syphilis: Clinical and laboratory characteristics. *Obstetrics & Gynecology, 97*(6), 947–53.

Houang, E. T., Ahmet, Z., & Lawrence, A. G. (1997). Successful treatment of four patients with recalcitrant vaginal trichomoniasis with a combination of zinc sulfate douche and metronidazole therapy. *Sexually Transmitted Diseases, 24*(2), 116–119.

Hwang, L., Ross, M., Zack, C., Bull, L., Rickman, K., & Holleman, M. (2000). Prevalence of sexually transmitted infections and associated risk factors among populations of drug abusers. *Clinical Infectious Diseases, 31*(4), 920–926.

Incidence of chlamydia high in young men. (April 2004). *The Clinical Advisor,* 16.

Ivey, J. B. (1997). The adolescent with pelvic inflammatory disease: Assessment and management. *The Nurse Practitioner, 22*(2), 78–91.

Jaworski, B., & Carey, M. (2001). Effects of a brief, theory-based STD-prevention program for female college students. *Journal of Adolescent Health, 29*(6), 417–425.

Jephcott, A. E. (1997). Microbiological diagnosis of gonorrhea. *Genitourinary Medicine, 73*(4), 245–252.

Kasten, M. J. (1999). Clindamycin, metronidazole, and chloramphenicol. *Mayo Clinic Proceedings*, 74(8), 825–833.

Kirby, P. K., Kiviat, N., Beckman, A., Wells, D., Sherwin, S., & Corey, L. (1988). Tolerance and efficacy of recombinant human interferon-γ in the treatment of refractory genital warts. *American Journal of Medicine, 85*, 183–188.

Klein, V., Cox, S., Mitchell, M., & Wendel, G. (1990). The Jarisch-Herxheimer reaction complicating syphilotherapy in pregnancy. *Obstetrics & Gynecology, 75*(3 Pt 1), 375–380.

Knapp, J. S., Wongba, C., & Limpakarnjanarat, K. (1997). Antimicrobial susceptibilities of strains of *Neisseria gonorrhoeae* in Bangkok, Thailand: 1994–1995. *Sexually Transmitted Diseases, 24*(3), 142–148.

Knodel, L. C., & Kraynak, M. A. (1997). Sexually transmitted diseases. In J. T. DiPiro, R. L. Talbert, G. C. Yee, G. R. Matzke, B. G. Wells, & L. M. Posey (Eds.), Pharmacotherapy: A pathophysiologic approach (pp. 2195–2219). Stamford, CT: Appleton & Lange.

Kohl, K., Farley, T., Ewell, J., & Scioneaux J. (1999). Usefulness of partner notification for syphilis control. *Sexually Transmitted Diseases, 26*(4), 201–207.

Kohler, C., Pickholtz, J., & Ballas, C. (2000). Neurosyphilis presenting as schizophrenia-like psychosis. *Neuropsychiatry, Neuropsychology, & Behavioral Neurology. 13*(4), 297–302.

Krebs, H. B. (1987). The use of topical 5-fluorouracil in the treatment of genital condylomas. *Obstetrics and Gynecology Clinics of North America, 14*, 559–568.

Keiger, J. N. (1995). Trichomoniasis in men: Old issues and new data. *Sexually Transmitted Diseases, 22*(2), 83–96.

Kumar, B., Gupta, S., & Muralidhar, S. (2001). Mucocutaneous manifestations of secondary syphilis in north Indian patients: A changing scenario? *Journal of Dermatology, 28*(3), 137–144.

Larsen, S., Steine, B., & Rudolph, A. (1995). Laboratory diagnosis and interpretation of tests for syphilis. *Clinical Microbiology Reviews, 8*(1), 1–21.

Lee, B., Feinberg, M., Abraham, J., & Murphy, A. (1992). Congenital malformations in an infant born to a woman treated with fluconazole. *Pediatric Infectious Disease Journal, 11*, 1062–1064.

Lopez-Zetina, J., Ford, W., Weber, M., Barna, S., Woerhle, T., Kerndt, P., & Monterroso, E. (2000). Predictors of syphilis seroreactivity and prevalence of HIV among street recruited injection drug users in Los Angeles County, 1994-6. *Sexually Transmitted Infections, 76*(6), 462–469.

Lukehart, S., & Holmes, K. (1998). Syphilis. In A.S. Fauci, B. Braunwald, & K.J. Isselbacher (Eds.), *Harrison's principles of internal medicine*. (pp. 1023–1033). New York: McGraw-Hill.

Lynch, C., Felder, T., Schwandt, R., & Shashy, R. (1999). Lymphogranuloma venereum presenting as a rectovaginal fistula. *Infectious Diseases in Obstetrics & Gynecology. 7*(4): 199–201.

Mabey, D., & Peeling, R. (2002). *Lymphogranuloma venereum. Sexually Transmitted Infections, 78*(2) 90–92.

Macsween, K. F., & Ridgway, G. L. (1998). ACP Broadsheet No 153; August 1998: The laboratory investigation of vaginal discharge. *Journal of Clinical Pathology*, 51(8), 564–567.

Meinking, T. L., Taplin, D., Herminda, J. L., Pardo, R., & Kerdel, F. A. (1995). The treatment of scabies with Invermectin. *New England Journal of Medicine, 333*(1), 26–30.

Mikamo, H., Kawazoe, K., Izumi, K., Watanabe, K., Ueno, K., & Tamaya, T. (1997). Comparative study on vaginal or oral treatment of bacterial vaginosis. *Chemotherapy, 43*(1), 60–68.

Morales, W. J., Schorr, S., & Albritton, J. (1994). Effect of metronidazole in patients with preterm birth in preceding pregnancy and bacterial vaginosis: A placebo-controlled, double-blind study. *American Journal of Obstetrics and Gynecology, 171*(2), 345–347.

Morse, S. A. (2001). New tests for bacterial sexually transmitted diseases. *Current Opinion in Infectious Diseases*, 14(1), 45–51.

Munoz, N., Bosch, F., deSanjose S., et al., for the International Agency for Research on Cancer, Multicenter Cervical Cancer Study Group. (2003). Epidemiologic classification of human papillomavirus types associated with cervical cancer. *New England Journal of Medicine, 348*(6), 518–527.

Neuhaus, G., Pavic, N., & Pletscher, M. (1991). Anaphylactic reaction after oral fluconazole. *BMJ, 302*, 1341.

Newton, E. R., Piper, J., & Peairs, W. (1997). Bacterial vaginosis and intraamniotic infection. *American Journal of Obstetrics and Gynecology, 176*(3), 672–677.

Nisson, D, (Ed). (2002). *2002 Mosby's drug consult.* St. Louis: Mosby. [Electronic version]. Retrived 12/2/2002 from http://online.statref.com

Nuttbrock, L., Rosenblum, A., Magura, S., McQuistion, H., & Joseph, H. (2000). The association between cocaine use and HIV/STDs among soup kitchen attendees in New York City. *Journal of Acquired Immune Deficiency Syndromes & Human Retrovirology, 25*(1), 86–91.

O'Farrell, N. (2001). Donovanosis: An update. *International Journal of STD & AIDS, 12*(7), 423–427.

O-Prasertsawat, P., & Bourlert, A. (1995). Comparative study of fluconazole and clotrimazole for the treatment of vulvovaginal candidiasis. *Sexually Transmitted Diseases, 22*(4), 228–230.

Paisarntantiwong, R., Brockmann, S., Clarke, L., Landesman, S., Feldman, J., & Minkoff, H. (1995). The relationship of vaginal trichomoniasis and pelvic inflammatory disease among women colonized with *Chlamydia trachomatis. Sexually Transmitted Diseases, 22*(6), 344–347.

Papagrigoriadis, S., & Rennie, J. (1998). Lymphogranuloma venereum as a cause of rectal strictures. *Postgraduate Medical Journal, 74*(869), 168–169.

Pearlman, M. D., Yashar, C., Ernst, S., & Solomon, W. (1996). An incremental dosing protocol for women with severe vaginal trichomoniasis and adverse reaction to metronidazole. *American Journal of Obstetrics and Gynecology, 174*(3), 934–936.

Platz-Christensen, J. J., Sundstrom, E., & Larsson, P-G. (1994). Bacterial vaginosis and cervical intraepithelial neoplasia. *Acta Obstetrica et Gynecologica Scandinavica, 73*, 586–588.

Priestley, C. J., Jones, B. M., Dhar, J., & Goodwin, L. (1997). What is normal vaginal flora? *Genitourinary Medicine, 73*(1), 23–28.

Rein, M. F., Shih, L. M., Miller, J. R., & Guerrant, R. L. (1996). Use of lactoferrin assay in the differential diagnosis of female genital tract infections and implications for the pathophysiology of bacterial vaginosis. *Sexually Transmitted Diseases, 23*(6), 517–521.

Reust, C., (2000). SOAP: Solutions to often asked problems. Chlamydia trachomatis testing. *Archives of Family Medicine. 9*(9), 885–886

Reynolds, M., & Wilson, J. (1996). Is trichomonas vaginalis still a market for other sexually transmitted infections in women? *International Journal of STD and AIDS, 7*(2), 131–132.

Rosemberg, S. K., Greenberg, M. D., & Reid, R. (1987). Sexually transmitted papillomaviral infection in men. *Obstetrics and Gynecology Clinics of North America, 14*, 495–512.

Rothenberg, R., Kimbrough, L., Lewis-Hardy, R., Heath, B., Williams, O., Tambe, P., Johnson, D., & Schrader, M. (2000). Social network methods for endemic foci of syphilis: A pilot project. *Sexually Transmitted Diseases* 27(1), 12–18.

Schaffer, S. (2004). Vaginitis and sexually transmitted diseases. In E. Q. Youngkin & M. S. Davis (Ed.), *Women's health: A primary care clinical guide* (3rd ed.). Upper Saddle River, NJ: Prentice Hall.

Scott, G. R. (2001) European guideline for the management of pediculosis pubis. European Branch of the International Union against Sexually Transmitted Infection and the European Office of the World Health Organization. *International Journal of STD & AIDS*, 12(3), 62.

Secor, R. M. C. (1997). Vaginal microscopy: Refining the nurse practitioner's technique. *Clinical Excellence for Nurse Practitioners, 1*(1), 29–34.

Shalev, E., Battino, S., Weiner, E., Colodner, R., & Keness, Y. (1996). Ingestion of yogurt containing *Lactobacillus acidophilus* compared with pasteurized yogurt as prophylaxis for recurrent candidal vaginitis and bacterial vaginosis. *Archives of Family Medicine, 5*(1), 593–596.

Sheffield, J., Sanchez, P., Morris, G., Maberry, M., Zeray, F., McIntire, D., & Wendel, G. (2002). Congenital syphilis after maternal treatment for syphilis during pregnancy. *American Journal of Obstetrics & Gynecology, 186*(3), 569–573.

Simms-Cendan, J. S. (1996). Metronidazole: Infectious diseases update. *Primary Care Update for OB/Gyns, 3*(5), 153–156.

Slavin, M. B., Benrubi, G. I., Parker, R., Griffin, C. R., & Magee, M. J. (1992). Single does oral fluconazole vs. intravaginal terconazole in treatment of candida vaginitis. *Journal of the Florida Medical Association, 79*(10), 693–696.

Sobel, J. D., Brooker, D., Stein, G. E., Thomason, J. L., Wermeling, D. P., Bradley, B., & Weinstein, L. (1995). Single oral does fluconazole compared with conventional clotrimazole topical therapy of Candida vaginitis: Fluconazole Vaginitis Study Group. *American Journal of Obstetrics and Gynecology, 172*(4, Pt. 1), 1263–1268.

Sobel, J. D., & Chaim, W. (1997). Treatment of *Torulopsis glabrata* vaginitis: Retrospective review of boric acid therapy. *Clinical Infectious Diseases, 24*(4), 649–652.

Sobel, J. D., Kapernick, P. S., Zervos, M., Reed, B. D., Wooton, T., Soper, D., Nvirjesy, P. Heine, M. W., Willems, J., Panzer, H., Wittes, H. (2001). Treatment of complicated Candida vaginitis: comparison of single and sequential doses of fluconazole. *American Journal of Obstetrics and Gynecology, 184*(2), 363–369.

Spinillo, A., Capuzzo, E., Egbe, T. O., Nicola, S., & Piazzi, G. (1995). *Torulopsis glabrata* vaginitis. *Obstetrics and Gynecology, 85*(6), 993–998.

Spinillo, A., Capuzzo, E., Gulminetti, R., Marone, P., Colonna, L., & Piazzi, G. (1997). Prevalence of and risk factors for fungal vaginitis caused by non-*albicans* species. *American Journal of Obstetrics and Gynecology, 176*(1) 138–141.

Steinhandler, L., Peipert, J.F., Herber, W., Montagno, A., & Cruichshank, C. (2002). Combination of bacterial vaginosis and leukorrhea as a predictor of cervical chlamydial or gonococcal infection. *American College of Obstetricians and Gynecologists*, 99(4), 603–607.

STDs that are transmitted orally, (May 2003). *The Clinical Advisor,* 64.

Swanson, J. M., (1999). The biopsychosocial burden of genital herpes: Evidence-based and other approaches to care. *Dermatology Nursing, 11*(4), 257–268.

Sweet, R. L. (1995). Role of bacterial vaginosis in pelvic inflammatory disease. Clinical Infectious Diseases, 20(suppl. 2), S271–S275.

Tidwell, B. H., Lushbaugh, W. B., Laughlin, M. D., Cleary, J. D., & Finley, R. W. (1994). A double-blind placebo-controlled trial of single-dose intravaginal versus single-dose oral metronidazole in the treatment of trichomonal vaginitis. *Journal of Infectious Diseases, 170*(1), 242–246.

Thomas, J., Eng, E., Earp, A., & Ellis, H. (2001). Trust and collaboration in the prevention of sexually transmitted diseases. *Public Health Reports, 116*(6), 540–547.

Tobin, M. J. (1995). Vulvovaginal candidiasis: Topical vs. oral therapy. *American Family Physician, 51*(7), 1715–1720.

Tracy, J. W., & Webster, L. T., Jr. (1995). Drugs used in the chemotherapy of protozoal infections: Trypanosomiasis, leishmaniasis, amebiasis, giardiasis, trichomoniasis, and other protozoal infections. In J. G. Hardman, A. G. Gillman, and L. E. Limbird (Eds.), Goodman & Gillmann's The Pharmacological basis of therapeutics (9th ed.) (pp 987–1008). New York: McGraw-Hill.

Venna, S., Fleischer, A. B., Feldman, S. R. (2001). Scabies and lice: Review of the clinical features and management principles. *Dermatology Nursing, 13*(4), 257–262, 265–266.

Washington, A. E., Arno, P. S., & Brooks, M. A. (1986). The economic cost of pelvic inflammatory disease. *JAMA, 255*(13), 1735–1738.

Weinberger, M. W., & Harger, J. H. (1993). Accuracy of the Papanicolaou smear in the diagnosis of asymptomatic infection with *Trichomonas vaginalis. Obstetrics and Gynecology, 82*(3), 425–429.

Weinstock, H., Dean, D., & Bolan, G. (1994). *Chlamydia trachomatis* infections. *Infectious Disease Clinics of North America, 8*(4), 797–819.

Winceslaus, S. J., & Calver, G. (1996). Recurrent bacterial vaginosis—an old approach to a new problem. *International Journal of STD and AIDS, 7*(4), 284–287.

Yeung-Yue, K. A., Brentjens, M. H., Lee, P. C., & Tyring, S. K. (2002). The management of herpes simplex virus infections. *Current Opinion in Infectious Diseases, 15*(2), 115–122.

Zhang, Z. (1996, September—October). Epidemiology of *Trichomonas vaginalis. Sexually Transmitted Diseases, 23*(5), 415–424.

CHAPTER ❖ 37

IMMUNE SYSTEM DISORDERS: HIV/AIDS, MONONUCLEOSIS AND ALLERGIC RESPONSES

C. Fay Parpart ◆ Denese Gomes

Immune system disorders occur when the immune system responds distressingly to certain specific, foreign substances and when infectious agents, allergens, or the immune system itself causes dysfunction or dysregulation. This chapter addresses in depth two conditions commonly encountered by primary care providers, human immunodeficiency virus (HIV)/acquired immune deficiency syndrome (AIDS) and allergic reactions. A short discussion of the treatment of a very common but usually self-limiting viral infection, infectious mononucleosis, is also included.*

HIV/AIDS

Minimal projections for HIV over the next few years are likely to be around 40,000 infections per year. The majority of these cases will be adults and adolescents (Osmond, 2003). This section addresses the treatment of HIV in the adult and adolescent population. The next section addresses the treatment of HIV in the pediatric population.

HIV is a retrovirus of the *Lentivirus* genus. Retroviruses are RNA viruses that replicate via DNA intermediates using the viral enzyme reverse transcriptase. After a long incubation period, HIV causes clinical syndromes, which are characterized by a protracted symptomatic phase. There are two types of HIV, 1 and 2. Although both types are known to cause AIDS, infection with HIV-1 is more common in the United States (Boucher & Larder, 1994; Hecht & Soloway, 1994).

HIV infections most often affect activated cells of the immune system, and particularly T-cell lymphocytes (often referred to as CD4 cells or T4 cells). HIV can also infect other cells such as glial cells in the brain, macrophages, Langerhans' cells (dendritic cells) in the skin, and chromaffin cells in the intestine (Boucher & Larder, 1994).

The overall effect of HIV infection is a severely compromised immune system. Recent findings suggest that the spread of the virus to organs other than lymphoid tissue occurs late in HIV disease, with the onset of AIDS-defining illnesses (Boucher & Larder, 1994). See Table 37–1.

ADULT AND ADOLESCENT POPULATION

Specific Considerations for Pharmacotherapy

Need for Drug Therapy and Rationale. Antiretroviral treatment of HIV infection has undergone great changes in recent years. Theoretically, the multiple steps in the replication of HIV provide many opportunities for antiviral action as noted in Table 37–2 (Lipsky, 1996). Although these multi-

*See also section on postexposure prophylaxis on page 845.

TABLE 37–1. Spectrum of HIV Infection

	Acute	Asymptomatic	Early Symptoms	AIDS
Time frame	4–6 weeks	Averages 10 years	Months to years	Months to years
Antibody status	(−)	(+)	(+)	(+/−)

At 3 months 90% of HIV-infected persons will have a (+) antibody test; at 6 months >95% of HIV-infected persons will have a (+) antibody test.

Source: From Miralles (1996).

ple steps have inspired the development of various medications that affect step 1, attachment of the virus to the cell, step 2, inhibition of reverse transcriptase, and step 6, inhibition of protein (viral subunits) processing, have been approved as therapies in the treatment of HIV infection. These agents are recommended to be utilized as combination therapies. The combination antiretroviral therapies have improved many patients' overall prognosis by inhibiting viral replication, as noted by significant changes in subsequent viral load testing. In addition, many patients also improve clinically when treated with combination antiretroviral therapies (Boucher & Larder, 1994; Goldschmidt & Dong, 1997).

Short- and Long-Term Goals of Pharmacotherapy. The short-term goals of treatment for HIV/AIDS are to decrease the viral load (burden), obtained by direct quantification of the virus (HIV RNA testing) in the patient's blood; to improve the immune status as indicated by the CD4 cell count; and to reduce or eliminate the constitutional symptoms, e.g., malaise, weight loss, and fever.

Long-term goals of treatment for HIV/AIDS include the prevention of HIV-related clinical symptoms and opportunistic infections, the management of medication-related toxicities, and the maintenance of a stable immune system.

Prevention and Nonpharmacologic Therapy for HIV/AIDS and Opportunistic Infections

Prevention. Inclusion of a nonjudgmental risk assessment about sexual behaviors and drug use into the clinician's history provides an opportunity for discussion about the patient's perception of risk and his or her plans for harm reduction.

Sexual behavior harm reduction includes the following:

1. Abstinence
2. Monogamous relationship with noninfected individual
3. Sexual behavior that does not involve an exchange of body fluids, e.g., hugging, erotic massage, self-masturbation while lying next to the partner, and showering together
4. Safer sex, including latex condom use from start to finish of anal or vaginal intercourse, use of latex barrier protection for oral sex, and providing educational materials about the choices involving sexual behavior and safer sex including instruction on proper condom use

Needle-sharing harm reduction includes the following:

1. Providing resources for drug treatment if the client is willing and ready
2. Providing patient educational material and instruction about transmission via blood exposure (American Medical Association [AMA], 1996; Coates, 1994; Makadon & Silian, 1995; Marks, 1994; Coates, DeCarlo, 1997; Stryker et al., 1995).

Nonpharmacologic Therapy. Many patients utilize a combination of traditional and alternative methodologies. Some of the complementary or supplemental therapies are noted in Table 37–3.

Time Frame for Initiating Pharmacotherapy. Some primary care providers seek specialty consultation or refer

TABLE 37–2. Opportunities for Antiviral Action on the Pathogenesis of HIV

1. Attachment of virus to the cell
2. Inhibition of reverse transcriptase, which creates DNA from viral RNA
3. Inhibition of Rnase H, which degrades viral RNA after viral DNA has been synthesized
4. Inhibition of viral integrase, which is used to integrate viral DNA into the cell's DNA
5. Inhibition of expression of the HIV gene once it is integrated into the host cell DNA, including the processes of transcription of more viral RNA and the translation to viral proteins
6. Inhibition of processing and post-translational modification to protein products of the virus

Source: From Lipsky (1996, p. 800).

TABLE 37–3. Complementary or Supplemental Therapies

Meditation	Acupuncture; acupressure
Counseling	Lymphatic massage
Reiki	Natural nutritional supplements
Homeopathic remedies	Aromatherapy
Color and light therapy	Healing touch; therapeutic touch
Sound therapy	Biofeedback
Feng shui	
Massage therapy	
Herbals	

Source: From Burroughs (1993); Moon (1997).

clients out for management shortly after the HIV diagnosis. Others choose to work with patients with HIV infection throughout the course of the disease. This is a decision for the provider and patient to make together (Hecht & Soloway, 1994). The Panel on Clinical Practices for Treatment of HIV Infection, convened by the Department of Health and Human Services (DHHS) and the Henry J. Kaiser Family Foundation, recommended that when possible a physician with extensive HIV experience should direct the treatment of patients with HIV infection. When this is not possible, the panel felt it is important that the provider have access to consultations with HIV experts.

When making decisions about initiation of pharmacotherapy, the CD4 cell count and viral load measurement should be performed on two occasions, ideally 1 week apart in the symptomatic patient and 1 month apart in the asymptomatic patient, to ensure accuracy of measurement and to determine whether these parameters are stable or changing (Japour, 1996).

It has been estimated that 50% of HIV infected persons will experience at least some symptoms associated with the acute retroviral syndrome or primary HIV infection (Table 37–4). Therefore, early diagnosis and potential intervention are contingent on providers maintaining a high level of suspicion for HIV infection in patients presenting with this spectrum of symptoms and obtaining an appropriate history (Carpenter, Fischel, Hammer, et al., 1996; Goldschmidt & Dong, 1997; Moore & Bartlett, 1996). The benefits and risks associated with initiation of pharmacotherapy during the acute phase and asymptomatic phase of HIV infection are noted in Table 37–5.

TABLE 37–4. Acute Retroviral Syndrome: Associated Signs and Symptoms

- Fever
- Lymphadenopathy
- Pharyngitis
- Rash
- Erythematous maculopapular rash with 5 to 10 mm lesions on face and trunk and sometimes extremities including palms and soles; mucocutaneous ulceration involving mouth, esophagus, or genitals
- Myalgia or arthralgia
- Diarrhea
- Headache
- Nausea and vomiting
- Hepatosplenomegaly
- Thrush
- Weight loss
- Neurologic symptoms:
  Meningoencephalitis or aseptic meningitis
  Peripheral neuropathy or radiculopathy
  Facial palsy
  Guillain-Barré syndrome
  Brachial neuritis
  Cognitive impairment or psychosis

Source: Adapted from Barlett & Gallant, 2003.

The HIV viral load and the CD4 T-cell count in conjunction with the clinical category are used as indicators for the initiation of antiretroviral therapy. Initiation of antiretroviral therapy for the asymptomatic HIV-infected patient continues to be under debate, and there is ongoing research in this area. Although clinical experts differ on when to initiate therapy, many providers follow the DHHS Guidelines and recommend antiretroviral treatment when the CD4 $\leq 350/mm^3$.

All patients diagnosed clinically or immunologically with advanced HIV disease (AIDS) as defined by the 1997 CDC HIV Classification System are recommended to initiate antiretroviral therapy (Panel on Clinical Practices for Treatment of HIV Infection, 2004; Goldschmidt & Dong, 1997).

Assessment Needed Prior to Therapy. The initial assessment following diagnosis of HIV infection includes a complete history and physical examination (Tables 37–6 and 37–7) and baseline laboratory and diagnostic workup (Table 37–8) (Hecht & Soloway, 1994).

Many patients are diagnosed with HIV infection secondary to the diagnosis of an AIDS-defining illness. Therefore, initiation of antiretroviral therapy may be delayed until the therapy for the acute illness is completed. In addition, a careful review of the history and physical examination and laboratory results for indications of underlying illness or increased potential for drug toxicities is recommended.

Patient/Caregiver Information. Patient education is paramount for successful antiretroviral therapy. Adherence to the medication plan is critical. Patient education materials are available from regional AIDS Education and Training Centers [national office—(301) 443-6364], national and state AIDS hotlines [United States, (800) 342-AIDS],

TABLE 37–5. Benefits and Risks Associated with Initiation of Pharmacotherapy During Acute Phase of HIV Infection or in the Asymptomatic Phase of HIV Infection

Benefits	Risks
Suppress viral replication	Adverse effects associated with drugs
Improve symptoms of acute infection	Potential for drug resistance
Alter the viral "set point"	Potential for indefinite use of drugs
Reduce the potential for viral mutations	Poor long-term prognosis in symptomatic patients
Better tolerance, fewer side effects	
Decreased immunosuppression	

Source: Adapted from Perrin & Kinloch-de Loes (1995); Fisher, E. J. (personal communication, March 1997).

TABLE 37–6. Review of Systems

Symptom	Possible Associated Condition(s)
Constitutional	
• Weight loss, fever, night sweats, fatigue	• Wasting syndrome,[a] opportunistic infection,[a] lymphoma[a]; acute HIV infection, tuberculosis[a]
Lymphatic	
• Lymphadenopathy	• HIV, Kaposi's sarcoma,[a] lymphoma,[a] mycobacteria[a]; acute HIV infection
HEENT	
• Sore/dry mouth White patches in mouth	• Thrush, oral hairy leukoplakia
• Acute unilateral vision loss or ↑ floaters	• Cytomegalovirus retinitis[a]
• Sinus/ear congestion	• Sinusitis
Respiratory	
• Dyspnea with or without exertion Cough Chest tightness or pain Gastrointestinal	• Pneumocystis pneumonia,[a] ordinary bacterial pneumonias,[b] tuberculosis[a]
• Dysphagia/odynophagia	• Candida esophagitis,[a] herpes or CMV esophagitis[a]
• Anorexia Nausea and vomiting Abdominal pain Constipation, diarrhea	• Cytomegalovirus,[a] cryptosporidium[a] +/ or microsporidium enteritis, or cholangitis; lymphoma,[a] *Mycobacterium avium,*[a] wasting syndrome
• Anorectal pain/sores	• Chronic herpes simplex[a]
Genitourinary	
• Hx abnormal Pap smear	• Cervical carcinoma[b]
• Painful sores	• Chronic herpes simplex[a]
• Vulvovaginal itch/discharge Symptoms of STD (VD)	• Candidiasis, other vaginitis/urethritis, STD
• Decreased libido	
Musculoskeletal	
• Myalgias, arthralgias	• HIV or zidovudine myopathy
Neurologic	
• Headache Seizure Focal symptoms Ataxia Decreased cognition (poor memory, trouble finding words)	• HIV encephalopathy (dementia),[a] CNS opportunistic infection,[a] lymphoma[a]; other HIV neurologic, acute HIV infection
• Pain, paresthesias, numbness	• Peripheral neuropathy
Skin	
• Rash	• Acute HIV infection, zoster, syphilis
• New lesion	• Kaposi's sarcoma[a]
• New or worsening dermatoses	• Dryness, seborrheic dermatitis, folliculitis, tineas, *Candida,* molluscum, psoriasis
• Bruising, petechiae	• HIV immune thrombocytopenia

[a]AIDS-defining condition.
[b]Possible AIDS-defining condition.

Source: Fisher (1995).

TABLE 37–7. HIV-Directed Physical Examination

Physical Finding	Possible Associated Condition(s)
Skin	
• Purplish lesion	• Kaposi's sarcoma[a]
• Common dermatoses	• Dryness, seborrheic dermatitis, folliculitis, tineas, *Candida,* molluscum, psoriasis
• Rash	• Zoster; acute HIV infection; syphilis
Eye (retina) (exam indicated if symptoms or very low immune function)	
• Exudates/hemorrhages	
• Smaller than disc, do not progress or affect vision	• Cotton wool spots (HIV retinopathy)
• Larger, progressive, often affect vision	• Cytomegalovirus retinitis[a]
Mouth	
• Redness, patchy or diffuse	• Thrush
• White exudates	
• Can be scraped off	• Thrush
• Cannot be scraped off	• Oral hairy leukoplakia
• Ulcer	• Herpes simplex,[b] aphthous or medication-induced ulcers, acute HIV infection
• Red or purple lesion	• Kaposi's sarcoma[a]
Lymphatic	
• Adenopathy	
• Relatively symmetric; axillary usually largest	• HIV lymphadenopathy; acute HIV infection
• Hard, fixed or disproportionately large	• Lymphoma,[a] Kaposi's sarcoma,[a] mycobacteria[a]
Lungs	
• Rales/wheezes Tachypnea	• Pneumocystis[a] or TB[a] (Note: lungs often clear), bacterial pneumonia,[b] pulmonary Kaposi's[a]
Abdomen	
• Hepatomegaly/splenomegaly	• *Mycobacteria,*[a] lymphoma[a] (Note: organomegaly usually of other cause)
• Mass	• Lymphoma[a]
• Tenderness	• Cytomegalovirus enterocolitis[a]; AIDS cholangiopathy/cholecystitis[a]
Anogenital	
• Cervical abnormality	• Dysplasia/carcinoma of cervix[b]
• Vulvovaginitis	• Candidiasis
• Ulcer	• Herpes simplex,[b] syphilis
• Rectal mass	• Lymphoma[a]
Neurologic	
• Decreased cognition Psychomotor slowing Ataxia Hypo- or hyperreflexia Hypesthesia/paresthesia Focal deficit	• HIV encephalopathy,[a] CNS opportunistic infection,[a] CNS lymphoma[a]; HIV myelopathy or neuropathy; acute HIV infection

Low immune function can be suspected from any one of the following physical findings: cachexia, thrush, oral hairy leukoplakia, retinal cotton wool spots, marked new facial seborrhea, or extragenital molluscum.

[a]AIDS-defining condition.

[b]Possible AIDS-defining condition.

Source: Fisher (1995).

AIDS service organizations, pharmaceutical companies, state and local health departments, and the National Institutes of Health [(301) 496-5717)]. The Internet offers chat rooms, educational forums, and access to the CDC (website: http://www.cdcnac.org), National Institutes of Health, and the U.S. Department of Health and Human Services, Public Health Service's HIV/AIDS Treatment Information Service (ATIS) (Email: atis @cdcnac.aspensys.com).

Outcomes Management

Selection of an Agent and Pharmacoeconomic Issues

Reverse Transcriptase Inhibitors. *Nucleoside/nucleotide analogues* interfere with DNA synthesis by inhibiting reverse transcriptase. Termination of DNA synthesis prevents the virus from replicating and therefore causes viral stasis. Currently, there are seven nucleosides: abacavir

TABLE 37–8. Laboratory, Skin Test, and X-Ray Evaluation Schedule

Baseline Tests	Routine Follow-up
CBC, diff, plt	Repeat every 3–6 months
Complete metabolic panel	Repeat annually or more frequently in patients with abnormal results and with administration of hepatoxic or nephrotoxic drugs
Viral load, CD4 & CD8 subsets, CD4/CD8 ratio	Repeat VL & T-cell subsets every 3–4 months if VL < 400/50; or VL 4–6 weeks after change or initiation of ART plan
Fasting lipid panel	Repeat every 3–4 months if on protease inhibitors
RPR (or VDRL)	Repeat every year
Toxoplasma IgG serology	Repeat every year if negative and CD4< 100
CMV IgG serology	Repeat every year if negative and CD4 < 200
Hep A Total serology	If non-reactive, offer Hep A vaccine
Hep B serology: HbsAg, sAB, and cAB	Repeat every year if negative; offer Hep B vac
Hep C serology	Repeat every year if negative
UA	Repeat every year
PPD	Repeat every if PPD negative
Pap smear	Repeat every six months
GC and Chlamydia screen	Repeat every 6 months
Chest x-ray	Repeat prn symptoms or if PPD +

Source: Adapted from Fisher (1995, p. 12) and Barlett (2003, p. 28–29).

(ABC), didanosine (DDI) emtricitabine (FTC), lamivudine (3TC), stavudine (d4t), zalcitabine (ddC), zidovudine (ZDV, AZT), and one nucleotide: tenofovir (TNF). Combination pills, Combivir (AZT and 3TC) and Trizivir (ABC, AZT and 3TC), are available to reduce pull burden. The reason for the continued development of drugs in this class is that all have limitations due to various toxicities and that they lack long-term efficacy, which may partly be due to development of resistance (American Foundation for AIDS Research [AmFAR], 2002).

Nonnucleoside Transcriptase Inhibitors. The three FDA-approved non-nucleoside reverse transcriptase inhibitors (NNRTIs) are delavirdine (Rescriptor), efavirenz (Sustiva), and nevirapine (Viramune emtricitabine (FTC) and tenofovir (TNF)). Due to its potent viral suppression, efavirenz is recommended as a first-line therapy option. The principal limitation of NNRTIs is the potential for rapid development of viral resistance.

Protease Inhibitors. Inhibition of the virally produced protease known as "HIV proteinase" provides another therapeutic category for the treatment of HIV infection. Two of the protein products of HIV are precursors that are cleaved to mature protein products. This cleavage is catalyzed by HIV proteinase. The released proteins are crucial for viral replication and include the protease itself as well as RT, integrase, and structural proteins. If these proteins are not cleaved from the precursor proteins, then HIV is noninfectious. Because the protease inhibitors (PIs) act at an entirely different site in the viral life cycle than the reverse transcriptase inhibitors, the PIs in combination with the nucleoside analogues demonstrate at least additive and often synergistic activity against HIV. Eight protease inhibitors (PIs) are available in the United States for treatment of HIV infection. The principal limitations of some PIs are poor bioavailability with gastrointestinal distress (saquinavir [second generation with improved bioavailability, 1998], gastrointestinal intolerance (ritonavir, amprenavir, fosamprenavir, Kaletra), nephrolithiasis (indinavir), and diarrhea (nelfinavir) (AmFAR, 2002; Panel on Clinical Practices for Treatment of HIV Infection, 2004). Long-term use of protease inhibitors has been associated with metabolic disorders—e.g., diabetes and lipid abnormalities. PIs are metabolized in the liver, and some are potent inhibitors of an important hepatic enzyme system (cytochrome P-450). Thus, there is the potential for drug-drug interactions with other compounds metabolized by or affecting this system (AmFAR, 2002).

Fusion Inhibitors. Fusion inhibitors are a specific type of entry inhibitors that prevent fusion between the HIV's outer envelope and the cell's outer membrane. Enfuvirtide (Fuzeon) was approved late in 2003. It is administered by sub-q injection twice a day. Currently, enfuvirtide is recommended for patients who have limited treatment options available. Several entry and fusion inhibitors are in various phases of research (Bartlett & Gallant, 2003)

Treatment Options. Combinations of antiretroviral medications require an understanding of the side effects and possible drug interactions as well as the combinations that have had favorable experience.

Dr. Anthony Japour (1996) and other experts suggest that treatment decisions should be based on a mutual agreement between the patient and the provider. The challenges of managing HIV disease include selection of antiretroviral drugs, offering prophylaxis against opportunistic diseases, treating the major complications of advanced HIV disease (AIDS), and providing comprehensive primary care.

Antiretroviral and prophylactic/suppressive agents' costs range from $10,000 to $20,000/ year. Some clients have a third-party payor, but others do not. Resources for financial assistance include the local health department's drug assistance program, community-based AIDS service organizations, research protocols, pharmaceutical companies' compassionate care programs, and local social service departments (Commonwealth of Virginia Department of Health, 2001; Wiese, 1997).

A change in pharmacotherapy should be recommended when a therapeutic failure, as defined by provider and patient, occurs. The *preferred goal of treatment* is no detectable virus as indicated by the plasma viral load test. *Modified goals of treatment* are a significant decrease in viral load, a stable CD4 cell count, or no new AIDS-defining illness. When making changes in therapy, consultation with a provider who has significant experience in HIV-related care is recommended. Resistance testing (genotype and/or phenotype) may be ordered by the specialist to guide decisions regarding therapy changes (Bartlett & Gallant, 2003).

Opportunistic Diseases. Prophylaxis and treatment of opportunistic infections remain important elements in managing HIV disease. The Centers for Disease Control and Prevention (CDC) guidelines for prevention of opportunistic infections are an excellent source of information about prophylaxis. Recommendations for treating specific opportunistic diseases and the major symptoms of HIV/AIDS are available from sources such as Fisher (1995), Goldschmidt and Dong (1997), AmFAR (2002), AIDS Clinical Trials Information Service (1-800-TRIALS-A; web site: http://www. actis.org), and Johns Hopkins University AIDS Service (web site: http://hopkins-aids.edu.)

Monitoring for Efficacy. HIV-infected patients with CD4 cell counts greater than 500 do not appear to be at any greater risk than other immunocompetent patients of developing unusual or serious illness. As HIV begins to weaken the immune system, patients develop innocuous, self-limited problems—e.g., more frequent outbreaks of herpes simplex and skin changes such as exacerbations of eczema, psoriasis, and seborrhea. Education can help patients distinguish these symptoms from the more potentially serious ones listed in Table 37–9.

When an immunocompromised patient with potentially serious symptoms presents, the primary care provider needs to determine the differential diagnosis, appropriate workup, and therapeutic interventions discussed earlier in this chapter (Hecht & Soloway, 1994).

Ongoing studies are being performed to help determine the optimal guidelines for monitoring viral load and CD4 cell count. Currently, the viral load and CD4 cell count should be monitored every 3 to 4 months if the CD4 cell count is less than 400 or every 4 to 6 weeks following initiation of treatment or changes in treatment regimen. Decreases in viral load measurements by threefold or 0.5 log can be interpreted as beneficial effects of therapies, whereas rises of threefold or 0.5 log or more can indicate progressive disease and possible pharmacotherapeutic failure (Goldsmith & Dong, 1997).

Followup Recommendations. The followup recommendations for clients with HIV infection are based on the clinical picture. Followup is needed every 3 to 6 months when the patient is asymptomatic, every 2 to 3 months when symptomatic and stable, and monthly when symptomatic with ongoing problems (Fisher, E. J., personal communication, March 1997).

POSTEXPOSURE PROPHYLAXIS

Although the risk of HIV infection to healthcare workers is small, even when there is a known exposure to body fluids of patient known to be HIV positive, postexposure prophylaxis (PEP) management has been shown to reduce the risk even more. The critical factor is timing of the prophylaxis, with most programs calling for initiation

TABLE 37–9. Symptoms Requiring Medical Attention

Fever greater than 103°F
Fever greater than 101°F for 3 days or more
Shortness of breath
Productive cough
Persistent headache
Seizures or loss of consciousness
Visual changes
Change in mental status
Localized weakness, paralysis, or change in balance or sensation
Persistent diarrhea
Unusual bleeding

Source: Adapted from Hecht & Soloway (1994, p. 53).

of treatment in high-risk situations within an hour of exposure. Although PEP is common in some hospitals, healthcare providers in primary care settings may not be aware of the necessity for such a program. The risk of HIV infection due to percutaneous (needle-stick) exposure to HIV-infected blood is 0.3%. If the volume of blood is large or the HIV titer is high, risk may be elevated. Mucous membrane and skin exposure to HIV-infected blood carries a risk of 0.1% or less. Zidovudine (ZDV) prophylaxis has been shown to reduce the risk by 79% after percutaneous exposure in a case-controlled study. Universal precautions remain the best defense against transmission of a variety of infectious agents. However, PEP programs can offer counseling to assist and inform healthcare providers exposed to body fluids from a patient of their options and risks. It is best if any healthcare worker exposed to body fluids is throroughly counseled by a PEP team member so that all options can be discussed. In some instances the support provided by the team is just as important as the drug therapy. CDC Prevention Guidelines address exposure to body fluids via percutaneous, mucous membrane and skin/blood exposure, and they rank options as "recommend PEP," "offer PEP," and "not offer PEP." Most PEP programs have team members on 24-hour call to respond to emerging problems immediately.

If you have questions about managing occupational exposures, call the National Clinicians' Post-Exposure Prophylaxis Hotline, (888) HIV-4911, (888) 448–4911.

HIV/AIDS IN CHILDREN

HIV infections in children and adults have several common physiologic mechanisms and several unique ones. Readers are encouraged to review the section in this chapter on adults with HIV infection for a general orientation to the condition.

Children's unique physiology changes the consideration for drug treatment. This section of the chapter addresses those differences. The majority of children with HIV infection and AIDS are managed by specialty providers because of their complex treatment needs. However, primary care providers are involved in the ongoing primary care of almost all children and need to be aware of the treatment, the unique acute care issues of this population, and the current state of knowledge regarding the presentations and treatment approaches for children with this condition. In addition, fewer than half of the parents or caregivers of these children reveal the nature of the illness to the child (Funck-Brentano Costagliola, Seibel, et al., 1997). The psychologic treatment and coping issues of both family and child play a central role in the treatment of children with HIV/AIDS. The primary care provider, working closely with a specialty provider, can be a central team member in the care of these children.

HIV is transmitted to children in several ways. The most prevalent is perinatal, or vertical, transmission. This mechanism is suspected to include transmission transplacentally in utero, during delivery by exposure to blood and vaginal secretions, and after delivery if there is ingestion of infected breast milk (Fahrner & Benson, 1996). Maternal, fetal, placental, obstetric, neonatal, and viral factors influence this mother-to-infant transmission. The second most common transmission is from contaminated blood and blood products and factors given between 1978 and 1985. The safeguards instituted in 1985 have eliminated almost all transmission caused by this mechanism. For a small number of children, sexual abuse is the overlooked cause of HIV transmission (Butz, Joyner, Friedman, & Hutton, 1998).

The vertically infected fetus has an immature immune system. Although the T-cell immune system is relatively well developed, their B-cell system is immature. This causes the infant to have trouble forming adequate antibodies, which can become problematic for some infants early in life. This mechanism puts them at higher susceptibility to bacterial infections than adults with HIV infection. Opportunistic infections such as *Pneumocystis carinii* pneumonia (PCP) are common.

Specific Considerations for Pharmacotherapy

Need for drug therapy and rationale. HIV is now being seen by many experts as a chronic disease that (though at times life-threatening) is also treatable (Fahrner & Benson, 1996). Since the majority of children with HIV have vertically transmitted conditions, their demographics parallel those of their mothers. Their care is often complicated by the treatment of one or more of their parents. A national study in 1994 dramatically changed the fabric of the HIV quilt for children. The double-blind clinical trial found zidovudine (AZT) given to the mother prenatally dramatically reduced the incidence of children born with HIV. The transmission rate for those who took the placebo was 26% and for those who took zidovudine was 8%. Studies are now underway to test altered dose and length of treatment patterns. The current data do suggest that even treatment late in pregnancy has some beneficial effect. Thus, treatment can be initiated at any time in pregnancy that an HIV-positive mother seeks prenatal care (Working Group on Antiretroviral Therapy and Medical Management of HIV-Infected Children, 2004). However, prenatal treatment is also a complex issue with unknown effects of prenatal AZT on mother, fetus, or newborn. Although data on children now 2 years old who were treated in the prenatal period show no untoward effects, the long-term effects are unknown. The current guidelines caution that the discussion of treatment options and recommendations should be noncoercive and that the final decision is the responsibility of the woman. A decision not to choose prenatal treatment should not result in punitive action or denial of care. On the other hand, the decision of the mother previously on multitherapy who chooses only to use AZT to avoid exposure of the fetus to other antiviral drugs during pregnancy should also be respected (Working Group on Antiretroviral Therapy and Medical Management of HIV-Infected children, 2004).

Treatment of HIV/AIDS in children has the same goals as in adults: to control the replication of the HIV virus, thus slowing the progression of the condition, and to treat the opportunistic infections and other associated problems that accompany this condition. In addition, most children need supportive therapy to control other complications of the condition.

Short- and Long-Term Goals of Pharmacotherapy. As in adults the short-term goals are to control the viral load (HIV RNA) and to improve immune status (CD4 count). The long-term goals are to delay disease progression, prevent opportunistic infections, and make a positive impact on the quality and length of life.

Prevention and Nonpharmacologic Therapy for HIV/AIDS and Opportunistic Infections

Prevention. Prevention of this condition can be accomplished by (1) prevention of spread of the disease in the mother (see adult section), (2) prenatal screening and treatment of HIV-positive mothers, (3) C-section (considered in patients with viral load > 1000), (4) education regarding the need for HIV-positive mothers to refrain from breastfeeding, and (5) continual efforts to assure the quality of blood products. In addition, there are many barriers to early initiation of prenatal care by at-risk mothers. Programs that address barriers to obtaining this care such as access, transportation, child care, and the stigma of being HIV-positive need to be implemented to facilitate women's receiving early prenatal care.

Prevention of opportunistic infections should be a major focus of anticipatory guidance for families with HIV-positive children. Primary care providers need to problem-solve with the adults in the family to achieve the optimal environment to prevent secondary infections. In addition, the child needs to be taught to avoid contact with the bodily fluids of others and to use good handwashing techniques. Prevention issues addressed in this chapter in the section on adults relative to sexuality and drug issues need to be discussed with young adolescents (Butz et al., 1998).

It is extremely important in this population to prevent the development of drug resistance. Lack of adherence to prescribed regimens or subtherapeutic levels of the medication could cause resistance. There are some data to the effect that development of resistance to one protease inhibitor may reduce the effectiveness of other protease inhibitors. Parents and adult caregivers need to realistically discuss the ability to carry out the proposed regimen. Liquid formulations of these drugs can be distasteful. Absorption of some drugs can be affected by food, and attempting to create a schedule for infants and young children may be very challenging. Other barriers such as family stressors may also challenge these families. In addition, if there are disclosure issues either to the child or the community, there may be consequences for drug schedules. Families may be hesitant to fill the prescription at the local pharmacy, may hide or relabel the medication in an attempt to maintain secrecy at home, or may skip the midday dose in order not to have to take the medication to school (Working Group, 2004). In addition, some families may be struggling with survival issues such as obtaining adequate food or housing or creating a safe environment. These issues may take priority over medication administration. The assessment of each family's stressors and support issues may be most effectively done by the primary care provider if a long-term relationship exists. Communication with the interdisciplinary team managing the HIV treatment is crucial.

Immunizations, a preventive strategy, should be aggressively used with HIV-positive children. Most of the routine childhood immunizations are given on schedule. Inactivated polio vaccine (IPV) should be used instead of oral polio vaccine (OPV) for the HIV-positive child and all other household contacts to protect both the child and other HIV-positive persons in the home.

Several additions to the routine immunization schedule are important for HIV-positive children. Influenza virus vaccines should be added. The first should be at or just after 6 months of age, with a second influenza vaccine given 1 month after the first and annual immunizations on the anniversary of the first influenza vaccine.

The pneumococcal vaccine (Prevnar) was licensed for use in the United States in 2000. The recommended schedule for all infants is at ages 2, 4, 6, and 12 to 15 months. Immunization is also recommended for children with HIV at 2 to 5 years of age if not previously vaccinated. For these children the following is recommended: two doses of conjugate vaccine (Prevnar) administered 2 months apart; and one dose of 23/valent polysaccharide vaccine (pneumovax) administered at least 2 months after the second conjugate vaccine. Children 5 years of age and older will continue to receive the 23/valent polysaccharide vaccine (Keyserling, 2002). The varicella vaccine continues to be studied in HIV-positive children (Butz et al., 1998; Fahrner & Benson, 1996; Gershon, Mervish, LaRussa, et al., 1997).

Nonpharmacologic Therapy for HIV/AIDS and Opportunistic Infections. Either mother or child may need nutritional support for associated problems such as failure to thrive. Each visit is an opportunity to monitor the child's growth and development. Growth charts need to be monitored closely for any sign of the child's falling out of his or her growth curve. Nutritional support is an important intervention that can impact immune function, quality of life, and bioactivity of antiretroviral drugs.

The child will need neurodevelopmental testing to address the neurologic impacts of the disease and may need special services in school for developmental delay or learning disability. An interdisciplinary team will be needed to address the physical, financial, and psychosocial issues common in families with a member who is HIV-positive. Close collaboration with the primary care provider will yield optimal care for the family.

Time Frame for Initiation of Therapy. The current protocol for treatment of known HIV-positive mothers is as follows:

Pregnancy should not preclude the use of antiretroviral therapy (ART) in women. The benefits of ART in a pregnant woman must be weighed against the risk of adverse events to the woman, fetus, and newborn. The AZT chemoprophylaxis regimen alone or in combination with other ARTs should be discussed with and offered to all HIV-infected, pregnant women. Women in the first trimester of pregnancy may decide to delay initiation of therapy until after 10 to 12 weeks of gestation, the period when the fetus is most susceptible to potential teratogenic effects of drugs. Women receiving ART in whom pregnancy is identified should be counseled about the risks and benefits of therapy during this period. Continuation of therapy should be considered.

Since opportunistic infections are the major threat to the HIV-exposed infant and young child, early initiation of prophylaxis is indicated. The CDC (Working group, 2004) has indicated that no prophylaxis of HIV-exposed infants is needed in the first 6 weeks of life due to the low incidence of the major opportunistic infection (PCP), the well-established adverse side effects of sulfa drugs in infants under 6 weeks, and the unknown interactions for infants on zidovudine during the first 6 weeks of life. Prophylaxis should be initiated at 6 weeks of life. If the HIV-exposed infant is determined to be HIV-infected or if the laboratory tests are inconclusive, prophylaxis with sulfa should be continued until 1 year (see the assessment section). After 1 year of age the continuation of sulfa will be determined by the CD4 count. From 1 to 5 years old, prophylaxis is continued if the CD4 count is less than 500 or the CD4% is less than 15%. From 6 to 12 years of age prophylaxis is continued if the CD4 count is less than 200 or CD4% less than 15%.

Assessment Needed Prior to Therapy. A complete history and physical examination (see Tables 37–7 and 37–8) using the systems appropriate for newborns, infants, children, and young adolescents should be done on each visit. Laboratory tests are crucial to the optimal treatment of this condition. HIV can be definitively diagnosed in most infants at 1 month of age, and for virtually all infants by 6 months of age. Positive HIV culture or DNA or RNA polymerase chain reactions (PCR) indicate HIV infection. HIV DNA PCR is the preferred test. HIV RNA may be more sensitive in HIV-exposed infants, but data are limited. HIV culture is more complex and expensive and may take 2 to 4 weeks to get results. Repeat testing should be done as soon as possible to confirm the diagnosis. In children of HIV-positive mothers testing should be done by 48 h of age. Testing is done at 48 h since 40% of infants can be identified at this time. Cord blood samples should not be used. For those who test negative, repeat testing needs to be done at 1 to 2 months of age and 3 to 6 months of age. Testing at 14 days of age is also common. A child is diagnosed with HIV if two virologic tests done on separate blood samples are positive (Working group, 2004). A child with no symptoms and two or more negative HIV tests done a month apart after 6 months of life can reasonably exclude HIV. Negative testing in an asymptomatic child at 18 months of life can definitely rule out HIV. The testing pattern used at Virginia Commonwealth University's HIV/AIDS Center is typical, testing at birth, 6 weeks, and 6 months with PCR DNA, and at 15 to 18 months with the HIV antibody test.

Patient/Caregiver Information. See the section on adults for a discussion of resources. The National Pediatric HIV Resource Center (800-362-0071) has useful resources for families. Families and caregivers with HIV-positive children will need continual and repeated instruction and support. Often families are dealing with the illness or death of the child's mother simultaneously. The primary care provider must know the ever-changing treatment picture for these children. Most providers accomplish this by keeping in close contact with the HIV center.

Outcomes Management

Selection of an Agent and Pharmacoeconomic Issues. See the section on adults for an introductory discussion of the current approaches to treatment of HIV, the categories of drugs (reverse transcriptase inhibitors including nucleoside analogues and non-nucleoside analogues as well as protease inhibitors) and an overview of treatment using these drugs.

Initial Treatment. Antiviral therapy is recommended for HIV-infected children with any clinical symptoms or any evidence of immune suppression. The consensus guidelines indicate most members would recommend starting treatment in HIV-positive children under 12 months of age as soon as the diagnosis is confirmed, regardless of clinical or immunologic status (Working group, 2004). It is felt that the sooner the treatment is started, the sooner the suppression can "get started." Frequently, children are symptomatic at a young age and the majority of those not symptomatic over 1 year of age have a CD4 lymphocyte percentage of 25%, which is indicative of immunosuppression (Butz et al., 1998; Working group, 2004). If therapy is deferred, the laboratory and clinical values should be monitored closely and treatment initiated with increasing HIV RNA levels, declining CD4 lymphocyte count, or clinical deterioration.

Combination therapy is recommended for infants, children, and adolescents who are treated with antiretroviral agents. When compared with monotherapy, combination therapy slows disease progression and improves survival, results in more sustained virological and immunological responses, and delays development of viral mutations that confer resistance to the drugs being used. The use of AZT alone is only appropriate in those infants who have an interdeterminate HIV status during the first 6 weeks of life. The Working Group (CDC, 1998b) has recommended that all antiviral drugs approved for treatment of HIV in adults may be used in children, when indicated, irrespective of labeling notations.

Changes in Treatment. The Working Group (2004) identified three main reasons to change therapy: First, if there is a failure of the current regimen evidenced by virologic, immunologic or clinical parameters; second, if toxicity or intolerance develops; or third, if new data suggest a superior drug regimen. Assessing the failure of treatment is complex (Working Group, 2004).

Changes in the antiretroviral regimen may be indicated based on immunological, virological, and/or clinical indications. They include:

- Change in immunologic classification
- Rapid decline in absolute CD4 count
- Minimally acceptable virologic response after 12 weeks of therapy
- Progressive neurodevelopmental deterioration or growth failure

For some children there may be unique considerations even when they meet the above criteria. Consultation with HIV specialists and reviewing the most recent recommendations for therapy is recommended before initiating such a change (Working Group, (2004).

Treatment of Opportunistic Infections. Numerous opportunistic infections need to be treated. The clinician needs to assess all illness of HIV-positive children quickly and treat it aggressively. The antibiotic choice for infections such as otitis media, sinusitis, or urinary tract infection needs to be based on cultures or the most likely organism. It is not appropriate to have a "wait and see" approach for any signs of infections such as fever, increased WBC, tachypnea, or malaise. *Candida* infections of the mouth or diaper area are common and should be treated appropriately (see Chapter 27). Whatever the condition, the HIV-positive child needs prompt treatment and close monitoring (Butz et al., 1998).

Monitoring for Efficacy

Signs and Symptoms. Clinical status, growth patterns, and neurodevelopmental status need to be evaluated routinely. Maintaining cognition and growth in the presence of stable laboratory values indicates effective treatment.

Physical Examination Findings. The continuing development and maturation of organ systems that metabolize and distribute drugs and the impact of the disease in multiple body systems mandate repeated physical examination. The absence of any clinical findings supports the effectiveness of treatment. Any deterioration in clinical status can be assumed to be a potential sign of ineffective treatment.

Laboratory Findings. The HIV-positive child needs close monitoring for any changes in virologic laboratory tests and any illnesses. Results substantiated by two repeated virologic tests may suggest treatment changes. CD4 counts should improve, or in some cases cease falling. The viral load (DNA HIV) should be undetectable or dramatically reduced. CD4 counts and HIV RNA testing (in children over 3 years) need to be done every 3 months.

In addition, all opportunistic infection indicators need to be followed closely. This may mean obtaining a wide variety of laboratory values. For example, complete blood counts, urine analysis and urine culture, blood or wound cultures, and respiratory function testing may all be indicated to monitor the specific clinical manifestations of a child.

Monitoring for Toxicity. See the Drug Table 106 for toxicity information. Each drug has a wide range of adverse effects. This is particularly true for drugs administered in the neonatal and early infancy period when there is limited information on pharmacokinetics, doses, and safety of these medications. If the child is responding to the treatment regimen and has mild to moderate adverse reactions, it will be up to the family (and in some instances the child) working with the professionals to determine when or if to change medications. Assess all other medications taken by the child for drug interactions. The Working Group (2004) recommends that all efforts need to be made to continue therapy in the presence of non-life-threatening toxicities. Adjunctive therapies such as granulocyte colony-simulating factor to combat neutropenia and erythropoietin or transfusions to combat anemia can be employed. The issue of quality of life in children with advanced disease needs to be considered by the caregiver and provider in formulating a plan (Working Group, 2004).

Followup Recommendations. It is recommended that children with HIV be followed up at least every 3 months when asymptomatic and more often when there are ongoing problems. In practice, asymptomatic children and adolescents are often followed every 2 months, with symptomatic and young children followed monthly. There may be a "mixed followup" model, where the child sees both the primary care provider and the specialists. Some HIV specialists assume the role of primary care provider. Providers offering primary care to these families need to be prepared to respond quickly to an ever-changing picture.

ALLERGIC REACTIONS

ALLERGIC RESPONSES

An allergy is defined as an adverse physiological reaction of immunologic origin. An allergic reaction must be associated with an antigen relationship between exposure to the antigen and the reaction. Two causes of allergic reactions that will be discussed in this section are (1) drugs and (2) insects. Food allergies will not be discussed, but treatment of food allergic reactions is the same as the treatment of drug and insect reactions. For information pertaining to atopic dermatitis, see Chapter 27 (Dermatologic Disorders); information about latex allergies may be found in Chapter 14.

ALLERGIC REACTIONS TO DRUGS

Allergic drug reactions account for approximately 6 to 10% of all observed adverse drug reactions. These data were obtained from hospital and insurance-provider records and therefore do not represent those reactions that are unreported. Because of the limited availability of in vitro and in vivo tests necessary for defining the immune mechanisms of drug reactions, many patients are incorrectly labeled as being allergic to one or more drugs (Bernstein, 1995; Guill, 1991). Therefore, it is important for the primary care provider to better understand the factors that predispose a patient to drug allergies and, in the case of a reaction, the steps to best manage the reaction.

A number of factors may increase the possibility of a patient's developing an allergic drug reaction. Such factors include (1) age, (2) atopy, (3) prior drug reactions, and (4) underlying disease. Treatment factors may also increase the chance of a patient developing a drug reaction. These include (1) a drug's molecular weight, (2) its metabolic breakdown products, (3) its ability to form haptens, (4) the route of administration (topical > oral), (5) the frequency of treatment (i.e., high doses over a long period of time), and (6) cross-sensitization between structurally homologous drugs (i.e., penicillins and cephalosporins) (Bernstein, 1995; Guill, 1991).

When a drug reaction does occur, some criteria that may be helpful in diagnosing such allergies are the following:

1. A reaction unlike any known pharmacologic reaction of the drug in question

2. A latent period of 7 to 10 days after the first administration of the drug
3. A recurrence of a similar reaction after a rechallenge of the same or a related drug (Breathnach, 1995; Guill, 1991).

Some signs and symptoms include urticaria, angioedema, cardiovascular or respiratory compromise, rhinitis, and nausea and vomiting. The eosinophilia may occur, but it is not necessary in the diagnosis of an immunologically mediated reaction (Guill, 1991).

Allergic drug reactions may involve either one organ system (i.e., dermatologic, renal, hematologic, hepatic, or lymphoid systems) or may be multisystem (i.e., anaphylaxis, serum sickness, drug fever, or vasculitis). Anaphylaxis is the most feared and most life-threatening of all allergic reactions (Guill, 1991).

The drugs that are the most common cause of allergic reactions include penicillins and their derivatives, sulfonamides, nonsteroidal antiinflammatory drugs (NSAIDs), and aspirin. Other examples of drugs that may cause allergic reactions include hydralazine, procainamide, isoniazid, antineoplastic agents, phenytoin, and allo-purinol (Adkinson, 1992; Bernstein, 1995; Breathnach, 1995; Guill, 1991).

Allergic reactions to insect stings or snake bites may also vary in intensity and type, depending on the location and number of cells degranulating their mediators. They may range from local irritation, which resolves in a day, to anaphylaxis. They can also range in presentation time of the reactions (i.e., minutes to several days). Other miscellaneous causes of allergic reactions, specifically anaphylaxis, include foods, such as nuts and seafood, exercise, and cold temperatures (Zieve, 1995).

SPECIFIC CONSIDERATIONS FOR PHARMACOTHERAPY

Need for Drug Therapy and Rationale

The approach to treatment of an established or presumed drug or insect allergic reaction depends on the severity of the reaction. In minor reactions, symptomatic relief is the main goal. Therapy may be delayed for hours to days, depending on the patient's discomfort. For patients who experience more severe reactions, such as anaphylaxis, immediate attention to managing the complication is necessary, since it may be fatal. In these cases, treatment with epinephrine should be initiated while the patient is still in the primary care provider's office (see Table 37–10).

TABLE 37–10. Epinephrine Dosing

	Epinephrine Dose
Children	0.01 mg/kg (0.1 mL/kg of 1:10,000) SC—may repeat every 15–20 min as needed
Adults	0.2–0.5 mg (0.2–0.5 mL of 1:1000) IM or SC—may repeat every 15–20 min as needed

If at home, the patient should be instructed to contact EMS in order to be immediately transported to the nearest emergency department.

Patients with a past history of anaphylaxis must have epinephrine available for emergencies at all times: at home, school, camp, on the ball field, or on the parade route if the patient is in a marching band. Anaphylactic reactions can occur at any time. A convenient way to be prepared is with epinephrine autoinjectors (EpiPen). Patients or parents accompanying children are strongly recommended to carry these devices with them. EpiPen is available for adults and children (see Table 37–11). Do not assume that all children need the EpiPen Jr. The dose in the EpiPen Jr. may not be sufficient for older children. All children over 44 lb need to use the adult EpiPen.

After the first dose of any of these products, the patient should be immediately transported to the emergency department, in case the reaction worsens and the patient requires intravenous therapy with epinephrine, aminophylline, dopamine, norepinephrine, and fluids.

Short- and Long-Term Goals of Pharmacotherapy

The short-term goal of treatment for an allergic reaction is the management of the signs and symptoms. The long-term goal is the consideration of immunotherapy in a patient with a known drug or insect sting allergy. An example of when this may be considered is in an HIV-infected patient who may require treatment or prophylaxis with trimethoprim-sulfamethoxazole and has a known allergic reaction to trimethoprim-sulfamethoxazole.

TABLE 37–11. EpiPen and EpiPen Jr. Dosing

EpiPen	Delivers 0.3 mg IM of epinephrine 1:1000 (2 mL)	May repeat every 20 min to 4 h
EpiPen Jr.	Delivers 0.15 mg IM of epinephrine 1:2000 (2 mL)	May repeat every 15 min for two doses, then every 4 h as needed

Nonpharmacologic Therapy for Allergic Reaction Therapy and Prevention

The following measures should be taken for allergic drug reaction therapy and prevention:

- Discontinue the drug immediately.
- Avoid rough clothing over affected areas.
- Bathe in cool water.
- Avoid scratching affected areas.

Preventive measures for individuals allergic to insect stings include the following:

- Outdoor activities that involve food should be engaged in cautiously.
- Keep garbage and food covered.
- Always wear long pants tucked into socks and shoes when in grass and field areas.
- Perfumes and brightly colored clothes should not be worn outdoors.
- Always apply insect repellant sprays.

Time Frame for Initiating Pharmacotherapy

For minor reactions, pharmacologic therapy may be deferred for hours to days, depending on the discomfort of the patient. In the case of severe reactions, the patient should be sent immediately to the emergency room for care, since intravenous drug therapy will probably be necessary.

Assessment Needed Prior to Therapy

The skin is the organ most commonly affected by allergic reactions; therefore, it should be examined carefully before determining an appropriate treatment. Exanthems, urticaria, angioedema, and contact dermatitis are the most common cutaneous reactions. The first signs of anaphylaxis are often flushing and pruritus. The cutaneous manifestations are most marked on the face, palms, and soles of the feet. Itching is most intense on the head, palms, and soles. Progression to hives and angioedema usually occurs (Wood, 1997). Respiratory symptoms can involve both the upper and lower airways.

Pulmonary manifestations, such as coughing, wheezing, dyspnea, and cyanosis, may also be the result of an allergic reaction. Patients with underlying airway disease may be at the highest risk due to lower airway complications (Wood, 1997). Given the possible seriousness of this type of manifestation, a lung examination should be immediately performed when an allergic reaction is suspected.

Other organ systems that may also be affected include the renal, hepatic, and hematologic systems, but this occurs more infrequently. Depending on the suspected drug, the provider may consider some blood tests, including a complete blood count (CBC), serum creatinine, BUN, or liver function tests.

There are no disease states that would preclude the treatment of an allergic reaction. If a patient is steroid-dependent secondary to asthma or an immunological disease (i.e., SLE, rheumatoid arthritis), the provider will need to consider a longer taper of corticosteroid therapy secondary to the adrenal suppression caused by chronic steroid therapy. Also, if the patient has a history of diabetes mellitus, steroid therapy may temporarily affect the patient's blood glucose control.

A thorough drug history is necessary before prescribing an antihistamine. Terfenadine and astemizole, two nonsedating antihistamines, have been associated with serious cardiac arrhythmias when they have been used in combination with drugs that inhibit the cytochrome P-450 system (i.e., erythromycin, cisapride, cimetidine).

Patient/Caregiver Information

When a patient is prescribed an antihistamine, the provider should always inform the patient of possible effects of the sedating antihistamines. If the patient has never taken a sedating antihistamine, the provider should recommend that the patient abstain from driving after the initial dose to allow for adequate assessment of the full sedating effect. Nonsedating antihistamines may also be considered, but they are also more expensive than the sedating antihistamines.

Patients with a past history of anaphylaxis must be reminded to have epinephrine available for emergencies at all times, especially on recreational outings. Anaphylatic reactions can occur at any time. Each year the provider needs to discuss with the patient and parents the different types of epinephrine available for self-administration, reassess the patient's plan for self-administration, and review the expiration date of any products the patient may have for emergency self-administration.

Advise all patients with a history of anaphylaxis to wear a medical alert identification. Provide a detailed plan for management of anaphylaxis to parents of an allergic child, and assess their ability to implement it. In addition, teach patients to identify early symptoms of a reaction and to seek medical attention early.

OUTCOMES MANAGEMENT

Selection of an Agent

Antihistamines are the mainstay of therapy for the palliative care of pruritis associated with allergic reactions. The main thing to consider is the patient's tolerance for a sedating antihistamine. If the patient cannot tolerate one of the sedating antihistamines, the healthcare provider may consider one of the available nonsedating formulations, which may be more expensive.

For those cases in which the reactions do not warrant intravenous therapy, but are severe enough that antihistamines are not effective, the provider may consider an oral corticosteroid, such as prednisone, for a short course. Dosing may vary, but a suggested dose would be prednisone 40 mg daily for 5 to 7 days. A corticosteroid may also block the late phase response of the allergic reaction.

Monitoring for Efficacy

If the patient is experiencing a minor allergic reaction, he or she should be considered to monitor the efficacy of treatment with antihistamines and/or corticosteroid therapy. The patient should watch for improvement or worsening of dermatologic manifestations, as well as any change in breathing ability. If no improvement or worsening of symptoms occurs, the patient should contact the provider immediately.

Monitoring for Toxicity

Patients using sedating antihistamines should monitor for any unacceptable amount of sedation, which may lead to decreased alertness. As stated previously, terfenadine and astemizole are associated with cardiac arrhythmias, which may occur if the patient is taking a higher than recommended dose or is taking it with a drug that may inhibit its metabolism. Because the arrhythmia is potentially fatal, the best thing a provider can do is to complete a thorough medication history before making any prescribing decisions.

Followup Recommendations

Once a drug allergic reaction has occurred, the primary care provider should emphasize to the patient the importance of informing potential prescribers (i.e., other healthcare providers, dentists) or pharmacists of the allergy. This information is critical in order to prevent the reaction from recurring.

As previously stated, a patient with a previous history of anaphylaxis should have an EpiPen or similar device available in case the patient is reexposed to whatever had initially caused the reaction (i.e., food, drug, insect). The patient may also consider some type of alert bracelet, which would be helpful if the patient is not conscious and requires immediate care. Avoidance is the key to the management of allergic reactions, but in the case of an allergic reaction, rapid assessment and management are necessary.

INFECTIOUS MONONUCLEOSIS

Infectious mononucleosis is a common acute, relatively benign, self-limited viral infection caused by the Epstein-Barr virus. The condition is uncommon in children under 5, rare before age 2, and seen often in adolescents (Schwartz, Bell, Brown, et al., 1996). This infection is thought to manifest with clinical symptoms only 50% of the time. It is hypothesized that persons who get the symptomatic disease have not been exposed prior to the second decade of life. This illness is characterized by nausea, pharyngitis, and often high fevers. Rapid onset of these symptoms is thought to be related to prolonged recovery (Dornbrand, Hoole, & Pickard, 1992). In most cases the acute symptoms last 7 to 10 days, but the fatigue can persist for several months. Persons who are immunosuppressed are particularly susceptible to this condition. The symptoms are thought to be caused by the changes in the B-lymphocytes. A rapid and sustained response results in the adenopathy and the atypical lymphocytosis characteristic of this condition.

SPECIFIC CONSIDERATIONS FOR PHARMACOTHERAPY

Need for Drug Therapy and Rationale

In most cases there is no need for specific drug treatment. Symptomatic treatment of fever or sore throat with acetaminophen or aspirin (in adults only) and local treatments such as throat gargles or lozenges are recommended. Antibiotics are needed only if there is a documented coexisting streptococcal pharyngitis (see Chapter 21). Avoidance of contact sports should be stressed (Cozad, 1996).

There are several controversial issues in the treatment of this condition. Although there is universal agreement that pharyngeal edema threatening respiratory function needs to be treated with corticosteroids and potentially hospitalization, the treatment of less severe symptoms with corticosteroids is not universally supported. Dornbrand et al. (1992) cite controlled studies that indicate corticosteroids lessen fever and pharyngitis, may result in an improved sense of well-being, and shorten the course of the condition but stop short of recommending use of this medication routinely. In addition, Ganzel, Goldman, and Padya (1996), in a retrospective review of 109 patients admitted to a hospital with severe airway obstruction, concluded that severe pharyngotonsilitis is more common than reported in the literature and recommended parental steroids in these cases.

Short- and Long-Term Goals of Pharmacotherapy

The short-term goal depends on the severity of the condition. For most it is the control of symptoms. For the severely ill patient it would be to maintain a functional airway. The long-term goal of treatment is return to normal functioning with no sequelae.

Time Frame for Initiating Treatment

Treatment for any compromised airway should be immediate. Initiation of any other treatment is based on symptoms.

Assessment Prior to Therapy

In addition to the history and physical examination routinely done with individuals presenting with upper respiratory symptoms, the provider needs to ask about immunosuppressed status, fever, and abdominal pain. In addition, the physical needs to include a thorough evaluation of the abdomen and close inspection of the skin. Lymphadenopathy is usually generalized.

Although a complete blood count is usually done and atypical lymphocytes are common, the definitive diagnosis is usually dependent on a positive "monospot." This laboratory test responds to the rise in heterophile antibodies, which occurs in the acute stage of this infection. The "monospot" can be negative in the first few days of the condition. Other specific serologic tests are possible but not used clinically (Avery & First, 1994).

Patient/Caregiver Information

See Chapter 21. Explain the course of the infection. The residual fatigue and malaise may be frustrating to the patient, especially the adolescent. They may need assistance in understanding their potentially slow recovery.

OUTCOMES MANAGEMENT

Selecting an Agent

Corticosteroids. Emergency treatment of patients at risk for airway obstruction is 1 mg/kg of prednisone daily for 3 days and tapered over 10 days. No other medication is common in the primary care setting. If antibiotics are used for coexisting streptococcal pharyngitis, penicillin or erythromycin is the drug of choice. Ampicillin should be avoided since it is thought to cause a "monorash."

Monitoring for Efficacy

The reduction of symptoms can be used to evaluate therapy, especially the enlarged tonsils and spleen. Laboratory work is usually not used to monitor efficiency since the monospot can be positive for an extended time.

Monitoring for Toxicity

The course of corticosteroids is short, and the normal side effects associated with a longer course usually are not a problem. Any untoward effects are unexpected and should be investigated.

Followup Recommendations

Monitor weekly until the patient is recovered and no splenomegaly exists. Refer for any toxicity, jaundice, or unexpected symptoms.

REFERENCES

Adkinson, N. F. (1992). Drug allergy. *JAMA, 268,* 771–773.

American Foundation for AIDS Research (AmFAR) (2002). *AIDS/HIV treatment directory.* New York: AmFAR.

American Medical Association (AMA). (1996). *A physician guide to HIV prevention.* Chicago: AMA.

Avery, M. E., & First, L. R. (1994). *Pediatric medicine* (2nd ed.). Baltimore: Williams & Wilkins.

Bartlett, J. & Gallant, J. (2003). 2003 Medical Management of HIV Infection. Baltimore: Johns Hopkins University.

Bernstein, J. A. (1995). Allergic drug reactions. *Postgraduate Medicine, 98,* 159–166.

Boucher, C. A., & Larder, B. A. (1994). *Viral variation and therapeutic strategies in HIV infection.* London: MediTech Media.

Breathnach, S. M. (1995). Management of drug eruptions: Part II. *Australian Journal of Dermatology, 36,* 187–191.

Burroughs, C. (1993). Alternative therapies for AIDS: An historical review. *The Gay Men's Health Crisis Newsletter of Experimental AIDS Therapies, 7, 11/12,* 2–4.

Butz, A. M., Joyner, M., Friedman, D. G., & Hutton, N. (1998). Primary care for children with Human Immunodeficiency Virus infection. *Journal of Pediatric Health Care, 12*(1), 10–19.

Coates, T. (1994). Report from the AIDS Conference. Care and prevention: Hand in hand. *Focus: A Guide to AIDS Research and Counseling, 9*(12), 1–4.

Cozad, J. (1996). Infectious mononucleosis. *Nurse Practitioner, 21*(3), 14–16.

Dornbrand, L., Hoole, A. J., & Pickard, C. G. (1992). *Manual of clinical problems in adult ambulatory care* (2nd ed.). Boston: Little, Brown.

Fahrner, R., & Benson, M. (1996). HIV infection and AIDS. In P. L. Jackson & J. A. Vessey (eds.), *Primary care of the child with a chronic condition* (2nd ed.). St. Louis: Mosby.

Fisher, E. J. (1995). *Clinician's guide to therapy of adults with HIV/AIDS.* Richmond: Virginia Commonwealth University HIV/AIDS Center.

Funck-Brentano, I., Costagliola, D., Seibel, N., Straub, E., Tardieu, M., & Blanche, S. (1997). Patterns of disclosure and perceptions of the human immunodeficiency virus in infected elementary school-age children. *Archives of Pediatric and Adolescent Medicine, 151*(10), 978–985.

Ganzel, T. M., Goldman, J. L., & Padhya, T. A. (1996). Otolaryngologic clinical patterns in pediatric infectious mononucleosis. *American Journal of Otolaryngology, 17*(6), 397–400.

Gershon, A. A., Mervish, N., LaRussa, P., Steinberg, S., Lo, S. H., Hodes, D., Fikrig, S., Bonagura, V., & Bakshi, S. (1997). Varicella-zoster virus infection in children with underlying human immunodeficiency virus infection. *Journal of Infectious Diseases, 176*(6), 1496–1500.

Goldschmidt, R. H., & Dong, B. J. (1997). Current report—HIV. Treatment of AIDS and HIV-related conditions—1997. *JABEFP, 10*(2), 144–167.

Guill, M. F. (1991). Allergic drug reactions: Identification and management. *Hospital Formulary, 26,* 582–589.

Hecht, F. M., & Soloway, B. (1994). *HIV infection: A primary care approach.* Waltham: Massachusetts Medical Society.

Japour, A. J. (1996). Measurement of HIV-1 RNA in clinical practice: An initial management algorithm. *Journal of the International Association of Physicians in AIDS Care, 2,* 16–19.

Lipsky, J. J. (1996). Antiretroviral drugs for AIDS. *Lancet, 348,* 800–803.

Makadon, H. J., & Silian, J. G. (1995). Prevention of HIV infection in primary care: Current practices, future possibilities. *Annals of Internal Medicine, 123*(9), 715–719.

Marks, R. (1994). The Brighton Conference and HIV prevention. *Focus: A Guide to AIDS Research and Counseling, 9*(12), 5–8.

Miralles, G. D. (1996). Virology and pathogenesis of HIV. In J. A. Bartlett (Ed.), *Care and management of patients with HIV infection* (pp. 14–17). Durham, NC: Glaxo Wellcome.

Moon, J. E. (1997). Collective for Environmental Design, POB 12161, Richmond, VA 23241.

Moore, R. D., & Bartlett, J. G. (1996). Combination antiretroviral therapy in HIV infection: An economic perspective. *PharmacoEconomics, 10*(2), 109–113.

Osmond, D. H. (2003). Epidemiology of HIV/AIDS in the United States. HIV InSite Knowledge Base Chapter. http://hivinsite.ucsf.edu.

Panel on Clinical Practices for Treatment of HIV Infection. (2004). Guidelines for the Use of Antiretroviral Agents in HIV-1-Infected Adults and Adolescents. Department of Health and Human Services (DHHS).

Schwartz, W. M., Bell, L. M., Brown, L., Clark, B. J., Kim, S. C., & Manno, C. S. (Eds.) (1996). *Clinical handbook of pediatrics.* Baltimore: Williams & Wilkins.

Stryker, J., Coates, T. J., DeCarlo, P., Haynes-Sanstad, K., Shriver, M., & Makadon, H. J. (1995). Prevention of HIV Infection. *JAMA, 272*(14), 1143–1148.

Tynell, E., Aurelius, E., Brazell, A., Jalander, I., Wood, M., Yao, Q. Y., Rickinson, A., Akerlund, B., & Anderson, J. (1996). Acyclovir and prednisolone treatment of acute infectious mononucleosis: A multicenter, double-blind, placebo-controlled study. *Journal of Infectious Diseases, 174*(2), 324–331.

Wiese, W. (1997). Developments in antiretroviral therapy for AIDS patients. *Internal Medicine, April,* 72–85.

Wood, R. (1997). Anaphylaxis in children. *Patient Care,* 161–183.

Working Group on Antroviral Therapy and Medical Management of HIV-Infected Children. (2004). Guidelines for the Use of Antiretroviral Agents in Pediatric HIV Infection. AIDSinfo Website. http://aidsinfo.nih.gov.

Zieve, P. D. (1995). *Handbook of ambulatory care.* Baltimore: Williams & Wilkins.

V ❖ Tables of Pharmacotherapeutic Agents

Tables of Pharmacotherapeutic Agents

BIBLIOGRAPHY

American Hospital Formulary Service (AHFS). (2004). *Drug information '04*. Bethesda, MD: American Society of Hospital Pharmacists.

Briggs, G.G., Freeman, R.K., & Yaffe, S.J. (2002). *Drugs in pregnancy and lactation* (6th ed.). Baltimore: Lippincott, Williams, and Wilkins.

Drug facts and comparisons. (2004). St. Louis: Facts and Comparisons.

Manufacturers' package inserts.

100. ANTI-INFECTIVE AGENTS
101. Amebicides

Drug and Dosage Forms	Spectrum of Activity and Usual Dosage Range	Administration Issues and Drug–Drug & Drug–Food Interactions	Common Adverse Drug Reactions (ADRs) and Pharmacokinetics	Contraindications, Pregnancy Category, and Lactation Issues
Iodoquinol Yodoxin Tablet: 210 mg 650 mg	**Spectrum of Activity** Entamoeba histolytica. **Treatment of intestinal amebiasis:** **Adults:** 650 mg tid pc × 20 d **Children:** 40 mg/kg/d up to max of 650 mg/dose tid × 20 d	Administration Issues Complete full course of therapy. Drug–Drug Interactions Iodoquinol may interfere with the effect of **levothyroxine** by increasing protein bound iodine levels.	ADRs Skin eruptions, nausea, vomiting, GI upset, blurred vision. Pharmacokinetics Poorly absorbed, metabolized in the liver, excreted in the feces.	Contraindications Hypersensitivity to iodine containing products. Pregnancy Category: C Lactation Issues Safety for use during breast feeding has not been established.
Paromomycin Humatin Capsule: 250 mg	**spectrum of Activity** Entamoeba histolytica, Cryptosporidium diarrhea. **Treatment of intestinal amebiasis:** **Adult: and children:** 25–35 mg/kg/d tid × 5–10	Administration Issues Complete full course of therapy; administer after meals to prevent gastric distress. Drug–Drug Interactions Rare due to lack of systemic absorption.	ADRs Skin eruptions, nausea, vomiting, GI upset. Pharmacokinetics Not absorbed systemically; excreted 100% unchanged in feces.	Contraindications Hypersensitivity to paromomycin; intestinal obstruction. Pregnancy Category: C Lactation Issues Safety for use during breast feeding has not been established.

102. Antibiotics

102.1 Cephalosporins: First Generation

Drug and Dosage Forms	Spectrum of Activity and Usual Dosage Range	Administration Issues and Drug—Drug & Drug—Food Interactions	Common Adverse Drug Reactions (ADRs) and Pharmacokinetics	Contraindications, Pregnancy Category, and Lactation Issues
Cephalexin Keflex, generics Tablet: 250 mg, 500 mg Capsule: 250 mg, 500 mg Powder for Oral Suspension: 100 mg/ml, 125 mg/5 ml, 250 mg/5 ml	**Antibacterial spectrum** Active against *S. aureus, S. pneumoniae,* and *S. pyogenes.* Majority of urinary isolates of community-acquired *E. coli, Klebsiella species,* and *P. mirabilis* are susceptible; not very active against *H. influenzae*; inactive against enterococci. **General indications** **Adults:** 250–500 mg q 6 h or × 10 to 14 d **If oral dose is > 4 gm/day, use parenteral drug** **Children:** 25–50 mg/kg/d divided qid × 10 to 14 d Otitis media: 75–100 mg/kg/d divided qid × 10 to 14 d **Prevention of bacterial endocarditis** Adults 2 gm (children 50 mg/kg) orally 1 h before procedure.	Administration Issues Complete full course of therapy; shake suspension well before administration; store suspension in the refrigerator; discard unused suspension after 14 d. Drug–Drug Interactions Cephalosporins may decrease the effectiveness of **oral contraceptives; probenecid** may increase cephalosporin plasma levels by competitively inhibiting renal excretion of cephalosporins.	ADRs Hypersensitivity reactions, urticarial rash, nausea, vomiting, diarrhea, superinfections. Pharmacokinetics Well absorbed from GI tract; does not readily enter CSF; use decreased dose with renal failure.	Contraindications Use with caution in patients with true penicillin allergy; 5–7% cross-sensitivity between penicillins and cephalosporins in allergic patients. Pregnancy Category: B Lactation Issues Excreted in breast milk in small quantities; use with caution in nursing mothers; modification and alteration of bowel flora in infants may cause side effects such as diarrhea.
Cefadroxil Duricef, various generics Tablet: 1 gm Capsule: 500 mg Powder for Oral Suspension: 125 mg/5 ml, 250 mg/5 ml, 500 mg/5 ml	**Antibacterial spectrum** Active against *S. aureus, S. pneumoniae,* and *S. pyogenes.* Majority of urinary isolates of community-acquired *E. coli, Klebsiella species,* and *P. mirabilis* are susceptible; not very active against *H. influenzae*; inactive against enterococci. **Uncomplicated urinary tract infection** **Adults:** 1–2 gm/d qd or divided bid × 7 to 10 d **Children:** 30 mg/kg/d divided bid × 7 to 10 d **Pharyngitis, tonsillitis, skin and soft tissue infections**	Administration Issues Complete full course of therapy; shake suspension well before administration; store suspension in the refrigerator; discard unused suspension after 14 d. Drug–Drug Interactions Cephalosporins may decrease the effectiveness of **oral contraceptives; probenecid** may increase cephalosporin plasma levels by competitively inhibiting renal excretion of cephalosporins.	ADRs Hypersensitivity reactions, urticarial rash, nausea, vomiting, diarrhea, superinfections. Pharmacokinetics Well absorbed from GI tract; does not readily enter CSF; use decreased dose with renal failure.	Contraindications Use with caution in patients with true penicillin allergy; 5–7% cross-sensitivity between penicillins and cephalosporins in allergic patients. Pregnancy Category: B Lactation Issues Excreted in breast milk in small quantities; use with caution in nursing mothers; modification and alteration of bowel flora in infants may cause side effects such as diarrhea.

(*continues on next page*)

102.1 Cephalosporins: First Generation *continued from previous page*

Drug and Dosage Forms	Spectrum of Activity and Usual Dosage Range	Administration Issues and Drug—Drug & Drug—Food Interactions	Common Adverse Drug Reactions (ADRs) and Pharmacokinetics	Contraindications, Pregnancy Category, and Lactation Issues
Cefadroxil *cont.*	**Adults:** 1 gm/d divided bid × 10 d **Children:** 30 mg/kg/d divided bid × 10 d **Prevention of bacterial endocarditis** Adults 2 gm (children 50 mg/kg) orally 1 h before procedure			
Cephradine Velosef, various generics Capsule: 250 mg, 500 mg Powder for Oral Suspension: 125 mg/5 ml, 250 mg/5 ml	**Antibacterial spectrum** Active against *S. aureus, S. pneumoniae*, and *S. pyogenes*. Majority of urinary isolates of community-acquired *E. coli, Klebsiella species*, and *P. mirabilis* are susceptible; not very active against *H. influenzae*; inactive against enterococci. **General indications** **Adults:** 250–500 mg q 6 h or 500–1000 mg q 12 h × 10 to 14 d **Children (Over 9 months):** 25–50 mg/kg/d divided q 6 to 12 h × 10 to 14 d Otitis media: 75–100 mg/kg/d divided q 6 to 12 h × 10 to 14 d	Administration Issues Complete full course of therapy; shake suspension well before administration; suspension stable for 7 days at room temperature and 14 days if refrigerated. Drug–Drug Interactions Cephalosporins may decrease the effectiveness of **oral contraceptives; probenecid** may increase cephalosporin plasma levels by competitively inhibiting renal excretion of cephalosporins.	ADRs Hypersensitivity reactions, urticarial rash, nausea, vomiting, diarrhea, superinfections. Pharmacokinetics Well absorbed from GI tract; does not readily enter CSF; use decreased dose with renal failure.	Contraindications Use with caution in patients with true penicillin allergy; 5–7% cross-sensitivity between penicillins and cephalosporins in allergic patients. Pregnancy Category: B Lactation Issues Excreted in breast milk in small quantities; use with caution in nursing mothers; modification and alteration of bowel flora in infants may cause side effects such as diarrhea.

102.2 Cephalosporins: Second Generation

Drug and Dosage Forms	Spectrum of Activity and Usual Dosage Range	Administration Issues and Drug–Drug & Drug–Food Interactions	Common Adverse Drug Reactions (ADRs) and Pharmacokinetics	Contraindications, Pregnancy Category, and Lactation Issues
Cefaclor Ceclor, various generics Capsule: 250 mg, 500 mg Tablet, extended release 375 mg, 500 mg Powder for Oral Suspension: 125 mg/5 ml, 187 mg/5 ml, 250 mg/5 ml, 375 mg/5 ml	**Spectrum of activity** Active against *S. aureus, S. pneumoniae, S. pyogenes, E. coli, Klebsiella species, M. catarrhalis*, and *P. mirabilis*. More active against ampicillin-susceptible *H. influenzae* than first generation cephalosporins but variable susceptibility against ampicillin-resistant strain of *H. influenzae*. Inactive against enterococci, *B. fragilis*, and many other gram-negative bacteria such as *Pseudomonas, Serratia*, and Enterobacter species. **General indications** 250–500 mg q 8 h × 10 to 14 d **Acute bronchitis or exacerbations of chronic bronchitis** 500 mg q12 h × 7 d **Pharyngitis and uncomplicated skin infections** 375 mg q 12h × 7 to 10 d **Children:** 20–40 mg/kg/d divided q 8 h × 10 to 14 d **Maximum children's dose is 1 gm/d.**	Administration Issues Complete full course of therapy; shake suspension well before administration; store suspension in the refrigerator; discard unused suspension 14 days after reconstitution. Administer tablets with food; do not crush, chew, or cut tablets. Drug–Drug Interactions Cephalosporins may decrease the effectiveness of **oral contraceptives; probenecid** may increase cephalosporin plasma levels by competitively inhibiting renal excretion of cephalosporins.	ADRs Hypersensitivity reactions, urticarial rash, nausea, vomiting, diarrhea, superinfections. Pharmacokinetics Does not readily enter CSF; use decreased dose with renal failure.	Contraindications Use with caution in patients with true penicillin allergy; 5–7% cross-sensitivity between penicillins and cephalosporins in allergic patients. Pregnancy Category: B Lactation Issues Excreted in breast milk in small quantities; use with caution in nursing mothers; modification/ alteration of bowel flora in infants may cause side effects such as diarrhea.
Cefuroxime Axetil Ceftin, generics Tablet: 125 mg, 250 mg, 500 mg Powder for Oral Suspension: 125 mg/5 ml, 250 mg/5 ml	**Spectrum of activity** Active against *S. aureus, S. pneumoniae*, and *S. pyogenes*. Active against *E. coli, Klebsiella species, M. catarrhalis*, and *P. mirabilis*. Active against beta-lactamase positive and beta-lactamase negative *H. influenzae*. Inactive against enterococci, *B. fragilis*, and many other gram-negative bacteria such as *Pseudomonas* and *Serratia*. **Pharyngitis/tonsillitis, bronchitis, and uncomplicated skin and skin structure infections**	Administration Issues **Tablets and suspension are not bioequivalent and cannot be substituted on a mg/kg basis** tablets can be taken without regard to meals; suspension must be taken with food; suspension may be stored at room temperature or in the refrigerator; discard unused suspension 10 days after reconstitution. Drug–Drug Interactions Cephalosporins may decrease the effectiveness of **oral contraceptives;**	ADRs Hypersensitivity reactions, urticarial rash, nausea, vomiting, diarrhea, superinfections. Pharmacokinetics Does not readily enter CSF; use decreased dose with renal failure; absorption increased with food.	Contraindications Use with caution in patients with true penicillin allergy; 5–7% cross-sensitivity between penicillins and cephalosporins in allergic patients. Pregnancy Category: B Lactation Issues Excreted in breast milk in small quantities; use with caution in nursing mothers; modification/alteration of bowel flora in infants may cause side effects such as diarrhea.

(*continues on next page*)

102.2 Cephalosporins: Second Generation *continued from previous page*

Drug and Dosage Forms	Spectrum of Activity and Usual Dosage Range	Administration Issues and Drug–Drug & Drug–Food Interactions	Common Adverse Drug Reactions (ADRs) and Pharmacokinetics	Contraindications, Pregnancy Category, and Lactation Issues
Cefuroxime Axetil *cont.*	**Adults and children ≥ 13 yr.:** 250–500 mg q 12 h × 10 d **Uncomplicated urinary tract infections** **Adults and children ≥ 13 yr.:** 125–250 mg q 12 h × 7 to 10 d **Uncomplicated gonococcal infections** **Adults and children ≥ 13 yr.:** 1000 mg as a single dose **Pharyngitis/tonsillitis** **Children 3 months to 12 yr.:** (dosage for suspension) 20 mg/kg/d divided q 12 h × 10 d Max dose: 500 mg/d **Uncomplicated skin infections and otitis media** **Children 3 months to 12 yr.:** (dosage for suspension) 30 mg/kg/d divided q 12 h × 10 d Max dose: 1000 mg/d	**probenecid** may increase cephalosporin plasma levels by competitively inhibiting renal excretion of cephalosporins.		
Cefprozil Cefzil Tablet: 250 mg, 500 mg Powder for Oral Suspension: 125 mg/5 ml, 250 mg/5 ml	**Spectrum of Activity** Active against *S. aureus, S. pneumoniae, S. pyogenes, E. coli, Klebsiella species, M. catarrhalis,* and *P. mirabilis.* Active against beta-lactamase positive and beta-lactamase negative *H. influenzae.* Inactive against enterococci, *B. fragilis,* and many other gram-negative bacteria such as *Pseudomonas* and *Serratia.* **Pharyngitis/tonsillitis and bronchitis** **Adults:** 500 mg q 12 to 24 h × 10 d **Children 2 to 12 yr.:** 15 mg/kg/d divided q 12 h × 10 d	Administration Issues Complete full course of therapy; shake suspension well before administration; store suspension in the refrigerator; discard unused suspension 14 days after reconstitution. Drug–Drug Interactions Cephalosporins may decrease the effectiveness of **oral contraceptives; probenecid** may increase cephalosporin plasma levels by competitively inhibiting renal excretion of cephalosporins.	ADRs Hypersensitivity reactions, urticarial rash, nausea, vomiting, diarrhea, superinfections. Pharmacokinetics Does not readily enter CSF; use decreased dose with renal failure; absorption increased with food.	Contraindications Use with caution in patients with true penicillin allergy; 5–7% cross-sensitivity between penicillins and cephalosporins in allergic patients. Pregnancy Category: B Lactation Issues Excreted in breast milk in small quantities; use with caution in nursing mothers; modification/ alteration of bowel flora in infants may cause side effects such as diarrhea.

	Uncomplicated skin and skin structure infections **Adults:** 250 mg q 12 h × 10 d or 500 mg q 12 to 24 h × 10 d **Children:** 20 mg/kg q 24 h × 10 d **Otitis media** **Children 6 months to 12 yr.:** 30 mg/kg/d divided q 12 h × 10 d			
Loracarbef Lorabid Capsule: 200 mg, 400 mg Powder for Oral Suspension: 100 mg/5 ml, 200 mg/5 ml	**Spectrum of Activity** Active against *S. aureus, S. pneumoniae, S. pyogenes, E. coli, Klebsiella species, M. catarrhalis*, and *P. mirabilis*. Active against beta-lactamase positive and beta-lactamase negative *H. influenzae*. Inactive against enterococci, *B. fragilis* and many other gram-negative bacteria such as *Pseudomonas* and *Serratia*. **Upper and lower respiratory tract infections, skin and soft tissue infections, uncomplicated UTI** **Adults and children ≥ 13 yr.:** 200–400 mg q 12 h × 7 to 14 d **Pharyngitis, tonsillitis, skin and soft tissue infections** **Children 6 months to 12 yr.:** 15–30 mg/kg/d divided q 12 h × 7 to 10 d **Acute Otitis Media (use suspension)** 30mg/kg/d divided q 12 h × 10 d	Administration Issues Complete full course of therapy; shake suspension well before administration; suspension may be kept at room temperature; discard unused suspension after 14 days; suspension is more rapidly absorbed than the capsules. Drug–Drug Interactions Cephalosporins may decrease the effectiveness of **oral contraceptives; probenecid** may increase cephalosporin plasma levels by competitively inhibiting renal excretion of cephalosporins.	ADRs Hypersensitivity reactions, urticarial rash, nausea, vomiting, diarrhea, superinfections. Pharmacokinetics Does not readily enter CSF; use decreased dose with renal failure; absorption increased with food.	Contraindications Use with caution in patients with true penicillin allergy; 5–7% cross-sensitivity between penicillins and cephalosporins in allergic patients. Pregnancy Category: B Lactation Issues Excreted in breast milk in small quantities; use with caution in nursing mothers; modification/alteration of bowel flora in infants may cause side effects such as diarrhea.

102.3 Cephalosporins: Third Generation

Drug and Dosage Forms	Spectrum of Activity and Usual Dosage Range	Administration Issues and Drug-Drug & Drug-Food Interactions	Common Adverse Drug Reactions (ADRs) and Pharmacokinetics	Contraindications, Pregnancy Category, and Lactation Issues
Cefdinir Omnicef Capsule: 300 mg Oral Suspension: 125 mg/5 mll	**Spectrum of activity** Active against *S. pyogenes*, penicillin-susceptible pneumococci, methicillin-susceptible *S. aureus, H. influenzae, M. catarrhalis, N. gonorrhoeae*, and many enteric gram-negative bacilli. No activity against methicillin-resistant *S. aureus* and *S. epidermidis, P. aeuruginosa*, enterococci, many anaerobes. **Acute exacerbations of chronic bronchitis/acute maxillary sinusitis, pharyngitis/tonsillitis/uncomplicated skin infections.** Adults and adolescents ≥ 13 yr.: The **total daily dose** for all infections is **600 mg**. Once-daily dosing for **10 days** is as effective as bid dosing; qd dosing has not been studied in **pneumonia or skin infections**; therefore, administer bid in those infections. Pharyngitis/tonsillitis can be treated for 5–10 days if using bid dosing. Children (6 months-12 yr.): The **total daily dose** for all infections is **14 mg/kg up to a max dose of 600 mg/day**; qd dosing for **10 days** is as effective as bid dosing. Once-daily dosing has not been studied in **skin infections**; therefore, administer twice daily in this infection. Pharyngitis/tonsillitis can be treated for 5–10 days if using bid dosing.	Administration Issues Complete full course of therapy. Both the capsules and oral suspension may be taken without regards to meals. Antacids containing magnesium or aluminum interfere with the absorption of cefdinir. If this type of antacid is required during cefdinir therapy, take cefdinir 2 hours before or after the antacid. If iron supplements are needed during cefdinir therapy, cefdinir should be taken 2 hours before or after the supplement or ion-fortified infant formula. Drug Interactions Cefdinir concentrations may be reduced by coadministration of **antacids. Iron supplements and foods fortified with iron** reduce the absorption of cefdinir by 80% and 30%, respectively. **Probenecid** may increase and prolong cephalosporin plasma levels.l	ADRs Hypersensitivity reactions, urticarial rash, nausea, vomiting, diarrhea, superinfections. Pharmacokinetics $T_{1/2}$ = 100 minutes Dose adjustment is needed for renal impairment.l	Contraindications Use with caution in patients with true penicillin allergy; 5–7% cross-sensitivity between penicillins and cephalosporins in allergic patients. Pregnancy Category: B Lactation Issues Excreted in breast milk in small quantities; use with caution in nursing mothers; modification/alteration of bowel flora in infants may cause side effects such as diarrhea.l

Cefditoren Pivoxil Spectracef Tablet: 200 mg	**Spectrum of activity** Active against *S. pyogenes*, penicillin-susceptible pneumococci, methicillin-susceptible *S. aureus, H. influenzae, M. catarrhalis, N. gonorrhoeae*, and many enteric gram-negative bacilli. No activity against methicillin-resistant *S. aureus* and *S. epidermidis, P. aeuruginosa*, enterococci, many anaerobes. **Acute exacerbations of chronic bronchitis/acute maxillary sinusitis, pharyngitis/tonsillitis/uncomplicated skin infections.** **Adults and adolescents ≥ 12 y.:** Acute exacerbations of chronic bronchitis: 400 mg bid × 10 d Pharyngitis/tonsillitis/uncomplicated skin infections 200 mg bid × 10 d	Administration Issues Complete full course of therapy. Take with meals. No dosage adjustment for mild renal impairment. Prescribe ≤ 200 mg bid in patients with moderate impairment and 200 mg qd in patients with severe impairment Drug Interactions Do not administer with **antacids** or **H2-receptor antagonists; probenecid** may increase and prolong cephalosporin plasma levels.	ADRs Hypersensitivity reactions, urticarial rash, nausea, vomiting, diarrhea, superinfections. Pharmacokinetics $T_{1/2}$ = 1.6 hours Dose adjustment is needed for moderate to severe renal impairment.	Contraindications Use with caution in patients with true penicillin allergy; 5–7% cross-sensitivity between penicillins and cephalosporins in allergic patients. In patients with carnitine deficiency or inborn errors of metabolism that may result in significant carnitine deficiency. Do not administer to patients with milk protein hypersensitivity. Pregnancy Category: B Lactation Issues Excreted in breast milk in small quantities; use with caution in nursing mothers; modification/alteration of bowel flora in infants may cause side effects such as diarrhea.

(continues on next page)

102.3 Cephalosporins: Third Generation *continued from previous page*

Drug and Dosage Forms	Spectrum of Activity and Usual Dosage Range	Administration Issues and Drug-Drug & Drug-Food Interactions	Common Adverse Drug Reactions (ADRs) and Pharmacokinetics	Contraindications, Pregnancy Category, and Lactation Issues
Cefpodoxime Proxetil Vantin Tablet: 100 mg, 200 mg Granules for Oral Suspension: 50 mg/5 ml, 100 mg/5 ml	**Spectrum of activity** Active against *S. pyogenes, S. agalactiae, S. pneumoniae*, beta-lactamase-positive and -negative *H. influenzae, M. catarrhalis, N. gonorrhoeae*, and many Enterobacteriaceae (not *Enterobacter, Serratia, or Morganella*). Modest activity against S. aureus with no activity for enterococci or MRSA. **Community-acquired pneumonia and bronchitis** Adults and children ≥ 13 yr.: 200 mg q 12 h × 10 to 14 d **Uncomplicated gonococcal infection** Adults and children ≥ 13 yr.: 200 mg as a single dose **Skin and skin structure infection** Adults and children ≥ 13 yr.: 400 mg q 12 h × 7 to 14 d **Pharyngitis/tonsillitis** Adults and children ≥ 13 yr.: 100 mg q 12 h × 10 d Children 6 months to 12 yr.: 10 mg/kg/d divided q 12 h × 10 d **Uncomplicated UTI** Adults and children ≥ 13 yr.: 100 mg q 12 h × 10 d **Acute otitis media** Children 6 months to 12 yr.: 10 mg/kg/d divided q 12 h × 10 d or 10 mg/kg q 24h × 10 d	Administration Issues Complete full course of therapy; give with food; administer with food to enhance absorption; shake suspension well before administration; store suspension in the refrigerator; discard unused suspension 14 days after reconstitution. Drug-Drug Interactions Cephalosporins may decrease the effectiveness of **oral contraceptives; probenecid** may increase cephalosporin plasma levels by competitively inhibiting renal excretion of cephalosporins.	ADRs Hypersensitivity reactions, urticarial rash, nausea, vomiting, diarrhea, superinfections. Pharmacokinetics Use decreased dose with renal failure.	Contraindications Use with caution in patients with true penicillin allergy; 5–7% cross-sensitivity between penicillins and cephalosporins in allergic patients. Pregnancy Category: B Lactation Issues Excreted in breast milk in small quantities; use with caution in nursing mothers; modification/alteration of bowel flora in infants may cause side effects such as diarrhea.

Ceftibutin Cedax Capsule: 400 mg Powder for Oral Suspension: 90 mg/5 ml, 180 mg/5 ml	**Spectrum of activity** Active against *S. pneumoniae* (penicillin-susceptible strains only), *S. pyogenes*, beta-lactamase producing strains of *H. influenzae* and *M. catarrhalis.* **Pharyngitis/tonsillitis, bronchitis, and otitis media** Adults and children ≥ 12 yr.: 400 mg qd × 10 d Children ≥ 12 yr.: 9 mg/kg qd × 10 d **Maximum children's dose is 400 mg/d**	Administration Issues Complete full course of therapy; shake suspension well before administration; store suspension in the refrigerator; discard unused suspension 14 days after reconstitution; give oral suspension at least 2 h before or 1 h after a meal. Drug-Drug Interactions Cephalosporins may decrease the effectiveness of oral contraceptives; probenecid may increase cephalosporin plasma levels by competitively inhibiting renal excretion of cephalosporins.	ADRs Hypersensitivity reactions, urticarial rash, nausea, vomiting, diarrhea, superinfections.	Contraindications Use with caution in patients with true penicillin allergy; 5–7% cross-sensitivity between penicillins and cephalosporins in allergic patients. Pregnancy Category: B Lactation Issues Excreted in breast milk in small quantities; use with caution in nursing mothers; modification/alteration of bowel flora in infants may cause side effects such as diarrhea.
Ceftriaxone Rocephin Powder for Injection: 250 mg, 500 mg, 1 gm, 2 gm	**Spectrum of activity** Ceftriaxone has activity as a single dose for uncomplicated gonococcal infections, chancroid, PID and as a one-time dose for the treatment of otitis media in children. **Uncomplicated gonococcal infections** Adults and children: 125 mg IM as a single dose plus 1 gram azithromycin in a single oral dose or doxycycline 100 mg q 12 h × 7 days **Children < 8 yr. should not receive doxycycline or any tetracycline antibiotic.** **Gonococcal conjunctivitis** **Adults:** 1 gm IM as a single dose with saline irrigation **Neonates:** 25–50 mg/kg (max = 125 mg) IV/IM as a single dose **Chancroid infection** **Adults: 250 mg IM as a single dose**	Administration Issues IM solutions reconstituted to 250 mg/ml concentration remain stable for 24 h at room temperature and 3 d refrigerated when reconstituted with sterile water for injection, 0.9% NaCl, dextrose 5%, bacteriostatic water, or 1% lidocaine solution without epinephrine. Drug-Drug Interactions Cephalosporins may decrease the effectiveness of **oral contraceptives; probenecid** may increase cephalosporin plasma levels by competitively inhibiting renal excretion of cephalosporins.	Pharmacokinetics Use decreased dose with renal failure. ADRs Hypersensitivity reactions, urticarial rash, nausea, vomiting, diarrhea, superinfections; may cause pain upon injection.	Contraindications Use with caution in patients with true penicillin allergy; 5–7% cross-sensitivity between penicillins and cephalosporins in allergic patients. Pregnancy Category: B Lactation Issues Excreted in breast milk in small quantities; use with caution in nursing mothers; modification/alteration of bowel flora in infants may cause side effects such as diarrhea.

102.3 Cephalosporins: Third Generation *continued from previous page*

Drug and Dosage Forms	Spectrum of Activity and Usual Dosage Range	Administration Issues and Drug-Drug & Drug-Food Interactions	Common Adverse Drug Reactions (ADRs) and Pharmacokinetics	Contraindications, Pregnancy Category, and Lactation Issues
Ceftriaxone *cont.*	**Pelvic inflammatory disease (outpatient treatment)** 250 mg IM as a single dose with doxycycline 100 mg q 12 h × 14 d with or without metronidazole 500 mg orally bid × 14 d **Otitis Media** **Children:** 50 mg/kg (max dose = 1 g) IM one time			

102.4 Fluoroquinolones

Drug and Dosage Forms	Spectrum of Activity and Usual Dosage Range	Administration Issues and Drug–Drug & Drug–Food Interactions	Common Adverse Drug Reactions (ADRs) and Pharmacokinetics	Contraindications, Pregnancy Category, and Lactation Issues
Ciprofloxacin Cipro, Cipro XR, generics Tablet: (Immediate Release) 100 mg, 250 mg, 500 mg, 750 mg Extended-Release Tablet: 500 mg, 1000 mg Suspension: 250 mg/5 mL, 500 mg/5 mL	**Spectrum of activity** Active against Enterobacteriaceae, *Enterobacter* sp., *Morganella morganil, N. gonorrhoeae, P. aeruginosa*, Proteus sp., *Serratia* sp.; also effective against *Mycobacterium avium*; less active against gram-positive organisms. **Mild to moderate urinary tract infections (uncomplicated)** 250 mg q 12 h × 7 to 14 d 500 mg XR × 3 d **Severe urinary tract infections** 500 mg q 12 h × 7 to 14 d 1000 XR q12 × 7 to 14d **Mild to moderate lower respiratory tract infections, bone and joint infections, skin/skin structure infections, infectious diarrhea, and typhoid fever** 500 mg q 12 h × 7 to 14 d	Administration Issues May be taken without regard to meals; do not take with antacids or products containing iron or zinc or take 2 h before or 2 h after taking such products; give with a full glass of water. Swallow XR tablet whole; do not split, crush or chew. IR and XR tablets are not interchangeable Drug–Drug/Drug–Food Interactions Ciprofloxacin may increase blood levels of **theophylline, cyclosporine, caffeine**, and **warfarin. Antacids and products containing calcium, magnesium, aluminum, dairy products, didanosine, iron salts, sucralfate**, and **zinc salts** interfere with the absorption of fluoroquinolones resulting in decreased serum levels. **Cimetidine** may interfere with the elimination of fluoroquinolones.	ADRs Nausea, abdominal discomfort, diarrhea, dizziness, photosensitivity, superinfections. **Use with caution in children < 18 yr. due to potential for cartilage damage and erosion.** Pharmacokinetics Well absorbed from GI tract; consider decreased dosage with renal impairment.	Contraindications Hypersensitivity to fluoroquinolones. Pregnancy Category: C Lactation Issues Excreted in breast milk with amount ingested by infant low.

	Severe lower respiratory tract infections, bone/joint infections, skin/skin structure infections 750 mg q 12 h × 7 to 14 d Bone/joint infections may require treatment for 4 to 6 weeks **Uncomplicated gonococcal infections** 500 mg as a single dose **Inhalation anthrax (post-exposure)** Adult 500 mg q 12 h × 60 d Pediatric 15 mg/kg/dose q 12 h × 60 d (not to exceed 500 mg per dose)			
Enoxacin Penetrex Tablet: 200 mg, 400 mg	**Spectrum of activity** Same as for ciprofloxacin for organisms confined to the urinary tract plus uncomplicated gonorrhea; no activity vs. *M. avium*. **Uncomplicated urinary tract infections** 200 mg q 12 h × 7 d **Complicated urinary tract infections** 400 mg q 12 h × 14 d	Administration Issues Take 1 h before or 2 h after meals; do not take with antacids or products containing iron or zinc; or take 2 h before or 2 h after product; give with a full glass of water. Drug–Drug/Drug–Food Interactions Enoxacin may increase blood levels of **theophylline, cyclosporine, caffeine**, and **warfarin. Antacids and products containing calcium, magnesium, aluminum, dairy products, didanosine, iron salts, sucralfate**, and **zinc salts** interfere with the absorption of fluoroquinolones resulting in decreased serum levels.	ADRs Nausea, abdominal discomfort, diarrhea, dizziness, photosensitivity, superinfections. **Use with caution in children < 18 yr. due to potential for cartilage damage and erosion.** Pharmacokinetics Well absorbed from GI tract; consider decreased dosage with renal impairment.	Contraindications Hypersensitivity to fluoroquinolones. Pregnancy Category: C Lactation Issues Excretion in breast milk is unknown; use with caution, decide whether to discontinue nursing or discontinue the drug.
Gatifloxacin Tequin Tablet: 200 mg, 400 mg	**Spectrum of activity** Active against *S. pneumoniae, S. aureus, H. influenzae, M. catarrhalis, N. gonorrhoeae, E. coli, K. pneumoniae*, or *P. mirabilis, M. pneumoniae, C. pneumoniae, L. pneumophila.*	Administration Issues Complete full course of therapy. Administer without regard to food, including milk and dietary supplements containing calcium. Administer ≥ 4 h before the administration of ferrous sulfate; dietary supplements containing zinc, magnesium, or iron; aluminum/magnesium-containing antacids; or didanosine buffered tablets, buffered solution, or	ADRs Headache, dizziness, nausea, vomiting, diarrhea, vaginitis. Pharmacokinetics $T_{1/2}$ = 7.8 hours Dose adjustment is needed renal impairment.	Contraindications Hypersensitivity to fluoroquinolones; tendinitis or tendon rupture associated with quinolone use. **Gatifloxacin has been shown to prolong the QT interval of the electrocardiogram in some patients. Avoid in patients with known prolongation of the QT interval, patients with uncorrected hypokalemia, and patients receiving**

(continues on next page)

102.4 Fluoroquinolones *continued from previous page*

Drug and Dosage Forms	Spectrum of Activity and Usual Dosage Range	Administration Issues and Drug–Drug & Drug–Food Interactions	Common Adverse Drug Reactions (ADRs) and Pharmacokinetics	Contraindications, Pregnancy Category, and Lactation Issues
Gatifloxacin *cont.*	**Acute exacerbations of chronic bronchitis/acute maxillary sinusitis, community-acquired pneumonia, UTIs, pyelonephtritis** **Acute exacerbations of chronic bronchitis:** 400 mg qd × 5 d **Acute sinusitis:** 400 mg qd × 10 d **Community-acquired pneumonia/complicated UTIs/acute pyelonephritis:** 400 mg qd × 7 to 14 d **Uncomplicated UTIs (cystitis):** 400 mg × 1 dose or 200 mg × 3 d **Uncomplicated urethral gonorrhea in men; enodcervical and rectal gonorrhea in women:** 400 mg × 1 dose	buffered powder for oral suspension, safety and efficacy in children < 18 years of age have not been established. Drug Interactions **The risk of life-threatening cardiac arrhythmias including torsades de pointes may be increased when given with antiarrhythmic agents**. Administer **sucralfate** ≥ 6 h after the quinolone. GI absorption of certain quinolones may be decreased by formation of an cation-quinolone complex. Avoid coadministration of **antacids, ddI and iron-salts**. **Cimetidine** may interfere with the elimination of the quinolones. **Probencid** may diminish urinary excretion of the quinolones.		**class IA (e.g., quinidine, procainamide) or class III (e.g., amiodarone, sotalol) antiarrhythmic agents**. Pregnancy Category: B Lactation Issues Because of the potential for serious adverse reactions in nursing infants, decide whether to discontinue nursing or to discontinue the drug.
Levofloxacin Levaquin Tablet: 250mg, 500mg, 750 mg	**Spectrum of activity** Active against *S. pneumoniae, H. influenzae, M. catarrhalis, S. aureus, K. pneumoniae, C. pneumoniae, L. pneumophila*, and urinary tract infections due to *E. cloacae, E. coli, P. mirabilis*, and *P. aeruginosa*. **Acute exacerbations of chronic bronchitis, community-acquired pneumonia, acute sinusitis** 500 mg q 24 h × 7–14 d **Complicated UTI/acute pyelonephritis** 250 mg q 24 h × 10 d **Complicated skin/skin structure** 750 mg q 24 × 7–14 d	Administration Issues May be taken without regard to meals; do not take with antacids or products containing iron or zinc or take 2 h before or 2 h after taking such products; give with a full glass of water. Drug–Drug/Drug–Food Interactions Levofloxacin may increase blood levels of **theophylline, cyclosporine, caffeine**, and **warfarin. Antacids and products containing calcium, magnesium, aluminum, dairy products, didanosine, iron salts, sucralfate**, and **zinc salts** interfere with the absorption of fluoroquinolones resulting in decreased serum levels. **Cimetidine** may interfere with the elimination of fluoroquinolones.	ADRs Nausea, abdominal discomfort, diarrhea, dizziness, photosensitivity, superinfections. **Use with caution in children < 18 yr. due to potential for cartilage damage and erosion.** Pharmacokinetics Well absorbed from GI tract; decrease dosage with renal impairment.	Contraindications Hypersensitivity to fluoroquinolones. Pregnancy Category: C Lactation Issues Excreted in breast milk with amount ingested by infant low.

Lomefloxacin Maxaquin Tablet: 400 mg	**Spectrum of activity** Active against *H. influenzae, M. catarrhalis*, and urinary tract infections caused by *E. coli, K. pneumoniae, P. aeruginosa*, and *S. saprophyticus*. Lomefloxacin is not indicated for empiric therapy of acute bacterial exacerbations of chronic bronchitis when *S. pneumoniae* may be a causative pathogen. **Uncomplicated urinary tract infections (other than *E. coli*)** 400 mg qd × 10 d **Uncomplicated cystitis in females caused by *E. coli*** 400 mg qd × 3 d **Complicated urinary tract infections** 400 mg qd × 14 d **Lower respiratory tract infections** 400 mg qd × 10 d **Uncomplicated gonococcal infections** 400 mg as a single dose	Administration Issues Do not take with antacids or products containing iron or zinc or take 2 h before or 2 h after taking such products; give with a full glass of water. Drug–Drug/Drug–Food Interactions Lomefloxacin may increase blood levels of **cyclosporine, caffeine**, and **warfarin. Antacids and products containing calcium, magnesium, aluminum, dairy products, didanosine, iron salts, sucralfate**, and **zinc salts** interfere with the absorption of fluoroquinolones resulting in decreased serum levels. **Cimetidine** may interfere with the elimination of fluoroquinolones. Lomefloxacin does **not** appear to alter theophylline or caffeine levels.	ADRs Nausea, abdominal discomfort, diarrhea, dizziness, photosensitivity, (severe) superinfections **Use with caution in children < 18 yr. due to potential for cartilage damage and erosion.** Pharmacokinetics Well absorbed from GI tract; consider decreased dosage with renal impairment.	Contraindications Hypersensitivity to fluoroquinolones. Pregnancy Category: C Lactation Issues Excretion in breast milk is unknown; use with caution, decide whether to discontinue nursing or discontinue the drug.
Moxifloxacin Avelox Tablet: 400 mg	**Spectrum of activity** Active against *S. pneumoniae, S. aureus, S. pyogenes, H. influenzae, M. catarrhalis, N. gonorrhoeae, M. pneumoniae, C. pneumoniae, L. pneumophila, H. parainfluenzae, K. pneumoniae.* **Acute exacerbations of chronic bronchitis/acute maxillary sinusitis, community-acquired pneumonia, uncomplicated skin/skin structure infections** **Acute exacerbations of chronic bronchitis:** 400 mg qd × 5 d **Acute sinusitis:** 400 mg qd × 10 d	Administration Issues Complete full course of therapy. Administer oral doses of moxifloxacin ≥ 4 h before or 8 h after antacids containing magnesium or aluminum, sucralfate, metal cations such as iron, multivitamin preparations with zinc, or didanosine (chewable/buffered tablets or pediatric powder for oral solution). Moxifloxacin may be administered without regard to food, including yogurt. Safety and efficacy in children < 18 years of age have not been established. Drug Interactions **The risk of life-threatening cardiac arrhythmias including torsades de pointes may be increased when given with antiarrhythmic agents**. A	ADRs/Abnormal Lab Values Headache, phototoxicity, dizziness, nausea, vomiting, diarrhea, bilirubin changes, decreases in hemoglobin, hematocrit. Pharmacokinetics $T_{1/2}$ = 12 hours; no dosage adjustment is required in renally impaired patients.	Contraindications Hypersensitivity to fluoroquinolones; tendinitis or tendon rupture associated with quinolone use. Pregnancy Category: B Lactation Issues Because of the potential for serious adverse reactions in nursing infants, decide whether to discontinue nursing or to discontinue the drug.

(*continues on next page*)

102.4 Fluoroquinolones *continued from previous page*

Drug and Dosage Forms	Spectrum of Activity and Usual Dosage Range	Administration Issues and Drug–Drug & Drug–Food Interactions	Common Adverse Drug Reactions (ADRs) and Pharmacokinetics	Contraindications, Pregnancy Category, and Lactation Issues
Moxifloxacin *cont.*	**Community-acquired pneumonia:** 400 mg qd × 7–14 d **Uncomplicated skin/skin structure infection:** 400 mg qd × 7 d	dminister **sucralfate** 6 h after the quinolone. GI absorption of certain quinolones may be decreased by formation of a cation-quinolone complex. Avoid coadministration of **antacids, ddI, and iron-salts**. **Cimetidine** may interfere with elimination, and **probencid** may diminish urinary excretion of quinolones.		
Norfloxacin Noroxin Tablet: 400 mg	**Spectrum of activity** Active against the following organisms found in urinary tract infections: *E. faecalis, E. coli, K. pneumoniae, P. mirabilis, P. aeruginosa, S. epidermidis, S. saprophyticus, E. aerogenes, E. cloacae, S. aureus, S. agalactiae.* Active against *N. gonorrhoeae* and prostatitis due to *E. coli.* **Treatment of uncomplicated urinary tract infections due to *E. coli, Klebsiella pneumonia*, or *Proteus mirabilis*** 400 mg q 12 h × 3 d Use 400 mg q 12 h × 7 to 10 d for UTI caused by other gram-negative organisms. **Uncomplicated gonococcal infections** 800 mg as a single dose **Prostatitis due to *E. coli*** 400 mg q 12 h × 28 d	Administration Issues Take 1 h before or 2 h after meals; do not take with antacids or products containing iron or zinc; give with a full glass of water. Drug–Drug/Drug–Food Interactions Norfloxacin may increase blood levels of **theophylline, cyclosporine, caffeine**, and **warfarin. Antacids and products containing calcium, magnesium, aluminum, dairy products, didanosine, iron salts, sucralfate**, and **zinc salts** interfere with the absorption of fluoroquinolones resulting in decreased serum levels. **Cimetidine** may interfere with the elimination of fluoroquinolones.	ADRs Nausea, abdominal discomfort, diarrhea, dizziness, photosensitivity, superinfections. **Use with caution in children < 18 yr. due to potential for cartilage damage and erosion.** Pharmacokinetics Consider decreased dosage with renal impairment.	Contraindications Hypersensitivity to fluoroquinolones. Pregnancy Category: C Lactation Issues Not detected in breast milk after a 20 mg dose.
Ofloxacin Floxin Tablet: 200 mg, 300 mg, 400 mg	**Spectrum of activity** Active against *H. influenzae, S. pneumoniae, N. gonorrhoeae, C. trachomatis,* and against urinary tract infections due to the following organisms: *E. coli, E. aerogenes, K. pneumoniae, P. mirabilis,*	Administration Issues Do not take with food; do not take with antacids or products containing iron or zinc; give with a full glass of water.	ADRs Nausea, abdominal discomfort, diarrhea, dizziness, photosensitivity, superinfections. **Use with caution in children < 18 yr. due to potential for cartilage damage and erosion.**	Contraindications Hypersensitivity to fluoroquinolones. Pregnancy Category: C

	P. aeruginosa and prostatitis due to *E. coli.* **Uncomplicated urinary tract infections due to *E. coli, Klebsiella pneumonia, Proteus mirabilis*** 200 mg q 12 h × 3 d Use 200 mg q 12 h × 7 d for UTI caused by other gram-negative organisms. **Complicated urinary tract infections** 200 mg q 12 h × 10 d **Prostatitis** 300 mg q 12 h × 6 weeks **Mild to moderate lower respiratory tract infections, bone/joint infections, skin/skin structure infections** 400 mg q 12 h × 10 d **Uncomplicated gonoccocal infectious of cervix, urethra and rectum** 400 mg as a single oral dose	Drug–Drug Interactions Ofloxacin may increase blood levels of **cyclosporine, caffeine**, and **warfarin. Antacids and products containing calcium, magnesium, aluminum, dairy products, didanosine, iron salts, sucralfate**, and **zinc salts** interfere with the absorption of fluoroquinolones, resulting in decreased serum levels. **Cimetidine** may interfere with the elimination of fluoroquinolones. Ofloxacin may not interfere with theophylline levels but data is inconclusive.	Pharmacokinetics Well absorbed from GI tract; consider decreased dosage with renal impairment.	Lactation Issues Breast milk concentrations have been found that are similar to plasma concentrations.
Sparfloxacin Zagam Tablet: 200 mg	**Spectrum of activity** Active against *S. pneumoniae, S. aureus, H. influenzae, M. catarrhalis, S. aureus, K. pneumoniae, C. pneumoniae, M. pneumoniae* **Community-acquired pneumonia** 400 mg day 1, followed by 200 mg qd × 9 d **Acute bacterial exacerbations of chronic bronchitis:** 400 mg day 1, followed by 200 mg qd × 9 d **Avoid exposure to direct or indirect sunlight and UV light during therapy and for 5 days after therapy; discontinue sparfloxacin at first sign or symptom of photoxicity reaction.**	Administration Issues Can be taken without regards to meals; vitamins and minerals containing iron, antacids products and sucralfate should be taken at least 4 h before or 4 h after sparfloxacin; give with a full glass of water; sparfloxacin may cause lightheadedness or dizziness. Drug–Drug Interactions **Antacids and products containing calcium, magnesium, aluminum, dairy products, didanosine, iron salts, sucralfate**, and **zinc salts** interfere with the absorption of fluoroquinolones resulting in decreased serum levels.	ADRs **photosensitivity**, nausea, headache, abdominal discomfort, diarrhea, dizziness, insomnia, superinfections, taste perversion. **Use with caution in children < 18 yr. due to potential for cartilage damage and erosion.** Pharmacokinetics Well absorbed from GI tract; consider decreased dosage with renal impairment.	Contraindications Hypersensitivity to fluoroquinolones; **Patients receiving QTC-prolonging antiarrhythmic drugs reported to cause torsades de pointes, such as class IA or Class III antiarrhythmic agents.** Pregnancy Category: C Lactation Issues Breast milk concentrations have been found that are similar to plasma concentrations.

(continues on next page)

102.4 Fluoroquinolones *continued from previous page*

Drug and Dosage Forms	Spectrum of Activity and Usual Dosage Range	Administration Issues and Drug–Drug & Drug–Food Interactions	Common Adverse Drug Reactions (ADRs) and Pharmacokinetics	Contraindications, Pregnancy Category, and Lactation Issues
Trovafloxacin Trovan Tablet: 100 mg, 200 mg	**Spectrum of activity** Active against *S. pneumoniae, S. aureus, H. influenzae, M. catarrhalis, S. aureus, K. pneumoniae, C. pneumoniae, C. trachomatis, N. gonorrhoeae, L. pneumophila, M. pneumoniae, B. fragilis, Peptostreptococcus species*, viridans group streptococci, *E. faecalis*, and urinary tract infections due to *E. coli.* **Trovafloxacin has been associated with severe liver injury leading to transplantation or death. Reserve trovafloxacin use in patients with serious life- or limb-threatening infections who receive their initial therapy in an in patient healthcare facility. Use exceeding two weeks is associated with increased risk of liver injury. Do not use trovafloxacin when safer alternative antimicrobial therapy will be effective.**	Administration Issues Can be taken without regards to meals; vitamins and minerals containing iron, antacids products and sucralfate should be taken at least 2 h before or 2 h after trovan; give with a full glass of water; trovan may cause lightheadedness or dizziness. Drug–Drug Interactions **Antacids and products containing calcium, magnesium, aluminum, dairy products, didanosine, iron salts, sucralfate**, and **zinc salts** interfere with the absorption of fluoroquinolones resulting in decreased serum levels.	ADRs dizziness, lightheadedness, nausea, abdominal discomfort, diarrhea, photosensitivity, headache, superinfections, liver toxicity. **Use with caution in children < 18 yr. due to potential for cartilage damage and erosion.** Pharmacokinetics Well absorbed from GI tract; no dosage adjustment necessary in patients with renal impairment.	Contraindications Hypersensitivity to fluoroquinolones. Pregnancy Category: C Lactation Issues Breast milk concentrations have been found that are similar to plasma concentrations.

102.5 Macrolides

Drug and Dosage Forms	Spectrum of Activity and Usual Dosage Range	Administration Issues and Drug–Drug & Drug–Food Interactions	Common Adverse Drug Reactions (ADRs) and Pharmacokinetics	Contraindications, Pregnancy Category, and Lactation Issues
Azithromycin Zithromax Capsule: 250 mg, 500 mg, 600 mg Suspension: 100 mg/5 ml, 200 mg/5 ml, 1 g/packet	**Antibacterial spectrum** Gram-positive organisms including *S. aureus, Streptococcus* sp., *Listeria monocytogenes*, and *Corynebacterium* sp.; gram-negative organisms including *M. catarrhalis, N. gonorrhoeae*, and *L. pneumophila*; other organisms such as *C. trachomatis, T. pallidum, M. pneumoniae, U. urealyticum*, and *E. histolytica*. Azithromycin is more active than erythromycin against *H. influenzae, M. catarrhalis*, and *Neisseria* species.	Administration Issues Complete full course of therapy; take at least 1 h before or 2 h after meals; shake suspension well prior to administration; store suspension in the refrigerator and use within 10 d of reconstitution. Drug–Drug Interactions Fever drug interactions compared to clarithromycin and erythromycin due to decreased hepatic metabolism.	ADRs Nausea, abdominal discomfort, diarrhea, superinfection. Pharmacokinetics Decreased absorption with food; distributes well into body tissues; poor penetration into the CNS; $T_{1/2}$ approximately 65 h; biliary excretion primarily as unchanged drug.	Contraindications Hypersensitivity to azithromycin or other macrolide antibiotics. Pregnancy Category: B Lactation Issues Excretion in breast milk is unknown; use with caution in nursing mothers.

	General Indications **Adults:** 500 mg as a single dose on day 1 followed by 250 mg once daily on days 2 through 5. **Children (≥ 6 months):** 10 mg/kg (not to exceed 500 mg/d) as a single dose on day 1 followed by 5 mg/kg (not to exceed 250 mg/d) on days 2 through 5 **Children (acute otitis media):** 30 mg/kg given as a single dose or 10 mg/kg once daily for 3 days or 10 mg/kg as a single close on the first day, followed by 5 mg/kg on days 2 through 5 **Chlamydial infection in adults/adolescents** 1 gm po as a single dose **Prevention of bacterial endocarditis** Adults 500 mg (children 15 mg/kg) orally 1 h before procedure	Concomitant use of **antacids** may decrease peak serum concentration of azithromycin.		
Clarithromycin Biaxin, Biaxin XL Tablet: 250 mg, 500 mg Extended-release tablets: 500 mg (Biaxin XL) Granules for Oral Suspension: 125 mg/5 ml, 250 mg/5 ml	**Spectrum of activity** Similar to azithromycin except clarithromycin has limited activity against *H. influenzae.* **General Indications** **Adults:** 250–500 mg q 12 h × 7–14 days or 2 × 500 mg (1000 mg) of XL Tablets × 7 d (Acute maxillary sinusifis generally treated for 14 d) **Children:** 15 mg/kg/d in divided doses q 12 h × 10 d **Prevention of bacterial endocarditis** Adults 500 mg (children 15 mg/kg) orally 1 h before procedure	Administration Issues Complete full course of therapy; may be taken without regard to meals; shake suspension well prior to administration; store suspension at room temperature and use within 14 d from reconstitution. Drug–Drug Interactions Concomitant use of clarithromycin with the following drugs may result in increased pharmacologic and toxic effects of **astemizole, carbamazepine, cisapride, cyclosporine, digoxin, disopyramide, ergot alkaloids, methylprednisolone, tacrolimus, terfenadine, theophylline, triazolam, warfarin**.	ADRs Naus ea, abdominal discomfort, diarrhea, superinfection, abnormal taste. Pharmacokinetics Distributes into body tissues; hepatic metabolism; renal excretion.	Contraindications Hypersensitivity to clarithromycin or other macrolide antibiotics; patients receiving terfenadine with preexisting cardiac abnormalities. Pregna ncy Category: C Lactation Issues Excretion in breast milk is unknown; use with caution in nursing mothers.

(*continues on next page*)

102.5 Macrolides *continued from previous page*

Drug and Dosage Forms	Spectrum of Activity and Usual Dosage Range	Administration Issues and Drug–Drug & Drug–Food Interactions	Common Adverse Drug Reactions (ADRs) and Pharmacokinetics	Contraindications, Pregnancy Category, and Lactation Issues
Clarithromycin *cont.*	**Treatment of Mycobacterium avium complex** 500 mg q 12 h × 26 weeks in combination with other antimycobacterial drugs **See Gastrointestinal chapter for use of clarithromycin in the treatment of *H. Pylori.***			
Dirithromycin Dynabec Tablet, enteric coated: 250 mg (delayed-release)	**Antibacterial spectrum** Gram-positive organisms including *S. aureus, Streptococcus* sp., and *Listeria monocytogenes*; gram-negative organisms including *M. catarrhalis* and *L. pneumophila*; other organisms such as *M. pneumoniae.* **General indications** **Adults and children ≥ 12 yr:** 500 mg once daily × 7 to 14 d	Administration Issues Complete full course of therapy; take with food or within 1 h of having eaten to decrease abdominal discomfort; do not cut, crush, or chew tablets. Drug–Drug Interactions The following interactions do not appear to occur or occur rarely, **however**, patients should be monitored appropriately. Dirithromycin may inhibit the metabolism of **terfenadine** and **astemizole** leading to serious cardiac dysrhythmias. Dirithromycin may inhibit the metabolism of **theophylline** leading to toxic adverse effects.	ADRs Nausea, abdominal discomfort, diarrhea, superinfection. Pharmacokinetics Achieves high tissue/plasma ratios; primarily excreted in the bile/feces with little hepatic metabolism.	Contraindications Hypersensitivity to dirithromycin or other macrolide antibiotics. Pregnancy Category: C Lactation Issues Excretion in breast milk is unknown; use with caution in nursing mothers.
Erythromycin Base E-mycin, generics Tablet, enteric coated: 250 mg, 333 mg, 500 mg Tablet, coated particles: PCE Dispertab: 333 mg, 500 mg Tablet, delayed release: generics 333 mg Tablet, film coated: Erythromycin Filmtabs 250 mg, 500 mg Capsule, delayed release, enteric coated: 250 mg	**Spectrum of activity** Similar to azithromycin except erythromycin has limited activity against *H. influenzae.* **General indications** **Adults:** 250–500 mg q 6 h × 10 days *or* 333 mg q 8 h × 10 d **Children:** 30–50 mg/kg/d in divided doses q 6–12 h × 10 d **Prophylaxis of rheumatic heart disease** 250 mg twice daily **Alternative drug in penicillin and tetracycline hypersensitivity for primary syphilis** 500 mg q 6 h × 14 d	Administration Issues Complete full course of therapy; take on empty stomach, however, may be taken with food if GI upset occurs; swallow tablets and capsules whole, do not crush tablets or enteric-coated pellets. Drug–Drug Interactions Concomitant use of erythromycin with the following drugs may result in increased pharmacologic and toxic effects of **astemizole, carbamazepine, cisapride, cyclosporine, digoxin, disopyramide, ergot alkaloids, methylprednisolone, tacrolimus, terfenadine, theophylline, triazolam, warfarin**.	ADRs Nausea, abdominal discomfort, diarrhea, superinfection. Pharmacokinetics Diffuses into body fluids including prostatic fluid, low concentrations found in cerebrospinal fluid; hepatic metabolism; biliary excretion.	Contraindications Hypersensitivity to erythromycin; preexisting liver disease. Pregnancy Category: B Lactation Issues Excreted in breast milk; erythromycin use is considered compatible with breast-feeding by the American Academy of Pediatrics.

	<u>Chlamydial infection</u> **Adults**: 500 mg qid for 7 d *or* 250 mg qid for 14 d *or* 666 mg q 8 h × 7 d *or* 333 mg q 8 h 14 d **Children:** 50 mg/kg/d in divided doses q 6–12h for 14 days (conjunctivitis) or 21 d (pneumonia) **<u>Legionnaire's disease</u>** 1–4 gm in divided doses q 6 h × 21 days alone or combined with rifampin			
Erythromycin Estolate <u>Ilosone, generics</u> <u>Tablet:</u> 250 mg, 500 mg <u>Capsule:</u> 250 mg <u>Suspension:</u> 125 mg/5 ml 250 mg/5 ml	**<u>Spectrum of Activity</u>** See erythromycin. **<u>General indications</u>** **Adults:** 250–500 mg q 6 h × 10 d **Children:** 30–50 mg/kg/d in divided doses q 6 h × 10 d **<u>Prophylaxis of rheumatic heart disease</u>** 250 mg twice daily **<u>Chlamydial infection</u>** **Adults:** 500 mg q 6 h × 7 d **or** 250 mg q 6 h × 14 d **Children:** 50 mg/kg/d divided q 6 h × 14 d (conjunctivitis) or 21 d (pneumonia) **<u>Legionnaire's disease</u>** 1–4 gm in divided doses q 6 h × 21 d alone or in combination with rifampin	<u>Administration Issues</u> Complete full course of therapy; take on empty stomach, however, may be taken with food if GI upset occurs; shake suspension well prior to administration; store suspension in the refrigerator. <u>Drug–Drug Interactions</u> Concomitant use of erythromycin with the following drugs may result in increased pharmacologic and toxic effects of **astemizole, carbamazepine, cisapride, cyclosporine, digoxin, disopyramide, ergot alkaloids, methylprednisolone, tacrolimus, terfenadine, theophylline, triazolam, warfarin**.	<u>ADRs</u> Nausea, abdominal discomfort, diarrhea, superinfection, abnormal taste. Do not use erythromycin estolate in pregnant patients. <u>Pharmacokinetics</u> Diffuses into body fluids including prostatic fluid, low concentrations found in cerebrospinal fluid; hepatic metabolism; biliary excretion.	<u>Contraindications</u> Hypersensitivity to erythromycin; preexisting liver disease. <u>Pregnancy Category: B</u> <u>Lactation Issues</u> Excreted in breast milk; erythromycin use is considered compatible with breast-feeding by the American Academy of Pediatrics.

(*continues on next page*)

102.5 Macrolides *continued from previous page*

Drug and Dosage Forms	Spectrum of Activity and Usual Dosage Range	Administration Issues and Drug–Drug & Drug–Food Interactions	Common Adverse Drug Reactions (ADRs) and Pharmacokinetics	Contraindications, Pregnancy Category, and Lactation Issues
Erythromycin Stearate Erythrocin Stearate, Wyamycin S, various generics Tablet, film coated: 250 mg, 500 mg	**Spectrum of Activity** see erythromycin base **General indications** **Adults:** 250–500 mg q 6 h × 10 d **Children:** 30–50 mg/kg/ divided q 6 h × 10 d **Prophylaxis of rheumatic heart disease** 250 mg twice daily **Chlamydial infection** **Adults:** 500 mg q 6 h × 7 d *or* 250 mg q 6 h × 14 d **Children:** 50 mg/kg/d divided q 6 h × 14 d (conjunctivitis) or 21 d (pneumonia) **Legionnaire's disease** 1–4 gm in divided doses q 6 h × 21 days alone or in combination with rifampin	Administration Issues Complete full course of therapy; take on empty stomach, however, may be taken with food if GI upset occurs. Drug–Drug Interactions Concomitant use of erythromycin with the following drugs may result in increased pharmacologic and toxic effects of **astemizole, carbamazepine, cisapride, cyclosporine, digoxin, disopyramide, ergot alkaloids, methylprednisolone, tacrolimus, terfenadine, theophylline, triazolam, warfarin**.	ADRs Nausea, abdominal discomfort, diarrhea, superinfection, abnormal taste. Pharmacokinetics Diffuses into body fluids including prostatic fluid, low concentrations found in cerebrospinal fluid; hepatic metabolism; biliary excretion.	Contraindications Hypersensitivity to erythromycin. Pregnancy Category: B Lactation Issues Excreted in breast milk; erythromycin use is considered compatible with breast-feeding by the American Academy of Pediatrics.
Erythromycin Ethylsuccinate generics Tablet, chewable: 200 mg Tablet: 400 mg Suspension: 100 mg/2.5 ml, 200 mg/5 ml, 400 mg/5 ml	**Spectrum of Activity** See erythromycin base. **General indications** **Adults:** 400 mg q 6 h × 10 d **Children:** 30–50 mg/kg/d divided q 6 h × 10 d **Prophylaxis of rheumatic heart disease** 400 mg twice daily	Administration Issues Complete full course of therapy; take on empty stomach, however, may be taken with food if GI upset occurs; shake suspension well prior to administration; store suspension in the refrigerator. Drug–Drug Interactions Concomitant use of erythromycin with the following drugs may result in increased pharmacologic and toxic effects of **astemizole, carbamazepine, cisapride, cyclosporine, digoxin, disopyramide, ergot alkaloids,**	ADRs Nausea, abdominal discomfort, diarrhea, superinfection, abnormal taste. Pharmacokinetics Diffuses into body fluids including prostatic fluid, low concentrations found in cerebrospinal fluid; hepatic metabolism; biliary excretion.	Contraindications Hypersensitivity to erythromycin; preexisting liver disease. Pregnancy Category: B Lactation Issues Excreted in breast milk; erythromycin use is considered compatible with breast-feeding by the American Academy of Pediatrics.

	Chlamydial infection **Adults:** 800 mg q 6 h × 7 d *or* 400 mg q 6 h × 14 d **Children:** 50 mg/kg/d divided q 6 h × 14 d (conjunctivitis) or 21 d (pneumonia) **Legionnaire's disease** 1.6–4 gm in divided doses q 6 h × 21 d alone or in combination with rifampin	**methylprednisolone, tacrolimus, terfenadine, theophylline, triazolam, warfarin**.		
Troleandomycin Tao Capsule: 250 mg	**Spectrum of activity** *Streptococcus pyogenes* and *Streptococcus pneumoniae* **Streptococcal infections** **Adults:** 250–500 mg q 6 h × 10 d **Children:** 125–250 mg q 6 h × 10 d	Administration Issues Complete full course of therapy; take on empty stomach. Drug–Drug Interactions Troleandomycin may increase the effects of the following drugs by inhibiting their metabolism: **carbamazepine, ergot alkaloids, methylprednisolone, theophylline, triazolam**. Hepatotoxicity may occur with concomitant use of troleandomycin and **oral contraceptives**.	ADRs Nausea, abdominal discomfort, diarrhea, superinfection. Pharmacokinetics Acetylated ester of oleandomycin; biliary and renal excretion.	Contraindications Hypersensitivity to troleandomycin. Safety for use during pregnancy has not been established.

102.6 Penicillins

Drug and Dosage Forms	Spectrum of Activity and Usual Dosage Range	Administration Issues and Drug–Drug & Drug–Food Interactions	Common Adverse Drug Reactions (ADRs) and Pharmacokinetics	Contraindications, Pregnancy Category, and Lactation Issues
Penicillin G Potassium Pentids, generics Tablet: 200,000 units, 250,000 units, 400,000 units, 500,000 units, 800,000 units Powder for Oral Solution: 400,000 units/5 ml	**Antibacterial spectrum** Gram-positive staphylococcal and streptococcal organisms; inactive alone against serious *Streptococcus* group D (enterococcus). **General indications Adults:** 200,000–500,000 units q 6 to 8 h × 10 d **Children < 12 yr.:** 25,000–90,000 units/kg/d in 3 to 6 divided doses × 10 d	Administration Issues Give 1 h before or 2 h after meals; complete full course of therapy; store reconstituted liquid in the refrigerator, discard unused portion after 14 d. Drug–Drug Interactions Penicillins may decrease the effectiveness of **oral contraceptives;** the bacteriostatic action of **tetracyclines** may interfere with the bactericidal effects of penicillins.	ADRs: Hypersensitivity reactions, urticarial rash, nausea, diarrhea, superinfections. Pharmacokinetics: $T_{1/2}$ 30 min; 35% protein binding; renal excretion mostly unchanged.	Contraindications True penicillin allergy. Pregnancy Category: B Lactation Issues Penicillins are excreted in breast milk in low concentrations; nursing infants may develop diarrhea, candidiasis, or an allergic reaction.

(*continues on next page*)

102.6 Penicillins *continued from previous page*

Drug and Dosage Forms	Spectrum of Activity and Usual Dosage Range	Administration Issues and Drug–Drug & Drug–Food Interactions	Common Adverse Drug Reactions (ADRs) and Pharmacokinetics	Contraindications, Pregnancy Category, and Lactation Issues
Penicillin G Procaine Injection: 600,000 units/ml, 1,200,000 units/2 ml, 2,400,000 units/4 ml	**Antibacterial spectrum** Gram-positive staphylococcal and streptococcal organisms, *treponema pallidum* associated with syphilis. **Streptococcal and staphylococcal infections** **Adults and children:** 600,000–1,200,000 units daily IM × 10 to 14 d	Administration Issues Give by deep IM injection into the upper, outer quadrant of the buttocks, for infants and children the midlateral aspect of the thigh may be preferable; rotate injection site for repeated doses. Drug–Drug Interactions Penicillins may decrease the effectiveness of **oral contraceptives;** the bacteriostatic action of **tetracyclines** may interfere with the bactericidal effects of penicillins.	ADRs: Hypersensitivity reactions, urticarial rash, nausea, diarrhea, superinfections. Pharmacokinetics: IM: provides more prolonged but lower penicillin G concentrations than equivalent IM penicillin G potassium; peak serum concentrations in 1–4 h and detectable for 1–2 d; renal excretion mostly unchanged.	Contraindications True penicillin allergy. Pregnancy Category: B Lactation Issues Penicillins are excreted in breast milk in low concentrations; nursing infants may develop diarrhea, candidiasis, or an allergic reaction.
Penicillin G Benzathine Bicillin L-A, generic Injection: 300,000 units/ml, 600,000 units/ml, 1,200,000 units/2 ml, 2,400,000 units/4 ml	**Antibacterial spectrum** Gram-positive staphylococcal and streptococcal organisms; *treponema pallidum* associated with syphilis. **Streptococcal (Group A) Upper Respiratory tract infections** **Adults:** 1.2 million units IM as single injection **Older children:** 900,000 units IM as single injection (> 60 lbs) **Early syphilis-primary, secondary, or latent of < 1 year's duration** **Adults:** 2,400,000 units IM for one dose **Children and neonates:** 50,000 units/kg (up to 2.4 million units) IM for one dose **Syphilis of > 1 year's duration, latent syphilis or cardiovascular syphilis** **Adults:** 2.4 million units IM once weekly for 3 successive wk. **Children and neonates:** 50,000 units/kg (up to 2.4 million units) IM weekly for 3 successive wk.	Administration Issues Give by deep IM injection into the upper, outer quadrant of the buttocks, for infants and children the midlateral aspect of the thigh may be preferable; rotate injection site for repeated doses. Drug–Drug Interactions Penicillins may decrease the effectiveness of **oral contraceptives;** the bacteriostatic action of **tetracyclines** may interfere with the bactericidal effects of penicillins.	ADRs: Hypersensitivity reactions, urticarial rash, nausea, diarrhea, superinfections. Pharmacokinetics: IM; provides more prolonged but lower penicillin G concentrations than equivalent IM procaine penicillin G or penicillin G potassium; peak serum concentrations in 13–24 h and detectable for 1–4 weeks; renal excretion mostly unchanged.	Contraindications True penicillin allergy. Pregnancy Category: B Lactation Issues Penicillins are excreted in breast milk in low concentrations; nursing infants may develop diarrhea, candidiasis, or an allergic reaction.

Penicillin G Benzathine and Procaine Bicillin C-R, generic Injection: 150,000 units/ml penicillin G benzathine and 150,000 units/ml penicillin G procaine 300,000 units/ml penicillin G benzathine and 300,000 units/ml penicillin G procaine 600,000 units/ml penicillin G benzathine and 600,000 units/ml penicillin G procaine 1,200,000 units/ml penicillin G benzathine and 1,200,000 units/ml penicillin G procaine 900,000 units penicillin G benzathine and 300,000 units penicillin G procaine	**Antibacterial spectrum** Gram-positive streptococcal organisms; *treponema pallidum* associated with syphilis **Moderately severe to severe streptococcal infections (Streptococci A, C, G, H, L, and M) of the upper respiratory tract, skin, and soft tissue** **Adult and children > 60 lbs. or 27 kg:** 2.4 million units IM as a single dose **Children 30–60 lbs. or 14 to 27 kg:** 900,000–1,200,000 units IM as a single dose **Infants and children < 30 lbs. or 14 kg:** 600,000 units IM **Streptococcus pneumoniae infections (except meningitis)** **Adults:** 1.2 million units IM as a single dose **Children:** 600,000 units IM as a single dose; repeat q 2 to 3 d until patient has been afebrile for 48 h **Congenital syphilis** **Newborns:** 50,000 U/kg IM qd × 10 d	Administration Issues Give by deep IM injection into the upper, outer quadrant of the buttocks, for infants and children the midlateral aspect of the thigh may be preferable; rotate injection site for repeated doses. Drug–Drug interactions Penicillins may decrease the effectiveness of **oral contraceptives;** the bacteriostatic action of **tetracyclines** may interfere with the bactericidal effects of penicillins.	ADRs: Hypersensitivity reactions, urticarial rash, nausea, diarrhea, superinfections. Pharmacokinetics: Renal excretion mostly unchanged.	Contraindications True penicillin allergy; hypersensitivity to procaine. Pregnancy Category: B Lactation Issues Penicillins are excreted in breast milk in low concentrations; nursing infants may develop diarrhea, candidiasis, or an allergic reaction.
Penicillin V Potassium Veetids, generics Tablets: 250 mg, 500 mg Powder for Oral Solution: 125 mg/5 ml, 250 mg/5 ml	**Antibacterial spectrum** Gram-positive organisms including non-penicillinase-producing *S. aureus, S. epidermidis, Streptococcus* sp. Coverage also includes gram-positive anaerobes such as *Clostridium* sp. and *Peptostreptococcus* sp.; inactive against gram-negative organisms	Administration Issues May be given without regard to meals; complete full course of therapy; store reconstituted liquid in the refrigerator, discard unused portion after 14 d.	ADRs: Hypersensitivity reactions, urticarial rash, nausea, diarrhea, superinfections. Pharmacokinetics: $T_{1/2}$ 60 min; 85% protein binding; renal excretion mostly unchanged.	Contraindications True penicillin allergy. Pregnancy Category: B Lactation Issues Penicillins are excreted in breast milk in low concentrations; nursing infants may

(*continues on next page*)

102.6 Penicillins *continued from previous page*

Drug and Dosage Forms	Spectrum of Activity and Usual Dosage Range	Administration Issues and Drug–Drug & Drug–Food Interactions	Common Adverse Drug Reactions (ADRs) and Pharmacokinetics	Contraindications, Pregnancy Category, and Lactation Issues
Penicillin V Potassium *cont.*	**General indications** **Adults:** 250–500 mg q 6 to 8 h × 10 d **Children:** 25–50 mg/kg/d in divided doses q 6 to 8 h × 10 d	Drug–Drug Interactions Penicillins may decrease the effectiveness of **oral contraceptives;** the bacteriostatic action of **tetracyclines** may interfere with the bactericidal effects of penicillins.		develop diarrhea, candidiasis, or an allergic reaction.

102.7 Aminopenicillins

Drug and Dosage Forms	Spectrum of Activity and Usual Dosage Range	Administration Issues and Drug–Drug & Drug–Food Interactions	Common Adverse Drug Reactions (ADRs) and Pharmacokinetics	Contraindications, Pregnancy Category, and Lactation Issues
Amoxicillin Amoxil, generics Tablet: 500 mg, 875 mg Tablet, chewable: 125 mg, 200 mg, 250 mg, 400 mg Capsule: 250 mg, 500 mg Powder for Oral Suspension: Pediatric drops: 50 mg/ml 125 mg/5 ml 200 mg/5 ml 250 mg/5 ml 400 mg/5 ml	**Antibacterial spectrum** Gram-positive coverage is the same as penicillin G; gram-negative includes *E. Coli, P. mirabilis, N. gonorrhoeae, and H. influenzae* (beta-lactamase negative) **General indications (ears, nose, throat, skin/skin structure GU tract)** ***Mild to moderate infections*** **Adults and children ≥ 40 kg:** 500 mg q 12h or 250 mg q 8h **Children > 3 mos and < 40 kg:** 25 mg/kg/day divided q 12h or 20 mg/kg/day divided q 8h ***Severe infections*** **Adults and children ≥ 40 kg:** 875 q 12h or 500 q 8h **Children > 3 mos and < 40 kg:** 45 mg/kg/day divided q 12h or 40 mg/kg/day divided q 8h **Lower respiratory tract** **Adults and children ≥ 40 kg:** 875 q 12h or 500 q 8h	Administration Issues May be given without regards to meals; complete full course of therapy; discard any liquid form after 10 d if at room temperature and after 14 d if refrigerated. Drug–Drug Interactions Penicillins may decrease the effectiveness of **oral contraceptives**; the bacteriostatic action of **tetracyclines** may interfere with the bactericidal effects of penicillins.	ADRs Hypersensitivity reactions, urticarial rash, nausea, diarrhea, superinfections. Pharmacokinetics $T_{1/2}$60min; 20% protein binding; renal excretion mostly unchanged.	Contraindications True penicillin allergy. Pregnancy Category: B Lactation Issues Penicillins are excreted in breast milk in low concentrations; nursing infants may develop diarrhea, candidiasis, or an allergic reaction.

	Children > 3 mos and < 40 kg: 45 mg/kg/day divided q 12h or 40 mg/kg/day divided q 8h **Gonorrhea** **Adults:** 3 g as single oral dose			
Amoxicillin and Potassium Clavulanate Augmentin, generics Tablet, chewable: 125 mg amoxicillin/31.25 mg clavulanic acid 200 mg amoxicillin/28.55 mg clavulanic acid 250 mg amoxicillin/62.5 mg clavulanic acid 400 mg amoxicillin/57 mg clavulanic acid Tablet: 250 mg amoxicillin/125 mg clavulanic acid 500 mg amoxicillin/125 mg clavulanic acid 875 mg amoxicillin/125 mg clavulanic acid Powder for Oral Suspension: 125 mg amoxicillin/31.25 mg clavulanic acid per 5 ml 200 mg amoxicillin/28.55 mg clavulanic acid per 5 ml 250 mg amoxicillin/62.5 mg clavulanic acid per 5 ml 400 mg amoxicillin/57 mg clavulanic acid per 5 ml, (Augmentin ES-600) 600 mg amoxicillin 42.9 mg clavulanate per 5 ml	**Antibacterial spectrum** Similar to amoxicillin, but addition of clavulanate confers penicillinase resistance, thereby extending the spectrum to include *Klebsiella sp.*, beta lactamase producing strains of *H. influenzae, E. coli,* and methicillin-sensitive *S. aureus* Dosage is given as amoxicillin equivalent. Both the 250 mg and 500 mg tablets contain the same amount of clavulanic acid, so two 250 mg tablets **are not** equivalent to one 500 mg tablet In addition, the 250 mg tablet and the 250 mg chewable tablet do NOT contain the same amount of clavulanic acid and should not be substituted for each other, as they are not interchangeable. **Adults** 250–500 mg q 8 h *or* 875 mg q 12 h for 10 d **Otitis media, sinusitis, lower respiratory tract infections (children > 3 months old)** 45 mg/kg/d divided bid (use 200 mg/5ml or 400 mg/5ml suspension) or 40 mg/kg/d divided tid (use 125 mg/5 ml or 250 mg/5 ml suspension) **Less severe infections (children > 3 months old)** 25 mg/kg/d divided bid (use 200 mg/5ml or 400 mg/5 ml suspension)	Administration Issues Give with food to decrease nausea and diarrhea; complete full course of therapy; store reconstituted liquid in the refrigerator, discard unused portion after 10 d. Drug–Drug Interactions Penicillins may decrease the effectiveness of **oral contraceptives**; the bacteriostatic action of **tetracyclines** may interfere with the bactericidal effects of penicillins.	ADRs: Hypersensitivity reactions, urticarial rash, nausea, diarrhea, superinfections. Pharmacokinetics: $T_{1/2}$60min; 20% protein binding; renal excretion mostly unchanged.	Contraindications True penicillin allergy. Pregnancy Category: B Lactation Issues Penicillins are excreted in breast milk in low concentrations; nursing infants may develop diarrhea, candidiasis, or an allergic reaction.

(*continues on next page*)

102.7 Aminopenicillins *continued from previous page*

Drug and Dosage Forms	Spectrum of Activity and Usual Dosage Range	Administration Issues and Drug–Drug & Drug–Food Interactions	Common Adverse Drug Reactions (ADRs) and Pharmacokinetics	Contraindications, Pregnancy Category, and Lactation Issues
Amoxicillin and Potassium Clavulanate *cont.*	or 20 mg/kg/d divided tid (use 125 mg/5 ml or 250 mg/5 ml suspension)			
Ampicillin Various generics Capsule: 250 mg, 500 mg Powder for Oral Suspension: 125 mg/5 ml, 250 mg/5 ml	**Antibacterial spectrum** Gram-positive coverage is the same as penicillin G; gram-negative includes *E. Coli, P. mirabilis, N. gonorrhoeae, Shigella sp., H. influenzae.* **General indications** **Adults and children ≥ 20 kg:** 250–500 mg q 6 h × 10 to 14 **Children:** 50 mg/kg/d divided q 6 to 8 h × 10 to 14 d	Administration Issues For optimal absorption, give on empty stomach; complete full course of therapy; store reconstituted liquid in the refrigerator, discard unused portion after 14 d. Drug–Drug Interactions Penicillins may decrease the effectiveness of **oral contraceptives**; the bacteriostatic action of **tetracyclines** may interfere with the bactericidal effects of penicillins; concomitant use of **allopurinol** may increase the risk of an ampicillin-induced rash.	ADRs Hypersensitivity reactions, urticarial rash, nausea, diarrhea, superinfections. Pharmacokinetics: 40% absorbed in GI tract; $T_{1/2}$60min; 20% protein binding; renal excretion mostly unchanged.	Contraindications True penicillin allergy. Pregnancy Category: B Lactation Issues Penicillins are excreted in breast milk in low concentrations; nursing infants may develop diarrhea, candidiasis, or an allergic reaction.
Carbenicillin Indanyl Sodium Geocillin Tablet: 382 mg	**Antibacterial spectrum** *E. coli, P. mirabilis, Morganella morganii, Providencia rettgeri, Pseudomonas, Enterobacter*, and enterococcus. **Urinary tract infection** *E. coli, Proteus mirabilis, and Enterobacter* sp: 382–764 mg qid ×10 d *Pseudomonas* and enterococci: 764 mg qid × 10 d	Administration Issues For optimal absorption, give on empty stomach; complete full course of therapy. Drug–Drug Interactions Penicillins may decrease the effectiveness of **oral contraceptives**; the bacteriostatic action of **tetracyclines** may interfere with the bactericidal effects of penicillins.	ADRs: Hypersensitivity reactions, urticarial rash, nausea, diarrhea, superinfections. Pharmacokinetics $T_{1/2}$ = 60min; 50% protein binding; renal excretion mostly as unchanged drug.	Contraindications True penicillin allergy. Pregnancy Category: B Lactation Issues Penicillins are excreted in breast milk in low concentrations; nursing infants may develop diarrhea, candidiasis, or an allergic reaction.

102.8 Penicillinase-Resistant Penicillins

Drug and Dosage Forms	Spectrum of Activity and Usual Dosage Range	Administration Issues and Drug–Drug & Drug–Food Interactions	Common Adverse Drug Reactions (ADRs) and Pharmacokinetics	Contraindications, Pregnancy Category, and Lactation Issues
Cloxacillin Sodium Capsule: Cloxapen, Tegopen, generics: 250 mg, 500 mg Powder for Oral Solution: Tegopen, generics: 125 mg/5 ml	**Antibacterial spectrum** Penicillinase-producing *Staphylococcus* sp.; less effective than penicillin G against non-penicillinase-producing staphylococci and other gram positive organisms; inactive against gram-negative organisms. **Mild to moderate upper respiratory and localized skin and soft tissue infections** **Adults and children > 20 kg:** 250 mg q 6 h × 10 to 14 d **Children (< 20 kg):** 50 mg/kg/d divided q 6 h × 10 to 14 d **Severe infections (lower respiratory tract or disseminated infections)** **Adults and children > 20 kg:** 500 mg–1 gm q 6 h × 10 to 14 d **Children (< 20 kg):** 50–100 mg/kg/d divided q 6 h × 10 to 14 d	Administration Issues For optimal absorption, give on empty stomach; complete full course of therapy; store reconstituted liquid in the refrigerator, discard unused portion after 14 d. Drug–Drug Interactions Penicillins may decrease the effectiveness of **oral contraceptives;** the bacteriostatic action of **tetracyclines** may interfere with the bactericidal effects of penicillins.	ADRs Hypersensitivity reactions. Urticarial rash, nausea, diarrhea, superinfections. Pharmacokinetics $T_{1/2}$ 30–60 min; 95% protein binding; renal excretion mostly unchanged.	Contraindications True penicillin allergy. Pregnancy Category: B Lactation Issues Penicillins are excreted in breast milk in low concentrations; nursing infants may develop diarrhea, candidiasis, or an allergic reaction.
Dicloxacillin Sodium generics Capsules: Dynapen 125 mg, 250 mg, 500 mg Powder for Oral Suspension: 62.5 mg/5 ml	**Antibacterial spectrum** Penicillinase-producing *Staphylococcus* sp.; less effective than penicillin G against non-penicillinase-producing staphylococci and other gram-positive organisms; inactive against gram-negative organisms **Mild to moderate upper respiratory and localized skin and soft tissue infections** **Adults and children > 40 kg:** 125–250 mg q 6 h × 10 to 14 d **Children:** 12.5–25 mg/kg/d divided q 6 h × 10 to 14 d	Administration Issues For optimal absorption, give on empty stomach; complete full course of therapy; store reconstituted liquid in the refrigerator, discard unused portion after 14 d. Drug–Drug Interactions Penicillins may decrease the effectiveness of **oral contraceptives;** the bacteriostatic action of **tetracyclines** may interfere with the bactericidal effects of penicillins.	ADRs Hypersensitivity reactions, Urticarial rash, nausea, diarrhea, superinfections. Pharmacokinetics $T_{1/2}$ 30–60 min; 95% protein binding; renal excretion mostly unchanged.	Contraindications True penicillin allergy. Pregnancy Category: B Lactation Issues Penicillins are excreted in breast milk in low concentrations; nursing infants may develop diarrhea, candidiasis, or an allergic reaction.

(*continues on next page*)

102.8 Penicillinase-Resistant Penicillins *continued from previous page*

Drug and Dosage Forms	Spectrum of Activity and Usual Dosage Range	Administration Issues and Drug–Drug & Drug–Food Interactions	Common Adverse Drug Reactions (ADRs) and Pharmacokinetics	Contraindications, Pregnancy Category, and Lactation Issues
Dicloxacillin Sodium *cont.*	**Severe infections (lower respiratory tract or disseminated infections)** **Adults and children > 40 kg:** 250 mg q 6 h for 10 to 14 d **Children:** 25 mg/kg/d divided q 6 h × 10 to 14 d **Use in newborns is not recommended**.			
Oxacillin Sodium generics Capsule: 250 mg, 500 mg Powder for Oral Solution: 250 mg/5 ml	**Antibacterial spectrum** Penicillinase-producing *Staphylococcus* sp.; less effective than penicillin G against non-penicillinase-producing staphylococci and other gram-positive organisms; inactive against gram negative organisms. **Bacterial Infectious** **Adults and children > 40 kg:** 500 mg–1 gm q 4 to 6 h for a minimum of 7 d depending on severity of infection **Children:** 50–100 mg/kg/d divided q 6 h for a minimum of 7 d depending on severity of infection	Administration Issues For optimal absorption, give on empty stomach; complete full course of therapy; store reconstituted liquid in the refrigerator, discard unused portion after 14 d. Drug–Drug Interactions Penicillins may decrease the effectiveness of **oral contraceptives;** the bacteriostatic action of **tetracyclines** may interfere with the bactericidal effects of penicillins.	ADRs: Hypersensitivity reactions, Urticarial rash, nausea, diarrhea, superinfections. Pharmacokinetics: $T_{1/2}$ 30–60 min; 95% protein binding; renal excretion mostly unchanged.	Contraindications True penicillin allergy. Pregnancy Category: B Lactation Issues Penicillins are excreted in breast milk in low concentrations; nursing infants may develop diarrhea, candidiasis, or an allergic reaction.

102.9 Sulfonamides

Drug and Dosage Forms	Spectrum of Activity and Usual Dosage Range	Administration Issues and Drug–Drug & Drug–Food Interactions	Common Adverse Drug Reactions (ADRs) and Pharmacokinetics	Contraindications, Pregnancy Category, and Lactation Issues
Sulfadiazine Various generics Tablet: 500 mg	**Antibacterial spectrum** Gram-negative organisms (*E. coli, Klebsiella sp., Enterobacter sp., P. mirabilis, P. vulgaris*) and *S. aureus* in the urine; *Nocardia sp., C. trachomatis; H. ducreyi.*	Administration Issues Complete full course of therapy; take on an empty stomach with a full glass of water; avoid prolonged exposure to sunlight, wear protective clothing, and apply sunscreen.	ADRs Nausea, abdominal discomfort, headache, photosensitivity. Pharmacokinetics Good GI absorption; readily penetrates into CSF; hepatic metabolism; renal excretion.	Contraindications Hypersensitivity to sulfonamides or chemically related drugs such as sulfonylureas, thiazide diuretics, and sunscreens containing PABA.

	General indications **Adults:** 2–4 gm loading dose, followed by 2 to 4 gm/day in 3 to 6 divided doses × 7 to 14 d	Drug–Drug Interactions Sulfonamides may increase the pharmacological and toxic effects of the following drugs: **methotrexate, phenytoin, sulfonylureas, warfarin, probenecid.**		Pregnancy Safety for use during pregnancy has not been established; sulfonamides do cross the placenta achieving fetal levels approximately 70%–90% of maternal serum levels; do not use during pregnancy at term. Lactation Issues Sulfonamides are excreted in breast milk; according to the American Academy of Pediatrics, breastfeeding and sulfonamides are compatible; avoid sulfonamides and nursing in premature infants, infants with hyperbilirubinemia, and infants with G-6-PD deficiency.
Sulfamethoxazole generics Tablet: 500 mg	**Antibacterial spectrum** Gram-negative organisms (*E. coli, Klebsiella sp., Enterobacter sp., P. mirabilis, P. vulgaris*) and *S. aureus* in the urine; *Nocardia sp., C. trachomatis; H. ducreyi.* **General indications** **Adults:** 2 gm initially, followed by 1 gm 2 to 3 times daily for 7 to 14 days	Administration Issues Complete full course of therapy; take on an empty stomach with a full glass of water; avoid prolonged exposure to sunlight, wear protective clothing, and apply sunscreen; shake suspension well prior to administration. Drug–Drug Interactions Sulfonamides may increase the pharmacological and toxic effects of the following drugs: **methotrexate, phenytoin, sulfonylureas, warfarin.**	ADRs Nausea, abdominal discomfort, headache, photosensitivity. Pharmacokinetics Good GI absorption; readily penetrates into CSF; hepatic metabolism; renal excretion.	Contraindications Hypersensitivity to sulfonamides or chemically related drugs such as sulfonylureas, thiazide diuretics, and sunscreens containing PABA. Pregnancy Safety for use during pregnancy has not been established; sulfonamides do cross the placenta achieving fetal levels approximately 70%–90% of maternal serum levels; do not use during pregnancy at term. Lactation Issues Sulfonamides are excreted in breast milk; according to the American Academy of Pediatrics, breastfeeding and sulfonamides are compatible; avoid sulfonamides and nursing in premature infants, infants with hyperbilirubinemia, and infants with G-6-PD deficiency.
Sulfisoxazole generics Tablet: 500 mg	**Antibacterial spectrum** Gram-negative organisms (*E. coli, Klebsiella sp., Enterobacter sp., P. mirabilis, P. vulgaris*) and *S. aureus* in the urine; *Nocardia sp., C. trachomatis; H. ducreyi.*	Administration Issues Complete full course of therapy; take on an empty stomach with a full glass of water; avoid prolonged exposure to sunlight, wear protective clothing, and apply sunscreen; shake suspension well prior to administration.	ADRs Nausea, abdominal discomfort, headache, photosensitivity, blood dyscrasies.	Contraindications Hypersensitivity to sulfonamides or chemically related drugs such as sulfonylureas, thiazide diuretics, and sunscreens containing PABA. Pregnancy Category: C

(*continues on next page*)

102.9 Sulfonamides *continued from previous page*

Drug and Dosage Forms	Spectrum of Activity and Usual Dosage Range	Administration Issues and Drug–Drug & Drug–Food Interactions	Common Adverse Drug Reactions (ADRs) and Pharmacokinetics	Contraindications, Pregnancy Category, and Lactation Issues
Sulfisoxazole *cont.* Syrup/Suspension: 500 mg/5 ml	**General Indications** **Adults:** Loading dose: 2–4 gm Maintenance dose: 4–8 g/d in 4–6 divided doses × 7 to 14 d	Drug–Drug Interactions Sulfonamides may increase the pharmacological and toxic effects of the following drugs: **methotrexate, phenytoin, sulfonylureas, warfarin, probenecid.**	Pharmacokinetics Good GI absorption; readily penetrates into CSF; hepatic metabolism; renal excretion.	Safety for use during pregnancy has not been established; sulfonamides do cross the placenta achieving fetal levels approximately 70%–90% of maternal serum levels; do not use during pregnancy at term (Category D). Lactation Issues Sulfonamides are excreted in breast milk; according to the American Academy of Pediatrics, breastfeeding and sulfonamides are compatible; avoid sulfonamides and nursing in premature infants, infants with hyperbilirubinemia, and infants with G-6-PD deficiency.

102.10 Sulfonamide Combinations

Drug and Dosage Forms	Spectrum of Activity and Usual Dosage Range	Administration Issues and Drug–Drug & Drug–Food Interactions	Common Adverse Drug Reactions (ADRs) and Pharmacokinetics	Contraindications, Pregnancy Category, and Lactation Issues
Erythromycin Ethylsuccinate and Sulfisoxazole Pediazole, Eryzole, various generics Granules for Oral Suspension: 200 mg erythromycin ethylsuccinate/ 600 mg sulfisoxazole per 5 ml	**Antibacterial spectrum** Susceptible strains of *H. influenzae* **Treatment of otitis media, pharynaitis, bronchitis, sinusitis in children** 50 mg/kg/d erythromycin and 150 mg/kg/d of sulfisoxazole divided doses qid × 10 d Recommended dosage: <8 kg(<18 lb.): adjust dosage by body weight, qid	Administration Issues Complete full course of therapy; may be given without regard to meals; take with a full glass of water; store in the refrigerator; discard unused portion after 14 d; avoid prolonged exposure to sunlight, wear protective clothing, and apply sunscreen. Drug–Drug Interactions See monographs for erythromycin ethylsuccinate and sulfisoxazole for potential drug interactions.	ADRs Nausea, abdominal distress, diarrhea, abnormal taste, photosensitivity. Pharmacokinetics See monographs for erythromycin ethylsuccinate and sulfisoxazole.	Contraindications Hypersensitivity to sulfonamides or chemically related drugs such as sulfonylureas, thiazide diuretics, and sunscreens containing PABA; hypersensitivity to erythromycin; preexisting liver disease. Pregnancy Safety for use during pregnancy has not been established; sulfonamides do cross the placenta achieving fetal levels approximately 70%–90% of maternal serum levels; do not use during pregnancy at term.

	8 kg (18 lb.): 2.5 ml qid 16 kg (35 lb.): 5 ml qid 24 kg (53 lb.): 7.5 ml qid >45 kg(>100 lb.): 10 ml qid			Lactation Issues Sulfonamides are excreted in breast milk; according to the American Academy of Pediatrics, breastfeeding and sulfonamides and erythromycin are compatible; avoid sulfonamides and nursing in premature infants, infants with hyperbilirubinemia, and infants with G-6-PD deficiency.
Trimethoprim and Sulfamethoxazole (TMP-SMZ) Bactrim, Septra Bactrim DS, generics Tablet (Single strength) 80 mg trim/400 mg sulfa Tablets (Double-strength) 160 mg trim/ 800 mg sulfa Suspension: 40 mg trim/ 200 mg sulfa/ 5 ml	**Antibacterial spectrum** Urinary infections caused by *E. coli, Proteus* sp., *K. pneumoniae, Enterobacter* sp., and coagulase-negative *Staphylococcus* sp.; *H. influenzae, M. catarrhalis, S. pneumoniae, Shigella* sp., *Salmonella* sp., *Pneumocystis carinii.* **Treatment of urinary tract infection and otitis media** **Adults:** 1 DS tablet bid for 10 to 14 d **Children** (≥ 2 months): 8 mg/kg TMP/40 mg/kg SMZ per day divided q 12 h × 10 d **Treatment of travelers' diarrhea in adults** 1 DS tablet bid × 5 d **Acute exacerbation of chronic bronchitis in adults:** 1 DS tablet bid × 14 d **Treatment of Pneumocystis carinii pneumonia Adults:** 15–20 mg/kg TMP/100 mg/kg SMZ/d divided q 6 h × 21 d **Children:** (give for 21 days) 8 kg: 5 ml suspension/dose q 6 h 16 kg: 10 ml suspension/dose q 6 h 24 kg: 15 ml suspension/dose q 6 h 32 kg: 20 ml suspension/dose q 6 h **Dosage reduction is recommended for patients with renal insufficiency.**	Administration Issues Complete full course of therapy; take each oral dose with a full glass of water. Drug–Drug Interactions TMP-SMZ may increase the pharmacological effect of the following drugs leading to toxicity: **dapsone, methotrexate, phenytoin, digoxin, sulfonylureas, warfarin.** TMP-SMZ may decrease the effect of **cyclosporine.** Use of **zidovudine, azathioprine,** or **ganciclovir** and TMP-SMZ may have additive bone marrow depressant effects in patients with HIV.	ADRs Abdominal distress, nausea, rash, neutropenia. Pharmacokinetics Rapidly absorbed; $T_{1/2}$ is approximately 10 h; SMZ undergoes hepatic metabolism; renal excretion.	Contraindications Hypersensitivity to trimethoprim or sulfonamides; megaloblastic anemia due to folate deficiency; pregnancy at term and lactation; infants < 2 months old, G6 PD deficiency. Pregnancy Category: C Lactation Issues Not recommended for use in nursing infants due to possibility of sulfonamide-associated kernicterus.

102.11 Tetracyclines

Drug and Dosage Forms	Spectrum of Activity and Usual Dosage Range	Administration Issues and Drug–Drug & Drug–Food Interactions	Common Adverse Drug Reactions (ADRs) and Pharmacokinetics	Contraindications, Pregnancy Category, and Lactation Issues
Demeclocycline Declomycin Tablet: 150 mg, 300 mg Capsule: 150 mg	**Antibacterial spectrum** *S. pneumonia, some gram-negative organisms including E. coli, Klebsiella sp., E. aerogenes, Acinetobacter sp.*, Rickettsiae (Rocky Mountain spotted fever), *M. pneumoniae, Bacteriodes sp., C. trachomatis, Brucella sp., Ureaplasma urealyticum, Borrelia burgdorferi* (Lyme disease) **Second line agent in treating bacterial infections** **Adults:** 150 mg q 6 h *or* 300 mg q 12 h × 10 to 14 d	Administration Issues Complete full course of therapy; take on empty stomach at least 1 h before or 2 h after meals; avoid simultaneous dairy products, antacids, laxatives, or iron-containing products; avoid prolonged exposure to the sun or sunlamps. Drug–Drug Interactions **Antacids** containing calcium, magnesium, aluminum, zinc, and bismuth salts, **sucralfate**, and iron-containing products may decrease the absorption of tetracyclines. Tetracyclines may increase serum **digoxin** levels. Tetracyclines may decrease the effectiveness of **oral contraceptives**. Concomitant use of **penicillins** may decrease the effectiveness of tetracyclines.	ADRs Photosensitivity, nausea, vomiting, dizziness, superinfection, polyuria, polydipsia. Pharmacokinetics 65–90% protein binding; 40% excreted unchanged in the urine.	Contraindications Hypersensitivity to tetracyclines. Pregnancy Category: D Lactation Issues Excreted in breast milk; due to potential, serious adverse effects in nursing infants decide whether to discontinue the drug or nursing.
Doxycycline Doxycycline, Vibramycin, Various generics Tablets: 50 mg, 75 mg, 100 mg Capsule: 50 mg, 100 mg Capsule, coated pellets: 75 mg 100 mg Powder for Oral Suspension: 25 mg/5 ml Syrup: 50 mg/5 ml	**Antibacterial Spectrum** *S. pneumonia, some gram-negative organisms including E. coli, Klebsiella sp., E. aerogenes, Acinetobacter* sp., Rickettsiae (Rocky Mountain spotted fever), *M. pneumoniae, Bacteriodes sp., C. trachomatis, Brucella sp., Ureaplasma urealyticum, Borrelia burgdorferi* (Lyme disease), Plasmodium sp. (malaria). **General indications** **Adults** Usual dose: 200 mg on first day of treatment (100 mg bid), follow with 100 mg qd maintenance dose More severe infections: 100 mg q 12 h	Administration Issues Complete full course of therapy; shake suspension well before administration; may take without regards to meals; avoid simultaneous dairy products, antacids, laxatives, or iron-containing products; avoid prolonged exposure to the sun or sunlamps. Drug–Drug Interactions **Antacids** containing calcium, magnesium, aluminum, zinc, and bismuth salts, **sucralfate**, and iron-containing products may decrease the absorption of tetracyclines. Tetracyclines may increase serum **digoxin** levels. Tetracyclines may decrease the effectiveness of **oral contraceptives**. Concomitant use of **penicillins** may decrease the effectiveness of tetracyclines. Concomitant use of	ADRs Nausea, vomiting, diarrhea, photosensitivity, dizziness, superinfection. Pharmacokinetics Increased absorption with food; high lipid solubility and penetration into cerebrospinal fluid; 90% protein binding; fecal elimination.	Contraindications Hypersensitivity to tetracyclines. Pregnancy Category: D Lactation Issues Excreted in breast milk; due to potential, serious adverse effects in nursing infants decide whether to discontinue the drug or nursing.

		carbamazepine, phenytoin, and **barbiturates** may increase the metabolism of doxycycline.		
Minocycline Minocin, Various generics Tablets 50 mg, 75 mg, 100 mg Capsule: 50 mg 75 mg 100 mg Suspension: 50 mg/5 ml Capsule, Pellet filled: 50 mg, 75 mg, 100 mg	**Antibacterial spectrum** *S. pneumonia*, some gram-negative organisms including *E. coli, Klebsiella sp., E. aerogenes, Acinetobacter* sp., Rickettsiae (Rocky Mountain spotted fever), *M. pneumoniae, Bacteriodes sp., C. trachomatis, Brucella sp., Ureaplasma urealyticum, Borrelia burgdorferi* (Lyme disease). **General Indications** **Adults:** 200 mg initially, followed by 100 mg q 12 h **Children > 8 yr.:** 4 mg/kg follow with 2 mg/kg bid	Administration Issues Complete full course of therapy; shake suspension well before administration; may take without regards to meals; avoid simultaneous dairy products, antacids, laxatives, or iron-containing products; avoid prolonged exposure to the sun or sunlamps. Drug–Drug Interactions **Antacids** containing calcium, magnesium, aluminum, zinc, and bismuth salts, **sucralfate**, and iron-containing products may decrease the absorption of tetracyclines. Tetracyclines may increase serum **digoxin** levels. Tetracyclines may decrease the effectiveness of **oral contraceptives**. Concomitant use of **penicillins** may decrease the effectiveness of tetracyclines.	ADRs Nausea, vomiting, diarrhea, photosensitivity, dizziness, superinfection. Pharmacokinetics High lipid solubility and penetration into cerebrospinal fluid; 75% protein binding; biliary excretion.	Contraindications Hypersensitivity to tetracyclines. Pregnancy Category: D Lactation Issues Excreted in breast milk; due to potential, serious adverse effects in nursing infants decide whether to discontinue the drug or nursing.
Tetracycline generics Tablet: 250 mg, 500 mg Capsule: 100 mg, 250 mg, 500 mg Suspension: 125 mg/5 ml	**Antibacterial spectrum** *S. pneumonia, some gram-negative organisms including E. coli, Klebsiella sp., E. aerogenes, Acinetobacter* sp., Rickettsiae (Rocky Mountain spotted fever), *M. pneumoniae, Bacteriodes sp., C. trachomatis, Brucella sp., Ureaplasma urealyticum, Borrelia burgdorferi* (Lyme disease) **General Indications** **Adults:** 1–2 gm daily in 2 to 4 divided doses × 7 to 14 d **Children > 8 yr.**: 25–50 mg/kg divided qid × 7 to 14 d **Severe acne:** 500 mg bid initially, then 125–500 mg daily as a maintenance dose	Administration Issues Complete full course of therapy; shake suspension well before administration; take on empty stomach at least 1 h before or 2 h after meals; avoid simultaneous dairy products, antacids, laxatives, or iron-containing products; avoid prolonged exposure to the sun or sunlamps. Drug–Drug Interactions **Antacids** containing calcium, magnesium, aluminum, zinc, and bismuth salts, **sucraifate**, and iron-containing products may decrease the absorption of tetracyclines. Tetracyclines may increase serum **digoxin** levels. Tetracyclines may decrease the effectiveness of **oral contraceptives**. Concomitant use of **penicillins** may decrease the effectiveness of tetracyclines.	ADRs Nausea, vomiting, diarrhea, photosensitivity, dizziness, superinfection. Pharmacokinetics Decreased absorption with food; less CNS penetration than doxycycline; 65% protein binding; 60% excreted unchanged in the urine. Contraindications, Pregnancy Category, and Lactation Issues	Contraindications Hypersensitivity to tetracyclines. Pregnancy Category: D Lactation Issues Excreted in breast milk; due to potential, serious adverse effects in nursing infants decide whether to discontinue the drug or nursing.

102.12 Miscellaneous Antibiotics

Drug and Dosage Forms	Spectrum of Activity and Usual Dosage Range	Administration Issues and Drug-Drug & Drug-Food Interactions	Common Adverse Drug Reactions (ADRs)	Contraindications, Pregnancy Category and Lactation Issues
Linezolid Zyvox Tablet: 400 mg, 600 mg Powder for oral solution: 100 mg/5 mL	**Antibacterial spectrum** Vancomycin-resistant *E. faecium, S. aureus* (methicillin-susceptible and -resistant strains) or *S. pneumoniae* (penicillin-susceptible strains only), *S. pyogenes*, or *S. agalactiae.* Vancomycin-resistant Enterococcus faeceium: 600 mg q 12 h × 14 to 28 d Nosocomial pneumonia/complicated skin and skin-structure infections: 600 mg q 12 h × 10 to 14 d Uncomplicated skin/skin-structure infections: 400 mg q 12 h × 10 to 14 d	Administration Issues Linezolid may be taken with or without food. Avoid large quantities of food or beverages with high tyramine content while taking linezolid. Quantities of tyramine consumed should be <100 mg/meal. Each 5 ml of the 100 mg/5 ml oral suspension contains 20 mg phenylalanine. The other linezolid formulations do not contain phenylalanine. Educate patient to inform healthcare provider before ingesting medications containing pseudoephedrine or phenylpropanolamine, such as cold remedies and decongestants, in addition to serotonin reuptake inhibitors or other antidepressants. Drug Interactions Linezolid has the potential for interaction with adrenergic agents. Reduce and titrate initial doses of adrenergic agents, such as dopamine and epinephrine. Linezolid has the potential for interaction with serotonergic agents. Because there is limited experience with concomitant administration of linezolid and serotonergic agents, physicians should be alert to the possibility of signs and symptoms of serotonin syndrome. Drug-Food Interactions: Large quantities of foods or beverages with high tyramine content should be avoided while taking linezolid. Quantities of tyramine consumed should be < 100 mg/meal.	ADRs/Lab Abnormalities: Headache, dizziness, nausea, diarrhea, vomiting, myelosuppression (including anemia, leukopenia, pancytopenia, and thrombocytopenia), thrombocytopenia. Pharmacokinetics Absolute bioavailability of ≈ 100. The half-life is 4.4 to 5.5 h.	Contraindications Hypersensitivity to linezolid or any of the other product components. Pregnancy Category: C Lactation Issues: Exercise caution when administering to a nursing woman.

103. Antifungals

Drug and Dosage Forms	Spectrum of Activity and Usual Dosage Range	Administration Issues and Drug–Drug & Drug–Food Interactions	Common Adverse Drug Reactions (ADRs) and Pharmacokinetics	Contraindications, Pregnancy Category, and Lactation Issues
Clotrimazole Mycelex Troche: 10 mg	**Antifungal Spectrum** *C. albicans.* **Local treatment of oropharyngeal candidiasis** 1 troche 5 times/d × 14 d. **Prophylaxis in immunocompromised patients** 1 troche tid	Administration Issues Dissolve troche slowly in mouth to achieve maximal effect.	ADRs Abnormal LFTs, nausea, vomiting, unpleasant taste in mouth, pruritus. Pharmacokinetics Dosing every 3 h maintains effective salivary levels for most strains of *Candida.*	Contraindications Hypersensitivity to clotrimazole. Pregnancy Category: C Lactation Issues Fluconazole is excreted in breast milk; use in nursing mothers is not recommended.
Fluconazole Diflucan, generics Tablet: 50 mg, 100 mg, 150 mg, 200 mg Powder for Oral Suspension: 10 mg/ml, 40 mg/ml	**Antifungal spectrum** Various fungal infections including: *C. neoformans; Candida* sp., *Aspergillus* sp., *Coccidioides immitis.* **Treatment of vaginal candidiasis** 150 mg as a single dose **Oropharyngeal candidiasis** **Adults:** 200 mg on first day, followed by 100 mg once daily, continue treatment for 2 weeks to decrease likelihood of relapse **Esophageal candidiasis** **Adults:** 200 mg on first day, followed by 100 mg once daily, continue treatment for a minimum of 3 weeks and for at least 2 weeks following resolution of symptoms; doses up to 400 mg/d may be used **Candidal UTI** 50–200 mg/d **Systemic Candidal infections** **Adults:** 100–400 mg/day	Administration Issues Complete full course of therapy; shake suspension well prior to administration; store suspension in the refrigerator or at room temperature; discard unused suspension after 2 weeks. Drug–Drug Interactions **Cimetidine** and **rifampin** may decrease the serum level of fluconazole. **Hydrochlorothiazide** may increase the serum level of fluconazole. Fluconazole may increase or decrease the effect of **oral contraceptives**. Fluconazole may cause an increase in the pharmacological and toxic effects of the following drugs: **terfenadine, astemizole, loratadine, cyclosporine, tacrolimus, phenytoin, theophylline, sulfonylureas, warfarin, zidovudine, cisapride**.	ADRs headache, nausea, abdominal pain, diarrhea Adverse effects are reported to occur more frequently in HIV infected patients compared to non-HIV infected patients Pharmacokinetics Excellent GI absorption; $T_{1/2}$ is approximately 30 h; good CSF penetration; hepatic metabolism; approximately 80% of a dose is excreted unchanged in the urine.	Contraindications Hypersensitivity to fluconazole; use with caution in patients allergic to other azole antifungals. Pregnancy Category: C Lactation Issues Fluconazole is excreted in breast milk; use in nursing mothers is not recommended.

(continues on next page)

103. Antifungals *continued from previous page*

Drug and Dosage Forms	Spectrum of Activity and Usual Dosage Range	Administration Issues and Drug–Drug & Drug–Food Interactions	Common Adverse Drug Reactions (ADRs) and Pharmacokinetics	Contraindications, Pregnancy Category, and Lactation Issues
Fluconazole *cont.*	**Cryptococcal meningitis** **Adults:** 400 mg on first day, followed by 200 mg once daily, continue treatment for 10–12 weeks after CSF cultures are negative; doses up to 400 mg/day may be used. **Suppression of relapse of cryptococcal meningitis** **Adults:** 200 mg qd			
Griseofulvin Microsize Tablet: 250 mg, 500 mg Capsule: 125 mg, 250 mg Oral Suspension: 125 mg/5 ml	**Antifungal spectrum** Limited antifungal spectrum including: *Microsporidium* sp., *Epidermophyton* sp., and *Trichophyton* sp. **Treatment of tinea corporis, tinea cruris, and tinea capitis** **Adults:** 500 mg microsize or 330–375 mg ultramicrosize daily in single or divided doses **Children > 2 yr.:** 11 mg microsize/kg/d or 7.3 mg ultramicrosize/kg/d **Treatment of tinea pedis and tinea ungulum** **Adults:** 0.75 mg–1 gm microsize or 660–750 mg ultramicrosize daily in divided doses **Children > 2 yr.:** 11 mg microsize/kg/d or 7.3 mg ultramicrosize/kg/d	Administration Issues Complete full course of therapy; avoid prolonged exposure to the sun; shake suspension well prior to administration; store suspension at room temperature. Serum levels may be increased with a high fat content meal. Avoid alcohol. Drug–Drug Interactions Griseofulvin may decrease the effect of the following drugs: **warfarin, oral contraceptives, cyclosporine, and salicylates. Barbiturates** may decrease serum levels of griseofulvin. Disulfuram-type reaction may occur with alcohol.	ADRs Rash, urticaria, nausea, headache, abdominal discomfort, dizziness, photosensitivity. Pharmacokinetics Poor and inconsistent GI absorption.	Contraindications Hypersensitivity to griseofulvin; porphyria; hepatocellular failure. Pregnancy Category: C
Griseofulvin Ultramicrosize Tablet: 125 mg, 165 mg, 250 mg, 330 mg	**Antifungal spectrum** Limited antifungal spectrum including: *Microsporidium* sp., *Epidermophyton* sp., and *Trichophyton* sp.	Administration Issues Complete full course of therapy; avoid prolonged exposure to the sun; shake suspension well prior to administration; store suspension at room temperature. Avoid alcohol.	ADRs Rash, urticaria, nausea, headache, abdominal discomfort, dizziness, photosensitivity.	Contraindications Hypersensitivity to griseofulvin; porphyria; hepatocellular failure. Pregnancy Category: C

Grisactin Ultra 125 mg, 250 mg, 330 mg Gris-PEG 125 mg, 250 mg	**Treatment of tinea corporis, tinea cruris, and tinea capitis** **Adults:** 500 mg microsize or 330–375 mg ultramicrosize daily in single or divided doses **Children > 2 yr.:** 11 mg microsize/kg/d or 7.3 mg ultramicrosize/kg/d **Treatment of tinea pedis and tinea ungulum** **Adults:** 0.75 mg–1 gm microsize or 660–750 mg ultramicrosize daily in divided doses **Children > 2 yr.:** 11 mg microsize/kg/d or 7.3 mg ultramicrosize/kg/d	Drug–Drug Interactions Griseofulvin may decrease the effect of the following drugs: **warfarin, oral contraceptives, cyclosporine, and salicylates. Barbiturates** may decrease serum levels of griseofulvin. Disulfuram-type reaction may occur with alcohol.	Pharmacokinetics Enhanced GI absorption compared to microsize formulation.	
Itraconazole Sporanox Capsule: 100 mg Oral Solution: 10 mg/mL	**Antifungal spectrum** Various fungal infections including *Blastomycosis, Histomycosis, Aspergillosis,* and *Onychomycosis* **Blastomycosis and Histoplasmosis infections** 200 mg qd; may increase to 400 mg/d if needed for a minimum of 3 months Give doses > 200 mg/d in two divided doses **Aspergillosis infection** 200–400 mg/d. Give doses > 200 mg/d in two divided doses for a minimum of 3 months **Onychomycosis infection** 200 mg qd for 12 consecutive weeks	Administration Issues Complete full course of therapy; do not take with antacids; administer with a cola drink in HIV patients; take with a full meal. Drug–Drug Interactions Itraconazole may increase the pharmacological and toxic effects of the following drugs: **astemizole, loratadine, terfenadine, cyclosporine, quinidine, tacrolimus, warfarin, cisapride, phenytoin, sulfonylureas, triazolam, midazolam**. The following drugs may decrease the effect of itraconazole: **rifampin, phenytoin, H_2 antagonist (cimetidine, ranitidine), antacids, didanosine**.	ADRs Nausea, vomiting, diarrhea, rash, headache. Pharmacokinetics Absorption is dependent on an acidic environment; long $T_{1/2}$ approximately 20 h; extensive hepatic metabolism; renal excretion of inactive metabolites.	**Contraindications** **Do not administer itraconazole in patients with a history of CHF or evidence of cardiac dysfunction. Concomitant use of terfenadine, astemizole, cisapride, triazolam, or midazolam; hypersensitivity to itraconazole or other azole antifungals; treatment of onychomycosis in pregnant women.** Pregnancy Category: C Lactation Issues Excreted in breast milk; do not use in nursing mothers.
Ketoconazole Nizoral, generics Tablet: 200 mg	**Antifungal spectrum** Various fungal infections including: *Blastomyces dermatitidis, Candida* sp., *Coccidioides immitis, Histoplasma capsulatum, Paracoccidioides brasiliensis, Phialophora* sp., *Trichophyton* sp., *Epidermophyton* sp., and *Microsporidium* sp.	Administration Issues Complete full course of therapy; do not give within two hours of antacids. Take with food to decrease GI disturbances.	ADRs Nausea, vomiting, abdominal discomfort, headache, dizziness. Hepatotoxicity has occurred, including rare fatalities. Frequent measurement of LFTs is recommended.	Contraindications Hypersensitivity to ketoconazole. Pregnancy Category: C

(*continues on next page*)

103. Antifungals *continued from previous page*

Drug and Dosage Forms	Spectrum of Activity and Usual Dosage Range	Administration Issues and Drug–Drug & Drug–Food Interactions	Common Adverse Drug Reactions (ADRs) and Pharmacokinetics	Contraindications, Pregnancy Category, and Lactation Issues
Ketoconazole *cont.*	**General indications** **Adults:** 200 mg qd, for serious infections or if clinical response is insufficient, 400 mg qd may be used **Children > 2 yr.:** 3.3–6.6 mg/kg/d as a single dose **Minimum treatment for candidiasis is 1 to 2 weeks. Minimum treatment for other systemic mycoses is 6 months. Chronic mucocutaneous candidiasis usually requires maintenance therapy. Minimum treatment for recalcitrant dermatophyte infections is 4 weeks.**	Drug–Drug Interactions **Antacids, H_2 antagonists,** and **anticholinergics** may increase gastric pH and decrease ketoconazole absorption. Ketoconazole may increase the pharmacological and toxic effects of the following drugs: **warfarin, astemizole, loratadine, terfenadine, corticosteroids, cyclosporine, tacrolimus, sulfonylureas, midazolam**. Ketoconazole may decrease the effect of **theophylline. Isoniazid** and **rifampin** may decrease the serum concentration of ketoconazole.	Pharmacokinetics Acidic pH required for dissolution and absorption; negligible CSF penetration; hepatic metabolism; biliary and fecal elimination.	Lactation Issues Ketoconazole is probably excreted in breast milk; avoid use in nursing mothers.
Nystatin Mycostatin, Nilstat, various generics Tablet, film coated: 500,000 units Vaginal tablets 100,000 units Oral Suspension: 100,000 units/ml Troche: Mycostatin Pastilles 200,000 units Bulk Powder: (million units): 50, 100, 500 Bulk Powder: (billion units): 1, 2, 5	**Antifungal spectrum** *Candida* sp. including *Candida albicans.* **Intestinal Candida infections** **Adults:** 500,000–1 million units tid, continue for 48 h after clinical cure **Children:** 100,000 units qid, continue for 48 h after clinical cure **Oral Candida infections** **Adults and children** Suspension: 400,000 to 600,000 units qid Troches: 200,000 to 400,000 units 4–5 times/d; for as long as 14 d, if necessary Powder: Add 1/8 tsp (500,000 units) to ½ cup water and stir well. Administer qid; use immediately and do not store. Continue for 48 h after clinical cure.	Administration Issues Complete full course of therapy; continue therapy for at least two days after symptoms disappear. When using suspension for oral candidiasis, retain drug in mouth as long as possible before swallowing. For the troches, do not chew or swallow whole. Allow troches to dissolve slowly in mouth. Do not store the powder after reconstitution.	ADRs Nausea, vomiting. Pharmacokinetics Minimal oral absorption; fecal elimination.	Contraindications Hypersensitivity to nystatin. Pregnancy No adverse effects or complications have been attributed to nystatin in infants born to women treated with nystatin. Lactation Issues Excretion in human breast milk is unknown; use with caution in nursing mothers.
Terbinafine Lamisil	**Antifungal spectrum** *Trichophyton mentagrophytes* and *T. rubrum*			**Contraindications:** **Rare cases of hepatic failure leading to death or liver transplant have occurred with the use of terbinafine.**

Tablet: 250 mg	**Treatment of onychomycosis of the toenail/fingernail due to dermatophytes** Fingernail: 250 mg/d for 6 weeks Toenail: 250 mg/d for 12 weeks Optimal clinical cure is seen months after mycological cure and cessation of treatment.	Administration Issues Use medication for recommended treatment time. Safety and efficacy in children is not established. Drug Interactions: Terbinafine clearance is decreased by **cimetidine, terfenadine.** Terbinafine clearance is increased by **rifampin**. Terbinafine increases the clearance of **cyclosporine** and decreases the clearance of **caffeine**.	ADRs Diarrhea, dyspepsia, abdominal pain, nausea, rash, pruritus, LFT abnormalities, headache, taste and visual disturbances. Pharmacokinetics Terbinafine is well absorbed.	**Do not use in patients with chronic or active live disease. Pretreatment LFTs are advised. Hypersensitivity to terbinafine; pre-existing liver disease or renal impairment (CrCl < 50 ml/min)** Pregnancy Category: B Lactation Issues: Terbinafine is excreted in human breast milk; avoid in nursing mothers.
Voriconazole Vfend Tablets 50 mg, 200 mg Powder for Injection: 200 mg single dose vial Powder for oral suspension 40 mg/mL	**Antifungal spectrum** *Aspergillus fumigatus, Scedosporium apiospermum, Fusarium* sp. **Treatment of adults with invasive aspergillosis and infections due to *Fusarium* sp. and *S. apiospermum*** Therapy must be initiated with the specified loading dose regimen of IV voriconazole to achieve plasma concentrations on day 1 that are close to steady state. Recommended dosing regimen: Loading dose of 6 mg/kg IV every 12 h for 2 doses, followed by a maintenance dose of 4 mg/kg IV every 12 h. Once the patient can tolerate medication given by mouth, the oral tablet form may be used. Wt $\geq$ 40 kg: 200 mg every 12 h. Wt < 40 kg: 100 mg every 12 h. On the basis of high oral bioavailability, switching between IV and oral administration is appropriate when clinically indicated. Base duration of therapy on the severity of the patient's underlying disease, recovery from immunosuppression, and clinical response.	Administration Issues Tablets should be taken at least 1 h before or 1 h after a meal. Advise patients not drive at night while taking voriconazole. It may cause changes to vision, including blurring or photophobia. Advise patients to avoid potentially hazardous tasks, such as driving or operating machinery if they perceive any changes in vision. Patients should avoid strong, direct sunlight during drug therapy. **Women of childbearing potential should use effective contraception during treatment.** Drug Interactions Voriconazole may inhibit the metabolism and increase levels of the following drugs: **protease inhibitors, proton pump inhibitors, benzodiazepines, calcium channel blockers, pimozide, cyclosporine, ergot alkaloids, warfarin, quinidine, cisapride, HMG-CoA reductase inhibitors, sulfonylureas, tacrolimus, sirolimus, vinca alkaloids.** Voriconazole may increase the levels of **phenytoin, rifabutin, protease inhibitors, NNRTIs, proton pump inhibitors**. The following drugs may decrease voriconazole levels: barbiturates, **phenytoin, rifampin, rifabutin**. The following drugs may increase voriconazole levels: **cimetidine, protease inhibitors, NNRTIs**.	ADRs/Lab Abnormalities Abnormal vision, photophobia, fever, chills, headache, dizziness, nausea, diarrhea, vomiting, tachycardia, hyper- and hypotension, hallucinations, abdominal pain, LFT abnormalities, alkaline phosphatase increases. Pharmacokinetics The pharmacokinetics are nonlinear because of the saturation of its metabolism. IV voriconazole should be avoided in patients with moderate or severe renal impairment (Ccr below 50 mL/min), unless an assessment of the benefit/risk to the patient justifies the use of IV voriconazole.	Contraindications Known hypersensitivity to voriconazole or its excipients; use caution when prescribing voriconazole to patients with hypersensitivity to other azoles; coadministration of the CYP3A4 substrates, cisapride, pimozide, or quinidine with voriconazole is contraindicated because increased plasma concentrations of these drugs can lead to QT prolongation and rare occurrences of torsades de points; coadministration of voriconazole with sirolimus, rifampin, carbamazepine, long-acting barbiturates, rifabutin, or ergot alkaloids (ergotamine and dihydroergotamine). Pregnancy Category: D Lactation Issues Voriconazole should not be used by nursing mothers unless the benefit clearly outweighs the risk.

104. Antimalarials

Drug and Dosage Forms	Spectrum of Activity and Usual Dosage Range	Administration Issues and Drug–Drug & Drug–Food Interactions	Common Adverse Drug Reactions (ADRs) and Pharmacokinetics	Contraindications, Pregnancy Category, and Lactation Issues
Chloroquine Phosphate generics Tablet: 250 mg Tablet: 500 mg	**Antimalarial spectrum** *P. falciparum, P. malariae,* and *P. vivax.* **Treatment of acute malaria** **Adults:** 600 mg on day 1, followed by 300 mg 6 h later, 300 mg on day 2, and 300 mg on day 3 **Children:** 10 mg/kg on day 1, followed by 5 mg/kg 6 h later, 5 mg/kg on day 2, and 5 mg/kg on day 3 **Suppression of malaria** **Adults:** 300 mg once weekly starting one week prior to travel, continue weekly during travel, and for 4 weeks after leaving areas **Children:** 5 mg/kg (max 300 mg) once weekly starting one week prior to travel, continue weekly during travel, and for 4 weeks after leaving such areas **Treatment of extraintestinal amebiasis** **Adults:** 1 gm qd for 2 d, followed by 500 mg qd for 2 to 3 weeks **Combination therapy with an effective intestinal amebicide (paromomycin, metronidazole) should be used**.	Administration Issues Complete full course of therapy; take tablets on the same day each week for malaria suppression; do not take on an empty stomach. Drug–Drug Interactions **Cimetidine** may decrease the elimination of chloroquine. **Kaolin** may decrease the absorption of chloroquine.	ADRs Nausea, vomiting, headache, GI upset, visual disturbances (possibly leading to irreversible retinal damage with long term administration). Pharmacokinetics Readily absorbed from GI tract; 55% protein bound; long elimination half-life; renal excretion.	Contraindications: Retinal or visual field changes; hypersensitivity to chloroquine or related compounds. Pregnancy: Use only when clearly needed and potential benefit outweighs the potential hazards to the fetus. Lactation Issues Excreted in breast milk in low concentrations; use with caution in nursing mothers
Hydroxychloroquine Sulfate Plaquenil; various generics Tablet: 200 mg (equivalent to 155 mg hydroxychloroquine)	**Antimalarial spectrum** *P. falciparum, P. malariae,* and *P. vivax* **Hydroxychloroquine is not effective against chloroquine-resistant strains of** ***Plasmodium falciparum.***	Administration Issues Complete full course of therapy; take tablets on the same day each week for malaria suppression; do not take on an empty stomach.	ADRs Nausea, vomiting, headache, GI upset, visual disturbances (possibly leading to irreversible retinal damage with long term administration).	Contraindications Retinal or visual field changes; hypersensitivity to chloroquine or related compounds; long-term use in children.

	Treatment of acute malaria **Adults:** 620 mg on day 1, followed by 310 mg 6 h later, 310 mg on day 2, and 310 mg on day 3 **Children:** 10 mg/kg on day 1, followed by 5 mg/kg 6 h later, 5 mg/kg on day 2, and 5 mg/kg on day 3 **Suppression of malaria** **Adults:** 310 mg once weekly starting one week prior to travel, continue weekly during travel, and for 4 weeks after leaving such areas **Children:** 5 mg/kg (max 300 mg) once weekly starting one week prior to travel, continue weekly during travel, and for 4 weeks after leaving such areas	Drug–Drug Interactions **Cimetidine** may decrease the elimination of chloroquine. **Kaolin** may decrease the absorption of chloroquine.	Pharmacokinetics Readily absorbed from GI tract; 55% protein bound; long elimination half-life; renal excretion.	Pregnancy Use only when clearly needed and potential benefit outweighs the potential hazards to the fetus. Lactation Issues Excreted in breast milk in low concentrations; use with caution in nursing mothers.
Mefloquine HCl Larium, generics Tablet: 250 mg	**Antimalarial spectrum** *P. falciparum* (both chloroquine-sensitive and resistant strains) and *P. vivax* **Treatment of mild to moderate malaria in adults** Five tablets (1250 mg) as a single dose **Patients with acute *P. vivax* malaria treated with mefloquine are at high risk of relapse because mefloquine does not eliminate exoerythrocytic (hepatic phase) parasites. To avoid relapse after treatment with mefloquine, subsequently treat with primaquine**. **Suppression of malaria** **Adults:** 250 mg once weekly starting one week prior to travel, continue weekly during travel, and for 4 weeks after leaving such areas	Administration Issues Complete full course of therapy; take tablets on the same day each week for malaria suppression; do not take on an empty stomach; take with a full glass of water. Drug–Drug Interactions Concomitant use of mefloquine and **beta-adrenergic blockers (propranolol, atenolol), calcium channel antagonist (verapamil, diltiazem), quinidine, and quinine** may lead to abnormal cardiac conduction and arrhythmias. Mefloquine may decrease **valproic acid** serum levels increasing the risk of seizures. Concomitant mefloquine and **chloroquine** use may lead to increased risk of convulsions.	ADRs Nausea, vomiting, dizziness, headache, visual disturbances. Pharmacokinetics Long $T_{1/2}$ approximately 21 d; highly protein bound, > 95%; concentrates in blood erythrocytes; primarily cleared by the liver.	Contraindications Hypersensitivity to mefloquine and related compounds. Pregnancy Category: C Lactation Issues Excreted in breast milk in low concentrations; use with caution in nursing mothers.

(continues on next page)

104. Antimalarials *continued from previous page*

Drug and Dosage Forms	Spectrum of Activity and Usual Dosage Range	Administration Issues and Drug–Drug & Drug–Food Interactions	Common Adverse Drug Reactions (ADRs) and Pharmacokinetics	Contraindications, Pregnancy Category, and Lactation Issues
Mefloquine HCl *cont.*	**Children:** 15–19 kg, ¼ tablet; 20–30 kg, ½ tablet; 31–45 kg, ¾ tablet; > 45 kg, 1 tablet. Take appropriate dose once weekly starting one week prior to travel, continue weekly during travel, and for 4 weeks after leaving such areas			
Primaquine Phosphate Tablet: 26.3 mg (15 mg base)	**Antimalarial spectrum** *P. vivax, P. ovale*, and gametocytial forms of *P. falciparum*. **Treatment of malaria in combination with chloroquine phosphate** **Adults:** 26.3 mg (15 mg base) qd for 14 days during the last 2 weeks of chloroquine therapy **Children:** 0.5 mg/kg/d (0.3 mg base/kg/d max 15 mg base/dose) qd for 14 d during the last 2 weeks of chloroquine therapy	Administration Issues Complete full course of therapy; take with food or after meals to decrease GI upset. Drug–Drug Interactions Concomitant use of **quinacrine** and primaquine may lead to toxicities related to primaquine.	ADRs Nausea, vomiting, GI upset, anemia. Pharmacokinetics Elimination $T_{1/2}$ is approximately 4 h; low concentration in the tissues; reaches high concentrations in the liver, lungs, brain, and heart; excreted primarily as metabolites in the urine.	Contraindications Concomitant use of quinacrine and primaquine; patients predisposed to granulocytopenia (rheumatoid arthritis and lupus erythematosus); patients with G-6-PD deficiency. Pregnancy Use only when clearly needed and potential benefit outweighs the potential hazards to the fetus.
Pyrimethamine Daraprim Tablet: 25 mg	**Antimalarial spectrum** Susceptible strains of *Plasmodium* sp. **Treatment of malaria in combination with chloroquine or quinacrine** **Adults and children > 10 yr.:** 50 mg qd for 2 d **Children 4 to 10 yr.:** 25 mg qd for 2 d **After clinical cure, follow with suppressive regimen for 6 to 10 weeks**. **Suppression of malaria** **Adults and children > 10 yr.:** 25 mg once weekly for 6 to 10 weeks	Administration Issues Complete full course of therapy; take with food to avoid GI upset. Drug–Drug Interactions Concomitant use of pyrimethamine and **methotrexate, sulfonamides, or TMP-SMZ** may increase risk of folate deficiency and bone marrow suppression.	ADRs Nausea, vomiting, anemia. Pharmacokinetics Well absorbed orally, $T_{1/2}$ approximately 4 d; 87% protein bound; hepatically metabolized; some renal excretion.	Contraindications Hypersensitivity to pyrimethamine; documented megaloblastic anemia. Pregnancy Category: C Lactation Issues Excreted in breast milk; safety for use has not been established; decide whether to discontinue nursing or discontinue the drug.

	Children 4 to 10 yr.: 12.5 mg once weekly for 6 to 10 weeks **Infants and children < 4 yr.:** 6.25 mg once weekly for 6 to 10 weeks **Treatment of toxoplasmosis** **Adults:** Initially, 50–75 mg qd with 1–4 gm of a sulfapyrimidine; continue for 1 to 3 weeks, depending on response and tolerance; dosage of each drug may then be decreased by ½ and continued for an additional 4 to 5 weeks. **Children:** 1 mg/kg/d divided bid with a sulfapyrimidine; after 2 to 4 days, decrease dose by ½ and continue for 1 month.			
Quinine Sulfate Generics Tablet: 260 mg Capsule: 200 mg, 260 mg, 325 mg	**Antimalarial spectrum** *P. falciparum, P. malariae, P. ovale, and P. vivax.* **Chloroquine-resistant malaria** **Adults:** 650 mg q 8 h for 5 to 7 d **Children:** 25 mg/kg/d divided q 8 h for 5 to 7 d **Chloroquine-sensitive malaria** **Adults:** 600 mg q 8 h for 5 to 7 d **Children:** 10 mg/kg/d divided q 8 h for 5 to 7 d **Treatment of nocturnal leg cramps** 260–300 mg at bedtime; if needed, may be taken after the evening meal and at bedtime	Administration Issues Complete full course of therapy; take with food or after meals to decrease GI upset. Drug–Drug Interactions **Aluminum containing antacids** may decrease the absorption of quinine. Quinine may enhance the effect of **warfarin**; Quinine may also enhance the effect of **digoxin** leading to toxicity. Concomitant use of quinine and **mefloquine** may lead to abnormal cardiac conduction and arrhythmias. **Acetazolamide** and **sodium bicarbonate** may decrease urinary excretion of quinine leading to quinine accumulation.	ADRs Nausea, vomiting, GI upset, ringing in the ears (tinnitus), headache, vertigo, visual disturbances. Pharmacokinetics Readily absorbed orally; approximately 75% protein bound; hepatic metabolism; renal excretion.	Contraindications Hypersensitivity to quinine; glucose-6-phosphate dehydrogenase (G-6-PD) deficiency; optic neuritis; tinnitus; pregnancy. Pregnancy Category: X Lactation Issues Excreted in small amounts in breast milk; rule out G-6-PD deficiency in infant prior to quinine use in nursing mother.
Sulfadoxine and Pyrimethamine Fansidar	**Antimalarial spectrum** Chloroquine-resistant strains of *P. falciparum.*	Administration Issues Complete full course of therapy; take with food to avoid GI upset.	ADRs **Fatalities associated with the administration of sulfadoxine and pyrimethamine**	Contraindications Hypersensitivity to sulfonamides or pyrimethamine; documented mega

(continues on next page)

104. Antimalarials *continued from previous page*

Drug and Dosage Forms	Spectrum of Activity and Usual Dosage Range	Administration Issues and Drug–Drug & Drug–Food Interactions	Common Adverse Drug Reactions (ADRs) and Pharmacokinetics	Contraindications, Pregnancy Category, and Lactation Issues
Sulfadoxine and Pyrimethamine *cont.* Tablet: 500 mg sulfadoxine plus 25 mg pyrimethamine	**Treatment of malaria** **Adults and children > 45 kg:** 3 tablets orally as a single dose **Children:** **31–45 kg** - 2 tablets as a single dose **21–30 kg** - 1 and ½ tablet as a single dose **11–20 kg** - 1 tablet as a single dose **5–10 kg** - ½ tablet as a single dose **Continue weekly chloroquine prophylaxis after treatment with sulfadoxine/pyrimethamine**. **Suppression of malaria** **Adults:** 1 tablet at least 1–2 d prior to entering endemic area, followed by 1 tablet weekly, continuing for 4–6 weeks after leaving the endemic area **Children 9–14 yr.:** ¾ tablet at least 1–2 d prior to entering endemic area, followed by ¾ tablet weekly, continuing for 4–6 weeks after leaving the endemic area **Children 4–8 yr.:** ½ tablet at least 1–2 d prior to entering endemic area, followed by ½ tablet weekly, continuing for 4–6 weeks after leaving the endemic area **Children < 4 yr.:** ¼ tablet at least 1–2 days prior to entering endemic area, followed by ¼ tablet weekly, continuing for 4–6 weeks after leaving the endemic area	Drug–Drug Interactions Concomitant use of pyrimethamine and **methotrexate, sulfonamides, or TMP-SMZ** may increase risk of folate deficiency and bone marrow suppression. Sulfadoxine/pyrimethamine may decrease the effectiveness of **oral contraceptives**.	**have occurred because of severe reactions. Discontinue drug at first appearence of a skin rash, reduction in blood counts, or occurence of infection** Nausea, vomiting, anemia, photosensitivity. Pharmacokinetics $T_{1/2}$ mean for sulfadoxine is 169 h and pyrimethamine is 111 h; renal excretion.	loblastic anemia; infants < 2 yr.; pregnancy at term and nursing. Pregnancy Category: C Lactation Issues Both drugs are excreted in breast milk; discontinue use during nursing.

105. Antituberculosis Agents

Drug and Dosage Forms	Spectrum of Activity and Usual Dosage Range	Administration Issues and Drug—Drug & Drug—Food Interactions	Common Adverse Drug Reactions (ADRs) and Pharmacokinetics	Contraindications, Pregnancy Category, and Lactation Issues
Aminosalicylate Sodium Paser Granules, delayed-release: 4g	**Antimycobacterial spectrum** *Mycobacterium tuberculosis.* **Treatment of tuberculosis in combination with other agents** **Adults:** 1 packet tid **For multidrug resistant tuberculosis, continue combination drug therapy for 9 months or 6 months after sputum cultures are negative, whichever is longer.**	Administration Issues Complete full course of therapy with strict compliance; do not use if packet is swollen or the granules have lost their tan color. Advise pts that first signs of hypersensitivity include rash and fever. If symptoms develop, stop medication and call healthcare provider. Sprinkle granules on acidic foods or suspend them in a fruit drink. Skeleton of the granules may be seen in the stool. Drug–Drug Interactions Aminosalicylate sodium may decrease the GI absorption of **vitamin B_{12}** Absorption of digoxin may be reduced when given concomitantly.	ADRs Nausea, vomiting, GI upset, diarrhea, hypersensitivity. Pharmacokinetics > 80% excreted by the kidneys.	Contraindications Hypersensitivity to drug, severe renal disease Pregnancy Category: C Lactation Issues Excreted in breast milk
Clofazimine Lamprene Capsules 50 mg, 100 mg	**Antibacterial spectrum** *Mycobacterium avium-intracelllulare* (MAC). **Treatment of MAC** 100 mg qd to tid	Administration Issues Complete full course of therapy; take with food; reversible red to brownish black skin discoloration may occur.	ADRs Pigmentation changes, rash, dryness, abdominal distress, diarrhea, nausea. Pharmacokinetics Highly lipophilic and deposits in fatty tissue; $T_{1/2}$ after repeated dosing is 70 days.	Pregnancy Category: C Lactation Issues Excreted in breast milk, do not use in nursing mothers unless clearly indicated.
Cycloserine Seromycin Pulvules Capsule: 250 mg	**Antimycobacterial spectrum** *Mycobacterium tuberculosis.* **Treatment of tuberculosis in combination with other agents.** **Adults:** Initially, 250 mg q 12 h for 2 weeks increasing up to 1 gm/d in 1 to 3 divided doses; maintain blood concentrations < 30 mcg/ml **Children:** 10–20 mg/kg/d up to max of 1 gm/d in 2 divided doses	Administration Issues Complete full course of therapy with strict compliance; avoid concurrent alcohol use; may cause drowsiness. **Administration of pyridoxine (VitB_6)** 100–300 mg/day is recommended to avoid neurotoxic side effects. Drug–Drug Interactions Concurrent **alcohol** use with cycloserine may increase the potential for epileptic episodes. **Isoniazid** may increase cycloserine CNS side effects, such as dizziness. Cycloserine may increase the effect of **phenytoin** leading to toxicity.	ADRs Drowsiness, headache, depression, seizures. Pharmacokinetics Widely distributes into body fluids with cerebrospinal fluids similar to plasma concentrations; 35% of dose is metabolized hepatically; renal excretion.	Contraindications Hypersensitivity to cycloserine; epilepsy; depression; severe anxiety or psychosis; severe renal insufficiency; excessive concurrent alcohol use. Pregnancy Category: C Lactation Issues Because of potential for serious adverse events in infants, decided whether to discontinue nursing or discontinue the drug.

(continues on next page)

105. Antituberculosis Agents *continued from previous page*

Drug and Dosage Forms	Spectrum of Activity and Usual Dosage Range	Administration Issues and Drug—Drug & Drug—Food Interactions	Common Adverse Drug Reactions (ADRs) and Pharmacokinetics	Contraindications, Pregnancy Category, and Lactation Issues
Cycloserine *cont.*	**For multidrug resistant tuberculosis, continue combination drug therapy for 9 months or 6 months after sputum cultures are negative, whichever is longer.**			
Ethambutol Myambutol Tablet: 100 mg, 400 mg	**Antimycobacterial spectrum** *Mycobacterium tuberculosis.* **Initial treatment of tuberculosis in combination with other agents** **Adults:** 15–25 mg/kg/d as a single dose (max. 2.5 gm) **Children:** 15–25 mg/kg/d as a single dose (max 2.5 gm) **Twice weekly TB regimen** **Adults:** 50 mg/kg (max 2.5 gm/dose) **Children:** 50 mg/kg (max 2.5 gm/dose) **Three times/week TB regimen** **Adults:** 25–30 mg/kg (max 2.5 gm/dose) **Children:** 25–30 mg/kg (max 2.5 gm/dose) **Not recommended for use in children < 13 yr.** **Retreatment of tuberculosis in combination with other agents** **Adults:** 25 mg/kg/d as a single dose, after 60 d, decrease dose to 15 mg/kg/d as a single dose	Administration Issues Complete full course of therapy with strict compliance; take with food if GI upset occurs; notify your physician, nurse, or pharmacist if visual changes occur. Ethambutol not recommended for children whose visual acuity cannot be monitored (<6 yr). Monthly eye exams are recommended with a 25 mg/kg/d dose Drug—Drug Interactions Aluminum salts (antacids, sucralfate) may decrease the absorption of ethambutol.	ADRs Visual changes, rash, nausea, vomiting, headache, dizziness. Pharmacokinetics Absorption unaffected by food; cerebrospinal fluid concentrations are 10%–50% of serum concentrations; approximately 20% of a dose is metabolized in the liver; predominately excreted renally, some fecal excretion.	Contraindications Hypersensitivity to ethambutol; known optic neuritis, unless clinical judgment determines that it may be used. Pregnancy The effect of ethambutol in combination with other agents on the fetus is unknown; administration to pregnant women has produced no detectable effect upon the fetus; use only when clearly needed and when the potential benefits outweigh potential hazards to the fetus.

	For multidrug resistant tuberculosis, continue combination drug therapy for 9 months or 6 months after sputum cultures are negative, whichever is longer.			
Ethionamide Trecator-SC Tablet: 250 mg	**Antimycobacterial Spectrum** *Mycobacterium tuberculosis* **Treatment of tuberculosis in combination with other agents** **Adults:** 15–20 mg/kg/d taken qd up to a max of 1 gm/d **Children:** 10–20 mg/kg/d divided bid to tid up to max of 1 gm or 15 mg/kg/24 hrs as a single daily dose **For multidrug resistant tuberculosis, continue combination drug therapy for 9 months or 6 months after sputum cultures are negative, whichever is longer.**	Administration Issues Complete full course of therapy with strict compliance; may take with food if GI upset occurs; metallic taste may occur. **Administration of pyridoxine (VitB$_6$)** 25–50 mg daily is recommended to avoid ethionamide-associated peripheral neuropathy.	ADRs Nausea, vomiting, GI upset, diarrhea, depression, drowsiness, asthenia. Pharmacokinetics $T_{1/2}$ is approximately 3 h; widely distributes into body fluids including cerebrospinal fluid; hepatic metabolism; renal excretion.	Contraindications Hypersensitivity to ethionamide; severe hepatic disease. Pregnancy Teratogenic effects have been demonstrated in animals receiving doses in excess of recommended human doses; use only when clearly needed and when the potential benefits outweigh potential hazards to the fetus. Lactation Issues Excretion in breast milk is unknown; use with caution in nursing mothers.
Isoniazid Laniazid, various generics Tablet: 50 mg, 100 mg, 300 mg Syrup: 50 mg/5 mL	**Antimycobacterial spectrum** *Mycobacterium tuberculosis.* **Treatment of tuberculosis in combination with other agents** **Adults:** 5 mg/kg/d as a single dose (max. 300 mg/d) **Children and infants:** 10–20 mg/kg/d as a single dose (max. of 300 mg/d) **Twice weekly TB regimen** **Adults:** 15 mg/kg, max 900 mg/dose **Children:** 20–40 mg/kg; max 900 mg/dose	Administration Issues Complete full course of therapy with strict compliance; take on an empty stomach; minimize daily alcohol use with isoniazid. **Administration of pyridoxine (VitB$_6$)** 25–50 mg daily is recommended to avoid isoniazid-associated peripheral neuropathy. Drug—Drug Interactions **Alcohol** increases the risk of isoniazid-induced hepatitis. Isoniazid may increase the effect of the following drugs leading to toxicity: **carbamazepine, phenytoin, warfarin, benzodiazepines**. Concomitant use of isoniazid and **ketoconazole** may lead to decreased serum levels of ketoconazole and antifungal treatment failure. Concomitant use of isoniazid and **cycloserine** may lead to increased cycloserine associated CNS toxicity.	ADRs **Severe and sometimes fatal hepatitis associated with INH therapy may occur or develop even after many months of therapy. Carefully moniter LFTs and interview patients regularly to assess for signs and symptoms of liver damage.** Peripheral neuropathy, (numbness and tingling of extremities), nausea, vomiting, GI upset, severe and sometimes fatal hepatitis. Pharmacokinetics Decreased oral absorption with food; distributes readily into cerebrospinal fluid; metabolized hepatic by acetylation; renal excretion.	Contraindications Patients with previous isoniazid-associated hepatic injury; hypersensitivity to isoniazid. Pregnancy Category: C Lactation Issues Excreted in breast milk; use with caution in nursing mothers.

(*continues on next page*)

105. Antituberculosis Agents *continued from previous page*

Drug and Dosage Forms	Spectrum of Activity and Usual Dosage Range	Administration Issues and Drug—Drug & Drug—Food Interactions	Common Adverse Drug Reactions (ADRs) and Pharmacokinetics	Contraindications, Pregnancy Category, and Lactation Issues
Isoniazid *cont.*	**Three times/week TB regimen:** **Adults:** 15 mg/kg; max 900 mg/dose **Children:** 20–40 mg/kg; max 900 mg/dose **Prevention of tuberculosis** **Adults:** 300 mg/d as a single dose **Children and infants:** 10 mg/kg/d as a single dose up to a max of 300 mg/d **Continue isoniazid therapy in combination with rifampin for 6 months with pyrazinamide for the first 2 months only. For multidrug resistant tuberculosis, continue combination drug therapy for 9 months or 6 months after sputum cultures are negative, whichever is longer.**			
Isoniazid and Rifampin Combination Capsule: Rifamate (150 mg isoniazid/300 mg rifampin) Tablets: Rifater (50 mg INH, 120 mg rifampin, 300 mg pyrazinamide)	**Antimicrobial spectrum** Isoniazid: *M. tuberculosis* Pyrazinamide: *M. tuberculosis* Rifampin: *M. tuberculosis, N. meningitidis, H. influenzae, S. aureus, S. epidermidis* **Treatment of tuberculosis in combination with other agents** 2 Rifamate capsules daily as a single dose *or* Rifater (Adults) 4 tablets once a day (if ≤ 97 lbs) 5 tablets once a day (if 98–120 lbs) 6 tablets once a day (≤ 121 lbs) **Continue combination therapy for 6 months with pyrazinamide for the first 2 months only. For multi-drug**	Administration Issues Complete full course of therapy with strict compliance; take on an empty stomach; may cause reddish-orange discoloration of the urine, stool, sweat, and tears; may permanently discolor contact lenses; minimize daily alcohol use with isoniazid. Drug—Drug Interactions See isoniazid and rifampin.	ADRs See adverse events for isoniazid and rifampin. Pharmacokinetics Distributes readily into cerebrospinal fluid; extensive hepatic metabolism; renal excretion.	Contraindications Patients with previous isoniazid-associated hepatic injury; hypersensitivity to isoniazid; hypersensitivity to rifampin. Pregnancy Category: C Lactation Issues Excreted in breast milk; decide whether to discontinue nursing or discontinue the drug.

	resistant tuberculosis, continue combination drug therapy for 9 months or 6 months after sputum cultures are negative, whichever is longer.			
Pyrazinamide Tablet: 500 mg	**Antimycobacterial spectrum** *M. tuberculosis* **Treatment of tuberculosis in combination with other agents** **Adults:** 15–30 mg/kg once daily, (max. 2 gm/day) **Children:** 15–30 mg/kg once daily (max. 2 gm/d) **Twice weekly TB regimen** **Adults:** 50–70 mg/kg; max 4 gm/d **Children:** 50–70 mg/kg; max 4 gm/d **Three times/week TB regimen** **Adults:** 50–70 mg/kg; max 3 gm/d **Children:** 50–70 mg/kg; max 3 gm/d **Continue isoniazid/rifampin combination therapy for 6 months with pyrazinamide for the first 2 months only.**	Administration Issues Complete full course of therapy with strict compliance.	ADRs Fever, gout attack, nausea, vomiting, arthralgia. Pharmacokinetics $T_{1/2}$ is approximately 10 h; widely distributes into body tissues including cerebrospinal fluid.	Contraindications Severe hepatic damage; hypersensitivity to pyrazinamide; acute gout. Pregnancy Category: C Lactation Issues Excreted in breast milk; use with caution in nursing mothers.
Rifabutin Mycobutin Capsule: 150 mg	**Antimycobacterial spectrum** *M. avium*, *M. intracellulare*, and *M. tuberculosis.* **Prevention of disseminated Mycobacterium avium complex disease in HIV affected patients** 300 mg once daily or 150 mg bid with food if GI upset occurs.	Administration Issues Complete full course of therapy; administer with food if GI upset occurs; may cause reddish-orange discoloration of the urine, stool, sweat, and tears; may permanently discolor contact lenses. Drug—Drug Interactions Rifabutin has less hepatic enzyme inducing capabilities compared to rifampin.	ADRs Rash, GI upset, anemia, leukopenia, neutropenia. Pharmacokinetics $T_{1/2}$ approximately 45 h; distributes readily into body tissues; hepatic metabolism; fecal and renal excretion; pharmacokinetic parameters may be variable in	Contraindications Hypersensitivity to rifabutin or rifampin. Pregnancy Category: B Lactation Issues Excretion in breast milk is unknown; because of potential for serious adverse events in infants, decide whether to discontinue nursing or discontinue the drug.

(*continues on next page*)

105. Antituberculosis Agents *continued from previous page*

Drug and Dosage Forms	Spectrum of Activity and Usual Dosage Range	Administration Issues and Drug—Drug & Drug—Food Interactions	Common Adverse Drug Reactions (ADRs) and Pharmacokinetics	Contraindications, Pregnancy Category, and Lactation Issues
Rifabutin *cont.*		The significance of potential drug interactions similar to rifampin is unknown. Rifabutin may decrease the serum level of **zidovudine**. Rifabutin may decrease the effectiveness of **oral contraceptives**.	symptomatic HIV patients compared to healthy volunteers.	
Rifampin Rifadin, generics <u>Capsule:</u> 150 mg, 300 mg	**<u>Antimicrobial spectrum</u>** *M. tuberculosis, N. meningitidis, H. influenzae, S. aureus, S. epidermidis.* **<u>Treatment of tuberculosis in combination with other agents</u>** **Adults:** 10 mg/kg/d as a single dose (max. 600 mg/d) **Children/infants:** 10–20 mg/kg/d as a single dose (max. 600 mg/d) **<u>Twice weekly TB regimen</u>** **Adults:** 10 mg/kg, max 600 mg/d **Children:** 10–20 mg/kg; max 600 mg/d **<u>Three times/week TB regimen</u>** **Adults:** 10 mg/kg; max 600 mg/d **Children:** 10–20 mg/kg; max 600 mg/d **Continue rifampin therapy in combination with isoniazid for 6 months with pyrazinamide for the first 2 months only.** **For multidrug resistant tuberculosis, continue combination drug therapy for 9 months or 6 months after sputum cultures are negative, whichever is longer.**	<u>Administration Issues</u> Complete full course of therapy with strict compliance; take on an empty stomach; may cause reddish-orange discoloration of the urine, stool, sweat, and tears; may permanently discolor contact lenses. <u>Drug—Drug Interactions</u> Rifampin is a potent inducer of hepatic metabolism and may decrease the effectiveness of the following drugs: **benzodiazepines, beta-blockers, oral contraceptives, corticosteroids, cyclosporine, phenytoin, carbamazepine, quinidine, sulfonylureas, theophylline, digoxin, ketoconazole, warfarin**. An extemporaneous oral suspension may be prepared by: 1. emptying the contents of 4 rifampin 300 mg capsules into a 4 oz. amber bottle 2. adding 20 ml of simple syrup 3. shaking vigorously 4. adding 100 ml simple syrup, shaking again The suspension is stable for 4 weeks at room temperature or in the refrigerator.	<u>ADRs</u> Flu-like symptoms (fever, chills, malaise), nausea, vomiting, GI upset, rash. <u>Pharmacokinetics</u> Food decreases oral absorption; distributes readily into cerebrospinal fluid; metabolized hepatically by deacetylation; renal excretion.	<u>Contraindications</u> Hypersensitivity to rifampin. <u>Pregnancy Category: C</u> <u>Lactation Issues</u> Excreted in breast milk; decide whether to discontinue nursing or discontinue the drug.

Rifampin cont.	**Contact with invasive *Haemophilus influenzae*** **Adults:** 600 mg qd as a single dose for 4 consecutive days **Children:** 10–20 mg/kg/d as a single dose to a max of 600 mg/d for 4 consecutive days **Close contact—meningococcal exposure** **Adults:** 600 mg q 12 h for 4 doses **Children:** 10 mg/kg q 12 h for 4 doses **Eradicate nasal carriage of *S. aureus*** 600 mg once daily with dicloxacillin 500 mg four times daily or SMZ-TMP DS one tablet twice daily for 10 d			
Streptomycin Cake, lypholized: 1 g	**Antimicrobial spectrum** *M. tuberculosis, N. meningitidis, H. influenzae, S. aureus, S. epidermidis.* **Treatment of tuberculosis in combination with other agents** **Adults:** 15 mg/kg qd, max 1 gm streptomycin combined with appropriate additional antitubercular drugs **Children:** 20–40 mg/kg/d (max. 1 g) **Twice weekly TB regimen** **Adults:** 25–30 mg/kg, max 1.5 gm IM **Children:** 25–30 mg/kg; max 1.5 gm IM **Three times/week TB regimen** **Adults:** 25–30 mg/kg, max 1 gm IM **Children:** 25–30 mg/kg; max 1 gm IM	Administration Issues Complete full course of therapy with strict compliance. Elderly patients should have a smaller daily dose of streptomycin. Drug is usually administered as a single daily IM dose. Patient should report any unusual symptoms of hearing loss, dizziness, roaring noises or fullness in ear. Drug Interactions **Streptomycin** may increase or prolong the effects of depolarizing and nondepolarizing neuromuscular blocking agents. Increased nephrotoxicity may occur with concurrent use of **amphotericin** and **loop diuretics**.	ADRs **Risk of neurotoxic reactions is sharply increased in patients with impaired renal function or prerenal azotenia. Monitor renal function carefully. Ototoxicity (auditory and vestibular), nephrotoxicity, nausea, vomiting, headache, tremor, weakness.** Pharmacokinetics Almost completely excreted as unchanged drug in urine; no metabolism.	Contraindications Hypersensitivity to aminoglycosides. Use with Caution: In patients with pre-existing vertigo, hearing loss, neuromuscular disorders. Pregnancy Category: There are reports of total irreversible bilateral congenital deafness in children whose mother received streptomycin during pregnancy. Lactation Issues Excreted in breast milk; decide whether to discontinue nursing or discontinue the drug.

106. Antiviral Agents

106.1 Agents for Herpes simplex and Herpes zoster

Drug and Dosage Forms	Spectrum of Activity and Usual Dosage Range	Administration Issues and Drug–Drug & Drug–Food Interactions	Common Adverse Drug Reactions (ADRs) and Pharmacokinetics	Contraindications, Pregnancy Category, and Lactation Issues
Acyclovir Zovirax Tablet: 400 mg, 800 mg Capsule: 200 mg Suspension: 200 mg/5 ml	**Antiviral spectrum** Herpes simplex virus type 1 (HSV-1), herpes simplex virus type 2 (HSV-2), varicella-zoster virus (VZV), Epstein-Barr virus, and cytomegalovirus (CMV) **Treatment of initial genital herpes episode** 200 mg q 4 h while awake for 5 doses/day × 10 d **or** 400 mg tid × 10 d **Chronic suppressive therapy for recurrent genital herpes** 400 mg bid for up to 12 months followed by reevaluation; alternative regimens include 200 mg 3 to 5 times daily **Intermittent therapy for genital herpes** 200 mg q 4 h while awake for 5 doses/d for 5 d **or** 400 mg tid for 5 d **or** 800 mg bid for 5 d; initiate therapy at the earliest sign or symptom of recurrence **Treatment of acute herpes zoster attack** 800 mg q 4 h for 5 doses/d for 7 to 10 d **Treatment of chickenpox** 20 mg/kg (not to exceed 800 mg) qid × 5 d **Dosage reduction is recommended for patients with renal insufficiency.**	Administration Issues Complete full course of therapy; acyclovir is not a cure for HSV; may take without regard to meals; avoid sexual intercourse when visible herpes lesions are present. Drug–Drug Interactions Concurrent acyclovir and **zidovudine** use may increase the potential for severe drowsiness and lethargy. The clearance of acyclovir may be decreased and half-life increased by **probenecid**.	ADRs Nausea, vomiting. Pharmacokinetics Low oral bioavailability that decreases with increasing doses; absorption unaffected by food; widely distributes into body fluids and tissues including cerebrospinal fluid; primarily eliminated as unchanged drug by the kidneys.	Contraindications Hypersensitivity to acyclovir. Pregnancy Category: C Lactation Issues Excreted in breast milk, use with caution in nursing mothers.
Famciclovir Famvir Tablet: 125 mg, 250 mg, 500 mg	**Antiviral Spectrum** Herpes simplex virus type 1 (HSV-1), herpes simplex virus type 2 (HSV-2), varicella-zoster virus (VZV) **Treatment of acute herpes zoster (shingles)**	Administration Issues Complete full course of therapy; may take without regard to meals. Patients should begin therapy as soon as herpes zoster is diagnosed.	ADRs Headache, nausea, fatigue. Pharmacokinetics Transformed to active compound penciclovir; $T_{1/2}$ is approximately 2 h; metabolism is extrahepatic; 70%–90% renal excreted.	Contraindications Hypersensitivity to famciclovir. Pregnancy Category: B Lactation Issues Excreted in breast milk of lactating rats in concentrations higher than serum

	500 mg q 8 h × 7 d; begin treatment promptly as soon as herpes zoster is diagnosed; most effective when therapy is started within 48 h of the onset of zoster rash **Treatment of initial genital herpes episode** 250 mg tid for 7–10 d **Chronic suppressive therapy for recurrent genital herpes** 250 mg bid for up to 12 months followed by reevaluation **Genital herpes (recurrent episodes)** 125 mg bid for 5 days. Initiate therapy at first signs/symptoms **Dosage reduction is recommended for patients with renal insufficiency.**	Drug–Drug Interactions **Probenecid** may decrease the renal excretion of famciclovir. **Digoxin** plasma levels may be increased by famciclovir.		famciclovir concentrations; excretion in human breast milk is unknown; because of potential for tumorigenicity in rats, one must decide whether to discontinue the drug or discontinue nursing, taking into account the drug's importance to the mother.
Valacyclovir Valtrex Tablet: 500 mg, 1 gm	**Antiviral spectrum** Herpes simplex virus type 1 (HSV-1), herpes simplex virus type 2 (HSV-2), varicella-zoster virus (VZV). **Treatment of acute herpes zoster (shingles)** 1 gm q 8 h × 7 d; begin treatment promptly as soon as herpes zoster is diagnosed; most effective when therapy is started within 48 h of the onset of zoster rash **Treatment of initial genital herpes episode** 1 gm bid for 7–10 d **Chronic suppressive therapy for recurrent genital herpes** 1 gm qd or 500 mg qd in patients with a history of 9 or fewer recurrences per year. **Recurrent genital herpes** 500 mg bid × 3 d; initiate therapy at the first signs/symptoms of herpes **Dosage reduction is recommended for patients with renal insufficiency.**	Administration Issues Complete full course of therapy; may take without regard to meals. Drug–Drug Interactions **Probenecid and cimetidine** may decrease the renal excretion of valacyclovir.	ADRs Nausea. Pharmacokinetics Transformed to active compound acyclovir; $T_{1/2}$ is approximately 2 to 3 h; limited hepatic metabolism; primarily excreted renally with some fecal excretion.	Contraindications Hypersensitivity to valacyclovir or acyclovir. Pregnancy Category: B Lactation Issues Excretion of valacyclovir in human breast milk is unknown; use with caution in nursing mothers; consider temporary discontinuation of breastfeeding.

106.2 Nucleoside and Nucleotide Reverse Transcriptase Inhibitors

Drug and Dosage Forms	Spectrum of Activity and Usual Dosage Range	Administration Issues and Drug–Drug & Drug–Food Interactions	Common Adverse Drug Reactions (ADRs) and Pharmacokinetics	Contraindications, Pregnancy Category, and Lactation Issues
Abacavir Ziagen Tablet: 300 mg Oral solution: 20 mg/mL	**HIV infection: In combination with other antiretroviral agents for the treatment of human immunodeficiency virus type 1 (HIV-1) infection.** **Adults:** 300 mg bid in combination with other antiretroviral agents **Children (3 months to up to 16 years of age):** 8 mg/kg bid (up to a max. of 300 mg twice daily) in combination with other antiretroviral agents	Administration Issues Dispense the Medication Guide and Warning Card that provide information about recognition of hypersensitivity reactions with each new prescription and refill. Abacavir may be taken with or without food. Systemic exposure to abacavir was comparable after administration of oral solution and tablets. Therefore, these products may be used interchangeably. **Advise patients of the possibility of a hypersensitivity reaction to abacavir that may result in death. Instruct patients to discontinue abacavir and seek medical evaluation immediately if they develop signs or symptoms of hypersensitivity instruct patients not to reintroduce abacavir without medical consultation and to undertake reintroduction of abacavir only if medical care can be readily accessed by the patient or others.** Drug Interactions **Ethanol:** Ethanol decreases the elimination of abacavir, causing an increase in overall exposure because of their common metabolic pathway. **Methadone:** Coadministration increased oral methadone clearance by 22% (90% CI 6% to 42%). This alteration will not result in a methadone dose modification in the majority of patients; however, an increased methadone dose may be required in a small number of patients.	ADRs/Lab Abnormalities **Fatal hypersensitivity reaction (see below)**, nausea, diarrhea, vomiting, insomnia, asthenia, headache, elevations in creatine kinase and serum amylase, hypertriglyceridemia. **Lactic acidosis/severe hepatomegaly with steatosis:** Lactic acidosis and severe hepatomegaly with steatosis, including fatal cases, have been reported with the use of nucleoside analogs alone or in combination with other antiretrovirals. **Hypersensitivity reactions:** Fatal hypersensitivity reactions have been associated with abacavir therapy. Discontinue abacavir in patients developing signs or symptoms of hypersensitivity (e.g., fever, rash, fatigue; GI symptoms such as nausea, vomiting, diarrhea, abdominal pain; respiratory symptoms such as pharyngitis, dyspnea, cough) as soon as a hypersensitivity reaction is first suspected; seek medical evaluation immediately. Pharmacokinetics Abacavir is rapidly and extensively absorbed after oral administration. The mean absolute bioavailability of the tablet is 83%.	Contraindications Hypersensitivity to any of the components of the product. **If symptoms of hypersensitivity develop, stop the medication and do not restart**. Pregnancy Category: C Lactation Issues: The Centers for Disease Control and Prevention recommend that HIV-infected mothers not breastfeed their infants to avoid risking postnatal transmission of HIV infection.
Didanosine (ddI) Videx, Videt EC	**Treatment of HIV Infection** Chewable tablets: **Adults/Adolescents ≥ 60 kg:**	Administration Issues Take on an empty stomach; do not share medication; do not exceed recommended	ADRs Peripheral neuropathy, pancreatitis, diarrhea, nausea.	Contraindications Hypersensitivity to didanosine or other components of the product.

Tablet, buffered, chewable: 25 mg, 50 mg, 100 mg, 150 mg, 200 mg Powder for Oral solution, buffered 100 mg, 167 mg, 250 mg, 375 mg Powder for Oral solution, Pediatric must be mixed with an antacid before dispensing; final concentration = 10 mg/ml Capsules, delayed release: 125 mg, 200 mg, 250 mg, 400 mg	200 mg bid or 400 mg qd (2 & 200 mg) **Adults/Adolescents < 60 kg:** 125 mg bid or 250 mg qd **Children:** 120 mg/m^2 bid **Take 2 tablets at each dose to ensure adequate gastric pH buffering; children < 1 year may use 1 tablet at each dose.** Powder **Adults/Adolescents ≥ 60 kg:** 250 mg bid **Adults/Adolescents < 60 kg:** 167 mg bid **Children:** 120 mg/m^2 bid Videx EC (Adults) ≥ 60 kg: 400 mg qd < 60 kg: 250 mg qd	dose; take 2 tablets at each dose; chew tablets thoroughly; tablets may be manually crushed prior to administration or dispersed in at least 1 ounce of water; after mixing oral solution, drink entire liquid immediately; shake pediatric solution well prior to administration; pediatric solution is stable for 30 days in the refrigerator Capsules should be take on an empty stomach and swallowed infact. Drug–Drug Interactions Didanosine may decrease GI absorption of **itraconazole, ketoconazole, dapsone, fluoroquinolones**, and **tetracyclines**; separate dosing by at least 2 h. Separate the dosing of ddl and **delavirdine** and **protease inhibitors** by at least 2 h. Concomitant use of ddl with the following drugs may increase the risk of peripheral neuropathy: **dapsone, zalcitabine, ethionamide, hydralazine, isoniazid, metronidazole, nitrofurantoin, phenytoin**. Drug–Food Interactions: Administration with food decreases ddl absorption by as much as 50%; take ddl on an empty stomach (1 h before or 2 h after meal).	Pharmacokinetics Rapidly degraded at acidic pH, all oral formulations contain buffering agents to increase gastric pH; food decreases oral absorption; renal elimination by filtration and secretion. Warning **Fatal and nonfatal pancreatitis has occurred during therapy with ddl. Fatal lactic acidosis has been reported in patients receiving the combination of ddl and stavudine. Dose modification is needed with renal impairment.**	Pregnancy Category: B Lactation Issues Excretion in breast milk is unknown; HIV infected females should not breastfeed to avoid postnatal transmission of HIV to a child who may not be infected.
Emtricitabine Emtriva Capsules: 200 mg	**HIV infection: In combination with other antiretroviral agents for the treatment of human immunodeficiency virus type 1 (HIV-1) infection.** **Adults:** 200 mg qd in combination with other antiretroviral agents. **Renal function impairment:** The dosing interval of emtricitabine should be adjusted in patients with baseline creatinine clearance less than 50 mL/min. See package labeling for dosing guidelines.	Administration Issues May be taken with or without food. Drug Interactions None reported	ADRs/Lab Abnormalities: Headache, diarrhea, nausea, rash **Lactic acidosis/severe hepatomegaly with steatosis:** Lactic acidosis and severe hepatomegaly with steatosis, including fatal cases, have been reported with the use of nucleoside analogs alone or in combination with other antiretrovirals. Pharmacokinetics Emtricitabine is rapidly and extensively absorbed following oral administration with peak plasma concentrations occurring at 1 to 2 hours postdose.	Contraindications Hypersensitivity to any of the components of the product Pregnancy Category: B Lactation Issues: The Centers for Disease Control and Prevention recommend that HIV-infected mothers not breastfeed their infants to avoid risking postnatal transmission of HIV infection.

(continues on next page)

106.2 Nucleoside and Nucleotide Reverse Transcriptase Inhibitors *continued from previous page*

Drug and Dosage Forms	Spectrum of Activity and Usual Dosage Range	Administration Issues and Drug–Drug & Drug–Food Interactions	Common Adverse Drug Reactions (ADRs) and Pharmacokinetics	Contraindications, Pregnancy Category, and Lactation Issues
Lamivudine (3TC) Epivir Tablet: 150 mg, 300 mg Solution: 5 mg/ml, 10 mg/ml Combination tablet: *Combivir:* 150 mg, lamivudine plus 300 mg zidovudine *Trizivir:* 150 mg lamivudine, 300 mg zidovudine, 300 mg abacavir	**Treatment of HIV Infection** **Adults/children > 12 yr.:** 150 mg bid or 300 mg qd For adults with low body weight (<50 kg), use 2 mg/kg bid **Children 3 months to 12 yr.:** 4 mg/kg bid **Combivir:** 1 tablet bid **Trizivir:** 1 tablet bid	Administration Issues May take without regard to meals; do not share medication; do not exceed recommended dose; oral solution may be stored in the refrigerator or at room temperature. Pharmacokinetics: **TMP/SMX** may increase lamivudine blood levels. Lamivudine may increase **zidovudine** blood levels.	ADRs Headache, pancreatitis (higher incidence in children), rash, abdominal pain, increased LFTs. **Abacavir has been associated with fatal hypersensitivity reactions (see abacavir section).** Pharmacokinetics Rapid GI absorption; limited metabolism; primarily excreted renally as unchanged drug. **Fatal lactic acidosis has been reported.** **Dosage reduction is recommended for patients with renal insufficiency.**	Contraindications Hypersensitivity to lamivudine. Pregnancy Category: C Lactation Issues Excretion in breast milk is unknown; HIV infected females should not breastfeed to avoid postnatal transmission of HIV to a child who may not be infected.
Stavudine (d4T) Zerit, Zerit XR Capsule: 15 mg, 20 mg, 30 mg, 40 mg Zerit XR capsules, extended-release 37.5 mg, 50 mg, 75 mg, 100 mg Solution: 1 mg/ml	**Treatment of HIV Infection** **Adults/Adolescents ≥ 60 kg:** 40 mg bid **Adults/Adolescents < 60 kg** 30 mg bid **Pediatric Dose:** 1 mg/kg bid (up to 30 kg) Extended-release capsules Adults ≥ 60 kg: give 100 mg qd Adults < 60 kg: give 75 mg qd Children: XR capsules have not been studied in children	Administration Issues May take without regard to meals. **Temporarily discontinue stavudine therapy if peripheral neuropathy (tingling, numbness, pain of hands or feet) develops; if symptoms resolve completely, resume therapy at one-half the treatment dose based on patient kg weight.**	ADRs Peripheral neuropathy (dose related), headache, diarrhea, skin rash. **Fatal lactic acidosis has been reported. Dosage reduction is recommended for patients with renal insufficiency.** Pharmacokinetics: Rapid absorption; $T_{1/2}$ is approximately 1 to 1.5 h.	Contraindications Hypersensitivity to stavudine. Pregnancy Category: C Lactation Issues Excretion in human breast milk is unknown; HIV infected females should not breastfeed to avoid postnatal transmission of HIV to a child who may not be infected.
Tenofovir Viread Tablet: 300 mg	**HIV infection: In combination with other antiretroviral agents for the treatment of human immunodeficiency virus type 1 (HIV-1) infection.** 300 mg once daily taken orally with a meal. **Renal function impairment:** Do not administer tenofovir to patients with renal insufficiency (Ccr < 60	Administration Issues When administered with didanosine, give tenofovir 2 h before or 1 h after didanosine administration. Instruct patients not to breastfeed if they are taking tenofovir. Take tenofovir with a meal. The most common side effects of tenofovir are diarrhea, nausea, vomiting, and flatulence.	ADRs/Lab Abnormalities Nausea, diarrhea, vomiting, and flatulence, asthenia, headache, elevations in creatine kinase and serum amylase, hypertriglyceridemia. **Lactic acidosis/severe hepatomegaly with steatosis:** Lactic acidosis and severe hepatomegaly with steatosis, including fatal cases, have	Contraindications Hypersensitivity to any of the components of the product. Pregnancy Category: B Lactation Issues The Centers for Disease Control and Prevention recommend that HIV-infected mothers not breastfeed their infants to

	mL/min) until data become available describing the disposition of tenofovir in these patients.	Drug Interactions When administered with tenofovir, C_{max} and AUC of **didanosine** (administered as the buffered formulation) increased by 28% and 44%, respectively. Monitor patients taking tenofovir and didanosine concomitantly for long-term didanosine-associated adverse events.	been reported with the use of nucleoside analogs alone or in combination with other antiretrovirals. Pharmacokinetics In vitro studies indicate that neither tenofovir disoproxil nor tenofovir are substrates of CYP450 enzymes.	avoid risking postnatal transmission of HIV infection.
Zalcitabine (ddC) Hivid Tablet: 0.375 mg, 0.75 mg Syrup: 0.1 mg/ml (investigational)	**Treatment of HIV infection** **Adults** 0.75 mg tid **Pediatric usual dose** 0.01 mg/kg q 8h (dosage range 0.005 to 0.01 mg/kg q 8h) **Temporarily discontinue zalcitabine therapy if peripheral neuropathy (tingling, numbness, pain of hands or feet) develops; if symptoms resolve completely, resume therapy at one-half the treatment dose based on patient kg weight.**	Administration Issues Take on an empty stomach; do not share medication; do not exceed recommended dose. Drug–Drug Interactions Concomitant administration of **aluminum/magnesium containing antacids** and **sucralfate** may decrease oral absorption of zalcitabine. Concomitant use of zalcitabine with the following drugs may increase the risk of peripheral neuropathy: **dapsone, didanosine, ethionamide, hydralazine, isoniazid, metronidazole, nitrofurantoin, phenytoin**. Clearance of zalcitabine may be decreased by: **probenecid, cimetidine, amphotericin, foscarnet and aminoglycosides**. Concomitant zalcitabine and **pentamidine** use may increase the risk of pancreatitis.	ADRs Peripheral neuropathy, fatigue, rash, stomatitis. **Fatal lactic acidosis has been reported.** **Dosage reduction is recommended for patients with renal insufficiency.** Pharmacokinetics Good GI tract absorption; food decreases oral absorption; no significant hepatic metabolism.	Contraindications Hypersensitivity to zalcitabine. Pregnancy Category: C Lactation Issues Excretion in breast milk is unknown; HIV infected females should not breastfeed to avoid postnatal transmission of HIV to a child who may not be infected.
Zidovudine (AZT, ZDV) Retrovir Capsule: 100 mg Tablet: 300 mg Syrup: 50 mg/5 ml	**Treatment of HIV infection** **Adults/Adolescents:** 200 mg tid or 300 mg bid **Children 6 weeks-12 yr.:** 160 mg/m^2 every 8 hours, not to exceed 200 mg q 8 h	Administration Issues May take without regard to meals; do not share medication; do not exceed recommended dose. Drug–Drug Interactions The following drugs may decrease zidovudine serum levels: **APAP, clarithromycin, rifampin**. The following drugs may increase zidovudine serum levels: **fluconazole, interferon beta-1b, probenecid, trimethoprim, phenytoin**. Concurrent use of zidovudine and **TMP-SMZ, ganciclovir,**	ADRs anemia, granulocytopenia, nausea, headache, fatigue confusion **Monitor hematologic indices (WBC, hemoglobin) q 2 weeks, discontinue therapy for severe anemia hemoglobin < 7.5 gm/dl or granulocytopenia WBC < 750/mm³ or reduction of > 50% from baseline.** Pharmacokinetics Rapid absorption in GI tract; hepatic metabolism; renal excretion.	Contraindications Hypersensitivity to zidovudine Pregnancy Category: C Lactation Issues Excretion in breast milk is unknown; HIV infected females should not breast feed to avoid postnatal transmission of HIV to a child who may not be infected.

(*continues on next page*)

106.2 Nucleoside and Nucleotide Reverse Transcriptase Inhibitors *continued from previous page*

Drug and Dosage Forms	Spectrum of Activity and Usual Dosage Range	Administration Issues and Drug–Drug & Drug–Food Interactions	Common Adverse Drug Reactions (ADRs) and Pharmacokinetics	Contraindications, Pregnancy Category, and Lactation Issues
Zidovudine (AZT, ZDV) ***cont.*** Combination tablet: Combivir: 150 mg lamivudine plus 300 mg zidovudine (see lamivudine for dosing) Trizivir: See lamivudine Section.		**flucytosine**, and **interferon alfa** may increase the risk of hematological toxicities such as anemia. **Ribavirin** may inhibit the activation of zidovudine. Concurrent zidovudine and **acyclovir** or **valacyclovir** use may increase the potential for severe drowsiness and lethargy.		

106.3 Non-nucleoside Reverse Transcriptase Inhibitors

Drug and Dosage Forms	Spectrum of Activity and Usual Dosage Range	Administration Issues and Drug–Drug & Drug–Food Interactions	Common Adverse Drug Reactions (ADRs) and Pharmacokinetics	Contraindications, Pregnancy Category, and Lactation Issues
Delavirdine (DLV) Rescriptor Tablet: 100 mg, 200 mg	**Treatment of HIV infection in combination with appropriate antiviral therapy** **Adults/adolescents:** 400 mg tid	Administration Issues May take with food; take 1 h before or 1 h after ddl or antacids; tablets can be dissolved in water and the resulting dispersion taken promptly; patients with achlorhydria should take delavirdine with an acidic beverage. Drug–Drug Interactions Coadministration of delavirdine with the following agents may result in potentially serious or life-threatening adverse events due to delavirdine being an inhibitor of CYP3A and CYP2C9 hepatic metabolism: **terfenadine, astemizole, clarithromycin, dapsone, rifabutin, benzodiazepines, cisapride, calcium channel blockers, ergot derivatives, protease inhibitors, quinidine, warfarin.** Delavirdine concentrations may be increased by the following drugs: fluoxetine, ketoconazole, The following drugs may decrease delavirdine concentrations: **antacids, anticonvulsants, rifampin, rifabutin, ddl.**	ADRs Headache, fatigue, GI complaints, rash (may be severe). Pharmacokinetics Rapidly absorbed.	Contraindications Hypersensitivity to delavirdine or other components of the product. Pregnancy Category: C Lactation Issues: HIV-infected females should not breast-feed to avoid postnatal transmission of HIV to a child who may not be infected.

Efavirenz Sustiva Capsules: 50 mg, 100 mg, 200 mg Tablets: 600 mg	**HIV infection** **In combination with other antiretroviral agents for the treatment of human immunodeficiency virus type 1 (HIV-1) infection.** **Adults:** The recommended dosage is 600 mg qd in combination with a protease inhibitor or nucleoside analog reverse transcriptase inhibitors (NRTIs). **Children:** It is recommended that efavirenz be taken on an empty stomach, preferably at bedtime. The recommended dose for pediatric patients ≥ 3 years of age and weighing between 10 and 40 kg (22 and 88 lbs) is: 10 to < 15 kg, give 200 mg qd 15 to < 20 kg, give 250 mg qd 20 to < 25 kg, give 300 mg qd 25 to < 32.5 kg, give 350 mg qd 32.5 to < 40 kg, give 400 mg qd ≥ 40 kg, give 600 mg qd	Administration Issues It is recommended that efavirenz be taken on an empty stomach, preferably at bedtime. The increased efavirenz concentration observed following administration of efavirenz with food may lead to an increase in frequency of adverse events. Efavirenz may interact with some drugs; therefore, advise patients to report the use of any prescription or nonprescription medication, as well as any natural product, particularly St. John's wort, to their healthcare provider. In order to improve the tolerability of nervous system side effects, bedtime dosing is recommended. Drug Interactions **P450 system:** Efavirenz induces CYP3A4 in vivo. Other compounds that are substrates of CYP3A4 may have decreased plasma concentrations when coadministered with efavirenz. Drugs that induce CYP3A4 activity (e.g., **phenobarbital, rifampin, rifabutin, St. John's wort**) would be expected to increase the clearance of efavirenz resulting in lowered plasma concentrations. Efavirenz may decrease the concentration of **saquinavir, amprenavir, indinavir, methadone, azoles, phenytoin, phenobarbital, carbamazepine**.	ADRs Rash, nausea, nervous system symptoms, and psychiatric symptoms including dizziness, insomnia, impaired concentration, somnolence abnormal dreams, and hallucinations. Pharmacokinetics Efavirenz has a terminal half-life of 52 to 76 h after single doses and 40 to 55 h after multiple doses.	Contraindications Hypersensitivity to any of the components of the product. Do not administer concurrently with cisapride, midazolam, triazolam, or ergot derivatives. Competition for CYP3A4 by efavirenz could result in inhibition of metabolism of these drugs and create the potential for serious or life-threatening adverse events (e.g., cardiac arrhythmias, prolonged sedation, respiratory depression). Pregnancy Category: C Lactation Issues The Centers for Disease Control and Prevention recommend that HIV-infected mothers not breastfeed their infants to avoid risking postnatal transmission of HIV infection. Instruct mothers not to breastfeed during efavirenz treatment.
Nevirapine (NPV) Viramune Tablet: 200 mg Suspension: 50 mg/5 mL	**Treatment of HIV infection in combination with appropriate antiviral therapy** **Adults/adolescents** Initial therapy: 200 mg qd × 14 d. If no rash or untoward effects, increase to maintenance therapy.	Administration Issues May be administered with food; may be given concurrently with ddI. Drug Interactions: Nevirapine concentrations may be decreased by **rifampin** and **rifabutin.** Nevirapine may decrease the concentrations of **protease inhibitors** and **oral contraceptives**.	ADRs Skin rash (may be severe), sedative effects, headache, diarrhea, nausea. Pharmacokinetics Well absorbed; extensively metabolized by the cytochrome P-450 system; half-life decreases over a 2–4 week period with chronic dosing due to autoinduction (i.e., $T_{1/2}$ initially 45 h and decreases to 23 h).	Contraindications Hypersensitivity to nevirapine. Pregnancy Category: C Lactation Issues HIV-infected females should not breastfeed to avoid postnatal transmission of HIV to a child who may not be infected.

(*continues on next page*)

106.3 Non-nucleoside Reverse Transcriptase Inhibitors *continued from previous page*

Drug and Dosage Forms	Spectrum of Activity and Usual Dosage Range	Administration Issues and Drug–Drug & Drug–Food Interactions	Common Adverse Drug Reactions (ADRs) and Pharmacokinetics	Contraindications, Pregnancy Category, and Lactation Issues
Nevirapine (NPV) ***cont.***	Maintenance: 200 mg bid in combination with nucleoside analog antiretroviral agents **Pediatric Dose** 2 months to 8 years: 4 mg/kg qd × 14 d followed by 7 mg/kg bid ≥ 8 *years*: 4 mg/kg qd × 14 d followed by 4 mg/kg bid **Total daily dose should not exceed 400 mg for any patient**.			

106.4 Protease Inhibitors

Drug and Dosage Forms	Spectrum of Activity and Usual Dosage Range	Administration Issues and Drug-Drug & Drug-Food Interactions	Common Adverse Drug Reactions (ADRs) and Pharmacokinetics	Contraindications, Pregnancy Category and Lactation Issues
Atazanavir Reyataz Capsules: 100 mg, 150 mg, 200 mg	**HIV infection:** **In combination with other antiretroviral agents for the treatment of HIV-1 infection.** Adults 400 mg (two 200 mg capsules) QD Concomitant therapy: When coadministered with 600 mg efavirenz, 300 mg atazanavir and 100 mg ritonavir be given with efavirenz	Administration Issues Take with food. Do not co administer atazanavir without ritonavir with efavirenz. When coadministered with didanosine buffered formulations, give atazanavir (with food) 2 hours before or 1 hour after didanosine. Atazanavir may interact with some drugs; therefore, advise patients to report to their doctor the use of any other prescription, nonprescription medication, or herbal products, particularly St. John's wort. Inform patients that asymptomatic elevations in indirect bilirubin have occurred in patients receiving atazanavir. This may be accompanied by yellowing of the skin or whites of the eyes.	ADRs/Lab Abnormalities: Hyperbilirubinemia, nausea, headache, abdominal pain, diarrhea, vomiting, rash Hepatic function impairment: Give with extreme caution in patients with mild to moderate hepatic insufficiency. Consider a dose reduction to 300 mg once daily for patients with moderate hepatic insufficiency. Monitor LFTs in patients with a history of hepatitis B or C. Pharmacokinetics Atazanavir is extensively metabolized in humans. Administration of atazanavir with food enhances bioavailability and reduces pharmacokinetic variability.	Contraindications Hypersensitivity to any of the components of the product. Co administration is contraindicated with drugs (e.g., midazolam, triazolam, ergot derivatives, cisapride, pimozide) that are highly dependent on CYP3A for clearance and for which elevated plasma concentrations are associated with serious and/or life-threatening events. Pregnancy Category: B Lactation Issues: The Centers for Disease Control and Prevention recommend that HIV-infected mothers not breastfeed their infants to

		Drug Interactions The following drugs may decrease Atazanavir levels: **rifampin, proton pump inhibitors, St. John's wort, didanosine, (buffered formulation only), efavirenz, antacids and buffered medications** Atazanavir may increase the concentrations of the following drugs: **ergot derivatives, benzodiazepines (midazolam, triazolam) HMG-CoA Reductase inhibitors, pimozide, antiarrhythmics, warfarin, tricyclic antidepressants, rifabutin, calcium channel blockers, sildenafil, saquinavir, immunosuppressants (cyclosporine, sirolimus, tacrolimus)**		avoid risking postnatal transmission of HIV infection.
Fosamprenavir Lexiva Tablets: 700 mg	**HIV infection: In combination with other antiretroviral agents for the treatment of HIV-1 infection.** **Therapy-naive patients:** 1400 mg BID (without ritonavir) OR 1400 mg QD plus ritonavir 200 mg once daily OR 700 mg BID plus ritonavir 100 mg BID **Protease inhibitor (PI)-experienced patients:** 700 mg BID plus ritonavir 100 mg twice daily. QD administration of fosamprenavir plus ritonavir is not recommended in PI-experienced patients. Adjustment of ritonavir dose when fosamprenavir plus ritonavir are administered with efavirenz: An additional 100 mg/day (300 mg total) of ritonavir is recommended when efavirenz is administered with fosamprenavir plus ritonavir once daily.	Administration Issues May be taken with or without food. Advise patients to inform their health care provider if they have a sulfa allergy. The potential for cross-sensitivity between drugs in the sulfonamide class and fosamprenavir is unknown. Fosamprenavir may interact with many drugs; therefore, advise patients to report to their health care provider the use of any other prescription or nonprescription medication or herbal products, particularly St. John's wort. Drug Interactions **Drug interactions:** Serious and/or life-threatening drug interactions could occur between fosamprenavir and amiodarone, lidocaine (systemic), tricyclic antidepressants, and quinidine. Concentration monitoring of these agents is recommended if these agents are used concomitantly with fosamprenavir The following drugs may decrease fosamprenavir levels: **rifampin, proton pump inhibitors, St. John's wort,**	ADRs: Diarrhea, nausea, vomiting, headache, rash Pharmacokinetics Fosamprenavir is a prodrug that is rapidly hydrolyzed to amprenavir. After administration of a single dose of fosamprenavir to HIV-1-infected patients, the time to peak amprenavir concentration (T_{max}) occurred between 1.5 and 4 hours(median 2.5 hours).	Contraindications Previously demonstrated clinically significant hypersensitivity to any of the components of this product or to amprenavir; coadministration with dihydroergotamine, ergonovine, ergotamine, methylergonovine, cisapride, pimozide, midazolam, or triazolam. If fosamprenavir is coadministered with ritonavir, the antiarrhythmic agents flecainide and propafenone also are contraindicated. Pregnancy Category: B Lactation Issues: The Centers for Disease Control and Prevention recommend that HIV-infected mothers not breastfeed their infants to avoid risking postnatal transmission of HIV infection.

(*continues on next page*)

106.4 Protease Inhibitors *continued from previous page*

Drug and Dosage Forms	Spectrum of Activity and Usual Dosage Range	Administration Issues and Drug-Drug & Drug-Food Interactions	Common Adverse Drug Reactions (ADRs) and Pharmacokinetics	Contraindications, Pregnancy Category and Lactation Issues
Fosamprenavir *cont.*	**Hepatic function impairment:** Use fosamprenavir with caution, at a reduced dosage of 700 mg BID in patients with mild or moderate hepatic impairment	**efavirenz, antacids, ranitidine, H2-antagonists, methadone, saquinavir** Fosamprenavir may increase the concentrations of the following drugs: **ergot derivatives, benzodiazepines, HMG-CoA Reductase inhibitors, pimozide, antiarrhythmics, tricyclic antidepressants, rifabutin, calcium channel blockers, sildenafil, vardenafil, immunosuppressants (cyclosporine, tacrolimus),**		
Amprenavir Agenerase Capsule: 50 mg 150 mg Oral solution: 15 mg/mL	**HIV infection: In combination with other antiretroviral agents for the treatment of human immunodeficiency virus type 1 (HIV-1) infection.** **Adults** 1200 mg (eight 150 mg capsules) bid in combination with other antiretroviral agents **Pediatric patients** ***Capsules*** For adolescents (13 to 16 years): 1200 mg (eight 150 mg capsules) bid in combination with other antiretroviral agents. For patients between 4 and 12 years of age or for patients 13 to 16 years of age with weight of < 50 kg: 20 mg/kg bid or 15 mg/kg tid (to a maximum daily dose of 2400 mg) in combination with other antiretroviral agents. ***Oral solution*** The recommended dose for patients between 4 and 12 years of age or for patients 13 to 16 years of age with weight < 50 kg is 22.5 mg/kg (1.5 ml/kg) bid or	Administration Issues Amprenavir may be taken with or without food; however, a high-fat meal decreases the absorption of amprenavir and should be avoided. Advise adult and pediatric patients not to take supplemental vitamin E since the vitamin E content of amprenavir capsules and oral solution exceeds the Reference Daily Intake (adults, 30 IU; pediatrics, 10 IU). Amprenavir capsules and oral solution are not interchangeable on a mg per mg basis Drug Interactions Serious or life-threatening drug interactions could occur between amprenavir and **amiodarone, lidocaine tricyclic antidepressants, and quinidine**. Do not use **rifampin** in combination with amprenavir because it reduces plasma concentrations and AUC of amprenavir by ≈ 90. Use particular caution when prescribing **sildenafil** in patients receiving amprenavir. Coadministration of amprenavir with sildenafil is expected to substantially increase sildenafil concentrations and may result in an increase in sildenafil-associated adverse events, including hy-	ADRs/Lab Abnormalities Nausea, vomiting, diarrhea, and abdominal pain, skin rash, paresthesias, hyperglycemia, hypertriglyceridemia, hypercholesterolemia. Pharmacokinetics Amprenavir is metabolized in the liver by the cytochrome CYP3A4 enzyme system.	Contraindications Hypersensitivity to any of the components of the product. Pregnancy Category: C Lactation Issues: The Centers for Disease Control and Prevention recommend that HIV-infected mothers not breastfeed their infants to avoid risking postnatal transmission of HIV infection.

	17 mg/kg (1.1 ml/kg) tid (to a maximum daily dose of 2800 mg) in combination with other antiretroviral agents.	potension, visual changes, and priapism. Amprenavir may increase the plasma concentrations of **anticonvulsants, antihistamines, benzodiazepines, calcium channel blockers, ergot alkaloids, HMG-CoA reductase inhibitors, tricyclic antidepressants, warfarin**.		
Indinavir* Crixivan Capsule: 200 mg, 100 mg, 333 mg, 400 mg * Frequently dosed with ritonavir to simplify administration and raise drug levels	**Treatment of HIV infection in combination with appropriate Therapy** Adults/adolescents: 800 mg q 8 h Cirrhosis Reduce dose to 600 mg q 8 h in patients with mild-moderate hepatic insufficiency	Administration Issues Do not take with food, take with water 1 h before or 2 h after a meal, or can take with a light meal; do not share medication; do not exceed recommended dose; store capsules in the original container and keep desiccant in the bottle; adequate hydration required to minimize risk of nephrolithiasis; if co-administered with ddl give at least 2 h apart on an empty stomach. Drug-Drug Interactions Indinavir may decrease the hepatic metabolism of the following drugs leading to toxicity: **astemizole, terfenadine, cisapride, triazolam, midazolam, clarithromycin, isoniazid, corticosteroids, rifabutin, zidovudine, stavudine**. The following drugs may decrease serum levels of indinavir: **ddl, fluconazole, itraconazole, rifampin, rifabutin**. The following drugs may increase serum levels of indinavir: **ketoconazole, clarithromycin, quinidine, zidovudine**.	ADRs Abdominal discomfort, nausea, diarrhea, headache, asymptomatic hyperbilirubinemia (10%), nephrolithiasis (4%). Pharmacokinetics Food, especially high fat and protein, decreases oral absorption; extensively metabolized by the cytochrome P-450 system.	Contraindications Hypersensitivity to indinavir. Pregnancy Category: C Lactation Issues Excretion in breast milk is unknown; HIV infected females should not breastfeed to avoid postnatal transmission of HIV to a child who may not be infected.
Lopinavir/Ritonavir Kaletra Capsule: 133.3 mg Lopinavir+ 33.3 mg ritonavir Oral Solution: 80 mg Lopinavir+ 20 mg ritonavir/mL	**HIV infection: In combination with other antiretroviral agents for the treatment of human immunodeficiency virus type 1 (HIV-1) infection.** **Adults** 400/100 mg of lopinavir/ritonavir (3 capsules or 5 mL) bid with food. ***Concomitant therapy with efavirenz or nevirapine:***	Administration Issues Take with food to enhance absorption. Lopinavir/ritonavir may interact with some drugs; therefore, advise patients to report to their healthcare professional the use of any other prescription or nonprescription medication or herbal product, particularly **St. John's wort.** Patients taking didanosine should take didanosine 1 h before or 2 h after lopinavir/ritonavir. Advise patients receiving sildenafil that they may be at an increased risk of silde	ADRs/Lab Abnormalities Nausea, vomiting, diarrhea, and abdominal pain, paresthesias, hypertriglyceridemia, hypercholesterolemia. Pharmacokinetics Lopinavir is extensively metabolized by the hepatic cytochrome P-450 system, almost exclusively by the CYP3A isozyme. Ritonavir is a potent CYP3A inhibitor that inhibits the metabolism of	Contraindications Hypersensitivity to any of the components of the product. Coadministration of lopinavir/ritonavir is contraindicated with drugs that are highly dependent on CYP3A or CYP2D6 for clearance and for which elevated plasma concentrations are associated with serious and/or life-threatening events. These drugs include the following: **flecainide, propafenone, dihydroergotamine, ergonovine,**

(continues on next page)

106.4 Protease Inhibitors *continued from previous page*

Drug and Dosage Forms	Spectrum of Activity and Usual Dosage Range	Administration Issues and Drug-Drug & Drug-Food Interactions	Common Adverse Drug Reactions (ADRs) and Pharmacokinetics	Contraindications, Pregnancy Category and Lactation Issues
Lopinavir/Ritonavir *cont.*	Consider a dose increase to 533/133 mg lopinavir/ritonavir (4 capsules or 6.5 mL) bid with food when used in combination with efavirenz or nevirapine. **Children (6 months to 12 years of age)** Oral solution dose: 12/3 mg/kg for those weighing 7 to less than 15 kg and 10/2.5 mg/kg for those 15 to 40 kg bid with food, up to a maximum dose of 400/100 mg, in children greater than 40 kg (5 mL or 3 capsules), bid. ***Concomitant therapy with efavirenz or nevirapine:*** Consider a dose increase of lopinavir/ritonavir oral solution to 13/3.25 mg/kg for those weighing 7 to less than 15 kg and 11/2.75 mg/kg for those 15 to 45 kg bid with food, up to a maximum dose of 533/133 mg in children over 45 kg bid.	nafil-associated adverse events, including hypotension, visual changes, and sustained erection, and to promptly report any symptoms to their doctor. Drug Interactions Use particular caution when prescribing **sildenafil** in patients receiving Lopinavir/ritonavir. Lopinavir/ritonavir may increase the plasma concentrations of **benzodiazepines, calcium channel blockers, HMG-CoA reductase inhibitors, azoles, pimozide, antiarrhythmics, clarithromycin, disulfuram, ergot derivatives, protease inhibitors, immunosuppressants, rifabutin, buproprion, clozapine, desipramine, piroxicam, quinidine.** Lopinavir/ritonavir may decrease the plasma concentrations **of narcotic analgesics, oral contraceptives, warfarin, theophylline, zolpidem**. Lopinavir/ritonavir levels may be decreased when used with **anticonvulsants, corticosteroids, efavirenz, nevirapine, rifabutin, rifampin, St. John's wort.**	lopinavir, and therefore increases plasma levels of lopinavir.	**ergotamine, methylergonovine, pimozide, midazolam, cisapride, triazolam.** Pregnancy Category: C Lactation Issues The Centers for Disease Control and Prevention recommend that HIV-infected mothers not breastfeed their infants to avoid risking postnatal transmission of HIV infection.
Nelfinavir Viracept Tablet: 250 mg, 625 mg Powder for oral suspension: 50 mg/level scoop (200 mg/level tsp)	**Treatment of HIV infection in combination with an appropriate therapy** Pediatric dose: 20 to 30 mg/kg/dose tid Adults/Adolescents 1250 mg (five 250 mg tablets or two 625 mg tablets) BID or 750 mg (three 250 mg tablets) 3 times/day	Administration Issues Give with meal or light snack. For oral solution: Powder may be mixed with water, milk, pudding, ice cream or formula (for up to 6 h), do not mix with any acidic food or juice because of resulting poor taste. Do not add water to bottles of oral powder— use special scoop provided for measuring purposes. Tablets readily dissolve in water and produce a dispersion that can be mixed with milk, chocolate milk. Tablets can also be crushed and administered with pudding.	ADRs Diarrhea, rash, abdominal pain, asthenia. Pharmacokinetics Extensively metabolized by the cytochrome P-450 system.	Contraindications Hypersensitivity to nelfinavir. Pregnancy Category: B Lactation Issues HIV-infected females should not breastfeed to avoid postnatal transmission of HIV to a child who may not be infected.

		Drug-Drug Interactions Nelfinavir concentrations may be decreased by **anticonvulsants, rifabutin, rifampin**. The following drugs may increase concentrations of nelfinavir: **Indinavir** and **ritonavir**. Nelfinavir may increase the concentrations of **rifabutin** (significantly), **terfenadine, astemizole**. Nelfinavir may decrease the concentrations of oral contraceptives, zidovudine, and lamivudine.		
Ritonavir Norvir Capsule: 100 mg Solution: 80 mg/ml	**Treatment of HIV infection in combination with an appropriate therapy** **Adults/adolescents:** 600 mg bid with food; therapy may be initiated slowly beginning with 300 mg bid to avoid GI upset **Pediatric dose:** 400 mg/m^2 bid; to minimize GI effects start therapy at 250 mg/ m^2 bid and increase stepwise to full dose over 5 d as tolerated.	Administration Issues Take with food; do not share medication; do not exceed recommended dose; store capsules and solution in the refrigerator; solution stored outside the refrigerator should be used within 30 days; the solution may be mixed with chocolate milk or Ensure within 1 hour of administration to improve taste. Drug-Drug Interactions Ritonavir may decrease the metabolism of the following drugs leading to toxicity: **tricyclic antidepressants, fluconazole, itraconazole, corticosteroids, erythromycin, warfarin, calcium channel blockers, astemizole, terfenadine, cisapride, benzodiazepines, antiarrhythmics, rifabutin, saquinavir**. Ritonavir may decrease serum levels of the following drugs: **ddI, clarithromycin, sulfamethoxazole, theophylline, zidovudine, atovaquone, metoclopramide**. Serum levels of ritonavir may be increased by **fluconazole, clarithromycin**, and **fluoxetine. Rifampin** may decrease serum levels of ritonavir.	ADRs Nausea, diarrhea, vomiting, anorexia, abdominal discomfort, numbness and tingling of hands and feet. Pharmacokinetics Extensively metabolized by the cytochrome P-450 system.	Contraindications Hypersensitivity to ritonavir; do not coadminister ritonavir with benzodiazepines, astemizole, terfenadine, cisapride, and amiodarone as toxicity may occur due to decreased hepatic metabolism of the drug by ritonavir. Pregnancy Category: B Lactation Issues Excretion in breast milk is unknown; HIV-infected females should not breastfeed to avoid postnatal transmission of HIV to a child who may not be infected.
Saquinavir* Invirase, Fortovase Capsule: hard gel (Invirase) 200 mg	**Treatment of HIV infection in combination or appropriate therapy** **Invirase**	Administration Issues : Invirase may take without regard to meals; do not share medication; do not exceed recommended dose; take within 2 h after a full meal	ADRs Diarrhea, GI upset, nausea, fatigue, photosensitization.	Contraindications Hypersensitivity to saquinavir; photosensitization may occur.

(continues on next page)

106.4 Protease Inhibitors *continued from previous page*

Drug and Dosage Forms	Spectrum of Activity and Usual Dosage Range	Administration Issues and Drug-Drug & Drug-Food Interactions	Common Adverse Drug Reactions (ADRs) and Pharmacokinetics	Contraindications, Pregnancy Category and Lactation Issues
Saquinavir *cont.* Capsule, soft gelatin: 200 mg (Fortovase) *Both Invirase and fortovase are dosed with ritonavir to simplify administration and raise drug levels.	**Adults/adolescents:** 1000 mg bid plus 100 mg ritonavir bid **Fortovase** 1000 mg bid plus 100 mg ritonavir bid **Invirase** 1000 mg Invirase-bid plus 100 mg ritonavir bid Unapproved Use 1600 mg saquinavir QD plus 100 mg ritonavir QD	Fortovase: Take with meals or up to 2 h after meal. Invirase given with ritonavir achieves similar drug concentrations as Fortovase boosted with ritonavir. **Invirase plus ritonavir preferred combination due to smaller capsule size, easier storage, and less GI toxicity.** Drug-Drug Interactions Saquinavir concentrations may be decreased by the following drugs: **rifampin, rifabutin, phenytoin, carbamazepine, phenobarbital** and **nevirapine**. Saquinavir may inhibit the metabolism of **terlenadine** and **astemizole** leading to drug accumulation and potential arrhythmias. Saquinavir may inhibit the metabolism of the following drugs leading to toxicity: **calcium channel blockers, quinidine, benzodiazepines**. Serum levels of saquinavir may be increased by **ketoconazole, clarithromycin.**	Pharmacokinetics Enhanced bioavailability in HIV patients when given with food; hepatic metabolism via cytochrome P-450 system. Invirase given with ritonavir achieves similar drug concentrations as Fortovase boosted with ritonavir. Invirase plus ritonavir preferred combination due to smaller capsule size, easier storage, and less GI toxicity.	Pregnancy Category: B Lactation Issues Excretion in breast milk is unknown; HIV-infected females should not breastfeed to avoid postnatal transmission of HIV to a child who may not be infected.

106.5 Fusion Inhibitors

Drug and Dosage Forms	Spectrum of Activity and Usual Dosage Range	Administration Issues and Drug-Drug	Common Adverse Drug Reactions (ADRs)	Contraindications, Pregnancy Category and Lactation Issues
Enfuvirtide Fuzeon Powder for Injection 90 mg (reconstituted)	**In combination with other antiretroviral agents for the treatment of HIV-1 infection in treatment-experienced patients with evidence of HIV-1 replication despite ongoing antiretroviral therapy.** **Adults:** 90 mg (1 mL) twice daily injected SC into the upper arm, anterior thigh, or abdomen.	Administration Issues Inject SC in the upper arm, anterior thigh, or abdomen. Give each injection at a site different from the preceding injection site. Do not inject enfuvirtide into moles, scar tissue, bruises, or the navel. Enfuvirtide contains no preservatives. Once reconstituted, inject immediately or keep refrigerated in the original vial; use within 24 hours. The subsequent dose can be reconstituted in advance, stored	ADRs: The most common adverse events are local injection site reactions. Manifestations may include pain and discomfort, induration, erythema, nodules and cysts, pruritus, and ecchymosis. Other ADRS: diarrhea (26.8%), nausea (20.1%), and fatigue (16.1%) An increased rate of bacterial pneumonia was observed in subjects treated with	Contraindications Hypersensitivity to any of the components of the product. Pregnancy Category: B Lactation Issues: The Centers for Disease Control and Prevention recommend that HIV-infected mothers not breastfeed their infants to avoid risking postnatal transmission of HIV infection.

	Children (6-16 yrs): 2 mg/kg twice daily up to a maximum dose of 90 mg twice daily injected SC.	in the refrigerator in the original vial, and used within 24 hours. Bring refrigerated reconstituted solution to room temperature before injection. Inform patients that injection site reactions commonly occur. Patients need to understand how to appropriately inject enfuvirtide and how to carefully monitor for signs or symptoms of cellulitis or local infection. Instruct patients when to contact their health care provider about these reactions. Drug Interactions No known drug interactions.	enfuvirtide. Carefully monitor patients for signs and symptoms of pneumonia Hypersensitivity reactions have been associated with enfuvirtide therapy and may recur on rechallenge. Pharmacokinetics Absorption of the 90 mg dose was comparable when injected into the subcutaneous tissue of the abdomen, thigh, or arm.	

106.6 Agents for Cytomegalovirus

Drug and Dosage Forms	Spectrum of Activity and Usual Dosage Range	Administration Issues and Drug–Drug & Drug–Food Interactions	Common Adverse Drug Reactions (ADRs) and Pharmacokinetics	Contraindications, Pregnancy Category, and Lactation Issues
Ganciclovir Cytovene Capsule: 250 mg, 500 mg	**Antiviral spectrum** Cytomegalovirus (CMV), herpes simplex virus type 1 (HSV-1), herpes simplex virus type 2 (HSV-2), varicella-zoster virus (VZV), Epstein-Barr virus, and hepatitis B virus. **Maintenance therapy following induction treatment of CMV retinitis** 1000 mg tid with food or 500 mg q 3 h while awake for 6 doses/d Dose should be modified in patients with renal impairment.	Administration Issues Complete full course of therapy; ganciclovir is not a cure for CMV retinitis and disease may progress during or after therapy; regular ophthalmologic exams are necessary; effective contraception should be used for males and females during ganciclovir therapy. Drug–Drug Interactions Concomitant use of ganciclovir with the following drugs may increase the potential for hematological disorders: **zidovudine, dapsone, flucytosine, amphotericin B, TMP-SMZ, chemotherapy agents**. Concomitant use of ganciclovir and **imipenemcilastatin** may increase the risk for seizures. Concomitant use of ganciclovir and **cyclosporine** or **amphotericin B** may increase the risk of nephrotoxicity. **Probenecid** may decrease renal excretion of ganciclovir. Concomitant use of ganciclovir with **zidovudine** or **didanosine** may increase	ADRs Asthenia, headache, hematological disorders (anemia, neutropenia), photosensitization, infertility. Pharmacokinetics Poor GI tract absorption with and without food; cerebrospinal fluid concentrations ranged from 25%–70% of plasma concentrations.	Contraindications Hypersensitivity to ganciclovir or acyclovir. Pregnancy Category: C Lactation Issues Excreted in breast milk; due to possible carcinogenic and teratogenic effects to infants, discontinue nursing while receiving ganciclovir.

(*continues on next page*)

106.6 Agents for Cytomegalovirus *continued from previous page*

Drug and Dosage Forms	Spectrum of Activity and Usual Dosage Range	Administration Issues and Drug–Drug & Drug–Food Interactions	Common Adverse Drug Reactions (ADRs) and Pharmacokinetics	Contraindications, Pregnancy Category, and Lactation Issues
Ganciclovir *cont.*		serum levels of zidovudine and didanosine while decreasing serum levels of ganciclovir.		
Valganciclovir Valcyte Tablet: 450 mg	**For the treatment of CMV retinitis in patients with acquired immunodeficiency syndrome (AIDS)** **CMV retinitis (normal renal function)** Induction dose: 900 mg (two 450 mg tablets) bid for 21 days with food. Maintenance dose: Following induction treatment, or in patients with inactive CMV retinitis, the recommended dosage is 900 mg (two 450 mg tablets) qd with food. ***Strict adherence to dosage recommendations is essential to avoid overdose. Valganciclovir tablets cannot be substituted for ganciclovir capsules on a one-to-one basis.***	Administration Issues Take with food to maximize bioavailability. Exercise caution in the handling of valganciclovir tablets. Do not break or crush tablets. Because valganciclovir is considered a potential teratogen and carcinogen in humans, observe caution in handling broken tablets. Avoid direct contact of broken or crushed tablets with skin or mucous membranes. If such contact occurs, wash thoroughly with soap and water and rinse eyes thoroughly with plain water. Valganciclovir tablets cannot be substituted for ganciclovir capsules on a one-to-one basis. Patients switching from ganciclovir capsules should be advised of the risk of overdosage if they take more than the prescribed number of valganciclovir tablets. **Advise women of childbearing potential to use effective contraception during valganciclovir treatment. Similarly, advise men to practice barrier contraception during and for at least 90 days following treatment with valganciclovir tablets.** Drug Interactions Concomitant use with cytotoxic drugs may increase the potential for hematological disorders. Concomitant use of the following drugs may increase the AUC of valganciclovir: **probenecid, zidovudine**. Increase in SCr may occur if valganciclovir is given with nephrotoxic drugs such as **amphotericin** and **cyclosporine**.	ADR/Lab Abnormalities Diarrhea, nausea, vomiting, abdominal pain, pyrexia neutropenia, anemia, headache, convulsions, sedation, dizziness, ataxia, or confusion, insomnia, peripheral neuropathy. Pharmacokinetics The absolute bioavailability of ganciclovir from valganciclovir tablets following administration with food was 60. Dosage adjustment is required according to creatinine clearance.	Contraindications Hypersensitivity to valganciclovir or ganciclovir. **Warning:** The clinical toxicity of valganciclovir, which is metabolized to ganciclovir, includes granulocytopenia, anemia, and thrombocytopenia. In animal studies, ganciclovir was carcinogenic, teratogenic, and caused aspermatogenesis. Pregnancy Category: C Lactation Issues Because of potential for serious adverse events in nursing infants, mothers should be instructed not to breastfeed if they are receiving valganciclovir tablets. In addition, the Centers for Disease Control and Prevention recommend that HIV-infected mothers not breastfeed their infants to avoid risking postnatal transmission of HIV.

106.7 Miscellaneous Antiviral Agents

Drug and Dosage Forms	Spectrum of Activity and Usual Dosage Range	Administration Issues and Drug–Drug & Drug–Food Interactions	Common Adverse Drug Reactions (ADRs) and Pharmacokinetics	Contraindications, Pregnancy Category, and Lactation Issues
Amantadine Symmetrel generics Capsule: 100 mg Tablet: 100 mg Syrup: 50 mg/5 ml	**Antiviral spectrum** Influenza A virus. **Prophylaxis of Influenza A virus** **Adults and children > 9 yr.**: 200 mg qd or 100 mg bid for at least 10 days following a known exposure ≥ **65 yrs:** 100 mg qd **Children 1 to 9 yr.:** 4.4–8.8 mg/kg/d qd or in two divided doses, do not exceed 150 mg/d for at least 10 d following a known exposure **Begin therapy in anticipation of contact or as soon as possible after exposure. For symptomatic management, start as soon as possible after onset of symptoms and continue for 24–48 h after symptoms resolve. Dosage reduction is recommended for patients with renal insufficiency.**	Administration Issues Complete full course of therapy. Drug–Drug Interactions Concomitant use of amantadine and **anticholinergic drugs** may predispose to certain side effects (confusion, dry mouth, constipation, decreased urination, blurred vision).	ADRs Nausea, dizziness, insomnia, confusion, dry mouth, constipation, decreased urination, blurred vision. Pharmacokinetics Readily absorbed in GI tract; no metabolism occurs; renal excretion as unchanged drug.	Contraindications Hypersensitivity to amantadine. Pregnancy Category: C Lactation Issues Amantadine is excreted in breast milk; use with caution in nursing mothers.
Oseltamivir Tamiflu Capsule: 75 mg Powder for oral suspension: 12 mg/mL	**Influenza infection** Treatment: Treatment of uncomplicated acute illness due to influenza infection in patients > 1 year of age who have been symptomatic for ≤ 2 d. **Prophylaxis:** For prophylaxis of influenza in adults and adolescents ≥ 13 years of age. Treatment of influenza **Adults and adolescents 13 yr.:** 75 mg bid × 5 d. Begin treatment within 2 d of onset of symptoms of influenza. **Children:** The recommended oral dose of oseltamivir oral suspension for children ≥ 1 year of age or adults who cannot swallow a capsule is:	Administration Issues Oseltamivir may be taken without regard to food. However, when taken with food, tolerability may be enhanced. Instruct patients to begin treatment with oseltamivir as soon as possible after the first appearance of flu symptoms. Instruct patients to take any missed doses as soon as they remember, except if it is near the next scheduled dose (within 2 h), and then to continue to take oseltamivir at the usual times. Oseltamivir is not a substitute for a flu shot. Advise patients to continue receiving an annual flu shot according to guidelines on immunization practices. Drug Interactions None reported.	ADRs Nausea, vomiting, diarrhea, bronchitis, abdominal pain, dizziness, headache. Pharmacokinetics Oseltamivir phosphate is readily absorbed from the GI tract after oral administration.	Contraindications Hypersensitivity to any of the components of the product. Pregnancy Category: C Lactation Issues Use oseltamivir only if the potential benefit for the lactating mother justifies the potential risk to the breastfed infant.

(continues on next page)

106.7 Miscellaneous Antiviral Agents *continued from previous page*

Drug and Dosage Forms	Spectrum of Activity and Usual Dosage Range	Administration Issues and Drug–Drug & Drug–Food Interactions	Common Adverse Drug Reactions (ADRs) and Pharmacokinetics	Contraindications, Pregnancy Category, and Lactation Issues
Oseltamivir *cont.*	≤ 15 kg, give 30 mg bid × 5 d > 15–23 kg, give 45 mg bid × 5 d > 23–40 kg, give 60 mg bid × 5 d > 40 kg, give 75 mg bid × 5 d Influenza prophylaxis **Adults and adolescents 13 yr. following close contact with an infected individual:** 75 mg qd for at least 7 days Therapy should begin within 2 d of exposure. The recommended dose for prophylaxis during a community outbreak of influenza is 75 mg qd. Safety and efficacy have been demonstrated for ≤ 6 weeks. The duration of protection lasts for as long as dosing is continued.			
Rimantadine Flumadine Tablet: 100 mg Syrup: 50 mg/5 ml	**Antiviral spectrum** Influenza A virus. **Prophylaxis of Influenza A virus** **Adults and children ≥ 10yr.:** 100 mg bid **Children 1 to 9 yr.:** 5 mg/kg/d qd, do not exceed 150 mg/d **Treatment of Influenza A virus** **Adults:** 100 mg bid × 7 to 10 d from the initial onset of symptoms **In patients with severe hepatic disease, renal failure, or elderly nursing home residents, a dose reduction to 100 mg daily is recommended.**	Administration Issues Complete full course of therapy. Drug–Drug Interactions **Aspirin** and **acetaminophen** may decrease rimantadine serum concentrations. **Cimetidine** may decrease hepatic metabolism of rimantadine.	ADRs Insomnia, dizziness, nausea, vomiting. Pharmacokinetics $T_{1/2}$ is approximately 32 h; extensive hepatic metabolism; < 25% of dose excreted renally as unchanged drug.	Contraindications Hypersensitivity to amantidine or rimantadine. Pregnancy Category: C Lactation Issues Rimantadine should not be used in nursing mothers; adverse events were noted in offspring of rats during the nursing period.
Zanamivir Relenza Blisters of powder for inhalation: 5 mg	**Influenza treatment** Treatment of uncomplicated acute illness due to influenza A and B virus in adults and children ≥ 7 yr. who have been symptomatic for ≤ 2 d.	Administration Issues Instruct patients in use of the delivery system. Include a demonstration whenever possible. Have the patient read and carefully follow the accompanying Patient's Instructions for Use. Effective and	ADRs Diarrhea, nausea, nasal signs and symptoms, bronchitis, sinusitis, cough, dizziness, headache, infections of the ear, nose, and throat.	Contraindications Hypersensitivity to any of the components of the product.

	Patients ≥ 7 yr.: 2 inhalations (one 5 mg blister per inhalation for a total dose of 10 mg) bid (≈ 12 h apart) for 5 d. Two doses should be taken on the first day of treatment whenever possible, provided there is ≥ 2 h between doses. On subsequent days, doses should be ≈ 12 h apart (e.g., morning and evening) at approximately the same time each day. Patients scheduled to use an inhaled bronchodilator at the same time as zanamivir should use their bronchodilator before taking zanamivir. *Zanamivir is for administration to the respiratory tract by oral inhalation only, using the Diskhaler device provided. Instruct patients in the use of the delivery system. Include a demonstration whenever possible. If zanamivir is prescribed for children, it should be used only under adult supervision and instruction, and the supervising adult should first be instructed by a healthcare professional.*	safe use of zanamivir requires proper use of the *Diskhaler* to inhale the drug. Advise patients to finish the entire 5 d course of treatment even if they start to feel better sooner. Patients should be advised of the risk of bronchospasm, especially in the setting of underlying airways disease, and should stop zanamivir and contact their healthcare provider if they experience increased respiratory symptoms during treatment such as worsening wheezing, shortness of breath, or other signs or symptoms of bronchospasm. If a decision is made to prescribe zanamivir for a patient with asthma or COPD, the patient should be made aware of the risks and should have a fast-acting bronchodilator available. Patients scheduled to take inhaled bronchodilators at the same time as zanamivir should be advised to use their bronchodilators before taking zanamivir. Drug Interactions None reported.	Allergic-like reactions, including oropharyngeal edema and serious skin rashes, have been reported in postmarketing experience with zanamivir. Stop zanamivir and institute appropriate treatment if an allergic reaction occurs or is suspected. Pharmacokinetics Approximately 4% to 17% of the inhaled dose is systemically absorbed. Peak serum concentrations ranged from 17 to 142 ng/mL within 1 to 2 hours after a 10 mg dose.	Precautions: Safety and efficacy have not been demonstrated in patients with underlying chronic pulmonary disease. In particular, this product has not been shown to be effective and may carry risk in patients with severe or decompensated chronic obstructive pulmonary disease or asthma, and serious adverse events have been reported in such patients. Therefore, zanamivir is not generally recommended for treatment of patients with underlying airways disease such as asthma or COPD. Pregnancy Category: C Lactation Issues Exercise caution when zanamivir is administered to a nursing mother.

107. Urinary Anti-Infectives

Drug and Dosage Forms	Spectrum of Activity and Usual Dosage Range	Administration Issues and Drug–Drug & Drug–Food Interactions	Common Adverse Drug Reactions (ADRs) and Pharmacokinetics	Contraindications, Pregnancy Category, and Lactation Issues
Cinoxacin Cinobac, generics Capsule: 250 mg, 500 mg	**Antibacterial spectrum** Gram-negative organisms including *E. coli, Proteus sp., Providencia rettgeri, Klebsiella* sp., and *Enterobacter* sp. **Treatment of urinary tract infections by susceptible gram-negative organisms** **Adults:** 1 gm/d in 2 to 4 divided doses for 7 to 14 d **Prophylaxis of urinary tract infection** 250 mg at bedtime for up to 5 months in women with a history of recurrent urinary tract infections	Administration Issues Complete full course of therapy; may take without regard to meals; take with fluids liberally; avoid prolonged exposure to sunlight, wear protective clothing, and apply sunscreen. Drug–Drug Interactions **Probenecid** inhibits renal excretion of cinoxacin. Consider possible drug interactions of other **quinolone** and **fluoroquinolone** antibiotics when using cinoxacin.	ADRs Nausea, vomiting, headache, dizziness, rash, photosensitivity. Pharmacokinetics Rapid absorption; concentrates in the urine where approximately 97% of an oral dose is excreted in 24 h. **Dosage reduction is recommended for patients with renal insufficiency.**	Contraindications Hypersensitivity to cinoxacin or other quinolones. Pregnancy Category: B Lactation Issues Due to the potential for adverse effects in infants, decide whether to discontinue nursing or discontinue the drug.
Methenamine Hippurate Hiprex, Urex Tablet: 1 gm	**Antibacierial spectrum** *E. coli*, enterococcal sp., and staphylococcal sp. **Prophylaxis or suppression/elimination of frequently recurring urinary tract infections** **Adults and children > 12 yr.:** 1 gm bid **Children 6 to 12 yr.:** 0.5 to 1 gm bid	Administration Issues Complete full course of therapy; cranberry juice or vitamin C may be used to acidify the urine and increase the efficacy of methenamine; take with food to decrease GI upset; drink fluids liberally to ensure adequate urine flow. Drug–Drug Interactions Concurrent use of methenamine and **sulfonamides** may cause the formation of an insoluble precipitate in the urine. **Urinary alkalinizers (milk products, sodium bicarbonate, acetazolamide)** may decrease the efficacy of methenamine by inhibiting its conversion to formaldehyde.	ADRs Nausea, vomiting, abdominal discomfort, bladder irritation. Pharmacokinetics Rapid absorption; 10% to 25% hepatic metabolism; concentrates in the urine; 90% excreted in the urine in 24 h.	Contraindications Hypersensitivity to methenamine; renal insufficiency; concurrent sulfonamide use; severe dehydration; severe hepatic insufficiency. Pregnancy Category: C Lactation Issues Excreted in breast milk; no adverse effects in nursing infants have been reported; use with caution in nursing mothers.
Methenamine Mandelate generics Tabets 0.5 g, 1 g	**Antibacterial spectrum** *E. coli*, enterococcal sp., and staphylococcal sp. **Prophylaxis or suppression/elimination of frequently recurring urinary tract infections**	Administration Issues Complete full course of therapy; cranberry juice or vitamin C may be used to acidify the urine and increase the efficacy of methenamine; take with food to decrease GI upset; drink fluids liberally to ensure adequate urine flow.	ADRs Nausea, vomiting, abdominal discomfort, bladder irritation. Pharmacokinetics Rapid absorption; 10% to 25% hepatic metabolism; concentrates in the urine; 90% excreted in the urine in 24 h.	Contraindications Hypersensitivity to methenamine; renal insufficiency; concurrent sulfonamide use; severe dehydration; severe hepatic insufficiency. Pregnancy Category: C

Tablet, enteric coated: generics 0.5 gm, 1 gm Suspension: 0.5 gm/5 ml	**Adults:** 1 gm qid with meals and at bedtime **Children 6 to 12 years:** 0.5 gm qid with meals and at bedtime **Children ≤ 6 years:** 0.25 gm/ 14 kg qid with meals and at bedtime	Drug–Drug Interactions Concurrent use of methenamine and *sulfonamides* may cause the formation of an insoluble precipitate in the urine. **Urinary alkalinizers (milk products, sodium bicarbonate, acetazolamide)** may decrease the efficacy of methenamine by inhibiting its conversion to formaldehyde.		Lactation Issues Excreted in breast milk; no adverse effects in nursing infants have been reported; use with caution in nursing.
Nalidixic Acid NegGram Caplet: 250 mg, 500 mg, 1 gm Suspension: 250 mg/5 ml	**Antibacterial spectrum** Gram-negative organisms including *E. coli, Proteus sp., Providencia rettgeri, Klebsiella* sp., and *Enterobacter* sp. **Treatment of urinary tract infections by susceptible gram-negative organisms** **Adults:** Initial therapy at 1 gm qid × 7 to 14 d; a maintenance therapy of 2 gm/d may be used after the initial treatment period **Children 3 months to ≤ 12 yr.:** Initial therapy at 55 mg/kg/d divided qid doses × 7 to 14 d; a maintenance therapy of 33 mg/kg/d may be used after the initial treatment period	Administration Issues Complete full course of therapy; take with food to avoid GI upset; avoid prolonged exposure to sunlight, wear protective clothing, and apply sunscreen. Nalidixic acid has been shown to cause erosion of cartilage in weight-bearing joints in animals, no joint lesions have been reported in humans, use with caution in prepubertal children. Drug–Drug Interactions Nalidixic acid may displace **warfarin** from protein-binding sites, increasing the therapeutic effect of warfarin. **Nitrefurantoin** may antagonize the antibiotic effect of nalidixic acid.	ADRs Photosensitivity, drowsiness, headache, abdominal discomfort, nausea. Pharmacokinetics Well absorbed in GI tract; 95% protein bound; $T_{1/2}$ in urine is 6 hours; hepatic metabolism; renal excretion.	Contraindications Hypersensitivity to nalidixic acid; history of convulsive disorders. Pregnancy Category: B Lactation Issues Data is scant; however, nalidixic acid is excreted in breast milk; one report of hemolytic anemia in nursing infant; use with caution in nursing mothers.
Nitrofurantoin Furadantin Suspension: 25 mg/5 ml	**Antibacterial spectrum** Gram-positive organisms including *S. aureus* and *S. saprophyticus*; gram-negative organisms including *E. coli, Klebsiella* sp., and *Enterobacter* sp., *Enterococcus faecalis.* **Treatment of urinary tract infections** **Adults:** 50–100 mg qid with meals and at bedtime × 7 to 10 d **Children:** 5–7 mg/kg/ d divided qid × 7 to 10 d	Administration Issues Complete full course of therapy; take with food or milk to decrease upset stomach; may cause brownish discoloration of the urine. Drug–Drug Interactions **Antacids** and **magnesium salts** may decrease the absorption of nitrofurantoin. **Probenecid** may decrease the elimination of nitrofurantoin.	ADRs Nausea, vomiting, anorexia, abdominal discomfort. Pharmacokinetics Food enhanced absorption from GI tract; metabolized by body tissues; concentrates in the urine; renal excretion.	Contraindications Hypersensitivity to nitrofurantoin; renal function impairment, anuria, or oliguria; pregnant women at term, during labor and delivery, or when onset of labor is imminent; infants < 1 month of age. Pregnancy Category: B Lactation Issues Safety for use in nursing mothers not established.

(*continues on next page*)

107. Urinary Anti-Infectives *continued from previous page*

Drug and Dosage Forms	Spectrum of Activity and Usual Dosage Range	Administration Issues and Drug–Drug & Drug–Food Interactions	Common Adverse Drug Reactions (ADRs) and Pharmacokinetics	Contraindications, Pregnancy Category, and Lactation Issues
Nitrofurantoin *cont.*	**Suppressive of urinary tract infections** **Adults:** 50–100 mg q hs **Children:** 1 mg/kg/d qd or divided bid			
Nitrofurantoin Macrocrystals Macrodantin, generics Capsule: 50 mg, 100 mg Capsule: Macrobid 100 mg (as 25 mg macrocrystals, 75 mg monohydrate)	**Antibacterial spectrum** Gram-positive organisms including *S. aureus* and *S. saprophyticus*; gram-negative organisms including *E. coli, Klebsiella* sp., and *Enterobacter* sp., *Enterococcus faecalis.* **Treatment of urinary tract infections** **Adults:** 50–100 mg qid with meals and at bedtime or Macrobid 100 mg bid with meals × 7 to 10 d **Children:** 5–7 mg/kg/d divided qid × 7 to 10 d	Administration Issues Complete full course of therapy; take with food or milk to decrease upset stomach; may cause brownish discoloration of the urine. Drug–Drug Interactions **Antacids** and **magnesium salts** may decrease the absorption of *nitrofurantoin.* **Probenecid** may decrease the elimination of nitrofurantoin.	ADRs Nausea, vomiting, anorexia, abdominal discomfort. Pharmacokinetics Slower dissolution and absorption compared to nitrofurantoin; food enhances absorption from GI tract; metabolized by body tissues; concentrates in the urine; renal excretion.	Contraindications Hypersensitivity to nitrofurantoin; renal function impairment, anuria, or oliguria; pregnant women at term, during labor and delivery, or when onset of labor is imminent; infants < 1 month of age. Pregnancy Category: B Lactation Issues Excreted in breast milk; safety for use in nursing mothers has not been established.
Trimethoprim Proloprim, generics Tablet: 100 mg, 200 mg Solution 50 mg/5 mL	**Antibacterial spectrum** Urinary infections caused by *E. coli, P. mirabilis, K. pneumoniae, Enterobacter* sp., and coagulase-negative *Staphylococcus* sp. **Treatment of urinary tract infection** 100 mg q 12 h or 200 mg q 24 h × 10 d **Dosage reduction is recommended for patients with renal insufficiency.**	Administration Issues Complete full course of therapy. Drug–Drug Interactions Trimethoprim may increase the pharmacological effects of **phenytoin**, leading to toxicity.	ADRs Rash, pruritus, abdominal distress, superinfection, photosensitivity. Pharmacokinetics Rapidly absorbed; $T_{1/2}$ is approximately 10 hours; minimal hepatic metabolism; renal excretion.	Contraindications Hypersensitivity to trimethoprim; megaloblastic anemia due to folate deficiency. Pregnancy Category: C Lactation Issues Excreted in breast milk; use with caution.

108. Drugs for Parasitic Infections

Drug and Dosage Forms	Spectrum of Activity and Usual Dosage Range	Administration Issues and Drug–Drug & Drug–Food Interactions	Common Adverse Drug Reactions (ADRs) and Pharmacokinetics	Contraindications, Pregnancy Category, and Lactation Issues
Mebendazole Vermox, generics Tablet, chewable: 100 mg	**Antibacterial spectrum** Trichuris trichiura (whipworm), Enterobius vermicularis (pinworm), Ascaris lumbricoides (roundworm), Ancylostoma duodenale (common hookworm), Necator americanus (American hookworm). **General indications** **Adults and children:** 100 mg each morning and evening for 3 consecutive days **Treatment of enterobiasis (pinworm) infection** 100 mg given as a single dose	Administration Issues Complete full course of therapy; chew or crush tablet and mix with food; if one family member has a pinworm infection, treat all family members in close contact with the patient; to prevent reinfection, disinfect toilet facilities daily, change and launder undergarments, bed linens, towels, and nightclothes daily. **If the patient is not cured 3 weeks after treatment, a second treatment course is recommended.**	ADRs Abdominal discomfort, diarrhea. Pharmacokinetics Poorly absorbed; minimal metabolism; fecal excretion.	Contraindications Hypersensitivity to mebendazole. Pregnancy Category: C Lactation Issues Safety for use in nursing mothers has not been established.
Niclosamide Niclocide Tablet, chewable: 500 mg	**Antibacterial spectrum** *Taenia saginata* (beef tapeworm), *Diphyllobothrium latum* (fish tapeworm), *Hymenolepis nana* (dwarf tapeworm). **Treatment of *Taenia saginata* (beef tapeworm), *Diphyllobothrium latum* (fish tapeworm) infections** **Adults:** 4 tablets as a single dose **Children > 34 kg:** 3 tablets as a single dose **Children 11–34 kg:** 2 tablets as a single dose **Treatment of *Hymenolepis nana* (dwarf tapeworm) infections** **Adults:** 4 tablets qd for 7 d **Children > 34 kg:** 3 tablets on the first day, then 2 tablets qd for the next 6 d **Children 11–34 kg:** 2 tablets on the first day, then 1 tablet qd for the next 6 d	Administration Issues Complete full course of therapy; take after a light meal; chew tablet, then swallow with a small amount of water **Detection of tapeworm segments in the stool on the seventh day of treatment indicates treatment failure; give a second course of treatment; a patient is not considered cured unless the stool is negative for a minimum of 3 months.**	ADRs Nausea, vomiting, abdominal discomfort, diarrhea, dizziness.	Contraindications Hypersensitivity to niclosamide. Pregnancy Category: B Lactation Issues Safety for use in nursing mothers has not been established.

(continues on next page)

108. Drugs for Parasitic Infections *continued from previous page*

Drug and Dosage Forms	Spectrum of Activity and Usual Dosage Range	Administration Issues and Drug–Drug & Drug–Food Interactions	Common Adverse Drug Reactions (ADRs) and Pharmacokinetics	Contraindications, Pregnancy Category, and Lactation Issues
Praziquantel Biltricide Tablet: 600 mg	**Antibacterial spectrum** *Schistosoma sp., Clonorchis sinensis* and *Opisthorchis viverrini* (liver flukes). **Treatment of schistosomiasis** 20 mg/kg for 3 doses given on the same day; the interval between doses should not be < 4 and not > 6 h **Treatment of liver flukes** 25 mg/kg for 3 doses given on the same day; the interval between doses should not be < 4 and not > 6 h	Administration Issues Complete full course of therapy; take with liquids during meals; do not chew tablets.	ADRs Headache, dizziness, abdominal discomfort. Pharmacokinetics Rapid absorption; undergoes first-pass hepatic metabolism, renal excretion.	Contraindications Hypersensitivity to praziquantel; do not treat ocular cysticercosis with praziquantel. Pregnancy Category: B Lactation Issues Excreted in breast milk; do not nurse on the day of treatment and for 72 h thereafter.
Pyrantel Antiminth, Pin-Rid, generics Capsule: 180 mg Suspension/liquid: 50 mg/ml	**Antibacterial spectrum** *Enterobius vermicularis* (pinworm), *Ascaris lumbricoides* (roundworm). **Treatment of *Enterobius vermicularis* (pinworm) and *Ascaris lumbricoides* (roundworm) infections** 11 mg/kg as a single dose; maximum total dose is 1 gm	Administration Issues May take with food, milk, juice, or on an empty stomach anytime during the day; if one family member has a pinworm infection, treat all family members in close contact with the patient; to prevent reinfection, disinfect toilet facilities daily, change and launder undergarments, bed linens, towels, and nightclothes daily.	ADRs Anorexia, nausea, vomiting, abdominal discomfort, diarrhea. Pharmacokinetics Poorly absorbed; minimal metabolism.	Contraindications Hepatic disease; pregnancy. Pregnancy Do not use during pregnancy unless otherwise directed by a physician.
Thiabendazole Mintezol Tablet, chewable: 500 mg Suspension: 500 mg/5 ml	**Antibacterial spectrum** *Trichuris trichiura* (whipworm), *Enterobius vermicularis* (pinworm), *Ascaris lumbricoides* (roundworm), *Ancylostoma duodenale* (common hookworm), *Necator americanus* (American hookworm), *Strongyloides stercoralis* (threadworm), *Ancylostoma braziliense* (dog and cat hookworm), *Toxocara sp.* (ascarids). **Treatment of strongyloidiasis** **Adults and children < 68 kg:** 22 mg/kg/dose bid for 2 consecutive days **Adults and children ≥ 68 kg:** 1.5 gm/dose bid for 2 consecutive days	Administration Issues Complete full course of therapy; take with food; chew tablets thoroughly before swallowing; if one family member has a pinworm infection, treat all family members in close contact with the patient; to prevent reinfection, disinfect toilet facilities daily, change and launder undergarments, bed linens, towels, and nightclothes daily. **Thiabendazole is considered second-line therapy when other agents are not available for treatment of hookworm, round worm, and whipworm infections.**	ADRs Dizziness, headache, drowsiness, anorexia, nausea, vomiting, diarrhea. Pharmacokinetics Rapid absorbtion; almost completely metabolized; renal excretion mostly as metabolites.	Contraindications Hypersensitivity to thiabendazole. Pregnancy Category: C Lactation Issues Excretion in breast milk is unknown; due to the potential for adverse effects in infants, decide whether to discontinue nursing or discontinue the drug.

	<u>Treatment of cutaneous larva migrans (creeping eruption)</u> **Adults and children < 68 kg:** 22 mg/kg/dose bid for 5 consecutive days, repeat in 2 d if active lesions persist **Adults and children ≥ 68 kg:** 1.5 gm/dose bid for 5 consecutive days, repeat in 2 d if active lesions persist Maximum daily dose is 3 gm			

109. Miscellaneous Antimicrobial Agents

Drug and Dosage Forms	Spectrum of Activity and Usual Dosage Range	Administration Issues and Drug–Drug & Drug–Food Interactions	Common Adverse Drug Reactions (ADRs) and Pharmacokinetics	Contraindications, Pregnancy Category, and Lactation Issues
Atovaquone Mepron Suspension: 750 mg/5 ml	**Antibacterial spectrum** *Pneumocystis carinii.* **Treatment of mild to moderate *Pneumocystis carinii* pneumonia in patients who are intolerant to TMP-SMZ** **Treatment of PCP** 750 mg bid with food for 7 days **Prevention of PCP** 1500 mg qd with a meal	Administration Issues Complete full course of therapy; take with food; do not exceed recommended dose. Drug–Drug Interactions **Rifampin** and **rifabutin** may decrease serum levels of atovaquone. Atovaquone may decrease protein binding of other highly bound drugs (**warfarin**) leading to toxicity.	ADRs Rash, nausea, diarrhea, headache. Pharmacokinetics Bioavailability increases with food; highly protein bound; $T_{1/2}$ is approximately 65 hours; fecal elimination.	Contraindications Hypersensitivity to atovaquone. Pregnancy Category: C Lactation Issues Excretion in breast milk is unknown; HIV-infected females should not breastfeed to avoid postnatal transmission of HIV to a child who may not be infected.
Dapsone Tablet: 25 mg, 100 mg	**Antibacterial spectrum** *Mycobacterium leprae, Pneumocystis carinii.* **Treatment of dermatitis herpetiformis** **Adults:** Initiate with 50 mg qd, increase dose upward to achieve resolution of skin lesions, usual dosage range is 50–300 mg qd; use minimal dose that achieves desired effect, the average time for dosage reduction is 8 months; therapy may be discontinued with the average time for dosage elimination being 29 months **Children:** Initiate with 1–2 mg/kg/d, increasing to desired response, maximum daily dose is 100 mg/d; continue therapy for a minimum of 3 years	Administration Issues Complete full course of therapy; avoid prolonged exposure to sunlight, wear protective clothing, and apply sunscreen. Drug–Drug Interactions The following drugs may decrease the effect of dapsone leading to treatment failure: **didanosine, para-aminobenzoic acid, rifampin, rifabutin**. The toxicity of dapsone may be increased by **folic acid antagonists (pyrimethamine, methotrexate), probenecid, and trimethoprim**.	ADRs Photosensitivity, hemolytic anemia, drug-induced lupus, erythematosus, nausea, vomiting, albuminuria. Pharmacokinetics Rapid absorption; highly protein bound; $T_{1/2}$ is approximately 28 h; appreciable tissue levels found 3 weeks after therapy is completed; hepatic metabolism; renal excretion.	Contraindications Hypersensitivity to dapsone. Pregnancy Category: C Lactation Issues Excreted in breast milk in substantial amounts; due to the potential for adverse effects in infants, decide whether to discontinue nursing or discontinue the drug.

Clindamycin Cleocin, various generics Capsules (as the hydrochloride salt): 75 mg, 150 mg, 300 mg Granules for Oral Solution (as the palmitate salt): 75 mg/5 ml	**Antibacterial spectrum** *S. aureus, S. epidermidis, S. pneumoniae, C. diphtheriae*; Anaerobic organisms including *Bacteriodes* sp., *Fusobacterium, Propionibacterium* (C acnes), and *Clostridium perfringens.* **General indications (use higher doses for more severe infections)** **Adults:** 150–450 mg q 6 h × 10 to 14 d **Children:** 8–20 mg/kg/d (as the hydrochloride salt) divided q 6 to 8 h × 10 to 14 d 8–25 mg/kg/d (as the palmitate salt) divided q 6 to 8 h × 10 to 14 d In children ≤ 10 kg, give 37.5 mg tid as the minimum dose	Administration Issues Complete full course of therapy; may be taken without regard to meals; notify your health care professional if diarrhea develops. **Limit clindamycin use to serious infections to avoid pseudomembranous colitis.** Drug–Drug Interactions **Erythromycin** may antagonize the antibiotic effect of clindamycin. The effect of **nondepolarizing, neuromuscular blocking agents** may be enhanced by clindamycin.	ADRs Nausea, vomiting, diarrhea (3.4%–30%), potentially pseudomembranous colitis. Pharmacokinetics Poor CNS penetration; 85% hepatic elimination with increased half-life in hepatic disease.	Contraindications Hypersensitivity to clindamycin; treatment of minor bacterial or viral infections. Pregnancy Category: Safety has not been established. Lactation Issues Excreted in breast milk; nursing is probably best discontinued when taking clindamycin.
Furazolidone Furoxone Tablet: 100 mg Liquid: 50 mg/15 ml	**Antibacterial spectrum** GI tract organisms including *E. coli, Staphylococcus* sp., *Salmonella* sp., *Proteus* sp., *Aerobacter aerogenes, Vibrio cholerae, Giardia lamblia.* **Treatment of diarrhea and enteritis caused by susceptible organisms** **Adults:** 100 mg qid × 7 d **Children ≥ 5years:** 25–50 mg qid **1 to 4 years:** 17–25 mg qid **1 month to 1 year:** 8–17 mg qid Continue treatment × 7 d	Administration Issues Complete full course of therapy; avoid ingestion of alcohol during and 4 d after treatment; avoid tyramine-containing foods (cheese, wine) during treatment; may discolor urine. Drug–Drug Interactions Furazolidine may increase the potential for a hypertensive reaction with the following drugs: **monoamine oxidase inhibitors, amphetamines, sympathomimetics, tricyclic antidepressants, levodopa**. Furazolidine may increase the toxic effects of **meperidine** leading to agitation, seizures, and coma. Furazolidine and **alcohol** may cause a disulfiram-like reaction with vomiting.	ADRs Hypotension, rash, urticaria, nausea, headache, hypoglycemia. Pharmacokinetics Extensive metabolism believed to be through the intestines; urinary excretion.	Contraindications Hypersensitivity to furazolidone; infants < 1 month. Pregnancy Category: C Lactation Issues Excretion in breast milk is unknown; safety for use in nursing mothers has not been established.

(*continues on next page*)

109. Miscellaneous Antimicrobial Agents *continued from previous page*

Drug and Dosage Forms	Spectrum of Activity and Usual Dosage Range	Administration Issues and Drug–Drug & Drug–Food Interactions	Common Adverse Drug Reactions (ADRs) and Pharmacokinetics	Contraindications, Pregnancy Category, and Lactation Issues
Kanamycin Sulfate Kantrex Capsule: 500 mg	**Antibacterial spectrum** bacteria of the intestinal tract. **Suppression of intestinal bacteria** 1 gm every hour for 4 h, followed by 1 gm every 6 h for 36 to 72 h	Administration Issues Complete full course of therapy; notify your healthcare professional if ringing of the ears occurs. Drug–Drug Interactions Oral aminoglycosides may decrease the absorption of the following drugs: **digoxin, methotrexate, vitamin A**. Oral aminoglycosides may increase the effect of **warfarin** by decreasing the absorption of dietary vitamin K.	ADRs Nausea, vomiting, diarrhea, ototoxicity, muscle weakness, superinfection. Pharmacokinetics Poor systemic absorption; elimination of intestinal bacteria persists for 48–72 h; fecal elimination.	Contraindications Presence of intestinal obstruction; hypersensitivity to aminoglycosides. Pregnancy Category: D Lactation Issues Aminoglycosides are excreted in breast milk; potentially serious adverse reactions may occur in nursing infants; decide whether to discontinue nursing or to discontinue the drug.
Methylene Blue Urolene Blue Tablet: 65 mg	**Antibacterial spectrum** Mild genitourinary antiseptic. **Genitourinary antiseptic or treatment of chronic urolithiasis** 65–100 mg tid **Maintenance therapy in chronic methemoglobinemia** 100–300 mg daily	Administration Issues Complete full course of therapy; take with meals and a glass of water.	ADRs Blue-green urine, stool, and possible skin discoloration, nausea, vomiting, diarrhea, bladder irritation. Pharmacokinetics Well absorbed from GI tract; reduced to leukomethylene blue in tissues; renal excretion.	Contraindications Renal insufficiency; hypersensitivity to methylene blue; G-6-PD deficient patients. Pregnancy: Safety of methylene blue in pregnancy has not been established.

Metronidazole Flagyl, Protostat, Flagyl ER, generics Tablet: 250 mg, 500 mg Tablet, extended-release: 750 mg Capsule: 375 mg Gel, vaginal: 0.75%	**Antibacterial spectrum** Anaerobic organisms including *Bacteroides* sp., *Clostridium* sp., *Peptostreptococcus* sp., and *Fusobacterium* sp.; *C. difficile* colitis; adjunct therapy in the treatment of *Helicobacter pylori*; bacterial vaginosis and giardiasis. **General indications** 250 mg tid or 500 mg bid × 7 to 14 d **Trichomoniasis** **Adults:** 2 gm as a single dose or 500 mg tid × 7 d **Children:** 15 mg/kg/d divided q 8 h × 7 d **Bacterial vaginosis** 500 mg bid for 7 d or 2 gm as a single dose or vaginal gel 5 gm intravaginally bid for 5 d or 750 mg ER qd × 7 d **Giardiasis** **Adults:** 250 mg tid × 7 d **Children:** 15 mg/kg/d divided q 8 h × 7 d **Treatment of *Helicobacter pylori*** 250 mg tid × 14 d with bismuth subsalicylate 525 mg qid × 14 d and tetracycline 500 mg qid or amoxicillin 500 mg bid × 14 d **Antibiotic-associated pseudomembranous colitis produced by *C. difficile*** 250 mg qid or 500 mg tid × 7 to 14 d **Treatment of intestinal amebiasis** **Adults:** 750 mg q 8 h × 5 to 10 d	Administration Issues Complete full course of therapy; may take with food if GI upset occurs; avoid alcoholic beverages including beer; refrain from sexual intercourse during treatment of trichomoniasis to avoid reinfection. **Take Flagyl ER under fasting conditions ≥ 1 h before or 2 h after meals.** Drug–Drug Interactions **Barbiturates** may decrease the effectiveness of metronidazole. **Cimetidine** may increase metronidazole serum concentrations. Metronidazole may increase the pharmacological and toxic effects of the following drugs: **warfarin, phenytoin, lithium**. Concomitant use of **ethanol** and metronidazole may produce flushing, nausea, vomiting, palpitations, and tachycardia.	ADRs Dizziness, nausea, abdominal discomfort, diarrhea, metallic taste, superinfection. Pharmacokinetics Achieves therapeutic levels in cerebrospinal fluid (50% of serum concentration); hepatic metabolism; renal excretion.	Contraindications Hypersensitivity to metronidazole; pregnancy during first trimester. Pregnancy Category: B Avoid metronidazole use during the first trimester of pregnancy. Lactation Issues Excreted in breast milk; nursing mothers should express and discard any breast milk produced while on the drug and resume nursing 24 to 48 h after the drug is discontinued.

(*continues on next page*)

109. Miscellaneous Antimicrobial Agents *continued from previous page*

Drug and Dosage Forms	Spectrum of Activity and Usual Dosage Range	Administration Issues and Drug–Drug & Drug–Food Interactions	Common Adverse Drug Reactions (ADRs) and Pharmacokinetics	Contraindications, Pregnancy Category, and Lactation Issues
Metronidazole *cont.*	**Children:** 35–50 mg/kg/d up to max of 750 mg/dose divided q 8 h × 5 to 10 d			
Neomycin Sulfate generics Tablet: 500 mg Oral Solution: 125 mg/5 ml	**Antibacterial spectrum** bacteria of the intestinal tract. **Preoperative prophylaxis for elective colorectal surgery** 1 gm given in combination with erythromycin 1 gm at 19 h, 18 h, and 9 h prior to procedure	Administration Issues Complete full course of therapy; notify your physician, nurse, or pharmacist if ringing of the ears occurs. Drug–Drug Interactions Oral aminoglycosides may decrease the absorption of the following drugs: **digoxin, methotrexate, vitamin A**. Oral aminoglycosides may increase effect of **warfarin** by decreasing absorption of dietary vitamin K.	ADRs Nausea, vomiting, diarrhea, ototoxicity, muscle weakness, superinfection. Pharmacokinetics Poor systemic absorption; elimination of intestinal bacteria persists for 48–72 h; fecal elimination.	Contraindications Presence of intestinal obstruction; hypersensitivity to aminoglycosides. Pregnancy Category: D Lactation Issues Aminoglycosides are excreted in breast milk; potential serious adverse reactions may occur in nursing infants; decide whether to discontinue nursing or to discontinue the drug.
Pentamidine Isethionate NebuPent, generics Aerosol: 300 mg	**Antibacterial spectrum** *Pneumocystis carinii* **Prophylaxis of *Pneumocystis carinii* pneumonia** 300 mg once q 4 weeks via nebulization in the Respirgard® II nebulizer	Administration Issues Reconstitute one vial with 6 ml Sterile Water for Injection, USP only, use of saline solution will cause the drug to precipitate; do not mix pentamidine solution with any other drugs for nebulization; the reconstituted solution is stable for 48 h in the original vial.	ADRs Fatigue, metallic taste, shortness of breath, decreased appetite, dizziness, hypotension, hypoglycemia, hyperglycemia. Pharmacokinetics Plasma concentrations via nebulization are substantially lower compared to intravenous dosing; renal excretion.	Contraindications Anaphylactic reaction to inhaled or intravenous pentamidine. Pregnancy Category: C Lactation Issues HIV-infected females should not breastfeed to avoid postnatal transmission of HIV to a child who may not be infected.

Vancomycin Vancocin Pulvules 125 mg, 250 mg Powder for Oral Solution: 1 gm bottle, 10 gm bottle **The parenteral product may be given orally.**	**Antibacterial spectrum** *C. difficile.* **Antibiotic-associated pseudomembranous colitis produced by *C. difficile* or *Staphylococcus sp.*** **Adults:** 125 mg qid × 7 to 14 d or 500 mg to 2 gm/day given in 3 to 4 divided doses for 7 to 10 days **Children:** 40 mg/kg/d divided qid × 7 to 10 d. Do not exceed 2 gm/d **Neonates:** 10 mg/kg/d divided qid × 7 to 10 d	Administration Issues Complete full course of therapy. Oral vancomycin is not effective for other types of infection. Metronidazole is the preferred agent for mild to moderate cases of *C difficile* colitis. Drug–Drug Interactions Rare due to lack of systemic absorption.	ADRs Rare due to lack of systemic absorption, superinfection. Pharmacokinetics Very poor systemic absorption; fecal elimination.	Contraindications Hypersensitivity of vancomycin Pregnancy Category: C Lactation Issues Limited systemic absorption with orally administered vancomycin; however, use with caution in nursing mothers.

200. CARDIOVASCULAR

201. Antianginal Agents

Drug and Dosage Forms	Usual Dosage Range	Administration Issues and Drug-Drug & Drug-Food Interactions	Common Adverse Drug Reactions (ADRs) and Pharmacokinetics	Contraindications, Pregnancy Category, and Lactation Issues
Isosorbide Dinitrate Dilatrate-SR, Isordil, Sorbitrate Sublingual Tablets 2.5 mg, 5 mg, 10 mg Chewable Tablets 5 mg, 10 mg Tablets 5 mg, 10 mg, 20 mg, 30 mg, 40 mg Sustained Release Tablets 40 mg Sustained Release Capsules 40 mg	**Prevention and treatment of angina pectoris** Sublingual tablets 2.5–5 mg initially and titrate to relief of angina Chewable tablets 5–10 mg initially and titrate to relief of angina Oral tablets Initial dose: 5–20 mg tid maintenance dose: 10–40 mg tid SR tablets/capsules 40–80 mg qd, bid, or tid as needed	Administration Issues Safety and efficacy have not been established in children; tolerance may develop—adjust dosing schedule to allow a "nitrate-free" period; do not crush or chew sustained release or sublingual tablets; do not crush chewable tablets before administering. Drug–Drug Interactions Severe hypotension may occur in patients who drink **alcohol;** orthostatic hypotension may occur in patients taking certain **calcium channel blockers** (e.g., nifedipine).	ADRs Headache, GI upset, flushing, hypotension, rash. Pharmacokinetics Absorption = 100%; SR onset = 4 hours, duration = 6–8 hours; sublingual onset = 2–5 minutes, duration = 1–3 hours; regular release onset = 20–40 minutes, duration = 4–6 hours; hepatically metabolized; 60% protein binding.	Contraindications hypersensitivity to nitrates; severe anemia; closed angle glaucoma; orthostatic hypotension; head trauma or cerebral hemorrhage Pregnancy Category: C Lactation Issues it is not known whether nitrates are excreted in breast milk
Isosorbide Mononitrate Imdur, ISMO, Monoket Tablets 10 mg, 20 mg Extended Release Tablets 60 mg	**Prevention of angina pectoris** Regular release tablets 20 mg bid given 7 h apart Extended release tablets: 30–120 mg qd	Administration Issues Safety and efficacy have not been established in children; tolerance may develop—adjust dosing schedule to allow a "nitrate-free" period; do not crush or chew extended release tablets but may break tablets. Drug–Drug Interactions Severe hypotension may occur in patients who drink **alcohol;** orthostatic hypotension may occur in patients taking certain **calcium channel blockers** (e.g., nifedipine).	ADRs Headache, GI upset, flushing, hypotension, rash. Pharmacokinetics Absorption = 100%; hepatically metabolized; 60% protein binding; onset 30–60 min	Contraindications Hypersensitivity to nitrates; severe anemia; closed angle glaucoma; orthostatic hypotension; head trauma or cerebral hemorrhage. Pregnancy Category: C Lactation Issues It is not known whether nitrates are excreted in breast milk.
Nitroglycerin Sublingual Nitrostat Tablets 0.15 mg, 0.3 mg, 0.4 mg, 0.6 mg	**Prophylaxis of angina pectoris** 1 tablet under tongue or between cheek and gum 5 to 10 minutes before activities that may precipitate an anginal attack	Administration Issues Safety and efficacy have not been established in children; decreased absorption may occur in patients with a dry mouth.	ADRs Headache, flushing, hypotension, rash, local burning or tingling sensation.	Contraindications Hypersensitivity to nitrates; severe anemia; closed angle glaucoma; orthostatic hypotension; head trauma or cerebral hemorrhage. Pregnancy Category: C

	Treatment of acute anginal attack 1 tablet immediately—may repeat every 5 minutes up to 3 tablets in 15 minutes; if no relief, call physician or EMS	Drug–Drug Interactions Severe hypotension may occur in patients who drink **alcohol;** orthostatic hypotension may occur in patients taking certain **calcium channel blockers** (e.g., nifedipine).	Pharmacokinetics Absorption = 100%; onset = 1–3 minutes; duration = 30–60 minutes.	Lactation Issues It is not known whether nitrates are excreted in breast milk.
Nitroglycerin, Sustained-Release Nitrong, Nitro-Bid, Nitrocine Timecaps, Nitroglyn Sustained Release Tablets 2.6 mg, 6.5 mg, 9 mg Sustained Release Capsules 2.5 mg, 6.5 mg, 9 mg, 13 mg	**Prevention of angina pectoris** Maintenance dose: 2.5–13 mg bid Maximum dose: 26 mg bid	Administration Issues Safety and efficacy have not been established in children; tolerance may develop—adjust dosing schedule to allow a "nitrate-free" period; do not crush or chew extended release tablets. Drug–Drug Interactions Severe hypotension may occur in patients who drink **alcohol;** orthostatic hypotension may occur in patients taking certain **calcium channel blockers** (e.g., nifedipine).	ADRs Headache; GI upset; flushing; hypotension; rash. Pharmacokinetics Absorption = 100%; onset = 20–45 minutes; duration = 3–8 h.	Contraindications Hypersensitivity to nitrates; severe anemia; closed angle glaucoma; orthostatic hypotension; head trauma or cerebral hemorrhage. Pregnancy Category: C Lactation Issues It is not known whether nitrates are excreted in breast milk.
Nitroglycerin, Topical Nitro-Bid, Nitrol Ointment: 2%	**Prevention and treatment of angina pectoris** Initial dose: 1/2 inch q 6–8 h Maximum dose: 2 inches q 6–8 h "Wipe off" (or do not give) at midnight to allow a "nitrate-free" period.	Administration Issues Safety and efficacy have not been established in children; tolerance may develop—adjust dosing schedule to allow a "nitrate-free" period; apply to non-hairy area; do not apply to distal parts of extremities; avoid areas with cuts or irritations. Drug–Drug Interactions Severe hypotension may occur in patients who drink **alcohol;** orthostatic hypotension may occur in patients taking certain **calcium channel blockers** (e.g., nifedipine).	ADRs Headache, flushing, hypotension, rash, topical allergic reactions, erythematous, vesicular and pruritic lesions. Pharmacokinetics Absorption = 100%; onset = 30–60 minutes; duration = 2–12 h.	Contraindications Hypersensitivity to nitrates; severe anemia; closed angle glaucoma; orthostatic hypotension. Pregnancy Category: C Lactation Issues It is not known whether nitrates are excreted in breast milk.
Nitroglycerin, Transdermal Deponit, Minitran, Nitro-Dur, Nitrodisc, Transderm-Nitro Patch: 0.1 mg/hr, 0.2 mg/hr, 0.3 mg/hr, 0.4 mg/hr, 0.6 mg/hr, 0.8 mg/hr	**Prevention of angina pectoris** Initial dose: 0.2–0.4 mg/hr qd Maximum dose: 0.8 mg/hr qd Remove for at least 12–14 h to allow a "nitrate-free" period.	Administration Issues Safety and efficacy have not been established in children; tolerance may develop—adjust dosing schedule to allow a "nitrate-free" period; apply to non-hairy area; do not apply to distal parts of extremities; avoid areas with cuts or irritations; should not be used for acute anginal attacks.	ADRs Headache, flushing, hypotension, rash, contact dermatitis. Pharmacokinetics Absorption = 100%; onset = 30–60 minutes; duration is up to 24 h.	Contraindications Hypersensitivity to nitrates; severe anemia; closed angle glaucoma; orthostatic hypotension; allergy to adhesives. Pregnancy Category: C Lactation Issues It is not known whether nitrates are excreted in breast milk.

(continues on next page)

201. Antianginal Agents *continued from previous page*

Drug and Dosage Forms	Usual Dosage Range	Administration Issues and Drug-Drug & Drug-Food Interactions	Common Adverse Drug Reactions (ADRs) and Pharmacokinetics	Contraindications, Pregnancy Category, and Lactation Issues
Nitroglycerin, Transdermal *cont.*		Drug–Drug Interactions Severe hypotension may occur in patients who drink **alcohol;** orthostatic hypotension may occur in patients taking certain **calcium channel blockers** (e.g., nifedipine).		
Nitroglycerin, Translingual Nitrolingual Spray 0.4 mg per metered dose	**Prophylaxis of angina pectoris** 1–2 sprays onto or under tongue 5–10 minutes before activities that may precipitate an anginal attack. **Treatment of an acute anginal attack:** 1–2 sprays onto or under tongue q 5 minutes up to 3 doses in 15 minutes; if no relief, call physician or EMS	Administration Issues Safety and efficacy have not been established in children; should not be inhaled. Drug–Drug Interactions Severe hypotension may occur in patients who drink **alcohol;** orthostatic hypotension may occur in patients taking certain **calcium channel blockers** (e.g., nifedipine).	ADRs Headache, flushing, hypotension, rash, local burning or tingling sensation. Pharmacokinetics Absorption = 100%; onset = 2 minutes; **duartion** = 30–60 minutes.	Contraindications Hypersensitivity to nitrates; severe anemia; closed angle glaucoma; orthostatic hypotension. Pregnancy Category: C Lactation Issues It is not known whether nitrates are excreted in breast milk.
Nitroglycerin, Transmucosal Nitrogard Controlled Release Buccal Tablets 1 mg, 2 mg, 3 mg	**Prevention of angina pectoris:** 1 mg q 3–5 h while awake Place tablet between lip and gum above incisors or between cheek and gum.	Administration Issues Safety and efficacy have not been established in children; tolerance may develop—adjust dosing schedule to allow a "nitrate-free" period; do not crush or chew extended release tablets. Drug–Drug Interactions Severe hypotension may occur in patients who drink **alcohol;** orthostatic hypotension may occur in patients taking certain **calcium channel blockers** (e.g., nifedipine).	ADRs Headache; flushing; hypotension; rash; local burning or tingling sensation. Pharmacokinetics Absorption = 100%; onset = 1–2 minutes; duration = 3–5 h.	Contraindications Hypersensitivity to nitrates; severe anemia; closed angle glaucoma; orthostatic hypotension. Pregnancy Category: C Lactation Issues It is not known whether nitrates are excreted in breast milk.

202. Antiarrhythmic Agents

Drug and Dosage Forms	Usual Dosage Range	Administration Issues and Drug-Drug & Drug-Food Interactions	Common Adverse Drug Reactions (ADRs) and Pharmacokinetics	Contraindications, Pregnancy Category, and Lactation Issues
Amiodarone Cordarone Tablet: 200 mg	**Life-threatening recurrent ventricular fibrillation hemodynamically unstable ventricular tachycardia, atrial fib/flutter** Loading dose 800–1600 mg/d in divided doses for 1–3 weeks Maintenance dose: 200–600 mg/d (use lowest effective dose)	Administration Issues Safety and efficacy in children have not been established; administer with meals to minimized GI upset. Drug-Drug Interactions Amiodarone may potentiate the effect of **warfarin;** amiodarone may increase **digoxin, theophylline, phenytoin, methotrexate, procainamide, quinidine, flecainide, and cyclosporine concentrations.**	ADRs Proarrhythmia, corneal microdeposits, pulmonary toxicity, hypothyroidism or hyperthyroidism, photosensitivity, pulmonary fibrosis, worsening congestive heart failure, elevated liver enzymes (AST, ALT), blue discoloration of the skin, GI upset, dizziness, ataxia, tremor, fatigue, paresthesias. Pharmacokinetics Absorption = 50%; v_d = 60 l/kg; 96% protein binding; hepatically metabolized; $T_{1/2}$ = 40–55 d.	Contraindications Severe sinus node dysfunction; second- or third-degree heart block in the absence of a pacemaker; hypersensitivity to amiodarone. Pregnancy Category: D Lactation Issues Amiodarone is excreted in breast milk; either the drug or nursing should be discontinued.
Disopyramide Norpace Capsules: 100 mg, 150 mg Capsules, Extended Release: 100 mg, 150 mg	**Life-threatening ventricular arrhythmias, atrial fibrillation:** Patients with moderate renal insufficiency, hepatic insufficiency or adults < 50 kg 400 mg/day (q 6 h with regular release capsules and q 12 h with extended release capsules) **Adults > 50 kg** 400–800 mg/d in divided doses **Children (in divided doses):** <1 year: 10–30 mg/kg/d 1–4 years: 10–20 mg/kg/d 4–12 years: 10–15 mg/kg/d 12–18 years: 6–15 mg/kg/d	Administration issues: Correct hypokalemia or hyperkalemia before instituting therapy. Drug-Drug Interactions: Disopyramide may increase **digoxin** concentrations; **erythromycin** may increase disopyramide levels; **phenytoin** and **rifampin** may decrease disopyramide levels; disopyramide may decrease the effect of **warfarin.**	ADRs Dry mouth, urinary hesitancy and retention, constipation, blurred vision, hypotension, congestive heart failure, dizziness, fatigue, headache, GI upset, rash, muscle pain or weakness. Pharmacokinetics Absorption = 90%; 50% excreted in urine as unchanged drug; $T_{1/2}$ = 4–10 h; $T_{1/2}$ prolonged with impaired renal function ($T_{1/2}$ = 8–18 h).	Contraindications Hypersensitivity to disopyramide; pre-existing second-or third-degree heart block (if no pacemaker present); congenital QT prolongation; sick sinus syndrome. Pregnancy Category: C Lactation Issues Disopyramide is present in breast milk; either the drug or nursing should be discontinued.
Flecainide Tambocor Tablets: 50 mg, 100 mg, 150 mg	**Prevention of paroxysmal atrial flutter, atrial fibrillation or supraventricular tachycardia with disabling symptoms without structural heart disease**	Administration Issues Safety and efficacy in children < 18 years of age have not been established.	ADRs Proarrhythmia; dizziness; dyspnea; headache; nausea; fatigue; palpitations; chest pain; tremor; asthenia; constipation; edema; GI upset; worsening congestive heart failure.	Contraindications Hypersensitivity to flecainide; pre-existing second-or third-degree heart block in the absence of a pacemaker; cardiogenic shock, coronary artery disease, and heart failure. Pregnancy Category: C

(*continues on next page*)

202. Antiarrhythmic Agents *continued from previous page*

Drug and Dosage Forms	Usual Dosage Range	Administration Issues and Drug-Drug & Drug-Food Interactions	Common Adverse Drug Reactions (ADRs) and Pharmacokinetics	Contraindications, Pregnancy Category, and Lactation Issues
Flecainide *cont.*	Initial dose: 50 mg q 12 h Maintenance dose: 50–100 mg q 12 h maximum dose = 300 mg/d Initial dose: 100 mg q 12 h Maintenance dose: 100–150 mg q 12 h maximum dose = 400 mg/d	Drug-Drug Interactions **Phenytoin** and **rifampin** may decrease tocainide concentrations; flecainide may increase **digoxin** concentrations; smoking increases flecainide clearance; **cimetidine** may increase flecainide concentrations; additive effects occur when given with other negative inotropic agents (**beta blockers, verapamil**); **amiodarone** may increase plasma levels; use caution in coadministration of disopyramide.	Pharmacokinetics Absorption = 100%; 40% protein binding; $T_{1/2}$ = 12–27 h; accumulation may occur with renal or hepatic impairment.	Lactation Issues Flecainide is excreted in breast milk; either the drug or nursing should be discontinued.
Mexiletine Mexitil Capsule: 150 mg, 200 mg, 250 mg	**Life-threatening ventricular arrhythmias** Initial dose: 200 mg q 8 h Maintenance dose: 200–400 mg q 8 h maximum dose = 1200 mg/d Patients with hepatic impairment may be controlled with lower dosages.	Administration Issues Take with food or an antacid to minimize GI upset; safety and efficacy in children have not been established. Drug-Drug Interactions Mexiletine may increase theophylline concentration; rifampin and phenytoin may lower mexiletine concentrations.	ADRs Proarrhythmia, GI upset, tremor, lightheadedness, headache, coordination difficulties, palpitations, chest pain, worsening congestive heart failure, diarrhea, constipation, dry mouth, tremor. Pharmacokinetics Absorption = 90%; 50–60% protein binding; hepatically metabolized; $T_{1/2}$ = 10–12 h (prolonged with hepatic impairment).	Contraindications Hypersensitivity to mexiletine; pre-existing second or third-degree heart block in the absence of a pacemaker; cardiogenic shock. Pregnancy Category: C Lactation Issues Mexiletine is excreted in breast milk; either the drug or nursing should be discontinued.
Moricizine Ethmozine Tablet: 200 mg, 250 mg, 300 mg	**Life-threatening ventricular arrhythmias** 600–900 mg/d divided q 8 h In patients with hepatic or renal impairment, start with doses ≤ 600 mg/d.	Administration issues Administering after meals slows the rate of absorption but does not decrease the extent of absorption; safety and efficacy in children < 18 years of age have not been established. Drug-Drug Interactions Cimetidine increases moricizine concentrations; moricizine decreases theophylline concentrations 44–66%.	ADRs Proarrhythmia, palpitations, dizziness, headache, fatigue, nausea, dyspnea. Pharmacokinetics Significant first-pass metabolism; large V_d (≥ 300L); 95% protein binding; mainly hepatically metabolized; < 1% excreted unchanged in urine; induces its own metabolism; $T_{1/2}$ = 1.5–3.5 h.	Contraindications Hypersensitivity to moricizine; pre-existing second-or third-degree heart block; bifasicular block unless a pacemaker is present. Pregnancy Category: B Lactation Issues Moricizine is present in breast milk; because of the potential for serious adverse effects, either the drug or nursing should be discontinued.

Procainamide Pronestyl, Procan SR Regular release tablet: 250 mg, 375 mg, 500 mg Regular release capsule: 250 mg, 375 mg, 500 mg Sustained release tablet: 250 mg, 500 mg, 750 mg, 1000 mg	**Life-threatening ventricular arrhythmias or atrial fib/flutter** 50 mg/kg/d (q 3 h with regular release products and q 6 h with SR products) **Children (suggested dosing):** 15–50 mg/kg/d in divided doses q 3–6 h (maximum 4 grams/d)	Administration Issues Patients > 50 years of age, or patients with renal, hepatic, or cardiac insufficiency may require lower doses or longer dosing intervals; safety and efficacy in children have not been established. Drug-Drug Interactions **Beta blockers, cimetidine, ranitidine,** and trimethoprim may increase procainamide concentrations. **Therapeutic range = 4–12 mcg/ml.**	ADRs Proarrhythmia, lupus erythematosus, neutropenia, thrombocytopenia, rash, GI upset, dizziness. Pharmacokinetics Well absorbed; $T_{1/2} \approx 1-3$ h; metabolized to N-acetyl procainamide (NAPA), which is renally eliminated.	Contraindications Hypersensitivity to procainamide; complete heart block; lupus erythematosus; torsades de pointes. Pregnancy Category: C Lactation Issues Procainamide and NAPA are present in breast milk; either the drug or nursing should be discontinued.
Propafenone Rythmol Tablet: 150 mg, 300 mg	**Life-threatening ventricular arrhythmias or atrial fib/flutter** Initial dose: 150 mg q 8 h Maintenance dose: 150–300 mg q 8 h Usual max dose 900 mg/d. Allow 3–4 days between dosage adjustments.	Administration Issues Safety and efficacy in children have not been established. Drug-Drug Interactions **Cimetidine** may increase propafenone concentrations; **rifampin** may decrease propafenone concentrations; propafenone may potentiate the effects of **warfarin; propafenone** may increase **digoxin** and **cyclosporine** concentrations and may increase plasma levels and pharmacologic effects of **beta blockers.**	ADRS Proarrhythmia, dizziness, unusual taste, first-degree AV block, intraventricular conduction delay, nausea, vomiting, constipation, headache, worsening congestive heart failure, palpitations. Pharmacokinetics Absorption = 100%; undergoes extensive first-pass metabolism; absolute bioavailability = 3–20%; hepatically metabolized; $T_{1/2} = 2-10$ h; metabolites renally eliminated.	Contraindications Hypersensitivity to propafenone; uncontrolled congestive heart failure; pre-existing second-or third-degree heart block or sick sinus syndrome in the absence of a pacemaker; bradycardia; marked hypotension; bronchospastic disease; electrolyte imbalance. Pregnancy Category: C Lactation Issues It is not known whether propafenone is excreted in breast milk; either the drug or nursing should be discontinued.
Quinidine Quinidex, Quinaglute Dura-Tabs, Cardioquin Regular release tablet: quinidine sulfate 200 mg, 300 mg quinidine polygalacturonate 275 mg Sustained release tablet: quinidine sulfate 300 mg quinidine gluconate 324 mg	**Atrial flutter; atrial fibrillation; ventricular tachycardia** Regular release tablets: 200–300 mg tid to qid Sustained release tablets: 300–600 mg q 8–12 h **Children (suggested dosing): 30 mg/kg/d or 900 mg/m^2/d in divided doses**	Administration Issues Take with food to minimize GI upset; safety and efficacy in children have not been established. Drug-Drug Interactions Hepatic enzyme inducers (**phenytoin, rifampin, phenobarbital**) may decrease quinidine concentrations; hepatic enzyme inhibitors (**cimetidine**) may increase quinidine concentrations; quinidine increases **digoxin** concentrations; **verapamil** increases quinidine concentrations; quinidine may potentiate the anticoagulant effect of **warfarin.** Therapeutic range: 2–5 mcg/mL	ADRS Proarrhythmia, QT prolongation (torsades de pointes), GI upset, diarrhea, drug fever, rash, photosensitivity, ringing in the ears. Pharmacokinetics Absorption = 70%; 80–90% protein binding; 60–80% hepatically metabolized; $T_{1/2} = 4-10$ h.	Contraindications Hypersensitivity to quinidine, myasthenia gravis, complete heart block or severe intraventricular conduction defects, history of drug-induced torsades de pointes or long QT syndrome; thrombocytopenia purpura. Pregnancy Category: C Lactation Issues Quinidine is excreted in breast milk; use with caution; the American Academy of Pediatrics considers quinidine to be compatible with breastfeeding.

(continues on next page)

202. Antiarrhythmic Agents *continued from previous page*

Drug and Dosage Forms	Usual Dosage Range	Administration Issues and Drug-Drug & Drug-Food Interactions	Common Adverse Drug Reactions (ADRs) and Pharmacokinetics	Contraindications, Pregnancy Category, and Lactation Issues
Sotalol Betapace Tablet: 80 mg. 160 mg, 240 mg	**Ventricular arrhythmias:** Initial dose: 80 mg bid Max dose: 320 mg/d Renal insufficiency: CrCl 30–60 mL/min: dosing interval = q 24 h CrCl 10–30 mL/min: dosing interval = q 36–48 h CrCl < 10 mL/min: individual dose	Administration Issues Food decreases the absorption of sotalol approximately 20%; therapy should not be abruptly discontinued; safety and efficacy have not been established in children. Drug-Drug Interactions Additive effects when given with other **negative inotropes** or **antihypertensive agents.**	ADRs Proarrhythmia; bradycardia; hypotension; worsening CHF; PVD; bronchospasm (in susceptible individuals); impotence; masking the signs of hypoglycemia; GI upset; dizziness; fatigue; sleep disturbance; increased triglycerides, total and LDL cholesterol; decreased HDL cholesterol. Pharmacokinetics No protein binding; $T_{1/2}$ = 12 h.	Contraindications Hypersensitivity to beta blocking agents; symptomatic bradycardia; greater than first-degree heart block; CHF (relative); asthma. Pregnancy Category: B Lactation Issues Sotalol is excreted in breast milk; either the drug or nursing should be discontinued.
Tocainide Tonocard Tablet: 400 mg, 600 mg	**Life-threatening ventricular arrhythmias** Initial dose: 400 mg q 8 h Maintenance dose: 400–600 mg q 8 h Patients with renal or hepatic impairment may be controlled with lower doses.	Administration Issues Hypokalemia should be corrected prior to initiating tocainide. Drug-Drug Interactions **Cimetidine** and **rifampin** may decrease tocainide concentrations.	ADRS Proarrhythmia, dizziness, vertigo, nausea, paresthesia, tremor, drowsiness, worsening congestive heart failure, blood dyscrasias, pulmonary fibrosis. Pharmacokinetics Absorption = 100%; $T_{1/2}$ = 15 hours (prolonged in severe renal impairment).	Contraindications Hypersensitivity to tocainide or amide-Type local anesthetics; second-or third-degree heart block in the absence of a pacemaker. Pregnancy Category: C Lactation Issues Tocainide is excreted into breast milk; either the drug or nursing should be discontinued.

203. Anticoagulants

Drug and Dosage Forms	Usual Dosage Range	Administration Issues and Drug–Drug & Drug–Food Interactions	Common Adverse Drug Reactions (ADRs) and Pharmacokinetics	Contraindications, Pregnancy Category, and Lactation Issues
Warfarin Coumadin, Panwarfarin, Sofarin Tablet: 1 mg, 2 mg, 2.5 mg, 3 mg, 4 mg, 5 mg, 6 mg, 7.5 mg, 10 mg	**Prophylaxis and treatment of deep venous thrombosis (DVT) or pulmonary embolism (PE) and atrial fibrillation with embolization; prophylaxis of systemic embolism after myocardial infarction (MI):** titrate dose to international normalized ratio (INR) between 2–3 **Prophylaxis of systemic embolism in valves:** titrate dose to international normalized ratio (INR) between 2.5–3.5 Usual dosage range: 1–10 mg/d	Administration Issues Safety and efficacy have not been established in children < 18 years of age. Drug–Drug Interactions **NSAIDs** and **salicylates** may increase the risk of bleeding; hepatic enzyme inducers (**phenytoin, carbamazepine, rifampin, phenobarbital**) may decrease the anticoagulant effect; **amiodarone, TMP/SMZ, erythromycin, ciprofloxacin, metronidazole, fluconazole, ketoconazole, quinidine, omeprazole, gemfibrozil,** and **acetaminophen** may potentiate the anticoagulant effect.	ADRs Bleeding (major and minor); GI upset, rash. Pharmacokinetics Absorption = 100%; 95% protein binding; hepatically metabolized to inactive metabolites that are renally eliminated; $T_{1/2}$ = 36 h.	Contraindications Pregnancy; hemorrhagic tendencies; active bleeding; uncontrolled, malignant hypertension; history of warfarin-induced necrosis. Pregnancy Category: X Lactation Issues Warfarin is excreted in breast milk in an inactive form; infants nursed by warfarin-treated mothers had no change in prothrombin time (PT).

204. Antihyperlipidemic Agents

204.1 Bile Acid Sequestrants

Drug and Dosage Forms	Usual Dosage Range	Administration Issues and Drug-Drug & Drug-Food Interactions	Common Adverse Drug Reactions (ADRs) and Pharmacokinetics	Contraindications, Pregnancy Category, and Lactation Issues
Cholestyramine Questran, Questran Light, Prevalite Questran powder: 49 grams/ 9 grams of powder Questran Light powder: 4 grams/ 5 grams of powder	**Hyperlipidemia:** Powder: 4 grams 1–6 qd Tablets: Initial dose: 4 grams qd to bid Maintenance dose: 8–16 grams bid	Administration Issues Take before meals; powder form should be mixed with fluid; other medications should be taken 1 h before or 4–6 h after taking cholestyramine; swallow tablets whole—do not crush or chew. Drug-Drug Interactions Bile acid resins may interfere with the absorption of **warfarin, digoxin, gemfibrozil, glipizide, propranolol, tetracyclines; thiazide diuretics, thyroid hormone,** and **vitamins A, D, E and K, aspirin, penicillin.**	ADRs Constipation; abdominal pain, bloating or cramping; transient increases in AST, ALT and alkaline phosphatase; increased triglycerides. Pharmacokinetics Not significantly absorbed from the GI tract.	Contraindications Hypersensitivity to bile acid resins; complete biliary obstruction. Pregnancy Category: Safety for use during pregnancy has not been established. Lactation Issues Use caution when nursing—the potential lack of proper vitamin absorption may have an effect on nursing infants.
Colestipol Colestid Granules: 5 gm colestipol/ 7.5 gm powder Tablet: 1 gram	**hyperlipidemia:** Granules Initial dose: 5 grams qd to bid Maintenance dose: 5–30 grams qd or in divided doses **Tablets:** Initial dose: 2 grams qd to bid Maintenance dose: 2–16 grams qd or in divided doses	Administration Issues Take before meals; powder form should be mixed with fluid; other medications should be taken 1 h before or 4–6 h after taking colestipol; swallow tablets whole—do not crush or chew. Drug-Drug Interactions Bile acid resins may interfere with the absorption of **warfarin, digoxin, gemfibrozil, glipizide, propranolol, tetracyclines; thiazide diuretics, thyroid hormone,** and **vitamins A, D, E and K.**	ADRs Constipation, abdominal pain, bloating or cramping, transient increases in AST, ALT and alkaline phosphatase, increased triglycerides. Pharmacokinetics Not significantly absorbed from the GI tract.	Contraindications Hypersensitivity to bile acid resins; complete biliary obstruction. Pregnancy Category: Safety for use during pregnancy has not been established. Lactation Issues Use caution when nursing—the potential lack of proper vitamin absorption may have an effect on nursing infants.
Colesevelam Welchol Tablet: 625 mg	**Hyperlipidemia:** 3 tablets bid or 6 tablets qd, may increase to 7 tablets qd	Administration Issues Can be used alone or in combination with HMG-CoA reductase inhibitors; administer with food and liquids. Drug-Drug Interactions May decrease blood levels of sustained-release form of **verapmail;** other interactions not yet documented likely to occur (see cholestyramin).	ADRs Constipation, dyspepsia. Pharmacokinetics: Not significantly absorbed from the GI tract.	Contraindications Hypersensitivity, bowel obstruction. Pregnancy Category: B Lactation Issues Use with caution when nursing—the potential lack of proper vitamin absorption may have an effect on nursing infants.

204.2 HMG-CoA Reductase Inhibitors

Drug and Dosage Forms	Usual Dosage Range	Administration Issues and Drug-Drug & Drug-Food Interactions	Common Adverse Drug Reactions (ADRs) and Pharmacokinetics	Contraindications, Pregnancy Category, and Lactation Issues
Atorvastatin Lipitor Tablet: 10 mg, 20 mg, 40 mg	**Hypercholesterolemia:** Initial dose: 10 mg/d Dose range: 10–80 mg/d	Administration Issues May be given without regard to food. Drug-Drug Interactions Atorvastatin may potentiate the anticoagulant effects of **warfarin;** concurrent use with **erythromycin, gemfibrozil,** or **niacin** may lead to severe myopathy or rhabdomyolysis; coadministration with **Maalox TC** may decrease atorvastatin levels.	ADRs Increased serum transaminases (AST, ALT), headache, myalgia, rash, flatulence, dyspepsia. Pharmacokinetics 98% protein binding, undergoes hepatic recycling, $T_{1/2} = 14$ h.	Contraindications Hypersensitivity to HMG-CoA reductase inhibitors; active liver disease or unexplained persistent elevated liver function tests; pregnancy; lactation; use with caution in patients who consume excessive amounts of alcohol. Pregnancy Category: X Lactation Issues: Women taking HMG-CoA reductase inhibitors should not nurse while taking these agents.
Fluvastatin Lescol Capsule: 20 mg, 40 mg	**Hypercholesterolemia:** 20–40 mg/d as a single dose in the evening	Administration Issues Safety and efficacy in children < 18 years of age have not been established; dose should be taken in the evening. Drug-Drug Interactions Fluvastatin may potentiate the anticoagulant effects of **warfarin;** concurrent use with **gemfibrozil** may lead to severe myopathy or rhabdomyolysis; **rifampin** may decrease fluvastatin levels.	ADRs Increased serum transaminases (AST, ALT), GI upset, muscle pain, headache, rash, photosensitivity, lens opacities (association unknown). Pharmacokinetics Extensive first pass metabolism; $T_{1/2} = 1.2$ h; 98% protein binding.	Contraindications Hypersensitivity to HMG-CoA reductase inhibitors; active liver disease or unexplained persistent elevated liver function tests; pregnancy; lactation. Pregnancy Category: X Lactation Issues Women taking HMG-CoA reductase inhibitors should not nurse while taking these agents.
Lovastatin Mevacor Tablet: 10 mg, 20 mg, 40 mg	**Hypercholesterolemia; atherosclerosis:** 20–80 mg/d in single or divided doses Maximum recommended dose in patients taking immunosuppressive agents: 20 mg/d.	Administration Issues Safety and efficacy in children < 18 years of age have not been established; dose should be taken with the evening meal. Drug-Drug Interactions Lovastatin may potentiate the anticoagulant effects of **warfarin;** concurrent use with **gemfibrozil, cyclosporine, erythromycin** or **niacin** may lead to severe myopathy or rhabdomyolysis.	ADRs Increased serum transaminases (AST, ALT), GI upset, muscle pain, headache, rash, photosensitivity, lens opacities (association unknown). Pharmacokinetics Extensive first pass metabolism, 95% protein binding.	Contraindications Hypersensitivity to HMG-CoA reductase inhibitors; active liver disease or unexplained persistent elevated liver function tests; pregnancy; lactation. Pregnancy Category: X Lactation Issues: Women taking HMG-CoA reductase inhibitors should not nurse while taking these agents.

(continues on next page)

204.2 HMG-CoA Reductase Inhibitors *continued from previous page*

Drug and Dosage Forms	Usual Dosage Range	Administration Issues and Drug-Drug & Drug-Food Interactions	Common Adverse Drug Reactions (ADRs) and Pharmacokinetics	Contraindications, Pregnancy Category, and Lactation Issues
Lovastatin *cont.*		Drug-Food Interactions Administering lovastatin with food increases its bioavailability.		
Pravastatin Pravachol Tablet: 10 mg, 20 mg, 40 mg	**Hypercholesterolemia:** 10–40 mg/d as a single dose in the evening	Administration Issues May be taken without regards to meals; safety and efficacy in children < 18 years of age have not been established; dose should be taken in the evening. Drug-Drug Interactions Pravastatin may potentiate the anticoagulant effects of **warfarin; bile acid resins** decrease the absorption of pravastatin; concurrent use with **gemfibrozil** may lead to severe myopathy or rhabdomyolysis.	ADRs Increased serum transaminases (AST, ALT); GI upset; muscle pain; headache; rash; photosensitivity; lens opacities (association unknown). Pharmacokinetics Extensive first pass metabolism; 50% protein binding.	Contraindications Hypersensitivity to HMG-CoA reductase inhibitors; active liver disease or unexplained persistent elevated liver function tests; pregnancy; lactation. Pregnancy Category: X Lactation Issues Women taking HMG-CoA reductase inhibitors should not nurse while taking these agents.
Simvastatin Zocor Tablet: 5 mg 10 mg 20 mg 40 mg	**Hypercholesterolemia:** 5–80 mg/d as a single dose in the evening	Administration Issues Safety and efficacy in children < 18 years of age have not been established; dose should be taken in the evening. Drug-Drug Interactions Simvastatin may potentiate the anticoagulant effects of **warfarin;** concurrent use with **gemfibrozil** may lead to severe myopathy or rhabdomyolysis.	ADRs Increased serum transaminases (AST, ALT); GI upset; muscle pain; headache; rash; photosensitivity; lens opacities (association unknown). Pharmacokinetics Extensive first pass metabolism; 95% protein binding.	Contraindications Hypersensitivity to HMG-CoA reductase inhibitors; active liver disease or unexplained persistent elevated liver function tests; pregnancy; lactation. Pregnancy Category: X Lactation Issues Women taking HMG-CoA reductase inhibitors should not nurse while taking these agents.

204.3 Miscellaneous Antihyperlipidemic Agents

Drug and Dosage Forms	Usual Dosage Range	Administration Issues and Drug-Drug & Drug-Food Interactions	Common Adverse Drug Reactions (ADRs) and Pharmacokinetics	Contraindications, Pregnancy Category, and Lactation Issues
Gemfibrozil Lopid Capsule: 300 mg Tablet: 600 mg	**Hypertriglyceridemia:** 600 mg bid given 30 minutes before the morning and evening meals	Administration Issues Safety and efficacy in children have not been established. Drug-Drug Interactions Gemfibrozil may potentiate the anticoagulant effects of **warfarin;** concurrent use with **HMG-CoA reductase inhibitors** may lead to severe myopathy or rhabdomyolysis.	ADRS GI upset; fatigue; increased liver function tests (AST, ALT, LDH, bilirubin, alkaline phosphatase); increased risk of cholelithiasis. Pharmacokinetics 99% protein binding, metabolized by the liver, $T_{1/2} = 1.4$ h.	Contraindications Hypersensitivity to gemfibrozil; hepatic or severe renal insufficiency; preexisting gallbladder disease. Pregnancy Category: sB Lactation Issues Due to the potential for tumorigenicity, either the drug or nursing should be discontinued.
Nicotinic Acid (Niacin) Slo-Niacin, Nicobid Tempules, Nicotinex, Niaspan Tablet: 25 mg, 50 mg, 100 mg, 250 mg, 500 mg Tablet, timed/controlled release: 250 mg, 500 mg, 750 mg Capsule, timed release: 125 mg, 250 mg, 300 mg, 400 mg, 500 mg Elixir: 50 mg/ 5 mL Tablets, extended released (Niaspan) 500 mg, 750 mg, 1000mg	**Hyperlipidemia:** Initial dose: 50 mg bid (titrate slowly to decrease the incidence of adverse effects) Maintenance dose: 3–6 grams/d given in 2–3 divided doses Maximum dose: 8 grams/day Niaspan Week 1 375 qhs Week 2 500 qhs Week 3 750 qhs Week 4 1000 qhs Week 4–7 1500 qhs Week 8 and beyond 2000 qhs	Administration Issues Take with meals to minimize GI upset; aspirin taken 30–60 minutes before niacin may decrease cutaneous flushing. Drug-Drug Interactions Concurrent use with statins may lead to severe myopathy or rhabdomyolysis.	ADRs Cutaneous flushing; GI upset; glucose intolerance; hyperuricemia; doses >2 g/d may result in hepatotoxicity—this is more common with SR products with severe cases resulting in fulminant hepatic failure and liver transplantation. Pharmacokinetics Completely absorbed from GI tract; mainly excreted in urine.	Contraindications Active peptic ulcer disease; use with caution in patients predisposed to gout, those with gallbladder disease, hepatic dysfunction or diabetes severe hypotension. Pregnancy Category: C Lactation Issues Niacin is excreted in breast milk.

205. Antihypertensive Agents

205.1 Angiotensin-Converting Enzyme Inhibitors

Drug and Dosage Forms	Usual Dosage Range	Administration Issues and Drug-Drug & Drug-Food Interactions	Common Adverse Drug Reactions (ADRs) and Pharmacokinetics	Contraindications, Pregnancy Category, and Lactation Issues
Benazepril Lotensin Tablet: 5 mg, 10 mg, 20 mg, 40 mg Combinations: w/ varying strengths of HCTZ and benazepril (combinations should not be used as initial therapy for HTN)	**Hypertension:** Initial dose: 10 mg qd Max dose: 40 mg qd Patients taking diuretics: Initial dose: 5 mg qd CrCl < 30 ml/min Initial dose: 5 mg qd	Administration Issues Discontinue as soon as possible if pregnancy is detected; safety and efficacy have not been established in children. Drug-Drug Interactions Concomitant use of **potassium sparing diuretics** or **potassium supplements** may result in hyperkalemia; may increase **lithium** concentrations; increased risk of hypersensitivity reactions when given with **allopurinol;** may increase **digoxin** concentrations; **phenothiazine** may increase the effects of ACEIs; NSAIDs may decrease the effects of ACEIs.	ADRs Hypotension; hyperkalemia; cough; rash; dysgeusia; renal insufficiency; bone marrow suppression; angioedema (rare). Pharmacokinetics Onset = 1 h; duration = 24 hours; >95% protein bound; $T_{1/2}$ = 10–11 h (prolonged in renal insufficiency).	Contraindications Hypersensitivity to angiotensin converting enzyme inhibitors. Pregnancy Category: C (first trimester); D (second and third trimester) Lactation Issues Benazepril is excreted in breast milk; either the drug or nursing should be discontinued.
Captopril Capoten Tablet: 12.5 mg, 25 mg, 50 mg, 100 mg Combinations: w/ varying strengths of HCTZ and captopril (combinations should not be used as initial therapy for HTN)	**Hypertension:** Initial dose: 12.5 mg tid Maximum dose: 50 mg tid **Heart failure and left ventricular dysfunction after myocardial infarction:** Initial dose: 6.25 mg tid Max dose: 50 mg tid **Diabetic nephropathy:** Initial dose: 12.5 mg tid Max dose: 25 mg tid	Administration Issues Food decreases the absorption of captopril—take on an empty stomach; discontinue as soon as possible if pregnancy is detected; safety and efficacy have not been established in children. Drug-Drug Interactions Concomitant use of **potassium-sparing diuretics** or **potassium supplements** may result in hyperkalemia; may increase **lithium** concentrations; increased risk of hypersensitivity reactions when given with **allopurinol;** may increase **digoxin** concentrations; **phenothiazine** may increase the effects of ACEIs; NSAIDs may decrease the effects of ACEIs; **antacids** may decrease the absorption of captopril.	ADRs Hypotension; hyperkalemia; cough; rash; dysgeusia; renal insufficiency; bone marrow suppression; angioedema (rare). Pharmacokinetics Onset = 15 minutes; food decreases absorption; protein binding = 25–30% $T_{1/2} < 2$ h (prolonged in renal insufficiency).	Contraindications Hypersensitivity to angiotensin converting enzyme inhibitors. Pregnancy Category: C (first trimester); D (second and third trimester) Lactation Issues Captopril is excreted in breast milk; either the drug or nursing should be discontinued.
Enalapril Vasotec	**Hypertension:** Initial dose: 5 mg qd Maximum dose: 40 mg qd	Administration Issues Discontinue as soon as possible if pregnancy is detected; safety and efficacy have not been established in children.	ADRs Hypotension; hyperkalemia; cough; rash; dysgeusia; renal insufficiency; bone marrow suppression; angioedema (rare).	Contraindications Hypersensitivity to angiotensin-converting enzyme inhibitors.

Tablet: 2.5 mg, 5 mg, 10 mg, 20 mg Combinations: 25 mg HCTZ/10 mg enalapril (do not use combination as initial therapy for HTN)	Patients taking diuretics Initial dose: 2.5 mg qd CrCl < 30 ml/min or hyponatremia Initial dose: 2.5 mg qd **Heart failure:** Initial dose: 2.5 mg bid Max dose: 20 mg bid **Asymptomatic left ventricular dysfunction:** Initial dose: 2.5 mg bid Max dose: 10 mg bid	Drug-Drug Interactions Concomitant use of **potassium-sparing diuretics** or **potassium supplements** may result in hyperkalemia; may increase **lithium** concentrations; increased risk of hypersensitivity reactions when given with **allopurinol;** may increase **digoxin** concentrations; **phenothiazine** may increase the effects of ACEIs; NSAIDs may decrease the effects of ACEIs.	Pharmacokinetics Onset = 1 h; duration = 24 h; $T_{1/2}$ = 1.3 h.<	Pregnancy Category: C (first trimester); D (second and third trimester) Lactation Issues Enalapril is excreted in breast milk; either the drug or nursing should be discontinued.
Fosinopril Monopril Tablet: 10 mg, 20 mg	**Hypertension:** Initial dose: 10 mg qd Max dose: 80 mg qd Patients taking diuretics: Initial dose: 5 mg qd **Heart failure:** Initial dose: 5 mg qd Max dose: 40 mg qd	Administration Issues Discontinue as soon as possible if pregnancy is detected; safety and efficacy have not been established in children. Drug-Drug Interactions Concomitant use of **potassium-sparing diuretics** or **potassium supplements** may result in hyperkalemia; may increase **lithium** concentrations; increased risk of hypersensitivity reactions when given with **allopurinol;** may increase **digoxin** concentrations; **phenothiazine** may increase the effects of ACEIs; NSAIDs may decrease the effects of ACEIs.	ADRs Hypotension; hyperkalemia; cough; rash; dysgeusia; renal insufficiency; bone marrow suppression; angioedema (rare). Pharmacokinetics Onset = 1 h; duration = 24 hours; = 24 hours; protein binding = 95%; $T_{1/2}$ = 12 h (prolonged in renal insufficiency).	Contraindications Hypersensitivity to angiotensin converting enzyme inhibitors. Pregnancy Category: C (first trimester); D (second and third trimester) Lactation Issues Fosinopril is excreted in breast milk; either the drug or nursing should be discontinued.
Lisinopril Prinivil, Zestril Tablet: 2.5 mg, 5 mg, 10 mg, 20 mg, 40 mg Combinations: w/ varying strengths of HCTZ and 20 mg lisinopril (combinations should not be used as initial therapy for HTN)	**Hypertension:** Initial dose: 10 mg qd Max dose: 40 mg qd Patients taking diuretics Initial dose: 5 mg qd Patients with renal insufficiency: CrCl 10–30 ml/min: 5 mg qd CrCl < 10 ml/min: 2.5 mg qd **Heart failure:** Initial dose: 5 mg qd Max dose: 20 mg qd	Administration Issues Discontinue as soon as possible if pregnancy is detected; safety and efficacy have not been established in children. Drug-Drug Interactions Concomitant use of **potassium-sparing diuretics** or **potassium supplements** may result in hyperkalemia; may increase **lithium** concentrations; increased risk of hypersensitivity reactions when given with **allopurinol;** may increase **digoxin** concentrations; **phenothiazine** may increase the effects of ACEIs; NSAIDs may decrease the effects of ACEIs.	ADRs Hypotension; hyperkalemia; cough; rash; dysgeusia; renal insufficiency; bone marrow suppression; angioedema (rare). Pharmacokinetics Onset = 1 h; duration = 24 h; 100% excreted in urine; $T_{1/2}$ = 12 h (prolonged in renal insufficiency).	Contraindications Hypersensitivity to angiotensin-converting enzyme inhibitors. Pregnancy Category: C (first trimester); D (second and third trimester) Lactation Issues It is not known if lisinopril is excreted in breast milk; either the drug or nursing should be discontinued.

(*continues on next page*)

205.1 Angiotensin-Converting Enzyme Inhibitors *continued from previous page*

Drug and Dosage Forms	Usual Dosage Range	Administration Issues and Drug-Drug & Drug-Food Interactions	Common Adverse Drug Reactions (ADRs) and Pharmacokinetics	Contraindications, Pregnancy Category, and Lactation Issues
Lisinopril *cont.*	Patients with hyponatremia or CrCl < 30 ml/min initial dose: 2.5 mg qd **Acute myocardial infarction:** Initial dose: 5 mg qd Max dose: 10 mg qd for 6 weeks			
Moexipril Univasc Tablet: 7.5 mg, 15 mg	**Hypertension:** Initial dose: 7.5 mg qd Max dose: 30 mg qd Patients taking diuretics: Initial dose: 3.75 mg qd CrCl < 40 ml/min: Initial dose: 3.75 mg qd Max dose: 15 mg qd	Administration Issues Food decreases the absorption of moexipril—take on an empty stomach; discontinue as soon as possible if pregnancy is detected; safety and efficacy have not been established in children. Drug-Drug Interactions Concomitant use of **potassium-sparing diuretics** or **potassium supplements** may result in hyperkalemia; may increase **lithium** concentrations; increased risk of hypersensitivity reactions when given with **allopurinol;** may increase **digoxin** concentrations; **phenothiazine** may increase the effects of ACEIs; NSAIDs may decrease the effects of ACEIs.	ADRs Hypotension; hyperkalemia; cough; rash; dysgeusia; renal insufficiency; bone marrow suppression; angioedema (rare). Pharmacokinetics Onset = 1 h; duration = 24 h; protein binding = 50%; $T_{1/2}$ = 2–9 hours (prolonged in renal insufficiency).	Contraindications Hypersensitivity to angiotensin converting enzyme inhibitors. Pregnancy Category: C (first trimester); D (second and third trimester) Lactation Issues It is not known if moexipril is excreted in breast milk; either the drug or nursing should be discontinued.
Perindopril Aceon Tablet: 2 mg, 4 mg, 8 mg	**Hypertension and heart failure** Initial dose: 4 mg daily Maintenance: 4–8 mg daily (max 16 mg)	Administration Issues Discontinue as soon as possible if pregnancy is detected; safety and efficacy have not been established in children. Drug-Drug Interactions Concomitant use of **potassium-sparing diuretics** or **potassium supplement** may result in hyperkalemia; indomethacin and other NSAIDs may decrease the effects of ACEIs	ADRs Hypotension; hyperkalemia; cough; rash; dysgeusia; renal insufficiency; angioedema (rare) Pharmacokinetics: 60% protein binding; renal elimination	Contraindications Hypersensitivity to angiotensin converting enzyme inhibitors Pregnancy Category: NR Lactation Issues: Unknown; however, use with caution when nursing—the potential lack of proper vitamin absorption may have an effect on nursing infants
Quinapril Accupril	**Hypertension:** Initial dose: 10 mg qd Max dose: 80 mg/d	Administration Issues Discontinue as soon as possible if pregnancy is detected; safety and efficacy have not been established in children.	ADRs Hypotension; hyperkalemia; cough; rash; dysgeusia; renal insufficiency; bone marrow suppression; angioedema (rare).	Contraindications Hypersensitivity to angiotensin-converting enzyme inhibitors.

Tablet: 5 mg, 10 mg, 20 mg, 40 mg	Patients taking diuretics: Initial dose: 5 mg qd Patients with renal insufficiency: CrCl 30–60 ml/min: 5 mg qd CrCl 10–30 ml/min: 2.5 mg qd **Heart failure:** Initial dose: 5 mg bid Max dose: 40 mg/d, divided bid Patients with hyponatremia or CrCl 10–30 ml/min initial dose: 2.5 mg bid	Drug-Drug Interactions Concomitant use of **potassium-sparing diuretics** or **potassium supplements** may result in hyperkalemia; may increase **lithium** concentrations; increased risk of hypersensitivity reactions when given with **allopurinol;** may increase **digoxin** concentrations; **phenothiazine** may increase the effects of ACEIs; NSAIDs may decrease the effects of ACEIs.	Pharmacokinetics Onset = 1 h; duration = 24 h; protein binding = 97%; $T_{1/2}$ = 2 h (prolonged in renal insufficiency). ADRs Hypotension; hyperkalemia; cough; rash; dysgeusia; renal insufficiency; bone marrow suppression; angioedema (rare).	Pregnancy Category: C (first trimester); D (second and third trimester) Lactation Issues It is not known if quinapril is excreted in breast milk; either the drug or nursing should be discontinued.
Ramipril Altace Capsule: 1.25 mg, 2.5 mg, 5 mg, 10 mg	**Hypertension:** Initial dose: 2.5 mg qd Max dose: 20 mg/d CrCl < 40 ml/min: Initial dose: 1.25 mg qd **Heart failure:** Initial dose: 2.5 mg bid Max dose: 5 mg bid CrCl < 40 ml/min Initial dose: 1.25 mg qd Max dose: 2.5 mg bid Patients taking diuretics: Initial dose: 1.25 mg qd	Administration Issues Discontinue as soon as possible if pregnancy is detected; safety and efficacy have not been established in children. Drug-Drug Interactions Concomitant use of **potassium-sparing diuretics** or **potassium supplements** may result in hyperkalemia; may increase **lithium** concentrations; increased risk of hypersensitivity reactions when given with **allopurinol;** may increase **digoxin** concentrations; **phenothiazine** may increase the effects of ACEIs; NSAIDs may decrease the effects of ACEIs.	Pharmacokinetics Onset = 1–2 h; duration = 24 h; protein binding = 73%; $T_{1/2}$ = 13–17 h (prolonged in renal insufficiency).	Contraindications Hypersensitivity to angiotensin-converting enzyme inhibitors. Pregnancy Category: C (first trimester); D (second and third trimester) Lactation Issues It is not known if ramipril is excreted in breast milk; either the drug or nursing should be discontinued.

205.2 Angiotensin II Antagonists

Drug and Dosage Forms	Usual Dosage Range	Administration Issues and Drug-Drug & Drug-Food Interactions	Common Adverse Drug Reactions (ADRs) and Pharmacokinetics	Contraindications, Pregnancy Category, and Lactation Issues
Candesartan Atacand Tablet: 4 mg, 8 mg 16 mg, 32 mg	**Hypertension:** Initial dose: 8 mg qd (lower doses in patients receiving diuretics) Maintenance dose: 4–32 mg qd	Administration Issues Discontinue as soon as possible if pregnancy is detected; safety and efficacy have not been established in children. Drug-Drug Interactions Additive antihypertensive effects (e.g., diuretics), antihypertensive effects may be blunted by NSAIDs.	ADRs Dizziness, headache, orthostatic, hypotension, back pain. Pharmacokinetics 15% absorption, minimal penetration of the blood-brain barrier; >99% protein binding; excreted mostly unchanged in urine and feces (via bile); $T_{1/2} = 9$ h.	Contraindications Hypersensitivity, pregnancy, or lactation. Pregnancy Category: C (first trimester); D (second and third trimesters) Lactation Issues It is not known if candasartan is excreted in breast milk; either the drug or nursing should be discontinued.
Irbesartan Avapro Tablet: 75 mg, 150 mg, 300 mg	**Hypertension:** Initial dose: 150 mg qd (lower doses in patients receiving diuretics) Maintenance dose: 75–300 mg qd	Administration Issues Discontinue as soon as possible if pregnancy is detected; safety and efficacy have not been established in children. Drug-Drug Interactions Additive antihypertensive effects (e.g., diuretics), antihypertensive effects may be blunted by NSAIDs and phenobarbital.	ADRs Dizziness, fatigue, headache, hypotension, diarrhea, drug-induced hepatitis, impaired renal function, hyperkalemia. Pharmacokinetics 60–80% absorption; some hepatic metabolism, some biliary excretion, some elimination as unchanged drug in urine; $T_{1/2} = 11–15$ h.	Contraindications: Hypersensitivity, pregnancy, or lactation. Pregnancy Category: C (first trimester); D (second and third trimesters) Lactation Issues It is not known if irbesartan is excreted in breast milk; either the drug or nursing should be discontinued.
Telmisartan Micardis Tablet: 20 mg, 40 mg, 80 mg	**Hypertension:** Initial dose: 40 mg qd Maintenance dose: 40–80 mg qd	Administration Issues Discontinue as soon as possible if pregnancy is detected; safety and efficacy have not been established in children. Drug-Drug Interactions Additive antihypertensive effects (e.g., diuretics), antihypertensive effects may be blunted by NSAIDs, may increase serum digoxin levels.	ADRs Dizziness, orthostaic hypotension, diarrhea, back pain. Pharmacokinetics 42–58% absorbed; > 99.5% protein binding; excreted mostly unchanged in feces via biliary excretion; 11% metabolized by liver; $T_{1/2} = 24$ h.	Contraindications Hypersensitivity, pregnancy, or lactation. Pregnancy Category: C (first trimester); D (second and third trimesters) Lactation Issues It is not known if telmisartan is excreted in breast milk; either the drug or nursing should be discontinued.
Losartan Cozaar Tablet: 25 mg 50 mg	**Hypertension and heart failure:** Initial dose: 50 mg qd Maintenance dose: 50–100 mg qd	Administration Issues Discontinue losartan as soon as possible if pregnancy is detected; safety and efficacy have not been established in children.	ADRs Dizziness; cough; diarrhea; GI upset; insomnia; nasal congestion.	Contraindications Hypersensitivity to losartan. Pregnancy Category: C (first trimester); D (second and third trimester)

	Patients taking diuretics or with hepatic failure: Initial dose: 25 mg qd	Drug-Drug Interactions **Cimetidine** increases losartan concentrations; **phenobarbital** decreases losartan concentrations.	Pharmacokinetics Well absorbed; extensive first pass metabolism to an active metabolite; both losartan and its active metabolite are highly protein bound (>98%).	Lactation Issues It is not known if losartan is excreted in breast milk; either the drug or nursing should be discontinued.
Valsartan Diovan Capsule: 80 mg 160 mg	**Hypertension and heart failure:** Initial dose: 80 mg qd Maintenance dose: 80 to 320 mg qd	Administration Issues Discontinue valsartan as soon as possible if pregnancy is detected; safety and efficacy have not been established in children. Drug-Drug Interactions None reported.	ADRs Dizziness; cough; diarrhea; GI upset; insomnia; nasal congestion.	Contraindications Hypersensitivity to losartan. Pregnancy Category: C (first trimester); D (second and third trimester) Lactation Issues It is not known if losartan is excreted in breast milk; either the drug or nursing should be discontinued.

205.3 Centrally and Peripherally Acting Antiadrenergic Agents

Drug and Dosage Forms	Usual Dosage Range	Administration Issues and Drug-Drug & Drug-Food Interactions	Common Adverse Drug Reactions (ADRs) and Pharmacokinetics	Contraindications, Pregnancy Category, and Lactation Issues
Clonidine Catapres Tablet: 0.1 mg, 0.2 mg, 0.3 mg Combinations: 15 mg chlorthalidone and varying strengths of clonidine (do not use combinations as initial therapy for HTN) Transdermal Patch: TTS-1 (0.1 mg/day), TTS-2 (0.2 mg/day), TTS-3 (0.3 mg/day)	**Hypertension:** **Adults (oral):** Initial dose: 0.1 mg bid Maintenance dose: 0.2–0.8 mg daily in divided doses Max dose: 2.4 mg/d **Children (oral):** 5–25 mcg/kg/d, divided q 6 h **Adults (transdermal patch):** 0.1–0.6 mg/d reapplied q 7 d **Alcohol withdrawal:** 0.3–0.6 mg q 6 h **Smoking cessation:** Oral: 0.15–0.4 mg qd Transdermal patch: 0.2 mg/d	Administration Issues Abrupt discontinuation may result in rebound hypertension—clonidine should be tapered gradually; safety and efficacy have not been established in children. Drug-Drug Interactions Concomitant use of **beta blockers** may result in paradoxical hypertension; **tricyclic antidepressants** may block the antihypertensive effects of clonidine.	ADRs Dry mouth; drowsiness; dizziness; sedation; constipation; impotence; contact dermatitis (with transdermal patch). Pharmacokinetics Oral: Onset = 30–60 minutes; 50% metabolized by the liver; $T_{1/2}$ = 12–16 h (prolonged in renal insufficiency); minimal amount removed by dialysis. Transdermal patch: Therapeutic levels are reached in 2–3 days; $T_{1/2}$ = 19 h.	Contraindications Hypersensitivity to clonidine or any component of transdermal system. Pregnancy Category: C Lactation Issues Clonidine is excreted in breast milk; use with caution in nursing mothers.

(continues on next page)

205.3 Centrally and Peripherally Acting Antiadrenergic Agents *continued from previous page*

Drug and Dosage Forms	Usual Dosage Range	Administration Issues and Drug-Drug & Drug-Food Interactions	Common Adverse Drug Reactions (ADRs) and Pharmacokinetics	Contraindications, Pregnancy Category, and Lactation Issues
Guanabenz Wytensin Tablet: 4 mg, 8 mg	**Hypertension:** Initial dose: 4 mg bid Max dose: 32 mg bid	Administration Issues Allow 1–2 weeks before adjusting dose; rebound hypertension rarely occurs with abrupt discontinuation; safety and efficacy have not been established in children < 12 years of age.	ADRs Dry mouth; drowsiness; dizziness; sedation; headache; constipation; impotence. Pharmacokinetics $T_{1/2}$ = 6 h (prolonged in hepatic and renal insufficiency).	Contraindications Hypersensitivity to guanabenz. Pregnancy Category: C Lactation Issues It is not known if guanabenz is excreted in breast milk; either the drug or nursing should be discontinued.
Guanfacine Tenex Tablet: 1 mg, 2 mg	**Hypertension:** Initial dose: 1 mg q hs Maintenance dose: 1–2 mg q hs	Administration Issues Administer at bedtime to minimize daytime somnolence; allow 3–4 weeks before adjusting dose; rebound HTN rarely occurs with abrupt discontinuation—when it does occur, it does so after 2–4 d, which is delayed compared to clonidine; safety and efficacy have not been established in children < 12 years of age.	ADRs Dry mouth; drowsiness; dizziness; sedation; headache; constipation; impotence. Pharmacokinetics Protein binding = 70%; 50% excreted unchanged in urine; $T_{1/2}$ = 17 h.	Contraindications Hypersensitivity to guanfacine. Pregnancy Category: B Lactation Issues Guanfacine is excreted in breast milk; use with caution in nursing mothers.
Methyldopa Aldomet Tablet: 125 mg, 250 mg 500 mg Oral Suspension: 250 mg/ 5 mL	**Hypertension:** **Adults:** Initial dose: 250 mg bid to tid Maintenance dose: 500 mg–3000 mg in 2–4 divided doses **Children:** Initial dose: 10 mg/kg daily in 2–4 divided doses Max dose: 65 mg/kg up to 3000 mg	Administration Issues Allow two days for maximum response before adjusting dosage. Drug-Drug Interactions Methyldopa may potentiate the effects of **levodopa, lithium, haloperidon, MAO inhibitors,** and **sympathomimetics;** paradoxical hypertension may occur with concomitant administration of **propranolol;** methyldopa may decrease the metabolism of **tolbutamide.**	ADRs Sedation; orthostatic hypotension; edema; GI upset; dry mouth; abnormal LFTs; hemolytic anemia; rash; lupus-like syndrome; amenorrhea; gynecomastia; impotence; nasal stuffiness. Pharmacokinetics $T_{1/2}$ = 105 minutes (prolonged in renal insufficiency).	Contraindications Hypersensitivity to methyldopa; active hepatitis or cirrhosis; coadministration with MAO inhibitors. Pregnancy Category: B Lactation Issues Methyldopa is excreted in breast milk.
Guanadrel Hylorel Tablet: 10 mg, 25 mg	**Hypertension:** Initial dose: 5 mg bid Maintenance dose: 20–75 mg/d in 2–4 divided doses Renal impairment (initial dose): CrCl = 30–60 ml/min: 5 mg qd CrCl < 30 ml/min: 5 mg qod	Administration Issues Safety and efficacy have not been established in children. Drug-Drug Interactions **Beta blockers** and **vasodilators** may potentiate the effects of guanadrel; **phenothiazines, sympathomimetics**	ADRs Orthostatic hypotension; dizziness; GI upset; impotence; fluid retention; congestive heart failure; asthma in susceptible individuals. Pharmacokinetics $T_{1/2}$ = 10 h.	Contraindications Hypersensitivity to guanadrel; pheochromocytoma; congestive heart failure; use of MAO inhibitors. Pregnancy Category: B

		and **tricyclic antidepressants** may inhibit the antihypertensive effects of guanadrel.		Lactation Issues It is not known if guanadrel is excreted in breast milk; either the drug or nursing should be discontinued.
Guanethidine Ismelin Tablet: 10 mg, 25 mg Combinations: 25 mg HCTZ/ 10 mg guanethidine (do not use combination as initial therapy in HTN)	**Hypertension:** **Adults:** Initial dose: 10 mg qd Maintenance dose: 10–50 mg qd **Children:** Initial dose: 0.2 mg/kg/d Max dose: 3 mg/kg/d	Administration Issues Allow 1–2 weeks before adjusting dose; safety and efficacy have not been established in children. Drug-Drug Interactions The antihypertensive effect of guanethidine may be inhibited by **haloperidol, methylphenidate, MAO inhibitors, phenothiazines, sympathomimetics, thioxanthenes,** and **tricyclic antidepressants;** concomitant use with **minoxidil** may result in profound orthostatic hypotension.	ADRs Orthostatic hypotension; dizziness; GI upset; impotence; fluid retention; congestive heart failure; asthma in susceptible individuals. Pharmacokinetics $T_{1/2} = 4–8$ d.	Contraindications Hypersensitivity to guanethidine; pheochromocytoma; congestive heart failure; use of MAO inhibitors. Pregnancy Category: C Lactation Issues Guanethidine is excreted in breast milk; either the drug or nursing should be discontinued.
Reserpine Tablet: 0.1 mg, 0.25 mg Combinations: w/ varying strengths of HCTZ, polythiazide, chlorothiazide, hydroxyflumethazide, chlorthalidone, methy- clothiazide and reserpine (do not use combinations as initial therapy for HTN)	**Hypertension:** **Adults:** 0.1–0.25 mg qd **Children:** Initial dose: 20 mcg/kg qd Max dose: 0.25 mg qd	Administration Issues Safety and efficacy have not been established in children < 12 years of age (use in children is not recommended). Drug-Drug Interactions **Tricyclic antidepressants** may block the antihypertensive effect of reserpine; concomitant use of **MAO inhibitors** may cause excitation and hypertension; concomitant use with **digitalis glycosides** may predispose patients to arrhythmias.	ADRs GI upset; increased gastric acid secretion; depression; drowsiness; nasal congestion; impotence. Pharmacokinetics Protein binding = 96%; $T_{1/2} = 33$ h.	Contraindications Hypersensitivity to reserpine; history of mental depression; active peptic ulcer disease; ulcerative colitis. Pregnancy Category: C Lactation Issues Reserpine is excreted in breast milk; either the drug or nursing should be discontinued.
Doxazosin Cardura Tablet: 1 mg, 2 mg, 4 mg, 8 mg	**Hypertension:** Initial dose: 1 mg q hs Max dose: 16 mg/d **Benign prostatic hypertrophy (BPH):** Initial dose: 1 mg q hs Max dose: 8 mg/d	Administration Issues Safety and efficacy have not been established in children; administer at bedtime to minimize adverse effects. Drug-Drug Interactions The antihypertensive effect of **clonidine** may be decreased.	ADRs Orthostatic hypotension; palpitations; GI upset; headache; peripheral edema; impotence. Pharmacokinetics Protein binding = 98%; $T_{1/2} = 22$ h.	Contraindications Hypersensitivity to prazosin, terazosin or doxazosin. Pregnancy Category: C Lactation Issues Doxazosin is excreted in breast milk; use caution in nursing mothers.
Prazosin Minipress	**Hypertension:**	Administration Issues Take the first dose at bedtime; safety and efficacy not established in children.	ADRs "First dose syncope"; orthostatic hypotension; palpitations; GI upset; headache; peripheral edema; impotence.	Contraindications Hypersensitivity to prazosin, terazosin, or doxazosin.

(continues on next page)

205.3 Centrally and Peripherally Acting Antiadrenergic Agents *continued from previous page*

Drug and Dosage Forms	Usual Dosage Range	Administration Issues and Drug-Drug & Drug-Food Interactions	Common Adverse Drug Reactions (ADRs) and Pharmacokinetics	Contraindications, Pregnancy Category, and Lactation Issues
Prazosin *cont.* Capsule: 1 mg, 2 mg, 5 mg Combinations: 0.5 mg polythiazide and varying strengths of prazosin (do not use combinations as initial therapy in HTN)	**Adults:** Initial dose: 1 mg bid to tid Max dose: 20 mg/d **Children:** 0.5–7 mg tid	Drug-Drug Interactions The antihypertensive effect of **clonidine** may be decreased; **indomethacin** may decrease the antihypertensive effect of prazosin; **verapamil** may increase serum prazosin concentrations; **beta blockers** may enhance the first dose syncope effect of prazosin.	Pharmacokinetics Protein binding = 92–97%; extensively metabolized; $T_{1/2}$ = 2–3 h (prolonged in renal insufficiency).	Pregnancy Category: C Lactation Issues Prazosin is excreted in breast milk; use caution in nursing mothers.
Tamulosin Flomax Capsule: 0.4 mg	**Benign prostatic hypertrophy (BPH):** Initial dose: 0.4 mg/d Max dose: 0.8 mg/d	Administration Issues Take ½ h after same meal each day; increase to 0.8 mg/d if response inadequate after 2–4 weeks; if dosing interrupted for several days, restart at 0.4 mg/d; prostate cancer should be ruled out prior to administration. Drug-Drug Interactions **Cimetidine** may interfere with the hepatic clearance of tamulosin; **warfarin** and tamulosin may alter hepatic metabolism of each other.	ADRs Abnormal ejaculate; decreased libido; priapism; postural hypotension; dizziness; syncope; rhinitis; cough; sinusitis; somnolence; amblyopia; nausea; diarrhea; elevated serum transaminases (ALT, AST); decreased RBC. Pharmacokinetics Bioavailability nearly 100%; decreased by food; protein binding 99%; extensive hepatic metabolism; 76% renally excreted; $T_{1/2}$ = 14–15 h in elders; decrease dose in severe hepatic dysfunction; no dose adjustment in renal dysfunction except not studied in patients with CrCl < 10 mL/min	Contraindications Hypersensitivity to tamulosin. Pregnancy Category: B Not indicated for use in women. Lactation Issues Not indicated for use in women.
Terazosin Hytrin Tablets: 1 mg, 2 mg, 5 mg, 10 mg Capsule: 1 mg, 2 mg, 5 mg, 10 mg	**Hypertension:** Initial dose: 1 mg q hs Maintenance dose: 1–5 mg/d Max dose: 20 mg/d **Benign prostatic hypertrophy (BPH):** Initial dose: 1 mg q hs Max dose: 20 mg/d	Administration Issues Take the first dose at bedtime; safety and efficacy have not been established in children. Drug-Drug Interactions The antihypertensive effect of **clonidine** may be decreased.	ADRs Orthostatic hypotension; palpitations; GI upset; headache; peripheral edema; impotence. Pharmacokinetics Protein binding = 90–94%; $T_{1/2}$ = 9–12 h.	Contraindications Hypersensitivity to prazosin, terazosin, or doxazosin. Pregnancy Category: C Lactation Issues It is not known if terazosin is excreted in breast milk; use caution in nursing mothers.

205.4 Alpha/Beta Adrenergic Blocking Agents

Drug and Dosage Forms	Usual Dosage Range	Administration Issues and Drug-Drug & Drug-Food Interactions	Common Adverse Drug Reactions (ADRs) and Pharmacokinetics	Contraindications, Pregnancy Category, and Lactation Issues
Carvedilol Coreg Tablet: 3.125 mg, 6.25 mg, 12.5 mg, 25 mg	**Hypertension and heart failure:** Initial dose: 6.25 mg bid Max dose: 50 mg/d	Administration Issues Take with food; therapy should not be abruptly discontinued; use with caution in patients with hepatic impairment. Drug-Drug Interactions Additive effects when given with other **negative inotropes** or **antihypertensive agents;** carvedilol may increase **digoxin** levels; **cimetidine** increases carvedilol levels; **rifampin** decreases carvedilol levels.	ADRs Bradycardia; hypotension; worsening congestive heart failure (CHF); worsening peripheral vascular disease (PVD); bronchospasm (in susceptible individuals); impotence; masking the signs of hypoglycemia; GI upset; dizziness; fatigue; increased cholesterol levels; increased liver function tests. Pharmacokinetics Protein binding $>$ 98%; $T_{1/2}$ = = 5–11 h.	Contraindications Hypersensitivity to carvedilol; symptomatic bradycardia; greater than first-degree heart block; NYHA Class IV heart failure; asthma. Pregnancy Category: C Lactation Issues It is not known if carvedilol is excreted in breast milk; either the drug or nursing should be discontinued.
Labetalol Normodyne, Trandate Tablet: 100 mg, 200 mg, 300 mg	**Hypertension:** Initial dose: 100 mg bid Maintenance dose: 200–400 mg bid Max dose: 2400 mg/d	Administration Issues Therapy should not be abruptly discontinued; safety and efficacy have not been established in children. Drug-Drug Interactions Additive effects when given with other **negative inotropes** or **antihypertensive agents; cimetidine** may increase the bioavailability of labetalol.	ADRs Bradycardia; hypotension; worsening congestive heart failure (CHF); worsening peripheral vascular disease (PVD); bronchospasm (in susceptible individuals); impotence; masking the signs of hypoglycemia; GI upset; dizziness; fatigue. Pharmacokinetics Protein binding = 50%; $T_{1/2}$ = 5–8 h.	Contraindications Hypersensitivity to beta blocking agents; symptomatic bradycardia; greater than first-degree heart block; CHF (relative); asthma. Pregnancy Category: C Lactation Issues Labetalol is excreted in breast milk; use with caution in nursing mothers.

205.5 Beta-Adrenergic Blocking Agents

Drug and Dosage Forms	Usual Dosage Range	Administration Issues and Drug-Drug & Drug-Food Interactions	Common Adverse Drug Reactions (ADRs) and Pharmacokinetics	Contraindications, Pregnancy Category, and Lactation Issues
Acebutolol Sectral Capsule: 200 mg, 400 mg	**Hypertension:** Initial dose: 400 mg qd Max dose: 1200 mg/d Renal insufficiency: CrCl < 50 mL/min: reduce dose by 50% CrCl < 25 mL/min: reduce dose by 75% Elderly patients may require lower maintenance doses.	Administration Issues Therapy should not be abruptly discontinued; safety and efficacy have not been established in children. Drug-Drug Interactions Additive effects when given with other **negative inotropes** or **antihypertensive agents.**	ADRs Bradycardia; hypotension; worsening CHF; worsening PVD; bronchospasm (in susceptible individuals); impotence; masking the signs of hypoglycemia; GI upset; dizziness; fatigue; sleep disturbance.	Contraindications Hypersensitivity to beta blocking agents; symptomatic bradycardia; greater than first-degree heart block; CHF (relative); asthma. Pregnancy Category: B

(*continues on next page*)

205.5 Beta-Adrenergic Blocking Agents *continued from previous page*

Drug and Dosage Forms	Usual Dosage Range	Administration Issues and Drug-Drug & Drug-Food Interactions	Common Adverse Drug Reactions (ADRs) and Pharmacokinetics	Contraindications, Pregnancy Category, and Lactation Issues
Acebutolol *cont.*			Pharmacokinetics Protein binding = 26%; does not enter the CNS; $T_{1/2}$ = 3–4 h.	Lactation Issues Acebutolol is excreted in breast milk; either the drug or nursing should be discontinued.
Atenolol Tenormin Tablet: 25 mg, 50 mg, 100 mg Combinations: 25 mg chlorthalidone w/varying strengths of atenolol (do not use combinations as initial therapy for HTN)	**Hypertension:** 50–100 mg qd **Angina:** 50–200 mg qd Renal insufficiency: CrCl 15–35 mL/min: max dose = 50 mg qd CrCl < 15 mL/min: max dose = 50 mg qod Hemodialysis: 50 mg after dialysis	Administration Issues Therapy should not be abruptly discontinued; safety and efficacy have not been established in children. Drug-Drug Interactions Additive effects when given with other **negative inotropes** or **antihypertensive agents.**	ADRs Bradycardia; hypotension; worsening CHF, worsening PVD; bronchospasm (in susceptible individuals); impotence; masking the signs of hypoglycemia; GI upset; dizziness; fatigue; sleep disturbance; increased triglycerides, total, and LDL cholesterol; decreased HDL cholesterol. Pharmacokinetics Protein binding = 6–16%; does not enter the CNS; $T_{1/2}$ = 6–9 h.	Contraindications Hypersensitivity to beta blocking agents; symptomatic bradycardia; greater than first degree heart block; CHF (relative); bronchospastic lung disease (asthma). Pregnancy Category: C Lactation Issues Atenolol is excreted in breast milk; either the drug or nursing should be discontinued.
Betaxolol Kerlone Tablet: 10 mg, 20 mg	**Hypertension:** 10–20 mg qd Consider starting with 5 mg qd in elderly patients.	Administration Issues Therapy should not be abruptly discontinued; safety and efficacy have not been established in children. Drug-Drug Interactions Additive effects when given with other **negative inotropes** or **antihypertensive agents.**	ADRs Bradycardia; hypotension; worsening CHF; worsening PVD; bronchospasm (in susceptible individuals); impotence; masking the signs of hypoglycemia; GI upset; dizziness; fatigue; sleep disturbance; increased triglycerides, total, and LDL cholesterol; decreased HDL cholesterol. Pharmacokinetics Protein binding = 50%; $T_{1/2}$ = 14–22 h.	Contraindications Hypersensitivity to beta blocking agents; symptomatic bradycardia; greater than first-degree heart block; CHF (relative); asthma. Pregnancy Category: C Lactation Issues Betaxolol is excreted in breast milk; either the drug or nursing should be discontinued.
Bisoprolol Zebeta Tablet: 5 mg 10 mg	**Hypertension and heart failure:** 5–20 mg qd Renal insufficiency: CrCl < 40 mL/min: initial dose = 2.5 mg qd	Administration Issues Therapy should not be abruptly discontinued; safety and efficacy have not been established in children. Drug-Drug Interactions Additive effects when given with other **negative inotropes** or **antihypertensive agents.**	ADRs Bradycardia; hypotension; worsening CHF; worsening PVD; bronchospasm (in susceptible individuals); impotence; masking the signs of hypoglycemia; GI upset; dizziness; fatigue; sleep disturbance.	Contraindications Hypersensitivity to beta blocking agents; symptomatic bradycardia; greater than first-degree heart block; CHF (relative); asthma. Pregnancy Category: C

Combinations: 6.25 mg HCTZ w/varying strengths of bisoprolol (do not use combinations as initial therapy for HTN)			Pharmacokinetics Protein binding = 30%; $T_{1/2}$ = 9–12 h.	Lactation Issues Bisoprolol is excreted in breast milk; either the drug or nursing should be discontinued.
Carteolol Cartrol Tablet: 2.5 mg, 5 mg	**Hypertension:** 2.5–10 mg qd Renal insufficiency: CrCl 20–60 mL/min: dosing interval = qod CrCl < 20 mL/min: dosing interval = q 3 d	Administration Issues Therapy should not be abruptly discontinued; safety and efficacy have not been established in children. Drug-Drug Interactions Additive effects when given with other **negative inotropes** or **antihypertensive agents.**	ADRs Bradycardia; hypotension; worsening CHF; worsening PVD; bronchospasm (in susceptible individuals); impotence; masking the signs of hypoglycemia; GI upset; dizziness; fatigue; sleep disturbance. Pharmacokinetics Protein binding = 23–30%; does not enter the CNS; $T_{1/2}$ = 6 h.	Contraindications Hypersensitivity to beta blocking agents; symptomatic bradycardia; greater than first-degree heart block; CHF (relative); asthma. Pregnancy Category: C Lactation Issues It is not known if carteolol is excreted in breast milk; either the drug or nursing should be discontinued.
Metoprolol Lopressor, Toprol XL Tablet: 50 mg, 100 mg Extended Release Tablets: 50 mg, 100 mg, 200 mg	**Hypertension, angina, myocardial infarction, and heart failure:** Immediate release tablets: Initial dose: 50 mg bid Max dose: 400 mg/d Extended release tablets: Initial dose: 50 mg qd Max dose: 400 mg/d	Administration Issues Food increases the absorption of metoprolol; therapy should not be abruptly discontinued; safety and efficacy have not been established in children. Drug-Drug Interactions Additive effects when given with other **negative inotropes** or **antihypertensive agents; cimetidine** may decrease the metabolism of metoprolol.	ADRs Bradycardia; hypotension; worsening CHF; worsening PVD; bronchospasm (in susceptible individuals); impotence; masking the signs of hypoglycemia; GI upset; dizziness; fatigue; sleep disturbance; increased triglycerides, total, and LDL cholesterol; decreased HDL cholesterol. Pharmacokinetics Protein binding = 12%; readily enters into the CNS; $T_{1/2}$ = 3–7 h.	Contraindications Hypersensitivity to beta blocking agents; symptomatic bradycardia; greater than first-degree heart block; CHF (relative); asthma. Pregnancy Category: C Lactation Issues Metoprolol is excreted in breast milk; either the drug or nursing should be discontinued.
Nadolol Corgard Tablet: 20mg, 40 mg, 80 mg, 120 mg, 160 mg Combinations: w/ varying strengths of nadolol and 5 mg bendroflumethiazide (combinations should not be used as initial therapy for HTN)	**Hypertension:** Initial dose: 40 mg qd Max dose: 320 mg/d **Angina:** Initial dose: 40 mg qd Max dose: 240 mg/d Renal insufficiency: CrCl 31–50 mL/min: dosing interval = 24–36 h CrCl 10–30 mL/min: dosing interval = 24–48 h CrCl < 10 mL/min: 40–60 h	Administration Issues Therapy should not be abruptly discontinued; safety and efficacy have not been established in children. Drug-Drug Interactions Additive effects when given with other **negative inotropes** or **antihypertensive agents.**	ADRs Bradycardia; hypotension; worsening CHF; worsening PVD; bronchospasm (in susceptible individuals); impotence; masking the signs of hypoglycemia; GI upset; dizziness; fatigue; sleep disturbance; increased triglycerides, total and LDL cholesterol; decreased HDL cholesterol Pharmacokinetics Protein binding = 30%; does not enter the CNS; $T_{1/2}$ = 20–24 h.	Contraindications Hypersensitivity to beta blocking agents; symptomatic bradycardia; greater than first-degree heart block; CHF (relative); asthma. Pregnancy Category: C Lactation Issues Nadolol is excreted in breast milk; either the drug or nursing should be discontinued.

(continues on next page)

205.5 Beta-Adrenergic Blocking Agents *continued from previous page*

Drug and Dosage Forms	Usual Dosage Range	Administration Issues and Drug-Drug & Drug-Food Interactions	Common Adverse Drug Reactions (ADRs) and Pharmacokinetics	Contraindications, Pregnancy Category, and Lactation Issues
Penbutolol Levatol Tablet: 20 mg	**Hypertension:** 20 mg qd Max dose = 80 mg	Administration Issues Therapy should not be abruptly discontinued; safety and efficacy have not been established in children. Drug-Drug Interactions Additive effects when given with other **negative inotropes** or **antihypertensive agents.**	ADRs Bradycardia; hypotension; worsening CHF; worsening PVD; bronchospasm (in susceptible individuals); impotence; masking the signs of hypoglycemia; GI upset; dizziness; fatigue; sleep disturbance; increased triglycerides, total and LDL cholesterol; decreased HDL cholesterol. Pharmacokinetics Protein binding = 80–98%; $T_{1/2}$ = 5 h.	Contraindications Hypersensitivity to beta blocking agents; symptomatic bradycardia; greater than first-degree heart block; CHF (relative); asthma. Pregnancy Category: C Lactation Issues It is not known if penbutolol is excreted in breast milk; either the drug or nursing should be discontinued.
Pindolol Visken Tablet: 5 mg, 10 mg	**Hypertension:** Initial dose: 5 mg bid Max dose: 60 mg/d	Administration Issues Therapy should not be abruptly discontinued; safety and efficacy have not been established in children. Drug-Drug Interactions Additive effects when given with other **negative inotropes** or **antihypertensive agents.**	ADRs Bradycardia; hypotension; worsening CHF; worsening PVD; bronchospasm (in susceptible individuals); impotence; masking the signs of hypoglycemia; GI upset; dizziness; fatigue; sleep disturbance. Pharmacokinetics Protein binding = 40%; $T_{1/2}$ = 3–4 h.	Contraindications Hypersensitivity to beta blocking agents; symptomatic bradycardia; greater than first-degree heart block; CHF (relative); asthma. Pregnancy Category: B Lactation Issues Pindolol is excreted in breast milk; either the drug or nursing should be discontinued.
Propranolol Inderal Tablet: 10 mg, 20 mg, 40 mg, 60 mg, 80 mg, 90 mg Sustained Release Capsules: 60 mg, 80 mg, 120 mg, 160 mg Solution: 4 mg/ml, 8 mg/ml, 80 mg/ml	**Hypertension:** Immediate release tablets: Initial dose: 40 mg bid Sustained release capsules: Initial dose: 80 mg qd Max dose: 640 mg/d **Angina/myocardial infarction:** Initial dose: 80 mg bid (immediate release tablets) 160 mg qd (SR capsules) Max dose: 320 mg/d	Administration Issues Food increases the absorption of propranolol; therapy should not be abruptly discontinued; safety and efficacy have not been established in children. Drug-Drug Interactions Additive effects when given with other **negative inotropes** or **antihypertensive agents; cimetidine** may decrease the metabolism of propranolol; **bile acid resins** may decrease the absorption of propranolol.	ADRs Bradycardia; hypotension; worsening CHF; worsening PVD; bronchospasm (in susceptible individuals); impotence; masking the signs of hypoglycemia; GI upset; dizziness; fatigue; sleep disturbance; increased triglycerides, total and LDL cholesterol; decreased HDL cholesterol. Pharmacokinetics Protein binding = 90%; readily enters the CNS; $T_{1/2}$ = 3–5 h.	Contraindications Hypersensitivity to beta blocking agents; symptomatic bradycardia; greater than first-degree heart block; CHF (relative); asthma. Pregnancy Category: C Lactation Issues Propranolol is excreted in breast milk; either the drug or nursing should be discontinued.

Combinations: w/ varying strengths of HCTZ and propranolol (combinations should not be used as initial therapy for HTN)	**Migraine prophylaxis:** Initial dose: 40 mg bid (immediate release tablets) Initial dose: 80 mg qd (sustained release capsules) Max dose: 240 mg/d **Essential tremor:** Initial dose: 40 mg bid Max dose: 320 mg/d **Traumatic Brain Injury** 5 mg bid, increase 5 mg q 5 d up to 45 mg			
Timolol Blocadren Tablet: 5 mg, 10 mg, 20 mg	**Hypertension:** Initial dose: 10 mg bid Max dose: 60 mg/d **Myocardial infarction:** 10 mg bid **Migraine prophylaxis:** Initial dose: 10 mg bid Max dose: 30 mg/d	Administration Issues Therapy should not be abruptly discontinued; safety and efficacy have not been established in children. Drug-Drug Interactions Additive effects when given with other **negative inotropes** or **antihypertensive agents.**	ADRs Bradycardia; hypotension; worsening congestive heart failure (CHF); worsening peripheral vascular disease (PVD); bronchospasm (in susceptible individuals); impotence; masking the signs of hypoglycemia; GI upset; dizziness; fatigue; sleep disturbance; increased triglycerides, total and LDL cholesterol; decreased HDL cholesterol. Pharmacokinetics Protein binding = 10%; $T_{1/2}$ = 4 h.	Contraindications Hypersensitivity to beta blocking agents; symptomatic bradycardia; greater than first-degree heart block; CHF (relative); asthma. Pregnancy Category: C Lactation Issues Timolol is excreted in breast milk; either the drug or nursing should be discontinued.

205.6 Calcium Channel Blockers

Drug and Dosage Forms	Usual Dosage Range	Administration Issues and Drug-Drug & Drug-Food Interactions	Common Adverse Drug Reactions (ADRs) and Pharmacokinetics	Contraindications, Pregnancy Category, and Lactation Issues
Amlodipine Norvasc Tablet: 2.5 mg 5 mg 10 mg	**Hypertension:** 2.5–10 mg qd **Chronic stable and vasospastic angina:** 5–10 mg qd	Administration Issues Safety and efficacy have not been established in children. Drug-Drug Interactions Additive myocardial depression may occur in patients taking beta blockers.	ADRs Hypotension, peripheral edema, tachycardia, flushing, headache, GI upset. Pharmacokinetics Absorption = 80–90%; extensive first pass metabolism; hepatically metabolized; 93% protein bound; $T_{1/2}$ = 30–50 h.	Contraindications Hypersensitivity to amlodipine; hypotension; sick sinus syndrome; second-or third-degree AV block. Pregnancy Category: C Lactation Issues It is not known if amlodipine is excreted in breast milk.

(*continues on next page*)

205.6 Calcium Channel Blockers *continued from previous page*

Drug and Dosage Forms	Usual Dosage Range	Administration Issues and Drug-Drug & Drug-Food Interactions	Common Adverse Drug Reactions (ADRs) and Pharmacokinetics	Contraindications, Pregnancy Category, and Lactation Issues
Bepridil Vascor Tablet: 200 mg, 300 mg, 400 mg	**Chronic stable angina:** 200–400 mg qd Max dose = 400 mg/day	Administration Issues Due to the risk of serious ventricular arrhythmias, use should be reserved to patients who fail to respond to or who are intolerant of other anti-anginals; safety and efficacy have not been established in children. Drug-Drug Interactions Additive myocardial depression may occur in patients taking beta blockers.	ADRs Hypotension, flushing, headache, GI upset, drowsiness, arrhythmias, prolonged QT interval. Pharmacokinetics Absorption = 100%; onset = 60 minutes; hepatically metabolized; > 99% protein bound; $T_{1/2}$ = 24 h.	Contraindications Hypersensitivity to bepridil; hypotension; sick sinus syndrome; second-or third-degree AV block; ventricular arrhythmias; prolonged QT interval; uncompensated heart failure. Pregnancy Category: C Lactation Issues Bepridil is excreted in breast milk.
Diltiazem Cardizem, Dilacor XR Tablet: 30 mg, 60 mg, 90 mg, 120 mg Sustained Release Capsule: 60 mg, 90 mg, 120 mg, 180 mg, 240 mg, 300 mg	**Hypertension, chronic stable and vasospastic angina:** Regular release tablets: 30–120 mg tid or qid Sustained release capsules (Cardizem SR): 60–240 mg bid Sustained release capsules (Cardizem CD, Dilacor XR): 120–480 mg qd	Administration Issues Do not crush or chew extended release capsules; Dilacor XR should be taken on an empty stomach; safety and efficacy have not been established in children. Drug-Drug Interactions Additive myocardial depression may occur in patients taking beta blockers; **cimetidine** and **ranitidine** may increase diltiazem levels.	ADRs Hypotension, peripheral edema, bradycardia, flushing, headache, GI upset, congestive heart failure. Pharmacokinetics Absorption = 80–90%; onset = 30–60 minutes; hepatically metabolized; 70–80% protein bound; $T_{1/2}$ = 3.5–7 h.	Contraindications Hypersensitivity to diltiazem; hypotension; sick sinus syndrome; second-or third-degree AV block; acute MI; CHF. Pregnancy Category: C Lactation Issues Diltiazem is excreted in breast milk.
Felodipine Plendil Extended Release Tablet: 2.5 mg, 5 mg, 10 mg	**Hypertension:** 2.5–10 mg qd	Administration Issues Avoid grapefruit products before and after dosing; do not crush or chew extended release tablets; safety and efficacy have not been established in children. Drug-Drug Interactions Additive myocardial depression may occur in patients taking **beta blockers; cimetidine** and **ranitidine** may increase felodipine levels.	ADRs Hypotension, peripheral edema, tachycardia, flushing, headache, GI upset. Pharmacokinetics Absorption = 100%; onset = 2–5 hours; hepatically metabolized; >99% protein bound; $T_{1/2}$ = 11–16 h.	Contraindications Hypersensitivity to felodipine; hypotension; sick sinus syndrome; second-or third-degree AV block Pregnancy Category: C Lactation Issues It is not known if felodipine is excreted in breast milk.
Isradipine Dynacirc	**Hypertension:** 2.5–10 mg bid	Administration Issues Safety and efficacy have not been established in children.	ADRs Hypotension, peripheral edema, tachycardia, flushing, headache, GI upset.	Contraindications Hypersensitivity to isradipine; hypotension; sick sinus syndrome; second-or third-degree AV block.

Capsule: 2.5 mg, 5 mg		Drug-Drug Interactions Additive myocardial depression may occur in patients taking **beta blockers.**	Pharmacokinetics Absorption = 90–95%; onset = 2 h; hepatically metabolized; 95% protein bound; $T_{1/2}$ = 8 h.	Pregnancy Category: C Lactation Issues It is not known if isradipine is excreted in breast milk.
Nicardipine Cardene Capsule: 20 mg, 30 mg Sustained Release Capsule: 45 mg, 60 mg	**Hypertension:** Regular release capsules: 20–40 mg tid Sustained release capsules: 30–60 mg bid **Angina:** 20–40 mg tid	Administration Issues Do not crush or chew extended release capsules; lower doses may be required in patients with hepatic insufficiency. Drug-Drug Interactions Additive myocardial depression may occur in patients taking **beta blockers.**	ADRs Hypotension, peripheral edema, tachycardia, flushing, headache, GI upset. Pharmacokinetics Absorption = 100%; onset = 20 minutes; hepatically metabolized; >95% protein bound; $T_{1/2}$ = 2–4 h.	Contraindications Hypersensitivity to nicardipine; hypotension; sick sinus syndrome; second-or third-degree AV block; advanced aortic stenosis. Pregnancy Category: C Lactation Issues Nicardipine is excreted in breast milk.
Nifedipine Adalat, Procardia Capsule: 10 mg, 20 mg Sustained Release Tablet: 30 mg, 60 mg, 90 mg	**Hypertension:** Regular release capsules: 10–20 mg tid or qid Sustained release tablets: 30–120 mg qd **Chronic stable and vasospastic angina:** Regular release capsules: 10–20 mg tid or qid Sustained release tablets: 30–90 mg qd	Administration Issues Do not crush or chew extended release tablets. Drug-Drug Interactions Additive myocardial depression may occur in patients taking **beta blockers.**	ADRs Hypotension, peripheral edema, tachycardia, flushing, headache, GI upset. Pharmacokinetics Absorption = 90%; onset = 20 minutes; hepatically metabolized; 92–98% protein bound; $T_{1/2}$ = 2–5 h.	Contraindications Hypersensitivity to nifedipine; hypotension; sick sinus syndrome; second-or third-degree AV block. Pregnancy Category: C Lactation Issues An insignificant amount of nifedipine is excreted in breast milk.
Nisoldipine Sular Extended Release Tablet: 10 mg, 20 mg, 30 mg, 40 mg	**Hypertension:** 10–60 mg qd	Administration Issues Avoid administration with a high fat meal; avoid grapefruit products before and after dosing; do not crush or chew extended release tablets; lower doses may be required in patients > 65 years or in patients with hepatic insufficiency. Drug-Drug Interactions Additive myocardial depression may occur in patients taking **beta blockers.**	ADRs Hypotension, peripheral edema, tachycardia, flushing, headache, GI upset. Pharmacokinetics Absorption = 80–90%; extensive first pass metabolism; hepatically metabolized; >99% protein bound; $T_{1/2}$ = 7–12 h.	Contraindications Hypersensitivity to nisoldipine; hypotension; sick sinus syndrome; second-or third-degree AV block. Pregnancy Category: C Lactation Issues It is not known if nisoldipine is excreted in breast milk.

(*continues on next page*)

205.6 Calcium Channel Blockers *continued from previous page*

Drug and Dosage Forms	Usual Dosage Range	Administration Issues and Drug-Drug & Drug-Food Interactions	Common Adverse Drug Reactions (ADRs) and Pharmacokinetics	Contraindications, Pregnancy Category, and Lactation Issues
Verapamil Calan, Covera-HS, Isoptin, Verelan Tablet: 40 mg, 80 mg, 120 mg Sustained Release Tablet: 120 mg, 180 mg, 240 mg Extended Release Tablet: 180 mg. 240 mg Sustained Release Capsule: 180 mg, 240 mg, 360 mg	**Hypertension:** Regular release tablets: 40–160 mg tid SR tablets and capsules: 120–480 mg qd (doses > 240 mg should be given divided bid) **Angina:** 40–120 mg tid **Atrial fibrillation, atrial flutter, supraventricular tachycardia:** 240–480 mg, divided, tid or qid	Administration Issues Do not crush or chew extended release tablets and capsules. Drug-Drug Interactions Additive myocardial depression may occur in patients taking **beta blockers;** increased **digoxin** and **quinidine** levels may occur with concomitant administration.	ADRs Hypotension, peripheral edema, bradycardia, flushing, headache, GI upset, congestive heart failure, constipation. Pharmacokinetics Absorption = 90%; onset = 30 minutes; hepatically metabolized; 83–92% protein bound; $T_{1/2}$ = 3–7 h.	Contraindications Hypersensitivity to verapamil; hypotension; sick sinus syndrome; second-or third-degree AV block; uncompensated heart failure. Pregnancy Category: C Lactation Issues Verapamil is excreted in breast milk.

205.7 Vasodilators

Drug and Dosage Forms	Usual Dosage Range	Administration Issues and Drug-Drug & Drug-Food Interactions	Common Adverse Drug Reactions (ADRs) and Pharmacokinetics	Contraindications, Pregnancy Category, and Lactation Issues
Hydralazine Apresoline Tablet: 10 mg, 25 mg, 50 mg, 100 mg Combinations: w/ varying strengths of HCTZ, hydralazine and reserpine (do not use combinations as initial therapy for HTN)	**Hypertension:** **Adults:** Initial dose: 10 mg qid Max dose: 300 mg/d, divided **Children:** Initial dose: 0.75 mg/kg/d qid Max dose: 7.5 mg/kg/d or 200 mg/d	Administration Issues Taking hydralazine with food increases absorption; take with meals; safety and efficacy have not been established in children. Drug-Drug Interactions **Metoprolol** and **propranolol** may increase hydralazine concentrations; hydralazine may increase **metoprolol** and **propranolol** concentrations; **indomethacin** may decrease the effects of hydralazine.	ADRs Reflex tachycardia; peripheral edema; headache; GI upset; palpitations; lupus-like syndrome. Pharmacokinetics Protein binding = 87%; extensive hepatic metabolism; $T_{1/2}$ = 3–7 h.	Contraindications Hypersensitivity to hydralazine; coronary artery disease; rheumatic mitral valve disease. Pregnancy Category: C Lactation Issues Hydralazine is excreted in breast milk; according to the American Academy of Pediatrics, hydralazine is compatible with breastfeeding.

Minoxidil Loniten Tablet: 2.5 mg, 10 mg	**Hypertension:** **Adults:** Initial dose: 2.5 mg qd Max dose: 100 mg/d **Children:** Initial dose: 0.2 mg/kg/d Max dose: 50 mg/day	Administration Issues Allow at least 3 days before titrating dosage; safety and efficacy have not been established in children. Drug-Drug Interactions Concomitant use with **guanethidine** may result in profound orthostatic hypotension.	ADRs Reflex tachycardia; peripheral edema; GI upset; headache; hirsutism; pericardial effusion. Pharmacokinetics No protein binding; metabolites are renally eliminated; $T_{1/2} = 4.2$ h.	Contraindications Hypersensitivity to minoxidil; coronary artery disease; pheochromocytoma; acute myocardial infarction. Pregnancy Category: C Lactation Issues Minoxidil is excreted in breast milk; either the drug or nursing should be discontinued.

206. Antiplatelet Agents

Drug and Dosage Forms	Usual Dosage Range	Administration Issues and Drug-Drug & Drug-Food Interactions	Common Adverse Drug Reactions (ADRs) and Pharmacokinetics	Contraindications, Pregnancy Category, and Lactation Issues
Dipyridamole Persantine Tablet: 25 mg, 50 mg, 75 mg	**Adjunct to warfarin in the prevention of postoperative thromboembolic complications of cardiac valve replacement** 75–100 mg qid along with warfarin therapy	Administration Issues Safety and efficacy in children < 12 years have not been established.	ADRs Hypotension; dizziness; GI upset; headache; rash; flushing. Pharmacokinetics $T_{1/2}$ = 10 h; highly protein bound; metabolized by the liver and excreted in bile.	Contraindications Hypersensitivity to dipyridamole. Pregnancy Category: B Lactation issues Dipyridamole is excreted in breast milk; use with caution in nursing women.
Cilostazol Pletal Tablet: 50 mg, 100 mg	**Intermittent claudication** 100 mg bid (50 mg bid. if receiving inhibitors of cilostazol metabolism)	Administration Issues: Give 30 minutes before or at least 2 h after food. Drug-Drug Interactions Concurrent administration of **ketoconazole, itraconazole, erythromycin, diltiazem, fluconazole, miconazole, fluvoxamine, fluoxetine, nefazodone, sertraline,** or **omeprazole** decreases metabolism and increases levels and activity of cilostazol.	ADRs Headache, dizziness, palpitations, tachycardia, diarrhea. Pharmacokinetics: Slowly absorbed after oral administration; 95–98% protein binding; extensively metabolized by liver (two active metabolites); $T_{1/2}$ = 11–13 h	Contraindications Hypersensitivity, heart failure, lactation. Pregnancy Category: C Lactation Issues: Contraindicated.
Clopidogrel Plavix Tablet: 75 mg	**Reduction of atherosclerotic events (e.g., MI, stroke, vascular death) in patients at risk; postintracoronary stent placement** 75 mg qd (300 mg loading dose for those post-stent placement)	Administration Issues May give without regard to meals. Drug-Drug Interactions Concurrent platelet inhibitors (e.g., **abciximab, tirofiban, aspirin, NSAIDs), heparin, thrombolytic agents, ticlopidine, warfarin** (increased risk of bleeding). May inhibit metabolism and increase the effect of **phenytoin, tolbutamide, tamoxifen, warfarin, torsemide, fluvastatin,** and many **NSAIDs.**	ADRs GI bleeding depression, dizziness, fatigue, headache, epistatis, cough, dyspnea, chest pain, edema, hypertension, abdominal pain, diarrhea, dyspepsia, gastritis, puritius, purpura, rash, neutropenia (rare) athralgia, back pain. Pharmacokinetics Well absorbed; 98% protein bound; Rapidly metabolized in liver its active metabolite, which is eliminated 50% in urine and 45% in feces; $T_{1/2}$ = 8 h	Contraindications Hypersensitivity, active (peptic ulcer, intracoastal, hemorrhage) pathologic bleeding. Pregnancy Category: B Lactation Issues Clopidogrel may be excreted into breast milk. Consider risk versus benefit.

Ticlopidine Ticlid Tablet: 250 mg	**To reduce the risk of stroke in patients who are intolerant of aspirin, who have experienced stroke precursors or have had a completed thrombotic stroke.** 250 mg bid with food	Administration Issues: Safety and efficacy in patients < 18 years of age have not been established; take with food to minimized GI upset. **CBCs should be done every 2 weeks through the third month of treatment.** Drug-Drug Interactions Administering ticlopidine with **antacids** may decrease its absorption; **cimetidine** may increase the concentration of ticlopidine; **aspirin** may potentiate the effects of ticlopidine; ticlopidine increases **theophylline** levels and decreases **digoxin** levels. Drug-Food Interactions Administering with food increases the bioavailability approximately 20%.	ADRs GI upset; diarrhea; rash; vomiting; **neutropenia;** increased risk of bleeding, increased liver function tests (AST, ALT, alkaline phosphatase). Pharmacokinetics: Absorption = 80%; $T_{1/2}$ = 4–5 days; protein binding = 98%; extensively metabolized by the liver to inactive metabolites.	Contraindications Hypersensitivity to ticlopidine; neutropenia; thrombocytopenia; active bleeding; severe liver impairment. Pregnancy Category: B Lactation issues Due to the potential risk for serious adverse effects, either the drug or nursing should be discontinued.

207. Cardiac Glycosides

Drug and Dosage Forms	Usual Dosage Range	Administration Issues and Drug-Drug & Drug-Food Interactions	Common Adverse Drug Reactions (ADRs) and Pharmacokinetics	Contraindications, Pregnancy Category, and Lactation Issues
Digoxin Lanoxin, Lanoxicaps Tablet 0.125 mg, 0.25 mg, 0.5 mg Capsule 0.05 mg, 0.1 mg, 0.2 mg Pediatric Elixir: 0.05 mg per ml	**Heart failure, atrial fibrillation, and atrial flutter** Oral loading dose: 0.01–0.02 mg/kg (using lean body weight). Give 50% to start. Give remaining 50% in two equal doses at 6–8 h intervals Assess for toxicity before each dose. Maintenance dose: Tablets: 0.625 mg to 0.5 mg daily based on size and renal function Capsules: 0.05 to 0.2 mg daily based on size and renal function	Administration Issues Bioavailability may vary among products. Drug–Drug Interactions The following drugs may increase digoxin levels: **amiodarone, quinidine, verapamil, antibiotics, propafenone, omeprazole, ibuprofen, indomethacin, captopril, itraconazle.** The following drugs may decrease digoxin levels: **cholestyramine, colestipol, antacids, rifampin, sucralfate, hydantoins, barbiturates.** Therapeutic range: 0.5 to 2 ng/ml.	ADRs Anorexia, nausea, vomiting, diarrhea, headache, visual disturbances (blurred, green or yellow vision, or halo effect), altered mental status, cardiac arrhythmias, gynecomastia, rash, eosinophilia, thrombocytopenia. Hypokalemia, hypomagnesemia, and hypercalcemia may predispose to cardiac arrhythmias. Pharmacokinetics Absorption: tablets 60%–80%; elixir 70%–85%; capsules 90%–100%; distributed into myocardium, skeletal muscle, liver and kidney; crosses blood brain barrier and placenta; correlates with lean body weight; primarily excreted by the kidney; not removed by dialysis.	Contraindications Ventricular fibrillation, ventricular tachycardia, presence of digoxin toxicity, beriberi heart disease, hypersensitivity to digoxin, hypersensitive carotid sinus syndrome. Pregnancy Category: C Lactation Issues Digoxin is excreted in breast milk; safety has not been established.
Digitoxin Crystodigin Tablet 0.05 mg, 0.1 mg	**Heart failure, atrial fibrillation, and atrial flutter** Rapid loading: 0.6 mg followed by 0.4 mg followed by 0.2 mg separated by 4–6 hours Slow loading: 0.2 mg bid for 4 d Maintenance dose: 0.05–0.3 mg daily **Children** Loading dose: < 1 year: 0.045 mg/kg 1–2 years: 0.04 mg/kg > 2 years: 0.03 mg/kg Maintenance dose: one-tenth of loading dose	Drug–Drug Interactions The following drugs may increase digitoxin levels: **amiodarone, quinidine, verapamil, antibiotics, propafenone, omeprazole, ibuprofen, indomethacin, captopril, itraconazle.** The following drugs may decrease digitoxin levels: **cholestyramine, colestipol, antacids, rifampin, sucralfate, hydantoins, barbiturates.** Therapeutic range: 14–26 ng/ml.	ADRs Anorexia, nausea, vomiting, diarrhea, headache, visual disturbances (blurred, green or yellow vision, or halo effect), altered mental status, cardiac arrhythmias, gynecomastia, rash, eosinophilia, thrombocytopenia. Pharmacokinetics Almost completely absorbed; distributed into myocardium, skeletal muscle, liver and kidney; metabolized by the liver primarily to inactive metabolites; not removed by dialysis.	Contraindications Ventricular fibrillation, ventricular tachycardia, presence of digitoxin toxicity, beriberi heart disease, hypersensitivity to digitoxin, hypersensitive carotid sinus syndrome. Pregnancy Category: C Lactation Issues It is not known whether digitoxin is excreted in breast milk.

208. Diuretics

208.1 Carbonic Anhydrase Inhibitors

Drug and Dosage Forms	Usual Dosage Range	Administration Issues and Drug-Drug & Drug-Food Interactions	Common Adverse Drug Reactions (ADRs) and Pharmacokinetics	Contraindications, Pregnancy Category, and Lactation Issues
Acetazolamide Diamox Tablet: 125 mg, 250 mg Sustained Released Capsule: 500 mg	**Open angle glaucoma:** 250–1000 mg in divided doses **Closed angle glaucoma:** (short term) 250 mg q 4 hours **Children:** 10–15 mg/kg/d divided, q 6–8 h **Diuresis:** 5 mg/kg (usually 250–375 mg) daily **Epilepsy:** 8–30 mg/kg/d (375–1000 mg daily), divided **Acute mountain sickness:** 500–1000 mg , divided; should initiate 24–48 h before ascent and continue for 48 h while at high altitude or longer to control symptoms	Administration Issues Increasing the dose does not appear to increase diuresis. Drug-Drug Interactions Acetazolamide may increase **cyclosporine** levels; may decrease **primidone** levels; concurrent use with **salicylates** may result in accumulation and toxicity of acetazolamide.	ADRs Hypokalemia, GI upset, paresthesias, bone marrow suppression, urticaria, rash, photosensitivity, metabolic acidosis. Pharmacokinetics Tablets: Onset = 1–1.5 h; Peak = 1–4 h; Duration = 8–12 h. SR capsules: Onset = 2 h; Peak = 3–6 h; Duration = 18–24 h.	Contraindications Hypersensitivity to acetazolamide. Pregnancy Category: C Lactation Issues Safety has not been established.
Dichlorphenamide Daranide Tablet: 50 mg	**Glaucoma:** Initial dose: 100–200 mg followed by 100 mg q 12 h Maintenance dose: 25–50 mg qd to tid	Drug-Drug Interactions Concurrent use with **salicylates** may result in accumulation and toxicity of dichlorphenamide.	ADRs xHypokalemia, GI upset, paresthesias, bone marrow suppression, urticaria, rash, photosensitivity, metabolic acidosis. Pharmacokinetics Onset = 1 h; Peak = 2–4 h; Duration = 6–12 h.	Contraindications Use caution in patients with severe respiratory acidosis, pulmonary obstruction, or emphysema (may impair ventilation). Pregnancy Category: C Lactation Issues Safety has not been established.
Methazolamide Neptazane Tablet: 25 mg 50 mg	**Glaucoma:** 50–100 mg 2 to 3 times daily	Drug-Drug Interactions Concurrent use with **salicylates** may result in accumulation and toxicity of methazolamide.	ADRs Hypokalemia, GI upset, paresthesias, bone marrow suppression, urticaria, rash, photosensitivity, metabolic acidosis. Pharmacokinetics Onset = 2–4 h; Peak = 6–8 h; Duration = 10–18 h.	Contraindications Use in patients with hepatic dysfunction may precipitate hepatic coma. Pregnancy Category: C Lactation Issues Safety has not been established.

208.2 Loop Diuretics

Drug and Dosage Forms	Usual Dosage Range	Administration Issues and Drug-Drug & Drug-Food Interactions	Common Adverse Drug Reactions (ADRs) and Pharmacokinetics	Contraindications, Pregnancy Category, and Lactation Issues
Bumetanide Bumex Tablet: 0.5 mg, 1 mg, 2 mg	**Edema:** Initial dose: 0.5–2 mg/d Max dose: 10 mg/d	Administration Issues Take early in the day to avoid nocturia Drug-Drug Interactions Additive effect with **thiazide** and **thiazide-like diuretics; salicylates** and **NSAIDs** may decrease efficacy of loop diuretics; may increase **lithium** levels.	ADRs Dehydration; hyponatremic, hypochloremic; hypokalemia; hypomagnesemia; hypocalcemia; hyperuricemia; increased triglycerides, LDL and total cholesterol; decreased HDL cholesterol; photosensitivity; hypotension; GI upset; pancreatitis; thrombocytopenia. Pharmacokinetics $T_{1/2}$ = 60–90 minutes; onset = 30 minutes; duration = 4–6 h.	Contraindications Severe electrolyte depletion until improved or corrected; anuria; hypersensitivity to bumetanide or sulfonylureas. Pregnancy Category: C Lactation Issues It is unknown if bumetanide is excreted in breast milk.
Ethacrynic Acid Edecrin Tablet: 25 mg, 50 mg	**Ascites, CHF, nephrotic syndrome, acute pulmonary edema:** Initial dose: 50–200 mg/d Max dose: 200 mg bid **Children:** Initial dose: 25 mg/d then titrate to response	Administration Issues Take early in the day to avoid nocturia. Drug-Drug Interactions Additive effect with **thiazide** and **thiazide-like diuretics; salicylates** and **NSAIDs** may decrease efficacy of loop diuretics; may increase **lithium** levels.	ADRs Severe, watery diarrhea; dehydration; hyponatremia; hypokalemia; hypochloremic alkalosis, hypomagnesemia; hypocalcemia; hyperuricemia; ototoxicity, increased triglycerides, LDL and total cholesterol; decreased HDL cholesterol; photosensitivity; hypotension; GI upset; pancreatitis. Pharmacokinetics Absorption = 100%; $T_{1/2}$ = 60 minutes; onset = 30 minutes; duration = 6–8 h.	Contraindications Anuria; hypersensitivity to ethacrynic acid; not recommended for use in children. Pregnancy Category: B Lactation Issues: It is unknown if ethacrynic acid is excreted in breast milk.
Furosemide Lasix Tablet: 20 mg, 40 mg, 80 mg Oral Solution: 10 mg/ml, 40 mg/5 ml	**Edema:** Initial dose: 20–40 mg/d Max dose: 600 mg/d **Hypertension:** Initial dose: 20–40 mg/d **Children:** Initial dose: 2 mg/kg/d Maintenance dose: 0.5–2 mg/kg bid Max dose: 6 mg/kg/d	Administration Issues Take early in the day to avoid nocturia. Drug-Drug Interactions Additive effect with **thiazide** and **thiazide-like diuretics; salicylates** and **NSAIDs** may decrease efficacy of loop diuretics; may increase **lithium** levels.	ADRs Dehydration; ototoxicity; hyponatremic, hypokalemia; hypomagnesemia; alkalosis, hypocalcemia; hyperuricemia; glucose intolerance; increased triglycerides, LDL and total cholesterol; decreased HDL cholesterol; photosensitivity; hypotension; GI upset; pancreatitis. Pharmacokinetics $T_{1/2}$ = 120 minutes; onset = 60 minutes; duration = 6–8 h.	Contraindications Anuria; hypersensitivity to furosemide or sulfonylureas. Pregnancy Category: C Lactation Issues Furosemide is excreted in breast milk.

Torsemide Demadex Tablet: 5 mg, 10 mg, 20 mg, 100 mg	**CHF:** Initial dose: 10–20 mg/d Max dose: 200 mg/d **Chronic renal failure:** Initial dose: 20 mg/d Max dose: 200 mg/d **Hepatic cirrhosis:** Initial dose: 5–10 mg/d Max dose: 40 mg/d **Hypertension:** Initial dose: 5 mg/d Max dose: 10 mg/d	Administration Issues Take early in the day to avoid nocturia; may be taken without regards to meals. Drug-Drug Interactions Additive effect with **thiazide** and **thiazide-like diuretics; salicylates** and **NSAIDs** may decrease efficacy of loop diuretics; may increase **lithium** levels.	ADRs Dehydration; ototoxicity; hyponatremic alkalosis; hypokalemia; hypomagnesemia; hypocalcemia; hyperuricemia; increased triglycerides, LDL and total cholesterol; decreased HDL cholesterol; photosensitivity; hypotension; GI upset. Pharmacokinetics $T_{1/2}$ = 210 minutes; onset = 60 minutes; duration = 6–8 h.	Contraindications Anuria; hypersensitivity to torsemide or sulfonylureas. Pregnancy Category: B Lactation Issues It is unknown if torsemide is excreted in breast milk.

208.3 Potassium-Sparing Diuretics

Drug and Dosage Forms	Usual Dosage Range	Administration Issues and Drug-Drug & Drug-Food Interactions	Common Adverse Drug Reactions (ADRs) and Pharmacokinetics	Contraindications, Pregnancy Category, and Lactation Issues
Amiloride Midamor Tablet: 5 mg Combinations: 5 mg amiloride and 50 mg HCTZ (do not use combinations as initial therapy of edema or HTN)	**Adjunctive therapy with a thiazide or loop diuretic in CHF and HTN; maintain normal potassium level in patients who develop hypokalemia with diuretic therapy** Initial dose: 5 mg Max dose: 20 mg/d	Administration Issues Take with food or milk; avoid salt substitutes and excessive ingestion of foods high in potassium. Drug-Drug Interactions **Potassium supplements, other potassium-sparing diuretics,** and **ACE inhibitors** may potentiate hyperkalemia; **NSAIDs** may decrease the effectiveness of amiloride; may decrease **digoxin** concentrations.	ADRs Hyperkalemia; dehydration; headache; GI upset; dizziness; impotence; weakness; hypotension; cough; dyspnea; may reactivate peptic ulcer disease. Pharmacokinetics Onset = 2 h; duration = 24 h; $T_{1/2}$ = 6–9 h.	Contraindications Hypersensitivity to amiloride; potassium > 5.5, renal impairment; patients receiving spironolactone or triamterene. Pregnancy Category: B Lactation Issues It is not known whether amiloride is excreted in breast milk.
Spironolactone Aldactone Tablet: 25 mg, 50 mg, 100 mg Combinations: w/varying strengths of spironolactone and HCTZ (do not use combinations as initial therapy of edema or HTN)	**Hyperaldosteronism:** 100–400 mg/d **Edema:** 25–200 mg/d (continue therapy at least 5 days before making a dosage adjustment) **Children:** 3.3 mg/kg/d qd or in divided doses	Administration Issues Take with food or milk; avoid salt substitutes and excessive ingestion of foods high in potassium. Drug-Drug Interactions Spironolactone may increase **digoxin** levels; **potassium supplements, ACE inhibitors,** and **other potassium-sparing diuretics** may result in hyperkalemia; **salicylates** may decrease the diuretic effect of spironolactone.	ADRs Hyperkalemia; gynecomastia; irregular menses or amenorrhea; postmenopausal bleeding; hirsutism; hyperchloremic metabolic acidosis in decompensated hepatic cirrhosis; hyponatremia; drowsiness. Pharmacokinetics onset = 24–48 h; 98% protein binding; $T_{1/2}$ = 20 h; active metabolite (canrenone) has $T_{1/2}$ = 10–35 h.	Contraindications Anuria; potassium > 5.5; renal impairment. Pregnancy Category: D Lactation Issues The American Academy of Pediatricians considers spironolactone safe for use during breastfeeding.

(*continues on next page*)

208.3 Potassium-Sparing Diuretics *continued from previous page*

Drug and Dosage Forms	Usual Dosage Range	Administration Issues and Drug-Drug & Drug-Food Interactions	Common Adverse Drug Reactions (ADRs) and Pharmacokinetics	Contraindications, Pregnancy Category, and Lactation Issues
Spironolactone *cont.*	**Hypertension:** Initial dose: 50–100 mg/d in single or divided doses (continue for 2 weeks before making a dosage adjustment) **Hypokalemia:** 25–100 mg/d	Drug-Food Interactions Administering spironolactone with food appears to increase its absorption. Drug-Laboratory Interaction Spironolactone and its metabolites may falsely elevate **digoxin** levels when measured using radioimmunoassay..		
Triamterene Dyrenium Capsule: 50 mg, 100 mg Combinations: w/varying strengths of triamterene and HCTZ (do not use combinations as initial therapy of edema or HTN)	**Edema:** Usual starting dose: 100 mg bid pc Max dose: 300 mg qd	Administration Issues Take with food or milk; avoid salt substitutes and excessive ingestion of foods high in potassium. Drug-Drug Interactions **Indomethacin** may increase risk of acute renal failure; may increase **amantadine** levels; increase potassium with **potassium supplements** and **angiotensin converting enzyme inhibitors; cimetidine** may increase triamterene levels.	ADRs Hyperkalemia, thrombocytopenia, megaloblastic anemia, rash, photosensitivity, GI upset, fatigue, weakness, dizziness, headache, dry mouth, metabolic acidosis, glucose intolerance, renal stones. Pharmacokinetics Onset = 2–4 h; duration = 12–16 h; $T_{1/2}$ = 3 h.	Contraindications Potassium > 5.5; renal impairment; severe hepatic disease. Pregnancy Category: B Lactation Issues Appears in breast milk in animals; if the drug is essential, patient should stop nursing.

208.4 Thiazide and Thiazide-Like Diuretics

Drug and Dosage Forms	Usual Dosage Range	Administration Issues and Drug-Drug & Drug-Food Interactions	Common Adverse Drug Reactions (ADRs) and Pharmacokinetics	Contraindications, Pregnancy Category, and Lactation Issues
Bendroflumethiazide Naturetin Tablet: 5 mg, 10 mg Combinations: reserpine, nadolol (combinations should not be used as initial therapy for edema or HTN)	**Edema:** Initial dose: up to 20 mg qd or divided bid Maintenance dose: 2.5–5.0 mg qd **Hypertension:** Initial dose: 5–20 mg qd Maintenance dose: 2.5–15 mg/d	Administration Issues Safety / efficacy not established in children; take early in the day to avoid nocturia; ineffective if CrCl <30 mL/min; allow 2–4 weeks for maximum antihypertensive effect. Drug-Drug Interactions May increase **lithium** levels; may decrease effectiveness of **anti-gout agents, sulfonylureas,** and **insulin;** additive effects with **loop diuretics;**	ADRs Dehydration; hypotension; hypokalemia; hypomagnesemia; hypercalcemia; hyponatremia, alkalosis; hyperuricemia; glucose intolerance; transient negative effects on lipids, photosensitivity; impotence; GI upset. Pharmacokinetics Absorption = 100%; excreted unchanged in urine within 24 h.	Contraindications Hypersensitivity to thiazide diuretics or sulfonamide derivatives; anuria; pregnancy. Pregnancy Category: C Lactation Issues It is not known whether bendroflumethiazide is excreted in breast milk; some manufacturers state that women receiving thiazide diuretics should not nurse.

		NSAIDs may decrease the effectiveness of thiazide diuretics; may increase hypersensitivity reactions to **allopurinol; bile acid resins** may decrease the absorption of thiazide diuretics.		
Benzthiazide Exna Tablet: 50 mg	**Edema:** Initial dose: 50–200 mg qd Maintenance dose: 50–150 mg qd If dose > 100 mg, give bid following morning and evening meal. **Hypertension:** Initial dose: 50 mg bid max dose: 200 mg qd	Administration Issues Safety /efficacy not established in children; take early in the day to avoid nocturia; ineffective if CrCl <30 mL/min; allow 2–4 weeks for maximum antihypertensive effect. Drug-Drug Interactions May increase **lithium** levels; may decrease effectiveness of **anti-gout agents, sulfonylureas** and **insulin;** additive effects with **loop diuretics; NSAIDs** may decrease the effectiveness of thiazide.	ADRs Dehydration; hypotension; hypokalemia; hypomagnesemia; hypercalcemia; hyponatremia, alkalosis; hyperuricemia; glucose intolerance; transient negative effects on lipids, photosensitivity; impotence; GI upset. Pharmacokinetics Absorption = 100%; excreted unchanged in urine within 24 h.	Contraindications Hypersensitivity to thiazide diuretics or sulfonamide derivatives; anuria; pregnancy. Pregnancy Category: C Lactation Issues It is not known whether benzthiazide is excreted in breast milk; some manufacturers state that women receiving thiazide diuretics should not nurse.
Hydrochlorothiazide HydroDIURIL, Apo-hydro Tablet: 25mg, 50mg, 100mg Solution: 50 mg/5ml 100mg/ml	**Edema:** Initial dose: 25–200 mg PO qd. Maintenance dose: 25–100 mg PO qd. **Hypertension:** 25–50 mg PO qd.	Drug-Drug Interaction Potentiates other antihypertensive drugs; binds with **cholestyramine** and **colestipol** preventing absorption: potentiates hyperglycaemic, hypotensive, and hyperuricemic effects of **diazoxide, insulin,** or **sulfonylureas:** reduce renal clearance of lithium raising **lithium** levels: decrease therapeutic efficacy of **methenamine.**	ADRs CNS: dizziness, vertigo, headache, paresthesia, weakness, restlessness. CV: volume depletion and dehydration, orthostatic hypotension, allergic myocarditis, vasculitis. GI: polyuria, urinary frequency, renal failure, interstitial nephritis. Hematologic: aplastic anemia, agranulocytosis, leukopenia, thrombocytopenia, haemolytic anemia. Hepatic: jaundice. Musculoskeletal: muscle cramps. Skin: dermatitis, photosensitivity, rash, purpura, alopecia.	Contraindications Anuria, hypersensitivity to thiazides or sulfonamide drugs; use cautiously in patients with impaired renal or hepatic function or progressive hepatic disease. Pregnancy Category: D Lactation Issues: Excreted into breast milk in small amounts; considered compatible with breastfeeding.

300. CENTRAL NERVOUS SYSTEM (CNS) AGENTS
301. Acetaminophen

Drug and Dosage Forms	Usual Dosage Range	Administration Issues and Drug–Drug & Drug–Food Interactions	Common Adverse Drug Reactions (ADRs) and Pharmacokinetics	Contraindications, Pregnancy Category, and Lactation Issues
Acetaminophen (APAP) Acephen, Anacin-3, Panadol, Tempra, Tylenol, various generics <u>Tablets, chewable</u> 80 mg, 160 mg <u>Tablets</u> 325 mg, 500 mg, 650 mg <u>Tablets, Extended release</u> 650 mg <u>Caplets</u> 160 mg, 500 mg, 650 mg <u>Capsules</u> 325 mg, 500 mg <u>Capsules, sprinkle</u> 80 mg, 160 mg <u>Gelcaps</u> 500 mg <u>Elixir</u> 80 mg/2.5 mL, 80 mg/5 mL, 120 mg/5 mL, 160 mg/5 mL <u>Liquid</u> 160 mg/5 mL; 500 mg/15 mL <u>Solution (drops)</u> 80 mg/1.66 mL, 100 mg/mL <u>Suspension</u> 32 mg/mL; 80 mg/mL <u>Syrup</u> 16 mg/mL <u>Suppositories</u> 80 mg, 120 mg, 125 mg, 300 mg, 325 mg, 650 mg	**Analgesic/antipyretic** <u>Oral</u> **Adults:** 325–650 mg q 4–6 h or 1 g 3–4 times daily. Do not exceed 4 g/d **Pediatrics** (dose given 4–5 times daily, max of 5 doses): 10 mg/kg or the following: 0–3 months: 40 mg 4–11 months: 80 mg 1–2 years: 120 mg 2–3 years: 160 mg 4–5 years: 240 mg 6–8 years: 320 mg 9–10 years: 400 mg 11 years: 480 mg **Warning: when prescribing liquid/solution/ suspension for pediatric patients, write the dose based on "mgs/dose" and NOT "mLs/dose." Hepatotoxicity has occurred due to accidental overdosing of infants/children.** <u>Suppositories</u> **Adults:** 650 mg q 4–6 h Max of 4 gm daily **Pediatrics:** 3–6 years: 120 mg q 4–6 h Max of 720 mg/d 6–12 years: 325 mg q 4–6 h Max of 2.6 g/d **Unlabeled Use:** prophylactic use in children receiving DTP vaccination	<u>Administration Issues</u> If pain persists longer than 5 days, consult physician. <u>Drug–Drug Interactions</u> **Increased toxic or pharmacologic effects of APAP:** alcohol (chronic); barbiturates, carbamazepine, hydantoins, propranolol, rifampin, sulfinpyrazone. **Decreased effect of APAP:** charcoal **Increased effect on warfarin** (possible increase in the INR)	<u>ADRs</u> Very few adverse reactions <u>Infrequent:</u> hemolytic anemia, neutropenia, leukopenia, pancytopenia, thrombocytopenia, skin rash, fever, hypoglycemia, jaundice <u>Overdose:</u> nausea, vomiting, drowsiness, confusion, liver tenderness, low blood pressure, cardiac arrhythmias, jaundice, acute hepatic and renal failure <u>Pharmacokinetics</u> Rapid onset (0.5–2 h); hepatically metabolized (toxic metabolite is metabolized by conjugation with hepatic glutathione); $T_{1/2} = 1-3$ h or 2.2–5 h in patients with cirrhosis	<u>Contraindications</u> Hypersensitivity to APAP. <u>Precautions</u> Use cautiously in those with hepatic dysfunction, chronic alcohol use. <u>Pregnancy/Lactation Issues</u> Used in all trimesters of pregnancy with no known harm to fetus. Excreted in breast milk, but no known harm to infant.

302. Narcotic Agonists

302.1 Phenanthrenes

Drug and Dosage Forms	Usual Dosage Range	Administration Issues and Drug–Drug & Drug–Food Interactions	Common Adverse Drug Reactions (ADRs) and Pharmacokinetics	Contraindications, Pregnancy Category, and Lactation Issues
Codeine Sulfate (CII) various generics Tablets 15 mg, 30 mg, 60 mg Soluble Tablets 15 mg, 30 mg, 60 mg, (30 mg, 60 mg—also available as codeine phosphate)	**Moderate to severe pain** 15–60 mg every 4–6 h prn Max dose is 360 mg/d. **Pediatrics** (>1 yr old): 0.5 mg/kg q 4–6 h prn Antitussive 10–20 mg q 4–6 h prn Max dose is 120 mg/d. **Pediatrics** (2–6 yrs): 2.5–5 mg q 4–6 h Max dose is 30 mg/d. **Pediatrics** (6–12 yrs): 5–10 mg q 4–6 h Max dose is 60 mg/d.	Administration Issues Take with food if GI upset occurs. Drug–Drug Interactions **Increased level/effect of:** warfarin; barbiturates, alcohol, other CNS depressants (increased respiratory/CNS depressant effect); chlorpromazine (increased toxic effects); cimetidine (increased CNS toxicity). **Drug dependence, tolerance** Narcotics have abuse potential although this potential is low if used for medical reasons. Prolonged use of these agents can lead to tolerance, thereby requiring increased doses. If medication is to be withdrawn, it should be tapered to prevent withdrawal symptoms.	ADRs Lightheadedness, dizziness, sedation, nausea, vomiting, sweating, constipation, drowsiness Pharmacokinetics Onset of action = 10–30 min; duration of action = 4–6 h; extensive hepatic metabolism; $T_{1/2}$ = 3 h; renal elimination of metabolites.	Contraindications Hypersensitivity to codeine, diarrhea caused by poisoning, acute bronchial asthma, upper airway obstruction. Precautions Use cautiously in patients with hepatic or renal dysfunction, acute abdominal conditions, in elderly or debilitated patients, patients with respiratory conditions, cardiovascular or seizure disorders, hypothyroidism, Addison's disease, acute alcoholism, DTs, prostatic hypertrophy. Pregnancy category: C Lactation Issues Use cautiously. Excreted in breast milk although no significant effects seen on infant.
Hydromorphone (CII) Dilaudid, various generics Tablets 2 mg, 4 mg, 8 mg Suppositories 3 mg Liquid 5 mg/5 ml	**Moderate to severe pain** Oral: 2 mg q 4–6 h. May use 4 mg q 4–6 h for severe pain. Rectal: 3 mg every 6–8 h	Administration issues Take with food if GI upset occurs. Safety/efficacy in children is not established. Drug–Drug Interactions **Increased level/effect of:** warfarin; barbiturates, alcohol, other CNS depressants (increased respiratory/CNS depressant effect); chlorpromazine (increased toxic effects); cimetidine (increased CNS toxicity). **Drug dependence, tolerance:** Narcotics have abuse potential, although this potential is low if used for medical reasons. Prolonged use of these agents can lead to tolerance, thereby requiring increased doses. If medication is to be withdrawn, it should be tapered to prevent withdrawal symptoms.	ADRs Lightheadedness, dizziness, sedation, nausea, vomiting, sweating, constipation, drowsiness. Pharmacokinetics Onset of action = 15–30 min; duration of action = 4–5 h; extensive hepatic metabolism; $T_{1/2}$ = 2–3 h; renal elimination of metabolites.	Contraindications Hypersensitivity to hydrocodone, diarrhea caused by poisoning, acute bronchial asthma, upper airway obstruction. Precautions Use cautiously in patients with hepatic or renal dysfunction, acute abdominal conditions, in elderly or debilitated patients, patients with respiratory conditions, cardiovascular or seizure disorders, hypothyroidism, Addisons disease, acute alcoholism, DTs, prostatic hypertrophy. Pregnancy Category: C Lactation Issues Use cautiously. Excreted in breast milk, although no significant effects seen on infant.

(continues on next page)

302.1 Phenanthrenes continued from previous page

Drug and Dosage Forms	Usual Dosage Range	Administration Issues and Drug–Drug & Drug–Food Interactions	Common Adverse Drug Reactions (ADRs) and Pharmacokinetics	Contraindications, Pregnancy Category, and Lactation Issues
Levorphanol (CII) Levo-Dromoran Tablets 2 mg	**Moderate to severe pain** 2 mg q 8–12 h prn	Administration Issues Take with food if GI upset occurs. Drug–Drug Interactions **Increased level/effect of:** warfarin; barbiturates, alcohol, other CNS depressants (increased respiratory/CNS depressant effect); chlorpromazine (increased toxic effects); cimetidine (increased CNS toxicity). **Drug dependence, tolerance:** Narcotics have abuse potential, although this potential is low if used for medical reasons. Prolonged use of these agents can lead to tolerance, thereby requiring increased doses. If medication is to be withdrawn, it should be tapered to prevent withdrawal symptoms.	ADRs Lightheadedness, dizziness, sedation, nausea, vomiting, sweating, constipation, drowsiness. Pharmacokinetics Onset of action = 30–90 min; duration of action = 6–8 h; extensive hepatic metabolism; $T_{1/2}$ = 12–16 h; renal elimination of metabolites.	Contraindications Hypersensitivity to levorphanol, diarrhea caused by poisoning, acute bronchial asthma, upper airway obstruction. Precautions Use cautiously in patients with hepatic or renal dysfunction, acute abdominal conditions, in elderly or debilitated patients, patients with respiratory conditions, cardiovascular or seizure disorders, hypothyroidism, Addison's disease, acute alcoholism, DTs, prostatic hypertrophy. Pregnancy Category: C Lactation Issues Use cautiously. Excreted in breast milk, although no significant effects seen on infant.
Morphine (CII) MSIR, Roxanol, RMS, various generics Soluble tablets 10 mg, 15 mg, 30 mg Tablets 15 mg, 30 mg Tablets, controlled-release 15 mg, 30 mg, 60 mg, 100 mg, 200 mg Tablets, extended-release 15 mg, 30 mg, 60 mg, 100 mg Capsules 15 mg, 30 mg Capsules, extended release 30 mg, 60 mg, 90 mg, 120 mg Capsules, sustained-release pellets 20 mg, 30 mg, 50 mg, 60 mg, 100 mg	**Moderate to severe acute or chronic pain** Oral: 10–30 mg q 4 h Immediate Release 5–30 mg q 4 h as directed Controlled Release 30 mg q 8–12 h; titrate as needed Rectal 10–30 mg q 4 h prn **Elderly or debilitated:** use smaller initial doses to prevent respiratory depression.	Administration Issues Take with food if GI upset occurs. Do not crush or chew controlled release products. Drug–Drug Interactions **Increased level/effect of:** warfarin; barbiturates, alcohol, other CNS depressants (increased respiratory/CNS depressant effect); chlorpromazine (increased toxic effects); cimetidine (increased CNS toxicity). **Drug dependence, tolerance** Narcotics have abuse potential, although this potential is low if used for medical reasons. Prolonged use of these agents can lead to tolerance, thereby requiring increased doses. If medication is to be withdrawn, it should be tapered to prevent withdrawal symptoms.	ADRs Lightheadedness, dizziness, sedation, nausea, vomiting, sweating, constipation, drowsiness. Pharmacokinetics Onset of action = 15–60 min; duration of action = 3–7 h; extensive hepatic metabolism; $T_{1/2}$ = 1.5–2 h; renal elimination of metabolites.	Contraindications Hypersensitivity to morphine, diarrhea caused by poisoning, acute bronchial asthma, upper airway obstruction. Precautions Use cautiously in patients with hepatic or renal dysfunction, acute abdominal conditions, in elderly or debilitated patients, patients with respiratory conditions, cardiovascular or seizure disorders, hypothyroidism, Addison's disease, acute alcoholism, DTs, prostatic hypertrophy. Pregnancy Category: C Lactation Issues Use cautiously. Excreted in breast milk, although no significant effects seen on infant.

Solution 10 mg/5 mL, 20 mg/5 mL, 20 mg/1 mL, 100 mg/5 mL Suppositories 5 mg, 10 mg, 20 mg, 30 mg				
Oxycodone (CII) Roxicodone, OxyContin, Roxicodone intensol, Oxycodone Capsule: 5 mg Tablets: 5 mg, 15 mg, 30 mg Tablets, extended release: 10 mg, 20 mg, 40 mg, 80 mg, 160 mg Solution 5 mg/5 mL Concentrate 20 mg/1 mL	**Moderate to severe pain** 5 mg q 4–6 h prn. May titrate dose as needed/tolerated. Extended Release: After an established dose is made with the immediate release product, may switch to the extended-release product and use q 12 hr prn. May titrate dose as needed/tolerated.	Administration Issues Take with food if GI upset occurs. Not recommended for children. Drug–Drug Interactions **Increased level/effect of:** warfarin; barbiturates, alcohol, other CNS depressants (increased respiratory/CNS depressant effect); chlorpromazine (increased toxic effects); cimetidine (increased CNS toxicity). **Drug dependence, tolerance** Narcotics have abuse potential, although this potential is low if used for medical reasons. Prolonged use of these agents can lead to tolerance, thereby requiring increased doses. If medication is to be withdrawn, it should be tapered to prevent withdrawal symptoms.	ADRs Lightheadedness, dizziness, sedation, nausea, vomiting, sweating, constipation, drowsiness. Pharmacokinetics Onset of action = 15–30 min; duration of action = 4–6 h; extensive hepatic metabolism; $T_{1/2}$—no data available; renal elimination of metabolites.	Contraindications Hypersensitivity to oxycodone, diarrhea caused by poisoning, acute bronchial asthma, upper airway obstruction. Precautions Use cautiously in patients with hepatic or renal dysfunction, acute abdominal conditions, in elderly or debilitated patients, patients with respiratory conditions, cardiovascular or seizure disorders, hypothyroidism, Addison's disease, acute alcoholism, DTs, prostatic hypertrophy. Pregnancy Category: C Lactation Issues Use cautiously. Excreted in breast milk, although no significant effects seen on infant.
Oxymorphone (CII) Numorphan Suppositories 5 mg	**Moderate to severe pain** 5 mg q 4–6 h. May titrate dose in nondebilitated patients if pain not relieved.	Administration Issues Take with food if GI upset occurs. Refrigerate suppositories. Safety/efficacy not established in children <12 yrs. Drug–Drug Interactions **Increased level/effect of:** warfarin; barbiturates, alcohol, other CNS depressants (increased respiratory/CNS depressant effect); chlorpromazine (increased toxic effects); cimetidine (increased CNS toxicity). **Drug dependence, tolerance** Narcotics have abuse potential, although this potential is low if used for medical reasons. Prolonged use of these agents can lead to tolerance, thereby requiring increased doses. If medication is to be withdrawn, it should be tapered to prevent withdrawal symptoms.	ADRs Lightheadedness, dizziness, sedation, nausea, vomiting, sweating, constipation, drowsiness. Pharmacokinetics Onset of action = 5–10 min; duration of action = 3–6 h; extensive hepatic metabolism; $T_{1/2}$—no data available; renal elimination of metabolites.	Contraindications Hypersensitivity to oxymorphone, diarrhea caused by poisoning, acute bronchial asthma, upper airway obstruction. Precautions Use cautiously in patients with hepatic or renal dysfunction, acute abdominal conditions, in elderly or debilitated patients, patients with respiratory conditions, cardiovascular or seizure disorders, hypothyroidism, Addison's disease, acute alcoholism, DTs, prostatic hypertrophy. Pregnancy Category: C Lactation Issues Use cautiously. Excreted in breast milk, although no significant effects seen on infant.

302.2 Phenylpiperidines

Drug and Dosage Forms	Usual Dosage Range	Administration Issues and Drug–Drug & Drug–Food Interactions	Common Adverse Drug Reactions (ADRs) and Pharmacokinetics	Contraindications, Pregnancy Category, and Lactation Issues
Actiq Fentanyl (C II) Duragesic, Actiq Transdermal system (Duragesic) 25 mcg/hr, 50 mcg/hr, 75 mcg/hr, 100 mcg/hr Oral Transmucosal (Actiq) 200 mcg, 400 mcg, 600 mcg, 800 mcg, 1200 mcg, 1600 mcg	**Moderate to severe chronic pain** Individualize dose. Apply patch every 72 hrs. If switching from another narcotic analgesic, convert daily dose to oral morphine equivalent and choose transdermal dose as follows: 45–134 mg/d: 25 mcg/hr 135–224 mg/d: 50 mcg/hr 225–314 mg/d: 75 mcg/hr 315–404 mg/d: 100 mcg/hr 405–494 mg/d: 125 mcg/hr 495–584 mg/d: 150 mcg/hr 585–674 mg/d: 175 mcg/hr 675–764 mg/d: 200 mcg/hr 765–854 mg/d: 225 mcg/hr etc Breakthrough cancer pain (Actiq only) Individualize dose.	Administration Issues Apply patch to nonirritated clean, dry portion of skin. Clip hair at site of application (do not shave). To cleanse the site use clear water (avoid irritating the skin prior to application). Drug–Drug Interactions: **Increased level/effect of:** warfarin; barbiturates, alcohol, other CNS depressants (increased respiratory/CNS depressant effect); chlorpromazine (increased toxic effects); cimetidine (increased CNS toxicity). Drug dependence, tolerance: Narcotics have abuse potential, although this potential is low if used for medical reasons. Prolonged use of these agents can lead to tolerance, thereby requiring increased doses. If medication is to be withdrawn, it should be tapered to prevent withdrawal symptoms	ADRs Lightheadedness, dizziness, sedation, nausea, vomiting, sweating, constipation, drowsiness. Pharmacokinetics Duration of action = 72 h (transdermal system); extensive hepatic metabolism; $T_{1/2}$ = 1.5–6 h; renal elimination of metabolites.	Contraindications Hypersensitivity to fentanyl, diarrhea caused by poisoning, acute bronchial asthma, upper airway obstruction. Precautions Use cautiously in patients with hepatic or renal dysfunction, acute abdominal conditions, in elderly or debilitated patients, patients with respiratory conditions, cardiovascular or seizure disorders, hypothyroidism, Addison's disease, acute alcoholism, DTs, prostatic hypertrophy. Pregnancy Category: C Lactation Issues Use cautiously. Excreted in breast milk, although no significant effects seen on infant.
Meperidine (C II) Demerol, various generics Tablets 50 mg, 100 mg Syrup 50 mg/5 mL	**Moderate to severe pain** 50–150 mg q 3–4 h prn	Administration Issues: Take with food if GI upset occurs. Drug–Drug Interactions: Increased level/effect of: warfarin; barbiturates, alcohol, other CNS depressants (increased respiratory/CNS depressant effect); chlorpromazine (increased toxic effects); cimetidine (increased CNS toxicity); MAO inhibitors (increased risk of hypertensive crisis). **Drug dependence, tolerance:** Narcotics have abuse potential, although this potential is low if used for medical reasons. Prolonged use of these agents can lead to tolerance, thereby requiring increased doses. If medication is to be withdrawn, it should be tapered to prevent withdrawal symptoms.	ADRs Lightheadedness, dizziness, sedation, nausea, vomiting, sweating, constipation, drowsiness. Pharmacokinetics: Onset of action = 10–45 min; duration of action = 2–4 h; extensive hepatic metabolism (active metabolite: normeperidine); $T_{1/2}$ = 3–4 h ($T_{1/2}$ of metabolite = 15–30 h); renal elimination of metabolite. Decrease dose in elderly by 50% with concurrent phenothiazine use. Reduce dose in renal impairment.	Contraindications Hypersensitivity, diarrhea caused by poisoning, acute bronchial asthma, upper airway obstruction. Precautions Use cautiously in patients with hepatic or renal dysfunction, acute abdominal conditions, in elderly or debilitated patients, patients with respiratory conditions, cardiovascular or seizure disorders, hypothyroidism, Addison's disease, acute alcoholism, DTs, prostatic hypertrophy. Pregnancy Category: C Lactation Issues Use cautiously. Excreted in breast milk, although no significant effects seen on infant.

302.3 Diphenylheptanes

Drug and Dosage Forms	Usual Dosage Range	Administration Issues and Drug–Drug & Drug–Food Interactions	Common Adverse Drug Reactions (ADRs) and Pharmacokinetics	Contraindications, Pregnancy Category, and Lactation Issues
Methadone (C II) Dolophine, various generics Tablets 5 mg, 10 mg Dispersible Tablets 40 mg Solution: 5 mg/5 mL 10 mg/5 mL Concentrate: 10 mg/ mL	Severe pain 2.5–10 mg q 3–4 h prn **Heroin detoxification treatment:** 15–20 mg daily for not more than 21 d. Repeated courses may not start earlier than 4 weeks after completion of previous course. May titrate to higher dose if withdrawal symptoms are not suppressed. Maintain dose to suppress withdrawal symptoms for 2–3 d, then gradually decrease dose on a daily or every 2 d schedule.	Administration Issues: Take with food if GI upset occurs. Not recommended for children. Drug–Drug Interactions **increased level/effect of:** warfarin; barbiturates, alcohol, other CNS depressants (increased respiratory/CNS depressant effect); chlorpromazine (increased toxic effects); cimetidine (increased CNS toxicity). **Drug dependence, tolerance:** Narcotics have abuse potential, although this potential is low if used for medical reasons. Prolonged use of these agents can lead to tolerance, thereby requiring increased doses. If medication is to be withdrawn, it should be tapered to prevent withdrawal symptoms.	ADRs Lightheadedness, dizziness, sedation, nausea, vomiting, sweating, constipation, drowsiness. Pharmacokinetics: Onset of action = 30–60 min; duration of action = 4–6 h; extensive hepatic metabolism; $T_{1/2}$ = 15–30 h; renal elimination of metabolites.	Contraindications Hypersensitivity, diarrhea caused by poisoning, acute bronchial asthma, upper airway obstruction. Precautions Use cautiously in patients with hepatic or renal dysfunction, acute abdominal conditions, in elderly or debilitated patients, patients with respiratory conditions, cardiovascular or seizure disorders, hypothyroidism, Addison's disease, acute alcoholism, DTs, prostatic hypertrophy. Pregnancy Category: C Lactation Issues Use cautiously. Excreted in breast milk, although no significant effects seen on infant.
Propoxyphene (C IV) Darvon, various generics Capsules 65 mg Propoxyphene napsylate Darvon-N Tablets 100 mg Suspension 10 mg/1 mL	**Mild to moderate pain** Propoxyphene: 65 mg q 4 h prn. Max dose is 390 mg/d. Propoxyphene Napsylate: 100 mg (equivalent to 65 mg propoxyphene) q 4 h prn. Max dose is 600 mg/d. **Elderly or debilitated patients** (renal or hepatic dysfunction): use smaller daily doses.	Administration Issues Take with food if GI upset occurs. Not recommended for children. Drug–Drug Interactions **Increased level/effect of:** warfarin; barbiturates, alcohol, other CNS depressants (inc respiratory/CNS depressant effect); chlorpromazine (inc toxic effects); cimetidine (inc CNS toxicity); carbamazepine (inc toxicity) decreased level/effect of propoxyphene: charcoal, smoking. **Drug dependence, tolerance:** Narcotics have abuse potential although this potential is low if used for medical reasons. Prolonged use of these agents can lead to tolerance, thereby requiring increased doses. If medication is to be withdrawn, it should be tapered to prevent withdrawal symptoms.	ADRs Dizziness, sedation, nausea, vomiting. Pharmacokinetics Onset of action = 30–60 min; duration of action = 4–6 h; extensive hepatic metabolism; $T_{1/2}$ = 6–12 h; renal elimination of metabolites.	Contraindications Hypersensitivity to ingredients. Precautions Use cautiously in patients with hepatic or renal dysfunction, in elderly or debilitated patients, patients with respiratory conditions. Pregnancy Issues Safety not established. Use cautiously. Lactation Issues Use cautiously. Excreted in breast milk, although no significant effects seen on infant.

302.4 Narcotic Agonists-Antagonists Combinations

Drug and Dosage Forms	Usual Dosage Range	Administration Issues and Drug–Drug & Drug–Food Interactions	Common Adverse Drug Reactions (ADRs) and Pharmacokinetics	Contraindications, Pregnancy Category, and Lactation Issues
Pentazocine & Naloxone (C IV) Talwin NX Tablets 50 mg/0.5 mg	**Moderate to Severe Pain** 50 mg of pentazocine q 3–4 h, initially. May titrate to 100 mg if necessary. Max dose is 600 mg/d.	Administration Issues Avoid alcohol use. Safety/efficacy not established for children < 12 yrs. Drug–Drug Interactions **Increased effect of:** alcohol, other CNS depressants. **Dependence, tolerance:** Psychological and physical dependence have occurred with prolonged use of this agent. Withdrawal symptoms have been associated with abrupt discontinuation.	ADRs Nausea, dizziness, lightheadedness, vomiting, euphoria, sedation, constipation. Pharmacokinetics: Extensively hepatically metabolized.	Contraindications Hypersensitivity Precautions: Use cautiously in patients with severe renal or hepatic dysfunction, or respiratory dysfunction. Use cautiously in patients previously receiving narcotic agonist—this may precipitate withdrawal. Pregnancy Category: C Lactation Issues: Safety not established.
Pentazocine & Aspirin (C IV) Talwin Compound Caplets Tablets 12.5 mg/325 mg	**Moderate to Severe Pain** 2 tablets tid to qid	Administration Issues Avoid alcohol use. Safety/efficacy not established for children < 12 yrs. Aspirin use in children with fever has been associated with Reye's syndrome. Drug–Drug Interactions **increased effect of:** alcohol, other CNS depressants. Aspirin **Increased level/effect of:** alcohol (GI effects); anticoagulants (bleeding effects); methotrexate, valproic acid, sulfonylureas (inc hypoglycemic effect). **Decreased level/effect of:** ACE inhibitors, beta blockers, diuretics (decreased antihypertensive effect); probenecid & sulfinpyrazone (decreased uricosuric effect). **Drug–Lab Interactions** **Aspirin:** false negative or positive urine glucose tests, uric acid levels (inc with salicylate	ADRs Nausea, dizziness, lightheadedness, vomiting, euphoria, sedation, constipation. **Aspirin:** Most frequent: nausea, dyspepsia, heartburn, GI bleeding, hives, rash, prolonged bleeding time, thrombocytopenia, aspirin intolerance (bronchospasm, rhinitis), "Salicylism": dizziness, tinnitus, difficulty hearing, nausea, vomiting, diarrhea, confusion, CNS depression, headache, sweating, hyperventilation, lassitude. Pharmacokinetics: Aspirin: hepatically metabolized.	Contraindications Hypersensitivity Aspirin: hemophilia, bleeding ulcers, hemorrhagic states. Precautions: Use cautiously in patients with severe renal or hepatic dysfunction, or respiratory dysfunction. Use cautiously in patients previously receiving narcotic agonist—this may precipitate withdrawal. Aspirin: Use cautiously in patients with asthma, nasal polyposis, chronic urticaria (inc risk of hypersensitivity); chronic renal insufficiency, PUD, bleeding disorders. Pregnancy Category: C Aspirin: Category D Lactation Issues: Safety not established.

<table>
<tr><td></td><td></td><td>levels < 10 mg/dL; decreased with salicylate levels > 10 mg/dL), falsely elevated urine vanillymandelic acid tests.

Dependence, tolerance:
Psychological and physical dependence have occurred with prolonged use of this agent. Withdrawal symptoms have been associated with abrupt discontinuation.</td><td></td><td></td></tr>
<tr><td>Pentazocine & Acetaminophen (C IV)
Talacen Caplets

Tablets
25 mg/650 mg</td><td>Moderate to Severe Pain
1 tablet q 4 h up to 6 tablets daily.

Acetaminophen
max. daily dose: 4 gm</td><td>Administration Issues
Avoid alcohol use. Safety/efficacy not established for children < 12 yrs.

Drug–Drug Interactions
Increased effect of:
alcohol, other CNS depressants.

Acetaminophen:
Increased toxic effect of APAP:
alcohol (chronic); barbiturates, carbamazepine, hydantoins, rifampin, sulfinpyrazone.

Decreased effect of APAP:
charcoal

Dependence, tolerance:
Psychological and physical dependence have occurred with prolonged use of this agent. Withdrawal symptoms have been associated with abrupt discontinuation.</td><td>ADRs
Nausea, dizziness, lightheadedness, vomiting, euphoria, sedation, constipation.

Acetaminophen:
Very few adverse reactions

Pharmacokinetics:
APAP:
rapid onset (0.5–2 h); hepatically metabolized (toxic metabolite is metabolized by conjugation with hepatic glutathione); $T_{1/2}$ = 1–3 h or 2.2–5 h in patients with cirrhosis.</td><td>Contraindications
Hypersensitivity.

Precautions:
Use cautiously in patients with severe renal or hepatic dysfunction, or respiratory dysfunction. Use cautiously in patients previously receiving narcotic agonist—this may precipitate withdrawal.

Pregnancy Category: C
Near term or prolonged use: Category D

Lactation Issues:
Safety not established.</td></tr>
<tr><td>Butorphanol (C IV)
Stadol NS

Nasal Spray:
10 mg/mL</td><td>Moderate to Severe Pain
1–2 mg q 3–4 h prn. Give 1 mg then wait 60 minutes before the next 1 mg if full pain relief not achieved.

Elderly or debilitated:
1 mg may repeat in 90–120 min if full effect not reached. Give q 6–8 h prn.

Unlabeled Use:
pain associated with migraine headache.</td><td>Administration Issues
Avoid alcohol use. Safety/efficacy in those < 18 yrs not established. Half-life is prolonged in the elderly. These patients may be more prone to adverse effects.

Drug–Drug Interactions
Increased effect of:
barbiturates, alcohol, other CNS depressants.</td><td>ADRs
Vasodilatation, palpitations, hypertension, anorexia, constipation, insomnia, tremor, convulsion, delusions, depression, nasal congestion, dyspnea, epistaxis, nasal irritation, pharyngitis, rhinitis, cough.

Pharmacokinetics
Onset of action = 15 min; duration of action = 4–5 h; $T_{1/2}$ = 2.9–9.2 h; extensively metabolized; renal or fecal elimination of metabolites.</td><td>Contraindications
Hypersensitivity.

Precautions
Use cautiously in patients with severe respiratory, cardiovascular, hepatic or renal dysfunction.

Pregnancy Category: C

Lactation Issues:
Use cautiously, excreted in breast milk; however, amount to infant may be negligible.</td></tr>
</table>

303. Narcotic Combinations

Drug and Dosage Forms	Usual Dosage Range	Administration Issues and Drug–Drug & Drug–Food Interactions	Common Adverse Drug Reactions (ADRs) and Pharmacokinetics	Contraindications, Pregnancy Category, and Lactation Issues
Acetaminophen (C, various) w/Codeine Capital w/Codeine, Tylenol w/Codeine No. 2, No. 3, No. 4; Phenaphen w/Codeine No. 3, Margesic No. 3, various generics Solution/Elixer 120 mg/ 12 mg/5 mL Tablets 300 mg/15 mg 325 mg/30 mg 300 mg/30 mg 650 mg/30 mg 300 mg/60 mg 325 mg/60 mg	**Moderate to Severe Pain** 1–4 tablets q 4 h prn (codeine content 15 mg) 0.5–2 tablets q 4 h prn (codeine content 30 mg) 1 tablet q 4 h prn (codeine content 60 mg or APAP content 650 mg) 15 mL q 4 h prn (for solution) Maximum Acetaminophen daily dose = 4 g.	Administration Issues Take with food if GI upset occurs. Drug–Drug Interactions **increased level/effect of:** warfarin; barbiturates, alcohol, other CNS depressants (inc respiratory/CNS depressant effect); chlorpromazine (inc toxic effects); cimetidine (inc CNS toxicity). Acetaminophen: **increased toxic effect of APAP:** alcohol (chronic); barbiturates, carbamazepine, hydantoins, rifampin, sulfinpyrazone **decreased effect of APAP:** charcoal. **Drug dependence, tolerance:** Narcotics have abuse potential, although this potential is low if used for medical reasons. Prolonged use of these agents can lead to tolerance, thereby requiring increased doses. If medication is to be withdrawn, it should be tapered to prevent withdrawal symptoms.	ADRs Lightheadedness, dizziness, sedation, GI effects, sweating, constipation, drowsiness. Acetaminophen: Very few adverse reactions	Contraindications Hypersensitivity, diarrhea caused by poisoning, acute bronchial asthma, upper airway obstruction. Precautions Use cautiously in patients with hepatic or renal dysfunction, acute abdominal conditions, in elderly or debilitated patients, patients with respiratory conditions, cardiovascular or seizure disorders, hypothyroidism, Addison's disease, acute alcoholism, DTs, prostatic hypertrophy. Pregnancy Category: C Near term or prolonged use: Category D Lactation Issues Use cautiously. Excreted in breast milk, although no significant effects seen on infant.
Aspirin w/Codeine (C III) Empirin w/Codeine No. 3 or No. 4, various generics Tablets 325 mg/30 mg, 325 mg/60 mg	**Moderate to severe pain** 1–2 tablets q 4 h prn (codeine content 30 mg) 1 tablet q 4 h prn (codeine content 60 mg)	Administration Issues Take with food if GI upset occurs. Aspirin use in children with fever has been associated with Reye's syndrome. Drug–Drug Interactions **increased level/effect of:** warfarin; barbiturates, alcohol, other CNS depressants (inc respiratory/CNS depressant effect); chlorpromazine (inc toxic effects); cimetidine (inc CNS toxicity).	Pharmacokinetics See individual agents. ADRs Lightheadedness, dizziness, sedation, GI effects, sweating, constipation, drowsiness. Aspirin: nausea, dyspepsia, heartburn, GI bleeding, hives, rash, prolonged bleeding time, thrombocytopenia, aspirin intolerance (bronchospasm, rhinitis), "Salicylism": dizziness, tinnitus, difficulty hearing, nau-	Contraindications Hypersensitivity, diarrhea caused by poisoning, acute bronchial asthma, upper airway obstruction. Aspirin: hemophilia, bleeding ulcers, hemorrhagic states. Precautions Use cautiously in patients with hepatic or renal dysfunction, acute abdominal conditions, in elderly or debilitated patients, patients with respiratory conditions, car-

		Aspirin: **Increased level/effect of:** alcohol (GI effects); anticoagulants (bleeding effects); methotrexate, valproic acid, sulfonylureas (inc hypoglycemic effect) **Decreased level/effect of:** ACE inhibitors, beta blockers, diuretics (decreased antihypertensive effect); probenecid & sulfinpyrazone (decreased uricosuric effect). Drug–Lab Interactions: Aspirin: see table 307. **Drug dependence, tolerance:** Narcotics have abuse potential although this potential is low if used for medical reasons. Prolonged use can lead to tolerance, thereby requiring increased doses. If medication is to be withdrawn, it should be tapered to prevent withdrawal symptoms.	sea, vomiting, diarrhea, confusion, CNS depression, headache, sweating, hyperventilation, lassitude. Pharmacokinetics See individual agents.	diovascular or seizure disorders, hypothyroidism, Addison's disease, acute alcoholism, DTs, prostatic hypertrophy. Aspirin: Use cautiously in patients with asthma, nasal polyposis, chronic urticaria (inc risk of hypersensitivity); chronic renal insufficiency, PUD, bleeding disorders. Pregnancy Category: C Aspirin: Category D Lactation Issues Use cautiously. Excreted in breast milk, although no significant effects seen on infant.
Acetaminophen, (C, various) Codeine, Caffeine, Butalbital Fioricet w/Codeine Tablet 325 mg APAP plus, 30 mg Codeine plus, 40 mg Caffeine plus, 50 mg Butalbital	**Moderate to severe pain** 1–2 tablets q 4 h prn (up to 6 tablets a day) Acetaminophen Max daily dose = 4 gm.	Administration Issues Take with food if GI upset occurs. Drug–Drug Interactions **increased level/effect of:** warfarin; barbiturates, alcohol, other CNS depressants (inc respiratory/CNS depressant effect); chlorpromazine (inc toxic effects); cimetidine (inc CNS toxicity). Acetaminophen: **Increased toxic effect of APAP:** alcohol (chronic); barbiturates, carbamazepine, hydantoins, rifampin, sulfinpyrazone. **Decreased effect of APAP:** charcoal. Caffeine: **Decreased effect/levels of caffeine:** smoking	ADRs Lightheadedness, dizziness, sedation, GI effects, sweating, constipation, drowsiness. Acetaminophen: Very few adverse reactions Caffeine: Insomnia, restlessness, tremor, excitement, anxiety, headaches, GI effects, palpitations, diuresis, withdrawal headaches after abrupt discontinuation (500–600 mg/d of caffeine) Pharmacokinetics See individual agents.	Contraindications Hypersensitivity, diarrhea caused by poisoning, acute bronchial asthma, upper airway obstruction. Precautions Use cautiously in patients with hepatic or renal dysfunction, acute abdominal conditions, in elderly or debilitated patients, patients with respiratory conditions, cardiovascular or seizure disorders, hypothyroidism, Addison's disease, acute alcoholism, DTs, prostatic hypertrophy. Pregnancy Category: C Lactation Issues Use cautiously. Excreted in breast milk, although no significant effects seen on infant.

(*continues on next page*)

303. Narcotic Combinations *continued from previous page*

Drug and Dosage Forms	Usual Dosage Range	Administration Issues and Drug–Drug & Drug–Food Interactions	Common Adverse Drug Reactions (ADRs) and Pharmacokinetics	Contraindications, Pregnancy Category, and Lactation Issues
Acetaminophen, (C, various) Codeine, Caffeine, Butalbital *cont.*		**Increased effect/levels of caffeine:** cimetidine, oral contraceptives, disulfiram, fluoroquinolones. **Drug dependence, tolerance:** Narcotics have abuse potential, although this potential is low if used for medical reasons. Prolonged use can lead to tolerance, thereby requiring increased doses. If medication is to be withdrawn, it should be tapered to prevent withdrawal symptoms.		
Aspirin, Codeine, Caffeine, Butalbital (C III) Fiorinal w/Codeine Tablets 325 mg aspirin plus, 30 mg codeine plus, 40 mg caffeine plus, 50 mg butalbital	**Moderate to severe pain** 1–2 tablets q 4 h prn (up to 6 tablets a day)	Administration Issues Take with food if GI upset occurs. Aspirin use in children with fever has been associated with Reye's syndrome. Drug–Drug Interactions **increased level/effect of:** warfarin; barbiturates, alcohol, other CNS depressants (inc respiratory/CNS depressant effect); chlorpromazine (inc toxic effects); cimetidine (inc CNS toxicity). Aspirin: **Increased level/effect of:** alcohol (GI effects); anticoagulants (bleeding effects); methotrexate, valproic acid, sulfonylureas (inc hypoglycemic effect) **decreased level/effect of:** ACE inhibitors, beta blockers, diuretics (decreased antihypertensive effect); probenecid and sulfinpyrazone (decreased uricosuric effect). Caffeine: **Increased effect/levels of caffeine:** cimetidine, oral contraceptives, disulfiram, fluoroquinolones.	ADRs lightheadedness, dizziness, sedation, nausea, vomiting, sweating, constipation, drowsiness Aspirin: nausea, dyspepsia, heartburn, GI bleeding, hives, rash, prolonged bleeding time, thrombocytopenia, aspirin intolerance (bronchospasm, rhinitis), "Salicylism": dizziness, tinnitus, difficulty hearing, nausea, vomiting, diarrhea, confusion, CNS depression, headache, sweating, hyperventilation, lassitude. Caffeine: insomnia, restlessness, tremor, excitement, anxiety, headaches, GI effects, palpitations, diuresis, withdrawal headaches after abrupt discontinuation (500–600 mg/d of caffeine). Pharmacokinetics See individual agents.	Contraindications Hypersensitivity, diarrhea caused by poisoning, acute bronchial asthma, upper airway obstruction. Aspirin: hemophilia, bleeding ulcers, hemorrhagic states. Precautions Use cautiously in patients with hepatic or renal dysfunction, acute abdominal conditions, in elderly or debilitated patients, patients with respiratory conditions, cardiovascular or seizure disorders, hypothyroidism, Addison's disease, acute alcoholism, DTs, prostatic hypertrophy. Aspirin: Use cautiously in patients with asthma, nasal polyposis, chronic urticaria (inc risk of hypersensitivity); chronic renal insufficiency, PUD, bleeding disorders. Pregnancy Category: C Aspirin: Category D

		Decreased effect/levels of caffeine: smoking. **Drug dependence, tolerance:** Narcotics have abuse potential, although this potential is low if used for medical reasons. Prolonged use can lead to tolerance, thereby requiring increased doses. If medication is to be withdrawn, it should be tapered to prevent withdrawal symptoms.		Lactation Issues Use cautiously. Excreted in breast milk, although no significant effects seen on infant.
Acetaminophen, Hydrocodone (C III) Lortab, Bancap, Ceta-Plus, Co-Gesic, Duocet, Dolacte, Hydrocet, Vicodin, Lorcet, various generics, others Tablets/Capsules 325 mg/5 mg 400 mg/5 mg 325 mg/7.5 mg 400 mg/7.5 mg 325 mg/10 mg 400 mg/10 mg 500 mg/10 mg 500 mg/2.5 mg 500 mg/5 mg 500 mg/7.5 mg 650 mg/7.5 mg 750 mg/7.5 mg 650 mg/10 mg Elixir 167 mg/2.5 mg/5 mL	**Moderate to severe pain** 15 mL q4–6 h prn (solution) 1–2 tablets q 4–6 h prn (up to 8 tablets a day) 1 tablet q 4–6 h prn (hydrocodone content 7.5 mg or higher) Max dose of 5 tablets a day if APAP content is 750 mg Acetaminophen: max dose is 4 gm.	Administration Issues Take with food if GI upset occurs. Drug–Drug Interactions **Increased level/effect of:** warfarin; barbiturates, alcohol, other CNS depressants (inc respiratory/CNS depressant effect); chlorpromazine (inc toxic effects); cimetidine (inc CNS toxicity). Acetaminophen: **Increased toxic effect of APAP:** alcohol (chronic); barbiturates, carbamazepine, hydantoins, rifampin, sulfinpyrazone. **Decreased effect of APAP:** charcoal. **Drug dependence, tolerance:** Narcotics have abuse potential, although this potential is low if used for medical reasons. Prolonged use can lead to tolerance, thereby requiring increased doses. If medication is to be withdrawn, it should be tapered to prevent withdrawal symptoms.	ADRs Lightheadedness, dizziness, sedation, nausea, vomiting, sweating, constipation, drowsiness. Acetaminophen: Very few adverse reactions Pharmacokinetics See individual agents.	Contraindications Hypersensitivity, diarrhea caused by poisoning, acute bronchial asthma, upper airway obstruction. Precautions Use cautiously in patients with hepatic or renal dysfunction, acute abdominal conditions, in elderly or debilitated patients, patients with respiratory conditions, cardiovascular or seizure disorders, hypothyroidism, Addison's disease, acute alcoholism, DTs, prostatic hypertrophy. Pregnancy Category: C Lactation Issues Use cautiously. Excreted in breast milk, although no significant effects seen on infant.
Aspirin, Hydrocodone (C III) Azdone, Damason, Lortab, ASA, Panasal Tablets 500 mg/5 mg	**Moderate to severe pain** 1–2 tablets q 4–6 h prn; up to 8 tablets a day.	Administration Issues Take with food if GI upset occurs. Aspirin use in children with fever has been associated with Reye's syndrome.	ADRs Lightheadedness, dizziness, sedation, nausea, vomiting, sweating, constipation, drowsiness.	Contraindications Hypersensitivity, diarrhea caused by poisoning, acute bronchial asthma, upper airway obstruction.

(continues on next page)

303. Narcotic Combinations *continued from previous page*

Drug and Dosage Forms	Usual Dosage Range	Administration Issues and Drug–Drug & Drug–Food Interactions	Common Adverse Drug Reactions (ADRs) and Pharmacokinetics	Contraindications, Pregnancy Category, and Lactation Issues
Aspirin, Hydrocodone (C III) ***cont.***		Drug–Drug Interactions **Increased level/effect of:** warfarin; barbiturates, alcohol, other CNS depressants (inc respiratory/CNS depressant effect); chlorpromazine (inc toxic effects); cimetidine (inc CNS toxicity). Aspirin: **Increased level/effect of:** alcohol (GI effects); anticoagulants (bleeding effects); methotrexate, valproic acid, sulfonylureas (inc hypoglycemic effect). **Decreased level/effect of:** ACE inhibitors, beta blockers, diuretics (decreased antihypertensive effect); probenecid & sulfinpyrazone (decreased uricosuric effect). Drug–Lab Interactions Aspirin: See table 307. **Drug dependence, tolerance:** Narcotics have abuse potential, although this potential is low if used for medical reasons. Prolonged use can lead to tolerance, thereby requiring increased doses. If medication is to be withdrawn, it should be tapered to prevent withdrawal symptoms.	Aspirin: nausea, dyspepsia, heartburn, GI bleeding, hives, rash, prolonged bleeding time, thrombocytopenia, aspirin intolerance (bronchospasm, rhinitis), "Salicylism": dizziness, tinnitus, difficulty hearing, nausea, vomiting, diarrhea, confusion, CNS depression, headache, sweating, hyperventilation, lassitude Pharmacokinetics See individual agents.	Aspirin: hemophilia, bleeding ulcers, hemorrhagic states. Precautions Use cautiously in patients with hepatic or renal dysfunction, acute abdominal conditions, in elderly or debilitated patients, patients with respiratory conditions, cardiovascular or seizure disorders, hypothyroidism, Addison's disease, acute alcoholism, DTs, prostatic hypertrophy. Aspirin: Use cautiously in patients with asthma, nasal polyposis, chronic urticaria (inc risk of hypersensitivity); chronic renal insufficiency, PUD, bleeding disorders. Pregnancy Category: C Aspirin: Category D Lactation Issues Use cautiously. Excreted in breast milk, although no significant effects seen on infant.
Acetaminophen, Dihydrocodeine, Caffeine (C III) DHC Plus Capsules Capsules 356.4 mg APAP plus 16 mg dihydrocodeine plus 30 mg caffeine	**Moderate to severe pain** 2 capsules q 4 h prn Acetaminophen: Max daily dose is 4 gm.	Administration Issues Take with food if GI upset occurs. Drug–Drug Interactions **Increased level/effect of:** warfarin; barbiturates, alcohol, other CNS depressants (inc respiratory/CNS depressant effect); chlorpromazine (inc toxic effects); cimetidine (inc CNS toxicity).	ADRs Lightheadedness, dizziness, sedation, nausea, vomiting, sweating, constipation, drowsiness. Acetaminophen: very few adverse reactions. Caffeine: insomnia, restlessness, tremor, excitement, anxiety, headaches, GI effects, pal-	Contraindications Hypersensitivity, diarrhea caused by poisoning, acute bronchial asthma, upper airway obstruction. Precautions Use cautiously in patients with hepatic or renal dysfunction, acute abdominal conditions, in elderly or debilitated patients, patients with respiratory conditions, cardiovascular or seizure disorders, hy-

		Acetaminophen: **Increased toxic effect of APAP:** alcohol (chronic); barbiturates, carbamazepine, hydantoins, rifampin, sulfinpyrazone. **Decreased effect of APAP:** charcoal. Caffeine: **Increased effect/levels of caffeine:** cimetidine, oral contraceptives, disulfiram, fluoroquinolones. **Decreased effect/levels of caffeine:** smoking. **Drug dependence, tolerance:** Narcotics have abuse potential, although this potential is low if used for medical reasons. Prolonged use can lead to tolerance, thereby requiring increased doses. If medication is to be withdrawn, it should be tapered to prevent withdrawal symptoms.	pitations, diuresis, withdrawal headaches after abrupt discontinuation (500–600 mg/d of caffeine). Pharmacokinetics See individual agents.	pothyroidism, Addison's disease, acute alcoholism, DTs, prostatic hypertrophy. Pregnancy Category: C Lactation Issues Use cautiously. Excreted in breast milk, although no significant effects seen on infant.
Aspirin, Dihydrocodeine, Caffeine (C III) Synalogos-DC Capsules 356.4 mg aspirin plus 16 mg dihydrocodeine plus 30 mg caffeine	**Moderate to severe pain** 2 capsules q 4 h prn	Administration Issues Take with food if GI upset occurs. Aspirin use in children with fever has been associated with Reye's syndrome. Drug–Drug Interactions **Increased level/effect of:** warfarin; barbiturates, alcohol, other CNS depressants (inc respiratory/CNS depressant effect); chlorpromazine (inc toxic effects); cimetidine (inc CNS toxicity). Aspirin: **Increased level/effect of:** alcohol (GI effects); anticoagulants (bleeding effects); methotrexate, valproic acid, sulfonylureas (inc hypoglycemic effect) **Decreased level/effect of:** ACE inhibitors, beta blockers, diuretics (decreased antihypertensive effect);	ADRs Lightheadedness, dizziness, sedation, nausea, vomiting, sweating, constipation, drowsiness. Aspirin: nausea, dyspepsia, heartburn, GI bleeding, hives, rash, prolonged bleeding time, thrombocytopenia, aspirin intolerance (bronchospasm, rhinitis), "Salicylism": dizziness, tinnitus, difficulty hearing, nausea, vomiting, diarrhea, confusion, CNS depression, headache, sweating, hyperventilation, lassitude. Caffeine: insomnia, restlessness, tremor, excitement, anxiety, headaches, GI effects, palpitations, diuresis, withdrawal headaches after abrupt discontinuation (500–600 mg/d of caffeine).	Contraindications Hypersensitivity, diarrhea caused by poisoning, acute bronchial asthma, upper airway obstruction. Aspirin: hemophilia, bleeding ulcers, hemorrhagic states. Precautions Use cautiously in patients with hepatic or renal dysfunction, acute abdominal conditions, in elderly or debilitated patients, patients with respiratory conditions, cardiovascular or seizure disorders, hypothyroidism, Addison's disease, acute alcoholism, DTs, prostatic hypertrophy. Aspirin: Use cautiously in patients with asthma, nasal polyposis, chronic urticaria (inc risk

(*continues on next page*)

303. Narcotic Combinations *continued from previous page*

Drug and Dosage Forms	Usual Dosage Range	Administration Issues and Drug–Drug & Drug–Food Interactions	Common Adverse Drug Reactions (ADRs) and Pharmacokinetics	Contraindications, Pregnancy Category, and Lactation Issues
Aspirin, Dihydrocodeine, Caffeine (C III) *cont.*		probenecid & sulfinpyrazone (decreased uricosuric effect). Caffeine: **Increased effect/levels of caffeine:** cimetidine, oral contraceptives, disulfiram, fluoroquinolones. **Decreased effect/levels of caffeine:** smoking. Drug–Lab Interactions Aspirin: see table 307. **Drug dependence, tolerance:** Narcotics have abuse potential, although this potential is low if used for medical reasons. Prolonged use can lead to tolerance, thereby requiring increased doses. If medication is to be withdrawn, it should be tapered to prevent withdrawal symptoms.	Pharmacokinetics See individual agents.	of hypersensitivity); chronic renal insufficiency, PUD, bleeding disorders. Pregnancy Category: C Aspirin: Category D Lactation Issues Use cautiously. Excreted in breast milk, although no significant effects seen on infant.
Acetaminophen, Oxycodone (C II) Percocet, Roxicet, Tylox, various generics Tablets 325 mg/2.5 mg, 325 mg/5 mg, 500 mg/7.5 mg, 650 mg/10 mg Capsules 500 mg/5 mg Solution 325 mg/5 mg (5 mL)	**Moderate to severe pain** 1 tablet or capsule q 6 h prn 5 mL every 6 hrs prn Acetaminophen: Maximum daily dose is 4 gm.	Administration Issues Take with food if GI upset occurs. Drug–Drug Interactions **Increased level/effect of:** warfarin; barbiturates, alcohol, other CNS depressants (inc respiratory/CNS depressant effect); chlorpromazine (inc toxic effects); cimetidine (inc CNS toxicity). Acetaminophen: **Increased toxic effect of APAP:** alcohol (chronic); barbiturates, carbamazepine, hydantoins, rifampin, sulfinpyrazone. **Decreased effect of APAP:** charcoal.	ADRs Lightheadedness, dizziness, sedation, nausea, vomiting, sweating, constipation, drowsiness. Acetaminophen: very few adverse reactions. Pharmacokinetics See individual agents.	Contraindications Hypersensitivity, diarrhea caused by poisoning, acute bronchial asthma, upper airway obstruction. Precautions Use cautiously in patients with hepatic or renal dysfunction, acute abdominal conditions, in elderly or debilitated patients, patients with respiratory conditions, cardiovascular or seizure disorders, hypothyroidism, Addison's disease, acute alcoholism, DTs, prostatic hypertrophy. Pregnancy Category: C Lactation Issues Use cautiously. Excreted in breast milk, although no significant effects seen on infant.

		Drug dependence, tolerance: Narcotics have abuse potential, although this potential is low if used for medical reasons. Prolonged use can lead to tolerance, thereby requiring increased doses. If medication is to be withdrawn, it should be tapered to prevent withdrawal symptoms.		
Aspirin, Oxycodone (C II) Percodan, Percodan-Demi, Roxiprin, various generics Tablets 325 mg/2.25 mg oxycodone HCL/ 0.19 mg oxycodone terephthalate 325 mg/4.5 mg oxycodone HCL/0.38 mg oxycodone terephthalate	**Moderate to severe pain** 1–2 tablets q 6 h prn	Administration Issues Take with food if GI upset occurs. Aspirin use in children with fever has been associated with Reye's syndrome. Drug–Drug Interactions **Increased level/effect of:** warfarin; barbiturates, alcohol, other CNS depressants (inc respiratory/CNS depressant effect); chlorpromazine (inc toxic effects); cimetidine (inc CNS toxicity). Aspirin: **Increased level/effect of:** alcohol (GI effects); anticoagulants (bleeding effects); methotrexate, valproic acid, sulfonylureas (inc hypoglycemic effect) **Decreased level/effect of:** ACE inhibitors, beta blockers, diuretics (decreased antihypertensive effect); probenecid & sulfinpyrazone (decreased uricosuric effect) Drug–Lab Interactions Aspirin: see table 307. **Drug dependence, tolerance:** Narcotics have abuse potential, although this potential is low if used for medical reasons. Prolonged use can lead to tolerance, thereby requiring increased doses. If medication is to be withdrawn, it should be tapered to prevent withdrawal symptoms.	ADRs Lightheadedness, dizziness, sedation, nausea, vomiting, sweating, constipation, drowsiness. Aspirin: nausea, dyspepsia, heartburn, GI bleeding, hives, rash, prolonged bleeding time, thrombocytopenia, aspirin intolerance (bronchospasm, rhinitis), "Salicylism": dizziness, tinnitus, difficulty hearing, nausea, vomiting, diarrhea, confusion, CNS depression, headache, sweating, hyperventilation, lassitude. Pharmacokinetics See individual agents.	Contraindications Hypersensitivity, diarrhea caused by poisoning, acute bronchial asthma, upper airway obstruction. Aspirin: hemophilia, bleeding ulcers, hemorrhagic states. Precautions Use cautiously in patients with hepatic or renal dysfunction, acute abdominal conditions, in elderly or debilitated patients, patients with respiratory conditions, cardiovascular or seizure disorders, hypothyroidism, Addison's disease, acute alcoholism, DTs, prostatic hypertrophy. Aspirin: Use cautiously in patients with asthma, nasal polyposis, chronic urticaria (inc risk of hypersensitivity); chronic renal insufficiency, PUD, bleeding disorders. Pregnancy Category: C Aspirin: Category D Lactation Issues Use cautiously. Excreted in breast milk, although no significant effects seen on infant.

(*continues on next page*)

303. Narcotic Combinations *continued from previous page*

Drug and Dosage Forms	Usual Dosage Range	Administration Issues and Drug–Drug & Drug–Food Interactions	Common Adverse Drug Reactions (ADRs) and Pharmacokinetics	Contraindications, Pregnancy Category, and Lactation Issues
Meperidine, Promethazine (C II) Mepergan Fortis Capsules 50 mg/25 mg	**Moderate to severe pain** 1 capsule q 4–6 h prn	Administration Issues Take with food if GI upset occurs. Limit use in children because of the possibility of extrapyramidal reactions. Drug–Drug Interactions Meperidine: **Increased level/effect of:** warfarin; barbiturates, alcohol, other CNS depressants (inc respiratory/CNS depressant effect); chlorpromazine (inc toxic effects); cimetidine (inc CNS toxicity); **MAO inhibitors (hypertensive crisis).** Promethazine: **Increased effect:** CNS effects (alcohol); EPS effect (fluoxetine, lithium); sedation/hypotension (meperidine). **Increased level of:** TCAs, valproic acid, phenytoin (or decreased level), propranolol (also increases level of antipsychotic). **Decreased level of antipsychotic:** aluminum antacids, barbiturates, carbamazepine, charcoal. **Decreased effect of antipsychotic:** anticholinergics. **Drug dependence, tolerance:** Narcotics have abuse potential, although this potential is low if used for medical reasons. Prolonged use can lead to tolerance, thereby requiring increased doses. If medication is to be withdrawn, it should be tapered to prevent withdrawal symptoms.	ADRs Lightheadedness, dizziness, sedation, nausea, vomiting, sweating, constipation, drowsiness. Promethazine: sedation, anticholinergic effects (dry mouth, constipation, urinary retention, blurred vision, miosis), pseudoparkinsonism, dystonias, orthostatic hypotension. (For other ADRs see table 312.1). Pharmacokinetics See individual agents.	Contraindications Hypersensitivity, diarrhea caused by poisoning, acute bronchial asthma, upper airway obstruction. Promethazine: comatose or severely depressed states, concomitant use of large amounts of other CNS depressants; bone marrow depression, liver damage, cerebral arteriosclerosis, coronary artery disease. Precautions Use cautiously in patients with hepatic or renal dysfunction, acute abdominal conditions, in elderly or debilitated patients, patients with respiratory conditions, cardiovascular or seizure disorders, hypothyroidism, Addison's disease, acute alcoholism, DTs, prostatic hypertrophy. Promethazine: use cautiously in patients with hyperthyroidism; do not use 48 hrs prior to myelography; do not abruptly withdraw therapy. Pregnancy Category: C. Safety not established for promethazine. Lactation Issues Use cautiously. Excreted in breast milk, although no significant effects seen on infant.

Acetaminophen, Propoxyphene (C IV) Darvocet-N, Propacet, various generics Tablets 325 mg/50 mg (as napsylate), 650 mg/100 mg (as napsylate), 650 mg/65 mg	**Mild to Moderate pain** 2 tablets q 4 h prn 1 tablet q 4 h prn (propoxyphene napsylate content 100 mg, or propoxyphene content 65 mg) Acetaminophen: Max daily dose is 4 gm.	Administration Issues Take with food if GI upset occurs. Drug–Drug Interactions **Increased level/effect of:** warfarin; barbiturates, alcohol, other CNS depressants (inc respiratory/CNS depressant effect); chlorpromazine (inc toxic effects); cimetidine (inc CNS toxicity). Acetaminophen: **Increased toxic effect of APAP:** alcohol (chronic); barbiturates, carbamazepine, hydantoins, rifampin, sulfinpyrazone. **Decreased effect of APAP:** charcoal. **Drug dependence, tolerance:** Narcotics have abuse potential, although this potential is low if used for medical reasons. Prolonged use can lead to tolerance, thereby requiring increased doses. If medication is to be withdrawn, it should be tapered to prevent withdrawal symptoms.	ADRs Lightheadedness, dizziness, sedation, nausea, vomiting, sweating, constipation, drowsiness. Acetaminophen: very few adverse reactions Pharmacokinetics See individual agents.	Contraindications Hypersensitivity, diarrhea caused by poisoning, acute bronchial asthma, upper airway obstruction. Precautions Use cautiously in patients with hepatic or renal dysfunction, acute abdominal conditions, in elderly or debilitated patients, patients with respiratory conditions, cardiovascular or seizure disorders, hypothyroidism, Addison's disease, acute alcoholism, DTs, prostatic hypertrophy. Pregnancy Category: C Lactation Issues Use cautiously. Excreted in breast milk, although no significant effects seen on infant.
Aspirin, Propoxyphene, Caffeine (C IV) Darvon, various generics Capsules 389 mg aspirin plus 65 mg propoxyphene plus 32.4 mg caffeine	**Mild to Moderate pain** 1 capsule q 4 h prn	Administration Issues Take with food if GI upset occurs. Aspirin use in children with fever has been associated with Reye's syndrome. Drug–Drug Interactions **Increased level/effect of:** warfarin; barbiturates, alcohol, other CNS depressants (inc respiratory/CNS depressant effect); chlorpromazine (inc toxic effects); cimetidine (inc CNS toxicity). Aspirin: **Increased level/effect of:** alcohol (GI effects); anticoagulants (bleeding effects); methotrexate, valproic acid, sulfonylureas (inc hypoglycemic effect).	ADRs Lightheadedness, dizziness, sedation, nausea, vomiting, sweating, constipation, drowsiness. Aspirin: nausea, dyspepsia, heartburn, GI bleeding, hives, rash, prolonged bleeding time, thrombocytopenia, aspirin intolerance (bronchospasm, rhinitis), "Salicylism": dizziness, tinnitus, difficulty hearing, nausea, vomiting, diarrhea, confusion, CNS depression, headache, sweating, hyperventilation, lassitude.	Contraindications Hypersensitivity, diarrhea caused by poisoning, acute bronchial asthma, upper airway obstruction. Aspirin: hemophilia, bleeding ulcers, hemorrhagic states. Precautions Use cautiously in patients with hepatic or renal dysfunction, acute abdominal conditions, in elderly or debilitated patients, patients with respiratory conditions, cardiovascular or seizure disorders, hypothyroidism, Addison's disease, acute alcoholism, DTs, prostatic hypertrophy.

(continues on next page)

303. Narcotic Combinations *continued from previous page*

Drug and Dosage Forms	Usual Dosage Range	Administration Issues and Drug–Drug & Drug–Food Interactions	Common Adverse Drug Reactions (ADRs) and Pharmacokinetics	Contraindications, Pregnancy Category, and Lactation Issues
Aspirin, Propoxyphene, Caffeine (C IV) ***cont.***		**Decreased level/effect of:** ACE inhibitors, beta blockers, diuretics (decreased antihypertensive effect); probenecid & sulfinpyrazone (decreased uricosuric effect). Drug–Lab Interactions Aspirin: see table 307. **Drug dependence, tolerance:** Narcotics have abuse potential, although this potential is low if used for medical reasons. Prolonged use can lead to tolerance, thereby requiring increased doses. If medication is to be withdrawn, it should be tapered to prevent withdrawal symptoms.		Aspirin: Use cautiously in patients with asthma, nasal polyposis, chronic urticaria (inc risk of hypersensitivity); chronic renal insufficiency, PUD, bleeding disorders. Pregnancy Category: C Aspirin: Category D Lactation Issues Use cautiously. Excreted in breast milk, although no significant effects seen on infant.

304. Nonnarcotic Analgesic Combinations

Drug and Dosage Forms	Usual Dosage Range	Administration Issues and Drug–Drug & Drug–Food Interactions	Common Adverse Drug Reactions (ADRs) and Pharmacokinetics	Contraindications, Pregnancy Category, and Lactation Issues
Acetaminophen, Aspirin, Caffeine Saleto (with salicylamide), Gelpirin, Excedrin, Goody's Extra Strength Powders, various generics *With antacids* (to minimize GI effects): Supac, Buffets, Vanquish Tablets 115 mg/210 mg/16 mg 125 mg/240 mg/32 mg 160 mg/230 mg/33 mg 162 mg/227 mg/32.4 mg 194 mg/227 mg/33 mg 250 mg/250 mg/65 mg Powders 260 mg/520 mg/32.5 mg	**Minor Aches/Pains** Adults: 1–2 tablets or 1 powder packet every 2–6 hrs as needed. Acetaminophen: Max daily dose is 4 gm.	Administration Issues If pain persists longer than 5 d, consult physician. Take with food. Safety/efficacy not established in those <12 yrs old. Aspirin use in children with fever has been associated with Reye's syndrome. Drug–Drug Interactions See individual agents.	ADRs and Pharmacokinetics See individual agents.	Contraindications Hypersensitivity; hemophilia, bleeding ulcers, hemorrhagic states. Precautions Use cautiously in those with hepatic dysfunction, chronic alcohol use. Use cautiously in patients with asthma, nasal polyposis, chronic urticaria (inc risk of hypersensitivity); chronic renal or hepatic dysfunction, PUD, bleeding disorders. Pregnancy Category: D Lactation Issues Safety not established.
Acetaminophen, Magnesium salicylate, Pamabrom (used as a diuretic) Maximum Pain Relief Pamprin Tablets 250 mg/250 mg/25 mg	**Minor Aches/Pains** Adults: 1–2 tablets every 2–6 hrs as needed. Acetaminophen: Max daily dose is 4 gm.	Administration Issues If pain persists longer than 5 days, consult physician. Take with food. Safety/efficacy not established in children. Drug–Drug Interactions See individual agents.	ADRs and Pharmacokinetics See individual agents.	Contraindications Hypersensitivity; hemophilia, bleeding ulcers, hemorrhagic states. Precautions Use cautiously in those with hepatic dysfunction, chronic alcohol use. Use cautiously in patients with asthma, nasal polyposis, chronic urticaria (inc risk of hypersensitivity); chronic renal or hepatic dysfunction, PUD, bleeding disorders. Pregnancy Category: D Lactation Issues Safety not established.
Acetaminophen, Caffeine Aspirin-Free Excedrin, Bayer Select *With pyrilamine* (an antihistamine for sedation): Midol Maximum Strength Caplets 500 mg/65 mg, 500 mg/60 mg	**Minor Aches/Pains:** Adults: 1–2 caplets every 2–6 hrs as needed. Acetaminophen: Max daily dose is 4 gm.	Administration Issues If pain persists longer than 5 days, consult physician. Drug–Drug Interactions See individual agents.	ADRs and Pharmacokinetics See individual agents.	Contraindications Hypersensitivity. Precautions Use cautiously in those with hepatic dysfunction, chronic alcohol use.

(continues on next page)

304. Nonnarcotic Analgesic Combinations *continued from previous page*

Drug and Dosage Forms	Usual Dosage Range	Administration Issues and Drug–Drug & Drug–Food Interactions	Common Adverse Drug Reactions (ADRs) and Pharmacokinetics	Contraindications, Pregnancy Category, and Lactation Issues
Acetaminophen, Caffeine *cont.*				Pregnancy/Lactation Issues Used in all trimesters of pregnancy with no known harm to fetus. Excreted in breast milk, but no known harm to infant.
Acetaminophen, Pamabrom (used as a diuretic) Premsyn PMS, Bayer Select Maximum Strength Menstrual Caplets *With pyridoxine:* Lurline *With pyrilamine* (an antihistamine for sedation): Multi-Symptom Pamprin, Maximum Strength Midol Caplets 500 mg/25 mg Tablets 500 mg/25 mg	**Minor Aches/Pains** Adults: 1–2 tablets or caplets every 2–6 h as needed.	Administration Issues If pain persists longer than 5 days, consult physician. Drug–Drug Interactions See individual agents.	ADRs and Pharmacokinetics See individual agents.	Contraindications Hypersensitivity. Precautions Use cautiously in those with hepatic dysfunction, chronic alcohol use. Pregnancy/Lactation Issues Used in all trimesters of pregnancy with no known harm to fetus. Excreted in breast milk, but no known harm to infant.
Acetaminophen, antacid combinations (to minimize GI effects) Aspirin Free Excedrin, Extra Strength Tylenol Headache Plus Caplets Caplets 500 mg	**Minor Aches/Pains** Adults: 1–2 caplets every 2–6 h as needed.	Administration Issues If pain persists longer than 5 days, consult physician. Drug–Drug Interactions See individual agents.	ADRs and Pharmacokinetics See individual agents.	Contraindications Hypersensitivity. Precautions Use cautiously in those with hepatic dysfunction, chronic alcohol use. Pregnancy/Lactation Issues Used in all trimesters of pregnancy with no known harm to fetus. Excreted in breast milk, but no known harm to infant.
Aspirin, Caffeine Anacin or Maximum Strength Anacin, Gensan *With salicylamide* (added analgesia): BC Tablets or Powder *With antacids* (to minimize GI effects): Cope Tablets	**Minor Aches/Pains** Adults: 1–2 tablets or 1 powder packet every 2–6 h as needed.	Administration Issues Take with food. Safety/efficacy not established in those <12 yrs old. Aspirin use in children with fever has been associated with Reye's syndrome. Drug–Drug Interactions See individual agents.	ADRs and Pharmacokinetics See individual agents.	Contraindications Hypersensitivity, hemophilia, bleeding ulcers, hemorrhagic states. Precautions Use cautiously in patients with asthma, nasal polyposis, chronic urticaria (inc risk of hypersensitivity); chronic renal or hepatic dysfunction, PUD, bleeding disorders.

Tablets 325 mg/16 mg, 400 mg/32 mg, 421 mg/32 mg, 500 mg/32 mg, 650 mg/32 mg, 742 mg/36 mg				Pregnancy Category: D Lactation Issues Safety not established.
Aspirin, Meprobamate (for sedative properties) Equagesic Tablets Tablets 325 mg/200 mg	**Minor Aches/Pains** Adults: 1–2 tablets every 2–6 h as needed.	Administration Issues Take with food. Safety/efficacy not established in those <12 yrs old. Aspirin use in children with fever has been associated with Reye's syndrome. Drug–Drug Interactions See individual agents.	ADRs and Pharmacokinetics See individual agents.	Contraindications Hypersensitivity, hemophilia, bleeding ulcers, hemorrhagic states, acute intermittent porphyria. Precautions Use cautiously in patients with asthma, nasal polyposis, chronic urticaria (inc risk of hypersensitivity); chronic renal or hepatic dysfunction, PUD, bleeding disorders. Meprobamate: Drug dependency is observed (avoid prolonged use); abrupt discontinuation may precipitate withdrawal. Use cautiously in patients with seizure disorders. Use cautiously in patients with severe renal or hepatic dysfunction. Pregnancy Category: D. Meprobamate: should not be used in pregnant women—increased risk of congenital malformations during the first trimester. Lactation Issues Safety not established.
Magnesium Salicylate, Phenyltoloxamine (an antihistamine for sedation) Mobigesic, Magsal Tablets 325 mg/30 mg, 600 mg/25 mg	**Minor Aches/Pains** Adults: 1–2 tablets every 2–6 h as needed	Administration Issues Take with food. Safety/efficacy not established in children. Drug–Drug Interactions See individual agents.	ADRs and Pharmacokinetics See individual agents.	Contraindications Hypersensitivity, hemophilia, bleeding ulcers, hemorrhagic states. Precautions Use cautiously in patients with asthma, nasal polyposis, chronic urticaria (inc risk of hypersensitivity); chronic renal or hepatic dysfunction, PUD, bleeding disorders. Pregnancy Category: D Lactation Issues Safety not established.

305. Nonnarcotic Analgesic Combinations with Barbiturates

Drug and Dosage Forms	Usual Dosage Range	Administration Issues and Drug–Drug & Drug–Food Interactions	Common Adverse Drug Reactions (ADRs) and Pharmacokinetics	Contraindications, Pregnancy Category, and Lactation Issues
Acetaminophen, Caffeine, Butalbital (a barbiturate for sedation) Esgic, Fioricet, Repan, Anoquan, Amaphen, Butace, Endolor, Femcet, various generics Tablets 325 mg/40 mg/50 mg Capsules 325 mg/40 mg/50 mg	**Mild to Moderate Pain** Adults: 1–2 every 4 h as needed	Administration Issues May produce irritability, excitability or aggression in children. Safety/efficacy not established for < 6 yrs old. Drug–Drug Interactions See individual agents.	ADRs and Pharmacokinetics See individual agents. Elderly: may observe paradoxical excitement. Precautions: **Drug abuse and dependence:** Prolonged use at high doses leads to physical dependence. If dependent on barbiturate, slowly withdraw over several weeks. May use long-acting barbiturate (phenobarbital) at dose of 30 mg per every 100–200 mg of butalbital to help prevent withdrawal symptoms.	Contraindications Hypersensitivity. Precautions Use cautiously in those with hepatic dysfunction, chronic alcohol use **Barbiturate** Contraindications Hypersensitivity; manifest or latent porphyria, severe hepatic, renal, or respiratory dysfunction; previous addiction to sedative/hypnotic. Pregnancy Category: D Lactation Issues Use cautiously in nursing mothers, sedation has been reported in infants
Acetaminophen, Butalbital (a barbiturate for sedation) Phrenilin, Bancap, Triaprin, Sedapap-10, Phrenilin Forte Tablets 325 mg/50 mg, 650 mg/50 mg Capsules 325 mg/50 mg, 650 mg/50 mg	**Mild to Moderate Pain** Adults: 1–2 every 4 h as needed	Administration Issues May produce irritability, excitability or aggression in children. Safety/efficacy not established for < 6 yrs old. Drug–Drug Interactions See individual agents.	ADRs and Pharmacokinetics See individual agents. Elderly: may observe paradoxical excitement. Precautions **Drug abuse and dependence:** Prolonged use at high doses leads to physical dependence. If dependent on barbiturate, slowly withdraw over several weeks. May use long-acting barbiturate (phenobarbital) at dose of 30 mg per every 100–200 mg of butalbital to help prevent withdrawal symptoms.	Contraindications Hypersensitivity. Precautions Use cautiously in those with hepatic dysfunction, chronic alcohol use. **Barbiturate** Contraindications Hypersensitivity; manifest or latent porphyria, severe hepatic, renal, or respiratory dysfunction; previous addiction to sedative/hypnotic. Pregnancy Category: D Lactation Issues Use cautiously in nursing mothers, sedation has been reported in infants.
Aspirin, Caffeine, Butalbital (a barbiturate for sedation)	**Mild to Moderate Pain** Adults: 1–2 every 4 h as needed.	Administration Issues Take with food. May produce irritability, excitability or aggression in children.	ADRs and Pharmacokinetics See individual agents.	Contraindications Hypersensitivity, hemophilia, bleeding ulcers, hemorrhagic states.

Florinal, Florgen PF, Lanorinal, various generics Tablets 325 mg/40 mg/50 mg, 650 mg/40 mg/50 mg Capsules 325 mg/40 mg/50 mg		Safety/efficacy not established in those < 6 yrs old. Aspirin use in children with fever has been associated with Reye's syndrome. Drug–Drug Interactions See individual agents.	Elderly: may observe paradoxical excitement. Precautions **Drug abuse and dependence:** Prolonged use at high doses leads to physical dependence. If dependent on barbiturate, slowly withdraw over several weeks. May use long-acting barbiturate (phenobarbital) at dose of 30 mg per every 100–200 mg of butalbital to help prevent withdrawal symptoms.	Precautions Use cautiously in patients with asthma, nasal polyposis, chronic urticaria (inc risk of hypersensitivity); chronic renal or hepatic dysfunction, PUD, bleeding disorders. Pregnancy Category: D Lactation Issues Safety not established. Use cautiously if at all.
Aspirin, Butalbital (a barbiturate for sedation) BAC, Axotal Tablets 650 mg/50 mg	**Mild to Moderate Pain** Adults: 1–2 every 4 h as needed.	Administration Issues Take with food. May produce irritability, excitability or aggression in children. Safety/efficacy not established for < 6 yrs old. Aspirin use in children with fever has been associated with Reye's syndrome. Drug-Drug Interactions See individual agents.	ADRs and Pharmacokinetics See individual agents. Elderly: may observe paradoxical excitement. Precautions **Drug abuse and dependence:** Prolonged use at high doses leads to physical dependence. If dependent on barbiturate, slowly withdraw over several weeks. May use long-acting barbiturate (phenobarbital) at dose of 30 mg per every 100–200 mg of butalbital to help prevent withdrawal symptoms.	Contraindications Hypersensitivity, hemophilia, bleeding ulcers, hemorrhagic states. Precautions Use cautiously in patients with asthma, nasal polyposis, chronic urticaria (inc risk of hypersensitivity); chronic renal or hepatic dysfunction, PUD, bleeding disorders. Pregnancy Category: D Lactation Issues Safety not established. Use cautiously if at all.

306 Nonsteroidal Anti-Inflammatory Agents

306.1 Propionic Acids

Drug and Dosage Forms	Usual Dosage Range	Administration Issues and Drug–Drug & Drug–Food Interactions	Common Adverse Drug Reactions (ADRs) and Pharmacokinetics	Contraindications, Pregnancy Category, and Lactation Issues
Fenoprofen Nalfon, various generics Capsules 200 mg, 300 mg Tablets 600 mg	**Rheumatoid arthritis or osteoarthritis** 300–600 mg tid to qid **Mild to moderate pain** 200 mg q 4–6 h prn **Maximum adult daily dose:** 3200 mg	Administration Issues Take with food, avoid alcohol and aspirin use. Safety/efficacy in children not established. Drug–Drug Interactions **Increased levels/effects of:** anticoagulants, cyclosporine (inc renal toxic effects), digoxin, dipyridamole, hydantoins, lithium. **Decreased levels/effects of:** ACE inhibitors, beta blockers, diuretics, (antihypertensive effect). **Increased levels/effects of NSAID: probenecid.**	ADRs Nausea, vomiting, diarrhea, constipation, abdominal distress, dyspepsia, dizziness, headache, drowsiness, rash. Less frequent: GI ulceration, cholestatic hepatitis, pancreatitis, hematuria, proteinuria, elevated BUN, increased serum creatinine, renal insufficiency/failure. Elderly patients: May be more prone to adverse effects. Pharmacokinetics Antirheumatic action onset = 2 d; hepatically metabolized; $T_{1/2}$ = 2–3 hrs; renal elimination of metabolites.	Contraindications Hypersensitivity to this or aspirin; preexisting renal disease. Precautions Use cautiously in patients with PUD, severe renal or hepatic dysfunction, bleeding disorders. Pregnancy Category: B Lactation Issues Excreted in breast milk—do not use in nursing mothers.
Flurbiprofen Ansaid Tablets 50 mg, 100 mg	**Rheumatoid arthritis or osteoarthritis** 200–300 mg/d in 2–4 divided doses, initially. Max single dose is 100 mg and max daily dose is 300mg.	Administration Issues Take with food; avoid alcohol and aspirin use. Safety/efficacy in children is not established. Drug–Drug Interactions **Increased levels/effects of:** anticoagulants, cyclosporine (inc renal toxic effects), digoxin, dipyridamole, hydantoins, lithium. **Decreased levels/effects of:** ACE inhibitors, beta blockers, diuretics, (antihypertensive effect). **Increased levels/effects of NSAID: probenecid.**	ADRs Most frequent: Nausea, vomiting, diarrhea, constipation, abdominal distress, dyspepsia, dizziness, headache, drowsiness, rash. Less frequent: See Fenoprofen. Elderly patients: May be more prone to adverse effects Pharmacokinetics: Hepatically metabolized; $T_{1/2}$ = 5.7 h; renal elimination of metabolites.	Contraindications Hypersensitivity to this or aspirin; preexisting renal disease. Precautions Use cautiously in patients with PUD, severe renal or hepatic dysfunction, bleeding disorders. Pregnancy Category: B Lactation Issues Excreted in breast milk—do not use in nursing mothers
Ibuprofen Motrin, Advil, Bayer Select, Genpril, Haltran, Menadol, Midol IB, Nuprin, various generics	**Rheumatoid arthritis or osteoarthritis** 300 mg qid or 400–800 mg tid to qid **Pediatrics: 30–70 mg/kg/d tid to qid**	Administration Issues: Take with food; avoid alcohol and aspirin use; OTC use: Do not use for >3 days for fever or >10 days for pain—consult physician if those symptoms last longer.	ADRs: Nausea, vomiting, diarrhea, constipation, abdominal distress, dyspepsia, dizziness, headache, drowsiness, rash.	Contraindications Hypersensitivity to this or aspirin; preexisting renal disease. Precautions

Tablets 100 mg, 200 mg, 300 mg, 400 mg, 600 mg, 800 mg Tablets, chewable 50 mg, 100 mg Suspension 100 mg/5 mL, 100 mg/2.5 mL Oral Drops 40 mg/mL Capsules 200 mg	**Mild to Moderate Pain** 400 mg q 4–6 h prn **Primary Dysmenorrhea** 400 mg q 4 h prn **OTC use (mild pain, dysmenorrhea, fever reduction)** 200 mg q 4–6 h prn (May increase to 400 mg q 4–6 h prn) **Max adult dose is 3200 mg.** **Pediatrics (fever reduction in 6 months to 12 yrs old):** Temp ≤ 102.5F: 5 mg/kg q 6–8 hrs prn Temp> 102.5F: 10 mg/kg q 6–8 h prn **Max pediatric dose: 40mg/kg/d.**	Drug–Drug Interactions **Increased levels/effects of:** anticoagulants, cyclosporine (inc renal toxic effects), digoxin, dipyridamole, hydantoins, lithium. **Decreased levels/effects of:** ACE inhibitors, beta blockers, diuretics, (antihypertensive effect). **Increased levels/effects of NSAID: probenecid.**	Less frequent: See Fenoprofen. Elderly patients: May be more prone to adverse effects. Pharmacokinetics: Analgesic onset of action = 0.5 hrs; analgesic duration of action = 4–6 h; antirheumatic onset of action = within 7 d; hepatically metabolized; $T_{1/2}$ = 1.8–2.5 h; renal elimination of metabolites.	Use cautiously in patients with PUD, severe renal or hepatic dysfunction, bleeding disorders. Pregnancy Category: B Lactation Issues Excreted in breast milk—do not use in nursing mothers.
Ketoprofen Orudis KT, Actron, Orudis, Oruvail, various generics Tablets 12.5 mg Capsules 25 mg, 50 mg, 75 mg Capsules, extended release 100 mg, 150 mg, 200 mg	**Rheumatoid arthritis or osteoarthritis** 150–300 mg/d divided tid to qid Extended Release formulation: 200 mg qd **Elderly, debilitated patients, or those with renal dysfunction:** 75–150 mg/d divided tid to qid. May titrate slowly if needed. **Max adult dose is 300 mg/d.** **Mild to moderate pain or primary dysmenorrhea** 25–50 mg q 6–8 h prn. Use smaller doses for elderly, debilitated or small patients, and those with renal or hepatic disease. **OTC use (mild pain, fever reduction): 12.5 mg q 4–6 h prn. May repeat dose after 1 hr if pain or fever persists. Do not exceed 25 mg in 4–6 h.**	Administration Issues Take with food, avoid alcohol and aspirin use. Not recommended for those <16 yrs old. Drug–Drug Interactions **Increased levels/effects of:** anticoagulants, cyclosporine (inc renal toxic effects), digoxin, dipyridamole, hydantoins, lithium. **Decreased levels/effects of:** ACE inhibitors, beta blockers, diuretics, (antihypertensive effect). **Decreased levels/effects of NSAID: probenecid.**	ADRs Nausea, vomiting, diarrhea, constipation, abdominal distress, dyspepsia, dizziness, headache, drowsiness, rash. Less frequent: See Fenoprofen. Elderly patients: May be more prone to adverse effects. Pharmacokinetics: Hepatically metabolized; $T_{1/2}$ = 2–4 hrs; renal elimination of metabolites.	Contraindications Hypersensitivity to this or aspirin; preexisting renal disease. Precautions Use cautiously in patients with PUD, severe renal or hepatic dysfunction, bleeding disorders. Pregnancy Category: B Lactation Issues Excreted in breast milk—do not use in nursing mothers.

(continues on next page)

306.1 Propionic Acids *continued from previous page*

Drug and Dosage Forms	Usual Dosage Range	Administration Issues and Drug–Drug & Drug–Food Interactions	Common Adverse Drug Reactions (ADRs) and Pharmacokinetics	Contraindications, Pregnancy Category, and Lactation Issues
Naproxen Naprosyn, Napron X, EC-Naprosyn, Naprelan, various generics Tablets 250 mg, 375 mg, 500 mg Tablets, delayed release 375 mg, 500 mg Suspension 125 mg/5 mL **Naproxen Sodium** Anaprox, Aleve, various generics Tablets 220 mg (200 mg of naproxen), 275 mg (250 mg naproxen), 550 mg (500 mg naproxen) Tablets, controlled release 421.5 mg (375 mg naproxen), 550 mg (500 mg naproxen)	**Rheumatoid arthritis, osteoarthritis, ankylosing spondylitis** **Naproxen:** 250–500 mg bid. May titrate to 1.5 g/d if needed for a limited period of time. Delayed release: 375–500 mg bid Controled release: 750–1000 mg qd Max dose is 1000 mg/d **Naproxen sodium:** 275–550 mg bid. May titrate to 1.65 g/d for limited periods of time. Pediatrics: 10 mg/kg divided bid. For the suspension: 13 kg: 2.5 mL twice daily 25 kg: 5 mL twice daily 38 kg: 7.5 mL twice daily **Acute gout** Naproxen: 750 mg followed by 250 mg q 8 h until attack is over. Naproxen sodium: 825 mg followed by 275 mg q 8 hrs until attack is over. Controlled release: 1000–1500 mg once daily on first day, then 1000 mg daily until attack is over. **Mild to moderate pain, dysmenorrhea, acute tendinitis, and bursitis** Naproxen: 500 mg followed by 250 mg q 6–8 hrs. Max dose is 1.25 g/d. Naproxen sodium: 550 mg followed by 275 mg q 6–8 h. Max dose is 1.375 g/d.	Administration Issues Take with food, avoid alcohol and aspirin use. Do not break, crush, or chew extended release products. Safety and efficacy in children <12 years of age has not been established. Drug–Drug Interactions **Increased levels/effects of:** anticoagulants, cyclosporine (inc renal toxic effects), digoxin, dipyridamole, hydantoins, lithium. **Decreased levels/effects of:** ACE inhibitors, beta blockers, diuretics, (antihypertensive effect). **increased levels/effects of NSAID:** probenecid.	ADRs Nausea, vomiting, diarrhea, constipation, abdominal distress, dyspepsia, dizziness, headache, drowsiness, rash. Less frequent: See Fenoprofen. Elderly patients: May be more prone to adverse effects. Pharmacokinetics: Analgesic onset of action = 1 h; analgesic duration of action = 7 h; antirheumatic onset of action = within 14 d; hepatically metabolized; $T_{1/2}$ = 1.2–15 h; renal elimination of metabolites.	Contraindications Hypersensitivity to this or aspirin; preexisting renal disease. Precautions Use cautiously in patients with PUD, severe renal or hepatic dysfunction, bleeding disorders. Pregnancy Category: B Lactation Issues Excreted in breast milk—do not use in nursing mothers.

	Controlled release: 1000 mg once daily. May titrate to 1500 mg/d for limited period of time as needed. **OTC analgesic use:** 200 mg q 8–12 h prn. May initiate therapy with 400 mg then follow with above schedule. Max dose is 600 mg/d unless otherwise directed by a health-care professional. **Elderly:** Max = 200 mg **q 12 h**			
Oxaprozin Daypro, Daypro ALTA Caplets 600 mg Tablets 600 mg Daypro ALTA Tablets: 678 oxaprozin phosphate (equivalent to 600 mg Oxaprozin)	**Rheumatoid arthritis or osteoarthritis:** 1200 mg qd. May initiate with 600 mg qd for smaller, elderly, or debilitated patients. **Max dose is 1800 mg/d, divided**	Administration Issues Take with food, avoid alcohol and aspirin use. Safety/efficacy in children is not established. Drug–Drug Interactions **Increased levels/effects of:** anticoagulants, cyclosporine (inc renal toxic effects), digoxin, dipyridamole, hydantoins, lithium. **Decreased levels/effects of:** ACE inhibitors, beta blockers, diuretics, (antihypertensive effect). **Increased levels/effects of NSAID:** probenecid.	ADRs Nausea, vomiting, diarrhea, constipation, abdominal distress, dyspepsia, dizziness, headache, drowsiness, rash. Less frequent: See Fenoprofen. Elderly patients: May be more prone to adverse effects. Pharmacokinetics Antirheumatic onset of action = within 7 d; hepatically metabolized; $T_{1/2}$ = 42–50 h; renal elimination of metabolites.	Contraindications Hypersensitivity to this or aspirin; preexisting renal disease. Precautions Use cautiously in patients with PUD, severe renal or hepatic dysfunction, bleeding disorders. Pregnancy Category: B Lactation Issues Excreted in breast milk—do not use in nursing mothers.

306.2 Acetic Acids

Drug and Dosage Forms	Usual Dosage Range	Administration Issues and Drug–Drug & Drug–Food Interactions	Common Adverse Drug Reactions (ADRs) and Pharmacokinetics	Contraindications, Pregnancy Category, and Lactation Issues
Diclofenac Sodium Voltaren, Cataflam, generics Tablets 50 mg Tablets, delayed release (enteric coated) 25 mg, 50 mg, 75 mg	**Osteoarthritis** 100–150 mg/d bid to tid **Rheumatoid arthritis** 150–200 mg/d tid to qid **Chronic therapy for OA or RA** Extended-release tablets: 100 mg/d	Administration Issues Take with food, avoid alcohol and aspirin use. Safety/efficacy in children is not established. Drug–Drug Interactions **Increased levels/effects of:** anticoagulants, cyclosporine (inc renal toxic effects), digoxin, dipyridamole, hydantoins, lithium.	ADRs Nausea, vomiting, diarrhea, constipation, abdominal distress, dyspepsia, dizziness, headache, drowsiness, rash. Less frequent: GI ulceration, cholestatic hepatitis, pancreatitis, hematuria, proteinuria, elevated BUN, increased serum creatinine, renal insufficiency/failure.	Contraindications Hypersensitivity to this or aspirin; preexisting renal disease. Precautions Use cautiously in patients with PUD, severe renal or hepatic dysfunction, bleeding disorders.

(*continues on next page*)

306.2 Acetic Acids *continued from previous page*

Drug and Dosage Forms	Usual Dosage Range	Administration Issues and Drug–Drug & Drug–Food Interactions	Common Adverse Drug Reactions (ADRs) and Pharmacokinetics	Contraindications, Pregnancy Category, and Lactation Issues
Diclofenac Sodium *cont.* Tablets, extended-release 100 mg	**Ankylosing spondylitis** 100–125 mg/d in 4–5 divided doses **Moderate pain or primary dysmenorrhea** 50 mg tid. May initiate therapy with 100 mg followed by 50 mg tid **Max dose is 200 mg/d.**	**Decreased levels/effects of:** ACE inhibitors, beta blockers, diuretics, (antihypertensive effect). **Increased levels/effects of NSAID:** probenecid.	Elderly patients: May be more prone to adverse effects. Pharmacokinetics: Hepatically metabolized; $T_{1/2} = 1-2$ h; renal elimination of metabolites.	Pregnancy Category: B Lactation Issues Excreted in breast milk—do not use in nursing mothers.
Diclofenac plus Misoprostol Arthrotec Tablets 50 mg/200 mcg, 75 mg/200 mcg	**Treatment of the signs and symptoms of osteoarthritis or rheumatoid arthritis in patients at high risk for developing NSAID-induced gastric or duodenal ulcers:** **Osteoarthritis** 50/200 mg tid or, if intolerant, 50/200 mg bid or 75/200 mg bid **Rheumatoid arthritis** 50/200 mg 3–4 times daily or, if intolerant, 50/200 mg bid or 75/200 mg bid Lower doses are less effective at preventing ulcers.	Administration Issues **Do not administer in women with childbearing potential unless the patient requires NSAID therapy and is at high risk for developing ulcers. Patient must have a negative serum pregnancy test within 2 weeks of beginning therapy and must capable of complying with effective contraceptive measures.** Should be administered with meals. and at bedtime. Do not take concurrently with antacids. Do not administer more than 200 mcg of misoprostol at any one time; do not exceed 800 mcg/day of misoprostol. **Patient Education** Advise patient to report any signs or symptoms of GI ulceration or bleeding, skin rash, weight gain or swelling. Stop therapy and seek medical attention is signs of liver toxicity occur. Drug Interactions. See individual drugs.	ADRs Most frequent: Refer to Diclofenac section. Misoprostol: abdominal pain, diarrhea, dyspepsia, nausea Pharmacokinetics Diclofenac-refer to diclofenac section Misoprostol terminal $T_{1/2} = 20-40$ minutes; extensively absorbed	Contraindications Pregnancy, vaginal bleeding, hypersensitivity to diclofenac or other NSAIDS. Pregnancy Category Dicolfenac: C **Misoprostol: X** Lactation Issues Do not use in nursing mothers.
Etodolac Lodine Lodine XL, generics Capsules: 200 mg, 300 mg	Arthritis Recommended starting dose is 300 mg 2 or 3 times/day or 400 or 500 mg BID.	Administration Issues: Take with food, avoid alcohol and aspirin use. Safety/efficacy in children is not established.	ADRs Most frequent: Nausea, vomiting, diarrhea, constipation, abdominal distress, dyspepsia, dizziness, headache, drowsiness, rash.	Contraindications Hypersensitivity to this or aspirin; preexisting renal disease.

Tablets 400 mg, 500 mg Tablets, Extended-release 400 mg, 500 mg, 600 mg	Adjust dose up or down depending upon the response. **Moderate pain:** 200–400 mg q 6–8 h prn (Immediate-release, only) **Max dose is 1200 mg/d.** Patients ≤ 60 kg: Do not exceed 20 mg/kg.	Drug–Drug Interactions: **Increased levels/effects of:** anticoagulants, cyclosporine (inc renal toxic effects), digoxin, dipyridamole, hydantoins, lithium **Decreased levels/effects of:** ACE inhibitors, beta blockers, diuretics, (antihypertensive effect). **Increased levels/effects of NSAID:** probenecid.	Less frequent: See Diclofenac. Elderly patients: May be more prone to adverse effects. Pharmacokinetics Analgesic onset of action = 0.5 hrs; analgesic duration of action = 4–12 h; hepatically metabolized; $T_{1/2}$ = 7.3 h; renal elimination of metabolites.	Precautions Use cautiously in patients with PUD, severe renal or hepatic dysfunction, bleeding disorders. Pregnancy Category: B Lactation Issues Excreted in breast milk—do not use in nursing mothers.
Indomethacin Indocin, Indochron E-R, various generics Capsules 25 mg, 50 mg Capsules, sustained release 75 mg Suspension 25 mg/5 mL Suppositories 50 mg	**Rheumatoid arthritis, osteoarthritis, ankylosing spondylitis** 25 mg bid to tid. Titrate by 25–50 mg/d q 7 d prn up to 200 mg/d Sustained release: 75 mg qd to bid **Acute bursitis or tendinitis** 75–150 mg daily in 3–4 divided doses for 7–14 d **Acute gout** 50 mg tid until attack is over (3–5 days). **Unlabeled uses** to prevent premature labor (not for long periods of time); topical eye drops 0.5% and 1% used to treat cystoid macular edema. **Max dose is 200 mg/d (150 mg of SR capsules).**	Administration Issues Take with food, avoid alcohol and aspirin use. Not recommended for those <14 yrs except when need outweighs risk. Drug–Drug Interactions: **Increased levels/effects of:** anticoagulants, cyclosporine (inc renal toxic effects), digoxin, dipyridamole, hydantoins, lithium. **Decreased levels/effects of:** ACE inhibitors, beta blockers, diuretics, (antihypertensive effect). **Increased levels/effects of NSAID:** probenecid.	ADRs Most frequent: Nausea, vomiting, diarrhea, constipation, abdominal distress, dyspepsia, dizziness, headache, drowsiness, rash. Less frequent: See Diclofenac. Elderly patients: May be more prone to adverse effects. Pharmacokinetics 90% protein bound; analgesic onset of action = 0.5 h; analgesic duration of action = 4–6 h; antirheumatic onset of action = within 7 d; $T_{1/2}$ = 4.5 h; renal elimination of metabolites.	Contraindications Hypersensitivity to this or aspirin; preexisting renal disease. Precautions Use cautiously in patients with PUD, severe renal or hepatic dysfunction, bleeding disorders. Pregnancy Category: B Lactation Issues Excreted in breast milk—do not use in nursing mothers.
Ketorolac Toradol, generics Tablets 10 mg Injection 15 mg/mL, 30 mg/mL	**Short-term (<5d) management of pain** Oral: 10 mg q 4–6 h prn Max oral = 40 mg/d **Continuation treatment to IM therapy for the management of moderately severe pain that requires analgesia at the opioid level:**	Administration Issues Take with food, avoid alcohol and aspirin use. Safety/efficacy in children is not established. Drug–Drug Interactions **Increased levels/effects of:** anticoagulants, cyclosporine (inc renal toxic effects), digoxin, dipyridamole, hydantoins, lithium.	ADRs Most frequent: **Serious GI bleeding and ulceration may occur,** nausea, vomiting, diarrhea, constipation, abdominal distress, dyspepsia, dizziness, headache, drowsiness, rash.	Contraindications Hypersensitivity to this or aspirin; preexisting renal disease. Precautions Use cautiously in patients with PUD, severe renal or hepatic dysfunction, bleeding disorders. Pregnancy Category: B

(continues on next page)

306.2 Acetic Acids *continued from previous page*

Drug and Dosage Forms	Usual Dosage Range	Administration Issues and Drug–Drug & Drug–Food Interactions	Common Adverse Drug Reactions (ADRs) and Pharmacokinetics	Contraindications, Pregnancy Category, and Lactation Issues
Ketorolac *cont.*	20 mg as first dose, followed by 10 mg every 4–6 h for those patients who received 60 mg IM, 30 mg IV or multiple 30 mg IM doses. **Max Dose is 40 mg/d (oral) or 120 mg/d (IM). DO NOT EXCEED 5 DAYS OF THERAPY.** **Elderly, debilitated (those with renal dysfunction), or small patients:** 10 mg first dose followed by 10 mg q 4–6 h for those who received 30 mg IM, 15 mg IV, or 15 mg IM multiple dosing.	**Decreased levels/effects of:** ACE inhibitors, beta blockers, diuretics, (antihypertensive effect). **Increased levels/effects of NSAID:** probenecid.	Less frequent: See Diclofenac. Elderly patients: May be more prone to adverse effects. Pharmacokinetics 90% protein bound; $T_{1/2} = 2.4–8.6$ h; renal elimination of metabolites.	Lactation Issues Excreted in breast milk—do not use in nursing mothers
Nabumetone Relafen, generics Tablets 500 mg, 750 mg	**Rheumatoid arthritis or osteoarthritis** 1000 mg qd. May titrate to 1500–2000 mg/d in 1–2 divided doses **Max dose is 2000 mg/d.**	Administration Issues Take with food, avoid alcohol and aspirin use. Safety/efficacy in children not established. Drug–Drug Interactions **Increased levels/effects of:** anticoagulants, cyclosporine (inc renal toxic effects), digoxin, dipyridamole, hydantoins, lithium. **Decreased levels/effects of:** ACE inhibitors, beta blockers, diuretics, (antihypertensive effect). **Increased levels/effects of NSAID:** probenecid.	ADRs Most frequent: Nausea, vomiting, diarrhea, constipation, abdominal distress, dyspepsia, dizziness, headache, drowsiness, rash. Less frequent: See Diclofenac. Elderly patients: May be more prone to adverse effects. Pharmacokinetics 90% protein bound; inactive prodrug that must be converted to an active metabolite; $T_{1/2} = 22.5–30$ h (active metabolite); renal elimination of metabolites.	Contraindications Hypersensitivity to this or aspirin; preexisting renal disease. Precautions Use cautiously in patients with PUD, severe renal or hepatic dysfunction, bleeding disorders. Pregnancy Category: B Lactation Issues Excreted in breast milk—do not use in nursing mothers.
Sulindac Clinorll, various generics Tablets 150 mg, 200 mg	**Rheumatoid arthritis, osteoarthritis or ankylosing spondylitis** 150 mg bid **Acute subacromial bursitis, tendinitis, or acute gouty arthritis** 200 mg bid for 7–14 d (bursitis or tendinitis) or 7 d (for gout).	Administration Issues Take with food; avoid alcohol and aspirin use. Drug–Drug Interactions **Increased levels/effects of:**	ADRs Most frequent: Nausea, vomiting, diarrhea, constipation, abdominal distress, dyspepsia, dizziness, headache, drowsiness, rash.	Contraindications Hypersensitivity to this or aspirin; preexisting renal disease. Precautions Use cautiously in patients with PUD, severe renal or hepatic dysfunction, bleeding disorders.

	Max dose is 400 mg/d.	anticoagulants, cyclosporine (inc renal toxic effects), digoxin, dipyridamole, hydantoins, lithium. **Decreased levels/effects of:** ACE inhibitors, beta blockers, diuretics, (antihypertensive effect). **Increased levels/effects of NSAID:** probenecid.	Less frequent: See Diclofenac. Elderly patients: May be more prone to adverse effects. Pharmacokinetics Antirheumatic onset of action = within 7 d; $T_{1/2}$ = 7.8 h.	Pregnancy Category: B Lactation Issues Excreted in breast milk—do not use in nursing mothers. Pediatrics Safety/efficacy not established.
Tolmetin Tolectin Tablets 200 mg, 600 mg Capsules 400 mg	**Rheumatoid arthritis or osteoarthritis** 400 mg tid/ May titrate up to 1800 mg/d divided tid **Pediatrics (≥ 2 yrs):** 20 mg/kg/d in 3–4 divided doses. May titrate up to 30 mg/kg/d if needed **Max dose is 2000 mg/d.**	Administration Issues Take with food; avoid alcohol and aspirin use. Drug–Drug Interactions **Increased levels/effects of:** anticoagulants, cyclosporine (inc renal toxic effects), digoxin, dipyridamole, hydantoins, lithium. **Decreased levels/effects of:** ACE inhibitors, beta blockers, diuretics, (antihypertensive effect). **Increased levels/effects of NSAID:** probenecid.	ADRs Most frequent: Nausea, vomiting, diarrhea, constipation, abdominal distress, dyspepsia, dizziness, headache, drowsiness, rash. Less frequent: See Diclofenac. Elderly patients: May be more prone to adverse effects. Pharmacokinetics 90% protein bound; antirheumatic onset of action = within 7 d; $T_{1/2}$ = 1–1.5 h; renal elimination of metabolites.	Contraindications Hypersensitivity to this or aspirin; preexisting renal disease. Precautions Use cautiously in patients with PUD, severe renal or hepatic dysfunction, bleeding disorders. Pregnancy Category: B Lactation Issues Excreted in breast milk—do not use in nursing mothers.

306.3 Fenamates and Oxicams

Drug and Dosage Forms	Usual Dosage Range	Administration Issues and Drug–Drug & Drug–Food Interactions	Common Adverse Drug Reactions (ADRs) and Pharmacokinetics	Contraindications, Pregnancy Category, and Lactation Issues
Meclofenamate Meclomen, various generics Capsules 50 mg, 100 mg	**Rheumatoid arthritis or osteoarthritis** 200–400 mg/d in 3–4 divided doses **Mild to moderate pain** 50 mg q 4–6 h. May titrate to 100 mg q 4–6 h pm	Administration Issues Take with food; avoid alcohol and aspirin use; not recommended for those <14 yrs old. Drug–Drug Interactions **Increased levels/effects of:** anticoagulants, cyclosporine (inc renal toxic effects), digoxin, dipyridamole, hydantoins, lithium.	ADRs Most frequent: Nausea, vomiting, diarrhea, constipation, abdominal distress, dyspepsia, dizziness, headache, drowsiness, rash. Less frequent: GI ulceration, cholestatic hepatitis, pancreatitis, hematuria, proteinuria, elevated	Contraindications Hypersensitivity to this or aspirin; preexisting renal disease. Precautions Use cautiously in patients with PUD, severe renal or hepatic dysfunction, bleeding disorders. Pregnancy Category: B

(continues on next page)

306.3 Fenamates and Oxicams *continued from previous page*

Drug and Dosage Forms	Usual Dosage Range	Administration Issues and Drug–Drug & Drug–Food Interactions	Common Adverse Drug Reactions (ADRs) and Pharmacokinetics	Contraindications, Pregnancy Category, and Lactation Issues
Meclofenamate *cont.*	**Primary dysmenorrhea, excessive menstrual blood loss** 100 mg tid for up to 6 days. Start with onset of bleeding. **Max dose is 400 mg/d.**	**Decreased levels/effects of:** ACE inhibitors, beta blocker, diuretics, (antihypertensive effect). **Increased levels/effects of NSAID:** probenecid.	BUN, increased serum creatinine, renal insufficiency/failure. Elderly patients: May be more prone to adverse effects. Pharmacokinetics Antirheumatic onset of action = within a few days; hepatically metabolized; $T_{1/2}$ = 2–3.3 h; renal elimination of metabolites.	Lactation Issues Excreted in breast milk—do not use in nursing mothers.
Mefenamic acid Ponstel Capsules 250 mg	**Moderate pain (≤ 1 week duration)** 500 mg initially, then 250 mg q 6 h as needed **Primary dysmenorrhea** 500 mg initially, then 250 mg q 6 h for 2–3 days. Start with onset of bleeding. **Max dose is 1000 mg/d.**	Administration Issues Take with food; avoid alcohol and aspirin use; not recommended for those <14 yrs old. Drug–Drug Interactions **Increased levels/effects of:** anticoagulants, cyclosporine (inc renal toxic effects), digoxin, dipyridamole, hydantoins, lithium. **Decreased levels/effects of:** ACE inhibitors, beta blockes, diuretics, (antihypertensive effect). **Increased levels/effects of NSAID:** probenecid.	ADRs Most frequent: Nausea, vomiting, diarrhea, constipation, abdominal distress, dyspepsia, dizziness, headache, drowsiness, rash. Less frequent: GI ulceration, cholestatic hepatitis, pancreatitis, hematuria, proteinuria, elevated BUN, increased serum creatinine, renal insufficiency/failure, **autoimmune hemolytic anemia associated with >12months of therapy.** Elderly patients: May be more prone to adverse effects. Pharmacokinetics $T_{1/2}$ = 2–4 hrs; renal elimination of metabolites.	Contraindications Hypersensitivity to this or aspirin; preexisting renal disease. Precautions Use cautiously in patients with PUD, severe renal or hepatic dysfunction, bleeding disorders. Pregnancy Category: B Lactation Issues Excreted in breast milk—do not use in nursing mothers.
Meloxicam Mobic Tablets 7.5 mg, 15mg	Osteoarthritis 7.5 – 15 mg once daily Max daily dose 15mg. Rheumatoid arthritis Optimal dosage has not been established. 7.5 – 15 mg qd for 3 weeks has been studied.	Administration Issues Can be administered with or without food. Drug–Drug Interactions NSAIDs class effect	ADRs Elevated liver enzymes, GI, dizziness, headache, rash, edema. Pharmacokinetics $T_{1/2}$ = 12–20 h; renally eliminated; 99.4% protein bound to plasma proteins.	Contraindications Asthma, nasal polyps, salicylate hypersensitivity, urticaria, GI bleed. Pregnancy Category: C Lactation Issues Do not use in nursing mothers.

Piroxicam Feldene, various generics Capsules 10 mg, 20 mg	**Osteoarthritis and rheumatoid arthritis** Initial and maintenance dose is 10 to 20 mg/d; may divide bid **Max dose is 20mg/d.**	Administration Issues Take with food; avoid alcohol and aspirin use; safety/efficacy in children is not established. Drug–Drug Interactions **Increased levels/effects of:** anticoagulants, cyclosporine (inc renal toxic effects), digoxin, dipyridamole, hydantoins, lithium. **Decreased levels/effects of:** ACE inhibitors, beta blockes, diuretics, (antihypertensive effect). **Increased levels/effects of NSAID:** probenecid.	ADRs Most frequent: Nausea, vomiting, diarrhea, constipation, abdominal distress, dyspepsia, dizziness, headache, drowsiness, rash. Less frequent: GI ulceration, cholestatic hepatitis, pancreatitis, hematuria, proteinuria, elevated BUN, increased serum creatinine, renal insufficiency/failure, **autoimmune hemolytic anemia associated with >12months of therapy.** Elderly patients: May be more prone to adverse effects. Pharmacokinetics Onset of antirheumatic action is 7–12 d; $T_{1/2} = 30-86$ h; renal elimination of metabolites.	Contraindication Hypersensitivity to this or aspirin; preexisting renal disease. Precautions Use cautiously in patients with PUD, severe renal or hepatic dysfunction, bleeding disorders. Pregnancy Category: C Lactation Issues Excreted in breast milk—do not use in nursing mothers.

306.4 Central Analgesics

Drug and Dosage Forms	Usual Dosage Range	Administration Issues and Drug-Drug & Drug-Food Interactions	Common Adverse Drug Reactions (ADRs) and Pharmacokinetics	Contraindications, Pregnancy Category, and Lactation Issues
Tramadol Ultram, generics Tablets 50 mg **Tramadol/APAP** Ultracet Tablets 37.5 mg/325 mg	**Moderate to moderately severe pain** 50–100 mg q 4–6 h **Elderly patients (>75 yrs):** 300 mg/d divided in 4–6 doses **Renal impairment** (CrCl <30 mL/min): 100 mg q 12 h **Hepatic dysfunction** (cirrhosis): 50 mg q 12 h **Max dose is 400 mg/d.** **Moderate Pain (Ultracet)** 2 tabs prn of 4–6 h	Administration Issues Safety/efficacy not established in those <16 yrs old; tramadol may impair physical or mental abilities. **Use in opioid dependence:** Do not use in patients dependent on opioids—will precipitate opioid withdrawal. Drug-Drug Interactions **Increased level/effect of tramadol:** MAO inhibitors (increased toxicity). **Decreased level/effect of tramadol:** carbamazepine.	ADRs Dizziness, vertigo, nausea, constipation, headache, somnolence, vomiting, pruritus, CNS stimulation, asthenia, sweating, dyspepsia, dry mouth, diarrhea. Pharmacokinetics 20% protein bound; renal elimination of metabolites; $T_{1/2} = 6-7$ h.	Contraindications Hypersensitivity; acute alcohol, hypnotic, centrally acting analgesic, opioid, or psychotropic intoxication. Precautions Use cautiously in patients with seizure disorders, severe renal or hepatic dysfunction. Pregnancy Category: C Lactation Issues Use cautiously, safety not established.

306.5 Selective COX-2 Inhibitors

Drug and Dosage Forms	Usual Dosage Range	Administration Issues and Drug-Drug & Drug-Food Interactions	Common Adverse Drug Reactions (ADRs) and Pharmacokinetics	Contraindications, Pregnancy Category, and Lactation Issues
Celebrex Celebrex Capsules 100 mg, 200 mg, 400 mg	**Osteoarthritis** 200 mg qd or 100 mg bid **Rheumatoid arthritis** 100–200 mg bid **Acute pain and primary dysmenorrhea** 400 mg × 1 dose on day 1; may give an additional 200 mg prn on day 1. Follow with 200 mg bid prn Reduce dose by 50% in moderate hepatic impairment.	Administration Issues Take with a full glass of water and remain sitting for at least 10 minutes. If upset stomach occurs, take with food or milk. Drug-Drug Interactions Class effects; fluconazole may increase celebrex levels.	ADRs Most frequent: GI, elevated liver enzymes, dizziness, pharyngitis, sinusitis, infection. Pharmacokinetics $T_{1/2}$ = 11 h; renally eliminated; 97% protein bound to plasma proteins.	Contraindications Asthma, nasal polyps, salicylate hypersensitivity, uritcaria, GI bleed, anemia (caution). Pregnancy Category: C Lactation Issues Do not use in nursing mothers.
Rofecoxib Vioxx Tablets 12.5 mg, 25 mg, 50 mg Suspension 12.5 mg/5 mL 25 mg/5 mL	**Osteoarthritis** Starting dose = 12.5 mg qd, may use up to 25 mg qd. Maximum daily dose is 25 mg qd **Rheumatoid arthritis** 25 mg qd. Maximum daily dose is 25 mg qd. **Acute pain and primary dysmenorrhea** 50 mg qd. Maximum daily dose is 50 mg qd. Do not use longer than 5 days of chronic dosing. Adjust dose in hepatic impairment.	Administration Issues Take with a full glass of water and remain sitting for at least 10 minutes. If upset stomach occurs, take with food or milk. Drug-Drug Interactions Class effects; rifampin may decrease levels of rofecoxib; rofecoxib may increase theophylline levels.	ADRs Most frequent: GI, elevated liver enzymes, dizziness, headache, rash, lower extremity edema. Pharmacokinetics $T_{1/2}$ = 17 h; renally eliminated; 87% protein bound to plasma proteins.	Contraindications Asthma, nasal polyps, salicylate hypersensitivity, uritcaria, GI bleed. Pregnancy Category: C Lactation Issues Do not use in nursing mothers.
Valdecoxib Bextra Tablets 10 mg, 20 mg	**Osteoarthritis** 10 mg qd **Rheumatoid arthritis** 10 mg qd **Primary dysmenorrhea** 20 mg bid prn Adjust dose in hepatic impairment.	Administration Issues Take with a full glass of water and remain sitting for at least 10 minutes. If upset stomach occurs, take with food or milk. Drug-Drug Interactions Class effect; fluconazole and ketoconazole may increase levels of valdecoxib.	ADRs Most frequent: Endoscopic peptic ulcers, GI, elevated liver enzymes, dizziness, headache, rash, lower extremity edema. Pharmacokinetics $T_{1/2}$ = 8–11 h; renally eliminated; 98% protein bound to plasma proteins.	Contraindications Asthma, nasal polyps, salicylate hypersensitivity, uritcaria, GI bleed, acute bronchospasm. Pregnancy Category: C Lactation Issues Do not use in nursing mothers.

307. Salicylates

Drug and Dosage Forms	Usual Dosage Range	Administration Issues and Drug–Drug & Drug–Food Interactions	Common Adverse Drug Reactions (ADRs) and Pharmacokinetics	Contraindications, Pregnancy Category, and Lactation Issues
Aspirin Bayer, Aspergum, Empirin, Genprin, Ecotrin, Easprin, various generics Tablets, chewable 81 mg Tablets, enteric coated 165 mg, 325 mg, 500 mg, 650 mg, 975 mg Tablets 325 mg, 500 mg Gum tablets 227.5 mg Tablets, controlled release 650 mg, 800 mg Suppositories 120 mg, 200 mg, 300 mg, 600 mg **Aspirin, buffered** Bufferin, Buffex, Wesprin Buffered, Ascriptin, Alka Seltzer with Aspirin, various generics Contain small amounts of antacids (calcium carbonate, magnesium oxide, magnesium carbonate, aluminum glycinate, magnesium carbonate, magnesium or aluminum hydroxides Tablets 325 mg, 500 mg Tablets, coated 325 mg, 500 mg Tablets, effervescent 325 mg, 500 mg	**Minor aches/pains** 325–650 mg every 4 hrs as needed. Extra strength products: 500 mg of 3 h 1000 mg q 6 h as needed. **Arthritis/other rheumatic conditions** 3.2–6 g/d in divided doses **Pediatrics:** 60–110 mg/kg/d in divided doses (q 6–8 h). Start at 60 mg/kg/d and titrate by 20 mg/kg/d after 5–7 days prn by 10 mg/kg/d after another 5–7 days prn **Acute rheumatic fever** 5–8 g/d in divided doses **Pediatrics:** 100 mg/kg/d for 2 weeks, then decrease to 75 mg/kg/d for 4–6 weeks **Transient ischemic attacks** 1300 mg/d in divided doses. May use smaller doses if not tolerated. **Myocardial infarction prophylaxis:** 81–325 mg/d (optimal dose has not been established; individualize). **Pediatric analgesic or antipyretic** 10–15 mg/kg/dose of 4 h up to 60–80 mg/kg/d. **DO NOT USE IN CHILDREN WITH CHICKEN POX OR FLU SYMPTOMS DUE TO POSSIBILITY OF REYE'S SYNDROME.** **Kawasaki disease** 80–180 mg/kg/d for acute febrile period, then reduce to 10 mg/kg/d	Administration Issues Take with food; Safety /efficacy not established in those <12 yrs old. **Aspirin use in children with fever has been associated with Reye's syndrome.** Drug–Drug Interactions **Increased level/effect of:** alcohol (GI effects); anticoagulants (bleeding effects); methotrexate, valproic acid, sulfonylureas (inc hypoglycemic effect) **Decreased level/effect of:** ACE inhibitors, beta blockers, diuretics (decreased antihypertensive effect); probenecid & sulfinpyrazone (decreased uricosuric effect). Drug–Lab Interactions False negative or positive urine glucose tests, uric acid levels (inc with salicylate levels <10 mg/dL; decreased with salicylate levels >10 mg/dL), falsely elevated urine vanillymandelic acid tests.	ADRs Nausea, dyspepsia, heartburn, GI bleeding, hives, rash, prolonged bleeding time, thrombocytopenia, aspirin intolerance (rhinitis, (bronchospasm) "Salicylism": dizziness, tinnitus, difficulty hearing, nausea, vomiting, diarrhea, confusion, CNS depression, headache, sweating, hyperventilation, lassitude. Pharmacokinetics 90% protein bound; hepatically metabolized; renal elimination of metabolites; $T_{1/2}$ of aspirin = 15–20 min; $T_{1/2}$ of salicylic acid = 2–3 h at low doses (may exceed 20 h at antiinflammatory doses).	Contraindications Hypersensitivity, hemophilia, bleeding ulcers, hemorrhagic states. Precautions Use cautiously in patients with asthma, nasal polyposis, chronic urticaria (inc risk of hypersensitivity); chronic renal or hepatic dysfunction, PUD, bleeding disorders. Pregnancy Category: D Lactation Issues Safety not established. Use cautiously if at all.

(continues on next page)

307. Salicylates *continued from previous page*

Drug and Dosage Forms	Usual Dosage Range	Administration Issues and Drug–Drug & Drug–Food Interactions	Common Adverse Drug Reactions (ADRs) and Pharmacokinetics	Contraindications, Pregnancy Category, and Lactation Issues
Choline Salicylate Arthropan Liquid 870 mg/5 mL	**Minor aches/pains** Adults or children (>12 yrs): 870 mg q 3–4 h. Max is 6 doses/day. **Rheumatoid arthritis** Adults or children (>12 yrs): 5–10 mL up to 4 times per day.	Administration Issues Take with food; Safety/ efficacy not established in those <12 yrs old. **Aspirin use in children with fever has been associated with Reye's syndrome.** Drug–Drug Interactions **Increased level/effect of:** alcohol (GI effects); anticoagulants (bleeding effects); methotrexate, valproic acid, sulfonylureas (inc hypoglycemic effect) **Decreased level/effect of:** ACE inhibitors, beta blockers, diuretics (decreased antihypertensive effect); probenecid & sulfinpyrazone (decreased uricosuric effect). Drug–Lab Interactions See aspirin.	ADRs (fewer GI effects than aspirin): Nausea, dyspepsia, heartburn, GI bleeding, hives, rash, prolonged bleeding time, thrombocytopenia, aspirin intolerance (rhinitis bronchospasm), "Salicylism": dizziness, tinnitus, difficulty hearing, nausea, vomiting, diarrhea, confusion, CNS depression, headache, sweating, hyperventilation, lassitude. Pharmacokinetics 90% protein bound; renal elimination of metabolites; $T_{1/2}$ of salicylic acid = 2–3 h at low doses (may exceed 20 h at antiinflammatory doses).	Contraindications Hypersensitivity, hemophilia, bleeding ulcers, hemorrhagic states. Precautions Use cautiously in patients with asthma, nasal polyposis, chronic urticaria (inc risk of hypersensitivity); chronic renal or hepatic dysfunction, PUD, bleeding disorders. Pregnancy Category: D Lactation Issues Safety not established. Use cautiously if at all.
Diflunisal Dolobid, generics Tablets 250 mg, 500 mg	**Mild to moderate pain** 1 g initially, followed by 500 mg q 8–12 h. **Elderly or debilitated patients:** 500 mg initially, followed by 250 mg q 8–12 h **Osteoarthritis/rheumatoid arthritis** 500–1000 mg daily in 2 divided doses. **Max dose 1500 mg daily.**	Administration Issues Take with food; do not crush or chew tablets; do not take with aspirin or acetaminophen; Safety/efficacy in children <12 yrs not established. **Use in children with fever has been associated with Reye's syndrome.** Drug–Drug Interactions **Increased levels/effects of:** acetaminophen, oral anticoagulants, indomethacin, hydrochlorothiazide. **Decreased levels/effects of:** sulindac.	ADRs Nausea, dyspepsia, diarrhea, headache, insomnia, rash, tinnitus. Pharmacokinetics Onset of action = 1 h; 99% protein bound; renal elimination of metabolites; $T_{1/2}$ = 8–12 h.	Contraindications Hypersensitivity to this or aspirin. Precautions Use cautiously in those with asthma, nasal polyposis, chronic urticaria (inc risk of hypersensitivity); severe chronic, renal, or hepatic dysfunction, PUD, bleeding disorders. Pregnancy Category: C Lactation Issues Use cautiously if at all; it is excreted In breast milk
Magnesium salicylate Doan's, Magan, Mobidin	**Minor aches/pains** 650 mg q 4 h or 1090 mg tid. May increase to 3.6–4.8 g/d in 3–4 divided doses.	Administration Issues Take with food; safety/ efficacy not established in children.	ADRs (fewer GI effects than aspirin): Nausea, dyspepsia, heartburn, GI bleeding, hives, rash, prolonged bleeding time,	Contraindications Hypersensitivity, hemophilia, bleeding ulcers, hemorrhagic states.

Caplets 325 mg, 500 mg Tablets 545 mg, 600 mg		Drug–Drug Interactions **Increased level/effect of:** alcohol (GI effects); anticoagulants (bleeding effects); methotrexate, valproic acid, sulfonylureas (inc hypoglycemic effect) **Decreased level/effect of:** ACE inhibitors, beta blockers, diuretics (decreased antihypertensive effect); probenecid & sulfinpyrazone (decreased uricosuric effect). Drug–Lab Interactions See aspirin.	thrombocytopenia, aspirin intolerance (rhinitis, bronchospasm). "Salicylism": dizziness, tinnitus, difficulty hearing, nausea, vomiting, diarrhea, confusion, CNS depression, headache, sweating, hyperventilation, lassitude. Pharmacokinetics 90% protein bound; renal elimination of metabolites; $T_{1/2}$ of salicylic acid = 2–3 h at low doses (may exceed 20 hrs at antiinflammatory doses).	Precautions Use cautiously in patients with asthma, nasal polyposis, chronic urticaria (inc risk of hypersensitivity); chronic renal or hepatic dysfunction, PUD, bleeding disorders. Pregnancy Category: D Lactation Issues Safety not established. Use cautiously if at all.
Salicylate Combinations (choline salicylate & magnesium salicylate) Trilisate Tablets 500 mg, 750 mg, 1000 mg Liquid 500 mg/5 mL	**Minor aches/pains** 500–750 mg q 3 h or 1000 mg q 6 h prn	Administration Issues Take with food; safety/ efficacy not established in those <12 yrs old. **Aspirin use in children with fever has been associated with Reye's syndrome.** Drug–Drug Interactions **Increased level/effect of:** alcohol (GI effects); anticoagulants (bleeding effects); methotrexate, valproic acid, sulfonylureas (inc hypoglycemic effect). **Decreased level/effect of:** ACE inhibitors, beta blockers, diuretics (decreased antihypertensive effect); probenecid & sulfinpyrazone (decreased uricosuric effect). Drug–Lab Interactions See aspirin.	ADRs (fewer GI effects than aspirin): nausea, dyspepsia, heartburn, GI bleeding, hives, rash, prolonged bleeding time, thrombocytopenia, aspirin intolerance (rhinitis, bronchospasm), "Salicylism": dizziness, tinnitus, difficulty hearing, nausea, vomiting, diarrhea, confusion, CNS depression, headache, sweating, hyperventilation, lassitude. Pharmacokinetics Oral; 90% protein bound; renal elimination of metabolites; $T_{1/2}$ of salicylic acid = 2–3 h at low doses (may exceed 20 hrs at antiinflammatory doses).	Contraindications Hypersensitivity, hemophilia, bleeding ulcers, hemorrhagic states Precautions Use cautiously in patients with asthma, nasal polyposis, chronic urticaria (inc risk of hypersensitivity); chronic renal or hepatic dysfunction, PUD, bleeding disorders. Pregnancy Category: D Lactation Issues Safety not established. Use cautiously if at all.
Salsalate Disalcid, Amigesic, Argesic-SA, Salflex, Salsitab, Artha-G, various generics Capsules 500 mg	**Minor aches/pains, arthritis:** 3000 mg/d in divided doses (2 to 4 times daily)	Administration Issues Take with food; Safety/efficacy not established in children. Drug–Drug Interactions	ADRs (fewer GI effects than aspirin): Nausea, dyspepsia, heartburn, GI bleeding, hives, rash, prolonged bleeding time, thrombocytopenia, aspirin intolerance (rhinitis, bronchospasm), "Salicylism": dizziness, tinnitus, difficulty hearing, nausea, vomit	Contraindications Hypersensitivity, hemophilia, bleeding ulcers, hemorrhagic states. Precautions Use cautiously in patients with asthma, nasal polyposis, chronic urticaria (inc risk

(*continues on next page*)

307. Salicylates *continued from previous page*

Drug and Dosage Forms	Usual Dosage Range	Administration Issues and Drug–Drug & Drug–Food Interactions	Common Adverse Drug Reactions (ADRs) and Pharmacokinetics	Contraindications, Pregnancy Category, and Lactation Issues
Salsalate *cont.* Tablets 500 mg, 750 mg		**Increased level/effect of:** alcohol (GI effects); anticoagulants (bleeding effects); methotrexate, valproic acid, sulfonylureas (inc hypoglycemic effect). **Decreased level/effect of:** ACE inhibitors, beta blockers, diuretics (decreased antihypertensive effect); probenecid & sulfinpyrazone (decreased uricosuric effect). Drug–Lab Interactions See aspirin.	ing, diarrhea, confusion, CNS depression, headache, sweating, hyperventilation, lassitude. Pharmacokinetics Insoluble in gastric secretions, not absorbed until it reaches small intestine; 90% protein bound; renal elimination of metabolites; $T_{1/2}$ of salicylic acid = 2–3 h at low doses (may exceed 20 h at antiinflammatory doses).	of hypersensitivity); chronic renal or hepatic dysfunction, PUD, bleeding disorders. Pregnancy Category: C Lactation Issues Safety not established. Use cautiously if at all.
Sodium Salicylate various generics Tablets, enteric coated 325 mg, 650 mg	**Minor aches/pains:** 325–650 mg q 4 h	Administration Issues Take with food; Safety/ efficacy not established in children. **Salicylate use in children with fever has been associated with Reye's syndrome.** Drug–Drug Interactions **Increased level/effect of:** alcohol (GI effects); anticoagulants (bleeding effects); methotrexate, valproic acid, sulfonylureas (inc hypoglycemic effect). **Decreased level/effect of:** ACE inhibitors, beta blockers, diuretics (decreased antihypertensive effect); probenecid & sulfinpyrazone (decreased uricosuric effect). Drug–Lab Interactions See aspirin.	ADRs (fewer GI effects than aspirin): Nausea, dyspepsia, heartburn, GI bleeding, hives, rash, prolonged bleeding time, thrombocytopenia, aspirin intolerance (rhinitis, bronchospasm), "Salicylism": dizziness, tinnitus, difficulty hearing, nausea, vomiting, diarrhea, confusion, CNS depression, headache, sweating, hyperventilation, lassitude. Pharmacokinetics 90% protein bound; renal elimination of metabolites; $T_{1/2}$ of salicylic acid = 2–3 h at low doses (may exceed 20 h at antiinflammatory doses)	Contraindications Hypersensitivity, hemophilia, bleeding ulcers, hemorrhagic states. Precautions Use cautiously in patients with asthma, nasal polyposis, chronic urticaria (inc risk of hypersensitivity); chronic renal or hepatic dysfunction, PUD, bleeding disorders. Pregnancy Category: D Lactation Issues Safety not established. Use cautiously if at all.

308. Anticonvulsants

308.1 Barbiturates

Drug and Dosage Forms	Usual Dosage Range	Administration Issues and Drug–Drug & Drug–Food Interactions	Common Adverse Drug Reactions (ADRs) and Pharmacokinetics	Contraindications, Pregnancy Category, and Lactation Issues
Mephobarbital Mebaral Tablets 32 mg, 50 mg, 100 mg	**Tonic/clonic, cortical focal** 400–600 mg/d in 3–4 divided doses **Pediatrics:** <5 yrs: 16–32 mg 3–4 times daily; >5 yrs: 32–64 mg 3–4 times daily **Elderly or debilitated patients (hepatic/renal dysfunction):** 16–32 mg 2–3 times daily. Titrate to higher doses as needed/tolerated	Administration Issues When replacing another anticonvulsant, slowly titrate this agent, while decreasing the other agent; may produce irritability, excitability, or aggression in children. Drug–Drug Interactions **Decreased levels of:** anticoagulants, beta blockers, carbamazepine, clonazepam, oral contraceptives, corticosteroids, doxycycline, doxorubicin, felodipine, quinidine, verapamil, theophylline. **Increased effect of:** alcohol and possibly narcotics (CNS effects), acetaminophen (liver toxicity). **Increased effect of barbiturates:** MAO inhibitors, valproic acid. **Unknown effects (monitor patient closely):** hydantoins.	ADRs Somnolence, agitation, confusion, ataxia, nightmares, nervousness, hallucinations, bradycardia, hypotension, nausea, vomiting, skin rashes, angioedema, exfoliative dermatitis. Elderly Patients: May observe paradoxical excitement. Pharmacokinetics Onset of action = 30–60 min; hepatically metabolized; $T_{1/2}$ = 11–67 h; duration of action = 10–16 h.	Contraindications Hypersensitivity; manifest or latent porphyria, severe hepatic, renal, or respiratory dysfunction; previous addiction to sedative/hypnotic. Precautions **Drug abuse and dependence:** Prolonged use at high doses leads to physical dependence. If dependent on barbiturate, slowly withdraw over several weeks. May use long-acting barbiturate (phenobarbital) at dose of 30 mg per every 100–200 mg of mephobarbital to help prevent withdrawal symptoms. Pregnancy Category: D Lactation Issues Use cautiously in nursing mothers, sedation has been reported in infants.
Phenobarbital Solfoton, various generics Tablets 15 mg, 16 mg, 30 mg, 60 mg, 100 mg Capsules 16 mg Elixir 15 mg/5 mL, 20 mg/ 5 mL	**Tonic/clonic, cortical focal** 60–100 mg/d in 2–3 divided doses **Pediatrics:** 3–6 mg/kg/d in 2–3 divided doses **Elderly or debilitated patients (hepatic/renal dysfunction):** Use lower initial dose and greater dosing intervals. Titrate to higher doses as needed/tolerated. **Traumatic brain injury** 60–200 mg qd	Administration Issues When replacing another anticonvulsant, slowly titrate this agent, while decreasing the other agent; may produce irritability, excitability, or aggression in children. Drug–Drug Interactions **Decreased levels of:** anticoagulants, beta blockers, carbamazepine, clonazepam, oral contraceptives, corticosteroids, doxycycline, doxorubicin, felodipine, quinidine, verapamil, theophylline. **Increased effect of:** alcohol and possibly narcotics (CNS effects), acetaminophen (liver toxicity).	ADRs Somnolence, agitation, confusion, ataxia, nightmares, nervousness, hallucinations, bradycardia, hypotension, nausea, vomiting, skin rashes, angioedema, exfoliative dermatitis. Elderly Patients: May observe paradoxical excitement. Pharmacokinetics Onset of action = 30–60 min; hepatically metabolized; $T_{1/2}$ = 53–118 h; duration of action = 10–16 h. Therapeutic plasma **levels = 15–40 mcg/mL.**	Contraindications Hypersensitivity; manifest or latent porphyria, severe hepatic, renal, or respiratory dysfunction; previous addiction to sedative/hypnotic. Precautions **Drug abuse and dependence:** Prolonged use at high doses leads to physical dependence. If dependent on barbiturate, slowly withdraw over several weeks. Pregnancy Category: D

(continues on next page)

308.1 Barbiturates *continued from previous page*

Drug and Dosage Forms	Usual Dosage Range	Administration Issues and Drug–Drug & Drug–Food Interactions	Common Adverse Drug Reactions (ADRs) and Pharmacokinetics	Contraindications, Pregnancy Category, and Lactation Issues
Phenobarbital *cont.*		**Increased effect of barbiturates:** MAO inhibitors, valproic acid. **Unknown effects (monitor patient closely):** hydantoins.		Lactation Issues Use cautiously in nursing mothers, sedation has been reported in infants.
Primidone Mysoline, various generics Tablet: 50 mg, 250 mg Suspension 250 mg/5 mL	**Tonic/clonic, psychomotor, focal** Initially, 100–125 mg at bedtime Titrate by 100–125 mg/d q 3 days up to max of 500 mg qid **Pediatrics (<8 yrs):** Initially, 50 mg at bedtime. Titrate by 50 mg/d q 3 days up to 125–250 mg tid or 10–25 mg/kg/d in divided doses. **Note:** Full therapeutic effect may not be seen for several weeks.	Administration Issues When replacing another anticonvulsant, slowly titrate this agent, while decreasing the other agent. May take with food if GI upset occurs **Due to bioequivalence differences, brand interchange is not recommended.** Drug–Drug Interactions **Decreased levels of primidone:** acetazolamide, carbamazepine, succinimides. **Increased levels of primidone:** hydantoins, isoniazid. **Increased levels of:** carbamazepine.	ADRs Drowsiness, dizziness, ataxia, vertigo, nystagmus, nausea, vomiting, anorexia, thrombocytopenia, megaloblastic anemia (responsive to folic acid), impotence, skin rash. Pharmacokinetics Hepatically metabolized to PEMA and phenobarbital (both active metabolites); $T_{1/2}$ = 5–15 h (primidone); $T_{1/2}$ = 10–18 h (PEMA); $T_{1/2}$ = 53–140 h (phenobarbital). **Therapeutic concentrations:** **5–12 mcg/mL (primidone), 15–40 mcg/mL (phenobarbital).**	Contraindications Hypersensitivity to primidone or phenobarbital; acute intermittent porphyria. Precaution: Abrupt withdrawal may precipitate status epilepticus. Pregnancy Issue: Reports of fetal malformation; greater risk to fetus if medication is discontinued during pregnancy. Lactation Issues Women should not nurse.

308.2 Benzodiazepines

Drug, and Dosage Forms	Usual Dosage Range	Administration Issues and Drug–Drug & Drug–Food Interactions	Common Adverse Drug Reactions (ADRs) and Pharmacokinetics	Contraindications, Pregnancy Category, and Lactation Issues
Clonazepam (CIV) Klonopin Tablets 0.5 mg, 1 mg, 2 mg	**Absence, myoclonic, akinetic** 0.5 mg tid. Titrate by 0.5–1 mg/d every 3 days as needed to max dose of 20 mg/d. **Pediatrics (<10 yrs):** 0.01–0.03 mg/kg/d in 2–3 divided doses. Titrate by 0.25–0.5 mg/d q 3 days as needed to max dose of 0.1–0.2 mg/kg/d	Administration Issues When replacing another anticonvulsant, slowly titrate this agent, while decreasing the other agent; not recommended for children <9 yrs old. Drug–Drug Interactions **Increased level of BZ:** cimetidine, oral contraceptives, disulfiram, fluoxetine, isoniazid, ketoconazole,	ADRs Drowsiness, ataxia, confusion (especially in elderly). Dependence: Abrupt discontinuation can precipitate withdrawal symptoms (e.g., anxiety, flu-like illness, concentration difficulties, fatigue, anorexia, restlessness, confusion, psychosis, paranoid delusions, grand mal	Contraindications Hypersensitivity, psychoses, acute narrow-angle glaucoma, clinical or biochemical evidence of significant liver disease. Pregnancy Category None, but avoid in pregnant women.

	Unlabeled uses: leg movements during sleep (0.5–2 mg/night); Parkinsonian dysarthria (0.25–0.5 mg/d); acute manic episodes of bipolar disorder (0.75–16 mg/d); multifocal tic disorders (1.5–12 mg/d); adjunctive treatment for schizophrenia (0.5–2 mg/d); neuralgias (2–4 mg/d) **Traumatic brain injury** 0.5–20 mg/d	metoprolol, propoxyphene, propranolol, valproic acid. **Increased CNS effects:** alcohol, barbiturates, narcotics. **Increased levels of:** digoxin, phenytoin (possibly). **Decreased level or effect of BZ:** rifampin (decreased level); theophylline (decreased effect).	seizures). Withdrawal can occur after as little as 4–6 weeks of therapy. Clonidine, propranolol, carbamazepine have been used as adjuncts in withdrawal. Drug Discontinuation: gradual decrease over 4–8 weeks. Pharmacokinetics $T_{1/2}$ = 18–50 h; speed of onset = intermediate; renal elimination.	Lactation Issues Excreted in breast milk—do not give to nursing mothers.
Clorazepate dipotassium (CIV) Tranxene, Tranxene-SD, Tranxene-SD-Half, Gen-Xene, various generics Capsules 3.75 mg 7.5 mg, 15 mg Tablets 3.75 mg, 7.5 mg, 15 mg Tablet, single dose 11.25 mg, 22.5 mg	**Adjunctive therapy for partial seizures** 7.5 mg tid. Titrate by 7.5 mg/d every week to max dose of 90 mg/d **Pediatrics (<12 yrs):** 7.5 mg bid. Titrate by ≤ 7.5 mg/d each week to max of 60 mg/d.	Administration Issues When replacing another anticonvulsant, slowly titrate this agent, while decreasing the other agent; not recommended for children <9 yrs old. Drug–Drug Interactions **Increased level of BZ:** cimetidine, oral contraceptives, disulfiram, fluoxetine, isoniazid, ketoconazole, metoprolol, propoxyphene, propranolol, valproic acid. **Increased CNS effects:** alcohol, barbiturates, narcotics. **Increased levels of:** digoxin, phenytoin (possibly). **Decreased level or effect of BZ:** rifampin (decreased level); theophylline (decreased effect).	ADRs Drowsiness, ataxia, confusion (especially in elderly). Dependence: Abrupt discontinuation can precipitate withdrawal symptoms (e.g., anxiety, flu-like illness, concentration difficulties, fatigue, anorexia, restlessness, confusion, psychosis, paranoid delusions, grand mal seizures). Withdrawal can occur after as little as 4–6 weeks of therapy. Clonidine, propranolol, carbamazepine have been used as adjuncts in withdrawal. Drug Discontinuation: gradual decrease over 4–8 weeks. Pharmacokinetics $T_{1/2}$ = 30–100 h (includes $T_{1/2}$ of metabolite); speed of onset = fast.	Contraindications Hypersensitivity, psychoses, acute narrow-angle glaucoma, clinical or biochemical evidence of significant liver disease. Pregnancy Category None, but avoid in pregnant women. Lactation Issues Excreted in breast milk—do not give to nursing mothers.
Diazepam (CIV) Valium, Valrelease, Zetran, various generics Tablets 2 mg, 5 mg, 10 mg Capsule, sustained release 15 mg	**Adjunctive therapy in convulsive disorders** 2–10 mg 2–4 times daily (sustained release preparation: 15–30 mg qd) **Pediatrics (>6 mos):** 1–2.5 mg 3–4 times daily. Titrate as needed/tolerated	Administration Issues Do not crush or chew sustained release products. Concentrated solution (5 mg/mL) should be diluted in liquid or semi-solid foods. When replacing another anticonvulsant, slowly titrate this agent, while decreasing the other agent; not recommended for <6 mos old.	ADRs Drowsiness, ataxia, confusion (especially in elderly). Dependence: Abrupt discontinuation can precipitate withdrawal symptoms (e.g., anxiety, flu-like illness, concentration difficulties, fatigue, anorexia, restlessness, confusion, psychosis, paranoid delusions, grand mal seizures). Withdrawal can occur after as	Contraindications Hypersensitivity, psychoses, acute narrow-angle glaucoma. Pregnancy Category: D Lactation Issues Excreted in breast milk—do not give to nursing mothers.

(continues on next page)

308.2 Benzodiazepines *continued from previous page*

Drug, and Dosage Forms	Usual Dosage Range	Administration Issues and Drug–Drug & Drug–Food Interactions	Common Adverse Drug Reactions (ADRs) and Pharmacokinetics	Contraindications, Pregnancy Category, and Lactation Issues
Diazepam (CIV) *cont.* Oral solution 5 mg/5 mL, 5 mg/mL	**Elderly or debilitated patients:** 2–2.5 mg 1–2 times daily. Titrate slowly as needed/tolerated	Drug–Drug Interactions **Increased level of BZ:** cimetidine, oral contraceptives, disulfiram, fluoxetine, isoniazid, ketoconazole, metoprolol, propoxyphene, propranolol, valproic acid. **Increased CNS effects:** alcohol, barbiturates, narcotics. **Increased levels of:** digoxin, phenytoin (possibly). **Decreased level or effect of BZ:** rifampin (decreased level); theophylline (decreased effect).	little as 4–6 weeks of therapy. Clonidine, propranolol, carbamazepine have been used as adjuncts in withdrawal. Drug Discontinuation: gradual decrease over 4–8 weeks. Pharmacokinetics $T_{1/2}$ = 20–80 h; speed of onset = very fast.	

308.3 Hydantoins

Drug and Dosage Forms	Usual Dosage Range	Administration Issues and Drug–Drug & Drug–Food Interactions	Common Adverse Drug Reactions (ADRs) and Pharmacokinetics	Contraindications, Pregnancy Category, and Lactation Issues
Ethotoin Peganone Tablets 250 mg	**Tonic/clonic or psychomotor** 250 mg 3–4 times daily, initially. Titrate to 2–3 g/d over several days. **Pediatrics:** 250 mg 1–3 times daily. Titrate to 500–1000 mg/d (some may require 2–3 g/d)	Administration Issues May take with food to avoid GI upset. Draw serum levels just prior to next dose. Maintain good oral hygiene. When replacing another anticonvulsant, slowly titrate this agent, while decreasing the other agent. Drug–Drug Interactions **Increased levels and/or effects of hydantoin:** allopurinol, amiodarone, benzodiazepines, cimetidine, ethanol (acute), fluconazole, isoniazid, metronidazole, miconazole, omeprazole, sulfonamides & trimethoprim, valproic acid, TCAs, salicylates, chlorpheniramine, ibuprofen, phenothiazines.	ADRs Nystagmus, ataxia, confusion, slurred speech, fatigue, drowsiness, tremor, headache, nervousness, diplopia, irritability, nausea, vomiting, diarrhea, constipation, thrombocytopenia, leukopenia, granulocytopenia, anemias, gingival hyperplasia, hepatitis, dermatologic reactions, osteomalacia. Overdose: Far-lateral nystagmus (>20 mcg/mL), ataxia (>30 mcg/mL), dysarthria, decreased level of consciousness (>40 mcg/mL).	Contraindications Hypersensitivity; hepatic abnormalities; hematologic disorders. Precautions Abrupt withdrawal of medication may precipitate status epilepticus; some patients are genetically predisposed to slowed metabolism, monitor carefully; use cautiously in patients with hepatic dysfunction. Pregnancy Issues Reports of fetal malformation; greater risk to fetus if medication is discontinued during pregnancy. Lactation Issues Women should not nurse.

		Decreased levels and/or effects of hydantoin: barbiturates, carbamazepine, ethanol (chronic), rifampin, theophylline, antacids, sucralfate, charcoal, antineoplastics, folic acid, loxapine, pyridoxine, nitrofurantoin, influenza virus vaccine. **Decreased levels and/or effects of:** amiodarone, acetaminophen (leads to inc risk of hepatotoxicity), carbamazepine, digoxin, corticosteroids disopyramide, doxycycline, estrogens & oral contraceptives, haloperidol, mexiletine, quinidine, theophylline, valproic acid, cyclosporine, furosemide, levodopa, phenothiazines, sulfonylureas. **Increased effect (toxicity) of:** lithium, meperidine, primidone, warfarin. Drug–Food Interaction **Decreased effect of hydantoin:** enteral feedings.	Pharmacokinetics Saturable hepatic metabolism to inactive metabolites; $T_{1/2} = 3-9$ h when level is < 8 mcg/mL. **Therapeutic plasma levels = 15–50 mcg/mL.**	
Mephenytoin Mesantoin Tablets 100 mg	**Tonic/clonic or psychomotor (refractory to other agents); focal; Jacksonian:** 50–100 mg/d, initially. Titrate each week by 50 or 100 mg/d to a range of 200–600 mg/d **Pediatrics:** Initiate therapy as above. Titrate to range of 100–400 mg/d.	Administration Issues May take with food to avoid GI upset. Draw serum levels just prior to next dose. Maintain good oral hygiene. When replacing another anticonvulsant, slowly titrate this agent, while decreasing the other agent. Drug–Drug Interactions **Increased levels and/or effects of hydantoin:** allopurinol, amiodarone, benzodiazepines, cimetidine, ethanol (acute), fluconazole, isoniazid, metronidazole, miconazole, omeprazole, sulfonamides & trimethoprim, valproic acid, TCAs, salicylates, chlorpheniramine, ibuprofen, phenothiazines. **Decreased levels and/or effects of hydantoin:** barbiturates, carbamazepine, ethanol (chronic), rifampin, theophylline,	ADRs Nystagmus, ataxia, confusion, slurred speech, fatigue, drowsiness, tremor, headache, nervousness, diplopia, irritability, nausea, vomiting, diarrhea, constipation, thrombocytopenia, leukopenia, granulocytopenia, anemias, gingival hyperplasia, hepatitis, dermatologic reactions, osteomalacia. Overdose: Far-lateral nystagmus (>20 mcg/mL), ataxia (>30 mcg/mL), dysarthria, decreased level of consciousness (>40 mcg/mL). Pharmacokinetics Absorption varies depending on formulation; saturable hepatic metabolism to inactive metabolites; $T_{1/2} = 6-24$ h when level is <10 mcg/mL.	Contraindications Hypersensitivity. Precautions Abrupt withdrawal of medication may precipitate status epilepticus; some patients are genetically predisposed to slowed metabolism, monitor carefully; use cautiously in patients with hepatic dysfunction. Pregnancy Issues Reports of fetal malformation; greater risk to fetus if medication is discontinued during pregnancy. Lactation Issues Women should not nurse.

(*continues on next page*)

308.3 Hydantoins *continued from previous page*

Drug and Dosage Forms	Usual Dosage Range	Administration Issues and Drug–Drug & Drug–Food Interactions	Common Adverse Drug Reactions (ADRs) and Pharmacokinetics	Contraindications, Pregnancy Category, and Lactation Issues
Mephenytoin *cont.*		antacids, sucralfate, charcoal, antineoplastics, folic acid, loxapine, pyridoxine, nitrofurantoin, influenza virus vaccine. **Decreased levels and/or effects of:** amiodarone, acetaminophen (inc risk of hepatotoxicity), carbamazepine, digoxin, corticosteroids, disopyramide, doxycycline, estrogens & oral contraceptives, haloperidol, mexiletine, quinidine, theophylline, valproic acid, cyclosporine, furosemide, levodopa, phenothiazines, sulfonylureas. **Increased effect (toxicity) of:** lithium, meperidine, primidone, warfarin. Drug–Food Interaction **Decreased effect of hydantoin:** enteral feedings.	**Therapeutic plasma levels = 10–20 mcg/mL; at these levels, time to eliminate 50% of the drug is extended (20–60 h).**	
Phenytoin Dilantin, Diphenylan, various generics **Phenytoin** Chewable tablets 50 mg Suspension 30 mg/5 mL, 125 mg/5 mL **Phenytoin Sodium** Capsules: 30 mg (27.6 mg phenytoin), 100 mg (92 mg phenytoin), 200 mg, 300 mg Capsules, Extended-release, 30 mg (27.6 mg phenytoin), 100 mg (92 mg phenytoin)	**Tonic/clonic or psychomotor** 100 mg tid initially. Titrate 100 mg/week as needed (some need 600 mg/d). **Pediatrics:** 5 mg/kg/d in 2–3 divided doses. Titrate to max of 300 mg/d as needed Single daily dose: Once the patient is controlled on 100 mg tid, 300 mg may be given as a single dose (must use extended-release capsules). **Unlabeled Use:** trigeminal neuralgia (tic douloureux). **Traumatic brain injury** 100–600 mg qd	Administration Issues May take with food to avoid GI upset. Draw serum levels just prior to next dose. Maintain good oral hygiene. When replacing another anticonvulsant, slowly titrate this agent, while decreasing the other agent. **Due to bioequivalence differences, brand interchange is not recommended.** Drug–Drug Interactions **Increased levels and/or effects of hydantoin:** allopurinol, amiodarone, benzodiazepines, cimetidine, ethanol (acute), fluconazole, isoniazid, metronidazole, miconazole, omeprazole, sulfonamides & trimethoprim, valproic acid, TCAs, salicy-	ADRs Nystagmus, ataxia, confusion, slurred speech, fatigue, drowsiness, tremor, headache, nervousness, diplopia, irritability, nausea, vomiting, diarrhea, constipation, thrombocytopenia, leukopenia, granulocytopenia, anemias, gingival hyperplasia, hepatitis, dermatologic reactions, osteomalacia. Overdose: Far-lateral nystagmus (>20 mcg/mL), ataxia (>30 mcg/mL), dysarthria, decreased level of consciousness (>40 mcg/mL). Pharmacokinetics Absorption varies depending on formulation; saturable hepatic metabolism to in-	Contraindications Hypersensitivity; sinus bradycardia; second/third degree AV block; Adams-Stokes syndrome. Precautions Abrupt withdrawal of medication may precipitate status epilepticus; some patients are genetically predisposed to slowed metabolism, monitor carefully; use cautiously in patients with hepatic dysfunction, hypotension, or severe myocardial insufficiency. Pregnancy Issues Reports of fetal malformation; greater risk to fetus if medication is discontinued during pregnancy.

Phenytoin sodium with phenobarbital Capsules 100 mg/16 mg (respectively), 100 mg/32 mg (respectively) Phenytoin sodium contains 92% phenytoin.		lates, chlorpheniramine, ibuprofen, phenothiazines. **Decreased levels and/or effects of hydantoin:** barbiturates, carbamazepine, ethanol (chronic), rifampin, theophylline, antacids, sucralfate, charcoal, antineoplastics, folic acid, loxapine, pyridoxine, nitrofurantoin, influenza virus vaccine. **Decreased levels and/or effects of:** amiodarone, acetaminophen (leads to inc risk of hepatotoxicity), carbamazepine, digoxin, corticosteroids, disopyramide, doxycycline, estrogens & oral contraceptives, haloperidol, mexiletine, quinidine, theophylline, valproic acid, cyclosporine, furosemide, levodopa, phenothiazines, sulfonylureas. **Increased effect (toxicity) of:** lithium, meperidine, primidone, warfarin. Drug–Food Interaction **Decreased effect of hydantoin:** enteral feedings.	active metabolites; $T_{1/2} = 6-24$ hrs when level is <10 mcg/mL. **Therapeutic plasma levels = 10–20 mcg/mL; at these levels, time to eliminate 50% of the drug is extended (20–60 h).**	Lactation Issues Women should not nurse.

308.4 Oxazolidinediones

Drug and Dosage Forms	Usual Dosage Range	Administration Issues and Drug–Drug & Drug–Food Interactions	Common Adverse Drug Reactions (ADRs) and Pharmacokinetics	Contraindications, Pregnancy Category, and Lactation Issues
Trimethadione Tridione Chewable tablets 150 mg Capsules 300 mg Solution 40 mg/mL	**Absence** 300 mg tid initially. Titrate by 300 mg/d each week as needed to range of 900–2400 mg/d **Pediatrics** 300–900 mg/d in 3–4 divided doses	Administration Issues When replacing another anticonvulsant, slowly titrate this agent, while decreasing the other agent. May take with food to decrease GI upset. Drug–Drug Interactions None known.	ADRs Drowsiness, headache, irritability, myasthenia-like syndrome, personality changes, nausea, vomiting, anorexia, rash, erythema multiforme, exfoliative dermatitis, photosensitivity, aplastic anemia, pancytopenia, hypoplastic anemia, proteinuria, hepatitis, lupus erythematosus. Pharmacokinetics Renal elimination of metabolite; $T_{1/2} = 16-24$ h.	Contraindications Hypersensitivity. Precautions Use cautiously in patients with hepatic or renal dysfunction, acute intermittent porphyria. Pregnancy Issues Reports of fetal malformation; greater risk to fetus if medication is discontinued during pregnancy. Lactation Issues Women should not nurse.

308.5 Succinimides

Drug and Dosage Forms	Usual Dosage Range	Administration Issues and Drug–Drug & Drug–Food Interactions	Common Adverse Drug Reactions (ADRs) and Pharmacokinetics	Contraindications, Pregnancy Category, and Lactation Issues
Ethosuximide Zarontin, generic Capsules 250 mg Syrup 250 mg/5 mL	**Absence** **Adults/pediatrics** (>6 yrs): 500 mg/d, initially. Titrate by 250 mg/d every 4–7 days as needed. Doses >1.5 g/d require strict supervision. **Pediatrics** (3–6 yrs): 250 mg/d initially. Titrate as above.	Administration Issues When replacing another anticonvulsant, slowly titrate this agent, while decreasing the other agent; may take with food to decrease GI upset; give bid to decrease side effects. Drug–Drug Interactions: **Increased and decreased levels (both) of:** valproic acid.	ADRs Drowsiness, ataxia, dizziness, confusion, nervousness, other psychological changes, nausea, vomiting, cramps, anorexia, diarrhea, weight loss, abdominal pain, constipation, eosinophilia, granulocytopenia, leukopenia, agranulocytosis (monitor blood counts during therapy), rash. Pharmacokinetics Extensively metabolized; $T_{1/2}$ = 30–60 min. **Therapeutic serum levels = 40–100 mcg/mL.**	Contraindications Hypersensitivity. Precautions Use cautiously in patients with renal or hepatic dysfunction (monitor renal and hepatic function). Pregnancy Issues Reports of fetal malformation; greater risk to fetus if medication is discontinued during pregnancy. Lactation Issues Women should not nurse.
Methsuximide Celontin Kapseals Capsules 150 mg, 300 mg	**Absence (refractory to other agents)** 300 mg/d initially. Titrate by 300 mg/d each week as needed to max of 1.2 g/d. **Pediatrics:** 150 mg/d initially. Titrate as above.	Administration Issues When replacing another anticonvulsant, slowly titrate this agent, while decreasing the other agent. May take with food to decrease GI upset. Drug–Drug Interactions **Increased levels of:** hydantoins. **Decreased levels of:** barbiturates, primidone. **Increased and decreased levels (both) of:** valproic acid.	ADRs Drowsiness, ataxia, dizziness, confusion, nervousness, other psychological changes, nausea, vomiting, cramps, anorexia, diarrhea, weight loss, abdominal pain, constipation, eosinophilia, granulocytopenia, leukopenia, agranulocytosis (monitor blood counts during therapy), rash, gum hypertrophy. Pharmacokinetics Extensively metabolized; $T_{1/2}$ = 2.6–4 h.	Contraindications Hypersensitivity. Precautions Use cautiously in renal or hepatic dysfunction (monitor renal and hepatic function); if used alone in mixed epilepsy—may increase frequency of tonic/clonic seizures. Pregnancy Issues Reports of fetal malformation; greater risk to fetus if medication is discontinued during pregnancy. Lactation Issues Women should not nurse.

308.6 Miscellaneous Anticonvulsants

Drug and Dosage Forms	Usual Dosage Range	Administration Issues and Drug-Drug & Drug-Food Interactions	Common Adverse Drug Reactions (ADRs) and Pharmacokinetics	Contraindications, Pregnancy Category, and Lactation Issues
Acetazolamide Diamox, AK-Zol, various generics Tablets 125 mg, 250 mg	**Catemenial epilepsy** 8–30 mg/kg/d in 2 divided doses (range: 375–1000 mg/d)	Administration Issues When replacing another anticonvulsant, slowly titrate this agent, while decreasing the other agent. Do not use sustained-release product. Drug-Drug Interactions **Increased levels/effects of:** cyclosporine, salicylates. **Increased levels/effects of acetazolamide:** salicylates, diflunisal. **Decreased levels/effects of:** primidone.	ADRs Anorexia, nausea, vomiting, constipation, melena, diarrhea, hematuria, glycosuria, urinary frequency, renal colic, renal calculi, polyuria, weakness, malaise, fatigue, nervousness, drowsiness, ataxia, disorientation, rash (including Stevens Johnson Syndrome), urticaria, pruritus, photosensitivity, bone marrow suppression, thrombocytopenia, hemolytic anemia, thrombocytopenic purpura, weight loss, fever, acidosis, decreased libido, impotence, electrolyte imbalance, hepatic insufficiency. Pharmacokinetics Peak effect 1–4 h; duration 8–12 h.	Contraindications Hypersensitivity to sulfonamides; decreased sodium/potassium levels; severe renal or hepatic dysfunction. Pregnancy Issues Reports of fetal malformation; greater risk to fetus if medication is discontinued during pregnancy. Lactation Issues Women should not nurse.
Carbamazepine Tegretol, Atretol, Epitol, Depitol, Carbatrol, Tegretol RX, various generics Tablets, chewable 100 mg Tablets 200 mg Tablets, extended release 100 mg, 200 mg, 400 mg Capsules, extended release 200 mg, 300 mg Suspension 100 mg/5 mL 200 mg/10 mL	**Tonic/clonic** 100–200 mg bid initially. Titrate by 200 mg/d each week (use 3–4 times daily regimen) up to 1200 mg/d (>15 yrs old), or 1000 mg/d (12–15 yrs), or 1600–2400 mg/d (adults) **Pediatrics** (6–12 yrs): 100 mg twice daily, initially. Titrate by 100 mg/d each week (use 3–4 times daily regimen) up to 1000 mg/d or 10–35 mg/kg/d **Trigeminal neuralgia** 100 mg twice daily, initially. Titrate by 200 mg/d as needed. **Suspension:** daily dose (including initial dose) is given in 4 divided doses. **Unlabeled uses:** bipolar disorder, unipolar depression, schizoaffective illness, alcohol or cocaine	Administration Issues When replacing another anticonvulsant, slowly titrate this agent, while decreasing the other agent, safety/efficacy not established in those <6 yrs old; avoid storing in hot homid conditions; do not combine suspensions with other liquids. Drug-Drug Interactions **Decreased levels/effects of:** TCAs, felbamate, valproic acid, anticoagulants, oral contraceptives, haloperidol, succinimides. **Decreased levels/effects of carbamazepine:** theophylline, hydantoins, barbiturates, charcoal. **Increased levels/effects of:** theophylline (possibly). **Increased levels/effects of carbamazepine:**	ADRs Dizziness, drowsiness, unsteadiness, nausea, vomiting, aplastic anemia, leukopenia, agranulocytosis, other hematologic effects, abnormal LFTs, hepatitis, rash, Stevens-Johnson syndrome, SIADH, congestive heart failure, hypotension, arrhythmias. Pharmacokinetics 76% protein bound; hepatically metabolized to carbamazepine epoxide; $T_{1/2}$ = 12–17 hrs (after continued dosing); renal elimination of metabolites; autoinduction **Therapeutic plasma concentrations = 4–12 mcg/mL**	Contraindications Hypersensitivity to this or TCAs, history of bone marrow suppression, concomitant use of MAO inhibitors. Precautions Closely monitor CBC and LFTs; use cautiously in patients with cardiac, hepatic, or renal dysfunction. May exacerbate atypical absence and myoclonic seizures. Pregnancy Issues Reports of fetal malformation; greater risk to fetus if medication is discontinued during pregnancy. Lactation Issues Women should not nurse.

(continues on next page)

308.6 Miscellaneous Anticonvulsants *continued from previous page*

Drug and Dosage Forms	Usual Dosage Range	Administration Issues and Drug-Drug & Drug-Food Interactions	Common Adverse Drug Reactions (ADRs) and Pharmacokinetics	Contraindications, Pregnancy Category, and Lactation Issues
Carbamazepine *cont.*	or benzodiazepine withdrawal, restless leg syndrome.	cimetidine, diltiazem, isoniazid, macrolides (not azithromycin), propoxyphene, verapamil, terfenadine, fluoxetine, fluvoxamine, valproic acid.		
Felbamate Felbatol Tablets 400 mg, 600 mg Suspension 600 mg/5 mL	**Partial with/without secondary generalization or Lennox-Gastaut syndrome:** (>14 yrs old) Monotherapy: 1200 mg/d in 3–4 divided doses. Titrate by 600 mg/d q 2 weeks up to 3600 mg/d as needed/tolerated. Conversion to monotherapy: 1200 mg/d divided tid to qid; reduce current AEDs by 1/3. Titrate felbamate to 2400 mg/d after 1 week; reduce current AEDs by 1/3. Titrate felbamate to 3600 mg/d after 1 week; reduce other AEDs as clinically indicated. Adjunctive therapy: Follow above directions, except reduce current AEDs by 20% initially, then as clinically indicated. **Elderly or debilitated patients:** Use lower doses and greater dosage intervals; titrate more slowly. **Pediatrics with Lennox-Gastaut Syndrome** (2–14 yrs old): 15 mg/kg/d divided tid to qid. Reduce present antiepileptics by 20%. Titrate felbamate by 15 mg/kg/d q week up to 45 mg/kg/d.	Administration Issues Patients should wear protective clothing to prevent photosensitivity. When replacing another anticonvulsant, slowly titrate this agent, while decreasing the other agent. Do not abruptly discontinue this medication. Drug-Drug Interactions **Increased levels of:** phenytoin, valproic acid, carbamazepine epoxide, warfarin, phenobarbital. **Decreased levels of:** carbamazepine. **Decreased levels of felbamate:** phenytoin, carbamazepine.	** **BECAUSE OF THE REPORTS OF APLASTIC ANEMIA, THE FDA HAS RECOMMENDED THAT FELBAMATE BE DISCONTINUED IN ALL PATIENTS UNLESS DISCONTINUATION WOULD POSE A SERIOUS THREAT TO THE PATIENT.** Restrict use to patients in whom benefit out weighs possible risk of a plastic anemia or hepatic failure. Educate patients on early signs and symptoms of serious side effects. ADRs Fatigue, headache, somnolence, dizziness, insomnia, nausea, dyspepsia, vomiting, anorexia, aplastic anemia, hepatic failure. Pharmacokinetics 22–25% protein bound; $T_{1/2} = 20-23$ h. Therapeutic plasma levels have not been established.	Contraindications Hypersensitivity to this or other carbamates. Precautions Use cautiously in patients with severe hepatic or renal dysfunction; monitor blood levels of other concomitant anticonvulsants due to drug interactions; monitor closely for signs of aplastic anemia, hepatic failure. Pregnancy Category: C Lactation Issues Felbamate is found in breast milk although effects unknown; women should not nurse.
Gabapentin Neurontin	**Add-on therapy for partial seizures with/without secondary generalization**	Administration Issues When replacing another anticonvulsant, slowly titrate this agent, while decreasing the other agent.	ADRs Somnolence, dizziness, ataxia, fatigue, nystagmus.	Contraindications Hypersensitivity.

Capsules 100 mg, 300 mg, 400 mg Tablets 600 mg, 800 mg Solution 250 mg/5 mL	300 mg day 1, 300 mg twice daily on day 2, 300 mg 3 times daily on day 3. Titrate further by 300–400 mg a day up to 1800 mg/d. Higher doses (2400–10,000 mg) have been used and well-tolerated. Pediatrics (3–12 years): Initially, 10–15 mg/kg/d divided tid; titrate to effective dose over 3 days. The effective dose in patients 3–4 years is 40 mg/kg/day divided tid. For pts ≥ 5 years, dose 25–35 mg/kg/day and divide tid. **Renal Impairment:** CrCl: >60 ml/min: 400 mg tid 30–60 ml/min: 300 mg bid 15–30 ml/min: 300 mg qd <15 ml/min: 300 mg qod Hemodialysis: 200–300 mg following each hemodialysis session	Drug-Drug Interactions **Decreased levels of gabapentin:** antacids.	Other (<1%): leukopenia, anemia, purpura. Pharmacokinetics Bioavailability is decreased with increasing doses; not protein bound; primarily RENALLY ELIMINATED as unchanged drug; $T_{1/2}$ = 5–7 h (prolonged by renal insufficiency). Therapeutic plasma levels have not been established.	Pregnancy Category: C. Lactation Issues Women should not nurse. Pediatrics Safety/efficacy not established in <12 yrs old.
Lamotrigine Lamictal Tablets 25 mg, 100 mg, 150 mg, 200 mg Tablets, chewable, dispersible 2 mg, 5 mg, 25 mg (may be swallowed whole)	**Adjunctive therapy for partial seizures** On enzyme inducing anti-epileptics (but not valproate): 50 mg once daily for 2 weeks, then 50 mg twice daily for 2 weeks. Usual maintenance dose is 300–500 mg/d in 2 divided doses On valproic acid: 25 mg every other day for 2 weeks, then 25 mg once daily for 2 weeks. Titrate after this to max of 150 mg/d	Administration Issues When replacing another anticonvulsant, slowly titrate this agent, while decreasing the other agent, safety/efficacy in <16 yrs old not established. Drug-Drug Interactions **Decreased levels/effect of lamotrigine:** carbamazepine, phenobarbital, primidone, phenytoin. **Increased levels/effect of:** carbamazepine. **Increased levels of lamotrigine:** valproic acid. **Decreased levels/effect of:** valproic acid.	ADRs Somnolence, dizziness, diplopia, ataxia, blurred vision, headache, nausea, vomiting, **rash (severe, potentially life-threatening, including Stevens-Johnson syndrome).** Risk of serious skin rash higher in children Pharmacokinetics 55% protein bound; hepatically metabolized; $T_{1/2}$ = 25–33 h (on no other antiepileptics); $T_{1/2}$ = 12–14 h (on enzyme inducing antiepileptics); $T_{1/2}$ = 48–70 h (on valproic acid). Therapeutic plasma 3–14 mcg/mL.	Contraindications Hypersensitivity. Precautions Use cautiously in patients with severe renal or hepatic dysfunction; rash risk increased with large doses rapid titration. Pregnancy Category: C. Lactation Issues Women should not nurse

(*continues on next page*)

308.6 Miscellaneous Anticonvulsants *continued from previous page*

Drug and Dosage Forms	Usual Dosage Range	Administration Issues and Drug-Drug & Drug-Food Interactions	Common Adverse Drug Reactions (ADRs) and Pharmacokinetics	Contraindications, Pregnancy Category, and Lactation Issues
Levetiracetam Keppra Tablets 250 mg, 500 mg, 750 mg Oral solutions 100 mg/mL	**Partial seizures** Start at 500 mg per day and increase to 3000 mg, given bid	Administration Issues Give bid; some patients respond to initial doses, reduce dose in patient with renal failure. Drug-Drug Interactions None.	ADRs Most frequent: somnolence, asthenia, dizziness, nervousness, headache, upper respiratory tract infections. Pharmacokinetics 66% excreted unchanged in urine; not metabolized by CYP-450 isoenzymes.	Contraindications Hypersensitivity to the drug or any of its ingredients Pregnancy Category: C Lactation Issues Use with caution in nursing mothers.
Oxycarbazepine Trileptal Tablets 150 mg, 300mg, 600 mg Suspension 300 mg/5 mL	**Partial seizures, primary tonic-clonic seizures, Nonepilespy bipolar, trigeminal neuralgia** Adults: 600 mg bid, increase by 300 to 600 mg bid every week; maintenance dose in adults is 1200–2400 mg/day, divided bid. Pediatrics: 8 to 10 mg/kg/day initial; 20 to 50 mg/kg/day maintenance	Administration Issues When replacing carbamazepine, increase dose by 1.5 times. Drug-Drug Interactions **Decreased MHD AUC** by carbamazepine, phenytoin, and phenobarbital. **Decreased levels of:** oral contraceptives.	ADRs Most frequent: similar to carbamazepine, more hyponatremia than carbamazepine; 33% cross reactivity with carbamazepine. Pharmacokinetics Metabolized to monohydrate derivative (MHD), which is the active form. Decrease dose in patients with renal impairment.	Contraindications Known hypersensitivity to oxcarbazepine or any of its components Pregnancy Category: C Lactation Issues Women should not nurse.
Tiagabine Gabatril Filmtabs 2 mg, 4 mg, 12 mg, 16 mg, 20 mg	**Adjunctive therapy for partial seizures** **Adults (>18 years):** Initiate at 4 mg qd; Total daily dose may be increased by 4 to 8 mg at weekly intervals until clinical response or max of 56 mg/d achieved. Give total daily dose in 2 to 4 divided doses. **Children (12–18 years):** Initiate at 4 mg qd. The total daily dose may be increased by 4 mg at beginning of week 2; thereafter, weekly increases of 4 to 8 mg up to a max of 32 mg/d may be done. Give total daily dose in 2 to 4 divided doses.	Administration Issues Should be taken with food; may cause dizziness or somnolence. Drug-Drug Interactions Clearance is 60% **greater** when given with carbamazepine, phenytoin, and phenobarbital.	ADRs Dizziness, somnolence, confusion, asthenia, nervousness, tremor, nausea, diarrhea, pharyngitis, rash. Pharmacokinetics $T_{1/2} = 7–9$ h; hepatic metabolism.	Contraindications Hypersensitivity. Precautions Abrupt withdrawal of medication may precipitate status epilepticus. Pregnancy Category: C Lactation Issues Excreted in breast milk; use cautiously.
Topiramate Topamax	**Adjunctive therapy for partial seizures in adults** Recommended dose is 200 mg bid; use the following titration schedule:	Administration Issues Do not break tablets; can be taken without regard to meals; safety/efficacy in children not established.	ADRs Asthenia, back pain, chest pain, ataxia, somnolence, dizziness, psychomotor slowing, speech disorders, nervousness,	Contraindications Hypersensitivity. Pregnancy Category: C

Tablets 25 mg, 50 mg, 100 mg, 200 mg Capsules, sprinkle 15 mg, 25 mg	Week / AM dose / PM dose 1 / none / 50 mg 2 / 50 mg / 50 mg 3 / 50 mg / 100 mg 4 / 100 mg / 100 mg 5 / 100 mg / 150 mg 6 / 150 mg / 150 mg 7 / 150 mg / 200 mg 8 / 200 mg / 200 mg	Drug-Drug Interactions May **increase** phenytoin concentrations and may **increase** the CNS effect of alcohol/ CNS depressants. **Decreased levels/effects of topiramate** may occur with phenytoin, carbamazepine, valproic acid; topiramate may **decrease effectiveness** of oral contraceptives and digoxin; avoid use with carbonic anhydrase inhibitors.	nystagmus, paresthesia, depression, rash, nausea, breast pain, dysmenorrhea, diplopia, weight decrease, fatigue. Pharmacokinetics $T_{1/2}$ = 18–27 h; decrease dose for moderate to severe renal impairment.	Lactation Issues It is not known if topiramate is excreted in breast milk.
Valproic Acid Depakene, various generics Capsules 250 mg Syrup 250 mg/5 mL (sodium valproate) **Divalproex Sodium** Depakote Tablets, delayed release 125 mg, 250 mg, 500 mg Tablets, extended release 500 mg Capsules, sprinkle 125 mg	**Absence** 15 mg/kg/d. Titrate by 5–10 mg/kg/d as needed/tolerated to max of 60 mg/kg/d. Doses > 250 mg should be divided. **Mania (bipolar disorder)** 750 mg in divided doses. Titrate as needed/ tolerated to max of 60 mg/kg/d. **Elderly or debilitated patients (hepatic/renal dysfunction):** Use lower initial doses and greater dosing intervals. Titrate to higher doses as needed/tolerated **Prophylaxis of migraine headache** 250 mg bid. Some patients may benefit from doses up to 1000 mg/d	Administration Issues When replacing another anticonvulsant, slowly titrate this agent, while decreasing the other agent. May take with food to decrease GI upset. Do not chew tablets or capsules; May sprinkle contents of capsule on soft food. Drug-Drug Interactions **Increased levels/effects of valproic acid:** cimetidine, felbamate, chlorpromazine, salicylates. **Increased levels/effects of:** zidovudine, warfarin, phenobarbital, primidone, lamotrigine, ethosuximide, clozapine, phenytoin, benzodiazepines, alcohol, other CNS depressants. **Decreased levels/effects of valproic acid:** charcoal, rifampin, carbamazepine, clonazepam, lamotrigine, phenytoin. **Decreased levels/effects of:** ethosuximide.	ADRs Nausea, vomiting, indigestion, diarrhea, anorexia, sedation, tremor, ataxia, headache, nystagmus, diplopia, dizziness, incoordination, depression, aggression, psychosis, hyperactivity, rash, photosensitivity, transient hair loss, Stevens-Johnson syndrome, thrombocytopenia, leukopenia, anemia, bone marrow suppression, acute intermittent porphyria, increased LFTs, hepatotoxicity, irregular menses, breast enlargement, abnormal thyroid function tests, hyperammonemia, pancreatitis, lupus erythematosus, fever, hearing loss. Pharmacokinetics Equivalent doses of divalproex sodium and valproic acid deliver equivalent quantities of valproate ion; 90% protein bound; hepatically metabolized; $T_{1/2}$ = 9–16 h (up to 18 h in patients with cirrhosis; 10–67 h for children <10 days old) **Therapeutic plasma concentrations = 50–100 mcg/mL.**	Contraindications Hypersensitivity; severe hepatic dysfunction. Precautions Monitor closely for hepatotoxicity, thrombocytopenia. Use cautiously in patients with severe hepatic/renal dysfunction. Pregnancy Category: D Lactation Issues Women should not nurse.
Zonisamide Zonegran Capsules 25 mg, 50 mg, 100 mg (may be used as a sprinkle)	**Partial seizures, primary tonic clonic seizures, myoclonic seizure, absence seizures, other generalized seizures** Adults: Initial dose 100 mg/d. After 2 weeks, the dose may be increased to 200 mg/d for	Administration Issues Administer zonisamide once or twice daily, except during the 100 mg dosage initiation; may be taken with or without food, use caution in patients with renal or hepatic disease.	ADRs Most Frequent: CNS depression, (e.g., somnolence, dizziness, headache, agitation, difficulty concentrating [higher incidence with rapid titration], nausea, anorexia, weight	Contraindications Hypersensitivity to sulfonamides or zonisamide Pregnancy Category: C Lactation Issues Use only if benefits outweigh risks.

(continues on next page)

308.6 Miscellaneous Anticonvulsants *continued from previous page*

Drug and Dosage Forms	Usual Dosage Range	Administration Issues and Drug-Drug & Drug-Food Interactions	Common Adverse Drug Reactions (ADRs) and Pharmacokinetics	Contraindications, Pregnancy Category, and Lactation Issues
Zonisamide *cont.*	at least 2 weeks. It can be increased to 300 and 400 mg/day, with the dose stable for at least 2 weeks to achieve steady-state at each level.	Drug-Drug Interactions **Decreased levels:** carbamazepine, phenytoin, and phenobarbital. **Increased levels:** valproate.	loss, rash (sulfonamide allergic patients), renal stones, decreased sweating. Pharmacokinetics Because of the long half-life of zonisamide, up to 2 weeks may be required to achieve steady-state levels upon reaching a stable dose or following dosage adjustment. Excreted 35% renally, unchanged, 50% metabolized by CYP3A4, 15% metabolized by acetylation.	

309. Anxiolytics

309.1 Benzodiazepines

Drug and Dosage Forms	Usual Dosage Range	Administration Issues and Drug–Drug & Drug–Food Interactions	Common Adverse Drug Reactions (ADRs) and Pharmacokinetics	Contraindications, Pregnancy Category, and Lactation Issues
Alprazolam (CIV) Xanax, generics Tablets 0.25 mg, 0.5 mg, 1 mg, 2 mg Intensol solution 1 mg/mL	**Anxiety disorders** Starting dose of 0.25–0.5 mg tid. Slowly titrate up to maximum of 4 mg/d. **Elderly patients:** starting dose of 0.25 mg 2–3 times daily. **Panic disorder with or without agoraphobia** Initially 0.5 mg tid. Titrate by ≤1 mg/d q 3–4 days up to 10 mg/d if needed. **Elderly patients:** starting dose of 0.25 mg 2–3 times daily. **Unlabeled uses:** agoraphobia & social phobia (2–8 mg/d), depression (0.25–3 mg/d), premenstrual syndrome (0.25–3 mg/d).	Administration Issues Safety/efficacy in children <18 yrs old not established. Drug–Drug Interactions: **Increased level of BZ:** cimetidine, oral contraceptives, disulfiram, fluoxetine, isoniazid, ketoconazole, metoprolol, propoxyphene, propranolol, valproic acid. **Increased CNS effects:** alcohol, barbiturates, narcotics. **Increased levels of:** digoxin, phenytoin (possibly). **Decreased level or effect of BZ:** rifampin (decreased level); theophylline (decreased effect).	ADRs Drowsiness, ataxia, confusion. Dependence: prolonged use can lead to dependence; abrupt discontinuation can precipitate withdrawal symptoms (e.g., anxiety, flu-like illness, concentration difficulties, fatigue, anorexia, restlessness, confusion, psychosis, paranoid delusions, grand mal seizures). Withdrawal can occur after as little as 4–6 weeks of therapy. Drug Discontinuation: Slow taper by 0.5 mg/d at most every 3 days or as tolerated. May take weeks or months to fully discontinue drug. Pharmacokinetics: $T_{1/2}$ = 12–15 h; renal elimination.	Contraindication: Hypersensitivity, psychoses, acute narrow-angle glaucoma. Pregnancy Category: D Lactation Issues: Excreted in breast milk—do not give to nursing mothers.
Chlordiazepoxide (CIV) Librium, Mitran, Reposans-10, Libritabs, various generics Capsules 5 mg, 10 mg, 25 mg	**Anxiety disorders** Mild/moderate: 5 or 10 mg tid to qid Severe: 20 or 25 mg 3–4 times daily Elderly patients: 5 mg 2–4 times daily Children (>6 yrs old): 5 mg 2–4 times daily or 0.5 mg/kg/d q 6–8 hours **Acute alcohol withdrawal syndrome** 50–100 mg followed by repeated doses as needed (up to 300 mg/d). Reduce to maintenance dose as soon as possible. Elderly patients: 25–50 mg initially. **Unlabeled uses:** Also used for irritable bowel syndrome.	Administration Issues Not recommended for children <6 yrs old. Drug–Drug Interactions **Increased level of BZ:** cimetidine, oral contraceptives, disulfiram, fluoxetine, isoniazid, ketoconazole, metoprolol, propoxyphene, propranolol, valproic acid. **Increased CNS effects:** alcohol, barbiturates, narcotics. **Increased levels of:** digoxin, phenytoin (possibly). **Decreased level or effect of BZ:** rifampin (decreased level); theophylline (decreased effect).	ADRs Drowsiness, ataxia, confusion. Dependence: Prolonged use can lead to dependence; abrupt discontinuation can precipitate withdrawal symptoms (e.g., anxiety, flu-like illness, concentration difficulties, fatigue, anorexia, restlessness, confusion, psychosis, paranoid delusions, grand mal seizures). Withdrawal can occur after as little as 4–6 weeks of therapy. Drug Discontinuation: gradual decrease over 4–8 weeks Pharmacokinetics $T_{1/2}$ = 5–30 hrs; renal elimination.	Contraindications Hypersensitivity, psychoses, acute narrow-angle glaucoma. Pregnancy Category: D Lactation Issues Excreted in breast milk—do not give to nursing mothers.

(continues on next page)

309.1 Benzodiazepines *continued from previous page*

Drug and Dosage Forms	Usual Dosage Range	Administration Issues and Drug–Drug & Drug–Food Interactions	Common Adverse Drug Reactions (ADRs) and Pharmacokinetics	Contraindications, Pregnancy Category, and Lactation Issues
Clorazepate dipotassium (CIV) Tranxene, Tranxene-SD, Tranxene-SD-Half, Gen-Xene, various generics Capsules 3.75 mg, 7.5 mg, 15 mg Tablets 3.75 mg, 7.5 mg, 15 mg Tablet, single dose 11.25 mg, 22.5 mg	**Anxiety disorders** Initially: 15 mg bid; titrate to 60 mg/d if needed **Elderly patients:** 3.75–7.5 mg bid initially; titrate based on response **Acute alcohol withdrawal** Day 1: 30 mg followed by 30–60 mg, divided Day 2: 45–90 mg, divided Day 3: 22.5–45 mg, divided Day 4: 15–30 mg, divided Then reduce dose to 7.5–15 mg daily; discontinue drug when patient stable **Unlabeled uses:** also used in irritable bowel syndrome.	Administration Issues May give daily dose at bedtime; not recommended for children <9 yrs old. Drug–Drug Interactions **Increased level of BZ:** cimetidine, oral contraceptives, disulfiram, fluoxetine, isoniazid, ketoconazole, metoprolol, propoxyphene, propranolol, valproic acid. **Increased CNS effects:** alcohol, barbiturates, narcotics. **Increased levels of:** digoxin, phenytoin (possibly). **Decreased level or effect of BZ:** rifampin (decreased level); theophylline (decreased effect).	ADRs Drowsiness, ataxia, confusion. Dependence: prolonged use can lead to dependence; abrupt discontinuation can precipitate withdrawal symptoms (e.g., anxiety, flu-like illness, concentration difficulties, fatigue, anorexia, restlessness, confusion, psychosis, paranoid delusions, grand mal seizures). Withdrawal can occur after as little as 4–6 weeks of therapy. Drug Discontinuation: gradual decrease over 4–8 weeks Pharmacokinetics $T_{1/2}$ = 30–100 hrs; renal elimination.	Contraindications Hypersensitivity, psychoses, acute narrow-angle glaucoma, clinical or biochemical evidence of significant liver disease. Pregnancy Category: none, but avoid in pregnant women. Lactation Issues Excreted in breast milk—do not give to nursing mothers.
Diazepam (CIV) Valium, Valrelease, Zetran, various generics Tablets 2 mg, 5 mg, 10 mg Capsule sustained release 15 mg Oral Solution 5 mg/5 mL, 5 mg/mL	**Anxiety disorders or short-term relief of anxiety symptoms** 2–10 mg 2–4 times daily (individualize dose); 15–30 mg/d of sustained release product **Acute alcohol withdrawal** 10 mg 3–4 times during first 24 hours, decrease to 5 mg 3–4 times daily prn **Muscle relaxant** 2–10 mg tid to qid **Elderly or debilitated patients:** 2–2.5 mg 1–2 times daily initially. Titrate slowly to avoid adverse effects. **Pediatrics:** 1–2.5 mg tid to qid initially. Titrate slowly prn. As a muscle relaxant: 0.12–0.8 mg/kg/d divided in 3–4 doses.	Administration Issues Do not crush or chew sustained release products. Concentrated solution (5 mg/mL) should be diluted in liquid or semi-solid foods, not recommended for children <6 mos old. Drug Interactions **Increased level of BZ:** cimetidine, oral contraceptives, disulfiram, fluoxetine, isoniazid, ketoconazole, metoprolol, propoxyphene, propranolol, valproic acid. **Increased CNS effects:** alcohol, barbiturates, narcotics. **Increased levels of:** digoxin, phenytoin (possibly).	ADRs Drowsiness, ataxia, confusion. Dependence: prolonged use can lead to dependence; abrupt discontinuation can precipitate withdrawal symptoms (e.g., anxiety, flu-like illness, concentration difficulties, fatigue, anorexia, restlessness, confusion, psychosis, paranoid delusions, grand mal seizures). Withdrawal can occur after as little as 4–6 weeks of therapy. Drug Discontinuation: gradual decrease over 4–8 weeks. Pharmacokinetics: $T_{1/2}$ = 20–80 h; renal elimination.	Contraindications Hypersensitivity, psychoses, acute narrow-angle glaucoma. Pregnancy Category: D Lactation Issues Excreted in breast milk—do not give to nursing mothers.

	Unlabeled uses: panic attacks, irritable bowel syndrome.	**Decreased level or effect of BZ:** rifampin (decreased level); theophylline (decreased effect).		
Lorazepam (CIV) Ativan, various generics Tablets 0.5 mg, 1 mg, 2 mg Concentrated Oral Solution 2 mg/mL	**Anxiety disorders, short-term relief of symptoms of anxiety, or anxiety associated with depressive symptoms** 2–3 mg given 2–3 times daily (dose range is 1–10 mg/d) **Elderly or debilitated patients:** 1–2 mg/d in divided doses. Titrate slowly and as needed. **Unlabeled uses:** acute alcohol withdrawal syndrome, irritable bowel syndrome.	Administration Issues Safety/efficacy in children <18 yrs old not established. Drug–Drug Interactions **Increased level of BZ:** cimetidine, oral contraceptives, disulfiram, fluoxetine, isoniazid, ketoconazole, metoprolol, propoxyphene, propranolol, valproic acid. **Increased CNS effects:** alcohol, barbiturates, narcotics. **Increased levels of:** digoxin, phenytoin (possibly). **Decreased level or effect of BZ:** rifampin (decreased level); theophylline (decreased effect).	ADRs Drowsiness, ataxia, confusion. Dependence: prolonged use can lead to dependence; abrupt discontinuation can precipitate withdrawal symptoms (e.g., anxiety, flu-like illness, concentration difficulties, fatigue, anorexia, restlessness, confusion, psychosis, paranoid delusions, grand mal seizures). Withdrawal can occur after as little as 4–6 weeks of therapy. Drug Discontinuation: gradual decrease over 4–8 weeks. Pharmacokinetics $T_{1/2}$ = 10–20 h; renal elimination.	Contraindications Hypersensitivity, psychoses, acute narrow-angle glaucoma. Pregnancy Category: D Lactation Issues Excreted in breast milk—do not give to nursing mothers.
Oxazepam (CIV) Serax, various generics Capsules 10 mg, 15 mg, 30 mg Tablets 15 mg	**Anxiety disorders** Mild/Moderate 10–15 mg 3–4 times daily Severe anxiety, agitation or anxiety associated with depression: 15–30 mg 3–4 times daily **Alcoholics with acute inebriation, tremulousness or anxiety on withdrawal** 15 mg 3–4 times daily **Anxiety, tension, irritability, and agitation in elderly patients** 10 mg tid. May increase to 15–30 mg 3–4 times daily if needed—do so cautiously. **Unlabeled uses:** Also used for irritable bowel syndrome.	Administration Issues Safety/efficacy for <12 yrs old not established. Drug–Drug Interactions **Increased level of BZ:** cimetidine, oral contraceptives, disulfiram, fluoxetine, isoniazid, ketoconazole, metoprolol, propoxyphene, propranolol, valproic acid. **Increased CNS effects:** alcohol, barbiturates, narcotics. **Increased levels of:** digoxin, phenytoin (possibly). **Decreased level or effect of BZ:** rifampin (decreased level); theophylline (decreased effect).	ADRs Drowsiness, ataxia, confusion (especially in elderly). Dependence: prolonged use can lead to dependence; abrupt discontinuation can precipitate withdrawal symptoms (e.g., anxiety, flu-like illness, concentration difficulties, fatigue, anorexia, restlessness, confusion, psychosis, paranoid delusions, grand mal seizures). Withdrawal can occur after as little as 4–6 weeks of therapy. Drug Discontinuation: gradual decrease over 4–8 weeks. Pharmacokinetics $T_{1/2}$ = 5–20 h; renal elimination.	Contraindications Hypersensitivity, psychoses, acute narrow-angle glaucoma. Pregnancy Category: D Lactation Issues Excreted in breast milk—do not give to nursing mothers.

309.2 Miscellaneous Anxiolytics

Drug and Dosage Forms	Usual Dosage Range	Administration Issues and Drug–Drug Interactions	Common Adverse Drug Reactions (ADRs) and Pharmacokinetics	Contraindications, Pregnancy Category, and Lactation Issues
Buspirone BuSpar, generics Tablets 5 mg, 7.5 mg, 10 mg, 15 mg, 30 mg	**Anxiety disorders or short term relief of symptoms of anxiety** Initial dose: 5 mg tid. Titrate by 5 mg/d every 2–3 days as needed. Max dose is 60 mg/d Elderly patients: 5 mg bid. Titrate as above, as needed. **Unlabeled use:** 25 mg/d used in decreasing the symptoms of premenstrual syndrome **Traumatic brain injury** 5 mg bid; increase by 5 mg q 5 d up to 45 mg	Drug–Drug Interactions **Increased level of:** haloperidol. **Hypertensive crisis:** MAOIs.	ADRs Dizziness, lightheadedness, excitement, drowsiness, nervousness, nausea. headache. Pharmacokinetics 95% protein bound; $T_{1/2} = 2-11$ h; optimal therapeutic effect seen 3–4 weeks.	Contraindications Hypersensitivity. Pregnancy Category: B Lactation Issues Unknown extent of excretion in breast milk. Use cautiously in nursing mothers. Other Precautions May bind to dopamine receptors, monitor for extrapyramidal symptoms, tardive dyskinesia.
Doxepin Adapin, Sinequan, various generics Capsules 10 mg, 25 mg, 50 mg, 75 mg, 100 mg, 150 mg Liquid concentrate 10 mg/1 mL	**Anxiety** 75 mg/d at bedtime starting dose. Titrate up to 300 mg/d in 2–3 divided doses. Single dose ≤ 150 mg. **Elderly patients:** 10–25 mg at bedtime starting dose. Titrate by 10–25 mg every 3–5 days to 75 mg/d. **Unlabeled uses:** 50–300 mg/d used for chronic pain (migraine, chronic tension headache, diabetic neuropathy, tic douloureux, cancer pain, peripheral neuropathy with pain, postherpetic neuralgia, arthritic pain), 10–30 mg/d used in chronic urticaria and angioedema, nocturnal pruritis in atopic eczema. Also used in peptic ulcer disease.	Administration issues Maintenance doses may be given once daily at bedtime to reduce daytime sedation. Concentrate: protect from light, dilute in juice or other liquid prior to administration; Not recommended for children < 12 yrs old. Drug–Drug Interactions **Hypertensive crisis:** clonidine, MAO inhibitors; can occur weeks after MAO inhibitor discontinued. **Increased TCA level:** cimetidine, ethanol, fluoxetine, haloperidol, oral contraceptives, phenothiazines. **Decreased TCA level:** barbiturates, phenytoin, chronic ethanol ingestion. **Increased level of:** phenytoin, warfarin. **Increased effect:** anticholinergic agents, ethanol or sedatives (increased CNS effects), thyroid hormones (increased effect of both drugs).	ADRs Dry mouth, urinary retention, blurred vision, constipation, orthostatic hypotension, tachycardia, palpitations, arrhythmias, sedation, seizures, confusion (esp. elderly), hallucinations, anxiety, nervousness, agitation, panic, hypomania, mania, nausea, vomiting, anorexia, constipation or diarrhea, flatulence, abdominal cramps, sexual dysfunction (increased or decreased libido; impotence, painful ejaculation). Pharmacokinetics >90% protein bound, lipid soluble, $T_{1/2} = 8-24$ h; time to maximal clinical benefit $= 2-4$ weeks. **Therapeutic plasma level = 100–200 ng/mL** (plasma levels and therapeutic effect are subject to wide interpatient variability).	Contraindications Any hypersensitivity to a TCA, concomitant use of MAO inhibitors, patients with glaucoma or tendency to urinary retention. Precautions Use with caution in patients with severe cardiovascular disease, seizure disorders. Patients with schizophrenia may experience worsening psychosis; patients with bipolar disorder may experience a switch to mania. Dosage reductions necessary in patients with hepatic or severe renal dysfunction. Pregnancy Category: C Lactation issues TCAs are excreted into breast milk. Use with caution in nursing mothers.

		Decreased effect of: guanethidine, methyldopa.		
Hydroxyzine Atarax, Anaxinal, Vistaril, various generics Tablets 10 mg, 25 mg, 50 mg, 100 mg Capsules 25 mg, 50 mg, 100 mg Syrup 10 mg/5 mL Suspension 25 mg/5 mL	**Symptomatic relief of anxiety/tension associated with psychoneurosis or organic disease states** 50–100 mg qid **Pediatrics (> 6 yrs):** 50–100 mg/d in divided doses **Pediatrics (< 6 yrs):** 50 mg/d divided **Pruritus due to allergic conditions (chronic urticaria, atopic/contact dermatoses, histamine-mediated pruritus)** 25 mg 3–4 times daily **Pediatrics (> 6 yrs):** 50–100 mg/d in divided doses **Pediatrics (< 6 yrs):** 50 mg/d in divided doses **Elderly patients:** 10 mg tid to qid	Drug–Drug Interactions **Increased CNS depressant effects:** alcohol, narcotics, barbiturates.	ADRs Drowsiness, dry mouth. Pharmacokinetics $T_{1/2}$ = 3 hrs; hepatic metabolism.	Contraindications Hypersensitivity. Pregnancy Category: C Lactation Issues Safety not established—do not use in lactating women.
Meprobamate (CIV) Equanil, Miltown, Neuramate, Miltown 600, Meprospan, various generics Tablets 200 mg, 400 mg	Anxiety disorders or short term relief of symptoms of anxiety 400 mg 3–4 times daily; max dose is 2400 mg/d (using SR capsules: 400–800 mg twice daily) Elderly or pediatric (6–12 yrs) patients: 100–200 mg 2–3 times daily	Administration Issues Safety/efficacy not established in children < 6 years old. Drug–Drug Interactions **increased CNS depressant effects:** alcohol, barbiturates, narcotics, and others.	ADRs Itching, urticarial erythematous maculopapular rash, drowsiness, ataxia, dizziness, slurred speech, headache, nausea, vomiting, diarrhea. Pharmacokinetics 15% protein binding; $T_{1/2}$ = 24–48 h during chronic administration; extensive hepatic metabolism.	Contraindications Hypersensitivity, acute intermittent porphyria. Other Precautions Drug dependency is observed (avoid prolonged use); abrupt discontinuation may precipitate withdrawal. Use cautiously in patients with seizure disorders. Use cautiously in patients with severe renal or hepatic dysfunction. Pregnancy Category: D Lactation Issues Meprobamate is excreted in breast milk—use cautiously in nursing mothers.

310. Sedatives/Hypnotics

310.1 Barbiturates

Drug and Dosage Forms	Usual Dosage Range	Administration Issues and Drug—Drug & Drug—Food Interactions	Common Adverse Drug Reactions (ADRs) and Pharmacokinetics	Contraindications, Pregnancy Category, and Lactation Issues
Butabarbital (CIII) Butisol Sodium, various generics Tablets 15 mg, 30 mg, 50 mg, 100 mg Elixir 30 mg/5 mL	**Short-term (< 2 weeks) treatment of insomnia** 50–100 mg at bedtime **Elderly or debilitated patients (hepatic/renal dysfunction):** 30–50 mg at bedtime. Titrate to higher dose as needed/tolerated **Sedation** 15–30 mg 3–4 times daily (use smaller dose in elderly or debilitated patients)	Administration Issues May produce irritability, excitability, or aggression in children. Drug–Drug Interactions **Decreased levels of:** anticoagulants, beta blockers, carbamazepine, clonazepam, oral contraceptives, corticosteroids, doxycycline, doxorubicin, felodipine, quinidine, verapamil, theophylline. **Increased effect of:** alcohol & possibly narcotics (CNS effects), acetaminophen (liver toxicity). **Increased effect of barbiturates:** MAO inhibitors, valproic acid. **Unknown effects (monitor patient closely):** hydantoins.	ADRs Somnolence, agitation, confusion, ataxia, nightmares, nervousness, hallucinations, bradycardia, hypotension, nausea, vomiting, skin rash. Elderly Patients: may observe paradoxical excitement. Precautions **Drug abuse and dependence:** Prolonged use at high doses leads to physical dependence. If dependent on barbiturate, slowly withdraw over several weeks. May use long-acting barbiturate (phenobarbital) at dose of 30 mg per every 100–200 mg of mephobarbital to help prevent withdrawal symptoms. Pharmacokinetics Onset of action = 45–60 min; $T_{1/2}$ = 66–140 h; duration of action = 6–8 h.	Contraindications Hypersensitivity; manifest or latent porphyria, severe hepatic, renal, or respiratory dysfunction; previous addiction to sedative/hypnotic. Pregnancy Category: D Lactation Issues Use cautiously in nursing mothers; sedation has been reported in infants.
Mephobarbital (CIV) Mebaral Tablets 32 mg, 50 mg, 100 mg	**Sedative** 32–100 mg 3–4 times daily **Pediatrics:** 16–32 mg 3–4 times daily **Elderly or debilitated patients (hepatic/renal dysfunction):** 16–32 mg 2–3 times daily. Titrate to higher doses as needed/tolerated.	Administration Issues May produce irritability, excitability, or aggression in children. Drug–Drug Interactions **Decreased levels of:** anticoagulants, beta blockers, carbamazepine, clonazepam, oral contraceptives, corticosteroids, doxycycline, doxorubicin, felodipine, quinidine, verapamil, theophylline. **Increased effect of:** alcohol and possibly narcotics (CNS effects), acetaminophen (liver toxicity). **Increased effect of barbiturates:** MAO inhibitors, valproic acid.	ADRs Somnolence, agitation, confusion, ataxia, nightmares, nervousness, hallucinations, bradycardia, hypotension, nausea, vomiting, skin rash. Elderly Patients: may observe paradoxical excitement. Precautions **Drug abuse and dependence:** Prolonged use at high doses leads to physical dependence. If dependent on barbiturate, slowly withdraw over several weeks. May use long-acting barbiturate (phenobarbital) at dose of 30 mg per every 100–200 mg of mephobarbital to help prevent withdrawal symptoms.	Contraindications Hypersensitivity; manifest or latent porphyria, severe hepatic, renal, or respiratory dysfunction; previous addiction to sedative/hypnotic. Pregnancy Category: D Lactation Issues Use cautiously in nursing mothers; sedation has been reported in infants.

		Unknown effects (monitor patient closely): hydantoins.	Pharmacokinetics Onset of action = 30 → 60 min; min; $T_{1/2}$ = 11–67 h; duration of action = 10–16 h.	
Pentobarbital (CII) Nembutal Sodium, various generics Capsules 50 mg, 100 mg Suppositories 30 mg, 60 mg, 120 mg, 200 mg Elixir 20 mg/5 mL	**Short-term (< 2 weeks) treatment of insomnia** 100 mg at bedtime (120–200 mg by suppository) **Sedative** 20 mg tid to qid **Pediatrics:** 2–6 mg/kg/d orally for sedative dose or hypnotic dose) Rectal administration: 12–14 yrs: 60–120 mg 5–12 yrs: 60 mg 1–4 yrs: 30–60 mg 2 months–1 yr: 30 mg **Elderly or debilitated patients (hepatic/renal dysfunction):** Use smaller doses and greater dosing intervals (for sedative dose). Titrate dose as needed/tolerated.	Administration Issues May produce irritability, excitability, or aggression in children. Drug–Drug Interactions **Decreased levels of:** anticoagulants, beta blockers, carbamazepine, clonazepam, oral contraceptives, corticosteroids, doxycycline, doxorubicin, felodipine, quinidine, verapamil, theophylline. **Increased effect of:** alcohol and possibly narcotics (CNS effects), acetaminophen (liver toxicity). **Increased effect of barbiturates:** MAO inhibitors, valproic acid. **Unknown effects (monitor patient closely):** hydantoins.	ADRs Somnolence, agitation, confusion, ataxia, nightmares, nervousness, hallucinations, bradycardia, hypotension, nausea, vomiting, skin rash. Elderly Patients: may observe paradoxical excitement. Precautions **Drug abuse and dependence:** Prolonged use at high doses leads to physical dependence. If dependent on barbiturate, slowly withdraw over several weeks. May use long-acting barbiturate (phenobarbital) at dose of 30 mg per every 100–200 mg of pentobarbital to help prevent withdrawal symptoms. Pharmacokinetics Onset of action = 10–15 min; $T_{1/2}$ = 15–50 h; duration of action = 3–4 h.	Contraindications Hypersensitivity; manifest or latent porphyria, severe hepatic, renal, or respiratory dysfunction; previous addiction to sedative/hypnotic. Pregnancy Category: D Lactation Issues Use cautiously in nursing mothers; sedation has been reported in infants.
Phenobarbital (CIV) Solfoton, various generics Tablets 15 mg, 16 mg, 30 mg, 60 mg, 90 mg, 100 mg Capsules 16 mg Elixir 15 mg/5 mL, 20 mg/5 mL	**Short-term (< 2 weeks) treatment of insomnia** 100–200 mg at bedtime **Pediatrics: 3–6 mg/kg/d** **Sedative** 15–40 mg 2–3 times daily. Titrate as needed (max dose is 400 mg/d). **Pediatrics: 8–32 mg/d** **Elderly or debilitated patients (hepatic/renal dysfunction):** Use smaller doses and greater dosing intervals (for sedative dose). Titrate dose prn.	Administration Issues May produce irritability, excitability, or aggression in children. Drug–Drug Interactions **Decreased levels of:** anticoagulants, beta blockers, carbamazepine, clonazepam, oral contraceptives, corticosteroids, doxycycline, doxorubicin, felodipine, quinidine, verapamil, theophylline. **Increased effect of:** alcohol and possibly narcotics (CNS effects), acetaminophen (liver toxicity).	ADRs Somnolence, agitation, confusion, ataxia, nightmares, nervousness, hallucinations, bradycardia, hypotension, nausea, vomiting, skin rash. Elderly Patients: may observe paradoxical excitement. Precautions **Drug abuse and dependence:** Prolonged use at high doses leads to physical dependence. If dependent on barbiturate, slowly withdraw over several weeks.	Contraindications Hypersensitivity; manifest or latent porphyria, severe hepatic, renal, or respiratory dysfunction; previous addiction to sedative/hypnotic. Pregnancy Category: D Lactation Issues Use cautiously in nursing mothers; sedation has been reported in infants.

(continues on next page)

310.1 Barbiturates *continued from previous page*

Drug and Dosage Forms	Usual Dosage Range	Administration Issues and Drug—Drug & Drug—Food Interactions	Common Adverse Drug Reactions (ADRs) and Pharmacokinetics	Contraindications, Pregnancy Category, and Lactation Issues
Phenobarbital (CIV) *cont.*		**Increased effect of barbiturates:** MAO inhibitors, valproic acid. **Unknown effects (monitor patient closely):** hydantoins.	Pharmacokinetics Onset of action = 30 → 60 min; $T_{1/2}$ = 53–118 h; duration of action = 10–16 h.	
Secobarbital (CII) Seconal Sodium Pulvules, various generics Capsules 100 mg	**Short-term (< 2 weeks) treatment of insomnia** 100 mg at bedtime **Elderly or debilitated patients (hepatic/renal dysfunction):** Use smaller doses and greater dosing intervals (for sedative dose). Titrate dose as needed/tolerated.	Administration Issues May produce irritability, excitability, or aggression in children. Drug–Drug Interactions **Decreased levels of:** anticoagulants, beta blockers, carbamazepine, clonazepam, oral contraceptives, corticosteroids, doxycycline, doxorubicin, felodipine, quinidine, verapamil, theophylline. **Increased effect of:** alcohol and possibly narcotics (CNS effects), acetaminophen (liver toxicity). **Increased effect of barbiturates:** MAO inhibitors, valproic acid. **Unknown effects (monitor patient closely):** hydantoins.	ADRs Somnolence, agitation, confusion, ataxia, nightmares, nervousness, hallucinations, bradycardia, hypotension, nausea, vomiting, skin rash. Elderly Patients: may observe paradoxical excitement. Precautions **Drug abuse and dependence:** Prolonged use at high doses leads to physical dependence. If dependent on barbiturate, slowly withdraw over several weeks. May use long-acting barbiturate (phenobarbital) at dose of 30 mg per every 100–200 mg of secobarbital to help prevent withdrawal symptoms. Pharmacokinetics Onset of action = 10–15 min; $T_{1/2}$ = 15–40 h; duration of action = 3–4 h.	Contraindications Hypersensitivity; manifest or latent porphyria, severe hepatic, renal, or respiratory dysfunction; previous addiction to sedative/hypnotic. Pregnancy Category: D Lactation Issues Use cautiously in nursing mothers; sedation has been reported in infants.

310.2 Benzodiazepines

Drug and Dosage Forms	Usual Dosage Range	Administration Issues and Drug–Drug & Drug–Food Interactions	Common Adverse Drug Reactions (ADRs) and Pharmacokinetics	Contraindications, Pregnancy Category, and Lactation Issues
Estazolam (CIV) Pro Som, various generics Tablets 1 mg, 2 mg	**Insomnia** 1 mg at bedtime; some require 2 mg **Debilitated or small elderly patients:** 0.5 mg at bedtime; titrate slowly	Administration Issues Safety/efficacy in children <18 yrs old not established. Drug–Drug Interactions **Increased level of BZ:** cimetidine, oral contraceptives, disulfiram, fluoxetine, isoniazid, ketoconazole, metoprolol, propoxyphene, propranolol, valproic acid. **Increased CNS effects:** alcohol, barbiturates, narcotics. **Increased levels of:** digoxin, phenytoin (possibly). **Decreased level or effect of BZ:** rifampin (decreased level); theophylline (decreased effect).	ADRs Drowsiness, ataxia, confusion (especially in elderly), nervousness. Dependence: Prolonged use can lead to dependence; abrupt discontinuation can precipitate withdrawal symptoms (e.g., anxiety, flu-like illness, concentration difficulties, fatigue, anorexia, restlessness, confusion, psychosis, paranoid delusions, grand mal seizures). Withdrawal can occur after as little as 4–6 weeks of therapy. Drug discontinuation: Slow taper of drug suggested if patient has received long course of therapy. Pharmacokinetics >90% protein bound; time to peak levels: 2 h; $T_{1/2} = 10-24$ h; renal elimination.	Contraindications Hypersensitivity. Pregnancy Category: X Lactation Issues Excreted in breast milk—do not give to nursing mothers.
Flurazepam (CIV) Dalmane, various generics Capsules 15 mg, 30 mg	**Insomnia** 30 mg at bedtime **Elderly or debilitated patients:** 15 mg at bedtime; titrate as needed	Administration Issues Safety/efficacy in children <15 yrs old not established. Drug–Drug Interactions **Increased level of BZ:** cimetidine, oral contraceptives, disulfiram, fluoxetine, isoniazid, ketoconazole, metoprolol, propoxyphene, propranolol, valproic acid. **Increased CNS effects:** alcohol, barbiturates, narcotics. **Increased levels of:** digoxin, phenytoin (possibly). **Decreased level or effect of BZ:** rifampin (decreased level); theophylline (decreased effect).	ADRs Drowsiness, ataxia, confusion (especially in elderly), nervousness. Dependence: Prolonged use can lead to dependence; abrupt discontinuation can precipitate withdrawal symptoms (e.g., anxiety, flu-like illness, concentration difficulties, fatigue, anorexia, restlessness, confusion, psychosis, paranoid delusions, grand mal seizures). Withdrawal can occur after as little as 4–6 weeks of therapy. Drug discontinuation: Slow taper of drug suggested if patient has received long course of therapy.	Contraindications Hypersensitivity. Pregnancy Category: X Contraindicated in pregnancy Lactation Issues Excreted in breast milk—do not give to nursing mothers.

(continues on next page)

310.2 Benzodiazepines *continued from previous page*

Drug and Dosage Forms	Usual Dosage Range	Administration Issues and Drug–Drug & Drug–Food Interactions	Common Adverse Drug Reactions (ADRs) and Pharmacokinetics	Contraindications, Pregnancy Category, and Lactation Issues
Flurazepam (CIV) ***cont.***			Pharmacokinetics >90% protein bound; time to peak levels: 0.5–1 h; $T_{1/2}$ = 50–100 h; renal elimination.	
Quazepam (CIV) Doral Tablets 7.5 mg, 15 mg	**Insomnia** 15 mg at bedtime; some only require 7.5 mg at bedtime **Elderly or debilitated patients:** may initiate at 15 mg at bedtime; attempt to reduce dose after first 2–3 nights	Administration Issues Safety/efficacy in children <18 yrs old not established. Drug–Drug Interactions **Increased level of BZ:** cimetidine, oral contraceptives, disulfiram, fluoxetine, isoniazid, ketoconazole, metoprolol, propoxyphene, propranolol, valproic acid. **Increased CNS effects:** alcohol, barbiturates, narcotics. **Increased levels of:** digoxin, phenytoin (possibly). **Decreased level or effect of BZ:** rifampin (decreased level); theophylline (decreased effect).	ADRs Drowsiness, ataxia, confusion (especially in elderly), nervousness. Dependence: Prolonged use can lead to dependence; abrupt discontinuation can precipitate withdrawal symptoms (e.g., anxiety, flu-like illness, concentration difficulties, fatigue, anorexia, restlessness, confusion, psychosis, paranoid delusions, grand mal seizures). Withdrawal can occur after as little as 4–6 weeks of therapy. Drug discontinuation: Slow taper of drug suggested if patient has received long course of therapy. Pharmacokinetics >90% protein bound; time to peak levels: 2 h; $T_{1/2}$ = 25–41 h; renal elimination.	Contraindications Hypersensitivity, suspected or established sleep apnea. Pregnancy Category: X Lactation Issues Excreted in breast milk—do not give to nursing mothers.
Temazepam (CIV) Restoril, various generics Capsules 7.5 mg, 15 mg, 30 mg	**Insomnia** 15 mg at bedtime; titrate to 30 mg if needed **Elderly or debilitated patients:** 15 mg at bedtime	Administration Issues Safety/efficacy in children <18 yrs old not established. Drug–Drug Interactions **Increased level of BZ:** cimetidine, oral contraceptives, disulfiram, fluoxetine, isoniazid, ketoconazole, metoprolol, propoxyphene, propranolol, valproic acid. **Increased CNS effects:** alcohol, barbiturates, narcotics.	ADRs Drowsiness, ataxia, confusion (especially in elderly), nervousness. Dependence: Prolonged use can lead to dependence; abrupt discontinuation can precipitate withdrawal symptoms (e.g., anxiety, flu-like illness, concentration difficulties, fatigue, anorexia, restlessness, confusion, psychosis, paranoid delusions, grand mal seizures). Withdrawal can occur after as little as 4–6 weeks of therapy.	Contraindications Hypersensitivity. Pregnancy Category: X Lactation Issues Excreted in breast milk—do not give to nursing mothers.

		Increased levels of: digoxin, phenytoin (possibly). **Decreased level or effect of BZ:** rifampin (decreased level); theophylline (decreased effect).	Drug discontinuation: Slow taper of drug suggested if patient has received long course of therapy. Pharmacokinetics >90% protein bound; time to peak levels: 2–4 h; $T_{1/2}$ = 10–17 h; renal elimination.	
Triazolam (CIV) Halcion, various generics Tablets 0.125 mg, 0.25 mg	**Insomnia** 0.125–0.5 mg at bedtime **Elderly or debilitated patients:** 0.125 mg at bedtime initially; titrate slowly by 0.125 mg/d if needed	Administration Issues Safety/efficacy in children <18 yrs old not established. Drug–Drug Interactions **Increased level of BZ:** cimetidine, oral contraceptives, disulfiram, fluoxetine, isoniazid, ketoconazole, metoprolol, propoxyphene, propranolol, valproic acid. **Increased CNS effects:** alcohol, barbiturates, narcotics. **Increased levels of:** digoxin, phenytoin (possibly). **Decreased level or effect of BZ:** rifampin (decreased level); theophylline (decreased effect).	ADRs Drowsiness, ataxia, confusion (especially in elderly), nervousness, anterograde amnesia. Dependence: Prolonged use can lead to dependence; abrupt discontinuation can precipitate withdrawal symptoms (e.g., anxiety, flu-like illness, concentration difficulties, fatigue, anorexia, restlessness, confusion, psychosis, paranoid delusions, grand mal seizures). Withdrawal can occur after as little as 4–6 weeks of therapy. Drug discontinuation: Slow taper of drug suggested if patient has received long course of therapy. Pharmacokinetics >90% protein bound; time to peak levels: 0.5–2 h; $T_{1/2}$ = 1.5–5.5 h; renal elimination.	Contraindications Hypersensitivity. Pregnancy Category: X Lactation Issues Excreted in breast milk—do not give to nursing mothers.

310.3 Miscellaneous Nonbarbiturates

Drug and Dosage Forms	Usual Dosage Range	Administration Issues and Drug–Drug Interactions	Common Adverse Drug Reactions (ADRs) and Pharmacokinetics	Cotraindications, Pregnancy Category, and Lactation Issues
Acetylcarbromal Paxarel Tablets 250 mg	**Sedative** 250–500 mg 2–3 times daily **Pediatrics:** no specific recommendations; give smaller doses proportionally based on age and weight.	Administration Issues Avoid alcohol use.	ADRs Drowsiness (particularly with high doses). Overdose: result from bromide accumulation and its displacement of chloride in body fluids. Symptoms: narcosis, respiratory depression, mental disturbances, dizziness,	Contraindications Hypersensitivity to bromides. Precautions May be habit forming. Pregnancy Category Unknown

(*continues on next page*)

310.3 Miscellaneous Nonbarbiturates *continued from precious page*

Drug and Dosage Forms	Usual Dosage Range	Administration Issues and Drug–Drug Interactions	Common Adverse Drug Reactions (ADRs) and Pharmacokinetics	Cotraindications, Pregnancy Category, and Lactation Issues
Acetylcarbromal cont.			irritability, dermatitis, headache, constipation, others. Pharmacokinetics No Data.	Lactation Issues Excreted in breast milk—women should not nurse.
Chloral Hydrate Noctec, Aquachloral Supprettes, various generics Capsules 250 mg, 500 mg Syrup 250 mg/5 mL, 500 mg/5 mL Suppositories 324 mg, 500 mg, 648 mg	**Nocturnal sedation: postoperative adjunct to oplates and analgesics for control of pain, alcohol withdrawal syndrome** Hypnotic 500–1000 mg at bedtime (15–30 min prior) Sedative 250 mg tid pc **Max dose = 2 g/d.** **Pediatrics:** Hypnotic: 50 mg/kg/d up to 1g/dose; may use divided doses Sedative: 25 mg/kg/d up to 500 mg/dose; may use divided doses	Administration Issues Give with a full glass of liquid. Syrup should be mixed in 1/2 glass of water, fruit juice, or ginger ale. Drug–Drug Interactions **Increased levels/effects of:** alcohol, CNS depressants, oral anticoagulants, furosemide. **Decreased levels/effects of:** phenytoin.	ADRs Somnambulism, disorientation, excitement, delirium, ataxia, dizziness, nightmares, malaise, headache, mental confusion, rash, hives, erythema, urticaria, nausea, vomiting, flatulence, diarrhea, unpleasant taste in mouth. Drug abuse and dependence may be habit forming if taken at high doses and prolonged intervals; withdrawal symptoms have occurred with acute discontinuation of this medication. Discontinue medication in manner similar to barbiturate withdrawal. Pharmacokinetics Onset of action is 30 min; $T_{1/2} = 7-10$ h; renal elimination of metabolites.	Contraindications Hypersensitivity; severe hepatic, renal, cardiac dysfunction; gastritis. Precautions Use cautiously in patients with acute intermittent porphyria. Pregnancy Category: C Lactation Issues Excreted in breast milk; use cautiously.
Glutethimide various generics Tablets 250 mg	**Short-term relief of insomnia** 250–500 mg at bedtime **Elderly or debilitated patients:** do not exceed 500 mg/d.	Administration Issues Do not administer for longer than 3–7 days; safety/ efficacy not established in children. Drug–Drug Interaction **Decreased levels/effects of:** oral anticoagulants. **Increased levels/effects of:** alcohol, CNS depressants.	ADRs Drowsiness, hangover, rash, nausea. Drug abuse and Dependence May be habit forming if taken at high doses and prolonged intervals. Withdrawal symptoms have occurred after abrupt discontinuation. Pharmacokinetics 50% protein bound; onset of action is 30 min; duration of action $= 4-8$ h; $T_{1/2} = 10-12$ h; renal elimination.	Contraindications Hypersensitivity; porphyria. Pregnancy Category: C Lactation Issues Do not nurse while taking this drug.

Zaleplon Sonata Capsules 5 mg, 10 mg	**Short-term treatment of insomnia:** Nonelderly adults 10 mg at bedtime. For certain low-weight individuals, 5 mg may be a sufficient dose. Although the risk of certain adverse events associated with zaleplon appears to be dose dependent, the 20 mg dose has been shown to be adequately tolerated and may be considered for the occasional patient who does not benefit from a trial of a lower dose.	Administration Issues Take zaleplon immediately before bedtime or after going to bed and experiencing difficulty falling asleep. Hypnotics should generally be limited to 7 to 10 days of use, and reevaluation of the patient is recommended if they are to be taken for >2 to 3 weeks. Use 5 mg dose in patients with hepatic impairment. Drug–Drug Interactions **Increased levels of zaleplon** with cimetidine. Use 5mg dose initially if giving these drug concomitantly. Drug–Food Interactions Do not take with or immediately after a high-fat/heavy meal.	ADRs Most Frequent: Somnolence, dizziness, nervousness, nausea, headache, short-term memory impairment. Pharmacokinetics $T_{1/2}$ 1 h.	Contraindications None known Pregnancy Category: C Lactation Issues Do not use in nursing mothers.
Zolpidem Ambien Tablets 5 mg, 10 mg	**Short-term treatment of insomnia** 10 mg at bedtime (max dose is 10 mg/d) **Elderly or debilitated patients:** 5 mg at bedtime	Administration Issues For faster onset of sleep, do not administer with food. Use only for 7–10 days; safety/efficacy not established in those <18 yrs. Drug–Drug Interactions Additive CNS effects with alcohol or other CNS depressants. Drug–Food Interaction Food decreases the absorption of zolpidem.	ADRs Daytime drowsiness, amnesia, dizziness, headache, nausea, vomiting, diarrhea. Elderly Patients closely monitor these patients for excessive sedation or impairment of motor or cognitive performance. Drug abuse and Dependence: Withdrawal symptoms may occur following abrupt discontinuation. Pharmacokinetics 92.5% protein bound; rapid onset of action; $T_{1/2}$ = 1.0–5.5 h; renal elimination.	Contraindications None Precautions Use cautiously in those with respiratory or severe hepatic dysfunction, or those with depression. Pregnancy Category: B Lactation Issues Not appreciably excreted in breast milk; however, use cautiously in nursing mothers.

310.4 Nonprescription Sleep Aids

Drug and Dosage Forms	Usual Dosage Range	Administration Issues and Drug–Drug & Drug–Food Interactions	Common Adverse Drug Reactions (ADRs) and Pharmacokinetics	Contraindications, Pregnancy Category, and Lactation Issues
Doxylamine Unisom Nighttime Sleep-Aid Tablets 25 mg	**Aid in relief of Insomnia** 25 mg at bedtime	Administration Issues Do not use for >2 weeks; safety/efficacy in children <12 yrs not established. Drug–Drug Interactions: **Increased effect of antihistamine:** MAO inhibitors (anticholinergic effects). **Increased effect of:** MAO inhibitors, alcohol, CNS depressants.	ADRs Urinary retention, blurred vision, dry mouth, drowsiness, irritability, thickening of bronchial secretions. Pharmacokinetics Rapid onset (15–30 minutes); duration of action 4–6 h renal elimination of metabolites.	Contraindications Hypersensitivity, asthma, glaucoma, prostate gland enlargement. Precautions Use carefully if operating heavy machinery, history of sleep apnea, hepatic dysfunction. Pregnancy Category: X. Lactation Issues Women should not nurse.
Diphenhydramine Dormin Caplets, Nytol, Sleep-eze 3, Sominex, Sleep Aid, Twilite, various generics Tablets 25 mg, 50 mg Capsules 25 mg, 50 mg	**Aid in relief of insomnia** 25–50 mg at bedtime	Administration Issues Do not use for >2 weeks; safety/efficacy in children <12 yrs not established. Drug–Drug Interactions **Increased effect of antihistamine:** MAO inhibitors (anticholinergic effects). **Increased effect of:** MAO inhibitors, alcohol, CNS depressants.	ADRs Urinary retention, blurred vision, dry mouth, drowsiness, irritability, thickening of bronchial secretions. Elderly Patients (>60yrs): more likely to experience confusion, dizziness, hypotension. Pharmacokinetics Rapid onset (15–30 minutes); duration of action 4–6 h renal elimination of metabolites.	Contraindications Hypersensitivity, asthma, glaucoma, prostate gland enlargement. Precautions Use carefully if operating heavy machinery, history of sleep apnea, hepatic dysfunction. Pregnancy Category: B. Lactation Issues Women should not nurse.
Diphenhydramine and Acetaminophen Extra-Strength Tylenol PM, Aspirin Free Anacin PM Caplets, Excedrin PM, others Tablets 25 mg/500 mg, 38 mg/500 mg, 50 mg/650 mg Capsules 25 mg/500 mg	**Aid in relief of insomnia and minor pain** 25–50 mg diphenhydramine and 500–650 mg acetaminophen at bedtime	Administration Issues Do not use for >2 weeks; safety/efficacy in children <12 yrs not established. Drug–Drug Interactions: Antihistamine: **Increased effect of antihistamine:** MAO inhibitors (anticholinergic effects) **Increased effect of:** MAO inhibitors, alcohol, CNS depressants.	ADRs Antihistamine: urinary retention, blurred vision, dry mouth, drowsiness, irritability, thickening of bronchial secretions. Elderly Patients (>60yrs): more likely to experience confusion, dizziness, hypotension. Acetaminophen: Very few adverse reactions.	Contraindications Hypersensitivity, asthma, glaucoma, prostate gland enlargement. Precautions Use carefully if operating heavy machinery, history of sleep apnea, hepatic dysfunction. Pregnancy Category: B. Consult physician before taking Lactation Issues Women should not nurse.

50 mg/500 mg <u>Powder</u> 50 mg/650 mg <u>Liquid</u> 8.3 mg/167 mg/5 mL 50 mg/1000 mg/30 mL		<u>Acetaminophen:</u> **Increased toxic effect of acetaminophen:** alcohol (chronic); barbiturates, carbamazepine, hydantoins, rifampin, sulfinpyrazone.	<u>Pharmacokinetics</u> See individual ingredients.	

311. Antidepressants

311.1 Tricyclic Antidepressants (TCAs)

Drug and Dosage Forms	Usual Dosage Range	Administration Issues and Drug–Drug Interactions	Common Adverse Drug Reactions (ADRs) and Pharmacokinetics	Contraindications, Pregnancy Category, and Lactation Issues
Amitriptyline Elavil, Endep, various generic forms Tablets 10 mg, 25 mg, 50 mg, 75 mg, 100 mg, 150 mg.	**Major Depression** starting dose of 50–100 mg/d at bedtime. Titrate by 25–50 mg q week to 150 mg/d. For severely depressed patients increase dose to 200–300 mg/d **Adolescent or elderly patients:** starting dose of 10–25 mg q hs. Titrate dose by 10–25 mg q week to 150 mg/d **Unlabeled uses:** 50–100 mg/d used for chronic pain. Also used in Bulimia nervosa.	Administration Issues Maintenance doses may be given once daily at bedtime to reduce daytime sedation. Drug–Drug Interactions **Hypertensive crisis:** clonidine, MAO inhibitors (can occur weeks after MAOI discontinued). **Increased TCA level:** cimetidine, ethanol, fluoxetine, haloperidol, oral contraceptives, phenothiazines. **Decreased TCA level:** barbiturates, phenytoin, chronic ethanol ingestion. **Increased level of:** phenytoin, warfarin. **Increased effect:** anticholinergic agents, ethanol or sedatives (increased CNS effects), thyroid hormones (increased effect of both drugs). **Decreased effect of:** guanethidine, methyldopa.	ADRs Dry mouth, urinary retention, blurred vision, constipation, orthostatic hypotension, tachycardia, sedation, confusion (esp. elderly), anxiety, nervousness, agitation, nausea, vomiting, anorexia, constipation or diarrhea, flatulence, abdominal cramps, sexual dysfunction (increased or decreased libido; impotence, painful ejaculation). Pharmacokinetics $T_{1/2} = 31-46$ h; time to maximal clinical benefit $= 2-4$ weeks; hepatic elimination (active metabolite = nortriptyline). **Therapeutic plasma level = 110–250 ng/mL** (plasma levels and therapeutic effect are subject to wide interpatient variability).	Contraindications Any hypersensitivity to a TCA, concomitant use of MAO inhibitors. Precautions Use with caution in patients with severe cardiovascular disease, seizure disorders. Patients with schizophrenia may experience worsening psychosis; patients with bipolar disorder may experience a switch to mania. Dosage reductions necessary in patients with hepatic or severe renal dysfunction. Pregnancy Category: C Lactation issues TCAs are excreted into breast milk. Use with caution.
Amoxapine Asendin, various generics Tablets 25 mg, 50 mg, 100 mg, 150 mg	**Major depression** 50 mg 2–3 times daily starting dose. Titrate to 100 mg 2–3 times daily within 1 week. If no effect with 300 mg/d for 2 weeks, increase dose to 400 mg/d in divided doses. **Elderly patients:** 25 mg 2–3 times daily starting dose. Titrate to 50 mg 2–3 times daily within 1	Administration Issues Maintenance doses may be given once daily at bedtime to reduce daytime sedation. Not recommended for children < 16 yrs old. Drug–Drug Interactions **Hypertensive crisis:** clonidine, MAO inhibitors (can occur weeks after MAOI discontinued).	ADRs Dry mouth, urinary retention, blurred vision, constipation, orthostatic hypotension, tachycardia, sedation, confusion (esp. elderly), anxiety, nervousness, agitation, nausea, vomiting, anorexia, constipation or diarrhea, flatulence, abdominal cramps, sexual dysfunction (increased or decreased libido; impotence, painful ejaculation).	Contraindications Any hypersensitivity to a TCA, concomitant use of MAO inhibitors. Precautions Due to its dopamine effects, patients may develop **neuroleptic malignant syndrome or tardive dyskinesia.** Use with caution in patients with severe cardiovascular disease, seizure disorders.

	week. If required, may titrate to 300 mg/d after 2 weeks.	**Increased TCA level:** cimetidine, ethanol, fluoxetine, haloperidol, oral contraceptives, phenothiazines. **Decreased TCA level:** barbiturates, phenytoin, chronic ethanol ingestion. **Increased level of:** phenytoin, warfarin. **Increased effect:** anticholinergic agents, ethanol or sedatives (increased CNS effects), thyroid hormones (increased effect of both drugs). **Decreased effect of:** guanethidine, methyldopa.	Pharmacokinetics $T_{1/2}$ = 8 h; time to maximal clinical benefit = 2–4 weeks **Therapeutic plasma level = 200–500 ng/mL** (plasma levels and therapeutic effect are subject to wide interpatient variability).	Patients with schizophrenia may experience worsening psychosis; patients with bipolar disorder may experience a switch to mania. Dosage reductions necessary in patients with hepatic or severe renal dysfunction. Pregnancy Category: C Lactation Issues TCAs are excreted into breast milk. Use with caution.
Clomipramine Anafranil, various generics Capsules 25 mg, 50 mg, 75 mg	**Obsessive–compulsive disorder** 25 mg/d starting dose. Titrate by 25 mg/d to 200 mg/d within 2 weeks. Max dose of 250 mg/d. **Children and Adolescents:** 25 mg/d at bedtime starting dose. Titrate within 2 weeks by 25 mg/d to the smaller of 3 mg/kg or 100 mg/d. Max dose of 3 mg/kg or 200 mg/d. **Unlabeled uses:** 25–200 mg/d used for chronic pain	Administration Issues Maintenance doses may be given once daily at bedtime to reduce daytime sedation; Not recommended for children < 10 yrs old. Drug–Drug Interactions **Hypertensive crisis:** clonidine, MAO inhibitors (can occur weeks after MAOI discontinued). **Increased TCA level:** cimetidine, ethanol, fluoxetine, haloperidol, oral contraceptives, phenothiazines. **Decreased TCA level:** barbiturates, phenytoin, chronic ethanol ingestion. **Increased level of:** phenytoin, warfarin. **Increased effect:** anticholinergic agents, ethanol or sedatives (increased CNS effects), thyroid hormones (increased effect of both drugs).	ADRs Dry mouth, urinary retention, blurred vision, constipation, orthostatic hypotension, tachycardia, sedation, confusion (esp. elderly), anxiety, nervousness, agitation, nausea, vomiting, anorexia, constipation or diarrhea, flatulence, abdominal cramps, sexual dysfunction (increased or decreased libido; impotence, painful ejaculation). Pharmacokinetics $T_{1/2}$ = 19–37 h; time to maximal clinical benefit = 2–4 weeks. **Therapeutic plasma level = 80–100 ng/mL** (plasma levels and therapeutic effect are subject to wide interpatient variability).	Contraindications Any hypersensitivity to a TCA, concomitant use of MAO inhibitors. Precautions Use with caution in patients with severe cardiovascular disease, seizure disorders. Patients with schizophrenia may experience worsening psychosis; patients with bipolar disorder may experience a switch to mania. Dosage reductions necessary in patients with hepatic or severe renal dysfunction. Pregnancy Category: C Lactation Issues TCAs are excreted into breast milk. Use with caution in nursing mothers.

(*continues on next page*)

311.1 Tricyclic Antidepressants (TCAs) *continued from previous page*

Drug and Dosage Forms	Usual Dosage Range	Administration Issues and Drug–Drug Interactions	Common Adverse Drug Reactions (ADRs) and Pharmacokinetics	Contraindications, Pregnancy Category, and Lactation Issues
Clomipramine *cont.*		**Decreased effect of:** guanethidine, methyldopa.		
Desipramine Norpramin, various generics Tablets 10 mg, 25 mg, 50 mg, 75 mg, 100 mg, 150 mg Capsules 25 mg, 50 mg	**Major depression** 75 mg/d at bedtime starting dose. Titrate by 50 mg/d every 3–4 days to 150–200 mg/d. Max dose is 300 mg/d. **Adolescent and elderly patients:** 10–25 mg at bedtime starting dose. Titrate by 10–25 mg every 3–4 days to 100–150 mg/d. **Unlabeled uses:** 50–200 mg/d for facilitation of cocaine withdrawal. Has also been used in bulimia nervosa. **Traumatic brain injury** 10 mg tid; up to 150 mg/d	Administration Issues Maintenance doses may be given once daily at bedtime to reduce daytime sedation. Not recommended for children <12 yrs old. Drug–Drug Interactions **Hypertensive crisis:** clonidine, MAO inhibitors; can occur weeks after MAOI discontinued. **Increased TCA level:** cimetidine, ethanol, fluoxetine, haloperidol, oral contraceptives, phenothiazines. **Decreased TCA level:** barbiturates, phenytoin, chronic ethanol ingestion. **Increased level of:** phenytoin, warfarin. **Increased effect:** anticholinergic agents, ethanol or sedatives (increased CNS effects), thyroid hormones (increased effect of both drugs). **Decreased effect of:** guanethidine, methyldopa.	ADRs Dry mouth, urinary retention, blurred vision, constipation, orthostatic hypotension, tachycardia, sedation, confusion (esp. elderly), anxiety, nervousness, agitation, nausea, vomiting, anorexia, constipation or diarrhea, flatulence, abdominal cramps, sexual dysfunction (increased or decreased libido; impotence, painful ejaculation). Pharmacokinetics $T_{1/2}$ = 12–24 h; time to maximal clinical benefit = 2–4 weeks. **Therapeutic plasma level = 125–300 ng/mL** (plasma levels and therapeutic effect are subject to wide interpatient variability).	Contraindications Any hypersensitivity to a TCA, concomitant use of MAO inhibitors. Precautions Use with caution in patients with severe cardiovascular disease, seizure disorders. Patients with schizophrenia may experience worsening psychosis; patients with bipolar disorder may experience a switch to mania. Dosage reductions necessary in patients with hepatic or severe renal dysfunction. Pregnancy Category: C Lactation Issues TCAs are excreted into breast milk. Use with caution.
Doxepin Adapin, Sinequan, various generics Capsules 10 mg, 25 mg, 50 mg, 75 mg, 100 mg, 150 mg	**Major depression or anxiety** 75 mg/d at bedtime starting dose. Titrate up to 300 mg/d in 2–3 divided doses. Single dose ≤ 150 mg. **Elderly patients:** 10–25 mg at bedtime starting dose. Titrate by 10–25 mg every 3–5 days to 75 mg/d.	Administration Issues Maintenance doses may be given once daily at bedtime to reduce daytime sedation. Concentrate: protect from light, dilute in juice or other liquid; Not recommended for children < 12 yrs old.	ADRs Dry mouth, urinary retention, blurred vision, constipation, orthostatic hypotension, tachycardia, sedation, confusion (esp. elderly), anxiety, nervousness, agitation, nausea, vomiting, anorexia, constipation or diarrhea, flatulence, abdominal cramps, sexual dysfunction	Contraindications Any hypersensitivity to a TCA, concomitant use of MAO inhibitors, patients with glaucoma or tendency to urinary retention. Precautions Use with caution in patients with severe cardiovascular disease, seizure disor-

Liquid concentrate 10 mg/1 mL	**Unlabeled uses:** 50–300 mg/d used for chronic pain; 10–30 mg/d used in chronic urticaria and angioedema, nocturnal pruritis in atopic eczema. Also used in peptic ulcer disease.	Drug–Drug Interactions **Hypertensive crisis:** clonidine, MAO inhibitors; can occur weeks after MAOI discontinued. **Increased TCA level:** cimetidine, ethanol, fluoxetine, haloperidol, oral contraceptives, phenothiazines. **Decreased TCA level:** barbiturates, phenytoin, chronic ethanol ingestion. **Increased level of:** phenytoin, warfarin. **Increased effect:** anticholinergic agents, ethanol or sedatives (increased CNS effects), thyroid hormones (increased effect of both drugs). **Decreased effect of:** guanethidine, methyldopa.	(increased or decreased libido; impotence, painful ejaculation). Pharmacokinetics $T_{1/2}$ = 8–24 h; time to maximal clinical benefit = 2–4 weeks. **Therapeutic plasma level = 100–200 ng/mL** (plasma levels and therapeutic effect are subject to wide interpatient variability).	ders. Patients with schizophrenia may experience worsening psychosis; patients with bipolar disorder may experience a switch to mania. Dosage reductions necessary in patients with hepatic or severe renal dysfunction. Pregnancy Category: C Lactation Issues TCAs are excreted into breast milk. Use with caution.
Imipramine Tofranil, Janimine, various generics Tablets 10 mg, 25 mg, 50 mg Capsules (imipramine pamoate-Tofranil PM) 75 mg, 100 mg, 125 mg, 150 mg	**Major depression** starting dose of 75 mg/d in divided doses or at bedtime. Titrate by 25 mg every 3–4 days up to 300 mg/d **Adolescent or elderly patients:** starting dose of 10–40 mg at bedtime. Titrate by 10–25 mg every 3–4 days up to 100 mg/d **Children:** starting dose of 1.5 mg/kg divided tid. Titrate by 1–1.5 mg/kg/d every 3–5 days to maximum of 5 mg/kg/d **Childhood enuresis >6 yrs old** 25 mg 1 hour before bedtime. Titrate by 25 mg/d each week up to 50 mg for children <12 yr and 75 mg for children >12	Administration Issues Maintenance doses may be given once daily at bedtime to reduce daytime sedation. Drug–Drug Interactions **Hypertensive crisis:** clonidine, MAO inhibitors; can occur weeks after MAOI discontinued. **Increased TCA level:** cimetidine, ethanol, fluoxetine, haloperidol, oral contraceptives, phenothiazines. **Decreased TCA level:** barbiturates, phenytoin, chronic ethanol ingestion. **Increased level of:** phenytoin, warfarin.	ADRs Dry mouth, urinary retention, blurred vision, constipation, orthostatic hypotension, tachycardia, sedation, confusion (esp. elderly), anxiety, nervousness, agitation, nausea, vomiting, anorexia, constipation or diarrhea, flatulence, abdominal cramps, sexual dysfunction (increased or decreased libido; impotence, painful ejaculation). Pharmacokinetics $T_{1/2}$ = 11–25 h; time to maximal clinical benefit = 2–4 weeks; hepatic elimination (active metabolite = desipramine). **Therapeutic plasma level = 200–350 ng/mL** (plasma levels and therapeutic effect are subject to wide interpatient variability).	Contraindications Any hypersensitivity to a TCA, concomitant use of MAO inhibitors. Precautions Use with caution in patients with severe cardiovascular disease, seizure disorders. Patients with schizophrenia may experience worsening psychosis; patients with bipolar disorder may experience a switch to mania. Dosage reductions necessary in patients with hepatic or severe renal dysfunction. Pregnancy Category: B Lactation Issues TCAs are excreted into breast milk. Use with caution in nursing mothers.

311.1 Tricyclic Antidepressants (TCAs) *continued from previous page*

Drug and Dosage Forms	Usual Dosage Range	Administration Issues and Drug–Drug Interactions	Common Adverse Drug Reactions (ADRs) and Pharmacokinetics	Contraindications, Pregnancy Category, and Lactation Issues
Imipramine *cont.*	**Unlabeled uses** 75–150 mg/d used in chronic pain; 25–75 mg/d used in panic disorder. Also used in bulimia nervosa.	**Increased effect:** anticholinergic agents, ethanol or sedatives (increased CNS effects), thyroid hormones (increased effect of both drugs). **Decreased effect of:** guanethidine, methyldopa.		
Nortriptyline Aventyl, Pamelor Capsules 10 mg, 25 mg, 50 mg, 75 mg Liquid 10 mg/5 mL	**Major depression** starting dose of 25 mg 3–4 times daily. Titrate every 3–4 days to 100–150 mg/d. **Elderly patients:** starting dose of 10–25 mg at bedtime. Titrate by 25 mg/d every 3–4 days up to 75 mg/d **Unlabeled uses:** 25–75 mg/d used in panic disorder. 50–125 mg/d used in premenstrual depression. 75 mg/d used in chronic urticaria and angioedema, nocturnal pruritis in atopic eczema **Traumatic brain injury** 25 mg q hs; up to 150 mg/d	Administration Issues Maintenance doses may be given once daily at bedtime to reduce daytime sedation. Not recommended for children. Drug–Drug Interactions **Hypertensive crisis:** clonidine, MAO inhibitors; can occur weeks after MAOI discontinued. **Increased TCA level:** cimetidine, ethanol, fluoxetine, haloperidol, oral contraceptives, phenothiazines. **Decreased TCA level:** barbiturates, phenytoin, chronic ethanol ingestion. **Increased level of:** phenytoin, warfarin. **Increased effect of:** anticholinergic agents, ethanol or sedatives (increased CNS effects), thyroid hormones (increased effect of both drugs). **Decreased effect of:** guanethidine, methyldopa.	ADRs Dry mouth, urinary retention, blurred vision, constipation, orthostatic hypotension, tachycardia, sedation, confusion (esp. elderly), anxiety, nervousness, agitation, nausea, vomiting, anorexia, constipation or diarrhea, flatulence, abdominal cramps, sexual dysfunction (increased or decreased libido; impotence, painful ejaculation). Pharmacokinetics $T_{1/2} = 18-44$ h; time to maximal clinical benefit $= 2-4$ weeks. **Therapeutic plasma level = 50–150 ng/mL** (plasma levels and therapeutic effect are subject to wide interpatient variability).	Contraindications Any hypersensitivity to a TCA, concomitant use of MAO inhibitors. Precautions Use with caution in patients with severe cardiovascular disease, seizure disorders. Patients with schizophrenia may experience worsening psychosis; patients with bipolar disorder may experience a switch to mania. Dosage reductions necessary in patients with hepatic or severe renal dysfunction. Pregnancy Category: C Lactation Issues TCAs are excreted into breast milk. Use with caution.
Protriptyline Vivactil, various generics	**Major depression** 15–40 mg/d in 3–4 divided doses starting dose. Titrate by 15 mg every 3–4 days to 60 mg/d	Administration Issues Maintenance doses may be given once daily at bedtime to reduce daytime sedation. Not recommended for children.	ADRs Dry mouth, urinary retention, blurred vision, constipation, orthostatic hypotension, tachycardia, sedation, confusion	Contraindications Any hypersensitivity to a TCA, concomitant use of MAO inhibitors.

Tablets 5 mg, 10 mg	**Adolescent and elderly patients:** 5 mg 1–3 times daily starting dose. Titrate by 5 mg/d every 3–7 days to 15–20 mg/d **Unlabeled use:** obstructive sleep apnea.	Drug–Drug Interactions **Hypertensive crisis:** clonidine, MAO inhibitors; can occur weeks after MAOI discontinued. **Increased TCA level of:** cimetidine, ethanol, fluoxetine, haloperidol, oral contraceptives, phenothiazines. **Decreased TCA level of:** barbiturates, phenytoin, chronic ethanol ingestion. **Increased level of:** phenytoin, warfarin. **Increased effect of:** anticholinergic agents, ethanol or sedatives (increased CNS effects), thyroid hormones (increased effect of both drugs). **Decreased effect of:** guanethidine, methyldopa.	(esp. elderly), anxiety, nervousness, agitation, nausea, vomiting, anorexia, constipation or diarrhea, flatulence, abdominal cramps, sexual dysfunction (increased or decreased libido; impotence, painful ejaculation). Pharmacokinetics $T_{1/2}$ = 67–89 h; time to maximal clinical benefit = 2–4 weeks. **Therapeutic plasma level = 100–200 ng/mL** (plasma levels and therapeutic effect are subject to wide interpatient variability).	Precautions Use with caution in patients with severe cardiovascular disease, seizure disorders. Patients with schizophrenia may experience worsening psychosis; patients with bipolar disorder may experience a switch to mania. Dosage reductions necessary in patients with hepatic or severe renal dysfunction. Pregnancy Category: C Lactation Issues TCAs are excreted into breast milk. Use with caution.
Trimipramine Surmontil Capsules 25 mg, 50 mg, 100 mg	**Major depression** 75 mg/d at bedtime starting dose. Titrate by 25–50 mg q 3 days to max dose of 200 mg/d. For severe depression, max dose of 300 mg/d **Adolescent and elderly patients:** 50 mg/d at bedtime starting dose. Titrate by 25 mg every 3 days to 100 mg/d **Unlabeled use:** 50 mg/d used in chronic urticaria and angioedema, nocturnal pruritis in atopic eczema. Also, has been used in peptic ulcer disease.	Administration issues Maintenance doses may be given once daily at bedtime to reduce daytime sedation. Not recommended for children. Drug–Drug Interactions **Hypertensive crisis:** clonidine, MAO inhibitors; can occur weeks after MAOI discontinued. **Increased TCA level:** cimetidine, ethanol, fluoxetine, haloperidol, oral contraceptives, phenothiazines. **Decreased TCA level:** barbiturates, phenytoin, chronic ethanol ingestion. **Increased level of:** phenytoin, warfarin. **Increased effect of:** anticholinergic agents, ethanol or sedatives (increased CNS effects), thyroid hormones (increased effect of both drugs). **Decreased effect of: guanethidine, methyldopa.**	ADRs Dry mouth, urinary retention, blurred vision, constipation, orthostatic hypotension, tachycardia, sedation, confusion (esp. elderly), anxiety, nervousness, agitation, nausea, vomiting, anorexia, constipation or diarrhea, flatulence, abdominal cramps, sexual dysfunction (increased or decreased libido; impotence, painful ejaculation). Pharmacokinetics $T_{1/2}$ = 7–30 h; time to maximal clinical benefit = 2–4 weeks. **Therapeutic plasma level = 180 ng/mL** (plasma levels and therapeutic effect are subject to wide interpatient variability).	Contraindications Any hypersensitivity to a TCA, concomitant use of MAO inhibitors. Precautions Use with caution in patients with severe cardiovascular disease, seizure disorders. Patients with schizophrenia may experience worsening psychosis; patients with bipolar disorder may experience a switch to mania. Dosage reductions necessary in patients with hepatic or severe renal dysfunction. Pregnancy Category: C Lactation Issues TCAs are excreted into breast milk. Use with caution.

311.2 Miscellaneous Antidepressants

Drug and Dosage Forms	Usual Dosage Range	Administration Issues and Drug–Drug Interactions	Common Adverse Drug Reactions (ADRs) and Pharmacokinetics	Contraindications, Pregnancy Category, and Lactation Issues
Buproprion Wellbutrin Tablets 75 mg, 100 mg Sustained Release 100 mg, 150 mg, 200 mg Extended-release tablets 100 mg, 150 mg, 300 mg	**Major depression** Starting dose of 100 mg bid. Titrate by 100 mg/d after 3 days to dose of 300 mg/d. Max dose is 450 mg/d; max single dose is 150 mg. **Elderly patients:** Starting dose of 50–100 mg/d. Titrate dose by 50–100 mg/d every 3–4 days as tolerated.	Administration Issues Safety/efficacy not yet established in those <18 years old. Drug–Drug Interactions Buproprion induces metabolism **Increased toxicity of:** levodopa; buproprion (with concurrent use of MAOIs). **Increased seizure potential:** other agents that decrease seizure threshold.	ADRs Dizziness, tachycardia, dry mouth, headache, sweating, tremor, sedation, insomnia, auditory disturbances, nausea, vomiting, constipation, weight loss, anorexia. Pharmacokinetics $T_{1/2}$ = 8–24 h; time to maximal clinical benefit = 2–4 weeks; hepatic elimination.	Contraindications Hypersensitivity; seizure disorder; current or prior diagnosis of bulimia or anorexia; concurrent use of MAOI within 14 days of stopping the MAOI. Pregnancy Category: B Lactation Issues Women should not nurse while receiving buproprion.
Maprotiline Ludiomil, various generics Tablets 25 mg, 50 mg, 75 mg	**Depressive illness associated with dysthymic disorder, manic-depression, and major depressive disorder** 75 mg/d at bedtime starting dose. Titrate after 2 weeks by 25 mg/d to 150 mg/d. Max dose 225 mg/d. **Elderly patients:** 25 mg/d at bedtime starting dose. Titrate by 25 mg/d every week to 50–75 mg/d.	Administration issues Maintenance doses may be given once daily at bedtime to reduce daytime sedation. Not recommended for children. Drug–Drug Interactions **Hypertensive crisis:** clonidine, MAO inhibitors; can occur weeks after MAO inhibitor discontinued. **Increased maprotiline level:** cimetidine, ethanol, fluoxetine, haloperidol, oral contraceptives, phenothiazines. **Decreased maprotiline level:** barbiturates, phenytoin, chronic ethanol ingestion. **Increased level of:** phenytoin, warfarin. **Increased effect:** anticholinergic agents, ethanol or sedatives (increased CNS effects), thyroid hormones (increased effect of both drugs). **Decreased effect of:** guanethidine, methyldopa.	ADRs Dry mouth, urinary retention, blurred vision, orthostatic hypotension, tachycardia, sedation, confusion (esp. elderly), hallucinations, anxiety, nervousness, agitation, nausea, vomiting, anorexia, constipation or diarrhea, flatulence, abdominal cramps, sexual dysfunction (increased or decreased libido; impotence, painful ejaculation). Pharmacokinetics $T_{1/2}$ = 21–25 h; time to maximal clinical benefit = 2–4 weeks. **Therapeutic plasma level = 200–300 ng/mL** (plasma levels and therapeutic effect are subject to wide interpatient variability).	Contraindications any hypersensitivity to tetracyclic; concomitant use of MAO inhibitors, known or suspected seizure disorder. Precautions Use with caution in patients with severe cardiovascular disease. Patients with schizophrenia may experience worsening psychosis; patients with bipolar disorder may experience a switch to mania. Dosage reductions necessary in patients with hepatic or severe renal dysfunction. Pregnancy Category: B Lactation Issues Maprotiline is excreted into breast milk. Use with caution.

Mirtazapine Remeron, Remeron SolTab Tablets 15 mg, 30 mg, 45 mg Tablets, orally disintegrating 15 mg, 30 mg, 45 mg	**Treatment of depression** Initial: 15 mg/d as a single dose May increase every 1–2 wk to max 45 mg/d. Use lower doses in geriatric patients.	Administration Issues Take in the evening, prior to sleep. Drug–Drug Interactions **Additive CNS effects** when taken with alcohol and benzodiazepines.	ADRs Somnolence, dry mouth, constipation, increased appetite, weight gain, abnormal dreams, dizziness. Pharmacokinetics $T_{1/2} = 20-40$ h; extensively metabolized.	Contraindications Any hypersensitivity to drug, concomitant use of MAO inhibitors. Precautions Use with caution in patients with severe cardiovascular disease. Patients with schizophrenia may experience worsening psychosis; patients with bipolar disorder may experience a switch to mania. Dosage reductions necessary in patients with hepatic or severe renal dysfunction. Pregnancy Category: C Lactation Issues It is not known if mirtazapine is excreted in breast milk. Use with caution.
Nefazodone Serzone Tablets 50 mg, 100 mg, 150 mg, 200 mg, 250 mg	**Major depression** starting dose of 100 mg twice daily. Titrate dose by 100–200 mg/d each week up to 600 mg/d. **Elderly patients** start with 50 mg twice daily. Titrate by 50–100 mg/d each week.	Administration Issues Safety/efficacy not established for those <18 years old. Drug–Drug Interactions **Hypertensive crisis:** with MAOIs. **Increased levels of:** astemizole, terfenadine, benzodiazepines, digoxin due to inhibition of metabolism. **Decreased levels** of propranolol and **increased levels** of nefazodone during concurrent use.	ADRs Postural hypotension, dizziness, drowsiness, insomnia, agitation, nausea, dry mouth, constipation, headache. Pharmacokinetics Rapidly absorbed but bioavailability is 20% due to first-pass metabolism; $T_{1/2} = 2-4$ h but with active metabolites $T_{1/2} = 11-24$ h; time to maximal benefit is 2–4 weeks.	Contraindications Hypersensitivity; coadministration with terfenadine or astemizole. Pregnancy Category: C Lactation Issues It is unknown if nefazodone and metabolites are excreted in breast milk. Use caution in nursing mothers.
Trazodone Desyrel, Desyrel Dividose, various generic forms Tablets 50 mg, 100 mg, 150 mg, 300 mg Tablet dividose 150 mg, 300 mg	**Major depression** starting dose of 50 mg tid. Titrate dose by 50 mg/d q 3–4 days. Max dose is 600 mg/d in 2 divided doses. **Elderly patients:** start at 25–50 mg at bedtime. Titrate dose by 25–50 mg q 3–4 d to 75–150 mg/d.	Administration Issues Safety/efficacy not established in children <18 yrs old. Drug–Drug Interactions **Increased CNS depressant activity:** alcohol, barbiturates, other CNS depressants.	ADRs Orthostatic tension, tachycardia, palpitations, drowsiness, fatigue, dizziness, tremors, anger, hostility, nightmares, confusion, nervousness, dry mouth, nausea, vomiting, constipation, bad taste in mouth, priapism, decreased libido, impotence, malaise, weight gain or loss musculoskeletal aches/pains.	Contraindications Hypersensitivity. Other Precautions Use cautiously in patients with preexisting cardiac disease—patients may be predisposed to cardiac arrhythmias. Pregnancy Category: C

(*continues on next page*)

311.2 Miscellaneous Antidepressants *continued from previous page*

Drug and Dosage Forms	Usual Dosage Range	Administration Issues and Drug–Drug Interactions	Common Adverse Drug Reactions (ADRs) and Pharmacokinetics	Contraindications, Pregnancy Category, and Lactation Issues
Trazodone *cont.*	**Traumatic brain injury** 50 mg, up to 150 mg q hs	**Increased levels of:** digoxin, phenytoin.	Pharmacokinetics $T_{1/2}$ = 4–9 h; time to maximal clinical benefit = 1–4 weeks. **Therapeutic plasma level = 800–1600 ng/mL** (plasma levels and therapeutic effect are subject to wide interpatient variability).	Lactation Issues Trazodone and metabolites have been found in breast milk. Use cautiously in nursing mothers.
Venlafaxine Effexor, Effexor XR Tablets 25 mg, 37.5 mg, 50 mg, 75 mg, 100 mg Extended release, capsules 37.5 mg, 75 mg, 150 mg	**Major Depression** Regular Release Tablets: starting dose of 75 mg/d in 2–3 divided doses. Titrate by 75 mg/d q 4d up to 225 mg/d or, for severely depressed patients, up to 350 mg/d. Max dose is 375 mg/d generally divided tid Extended Release Tablets 37.5 or 75 mg qd initially; increase at dosages of 75 mg/d at intervals of at least 4 d; max XR = 225 mg/d **Elderly patients:** 12.5–25 mg bid. Titrate by 25 mg/d as needed. **Hepatic dysfunction:** 50% dose reduction recommended. **Renal dysfunction:** 25% dose reduction with 50% dose reduction in patients undergoing hemodialysis.	Administrative Issues Safety/efficacy in those <18 years old not established. Extended release tablets can be taken in the morning or evening, but patients should consistently take venlafaxine at the same time every day. Patients stabilized on the regular release tablets can be converted to the nearest equivalent dose of the XR tablets. Drug–Drug Interactions **Hypertensive crisis:** with concurrent use of MAOIs. **Increased levels of venlafaxine by:** cimetidine (but does not appear to affect metabolite).	ADRs Hypertension, drowsiness, dry mouth, dizziness, insomnia, nervousness, anxiety, nausea, constipation, anorexia, abnormal ejaculation/orgasm, impotence, headache, asthenia. Pharmacokinetics $T_{1/2}$ = 5 h and for active metabolite it is 11 h; Time to maximal benefit is 2–4 weeks.	Contraindications Hypersensitivity. Pregnancy Category: C Lactation Issues Unknown whether venlafaxine is excreted in breast milk. Use caution in nursing mothers.

311.3 Monoamine Oxidase Inhibitors

Drug and Dosage Forms	Usual Dosage Range	Administration Issues and Drug–Drug & Drug–Food Interactions	Common Adverse Drug Reactions (ADRs) and Pharmacokinetics	Contraindications, Pregnancy Category, and Lactation Issues
Phenelzine Nardil Tablets 15 mg	**Atypical major depression** 15 mg tid. Titrate to 60 mg/d within a few days as tolerated. Max dose is 90 mg/d.	Drug–Drug Interactions **Increased effect of:** beta blockers (bradycardia); antidiabetic agents (hypoglycemia); meperidine (agitation, seizures, diaphoresis, fever, coma, death).	ADRs Orthostatic hypotension, disturbances in cardiac rate and rhythm, dizziness, vertigo, headache, overactivity, hyperreflexia, tremors, jitteriness, confusion, memory impairment, insomnia, weak-	Contraindications Hypersensitivity, pheochromocytoma, congestive heart failure, history of liver disease or abnormal LFTs, severe renal impairment, cardiovascular disease, cerebrovascular disease.

	Elderly patients: 7.5 mg/d starting dose. Titrate by 7.5–15 mg/d every 3–4 days to 60 mg/d **Unlabeled uses:** bulimia nervosa, panic disorder with agoraphobia and treatment of cocaine addiction	**Hypertensive crisis:** antidepressants (SSRIs, TCAs); levodopa, sympathomimetics, L-tryptophan. Drug–Food Interactions Tyramine-containing foods in combination with MAOI may result in hypertensive crisis: cheeses (camembert, cheddar, others); meat/fish (fermented sausages - bologna, pepperoni; pickled or spoiled herring; others); alcoholic beverages; fruit/vegetables (yeast extracts, others); other foods containing vasopressors (e.g., caffeine, chocolate).	ness, fatigue, drowsiness, agitation, constipation, nausea, diarrhea, abdominal pain, edema, dry mouth, blurred vision, rash, anorexia, weight gain. Pharmacokinetics Onset of activity 3–4 weeks; effects continue for up to 2 weeks after discontinuation; primarily renal route of elimination.	Other Precautions Use with caution in elderly due to increased morbidity from adverse effects. Pregnancy Category: Effects have not been established; use only when benefits far outweigh risks. Lactation Issues: Effects not well established, use with caution.
Tranylcypromine Parnate Tablets 10 mg	**Atypical reactive depression** 30 mg/d in divided doses. Titrate after 2 weeks by 10 mg/d to 60 mg/d. **Unlabeled uses:** bulimia nervosa, panic disorder with agoraphobia and treatment of cocaine addiction	Drug–Drug Interactions **Increased effect of:** beta blockers (bradycardia); antidiabetic agents (hypoglycemia); meperidine (agitation, seizures, diaphoresis, fever, coma, death). **Hypertensive crisis:** antidepressants (SSRIs, TCAs); levodopa, sympathomimetics, L-tryptophan. Drug–Food Interactions Tyramine-containing foods in combination with MAOI may result in hypertensive crisis: cheeses (camembert, cheddar, others); meat/fish (fermented sausages - bologna, pepperoni; pickled or spoiled herring; others); alcoholic beverages; fruit/vegetables (yeast extracts, others); other foods containing vasopressors (e.g., caffeine, chocolate).	ADRs Orthostatic hypotension, disturbances in cardiac rate and rhythm, dizziness, vertigo, headache, overactivity, hyperreflexia, tremors, jitteriness, confusion, memory impairment, insomnia, weakness, fatigue, drowsiness, agitation, constipation, nausea, diarrhea, abdominal pain, edema, dry mouth, blurred vision, rash, anorexia, weight gain. Pharmacokinetics Onset of activity 10 days; effects continue for up to 10 days after discontinuation; $T_{1/2} = 90-190$ minutes; primarily renal route of elimination.	Contraindications Hypersensitivity, pheochromocytoma, congestive heart failure, history of liver disease or abnormal LFTs, severe renal impairment, cardiovascular disease, cerebrovascular disease. Other Precautions Use with caution in elderly due to increased morbidity from adverse effects. Pregnancy Category Effects have not been established; use only when benefits far outweigh risks. Lactation Issues Effects not well established, use with caution. Tranylcypromine is excreted in breast milk.

311.4 Selective Serotonin Reuptake Inhibitors

Drug and Dosage Forms	Usual Dosage Range	Administration Issues and Drug–Drug Interactions	Common Adverse Drug Reactions (ADRs) and Pharmacokinetics	Contraindications, Pregnancy Category and Lactation Issues
Citalopram Celexa Tablets 10 mg, 20 mg, 40 mg Oral solution 2 mg/mL	**Treatment of depression** **Initial therapy:** 20 mg qd, Generally with an increase to a dose of 40 mg/day. Dose increases usually should occur in increments of 20 mg at intervals of no less than 1 week. Max dose: 40mg/day **Elderly/hepatic function impairment:** 20 mg/day is the recommended dose for most elderly patients and patients with hepatic impairment, with titration to 40 mg/day only for nonresponding patients.	Administration Issues Administer once daily in the morning or evening, with or without food. Safety and efficacy in children (<18 years of age) have not been established. May cause photosensitivity (sensitivity to sunlight). Avoid prolonged exposure to the sun and other ultraviolet light. Use sunscreens and wear protective clothing until tolerance is determined. Drug Interactions In vitro studies indicate that cytochrome P450 3A4 and 2C19 are the primary enzymes involved in metabolism of citalopram. Inhibitors of 3A4 (e.g., **azole antifungals, macrolide antibiotics**) and 2C19 (e.g., **omeprazole**) would be expected to increase plasma citalopram levels. Inducers of 3A4 (e.g., **carbamazepine**) would be expected to decrease citalopram levels. **Serotonin syndrome:** The serotonin syndrome is a complication of therapy with serotonergic drugs. It is most commonly observed when 2 drugs that potentiate serotonergic neurotransmission are used concurrently. When this problem occurs with SSRIs, it is most commonly in the setting of other concurrent medications such as MAOIs, which increase serotonin by different mechanisms. Other such drugs include **tryptophan, amphetamines or other psychostimulants, other antidepressants that increase 5-HT levels, buspirone, lithium, or dopamine agonists (e.g., amantadine, bromocriptine).**	ADRs Insomnia, somnolence, anxiety, tremor, fatigue, nausea, diarrhea, dry mouth, anorexia, abnormal ejaculation, upper respiratory tract infections. Pharmacokinetics $T_{1/2}$ 35 h.	Contraindications Hypersensitivity to SSRIs or any inactive ingredients; in combination with an MAO inhibitor, or within 14 days of discontinuing an MAOI. Pregnancy Category: C Lactation Issues Citalopram is excreted in breast milk. Exercise caution when SSRIs are administered to a nursing woman. Decide whether to discontinue nursing or discontinue the drug taking into account the importance of the drug to the mother.

Fluoxetine Prozac, Prozac weekly, Sarafem, generics Tablets 10 mg, 20 mg Pulvules 10 mg, 20 mg, 40 mg Capsules, Delayed-release 90 mg Liquid Solution 20 mg/5 mL Sarafem Pulvules 10 mg, 20 mg	**Major depression** 20 mg/d q am. Max dose: 80 mg/d Weekly dosing: Initiate Prozac weekly 7 d after the last 20 mg daily dose. **Obsessive–compulsive disorder** 20 mg/d to 60 mg/d q am Max dose: 80 mg/d **Traumatic brain injury** Initial dose: 5–10 mg qd Maintenance dose: 10–20 mg qd Sarafem for premenstrual dysphoric disorder (PMDD): 20 mg QD Max dose: 80 mg **Hepatic dysfunction or elderly:** Initiate at lower dose (i.e., 10 mg q am)	Administration Issues Administer dose in the morning to decrease nighttime insomnia. Drug–Drug Interactions **Hypertensive crisis:** MAO inhibitors (may be fatal). Avoid use within 14 days of stopping an MAOI; avoid starting MAOI within 5 weeks of stopping the SSRI. **Serotonin Syndrome:** MAOI, other antidepressants, buspirone, lithium, tryptophan, triptoins, dopamine agonists, psychostimulants. **Increased levels of:** carbamazepine, phenytoin, lithium. **Increased effect:** dextromethorphan (hallucinations occurred), L-tryptophan (headache, sweating, dizziness, agitation, nausea, vomiting). **Decreased effect of SSRI:** cyproheptadine.	ADRs: nervousness, insomnia, anxiety, asthenia, tremor, increased sweating, dizziness; decreased libido; drowsiness, fatigue, anorexia, weight loss, nausea, diarrhea, dyspepsia, constipation Pharmacokinetics $T_{1/2} = 48-96$ hrs; $T_{1/2}$ of active metabolite 48–216 hrs	Contraindications Hypersensitivity, in combination with MAOI, coadministration with astemizole or terfenadine Other precautions: Watch for precipitation of mania in bipolar patients. SSRIs may precipitate seizures in patients with seizure disorder Pregnancy Category: C Lactation Issues SSRIs are secreted in breast milk although no adverse effects have been noted in infants. Use caution in nursing women.
Fluvoxamine Luvox, generics Tablets 25 mg, 50 mg, 100 mg	**Obsessive–compulsive disorder** Initiate at 50 mg q hs (range 100–300 mg/d). Increase dose in 50 mg increments q 4 to 7 days as needed. Doses >100 mg/d should be divided in two doses **Hepatic dysfunction or elderly:** Initiate at lower dose (i.e., 25 mg q hs—50 mg tablets are scored)	Administration Issues Safety and efficacy in children <18 years old not established. Drug–Drug Interactions **Hypertensive crisis:** MAO inhibitors (may be fatal) Avoid use within 14 days of stopping an MAOI; avoid starting MAOI within 5 weeks of stopping the SSRI. **Serotonin Syndrome:** MAOIs, other antidepressants, buspirone, lithium, tryptophan triptoins, dopamine agonists, other psychostimulants. **Increased levels of:** theophylline, carbamazepine, warfarin.	ADRs Nervousness, anxiety, asthenia, tremor, increased sweating, dizziness; decreased libido; drowsiness or fatigue, anorexia, nausea, diarrhea, dyspepsia, constipation. Pharmacokinetics $T_{1/2} = 14-16$ h; 80% protein binding; renal route of elimination.	Contraindications Hypersensitivity, in combination with MAOI, coadministration with astemizole or terfenadine. Other precautions Watch for precipitation of mania in bipolar patients. SSRIs may precipitate seizures in patients with seizure disorder. Pregnancy Category: C Lactation Issues SSRIs are secreted in breast milk although no adverse effects have been noted in infants. Use caution in nursing women.

(*continues on next page*)

311.4 Selective Serotonin Reuptake Inhibitors *continued from previous page*

Drug and Dosage Forms	Usual Dosage Range	Administration Issues and Drug–Drug Interactions	Common Adverse Drug Reactions (ADRs) and Pharmacokinetics	Contraindications, Pregnancy Category and Lactation Issues
Fluvoxamine *cont.*		**Increased effect:** diltiazem (bradycardia), L-tryptophan (headache, sweating, dizziness, agitation, nausea, vomiting). **Increased effect of SSRI:** lithium, TCAs. **Decreased effect of SSRI:** smoking. **Increased risk of cardiac arrhythmias:** astemizole and terfenadine.		
Paroxetine Paxil, Paxil CR Tablets 10 mg, 20 mg, 30 mg, 40 mg Tablets, controlled-release 12.5 mg, 25 mg, 37.5 mg Suspension 10 mg/5 mL	**Major depression** Initiate at 20 mg q am (range 20–50 mg/d). Dose titration of 10 mg/d every week as needed. **Panic disorder** Initiate at 10 mg/QD (target dose 40 mg/d) Max dose 60 mg/d **Traumatic brain injury** 5 mg/d; may titrate up to 20–30 mg/d **Renal/hepatic dysfunction or elderly:** Initiate at 10 mg/d (range 10–40 mg/d)	Administration Issues Administer dose in the morning to decrease nighttime insomnia. Drug–Drug Interactions **Hypertensive crisis:** MAO inhibitors (may be fatal) Avoid use within 14 days of stopping an MAOI; avoid starting MAOI within 5 weeks of stopping the SSRI. **Serotonin Syndrome:** MAOIs, other antidepressants, buspirone, lithium, tryptophan, tripans, dopamine agonists, other psychostimulants. **Increased levels of:** phenytoin, warfarin. **Increased SSRI plasma levels:** cimetidine. **Increased effect:** L-tryptophan (headache, sweating, dizziness, agitation, nausea, vomiting).	ADRs Nervousness, insomnia, anxiety, asthenia, tremor, increased sweating, dizziness; decreased libido; drowsiness or fatigue may occur, anorexia, nausea, diarrhea, dyspepsia, constipation. Pharmacokinetics $T_{1/2}$ = 21 h.	Contraindications Hypersensitivity, in combination with MAOI, coadministration with astemizole or terfenadine. Other precautions Watch for precipitation of mania in bipolar patients. SSRIs may precipitate seizures in patients with seizure disorder. Pregnancy Category: C Lactation Issues SSRIs are secreted in breast milk although no adverse effects have been noted in infants. Use caution in nursing women.

		Decreased effect of SSRI: barbiturates, phenytoin.		
Sertraline Zoloft Tablets 25 mg, 50 mg, 100 mg Oral Concentrate 20 mg/mL	**Major depression** Initiate at 50 mg qd (range 50–200 mg/d). Dose titration of 50 mg/d every week as needed. **Panic disorder and Posttraumatic stress disorder** Initiate 25 mg QD; increase dose to 50 mg/d after one week **Premenstrual dysphoric disorder (PMDD)** Continuous: 50 mg QD (max 150 mg QD) Intermittent: 50 mg QD for last 14 days of menstrual cycle (max. 100 mg qd) **Pediatric OCD** 25 mg/d (6–12 yrs) or 50 mg/d (13–17 yrs) titrate to effect (max 200 mg) **Traumatic brain injury** 25 mg/d; may titrate up to 100 mg/d **Renal/hepatic dysfunction** Initiate at 25 mg/d (50 mg tablets are scored)	Administration Issues Administer dose in the morning to decrease nighttime insomnia. Dilute oral concentrate with 4 oz. of water or ginger ale, lemon-lime soda, lemonade, or orange juice; administer immediately after mixing. Drug–Drug Interactions **Hypertensive crisis:** MAO inhibitors (may be fatal). Avoid use within 14 days of stopping an MAOI; avoid starting MAOI within 5 weeks of stopping the SSRI. **Serotonin Syndrome:** MAOIs, other antidepressants, buspirone, lithium, tryptophan, tripans, dopamine agonists, other psychostimulants. **Increased levels of:** tolbutamide, lithium, warfarin.	ADRs Nervousness, insomnia, anxiety, asthenia, tremor, increased sweating, dizziness; decreased libido; drowsiness or fatigue may occur, Male sexual dysfunction: primary ejaculatory delay, anorexia, nausea, diarrhea, dyspepsia, constipation. Pharmacokinetics $T_{1/2} = 26–104$ hrs.	Contraindications Hypersensitivity, in combination with MAOI, coadministration with astemizole or terfenadine. Other precautions Watch for precipitation of mania in bipolar patients. SSRIs may precipitate seizures in patients with seizure disorder. Pregnancy Category: C Lactation Issues SSRIs are secreted in breast milk although no adverse effects have been noted in infants. Use with caution in nursing women.

312. Antipsychotic Agents

312.1 Phenothiazines

Drug and Dosage Forms	Usual Dosage Range	Administration Issues, Drug–Drug & Drug–Food Interactions	Common Adverse Drug Reactions (ADRs) and Pharmacokinetics	Contraindications, Pregnancy Category, and Lactation Issues
Chlorpromazine Thorazine, various generics Tablets 10 mg, 25 mg, 50 mg, 100 mg, 200 mg Capsules (sustained release) 30 mg, 75 mg, 150 mg, 200 mg, 300 mg Syrup 10 mg/5 mL Concentrate 30 mg/mL, 100 mg/mL Suppositories 25 mg, 100 mg	**Psychotic disorders** 10 mg tid to qid or 25 mg bid to tid. Titrate by 20–50 mg/d biweekly until desired response. Doses of 800 mg/d not unusual. **Elderly or debilitated:** 10–25 mg 1–2 times daily; slowly titrate as needed by 10–25 mg/d every 4–7 days **Pediatrics:** Oral dose: 0.5 mg/kg q 4–6 hrs rectal dose: 1 mg/kg q 6–8 hrs	Administration Issues To decrease daytime sedation, the daily dose may be given as a single dose at bedtime once appropriate dose has been established. Concentrates: Protect from light, dilute in juices or other liquid. Titrate oral doses to patient response; once psychosis is controlled, decrease dose to lowest dose required by patient; not recommended for those <6 mos old. Drug–Drug Interactions **Increased effect:** CNS effects (alcohol); EPS effect (fluoxetine, lithium); sedation/ hypotension (meperidine). **Increased level of:** TCAs, valproic acid, phenytoin (or decreased level), propranolol (also increases level of antipsychotic). **Decreased level of antipsychotic:** aluminum antacids, barbiturates, carbamazepine, charcoal. **Decreased effect of antipsychotic:** anticholinergics.	**ADRs** Sedation High: High Anticholinergic effects (dry mouth, constipation, urinary retention, blurred vision): Moderate. Extrapyramidal effects (pseudoparkinsonism, akathisia, dystonias): Moderate. Orthostatic hypotension: High. **Other ADRs** Arrhythmias, myocardial depression, headache, hypertension, lethargy, restlessness, weight gain, hyperactivity, breast enlargement, galactorrhea, menstrual irregularities, changes in libido, tardive dyskinesia (after prolonged therapy—may be irreversible); neuroleptic malignant syndrome. Pharmacokinetics $T_{1/2} = 10-20$ h; full therapeutic effect may not be seen for 6 weeks.	Contraindications Hypersensitivity, comatose, or severely depressed states, concomitant use of large amounts of other CNS depressants; bone marrow depression, liver damage, cerebral arteriosclerosis, coronary artery disease. Precautions Use cautiously in patients with: seizure disorders, impaired renal or hepatic dysfunction, hyperthyroidism; do not use 48 hrs prior to myelography; do not abruptly withdraw therapy. Pregnancy/Lactation issues Safety not established. Use only when benefits clearly outweigh risks to fetus/neonate.
Fluphenazine Prolixin, Permitil, various generics Tablets 1 mg, 2.5 mg, 5 mg, 10 mg Elixir 2.5 mg/5 mL Concentrate 5 mg/mL	**Psychotic disorders** 0.5–10 mg/d tid to qid (daily doses >3 mg not usually necessary) **Elderly or debilitated:** 1–2.5 mg daily; slowly titrate as needed Decanoate or Ethanate injection 12.5–25 mg initially q 3–4 weeks. Subsequent dose and interval based on response. Max dose is 100 mg. One study showed 20 mg/d of short acting agent is	Administration Issues To decrease daytime sedation, the daily dose may be given as a single dose at bedtime once appropriate dose has been established. Concentrates: Protect from light, dilute in juices or other liquid; Titrate oral doses to patient response; once psychosis is controlled, decrease dose to lowest dose required by patient; not generally recommended in children < 12 yrs old.	**ADRs** Sedation: Low. Anticholinergic effects (dry mouth, constipation, urinary retention, blurred vision): Low. Extrapyramidal effects (pseudoparkinsonism, akathisia, dystonias): High.	Contraindications Hypersensitivity, comatose or severely depressed states, concomitant use of large amounts of other CNS depressants; bone marrow depression, liver damage, cerebral arteriosclerosis, coronary artery disease. Precautions Use cautiously in patients with: seizure disorders, impaired renal or hepatic dysfunction, hyperthyroidism; do not use 48

Fluphenazine Enanthate or Deconate Prolixin Enanthate, Prolixin Deconate, various generics Injection 25 mg/mL	approximately equal to 25 mg of deconate q 3 weeks. **Traumatic Brain Injury** start at 0.5 mg bid	Drug–Drug Interactions **Increased effect:** CNS effects (alcohol); EPS effect (fluoxetine, lithium); sedation/ hypotension (meperidine). **Increased level of:** TCAs, valproic acid, phenytoin (or decreased level), propranolol (also increases level of antipsychotic). **Decreased level of antipsychotic:** aluminum antacids, barbiturates, carbamazepine, charcoal. **Decreased effect of antipsychotic:** anticholinergics.	Orthostatic hypotension: Low. **Other ADRs** Arrhythmias, myocardial depression, headache, hypertension, lethargy, restlessness, weight gain, hyperactivity, breast enlargement, galactorrhea, menstrual irregularities, changes in libido, tardive dyskinesia (after prolonged therapy—may be irreversible); neuroleptic malignant syndrome. Pharmacokinetics $T_{1/2} = 10-20$ h; full therapeutic effect may not be seen for 6 weeks.	hrs prior to myelography; do not abruptly withdraw therapy. Pregnancy/Lactation Issues Safety not established. Use only when benefits clearly outweigh risks to fetus/neonate.
Mesoridazine Serentil Tablets 10 mg, 25 mg, 50 mg, 100 mg Concentrate 25 mg/mL	**Psychotic disorders** 50 mg tid; titrate based on response to 100–400 mg/d **Elderly or debilitated patients:** 10 mg qd to bid; slow titration to max dose of 250 mg/d **Behavior problems in mental deficiency and chronic brain syndrome:** 25 mg tid; titrate to 75–300 mg/d **Psychoneurotic manifestations:** 10 mg tid; titrate to 30–150 mg/d	Administration Issues To decrease daytime sedation, the daily dose may be given as a single dose at bedtime once appropriate dose has been established. Concentrates: Protect from light, dilute in juices or other liquid. Titrate oral doses to patient response; once psychosis is controlled, decrease dose to lowest dose required by patient; not generally recommended for children < 12 yrs old. Drug–Drug Interactions **Increased effect:** CNS effects (alcohol); EPS effect (fluoxetine, lithium); sedation/hypotension (meperidine). **Increased level of:** TCAs, valproic acid, phenytoin (or decreased level), propranolol (also increases level of antipsychotic). **Decreased level of antipsychotic:** aluminum antacids, barbiturates, carbamazepine, charcoal. **Decreased effect of antipsychotic:** anticholinergics.	**ADRs** Sedation High: High. Anticholinergic effects (dry mouth, constipation, urinary retention, blurred vision): High. Extrapyramidal effects (pseudoparkinsonism, akathisia, dystonias): Low. Orthostatic hypotension : Moderate. **Other ADRs** Arrhythmias, myocardial depression, headache, hypertension, lethargy, restlessness, weight gain, hyperactivity, breast enlargement, galactorrhea, menstrual irregularities, changes in libido, tardive dyskinesia (after prolonged therapy—may be irreversible); neuroleptic malignant syndrome. Pharmacokinetics $T_{1/2} = 10-20$ h; full therapeutic effect may not be seen for 6 weeks.	Contraindications Hypersensitivity, comatose or severely depressed states, concomitant use of large amounts of other CNS depressants; bone marrow depression, liver damage, cerebral arteriosclerosis, coronary artery disease. Precautions Use cautiously in patients with: seizure disorders, impaired renal or hepatic dysfunction, hyperthyroidism; do not use 48 hrs prior to myelography; do not abruptly withdraw therapy. Pregnancy/Lactation Issues Safety not established. Use only when benefits clearly outweigh risks to fetus/neonate.

(*continues on next page*)

312.1 Phenothiazines *continued from previous page*

Drug and Dosage Forms	Usual Dosage Range	Administration Issues, Drug–Drug & Drug–Food Interactions	Common Adverse Drug Reactions (ADRs) and Pharmacokinetics	Contraindications, Pregnancy Category, and Lactation Issues
Perphenazine Trilafon, various generics Tablets 2 mg, 4 mg, 8 mg, 16 mg Concentrate 16 mg/5 mL	**Psychotic disorders** 4–16 mg tid **Elderly or debilitated patients:** 2–4 mg qd to bid; slowly titrate to max dose of 32 mg/d **Pediatrics:** (> 12 yrs old) 4 mg tid; slowly titrate as needed	Administration Issues To decrease daytime sedation, the daily dose may be given as a single dose at bedtime once appropriate dose has been established. Concentrates: Protect from light, dilute in juices or other liquid; titrate oral doses to patient response; once psychosis is controlled, decrease dose to lowest dose required by patient; not generally recommended for children < 12 yrs old. Drug–Drug Interactions **Increased effect:** CNS effects (alcohol); EPS effect (fluoxetine, lithium); sedation/ hypotension (meperidine). **Increased level of:** TCAs, valproic acid, phenytoin (or decreased level), propranolol (also increases level of antipsychotic). **Decreased level of antipsychotic:** Aluminum antacids, barbiturates, carbamazepine, charcoal. **Decreased effect of antipsychotic:** anticholinergics.	ADRs Sedation: Low. Anticholinergic effects (dry mouth, constipation, urinary retention, blurred vision): Low. Extrapyramidal effects (pseudoparkinsonism, akathisia, dystonias): High. Orthostatic hypotension: Low. **Other ADRs** Arrhythmias, myocardial depression, headache, hypertension, lethargy, restlessness, weight gain, hyperactivity, breast enlargement, galactorrhea, menstrual irregularities, changes in libido, tardive dyskinesia (after prolonged therapy—may be irreversible); neuroleptic malignant syndrome. Pharmacokinetics $T_{1/2}$ = 10–20 h; full therapeutic effect may not be seen for 6 weeks.	Contraindications Hypersensitivity, comatose or severely depressed states, concomitant use of large amounts of other CNS depressants; bone marrow depression, liver damage, cerebral arteriosclerosis, coronary artery disease. Precautions Use cautiously in patients with: seizure disorders, impaired renal or hepatic dysfunction, hyperthyroidism; do not use 48 hrs prior to myelography; do not abruptly withdraw therapy. Pregnancy/Lactation Issues Safety not established. Use only when benefits clearly outweigh risks to fetus/neonate.
Prochlorperazine Compazine, various generics Tablets 5 mg, 10 mg, 25 mg Capsules sustained release 10 mg, 15 mg, 30 mg Suppositories 2.5 mg, 5 mg, 25 mg	**Psychotic disorders** 5–10 mg tid to qid; slowly titrate to 50–75 mg/d for less severe conditions; slowly titrate to 100–150 mg/d for more severe conditions. **Elderly or debilitated patients:** 2.5–5 mg qd to bid; slowly titrate to max dose of 75 mg/d	Administration Issues To decrease daytime sedation, the daily dose may be given as a single dose at bedtime once appropriate dose has been established. Titrate oral doses to patient response; once psychosis is controlled, decrease dose to lowest dose required by patient; not recommended for children < 2 yrs old.	ADRs Sedation: Moderate. Anticholinergic effects (dry mouth, constipation, urinary retention, blurred vision): Low. Extrapyramidal effects (pseudoparkinsonism, akathisia, dystonias): High.	Contraindications Hypersensitivity, comatose, or severely depressed states, concomitant use of large amounts of other CNS depressants; bone marrow depression, liver damage, cerebral arteriosclerosis, coronary artery disease. Precautions Use cautiously in patients with: seizure disorders, impaired renal or hepatic dysfunction, hyperthyroidism; do not use 48

Syrup 5 mg/5 mL	**Pediatrics:** (2–12 yrs old) 2.5 mg bid to tid; slowly titrate to max dose of 20 mg/d (for 2–5 yrs old) or 25 mg/d (for 6–12 yrs old) **Nonpsychotic anxiety:** 5 mg tid to qid; max dose is 20 mg/d; max length of therapy is 12 weeks.	Drug–Drug Interactions **Increased effect:** CNS effects (alcohol); EPS effect (fluoxetine, lithium); sedation/ hypotension (meperidine). **Increased level of:** TCAs, valproic acid, phenytoin (or decreased level), propranolol (also increases level of antipsychotic). **Decreased level of antipsychotic:** aluminum antacids, barbiturates, carbamazepine, charcoal. **Decreased effect of antipsychotic:** anticholinergics.	Orthostatic hypotension: Low. **Other ADRs** Arrhythmias, myocardial depression, headache, hypertension, lethargy, restlessness, weight gain, hyperactivity, breast enlargement, galactorrhea, menstrual irregularities, changes in libido, tardive dyskinesia (after prolonged therapy—may be irreversible); neuroleptic malignant syndrome. Pharmacokinetics $T_{1/2} = 10-20$ h; full therapeutic effect may not be seen for 6 weeks.	hrs prior to myelography; do not abruptly withdraw therapy. Pregnancy/Lactation Issues Safety not established. Use only when benefits clearly outweigh risks to fetus/neonate.
Thioridazine Mellaril, various generics Tablets 10 mg, 15 mg, 25 mg, 50 mg, 100 mg, 150 mg, 200 mg Concentrate (either alcohol or water base) 30 mg/mL, 100 mg/mL Suspension 25 mg/5 mL, 100 mg/5 mL	**Psychotic disorders** 50–100 mg tid; slowly titrate to max dose of 800 mg/d **Elderly or debilitated patients:** 25 mg tid; slowly titrate to max dose of 200 mg/d **Pediatrics:** (2–12 yrs old) 10 mg 2–3 times daily; slowly titrate to doses of 0.5–3 mg/kg/d	Administration Issues To decrease daytime sedation, the daily dose may be given as a single dose at bedtime once appropriate dose has been established. Concentrates: Protect from light, dilute in juices or other liquid. Titrate oral doses to patient response; once psychosis is controlled, decrease dose to lowest dose required by patient; not recommended for children < 2 yrs old. Drug–Drug Interactions **Increased effect:** CNS effects (alcohol); EPS effect (fluoxetine, lithium); sedation/ hypotension (meperidine). **Increased level of:** TCAs, valproic acid, phenytoin (or decreased level), propranolol (also increases level of antipsychotic). **Decreased level of antipsychotic:** aluminum antacids, barbiturates, carbamazepine, charcoal. **Decreased effect of antipsychotic:** anticholinergics.	ADRs Sedation: High. Anticholinergic effects (dry mouth, constipation, urinary retention, blurred vision): High. Extrapyramidal effects (pseudoparkinsonism, akathisia, dystonias): Low. Orthostatic hypotension: Moderate. **Other ADRs** Arrhythmias, myocardial depression, headache, hypertension, lethargy, restlessness, weight gain, hyperactivity, breast enlargement, galactorrhea, menstrual irregularities, changes in libido, tardive dyskinesia (after prolonged therapy—may be irreversible); neuroleptic malignant syndrome. Pharmacokinetics $T_{1/2} = 10-20$ h; full therapeutic effect may not be seen for 6 weeks.	Contraindications Hypersensitivity, comatose, or severely depressed states, concomitant use of large amounts of other CNS depressants; bone marrow depression, liver damage, cerebral arteriosclerosis, coronary artery disease. Precautions Use cautiously in patients with: seizure disorders, impaired renal or hepatic dysfunction, hyperthyroidism; do not use 48 hrs prior to myelography; do not abruptly withdraw therapy. Pregnancy/Lactation Issues: Safety not established. Use only when benefits clearly outweigh risks to fetus/neonate.

(continues on next page)

312.1 Phenothiazines *continued from previous page*

Drug and Dosage Forms	Usual Dosage Range	Administration Issues, Drug–Drug & Drug–Food Interactions	Common Adverse Drug Reactions (ADRs) and Pharmacokinetics	Contraindications, Pregnancy Category, and Lactation Issues
Trifluoperazine Stelazine, various generics Tablets 1 mg, 2 mg, 5 mg, 10 mg Concentrate 10 mg/mL	**Psychotic disorders** 2–5 mg bid; slowly titrate to max dose of 40 mg/d as needed **Elderly or debilitated patients:** 0.5–1 mg qd to bid; slowly titrate to max dose of 40 mg/d **Pediatrics:** (6–12 yrs old—usually should be hospitalized) 1 mg qd to bid; slowly titrate to 15 mg/d as needed **Nonpsychotic anxiety** 1–2 mg bid. Max dose is 6 mg/d; max length of therapy is 12 weeks.	Administration Issues To decrease daytime sedation, the daily dose may be given as a single dose at bedtime once appropriate dose has been established. Concentrates: Protect from light, dilute in juices or other liquid. Titrate oral doses to patient response; once psychosis is controlled, decrease dose to lowest dose required by patient; not recommended for children < 6 yrs old. Drug–Drug Interactions **Increased effect:** CNS effects (alcohol); EPS effect (fluoxetine, lithium); sedation/ hypotension (meperidine). **Increased level of:** TCAs, valproic acid, phenytoin (or decreased level), propranolol (also increases level of antipsychotic). **Decreased level of antipsychotic:** aluminum antacids, barbiturates, carbamazepine, charcoal. **Decreased effect of antipsychotic:** anticholinergics.	ADRs Sedation : Low. Anticholinergic effects (dry mouth, constipation, urinary retention, blurred vision): Low. Extrapyramidal effects (pseudoparkinsonism, akathisia, dystonias): High. Orthostatic hypotension : Low. **Other ADRs** Arrhythmias, myocardial depression, headache, hypertension, lethargy, restlessness, weight gain, hyperactivity, breast enlargement, galactorrhea, menstrual irregularities, changes in libido, tardive dyskinesia (after prolonged therapy—may be irreversible); neuroleptic malignant syndrome. Pharmacokinetics $T_{1/2}$ = 10–20 h; full therapeutic effect may not be seen for 6 weeks.	Contraindications Hypersensitivity, comatose, or severely depressed states, concomitant use of large amounts of other CNS depressants; bone marrow depression, liver damage, cerebral arteriosclerosis, coronary artery disease. Precautions Use cautiously in patients with: seizure disorders, impaired renal or hepatic dysfunction, hyperthyroidism; do not use 48 hrs prior to myelography; do not abruptly withdraw therapy. Pregnancy/Lactation Issues Safety not established. Use only when benefits clearly outweigh risks to fetus/neonate.

312.2 Other Typical Antipsychotic Agents

Drug and Dosage Forms	Usual Dosage Range	Administration Issues and Drug–Drug Interactions	Common Adverse Drug Reactions (ADRs) and Pharmacokinetics	Contraindications, Pregnancy Category, and Lactation Issues
Haloperidol Haldol, Haldol Deconate, various generics Tablets 0.5 mg, 1 mg, 2 mg, 5 mg, 10 mg, 20 mg	**Psychotic disorders** **Mild conditions, elderly or debilitated patients:** 0.5–2 mg bid to tid; slowly titrate to max dose of 100 mg/d as needed	Administration Issues To decrease daytime sedation, the daily dose may be given as a single dose at bedtime once appropriate dose has been established. Concentrates: Protect from light, dilute in juices or other liquid.	**ADRs** **Rate of most common:** Sedation: Low.	Contraindications Hypersensitivity, comatose, or severely depressed states, concomitant use of large amounts of other CNS depressants; bone marrow depression, liver damage, cerebral arteriosclerosis, coronary artery disease.

Concentrate 2 mg/mL Injection (deconate) 50 mg/mL, 100 mg/mL	**Severe psychoses:** 3–5 mg bid to tid; slowly titrate to 100 mg/d as needed **Pediatrics:** (3–12 yrs old) 0.5 mg/d in 2–3 divided doses; slowly titrate as needed (range is 0.05–0.15 mg/kg/d) Deconate injection (IM): No more than 100 mg initially (equivalent to 10 mg/d oral haloperidol) q 4 weeks **Tourette's syndrome** Pediatrics: 0.05–0.75 mg/kg/d divided bid to tid **Hyperactive children** dose range is 0.05–0.15 mg/kg/d divided bid to tid **Traumatic brain injury** start at 0.5 mg bid	Titrate oral doses to patient response; once psychosis is controlled, decrease dose to lowest dose required by patient; not recommended for children <3 yrs old. Drug–Drug Interactions **Increased effect:** CNS effects (alcohol); EPS effect (fluoxetine, lithium); sedation/ hypotension (meperidine). **Increased level of:** TCAs, valproic acid, phenytoin (or decreased level), propranolol (also increases level of antipsychotic). **Decreased level of antipsychotic:** aluminum antacids, barbiturates, carbamazepine, charcoal. **Decreased effect of antipsychotic:** anticholinergics.	Anticholinergic effects (dry mouth, blurred vision, constipation, urinary retention): Low. Extrapyramidal effects (pseudoparkinsonism, akathisia, dystonias): High. Orthostatic hypotension: Low. **Other ADRs** Arrhythmias, myocardial depression, headache, hypertension, lethargy, restlessness, weight gain, hyperactivity, breast enlargement, galactorrhea, menstrual irregularities, changes in libido, tardive dyskinesia (after prolonged therapy—may be irreversible); neuroleptic malignant syndrome. Pharmacokinetics $T_{1/2} = 24$ h; full therapeutic effect may not be seen for 6 weeks.	Precautions Use cautiously in patients with: seizure disorders, impaired renal or hepatic dysfunction, hyperthyroidism; do not use 48 hrs prior to myelography; do not abruptly withdraw therapy. Pregnancy/Lactation Issues Safety not established. Use only when benefits clearly outweigh risks to fetus/neonate.
Loxapine Loxitane Capsules 5 mg, 10 mg, 25 mg, 50 mg Concentrate 25 mg/mL	**Psychotic disorders** 10 mg bid; titrate fairly rapidly over first 7–10 days until psychotic symptoms are controlled. Max dose is 250 mg/d. **Elderly or debilitated patients:** 5–10 mg 1–2 times daily; slowly titrate to max dose of 125 mg/d as needed	Administration Issues To decrease daytime sedation, the daily dose may be given as a single dose at bedtime once appropriate dose has been established. Concentrates: Protect from light, dilute in juices or other liquid. Titrate oral doses to patient response; once psychosis is controlled, decrease dose to lowest dose required by patient; not recommended for children <16 yrs old. Drug–Drug Interactions **Increased effect:** CNS effects (alcohol); EPS effect (fluoxetine, lithium); sedation/ hypotension (meperidine). **Increased level of:** TCAs, valproic acid, phenytoin (or decreased level), propranolol (also increases level of antipsychotic).	ADRs Sedation: Moderate. Anticholinergic effects (dry mouth, blurred vision, constipation, urinary retention): Low. Extrapyramidal effects (pseudoparkinsonism, akathisia, dystonias): High. Orthostatic hypotension: Moderate. **Other ADRs** Arrhythmias, myocardial depression, headache, hypertension, lethargy, restlessness, weight gain, hyperactivity, breast enlargement, galactorrhea, menstrual irregularities, changes in libido, tardive dyskinesia (after prolonged ther	Contraindications Hypersensitivity, comatose or severely depressed states, concomitant use of large amounts of other CNS depressants; bone marrow depression, liver damage, cerebral arteriosclerosis, coronary artery disease. Precautions Use cautiously in patients with: seizure disorders, impaired renal or hepatic dysfunction, hyperthyroidism; do not use 48 hrs prior to myelography; do not abruptly withdraw therapy. Pregnancy/Lactation Issues Safety not established. Use only when benefits clearly outweigh risks to fetus/neonate.

312.2 Other Typical Antipsychotic Agents *continued from previous page*

Drug and Dosage Forms	Usual Dosage Range	Administration Issues and Drug–Drug Interactions	Common Adverse Drug Reactions (ADRs) and Pharmacokinetics	Contraindications, Pregnancy Category, and Lactation Issues
Loxapine *cont.*		**Decreased level of antipsychotic:** aluminum antacids, barbiturates, carbamazepine, charcoal. **Decreased effect of antipsychotic:** anticholinergics.	apy—may be irreversible); neuroleptic malignant syndrome. Pharmacokinetics $T_{1/2}$ = 10–20 h; full therapeutic effect may not be seen for 6 weeks.	
Molindone Moban Tablets 5 mg, 10 mg, 25 mg, 50 mg, 100 mg Concentrate 20 mg/mL	**Psychotic disorders** 50–75 mg/d; titrate to 225 mg/d as needed **Elderly or debilitated patients:** 5–10 mg 1–2 times daily; slowly titrate to max dose of 112 mg/d as needed	Administration Issues To decrease daytime sedation, the daily dose may be given as a single dose at bedtime once appropriate dose has been established. Concentrates: Protect from light, dilute in juices or other liquid. Titrate oral doses to patient response; once psychosis is controlled, decrease dose to lowest dose required by patient; not recommended for children <12 yrs old. Drug–Drug Interactions **Increased effect:** CNS effects (alcohol); EPS effect (fluoxetine, lithium); sedation/ hypotension (meperidine). **Increased level of:** TCAs, valproic acid, phenytoin (or decreased level), propranolol (also increases level of antipsychotic). **Decreased level of antipsychotic:** aluminum antacids, barbiturates, carbamazepine, charcoal. **Decreased effect of antipsychotic:** anticholinergics.	ADRs Sedation: Low. Anticholinergic effects (dry mouth, blurred vision, constipation, urinary retention): Low. Extrapyramidal effects (pseudoparkinsonism, akathisia, dystonias): High. Orthostatic hypotension: Low. **Other ADRs** Arrhythmias, myocardial depression, headache, hypertension, lethargy, restlessness, weight gain, hyperactivity, breast enlargement, galactorrhea, menstrual irregularities, changes in libido, tardive dyskinesia (after prolonged therapy—may be irreversible); neuroleptic malignant syndrome. Pharmacokinetics $T_{1/2}$ = 10–20 h; full therapeutic effect may not be seen for 6 weeks.	Contraindications Hypersensitivity, comatose, or severely depressed states, concomitant use of large amounts of other CNS depressants; bone marrow depression, liver damage, cerebral arteriosclerosis, coronary artery disease. Precautions Use cautiously in patients with: seizure disorders, impaired renal or hepatic dysfunction, hyperthyroidism; do not use 48 hrs prior to myelography; do not abruptly withdraw therapy. Pregnancy/Lactation Issues Safety not established. Use only when benefits clearly outweigh risks to fetus/neonate.
Pimozide Orap Tablets 1 mg, 2 mg	**Tourette's syndrome refractory to traditional treatment** 1–2 mg/d bid. Titrate dose every other day to 10 mg/d or 0.2 mg/kg (whichever is less)	Administration Issues Perform baseline ECG and periodically through treatment. Titrate oral doses to patient response; once psychosis is controlled, decrease dose to lowest dose re-	ADRs Sedation: Moderate. Anticholinergic effects (dry mouth, blurred vision, constipation, urinary retention): Moderate.	Contraindications Hypersensitivity; treatment of simple tics or tics other than those associated with Tourette's; drug-induced tics; long QT syndrome; history of cardiac arrhyth-

		quired by patient; efficacy/safety in <12 yrs old not established. Drug–Drug Interactions **Increased effect (additive):** phenothiazines, TCAs or Type 1 antiarrhythmics (additive prolongation of QT interval); CNS depressants.	Extrapyramidal effects (pseudoparkinsonism, akathisia, dystonias): High. Orthostatic hypotension: Low. **Other ADRs** Arrhythmias, myocardial depression, headache, hypertension, lethargy, restlessness, weight gain, hyperactivity, breast enlargement, galactorrhea, menstrual irregularities, changes in libido, tardive dyskinesia (after prolonged therapy—may be irreversible); neuroleptic malignant syndrome. Pharmacokinetics $T_{1/2}$ = 55 h.	mias; severe toxic CNS depression or comatose states. Pregnancy Category: C Lactation Issues Should not be used in nursing mothers.
Thiothixene Navane, various generics Capsules 1 mg, 2 mg, 5 mg, 10 mg, 20 mg Concentrate 5 mg/mL	**Psychotic disorders** 2 mg tid; slowly titrate to 15 mg/d as needed **Severe psychoses:** 5 mg bid; slowly titrate to 60 mg/d as needed **Elderly or debilitated patients:** 1–2 mg qd to bid; slowly titrate to max dose of 30 mg/d as needed **Pediatrics:** (>12 yrs old) 2 mg tid; slowly titrate to 15 mg/d as needed	Administration Issues To decrease daytime sedation, the daily dose may be given as a single dose at bedtime once appropriate dose has been established. Concentrates: protect from light, dilute in juices or other liquid. Titrate oral doses to patient response; once psychosis is controlled, decrease dose to lowest dose required by patient; not recommended for children <12 yrs old. Drug–Drug Interactions **Increased effect:** CNS effects (alcohol); EPS effect (fluoxetine, lithium); sedation/ hypotension (meperidine). **Increased level of:** TCAs, valproic acid, phenytoin (or decreased level), propranolol (also increases level of antipsychotic). **Decreased level of antipsychotic:** aluminum antacids, barbiturates, carbamazepine, charcoal. **Decreased effect of antipsychotic:** anticholinergics.	ADRs Sedation: Low. Anticholinergic effects (dry mouth, blurred vision, constipation, urinary retention): Low. Extrapyramidal effects (pseudoparkinsonism, akathisia, dystonias): High. Orthostatic hypotension: Low. **Other ADRs** Arrhythmias, myocardial depression, headache, hypertension, lethargy, restlessness, weight gain, hyperactivity, breast enlargement, galactorrhea, menstrual irregularities, changes in libido, tardive dyskinesia (after prolonged therapy—may be irreversible); neuroleptic malignant syndrome. Pharmacokinetics $T_{1/2}$ = 10–20 h; full therapeutic effect may not be seen for 6 weeks.	Contraindications Hypersensitivity, comatose or severely depressed states, concomitant use of large amounts of other CNS depressants; bone marrow depression, liver damage, cerebral arteriosclerosis, coronary artery disease. Precautions Use cautiously in patients with: seizure disorders, impaired renal or hepatic dysfunction, hyperthyroidism; do not use 48 hrs prior to myelography; do not abruptly withdraw therapy. Pregnancy/Lactation Issues Safety not established. Use only when benefits clearly outweigh risks to fetus/neonate.

312.3 Atypical Antipsychotics

Drug and Dosage Forms	Usual Dosage Range	Administration Issues and Drug–Drug Interactions	Common Adverse Drug Reactions (ADRs) and Pharmacokinetics	Contraindications, Pregnancy Category, and Lactation Issues
Clozapine Clozaril Tablets 12.5 mg 25 mg, 100 mg	**Severely Ill schizophrenia; refractory to traditional therapy** 25 mg 1–2 times daily. Titrate by 25–50 mg/d each day as tolerated to 300–450 mg/d. Further dosage adjustments: ≤ 100 mg/d, no more frequently than 1–2 times each week. Max dose is 900 mg/d. **Traumatic brain injury** start 25 mg qd; may titrate up to 300–400 mg/d divided qd or bid	Administration Issues **Due to potential for agranulocytosis, monitor WBC and granulocyte count weekly:** WBC <3500 at baseline: do not start therapy. WBC <3500 or >3500 with substantial drop after starting therapy: repeat WBC and monitor. WBC 3000–3500, granulocyte count >1500: monitor WBC twice weekly. WBC <3000 and gran <1500: stop therapy, monitor for infection, restart therapy when WBC returns to baseline. WBC <2000, gran <1000: stop therapy, monitor closely, do not rechallenge. Dispense medication for 1 week at a time. Titrate oral doses to patient response; once psychosis is controlled, decrease dose to lowest dose required by patient; safety/efficacy not established for those <16 yrs old. Drug–Drug Interactions **Increased effect (additive effects):** anticholinergics; antihypertensives; CNS agents; bone marrow suppressing agents.	ADRs Sedation: High. Anticholinergic effects (dry mouth, constipation, urinary retention, blurred vision, miosis): High. Extrapyramidal effects (pseudoparkinsonism, akathisia, dystonias): Low. Orthostatic hypotension: High. **Others ADRs** Tachycardia, hypertension, dizziness, headache, tremor, syncope, nightmares, restlessness, agitation, seizures, constipation, nausea, agranulocytosis. Pharmacokinetics $T_{1/2}$ = 12 h (at steady-state dosing).	Contraindications Hypersensitivity; myeloproliferative disorders; history of severe granulocytopenia; concomitant administration of other bone-marrow suppressing agents; severe CNS depression or comatose states. Pregnancy Category: B Lactation Issues Should not be used in nursing mothers.
Olanzapine Zyprexa, Zyprexa, Zydis Tablets 2.5 mg, 5 mg, 7.5 mg, 10 mg, 15 mg, 20 mg Tablets, Orally Disintegrating 5 mg, 10 mg, 15 mg, 20 mg	**Psychotic disorders** 5–10 mg qd, initially. Target dose = 10 mg within several days. **Debilitated patients:** starting dose = 5 mg; increase with caution	Administration Issues Dose increases should be done at an interval of not less than 1 week, though doses >10 mg did not show an increase in efficacy. Give without regards to meals. Avoid alcohol. Drug Interactions Olanzapine concentrations are **decreased** by carbamazepine; olanzapine may have additive effect with **antihypertensive agents** and may cause **increased CNS effects** when given with other CNS drugs and alcohol. Olanzapine may **decrease** the effectiveness of levodopa and dopamine agonists.	ADRs Orthostatic hypotension, weight gain, somnolence, dizziness, headache, agitation, insomnia, rhinitis, constipation, nervousness, hostility, akathisia. Pharmacokinetics $T_{1/2}$ = 21–54 h.	Contraindications Hypersensitivity. Pregnancy Category: C Lactation Issues Should not be used in nursing mothers.

Quetiapine Seroquel Tablets 25 mg, 100 mg, 200 mg, 300 mg	**Psychotic disorders** 25 mg bid, initially, with increases in increments of 25–50 mg bid or tid on the second and third day, as tolerated. Target dose range of 300–400 mg/d divided bid or tid by day 4. Further dosage increments should be done at intervals of ≥ 2 d. **Elderly, debilitated, hepatic impairment:** consider slower rate of dose escalation	Administration Issues Patients should be advised of the risk of orthostatic hypotension during drug initiation and following any dose increase. Drug may cause somnolence and avoid the use of alcohol while taking this medication. Drug Interactions Phenytoin and thioridazine may increase the clearance of quetiapine. Cimetidine may **decrease** quetiapine clearance. Quetiapine may antagonize the effects of levodopa and dopamine agonists and may **decrease** clearance of lorazepam.	ADRs Headache, somnolence, dizziness, constipation, dry mouth, dyspepsia, postural hypotension, tachycardia, rash, asthenia. Pharmacokinetics $T_{1/2}$ = 6 h; extensively metabolized.	Contraindications Hypersensitivity to drug. Pregnancy Category: C Lactation Issues Should not be used in nursing mothers.
Risperidone Risperdal Tablets 0.25 mg, 0.5 mg, 1 mg, 2 mg, 3 mg, 4 mg Solution 1 mg/mL Tablets, orally disintegrating 0.5 mg 1 mg 2 mg	**Psychotic disorders** 1 mg bid initially. Titrate by 1–2 mg/d every 2–3 days to target of 3 mg twice daily. Continued dose adjustments made each week. Max dose is 16 mg/d. **Elderly or debilitated patients:** 0.5 mg twice daily initially. Titrate by 0.5 mg twice daily every 3–5 days as tolerated.	Administration Issues Titrate oral doses to patient response; once psychosis is controlled, decrease dose to lowest dose required by patient; safety and efficacy in children is not established. Drug–Drug Interactions **Increased level of risperidone:** SSRIs, quinidine, others that inhibit P450IID6. **Decreased effect of:** levodopa. **Decreased level of risperidone:** carbamazepine.	ADRs Sedation: Low. Anticholinergic effects (dry mouth, constipation, urinary retention, blurred vision, miosis): Low. Extrapyramidal effects (pseudoparkinsonism, akathisia, dystonias): Low or none. Orthostatic hypotension: Low. **Other ADRs** Tachycardia; potential for QT prolongation and arrhythmias at high doses (12–16 mg/d), headache, agitation, anxiety, insomnia, constipation, dyspepsia, nausea/vomiting, rash, dry skin, rhinitis tardive dyskinesia (after prolonged therapy—may be irreversible); neuroleptic malignant syndrome. Pharmacokinetics $T_{1/2}$ = 3 h (risperidone) & 21 h (metabolite); $T_{1/2}$ (in poor metabolizers) = 20 h & 30 h, respectively.	Contraindications Hypersensitivity. Precautions Use caution in patients with: seizure disorder. Reduce dose in patients with severe renal or hepatic dysfunction, or those predisposed to orthostatic hypotension. Pregnancy Category: C Lactation Issues Safety is not established; women should not nurse.

312.4 Psychotherapeutic Combinations

Drug and Dosage Forms	Usual Dosage Range	Administration Issues and Drug–Drug Interactions	Common Adverse Drug Reactions (ADRs) and Pharmacokinetics	Contraindications, Pregnancy Category, and Lactation Issues
Chlordiazepoxide/ Amitriptyline Limbitrol DS, various generics Tablets 5 mg/12.5 mg, 10 mg/25 mg	**Moderate/Severe Depression Associated with Moderate/Severe Anxiety** 10 mg chlordiazepoxide and 25 mg amitriptyline 3–4 times daily. May titrate to 6 times daily. **Elderly or Debilitated Patients:** 5 mg/12.5 mg 1–2 times daily. Titrate as tolerated and as needed.	Administration Issues Once symptoms are controlled, slowly decrease dose to find lowest effective dose. Give largest dose at bedtime; in some patients, may give total daily dose at bedtime; not recommended for <6 yrs old. Drug–Drug Interactions See individual agents.	ADRs TCA: dry mouth, orthostatic hypotension, sedation, others. Chlordiazepoxide: drowsiness, ataxia, confusion (especially in elderly). Dependence: Prolonged use can lead to dependence; abrupt discontinuation can precipitate withdrawal symptoms (e.g., anxiety, flu-like illness, concentration difficulties, fatigue, anorexia, restlessness, confusion, psychosis, paranoid delusions, grand mal seizures). Withdrawal can occur after as little as 4–6 weeks of therapy. Drug Discontinuation: gradual decrease over 4–8 weeks Pharmacokinetics See individual agents.	Contraindication Any hypersensitivity to a TCA or benzodiazepine, concomitant use of MAO inhibitors. Other Precautions Use with caution in patients with severe cardiovascular disease, seizure disorders. Patients with schizophrenia may experience worsening psychosis; patients with bipolar disorder may experience a switch to mania. Dosage reductions necessary in patients with hepatic or severe renal dysfunction. Pregnancy Category: D Lactation Issues Excreted in breast milk—women should not nurse.
Perphenazine/Amitriptyline Etrafon, Triavil, various generics Tablets 2 mg/10 mg, 2 mg/25 mg, 4 mg/10 mg, 4 mg/25 mg, 4 mg/50 mg	**Moderate/Severe Anxiety or Agitation and Depressed Mood; Schizophrenic Patients with Symptoms of Depression; Anxiety and Depression Associated with Chronic Physical Disease; Anxiety and Depression that are not Clearly Differentiated:** 2–4 mg perphenazine with 10–50 mg amitriptyline 3–4 times daily	Administration Issues Once symptoms are controlled, slowly decrease dose to find lowest effective dose; not generally recommended for children <12 yrs old. Drug–Drug Interactions See individual agents.	ADRs Amitriptyline: dry mouth, orthostatic hypotension, sedation, others. Perphenazine: Sedation, anticholinergic effects (dry mouth, constipation, urinary retention, blurred vision, miosis), extrapyramidal effects (pseudoparkinsonism, akathisia, dystonias), orthostatic hypotension, tardive dyskinesia (after prolonged therapy—may be irreversible); neuroleptic malignant syndrome.	Contraindications Any hypersensitivity to a TCA or perphenazine, concomitant use of MAO inhibitors, comatose or severely depressed states, concomitant use of large amounts of other CNS depressants; bone marrow depression, liver damage, cerebral arteriosclerosis, coronary artery disease. Precautions: Use with caution in patients with severe cardiovascular disease, seizure disorders, hyperthyroidism. Dosage reductions necessary in patients with hepatic or severe renal dysfunction. Do not use 48 hrs prior to myelography; do not abruptly withdraw therapy.

			Pharmacokinetics See individual agents.	Pregnancy Issues Safety not established. Use only when benefits clearly outweigh risks to fetus/neonate. Lactation Issues TCAs are excreted into breast milk. Use with caution in nursing mothers.

313. Miscellaneous Psychotherapeutic Agents

Drug and Dosage Forms	Usual Dosage Range	Administration Issues and Drug–Drug Interactions	Common Adverse Drug Reactions (ADRs) and Pharmacokinetics	Contraindications, Pregnancy Category, and Lactation Issues
Lithium Eskalith, Lithane, Lithotabs, Lithobid, Eskalith CR, Cibalith-S, various generics Tablets 300 mg (8.12 mEq lithium) Capsules 150 mg (4.06 mEq Li), 300 mg (8.12 mEq Li), 600 mg (16.24 mEq Li) Tablets, slow release or controlled release 300 mg (8.12 mEq Li), 450 mg (12.18 mEq Li) Syrup 300 mg/5 mL (8.12 mEq Li)	**Acute manic episodes** 600 mg tid or 900 mg bid of the extended release form or until reach target serum levels of 0.8 to 1.4 mg/L **Maintenance therapy:** 300 mg tid to qid or until reach target serum levels of 0.4 to 1.0 mg/L **Elderly patients:** 300 mg bid. Titrate by 300 mg/d each week until reach target clinical and/or serum level **Renal impairment:** CrCl = 10–50 mL/min: give 50–75% of dose CrCl<10 mL/min: give 25–50% of dose Monitor levels closely **Unlabeled uses:** improves neutrophil count in cancer-chemotherapy induced neutropenia and in AIDS patients taking zidovudine; prophylaxis of cluster headaches, premenstrual tension, bulimia, alcoholism, SIADH, tardive dyskinesia, hyperthyroidism, postpartum affective psychosis, corticosteroid-induced psychosis. **Traumatic brain injury** start 300 mg qd to bid; monitor levels	Administration Issues Give with food to decrease GI upset. Drink 8–12 glasses of water while taking medication and maintain normal diet (including sodium). Draw serum levels 8–12 hours after the last dose at steady-state (reached in 5–7 days). Evaluate clinical response when interpreting serum levels; do not rely on serum levels alone; safety/efficacy not established in children <12 yrs old. Other monitoring parameters: Serum levels, electrolytes, renal function, hydration status Drug–Drug Interactions **Decreased Li levels:** Acetazolamide, urinary alkalinizers, osmotic diuretics. **Increased Li levels:** Fluoxetine, loop and thiazide diuretics, NSAIDs. **Increased Li toxicity/effect:** carbamazepine, haloperidol, methyldopa. **Li increases the effect of:** tricyclic antidepressants, iodide salts, neuromuscular blocking agents. **Li decreased the effect of:** sympathomimetics.	**Dose-related adverse effects are decreased when serum levels are maintained less than 1.5 mEq/L. Mild to moderate toxicity may occur at levels of 1.5–2.5 mEq/L; moderate to severe reactions may occur at levels >2 mEq/L.** ADRs Fine hand tremor, polyuria, mild thirst, and nausea can occur during initial therapy but may persist throughout treatment. Other ADRs Hypotension, arrhythmias, headache, blackouts, seizures, slurred speech, dizziness, drowsiness, blurred vision, cog wheel rigidity, impaired cognition, hallucinations, anorexia, nausea, vomiting, diarrhea, dry mouth, dehydration, impotence, oliguria, glycosuria, albuminuria, polyuria, symptoms of nephrogenic diabetes, euthyroid goiter or hypothyroidism. Overdose: **Levels <2mEq/L:** diarrhea, vomiting, nausea, drowsiness, muscular weakness, lack of coordination. **Levels 2–3mEq/L:** giddiness, ataxia, blurred vision, tinnitus, vertigo, confusion, slurred speech, blackouts, muscle twitching of entire limbs, agitation. **Levels >3mEq/L:** seizures, arrhythmias, hypotension, peripheral vascular collapse, stupor, muscle twitching, spasticity, coma. Pharmacokinetics $T_{1/2}$ = 24 h (range 17–36 h); onset of action 5 to 14 d; sodium and lithium compete for reabsorption in the kidney—sodium depletion will make kidney reabsorb lithium causing lithium levels to rise.	Contraindications None. Precautions/Warnings Lithium toxicity is increased in patients with significant renal or cardiovascular disease, severe debilitation, dehydration, or sodium depletion or in patients receiving diuretics. Monitor patients closely. Pregnancy Category: D Lactation Issues 40% of Li dose is excreted in breast milk. Patients should not nurse while taking Lithium.

Methylphenidate (CII) Ritalin, Ritalin-SR, Ritalin LA, Metadate DC, Concerta, various generics Tablets 5 mg, 10 mg, 20 mg Tablets, extended release 10 mg, 18 mg, 20 mg, 27 mg, 36 mg, 54 mg Capsules, extended-release 10 mg, 20 mg, 30 mg, 40 mg Tablets, chewable 2.5 mg, 5 mg, 10 mg Tablets, sustained release 20 mg	**Attention deficit disorder or narcolepsy** **Adults:** 10 mg bid to tid. Titrate to range of 10–60 mg/d as needed by patient. Metadate CD/Ritalin LA Recommended starting dose is 20 mg QD. Titrate according to package insert **Pediatrics (6 years or older):** 5 mg bid. Titrate by 5–10 mg/d each week as needed and tolerated. Max dose is 60 mg/d Sustained release: May use when dose for 8 hours is established using regular release tablets. **Unlabeled uses:** treatment of depression in elderly, cancer, and post-stroke patients	Administration Issues Give medication before breakfast and lunch (30–45 minutes prior to meals). Discontinue medication occasionally to assess need for continued therapy; safety/efficacy in <6 yrs old not established. SR and Methylin ER tablets have a duration of approx. 8 hrs. and may be used in place of regular tablets when the 8-hr dosage of the SR tablet and Methylin ER corresponds to the titrated 8-hr dosage of the regular tablets. SR and ER tablets must be swalled whole, never crushed or chewed. Take the chewable tablets with at least 8 oz. of fluid. Concerta Administer once daily in the morning with or without food. Advise patients to swall capsule whole with a liquid. Do not chew, crush or divide capsules. Metadate CD Administer QD in the morning. Can be swallowed whole, or the capsule may be opened and contents sprinkled onto a small amount (1 tablespoon) of applesauce and given immediately. The capsule and contents should not be crushed or chewed. Drug–Drug Interactions **Increases effect of methylphenidate:** monoamine oxidase inhibitors (headache, hypertension, nausea, etc). Decreased effect of: guanethidine.	ADRs Nervousness, insomnia, dizziness, headache, dyskinesia, tachycardia, palpitations, hyper- or hypotension, anorexia, nausea, weight loss. ADRs common among pediatrics Anorexia, weight loss, insomnia, tachycardia. Other effects may occur (listed above). Drug dependence: chronic use/abuse can lead to drug dependence. Carefully supervise withdrawal of medication. Pharmacokinetics $T_{1/2}$ = 1–3 h (pharmacological effect is 4–6 h).	Contraindications Hypersensitivity; glaucoma; marked anxiety, tension, or agitation; motor tics or family history or diagnosis of Tourette's syndrome. Pregnancy Category Use only when benefits far outweigh risks to fetus. Lactation Issues Methylphenidate is excreted in breast milk; safety not established.
Pemoline (CIV) Cylert, Pem ADD Tablets 18.75 mg, 37.5 mg, 75 mg Chewable tablets 37.5 mg	**Attention deficit disorder** 37.5 mg/d each morning. Titrate each week by 18.75 mg/d as needed. Max dose is 112.5 mg/d. **Unlabeled use:** 50–200 mg used for narcolepsy and excessive daytime sleepiness	Administration Issues Interrupt therapy occasionally to assess need for continued therapy. Gradual onset of action—full clinical benefit may not be seen for 3–4 weeks; safety/efficacy in <6 yrs old not established. Drug–Drug Interactions None.	ADRs Insomnia, headache, dizziness, dyskinetic movements, abnormal oculomotor function, anorexia, nausea, asymptomatic elevated LFTs, hepatitis, jaundice, rash, growth suppression with prolonged use. Drug dependence chronic use/abuse can lead to drug dependence. Carefully supervise withdrawal of medication. Pharmacokinetics $T_{1/2}$ = 7–12 h.	Contraindications Hypersensitivity; hepatic insufficiency. Use cautiously in renal insufficiency. Pregnancy Category: B Lactation Issues Safety not established. Use cautiously.

314. Skeletal Muscle Relaxants

Drug and Dosage Forms	Usual Dosage Range	Administration Issues and Drug–Drug Interactions	Common Adverse Drug Reactions (ADRs) and Pharmacokinetics	Contraindications, Pregnancy Category, and Lactation Issues
Baciofen Lioresal, various generics Tablets 10 mg, 20 mg Tablets, orally disintegrating 10 mg, 20 mg	**Spasticity resulting from multiple sclerosis (flexor spasms, clonus, muscular rigidity)** 5 mg tid for 3 days; 10 mg tid for 3 days; 15 mg tid for 3 days; 20 mg tid for 3 days. May further titrate but do not exceed 80 mg/d. **Elderly or debilitated patients:** 5 mg 2–3 times daily. Titrate as needed/tolerated. **Unlabeled uses:** 40 mg/d for tic douloureux or tardive dyskinesia	Administration Issues Avoid alcohol use; safety/efficacy not established in those <12 yrs old. Drug–Drug Interactions **Increased effect of:** alcohol, other CNS depressants.	ADRs Drowsiness, depression, excitement, euphoria, hallucinations, tinnitus, ataxia, nystagmus, diplopia, dry mouth, anorexia, taste disorder, diarrhea, urinary retention, dysuria, impotence, rash, edema, weight gain, increased perspiration, elevated blood sugar, elevated AST. Pharmacokinetics Absorption may be dose-dependent (may decrease with increasing doses); $T_{1/2} = 3-4$ h.	Contraindications Hypersensitivity; skeletal muscle spasm resulting from rheumatic disorders, stroke, cerebral palsy, or Parkinson's disease. Precautions Taper drug upon discontinuation to decrease risk of withdrawal symptoms (hallucinations, psychosis); use cautiously in those with seizure disorders, psychotic disorders, autonomic dysreflexia. Pregnancy Category: C Lactation Issues May be excreted in breast milk. Use cautiously.
Carisoprodol Soma, various generics Tablets 350 mg	**As an adjunct to rest, physical therapy and other measures for the relief of discomfort associated with acute, painful musculoskeletal conditions** 350 mg 3–4 times a day. Take last dose at bedtime.	Administration Issues May take with food; not recommended for children <12 yrs old. Drug–Drug Interactions None known.	ADRs Drowsiness, dizziness, vertigo, ataxia, tremor, agitation, irritability, headache, insomnia, syncope, depression, tachycardia, postural hypotension, flushing, nausea, vomiting, hiccoughs, epigastric distress, allergic reactions, rash, erythema multiforme, cross reaction with meprobamate. Pharmacokinetics Onset of action = 30 min; duration of action = 4–6 h.	Contraindications Hypersensitivity to this or meprobamate; acute intermittent porphyria. Precautions Use cautiously in patients with severe renal or hepatic dysfunction. Pregnancy/Lactation Issues Safety not established. Use cautiously. It is excreted in breast milk.
Chlorphenesin Carbamate Maolate Tablets 400 mg	**As an adjunct to rest, physical therapy and other measures for the relief of discomfort associated with acute, painful musculoskeletal conditions** 800 mg tid. Maintenance dose: 400 mg qid. Not recommended for use longer than 8 weeks.	Administration Issues May take with food. Safety not established in children. Drug–Drug Interactions **Increased effect of:** alcohol, other CNS depressants.	ADRs Drowsiness, dizziness, confusion, nervousness, headache, insomnia, stimulation, nausea, epigastric distress, hypersensitivity reactions, leukopenia, thrombocytopenia, agranulocytosis, pancytopenia. Pharmacokinetics Rapidly absorbed; $T_{1/2} = 3.5$ h.	Contraindications Hypersensitivity. Precautions Use cautiously in patients with severe hepatic dysfunction; not recommended for use longer than 8 weeks. Pregnancy/Lactation Issues Safety not established. Use cautiously or not at all.

Chlorzoxazone Paraflex, Remular-S, Parafon Forte DSC, various generics Tablets 250 mg, 500 mg Caplets 250 mg, 500 mg	**As an adjunct to rest, physical therapy and other measures for the relief of discomfort associated with acute, painful musculoskeletal conditions** 250 mg 3–4 times daily. May increase to 500 mg 3–4 times daily or 750 mg 3–4 times daily.	Administration Issues May take with food. Avoid alcohol or other CNS depressants. Drug–Drug Interactions **Increased effect of:** alcohol, other CNS depressants.	ADRs Drowsiness, dizziness, lightheadedness, malaise, overstimulation, minor GI upset, rash, hypersensitivity reactions, liver toxicity (drug-induced hepatitis), urine discoloration. Pharmacokinetics Onset = 1 h; duration of action = 3–4 h.	Contraindications Hypersensitivity. Precautions Use cautiously in patients with hepatic dysfunction; if signs of liver toxicity are observed; discontinue use. Pregnancy/Lactation Issues Safety not established.
Cyclobenzaprine Flexeril, various generics Tablets 5 mg, 10 mg	**As an adjunct to rest, physical therapy and other measures for the relief of discomfort associated with acute, painful musculoskeletal conditions** 10 mg tid. Do not exceed 60 mg/d. Do not give for longer than 2–3 weeks. **Unlabeled use:** 10–40 mg/d useful adjunct in fibrositis syndrome	Administration Issues Avoid alcohol or other CNS depressants; safety/efficacy in children <15 yrs old not established. Drug–Drug Interactions **Increased levels/effects of:** anticholinergics, barbiturates (CNS effects), clonidine (hypertensive crisis), oral anticoagulants. **Decreased levels/effects of:** guanethidine, levodopa. **Increased levels/effects of cyclobenzaprine:** cimetidine, fluoxetine, oral contraceptives, phenothiazines. **Decreased levels/effects of cyclobenzaprine:** barbiturates (drug levels), charcoal, smoking.	ADRs Drowsiness, dizziness, fatigue, tiredness, asthenia, blurred vision, headache, nervousness, convulsions, ataxia, vertigo, dysarthria, tremors, decreased/increased libido, extrapyramidal reactions, tachycardia, vasodilatation, hypotension, dry mouth, nausea, constipation, dyspepsia, vomiting, anorexia, gastritis, urinary retention, impotence, gynecomastia, hepatitis, jaundice, rash, photosensitivity. Pharmacokinetics Onset of action = 1 h; duration of 12–24 h; $T_{1/2}$ = 1–3 days.	Contraindications Hypersensitivity; concomitant use of MAO inhibitors; acute recovery phase of myocardial infarction, other cardiac problems (CHF, arrhythmias, heart block); hyperthyroidism. Precautions Use cautiously in patients with urinary retention, angle-closure glaucoma, intraocular pressure; use only for short (2–3 weeks) periods of time. Pregnancy Category B Lactation Issues Not known if excreted in breast milk. Use cautiously.
Dantrolene Sodium Dantrium Capsules 25 mg, 50 mg, 100 mg	**Spasticity from upper motor neuron disorders (e.g., spinal cord injury, stroke, cerebral palsy, multiple sclerosis)** 25 mg once daily, initially. Titrate by 25 mg/d up to 100 mg 2–4 times daily every 4–7 days as needed/tolerated. **Pediatrics:** 0.5 mg/kg bid. Titrate by 0.5 mg/kg/d up to 3 mg/kg 2–4 times daily if needed. Do not exceed 100 mg 4 times daily.	Administration Issues Avoid alcohol or CNS depressant use. Safety/efficacy not established in those <5 yrs old. Drug–Drug Interactions **Increased effect/levels of dantrolene:** estrogens (potential for hepatotoxicity).	ADRs Drowsiness, dizziness, diarrhea, tachycardia, weakness, general malaise, fatigue. Pharmacokinetics Incomplete absorption; $T_{1/2}$ = 9 h.	Contraindications Hypersensitivity, active hepatic disease, where spasticity is utilized to sustain upright posture and balance in locomotion or to obtain or maintain increased function, treatment of skeletal muscle spasm resulting from rheumatic disorders. Precautions Use cautiously in patients with impaired pulmonary, cardiac, or hepatic function.

(*continues on next page*)

314. Skeletal Muscle Relaxants *continued from previous page*

Drug and Dosage Forms	Usual Dosage Range	Administration Issues and Drug–Drug Interactions	Common Adverse Drug Reactions (ADRs) and Pharmacokinetics	Contraindications, Pregnancy Category, and Lactation Issues
Dantrolene Sodium *cont.*		**Decreased effect/levels of dantrolene:** clofibrate, warfarin. **Increased effect/levels of:** verapamil, alcohol, CNS depressants.		Pregnancy/Lactation Issues Safety not established.
Diazepam (CIV) Valium, Valrelease, Zetran, various generics Tablets 2 mg, 5 mg, 10 mg Capsule sustained release 15 mg Oral Solution 5 mg/5 mL, 5 mg/mL	**As an adjunct to rest, physical therapy and other measures for the relief of discomfort associated with acute, painful musculoskeletal conditions** 2–10 mg 3–4 times daily. 15–30 mg daily of the sustained release product. **Elderly or debilitated patients:** 2–2.5 mg 1–2 times daily. Titrate as needed/tolerated. **Pediatrics (>6 months old):** 1–2.5 mg 3–4 times daily. Titrate as needed/tolerated.	Administration Issues Do not crush or chew sustained release products. Concentrated solution (5 mg/mL) should be diluted in liquid or semi-solid foods; not recommended for <6 mos old. Drug–Drug Interactions **Increased level of BZ:** cimetidine, oral contraceptives, disulfiram, fluoxetine, isoniazid, ketoconazole, metoprolol, propoxyphene, propranolol, valproic acid. **Increased CNS effects:** alcohol, barbiturates, narcotics. **Increased levels of:** digoxin, phenytoin (possibly). **Decreased level or effect of BZ:** rifampin (decreased level); theophylline (decreased effect).	ADRs Drowsiness, ataxia, confusion (especially in elderly). Dependence: Prolonged use can lead to dependence; abrupt discontinuation can precipitate withdrawal symptoms (anxiety, flulike illness, concentration difficulties, fatigue, anorexia, restlessness, confusion, psychosis, paranoid delusions, grand mal seizures). Withdrawal can occur after as little as 4–6 weeks of therapy. Clonidine, propranolol, carbamazepine have been used as adjuncts in withdrawal. Drug Discontinuation: gradual decrease over 4–8 weeks. Pharmacokinetics $T_{1/2}$ = 20–80 h; speed of onset = very fast.	Contraindications Hypersensitivity, psychoses, acute narrow-angle glaucoma. Pregnancy Category: D Lactation Issues Excreted in breast milk—do not give to nursing mothers.
Metaxalone Skelaxin Tablets 400 mg, 800 mg	**As an adjunct to rest, physical therapy and other measures for the relief of discomfort associated with acute, painful musculoskeletal conditions** 800 mg 3–4 times daily	Administration Issues Avoid alcohol or CNS depressants; Safety/efficacy not established for those <12 yrs old. Drug–Drug Interactions **Increased effect of:** alcohol or other CNS depressants.	ADRs Drowsiness, dizziness, headache, nervousness, irritability, nausea, vomiting, hypersensitivity (rash); leukopenia, hemolytic anemia, jaundice. Pharmacokinetics Onset = 1 h; duration = 4–6 h; $T_{1/2}$ = 2–3 h.	Contraindications Hypersensitivity; drug-induced hemolytic or other anemias; severe renal or hepatic dysfunction. Pregnancy/Lactation Issues Safety has not been established; use cautiously if at all.

Methocarbamol Robaxin, various generics Tablets 500 mg, 750 mg	**As an adjunct to rest, physical therapy and other measures for the relief of discomfort associated with acute, painful musculoskeletal conditions** 1.5 g qid, initially (first 48–72 h). Maintenance doses include: 1 g qid or 750 mg q 4 h.	Administration Issues Avoid alcohol or CNS depressants; safety/efficacy not established in those <12 yrs old. Drug–Drug Interactions **Increased effect of:** alcohol or other CNS depressants.	ADRs Lightheadedness, dizziness, drowsiness, headache, blurred vision, nausea, fever, rash, conjunctivitis, urticaria, pruritis, urine discoloration (brown, black, green). Pharmacokinetics Onset of action = 30 min; $T_{1/2}$ = 1–2 h.	Contraindications Hypersensitivity. Pregnancy/Lactation Issues Safety not established. Use cautiously if at all.
Orphenadrine Citrate Norflex, various generics Tablets 100 mg Tablets, sustained release 100 mg	**As an adjunct to rest, physical therapy and other measures for the relief of discomfort associated with acute, painful musculoskeletal conditions:** 100 mg bid **Unlabeled Use:** 100 mg at bedtime is useful for quinine-resistant leg cramps	Administration Issues Do not crush or chew sustained release preparations; safety/efficacy not established for children. Drug–Drug Interactions **Increased effects of orphenadrine:** amantadine (increased anticholinergic effects). **Increased effects of:** haloperidol (tardive dyskinesia). **Decreased effects of:** phenothiazines, haloperidol.	ADRs Dry mouth, tachycardia, constipation, urinary hesitancy, blurred vision, weakness, headache, dizziness, agitation, tremor, drowsiness, confusion, nausea, vomiting, urticaria. Pharmacokinetics Duration of action is 4–6 h; $T_{1/2}$ = 2–25 h.	Contraindications Hypersensitivity; glaucoma; pyloric/duodenal obstruction; peptic ulcers; prostatic hypertrophy; bladder obstruction; cardiospasm; myasthenia gravis. Precautions Use cautiously in those with cardiac disease. Long-term safety has not been established. Pregnancy Category: C Lactation Issues Use cautiously, unknown if excreted in breast milk.

314.1 Skeletal Muscle Relaxant Combinations

Drug and Dosage Forms	Usual Dosage Range	Administration Issues and Drug-Drug Interactions	Common Adverse Drug Reactions (ADRs) and Pharmacokinetics	Contraindications, Pregnancy Category, and Lactation Issues
Methocarbamol/Aspirin Robaxisal, various generics Tablets 400 mg/325 mg	**Adjunct to rest, physical therapy, and other therapy for relief of discomfort associated with acute, painful musculoskeletal conditions** 2 tabs 4 times daily	Administration Issues Take with food. Avoid alcohol or CNS depressants. Safety/efficacy not established in those <12 yrs old. Aspirin use in children with fever has been associated with Reye's syndrome. Drug-Drug Interactions See individual agents.	ADRs Methocarbamal: Lightheadedness, dizziness, drowsiness, headache, blurred vision, nausea, fever, rash, conjunctivitis, urticaria, pruritis, urine discoloration (brown, black, green). Aspirin: Nausea, dyspepsia, heartburn, GI bleeding, hives, rash, prolonged bleeding time, thrombocytopenia, aspirin intolerance (bronchospasm, rhinitis), "Salicylism":	Contraindications Hypersensitivity. Aspirin: hemophilia, bleeding ulcers, hemorrhagic states. Precautions Aspirin: Use cautiously in patients with asthma, nasal polyposis, chronic urticaria (inc risk of hypersensitivity); chronic renal insufficiency, PUD, bleeding disorders. Pregnancy/Lactation Issues Safety not established. Use cautiously if at all.

(*continues on next page*)

314.1 Skeletal Muscle Relaxant Combinations *continued from previous page*

Drug and Dosage Forms	Usual Dosage Range	Administration Issues and Drug-Drug Interactions	Common Adverse Drug Reactions (ADRs) and Pharmacokinetics	Contraindications, Pregnancy Category, and Lactation Issues
Methocarbamol/Aspirin *cont.*			dizziness, tinnitus, difficulty hearing, nausea, vomiting, diarrhea, confusion, CNS depression, headache, sweating, hyperventilation, lassitude. Pharmacokinetics See individual agents.	Aspirin: Category D
Carisoprodol/Aspirin Sodol Compound, Soma Compound, various generics Tablets 200 mg/325 mg	**Adjunct to rest, physical therapy, and other therapy for relief of discomfort associated with acute, painful musculoskeletal conditions** 1–2 tabs 4 times daily	Administration Issues Take with food. Not recommended for children <12 yrs old. Aspirin use in children with fever has been associated with Reye's syndrome. Drug-Drug Interactions See individual agents.	ADRs Carisoprodol: Drowsiness, dizziness, vertigo, ataxia, tremor, agitation, irritability, headache, insomnia, syncope, depression, tachycardia, postural hypotension, flushing, nausea, vomiting, hiccoughs, epigastric distress, allergic reactions, rash, erythema multiforme, cross reaction with meprobamate. Aspirin: Nausea, dyspepsia, heartburn, GI bleeding, hives, rash, prolonged bleeding time, thrombocytopenia, aspirin intolerance (bronchospasm, rhinitis), "Salicylism": dizziness, tinnitus, difficulty hearing, nausea, vomiting, diarrhea, confusion, CNS depression, headache, sweating, hyperventilation, lassitude. Pharmacokinetics See individual agents.	Contraindications Hypersensitivity to this or meprobamate; acute intermittent porphyria. Aspirin: Hemophilia, bleeding ulcers, hemorrhagic states. Precautions Use cautiously in patients with severe renal or hepatic dysfunction. Aspirin: Use cautiously in patients with asthma, nasal polyposis, chronic urticaria (inc risk of hypersensitivity); chronic renal insufficiency, PUD, bleeding disorders. Pregnancy/Lactation Issues Safety not established. Use cautiously. It is excreted in breast milk. Aspirin: Category D
Carisoprodol/Aspirin/ Codeine Soma Compound w/ Codeine Tablets 200 mg/325 mg/16 mg	**Adjunct to rest, physical therapy, and other therapy for relief of discomfort associated with acute, painful musculoskeletal conditions** 1–2 tabs 4 times daily	Administration Issues Take with food; carisoprodol not recommended for children <12 yrs old. Aspirin use in children with fever has been associated with Reye's syndrome. Drug-Drug Interactions See individual agents.	ADRs Carisoprodol: Ataxia, tremor, agitation, irritability, headache, insomnia, syncope, depression, tachycardia, postural hypotension, flushing, nausea, vomiting, hiccoughs, epigastric distress, allergic reactions, rash, erythema multiforme, cross reaction with meprobamate.	Contraindications Hypersensitivity to any ingredients or meprobamate; acute intermittent porphyria Codeine: diarrhea caused by poisoning, acute bronchial asthma, upper airway obstruction Aspirin: hemophilia, bleeding ulcers, hemorrhagic states.

			Codeine: Lightheadedness, dizziness, sedation, nausea, vomiting, sweating, constipation, drowsiness. Aspirin: Nausea, dyspepsia, heartburn, GI bleeding, hives, rash, prolonged bleeding time, thrombocytopenia, aspirin intolerance (bronchospasm, rhinitis), "Salicylism": dizziness, tinnitus, difficulty hearing, nausea, vomiting, diarrhea, confusion, CNS depression, headache, sweating, hyperventilation, lassitude. Pharmacokinetics See individual agents.	Precautions Use cautiously in patients with severe renal or hepatic dysfunction. Codeine: Use cautiously in patients with acute abdominal conditions, in elderly or debilitated patients, patients with respiratory conditions, cardiovascular or seizure disorders, hypothyroidism, Addison's disease, acute alcoholism, prostatic hypertrophy. Narcotics can lead to physical dependence when used for prolonged periods of time; withdrawal symptoms can occur following abrupt withdrawal. Aspirin: Use cautiously in patients with asthma, nasal polyposis, chronic urticaria (inc risk of hypersensitivity); chronic renal insufficiency, PUD, bleeding disorders. Pregnancy/Lactation Issues Safety not established. Use cautiously. It is excreted in breast milk. Codeine: Category C Aspirin: Category D
Chlorzoxazone/ Acetaminophen Chlorofon-F, Chlorzone Forte, Pargen Fortified, Flexaphen, Lobac, Mus-Lax, Skelex, various generics Tablets 250 mg/300 mg	**Adjunct to rest, physical therapy, and other therapy for relief of discomfort associated with acute, painful musculoskeletal conditions** 2 tabs 4 times daily	Administration Issues May take with food. Avoid alcohol or other CNS depressants. Drug-Drug Interactions See individual agents.	ADRs Chlorzoxazone: Drowsiness, dizziness, lightheadedness, malaise, overstimulation, minor GI upset, rash, hypersensitivity reactions, liver toxicity (drug-induced hepatitis), urine discoloration. Acetaminophen: Very few adverse reactions. Pharmacokinetics See individual agents.	Contraindications Hypersensitivity. Precautions Use cautiously in patients with hepatic dysfunction; if signs of liver toxicity are observed; discontinue use. Pregnancy/Lactation Issues Safety not established.
Orphenadrine Citrate/Aspirin/Caffeine Orphengesic, Norgesic, Orphengesic Forte, Norgesic Forte	**Adjunct to rest, physical therapy, and other therapy for relief of discomfort associated with acute, painful musculoskeletal conditions**	Administration Issues Do not crush or chew sustained release preparations. Safety/efficacy not established for children. Use not recommended. Aspirin use in children with	ADRs Orphenadrine: Dry mouth, tachycardia, constipation, urinary hesitancy, blurred vision, weakness, headache, dizziness, agitation, tremor,	Contraindications Hypersensitivity; glaucoma; pyloric/duodenal obstruction; peptic ulcers; prostatic hypertrophy; bladder obstruction; cardiospasm; myasthenia gravis. Aspirin:

(continues on next page)

314.1 Skeletal Muscle Relaxant Combinations *continued from previous page*

Drug and Dosage Forms	Usual Dosage Range	Administration Issues and Drug-Drug Interactions	Common Adverse Drug Reactions (ADRs) and Pharmacokinetics	Contraindications, Pregnancy Category, and Lactation Issues
Orphenadrine Citrate/Aspirin/Caffeine *cont.* Tablets 25 mg/385 mg/30 mg 50 mg/770 mg/60 mg	1–2 tabs 3–4 times daily (of the smaller dose); 1/2–1 tab 3–4 times daily (of the larger dose)	fever has been associated with Reye's syndrome. Drug-Drug Interactions Caffeine: **Decreased effect/levels of caffeine:** smoking. **Increased effect/levels of caffeine:** cimetidine, oral contraceptives, disulfiram, fluoroquinolones. Aspirin and Orphenadrine: see individual agents.	drowsiness, confusion, nausea, vomiting, urticaria. Caffeine: Insomnia, restlessness, excitement, nervousness, tremor, headaches, anxiety, nausea, vomiting, diarrhea, tachycardia, palpitations, diuresis, withdrawal headaches after abrupt discontinuation (500–600 mg/d of caffeine). Aspirin: Nausea, dyspepsia, heartburn, GI bleeding, hives, rash, prolonged bleeding time, thrombocytopenia, aspirin intolerance, (bronchospasm, rhinitis), "Salicylism": dizziness, tinnitus, difficulty hearing, nausea, vomiting, diarrhea, confusion, CNS depression, headache, sweating, hyperventilation, lassitude. Pharmacokinetics See individual agents.	hemophilia, bleeding ulcers, hemorrhagic states. Precautions Use cautiously in those with cardiac disease. Long-term safety has not been established. Aspirin: Use cautiously in patients with asthma, nasal polyposis, chronic urticaria (inc risk of hypersensitivity); chronic renal insufficiency, PUD, bleeding disorders. Pregnancy Category: C Aspirin: Category D Lactation Issues Use cautiously, unknown if excreted in breast milk.

315. Agents for Alzheimer's Dementia

Drug and Dosage Forms	Usual Dosage Range	Administration Issues and Drug–Drug & Drug–Food Interactions	Common Adverse Drug Reactions (ADRs) and Pharmacokinetics	Contraindications, Pregnancy Category, and Lactation Issues
Donepezil Aricept Tablets 5 mg, 10 mg	**Mild/moderate Alzheimer's dementia** Usual dose is 5–10 mg qd. Some evidence exists that doses >10mg may be beneficial in some patients. Do not increase to 10 mg until patients have been on daily dose of 5 mg for 4–6 weeks.	Administration Issues Take in evening, just prior to going to bed. May be taken without regard to food. Drug–Drug Interactions Donepezil may **decrease** the effectiveness of anticholinergics; ketoconazole and quindine may inhibit the metabolism of donepezil.	ADRs Headache, fatigue, nausea, diarrhea, muscle cramps, insomnia, dizziness. Pharmacokinetics $T_{1/2}$ = 70 h.	Contraindications Hypersensitivity to donepezil or to piperidine derivative. Pregnancy Category: C Lactation Issues It is not known whether donepezil is excreted in breast milk.
Ergoloid Mesylates Hydergine, various generics Tablets, sublingual 0.5 mg, 1 mg Tablets 0.5 mg, 1 mg Capsules 1 mg Liquid 1 mg/mL	**Age-related mental capacity decline (primary progressive, Alzheimer's, senile onset, or multi-infarct dementia)** 1 mg tid (alleviation of symptoms may take 3–4 weeks). Titrate dose based on clinical response and tolerance (range: 4.5–12 mg/d).	Administration Issues Do not crush or chew sublingual forms. Drug–Drug Interactions None known	ADRs Sublingual irritation, nausea, other GI disturbances. Pharmacokinetics Extensive first-pass metabolism (bioavailablity is 6%–25%; capsule has 12% higher bioavailability); $T_{1/2}$ = 2.6–5.1 h.	Contraindications Hypersensitivity; acute or chronic psychosis. Other Considerations Rule out delirium and dementiform illness secondary to systemic disease, primary neurological disease, or primary disturbance of mood. Periodically reassess patient for continued benefit.
Galantamine Reminyl Tablets 4 mg, 8 mg, 12 mg Liquid 4 mg/mL	**Mild/moderate Alzheimer's dementia** 4 mg bid initially. Titrate every 4 wks by 8 mg to 16–24 mg/d divided dose. Max dose: 24–32 mg/day.	Administration Issues Take with meals. Monitor for symptoms of active or occult GI bleeding esp. in those with PMH of ulcers or on NSAIDs If therapy is interrupted, should be restarted at lowest dose and titrated to previous dose. Drug–Drug Interactions **Increased effect of:** neuromuscular blocking agents during anesthesia **Increased effect of:** cholinergic agents **decreased effect of** anticholinergic agents.	ADRs Loss of appetite weight los$$$ diarrhea nausea vomiting syncopy. Pharmacokinetics $T_{1/2}$ = 7 h.	Contraindications Hypersensitivity. Use with care in patients with asthma or COPD. Pregnancy Category: B Lactation Issues Not Known.

(continues on next page)

315. Agents for Alzheimer's Dementia *continued from previous page*

Drug and Dosage Forms	Usual Dosage Range	Administration Issues and Drug–Drug & Drug–Food Interactions	Common Adverse Drug Reactions (ADRs) and Pharmacokinetics	Contraindications, Pregnancy Category, and Lactation Issues
Rivastigmine Exelon Capsules 1.5 mg, 3 mg, 4.5 mg, 6 mg Solution 2 mg/mL	**Mild/moderate Alzheimer's dementia** 1.5 mg bid initially. Titrate every 2 weeks by 1.5 mg to 3 to 6 mg bid. Max dose: 6 mg bid.	**Administration Issues** Take with meals. If therapy is interrupted, should be restarted at lowest dose and titrated to previous dose. **Drug–Drug Interactions** Increased effect of: neuromuscular blocking agents during anesthesia Increased effect of cholinergic agents. decreased effect of anticholinergic agents. **Drug–Food Interactions** None known.	ADRs Significant gastrointestinal adverse reactions, including nausea, vomiting, anorexia, dyspepsia, weight loss. For this reason, Exelon should be started at lowest dose. Pharmacokinetics $T_{1/2} = 1$ h.	Contraindications Hypersensitivity. Use with care in patients with asthma or COPD. Pregnancy Category:B Lactation Issues Not known.
Tacrine Cognex Capsules 10 mg, 20 mg, 30 mg, 40 mg	**Mild/moderate Alzheimer's dementia** 10 mg tid for 6 weeks, initially. Titrate by 40 mg/d every 6 weeks based on tolerance. Max dose is 160 mg/d. Rechallenging: If drug was stopped due to elevated transaminases (>5× upper limit of normal), may be rechallenged once LFTs have returned to normal. Follow titration as above.	Administration Issues Must monitor transaminases weekly (≤ 3× upper limit of normal: continue treatment; >3 but ≤ 5 upper limit of normal: decrease dose by 40 mg/d then increase dose once normal; >5 upper limit of normal: discontinue medication); safety/efficacy not established in any dementing disease found in children. Drug–Drug Interactions **Increased effect:** cholinergic agents **Decreased effect:** anticholinergic agents **Increased level of:** theophylline **Increased tacrine level:** cimetidine **Decreased tacrine level:** smoking. Drug–Food Interaction Food decreases levels of tacrine (take on empty stomach if possible).	ADRs Nausea, vomiting, diarrhea, dyspepsia, anorexia, increased transaminase levels, myalgia, ataxia. Pharmacokinetics $T_{1/2} = 2–4$ h; levels are higher in women (50%) due to lower activity of liver enzyme responsible for metabolism of tacrine.	Contraindications Hypersensitivity, previous treatment with tacrine that resulted in jaundice (total bilirubin > 3 mg/dL). Pregnancy Category: C Lactation Issues Should not be used in nursing mothers.

316. Agents for Gout

Drug and Dosage Forms	Usual Dosage Range	Administration Issues and Drug–Drug & Drug–Food Interactions	Common Adverse Drug Reactions (ADRs) and Pharmacokinetics	Contraindications, Pregnancy Category, and Lactation Issues
Allopurinol Zyloprim, various generics Tablets 100 mg, 300 mg	**Control of gout and hyperuricemia** To reduce incidence of gout flare-up: Initially, 100 mg/d, titrate q week by 100 mg/d. **Maintenance therapy:** 200–300 mg/d for mild gout; 400–600 mg/d for moderately severe tophaceous gout. Divide daily doses >300 mg into 2 doses. Max dose is 800 mg/d. **Prevention of uric acid nephropathy during vigorous therapy of neoplastic disease** 600–800 mg/d for 2–3 days **Pediatrics:** 300 mg/d (6–10 yrs old) or 150 mg/d (<6 yrs old). May also use 10 mg/kg/d divided q 6 h to max of 600 mg/d. Titrate dose after 48 hrs to minimum effective dose to maintain uric acid levels in normal range. **Recurrent calcium oxalate stones** 200–300 mg/d divided qd to bid **Renal impairment:** CrCl = 60 mL/min: 200 mg/d CrCl = 40 mL/min: 150 mg/d CrCl = 20 mL/min: 100 mg/d CrCl = 10 mL/min: 100 mg on alternate days. CrCl<10 mL/min: 100 mg 3 times weekly.	Administration Issues Drink 10–12 glasses of water daily. May take with food if GI upset occurs. When replacing a uricosuric, gradually reduce the uricosuric dose over several weeks while increasing allopurinol dose. Rarely indicated for children except in malignancies. Drug–Drug Interactions **Increased levels/effects of:** ampicillin, cyclophosphamide, theophylline, thiopurines. **Increased levels/effects of allopurinol:** ACE inhibitors, thiazide diuretics. **Decreased levels/effects of allopurinol:** uricosuric agents, aluminum salts.	ADRs Rash, dermatitis, urticaria, pruritus, nausea, vomiting, diarrhea, intermittent abdominal pain, gastritis, dyspepsia, increased liver function tests, leukopenia, leukocytosis, eosinophilia, thrombocytopenia, headache, somnolence, arthralgia, acute attacks of gout, fever myopathy, epistaxis, renal failure, alopecia. Pharmacokinetics $T_{1/2}$ = 1–2 h for allopurinol.	Contraindications Hypersensitivity; prior severe reactions to this agent. Precautions Use cautiously in those with severe renal impairment. Do not use to treat asymptomatic hyperuricemia. Monitor closely for signs of acute gout. Monitor liver and kidney function periodically. Pregnancy Category: C Lactation Issues Excreted in breast milk—use cautiously.
Colchicine various generics Tablets 0.5 mg, 0.6 mg	**Acute gouty arthritis** 1–1.2 mg at onset of symptoms, followed by 0.5–1.2 mg q 1–2 hrs until pain is relieved or nausea, vomiting or diarrhea occurs. Usual dose is 4–8 mg/attack.	Drug–Drug Interactions None known. Renal dosing: Dose should be adjusted with renal impairment.	ADRs Most frequent: Bone marrow depression, aplastic anemia, agranulocytosis, thrombocytopenia, peripheral neuritis, purpura, myopathy, alopecia, reversible azoospermia, der	Contraindications Hypersensitivity; serious GI, renal, hepatic, or cardiac disorders; blood dyscrasias.

(continues on next page)

316. Agents for Gout *continued from previous page*

Drug and Dosage Forms	Usual Dosage Range	Administration Issues and Drug–Drug & Drug–Food Interactions	Common Adverse Drug Reactions (ADRs) and Pharmacokinetics	Contraindications, Pregnancy Category, and Lactation Issues
Colchicine *cont.*	**Prevention of gouty arthritis** <1 attack/year: 0.5–0.6 mg/d for 3–4 days/week. >1 attack/year: 0.5–0.6 mg/d. More severe cases may require 1–1.8 mg/d Prior to surgery: 0.5–0.6 mg 3 times daily for 3 days prior to surgical procedure.		matoses, hypersensitivity, vomiting, diarrhea, abdominal pain, nausea. Pharmacokinetics $T_{1/2}$ = 12–30 min.	Precautions Use cautiously in the elderly or debilitated patients (severe hepatic or renal dysfunction); monitor blood counts periodically. Pregnancy Category: C Lactation Issues Use cautiously, not known if excreted in breast milk.
Probenecid Benemid, Probalan, various generics Tablets 500 mg	**Hyperuricemia associated with gout and gouty arthritis** 250 mg bid for 1 week, followed by 500 mg twice daily thereafter. **Renal impairment:** May need to titrate to 1500–2000 mg/d to achieve good uric acid excretion. If CrCl <30 mL/min, probenecid likely to be ineffective. **Maintenance doses:** When no attacks for 6 months, may decrease dose by 500 mg/d every 6 months. Monitor serum uric acid levels.	Administration Issues May take with food if GI upset occurs. Drink 6–8 glasses of water daily. Consider 3–7.5 g/d of sodium bicarbonate or potassium citrate to alkalinize the urine. Drug–Drug Interactions **Increased levels/effects of:** acyclovir, allopurinol, benzodiazepines, dapsone, methotrexate, NSAIDs, penicillamine, sulfonylureas, zidovudine. **Decreased levels/effects of probenecid:** salicylates.	ADRs Headache, anorexia, nausea, vomiting, urinary frequency, hypersensitivity, sore gums, flushing dizziness, anemia, hemolytic anemia, nephrotic syndrome, hepatic necrosis, aplastic anemia, exacerbation of gout, uric acid stones with or without hematuria, renal colic or costovertebral pain. Pharmacokinetics $T_{1/2}$ = 5–8 h (dose dependent and could be <5 and >8 h.	Contraindications Hypersensitivity; children <2 yrs; blood dyscrasias, uric acid kidney stones. **DO NOT START THERAPY UNTIL ACUTE GOUT ATTACK IS OVER.** Precautions Some renal adverse effects may be reduced by alkalinizing the urine. Use cautiously in those with PUD, severe renal or hepatic dysfunction. Pregnancy Issues Does cross placental barrier—use cautiously.
Probenecid and Colchicine ColBenemid, Proben-C, Col-Probenecid, various generics Tablets 500 mg/0.5 mg	**Chronic gouty arthritis** 1 tablet daily for 1 week followed by 1 tablet twice daily thereafter. **Renal impairment:** May need to titrate to 4 tablets/d to achieve good uric acid excretion. If CrCl <30 mL/min, probenecid likely to be ineffective.	Administration Issues May take with food if GI upset occurs. Drink 6–8 glasses of water daily. Consider 3–7.5 g/d of sodium bicarbonate or potassium citrate to alkalinize the urine. Do not use in those <2 yrs old. Drug–Drug Interactions **Increased levels/effects of:** acyclovir, allopurinol, benzodiazepines, dapsone, methotrexate, NSAIDs, penicillamine, sulfonylureas, zidovudine.	ADRs Probenecid Headache, anorexia, nausea, vomiting, urinary frequency, hypersensitivity, sore gums, flushing, exacerbation of gout, uric acid stones with or without hematuria, renal colic or costovertebral pain. Colchicine: Bone marrow depression, aplastic anemia, agranulocytosis, thrombocytopenia, peripheral neuritis, purpura, myopathy, alopecia, reversible azoospermia, dermatoses, hypersensitivity, vomiting, diarrhea, abdominal pain, nausea.	Contraindications Hypersensitivity; children <2 yrs; blood dyscrasias, uric acid kidney stones, serious GI, renal, hepatic, or cardiac disorders. Precautions Some renal adverse effects may be reduced by alkalinizing the urine. Use cautiously in those with PUD, severe renal or hepatic dysfunction. Use cautiously in the elderly; monitor blood counts periodically.

		Decreased levels/effects of probenecid: salicylates. Drug–Drug Interactions **Colchicine:** None known.	Pharmacokinetics See individual agents.	Pregnancy Issues Does cross placental barrier—use cautiously. Pregnancy Category: D Lactation Issues Not known if excreted in breast milk.
Sulfinpyrazone Anturane, various generics Tablets 100 mg, 200 mg Capsules 200 mg	**Chronic and intermittent gouty arthritis** Initially, 200–400 mg/d in 2 divided doses. Titrate to full maintenance dose within 1 week: 400 mg daily in 2 divided doses. May titrate further to 800 mg/d if needed.	Administration Issues May take with food if GI upset occurs. Drink 10–12 glasses of water daily. Consider 3–7.5 g/d of sodium bicarbonate or potassium citrate to alkalinize the urine. Drug–Drug Interactions **Increased levels/effects of:** acetaminophen (toxic effects), anticoagulants, tolbutamide. **Decreased levels/effects of:** acetaminophen (therapeutic effects), theophylline, verapamil. **Decreased levels/effects of sulfinpyrazone:** niacin, salicylates.	ADRs Upper GI disturbances. Less frequent: Blood dyscrasias, rash, bronchoconstriction (in those intolerant to aspirin). Pharmacokinetics $T_{1/2} = 2.2–3$ h.	Contraindications Hypersensitivity; active peptic ulcer or symptoms of GI inflammation or ulceration; blood dyscrasias Precautions Use cautiously in those with history of PUD. Monitor blood counts and renal function periodically. Pregnancy Issues Use cautiously—only when benefits clearly outweigh risks Pregnancy Category: C

317. Agents for Migraine

Note: Additional agents used for migraine and/or tension headaches include: ASA (table 307), APAP (table 301), Analgesics with Butalbital (table 305), Narcotic Analgesics (tables 302 and 303), and NSAIDs (table 306). For additional agents for migraine prophylaxis see: Valproic Acid (table 308.6), Propranolol and Timolol (table 205.5).

Drug and Dosage Forms	Usual Dosage Range	Administration Issues and Drug–Drug & Drug–Food Interactions	Common Adverse Drug Reactions (ADRs) and Pharmacokinetics	Contraindications, Pregnancy Category, and Lactation Issues
Almotriptan Malate Axert Tablets 6.25 mg, 12.5 mg	**For the acute treatment of migraine attacks with or without aura in adults** Doses of 6.25 and 12.5 mg were effective for the acute treatment of migraines in adults, with the 12.5 mg dose tending to be a more effective dose. **Hepatic/renal impairment:** Do not exceed the maximum daily dose of 12.5 mg over a 24-hour period, and use a starting dose of 6.25 mg.	Administration Issues If the headache returns, the dose may be repeated after 2 hours, but do not give more than 2 doses within a 24-hour period. Drug-Drug Interactions **Increase risk of vasospastic reaction** if given with ergot alkaloids, other 5-HT_1 agonists. **Use with or within 2 weeks following discontinuation of MAO inhibitors is contraindicated.** Observe patient carefully if given with an SSRI due to reports of weakness, hyperreflexia, and incoordination.	ADRs Chest, jaw, or neck tightness; acute MI, arrhythmias, death; cerebral hemorrhage, subarachnoid hemorrhage, stroke; hypertension; hypersensitivity reactions, photosensitivity. Pharmacokinetics $T_{1/2} \approx 3.1$ h.	Contraindications/Warnings Patients with ischemic heart disease (angina pectoris, history of MI, silent MI, strokes, transient ischemic attacks, silent ischemia, ischemic heart disease, or coronary artery vasospasm); concurrent use of (or use within 24 hours of) ergotamine-containing preparations, concurrent MAO inhibitor therapy (or within 2 weeks of discontinuing an MAO); within 24 hours of another 5-HT_1 agonist; hypersensitivity to the product or any of its ingredients; management of hemiplegic or basilar migraine; ischemic bowel disease. Pregnancy Category: C Lactation Issues Exercise caution when administering to a nursing woman.
Ergotamine Tartrate Ergostat, Medihaler, Ergotamine Tablets, sublingual 2 mg Aerosol 9 mg/mL	**To abort vascular headaches (migraine, migraine variant, cluster headache)** **Sublingual:** 1 tablet at onset of symptoms, take subsequent doses at 30 min intervals. Max of 3 tablets/d and 10 tablets/week. **Inhalation:** 1 inhalation, may repeat in 5 minutes if not relieved. Max of 6 inhalations/d or 15 inhalations/week.	Administration Issues Take with food. Continuous administration should not exceed 6 months. Need a drug-free period every 6 months for 3–4 weeks. Taper medication—do not abruptly discontinue medication. Not recommended for use in children. Drug–Drug Interactions **Increased vasoconstrictive effects in periphery: betablockers.** **Increased effects of ergot derivatives: macrolides.**	ADRs Nausea, vomiting, numbness and tingling of fingers/toes, muscle pain in extremities, weakness in legs, edema, itching, transient tachycardia or bradycardia. Pharmacokinetics $T_{1/2} = 2$ h.	Contraindications Hypersensitivity; pregnancy; peripheral vascular disease, hepatic or renal impairment, severe pruritus, coronary artery disease, hypertension, sepsis, malnutrition. Precautions Do not use for long periods of time (leads to ergotism, gangrene, drug dependence). Pregnancy Category: X Lactation Issues Do not use in nursing mothers—symptoms of ergotism (vomiting, diarrhea) have occurred in infants.

Frovatriptan Frova Tablets 2.5 mg	**For the acute treatment of migraine attacks with or without aura in adults** The recommended dosage is a single tablet (2.5 mg) taken orally with fluids. The total daily dose of frovatriptan should not exceed 3 tablets (3×2.5 mg/day).	Administration Issues If the headache recurs after initial relief, a second tablet may be taken, providing there is an interval of ≥ 2 hours between doses. Drug-Drug Interactions **Increased risk of vasospastic reaction** if given with ergot alkaloids, other 5-HT_1 agonists. Use with or within 2 weeks following discontinuation of MAO inhibitors is contraindicated. **Increase in AUC/Cmax of frovastatin** when given with oral contraceptives. Observe patient carefully if given with an SSRI due to reports of weakness, hyperreflexia, and incoordination.	ADRs Chest, jaw, or neck tightness; acute MI, arrhythmias, death; cerebral hemorrhage, subarachnoid hemorrhage, stroke; hypertension; hypersensitivity reactions, photosensitivity. Pharmacokinetics $T_{1/2} = 25.7$ h.	Contraindications/Warnings Peripheral vascular disease including but not limited to ischemic bowel disease, ischemic heart disease (angina pectoris, history of MI, silent MI, strokes, transient ischemic attacks, silent ischemia, ischemic heart disease or coronary artery vasospasm); uncontrolled hypertension, concurrent use of (or use within 24 hours of) ergotamine-containing preparations, concurrent MAO inhibitor therapy (or within 2 weeks of discontinuing an MAOI); within 24 hours of another 5-HT_1 agonist; hypersensitivity to the product or any of its ingredients; management of hemiplegic or basilar migraine; ischemic bowel disease. Pregnancy Category: C Lactation Issues Exercise caution when administering to a nursing woman.
Methysergide Maleate Sansert Tablets 2 mg	**Prophylaxis of vascular headaches** 4–8 mg daily. If no response after 3 weeks of therapy, discontinue treatment.	Administration Issues Take with food. Continuous administration should not exceed 6 months. Need a drug-free period every 6 months for 3–4 weeks. Taper medication—do not abruptly discontinue medication. Not recommended for use in children. Drug–Drug Interactions **Increased vasoconstrictive effects in periphery:** beta blockers.	ADRs Vasoconstriction of large and small arteries; postural hypotension, tachycardia, nausea, vomiting, diarrhea, heartburn, abdominal pain. insomnia, drowsiness, euphoria, dizziness, ataxia, weakness, lightheadedness, facial flush, telangiectasia, rash, hair loss, retroperitoneal fibrosis, peripheral edema, neutropenia, arthralgia, myalgia, weight gain. Pharmacokinetics Oral. No other data available.	Contraindications Hypersensitivity; pregnancy; peripheral vascular disease; severe arteriosclerosis, hypertension, coronary artery disease; phlebitis or cellulitis of the lower limbs; pulmonary disease; collagen diseases; impaired liver or renal function; valvular heart disease; debilitated states; serious infections. Precautions: Prolonged uninterrupted use is not recommended. Pregnancy Category: Contraindicated. Lactation Issues Do not use in nursing mothers—symptoms of ergotism (vomiting, diarrhea) have occurred in infants.

(*continues on next page*)

317. Agents for Migraine *continued from previous page*

Drug and Dosage Forms	Usual Dosage Range	Administration Issues and Drug–Drug & Drug–Food Interactions	Common Adverse Drug Reactions (ADRs) and Pharmacokinetics	Contraindications, Pregnancy Category, and Lactation Issues
Naratriptan HCl Amerge Tablets 1 mg, 2.5 mg	**For the acute treatment of migraine attacks with or without aura in adults** Single doses of 1 and 2.5 mg taken with fluid are effective for the acute treatment of migraine in adults. There is evidence that doses of 5 mg do not provide a greater effect than 2.5 mg. **Renal/hepatic function impairment:** The use of naratriptan is contraindicated in patients with severe renal impairment or severe hepatic impairment. In patients with mild-to-moderate renal or hepatic impairment, the maximum daily dose should not exceed 2.5 mg over a 24-hour period and a lower starting dose should be considered.	Administration Issues If the headache returns or if the patient has only partial response, the dose may be repeated once after 4 hours, for a maximum dose of 5 mg in a 24-hour period. Drug–Drug Interactions **Increased risk of vasospastic reaction** if given with ergot alkaloids, other 5-HT_1 agonists. **Use with or within 2 weeks following discontinuation of MAO inhibitors is contraindicated.** Observe patient carefully if given with an SSRI de to reports of weakness, hyperreflexia, and incoordination. A "serotonin syndrome" may occur if given with sibutramine. Co-administration is not recommended.	ADRs Chest, jaw, or neck tightness; acute MI, arrhythmias, death; cerebral hemorrhage, subarachnoid hemorrhage, stroke; hypertension; hypersensitivity reactions, photosensitivity. Pharmacokinetics $T_{1/2} = 5.5$ h.	Contraindications/Warnings Ischemic heart disease (angina pectoris, history of MI, silent MI, strokes, transient ischemic attacks, silent ischemia, ischemic heart disease, or coronary artery vasospasm); uncontrolled hypertension, concurrent use of (or use within 24-hours of) ergotamine-containing preparations, concurrent MAO inhibitor therapy (or within 2 weeks of discontinuing an MAOI); within 24 hours of another 5-HT_1 agonist; hypersensitivity to the product or any of its ingredients; management of hemiplegic or basilar migraine; ischemic bowel disease. Pregnancy Category: C Lactation Issues: Exercise caution when administering to a nursing woman.
Rizatriptan Benzoate Maxalt, Maxalt-MLT Tablets 5 mg, 10 mg Tablets, orally disintegrating 5 mg, 10 mg	**For the acute treatment of migraine attacks with or without aura in adults** Single doses of 5 and 10 mg are effective for the acute treatment of migraines in adults.	Administration Issues **Redosing:** Doses should be separated by at least 2 hours; no more than 30 mg should be taken in any 24-hour period. Drug-Drug Interactions **Increased risk of vasospastic reaction** if given with ergot alkaloids, other 5-HT_1 agonists. **Use with or within 2 weeks following discontinuation of MAO inhibitors is contraindicated.** Observe patient carefully if given with an SSR, due to reports of weakness, hyperreflexia, and incoordination. **A "serotonin syndrome" may** occur if given with sibutramine. Co-administration is not recommended.	ADRs Chest, jaw, or neck tightness; acute MI, arrhythmias, death; cerebral hemorrhage, subarachnoid hemorrhage, stroke; hypertension; hypersensitivity reactions, photosensitivity. Phenylketonurics: Inform phenylketonuric patients that rizatriptan orally disintegrating tablets contain phenylalanine (a component of aspartame). Pharmacokinetics $T_{1/2} = 2$ h.	Contraindications/Warnings Ischemic heart disease (angina pectoris, history of MI, silent MI, strokes, transient ischemic attacks, silent ischemia, ischemic heart disease, or coronary artery vasospasm); uncontrolled hypertension, concurrent use of (or use within 24 hours of) ergotamine-containing preparations, concurrent MAO inhibitor therapy (or within 2 weeks of discontinuing an MAOI); within 24 hours of another 5-HT_1 agonist; hypersensitivity to the product or any of its ingredients; management of hemiplegic or basilar migraine; ischemic bowel disease. Pregnancy Category: C

		Propranolol patients: In patients receiving propranolol, use the 5 mg dose of rizatriptan benzoate tablets, up to a maximum of 3 doses in 24 hours.		Lactation Issues Exercise caution when administering to a nursing woman.
Sumatriptan Imitrex Tablets 25 mg, 50 mg, 100 mg Injection 12 mg/mL Spray, nasal 5 mg, 20 mg	**Acute migraine with or without aura** Injection: 6 mg SC one time dose. Max of 12 mg/d (separate 2 doses by at least 1 hr). Oral: 25 mg per dose. Max of 100 mg per dose. May repeat dose after 2 hrs if no response. Max dose is 300 mg/d. Intranasal: A single dose of 5 mg, 10 mg, or 20 mg administered in 1 nostril is effective for the acute treatment of migraine in adults. If headache returns repeat × 1 after 2 hours, not to exceed daily dose of 40 mg.	Administration Issues Use the autoinjector for injections into SC area. Protect injection from light. Take medication as soon as symptoms appear. Safety/efficacy not established in children. Drug–Drug Interactions **Increased levels/effects of sumatriptan: MAO inhibitors, ergot-containing drugs.**	ADRs SC reactions: Dizziness, drowsiness, headache, anxiety, malaise, chest tightness, hypertension, hypotension, bradycardia, tachycardia, palpitations, transient ECG changes, weakness, neck pain, myalgia, muscle cramps, tingling, warm, feeling of heaviness, numbness, injection site reaction, flushing, jaw discomfort. Oral reactions: Confusion, photophobia, convulsions, drowsiness; dizziness, fatigue, chest discomfort, hypertension, hypotension, arrhythmia, angina, cerebral ischemia, diarrhea, dysphagia, GERD, constipation, feeling of heaviness, tightness, tingling, warm sensation, weakness. Pharmacokinetics SC: $T_{1/2} = 1.5–2$ h; oral: $T_{1/2} = 2.5$ h.	Contraindications Hypersensitivity; IV use; patients with ischemic heart disease, uncontrolled hypertension; concurrent use of MAO inhibitors or ergotamine derivatives; management of hemiplegic or basilar migraine. Precautions Use cautiously in patients with severe renal or hepatic dysfunction. Pregnancy Category: C Lactation Issues Excreted in breast milk—use cautiously in nursing mothers.
Zolmitriptan Zomig, Zomig ZMT Tablets 2.5 mg, 5 mg Tablets, orally disintegrating 2.5 mg Nasal spray 5 mg	**For the acute treatment of migraine attacks with or without aura in adults** **Tablets:** Initial recommended dose is ≤ 2.5 mg (achieved by manually breaking a 2.5 mg tablet in half) **Orally disintegrating tablets:** A single dose of 2.5 mg **Hepatic function impairment:** Administer zolmitriptan with caution in patients with liver disease, use doses <2.5 mg.	Administration Issues If the headache returns, the dose may be repeated after 2 hours, not to exceed 10 mg within a 24-hour period. Drug-Drug Interactions **Increased risk of vasospastic reaction** if given with ergot alkaloids, other 5-HT_1 agonists. **Use with or within 2 weeks following discontinuation of MAO inhibitors is contraindicated.** Observe patient carefully if given with an SSRI, due to reports of weakness, hyperreflexia, and incoordination.	ADRs Chest, jaw, or neck tightness; acute MI, arrhythmias, death; cerebral hemorrhage, subarachnoid hemorrhage, stroke; hypertension; hypersensitivity reactions, photosensitivity. Pharmacokinetics $T_{1/2}$-3 h.	Contraindications/Warnings Ischemic heart disease (angina pectoris, history of MI, silent MI, strokes, transient ischemic attacks, silent ischemia, ischemic heart disease or coronary artery vasospasm); uncontrolled hypertension, concurrent use of (or use within 24 hours of) ergotamine-containing preparations, concurrent MAO inhibitor therapy (or within 2 weeks of discontinuing an MAO); within 24 hours of another 5-HT_1 agonist; hypersensitivity to the product or any of its ingredients; management of hemiplegic or basilar migraine; ischemic bowel disease.

(*continues on next page*)

317. Agents for Migraine *continued from previous page*

Drug and Dosage Forms	Usual Dosage Range	Administration Issues and Drug–Drug & Drug–Food Interactions	Common Adverse Drug Reactions (ADRs) and Pharmacokinetics	Contraindications, Pregnancy Category, and Lactation Issues
Zolmitriptan *cont.*		**A "serotonin syndrome" may** occur if given with sibutramine. Co-administration is not recommended. **Co-administration with cimetidine** doubled the half-life and AUC of zolmitriptan.		Pregnancy Category: C Lactation Issues Exercise caution when administering to a nursing woman.

317.1 Combination Agents for Migraines

Drug and Dosage Forms	Usual Dosage Range	Administration Issues and Drug–Drug Interactions	Common Adverse Drug Reactions (ADRs) and Pharmacokinetics	Contraindications, Pregnancy Category, and Lactation Issues
Ergotamine and Caffeine Cafergot, Ercaf, Wigraine, Cafatine With belladona alkaloids and pentobarbital: Cafatine-PB Tablets 1 mg/100 mg with belladona alkaloids and pentobarbital (used as antiemetic and sedative, respectively) 1 mg/100 mg/0.125 mg/30 mg Suppositories 2 mg/100 mg	**For relief of vascular headaches** 2 tablets at first sign of symptoms, follow with 1 tablet every 1/2 hr as needed. Max dose is 6 tablets/attack or 10 tablets/week. For the 2 mg/100 mg dose: Follow above directions except the max dose is 2 tablets/attack.	Administration Issues Take with food. Continuous administration should not exceed 6 months. Need a drug free period every 6 months for 3–4 weeks. Taper medication—do not abruptly discontinue medication. Not recommended for use in children. Drug–Drug Interactions See individual agents.	ADRs Ergotamine: Nausea, vomiting, numbness and tingling of fingers/toes, muscle pain in extremities, weakness in legs, edema, itching, transient tachycardia or bradycardia. Caffeine: Insomnia, restlessness, excitement, nervousness, tremor, headaches, anxiety, nausea, vomiting, diarrhea, tachycardia, palpitations, diuresis, withdrawal headaches after abrupt discontinuation (500–600 mg/d of caffeine). Pharmacokinetics See individual agents.	Contraindications Hypersensitivity; pregnancy; peripheral vascular disease, hepatic or renal impairment, severe pruritus, coronary artery disease, hypertension, sepsis, malnutrition. Precautions Do not use for long periods of time (leads to ergotism, gangrene, drug dependence). Pregnancy Category: Contraindicated Lactation Issues Do not use in nursing mothers—symptoms of ergotism (vomiting, diarrhea) have occurred in infants.
Isometheptene Mucate/Dichloralphenazone/Acetaminophen Midrin, Isocom, Isopap, Migratine, various generics	**For relief of vascular headaches** 2 capsules at onset of symptoms, followed by 1 capsule q hr until relieved. Max of 5 capsules/12 hrs. **For relief of tension headaches** 1–2 capsules q 4 h up to 8 capsules/d	Drug–Drug Interactions **Increased effects of:** MAO inhibitors (hypertensive crisis).	ADRs Isometheptene/Dichloralphenazone: Dizziness, rash. Acetaminophen: Very few adverse reactions.	Contraindications Hypersensitivity; glaucoma, severe renal disease, hypertension, organic heart disease, hepatic disease, concurrent MAO inhibitor use.

<u>Capsules</u> 65 mg/100 mg/325 mg		**Increased toxic effect of acetaminophen:** alcohol (chronic); barbiturates, carbamazepine, hydantoins, rifampin, sulfinpyrazone. **Decreased effect of acetaminophen:** charcoal.	<u>Pharmacokinetics</u> **Data only available for acetaminophen** (see table 301).	<u>Precautions</u> Use cautiously in those with peripheral vascular disease and after recent cardiovascular attacks.

318. Agents for Parkinson's Disease

Drug and Dosage Forms	Usual Dosage Range	Administration Issues and Drug–Drug & Drug–Food Interactions	Common Adverse Drug Reactions (ADRs) and Pharmacokinetics	Contraindications, Pregnancy Category, and Lactation Issues
Amantadine Symadine, Symmetrel, various generics Capsules 100 mg Syrup 50 mg/5 mL	**Parkinson's** 100 mg bid when used alone. May titrate to 400 mg/d if needed/tolerated. **Concurrent therapy with levodopa:** 100 mg qd to bid while titrating levodopa dose **Elderly /debilitated:** 100 mg qd **Renal dysfunction (CrCl):** 80–100 ml/min: 100 mg bid 60 ml/min: 200 mg qod + 100 mg qod 40–50 ml/min: 100 mg/d 30 ml/min: 200 mg 2/week 20 ml/min: 100 mg 3/week ≤ 10 ml/min: 200 mg/week alternating with 10/week **Drug-induced extrapyramidal reactions:** 100 mg bid. May titrate to 100 mg tid if needed. **Traumatic brain injury** 50 mg bid up to 400 mg/d	Administration Issues Safety/efficacy not established in those <1 yr old. Drug–Drug Interactions **Increased effects of:** anticholinergic agents. **Increased levels of amantadine:** hydrochlorthiazide/ triamterene combination.	ADRs Nausea, dizziness, lightheadedness, insomnia, depression, anxiety, irritability, hallucinations, confusion, anorexia, dry mouth, constipation, ataxia, orthostatic hypotension, headache, livedo reticularis, peripheral edema. Elderly Patients: Use smaller doses Pharmacokinetics $T_{1/2}$ = 15 h (prolonged in elderly and those with renal dysfunction).	Contraindications Hypersensitivity. Precautions Do not abruptly discontinue medication due to precipitation of Parkinsonian crisis. Pregnancy Category: C Lactation Issues Excreted in breast milk. Use cautiously
Benztropine Cogentin, various generics Tablets 0.5 mg, 1 mg, 2 mg	**Adjunct in therapy of all forms of parkinsonism** 0.5–1 mg at bedtime. Titrate as needed/tolerated to 4–6 mg/d. May take as one daily dose or divide into 2–4 daily doses. **Drug-induced extrapyramidal reactions:** 1–2 mg 2–3 times daily initially for 1–2 weeks. Slowly withdraw medication to determine its continued need. If EPS recurs, reinstitute medication.	Administration Issues May take with food if GI upset occurs. If substituting another anticholinergic, gradually reduce other agent while gradually increasing this agent. Safety/efficacy not established in children. DO NOT USE IN THOSE <3 YRS. Drug–Drug Interactions **Decreased levels/effects of:** haloperidol, phenothiazines, levodopa. **Increased levels/effects of:** amantadine, digoxin, cannabinoids, barbiturates, alcohol.	ADRs Disorientation, confusion, memory loss, agitation, euphoria, excitement, dizziness, headache, drowsiness, dry mouth, acute suppurative parotitis, nausea, constipation, tachycardia, hypotension, blurred vision, mydriasis, urinary retention, muscle weakness, cramping, flushing, decreased sweating, impotence, skin rash. Elderly Patients (>60 yrs): More sensitive to CNS adverse effects. Use smaller doses.	Contraindications Hypersensitivity; angle-closure glaucoma; pyloric/duodenal obstruction; peptic ulcers; prostatic hypertrophy or bladder neck obstructions; achalasia; myasthenia gravis; megacolon. Precautions Use cautiously in those with arrhythmias, hypertension, hypotension, GI/GU obstructions. Not useful in patients with tardive dyskinesia—may actually aggravate symptoms. These agents may be abused—for the production of mood elevation or psychedelic experiences.

			Pharmacokinetics **No data available.**	Pregnancy Category: C Lactation Issues Use cautiously; effects on infant not known.
Biperiden Akineton Tablets 2 mg	**Adjunct in therapy of all forms of parkinsonism** 2 mg 3–4 times daily. May titrate to max of 16 mg/d as needed **Drug-induced extrapyramidal reactions:** 2 mg 1–3 times daily	Administration Issues May take with food if GI upset occurs. If substituting another anticholinergic: gradually reduce other agent while gradually increasing this agent; safety/efficacy not established in children. Drug–Drug Interactions **Decreased levels/effects of:** haloperidol, phenothiazines, levodopa. **Increased levels/effects of:** amantadine, digoxin, cannabinoids, barbiturates, alcohol.	ADRs Disorientation, confusion, memory loss, hallucinations, nervousness, euphoria, excitement, dizziness, headache, drowsiness, dry mouth, acute suppurative parotitis, nausea, vomiting, constipation, tachycardia, hypotension, blurred vision, mydriasis, urinary retention, muscle weakness, cramping, elevated temperature, flushing, decreased sweating, impotence, skin rash. Elderly Patients (>60 yrs): More sensitive to CNS adverse effects. Use smaller doses. Pharmacokinetics $T_{1/2}$ = 18.4–24.3 h.	Contraindications Hypersensitivity; angle-closure glaucoma; pyloric/duodenal obstruction; peptic ulcers; prostatic hypertrophy or bladder neck obstructions; achalasia; myasthenia gravis; megacolon. Precautions Use cautiously in those with arrhythmias, hypertension, hypotension, GI/GU obstructions. Not useful in patients with tardive dyskinesia—may actually aggravate symptoms. These agents may be abused—for the production of mood elevation or psychedelic experiences. Pregnancy Category: C Lactation Issues Use cautiously; effects on infant not known.
Bromocriptine Parlodel Snap tabs, Parlodel Tablets 2.5 mg Capsules 5 mg	**Parkinsonism** 1.25 mg bid with meals. Titrate every 2–4 weeks by 2.5 mg/d to 10–40 mg/d **Traumatic brain injury** 2.5 mg/d up to 30 mg/d	Administration Issues Take with food; take first dose lying down due to possibility of dizziness/fainting; safety/efficacy in children <15 yrs not established. Drug–Drug Interactions **Increased levels/effects of bromocriptine:** erythromycin, sympathomimetics. **Decreased levels/effects of bromocriptine:** phenothiazines.	ADRs Nausea, headache, dizziness, fatigue, lightheadedness, vomiting, nasal congestion, constipation, diarrhea, drowsiness, psychosis, hypotension, abdominal cramps. Pharmacokinetics $T_{1/2}$ = 6–8 h.	Contraindications Hypersensitivity to this or ergot derivatives; severe ischemic heart disease or peripheral vascular disease. Precautions Digital vasospasm has occurred in patients with acromegaly. Long-term treatment (20–100 mg/d) has resulted in pulmonary infiltrates, pleural effusion, pleural thickening (slowly reversible upon drug discontinuation). Pregnancy Category: B. Should discontinue medication once pregnancy is confirmed. Lactation Issues Prevents lactation—mothers should not nurse.

(continues on next page)

318. Agents for Parkinson's Disease *continued from previous page*

Drug and Dosage Forms	Usual Dosage Range	Administration Issues and Drug–Drug & Drug–Food Interactions	Common Adverse Drug Reactions (ADRs) and Pharmacokinetics	Contraindications, Pregnancy Category, and Lactation Issues
Carbidopa/Levodopa Sinemet, Sinemet CR, generics Tablets 10/100 mg, 25/100 mg, 25/250 mg Tablets, sustained release 25/100 mg, 50/200 mg Tablets, extended-release 25/100 mg 50/200 mg **Levodopa** Larodopa, Dopar Tablets 100 mg, 250 mg, 500 mg Capsules 100 mg, 250 mg, 500 mg **Carbidopa** Lodosyn Tablets 25 mg	**Levodopa** **Treatment of all forms of parkinsonism:** 0.5–1 g daily divided into 2 or more doses. Titrate by 0.75 g every 3–7 days as tolerated. Max dose is 8 g/d. **Carbidopa** **For use with levodopa:** Titrate carefully. Usually require 70–100 mg/d to saturate peripheral dopa decarboxylase. **Combination Product** If currently treated with levodopa, discontinue at least 8 days prior to initiation of combination product and reduce levodopa dose by 25%. Give 25 mg/100 mg (carbidopa/levodopa) tid or 10 mg/100 mg (carbidopa/levodopa) tid to qid. Titrate by 1 tablet daily every day or every other day as tolerated/needed. Max of 8 tablets daily. * When more carbidopa is required: use the 25 mg/100 mg tablet. * When more levodopa is required: use the 25 mg/250 mg tablet. **Sustained Release Combination:** 1 tablet bid at intervals not less than 6 hrs. Titrate q 3 days to 2–8 tablets/d at intervals of 4–8 hrs while awake. **Traumatic Brain Injury** 10/100 mg tid to 25/250 mg qid	Administration Issues Combination of carbidopa/levodopa is the preferred method, but some patients require individual drug titration. Peripheral dopa decarboxylase is saturated by carbidopa at approximately 70–100 mg/d May take a few weeks to months to see full effects. Give with food. Safety/efficacy not established for those <12 yrs old. Drug–Drug Interactions **Decreased levels/effects of levodopa:** anticholinergics, benzodiazepines, hydantoins, papaverine, pyridoxine, TCAs, methionine. **Increased levels/effects of levodopa:** antacids, MAO inhibitors. **Increased adverse effects of:** TCAs (by carbidopa). Drug–Food Interactions Protein-rich food reduces and delays peak plasma concentrations—causing fluctuations in response to levodopa.	ADRs Adventitious movements (choreiform, dystonic), anorexia, nausea, vomiting, dry mouth, abdominal pain, headache, dizziness, numbness, weakness, faintness, confusion, insomnia, nightmares, hallucinations, delusions, agitation, anxiety, malaise, fatigue, euphoria. Elderly Patients: often require smaller doses due to decrease in peripheral dopa decarboxylase. Pharmacokinetics **Levodopa:** $T_{1/2} = 1-3$ h. **Carbidopa:** Only given with levodopa to prolong $T_{1/2}$ of levodopa. Also increases urinary excretion of levodopa as unchanged drug.	Contraindications Hypersensitivity; narrow-angle glaucoma; concomitant use of MAO inhibitors (not selegiline); history of or suspected melanoma. Precautions Use cautiously in those with wide-angle glaucoma; use carefully to prevent "on-off" phenomenon by using lowest dose, reserving drug for severe cases, using drug holidays (5–14 days). Pregnancy/lactation Issues Safety not established. Use only when benefit far outweighs risk.
Diphenhydramine Benadryl, various generics Tablets 25 mg, 50 mg Capsules 25 mg, 50 mg	**Mild parkinsonism (e.g., drug induced) in combination with centrally acting anticholinergic agents; drug-induced extrapyramidal reactions in elderly unable to tolerate more potent agents** 25–50 mg 3–4 times daily	Administration Issues Safety/efficacy in children <12 yrs not established. Drug–Drug Interactions **Increased effect of antihistamine:** MAO inhibitors (anticholinergic effects).	ADRs Urinary retention, blurred vision, dry mouth, drowsiness, irritability, thickening of bronchial secretions. Elderly Patients (>60yrs): more sensitive to CNS adverse effects. Use smaller doses.	Contraindications Hypersensitivity, asthma, glaucoma, prostate gland enlargement. Precautions Use carefully if operating heavy machinery, history of sleep apnea, hepatic dysfunction.

Syrup 12.5 mg/ml	**Pediatrics (>9 kg):** 12.5–25 mg 3–4 times daily or 5 mg/kg/d. Max dose is 300 mg/d or 150 mg/m^2/day	**Increased effect of:** MAO inhibitors, alcohol, CNS depressants. **Decreased effect of:** levodopa, phenothiazines, haloperidol.	Pharmacokinetics Rapid onset (15–30 minutes); duration of action = 4–6 h.	Pregnancy Category: B. Lactation Issues Women should not nurse.
Entacapone Comtan Tablets 200 mg	**As an adjunct to levodopa/carbidopa to treat patients with idiopathic Parkinson's disease who experience the signs and symptoms of end-of-dose wearing-off** The recommended dose is one 200 mg tablet administered concomitantly with each levodopa/carbidopa dose. Maximum of 8 times daily (1600 mg/day).	Administration Issues Always administer in combination with levodopa/carbidopa. Entacapone has no antiparkinsonian effect of its own. Entacapone can be combined with the immediate- and sustained-release formulations of levodopa/carbidopa. Entacapone may be taken with or without food. Advise patients that drug will change color of urine to brownish orange. **Withdrawing patients from entacapone:** Rapid withdrawal or abrupt reduction in the entacapone dose could lead to emergence of signs and symptoms of Parkinson's disease and may lead to hyperpyrexia and confusion, a symptom complex resembling neuroleptic malignant syndrome. Drug–Drug Interaction Drugs metabolized by COMT (isoproterenol, epinephrine, norepinephrine, dopamine, dobutamine, methyldopa, apomorphine, isoetherine, bitolterol), as their interaction may result in increased heart rates, arrhythmias, and excessive changes in blood pressure.	ADRs Orthostatic hypotension, diarrhea, hallucinations, dyskinesia, rhabdomyolysis, respiratory effects, symptoms resembling malignant neuroleptic syndrome, use with caution in patients with biliary obstruction. Pharmacokinetics Not altered by age or renal function; effect of liver impairment unknown, drug is almost completely metabolized by glucuronidation; $T_{max} \approx 1$ h.	Contraindications/Warnings Hypersensitivity to the drug or its ingredients. Pregnancy Category: C Lactation Issues Exercise caution when entacapone is administered to nursing women.
Pergolide Permax Tablets 0.05 mg, 0.25 mg, 1 mg	**Adjunct to carbidopa/levodopa in the management of parkinsonism** 0.05 mg/d for first 2 days. Titrate by 0.1–0.15 mg q 3 days for the next 12 days of therapy. Titrate further by 0.25 mg/d q 3 days as needed/tolerated. Divide daily dose into 3 doses.	Administration Issues During dose titration, cautiously decrease dose of carbidopa/levodopa; safety/efficacy not established for children. Drug–Drug Interactions **Decreased effect of pergolide:** neuroleptics, metoclopramide.	ADRs Dyskinesia, dizziness, hallucinations, dystonia, confusion, somnolence, insomnia, anxiety, personality disorder, psychosis, orthostatic hypotension, vasodilatation, palpitation, syncope, arrhythmia, nausea, constipation, diarrhea, dyspepsia, anorexia, dry mouth, vomiting.	Contraindications Hypersensitivity to this or ergot derivatives. Precautions Use cautiously in patients with arrhythmias, those who are elderly, very ill, or at high risk for death.

(*continues on next page*)

318. Agents for Parkinson's Disease *continued from previous page*

Drug and Dosage Forms	Usual Dosage Range	Administration Issues and Drug–Drug & Drug–Food Interactions	Common Adverse Drug Reactions (ADRs) and Pharmacokinetics	Contraindications, Pregnancy Category, and Lactation Issues
Pergolide ***cont.***			Pharmacokinetics No data on $T_{1/2}$.	Pregnancy Category: B Lactation Issues Effects unknown; not recommended for mothers to nurse.
Pramipexole Mirapex Tablets 0.125 mg, 0.25 mg, 0.5 mg, 1 mg, 1.5 mg	**Signs and symptoms of Parkinson's disease** Suggested dosage schedule: Week / Dosage / Total daily dosage 1 / 0.125 mg tid / 0.375 mg 2 / 0.25 mg tid / 0. 75 mg 3 / 0.5 mg tid / 1.5 mg 4 / 0.75 mg tid / 2.25 mg 5 / 1 mg tid / 3 mg 6 / 1.25 mg tid / 3.75 mg 7 / 1.5 mg tid / 4.5 mg It is recommended that pramipexole be decreased over a 1 week period.	Administration Issues May be taken with food to decrease nausea; safety/efficacy in children not established; warn patients that they may experience postural hypotension. Drug–Drug Interactions Pramipexole may **increase** levodopa concentrations; pramipexole clearance may be **decreased** by verapamil, ciprofloxacin, cimetidine, diltiazem, quinidine; pramipexole may have **decreased effectiveness** if given with dopamine antagonists (phenothiazines, thioxanthenes, metoclopramide).	ADRs* Asthenia, dizziness, somnolence, insomnia, postural hypotension, extrapyramidal syndrome, hallucinations, confusion, constipation, dry mouth. * Some ADRs seen in patients also taking levodopa. Pharmacokinetics $T_{1/2}$ = 6 h; decrease dosage moderate to severe renal impairment.	Contraindications Hypersensitivity. Pregnancy Category: C Lactation Issues It is not known whether pramipexole is excreted in breast milk.
Procyclidine Kemadrin Tablets 5 mg	**Adjunct in therapy of all forms of parkinsonism** 2.5 mg tid. Titrate to 5 mg 3–4 times daily **Drug-induced extrapyramidal reactions** 2.5 mg tid. Titrate as needed/tolerated to 10–20 mg/d	Administration Issues May take with food if GI upset occurs. If substituting another anticholinergic: gradually reduce other agent while gradually increasing this agent; safety/efficacy not established in children. Drug–Drug Interactions **Decreased levels/effects of:** haloperidol, phenothiazines, levodopa. **Increased levels/effects of:** amantadine, digoxin, cannabinoids, barbiturates, alcohol.	ADRs Disorientation, confusion, memory loss, hallucinations, nervousness, euphoria, excitement, dizziness, headache, drowsiness, dry mouth, acute suppurative parotitis, nausea, vomiting, constipation, tachycardia, hypotension, blurred vision, mydriasis, urinary retention, muscle weakness, cramping, elevated temperature, flushing, decreased sweating, impotence, skin rash. Elderly Patients (>60 yrs): More sensitive to CNS adverse effects. Use smaller doses. Pharmacokinetics $T_{1/2}$ = 11.5–12.6 h.	Contraindications Hypersensitivity; angle-closure glaucoma; pyloric/duodenal obstruction; peptic ulcers; prostatic hypertrophy or bladder neck obstructions; achalasia; myasthenia gravis; megacolon. Precautions Use cautiously in those with arrhythmias, hypertension, hypotension, GI/GU obstructions. Not useful in patients with tardive dyskinesia—may actually aggravate symptoms. These agents may be abused—for the production of mood elevation or psychedelic experiences. Pregnancy Category: C Lactation Issues Use cautiously; effects on infant not known.

Ropinirole Requip Tablets 0.25 mg, 0.5 mg, 1 mg, 2 mg, 5 mg	**Signs and symptoms of Parkinson's disease** 0.25 mg tid initially then follow the titration schedule below: Week / Dosage / Total daily dose 1 / 0.25 mg tid / 0.75 mg 2 / 0.5 mg tid / 1.5 mg 3 / 0.75 mg tid / 2.25 mg 4 / 1 mg tid / 3 mg After week 4, dosage may be increased by 1.5 mg/d on a weekly basis up to a dose of 9 mg/d, and then by ≤ 3 mg/d weekly to total dose of 24 mg/d. Discontinue ropinirole gradually over a 7–day period. Decrease administration from tid to bid for 4 days then to qd for the remaining 3 days. **With levodopa:** Concurrent dose of levodopa may be decreased gradually as tolerated.	Administration Issues Can be taken without regards to food; administration with food may reduce nausea; safety/efficacy in children not established; warn patients that they may experience postural hypotension. Drug–Drug Interactions Ropinirole may **increase** levodopa concentrations; ropinirole clearance may be **decreased** by estrogens, tacrine, erythromycin, fluvoxamine, verapamil, ciprofloxacin, enoxacin, cimetidine, diltiazem, quinidine; ropinirole may have **decreased effectiveness** if given with dopamine antagonists (phenothiazines, thioxanthenes, metoclopramide).	ADRs* Fatigue, postural hypotension, syncope, dizziness, somnolence, nausea, vomiting, asthenia. * Some ADRs seen in patients also taking levodopa. Pharmacokinetics $T_{1/2} = 8$ h; titrate with caution in patients with impaired hepatic function.	Contraindications Hypersensitivity. Pregnancy Category: C Lactation Issues It is not known whether ropinirole is excreted in breast milk.
Selegiline Eldepryl, generics Tablets 5 mg Capsules 5 mg	**Adjunct to carbidopa/levodopa in the management of parkinsonism in patients who have exhibited deterioration in response to carbidopa/levodopa** 5 mg before breakfast and lunch. Attempt to reduce levodopa/carbidopa dose after 2–3 days of treatment with selegiline.	Administration Issues Do not exceed 10 mg/d. May need to decrease dose of levodopa by 10–30% due to increased side effects of levodopa after initiating therapy with selegiline; safety/efficacy not established in children. Drug–Drug Interactions **Increased adverse effects of (death has occurred):** fluoxetine, meperidine.	ADRs Dizziness, lightheadedness, fainting, confusion, vivid dreams, headache, increased tremor, nausea, vomiting, constipation, weight loss, anorexia, dysphagia, diarrhea, heartburn, orthostatic hypotension, hypertension, palpitations, urinary retention, prostatic hypertrophy, increased sweating, diaphoresis, facial hair, rash, photosensitivity, asthma, diplopia, dry mouth. Pharmacokinetics Extensively metabolized to 3 metabolites.	Contraindications Hypersensitivity; meperidine use. Precautions Do not use doses >10 mg/d (nonselectivity for MAO inhibition is lost). Pregnancy Category: C Lactation Issues Effects unknown, use cautiously.
Tolcapone Tasmar Tablets 100 mg, 200 mg	**Adjunct to levodopa and carbidopa for the treatment of the signs and symptoms of idiopathic Parkinson's disease** Initial dose of 100 mg tid. The recommended daily dose of tolcapone is 100 mg tid. If a patient fails to show the expected incremental benefit on the 200 mg dose after a total of 3 weeks of treat	Administration Issues **Before starting treatment with tolcapone, appropriate tests to exclude the presence of liver disease should be conducted.** Always administer in combination with levodopa/carbidopa. Tolcapone has no antiparkinsonian effect of its own. Tolcapone can be combined with the imme-	ADRs Orthostatic hypotension, diarrhea, hallucinations, dyskinesia, rhabdomyolysis, respiratory effects, symptoms resembling malignant neuroleptic syndrome, use with caution in patients with biliary obstruction.	Contraindications/Warnings Tolcapone therapy should not be initiated if any patient with liver disease or two SGPT/ALT or SGOT/AST values greater than the upper limit of normal. Pregnancy Category: C

(*continues on next page*)

318. Agents for Parkinson's Disease *continued from previous page*

Drug and Dosage Forms	Usual Dosage Range	Administration Issues and Drug–Drug & Drug–Food Interactions	Common Adverse Drug Reactions (ADRs) and Pharmacokinetics	Contraindications, Pregnancy Category, and Lactation Issues
Tolcapone *cont.*	ment (regardless of dose), drug should be discontinued. Hepatotoxicity greater at higher doses. Because of the **risk** of potentially fatal, **acute fulminant liver** failure, tolcapone should ordinarily be used in patients with Parkinson's disease on levodopa/carbidopa who are experiencing symptom fluctuations and are not responding satisfactorily to or are not appropriate candidates for other adjunctive therapies.	diate- and sustained-release formulations of levodopa/carbidopa. Drug–Drug Interactions Tolcapone may influence the pharmacokinetics of drugs metabolized by COMT. However, no effects were seen on the pharmacokinetics of the COMT substrate carbidopa. The effect of tolcapone on the pharmacokinetics of other drugs of this class, such as a-methyldopa and dobutamine, has not been evaluated. A dose reduction of such compounds should be considered when they are coadministered with tolcapone. **Effect of tolcapone on the metabolism of other drugs:** Coagulation parameters should be monitored when warfarin and tolcapone, are coadministered.	Pharmacokinetics Tolcapone is almost completely metabolized prior to excretion.	Lactation Issues Exercise caution when tolcapone is administered to nursing women.
Trihexyphenidyl Artane, Artane-Sequels, Trihexy-2, Trihexy-5, various generics Tablets 2 mg, 5 mg Capsules, sustained-release 5 mg Elixir 2 mg/5 mL	**Adjunct in therapy of all forms of parkinsonism** 1–2 mg/d in 3 divided doses; titrate by 2 mg/d every 3–5 days as needed/tolerated up to 6–10 mg/d. Some patients may need higher doses (12–15 mg/d)—divide higher doses in 4 equal doses. Concurrent use with levodopa: Generally use smaller doses (3–6 mg/d) **Drug-induced extrapyramidal reactions** 1 mg dose initially (determine effect). Titrate to 5–15 mg/d as needed/tolerated. **Sustained-release preparation:** Use after stabilized on immediate release. Substitute mg per mg. Give sustained release as one daily dose or divide into 2 doses given 12 h apart.	Administration Issues May take with food if GI upset occurs If substituting another anticholinergic: gradually reduce other agent while gradually increasing this agent; safety/efficacy. Drug–Drug Interactions **Decreased levels and/or effects of:** haloperidol, phenothiazines, levodopa. **Increased levels and/or effects of:** amantadine, digoxin, cannabinoids, barbiturates, alcohol.	ADRs Disorientation, confusion, memory loss, hallucinations, nervousness, euphoria, excitement, dizziness, headache, drowsiness, dry mouth, acute suppurative parotitis, nausea, vomiting, constipation, tachycardia, hypotension, blurred vision, mydriasis, urinary retention, muscle weakness, cramping, elevated temperature, flushing, decreased sweating, impotence, skin rash. Elderly Patients (>60 yrs): More sensitive to CNS adverse effects. Use smaller doses. Pharmacokinetics $T_{1/2}$ = 5.6–10.2 h.	Contraindications Hypersensitivity; angle-closure glaucoma; pyloric/duodenal obstruction; peptic ulcers; prostatic hypertrophy or bladder neck obstructions; achalasia; myasthenia gravis; megacolon. Precautions Use cautiously in those with arrhythmias, hypertension, hypotension, GI/GU obstructions. Not useful in patients with tardive dyskinesia—may actually aggravate symptoms. These agents may be abused—for the production of mood elevation or psychedelic experiences. Pregnancy Category: C Lactation Issues Use cautiously; effects on infant not known.

319. AGENTS FOR RHEUMATISM

Note: For additional agents see NSAIDs (table 306).

Drug and Dosage Forms	Usual Dosage Range	Administration Issues, Drug-Drug & Drug-Food Interactions	Common Adverse Drug Reactions (ADRs) and Pharmacokinetics	Contraindications, Pregnancy Category, and Lactation Issues
Adalimumab Humira Injectable: 40 mg/0.8 mL	**Treatment of rheumatoid arthritis.** 40 mg subcutaneous every other week. If not used as an adjuvant to MTX, then does may be increased to weekly.	Administration issues: Available in single dose pre-filled glass syringes fixed with 27 gauge needles. Must be refrigerated and protected from light. Do not freeze. Drug-Drug Interactions: When administered with MTX as a single dose, clearance is reduced by 27% and 44% after multiple doses.	ADRs: Serious, sometimes fatal infections have been reported. Pain at injection site, headache. Stop if numbness or tingling occurs. Lymphoma has been observed in patients treated with other drugs in this class. Pharmacokinetics: Binds to TNF-alpha and blocks interaction with the p55 and p75 cell surface TNF receptors. Also lyses surface TNF expressing cells in Vitro in the present of complement. Modulates biological responses that are induced or regulated by TNF, including changes in the levels of adhesion molecules responsible for leukocyte migration (ELAM-1, VCAM-1, and ICAM-1 with an IC_{50} of 1-2 $X10^{-10}M$) **Warning:** Black box warning regarding the risk for infection (tuberculosis) with the administration of the drug. Evaluate patients for latent TB infection with a tuberculin skin-test. Initiate treatment of latent TB infection prior to therapy with adalimumab.	Contraindications: Hypersensitivity to sodium phosphate, sodium citrate, citric acid, mannitol, or polysorbate 80. A current infection, or if patient has ever been diagnosed with an autoimmune disease. Not to be given if immunizations or surgery are planned. Pregnancy Category: B Lactation: Not approved.
Auranofin Ridaura Capsules 3 mg	**Rheumatoid arthritis** 6 mg daily in 1–2 divided doses. May titrate to 3 mg 3 times daily after 6 months if needed. **Pediatrics:** 0.1 mg/kg/d initially. Maintenance doses: 0.15 mg/kg/d. Max dose: 0.2 mg/kg/d **Unlabeled Uses:** pemphigus, psoriatic arthritis in those not tolerant to NSAIDs.	Administration Issues Safety/efficacy not established in children. Drug-Drug Interactions **Increased levels/effects of:** phenytoin.	ADRs Diarrhea, rash, stomatitis, anemia, elevated liver function test, leukopenia, proteinuria, thrombocytopenia, pulmonary effects. Pharmacokinetics $T_{1/2}$ = 26 days.	Contraindications Hypersensitivity; uncontrolled diabetes; severe debilitation, renal disease, hepatic dysfunction or history of hepatitis; uncontrolled CHF; systemic lupus erythematosus; agranulocytosis; blood dyscrasias; urticaria; eczema, colitis; pregnancy. Pregnancy Category: C; however, it is contraindicated. Lactation Issues Excreted in breast milk—discontinue nursing.

(continues on next page)

319. AGENTS FOR RHEUMATISM *continued from previous page*

Usual Dosage Range	Usual Dosage Range	Administration Issues, Drug-Drug & Drug-Food Interactions	Common Adverse Drug Reactions (ADRs) and Pharmacokinetics	Contraindications, Pregnancy Category, and Lactation Issues
Aurothioglucose Solganal Injection, suspension 50 mg/mL	**Rheumatoid arthritis** First dose = 10 mg, followed by 25 mg (2nd and 3rd dose), followed by 50 mg (4th and subsequent doses). Continue with 50 mg/week until 0.8–1 g has been given. Then continue 50 mg dose every 3–4 weeks. **Pediatrics:** 1/4 of adult dose based on body weight (not to exceed 25 mg/dose). **Unlabeled uses:** pemphigus, psoriatic arthritis in those not tolerant to NSAIDs.	Administration Issues Given by IM injection weekly in doctor's office. Observe patient (recumbent) for 15 minutes after administration. Safety/efficacy not established for those <6 yrs. Drug-Drug Interactions None known.	ADRs Most frequent (when cumulative dose is 300–500 mg): diarrhea, rash, stomatitis, anemia, elevated liver function test, leukopenia, proteinuria, thrombocytopenia, pulmonary effects. Pharmacokinetics $T_{1/2}$ = 3–27 days (first dose), 14–40 days (3rd dose); up to 168 days (11th dose).	Contraindications Hypersensitivity; uncontrolled diabetes; severe debilitation, renal disease, hepatic dysfunction or history of hepatitis; uncontrolled CHF; systemic lupus erythematosus; agranulocytosis; blood dyscrasias; urticaria; eczema, colitis; pregnancy. Pregnancy Category: C; it is contraindicated. Lactation Issues Excreted in breast milk—discontinue nursing.
Azathioprine Imuran Tablets 50 mg	**Rheumatoid arthritis** **Adults:** 1 mg/kg/d for 6–8 wk.; increase by 0.5 mg/kg q 4 wk. until response or up to 2.5 mg/kg/d **Elderly or renal impairment:** use a decreased dose	Administration Issues Response may take up to 3 months; do not have any vaccinations before checking with prescriber; report persistent sore throat, unusual bleeding or bruising or fatigue; take with food if GI upset occurs. Drug-Drug Interactions **Increased toxicity /effects of azathioprine:** allopurinol (decrease azathioprine dose to 1/3 to 1/4 of normal dose).	ADRs Fever, chills, nausea, vomiting, anorexia, diarrhea, thrombocytopenia, leukopenia, anemia, secondary infections, rash, pancytopenia, hepatotoxicity. Pharmacokinetics Extensively metabolized; $T_{1/2}$ (parent) = 12 min.	Contraindications Hypersensitivity to drug; pregnancy or lactation. Pregnancy Category: D; it is contraindicated. Lactation Issues Excreted in breast milk—discontinue nursing.
Etanercept Enbrel Injection 25 mg/5mL	**Rheumatoid arthritis (RA)** For reduction in signs and symptoms and inhibiting the progression of structural damage in moderately to severely active RA. It can be used in combination with methotrexate (MTX) in patients who do not respond adequately to MTX alone. **Polyarticular-course juvenile rheumatoid arthritis (JRA)** For reducing signs and symptoms of moderately to severely active polyarticular-course JRA in patients who have had an inadequate response to 1 or more	Administration Issues Have the patient/caregiver perform the first injection under the supervision of a qualified healthcare professional. Injection sites include thigh, abdomen, or upper arm. Rotate site and inject at least 1 inch from an old site. Refrigerate (36–46 degrees). Opened vials should be used within 45 days. Drug-Drug Interactions Use with Anakinra may result in higher rates of infections. Use of myelosuppressive antirheumatic agents may result in pancytopenia, including aplastic anemia.	ADRs Injection site reactions, headache, nausea, vomiting, dizziness, alopecia, cough, asthenia, abdominal pain, rash, dyspepsia, peripheral edema, stomatitis/oral ulceration. Malignancies, infections, were the most common serious adverse events observed. Infrequent serious adverse events observed in RA and psoriatic arthritis clinical trials:	Contraindications/Warnings Sepsis; hypersensitivity to etanercept or any of its components, agranulocytosis, bleeding, fever, hematological disease, latex hypersensitivity. Pregnancy Category: B Lactation Issues It is not known whether etanercept is excreted in breast milk or absorbed systemically after ingestion. Because many drugs and immunoglobulins are excreted in breast milk and because of the poten-

	disease-modifying antirheumatic drugs (DMARD). **Psoriatic arthritis** For reducing signs and symptoms of active arthritis in patients with psoriatic arthritis. It can be used in combination with MTX in patients who do not respond adequately to MTX alone. **Adults:** The recommended dose of etanercept for adult patients with RA or psoriatic arthritis is 25 mg given twice weekly as an SC injection, 72 to 96 hours apart. **Children (4 to 17 years of age):** 0.4 mg/kg (up to a maximum of 25 mg/dose) given SC twice weekly 72 to 96 hours apart. **Registration with the manufacturer required:** Enrollment information at: 1-888-436-2735		heart failure, MI, myocardial ischemia, cerebral ischemia, hypertension, hypotension, cholecystitis, pancreatitis, GI hemorrhage, bursitis, depression, dyspnea, deep vein thrombosis, pulmonary embolism, membranous glomerulonephropathy, polymyositis, thrombophlebitis, MS. Pharmacokinetics $T_{1/2}$ = 102 hours.	tial for serious adverse reactions in nursing infants from etanercept, decide whether to discontinue nursing or to discontinue the drug.
Gold Sodium Thiomalate Myochrisine, Aurolate Injection 25 mg/mL, 50 mg/mL	**Rheumatoid arthritis** First dose = 10 mg, followed by 25 mg (2nd dose), followed by 25–50 mg (3rd and subsequent doses). Continue with 25–50 mg/week until 1 g has been given. If clinical improvement before 1 g, may give dose q other week for weeks 2–20. Then continue 25–50 mg dose q 3–4 weeks. **Pediatrics:** Initially, 10 mg, then 1 mg/kg up to 50 mg for a single injection. Follow above schedule. **Unlabeled uses:** pemphigus, psoriatic arthritis in those not tolerant to NSAIDs.	Administration Issues Given by IM injection weekly in doctor's office. Observe patient (recumbent) for 15 minutes after administration. Safety/efficacy not established in children. Drug-Drug Interactions None known.	ADRs Most frequent (when cumulative dose is 400–800 mg): diarrhea, rash, stomatitis, anemia, elevated liver function test, leukopenia, proteinuria, thrombocytopenia, pulmonary effects. Pharmacokinetics $T_{1/2}$ = 3–27 days (first dose), 14–40 days (3rd dose); up to 168 days (11th dose).	Contraindications Hypersensitivity; uncontrolled diabetes; severe debilitation, renal disease, hepatic dysfunction or history of hepatitis; uncontrolled CHF; systemic lupus erythematosus; agranulocytosis; blood dyscrasias; urticaria; eczema, colitis; pregnancy. Pregnancy Category: C; it is contraindicated. Lactation Issues Excreted in breast milk—discontinue nursing.

(continues on next page)

319. AGENTS FOR RHEUMATISM *continued from previous page*

Usual Dosage Range	Usual Dosage Range	Administration Issues, Drug-Drug & Drug-Food Interactions	Common Adverse Drug Reactions (ADRs) and Pharmacokinetics	Contraindications, Pregnancy Category, and Lactation Issues
Hydroxychloroquine Plaquenil Tablets 200 mg	**Rheumatoid arthritis** Initially, 400–600 mg daily. When clinical improvement noted, decrease dose to 200–400 mg/d. **Systemic Lupus Erythematosus** 400 mg qd to bid **Pediatrics (for either indication):** 3–5 mg/kg/d up to a max of 400 mg/d in 1–2 divided doses. May titrate to 7 mg/kg/d if needed.	Administration Issues May take with food if GI upset occurs. Use cautiously, in children as they are more sensitive to toxic effects. Drug-Drug Interactions **Increased levels of:** digoxin. Reduced metabolism of metoprolol (CYP206).	ADRs Irritability, nervousness, emotional changes, nightmares, psychosis, headache, ataxia, dizziness, nystagmus, blurred vision, edema of cornea or retina, corneal opacities, retinal atrophy, abnormal pigmentation, optic disc atrophy, decreased visual acuity, bleaching of hair, alopecia, pruritus, skin pigmentation; skin eruptions (urticarial, others), non-light sensitive psoriasis, hemolysis in those with G-6-PD deficiency, anorexia, nausea, vomiting, diarrhea, abdominal cramps, skeletal muscle weakness, weight loss, lassitude, exacerbation, precipitation of porphyria, peripheral neuropathy. Pharmacokinetics Concentrates in liver, spleen, kidney, heart, and brain and is strongly bound in melanin-containing cells such as those in the eyes and skin; slow elimination.	Contraindications Hypersensitivity; retinal or visual field changes attributable to any 4-aminoquinoline compound; long-term therapy in children. Precautions Use cautiously in those with severe renal or hepatic dysfunction, or in alcoholics. Monitor complete blood counts periodically. Pregnancy Issues: Avoid use. Lactation Issues Not significantly excreted in breast milk; however, use cautiously.
Leflunomide Arava Tablets 10 mg, 20 mg, 100 mg	**Treatment of active RA in adults to reduce signs and symptoms and to retard structural damage as evidenced by x-ray erosions and joint space narrowing** **Loading dose:** Initiate therapy with a single oral 100 mg/day dose for 3 days. **Maintenance therapy:** 20 mg/day; doses > 20 mg/day are not recommended due to greater incidence of side effects. If dosing at 20 mg/day is not well tolerated clinically, the dose may be decreased to 10 mg/day.	Administration Issues/Monitoring Administer on an empty stomach or with food. Take dosage at the same time each day. NEVER stop drug without following the elimination procedure. Monitor liver enzymes; dose adjustments may be necessary. At minimum, perform ALT at baseline and monitor initially at monthly intervals, then if stable, at intervals determined by the individual clinical situation. Due to the prolonged half-life of the active metabolite of leflunomide, observe patients carefully after dose reduction since it may take several weeks for metabolite levels to decline.	ADRs Diarrhea, dyspepsia, nausea, vomiting, elevated hepatic enzymes, alopecia, maculopapular rash, pruritis, hypertension, headache, dizziness. Pharmacokinetics Peak levels of the active metabolite, M1, occurred between 6 to 12 h after dosing. Due to the very long half-life of M1 (2 weeks), a loading dose of 100 mg for 3 days was used in clinical studies to facilitate the rapid attainment of steady-state levels of M1.	Contraindications/Warnings Hypersensitivity to the drug or its ingredients. **Pregnancy must be excluded before the start of treatment with leflunomide. It is contraindicated in pregnant women, or women of child-bearing potential who are not using reliable contraception.** Pregnancy must be avoided during leflunomide treatment or prior to the completion of the drug elimination procedure after treatment. Pregnancy Category: X

	Drug elimination procedure: After discontinuation, a drug elimination procedure with cholestyramine is recommended to rapidly obtain levels of less than 0.02 mg/mL. Administer-cholestyramine 8 g 3 times daily for 11 days. (The 11 days do not need to be consecutive unless there is a need to lower the plasma level rapidly.) Verify plasma levels < 0.02 mg/L (0.02 mcg/ml) by 2 separate tests at least 14 days apart. If plasma levels are > 0.02 mg/L consider additional cholestyramine treatment. Without the drug elimination procedure, it may take ≤ 2 years to reach plasma M1 metabolite levels < 0.02 mg/L due to individual variation in drug clearance.	Drug-Drug Interactions Cholestyramine binds leflunomide and enhances clearance. **Increased side effects** may occur when leflunomide is given concomitantly with hepatotoxic substances.		Lactation Issues Leflunomide should not be used by nursing mothers.
Methotrexate Rheumatrex Dose Pack, Trexall various generics Tablets 2.5 mg, 5 mg, 7.5 mg, 10 mg, 15 mg	**Rheumatoid arthritis:** 2.5 mg every 12 h for 3 doses. This schedule is repeated weekly. 7.5 mg orally once weekly.	Administration Issues Drink plenty of fluid. Safety/efficacy for rheumatoid arthritis not established in children. Drug-Drug Interactions **Increased levels/effects of:** etretinate (increased hepatotoxicity). **Increased levels/effects of methotrexate:** probenecid, salicylates, sulfonamides, NSAIDs (MAY inc toxicity). **Decreased levels/effects of methotrexate:** folic acid, charcoal. Drug-Food Interaction Food may decrease absorption of MTX.	ADRs Elevated liver function tests, nausea, vomiting, thrombocytopenia, stomatitis, rash, pruritus, dermatitis, diarrhea, alopecia, leukopenia, pancytopenia, dizziness, anorexia, abdominal cramps, pulmonary toxicity, hepatotoxicity. Pharmacokinetics $T_{1/2}$ = 3–10 h; renally eliminated.	Contraindications Hypersensitivity; pregnant or lactating women; alcoholism; liver disease; immunodeficiency syndromes; preexisting blood dyscrasias. Precautions Monitor hematology liver and renal function every 1–2 months. Pregnancy Category: X Lactation Issues Contraindicated.

(*continues on next page*)

319. AGENTS FOR RHEUMATISM *continued from previous page*

Usual Dosage Range	Usual Dosage Range	Administration Issues, Drug-Drug & Drug-Food Interactions	Common Adverse Drug Reactions (ADRs) and Pharmacokinetics	Contraindications, Pregnancy Category, and Lactation Issues
Penicillamine Cuprimine, Depen Tablets, titratable 250 mg Capsules 125 mg, 250 mg	**Rheumatoid arthritis** **Adults:** Initial therapy: 125–250 mg as a single daily dose; increase at 1–3 month intervals by 125–250 mg/d as patient response and tolerance indicates. If satisfactory remission achieved, continue the dose. If no improvement after 3–4 months with 1–1.5 gm/d, discontinue drug. **Children (Juvenile RA*):** Initial: 3 mg/kg/d (≤ 250 mg/d) for 3 months, then 6 mg/kg/d (≤ 500 mg/d), divided bid for 3 months to a maximum of 10 mg/kg/d divided tid to qid *Non-FDA approved indication.	Administration Issues Take on an empty stomach, 1 hr before or 2 hr after meals and at least 1 hr apart from any other drug, food or milk; notify prescriber if skin rash, unusual bruising or bleeding, sore throat, unexplained coughing/wheezing, fever, or chills occur. Drug Interactions The absorption of penicillamine is **decreased** with coadministration with iron salts and antacid. Penicillamine may **decrease** digoxin serum levels. Penicillamine should not be coadministered with gold therapy, antimalarial, or cytotoxic drugs due to similar **serious hematologic and renal reactions.**	ADRs Fever, rash, urticaria, hypogeusia, arthralgia; edema of face, feet or lower limbs; chills, weight gain, sore throat, bloody or cloudy urine, aplastic or hemolytic anemia, leukopenia, thrombocytopenia, white spots on lips or mouth, proteinuria. Pharmacokinetics $T_{1/2}$ = 1.7–3.2 h.	Contraindications Hypersensitivity to drug; history of penicillamine-related aplastic anemia or agranulocytosis; renal insufficiency, pregnancy, breastfeeding. Pregnancy Category: D Lactation Issues Do not breastfeed.

Sulfasalazine Azulfidine Tablets 500 mg Tablet, enteric coated 500 mg	**Rheumatoid arthritis** 0.5 gm–1 gm orally per day for 1st week. Increase daily dose by 500 mg each week up to a maintenance dose of 2gm/day.	Administration Issues Maintain adequate fluid intake; take after meals; may cause an orange-yellow discoloration of urine and skin; may permanently stain contact lenses; avoid prolonged exposure to sunlight; do not take with antacids. Drug Interactions **Decreased effect** with iron and digoxin. **Increased effects/actions of:** oral anticoagulants, methotrexate, oral hypoglycemic agents. **Increased risk** of folate deficiency.	ADRs Fever, dizziness, headache, rash, photosensitivity, anorexia, nausea, diarrhea, reversible oligospermia, granulocytopenia, leukopenia, thrombocytopenia, aplastic anemia, hemolytic anemia. Pharmacokinetics 10–15% of dose is absorbed as unchanged drug from the small intestine, $T_{1/2} = 6–10$ h.	Contraindications Hypersensitivity to sulfasalazine or sulfa drugs, porphyria, GI or GU obstruction; hypersensitivity to salicylates, pregnancy. Precautions Use cautiously in those with severe renal or hepatic dysfunction, those with G-6-PD deficiency. Pregnancy Category: B (D at term) Lactation Issues Use cautiously.

400. EYE AND EAR PREPARATIONS

401. Ophthalmic Preparations

401.1 Agents for Glaucoma (for oral treatment see Carbonic Anhydrase Inhibitors, section 208.1)

Drug, Dosage Forms, and *Pharmacologic Action*	Usual Dosage Range	Administration Issues and Drug–Drug Interactions	Common Adverse Drug Reactions (ADRs)	Contraindications, Pregnancy Category, and Lactation Issues
Apraclonidine Iopidine Solution 0.5% *sympathomimetic*	Short term adjunctive therapy in patients on maximally tolerated medical therapy who require additional IOP reduction **0.5% solution** 1–2 drops in affected eye(s) tid	Administration Issues Do not touch tip of container to any surface; tachyphylaxis occurs in most patients—the benefit for most patients is < 1 month; safety and efficacy have not been established in children.	ADRs Hyperemia; pruritus; tearing; eye discomfort; lid edema; dry mouth; foreign body sensation; upper lid elevation; GI upset; bradycardia; insomnia, lethargy, dry nose.	Contraindications Hypersensitivity to apraclonidine or clonidine; concurrent monoamine oxidase inhibitor therapy. Pregnancy Category: C Lactation Issues It is not known whether apraclonidine is excreted in breast milk; use caution in nursing women
Betaxolol Betoptic, Betoptic S Solution 0.5% Suspension 0.25% *beta blocker*	Chronic open-angle glaucoma/ocular hypertension 1–2 drops in affected eye(s) bid	Administration Issues Shake suspension well before use; do not touch tip of container to any surface; safety and efficacy have not been established in children. Drug–Drug Interactions Additive effects may occur when given with oral **beta blockers** or **verapamil.**	ADRs Transient burning/stinging; tearing; bradycardia; hypotension; congestive heart failure; bronchospasm; masked symptoms of hypoglycemia; dizziness.	Contraindications Hypersensitivity to beta blockers; asthma; sinus bradycardia; second or third degree AV block; overt CHF Pregnancy Category: C Lactation Issues It is not known whether betaxolol is excreted in breast milk; either the drug or breast feeding should be discontinued
Bimatoprost Lumigan Solution: 0.03% *prostaglandin analog*	Chronic open-angle glaucoma/ocular hypertension who are intolerant of other IOP-lowering medications or insufficient response to other medications Instill 1 drop in the affected eye(s) once daily in the evening. No more than 1 dose per day.	Administration Issues Soft contact should be removed before administering medication and should not be reinserted for at least 15 minutes. Wait at least 5–10 minutes before using other ophthalmic medication. Wear eyeglasses and avoid exposure to bright light.	ADRs Conjunctival hyperemia, growth of eyelashes, ocular pruritis, headache, weakness, blepharitis, burning, cataract, dryness, eyelid redness, eyelash darkening, foreign body sensation, irritation, pain kertitis, visual disturbance, changes in skin pigmentation, tearing, eye discharge, photophobia.	Contraindications Hypersensitivity to bimatoprost or benzalkonium chloride. Pregnancy Category: C

Brinzolamide Azopt Solution 1% *topical carbonic anhydrase inhibitor*	Open-angle glaucoma or ocular hypertension 1 drop tid	Administration Issues Wait at least 10 minutes before using other ophthalmic medication.	ADRs Well tolerated. Potential for burning and stinging, but less than with dorzolamide.	Pregnancy Category: C
Brimonidine Alphagan Solution 0.15% Solution 0.2% *alpha-2 selective adrenergic agonist*	Open-angle glaucoma or ocular hypertension 1 drop into affected eye(s) bid-tid	Administration Issues Soft contact should be removed before administering medication and should not be reinserted for at least 15 minutes.	ADRs Conjunctival hyperemia, headaches, allergic reactions, fatigue/drowsiness	Pregnancy Category: B
Carbachol Isopto Carbachol, Carboptic Solution 0.75%, 1.5%, 2.25%, 3% *cholinergic agent & miotic, direct acting*	Glaucoma 2 drops in affected eye(s) tid	Administration Issues Do not touch tip of container to any surface; safety and efficacy have not been established in children. Drug–Drug Interactions Reports exist that both **topical NSAIDs** and acetylcholine are ineffective when used concurrently.	ADRs Transient stinging/burning; corneal clouding; ciliary spasm; headache; salivation; flushing; sweating; GI upset; hypotension; frequent urge to urinate, eye pain.	Contraindications Hypersensitivity to acetylcholine; conditions where pupillary constriction is undesirable; acute inflammatory disease of the anterior chamber. Pregnancy Category: C Lactation Issues It is not known whether carbachol is excreted in breast milk; either the drug or breast feeding should be discontinued.
Carteolol Ocupress Solution 1% *beta blocker*	Chronic open-angle glaucoma/ocular hypertension 1 drop in affected eye(s) bid	Administration Issues Do not touch tip of container to any surface; safety and efficacy have not been established in children. Drug–Drug Interactions Additive effects may occur when given with oral **beta blockers** or **verapamil.**	ADRs Transient burning/stinging; tearing; bradycardia; hypotension; congestive heart failure; bronchospasm; masked symptoms of hypoglycemia; dizziness.	Contraindications Hypersensitivity to beta blockers; asthma; sinus bradycardia; second or third degree AV block; overt CHF. Pregnancy Category: C Lactation Issues Carteolol is excreted in breast milk; either the drug or breastfeeding should be discontinued.

(*continues on next page*)

401.1 Agents for Glaucoma *continued from previous page*

Drug, Dosage Forms, and *Pharmacologic Action*	Usual Dosage Range	Administration Issues and Drug–Drug Interactions	Common Adverse Drug Reactions (ADRs)	Contraindications, Pregnancy Category, and Lactation Issues
Demecarium Humorsol Solution 0.125%, 0.25% *miotic, cholinesterase inhibitor*	Open-angle glaucoma, when shorter acting miotics have proved inadequate 1–2 drops in affected eye(s) frequency of administration may range from bid to twice weekly	Administration Issues Do not touch tip of container to any surface; wash hands immediately after administration; protect from heat; do not freeze. Drug–Drug Interactions Additive effects may occur when administered concurrently with systemic anticholinesterases.	ADRs Iris cysts (more common in children); burning; lacrimation; lid muscle twitching; browache; headache; blurring; retinal detachment; GI upset; urinary incontinence; sweating; salivation; myopia.	Contraindications Hypersensitivity to cholinesterase inhibitors; glaucoma associated with iridocyclitis; inflammatory disease of the iris or ciliary body; pregnancy. Pregnancy Category: C Lactation Issues It is not known whether demecarium is excreted in breast milk; either the drug or breast feeding should be discontinued.
Dipivefrin Propine Solution 0.1% *sympathomimetic*	Glaucoma 1 drop q 12 h	Administration Issues Do not touch tip of container to any surface; do not use while wearing soft contact lenses; when used with other miotics, instill the miotic first; safety and efficacy have not been established in children; avoid exposure to light and air; discolored or darkened solutions indicate loss of potency.	ADRs Transient stinging/burning; eye pain; browache; headache; watery eyes; ocular congestion, photophobia; blurred vision.	Contraindications Hypersensitivity to dipivefrin; narrow angle glaucoma. Pregnancy Category: B Lactation Issues: It is not known whether dipivefrin is excreted in breast milk; use caution in nursing women.
Dorzolamide Trusopt Solution 2% *carbonic anhydrase inhibitor*	Open-angle glaucoma/ocular hypertension 1 drop in affected eye(s) tid	Administration Issues Do not touch tip of container to any surface; if more than one topical ophthalmic drug is being used, administer the drugs at least ten minutes apart; safety and efficacy have not been established in children. Drug–Drug Interactions Additive effects may occur when administered concurrently with systemic carbonic anhydrase inhibitors.	ADRs Ocular burning/stinging; bitter taste; superficial punctate keratitis; blurred vision; tearing; dryness; photophobia; headache.	Contraindications Hypersensitivity to dorzolamide. Pregnancy Category: C Lactation Issues It is not known whether dorzolamide is excreted in breast milk; either the drug or breastfeeding should be discontinued.
Echothiophate Phospholine	Open-angle glaucoma; angle-closure glaucoma	Administration Issues Do not touch tip of container to any surface; administer one of the two daily	ADRs Iris cysts (more common in children); burning; lacrimation; lid muscle twitch-	Contraindications Hypersensitivity to cholinesterase inhibitors; glaucoma associated with irido-

Solution 0.03%, 0.06%, 0.125%, 0.25% *miotic, cholinesterase inhibitor*	1 drop in affected eye(s) frequency of administration may range from qod to bid	doses at bedtime to avoid inconvenience due to miosis; store in refrigerator to maintain potency for 6 months; must be reconstituted with diluent. Drug–Drug Interactions Additive effects may occur when administered concurrently with systemic anticholinesterases.	ing; browache; headache; blurring; retinal detachment; GI upset; urinary incontinence; sweating; salivation.	cyclitis; inflammatory disease of the iris or ciliary body; closed-angle glaucoma. Pregnancy Category: C Lactation Issues It is not known whether phospholine is excreted in breast milk; either the drug or breastfeeding should be discontinued.
Epinephrine Epifrin, Glaucon Solution 0.1%, 0.5%, 1%, 2% *sympathomimetic*	Glaucoma 1 drop into affected eye(s) qd to bid	Administration Issues Do not touch tip of container to any surface; do not use while wearing soft contact lenses; when used with other miotics, instill the miotic first; safety and efficacy have not been established in children	ADRs Transient stinging/burning; eye pain; browache; headache; watery eyes.	Contraindications Hypersensitivity to epinephrine; narrow or shallow angle glaucoma; aphakia. Pregnancy Category: C Lactation Issues It is not known whether epinephrine is excreted in breast milk; use caution in nursing women.
Latanoprost Xalatan Solution 0.005% (50 mcg/ml) *prostaglandin analog*	Elevated intraocular pressure in patients with open-angle glaucoma and ocular hypertension who have failed other medications one drop (1.5 mcg) in affected eye(s) qd in the evening. Do not exceed once daily dosage.	Administration Issues Inform patient about possibility of iris color change (increasing the amount of brown pigment); do not touch tip of container to any surface; remove contact lenses prior to administration and reinsert 15 minutes after administration; if using concomitantly with another ophthalmic drug, administer drugs at least 5 minutes apart; protect from light; refrigerate unopened bottle; once opened, container may be stored at room temperature for 6 weeks.	ADRs Blurred vision, burning; stinging; conjunctival hyperemia, foreign body sensation; itching; increased pigmentation of iris; punctate epithelial keratopathy, dry eye; eye pain; photophobia.	Contraindications Hypersensitivity to latanoprost. Pregnancy Category: C Lactation Issues It is not known whether latanoprost is excreted in breast milk; either the drug or breastfeeding should be discontinued.
Levobunolol AKBeta, Betagan, Levobunolol Solution 0.25%, 0.5% *beta blocker*	Chronic open-angle glaucoma/ocular hypertension 1 drop in affected eye(s) qd to bid	Administration Issues Do not touch tip of container to any surface; safety and efficacy have not been established in children. Drug–Drug Interactions Additive effects may occur when given with oral **beta blocker, quinidine** or **verapamil.**	ADRs Transient burning/stinging; tearing; bradycardia; hypotension; congestive heart failure; bronchospasm; masked symptoms of hypoglycemia; dizziness; headache, conjunctivitis; keratitis.	Contraindications Hypersensitivity to beta blockers; asthma; sinus bradycardia; second or third degree AV block; overt CHF; severe COPD. Pregnancy Category: C Lactation Issues It is not known whether levobunolol is excreted in breast milk; either the drug or breastfeeding should be discontinued.

(continues on next page)

401.1 Agents for Glaucoma *continued from previous page*

Drug, Dosage Forms, and *Pharmacologic Action*	Usual Dosage Range	Administration Issues and Drug–Drug Interactions	Common Adverse Drug Reactions (ADRs)	Contraindications, Pregnancy Category, and Lactation Issues
Metipranolol Optipranolol Solution 0.3% *beta blocker*	Chronic open-angle glaucoma/ocular hypertension 1 drop in affected eye(s) bid	Administration Issues Do not touch tip of container to any surface; safety and efficacy have not been established in children. Drug–Drug Interactions Additive effects may occur when given with oral **beta blocker, quinidine** or **verapamil.**	ADRs Transient burning/stinging; tearing; bradycardia; hypotension; congestive heart failure; bronchospasm; masked symptoms of hypoglycemia; dizziness.	Contraindications Hypersensitivity to beta blockers; asthma; sinus bradycardia; second or third degree AV block; overt CHF. Pregnancy Category: C Lactation Issues It is not known whether metipranolol is excreted in breast milk; either the drug or breastfeeding should be discontinued.
Physostigmine Eserine Ointment 0.25% *miotic, cholinesterase inhibitor*	Open-angle glaucoma apply small quantity to lower fornix in affected eye(s) up to tid	Administration Issues Do not touch tip of container to any surface; wash hands immediately after administration; safety and efficacy have not been established in children. Drug–Drug Interactions Additive effects may occur when administered concurrently with systemic anticholinesterases.	ADRs Iris cysts (more common in children); burning; lacrimation; lid muscle twitching; browache; headache; blurring; retinal detachment; GI upset; urinary incontinence; sweating; salivation; eye pain.	Contraindications Hypersensitivity to cholinesterase inhibitors; glaucoma associated with iridocyclitis; inflammatory disease of the iris or ciliary body. Pregnancy Category: C Lactation Issues It is not known whether physostigmine is excreted in breast milk; either the drug or breastfeeding should be discontinued.
Pilocarpine Isopto Carpine, Pilocar, Piloptic, Akarpine, Pilostat, Adsorbocarpine Solution 0.25%, 0.5%, 1%, 2%, 3%, 4%, 5%, 6%, 8%, 10% Gel 4% *cholinergic agent & miotic, direct acting*	Chronic simple glaucoma, chronic angle-closure glaucoma **solution:** 1–2 drops in affected eye(s) tid to qid **gel:** 1/2 inch in the lower conjunctival sac of affected eye(s) q hs	Administration Issues Do not touch tip of container to any surface; if other glaucoma medication is also used at bedtime, use drops at least 5 minutes before using the gel; safety and efficacy have not been established in children. Drug–Drug Interactions Reports exists that both **topical NSAIDs** and acetylcholine are ineffective when used concurrently.	ADRs Transient stinging/burning; tearing; ciliary spasm; headache; hypertension; tachycardia; salivation; sweating; GI upset.	Contraindications Hypersensitivity to acetylcholine; conditions where pupillary constriction is undesirable. Pregnancy Category: C Lactation Issues It is not known whether pilocarpine is excreted in breast milk; either the drug or breastfeeding should be discontinued.
Pilocarpine Ocular Therapeutic System Ocusert Pilo	Glaucoma/IOP reduction initial dose: 20 mcg/hr system q 7 days	Administration Issues Wash hands with soap and water before touching the system; discard contaminated systems and replace with a fresh	ADRs Conjunctival irritation; tearing; ciliary spasm; headache; hypertension; tachycardia; salivation; sweating; GI upset.	Contraindications Hypersensitivity to acetylcholine; conditions where pupillary constriction is undesirable.

Ocular Therapeutic System: 20 mcg/hr; 40 mcg/hr *miotic, direct acting*	maximum dose: 40 mcg/hr system q 7 days	unit; safety and efficacy have not been established in children. Drug–Drug Interactions Reports exists that both **topical NSAIDs** and acetylcholine are ineffective when used concurrently.	ADRs Transient burning/stinging; tearing; bradycardia; hypotension; congestive heart failure; bronchospasm; masked symptoms of hypoglycemia; dizziness.	Pregnancy Category: C Lactation Issues It is not known whether pilocarpine is excreted in breast milk; either the drug or breastfeeding should be discontinued.
Timolol Timoptic Solution 0.25%, 0.5% Gel 0.25%, 0.5% *beta blocker*	Chronic open-angle glaucoma/ocular hypertension/aphakic patients with glaucoma **solution** initial dose: 1 drop (0.25%) in affected eye(s) bid Maximum dose: 1 drop (0.5%) in affected eye(s) bid some patients may be maintained with qd dosing **gel** initial dose: apply (0.25%) to affected eye (s) qd maximum dose: apply (0.5%) to affected eye(s) qd	Administration Issues Shake gel once before use; administer other ophthalmics at least 10 minutes before the gel; do not touch tip of container to any surface; safety and efficacy have not been established in children. Drug–Drug Interactions Additive effects may occur when given with oral **beta blockers** or **verapamil.**	ADRs Transient burning/stinging; tearing; bradycardia; hypotension; congestive heart failure; bronchospasm; masked symptoms of hypoglycemia; dizziness.	Contraindications Hypersensitivity to beta blockers; asthma; sinus bradycardia; second or third degree AV block; overt CHF; severe COPD. Pregnancy Category: C Lactation Issues Timolol is excreted in breast milk; either the drug or breastfeeding should be discontinued.
Travoprost Travatan Solution 0.004% *prostaglandin analog*	Patients with chronic open-angle glaucoma/ocular hypertension who are intolerant of other IOP-lowering medications or insufficient response to other medications One drop each evening in affected eye(s)	Administration Issues Do not touch tip of container. Discard 6 weeks after removing form sealed pouch. If more than one ophthalmic product is used, products should be spaced 10 minutes apart.	ADRs Temporary or permanent changes in eye pigmentation and growth of eyelashes. These changes may occur over months or years and may not be immediately noticeable. Hyperemia, decreased visual acuity, foreign body sensation, pain, pruritis, chest pain, bradycardia, blood pressure changes, depression, headache, anxiety, hypercholesterolemia, dyspepsia, urinary incontinence, arthritis, blurred vision, conjunctivitis, pruritis, lid crusting, photophobia.	Contraindication Use with caution in patients with active intraocular inflammation (uveitis/iritis). Avoid if sensitive to benzalkonium chloride. Pregnancy Category: C Possible teratogenicity. Do not use in women who are regnant or who are attempting to become pregnant. Pregnant patients or healthcare workers should wash their hands thoroughly with soap and water after handling.

401.2 Ophthalmic Antibiotic Agents

Drug and Dosage Forms	Usual Dosage Range	Administration Issues and Drug–Drug Interactions	Common Adverse Drug Reactions (ADRs)	Contraindications, Pregnancy Category, and Lactation Issues
Bacitracin AK-Tracin Ointment 500 units/g	Superficial ocular infection due to strains of microorganisms susceptible to antibiotics 1/2 inch in affected eye(s) qd to bid	Administration Issues Do not touch tip of container to any surface; do not use while wearing soft contact lenses. Drug–Drug Interactions Sensitization from the topical use of an antibiotic may contraindicate the drug's later systemic use in serious infections.	ADRs Burning/stinging; itching.	Contraindications Hypersensitivity to bacitracin; vaccinia; varicella; mycobacterial infections of the eye; ocular fungal infection; use of steroid combinations after uncomplicated removal of a corneal foreign body. Pregnancy Category: C Lactation Issues It is not known if bacitracin is excreted in breast milk; either the drug or nursing should be discontinued.
Chloramphenicol AK-Chlor, Chloroptic, Chloromycetin Solution 0.5% (5 mg/mL) Ointment 1% (10 mg/g)	Superficial ocular infection due to strains of microorganisms susceptible to antibiotics **solution:** 1–2 drops in affected eye(s) q 3–4 h **ointment:** 1/2 inch in affected eye(s) q 3–4 h The dosing interval may be increased after the first 48 hours; treatment should continue for at least 48 hours after the eye appears normal.	Administration Issues Do not touch tip of container to any surface; do not use while wearing soft contact lenses. Drug–Drug Interactions Sensitization from the topical use of an antibiotic may contraindicate the drug's later systemic use in serious infections.	ADRs Burning/stinging; itching; bone marrow suppression (rare); headache, rash.	Contraindications Hypersensitivity to chloramphenicol; vaccinia; varicella; mycobacterial infections of the eye; ocular fungal infection; use of steroid combinations after uncomplicated removal of a corneal foreign body. Pregnancy Category: C Lactation Issues It is not known if chloramphenicol is excreted in breast milk; either the drug or nursing should be discontinued.
Ciprofloxacin Ciloxan Solution 3.5 mg/ml	Bacterial keratitis 2 drops in the affected eye(s) q 15 minutes for 6 h, then 2 drops in the affected eye(s) q 30 minutes for the remainder of the first day; on day 2, 2 drops in the affected eye(s) q hour; on days 3–14, 2 drops in the affected eye(s) q 4 h Bacterial conjunctivitis 1–2 drops in the affected eye(s) q 2 h while awake for 2 days, then 1–2 drops in the affected eye(s) q 4 h while awake for the next 5 days	Administration Issues Do not touch tip of container to any surface; do not use while wearing soft contact lenses. Drug–Drug Interactions Sensitization from the topical use of an antibiotic may contraindicate the drug's later systemic use in serious infections.	ADRs Burning/stinging; itching; white crystalline precipitates; crusting; foreign body sensation; bitter taste; tearing; photophobia.	Contraindications Hypersensitivity to fluoroquinolones; vaccinia; varicella; mycobacterial infections of the eye; ocular fungal infection; use of steroid combinations after uncomplicated removal of a corneal foreign body. Pregnancy Category: C Lactation Issues It is not known if ciprofloxacin is excreted in breast milk; either the drug or nursing should be discontinued.

Erythromycin Ilotycin Ointment 5 mg/g	Superficial ocular infection due to strains of microorganisms susceptible to antibiotics 1/2 inch in affected eye(s) qd to bid Trachoma 1/2 inch in the affected eye(s) bid for 2 months or 1/2 inch in the affected eye(s) for the first 5 days of each month for 6 months	Administration Issues Do not touch tip of container to any surface; do not use while wearing soft contact lenses. Drug–Drug Interactions Sensitization from the topical use of an antibiotic may contraindicate the drug's later systemic use in serious infections.	ADRs Burning/stinging; itching.	Contraindications Hypersensitivity to erythromycin; vaccinia; varicella; mycobacterial infections of the eye; ocular fungal infection; use of steroid combinations after uncomplicated removal of a corneal foreign body. Pregnancy Category: B Lactation Issues It is not known if erythromycin is excreted in breast milk; either the drug or nursing should be discontinued.
Gentamicin Garamycin, Genoptic, Gentacidin, Gentak Solution 3 mg/ml Ointment: 3 mg/g (0.3%)	Superficial ocular infection due to strains of microorganisms susceptible to antibiotics **solution:** 1–2 drops in affected eye(s) q 2–4 h; up to 2 drops q h for severe infections **ointment:** 1/2 inch in affected eye(s) bid to tid	Administration Issues Do not touch tip of container to any surface; do not use while wearing soft contact lenses. Drug–Drug Interactions Sensitization from the topical use of an antibiotic may contraindicate the drug's later systemic use in serious infections.	ADRs Burning/stinging; itching; conjunctival erythema; corneal ulcers.	Contraindications Hypersensitivity to gentamicin; vaccinia; varicella; mycobacterial infections of the eye; ocular fungal infection; use of steroid combinations after uncomplicated removal of a corneal foreign body. Pregnancy Category: C Lactation Issues It is not known if gentamicin is excreted in breast milk; either the drug or nursing should be discontinued.
Levofloxacin Quixin Solution 0.5%	For bacterial conjunctivitis: on days 1 and 2: instill 1–2 drops q 2 h into affected eye(s) while awake (up to 8 times per day) On days 3–7: 1–2 drops 4 h (up to q 4 times per day)	Administration Issues Do not touch tip of container. May be used in pediatric patients over 1 year of age. Do not use contact lenses while receiving medication.	ADRs Temporary burning and/or stinging. Fever, foreign body sensation, burning, itching, tearing, transient decrease in visual acuity.	Contraindications Hypersensitivity, mycobacterial infection of the eyes. Pregnancy Category: C
Norfloxacin Chibroxin Solution 3 mg/ml (0.3%)	Bacterial conjunctivitis 1–2 drops in the affected eye(s) qid for up to 7 days; in severe infections, 1–2 drops in the affected eye(s) q 2 h while awake may be used on the first 2 days of therapy	Administration Issues Do not touch tip of container to any surface; do not use while wearing soft contact lenses; safety and efficacy in infants < 1 year have not been established. Drug–Drug Interactions Sensitization from the topical use of an antibiotic may contraindicate the drug's later systemic use in serious infections.	ADRs Burning/stinging; itching; white crystalline precipitates; crusting; foreign body sensation; bitter taste; tearing; photophobia.	Contraindications Hypersensitivity to fluoroquinolones; vaccinia; varicella; mycobacterial infections of the eye; ocular fungal infection; use of steroid combinations after uncomplicated removal of a corneal foreign body. Pregnancy Category: C

(*continues on next page*)

401.2 Ophthalmic Antibiotic Agents *continued from previous page*

Drug and Dosage Forms	Usual Dosage Range	Administration Issues and Drug–Drug Interactions	Common Adverse Drug Reactions (ADRs)	Contraindications, Pregnancy Category, and Lactation Issues
Norfloxacin *cont.*				Lactation Issues It is not known if norfloxacin is excreted in breast milk; either the drug or nursing should be discontinued.
Ofloxacin Ocuflox Solution 3 mg/ml (0.3%)	Bacterial conjunctivitis; corneal ulcers 1–2 drops in the affected eye(s) q 2–4 h while awake for 2 days, then 1–2 drops in the affected eye(s) qid for up to 5 more days; for more severe infections, more frequent administration may be required	Administration Issues Do not touch tip of container to any surface; do not use while wearing soft contact lenses; safety and efficacy in infants < 1 year have not been established. Drug–Drug Interactions Sensitization from the topical use of an antibiotic may contraindicate the drug's later systemic use in serious infections.	ADRs Burning/stinging; itching; white crystalline precipitates; crusting; foreign body sensation; bitter taste; tearing; photophobia.	Contraindications Hypersensitivity to fluoroquinolones; vaccinia; varicella; mycobacterial infections of the eye; ocular fungal infection; use of steroid combinations after uncomplicated removal of a corneal foreign body. Pregnancy Category: C Lactation Issues It is not known if ofloxacin is excreted in breast milk; either the drug or nursing should be discontinued.
Polymyxin B Solution 25,000 units/mL	Superficial ocular infection due to strains of microorganisms susceptible to antibiotics **solution:** 1–2 drops in affected eye(s) bid to qid **ointment:** 1/2 inch in affected eye(s) q 3–4 h	Administration Issues Do not touch tip of container to any surface; do not use while wearing soft contact lenses; safety and efficacy in infants < 2 months have not been established. Drug–Drug Interactions Sensitization from the topical use of an antibiotic may contraindicate the drug's later systemic use in serious infections.	ADRs Burning/stinging; itching.	Contraindications Hypersensitivity to polymyxin; vaccinia; varicella; mycobacterial infections of the eye; ocular fungal infection; use of steroid combinations after uncomplicated removal of a corneal foreign body. Pregnancy Category: B Lactation Issues It is not known if polymyxin is excreted in breast milk; either the drug or nursing should be discontinued.
Sulfacetamide AK-Sulf, Bleph-10, Ocusulf-10, Sodium Sulamyd, Sulf-10, Cetamide Solution 10%, 15%, 30% Ointment 10%	Superficial ocular infection due to strains of microorganisms susceptible to antibiotics **solution:** 1–2 drops in the affected eye(s) q 1–4 h initially according to severity of infection; taper dose by increasing the time interval between doses	Administration Issues Do not touch tip of container to any surface; do not use while wearing soft contact lenses; safety and efficacy in children have not been established; protect from light.	ADRs Burning/stinging; itching; periorbital edema; rash; photosensitivity; headache; GI upset; bone marrow suppression (rare); rare occurrences of severe sensitivity reactions have been reported.	Contraindications Hypersensitivity to sulfonamides; infants < 2 months; epithelial herpes simplex keratitis; vaccinia; viral, mycobacterial or fungal infection of the ocular structures; after uncomplicated removal of a corneal foreign body. Pregnancy Category: C

	ointment: 1/2 inch in affected eye(s) tid to qid and q hs Trachoma **solution:** 2 drops in affected eye(s) q 2 h	Drug–Drug Interactions **Silver preparations** are incompatible with topical sulfonamides.		Lactation Issues Sulfacetamide is excreted in breast milk.
Sulfisoxazole Gantrisin Solution 4%	Superficial ocular infection due to strains of microorganisms susceptible to antibiotics 1–2 drops in affected eye(s) q 1–4 h initially according to severity of infection; taper dose by increasing the time interval between doses Trachoma 2 drops in affected eye(s) q 2 h	Administration Issues Do not touch tip of container to any surface; do not use while wearing soft contact lenses; safety and efficacy in children have not been established; protect from light. Drug–Drug Interactions **Silver preparations** are incompatible with topical sulfonamides.	ADRs Burning/stinging; itching; periorbital edema; photosensitivity; headache; rash; GI upset; bone marrow suppression (rare); rare occurrences of severe sensitivity reactions have been reported.	Contraindications Hypersensitivity to sulfonamides; infants < 2 months; epithelial herpes simplex keratitis; vaccinia; viral, mycobacterial or fungal infection of the ocular structures; after uncomplicated removal of a corneal foreign body. Pregnancy Category: B (Category D at term) Lactation Issues Sulfisoxazole is excreted in breast milk.
Tobramycin AKTob, Tobrex Solution 0.3% Ointment 3 mg/g	Superficial ocular infection due to strains of microorganisms susceptible to antibiotics **solution:** 1–2 drops in affected eye(s) q 4 h **ointment:** 1/2 inch in affected eye(s) bid to tid Therapy should be continued for at least 48 hours after the infection is controlled.	Administration Issues Do not touch tip of container to any surface; do not use while wearing soft contact lenses; safe and effective in children. Drug–Drug Interactions Sensitization from the topical use of an antibiotic may contraindicate the drug's later systemic use in serious infections.	ADRs Burning/stinging; itching; conjunctival erythema; corneal ulcers.	Contraindications Hypersensitivity to tobramycin; vaccinia; varicella; mycobacterial infections of the eye; ocular fungal infection; use of steroid combinations after uncomplicated removal of a corneal foreign body. Pregnancy Category: C Lactation Issues It is not known if tobramycin is excreted in breast milk; either the drug or nursing should be discontinued.

401.3 Ophthalmic Antifungal Agents

Drug and Dosage Forms	Usual Dosage Range for Specific Indications	Administration Issues and Drug Interactions	Common Adverse Drug Reactions (ADRs)	Contraindications, Pregnancy Category, and Lactation Issues
Natamycin Natacyn Suspension 5%	Fungal blepharitis, conjunctivitis 1 drop in the affected eye(s) 4–6 times daily for up to 7–10 days Fungal keratitis 1 drop in the affected eye(s) q 1–2 h for 3–4 days followed by 1 drop 6–8 times daily to complete 14–21 days or until resolution	Administration Issues Do not touch tip of container to any surface; shake well before use; safety and efficacy have not been established in children. Drug Interactions Increased toxicity with **topical corticosteroids** (concomitant use is contraindicated).	ADRs Blurred vision, eye pain, photophobia, one case of conjunctival chemosis and hyperemia, thought to be allergic in nature, has been reported.	Contraindications Hypersensitivity to natamcycin. Pregnancy Category: C Lactation Issues It is not known whether natamycin is excreted in breast milk; use caution in nursing women.

401.4 Ophthalmic Antiviral Agents

Drug and Dosage Forms	Usual Dosage Range	Administration Issues and Drug–Drug Interactions	Common Adverse Drug Reactions (ADRs)	Contraindications, Pregnancy Category, and Lactation Issues
Trifluridine Viroptic Solution 1%	Recurrent epithelial keratitis due to herpes simplex virus 1 and 2; superficial keratitis caused by herpes simplex virus that has not responded to topical idoxuridine or when adverse reactions to idoxuridine have occurred 1 drop in affected eye(s) q 2 h while awake for a maximum daily dose of 9 drops until the corneal ulcer has completely re-epithelialized; treat for an additional 7 days with 1 drop in the affected eye(s) q 4 h while awake (minimum 5 drops daily); do not exceed 21 days of treatment	Administration Issues Do not touch tip of container to any surface; corticosteroids are usually contraindicated in herpes simplex virus eye infections—if administered with topical corticosteroid therapy, consider corticosteroid-induced ocular side effects such as glaucoma or cataract formation and progression of bacterial or viral infection; solution must be stored in the refrigerator.	ADRs Burning/stinging; palpebral edema; superficial punctate keratitis; stromal edema.	Contraindications Hypersensitivity to trifluridine. Pregnancy Category: C Lactation Issues It is not known whether trifluridine is excreted in breast milk; either the drug or breastfeeding should be discontinued.
Vidarabine Vira-A Ointment 3%	Acute keratoconjunctivitis and recurrent epithelial keratitis due to herpes simplex virus 1 and 2; superficial keratitis caused by herpes simplex virus that has not responded to topical idoxuridine or when adverse reactions to idoxuridine have occurred	Administration Issues Do not touch tip of container to any surface; corticosteroids are usually contraindicated in herpes simplex virus eye infections—if administered with topical corticosteroid therapy, consider corticosteroid-induced ocular side effects such	ADRs Lacrimation; foreign body sensation; conjunctival infection; burning/irritation; superficial punctate keratitis; photophobia.	Contraindications Hypersensitivity to vidarabine; sterile trophic ulcers. Pregnancy Category: C

	1/2 inch in the affected eye(s) 5 times daily at 3 hour intervals; treat for an additional 7 days after re-epithelialization has occurred with 1/2 inch in the affected eye(s) bid to prevent recurrence	as glaucoma or cataract formation and progression of bacterial or viral infection.		Lactation Issues It is not known whether vidarabine is excreted in breast milk; either the drug or breastfeeding should be discontinued.

401.5 Ophthalmic Antiallergic Agents

Drug and Dosage Forms	Usual Dosage Ranges	Administration Issues and Drug—Drug Interactions	Common Adverse Drug Reactions (ADRs)	Contraindications, Pregnancy Category, and Lactation Issues
Azelastine HCL Optivar Solution 0.5 mg/mL	Allergic conjunctivitis 1 drop in each eye twice daily	Administration Issues Do not touch tip of container. Wait at least 10 minutes after instilling drops to insert soft contact lenses. Do not use contact lenses if eyes are red. May cause drowsiness, avoid tasks that require a high degree of attention (driving, heavy machinery operation). May be used in children $\geq$ 3 years of age.	ADRs Burning, stinging, headache, fatigue, bitter taste.	Contraindications Hypersensitivity to azelastine or benzalkonium chloride; use with caution if patient is receiving other CNS depressants. Pregnancy Category: C Lactation Excreted in breast milk.
Cromolyn Crolom Solution 4%	Conjunctivitis 1–2 drops in each eye 4–6 times daily at regular intervals	Administration Issues Do not touch tip of container to any surface; shake well before use; do not wear soft contact lenses during treatment with cromolyn; safety and efficacy have not been established in children < 4 years.	ADRs Ocular stinging/burning; tearing; itchy eyes.	Contraindications Hypersensitivity to cromolyn. Pregnancy Category: B Lactation Issues It is not known if cromolyn is excreted in breast milk; use caution in nursing women.
Levocabastine Livostin Suspension 0.05%	Allergic conjunctivitis 1 drop in the affected eye(s) qid for up to 2 weeks	Administration Issues Do not touch tip of container to any surface; shake well before use; do not wear soft contact lenses during treatment with levocabastine; safety and efficacy have not been established in children < 12 years.	ADRs Burning/stinging; headache; blurred vision; dry mouth; lacrimation/discharge.	Contraindications Hypersensitivity to levocabastine. Pregnancy Category: B Lactation Issues Levocabastine is excreted in breast milk; use caution in nursing women.

(continues on next page)

401.5 Ophthalmic Antiallergic Agents *continued from previous page*

Drug and Dosage Forms	Usual Dosage Ranges	Administration Issues and Drug–Drug Interactions	Common Adverse Drug Reactions (ADRs)	Contraindications, Pregnancy Category, and Lactation Issues
Lodoxamide Alomide Solution 0.1%	Vernal keratoconjunctivitis, conjunctivitis and keratitis **adults and children > 2 years:** 1–2 drops in the affected eye(s) qid for up to 3 months	Administration Issues Do not touch tip of container to any surface; do not wear soft contact lenses during treatment with lodoxamide; safety and efficacy have not been established in children < 2 years.	ADRs Burning/stinging; ocular pruritus; blurred vision; dry eye; tearing; foreign body sensation; headache.	Contraindications Hypersensitivity to lodoxamide. Pregnancy Category: B Lactation Issues It is not known if lodoxamide is excreted in breast milk; use caution in nursing women.
Ketotifen fumarate Zaditor Solution 0.025%	Allergic conjunctivitis 1 drop of 8–12 h	Administration Issues Do not use to treat irritation from the wearing of contact lenses. Do not touch tip of bottle. Wait at least 10 minutes after instilling drops to insert soft contact lenses. Do not wear contact lenses if the eyes remain red. Not for use in children < 3 years old.	ADRs Allergic reactions, burning, stinging, conjunctivitis, discharge, dry eyes, pain, itching, keratitis, photophobia.	Contraindications Sensitivity to ketotifen or benzalkonium chloride. Pregnancy Category: C Oral use has led to teratogenicity in animals.
Nedocromil Alocril Solution 2%	Allergic conjunctivitis 1–2 drops in the affected eye(s) bid	Administration Issues Do not use to treat irritation from the wearing of contact lenses. Do not touch tip of bottle. Wait at least 10 minutes after instilling drops to insert soft contact lenses. Do not wear contact lenses if the eyes remain red. Not for use in children < 3 years old.	ADRs Headache, unpleasant taste, irritation, stinging, burning, eye redness, photophobia.	Contraindication Sensitivity to nedocromil or benzalkonium chloride. Pregnancy Category: B Lactation Issue Drug is transferred into breast milk.
Olopatadine Patanol	Allergic conjunctivitis 1 drop into the affected eye(s) bid at 6–8h intervals	Administration Issues Do not use to treat irritation from the wearing of contact lenses. Do not touch tip of bottle.	ADRs Headaches, asthenia, blurred vision, burning or stinging, cold syndrome, dry eye, foreign body sensation, hyperemia,	Contraindication Sensitivity to olopadatine or benzalkonium chloride.

Solution 0.1%		Wait at least 10 minutes after instilling drops to insert soft contact lenses. Do not wear contact lenses if the eyes remain red. Not for use in children < 3 years old.	hypersensitivity, keratitis, lid edema, nausea, pharyngitis, pruritus, rhinitis, sinusitis, taste perversion.	Pregnancy Category: C Lactation Issue Drug is transferred into breast milk.

401.6 Ophthalmic Nonsteroidal Anti-Inflammatory Agents

Drug and Dosage Forms	Usual Dosage Range	Administration Issues	Common Adverse Drug Reactions (ADRs)	Contraindications, Pregnancy Category, and Lactation Issues
Diclofenac Voltaren Solution 0.1%	Postoperative inflammation following cataract extraction one drop into affected eye qid beginning 24 h post cataract surgery and continuing throughout the first 2 weeks of the postoperative period	Administration Issues Do not touch tip of container to any surface; safety and efficacy have not been established in children.	ADRs Burning/stinging, keratitis, ocular allergy, nausea, vomiting.	Contraindications Hypersensitivity to diclofenac or other NSAIDs; patients wearing soft contacts may experience ocular irritation. Pregnancy Category: B Lactation Issues It is not known if diclofenac is excreted in breast milk; use caution in nursing women.
Flurbiprofen Ocufen, various generics Solution 0.03%	Inhibition of intraoperative miosis instill one drop every 30 minutes beginning 2 h prior to surgery (total of 4 drops)	Administration Issues Do not touch tip of container to any surface; safety and efficacy have not been established in children.	ADRs Burning/stinging; increased bleeding tendency of ocular tissue in conjunction with ocular surgery.	Contraindications Hypersensitivity to flurbiprofen or other NSAIDs; epithelial herpes simplex keratitis (dendritic keratitis). Pregnancy Category: C Lactation Issues It is not known if flurbiprofen is excreted in breast milk; use caution in nursing women.
Ketorolac Acular Solution 0.5%	Relief of ocular itching caused by seasonal allergic conjunctivitis one drop (0.25 mg) qid Treatment of postoperative inflammation following cataract extraction one drop into affected eye qid beginning 24 h post cataract surgery and continu-	Administration Issues Do not touch tip of container to any surface; safety and efficacy have not been established in children.	ADRs Ocular irritation, allergic reactions, superficial keratitis, superficial ocular infections, eye dryness, corneal infiltrates, corneal ulcer, blurry vision.	Contraindications Hypersensitivity to ketorolac or other NSAIDs. Pregnancy Category: B (Category D in 3rd trimester)

(*continues on next page*)

401.6 Ophthalmic Nonsteroidal Anti-Inflammatory Agents *continued from previous page*

Drug and Dosage Forms	Usual Dosage Range	Administration Issues	Common Adverse Drug Reactions (ADRs)	Contraindications, Pregnancy Category, and Lactation Issues
Ketorolac *cont.*	ing throughout the first 2 weeks of the postoperative period			Lactation Issues It is not known if ketorolac is excreted in breast milk; use caution in nursing women.
Suprofen Profenal Solution 1%	Inhibition of intraoperative miosis On the day of surgery, instill 2 drops into conjunctival sac at 3, 2, and 1 hour(s) prior to surgery. Two drops may be instilled into conjunctival sac q 4 h while awake the day preceding surgery.	Administration Issues Do not touch tip of container to any surface; safety and efficacy have not been established in children.	ADRs Discomfort, itching, redness, allergy, iritis, pain, chemosis, photophobia, irritation.	Contraindications Hypersensitivity to suprofen or other NSAIDs; epithelial herpes simplex keratitis (dendritic keratitis). Pregnancy Category: C Lactation Issues Suprofen is excreted in breast milk after oral use and systemic absorption may occur following ocular administration, therefore use caution in nursing women.

401.7 Ophthalmic Steroidal Agents

Drug and Dosage Forms	Usual Dosage Range	Administration Issues	Common Adverse Drug Reactions (ADRs)	Contraindications, Pregnancy Category, and Lactation Issues
Dexamethasone AK-Dex, Decadron, Maxidex Solution 0.1% Suspension 0.1%, 0.5% Ointment 0.05%	Inflammatory ocular conditions; corneal injury; graft rejection after keratoplasty **solution and suspension:** 1–2 drops in the affected eye(s) q hour during the day and q 2 h at night initially; after response, reduce dose to 1 drop in the affected eye(s) q 4 h then tid to qid **ointment:** 1/2 inch in affected eye(s) tid to qid initially; after response, reduce dose to bid then qd Postoperative inflammation 1–2 drops in the affected eye(s) qid beginning 24 h after surgery and continue for 2 weeks	Administration Issues Shake suspension well before use; do not touch tip of container to any surface; relapse may occur if therapy is reduced too rapidly—taper over several days; safety and efficacy have not been established in children.	ADRs Elevated IOP; posterior subcapsular cataract formation; secondary ocular infection.	Contraindications Hypersensitivity to topical steroids; herpes simplex keratitis; ocular fungal or viral infection; ocular tuberculosis; after uncomplicated removal of a superficial corneal foreign body. Pregnancy Category: C Lactation Issues It is not known if topical steroids are excreted in breast milk; exercise caution when administering to a nursing woman.

Fluorometholone Fluor-Op, FML, Flarex Suspension 0.1%, 0.25% Ointment 0.1%	Inflammatory ocular conditions; corneal injury; graft rejection after keratoplasty **suspension:** 1–2 drops in the affected eye(s) q hour during the day and q 2 h at night initially; after response, reduce dose to 1 drop in the affected eye(s) q 4 hours then tid to qid **ointment:** 1/2 inch in affected eye(s) tid to qid initially; after response, reduce dose to bid then qd Postoperative inflammation 1–2 drops in the affected eye(s) qid beginning 24 h after surgery and continue for 2 weeks	Administration Issues Shake suspension well before use; do not touch tip of container to any surface; relapse may occur if therapy is reduced too rapidly—taper over several days; safety and efficacy have not been established in children.	ADRs Elevated IOP; posterior subcapsular cataract formation; secondary ocular infection.	Contraindications Hypersensitivity to topical steroids; herpes simplex keratitis; ocular fungal or viral infection; ocular tuberculosis; after uncomplicated removal of a superficial corneal foreign body. Pregnancy Category: C Lactation Issues It is not known if topical steroids are excreted in breast milk; exercise caution when administering to a nursing woman.
Medrysone HMS Suspension 1%	Inflammatory ocular conditions; corneal injury; graft rejection after keratoplasty 1–2 drops in the affected eye(s) q hour during the day and q 2 h at night initially; after response, reduce dose to 1 drop in the affected eye(s) q 4 h then tid to qid Postoperative inflammation 1–2 drops in the affected eye(s) qid beginning 24 h after surgery and continue for 2 weeks	Administration Issues Shake suspension well before use; do not touch tip of container to any surface; relapse may occur if therapy is reduced too rapidly—taper over several days; safety and efficacy have not been established in children.	ADRs Elevated IOP; posterior subcapsular cataract formation; secondary ocular infection.	Contraindications Hypersensitivity to topical steroids; herpes simplex keratitis; ocular fungal or viral infection; ocular tuberculosis; after uncomplicated removal of a superficial corneal foreign body. Pregnancy Category: C Lactation Issues It is not known if topical steroids are excreted in breast milk; exercise caution when administering to a nursing woman.
Prednisolone AK-Pred, Pred Forte, Econopred Plus, Pred Mild, generics Suspension 0.12%, 0.125%, 1% Solution 0.125%, 1%	Inflammatory ocular conditions; corneal injury; graft rejection after keratoplasty 1–2 drops in the affected eye(s) q hour during the day and q 2 h at night initially; after response, reduce dose to 1 drop in the affected eye(s) q 4 h then tid to qid Postoperative inflammation 1–2 drops in the affected eye(s) qid beginning 24 h after surgery and continue for 2 weeks	Administration Issues Shake suspension well before use; do not touch tip of container to any surface; relapse may occur if therapy is reduced too rapidly—taper over several days; safety and efficacy have not been established in children.	ADRs Elevated IOP; posterior subcapsular cataract formation; secondary ocular infection.	Contraindications Hypersensitivity to topical steroids; herpes simplex keratitis; ocular fungal or viral infection; ocular tuberculosis; after uncomplicated removal of a superficial corneal foreign body. Pregnancy Category: C Lactation Issues It is not known if topical steroids are excreted in breast milk; exercise caution when administering to a nursing woman.

(*continues on next page*)

401.7 Ophthalmic Steroidal Agents *continued from previous page*

Drug and Dosage Forms	Usual Dosage Range	Administration Issues	Common Adverse Drug Reactions (ADRs)	Contraindications, Pregnancy Category, and Lactation Issues
Rimexolone Vexol Suspension 1%	Inflammatory ocular conditions; corneal injury; graft rejection after keratoplasty 1–2 drops in the affected eye(s) q hour during the day and q 2 h at night initially; after response, reduce dose to 1 drop in the affected eye(s) q 4 h then tid to qid Postoperative inflammation 1–2 drops in the affected eye(s) qid beginning 24 h after surgery and continue for 2 weeks	Administration Issues Shake suspension well before use; do not touch tip of container to any surface; relapse may occur if therapy is reduced too rapidly—taper over several days; safety and efficacy have not been established in children.	ADRs Elevated IOP; posterior subcapsular cataract formation; secondary ocular infection.	Contraindications Hypersensitivity to topical steroids; herpes simplex keratitis; ocular fungal or viral infection; ocular tuberculosis; after uncomplicated removal of a superficial corneal foreign body. Pregnancy Category: C Lactation Issues It is not known if topical steroids are excreted in breast milk; exercise caution when administering to a nursing woman.

402. Otic Preparations

402.1 Antibiotics

Drug and Dosage Forms	Usual Dosage Range	Administration Issues and Patient Education	Common Adverse Drug Reactions (ADRs) and Contraindications
Chloramphenicol Chloromycetin Otic Solution 0.5%	**Treatment of superficial infections involving the external auditory canal:** 2–3 drops tid For serious infections, supplement with systemic antibiotics.	**FOR OTIC USE ONLY.** Do not touch dropper to ear; wash hands prior to use To allow drops to flow into ear, tilt head to side and: **Adults:** hold earlobe up and back **Children:** hold earlobe down and back	ADRs *Local irritation:* itching, burning, angioneurotic edema, urticaria, vesicular and maculopapular dermatitis indicate a sensitivity to chloramphenicol and constitute discontinuation of medication. *Superinfection:* prolonged use may result in overgrowth of nonsusceptible organisms and fungi (e.g., herpes simplex, vaccinia, varicella). ***Warnings:* Bone marrow hypoplasia has occurred; Ototoxicity more likely if medication enters the middle ear (i.e., perforated tympanic membrane).** Contraindications Hypersensitivity to any component; perforated tympanic membrane.
Ciprofloxacin HCl and hydrocortisone otic suspension Cipro-HC Otic Otic solution 2 mg Ciprofloxacin plus 10 mg hydrocortisone/mL	**Treatment of acute otitis externa in adult and pediatric patients, one year and older, due to susceptible strains of *Pseudomonas aeurugi-nosa, Staphylococcus aureus,* and *Proteus mirabilis*** For children (age 1 year and older) and adults, 3 drops of the suspension should be instilled into the affected ear bid for 7 days	**FOR OTIC USE ONLY.** SHAKE WELL IMMEDIATELY BEFORE USING. The suspension should be warmed by holding the bottle in the hand for 1–2 minutes to avoid the dizziness that may result from the instillation of a cold solution into the ear canal. The patient should lie with the affected ear upward and then the drops should be instilled. This position should be maintained for 30–60 seconds to facilitate penetration of the drops into the ear. Repeat, if necessary, for the opposite ear. Discard unused portion after therapy is completed.	ADRs Headache, itching. Contraindications Drug is contraindicated in persons with a history of hypersensitivity to hydrocortisone, ciprofloxacin, or any member of the quinolone class of antimicrobial agents. This nonsterile product should not be used if the tympanic membrane is perforated. Use of this product is contraindicated in viral infections of the external canal including varicella and herpes simplex infections.

(continues on next page)

402.1 Antibiotics *continued from previous page*

Drug and Dosage Forms	Usual Dosage Range	Administration Issues and Patient Education	Common Adverse Drug Reactions (ADRs) and Contraindications
Hydrocortisone 1% plus neomycin 5 mg/mL plus polymyxin B 10,000 U/mL Cortisporin Otic, Otosporin, others (Solution or suspension) **Hydrocortisone 0.5% plus polymyxin B 10,000 U/mL** Otobiotic Otic (Solution) **Hydrocortisone 1% plus neomycin 4.71 mg/mL** Coly-Mycin S Otic (Suspension)	**Treatment of superficial bacterial infections of the external auditory canal** solution or suspension: 4 drops tid to qid **Treatment of infections related to mastoidectomy and fenestration cavities** suspension only: 4 drops tid to qid	**FOR OTIC USE ONLY.** For the suspension—shake well for 10 seconds prior to use. Do not touch dropper to ear; wash hands prior to use. To allow drops to flow into ear, till head to side and: **Adults:** hold earlobe up and back **Children:** hold earlobe down and back	ADRs *Superinfection:* prolonged use may result in overgrowth of nonsusceptible organisms and fungi (e.g., herpes simplex, vaccinia, varicella). Contraindications Hypersensitivity to any component; perforated tympanic membrane; FOR OTIC USE ONLY.
Ofloxacin otic Floxcin Otic Otic solution 0.3% solution	**Ofloxacin otic solution is used to treat infections of the ear canal. It also is used to treat infections of the middle ear in patients with nonintact tympanic membranes (holes or tubes in the eardrums).** Adults and teenagers (12 years of age and older)—Place 10 drops in each affected ear bid for 10–14 days, depending on the infection. Children 1 to 12 years of age—Place 5 drops in each affected ear bid for 10 days. Children $<$ 1 year of age—Use and dose must be determined by your doctor.	**FOR OTIC USE ONLY.** Hold the bottle in your hands for 1–2 minutes to warm up the solution before putting it in your ear. Wash your hands with soap and water. Gently clean any discharge that can be removed easily from the outer ear. If you are using the eardrops for a middle ear infection—Drop the medicine into the ear canal. Then, gently press the tragus of the ear 4 times in a pumping motion. This will allow the drops to pass through the hole or tube in the eardrum and into the middle ear. If you are using the eardrops for an ear canal infection—Gently pull the outer ear up and back for adults (down and back for children) to straighten the ear canal. This will allow the eardrops to flow down into the ear canal. Keep the ear facing up for about 5 minutes to allow the medicine to come into contact with the infection.	ADRs Burning, itching, redness, skin rash, swelling, or other sign of irritation not present before use of this medicine. Contraindications Hypersensitivity to ofloxacin or any other quinolones or any other quinolones or any components of this medications.

		If both ears are being treated, turn over after 5 minutes, and repeat the application for the other ear. *To keep the medicine as germ-free as possible, do not touch the applicator tip to any surface (including the ear).* Also, keep the container tightly closed.		

402.2 Miscellaneous Otic Preparations

Drug and Dosage Forms	Usual Dosage Range	Ingredient Use(s)	Administration Issues & Patient Education	Common Adverse Drug Reactions (ADRs) and Contraindications
Acetic Acid (2%); Propylene Glycol Diacetate (3%); Benzethonium Chloride (0.02%); Sodium Acetate (0.015%) Acetasol; VoSol; Acetic Acid Otic (Solution)	**Minor Outer Ear Complaints** Insert saturated wick; keep moist for 24 h. Remove wick and instill 5 drops 3–4 times daily.	**Acetic Acid, Acetate, Benzethonium Chloride:** antibacterial or antifungal action	**For Otic Use ONLY** Do not touch dropper to ear; wash hands prior to use To allow drops to flow into ear, tilt head to side and: **Adults:** hold earlobe up and back **Children:** hold earlobe down and back	ADRs Local reactions (redness, itching). Contraindications Hypersensitivity to any ingredient.
Acetic Acid (2%); Aluminum Acetate Burow's Otic; Otic Domeboro; generic (Solution)	**Minor Outer Ear Complaints** Insert saturated wick; keep moist for 24 h. Remove wick and instill 4–6 drops every 2–3 hrs.	**Acetic Acid, Aluminum Acetate:** antibacterial or antifungal action	**For Otic Use ONLY** Do not touch dropper to ear; wash hands prior to use To allow drops to flow into ear, tilt head to side and: **Adults:** hold earlobe up and back **Children:** hold earlobe down and back	ADRs Local reactions (redness, itching). Contraindications Hypersensitivity to any ingredient.
Acetic Acid (Nonaqueous); Burow's Solution; Boric Acid; Propylene Glycol Star Otic (Solution)	**Minor Outer Ear Complaints** 2–3 drops in each ear before and after swimming or showering.	**Acetic Acid, Burow's Solution, Boric Acid:** antibacterial or antifungal activity	**For Otic Use ONLY** Do not touch dropper to ear; wash hands prior to use To allow drops to flow into ear, tilt head to side and: **Adults:** hold earlobe up and back **Children:** hold earlobe down and back	ADRs Local reactions (redness, itching). Contraindications Hypersensitivity to any ingredient.

(*continues on next page*)

402.2 Miscellaneous Otic Preparations *continued from previous page*

Drug and Dosage Forms	Usual Dosage Range	Ingredient Use(s)	Administration Issues & Patient Education	Common Adverse Drug Reactions (ADRs) and Contraindications
Benzocaine (1.4%); Antipyrine (5.4%); Glycerin Allergan Ear Drops; Antipyrine & Benzocaine Otic; Auralgan; Auroto; Otocalm (Solution)	**Minor Outer Ear Complaints** Fill ear canal with 2–4 drops; insert saturated cotton pledget. Repeat 3–4 times daily or once every 1–2 h.	**Benzocaine:** Local anesthetic **Antipyrine:** Analgesic **Glycerin:** solvent and vehicle. It is an emollient, hygroscopic and humectant	**For Otic Use ONLY** Do not touch dropper to ear; wash hands prior to use To allow drops to flow into ear, tilt head to side and: **Adults:** hold earlobe up and back **Children:** hold earlobe down and back	ADRs Local reactions (redness, itching). Contraindications Hypersensitivity to any ingredient.
Benzocaine (5%); Antipyrine (5%); Phenylephrine (0.25%); Propylene Glycol Tympagesic (Solution)	**Minor Outer Ear Complaints** Fill ear canal; plug with saturated cotton and repeat every 2–4 hrs.	**Benzocaine:** Local anesthetic **Antipyrine:** Analgesic **Phenylephrine:** Vasoconstrictor (decongestant)	**For Otic Use ONLY** Do not touch dropper to ear; wash hands prior to use To allow drops to flow into ear, tilt head to side and: **Adults:** hold earlobe up and back **Children:** hold earlobe down and back	ADRs Local reactions (redness, itching). Contraindications Hypersensitivity to any ingredient.
Benzocaine (20%); Benzothonium Chloride (0.1%); Glycerin (1%); PEG 300	**Minor Outer Ear Complaints** Fill canal with 4–5 drops; insert a cotton pledget. Repeat every 1–2 h.	**Benzocaine:** Local anesthetic **Benzothonium Chloride:** antibacterial or antifungal action	**For Otic Use ONLY** Do not touch dropper to ear; wash hands prior to use. To allow drops to flow into ear, tilt head to side and: **Adults:** hold earlobe up and back **Children:** hold earlobe down and back	ADRs Local reactions (redness, itching). Contraindications Hypersensitivity to any ingredient.
Benzocaine Americaine Otic; Otocain (Solution)		**Glycerin:** solvent and vehicle. It is an emollient, hygroscopic, and humectant	**For Otic Use ONLY** Do not touch dropper to ear; wash hands prior to use. To allow drops to flow into ear, tilt head to side and: **Adults:** hold earlobe up and back **Children:** hold earlobe down and back	ADRs Local reactions (redness, itching). Contraindications Hypersensitivity to any ingredient.

Boric Acid (2.75%); Isopropyl alcohol Auro-Dri; Dri/Ear; Ear-Dry (Solution)	**Minor Outer Ear Complaints** 3–8 drops in each ear.	**Boric Acid:** antibacterial or antifungal activity **Isopropyl Alcohol:** drying agent	**For Otic Use ONLY** Do not touch dropper to ear; wash hands prior to use. To allow drops to flow into ear, tilt head to side and: **Adults:** hold earlobe up and back **Children:** hold earlobe down and back	ADRs Local reactions (redness, itching). Contraindications Hypersensitivity to any ingredient.
Carbamide Peroxide (6.5%); Glycerin, Propylene Glycol; Sodium Stannate Debrox (Solution)	**Minor Outer Ear Complaints** 5–10 drops bid for up to 4 d	**Carbamide Peroxide:** emulsify/disperse ear wax **Glycerin:** solvent and vehicle. It is an emollient, hygroscopic, and humectant	**For Otic Use ONLY** Do not touch dropper to ear; wash hands prior to use. To allow drops to flow into ear, tilt head to side and: **Adults:** hold earlobe up and back **Children:** hold earlobe down and back	ADRs Local reactions (redness, itching). Contraindications Hypersensitivity to any ingredient.
Carbamide Peroxide (6.5%); Alcohol (6.3%); Glycerin, Polysorbate 20 Murine Ear (Solution)	**Minor Outer Ear Complaints** 5–10 drops bid for up to 4 d	**Carbamide Peroxide:** emulsify/disperse ear wax **Alcohol:** drying agent **Glycerin:** solvent and vehicle. It is an emollient, hygroscopic, and humectant	**For Otic Use ONLY** Do not touch dropper to ear; wash hands prior to use. To allow drops to flow into ear, tilt head to side and: **Adults:** hold earlobe up and back **Children:** hold earlobe down and back	ADRs Local reactions (redness, itching). Contraindications Hypersensitivity to any ingredient.
Carbamide Peroxide (6.5%); anhydrous glycerin base Auro Ear Drops (Solution)	**Minor Outer Ear Complaints** 5–10 drops bid for up to 4 d	**Carbamide Peroxide:** emulsify/disperse ear wax **Glycerin:** solvent and vehicle. It is an emollient, hygroscopic, and humectant	**For Otic Use ONLY** Do not touch dropper to ear; wash hands prior to use To allow drops to flow into ear, tilt head to side and: **Adults:** hold earlobe up and back **Children:** hold earlobe down and back	ADRs Local reactions (redness, itching). Contraindications Hypersensitivity to any ingredient.
Desonide (0.05%); Acetic Acid (2%); Propylene glycol Otic Tridesilon (Solution)	**Minor Outer Ear Complaints** 3–4 drops in ear 3–4 times daily. Or insert saturated wick and leave in until relief.	**Desonide:** anti-inflammatory and antipruritic effects **Acetic Acid:** antibacterial or antifungal activity	**For Otic Use ONLY** Do not touch dropper to ear; wash hands prior to use. To allow drops to flow into ear, tilt head to side and:	ADRs Local reactions (redness, itching). Contraindications Hypersensitivity to any ingredient.

(continues on next page)

402.2 Miscellaneous Otic Preparations *continued from previous page*

Drug and Dosage Forms	Usual Dosage Range	Ingredient Use(s)	Administration Issues & Patient Education	Common Adverse Drug Reactions (ADRs) and Contraindications
Desonide (0.05%); Acetic Acid (2%); Propylene glycol ***cont.***			**Adults:** hold earlobe up and back **Children:** hold earlobe down and back	
Hydrocortisone (1%); Acetic Acid (2%); Propylene glycol diacetate (3%); Sodium acetate (0.015%); Benzethonium Chloride (0.02%) VoSol HC; Acetasol HC (Solution)	**Minor Outer Ear Complaints** Insert saturated wick into ear; leave in ear for 24 h, keeping it moist with 3–5 drops every 4–6 h. Remove wick and instill 5 drops 3–4 times daily.	**Hydrocortisone:** anti-inflammatory and antipruritic effects **Acetic Acid, Acetate, Benzothonium Chloride:** antibacterial or antifungal action	**For Otic Use ONLY** Do not touch dropper to ear; wash hands prior to use To allow drops to flow into ear, tilt head to side and: **Adults:** hold earlobe up and back **Children:** hold earlobe down and back	ADRs Local reactions (redness, itching). Contraindications Hypersensitivity to any ingredient.
Hydrocortisone (1%); Alcohol (44%); Propylene glycol; Dermprotective Factor yerba santa; Benzyl Benzoate EarSol HC (Solution)	**Minor Outer Ear Complaints** 4–6 drops into ear 3–4 times daily	**Hydrocortisone:** anti-inflammatory and antipuritic effects **Alcohol:** drying agent	**For Otic Use ONLY** Do not touch dropper to ear; wash hands prior to use. To allow drops to flow into ear, tilt head to side and: **Adults:** hold earlobe up and back **Children:** hold earlobe down and back	ADRs Local reactions (redness, itching). Contraindications Hypersensitivity to any ingredient.
Hydrocortisone (1%); Acetic Acid glacial (2%); Propylene Glycol diacetate (3%); Sodium Acetate (0.015%); Benzothonium Chloride (0.02%); Citric Acid (0.2%) AA-HC (Solution)	**Minor Outer Ear Complaints** Insert saturated wick into ear; leave in ear for 24 h, keeping it moist with 3–5 drops every 4–6 h. Remove wick and instill 5 drops 3–4 times daily.	**Hydrocortisone:** anti-inflammatory and antipuritic effects **Acetic Acid, Acetate, Benzothonium Chloride, citric acid:** antibacterial or antifungal action	**For Otic Use ONLY** Do not touch dropper to ear; wash hands prior to use. To allow drops to flow into ear, tilt head to side and: **Adults:** hold earlobe up and back **Children:** hold earlobe down and back	ADRs Local reactions (redness, itching). Contraindications Hypersensitivity to any ingredient.
M-Cresyl Acetate (25%); Isopropanol (25%); Chlorobutanol (1%); Benzyl alcohol (1%); 5% Castor Oil; Propylene Glycol Cresylate (Solution)	**Minor Outer Ear Complaints** 2–4 drops as needed.	**M-Cresyl Acetate:** antibacterial or antifungal action	**For Otic Use ONLY** Do not touch dropper to ear; wash hands prior to use To allow drops to flow into ear, tilt head to side and: **Adults:** hold earlobe up and back **Children:** hold earlobe down and back	ADRs Local reactions (redness, itching). Contraindications Hypersensitivity to any ingredient.

Triethanolamine Polypeptide Oleate-Condensate (10%); Chlorobutanol (0.5%); Propylene glycol Cerumenex Drops (Solution)	**Minor Outer Ear Complaints** Fill ear canal; insert cotton plug. Allow to remain for 15–30 min; then flush ear canal.	**Triethanolamine:** emulsify and disperse ear wax	**For Otic Use ONLY** Do not touch dropper to ear; wash hands prior to use To allow drops to flow into ear, tilt head to side and: **Adults:** hold earlobe up and back **Children:** hold earlobe down and back	ADRs Local reactions (redness, itching). Contraindications Hypersensitivity to any ingredient.

500. Gastrointestinal Agents

501.1 Antacids

Drug and Dosage Forms	Usual Dosage Range	Administration Issues and Drug–Drug Interactions	Common Adverse Drug Reactions (ADRs)	Contraindications, Pregnancy Category, and Lactation Issues
Aluminum Carbonate Gel, Basic Basaljel Tablets, Capsules Equivalent to 500 mg of aluminum hydroxide Suspension Equivalent to 400 mg of aluminum hydroxide per 5 ml	**Antacid** tablets, capsules 1000 mg as often as q 2 h, up to 12 doses/day suspension: 10 ml in water or fruit juice as often as q 2 h, up to 12 doses/day **Hyperphosphatemia** tablets, capsules 1000 mg with meals and at bedtime suspension: 15–30 ml in water or fruit juice with meals and at bedtime	Administration Issues Antacid dosing should be staggered at least 2 hours from other drugs where a potential drug interaction may occur. Drug–Drug Interactions Antacids may interfere with drugs by increasing gastric pH or binding other drugs, thus decreasing absorption of drugs such as **tetracycline, digoxin, iron salts, isoniazid, allopurinol, ciprofloxacin, ofloxacin, ketoconazole, and itraconazole.**	ADRs Constipation. Warnings/Precautions Hypophosphatemia (anorexia, malaise, tremors, muscle weakness); aluminum toxicity (dementia) may occur with repeated dosing, especially in presence of renal insufficiency.	Contraindications Prolonged use of high doses in presence of low serum phosphate; hypersensitivity to aluminum salts; recent GI hemorrhage. Pregnancy Category: C Lactation Issues Safety not established, do not use in nursing mothers
Aluminum Hydroxide Gel Amphojel, Alu-Tab, Dialume, AlternaGEL, various generic Tablets 300 mg, 500 mg, 600 mg Capsules 400 mg, 500 mg Suspension 320 mg/5ml Suspension, concentrated 450 mg/5 ml 675 mg/5 ml liquid, concentrated: 600 mg/5 ml	**Antacid** tablets, capsules: 500–1800 mg 3–6 times daily, between meals and at bedtime suspension, liquid: 5–30 ml prn between meals and at bedtime **Hyperphosphatemia** tablets, capsules: 500–1800 mg 3 to 6 times daily, with meals and at bedtime suspension, liquid: 5–30 ml with meals and at bedtime	Administration Issues Antacid dosing should be staggered at least 2 hours from other drugs where a potential drug interaction may occur. Drug–Drug Interactions Antacids may interfere with drugs by increasing gastric pH or binding other drugs, thus decreasing absorption of drugs such as **tetracycline, digoxin, iron salts, isoniazid, allopurinol, ciprofloxacin, ofloxacin, ketoconazole, and itraconazole.**	ADRs Constipation. Warnings/Precautions Hypophosphatemia (anorexia, malaise, tremors, muscle weakness); aluminum toxicity (dementia) may occur with repeated dosing, especially in presence of renal insufficiency	Contraindications Prolonged use of high doses in presence of low serum phosphate; hypersensitivity to aluminum salts; recent GI hemorrhage. Pregnancy Category: C Lactation Issues Safety not established, do not use in nursing mothers

Calcium Carbonate Tablets Various generics: 500 mg, 600 mg, 650 mg, 1000 mg, 1250 mg Tablets, chewable Tums, Extra Strength Tums, various generics: 500 mg, 750 mg Amitone: 350 mg Mallamint: 420 mg Alka-Mints: 850 mg Tums Ultra: 1000 mg Rolaids Calcium Rich: 550 mg Gum tablets 500 mg Gum 300 mg, 450 mg Capsules 1250 mg, 1500 mg Suspension Various generics: 1250 mg/5 ml Lozenges Mylanta 600 mg (note: not an all-inclusive list)	**All doses are in terms of elemental calcium: 1 g calcium carbonate = 400 mg (20 mEq) elemental calcium** **Antacid:** 0.5–1.5 g 3 to 6 times a day as needed **Dietary supplementation:** 500 mg to 2 g divided bid-qid	Administration issues Antacid dosing should be staggered at least 2 hours from other drugs where a potential drug interaction may occur. Drug–Drug Interactions Antacids may interfere with drugs by increasing gastric pH or binding other drugs, thus decreasing absorption of drugs such as **tetracycline, iron salts, ciprofloxacin, ofloxacin, ketoconazole, and itraconazole.**	ADRs Constipation, flatulence. Warnings/Precautions Milk-alkali syndrome, hypercalcemia, and metabolic alkalosis; acid rebound may occur with repeated dosing.	Contraindications Hypercalcemia, renal calculi, hypophosphatemia. Pregnancy Category: C Lactation Issues Safety not established, do not use in nursing mothers.
Magaldrate (Aluminum Magnesium Hydroxide Sulfate) Suspension/liquid Riopan, Magaldrate, Iosopan 540 mg/5 ml	**Antacid** suspension/liquid: 5–10 ml between meals and at bedtime	Administration Issues Antacid dosing should be staggered at least 2 hours from other drugs where a potential drug interaction may occur Drug-Drug Interactions Antacids may interfere with drugs by increasing gastric pH or binding other drugs, thus decreasing absorption of drugs such as **tetracycline, digoxin, iron salts, isoniazid, allopurinol, ciprofloxacin, ofloxacin, ketoconazole, and itraconazole.**	ADRs Diarrhea, constipation, hypophosphatemia, hypermagnesemia and aluminum toxicity, especially in the presence of renal insufficiency.	Contraindications Colostomy or ileostomy, appendicitis, ulcerative colitis, diverticulitis. Pregnancy Category: C Lactation Issues Safety not established, do not use in nursing mothers.
Magnesium Hydroxide Phillips' Milk of Magnesia, various generics	**Antacid** Adults and children > 12: 2–4 tablets up to 4 times daily	Administration Issues Antacid dosing should be staggered at least 2 hours from other drugs where a	ADRs Diarrhea.	Contraindications Appendicitis, renal failure, fecal impaction, colostomy, ileostomy, intestinal

(*continues on next page*)

501.1 Antacids *continued from previous page*

Drug and Dosage Forms	Usual Dosage Range	Administration Issues and Drug–Drug Interactions	Common Adverse Drug Reactions (ADRs)	Contraindications, Pregnancy Category, and Lactation Issues
Magnesium Hydroxide *cont.* Tablets, chewable 311 mg Liquid 400 mg/5ml Liquid, concentrated 800 mg/5ml	5–15 ml liquid up to 4 times daily with water 2.5–7.5 ml liquid concentrate up to 4 times daily with water **Laxative** **adults and children > 12 years:** 30–60 ml/day or in divided doses **children** 6–12 years: 15–30 ml/day or in divided doses 2–5 years: 5–15 ml/day or in divided doses < 2 years: 0.5 ml/kg/dose	potential drug interaction may occur; chew tablets thoroughly and follow with glass of water. Drug–Drug Interactions Antacids may interfere with drugs by increasing gastric pH or binding other drugs, thus decreasing absorption of drugs such as **tetracycline, digoxin, iron salts, allopurinol, ciprofloxacin, ofloxacin, ketoconazole, and itraconazole.**	Warning/Precautions Hypermagnesemia characterized by hypotension, nausea, vomiting may occur with repeated dosing in patients with renal impairment (CrCl < 30 ml/min).	obstruction, hypersensitivity to any component. Pregnancy Category: B Lactation Issues Safety not established.
Magnesium Oxide Tablets Mag-Ox 400 mg Maox 420 mg Various generics: 500 mg Capsules Uro-Mag 140 mg	**Antacid** tablets: total daily dose is 400–840 mg with milk or water capsules: 140 mg tid to qid with milk or water **Laxative** 2–4 g at bedtime with full glass of water	Administration Issues Antacid dosing should be staggered at least 2 hours from other drugs where a potential drug interaction may occur. Drug–Drug Interactions Antacids may interfere with drugs by increasing gastric pH or binding other drugs, thus decreasing absorption of drugs such as **tetracycline, digoxin, iron salts, allopurinol, ciprofloxacin, ofloxacin, ketoconazole, and itraconazole.**	ADRs Diarrhea. Warnings/Precautions Hypermagnesemia characterized by hypotension, nausea, vomiting may occur with repeated dosing in patients with renal impairment (CrCl < 30 ml/min).	Contraindications Colostomy or ileostomy, appendicitis, ulcerative colitis, diverticulitis, heart block, myocardial damage, serious renal impairment, hepatitis, Addison's disease, hypersensitivity to any component. Pregnancy Category: B Lactation Issues Safety not established, do not use in nursing mothers.
Sodium Bicarbonate Soda Mint, various generic Tablets 325 mg, 520 mg, 650 mg	**Antacid** Tablet: 0.3–2 gm 1 to 4 times daily Not the antacid of choice for the elderly because of sodium content and potential for systemic alkalosis.	Administration Issues Antacid dosing should be staggered at least 2 hours from other drugs where a potential drug interaction may occur Drug–Drug Interactions Sodium bicarbonate may increase urinary pH inhibiting excretion of basic drugs such as **pseudoephedrine and amphetamines** and enhance the excretion of acidic drugs such as **salicylates and lithium.**	ADRs Belching, gastric distension. Warnings/Precautions Milk-alkali syndrome with hypercalcemia, and metabolic alkalosis; acid rebound may occur with repeat dosing; May worsen hypertension and heart failure due to sodium content.	Contraindications Alkalosis, hypernatremia, severe pulmonary edema, hypocalcemia, unknown abdominal pain. Pregnancy Category: C Lactation Issues Safety not established, do not use in nursing mothers.

501.2 Antacid Combination Products
Listed below is a representative sample of antacid combination products. Administration and dosage depends on the condition being treated and the agent being used. See individual products (section 501.1) for administration issues, interactions, ADRs, etc.
Aluminum Hydroxide and Magnesium Hydroxide RuLox, Mintox (chewable tablets) Maalox Suspension, RuLox Suspension, Maalox Therapeutic Concentrate Suspension
Calcium Carbonate and Magnesium Carbonate Mylanta Gelcaps
Calcium Carbonate and Simethicone Titralac Plus Tablets, Titralac Plus Liquid
Aluminum Hydroxide, Alginic Acid, Sodium Bicarbonate, and Magnesium Trisilicate Gaviscon, Double Strength Gaviscon-2, Foamicon (chewable tablets)
Aluminum Hydroxide, Magnesium Hydroxide, and Simethicone Gelusil Tablets, Mylanta Double Strength Tablets, Almacone Tablets, Mintox Plus Tablets (all are chewable tablets) Mylanta, RuLox Plus Suspension, Di-Gel Liquid, Mylanta Double Strength Liquid, Extra Strength Maalox Plus Suspension
Magnesium Hydroxide, Calcium Carbonate, and Simethicone Advanced Formula Di-Gel Chewable Tablets
Magaldrate and Simethicone Riopan Plus, Riopan Plus Double Strength (all are chewable tablets) Riopan Plus Suspension, Riopan Plus Double Strength Suspension
Sodium Bicarbonate, Acetaminophen, Citric Acid Bromo Seltzer Effervescent Granules
Sodium Bicarbonate, Citric Acid, Potassium Bicarbonate Gold Alka-Seltzer Effervescent Tablets
Sodium Bicarbonate, Citric Acid, and Aspirin Alka-Seltzer, Extra Strength Alka-Seltzer (effervescent tablets)

501.3 Gastrointestinal Anticholinergics/Antispasmodics

Drug and Dosage Forms	Usual Dosage Range	Administration Issues and Drug-Drug Interactions	Common Adverse Drug Reactions (ADRs) and Pharmacokinetics	Contraindications, Pregnancy Category, and Lactation Issues
Atropine Sulfate Tablets 0.4 mg Tablets, soluble 0.4 mg, 0.6 mg	**Indications include management of peptic ulcer; decrease motility (smooth muscle tone) in GI, biliary, and urinary tracts; irritable bowel syndrome; for antisecretory effects.** **Spastic conditions of the GI tract** **adults:** usual dose is 0.4 mg–0.6 mg q 4 to 6 hrs **children:** individualize dosage according to weight	Administration Issues Oral doses are usually given with meals and at bedtime. Monitor therapeutic response according to purpose for use. Anticholinergic agents are generally not well tolerated in the elderly, and their use should be avoided when possible. Drug-Drug Interactions Administration of atropine with **amantadine, tricyclic antidepressants (amitriptyline, imipramine), or phenothiazines** may result in increased anticholinergic side effects.	ADRs Palpitations, fatigue, delirium, headache, confusion, dry and hot skin, impaired GI motility, dry mouth, dry throat, dry nose, decreased diaphoresis; difficult urination, blurred vision, mydriasis, increased sensitivity to light; dysphagia. Pharmacokinetics Liver metabolism, renal excretion may be prolonged with renal dysfunction.	Contraindications Hypersensitivity to anticholinergic agents, hypersensitivity to atropine or any component of the formulation, narrow-angle glaucoma, adhesions between the iris and lens, tachycardia, unstable cardiovascular status in acute hemorrhage, obstructive GI disease, paralytic ileus, intestinal atony of the elderly or debilitated patient, severe ulcerative colitis, toxic megacolon, hepatic disease, obstructive uropathy, renal disease, myasthenia gravis, asthma, thyrotoxicosis, Mobitz type II block. Pregnancy Category: C Lactation Issues Passage of atropine into breast milk is controversial; American Academy of Pediatrics considers atropine to be usually compatible with breastfeeding; use with caution.
Belladonna (contains the anticholinergic alkaloids hyoscyamine, scopolamine, and other minor alkaloids) Belladonna tincture Liquid 27 to 33 mg belladonna alkaloids/100 ml	**Indications include adjunctive therapy in treatment of peptic ulcer disease; motion sickness; GI motility disturbances; irritable bowel syndrome; parkinsonism** **Gastrointestinal motility disorders** **adults:** 0.6–1 ml 3 to 4 times/day **children:** 0.03 ml/kg 3 times/day	Administration Issues Take 30 to 60 min before a meal. Monitor therapeutic response according to purpose for use. Anticholinergic agents are generally not well tolerated in the elderly, and their use should be avoided when possible. Drug–Drug Interactions Adminisration of belladonna liquid with **amantadine, tricyclic antidepressants (amitriptyline, imipramine), or phenothiazines** may result in increased anticholinergic side effects.	ADRs Palpitations, fatigue, delirium, headache, confusion, dry skin, constipation, dry mouth, dry throat, dry nose, decreased diaphoresis, increased sensitivity to light, dysphagia. Pharmacokinetics Little information is available on belladonna distribution, metabolism, and excretion.	Contraindications Hypersensitivity to anticholinergic agents; hypersensitivity to belladonna or any component of the formulation, narrow-angle glaucoma, elevated intraocular pressure, obstructive GI disease, obstructive uropathy, paralytic ileus, intestinal atony of the elderly or debilitated patient, significant hepatic or renal disease, pulmonary insufficiency, unstable cardiovascular status in acute hemorrhage, ulcerative colitis or toxic megacolon, reflux esophagitis, myasthenia gravis. Pregnancy Category: C

				Lactation Issues Belladonna is excreted into breast milk; use in nursing women is controversial (see Atropine). Belladonna is excreted in breast milk and may result in neonatal toxicity and decreased milk production; refrain from use in nursing women.
Clidinium Bromide Quarzan Capsules 2.5 mg, 5 mg	**Adjunctive therapy in the treatment of peptic ulcer disease; GI disorders; irritable bowel syndrome** **adults:** 2.5 mg–5 mg 3 or 4 times daily before meals and at bedtime **geriatric, debilitated:** 2.5 mg $$$lid before meals	Administration Issues Take 30 to 60 min before a meal. Monitor therapeutic response according to purpose for use. Anticholinergic agents are generally not well tolerated in the elderly, and their use should be avoided when possible. Drug–Drug Interactions Administration of clidinium bromide with **amantadine, tricyclic antidepressants (amitriptyline, imipramine), or phenothiazines** may result in increased anticholinergic side effects.	ADRs Allergic urticaria, palpitations, tachycardia, headache, drowsiness dizziness, confusion, dry mouth, constipation, nausea, vomiting, decreased diaphoresis, urinary hesitancy and retention, impotence, blurred vision, worsening of glaucoma. Pharmacokinetics Poor oral absorption; hepatic metabolism; renal and fecal excretion.	Contraindications Hypersensitivity to anticholinergic agents, hypersensitivity to clidinium bromide or any component of the formulation, narrow-angle glaucoma, elevated intraocular pressure, obstructive GI disease, obstructive uropathy, paralytic ileus, intestinal atony of the elderly or debilitated patient, significant hepatic or renal disease, pulmonary insufficiency, unstable cardiovascular status in acute hemorrhage, ulcerative colitis or toxic megacolon, reflux esophagitis, myasthenia gravis. Pregnancy Category: C Lactation Issues Clidinium is excreted into breast milk; no data available; use in nursing women is controversial (see Atropine).
Dicyclomine Bentyl, various generics Tablets 20 mg Capsules 10 mg, 20 mg Syrup 10 mg/5 ml	**Treatment of functional bowel/irritable bowel syndrome** **adult:** 20 mg qid, then increase to 40 mg qid **160 mg / day is the only oral dose shown to be effective; however side effects frequently occur at this dose** **children (≥ 6 months):** 5–10 mg 3 to 4 times daily	Administration Issues Take 30 to 60 min before a meal. Monitor therapeutic response according to purpose for use. Long-term use of antispasmodics should be avoided in the elderly. Drug-Drug Interactions Administration of dicyclomine with **amantadine, tricyclic antidepressants (amitriptyline, imipramine), or phenothiazines** may result in increased anticholinergic side effects.	ADRs Hypersensitivity reactions, allergic urticaria, palpitations, tachycardia, headache, drowsiness, dizziness, confusion, dry mouth, constipation, nausea, vomiting, decreased diaphoresis, urinary hesitancy and retention, impotence, blurred vision, mydriasis, apnea, dyspnea. Pharmacokinetics Well absorbed after oral administration; hepatic metabolism; ~ 80% renal elimination and <10% fecal excretion.	Contraindications Dicyclomine is contraindicated in infants < 6 months of age due to reports of respiratory distress and collapse. Hypersensitivity to anticholinergic agents, hypersensitivity to dicyclomine or any component of the formulation, narrow-angle glaucoma, elevated intraocular pressure, obstructive GI disease, obstructive uropathy, paralytic ileus, intestinal atony of the elderly or debilitated patient, significant hepatic or renal disease, pulmonary insufficiency, unstable cardiovascular status in acute hemorrhage, ulcerative colitis or toxic megacolon, reflux esophagitis, myasthenia gravis.

(*continues on next page*)

501.3 Gastrointestinal Anticholinergics/Antispasmodics *continued from previous page*

Drug and Dosage Forms	Usual Dosage Range	Administration Issues and Drug-Drug Interactions	Common Adverse Drug Reactions (ADRs) and Pharmacokinetics	Contraindications, Pregnancy Category, and Lactation Issues
				Pregnancy Category: B Lactation Issues Dicyclomine is excreted in breast milk and may result in infant toxicity, refrain from use in nursing women.
Glycopyrrolate Robinul, Robinul Forte Tablets Robinul 1 mg Robinul Forte 2 mg	**Adjunctive therapy in the treatment of peptic ulcer** **Adults** initial dosing: 1 mg tid or 2 mg bid to tid maintenance dosing: 1 mg bid **Use in children < 12 years for the treatment of peptic ulcer is not established.**	Administration Issues Take 30 to 60 min before a meal. Monitor therapeutic response according to purpose for use. Anticholinergic agents are generally not well tolerated in the elderly, and their use should be avoided when possible. Drug–Drug Interactions Administration of glycopyrrolate with **amantadine, tricyclic antidepressants (amitriptyline, imipramine), or phenothiazines** may result in increased anticholinergic side effects	ADRs Hypersensitivity reactions, allergic urticaria, palpitations, tachycardia, fatigue, delirium, headache, confusion, dry skin, constipation, dry mouth, dry throat, dry nose, decreased diaphoresis, increased sensitivity to light, gastroesophageal reflux. Pharmacokinetics Poor oral absorption; primarily renal excretion; some excretion in the bile.	Contraindications Hypersensitivity to anticholinergic agents, hypersensitivity to glycopyrrolate or any component of the formulation, narrow-angle glaucoma, elevated intraocular pressure, obstructive GI disease, obstructive uropathy, paralytic ileus, intestinal atony of the elderly or debilitated patient, significant hepatic or renal disease, pulmonary insufficiency, unstable cardiovascular status in acute hemorrhage, ulcerative colitis or toxic megacolon, reflux esophagitis, myasthenia gravis. Pregnancy Category: B Lactation Issues Glycopyrrolate excretion into breast milk is unknown; no data are available; use in nursing women is controversial (see atropine).
L-Hyoscyamine Sulfate Anaspaz, Levsin, generics Tablets 0.125 mg, 0.15 mg Capsules, time released 0.375 mg Tablet, sublingual 0.125 mg	**Indications include to aid in the control of gastric secretion, visceral spasm, hypermotility in spastic colitis, spastic bladder, pylorospasm; to relieve symptoms in functional intestinal disorders; adjunctive therapy in peptic ulcer; irritable bowel syndrome; neurogenic bowel disturbances; for antisecretory effects** **adults:** 0.125 mg–0.25 mg tid or qid orally or sublingually; or 0.375–0.75 mg in sustained-release form of 12 h	Administration Issues Take 30 to 60 min before a meal. Monitor therapeutic response according to purpose for use. Anticholinergic agents are generally not well tolerated in the elderly, and their use should be avoided when possible. Do not crush or chew extended release forms. Levbid tablets are scored and may be broken in half for dose titration; do not crush or chew.	ADRs Hypersensitivity reactions, allergic urticaria, palpitations, tachycardia, fatigue, delirium, headache, confusion, dry skin, constipation, dry mouth, dry throat, dry nose, urinary hesitancy or urinary retention, decreased diaphoresis. Pharmacokinetics Liver metabolism, renal excretion may be prolonged with renal dysfunction	Contraindications Hypersensitivity to anticholinergic agents, hypersensitivity to hyoscyamine or any component of the formulation, narrow-angle glaucoma, elevated intraocular pressure, obstructive GI disease, obstructive uropathy, paralytic ileus, intestinal atony of the elderly or debilitated patient, significant hepatic or renal disease, pulmonary insufficiency, unstable cardiovascular status in acute hemorrhage, ulcerative colitis or toxic megacolon, reflux esophagitis, myasthenia gravis.

Solution 0.125 mg/ml Tablets, extended release 0.375 mg Elixir 0.125 mg/5 ml Tablets, sustained release 0.375 mg Tablets, orally disintegrating 0.125 mg Oral spray 0.125 mg/spray Capsules, extended release 0.375 mg	**children:** individualize dosage according to weight	Drug–Drug Interactions Administration of hyoscyamine with **amantadine, tricyclic antidepressants (amitriptyline, imipramine), or phenothiazines** may result in increased anticholinergic side effects.		Pregnancy Category: C Lactation Issues Hyoscyamine is excreted into breast milk; breastfeeding is not recommended (see atropine).
Propantheline Bromide Pro-Banthine, various generics Tablets 7.5 mg, 15 mg	**Adjunctive therapy in the treatment of peptic ulcer** **adults:** 30 min 15 mg tid before meals and 30 mg at bedtime **geriatrics:** 7.5 mg tid before meals	Administration Issues Take 30 to 60 min before a meal. Monitor therapeutic response according to purpose for use. Anticholinergic agents are generally not well tolerated in the elderly, and their use should be avoided when possible. Drug–Drug Interactions Administration of propantheline with **amantadine, tricyclic antidepressants (amitriptyline, nortriptyline), or phenothiazines** may result in increased anticholinergic side effects.	ADRs Hypersensitivity reactions, allergic urticaria; dry skin, constipation, dry mouth, dry throat, dry nose, dysphagia; decreased diaphoresis. Pharmacokinetics Poor oral absorption; renal excretion.	Contraindications Hypersensitivity to anticholinergic agents, hypersensitivity to propantheline or any component of the formulation, narrow-angle glaucoma, elevated intraocular pressure, obstructive GI disease, obstructive uropathy, paralytic ileus, intestinal atony of the elderly or debilitated patient, significant hepatic or renal disease, pulmonary insufficiency, unstable cardiovascular status in acute hemorrhage, ulcerative colitis or toxic megacolon, reflux esophagitis, myasthenia gravis. Pregnancy Category: C Lactation Issues No data available (also see atropine).

501.4 Gastrointestinal Anticholinergic Combinations
Listed below are combination anticholinergic GI products and dosage forms available. Refer to the individual drugs for information on ADRs, etc.
Atropine, Scopolamine, Hyoscyamine, and Phenobarbital Barbidonna No. 2 Tablets, Barbidonna Tablets, Donnatal Capsules and Tablets, Hyosophen Tablets, Donnatal Extentabs
Belladonna Extract, Bulabarbital Sodium Bulibel Tablets, Elixir
Hyoscyamine Sulfate and Phenobarbital Bellacane Tablets
Clidinium Bromide and Chlordiazepoxide Librax (capsules)
Belladonna, Phenobarbital, and Ergotamine Tartrate Bellergal-S Tablets, Bellacane SR Tablets, Bel-Phen-Ergot SR Tablets

501.5 Agents for Ulcers and GERD

Drug and Dosage Forms	Usual Dosage Range	Administration Issues and Drug–Drug Interactions	Common Adverse Drug Reactions (ADRs) and Pharmacokinetics	Contraindications, Pregnancy Category, and Lactation Issues
Cimetidine Tagamet, generics Tablets 200 mg, 300 mg, 400 mg, 800 mg Liquid 300 mg/5 ml	**Duodenal and gastric ulcers, treatment** **adults and children > 12:** 800 mg q hs OR 300 mg qid with meals and q hs OR 400 mg bid (Continue treatment for 4–8 weeks unless healing is demonstrated by endoscopy) **Duodenal ulcers, maintenance** **adults and children > 12:** 400 mg q hs **Gastroesophageal reflux (GERD)** **adults and children > 12:** 800 mg bid OR 400 mg qid (continue treatment for 12 weeks; use beyond 12 weeks has not been established) **Hypersecretory conditions (Zollinger-Ellison syndrome)** **adults and children > 12:** 300 mg qid with meals and q h; may need to give more often than 4 times daily; individualize treatment; do not exceed 2400 mg/day. (Continue treatment as long as clinically indicated). **Heartburn, acid indigestion** **adults and children > 12:** 200 mg with water as symptoms occur, up to bid (400 mg in 24 hours)	Administration Issues Give antacids as needed for pain relief; separate antacid dosing from cimetidine by 1 hour if possible. Use not recommended for children < 12. Drug–Drug Interactions Cimetidine may inhibit the hepatic metabolism and increase the effect of drugs such as **metoprolol, labetalol, propranolol, warfarin, carbamazepine, phenytoin, theophylline, tricyclic antidepressants, sulfonylureas, and valproic acid.** Cimetidine may decrease the absorption of drugs such as **ketoconazole and itraconazole.**	ADRs Headache, dizziness, confusion, somnolence, gynecomastia, diarrhea. Pharmacokinetics Decrease dosage with renal impairment (CrCl < 50 ml/min).	Contraindications Patients hypersensitive to cimetidine, other H2 antagonists, or any component of the formulation. Pregnancy Category: B Lactation Issues Excreted in breast milk in high concentrations; use with caution; American Academy of pediatrics considers cimetidine compatible with breastfeeding.
Esomeprazole Magnesium Nexium Capsules, delayed-release 20 mg, 40 mg	**Erosive esophagitis treatment** 20 or 40 mg once daily for 4 to 8 weeks; may consider an additional 4–8 weeks of treatment if patient is not healed. **Maintenance** 20 mg once daily (clinical trials evaluated therapy for ≤ 6 months)	Administration Issues Do not break, crush, or chew capsule. Swallow capsule whole and take ≥ 1 hour before eating. Safety and efficacy have not been established in pediatric patients.	ADRs Headache, diarrhea, nausea, flatulence, abdominal pain, constipation, xerostomia. Pharmacokinetics Hepatic metabolism; 80% excreted in urine, 20% feces. Dose should not exceed 20 mg/day in severe liver impairment.	Contraindications Hypersensitivity to esomeprazole, lansoprazole, omeprazole, rabeprazole, or any component of the formulation. Pregnancy Category: B Lactation Issues Not known if drug is excreted in breast milk; contraindicated.

(*continues on next page*)

501.5 Agents for Ulcers and GERD *continued from previous page*

Drug and Dosage Forms	Usual Dosage Range	Administration Issues and Drug–Drug Interactions	Common Adverse Drug Reactions (ADRs) and Pharmacokinetics	Contraindications, Pregnancy Category, and Lactation Issues
Esomeprazole Magnesium Nexium *cont.*	**Symptomatic gastroesophageal reflux (GERD)** 20 mg once daily for 4 weeks; may consider an additional 4 weeks of treatment if symptoms do not resolve	Drug-Drug Interactions Esomeprazole may decrease the absorption of drugs such as **iron salts, ketoconazole, and digoxin** by altering gastric pH. Esomeprazole may increase the concentration of drugs such as **diazepam and penicillins.**		
Famotidine Pepcid, generics Tablet Pepcid AC Acid Controller 10mg Pepcid: 20 mg, 40 mg Tablets, chewable Pepcid AC: 10 mg Pepcid Complete: 10 mg (also contains 800 mg calcium carbonate and 165 mg magnesium hydroxide) Tablets, orally disintegrating Pepcid RPD: 20mg, 40 mg Gelcaps Pepcid AC: 10 mg Powder for oral suspension Pepcid 40 mg/5 ml	**Duodenal and gastric ulcers, treatment** **adults and children > 12** 40 mg q hs OR 20 mg bid (continue treatment for 4–8 weeks unless healing is demonstrated by endoscopy) **Duodenal ulcers, maintenance** **adults and children > 12:** 20 mg q hs **Gastroesophageal reflux (GERD):** **adults and children > 12:** 20 mg bid for up to 6 weeks (can treat up to 12 weeks; use beyond 12 weeks has not been established) **Hypersecretory conditions (Zollinger–Ellison syndrome):** **adults and children > 12:** 20 mg q 6 h; may need to give higher starting dose; individualize treatment; do not exceed 640 mg/day (continue treatment as long as clinically indicated) **Heartburn, acid indigestion:** **adults and children > 12:** 10 mg with water; up to bid (up to 20 mg in 24 hrs)	Administration Issues Give antacids as needed for pain relief; reconstituted suspension may be stored at room temperature, keep away from heat, discard unused portion 30 days after reconstitution. Use not recommended for children < 12. Drug–Drug Interactions Famotidine may decrease the absorption of drugs such as **ketoconazole** and **itraconazole.**	ADRs Headache, dizziness, diarrhea, constipation. Pharmacokinetics Decrease dosage with renal impairment (CrCl < 50 ml/min).	Contraindications Patients hypersensitive to famotidine, other H2 antagonists, or any component of the formulation. Some dosage forms of famotidine contain phenylalanine. Pregnancy Category: B Lactation Issues Famotidine is excreted into breast milk, but to a lesser degree than cimetidine or ranitidine (also see cimetidine).

Lansoprazole Prevacid Capsule, delayed, release: 15 mg, 30 mg Tablets, orally disintegration, delayed-release 15 mg, 30 mg Granules for oral suspension, delayed-release 15 mg, 30 mg	**Duodenal ulcer** **treatment:** 15 mg qd for 4 weeks **maintenance:** 15 mg qd **Gastric ulcer** **treatment:** 30 mg qd for ≤ 8 weeks **NSAID-associated gastric ulcer** **healing:** 30 mg qd for 8 weeks **to reduce risk:** 15 mg qd for ≤ 12 weeks **Erosive esophagitis** **treatment:** 30 mg qd for ≤ 8 weeks; continued treatment for an additional 8 weeks may be considered for recurrence or for patients that do not heal after the first 8 weeks of therapy maintenance: 15 mg qd **Gastroesophageal reflux (GERD)** 15 mg qd for up to 8 weeks **Hypersecretory conditions (Zollinger-Ellison syndrome)** 60 mg qd, but individualize treatment; doses up to 90 mg bid have been used (continue treatment as long as clinically indicated)	Administration Issues Do not chew or crush capsules or granules; take capsule before eating. If patient on sucralfate, give lansoprazole at least 30 minutes prior to sucralfate. Drug–Drug Interactions Lansoprazole may decrease the absorption of **ketoconazole, iron supplements, and digoxin** by altering gastric pH	ADRs: diarrhea, abdominal pain, headache Pharmacokinetics: extensive hepatic metabolism; primarily excreted by biliary/fecal route Consider dosage adjustment in patients with severe liver disease.	Contraindications: Hypersensitivity to lansoprazole or any component of the formulation. Pregnancy Category: B Lactation Issues Excretion in breast milk unknown/contraindicated.
Misoprostol Cytotec Tablet: 100 mcg, 200 mcg	**Prevention of NSAID-induced gastric ulcers** 200 mcg qid with food; if not tolerated, may use 100 mcg qid or 200 mcg bid with food	Administration Issues Take with meals and take the last dose of the day at bedtime.	ADRs: Diarrhea, abdominal pain, nausea, headache, dyspepsia, flatulence. Pharmacokinetics Rapid oral absorption; primarily renal elimination. Use with caution in patients with renal impairment and the elderly.	Contraindications Hypersensitivity to misoprostol, prostaglandins, or any component of the formulation; pregnancy. Pregnancy Category: X Lactation Issues Excretion in breast milk unknown; contraindicated because of the potential for severe diarrhea in nursing infants.
Nizatidine Tablet Axid AR: 75 mg	**Duodenal and gastric ulcers** **treatment:** 300 mg q hs OR 150 mg bid (continue treatment for 4–8 weeks unless healing is demonstrated by endoscopy)	Administration Issues Give antacids as needed for pain relief; separate antacid dosing from nizatidine by 1 h if possible	ADRs Headache, dizziness, somnolence, diarrhea, constipation, sweating.	Contraindications Patients hypersensitive to nizatidine, other H2 antagonists, or any component of the formulation.

(continues on next page)

501.5 Agents for Ulcers and GERD *continued from previous page*

Drug and Dosage Forms	Usual Dosage Range	Administration Issues and Drug–Drug Interactions	Common Adverse Drug Reactions (ADRs) and Pharmacokinetics	Contraindications, Pregnancy Category, and Lactation Issues
Nizatidine *cont.* Capsule Axid: 150 mg, 300 mg	**maintenance:** 150 mg q hs **Gastroesophageal reflux (GERD)** 150 mg bid (Use beyond 6 weeks not adequately studied)	Drug–Drug Interactions Nizatidine may decrease the absorption of drugs such as **ketoconazole** and **itraconazole.**	Pharmacokinetics Decrease dosage with renal impairment (CrCl < 50 ml/min).	Pregnancy Category: C Lactation Issues Nizatidine is excreted into breast milk; use with caution (also see cimetidine).
Omeprazole Prilosec, generics Capsule, delayed release 10 mg, 20 mg, 40 mg Tablets, delayed-release 20 mg	**Duodenal ulcer, treatment** 20 mg qd for 4 to 8 weeks **Gastric ulcer, treatment** 40 mg qd for 4 to 8 weeks **Gastroesophageal reflux (GERD)** 20 mg qd for 4 to 8 weeks **Hypersecretory conditions (Zollinger-Ellison syndrome)** 60 mg qd; individualize dosage; doses up to 120 mg bid have been used (continue treatment as long as clinically indicated) **Erosive esophagitis** **treatment:** 20 mg qd for 4 to 8 weeks **maintenance:** 20 mg qd	Administration Issues Do not open, chew, or crush capsule; swallow whole capsule; take capsule before eating. If patient on sucralfate, give omeprazole at least 30 minutes prior to sucralfate. Drug–Drug Interactions Omeprazole may decrease the absorption of **iron salts, ketoconazole, and digoxin** by altering gastric pH. Omeprazole may inhibit the metabolism of drugs such as **diazepam and warfarin,** increasing each drug's effect.	ADRs Diarrhea, nausea, vomiting, abdominal pain, headache, dizziness. Pharmacokinetics Extensive hepatic metabolism; primarily renal excretion.	Contraindications Hypersensitivity to omeprazole or any component of the formulation. Pregnancy Category: C Lactation Issues Use with caution in nursing mothers, excretion in breast milk is unknown; use should probably be avoided during breastfeeding.
Pantoprazole Sodium Protonix Tablets, delayed-release 20 mg, 40 mg	**Erosive esophagitis associated with gastroesophageal reflux** 40 mg once daily (or two 20 mg tablets) for ≤ 8 weeks; an additional 8 weeks may be used in patients who have not healed after an 8-weeks course; maintenance of healing: 40 mg qd–lower doses (20 mg qd) have been used successfully in mild GERD treatment and maintenance of healing.	Administration Issues Swallow tablets whole, with or without food. Do not split, chew, or crush tablets. Drug-Drug Interactions Pantoprazole may decrease the absorption of drugs such as **iron salts, ketoconazole, and digoxin** by altering gastric pH.	ADRs Headache, diarrhea, flatulence, abdominal pain, rash, eructation, insomnia, hyperglycemia. Pharmacokinetics Extensive hepatic metabolism; eliminated in urine (71%) and feces (18%).	Contraindications Hypersensitivity to pantoprazole or any component. Pregnancy Category: B Lactation Issues Excretion in breast milk unknown; do not use in nursing mothers.
Rabeprazole Sodium Aciphex	**Duodenal ulcers** 20 mg once daily after the morning meal for a period of ≤ 4 weeks	Administration Issues Swallow tablets whole. Do not split, chew, or crush tablets.	ADRs Headache.	Contraindications Hypersensitivity to rabeprazole, substituted benzimidazoles, or any component of the formulation.

Tablets, delayed-release 20 mg	**Erosive or ulcerative GERD** **treatment:** 20 mg qd for 4 to 8 weeks; consider an additional 8-week course if patient not healed after 8 weeks **maintenance:** 20 mg qd **Hypersecretory conditions, including Zollinger-Ellison syndrome** 60 mg once daily; individualize dose; continue for as long as clinically indicated; some patients may require divided doses; doses ≤ 100 mg/day and 60 mg bid have been administered; some patients have been treated continuously for ≤ 1 year	Drug-Drug Interactions Rabeprazole may decrease the absorption of drugs such as **ketoconazole or itraconazole.** Rabeprazole (in extremely high concentrations) may increase serum levels of **digoxin and cyclosporine.**	Pharmacokinetics Hepatic metabolism; 90% eliminated in urine.	Pregnancy Category: B Lactation Issues Excretion in breast milk unknown; do not use in nursing mothers.
Sucralfate Carafate Tablets 1 gm Suspension 1 gm/10 ml	**Treatment of duodenal ulcer, adults** tablets: 1 gm qid 1 hour ac and hs suspension: 10 ml qid 1 hour ac and hs (continue treatment for 4–8 weeks unless healing is demonstrated by endoscopy) **Maintenance therapy of duodenal ulcer, adults** tablets: 1 gm bid	Administration Issues Sucralfate should be taken on an empty stomach; do not take antacids 1/2 hour before or after taking sucralfate. Drug–Drug Interactions Sucralfate may decrease the effect of drugs such as **warfarin, digoxin, phenytoin, ketoconazole, quinidine, ciprofloxacin, ofloxacin, and norfloxacin.**	ADRs Constipation, diarrhea, nausea, vomiting, indigestion. Use with caution in chronic renal failure patients secondary to potential for aluminum accumulation. Pharmacokinetics Minimally absorbed from the GI tract (<5%); approximately 90% is excreted in the stool.	Contraindications Hypersensitivity to sucralfate or any component of the formulation. Pregnancy Category: B Lactation Issues It is not known if sucralfate is excreted in breast milk; use caution when sucralfate is administered to nursing mothers.
Ranitidine Zantac, Zantac 75, Zantac EFFERdose, Zantac GELdose Tablets 75 mg, 150 mg, 300 mg Tablet, effervescent 150 mg Capsules 150 mg, 300 mg Granules, effervescent 150 mg Syrup 150 mg/10 ml	**Duodenal and gastric ulcers** treatment: 300 mg q hs OR 150 mg bid (continue treatment for 4–8 weeks unless healing is demonstrated by endoscopy) **maintenance:** 150 mg q hs **Gastroesophageal reflux (GERD)** 150 mg bid (use beyond 6 weeks has not been adequately studied) **Hypersecretory conditions (Zollinger-Ellison syndrome)** 150 mg bid; may need to give more often; individualize treatment; doses up to 6 gm/day have been used (continue treatment as long as clinically indicated) **Erosive esophagitis** **treatment:** 150 mg qid **maintenance:** 150 mg bid	Administration Issues Give antacids as needed for pain relief; separate antacid dosing from ranitidine by 1 hour if possible Drug–Drug Interactions Ranitidine may increase the effect of drugs such as **sulfonylureas, warfarin, phenytoin, and triazolam.** Ranitidine may decrease the absorption of drugs such as **ketoconazole and itraconazole.**	ADRs Headache, dizziness, somnolence, diarrhea constipation. Pharmacokinetics Decrease dosage with renal impairment (CrCl < 50 ml/min).	Contraindications Patients hypersensitive to ranitidine, other H2 antagonists, or any component of the formulation. Pregnancy Category: B Lactation Issues Excreted in breast milk, use caution when administering to nursing mothers (also see cimetidine).

501.6 GI Stimulants

Drug and Dosage Forms	Usual Dosage Range	Administration Issues and Drug–Drug Interactions	Common Adverse Drug Reactions (ADRs) and Pharmacokinetics	Contraindications, Pregnancy Category, and Lactation Issues
Metoclopramide Reglan, various generics Tablet 5 mg, 10 mg Syrup 5 mg/5 ml Solution, concentrated 10 mg/ml	**Diabetic gastroparesis** 10 mg 30 minutes ac and hs for 2 to 8 weeks **Gastroesophageal reflux** 10 mg-15 mg up to 4 times daily 30 minutes ac and hs; 10 mg-20 mg may be given as a single dose prior to events known to provoke reflux symptoms **Elderly may require only 5 mg per dose**	Administration Issues Take 30 minutes before meals. May produce drowsiness or dizziness; observe caution while driving or performing tasks requiring alertness, coordination, or physical dexterity; notify physician if involuntary movements occur. Drug-Drug Interactions Metoclopramide may decrease the absorption of drugs such as **digoxin** and **cimetidine** and may increase the absorption of drugs such as **cyclosporine.** **Anticholinergic agents (hyoscyamine, tricyclic antidepressants)** may antagonize the effects of metoclopramide. Metoclopramide and **levodopa** have opposite effects on dopamine receptors; metoclopramide can increase the absorption of **levodopa** and increase the incidence of extrapyramidal symptoms. Metoclopramide may increase the hypertensive effects of **MAO Inhibitors (Isocarboxazid, phenelzine, and tranylcypromine).**	ADRs Drowsiness, dizziness, restlessness, fatigue, diarrhea, and extrapyramidal symptoms such as acute dystonic reactions, tardive dyskinesia, akathisia, and Parkinson-like symptoms including bradykinesia, tremor, cogwheel rigidity, mask-like facies. Pharmacokinetics Onset of action is 30–60 minutes following oral dose; dosage decrease needed with renal impairment (CrCl < 40 ml/min).	Contraindications Patients where stimulation of GI motility may be dangerous (mechanical obstruction or perforation, GI hemorrhage); pheochromocytoma; sensitivity or intolerance to metoclopramide or any component of the formulation; history of seizure disorder. Pregnancy Category: B Lactation Issues Metoclopramide is excreted into breast milk; there appears to be no risk to the nursing infant when the mother's dose is ≤ 45 mg/ day; use with caution in nursing mothers.

501.7 Digestive Enzymes

Drug and Dosage Forms	Usual Dosage Range	Administration Issues and Drug–Drug Interactions	Common Adverse Drug Reactions (ADRs) and Pharmacokinetics	Contraindications, Pregnancy Category, and Lactation Issues
Pancrelipase Tablets Viokase Tablets (lipase 8,000 units, protease 30,000 units, amylase 30,000 units)	**Enzyme replacement therapy in patients with cystic fibrosis, chronic pancreatitis, ductal obstructions, pancreatic insufficiency and for steatorrhea of malabsorption syndrome and postgastrectomy or post-GI surgery**	Administration Issues Swallow tablets / capsules whole; do not crush microspheres; if swallowing is difficult, give contents of capsule on applesauce or gelatin and swallow without chewing; do not inhale powder.	ADRs Nausea, diarrhea, abdominal cramps, constipation. Pharmacokinetics Absorption: none, acts locally in GI tract; excretion in feces; pancreatic lipase is inactivated at pH ≤ 4.	Contraindications Hypersensitivity to pork protein or enzymes; acute pancreatitis; acute exacerbations of chronic pancreatic disease.

Powder Viokase Powder (lipase 16,800 units, protease 70,000 units, amylase 70,000 units per 0.7 g) Capsules Kutrase Capsules (lipase 2,400 units, protease 30,000 units, amylase 30,000 units); Ku-Zyme Capsules (lipase 1,200 units, protease 15,000 units, amylase 15,000 units); Pancrease Capsules (lipase 4,500 units, protease 25,000 units, amylase 30,000 units); Pancrease MT 4 Capsules (lipase 4,500 units, protease 12,000 units, amylase 12,000 units) plus others	Adjust dosage according to the severity of pancreatic enzyme deficiency; estimate dosage by assessing which dose minimizes steatorrhea and maintains good nutritional status **capsules and tablets** **adults:** 4,000 units–48,000 units lipase with each meal and with snacks **children 7–12 years:** 4,000 units–12,000 units lipase with each meal and with snacks **children 1–6 years:** 4,000 units–8,000 units lipase with each meal and with snackes **children 6 months–1 year:** 2,000 units lipase per meal *powder* (in cystic fibrosis): 0.7 g with meals	Drug–Drug Interactions Administration with **antacids** may cause the enteric-coated capsules to dissolve in the stomach and inactivate the product. The effect of oral **iron supplements** may be decreased with concomitant use of pancreatic enzymes.		Pregnancy Category: C Lactation Issues It is unknown if pancrelipase is excreted in breast milk; use with caution in nursing mothers.
Pancreatin Donnazyme, Creon Tablets Donnazyme Tablets (Pancreatin 500 mg, lipase 1,000 units; protease 12,500 units; amylase 12,500 units) Capsules Creon Capsules (Pancreatin 300 mg, lipase 8,000 units, protease 13,000 units, amylase 30,000 units) plus others	**Enzyme replacement therapy in patients with cystic fibrosis, chronic pancreatitis, ductal obstructions, pancreatic insufficiency and for steatorrhea of malabsorption syndrome and postgastrectomy or post-GI surgery.** Adjust dosage according to the severity of pancreatic enzyme deficiency; estimate dosage by assessing which dose minimizes steatorrhea and maintains good nutritional status Take 1–2 tablets or capsules with meals or snacks. Adjust according to individual requirements for control of steatorrhea.	Administration Issues Swallow tablets/capsules whole; do not crush microspheres; if swallowing is difficult, give contents of capsule on applesauce or gelatin and swallow without chewing; do not inhale powder. Drug–Drug Interactions Administration with **antacids** may cause the enteric-coated capsules to dissolve in the stomach and inactivate the product. The effect of oral **iron supplements** may be decreased with concomitant use of pancreatic enzymes.	ADRs Nausea, diarrhea, abdominal cramps, constipation. Pharmacokinetics Absorption: none, acts locally in GI tract; excretion in feces; pancreatic lipase is inactivated at pH $\leq$ 4.	Contraindications Hypersensitivity to pork protein or enzymes; acute pancreatitis; acute exacerbations of chronic pancreatic disease. Pregnancy Category: C Lactation Issues It is unknown if pancreatin is excreted in breast milk; use with caution in nursing mothers.
Ursodiol Actigall, generics Capsule 300 mg	**Dissolution of gallbladder stones** 8–10 mg/kg/day given in 2 to 3 divided doses Safety of use beyond 24 months has not been established.	Administration Issues **Gallbladder stone dissolution with Ursodiol treatment requires months of therapy. Carefully select patients for therapy with Ursodiol and consider altemative therapies.**	ADRs Nausea, vomiting, abdominal pain, constipation, pruritus, rash. Pharmacokinetics Absorbed in small bowel; secreted into hepatic bile ducts and expelled into the duodenum in response to eating.	Contraindications Patients with calcified cholesterol stones, radiopaque stones, radiolucent bile pigment stones, compelling reasons for cholecystectomy, allergy to bile acids, chronic liver disease.

(*continues on next page*)

501.7 Digestive Enzymes *continued from previous page*

Drug and Dosage Forms	Usual Dosage Range	Administration Issues and Drug–Drug Interactions	Common Adverse Drug Reactions (ADRs) and Pharmacokinetics	Contraindications, Pregnancy Category, and Lactation Issues
Ursodiol *cont.*		Drug–Drug Interactions **Antacids and bile acid sequestrants (cholestyramine, colestipol)** may interfere with the action of ursodiol by decreasing its absorption.		Pregnancy Category: B Lactation Issues Excretion in breast milk is not known; use with caution in nursing mothers.

501.8 Antidiarrheals

Drug and Dosage Forms	Usual Dosage Range	Administration Issues and Drug–Drug Interactions	Common Adverse Drug Reactions (ADRs) and Pharmacokinetics	Contraindications, Pregnancy Category, and Lactation Issues
Bismuth Subsalicylate Pepto-Bismol, others Tablets, chewable 262 mg Caplets 262 mg Liquid 87 mg/5 ml, 262 mg/15 ml, 524 mg/15 ml	**Indigestion, diarrhea, nausea** **adults** 2 tablets or 30 ml; repeat dose q 30 min to 1 hour prn; do not exceed 8 doses in 24 hours **children** 9–12 years: 1 tablet or 15 ml 6–9 years: 2/3 tablet or 10 ml 3–6 years: 1/3 tablet or 5 ml repeat dose q 30 min to 1 hour prn do not exceed 8 doses in 24 hours	Administration Issues Shake liquid well; chew tablets thoroughly; stool may appear gray-black (may mask GI bleeding); separate dosing from other medication. Do not use in children who have a high fever. Consult healthcare professional if diarrhea persists for > 2 days or is accompanied by high fever. Drug–Drug Interactions Bismuth subsalicylate contains salicylate, concomitant use of **aspirin** may cause toxicity. Bismuth may decrease the GI absorption of **tetracycline.**	ADRs Temporary darkening of stools. Pharmacokinetics Absorption of bismuth is negligible; salicylate is absorbed, > 90% of salicylate excreted renally.	Contraindications Hypersensitivity to salicylates or any component of the formulation; history of severe GI bleeding; history of coagulopathy; pregnancy (third trimester); do not use in patients with influenza or chickenpox. Pregnancy Category: C/D (third trimester) Lactation Issues Breastfeeding is unsafe. Salicylate absorbed from bismuth subsalicylate appears in breast milk. Adverse effects in the infant are possible with prolonged ingestion of large doses of bismuth subsalicylate.
Difenoxin and Atropine Sulfate (CIV) Motofen Tablet 1 mg difenoxin 0.025 mg atropine sulfate	**Antidiarrheal** 2 tablets, then 1 tablet after each loose stool; 1 tablet every 3 to 4 hours as needed **Total dosage in 24 hours should not exceed 8 tablets.**	Administration Issues Studies in children < 12 years are inadequate to evaluate safety and efficacy. Consult healthcare professional if diarrhea persists for > 2 days. Drug–Drug Interactions Difenoxin may potentiate effects of **barbiturates, tranquilizers, narcotics, and alcohol.** Use of difenoxin with **MAO inhibitors such as phenelzine** may precipitate a hypertensive crisis.	ADRs Vomiting, nausea, dry mouth, dizziness, drowsiness, constipation, lightheadedness. Pharmacokinetics Hepatic metabolism; excreted in urine and feces.	Contraindications Diarrhea associated with toxigenic *E. coli*, *Salmonella* sp., or *Shigella* and pseudomembranous colitis; hypersensitivity to difenoxin, atropine, or any of the inactive ingredients; jaundice. Pregnancy Category: C Lactation Issues Serious adverse effects may occur in nursing infants; evaluate need for nursing versus need for antidiarrheal.

Diphenoxylate and Atropine Sulfate (CV) Lomotil, various generics Tablet 2.5 mg diphenoxylate 0.025 mg atropine sulfate Liquid 2.5 mg diphenoxylate 0.025 mg atropine sulfate per 5 ml	**Antidiarrheal** **Adults** Initial dose is 5 mg of diphenoxylate qid; individualize dosage to control symptoms; clinical improvement usually occurs within 48 hours **Reduce dosage as soon as initial control of symptoms is achieved. Total dosage in 24 hours should not exceed 8 tablets (20 mg of diphenoxylate)** **Children** In children 2 to 12 years of age, use liquid form only. The recommended initial dosage is 0.3 to 0.4 mg/kg daily, in 4 divided doses. Pediatric dosage is an approximation of an average dose recommendation which may be adjusted downward according to nutritional status and degree of dehydration. 9–12 years: 3.5–5 ml qid 6–8 years: 2.5–5 ml qid 5 years: 2.5–4.5 ml qid 4 years: 2–4 ml qid 3 years: 2–3 ml qid 2 years: 1.5–3 ml qid	Administration Issues Children should receive the liquid form only. Do not use in children < 2 years. Consult healthcare professional if diarrhea persists for > 2 days or if fever, palpitations, or abnormal distension occur. Drug–Drug Interactions Diphenoxylate may potentiate the depressant action of **barbiturates, tranquilizers, and alcohol.** Use of **MAO inhibitors (phenelzine)** and diphenoxylate may precipitate hypertensive crisis	ADRs Nausea, vomiting, dry mouth, dizziness, drowsiness, paralytic ileus. Pharmacokinetics Hepatic metabolism; excreted in urine and feces.	Contraindications Diarrhea associated with toxigenic *E. coli, Salmonella* sp., or *Shigella* and pseudomembranous enterocolitis. Hypersensitivity to diphenoxylate, atropine, or any component of the formulation, severe liver disease, jaundice, dehydration, narrow-angle glaucoma. Pregnancy Category: C Lactation Issues Use with caution in nursing mothers; probably excreted into breast milk.
Loperamide Imodium, Pepto Diarrhea Control, generics Tablet/Capsule 2 mg Liquid 1 mg/5 ml; 1 mg/ml	**Antidiarrheal** **adults** 4 mg followed by 2 mg after each loose stool; do not exceed 16 mg/day **children, first day** 8–12 years: 2mg tid 6–8 years: 2 mg bid 2–5 years: 1 mg tid **children, subsequent dosing** 1 mg/10 kg dose after each loose stool; total daily dosage should not exceed recommended dosages for the first day	Administration Issues Drink fluids to avoid dehydration. Do not exceed prescribed dosage. Not intended for use in children < 2 yrs old. Consult health-care professional if diarrhea persists for > 2 days or if abdominal pain or distension or fever occurs. Drug–Drug Interactions Loperamide may potentiate adverse effects of **CNS depressants, phenothiazines, and tricyclic antidepressants.**	ADRs Nausea, vomiting, dry mouth, dizziness, drowsiness, constipation. Pharmacokinetics Hepatic metabolism; excreted in urine and feces.	Contraindications Diarrhea associated with toxigenic *E. coli, Salmonella* sp., or *Shigella* and pseudomembranous colitis. Hypersensitivity to loperamide or any component of the formulation; bloody diarrhea; patients who must avoid constipation. Pregnancy Category: B Lactation Issues: Excretion in breast milk unknown, but American Academy of Pediatrics considers loperamide to be compatible with breastfeeding.

(*continues on next page*)

501.8 Antidiarrheals *continued from previous page*

Drug and Dosage Forms	Usual Dosage Range	Administration Issues and Drug–Drug Interactions	Common Adverse Drug Reactions (ADRs) and Pharmacokinetics	Contraindications, Pregnancy Category, and Lactation Issues
Antidiarrheal Combination Products Kaolin with Pectin, Kapectolin, various generics Suspension 90 g kaolin and 2 g pectin per 30 ml	**Antidiarrheal** adults 60–120 ml after each loose stool children (after each loose stool) 6–12 years: 30–60 ml 3–6 years: 15–30 ml	Administration Issues Shake suspension well; separate dosing from other medication. Consult health-care professional if diarrhea persists for > 2 days or if abdominal pain or distension or fever occurs. Drug–Drug Interactions May decrease the absorption of many orally administered medications.	ADRs Constipation, fecal impaction.	Contraindications Suspected obstructive bowel lesion, pseudomembranous colitis, diarrhea associated with bacteria toxins; hypersensitivity to kaolin/pectin products. Pregnancy Category: C Lactation Issues: Limited information available
Products with Attapulgite Tablet Diasorb: 750 mg Donnagel: 600 mg Caplets Kaopectate Maximum Strength 750 mg, generics Liquid Donnagel, Children's Kaopectate, generics: 600 mg/15 ml Diasorb: 750 mg/5 ml	**Antidiarrheal** **adults** 4 tablets (750 mg/tablet) or 20 ml (750 mg/5 ml) after each loose stool; do not exceed 3 doses/day **or** 2 tablets (600 mg/tablet) or 30 ml (600 mg/15 ml) after each loose stool; do not exceed 7 doses/day **children** 6–12 years: 2 tablets (750 mg/tablet) or 10 ml (750 mg/5 ml) after each loose stool; do not exceed 3 doses/day **or** 1 tablet (600 mg/tablet) or 15 ml (600 mg/15 ml) after each loose stool; do not exceed 7 doses/day 3–6 years: 1 tablet (750 mg/tablet) or 5 ml (750 mg/5 ml) after each loose stool; do not exceed 3 doses/day **or** 1/2 tablet (600 mg/tablet) or 7.5 ml (600 mg/15 ml) after each loose stool; do not exceed 7 doses/day	Administration Issues Shake suspension well; separate dosing from other medication. Consult health-care professional if diarrhea persists for > 2 days or if abdominal pain or distension or fever occurs. Drug–Drug Interactions May decrease the absorption of many orally administered medications.	ADRs Constipation (dose-related).	Contraindications Suspected obstructive bowel lesion, pseudomembranous colitis, diarrhea associated with bacteria toxins; previous hypersensitivity to attapulgite; suspected obstructive lesions of the bowel. Pregnancy Category: B Lactation Issues: No information available.

501.9 Laxatives

Drug and Dosage Forms	Usual Dosage Range	Administration Issues and Drug–Drug Interactions	Common Adverse Drug Reactions (ADRs) and Pharmacokinetics	Contraindications, Pregnancy Category, and Lactation Issues
Bisacodyl Dulcolax, various generics Tablet, enteric 5 mg Suppository 10 mg Tablet 5 mg Tablet, delayed release 10 mg	**Laxative** **adults** 5–15 mg po as a single dose once daily; 10 mg PR as a single dose once daily **children** tablet ≥ 12 years: 5–15 mg po as a single dose once daily 6 to < 12 years: 5 mg po once daily suppository 6 to < 12 years: 5 mg once daily	Administration Issues Swallow tablet whole, do not crush or chew; do not take within 1 hour of antacids, H2 antagonists, proton pump inhibitors, or milk.	ADRs Abdominal discomfort, cramps, nausea, diarrhea, electrolyte disturbances, loss of normal bowel function, and laxative dependence with excessive use. Pharmacokinetics Onset = 6–10 h (oral) or 0.25–1 h (rectal).	Contraindications Hypersensitivity to bisacodyl or any component of the formulation; abdominal pain, obstruction, nausea, or vomiting. Pregnancy Category: C Lactation Issues No information available.
Cascara Sagrada various generics Tablet 325 mg Liquid approximately 18% to 19% alcohol	**Laxative** **adults and children > 12 years** tablet: 1 tablet at bedtime liquid (aromatic fluid extract): 5 ml (range: 2–6 ml) singe daily dose	Administration Issues Administer with a full glass of water on an empty stomach for best results.	ADRs Abdominal discomfort, cramps, nausea, diarrhea, electrolyte disturbances, loss of normal bowel function, and laxative dependence with excessive use, may discolor urine. Pharmacokinetics Onset = 6–8 h; may take up to 24 hours.	Contraindications Nausea, vomiting, abdominal pain, fecal impaction, intestinal obstruction, GI bleeding, appendicitis, congestive heart failure, hypersensitivity to anthraquinone laxatives. Pregnancy Category: C Lactation Issues Cascara is excreted in breast milk, use with caution; American Academy of Pediatrics considers cascara to be compatible with breastfeeding.
Castor Oil Liquid castor oil Purge: 95% castor oil Emulsion Emulsoil: 95% castor oil Neoloid: 36.4% castor oil	**Preparation for rectal or bowel examination or surgery** **adults and children > 12 years (oral)** liquid 15–60 ml/day emulsified 36.4%: 45–60 ml/day 95%: 15–60 ml/day mixed with _ to 1 full glass liquid	Administration Issues Shake emulsion well before use; chill or administer with juice or carbonated beverage to improve palatability.	ADRs Abdominal discomfort, cramps nausea, diarrhea, electrolyte disturbances, loss of normal bowel function, and laxative dependence with excessive use; hypotension, dizziness. Pharmacokinetics Onset = 2–6 h.	Contraindications Intestinal obstruction fecal impaction. Pregnancy Category: X Use during pregnancy may induce premature labor due to irritant effect. Lactation Issues No information available.

501.9 Laxatives *continued from previous page*

Drug and Dosage Forms	Usual Dosage Range	Administration Issues and Drug–Drug Interactions	Common Adverse Drug Reactions (ADRs) and Pharmacokinetics	Contraindications, Pregnancy Category, and Lactation Issues
Castor Oil *cont.*	**children, 2–11 years (oral)** liquid 5–15 ml/day emulsified 36.4%: 15–30 ml/day 95%: 5–15 ml/day mixed with _ to 1 full glass liquid			
Docusate Calcium Surfak, various generics Capsules 240 mg Capsules, softgels 240 mg	**Laxative** **adults and children ≥ 12 years:** 240 mg daily until bowel movements normal	Administration Issues Give each dose with a full glass of water, milk, or fruit juice. Drug–Drug Interactions Do not give **mineral oil** with docusate calcium.	ADRs Abdominal discomfort, cramps; diarrhea. Pharmacokinetics Onset = 12–72 h.	Contraindications Hypersensitivity to docusate or any component of the formulation; concomitant use of mineral oil; intestinal obstruction, acute abdominal pain, nausea, or vomiting. Pregnancy Category: C Lactation Issues Excretion in breast milk is unknown, use with caution in nursing mothers.
Docusate Sodium Colace, Diocto, various generics Tablet 100 mg Capsules 50 mg, 100 mg, 250 mg Syrup 50 mg/15 ml, 60 mg/15 ml, 100 mg/30 ml Liquid 150 mg/15 ml	**Laxative** **adults and children ≥ 12 years** 50 mg–500 mg/d in 1–4 divided doses PR: Add 50 mg–100 mg docusate liquid to enema fluid **children (oral)** infants and children <3 years: 10–40 mg/day in 1–4 divided doses 3–6 years: 20–60 mg/day in 1–4 divided doses 6–12 years: 40–150 mg/day in 1–4 divided doses	Administration Issues Docusate liquid should be given in milk, fruit juice, or infant formula to mask taste. Drug–Drug Interactions Do not give **mineral oil** with docusate sodium.	ADRs Abdominal discomfort, cramps, diarrhea. Pharmacokinetics Onset = 12–72 h.	Contraindications Hypersensitivity to docusate or any component of the formulation; concomitant use of mineral oil; intestinal obstruction, acute abdominal pain, nausea, or vomiting. Pregnancy Category: C Lactation Issues Excretion in breast milk is unknown, use with caution in nursing mothers.
Glycerin Sani-Supp, Fleet Babylax, generics	**Laxative** **adult** 1 suppository rectally and retain 15–30 minutes	Administration Issues Retain suppository in rectum for 15 min; suppository does not have to melt to pro-	ADRs Rectal discomfort, rectal irritation, burning.	Contraindications Intestinal obstruction, abdominal pain, N/V, fecal impaction; hypersensitivity to any component in preparation.

Suppository glycerin/sodium stearate Liquid 4 ml per applicator	1 liquid applicator in rectum	duce laxative action; insert applicator stem with tip pointing towards navel and squeeze unit gently; a small portion of liquid will remain in applicator	Pharmacokinetics Onset = 15–60 min.	Pregnancy Category: C Lactation Issues No data are available.
Magnesium Citrate Citrate of Magnesia Liquid 300 ml	**Evacuation of bowel prior to certain surgical and diagnostic procedures or overdose situations** **adults and children ≥ 12 years** ½ to 1 full bottle (120–300 ml) **children** ≤ 6 years: 0.5 ml/kg up to a maximum of 200 ml repeated every 4–6 hours until stools are clear 6–12 years: 100–150 ml	Administration Issues Take with a glass of water, fruit juice, or citrus-flavored carbonated beverage to improve taste, chill before using; report severe abdominal pain to physician.	ADRs Dehydration, electrolyte imbalance (with repeated use), hypotension, abdominal cramps, diarrhea, gas. Pharmacokinetics Onset = 0.5–3 h.	Contraindications Renal failure, appendicitis, abdominal pain, intestinal impaction, obstruction or perforation, complications in gastrointestinal tract, patients with colostomy or ileostomy, ulcerative colitis, diverticulitis. Pregnancy Category: B Lactation Issues No data are available.
Magnesium Hydroxide Phillips' Milk of Magnesia Liquid, oral 400 mg/5 ml Liquid, oral concentrate 800 mg/5 ml Tablets 300 mg, 600 mg	**Laxative** **adults and children ≥ 12 years:** liquid: 30–60 ml/day (15–30 ml/day of liquid concentrate) or in divided doses tablet: 6–8 tablets before bedtime **children** liquid < 2 years: 0.5 ml/kg/dose 2–5 years: 5–15 ml/day (2.5–7.5 ml/day of liquid concentrate) or in divided doses 6–12 years: 15–30 ml/day (7.5–15 ml/day of liquid concentrate) or in divided doses tablet 2–5 years: 1–2 tablets before bedtime 6–11 years: 3–4 tablets before bedtime	Administration Issues Dilute in water or juice, shake well; should be followed by 8 ounces of water; taste can be improved by following each dose with citrus fruit juice. Drug–Drug Interactions Absorption of tetracyclines, digoxin, iron salts, isoniazid, or quinolones may be decreased.	ADRs Hypermagnesemia, diarrhea, abdominal cramps, hypotension. Pharmacokinetics Onset of action (laxative): 4–8 h; excretion in urine; feces (as unabsorbed drug).	Contraindications Hypersensitivity to any component of the formulation; patients with colostomy or an ileostomy, intestinal obstruction, fecal impaction, renal failure, appendicitis. Pregnancy Category: B Lactation Issues No information available.
Methylcellulose Citrucel, Citrucel Sugar Free	**Laxative** **adults and children ≥ 12 years** 1 heaping tablespoonful in 8 oz. of cold water 1 to 3 times daily	Administration Issues Take with a full glass of water. Use sugar-free preparation with caution in patients with phenylketonuria.	ADRs Abdominal discomfort, bloating. **Esophageal obstruction, swelling, or blockage may occur when insufficient**	Contraindications Hypersensitivity to methylcellulose or any component of the formulation; fecal impaction; GI obstruction.

(*continues on next page*)

501.9 Laxatives *continued from previous page*

Drug and Dosage Forms	Usual Dosage Range	Administration Issues and Drug–Drug Interactions	Common Adverse Drug Reactions (ADRs) and Pharmacokinetics	Contraindications, Pregnancy Category, and Lactation Issues
Methylcellulose *cont.* Powder Citrucel (2 gm methylcellulose/heaping tablespoon) Citrucel Sugar Free (2 gm methylcellulose, 52 mg phenylalanine/leveled scoop)	**children 6 to < 12 years:** ½ of adult dose in 8 oz of cold water once daily	Elderly may have insufficient fluid intake, which may predispose them to fecal impaction and bowel obstruction. Drug–Drug Interactions The absorption of drugs such as **digoxin, warfarin, nitrofurantoin, and salicylates** in the GI tract may be decreased by bulk-forming laxatives.	**liquid is administered with bulk-forming laxatives.** Pharmacokinetics Onset 12–72 h.	Pregnancy Category: B Lactation Issues: Excretion in breast milk unknown.
Mineral Oil Liquid Mineral Oil, various generics Emulsion Kondremul Plain	**Laxative** **adults and children ≥ 12 years:** 15 to 45 ml, take at bedtime; Kondremul, 30 to 75 ml **children 6 to < 12 years:** 5 to 15 ml; Kondremul, 10 to 25 ml.	Administration Issues Shake emulsion well before use. Mineral oil is preferably administered on an empty stomach. Drug–Drug Interactions The absorption of **fat-soluble vitamins (Vit A, E, D, K)** may be decreased by mineral oil. The absorption of **oral contraceptives and warfarin** may be decreased by mineral oil. Do not give **docusate products** with mineral oil.	ADRs Larger doses of mineral oil may cause anal seepage, resulting in itching, rectal inflammation, and perianal discomfort. Pharmacokinetics Onset = 6–8 h.	Contraindications Use with caution in debilitated, young, or elderly patients, aspiration upon reclining may cause lipid pneumonitis; intestinal obstruction fecal impaction. Pregnancy Category: C Lactation Issues No data are available.
Polycarbophil FiberCon, Mitrolan, Fiber Norm Tablet 500 mg, 625 mg Tablet, chewable 500 mg	**Laxative** **adults and children ≥ 12 years** 1 g 1 to 4 times daily or as needed; do not exceed 4 g in 24 h **children** 6 to < 12 years: 500 mg < 4 times daily or as needed; do not exceed 2 g in 24 h < 6 years: Products vary; consult product labeling for specific guidelines	Administration Issues Take with a full glass of water. Elderly may have insufficient fluid intake, which may predispose them to fecal impaction and bowel obstruction. Drug–Drug Interactions The absorption of drugs such as **digoxin, warfarin, nitrofurantoin, and salicylates** in the GI tract may be decreased by bulk-forming laxatives.	ADRs Abdominal discomfort, bloating. **Esophageal obstruction, swelling, or blockage may occur when insufficient liquid is administered with bulk-forming laxatives.** Pharmacokinetics Onset 12–72 h.	Contraindications Hypersensitivity to polycarbophil or any component of the formulation; fecal impaction; GI obstruction. Pregnancy Category: B Lactation Issues Excretion in breast milk unknown.
Psyllium Fiberall, Metamucil, Perdiem Fiber, Hydrocil Powder, effervescent Metamucil: 3.4 gm psyllium/dose	**Laxative** **adult:** 1–2 rounded teaspoonfuls or 1–2 packets or 1–2 wafers in 8 oz glass of liquid, 1–3 times/day	Administration Issues Take with a full glass of water; do not chew psyllium granules. Use sugar-free preparation with caution in patients with phenylketonuria Elderly may have insufficient fluid intake, which may predispose	ADRs Abdominal discomfort, bloating. **Esophageal obstruction, swelling, or blockage may occur when insufficient liquid is administered with bulk-forming laxatives.**	Contraindications Hypersensitivity to psyllium or any component of the formulation; fecal impaction; GI obstruction. Pregnancy Category: B

Granules Perdiem Fiber: 4.03 gm psyllium/tsp Wafer Fiberall: 3.4 gm psyllium/dose	**children 6–11 years:** ½ to 1 rounded teaspoonful in 4 oz glass of liquid 1–3 times/day	them to fecal impaction and bowel obstruction. Drug–Drug Interactions The absorption of drugs such as **digoxin, warfarin, nitrofurantoin, and salicylates** in the GI tract may be decreased by bulk-forming laxatives.	Pharmacokinetics Onset 12–72 h.	Lactation Issues Excretion in breast milk unknown.
Senna Senokot, generics Tablets (sennosides) Senokot, Senna-Gen: 8.6 mg SennakotXTRA: 17 mg Granules (sennosides) Senokot: 15 mg/5 ml Black-Draught: 20 mg/5 ml Syrup (sennosides) Senokot: 8.8 mg/5 ml Liquid Fletcher's Castoria: 33.3 mg/ml senna concentrate	**Laxative** standard senna concentrate **adults:** 1–2 tablets or ½–1 tsp once or twice daily (max 4 tablets or 2 tsp bid) granules: 1 teaspoon (sennosides 15 milligrams (mg)), preferably prior to bedtime once a day, up to a maximum of 2 teaspoons (30 mg) twice a day syrup: syrup forms of senna usually contain standardized senna extract in a concentration of 218 milligrams (mg) per 5-ml measure. The usual recommended oral dose is 10 to 15 mL (436 to 654 mg standardized senna extract) once a day (preferably at bedtime), up to a maximum of 30 mL/day for adults. tablets: sennosides 15 to 17 milligrams (mg) once a day, ideally before bedtime, up to a maximum of 34 to 50 mg twice a day **children** granules: 2–6 years: initial dosage is 0.25 teaspoon (3.75 mg sennosides) qd, preferably at bedtime. The maximum recommended dosage is 0.5 teaspoon (7.5 mg sennosides) bid. One teaspoon of senna granules contains 15 mg sennosides. 6–12 years: initial dosage is 0.5 teaspoon (7.5 mg sennosides) qd, preferably at bedtime. The maximum recom	Administration Issues Administer with a full glass of water on an empty stomach for best results.	ADRs Abdominal discomfort, cramps, nausea, diarrhea, electrolyte disturbances, loss of normal bowel function, and laxative dependence with excessive use; may discolor urine. Pharmacokinetics Onset = 6–10 h; may take up to 24 hours	Contraindications Hypersensitivity to anthraquinone laxatives; intestinal obstruction, acute intestinal inflammation, colitis ulcerosa, appendicitis, abdominal pain of unknown origin, and pregnancy. Use with caution in children <12 years of age. Pregnancy Category: C Lactation Issues Not excreted into breast milk to a significant degree. The American Academy of Pediatrics regards senna compatible with breastfeeding.

(continues on next page)

501.9 Laxatives *continued from previous page*

Drug and Dosage Forms	Usual Dosage Range	Administration Issues and Drug–Drug Interactions	Common Adverse Drug Reactions (ADRs) and Pharmacokinetics	Contraindications, Pregnancy Category, and Lactation Issues
Senna *cont.*	mended dosage is 1 teaspoon (15 mg sennosides) bid. syrup: 2–6 years: initial dosage is 0.5 to 0.75 teaspoon (4.4 to 6.6 mg sennosides) qd, preferably at bedtime. The maximum recommended dosage is 0.75 teaspoon (6.6 mg sennosides) bid. One teaspoon of syrup contains 8.8 mg sennosides. 6–12 years: initial dosage is 1 to 1.5 teaspoons (8.8 to 13.2 mg sennosides) qd, preferably at bedtime. The maximum recommended dosage is 1.5 teaspoons (13.2 mg sennosides) bid. tablets: 2–6 years: initial dosage is 4.3 mg sennosides qd, preferably at bedtime. The maximum recommended dosage is 8.6 mg sennosides bid. 6–12 years: initial dosage is 8.5 to 15 mg sennosides qd, preferably at bedtime. The maximum recommended dosage is 17 to 25 mg sennosides bid			
Sodium Phosphate and Sodium Biphosphate Fleet Phospho-Soda Solution, oral Monobasic sodium phosphate monohydrate 2.4 g and dibasic sodium phosphate heptahydrate 0.9 g per 5 ml	**Laxative** **adults and children ≥ 12 years** 20 to 45 ml/day **children** 10 to 11 years: 10 to 20 ml/day 5 to 9 years: 5 to 10 ml/day	Administration Issues Take on an empty stomach; dilute dose with 4 oz cool water, then follow dose with 8 oz water; do not repeat dose within 24 hours.	ADRs: Hypotension, dehydration, electrolyte imbalance (with repeated use), abdominal pain, nausea. Pharmacokinetics Onset = 0.5–3 h.	Contraindications Hypersensitivity to sodium phosphate salts or any component of the formulation; congenital megacolon, toxic megacolon, bowel obstruction, bowel perforation, congestive heart failure, ascites. Pregnancy Category: C Lactation Issues Use with caution in nursing women. henolphthalein intestinal obstruction fecal impaction.

501.10 Laxative Combinations
Listed below is a representative sample of laxative combination products. Administration and dosage depends on the condition being treated and the agent being used. See individual products (section 501.9) for administration issues, interactions, ADRs, etc.
Dialose Plus, various generics Capsule 100 mg docusate sodium/30 mg casanthranol
Doxidan Capsule 100 mg docusate sodium/30 mg casanthranol
Ex-lax Gentle Strength Caplets Caplet 65 mg docusate sodium/10 mg senna concentrate
Peri-Colace, various generics Capsule 100 mg docusate sodium/30 mg casanthranol Syrup 60 mg docusate sodium/30 mg casanthranol per 15 ml
Perdiem Overnight Relief Granules 3.25 g psyllium/0.74 g senna per rounded teaspoonful
Senokot-S Tablet 50 mg docusate sodium/8.6 mg senna concentrate

501.11 Enemas

Drug and Dosage Forms	Usual Dosage Range	Administration Issues and Drug–Drug Interactions	Common Adverse Drug Reactions (ADRs)	Contraindications, Pregnancy Category, and Lactation Issues
Miscellaneous Enemas Fleet: 7 g dibasic sodium phosphate and 19 g monobasic sodium phosphate per 118 ml Fleet Bisacodyl: 10 mg bisacodyl per 30 ml Fleet Mineral Oil: Mineral oil Therevac-SB: 283 mg docusate sodium in a base of soft soap, PEG, and 275 mg glycerin per 4 ml Therevac-Plus: 283 mg docusate sodium, 275 mg glycerin, and 20 mg benzocaine in a base of soft soap, PEG per 4 ml	**Laxative** **adults and children ≥ 12 years** Fleet and Fleet Mineral Oil: 118 ml Fleet Bisacodyl: 30 ml Therevac-SB and Therevac-Plus: 4 ml **children 2 to < 12 years** Fleet and Fleet Mineral Oil: 59 ml	Administration Issues For rectal use only. **Do not use enemas in children < 2 years.**	ADRs (Fleet Enema) Dehydration, hypotension, electrolyte imbalance (with repeated use), abdominal pain, nausea.	Contraindications (Fleet Enema) Hypersensitivity to sodium phosphate salts or any component of the formulation; congenital megacolon, toxic megacolon, bowel obstruction, bowel perforation, imperforate anus, congestive heart failure, ascites. Pregnancy Category (Fleet Enema): C Lactation Issues (Fleet Enema) Use with caution in nursing women.
Polyethylene Glycol-Electrolyte Solution Powder, for oral solution CoLyte GoLYTELY NuLytely MiraLax Oral Solution OCL	**Bowel cleansing prior to GI exam (CoLyte, GoLYTELY, NuLytely)** Drink 4 liters prior to GI exam; drink 8 oz every 10 minutes until 4 liters are consumed or the rectal effluent is clear; first bowel movement should occur approximately 1 hour after the start of administration. **Occasional constipation (MiraLax)** 17 g of powder (~ 1 heaping tablespoon) dissolved in 8 oz of water; once daily; do not use for > 2 weeks	Administration Issues Patient should fast for 3–4 hours prior to ingesting fluid; no solid foods should be given < 2 hours before solution is given; reconstitute solution with tap water; shake solution well prior to administration; store solution in the refrigerator; use solution within 48 hours after reconstitution; do not add flavorings or additional ingredients to solution before ingestion. Safety and efficacy for use in children have not been established. Drug–Drug Interactions Do not give oral medications within one hour of start of drinking solution, decreased drug absorption may occur due to laxative effect of solution.	ADRs Nausea, abdominal fullness, bloating, abdominal cramps.	Contraindications Hypersensitivity to polyethylene glycol or any component of the formulation; gastrointestinal obstruction, gastric retention, bowel perforation, toxic colitis, megacolon. Pregnancy Category: C Lactation Issues Excretion in breast milk unknown; use caution.

Lactulose Cephulac, Chronulac, Duphalac, various generics Syrup 10 gm / 15 ml	**Laxative** **adults:** 15–30 ml daily, increased to 60 ml/day if necessary **Prevention and treatment of portal-systemic encephalopathy** **adults** oral: 30 to 45 ml, 3 or 4 times/day; adjust dosage every day or two to produce 2 or 3 soft stools daily rectal: Rectal enemas may be extemporaneously compounded by mixing 300 ml of lactulose with 700 ml of water or normal saline; have patient retain enema for 30 to 60 minutes; repeat enema if needed every 4 to 6 hours **children** Little information on use in children and adolescents; goal is to produce 2 or 3 soft stools daily; for older children and adolescents, the total daily oral dose is 40 to 90 ml in divided doses.	Administration Issues May not see beneficial effects for 24–48 hours; diarrhea may indicate overdosage and responds to dose reduction; give with fruit juice, water, or milk to make more palatable. Drug–Drug Interactions **Neomycin and other antibiotics** may eliminate colonic bacteria necessary for the action of lactulose **Antacids** given with lactulose may inhibit the desired lactulose-induced decrease in colonic pH	ADRs: Gaseous distension with flatulence, belching, abdominal discomfort such as cramping; nausea; vomiting. Elderly, debilitated patients who receive lactulose for > 6 months should have serum electrolytes and carbon dioxide measured periodically. Pharmacokinetics Onset = 24–48 h.	Contraindications Patients requiring a low galactose diet; galactosemia; hypersensitivity to lactulose or any component of the formulation. Pregnancy Category: B Lactation Issues Excretion in breast milk is unknown; use with caution in nursing mothers; no data are available.

501.12 Agents for Crohn's Disease, Irritable Bowel Syndrome, and Ulcerative Colitis

Drug and Dosage Forms	Usual Dosage Range	Administration Issues and Drug–Drug Interactions	Common Adverse Drug Reactions (ADRs) and Pharmacokinetics	Contraindications, Pregnancy Category, and Lactation Issues
Balsalazide Disodium Colazal Capsules 750 mg	**Active ulcerative colitis** Take three 750 mg capsules 3 times a day for a total daily dose of 6.75 g for a duration of 8 weeks; some patients in clinical trials required treatment for 12 weeks; safety and efficacy beyond 12 weeks have not been established.	Administration Issues Do not chew or open capsules; take as directed; report abdominal pain, unresolved diarrhea, severe headache, or chest pain to prescriber.	ADRs Headache, abdominal pain, diarrhea, nausea. Pharmacokinetics: Onset of action is delayed; may require several days to weeks; azoreduced in colon to 5-aminosalicylic acid (active), 4-aminobenzoyl-beta-alanine (inert), and N-acetylated metabolites; primary effect is topical (colonic mucosa); primarily excreted in feces.	Contraindications: Hypersensitivity to salicylates, components of the formulation, or metabolites of balsalazide. Pregnancy Category: B Lactation Issues Excretion in breast milk unknown; use with caution in nursing mothers.

(continues on next page)

501.12 Agents for Crohn's Disease, Irritable Bowel Syndrome and Ulcerative Colitis *continued from previous page*

Drug and Dosage Forms	Usual Dosage Range	Administration Issues and Drug–Drug Interactions	Common Adverse Drug Reactions (ADRs) and Pharmacokinetics	Contraindications, Pregnancy Category, and Lactation Issues
Infliximab Remicade Powder for injection 100 mg	**Crohn's disease, moderate-to-severe** 5 mg/kg as a single infusion over a minimum of 2 hours **Crohn's disease, fistulizing** 5 mg/kg as an infusion over a minimum of 2 hours; dose repeated at 2 and 6 weeks after the initial infusion	Administration Issues Do not shake reconstituted vials; infusion of dose should begin within 3 hours of preparation; infuse over at least 2 hours; medications for the treatment of hypersensitivity reactions should be readily available.	ADRs **Tuberculosis, invasive fungal infections and other opportunistic infections have been observed in patients receiving infliximab. Some of these infections have been fatal. Evaluate patients for latent TB infection with a tuberculin skin test.** Headache, fatigue, fever, rash, nausea, diarrhea, abdominal pain, infusion reactions, upper respiratory tract infection, cough, sinusitis, pharyngitis, development of antinuclear antibodies, infections. Pharmacokinetics Onset of action ~ 2 weeks.	Contraindications Hypersensitivity to murine proteins or any component of the formulation; congestive heart failure. Pregnancy Category: B (manufacturer) Lactation Issues Excretion in breast milk unknown; because many immunoglobulins are secreted in milk and potential for serious adverse reactions exist, breastfeeding not recommended.
Mesalamine Asacol, Pentasa, generics Tablets, delayed release Asacol: 400 mg Capsules, controlled release Pentasa: 250 mg Suppositories Rowasa: 500 mg Rectal suspension Rowasa: 4 gm / 60 ml (contains potassium metabisulphite)	**Chronic inflammatory bowel disease, including ulcerative colitis and proctitis** tablets: 800 mg tid for 6 weeks capsules: 1 gm qid for up to 8 weeks suppositories: I suppository bid for 3 to 6 weeks; retain suppository for 1 to 3 hours retention enema: 60 ml rectally at bedtime, retained overnight, approximately 8 hours	Administration Issues Swallow tablet and capsule whole, do not chew or crush; remove foil from suppository before administration and avoid excessive handling; shake suspension enema well before administration; use with caution in patients with impaired hepatic or renal function; monitor CBC and renal function, particularly in elderly patients.	ADRs Pain, abdominal pain, eructation, pharyngitis. Pharmacokinetics Tablet and capsule formulations release mesalamine for topical action in GI tract; <30% is absorbed; metabolized in the liver to acetyl-5-aminosalicylic acid (active); intestinal metabolism may also occur; primarily excreted renally.	Contraindications Hypersensitivity to mesalamine, sulfasalazine, salicylates, or any component of the formulation; mesalamine rectal suspension should not be used in patients with a known history of sulfite hypersensitivity. Pregnancy Category: B Lactation Issues Use with caution in nursing mothers; excreted into breast milk.
Olsalazine Dipentum Capsule 250 mg	**Ulcerative colitis (maintenance of remission)** 500 mg bid	Administration Issues Take with food; take daily dose in two evenly divided doses.	ADRs Diarrhea, headache, nausea abdominal pain cramps.	Contraindications Hypersensitivity to olsalazine, salicylates, or any component of the formulation.

			Pharmacokinetics Olsalazine is converted to active mesalamine by bacteria in the colon; mesalamine exerts topical, local action in the colon; highly protein bound; primarily excreted in feces.	Pregnancy Category: C Lactation Issues Excretion in breast milk is unknown; use with caution in nursing mothers.
Sulfasalazine Tablet Azulfidine, generics 500 mg Tablets, enteric coated Azulfidine EN-tabs: 500 mg	**Treatment of ulcerative colitis** **adults:** initial therapy, 3 to 4 g daily in evenly divided doses; may be advisable to initiate therapy with lower dosage of 1 to 2 g daily in evenly divided doses; doses of 2 g daily in evenly divided doses may be used for maintenance therapy **children ≥ 2 years:** initially, 40–60 mg/kg/day in 3–6 divided doses; of 20–30 mg/kg/day in 4 divided doses may be used for maintenance therapy	Administration Issues Take after meals; orange-yellow discoloration of the urine or skin may occur; avoid prolonged exposure to sunlight, wear protective clothing, and apply sunscreen; drink plenty of water. Drug–Drug Interactions Sulfasalazine may decrease the absorption of **digoxin** and **folic acid** and may impair hepatic metabolism of sulfonylureas or alter plasma protein binding.	ADRs Anorexia, nausea, diarrhea, headache, rash photosensitivity, vomiting, reversible oligospermia Pharmacokinetics Metabolized to sulfapyridine and 5-aminosalicylic acid via colonic intestinal flora; primarily urine excretion.	Contraindications Hypersensitivity to sulfasalazine, sulfa drugs, salicylates, or any component of the formulation; porphyria; GI or GU obstruction; children < 2 years of age; pregnancy (at term). Pregnancy Category: B/D (near term) Lactation Issues Sulfapyridine is excreted into breast milk. American Academy of Pediatrics classifies sulfasalazine as a drug that should be given to nursing women with caution because significant adverse effects may occur in some nursing infants.
Tegaserod Zelnorm Tablet 2 mg, 6 mg	**Short-term treatment of constipation-predominate irritable bowel syndrome in women** Women: 6 mg BID before meals for 4 to 6 weeks; may consider continuing treatment for an additional 4 to 6 weeks in patients who respond initially. **Safety and efficacy in men has not been established.**	Administration Issues Take on an empty stomach, 30 minutes before meals. Drug-Drug Interactions No clinically significant interactions have been reported.	ADRs Headache, abdominal pain, diarrhea, nausea, flatulence, back pain, dizziness, migraine, arthropathy, leg pain. Pharmacokinetics GI metabolsim: hydrolysis in the stomach; Hepatic: oxidation, conjugation, and glucuronidation; significant first-pass effect; ~66% excreted as unchanged drug in feces, ~33% excreted as metabolites in urine.	Contraindications Hypersensitivity to tegaserod or any component of the formulation, severe renal impairment, moderate or severe hepatic impairment, history of bowel obstruction, symptomatic gallbladder disease, suspected sphincter of Oddi dysfunction, or abdominal adhesions. Treatment should not be started in patients with diarrhea or in those who experience diarrhea frequently. Pregnancy Category: B Lactation Issues Excretion in breast milk unknown/not recommended.

501.13 Antiflatulent Agents

Drug and Dosage Forms	Usual Dosage Range	Administration Issues and Drug–Drug Interactions	Common Adverse Drug Reactions (ADRs) and Pharmacokinetics	Contraindications, Pregnancy Category, and Lactation Issues
Charcoal CharcoCaps, various generics Capsules 260 mg	**Relief of intestinal gas, diarrhea, indigestion** 520 mg after meals or at first sign of discomfort; repeat as needed up to 4.16 g daily	Administration Issues Take charcoal 2 hours before or 1 hour after other medications. **Do not use in children < 3 years.** Charcoal will cause stools to turn black. Drug–Drug Interactions Charcoal may decrease the absorption of and actually remove drugs such as **acetaminophen, barbiturates, carbamazepine, digoxin, phenytoin, salicylates, theophylline, tricyclic antidepressants, and valproic acid** from the systemic circulation.	ADRs Vomiting, diarrhea with sorbitol, constipation. Pharmacokinetics Charcoal is not absorbed or metabolized; excreted in feces.	Contraindications Do not use charcoal with sorbitol in patients with fructose intolerance. Pregnancy Category: C Lactation Issues Does not enter breast milk/compatible.
Charcoal and Simethicone Flatulex Tablets 250 mg activated charcoal and 80 mg simethicone	**Antiflatulent** 1 tablet 3 times daily and at bedtime	Administration Issues Take charcoal 2 hours before or 1 hour after other medications; do not crush tablet. **Do not use in children < 3 years.** Charcoal will cause stools to turn black. Drug–Drug Interactions Charcoal may decrease the absorption of and actually remove drugs such as **acetaminophen, barbiturates, carbamazepine, digoxin, phenytoin, salicylates, theophylline, tricyclic antidepressants, and valproic acid** from the systemic circulation.	ADRs Vomiting, constipation, loose stools. Pharmacokinetics Simethicone is not absorbed after oral administration; charcoal is not absorbed or metabolized.	Contraindications Do not use charcoal with sorbitol in patients with fructose intolerance; hypersensitivity to simethicone or any component of the formulation. Pregnancy Category: C Lactation Issues No data are available.
Simethicone Mylanta Gas, Gas-X, Maximum Strength Mylanta Gas, Phazyme, Phazyme 125, Mylicon, various generics	**Antiflatulent** **Adult and children > 12:** 40 mg–125 mg qid after meals and at bedtime, not to exceed 500 mg/day	Administration Issues Take after meals and at bedtime; ensure that chewable tablets are chewed thoroughly and followed with a glass of water; shake drops well before use;	ADRs Loose stools. Pharmacokinetics Simethicone is not absorbed after oral administration	Contraindications Hypersensitivity to simethicone or any component of the formulation. Pregnancy Category: C

Tablets 60 mg, 95 mg Tablets chewable 40 mg, 80 mg, 125 mg, 150 mg Capsules 125 mg Drops 40 mg/0.6 ml Capsules, Softgel 125 mg	**Children** 2–12 years: 40 mg 4 times daily < 2 years: 20 mg (0.3 ml) qid up to 240 mg/d	drops can be mixed with 30 ml cool water, infant formula, or other suitable liquids		Lactation Issues No data are available.

502. Antiemetic/Antivertigo Agents

502.1 Anticholinergic Agents

Drug and Dosage Forms	Usual Dosage Range	Administration Issues and Drug–Drug Interactions	Common Adverse Drug Reactions (ADRs) and Pharmacokinetics	Contraindications, Pregnancy Category, and Lactation Issues
Buclizine Bucladin-S Softabs Tablets 50 mg	**Motion Sickness** 50 mg before departure; repeat q 4–6 hrs as needed up to 150 mg/d	Administration Issues Give dose 30 minutes prior to motion, then before meals and at bedtime for duration of journey. Tablets can be allowed to dissolve in mouth, can be chewed, or can be swallowed whole; safety/efficacy in children < 12 yrs not established Drug–Drug Interactions **Increased effect of antihistamine:** MAO inhibitors (anticholinergic effects) **Increased effect of:** MAO inhibitors, alcohol, CNS depressants	ADRs Urinary retention, blurred vision, dry mouth, drowsiness, irritability, thickening of bronchial secretions. Elderly (>60yrs): more likely to experience confusion, dizziness, hypotension. Pharmacokinetics Rapid onset (15–30 minutes); hepatically metabolized; duration of action = 4–6 h.	Contraindications Hypersensitivity, asthma, glaucoma, prostate gland enlargement Precautions Use carefully if operating heavy machinery, history of sleep apnea, hepatic dysfunction Pregnancy Category: B Lactation Issues Women should not nurse.
Cyclizine Marezine Tablets 50 mg	**Motion Sickness** 50 mg before departure; repeat q 4–6 hrs. Max daily dose is 200 mg Pediatrics (6–12 yrs): 25 mg up to 3 times daily	Administration Issues Give dose 30 minutes prior to motion, then before meals and at bedtime for duration of journey; safety/efficacy in children <12 yrs not established Drug–Drug Interactions **increased effect of antihistamine:** MAO inhibitors (anticholinergic effects) **increased effect of:** MAO inhibitors, alcohol, CNS depressants	ADRs Urinary retention, blurred vision, dry mouth, drowsiness, irritability, thickening of bronchial secretions. Elderly (>60yrs): more likely to experience confusion, dizziness, hypotension. Pharmacokinetics Onset = 30–60 minutes; duration of action = 4–6 h.	Contraindications Hypersensitivity, asthma, glaucoma, prostate gland enlargement. Precautions Use carefully if operating heavy machinery, history of sleep apnea, hepatic dysfunction Pregnancy Category: B Lactation Issues Women should not nurse.
Dimenhydrinate Calm-X, Dimetabs, Dramamine, Marmine, Triptone Caplets, various generics Tablets 50 mg Chewable tablets 50 mg Capsules 50 mg	**Motion Sickness:** 50–100 mg every 4–6 h; max dose is 400 mg/d Pediatrics (6–12 yrs): 25–50 mg every 6–8 h; max dose is 150 mg/d	Administration Issues Give dose 30 minutes prior to motion, then before meals and at bedtime for duration of journey; safety/efficacy in children <12 yrs not established. Drug–Drug Interactions **Increased effect of antihistamine:** MAO inhibitors (anticholinergic effects).	ADRs Urinary retention, blurred vision, dry mouth, drowsiness, irritability, thickening of bronchial secretions. Elderly (>60yrs): more likely to experience confusion, dizziness, hypotension. Pharmacokinetics Rapid onset (15–30 minutes); duration of action = 4–6 hrs.	Contraindications Hypersensitivity, asthma, glaucoma, prostate gland enlargement. Precautions Use carefully if operating heavy machinery, history of sleep apnea, hepatic dysfunction. Pregnancy Category: B

Liquid 15.62 mg/5 mL, 12.5 mg/4 mL, 12.5 mg/5 mL		**Increased effect of:** MAO inhibitors, alcohol, CNS depressants.		Lactation Issues Women should not nurse.
Diphenhydramine Benadryl, various generics Tablets 25 mg, 50 mg Capsules 25 mg, 50 mg Tablets, chewable 12.5 mg Liquid/Elixir/Syrup 12.5 mg/5 mL	**Motion sickness:** 25–50 mg 3–4 times daily **Pediatrics** (>9.1 kg): 12.5–25 mg 3–4 times daily; do not exceed 300 mg/d	Administration Issues Give dose 30 minutes prior to motion, then before meals and at bedtime for duration of journey; safety/efficacy in children <12 yrs not established. Drug–Drug Interactions **Increased effect of antihistamine:** MAO inhibitors (anticholinergic effects). **Increased effect of:** MAO inhibitors, alcohol, CNS depressants.	ADRs Urinary retention, blurred vision, dry mouth, drowsiness, irritability, thickening of bronchial secretions. Elderly (>60yrs): more likely to experience confusion, dizziness, hypotension. Pharmacokinetics Rapid onset (15–30 minutes); duration of action = 4–6 hrs.	Contraindications Hypersensitivity, asthma, glaucoma, prostate gland enlargement. Precautions Use carefully if operating heavy machinery, history of sleep apnea, hepatic dysfunction. Pregnancy Category: B Lactation Issues Women should not nurse.
Meclizine Antivert, Antrizine, RuVert-M, Bonine, Dizmiss, Meni-D, various generics Tablets 12.5 mg, 25 mg, 50 mg Chewable tablets 25 mg Capsules 25 mg	**Motion sickness:** 25–50 mg before departure; may repeat every 24 hrs for duration of journey **Vertigo:** 25–100 mg daily in 2–3 divided doses	Administration Issues Give dose 60 minutes prior to motion; safety/efficacy in children <12 yrs not established. Drug–Drug Interactions **Increased effect of antihistamine:** MAO inhibitors (anticholinergic effects) **Increased effect of:** MAO inhibitors, alcohol, CNS depressants.	ADRs Urinary retention, blurred vision, dry mouth, drowsiness, irritability, thickening of bronchial secretions. Elderly (>60yrs): more likely to experience confusion, dizziness, hypotension. Pharmacokinetics Oral; onset = 30–60 minutes; duration of action = 8–24 hrs.	Contraindications Hypersensitivity, asthma, glaucoma, prostate gland enlargement. Precautions Use carefully if operating heavy machinery, history of sleep apnea, hepatic dysfunction. Pregnancy Category: B Lactation Issues Women should not nurse.
Scopolamine, Transdermal Transderm-Scop Transdermal Therapeutic System 1.5 mg	**Control of nausea/vomiting associated with motion sickness** Apply 1 system behind the ear at least 4 h before antiemetic effect is required. Wear only 1 disk at a time.	Administration Issues Wash hands thoroughly after handling disk. Temporary dilation of pupils and blurred vision may occur if drug comes in contact with eyes. If therapy longer than 3 days is required, remove old disc and place a new one in hairless area behind ear. Do not use system in children.	ADRs Dry mouth, blurred vision, drowsiness. Pharmacokinetics System delivers 0.5 mg scopolamine/d over 3 d.	Contraindications Hypersensitivity to scopolamine, glaucoma. Pregnancy Category: C Lactation Issues It is not known whether drug is excreted in breast milk. Use caution in nursing women.

(continues on next page)

502.1 Anticholinergic Agents *continued from previous page*

Drug and Dosage Forms	Usual Dosage Range	Administration Issues and Drug–Drug Interactions	Common Adverse Drug Reactions (ADRs) and Pharmacokinetics	Contraindications, Pregnancy Category, and Lactation Issues
Trimethobenzamide Tigan, Trimazide, Tebamide, generics Capsules 100 mg, 250 mg Suppositories 100 mg, 200 mg	**Control of nausea/vomiting adults** oral: 250 mg tid to qid rectal: 200 mg tid to qid **Pediatrics (13.6–40.9 kg)** oral: 100–200 mg tid to qid rectal: 100–200 mg tid to qid **(<13.6 kg):** 100 mg tid to qid	None known	ADRs Drowsiness, dizziness, headache, disorientation, Parkinson-like symptoms, coma convulsions, depression, diarrhea, hypersensitivity reactions, rash. Pharmacokinetics Oral; onset = 10–40 minutes; duration of action = 3–4 h.	Contraindications Hypersensitivity to this or benzocaine or other local anesthetics; suppository use in premature infants or neonates. Pregnancy/Lactation Issues Safety has not been established; use cautiously.

502.2 Antidopaminergic Agents

See chlorpromazine, perphanazine, prochlorperazine, promethazine, thiethylperazine (Table 312) and metoclopramide (Table 501.6) for doses, ADRs, etc. of these agents as antiemetics.

502.3 Miscellaneous Agents

Drug and Dosage Forms	Usual Dosage Range	Administration Issues and Drug–Drug Interactions	Common Adverse Drug Reactions (ADRs) and Pharmacokinetics	Contraindications, Pregnancy Category, and Lactation Issues
Dronabinol (C III) Marinol Capsules 2.5 mg, 5 mg, 10 mg	**Treatment of nausea/vomiting associated with cancer chemotherapy** 5 mg/m^2 1–3 hrs prior to chemotherapy, then every 2–4 hrs after chemotherapy for a total of 4–6 doses/day. May titrate by 2.5 mg/m^2 to a max of 15 mg/m^2 per dose if needed. **Appetite stimulant in AIDS patients** 2.5 mg bid before lunch and supper. Titrate to 2.5 mg at lunch and 5 mg at supper if tolerated. Titrate to 10 mg/d if needed/tolerated. Max dose is 20 mg/d	Administration Issues Not recommended as an appetite stimulant in children with AIDS. Drug–Drug Interactions **increased levels/effects of:** amphetamines, sympathomimetics, anticholinergics, antihistamines, TCAs, alcohol, sedatives, hypnotics, psychomimetics, disulfiram, fluoxetine. **Decreased levels/effects of:** theophylline.	ADRs Palpitations, tachycardia, vasodilation, nausea, vomiting, diarrhea, euphoria, dizziness, paranoid reaction, somnolence, asthenia, amnesia, ataxia, confusion, hallucination. Elderly: Use cautiously due to increased sensitivity to psychoactive effects.	Contraindications Hypersensitivity to this, marijuana or sesame oil Precautions Use cautiously in patients with hypertension, heart disease, or psychiatric disorders Pregnancy Category: B Lactation Issues Excreted in breast milk—mothers should not nurse.

			Pharmacokinetics Onset of action is 0.5–1 hr; duration of action is 4–6 hrs (antiemetic effect) but may exceed 24 hrs (appetite stimulant effect). Drug Abuse & Dependence Highly abusable/addicting. Withdrawal can occur within 12 hrs of abrupt discontinuation of this medication (continues for 96 hrs). Therefore, gradual discontinuation is advised.	
Dolasetron Anzemet Tablets 50 mg, 100 mg	**Prevention of postoperative nausea and vomiting** **adults** 100 mg within 2 hrs. before surgery. **pediatrics (2–16 yrs)** 1.2 mg/kg within 2 hrs before surgery; max dose = 100 mg.	Administration Issues Safety/efficacy not established for those ≤ 2 yrs. Drug–Drug Interactions Clinically significant interactions are not known	ADRs Headache, asthenia, dizziness, diarrhea constipation, abdominal pain. **Acute ECG changes** Pharmacokinetics $T_{1/2}$ = 8.1 h.	Contraindications Hypersensitivity, markedly prolonged QTc or AV block, patients receiving class I or III antiarrhythmic agents. Pregnancy Category: B Lactation Issues: May be excreted in breast milk—use cautiously
Granisetron Kytril Tablets 1 mg Oral Solution 1 mg/5 ml	**Prevention of nausea/vomiting associated with emetogenic chemotherapy (including cisplatin)** Adult dosage of 2 mg QD or 1 mg BID, up to 1 hour before chemotherapy. In the 1 mg BID regimen, give 1 mg up to 1 hour before chemotherapy and the second 1 mg dose 12 hours after the first.	Administration Issues Safety/efficacy not established for those ≤ 2 yrs. Drug–Drug Interactions Clinically significant interactions are not known	ADRs Headache, asthenia, dizziness, diarrhea, constipation, abdominal pain. Pharmacokinetics $T_{1/2}$ = 6.23 hrs (may be prolonged in cancer patients).	Contraindications Hypersensitivity. Pregnancy Category: B Lactation Issues May be excreted in breast milk—use cautiously.
Ondansetron Zofran, Zofran ODT Tablets 4 mg, 8 mg, 24 mg Tablets, orally disintegrating 4 mg, 8mg Solution 4 mg/5 ml	**Nausea/vomiting associated with moderately emetogenic chemotherapy** 8 mg bid for 1–2 days after completion of chemotherapy **Pediatrics (4–11 yrs):** 4 mg tid for 1–2 days after completion of chemotherapy **Hepatic dysfunction:** do not exceed 8 mg/d	Administration Issues Safety/efficacy not established for those ≤ 3 yrs. Drug–Drug Interactions Clinically significant interactions are not known	ADRs Headache, fatigue, dizziness, diarrhea, constipation, abdominal pain. Pharmacokinetics $T_{1/2}$ = 3 hrs (4.5–6.2 hrs in elderly, but no difference in safety/efficacy).	Contraindications Hypersensitivity. Precautions Use cautiously in patients with severe hepatic dysfunction; those undergoing abdominal surgery. Pregnancy Category: B Lactation Issues May be excreted in breast milk—use cautiously.

600. HORMONES AND SYNTHETIC SUBSTANCES
601. Adrenal Corticosteroids
601.1 Glucocorticoids

Drug and Dosage Forms	Usual Dosage Range	Administration Issues and Drug–Drug Interactions	Common Adverse Drug Reactions (ADRs) and Pharmacokinetics	Contraindications, Pregnancy Category, and Lactation Issues
Betamethasone Celestone Tablets 0.6 mg Syrup 0.6 mg/5 mL	**Endocrine disorders (adrenal insufficiency), rheumatic disorders, collagen diseases (systemic lupus erythematosus), dermatologic diseases, allergic states, respiratory disease, hematologic disorders, neoplastic disease, edematous states, GI diseases, neurological diseases:** **MUST INDIVIDUALIZE DOSE:** 0.6–7.2 mg/d.	Administration Issues Use lowest possible dose. Take with food if GI upset occurs. Avoid abrupt withdrawal of therapy. Closely monitor growth and development of children who receive long-term corticosteroid therapy. Drug Interactions **Increased toxicity with:** cyclosporine, digoxin, diuretics. **Decreased levels/effects of:** anticholinesterases, isoniazid, salicylates. **Decreased levels/effects of corticosteroids:** barbiturates, hydantoins, rifampin. **Increased levels/effects of corticosteroids:** oral contraceptives, estrogens, ketoconazole.	ADRs Insomnia, increased appetite, indigestion, temporary mild blurred vision, erythema, itching, hyperglycemia, skin dryness, headache, impaired wound healing, acne, sodium retention, peptic ulcer. Elderly: Use cautiously. Use lower doses. Pharmacokinetics Hepatically metabolized; plasma $T_{1/2}$ = 300+ min; biologic $T_{1/2}$ = 36–54 h.	Contraindications Hypersensitivity; systemic fungal infections; administration of live virus vaccines in patients receiving immunosuppressives. Precautions Monitor closely for infection (these agents may mask signs of infection); avoid prolonged therapy (leads to adrenal suppression); monitor electrolytes, blood glucose, weight, and blood pressure. Use cautiously in those with PUD, hypertension, CHF, osteoporosis, convulsive disorders, myasthenia gravis, diabetes mellitus, hypothyroidism, cirrhosis. Pregnancy/Lactation Issues Use cautiously (only when benefits clearly outweigh risks), these do cross placental barrier and are excreted into breast milk.
Cortisone Cortone, various generics Tablets 5 mg, 10 mg, 25 mg	**Endocrine disorders (adrenal insufficiency), rheumatic disorders, collagen diseases (systemic lupus erythematosus), dermatologic diseases, allergic states, respiratory disease, hematologic disorders, neoplastic disease, edematous states, GI diseases, neurological diseases:** **MUST INDIVIDUALIZE DOSE:** 25–300 mg/d.	Administration Issues Use lowest possible dose. Take with food if GI upset occurs. Avoid abrupt withdrawal of therapy. Closely monitor growth and development of children who receive long-term corticosteroid therapy. Drug Interactions **Increased toxicity with:** cyclosporine, digoxin, diuretics. **Decreased levels/effects of:** anticholinesterases, isoniazid, salicylates. **Decreased levels/effects of corticosteroids:** barbiturates, hydantoins, rifampin.	ADRs Insomnia, increased appetite, indigestion, temporary mild blurred vision, erythema, itching, hyperglycemia, skin dryness, headache, impaired wound healing, acne, sodium retention, peptic ulcer. Pharmacokinetics Hepatically metabolized; plasma $T_{1/2}$ = 30 min; biologic $T_{1/2}$ = 8–12 h.	Contraindications Hypersensitivity; systemic fungal infections; administration of live virus vaccines in patients receiving immunosuppressives. Precautions Monitor closely for infection (these agents may mask signs of infection); avoid prolonged therapy (leads to adrenal suppression); monitor electrolytes, blood glucose, weight, and blood pressure. Use cautiously in those with PUD, hypertension, CHF, osteoporosis, convulsive disorders, myasthenia gravis, diabetes mellitus, hypothyroidism, cirrhosis.

		Increased levels/effects of corticosteroids: oral contraceptives, estrogens, ketoconazole.		Pregnancy/Lactation Issues Use cautiously (only when benefits clearly outweigh risks), these do cross placental barrier and are excreted into breast milk.
Dexamethasone Decadron, Hexadrol, various generics Tablets 0.25 mg, 0.5 mg, 0.75 mg, 1 mg, 1.5 mg, 2 mg, 4 mg, 6 mg Tablets, Therapeutic Pack Six 1.5 mg tablets Eight 0.75 mg tablets Elixir 0.5 mg/5 mL Oral Solution 0.5 mg/5 mL 0.5 mg/0.5 mL	**Endocrine disorders (adrenal insufficiency), rheumatic disorders, collagen diseases (systemic lupus erythematosus), dermatologic diseases, allergic states, respiratory disease, hematologic disorders, neoplastic disease, edematous states, GI diseases, neurological diseases:** **MUST INDIVIDUALIZE DOSE:** 0.75–9 mg/d initially. **Tapering schedule for acute self-limited allergic disorders or exacerbations of chronic allergic disorders:** First day: 1–2 mL IM injection; Second day: 4 tablets (0.75 mg) in 2 divided doses; Third day: 4 tablets in 2 divided doses; Fourth day: 2 tablets in 2 divided doses; Fifth day: 1 tablet; Sixth day: 1 tablet. **Suppression Test:** 1 mg at 11 p.m. Draw blood for plasma cortisol determination the following day at 8 a.m. For greater accuracy: give 0.5 mg every 6 hrs for 48 hrs, then measure 17-hydroxycorticosteroid excretion collected in a 24-hr urine sample.	Administration Issues Use lowest possible dose. Take with food if GI upset occurs. Avoid abrupt withdrawal of therapy. Closely monitor growth and development of children who receive long-term corticosteroid therapy. Drug Interactions **Increased toxicity with:** cyclosporine, digoxin, diuretics. **Decreased levels/effects of:** anticholinesterases, isoniazid, salicylates. **Decreased levels/effects of corticosteroids:** barbiturates, hydantoins, rifampin. **Increased levels/effects of corticosteroids:** oral contraceptives, estrogens, ketoconazole.	ADRs Insomnia, increased appetite, indigestion, temporary mild blurred vision, erythema, itching, hyperglycemia, skin dryness, headache, impaired wound healing, acne, sodium retention, peptic ulcer. Pharmacokinetics Hepatically metabolized; plasma $T_{1/2}$ = 110–210 min; biologic $T_{1/2}$ = 36–54 h.	Contraindications Hypersensitivity; systemic fungal infections; administration of live virus vaccines in patients receiving immunosuppressives. Precautions Monitor closely for infection (these agents may mask signs of infection); avoid prolonged therapy (leads to adrenal suppression); monitor electrolytes, blood glucose, weight, and blood pressure. Use cautiously in those with PUD, hypertension, CHF, osteoporosis, convulsive disorders, myasthenia gravis, diabetes mellitus, hypothyroidism, cirrhosis. Pregnancy/Lactation Issues Use cautiously (only when benefits clearly outweigh risks), these do cross placental barrier and are excreted into breast milk.
Hydrocortisone Cortef, various generics Tablets 5 mg, 10 mg, 20 mg Oral Suspension 10 mg/5 mL (as cypionate)	**Endocrine disorders (adrenal insufficiency), rheumatic disorders, collagen diseases (systemic lupus erythematosus), dermatologic diseases, allergic states, respiratory disease, hematologic disorders, neoplastic disease, edematous states, GI diseases, neurological diseases:** **MUST INDIVIDUALIZE DOSE:** 20–240 mg/d.	Administration Issues: Use lowest possible dose. Take with food if GI upset occurs. Avoid abrupt withdrawal of therapy. Closely monitor growth and development of children who receive long-term corticosteroid therapy. Drug Interactions **Increased toxicity with:** cyclosporine, digoxin, diuretics.	ADRs Insomnia, increased appetite, indigestion, temporary mild blurred vision, erythema, itching, hyperglycemia, skin dryness, headache, impaired wound healing, acne, sodium retention, peptic ulcer. Pharmacokinetics Hepatically metabolized; plasma $T_{1/2}$ = 80–118 min; biologic $T_{1/2}$ = 8–12 h.	Contraindications Hypersensitivity; systemic fungal infections; administration of live virus vaccines in patients receiving immunosuppressives. Precautions Monitor closely for infection (these agents may mask signs of infection); avoid prolonged therapy (leads to adrenal suppression); monitor electrolytes, blood glucose, weight, and blood pressure. Use

(continues on next page)

601.1 Glucocorticoids *continued from previous page*

Drug and Dosage Forms	Usual Dosage Range	Administration Issues and Drug–Drug Interactions	Common Adverse Drug Reactions (ADRs) and Pharmacokinetics	Contraindications, Pregnancy Category, and Lactation Issues
Hydrocortisone *cont.*		**Decreased levels/effects of:** anticholinesterases, isoniazid, salicylates. **Decreased levels/effects of corticosteroids:** barbiturates, hydantoins, rifampin. **Increased levels/effects of corticosteroids:** oral contraceptives, estrogens, ketoconazole.		cautiously in those with PUD, hypertension, CHF, osteoporosis, convulsive disorders, myasthenia gravis, diabetes mellitus, hypothyroidism, cirrhosis. Pregnancy/Lactation Issues Use cautiously (only when benefits clearly outweigh risks), these do cross placental barrier and are excreted into breast milk.
Methylprednisolone Medrol, various generics Tablets 2 mg, 4 mg, 8 mg, 16 mg, 24 mg, 32 mg	**Endocrine disorders (adrenal insufficiency), rheumatic disorders, collagen diseases (systemic lupus erythematosus), dermatologic diseases, allergic states, respiratory disease, hematologic disorders, neoplastic disease, edematous states, GI diseases, neurological diseases:** **MUST INDIVIDUALIZE DOSE:** 4–48 mg/d. Tapering schedule for acute self-limited allergic disorders or exacerbations of chronic allergic disorders: Dosepak 21 therapy—follow manufacturer's directions.	Administration Issues: Use lowest possible dose. Take with food if GI upset occurs. Avoid abrupt withdrawal of therapy. Closely monitor growth and development of children who receive long-term corticosteroid therapy. Drug Interactions **Increased toxicity with:** cyclosporine, digoxin, diuretics. **Decreased levels/effects of:** anticholinesterases, isoniazid, salicylates. **Decreased levels/effects of corticosteroids:** barbiturates, hydantoins, rifampin. **Increased levels/effects of corticosteroids:** oral contraceptives, estrogens, ketoconazole.	ADRs Insomnia, increased appetite, indigestion, temporary mild blurred vision, erythema, itching, hyperglycemia, skin dryness, headache, impaired wound healing, acne, sodium retention, peptic ulcer. Pharmacokinetics Hepatically metabolized; plasma $T_{1/2} = 78-188$ min; biologic $T_{1/2} = 18-36$ h.	Contraindications Hypersensitivity; systemic fungal infections; administration of live virus vaccines in patients receiving immunosuppressives. Precautions Monitor closely for infection (these agents may mask signs of infection); avoid prolonged therapy (leads to adrenal suppression); monitor electrolytes, blood glucose, weight, and blood pressure. Use cautiously in those with PUD, hypertension, CHF, osteoporosis, convulsive disorders, myasthenia gravis, diabetes mellitus, hypothyroidism, cirrhosis. Pregnancy/Lactation Issues Use cautiously (only when benefits clearly outweigh risks), these do cross placental barrier and are excreted into breast milk.
Prednisone Deltasone, Orasone, various generics Tablets 1 mg, 2.5 mg, 5 mg, 10 mg, 20 mg, 50 mg	**Endocrine disorders (adrenal insufficiency), rheumatic disorders, collagen diseases (systemic lupus erythematosus), dermatologic diseases, allergic states, respiratory disease, hematologic disorders, neoplastic**	Administration Issues Use lowest possible dose. Take with food if GI upset occurs. Avoid abrupt withdrawal of therapy. Closely monitor growth and development of children who receive long-term corticosteroid therapy.	ADRs Insomnia, increased appetite, indigestion, temporary mild blurred vision, erythema, itching, hyperglycemia, skin dryness, headache, impaired wound healing, acne, sodium retention, peptic ulcer.	Contraindications Hypersensitivity; systemic fungal infections; administration of live virus vaccines in patients receiving immunosuppressives.

Oral Solution 5 mg/5 mL; 5 mg/mL Syrup 5 mg/5 mL	**disease, edematous states, GI diseases, neurological diseases:** **MUST INDIVIDUALIZE DOSE:** 5–60 mg/d.	Drug Interactions **Increased toxicity with:** cyclosporine, digoxin, diuretics. **Decreased levels/effects of:** anticholinesterases, isoniazid, salicylates. **Decreased levels/effects of corticosteroids:** barbiturates, hydantoins, rifampin. **Increased levels/effects of corticosteroids:** oral contraceptives, estrogens, ketoconazole.	Pharmacokinetics Converted to prednisolone; $T_{1/2} = 2.5–3.5$ h.	Precautions Monitor closely for infection (these agents may mask signs of infection); avoid prolonged therapy (leads to adrenal suppression); monitor electrolytes, blood glucose, weight, and blood pressure. Use cautiously in those with PUD, hypertension, CHF, osteoporosis, convulsive disorders, myasthenia gravis, diabetes mellitus, hypothyroidism, cirrhosis. Pregnancy/Lactation Issues Use cautiously (only when benefits clearly outweigh risks), these do cross placental barrier and are excreted into breast milk.
Prednisolone Prelone, Delta-Cortef, various generics Tablets 5 mg Syrup 15 mg/5 mL 5 mg/5 mL	**Endocrine disorders (adrenal insufficiency), rheumatic disorders, collagen diseases (systemic lupus erythematosus), dermatologic diseases, allergic states, respiratory disease, hematologic disorders, neoplastic disease, edematous states, GI diseases, neurological diseases:** **MUST INDIVIDUALIZE DOSE:** 5–60 mg/d. Acute exacerbations of multiple sclerosis: 200 mg daily for 1 week followed by 80 mg every other day for 1 month.	Administration Issues Use lowest possible dose. Take with food if GI upset occurs. Avoid abrupt withdrawal of therapy. Closely monitor growth and development of children who receive long-term corticosteroid therapy. Drug Interactions **Increased toxicity with:** cyclosporine, digoxin, diuretics. **Decreased levels/effects of:** anticholinesterases, isoniazid, salicylates. **Decreased levels/effects of corticosteroids:** barbiturates, hydantoins, rifampin. **Increased levels/effects of corticosteroids:** oral contraceptives, estrogens, ketoconazole.	ADRs Insomnia, increased appetite, indigestion, temporary mild blurred vision, erythema, itching, hyperglycemia, skin dryness, headache, impaired wound healing, acne, sodium retention, peptic ulcer. Pharmacokinetics $T_{1/2} = 3.6$ h.	Contraindications Hypersensitivity; systemic fungal infections; administration of live virus vaccines in patients receiving immunosuppressives. Precautions Monitor closely for infection (these agents may mask signs of infection); avoid prolonged therapy (leads to adrenal suppression); monitor electrolytes, blood glucose, weight, and blood pressure. Use cautiously in those with PUD, hypertension, CHF, osteoporosis, convulsive disorders, myasthenia gravis, diabetes mellitus, hypothyroidism, cirrhosis. Pregnancy/Lactation Issues Use cautiously (only when benefits clearly outweigh risks), these do cross placental barrier and are excreted into breast milk.
Triamcinolone Aristocort, Kenacort, various generics Tablets 1 mg, 2 mg, 4 mg, 8 mg	**MUST INDIVIDUALIZE DOSE:** **Endocrine disorders (adrenal insufficiency):** 4–12 mg/d in addition to mineralocorticoid therapy.	Administration Issues Use lowest possible dose. Take with food if GI upset occurs. Avoid abrupt withdrawal of therapy. Closely monitor growth and development of	ADRs Insomnia, increased appetite, indigestion, temporary mild blurred vision, erythema, itching, hyperglycemia, skin dryness, headache, impaired wound healing, acne, sodium retention, peptic ulcer.	Contraindications Hypersensitivity; systemic fungal infections; administration of live virus vaccines in patients receiving immunosuppressives.

(*continues on next page*)

601.1 Glucocorticoids *continued from previous page*

Drug and Dosage Forms	Usual Dosage Range	Administration Issues and Drug–Drug Interactions	Common Adverse Drug Reactions (ADRs) and Pharmacokinetics	Contraindications, Pregnancy Category, and Lactation Issues
Triamcinolone *cont.* Syrup 4 mg/5 mL	**Rheumatic disorders, dermatological, and bronchial asthma:** 8–16 mg/d. **Collagen diseases (systemic lupus erythematosus):** 20–32 mg/d. **Allergic states:** 8–12 mg/d. **Respiratory diseases:** 16–48 mg/d. **Hematologic disorders:** 16–60 mg/d. **Neoplastic disease:** 16–40 mg/d up to 100 mg/d. Children may need 1–2 mg/kg. **Edematous states:** 16–20 mg/d up to 48 mg/d until diuresis occurs. **Tuberculous meningitis:** 32–48 mg/d.	children who receive long-term corticosteroid therapy. Drug Interactions **Increased toxicity with:** cyclosporine, digoxin, diuretics. **Decreased levels/effects of:** anticholinesterases, isoniazid, salicylates. **Decreased levels/effects of corticosteroids:** barbiturates, hydantoins, rifampin. **Increased levels/effects of corticosteroids:** oral contraceptives, estrogens, ketoconazole.	Pharmacokinetics Hepatically metabolized; plasma $T_{1/2}$ = 200+ min; biologic $T_{1/2}$ = 18–36 h.	Precautions Monitor closely for infection (these agents may mask signs of infection); avoid prolonged therapy (leads to adrenal suppression); monitor electrolytes, blood glucose, weight, and blood pressure. Use cautiously in those with PUD, hypertension, CHF, osteoporosis, convulsive disorders, myasthenia gravis, diabetes mellitus, hypothyroidism, cirrhosis. Pregnancy/Lactation Issues Use cautiously (only when benefits clearly outweigh risks), these do cross placental barrier and are excreted into breast milk.

601.2 Mineralocorticoids

Drug and Dosage Forms	Usual Dosage Range	Administration Issues and Drug–Drug Interactions	Common Adverse Drug Reactions (ADRs) and Pharmacokinetics	Contraindications, Pregnancy Category, and Lactation Issues
Fludrocortisone Florinef Tablets 0.1 mg	**Addison's disease:** 0.1 mg/d. May titrate to 0.2 mg/d if needed. If hypertension develops, decrease dose to 0.05 mg/d. **Pediatrics:** 0.05–0.1 mg/d. **Infants:** 0.1–0.2 mg/d. **Salt-losing adrenogenital syndrome:** 0.1–0.2 mg/d.	Administration Issues Use smallest dose. Take with food if GI upset occurs. Avoid abrupt withdrawal of therapy.	ADRs Edema, hypertension, CHF, enlargement of the heart, bruising, increased sweating, hives, allergic skin rash. Pharmacokinetics Hepatically metabolized; plasma $T_{1/2} = 3.5$ h; biological $T_{1/2} = 18-36$ h.	Contraindications Hypersensitivity; systemic fungal infections. Precautions Monitor closely for infection (these agents may mask signs of infection); monitor electrolytes, weight, and blood pressure. Monitor patients with Addison's disease closely for exaggerated side effects. Pregnancy Category: C Lactation Issues Use cautiously—is excreted into breast milk.

602. Androgens and Androgen Inhibitors

602.1 Androgens

Drug and Dosage Forms	Usual Dosage Range	Administration Issues and Drug–Drug Interactions	Common Adverse Drug Reactions (ADRs) and Pharmacokinetics	Contraindications, Pregnancy Category, and Lactation Issues
Fluoxymesterone Halotestin, various generics Tablets 2 mg, 5 mg, 10 mg	Males **Hypogonadism:** 5–20 mg/d Females **Breast cancer:** 10–40 mg/d in divided doses. **Prevention of postpartum breast pain and engorgement:** 2.5 mg shortly after delivery, then 5–10 mg/d in divided doses for 4–5 days.	Administration Issues Take with food if GI upset occurs. Use very cautiously in children due to the bone maturation effects. Drug–Drug Interactions **Increased level/effect of:** anticoagulants, imipramine (increased paranoid symptoms).	**ADRs** Most Frequent for Males: gynecomastia, excessive frequency and duration of penile erections, decreased ejaculatory volume, oligospermia (at high doses). Most Frequent for Females: amenorrhea, other menstrual irregularities, virilization, (deepening of voice, clitoral enlargement). Pharmacokinetics 56% bioavailable; 98% protein bound; hepatically metabolized; $T_{1/2} = 9.2$ h.	Contraindications Hypersensitivity; serious cardiac, hepatic or renal disease, men with carcinomas of the breast or prostate, pregnancy, allergy to mercury compounds. Precautions Monitor women for signs of virilization, monitor serum/urine calcium levels. Use cautiously in those with acute intermittent porphyria, hypercholesterolemia, elderly males (increased risk of prostatic hypertrophy and carcinoma). Pregnancy Category: X Lactation Issues Unknown if excreted in breast milk. Use cautiously if at all.
Methyltestosterone Android, Oreton Methyl, Testred, Virilon, various generics Tablets 10 mg, 25 mg Tablets, buccal 10 mg Capsules 10 mg	Males **Hypogonadism:** 10–40 mg/d orally. **Androgen deficiency:** 10–50 mg/d orally or 5–25 mg buccally. **Postpubertal cryptorchidism:** 30 mg/d orally. Females **Postpartum breast pain and engorgement:** 80 mg/d orally for 3–5 days. **Breast cancer:** 50–200 mg/d orally or 25–100 mg/d buccally.	Administration Issues Take with food if GI upset occurs. Buccal tablets should not be chewed or swallowed. They should dissolve between gum and cheek. Use very cautiously in children due to the bone maturation effects. Drug–Drug Interactions **Increased level/effect of:** anticoagulants, imipramine (increased paranoid symptoms).	**ADRs** Most Frequent for Males: gynecomastia, excessive frequency and duration of penile erections, decreased ejaculatory volume, oligospermia (at high doses) Most Frequent for Females: amenorrhea, other menstrual irregularities, virilization (deepening of voice, clitoral enlargement). Pharmacokinetics: 56% bioavailable (more bioavailable if given buccally); 98% protein bound; hepatically metabolized; $T_{1/2} = 2.5–3$ h.	Contraindications Hypersensitivity; serious cardiac, hepatic or renal disease, men with carcinomas of the breast or prostate, pregnancy, allergy to mercury compounds. Precautions Monitor women for signs of virilization, monitor serum/urine calcium levels. Use cautiously in those with acute intermittent porphyria, hypercholesterolemia, elderly males (increased risk of prostatic hypertrophy and carcinoma). Pregnancy Category: X Lactation Issues Unknown if excreted in breast milk. Use cautiously if at all.

Testosterone Transdermal System Testoderm, Androderm, Testoderm TTS Testoderm Patch 4 mg/24 hrs 6 mg/24 hrs Testoderm TTS 5mg/24 hrs Androderm Patch 2.5 mg/24 hrs Testosterone Gel AndroGel 1% Testion 1%	**Primary or Secondary Hypogonadism:** Testoderm: 6 mg/d. If scrotal area is small, use the 4 mg/d patch. Testoderm TTS One system is applied at about the same time each day. Testosterone gel Recommended starting dose is 5 g (to deliver 50 mg testosterone) applied once daily to clean, dry, in tact skin on the shoulders and upper arms or abdomen. **Androderm: 5 mg/d (2 patches worn daily). For nonvirilized patient may start with 2.5 mg/d.**	Administration Issues Use very cautiously in children due to the bone maturation effects. Testoderm: apply to scrotal skin. Place on clean, dry portion of scrotal skin. Dry shave the area. Androderm: apply to nonscrotal skin. Place on clean dry area of back, abdomen, upper arms or thighs. Do not apply gel to the genitals. Drug–Drug Interactions: **Increased level/effect of:** anticoagulants, imipramine (increased paranoid symptoms).	**ADRs** Most Frequent for Males: gynecomastia, excessive frequency and duration of penile erections, decreased ejaculatory volume, oligospermia (at high doses). Most Frequent for Females: amenorrhea, other menstrual irregularities, virilization (deepening of voice, clitoral enlargement). Pharmacokinetics Transdermal; peak levels achieved after 2–4 hrs; serum levels reach plateau after 3–4 weeks of therapy.	Contraindications Hypersensitivity; serious cardiac, hepatic, or renal disease, men with carcinomas of the breast or prostate, pregnancy, allergy to mercury compounds. Precautions Monitor women for signs of virilization, monitor serum/urine calcium levels. Use cautiously in those with acute intermittent porphyria, hypercholesterolemia, elderly males (increased risk of prostatic hypertrophy and carcinoma). Pregnancy Category: X Lactation Issues Unknown if excreted in breast milk. Use cautiously if at all.

602.2 Androgen Inhibitors

Drug and Dosage Forms	Usual Dosage Range	Administration Issues and Drug–Drug Interactions	Common Adverse Drug Reactions (ADRs) and Pharmacokinetics	Contraindications, Pregnancy Category, and Lactation Issues
Dutasteride Avodart Capsules 0.5 mg	**Benign prostatic hypertrophy (BPH):** 0.5 mg qd.	Administration Issues Dutasteride may be administered with or without food. Swallow the capsules whole. Drug-Drug Interactions Based on in vitro data, blood concentrations of dutasteride may increase in the presence of inhibitors of CYP3A4, such as **ritonavir, ketoconazole, verapamil, diltiazem, cimetidine, and ciprofloxacin.**	ADRs Abnormal ejaculate; decreased libido, impotence (sexual adverse events decrease with duration of treatment). Pharmacokinetics Extensive hepatic metabolism $T_{½}$ = 5 weeks No dose adjustment in renal dysfunction.	Contraindications/Warnings Women and children; known hypersensitivity to dutasteride, other 5α-reductase inhibitors, or any component of the preparation. Men treated with dutasteride should not donate blood until at least 6 months have passed following their last does to prevent pregnant women from receiving dutasteride through blood transfusion. Pregnancy Category: X Not indicated for use in women. Pregnant women should not handle dutasteride capsules since the drug may be absorbed through the skin. Lactation Issues Not indicated for use in women.

(continues on next page)

602.2 Androgen Inhibitors *continued from previous page*

Drug and Dosage Forms	Usual Dosage Range	Administration Issues and Drug–Drug Interactions	Common Adverse Drug Reactions (ADRs) and Pharmacokinetics	Contraindications, Pregnancy Category, and Lactation Issues
Finasteride Proscar, generic Tablets 1 mg, 5 mg	**Symptomatic Benign Prostatic Hyperplasia (BPH):** 5 mg once daily. Androgenic alopecia: 1 mg once daily	Drug-Drug Interactions **Increased levels/effects of:** theophylline. Drug-Lab Interaction PSA levels are decreased during therapy.	ADRs Impotence, decreased libido, decreased volume of ejaculate. Pharmacokinetics Hepatically metabolized; $T_{1/2} = 6$ h; renal elimination of metabolites.	Contraindications Hypersensitivity; pregnancy; lactation; children. Precautions Use cautiously in those with liver or severe renal dysfunction.

603. Contraceptives

603.1 Oral Contraceptives—Monophasic

Drug and Dosage Forms	Usual Dosage Range	Administration Issues and Drug–Drug Interactions	Common Adverse Drug Reactions (ADRs)	Contraindications, Pregnancy Category, and Lactation Issues
Norethindrone & Mestranol Genora 1/50, Nelova 1/50, Norethin 1/50, Norinyl 1 + 50, Ortho-Novum 1/50, Necon 1/50 Tablets 1 mg/50 mcg	**Contraception** Sunday start packs: Take first tablet on first Sunday after menstruation begins; if menstruation begins on Sunday, take the first tablet on that day. 21-day regimen: To start—take 1 tablet daily for 21 days starting on the 5th day of the menstruation period. After 7 days with no tablets, begin 21 day cycle again. 28-day regimen: Follow same schedule as above. These packs will have 7 inert tablets for the 7-day free period.	Administration Issues Take exactly as directed. Do not miss doses. If > 2 days are missed, use another means of contraception until 7 days of therapy have been adhered to. Follow schedule below for missed doses: If 1 dose is missed: may take 2 tablets the next day. If 2 doses are missed: take 2 tablets as soon as remembered with the next pill or take 2 tablets daily for the next 2 days. If 3 doses are missed: begin a new compact of tablets starting on day one of the cycle after the last pill was taken Drug–Drug Interactions **Increased levels/effects of:** TCAs, benzodiazepines (oxidative metabolism); beta blockers, caffeine, corticosteroids, theophyllines. **Decreased levels/effects of:** benzodiazepines, salicylates, clofibrate. **Decreased levels/effects of contraceptives:** antibiotics, barbiturates, hydantoins, rifampin.	ADRs Breakthrough bleeding, spotting, change in menstrual flow, amenorrhea, vaginal candidiasis, change in cervical secretions, nausea, vomiting, abdominal cramps, bloating, rash, headaches, depression, edema, weight change. Serious: thrombophlebitis, venous thrombosis, pulmonary embolism, coronary thrombosis, MI, cerebral thrombosis, arterial thromboembolism, cerebral hemorrhage, hypertension, gallbladder disease, hepatic adenomas, hepatocellular carcinoma, mesenteric thrombosis, Budd-Chiari syndrome.	Contraindications Hypersensitivity; thrombophlebitis, thromboembolic disorders, cerebral vascular disease, myocardial infarction, coronary artery disease, breast carcinoma or estrogen-dependent neoplasia, carcinoma of endometrium, hepatic adenomas/carcinomas, undiagnosed abnormal genital bleeding, pregnancy, cholestatic jaundice. Precautions Monitor cholesterol and glucose levels, blood pressure, for bleeding irregularities, thromboembolic events, development of pregnancy. Use cautiously in those patients with acute intermittent porphyria. Prolonged use (>5 yr.) should be done cautiously. Pregnancy Category: X Lactation Issues Some excreted in breast milk. Mother should not nurse or should not take these pills until infant is weaned.
Norethindrone & Ethinyl estradiol Ovcon, Genora, NEE, Nelova, Norinyl, Ortho-Novum, Brevicon, Modicon, Loestrin, Necon Tablets 1 mg/50 mcg 1 mg/35 mcg 0.5 mg/35 mcg 0.4 mg/35 mcg	**Contraception** Sunday start packs: take first tablet on first Sunday after menstruation begins; if menstruation begins on Sunday, take the first tablet on that day. 21-day regimen: To start—take 1 tablet daily for 21 days starting on the 5th day of the menstruation period. After 7 days with no tablets, begin 21 day cycle again.	Administration Issues Take exactly as directed. Do not miss doses. If > 2 days are missed, use another means of contraception until 7 days of therapy have been adhered to. Follow schedule below for missed doses: If 1 dose is missed: may take 2 tablets the next day. If 2 doses are missed: take 2 tablets as soon as remembered with the next pill or take 2 tablets daily for the	ADRs Breakthrough bleeding, spotting, change in menstrual flow, amenorrhea, vaginal candidiasis, change in cervical secretions, nausea, vomiting, abdominal cramps, bloating, rash, headaches, depression, edema, weight change.	Contraindications Hypersensitivity; thrombophlebitis, thromboembolic disorders, cerebral vascular disease, myocardial infarction, coronary artery disease, breast carcinoma or estrogen-dependent neoplasia, carcinoma of endometrium, hepatic adenomas/carcinomas, undiagnosed abnormal genital bleeding, pregnancy, cholestatic jaundice.

(*continues on next page*)

603.1 Oral Contraceptives—Monophasic *continued from previous page*

Drug and Dosage Forms	Usual Dosage Range	Administration Issues and Drug–Drug Interactions	Common Adverse Drug Reactions (ADRs)	Contraindications, Pregnancy Category, and Lactation Issues
Norethindrone & Ethinyl estradiol *cont.* 1.5 mg/30 mcg 1 mg/20 mcg	28-day regimen: Follow same schedule as above. These packs will have 7 inert tablets for the 7-day free period.	next 2 days. If 3 doses are missed: begin a new compact of tablets starting on day one of the cycle after the last pill was taken Drug–Drug Interactions **Increased levels/effects of:** TCAs, benzodiazepines (oxidative metabolism); beta blockers, caffeine, corticosteroids, theophyllines. **Decreased levels/effects of:** benzodiazepines, salicylates, clofibrate. **Decreased levels/effects of contraceptives:** antibiotics, barbiturates, hydantoins, rifampin.	Serious: thrombophlebitis, venous thrombosis, pulmonary embolism, coronary thrombosis, MI, cerebral thrombosis, arterial thromboembolism, cerebral hemorrhage, hypertension, gallbladder disease, hepatic adenomas, hepatocellular carcinoma, mesenteric thrombosis, Budd-Chiari syndrome.	Precautions Monitor cholesterol and glucose levels, blood pressure, for bleeding irregularities, thromboembolic events, development of pregnancy. Use cautiously in those patients with acute intermittent porphyria. Prolonged use (>5 yr.) should be done cautiously. Pregnancy Category: X Lactation Issues Some excreted in breast milk. Mother should not nurse or should not take these pills until infant is weaned.
Ethynodiol diacetate & Ethinyl estradiol Demulen Tablets 1 mg/50 mcg 1 mg/35 mcg	**Contraception** Sunday start packs: take first tablet on first Sunday after menstruation begins; if menstruation begins on Sunday, take the first tablet on that day. 21-day regimen: To start—take 1 tablet daily for 21 days starting on the 5th day of the menstruation period. After 7 days with no tablets, begin 21 day cycle again. 28-day regimen: Follow same schedule as above. These packs will have 7 inert tablets for the 7-day free period.	Administration Issues Take exactly as directed. Do not miss doses. If > 2 days are missed, use another means of contraception until 7 days of therapy have been adhered to. Follow schedule below for missed doses: If 1 dose is missed: may take 2 tablets the next day. If 2 doses are missed: take 2 tablets as soon as remembered with the next pill or take 2 tablets daily for the next 2 days. If 3 doses are missed: begin a new compact of tablets starting on day one of the cycle after the last pill was taken Drug–Drug Interactions **Increased levels/effects of:** TCAs, benzodiazepines (oxidative metabolism); beta blockers, caffeine, corticosteroids, theophyllines. **Decreased levels/effects of:** benzodiazepines, salicylates, clofibrate.	ADRs Breakthrough bleeding, spotting, change in menstrual flow, amenorrhea, vaginal candidiasis, change in cervical secretions, nausea, vomiting, abdominal cramps, bloating, rash, headaches, depression, edema, weight change. Serious: thrombophlebitis, venous thrombosis, pulmonary embolism, coronary thrombosis, MI, cerebral thrombosis, arterial thromboembolism, cerebral hemorrhage, hypertension, gallbladder disease, hepatic adenomas, hepatocellular carcinoma, mesenteric thrombosis, Budd-Chiari syndrome.	Contraindications Hypersensitivity; thrombophlebitis, thromboembolic disorders, cerebral vascular disease, myocardial infarction, coronary artery disease, breast carcinoma or estrogen-dependent neoplasia, carcinoma of endometrium, hepatic adenomas/carcinomas, undiagnosed abnormal genital bleeding, pregnancy, cholestatic jaundice. Precautions Monitor cholesterol and glucose levels, blood pressure, for bleeding irregularities, thromboembolic events, development of pregnancy. Use cautiously in those patients with acute intermittent porphyria. Prolonged use (>5 yr.) should be done cautiously. Pregnancy Category: X

		Decreased levels/effects of contraceptives: antibiotics, barbiturates, hydantoins, rifampin.		Lactation Issues Some excreted in breast milk. Mother should not nurse or should not take these pills until infant is weaned.
Norgestrel & Ethinyl estradiol Ovral, Lo/Ovral, Ogestrel, Low-Ogestrel Tablets 0.5 mg/50 mcg 0.3 mg/30 mcg	**Contraception** Sunday start packs: take first tablet on first Sunday after menstruation begins; if menstruation begins on Sunday, take the first tablet on that day. 21-day regimen: To start—take 1 tablet daily for 21 days starting on the 5th day of the menstruation period. After 7 days with no tablets, begin 21 day cycle again. 28-day regimen: Follow same schedule as above. These packs will have 7 inert tablets for the 7-day free period.	Administration Issues Take exactly as directed. Do not miss doses. If > 2 days are missed, use another means of contraception until 7 days of therapy have been adhered to. Follow schedule below for missed doses: If 1 dose is missed: may take 2 tablets the next day. If 2 doses are missed: take 2 tablets as soon as remembered with the next pill or take 2 tablets daily for the next 2 days. If 3 doses are missed: begin a new compact of tablets starting on day one of the cycle after the last pill was taken. Drug–Drug Interactions **Increased levels/effects of:** TCAs, benzodiazepines (oxidative metabolism); beta blockers, caffeine, corticosteroids, theophyllines. **Decreased levels/effects of:** benzodiazepines, salicylates, clofibrate. **Decreased levels/effects of contraceptives:** antibiotics, barbiturates, hydantoins, rifampin.	ADRs Breakthrough bleeding, spotting, change in menstrual flow, amenorrhea, vaginal candidiasis, change in cervical secretions, nausea, vomiting, abdominal cramps, bloating, rash, headaches, depression, edema, weight change. Serious: thrombophlebitis, venous thrombosis, pulmonary embolism, coronary thrombosis, MI, cerebral thrombosis, arterial thromboembolism, cerebral hemorrhage, hypertension, gallbladder disease, hepatic adenomas, hepatocellular carcinoma, mesenteric thrombosis, Budd-Chiari syndrome.	Contraindications Hypersensitivity; thrombophlebitis, thromboembolic disorders, cerebral vascular disease, myocardial infarction, coronary artery disease, breast carcinoma or estrogen-dependent neoplasia, carcinoma of endometrium, hepatic adenomas/carcinomas, undiagnosed abnormal genital bleeding, pregnancy, cholestatic jaundice. Precautions Monitor cholesterol and glucose levels, blood pressure, for bleeding irregularities, thromboembolic events, development of pregnancy. Use cautiously in those patients with acute intermittent porphyria. Prolonged use (>5 yr.) should be done cautiously. Pregnancy Category: X Lactation Issues Some excreted in breast milk. Mother should not nurse or should not take these pills until infant is weaned.
Norgestimate & Ethinyl estradiol Ortho-Cyclen Tablets 0.25 mg/35 mcg	**Contraception** Sunday start packs: take first tablet on first Sunday after menstruation begins; if menstruation begins on Sunday, take the first tablet on that day. 21-day regimen: To start—take 1 tablet daily for 21 days starting on the 5th day of the menstruation period. After 7 days with no tablets, begin 21 day cycle again.	Administration Issues Take exactly as directed. Do not miss doses. If > 2 days are missed, use another means of contraception until 7 days of therapy have been adhered to. Follow schedule below for missed doses: If 1 dose is missed: may take 2 tablets the next day. If 2 doses are missed: take 2 tablets as soon as remembered with the next pill or take 2 tablets daily for the next 2 days. If 3 doses are missed: begin	ADRs Breakthrough bleeding, spotting, change in menstrual flow, amenorrhea, vaginal candidiasis, change in cervical secretions, nausea, vomiting, abdominal cramps, bloating, rash, headaches, depression, edema, weight change. Serious: thrombophlebitis, venous thrombosis, pulmonary embolism, coronary thrombosis, MI, cerebral thrombosis, arterial	Contraindications Hypersensitivity; thrombophlebitis, thromboembolic disorders, cerebral vascular disease, myocardial infarction, coronary artery disease, breast carcinoma or estrogen-dependent neoplasia, carcinoma of endometrium, hepatic adenomas/carcinomas, undiagnosed abnormal genital bleeding, pregnancy, cholestatic jaundice.

(continues on next page)

603.1 Oral Contraceptives—Monophasic *continued from previous page*

Drug and Dosage Forms	Usual Dosage Range	Administration Issues and Drug–Drug Interactions	Common Adverse Drug Reactions (ADRs)	Contraindications, Pregnancy Category, and Lactation Issues
Norgestimate & Ethinyl estradiol *cont.*	28-day regimen: Follow same schedule as above. These packs will have 7 inert tablets for the 7-day free period. Titrate dose of contraceptives as needed by patient.	a new compact of tablets starting on day one of the cycle after the last pill was taken Drug–Drug Interactions **Increased levels/effects of:** TCAs, benzodiazepines (oxidative metabolism); beta blockers, caffeine, corticosteroids, theophyllines. **Decreased levels/effects of:** benzodiazepines, salicylates, clofibrate. **Decreased levels/effects of contraceptives:** antibiotics, barbiturates, hydantoins, rifampin.	thromboembolism, cerebral hemorrhage, hypertension, gallbladder disease, hepatic adenomas, hepatocellular carcinoma, mesenteric thrombosis, Budd-Chiari syndrome.	Precautions Monitor cholesterol and glucose levels, blood pressure, for bleeding irregularities, thromboembolic events, development of pregnancy. Use cautiously in those patients with acute intermittent porphyria. Prolonged use (>5 yr.) should be done cautiously. Pregnancy Category: X Lactation Issues Some excreted in breast milk. Mother should not nurse or should not take these pills until infant is weaned.
Desogestrel & Ethinyl estradiol Desogen, Ortho-Cept, Apri Tablets 0.15 mg/30 mcg 0.15 mg/20 mcg	**Contraception** Sunday start packs: take first tablet on first Sunday after menstruation begins; if menstruation begins on Sunday, take the first tablet on that day. 21-day regimen: To start—take 1 tablet daily for 21 days starting on the 5th day of the menstruation period. After 7 days with no tablets, begin 21 day cycle again. 28-day regimen: Follow same schedule as above. These packs will have 7 inert tablets for the 7-day free period.	Administration Issues Take exactly as directed. Do not miss doses. If > 2 days are missed, use another means of contraception until 7 days of therapy have been adhered to. Follow schedule below for missed doses: If 1 dose is missed: may take 2 tablets the next day. If 2 doses are missed: take 2 tablets as soon as remembered with the next pill or take 2 tablets daily for the next 2 days. If 3 doses are missed: begin a new compact of tablets starting on day one of the cycle after the last pill was taken Drug–Drug Interactions **Increased levels/effects of:** TCAs, benzodiazepines (oxidative metabolism); beta blockers, caffeine, corticosteroids, theophyllines. **Decreased levels/effects of:** benzodiazepines, salicylates, clofibrate.	ADRs Breakthrough bleeding, spotting, change in menstrual flow, amenorrhea, vaginal candidiasis, change in cervical secretions, nausea, vomiting, abdominal cramps, bloating, rash, headaches, depression, edema, weight change. Serious: thrombophlebitis, venous thrombosis, pulmonary embolism, coronary thrombosis, MI, cerebral thrombosis, arterial thromboembolism, cerebral hemorrhage, hypertension, gallbladder disease, hepatic adenomas, hepatocellular carcinoma, mesenteric thrombosis, Budd-Chiari syndrome.	Contraindications Hypersensitivity; thrombophlebitis, thromboembolic disorders, cerebral vascular disease, myocardial infarction, coronary artery disease, breast carcinoma or estrogen-dependent neoplasia, carcinoma of endometrium, hepatic adenomas/carcinomas, undiagnosed abnormal genital bleeding, pregnancy, cholestatic jaundice. Precautions Monitor cholesterol and glucose levels, blood pressure, for bleeding irregularities, thromboembolic events, development of pregnancy. Use cautiously in those patients with acute intermittent porphyria. Prolonged use (>5 yr.) should be done cautiously. Pregnancy Category: X Lactation Issues Some excreted in breast milk. Mother should not nurse or should not take these pills until infant is weaned.

		Decreased levels/effects of contraceptives: antibiotics, barbiturates, hydantoins, rifampin.		
Drospirenone & Ethinyl estradiol Yasmin Tablets 3 mg/30 mcg	**Contraception** Sunday start packs: take first tablet on first Sunday after menstruation begins; if menstruation begins on Sunday, take the first tablet on that day. 21-day regimen: To start—take 1 tablet daily for 21 days starting on the 5th day of the menstruation period. After 7 days with no tablets, begin 21 day cycle again. 28-day regimen: Follow same schedule as above. These packs will have 7 inert tablets for the 7-day free period. **Caution should be used in women at risk for hyperkalemia, given drospirenone's potassium-sparing effect.**	Administration Issues Take exactly as directed. Do not miss doses. If > 2 days are missed, use another means of contraception until 7 days of therapy have been adhered to. Follow schedule below for missed doses: If 1 dose is missed: may take 2 tablets the next day. If 2 doses are missed: take 2 tablets as soon as remembered with the next pill or take 2 tablets daily for the next 2 days. If 3 doses are missed: begin a new compact of tablets starting on day one of the cycle after the last pill was taken Drug–Drug Interactions **Increased levels/effects of:** TCAs, benzodiazepines (oxidative metabolism); beta blockers, caffeine, corticosteroids, theophyllines. **Decreased levels/effects of:** benzodiazepines, salicylates, clofibrate. **Decreased levels/effects of contraceptives:** antibiotics, barbiturates, hydantoins, rifampin.	ADRs Breakthrough bleeding, spotting, change in menstrual flow, amenorrhea, vaginal candidiasis, change in cervical secretions, nausea, vomiting, abdominal cramps, bloating, rash, headaches, depression, edema, weight change. Serious: thrombophlebitis, venous thrombosis, pulmonary embolism, coronary thrombosis, MI, cerebral thrombosis, arterial thromboembolism, cerebral hemorrhage, hypertension, gallbladder disease, hepatic adenomas, hepatocellular carcinoma, mesenteric thrombosis, Budd-Chiari syndrome.	Contraindications Hypersensitivity; thrombophlebitis, thromboembolic disorders, cerebral vascular disease, myocardial infarction, coronary artery disease, breast carcinoma or estrogen-dependent neoplasia, carcinoma of endometrium, hepatic adenomas/carcinomas, undiagnosed abnormal genital bleeding, pregnancy, cholestatic jaundice. Precautions Monitor cholesterol and glucose levels, blood pressure, for bleeding irregularities, thromboembolic events, development of pregnancy. Use cautiously in those patients with acute intermittent porphyria. Prolonged use (>5 yr.) should be done cautiously. Pregnancy Category: X Lactation Issues Some excreted in breast milk. Mother should not nurse or should not take these pills until infant is weaned.
Levonorgestrel & Ethinyl estradiol Levlen, Levora, Nordette, Aviane, Portia, Alesse Levlite Tablets 0.15 mg/30 mcg 0.10/20 mcg	**Contraception** Sunday start packs: take first tablet on first Sunday after menstruation begins; if menstruation begins on Sunday, take the first tablet on that day. 21-day regimen: To start—take 1 tablet daily for 21 days starting on the 5th day of the menstruation period. After 7 days with no tablets, begin 21 day cycle again.	Administration Issues Take exactly as directed. Do not miss doses. If > 2 days are missed, use another means of contraception until 7 days of therapy have been adhered to. Follow schedule below for missed doses: If 1 dose is missed: may take 2 tablets the next day. If 2 doses are missed: take 2 tablets as soon as remembered with the next pill or take 2 tablets daily for the next 2 days. If 3 doses are missed: begin	ADRs Breakthrough bleeding, spotting, change in menstrual flow, amenorrhea, vaginal candidiasis, change in cervical secretions, nausea, vomiting, abdominal cramps, bloating, rash, headaches, depression, edema, weight change. Serious: thrombophlebitis, venous thrombosis, pulmonary embolism, coronary thrombosis, MI, cerebral thrombosis, arterial	Contraindications Hypersensitivity; thrombophlebitis, thromboembolic disorders, cerebral vascular disease, myocardial infarction, coronary artery disease, breast carcinoma or estrogen-dependent neoplasia, carcinoma of endometrium, hepatic adenomas/carcinomas, undiagnosed abnormal genital bleeding, pregnancy, cholestatic jaundice.

(continues on next page)

603.1 Oral Contraceptives—Monophasic *continued from previous page*

Drug and Dosage Forms	Usual Dosage Range	Administration Issues and Drug–Drug Interactions	Common Adverse Drug Reactions (ADRs)	Contraindications, Pregnancy Category, and Lactation Issues
Levonorgestrel & Ethinyl estradiol *cont.*	28-day regimen: Follow same schedule as above. These packs will have 7 inert tablets for the 7-day free period.	a new compact of tablets starting on day one of the cycle after the last pill was taken Drug–Drug Interactions **Increased levels/effects of:** TCAs, benzodiazepines (oxidative metabolism); beta blockers, caffeine, corticosteroids, theophyllines. **Decreased levels/effects of:** benzodiazepines, salicylates, clofibrate. **Decreased levels/effects of contraceptives:** antibiotics, barbiturates, hydantoins, rifampin.	thromboembolism, cerebral hemorrhage, hypertension, gallbladder disease, hepatic adenomas, hepatocellular carcinoma, mesenteric thrombosis, Budd-Chiari syndrome.	Precautions Monitor cholesterol and glucose levels, blood pressure, for bleeding irregularities, thromboembolic events, development of pregnancy. Use cautiously in those patients with acute intermittent porphyria. Prolonged use (>5 yr.) should be done cautiously. Pregnancy Category: X Lactation Issues Some excreted in breast milk. Mother should not nurse or should not take these pills until infant is weaned.

603.2 Oral Contraceptives—Biphasic

Drug and Dosage Forms	Usual Dosage Range	Administration Issues and Drug–Drug Interactions	Common Adverse Drug Reactions (ADRs)	Contraindications, Pregnancy Category, and Lactation Issues
Norethindrone & Ethinyl estradiol Jenest-28, Nelova 10/11, Ortho-Novum 10/11, Necon 10/11 Tablets (1st phase) 0.5 mg/35 mcg (7 tabs) 0.5 mg/35 mcg (10 tabs) Tablets (2nd phase) 1 mg/35 mcg (14 tabs) 1 mg/35 mcg (11 tabs)	**Contraception** Follow directions contained in pack describing when cycle should start, etc.	Administration Issues Take exactly as directed. Do not miss doses. If > 2 days are missed, use another means of contraception until 7 days of therapy have been adhered to. Follow schedule below for missed doses: If 1 dose is missed: may take 2 tablets the next day. If 2 doses are missed: take 2 tablets as soon as remembered with the next pill or take 2 tablets daily for the next 2 days. If 3 doses are missed: begin a new compact of tablets starting on day one of the cycle after the last pill was taken.	ADRs Breakthrough bleeding, spotting, change in menstrual flow, amenorrhea, vaginal candidiasis, change in cervical secretions, nausea, vomiting, abdominal cramps, bloating, rash, headaches, depression, edema, weight change. Serious: thrombophlebitis, venous thrombosis, pulmonary embolism, coronary thrombosis, MI, cerebral thrombosis, arterial thromboembolism, cerebral hemorrhage, hypertension, gallbladder disease, hepatic adenomas, hepatocellular carci-	Contraindications Hypersensitivity; thrombophlebitis, thromboembolic disorders, cerebral vascular disease, myocardial infarction, coronary artery disease, breast carcinoma or estrogen-dependent neoplasia, carcinoma of endometrium, hepatic adenomas/carcinomas, undiagnosed abnormal genital bleeding, pregnancy, cholestatic jaundice. Precautions Monitor cholesterol and glucose levels, blood pressure, for bleeding irregularities, thromboembolic events, develop-

Desogestrel/Ethinyl estradiol Kariva, Micette Tablets (1st phase) 0.15 mg/20 mcg (21 tabs) Tablets (2nd phase) 10 mcg ethinyl estradiol (5 tabs)		Drug–Drug Interactions **Increased levels/effects of:** TCAs, benzodiazepines (oxidative metabolism); beta blockers, caffeine, corticosteroids, theophyllines. **Decreased levels/effects of:** benzodiazepines, salicylates, clofibrate. **Decreased levels/effects of contraceptives:** antibiotics, barbiturates, hydantoins, rifampin.	noma, mesenteric thrombosis, Budd-Chiari syndrome.	ment of pregnancy. Use cautiously in those patients with acute intermittent porphyria. Prolonged use (>5 yr.) should be done cautiously. Pregnancy Category: X Lactation Issues Some excreted in breast milk. Mother should not nurse or should not take these pills until infant is weaned.

603.3 Oral Contraceptives—Triphasic

Drug and Dosage Forms	Usual Dosage Range	Administration Issues and Drug–Drug Interactions	Common Adverse Drug Reactions (ADRs)	Contraindications, Pregnancy Category, and Lactation Issues
Norethindrone & Ethinyl estradiol Tri-Norinyl, Ortho-Novum 7/7/7 Tablets (1st phase) 0.5 mg/35 mcg (7 tabs) Tablets (2nd phase) 1 mg/35 mcg (9 tabs) 0.75 mg/35 mcg (7 tabs) Tablets (3rd phase) 0.5 mg/35 mcg (5 tabs) 1 mg/35 mcg (7 tabs)	**Contraception** Follow directions contained in pack describing when cycle should start, etc.	Administration Issues Take exactly as directed. Do not miss doses. If > 2 days are missed, use another means of contraception until 7 days of therapy have been adhered to. Follow schedule below for missed doses: If 1 dose is missed: may take 2 tablets the next day. If 2 doses are missed: take 2 tablets as soon as remembered with the next pill or take 2 tablets daily for the next 2 days. If 3 doses are missed: begin a new compact of tablets starting on day one of the cycle after the last pill was taken	ADRs Breakthrough bleeding, spotting, change in menstrual flow, amenorrhea, vaginal candidiasis, change in cervical secretions, nausea, vomiting, abdominal cramps, bloating, rash, headaches, depression, edema, weight change. Serious: thrombophlebitis, venous thrombosis, pulmonary embolism, coronary thrombosis, MI, cerebral thrombosis, arterial thromboembolism, cerebral hemorrhage, hypertension, gallbladder disease, hepatic adenomas, hepatocellular carcinoma, mesenteric thrombosis, Budd-Chiari syndrome.	Contraindications Hypersensitivity; thrombophlebitis, thromboembolic disorders, cerebral vascular disease, myocardial infarction, coronary artery disease, breast carcinoma or estrogen-dependent neoplasia, carcinoma of endometrium, hepatic adenomas/carcinomas, undiagnosed abnormal genital bleeding, pregnancy, cholestatic jaundice. Precautions Monitor cholesterol and glucose levels, blood pressure, for bleeding irregularities, thromboembolic events, development of pregnancy. Use cautiously in those patients with acute intermittent

(continues on next page)

603.3 Oral Contraceptives—Triphasic *continued from previous page*

Drug and Dosage Forms	Usual Dosage Range	Administration Issues and Drug–Drug Interactions	Common Adverse Drug Reactions (ADRs)	Contraindications, Pregnancy Category, and Lactation Issues
Norethindrone & Ethinyl estradiol *cont.*		Drug–Drug Interactions **Increased levels/effects of:** TCAs, benzodiazepines (oxidative metabolism); beta blockers, caffeine, corticosteroids, theophyllines. **Decreased levels/effects of:** benzodiazepines, salicylates, clofibrate. **Decreased levels/effects of contraceptives:** antibiotics, barbiturates, hydantoins, rifampin.		porphyria. Prolonged use (>5 yr.) should be done cautiously. Pregnancy Category: X Lactation Issues Some excreted in breast milk. Mother should not nurse or should not take these pills until infant is weaned.
Levonorgestrel & Ethinyl estradiol Tri-Levlen, Triphasil, Trivora Tablets (1st phase) 0.05 mg/30 mcg (6 tabs) Tablets (2nd phase) 0.075 mg/40 mcg (5 tabs) Tablets (3rd phase) 0.125 mg/30 mcg (10 tabs)	**Contraception** Follow directions contained in pack describing when cycle should start, etc.	Administration Issues Take exactly as directed. Do not miss doses. If > 2 days are missed, use another means of contraception until 7 days of therapy have been adhered to. Follow schedule below for missed doses: If 1 dose is missed: may take 2 tablets the next day. If 2 doses are missed: take 2 tablets as soon as remembered with the next pill or take 2 tablets daily for the next 2 days. If 3 doses are missed: begin a new compact of tablets starting on day one of the cycle after the last pill was taken Drug–Drug Interactions **Increased levels/effects of:** TCAs, benzodiazepines (oxidative metabolism); beta blockers, caffeine, corticosteroids, theophyllines. **Decreased levels/effects of:** benzodiazepines, salicylates, clofibrate. **Decreased levels/effects of contraceptives:** antibiotics, barbiturates, hydantoins, rifampin.	ADRs Breakthrough bleeding, spotting, change in menstrual flow, amenorrhea, vaginal candidiasis, change in cervical secretions, nausea, vomiting, abdominal cramps, bloating, rash, headaches, depression, edema, weight change. Serious: thrombophlebitis, venous thrombosis, pulmonary embolism, coronary thrombosis, MI, cerebral thrombosis, arterial thromboembolism, cerebral hemorrhage, hypertension, gallbladder disease, hepatic adenomas, hepatocellular carcinoma, mesenteric thrombosis, Budd-Chiari syndrome.	Contraindications Hypersensitivity; thrombophlebitis, thromboembolic disorders, cerebral vascular disease, myocardial infarction, coronary artery disease, breast carcinoma or estrogen-dependent neoplasia, carcinoma of endometrium, hepatic adenomas/carcinomas, undiagnosed abnormal genital bleeding, pregnancy, cholestatic jaundice. Precautions Monitor cholesterol and glucose levels, blood pressure, for bleeding irregularities, thromboembolic events, development of pregnancy. Use cautiously in those patients with acute intermittent porphyria. Prolonged use (>5 yr.) should be done cautiously. Pregnancy Category: X Lactation Issues Some excreted in breast milk. Mother should not nurse or should not take these pills until infant is weaned.

Norgestimate & Ethinyl estradiol Ortho Tri-Cyclen Tablets (1st phase) 0.18 mg/35 mcg (7 tabs) Tablets (2nd phase) 0.215 mg/35 mcg (7 tabs) Tablets (3rd phase) 0.25 mg/35 mcg (7 tabs) **Norethindrone acetate & Ethinyl estradiol** Estrostep Tablets (1st phase) 1 mg/20 mcg (5 tabs) Tablets (2nd phase) 1 mg/30 mcg (7 tabs) Tablets (3rd phase) 1 mg/35 mcg (9 tabs)	**Contraception** Follow directions contained in pack describing when cycle should start, etc.	Administration Issues Take exactly as directed. Do not miss doses. If > 2 days are missed, use another means of contraception until 7 days of therapy have been adhered to. Follow schedule below for missed doses: If 1 dose is missed: may take 2 tablets the next day. If 2 doses are missed: take 2 tablets as soon as remembered with the next pill or take 2 tablets daily for the next 2 days. If 3 doses are missed: begin a new compact of tablets starting on day one of the cycle after the last pill was taken Drug–Drug Interactions **Increased levels/effects of:** TCAs, benzodiazepines (oxidative metabolism); beta blockers, caffeine, corticosteroids, theophyllines. **Decreased levels/effects of:** benzodiazepines, salicylates, clofibrate. **Decreased levels/effects of contraceptives:** antibiotics, barbiturates, hydantoins, rifampin.	ADRs Breakthrough bleeding, spotting, change in menstrual flow, amenorrhea, vaginal candidiasis, change in cervical secretions, nausea, vomiting, abdominal cramps, bloating, rash, headaches, depression, edema, weight change. Serious: thrombophlebitis, venous thrombosis, pulmonary embolism, coronary thrombosis, MI, cerebral thrombosis, arterial thromboembolism, cerebral hemorrhage, hypertension, gallbladder disease, hepatic adenomas, hepatocellular carcinoma, mesenteric thrombosis, Budd-Chiari syndrome.	Contraindications Hypersensitivity; thrombophlebitis, thromboembolic disorders, cerebral vascular disease, myocardial infarction, coronary artery disease, breast carcinoma or estrogen-dependent neoplasia, carcinoma of endometrium, hepatic adenomas/carcinomas, undiagnosed abnormal genital bleeding, pregnancy, cholestatic jaundice. Precautions Monitor cholesterol and glucose levels, blood pressure, for bleeding irregularities, thromboembolic events, development of pregnancy. Use cautiously in those patients with acute intermittent porphyria. Prolonged use (>5 yr.) should be done cautiously. Pregnancy Category: X Lactation Issues Some excreted in breast milk. Mother should not nurse or should not take these pills until infant is weaned.

603.4 Oral Contraceptives—Progestin Only

Drug and Dosage Forms	Usual Dosage Range	Administration Issues and Drug–Drug Interactions	Common Adverse Drug Reactions (ADRs)	Contraindications, Pregnancy Category, and Lactation Issues
Norethindrone Micronor, Nor-QD Tablets 0.35 mg	**Contraception** Take 1 tablet daily beginning on the first day of menstruation. Take daily for every day of the year.	Administration Issues Take exactly as directed Do not miss doses. If > 2 days are missed, use another means of contraception until 7 days of therapy have been adhered to.	ADRs Headache, nervousness, dizziness, rash, acne, photosensitivity, weight gain, many days of bleeding, breakthrough bleeding, spotting, change in menstrual flow, amenorrhea, changes in cervical secretions, breast changes, mastalgia, scalp hair loss, hypertrichosis, edema, hirsutism.	Contraindications Hypersensitivity, thrombophlebitis, thromboembolic disorders, cerebral hemorrhage, impaired liver function, carcinoma of the breast or genital organs, undiagnosed vaginal bleeding, missed abortion, for use as a diagnostic test for pregnancy.

(continues on next page)

603.4 Oral Contraceptives—Progestin Only *continued from previous page*

Drug and Dosage Forms	Usual Dosage Range	Administration Issues and Drug–Drug Interactions	Common Adverse Drug Reactions (ADRs)	Contraindications, Pregnancy Category, and Lactation Issues
Norethindrone *cont.*		Follow the schedule below for missed doses: If 1 dose is missed: take as soon as remembered. If 2 doses are missed: do not make up doses. Discard the 2 tablets and start back on schedule. If 3 doses are missed: discontinue altogether. Drug–Drug Interactions **Decreased levels/effects of progestin:** aminoglutethimide, rifampin, carbamazepine, phenytoin.		Pregnancy Category: D Lactation Issues Small amounts excreted in breast milk—effects on infant not known.
Norgestrel Ovrette Tablets 0.075 mg	**Contraception** Take 1 tablet daily beginning on the first day of menstruation. Take daily for every day of the year.	Administration Issues Take exactly as directed Do not miss doses. If > 2 days are missed, use another means of contraception until 7 days of therapy have been adhered to. Follow the schedule below for missed doses: If 1 dose is missed: take as soon as remembered. If 2 doses are missed: do not make up doses. Discard the 2 tablets and start back on schedule. If 3 doses are missed: discontinue altogether. Drug–Drug Interactions **Decreased levels/effects of progestin:** aminoglutethimide, rifampin, carbamazepine, phenytoin.	ADRs Headache, nervousness, dizziness, rash, acne, photosensitivity, weight gain, many days of bleeding, breakthrough bleeding, spotting, change in menstrual flow, amenorrhea, changes in cervical secretions, breast changes, mastalgia, scalp hair loss, hypertrichosis, edema, hirsutism.	Contraindications Hypersensitivity, thrombophlebitis, thromboembolic disorders, cerebral hemorrhage, impaired liver function, carcinoma of the breast or genital organs, undiagnosed vaginal bleeding, missed abortion, for use as a diagnostic test for pregnancy. Pregnancy Category: D Lactation Issues Small amounts excreted in breast milk—effects on infant not known.

603.5 Contraceptive Implants

Drug and Dosage Forms	Usual Dosage Range	Administration Issues and Drug–Drug Interactions	Common Adverse Drug Reactions (ADRs)	Contraindications, Pregnancy Category, and Lactation Issues
Levonorgestrel Norplant, Norplant-Z Capsules (kit) 6 (each contains 36 mg) Norplant-Z (each contains 70 mg)	**Contraception:** Norplant All 6 capsules should be implanted during the 7 days of the onset of menses. Contraceptive protection should last 5 years. Norplant-Z All capsules should be implanted during the 7 days of the onset of menses. Contraceptive protection should last 7 years.	Administration Issues Surgically implanted. Implantation is subdermal in the mid-portion of the upper arm. Drug–Drug Interactions **Decreased levels/effects of progestin:** aminoglutethimide, rifampin, carbamazepine, phenytoin. Drug–Lab Interaction The following tests may be affected by progestins: hepatic function, coagulation, thyroid, metyrapone, and endocrine function.	ADRs Fluid retention, headache, nervousness, dizziness, rash, acne, weight gain, many days of bleeding, breakthrough bleeding, spotting, change in menstrual flow, amenorrhea, changes in cervical secretions, breast changes, mastalgia, scalp hair loss, hypertrichosis, edema, hirsutism.	Contraindications Hypersensitivity, thrombophlebitis, thromboembolic disorders, cerebral hemorrhage, impaired liver function, carcinoma of the breast or genital organs, undiagnosed vaginal bleeding, missed abortion, for use as a diagnostic test for pregnancy. Pregnancy Category: Implants should be removed if pregnancy occurs. Lactation Issues Small amounts excreted in breast milk—effects on infant not known.

603.6 Contraceptive Injections

Drug and Dosage Forms	Usual Dosage Range	Administration Issues and Drug–Drug Interactions	Common Adverse Drug Reactions (ADRs)	Contraindications, Pregnancy Category, and Lactation Issues
Medroxyprogesterone Depo-Provera Injection (suspension) 150 mg/mL	**Contraception:** 150 mg by IM injection every 3 months	Administration Issues Shake vial prior to administration to ensure complete suspension. Drug–Drug Interactions **Decreased levels/effects of progestin:** aminoglutethimide, rifampin, carbamazepine, phenytoin. Drug–Lab Interaction The following tests may be affected by progestins: hepatic function, coagulation, thyroid, metyrapone, and endocrine function.	ADRs Headache, nervousness, dizziness, rash, acne, weight gain, many days of bleeding, breakthrough bleeding, spotting, change in menstrual flow, amenorrhea, changes in cervical secretions, breast changes, mastalgia, scalp hair loss, hypertrichosis, edema, hirsutism.	Contraindications Hypersensitivity, thrombophlebitis, thromboembolic disorders, cerebral hemorrhage, impaired liver function, carcinoma of the breast or genital organs, undiagnosed vaginal bleeding, missed abortion, for use as a diagnostic test for pregnancy. Pregnancy Category: Implants should be removed if pregnancy occurs. Lactation Issues Small amounts excreted in breast milk—effects on infant not known.

(*continues on next page*)

603.6 Contraceptive Injections *continued from previous page*

Drug and Dosage Forms	Usual Dosage Range	Administration Issues and Drug–Drug Interactions	Common Adverse Drug Reactions (ADRs)	Contraindications, Pregnancy Category, and Lactation Issues
Medroxyprogesterone acetate & Estradiol cypionate Lunelle Injection 25 mg/5 mg/0.5 mL	**Contraception** 0.5 mL every 28–30 days	Shake vigorously.	Same as combination oral contraceptives	Same as combination oral contraceptives

603.7 Miscellaneous Contraceptives

Drug and Dosage Forms	Usual Dosage Range	Administration Issues and Drug–Drug & Drug-Food Interactions	Common Adverse Drug Reactions (ADRs) and Pharmacokinetics	Contraindications, Pregnancy Category, and Lactation Issues
Norelgestromin/ethinyl estradiol Transdermal System Ortho-Evra **Patch** Release Rate 0.15 mg norelgestromin, 0.02 mg ethinyl estradiol/24 hrs	**Contraception** This system uses a 28-day (4-week) cycle. A new patch is applied each week for 3 weeks (21 days total). Week 4 is patch-free. Withdrawal bleeding is expected to begin during this time. **The patient must choose 1 option:** **First day start:** For first day start, the woman should apply her first patch during the first 24 hours of her menstrual period. If therapy starts after day 1 of the menstrual cycle, a nonhormonal backup contraceptive (e.g., condoms, spermicide, diaphragm) should be used concurrently for the first 7 consecutive days of the first treatment cycle. **Sunday start:** For Sunday start, the woman should apply her first patch on the first Sunday after her menstrual period starts. She must use backup contraception for the first week of her first cycle. If the menstrual period begins on a Sunday, the first patch should be applied on	Administration Issues Apply every new patch on the same day of the week. This day is known as the "Patch Change Day." Wear only 1 patch at a time. On the day after week 4 ends, a new 4-week cycle is started by applying a new patch. Under no circumstances should there be more than a 7-day patch-free interval between dosing cycles. **Application:** Apply the patch to clean, dry, intact, healthy skin on the buttock, abdomen, upper outer arm, or upper torso in a place where it will not be rubbed by tight clothing. The patch should not be placed on skin that is red, irritated, or cut, nor should it be placed on the breasts. To prevent interference with the adhesive properties of the patch, no makeup, creams, lotions, powders, or other topical products should be applied to the skin area where the patch is or will be placed. Patch changes may occur at any time on the change day. Apply each new patch to a new spot on the skin to help avoid irri-	ADRs Same as combination oral contraceptive. Local reaction where applied. Pharmacokinetics: Since the patch is applied transdermally, first-pass metabolism (via the GI tract or liver) of norelgestromin and ethinyl estradiol that would be expected with oral administration is avoided.	Contraindications/Warnings: Same as combination oral contraceptives. Pregnancy Category: X Lactation Issues: Nursing mothers should use another form of contraception until child is weaned.

	that day and no backup contraception is needed.	tation, although they may be kept within the same anatomic area. Drug–Drug Interactions Same as with oral combination contraceptives.		
Etonogestrel/ethinyl estradiol Vaginal Ring NuvaRing **Ring** Release Rate 0.12 mg etonogestrel, 0.015 mg ethinyl estradiol/day	**Contraception** One etonogestrel/ethinyl estradiol vaginal ring is inserted in the vagina by the woman herself. This ring is to remain in place continuously for 3 weeks. It is removed for a 1-week break, during which a withdrawal bleed usually occurs. A new ring is inserted 1 week after the last ring was removed on the same day of the week as it was inserted in the previous cycle. The withdrawal bleed usually starts on day 2 to 3 after removal of the ring and may not have finished before the next ring is inserted. In order to maintain contraceptive effectiveness, insert the new ring 1 week after the previous one was removed even if menstrual bleeding has not finished.	Administration Issues **Insertion:** The user can choose the insertion position that is most comfortable to her—for example, standing with one leg up, squatting, or lying down. Compress the ring and insert into the vagina. The exact position of the contraceptive vaginal ring inside the vagina is not critical for its function. Insert the contraceptive vaginal ring on the appropriate day and leave in place for 3 consecutive weeks. **Removal:** The ring is removed 3 weeks later on the same day of the week as it was inserted and at about the same time. Remove the vaginal ring by hooking the index finger under the forward rim or by grasping the rim between the index and middle finger and pulling it out. Place the used ring in the sachet (foil pouch) and discard in a waste receptacle out of the reach of children and pets. Do not flush in the toilet. Drug–Drug Interactions Same as with oral combination contraceptives.	ADRs Same as combination oral contraceptive. Plus vaginitis, headache, upper respiratory tract infection, leukorrhea, sinusitis, weight gain, and nausea. Pharmacokinetics Etonogestrel released by the vaginal ring is rapidly absorbed. Bioavailability of etonogestrel after vaginal administration is $\approx$ 100%. Ethinyl estradiol released by the vaginal ring is rapidly absorbed. Bioavailability of ethinyl estradiol after vaginal administration is 55.6%, which is comparable to that with oral administration of ethinyl estradiol.	Contraindications/Warnings: Same as combination oral contraceptives Pregnancy Category: X Lactation Issues: Nursing mothers should use another form of contraception until child is weaned.

604. Antidiabetic Agents

604.1 Sulfonylureas

Drug and Dosage Forms	Usual Dosage Range	Administration Issues and Drug–Drug Interactions	Common Adverse Drug Reactions (ADRs) and Pharmacokinetics	Contraindications, Pregnancy Category, and Lactation Issues
Chlorpropamide Diabinese, various generics Tablets 100 mg, 250 mgl	**As adjunct to diet/exercise to control blood glucose in NIDDM (Type 2):** 250 mg/d, initially. May titrate to 500 mg/d if needed. Do not exceed 750 mg/d. **Elderly or debilitated patients:** 100–125 mg/d initially.	Administration Issues Take with food if GI upset occurs. Avoid alcohol. Drug–Drug Interactions **Increased hypoglycemic effect:** androgens, anticoagulants, chloramphenicol, clofibrate, fenfluramine, fluconazole, gemfibrozil, H_2 antagonists, magnesium salts, methyldopa, MAO inhibitors, phenylbutazone, probenecid, salicylates, sulfinpyrazone, sulfonamides, TCAs, urinary acidifiers, alcohol (acute use). **Increased levels/effects of:** digoxin. **Decreased hypoglycemic effect:** beta blockers, cholestyramine, diazoxide, hydantoins, rifampin, thiazide diuretics, urinary alkalinizers, activated charcoal, alcohol (chronic use).	ADRs Hypoglycemia, nausea, heartburn, epigastric fullness, allergic skin reactions, eczema, pruritus, erythema, disulfiram-like reactions (if taken with alcohol), elevated liver function tests, SIADH. Chlorpropamide has a higher incidence of side-effects than other sulfonylureas. Elderly Use cautiously—particularly susceptible to hypoglycemic effects. Also, elderly patients may not recognize symptoms of hypoglycemia. Pharmacokinetics Onset of action = 1 h; duration of action = up to 60 h; 80% metabolized in liver; renal elimination of metabolites; $T_{1/2}$ = 36 h (Agents with shorter $T_{1/2}$ are generally better choices for elderly patients).	Contraindications Hypersensitivity, diabetes complicated by ketoacidosis with or without coma; sole therapy of Type I diabetes; diabetes complicated by pregnancy. Precautions Monitor patients closely during periods of stress (e.g., infection, etc.) for poor glucose control. Use cautiously in those with severe hepatic or renal impairment. Pregnancy Category: C Lactation Issues Excreted in breast milk—do not give to nursing mothers.
Glipizide Glucotrol, Glucotrol XL, various generics Tablets 5 mg, 10 mg Tablets, extended release 2.5 mg, 5 mg, 10 mg	**As adjunct to diet/exercise to control blood glucose in NIDDM (Type 2):** 5 mg each morning, initially. May titrate by 2.5–5 mg/d every several days as needed. Max single daily dose is 15 mg; max daily dose is 40 mg. Elderly or debilitated patients: 2.5 mg/d initially.	Administration Issues Take 30 minutes prior to a meal. Avoid alcohol. Drug–Drug Interactions **Increased hypoglycemic effect:** androgens, anticoagulants, chloramphenicol, clofibrate, fenfluramine, fluconazole, ketoconazole, gemfibrozil, H_2 antagonists, magnesium salts, methyldopa, MAO inhibitors, phenylbutazone, probenecid, salicylates, sulfinpyrazone, sulfonamides, TCAs, urinary acidifiers, alcohol (acute use). **Increased levels/effects of:** digoxin	ADRs Hypoglycemia, nausea, heartburn, epigastric fullness, allergic skin reactions, eczema, pruritus, erythema, disulfiram-like reactions (if taken with alcohol), elevated liver function tests, SIADH. Other effects: increased effects on total cholesterol, total triglycerides, LDL, body weight (3–8 kg). Elderly: Use cautiously—particularly susceptible to hypoglycemic effects. Also, elderly patients may not recognize symptoms of hypoglycemia	Contraindications Hypersensitivity, diabetes complicated by ketoacidosis with or without coma; sole therapy of Type I diabetes; diabetes complicated by pregnancy. Precautions Monitor patients closely during periods of stress (e.g., infection, etc.) for poor glucose control. Use cautiously in those with severe hepatic or renal impairment. Pregnancy Category: C Lactation Issues Excreted in breast milk—do not give to nursing mothers.

		Decreased hypoglycemic effect: beta blockers, cholestyramine, diazoxide, hydantoins, rifampin, thiazide diuretics, urinary alkalinizers, charcoal, alcohol (chronic use).	Pharmacokinetics Onset of action = 1–1.5 h; duration of action = 10–16 h; hepatically metabolized; renal elimination of metabolites; $T_{1/2}$ = 2–4 h.	
Glimepiride Amaryl Tablets 1 mg, 2 mg, 4 mg	**As adjunct to diet/exercise to control blood glucose in NIDDM (Type 2):** 1–2 mg once daily, initially. May titrate by 1–2 mg/d each week up to 4 mg once daily if needed. Max dose is 8 mg/d. Combination therapy with insulin: 8 mg/d with low dose insulin.	Administration Issues Take with food if GI upset occurs. Avoid alcohol Drug–Drug Interactions **Increased hypoglycemic effect:** androgens, anticoagulants, chloramphenicol, clofibrate, fenfluramine, fluconazole, gemfibrozil, H_2 antagonists, magnesium salts, methyldopa, MAO inhibitors, phenylbutazone, probenecid, salicylates, sulfinpyrazone, sulfonamides, TCAs, urinary acidifiers, alcohol (acute use). **Increased levels/effects of:** digoxin. **Decreased hypoglycemic effect:** beta blockers, cholestyramine, diazoxide, hydantoins, rifampin, thiazide diuretics, urinary alkalinizers, charcoal, alcohol (chronic use).	ADRs Hypoglycemia, nausea, heartburn, epigastric fullness, allergic skin reactions, eczema, pruritus, erythema, disulfiram-like reactions (if taken with alcohol), elevated liver function tests, SIADH, photosensitivity. Other effects: increased effects on total cholesterol, total triglycerides, LDL, body weight (3–8 kg). Elderly: Use cautiously—particularly susceptible to hypoglycemic effects. Also, elderly patients may not recognize symptoms of hypoglycemia Pharmacokinetics Onset of action = 2–4 h; duration of action = 24 h; 80% metabolized in liver; renal elimination of metabolites; $T_{1/2}$ = 10 h.	Contraindications Hypersensitivity, diabetes complicated by ketoacidosis with or without coma; sole therapy of Type I diabetes; diabetes complicated by pregnancy. Precautions Monitor patients closely during periods of stress (e.g., infection, etc.) for poor glucose control. Use cautiously in those with severe hepatic or renal impairment. Pregnancy Category: C Lactation Issues Excreted in breast milk—do not give to nursing mothers.
Glyburide Diabeta, Micronase, Glynase Pres Tab, various generics Tablets 1.25 mg, 2.5 mg, 5 mg Tablets, micronized 1.5 mg, 3 mg, 6 mg	**As adjunct to diet/exercise to control blood glucose in NIDDM (Type 2):** Non-micronized: 2.5–5 mg/d, initially. May titrate by 2.5–5 mg/d every several days up to 20 mg/d if needed, though doses >10 mg/d rarely provide added glucose lowering. **Elderly or debilitated patients:** 1.25 mg/d initially.	Administration Issues Take with food if GI upset occurs. Avoid alcohol. Drug–Drug Interactions **Increased hypoglycemic effect:** androgens, anticoagulants, chloramphenicol, clofibrate, fenfluramine, fluconazole, ketoconazole, gemfibrozil, H_2 antagonists, magnesium salts, methyldopa, MAO inhibitors, phenylbutazone, probenecid, salicylates, sulfinpyrazone, sulfonamides, TCAs, urinary acidifiers, alcohol (acute use).	ADRs Hypoglycemia, nausea, heartburn, epigastric fullness, allergic skin reactions, eczema, pruritus, erythema, disulfiram-like reactions (if taken with alcohol), elevated liver function tests, SIADH, photosensitivity. Other effects: increased effects on total cholesterol, total triglycerides, LDL, body weight (3–8 kg).	Contraindications Hypersensitivity, diabetes complicated by ketoacidosis with or without coma; sole therapy of Type I diabetes; diabetes complicated by pregnancy. Precautions Monitor patients closely during periods of stress (e.g., infection, etc.) for poor glucose control. Use cautiously in those with severe hepatic or renal impairment. Pregnancy Category: C

(continues on next page)

604.1 Sulfonylureas *continued from previous page*

Drug and Dosage Forms	Usual Dosage Range	Administration Issues and Drug–Drug Interactions	Common Adverse Drug Reactions (ADRs) and Pharmacokinetics	Contraindications, Pregnancy Category, and Lactation Issues
Glyburide *cont.*	Micronized: 1.5–3 mg/d, initially. May titrate by 0.75–1.5 mg/d every several days up to 12 mg/d if needed. Doses >6 mg/d may be divided into 2 doses. **Elderly or debilitated patients:** 0.75 mg/d initially.	**Increased levels/effects of:** digoxin. **Decreased hypoglycemic effect:** beta blockers, cholestyramine, diazoxide, hydantoins, rifampin, thiazide diuretics, urinary alkalinizers, charcoal, alcohol (chronic use).	Elderly Use cautiously—particularly susceptible to hypoglycemic effects. Also, elderly patients may not recognize symptoms of hypoglycemia Pharmacokinetics Onset of action = 2–4 h (micronized = 1 h); duration of action = 24 h (for micronized and non-micronized); hepatically metabolized; renal elimination of metabolites; $T_{1/2}$ = 10 hrs (micronized = 4 h).	Lactation Issues Excreted in breast milk—do not give to nursing mothers.
Tolazamide Tolinase, various generics Tablets 100 mg, 250 mg, 500 mg	**As adjunct to diet/exercise to control blood glucose in NIDDM (Type 2):** 100–250 mg/d, initially. If fasting glucose <200 mg/dL, use 100 mg/d; if >200 mg/dL, use 250 mg/d. May titrate to 1000 mg/d if needed. Doses >500 mg/d should be divided in two daily doses. **Elderly or debilitated patients:** 100 mg/d	Administration Issues Take with food if GI upset occurs. Avoid alcohol Drug–Drug Interactions **Increased hypoglycemic effect:** androgens, anticoagulants, chloramphenicol, clofibrate, fenfluramine, fluconazole, ketoconazole, gemfibrozil, H_2 antagonists, magnesium salts, methyldopa, MAO inhibitors, phenylbutazone, probenecid, salicylates, sulfinpyrazone, sulfonamides, TCAs, urinary acidifiers, alcohol (acute use). **Increased levels/effects of:** digoxin **Decreased hypoglycemic effect:** beta blockers, cholestyramine, diazoxide, hydantoins, rifampin, thiazide diuretics, urinary alkalinizers, charcoal, alcohol (chronic use).	ADRs Hypoglycemia, nausea, heartburn, epigastric fullness, allergic skin reactions, eczema, pruritus, erythema, disulfiram-like reactions (if taken with alcohol), elevated liver function tests, SIADH, photosensitivity. Other effects increased effects on total cholesterol, total triglycerides, LDL, body weight (3–8 kg). Elderly Use cautiously—particularly susceptible to hypoglycemic effects. Also, elderly patients may not recognize symptoms of hypoglycemia. Pharmacokinetics Onset of action = 4–6 h; duration of action = 12–24 h; hepatically metabolized; renal elimination of metabolites; $T_{1/2}$ = 7 h.	Contraindications Hypersensitivity, diabetes complicated by ketoacidosis with or without coma; sole therapy of Type I diabetes; diabetes complicated by pregnancy. Precautions Monitor patients closely during periods of stress (e.g., infection, etc.) for poor glucose control. Use cautiously in those with severe hepatic or renal impairment. Pregnancy Category: C Lactation Issues Excreted in breast milk—do not give to nursing mothers.
Tolbutamide Orinase, various generics	**As adjunct to diet/exercise to control blood glucose in NIDDM (Type 2):**	Administration Issues Take with food if GI upset occurs. Avoid alcohol	ADRs Hypoglycemia, nausea, heartburn, epigastric fullness, allergic skin reactions,	Contraindications Hypersensitivity, diabetes complicated by ketoacidosis with or without coma; sole

Tablets 500 mg	250 mg each morning initially. May titrate to 2 gm/d. Max of 3 gm/d. (Doses >2 gm/d usually not therapeutically beneficial).	Drug–Drug Interactions **Increased hypoglycemic effect:** androgens, anticoagulants, chloramphenicol, clofibrate, fenfluramine, fluconazole, ketoconazole, gemfibrozil, H_2 antagonists, magnesium salts, methyldopa, MAO inhibitors, phenylbutazone, probenecid, salicylates, sulfinpyrazone, sulfonamides, TCAs, urinary acidifiers, alcohol (acute use). **Increased levels/effects of:** digoxin. **Decreased hypoglycemic effect:** beta blockers, cholestyramine, diazoxide, hydantoins, rifampin, thiazide diuretics, urinary alkalinizers, charcoal, alcohol (chronic use).	eczema, pruritus, erythema, disulfiram-like reactions (if taken with alcohol), elevated liver function tests, SIADH, photosensitivity. Other effects increased effects on total cholesterol, total triglycerides, LDL, body weight (3–8 kg). Elderly Use cautiously—particularly susceptible to hypoglycemic effects. Also, elderly patients may not recognize symptoms of hypoglycemia Pharmacokinetics Onset of action = 1 h; duration of action = 6–12 h; hepatically metabolized; renal elimination of metabolites; $T_{1/2}$ = 4.5–6.5 h.	therapy of Type I diabetes; diabetes complicated by pregnancy. Precautions Monitor patients closely during periods of stress (e.g., infection, etc.) for poor glucose control. Use cautiously in those with severe hepatic or renal impairment. Pregnancy Category: C Lactation Issues Excreted in breast milk—do not give to nursing mothers.

604.2 Miscellaneous Antidiabetic Agents

Drug and Dosage Forms	Usual Dosage Range	Administration Issues and Drug–Drug Interactions	Common Adverse Drug Reactions (ADRs) and Pharmacokinetics	Contraindications, Pregnancy Category, and Lactation Issues
Acarbose Precose Tablets 25 mg, 50 mg, 100 mg	**As monotherapy as an adjunct to diet to lower blood glucose in patients with NIDDM, or as adjunctive therapy with a sulfonylurea for control of blood glucose:** Initially, 25 mg tid. Titrate the dose by 25 mg 3 times daily every 8 week intervals based on 1-h postprandial glucose levels and tolerance up to 100 mg 3 times daily. Max dose is 100 mg 3 times daily for those > 60 kg; 50 mg 3 times daily for those < 60 kg.	Administration Issues Take with the start of each main meal. Patients must continue to follow regular diet and exercise program. Drug–Drug Interactions **Decreased effect of acarbose:** digestive enzymes, intestinal absorbents (e.g., charcoal).	ADRs Abdominal pain, diarrhea, flatulence. Pharmacokinetics < 2% absorbed from GI tract (51% excreted in feces); metabolized within the GI tract (some absorbed then excreted in urine); plasma $T_{1/2}$ = 2 h.	Contraindications Hypersensitivity; diabetic ketoacidosis; cirrhosis; inflammatory bowel disease; colonic ulcerations; partial intestinal obstruction; chronic intestinal diseases. Precautions Monitor patients closely during periods of stress (e.g., infection, etc) for poor glucose control. Use cautiously in those with severe renal impairment.

(continues on next page)

604.2 Miscellaneous Antidiabetic Agents *continued from previous page*

Drug and Dosage Forms	Usual Dosage Range	Administration Issues and Drug–Drug Interactions	Common Adverse Drug Reactions (ADRs) and Pharmacokinetics	Contraindications, Pregnancy Category, and Lactation Issues
Acarbose *cont.*				Pregnancy Category: B Lactation Issues May be excreted in breast milk—do not give to nursing mothers.
Glipizide/Metformin Metaglip Tablets 2.5 mg/250 mg 2.5 mg/500 mg 5 mg/500 mg	**Type 2 diabetes** **Initial therapy:** **As an adjunct to diet and exercise to improve glycemic control in patients with type 2 diabetes whose hyperglycemia cannot be satisfactorily managed with diet and exercise alone.** **Second-line therapy:** **When diet, exercise, and initial treatment with a sulfonylurea or metformin do not result in adequate glycemic control in patients with type 2 diabetes.** **Initial therapy:** The recommended starting dose of glipizide/metformin is 2.5 mg/250 mg once a day with a meal. For patients whose fasting plasma glucose (FPG) is 280 to 320 mg/dL, consider a starting dose of 2.5 mg/500 mg twice daily. Increase dosage in increments of 1 tablet per day every 2 weeks up to a maximum of 10 mg/1000 mg or 10 mg/2000 mg per day given in divided doses **Second-line therapy:** Starting dose is 2.5 mg/500 mg or 5 mg/500 mg twice daily with the morning and evening meals. Patients previously treated with combination therapy of glipizide (or another sulfonylurea) plus metformin may be switched to glipizide/metformin 2.5 mg/500 mg or 5 mg/500 mg; the starting dose should not exceed the daily dose of glipizide (or equivalent dose of another sulfonylurea) and metformin already being taken.	Administration Issues Closely monitor patients for signs and symptoms of hypoglycemia. Drug-Drug Interactions See Glipizide and Metformin.	ADRs Most Frequent: See Glipizide and Metformin. Pharmacokinetics: See Glipizide and Metformin.	Contraindications/Warnings Lactic acidosis is a rare, but serious, metabolic complication that can occur because of metformin accumulation during treatment with glipizide/metformin. When it occurs, it is fatal in approximately 50% of cases. See Glipizide and Metformin for other contraindications and warnings. Pregnancy Category: B Lactation Issues: See Glipizide and Metformin

Glyburide/Metformin Glucovance Tablets 1.25 mg/250 mg 2.5 mg/500 mg 5 mg/500 mg	**Type 2 diabetes** **Initial therapy:** **As an adjunct to diet and exercise, to improve glycemic control in patients with type 2 diabetes whose hyperglycemia cannot be satisfactorily managed with diet and exercise alone.** **Second-line therapy:** **When diet, exercise, and initial treatment with a sulfonylurea or metformin do not result in adequate glycemic control in patients with type 2 diabetes.** **Initial therapy:** Starting dose: 1.25 mg/250 mg once or twice daily with meals. Increase dosage in increments of 1.25 mg/250 mg/day every 2 weeks up to the minimum effective dose necessary to achieve adequate control of blood glucose. Do not use glyburide/metformin 5 mg/500 mg as initial therapy because of an increased risk of hypoglycemia. **Second-line therapy:** Starting dose: 2.5 mg/500 mg or 5 mg/500 mg twice daily with meals. Titrate the daily dose in increments of no more than 5 mg/500 mg up to the minimum effective dose to achieve adequate control of blood glucose or to a maximum dose of 20 mg/2000 mg/day.	Administration Issues Take with food or a snack. Drug-Drug Interactions See Glyburide and Metformin.	ADRs Most frequent See Glyburide and Metformin. Pharmacokinetics See Glyburide and Metformin.	Contraindications/Warnings Lactic acidosis is a rare, but serious, metabolic complication that can occur because of metformin accumulation during treatment with glyburide/metformin. When it occurs, it is fatal in approximately 50% of cases. See Glyburide and Metformin for other contraindications and warnings. Pregnancy Category: B Lactation Issues: See Glyburide and Metformin.
Metformin Glucophage, Glucophage XR Tablets 500 mg, 850 mg, 1000 mg Tablets, extended release XR 500 mg, 750 mg	**As an adjunct to diet/exercise or sulfonylurea for the control of blood glucose in NIDDM (Type 2 diabetes):** 250 mg or 500 mg qd, initially, increasing over 2 wks to at least 1 gm. Give increased doses bid. May also initiate therapy with 425 mg once daily. May titrate in increments of 425 mg/d every other week up to max of 2550 mg/d (in 2–3 divided doses).	Administration Issues Avoid alcohol. Take with food to help minimize GI effects. **Temporarily hold metformin, if possible, 24 to 48 h prior to undergoing radiologic studies involving parenteral administration of iodinated contrast materials—can restart metformin 48 h after study if kidney function at baseline.**	ADRs Diarrhea, nausea, vomiting, abdominal bloating, flatulence, anorexia, unpleasant metallic taste, asymptomatic subnormal serum vitamin B12 levels. Rare, but potentially fatal lactic acidosis	Contraindications Hypersensitivity; renal disease (SrCr > 1.5 mg/dL in men, > 1.4 mg/dL in women); acute or chronic metabolic acidosis (including diabetic ketoacidosis), acute MI, septicemia, elderly age > 80 yrs Precautions Monitor patients closely during periods of stress (e.g., infection, etc.) for poor glucose control; monitor for signs of lactic acidosis

(*continues on next page*)

604.2 Miscellaneous Antidiabetic Agents *continued from previous page*

Drug and Dosage Forms	Usual Dosage Range	Administration Issues and Drug–Drug Interactions	Common Adverse Drug Reactions (ADRs) and Pharmacokinetics	Contraindications, Pregnancy Category, and Lactation Issues
Metformin *cont.*	Extended release given once daily with evening meal (maximum daily dose 2000 mg given as once daily). **Elderly or debilitated patients:** Use smaller doses, do not titrate to maximum doses. Contraindicated in elderly age 80 yrs or older.	Drug–Drug Interactions **Increased effects of metformin:** furosemide, alcohol, cationic drugs (amiloride, digoxin, morphine, etc), cimetidine, iodinated contrast material, nifedipine. **Decreased levels/effects of:** furosemide, glyburide.	Other effects increased effects on triglycerides; decreased effects on cholesterol and LDL; no change or decrease in body weight. Elderly Use cautiously and use smaller doses, initially. Monitor renal function frequently. Not recommended in those > 80 years of age. Pharmacokinetics 50–60% bioavailable; > 90% protein bound; renal elimination of unchanged drug (no hepatic metabolism); $T_{1/2} = 6.2$ h.	Pregnancy Category: B Lactation Issues Excreted in breast milk—use cautiously.
Miglitol Glyset Tablets 25 mg, 50 mg, 100 mg	**As monotherapy as an adjunct to diet to lower blood glucose in patients with NIDDM, or as adjunctive therapy with a sulfonylurea for control of blood glucose:** Initially, 25 mg tid. Some may need to start at 25 mg qd to minimize GI effects, then gradually increase administration to tid. Maintenance Dose: 50 mg tid (After 4–8 weeks, increases dose to 50 mg tid; some may benefit from doses up to 100 mg tid)	Administration Issues Take drug with first bite of each main meal. Drug Interactions **Decreased effects/levels of:** digoxin, glyburide, metformin, propranolol, ranitidine. **Decreased effects of miglitol by:** digestive enzymes, intestinal adsorbents (charcoal).	ADRs Flatulence, diarrhea, abdominal pain, skin rash. Pharmacokinetics $T_{1/2} = 2$ h. Duration of action 4–6 hr.	Contraindications Hypersensitivity to product, diabetic ketoacidosis, inflammatory bowel disease, colonic ulceration, patients predisposed to intestinal obstruction. Precaution Not recommended in patients with SrCr > 2 mg/dL Pregnancy Category: B Lactation Issues Miglitol is excreted in low doses in breast milk; do not administer to nursing mothers.
Nateglinide Starlix Tablets 60 mg, 120 mg	**Monotherapy** **To lower blood glucose in patients with type 2 diabetes whose hyperglycemia cannot be adequately controlled by diet and exercise and who have not been chronically treated with other antidiabetic agents.** **Combination therapy:** **In patients whose hyperglycemia is inadequately controlled with metformin, nateglinide may be added to, but not substituted for, metformin.**	Administration Given 30 minutes prior to meals Drug Interactions: **increased effect:** Propranold, ASA. NSAIDs, **reduce affect:** Thiazides, corticosteroids, thyroid products.	ADRs Nausea, diarrhea, hypoglycemia. Pharmacokinetics Rapidly well absorbed: $T_{1/2} = 1.5$ h.	Contraindications Pts who have failed sulfonylureas Pregnancy Category: C Lactation Issues: It is unknown

	120 mg tid. Given 30 minutes prior to meals. May reduce dose to 60 mg tid for elderly			
Pioglitazone Actos Tablets 15 mg, 30 mg, 45 mg	**Type 2 diabetes: Monotherapy as an adjunct to diet and exercise to improve glycemic control in patients with type 2 diabetes. In combination with a sulfonylurea, metformin, or insulin when diet, exercise and the single agent do not result in adequate glycemic control.** Initiate with 15–30 mg daily. May increase to 45 mg after 8–12 weeks. Maximum dose: 45 mg qd.	Administration Issues Take with or without food. Administer once daily. When adding to insulin therapy, reduce insulin by 10–25%. **Hepatic Impairment:** Do not initiate pioglitazone if the patient exhibits clinical evidence of active liver disease or serum transaminase levels (ALT more than 2.5 times the ULN). Drug-Drug Interactions **Deceased effectiveness** of oral contraceptives..	ADRs Most Frequent: Upper respiratory infections, headache, myalgia, sinusitis, tooth disorders, pharyngitis. Pharmacokinetics: $T_{1/2} = 3–7$ h.	Contraindications Hypersensitivity to pioglitazone. Pregnancy Category: C Lactation Issues Do not administer to nursing mothers.
Repaglinide Prandin Tablets 0.5 mg, 1 mg, 2 mg	**As adjunct to diet/exercise to control blood glucose in NIDDM (Type 2) or in combination with metformin:** Initially, 0.5 mg before meals up to 4 mg before meals. Max dose = 16 mg/d.	Administration Issues Take before meals. Monitor LFTs frequently and evaluate patients clinically for signs/symptoms of hepatic failure. Drug Interactions **Increased effects of repaglinide:** ketoconazole, erythromycin **decreased action/effects of repaglinide**: troglitazone, rifamphin, barbiturates, carbamazepine	ADRs Hyperglycemia, hypoglycemia, nausea, diarrhea, arthralgia. Pharmacokinetics $T_{1/2} < 1$ h; well absorbed.	Contraindications Hypersensitivity to repaglinide, diabetic ketoacidosis, IDDM. Pregnancy Category: C Lactation Issues It is not known whether repaglinide is excreted in breast milk.
Rosiglitazone Avandia Tablets 2 mg, 4 mg, 8 mg	**Type 2 diabetes: Monotherapy as an adjunct to diet and exercise to improve glycemic control in patients with type 2 diabetes. In combination with a sulfonylurea, metformin, or insulin when diet, exercise and the single agent do not result in adequate glycemic control.** Initiate with 4 mg daily, may increase to bid after 8–12 weeks. Max dose: 8 mg/day.	Administration Issues Take with or without food. When adding to insulin therapy, reduce insulin by 10–25%. **Hepatic impairment:** Use with caution in patients with hepatic impairment. Do not initiate rosiglitazone therapy if the patient exhibits clinical evidence of active liver disease or increased serum transaminase levels (ALT more than 2.5 times the ULN) at start of therapy. Liver enzyme monitoring is recommended in all patients prior to initiation of therapy with rosiglitazone and periodically thereafter. Drug-Drug Interactions **Deceased effectiveness** of oral contraceptives.	ADRs Most Frequent: nausea, diarrhea, upper respiratory infections, headache, sinusitis, myalgias. Pharmacokinetics: $T_{1/2} = 3–4$ h.	Contraindications Hypersensitivity to rosiglitazone or any of their components. Pregnancy Category: C Lactation Issues Do not administer to nursing mothers.

(continues on next page)

604.2 Miscellaneous Antidiabetic Agents *continued from previous page*

Drug and Dosage Forms	Usual Dosage Range	Administration Issues and Drug–Drug Interactions	Common Adverse Drug Reactions (ADRs) and Pharmacokinetics	Contraindications, Pregnancy Category, and Lactation Issues
Rosiglitazone Maleate/ Metformin Avandamet Tablets 1 mg/500 mg 2 mg/500 mg 2 mg/1000 mg 4 mg/500 mg 4 mg/1000 mg	**Type 2 diabetes: As an adjunct to diet and exercise to improve glycemic control in patients with type 2 diabetes mellitus who are already treated with combination rosiglitazone and metformin or who are not adequately controlled on metformin alone.** Individualize the dosage of antidiabetic therapy with rosiglitazone/metformin on the basis of effectiveness and tolerability while not exceeding the maximum recommended daily dose of 8 mg/2000 mg.	Administration Issues Give rosiglitazone/metformin in divided doses with meals, with gradual dose escalation. After an increase in metformin dosage, dose titration is recommended if patients are not adequately controlled after 1 to 2 weeks. After an increase in rosiglitazone dosage, dose titration is recommended if patients are not adequately controlled after 8 to 12 weeks. Drug-Drug Interactions See Rosiglitazone and Metformin.	ADRs Most Frequent: See Rosiglitazone and Metformin. Pharmacokinetics See Rosiglitazone and Metformin.	Contraindications/Warnings Lactic acidosis is a rare, but serious, metabolic complication that can occur because of metformin accumulation during treatment with rosiglitazone/metformin. When it occurs, it is fatal in approximately 50% of cases. See Rosiglitazone and Metformin for other contraindications and warnings. Pregnancy Category: B Lactation Issues: See Rosiglitazone and Metformin.

604.3 Insulin

Drug and Dosage Forms	Usual Dosage Range	Administration Issues and Drug–Drug Interactions	Common Adverse Drug Reactions (ADRs) and Pharmacokinetics	Contraindications, Pregnancy Category, and Lactation Issues
Aspart Novolog Injection: 100 U/ml human insulin aspart-insulin analog	**Diabetes mellitus type 1** **Dosage must be individualized** One unit of aspart has the same glucose-lowering ability of human regular insulin but the effect is more rapid and of shorter duration **Adults:** 5–10 U 0–15 min before meals.	Administration Issues Use the same type and brand of syringe and insulin(s). Do not change order of mixing insulins (if applicable). When mixing insulins, draw up clear regular insulin first. Rotate injection sites. During periods of stress, monitor glucose (insulin requirements may increase). Store vial or cartridge in refrigerator. Discard unused insulin after 28 days. Drug–Drug Interactions **Decreased hypoglycemic effect:** oral contraceptives, corticosteroids, dextrothyroxine, diltiazem, dobutamine, epinephrine, smoking, thiazide diuretics, thyroid hormone.	ADRs Hypoglycemia, insulin allergy: (rarely: either local reactions or systemic reactions), lipoatrophy, breakdown of adipose tissue at the insulin injection site perhaps due to less pure insulins, lipohypertrophy, accumulation of SC fat at the injection site if the same site is used continuously. Pharmacokinetics Injection SC; onset of action 0.25 hr peak = 0.5–1.5 h; duration = 6–8 h.	Contraindications None Pregnancy: C Lactation Issues Unknown.

		Increased hypoglycemic effect: alcohol, anabolic steroids, beta-blockers, clofibrate, guanethidine, fenfluramine, MAO inhibitors, phenylbutazone, salicylates, sulfinpyrazone, tetracyclines.		
Lispro Humalog Injection 100 U/mL human insulin lispro (rDNA)	**Diabetes mellitus type 1** **Dosage must be individualized** One unit of lispro has the same glucose-lowering ability of human regular insulin but the effect is more rapid and of shorter duration **Adults:** 5–10 U 0–15 min before meals.	Administration Issues Use the same type and brand of syringe and insulin(s). Do not change order of mixing insulins (if applicable). When mixing insulins, draw up clear regular insulin first. Rotate injection sites. During periods of stress, monitor glucose (insulin requirements may increase). Store vial or cartridge in refrigerator. Discard unused insulin after 28 days. Drug–Drug Interactions **Decreased hypoglycemic effect:** oral contraceptives, corticosteroids, dextrothyroxine, diltiazem, dobutamine, epinephrine, smoking, thiazide diuretics, thyroid hormone. **Increased hypoglycemic effect:** alcohol, anabolic steroids, beta-blockers, clofibrate, guanethidine, fenfluramine, MAO inhibitors, phenylbutazone, salicylates, sulfinpyrazone, tetracyclines.	ADRs Hypoglycemia, insulin allergy: (rarely: either local reactions or systemic reactions), lipoatrophy, breakdown of adipose tissue at the insulin injection site perhaps due to less pure insulins, lipohypertrophy, accumulation of SC fat at the injection site if the same site is used continuously. Pharmacokinetics Injection SC; onset of action 0.25 hr peak = 0.5–1.5 h; duration = 6–8 h. (Designed to be peakless; however, peaks may occur depending on injection variables)	Contraindications None Precautions Monitor for insulin resistance (>100 u/d of insulin required). Pregnancy: C Monitor these patients closely, blood glucose may be more difficult to control. Lactation Issues Does not pass into breast milk. Breast-feeding may decrease insulin requirements.
Regular Insulin Regular Iletin, Humulin R, Novolin R, Velosulin Human, various generics Injection 100 U/mL human insulin Cartridge for PenFill 100 U/mL human insulin	**Diabetes mellitus type I, or type II:** **Dosage must be individualized:** **Adults/children:** 0.5–1 u/kg/day **Adolescents during a growth phase:** 0.8–1.2 u/kg/day	Administration Issues Use the same type and brand of syringe and insulin(s). Do not change order of mixing insulins (if applicable). When mixing insulins, draw up clear regular insulin first. Rotate injection sites. During periods of stress, monitor glucose (insulin requirements may increase). Store extra insulin in refrigerator; current Ågin-useÅh insulin can be kept at room temperature. Prefilled syringes should be refrigerated and are good for 7–14 days. Drug–Drug Interactions **Decreased hypoglycemic effect:** oral contraceptives, corticosteroids, dextrothyroxine, diltiazem, dobutamine, epi	ADRs Hypoglycemia, insulin allergy: (rarely: either local reactions or systemic reactions), lipoatrophy, breakdown of adipose tissue at the insulin injection site perhaps due to less pure insulins, lipohypertrophy, accumulation of SC fat at the injection site if the same site is used continuously. Pharmacokinetics Injection SC; onset of action = 0.5–1 h; peak effect = 2–6 h; duration of action = 6–8 h.	Contraindications None Precautions Monitor for insulin resistance (>100 u/d of insulin required). Pregnancy: Monitor these patients closely, blood glucose may be more difficult to control. Lactation Issues Does not pass into breast milk. Breast-feeding may decrease insulin requirements.

(continues on next page)

604.3 Insulin *continued from previous page*

Drug and Dosage Forms	Usual Dosage Range	Administration Issues and Drug–Drug Interactions	Common Adverse Drug Reactions (ADRs) and Pharmacokinetics	Contraindications, Pregnancy Category, and Lactation Issues
Regular Insulin *cont.*		nephrine, smoking, thiazide diuretics, thyroid hormone. **Increased hypoglycemic effect:** alcohol, anabolic steroids, beta-blockers, clofibrate, guanethidine, fenfluramine, MAO inhibitors, phenylbutazone, salicylates, sulfinpyrazone, tetracyclines.		
Isophane Insulin Suspension (NPH) NPH Iletin, NPH-N, Humulin N, Novolin N, various generics Injection 100 U/mL human insulin Cartridge for PenFill 100 U/mL human insulin	**Diabetes mellitus type 1, or type 2: Dosage must be individualized:** **Adults/Children:** 0.5–1 u/kg/day **Adolescents during a growth phase:** 0.8–1.2 u/kg/day	Administration Issues Use the same type and brand of syringe and insulin(s). Do not change order of mixing insulins (if applicable). When mixing insulins, draw up clear regular insulin first. Rotate injection sites. During periods of stress, monitor glucose (insulin requirements may increase). Store extra insulin in refrigerator; current "in-use" insulin can be kept at room temperature. Prefilled syringes should be refrigerated and are good for 7–14 days. Drug–Drug Interactions **Decreased hypoglycemic effect:** oral contraceptives, corticosteroids, dextrothyroxine, diltiazem, dobutamine, epinephrine, smoking, thiazide diuretics, thyroid hormone. **Increased hypoglycemic effect:** alcohol, anabolic steroids, beta-blockers, clofibrate, guanethidine, fenfluramine, MAO inhibitors, phenylbutazone, salicylates, sulfinpyrazone, tetracyclines.	ADRs Hypoglycemia, insulin allergy: (rarely: either local reactions or systemic reactions), lipoatrophy, breakdown of adipose tissue at the insulin injection site perhaps due to less pure insulins, lipohypertrophy, accumulation of SC fat at the injection site if the same site is used continuously. Pharmacokinetics Injection SC; onset of action = 1–1.5 h; peak effect = 4–12 h; duration of action = 24 h.	Contraindications None Precautions Monitor for insulin resistance (>100 u/d of insulin required). Pregnancy: Monitor these patients closely, blood glucose may be more difficult to control. Lactation Issues Does not pass into breast milk. Breastfeeding may decrease insulin requirements.
Insulin Zinc Suspension (Lente) Lente Iletin, Lente L, Humulin L, Novolin L Injection 100 U/mL human, insulin	**Diabetes mellitus type 1, or type 2: Dosage must be individualized:** **Adults/children:** 0.5–1 u/kg/day	Administration Issues Use the same type and brand of syringe and insulin(s). Do not change order of mixing insulins (if applicable). When mixing insulins, draw up clear regular insulin first. Rotate injection sites. During periods of stress, monitor glucose (insulin re-	ADRs Hypoglycemia, insulin allergy: (rarely: either local reactions or systemic reactions), lipoatrophy, breakdown of adipose tissue at the insulin injection site perhaps due to less pure insulins, lipohypertrophy, accumulation of SC fat at the injection site if the same site is used continuously.	Contraindications None Precautions Monitor for insulin resistance (>100 u/d of insulin required).

	Adolescents during a growth phase: 0.8–1.2 u/kg/day	quirements may increase). Store extra insulin in refrigerator; current "in-use" insulin can be kept at room temperature. Prefilled syringes should be refrigerated and are good for 7–14 days. Drug–Drug Interactions **Decreased hypoglycemic effect:** oral contraceptives, corticosteroids, dextrothyroxine, diltiazem, dobutamine, epinephrine, smoking, thiazide diuretics, thyroid hormone. **Increased hypoglycemic effect:** alcohol, anabolic steroids, beta-blockers, clofibrate, guanethidine, fenfluramine, MAO inhibitors, phenylbutazone, salicylates, sulfinpyrazone, tetracyclines.	Pharmacokinetics Injection SC; onset of action = 1–2.5 h; peak effect = 7–15 h; duration of action = 24 h.	Pregnancy: Monitor these patients closely, blood glucose may be more difficult to control. Lactation Issues Does not pass into breast milk. Breastfeeding may decrease insulin requirements.
Insulin Zinc Suspension, Extended (Ultralente) Ultralente U, Humulin U Ultralente	**Diabetes mellitus type 1, or type 2: Dosage must be individualized:** **Adults/Children:** 0.5–1 u/kg/day **Adolescents during a growth phase:** 0.8–1.2 u/kg/day	Administration Issues Use the same type and brand of syringe and insulin(s). Do not change order of mixing insulins (if applicable). When mixing insulins, draw up clear regular insulin first. Rotate injection sites. During periods of stress, monitor glucose (insulin requirements may increase). Store extra insulin in refrigerator; current "in-use" insulin can be kept at room temperature. Prefilled syringes should be refrigerated and are good for 7–14 days. Drug–Drug Interactions **Decreased hypoglycemic effect:** oral contraceptives, corticosteroids, dextrothyroxine, diltiazem, dobutamine, epinephrine, smoking, thiazide diuretics, thyroid hormone. **Increased hypoglycemic effect:** alcohol, anabolic steroids, beta-blockers, clofibrate, guanethidine, fenfluramine, MAO inhibitors, phenylbutazone, salicylates, sulfinpyrazone, tetracyclines.	ADRs Hypoglycemia, insulin allergy: (rarely: either local reactions or systemic reactions), lipoatrophy, breakdown of adipose tissue at the insulin injection site perhaps due to less pure insulins, lipohypertrophy, accumulation of SC fat at the injection site if the same site is used continuously. Pharmacokinetics Injection SC; onset: 4–8 h: peak effect = 10–30 h; duration of action >36 h.	Contraindications None Precautions Monitor for insulin resistance (>100 u/d of insulin required). Pregnancy: Monitor these patients closely, blood glucose may be more difficult to control. Lactation Issues Does not pass into breast milk. Breastfeeding may decrease insulin requirements.

(*continues on next page*)

604.3 Insulin *continued from previous page*

Drug and Dosage Forms	Usual Dosage Range	Administration Issues and Drug–Drug Interactions	Common Adverse Drug Reactions (ADRs) and Pharmacokinetics	Contraindications, Pregnancy Category, and Lactation Issues
Insulin Glargine Lantus Injection: 100 U/ml human insulin-insulin analog.	**Diabetes mellitus type 1, or type 2: Dosage must be individualized:** **Adults/Children:** 0.5–1 u/kg/day **Adolescents during a growth phase:** 0.8–1.2 u/kg/day **Caution!** Insulin Glargire is a clear solution. Do NOT mix with other insulins! Unrefrigerated vials and cartridges must be used within 28 days.	Administration Issues Stinging may occur at injection site. Use the same type and brand of syringe and insulin(s). Do not change order of mixing insulins (if applicable). When mixing insulins, draw up clear regular insulin first. Rotate injection sites. During periods of stress, monitor glucose (insulin requirements may increase). Store extra insulin in refrigerator; current "in-use" insulin can be kept at room temperature. Stinging may occur at injection site. **Drug–Drug Interaction:** **Decreased hypoglycemic effect:** oral contraceptives, corticosteroids, dextrothyroxine, diltiazem, dobutamine, epinephrine, smoking, thiazide diuretics, thyroid hormone. **Increased hypoglycemic effect:** alcohol, anabolic steroids, beta-blockers, clofibrate, guanethidine, fenfluramine, MAO inhibitors, phenylbutazone, salicylates, sulfinpyrazone, tetracyclines.	ADRs Hypoglycemia, insulin allergy: (rarely: either local reactions or systemic reactions), lipoatrophy, breakdown of adipose tissue at the insulin injection site perhaps due to less pure insulins, lipohypertrophy, accumulation of SC fat at the injection site if the same site is used continuously, stinging at injection site. Pharmacokinetics Injection SC; onset of action = 1–4 h; peak effect = 4 h; duration of action = >18–24 h. (Designed to be peakless; however, peaks may occur depending on injection variables)	Contraindications None Pregnancy: C Monitor these patients closely, blood glucose may be more difficult to control. Lactation: Unknown
Combination Isophane Insulin Suspension & Regular Insulin (50%/50%) Humulin 50/50 Injection 100 U/mL human insulin	**Diabetes mellitus type 1, or type 2: Dosage must be individualized:** **Adults/Children:** 0.5–1 u/kg/day **Adolescents during a growth phase:** 0.8–1.2 u/kg/day	Administration Issues Use the same type and brand of syringe and insulin(s). Do not change order of mixing insulins (if applicable). When mixing insulins, draw up clear regular insulin first. Rotate injection sites. During periods of stress, monitor glucose (insulin requirements may increase). Store extra insulin in refrigerator; current "in-use" insulin can be kept at room temperature. Prefilled syringes should be refrigerated and are good for 7–14 days. Drug–Drug Interactions **Decreased hypoglycemic effect:** oral contraceptives, corticosteroids, dextrothyroxine, diltiazem, dobutamine, epi-	ADRs Hypoglycemia, insulin allergy: (rarely: either local reactions or systemic reactions), lipoatrophy, breakdown of adipose tissue at the insulin injection site perhaps due to less pure insulins, lipohypertrophy, accumulation of SC fat at the injection site if the same site is used continuously. Pharmacokinetics **Regular:** Injection SC; onset of action = 0.5–1 h; peak effect = 5–10 h; duration of action = 6–8 h.	Contraindications None Precautions Monitor for insulin resistance (>100 u/d of insulin required). Pregnancy: Monitor these patients closely, blood glucose may be more difficult to control. Lactation Issues Does not pass into breast milk. Breastfeeding may decrease insulin requirements.

		nephrine, smoking, thiazide diuretics, thyroid hormone. **Increased hypoglycemic effect:** alcohol, anabolic steroids, beta-blockers, clofibrate, guanethidine, fenfluramine, MAO inhibitors, phenylbutazone, salicylates, sulfinpyrazone, tetracyclines.	**NPH:** Injection SC; onset of action = 1–1.5 h; peak effect = 4–12 h; duration of action = 24 h.	
Combination Isophane Insulin Suspension & Regular Insulin (70/30) Humulin 70/30, Novolin 70/30 <u>Injection</u> 100 U/mL human insulin <u>Cartridge for PenFill</u> 100 U/mL human insulin	**<u>Diabetes mellitus type 1, or type 2:</u>** **<u>Dosage must be individualized:</u>** **Adults/Children:** 0.5–1 u/kg/day **Adolescents during a growth phase:** 0.8–1.2 u/kg/day	<u>Administration Issues</u> Use the same type and brand of syringe and insulin(s). Do not change order of mixing insulins (if applicable). When mixing insulins, draw up clear regular insulin first. Rotate injection sites. During periods of stress, monitor glucose (insulin requirements may increase). Store extra insulin in refrigerator; current Ågin-useÅh insulin can be kept at room temperature. Prefilled syringes should be refrigerated and are good for 7–14 days. <u>Drug–Drug Interactions</u> **Decreased hypoglycemic effect:** oral contraceptives, corticosteroids, dextrothyroxine, diltiazem, dobutamine, epinephrine, smoking, thiazide diuretics, thyroid hormone. **Increased hypoglycemic effect:** alcohol, anabolic steroids, beta-blockers, clofibrate, guanethidine, fenfluramine, MAO inhibitors, phenylbutazone, salicylates, sulfinpyrazone, tetracyclines.	<u>ADRs</u> Hypoglycemia, insulin allergy: (rarely: either local reactions or systemic reactions), lipoatrophy, breakdown of adipose tissue at the insulin injection site perhaps due to less pure insulins, lipohypertrophy, accumulation of SC fat at the injection site if the same site is used continuously. <u>Pharmacokinetics</u> **Regular:** Injection SC; onset of action = 0.5–1 hr; peak effect = 5–10 hr; duration of action = 6–8 h. **NPH:** Injection SC; onset of action = 1–1.5 hr; peak effect = 4–12 h; duration of action = 24 h.	<u>Contraindications</u> None <u>Precautions</u> Monitor for insulin resistance (>100 u/d of insulin required). <u>Pregnancy:</u> Monitor these patients closely, blood glucose may be more difficult to control. <u>Lactation Issues</u> Does not pass into breast milk. Breastfeeding may decrease insulin requirements.

605. Estrogen and Progestin Products

605.1 Estrogens

Drug and Dosage Forms	Usual Dosage Range	Administration Issues and Drug–Drug Interactions	Common Adverse Drug Reactions (ADRs) and Pharmacokinetics	Contraindications, Pregnancy Category, and Lactation Issues
Conjugated Estrogens Premarin Tablets 0.3 mg, 0.45 mg, 0.625 mg, 0.9 mg, 1.25 mg, 2.5 mg	**Use cyclical pattern of therapy (3 weeks on, 1 week off) unless otherwise specified.** **Vasomotor symptoms associated with menopause, female castration or primary ovarian failure:** 1.25 mg/d initially. Titrate to patient response. **Atrophic vaginitis, kraurosis vulvae:** 0.3–1.25 mg/d. **Hypogonadism:** 2.5–7.5 mg/d in divided doses for 20 days, followed by rest period of 10 days. **Breast cancer:** 10 mg tid for 3 months (do not use cyclical therapy). **Prostatic carcinoma:** 1.25–2.5 mg tid (do not use cyclical therapy). **Osteoporosis:** 0.625 mg/d. **Stress urinary incontinence** 0.3 to 1.25 mg qd continuous or cyclic (days 1–25).	Administration Issues Avoid prolonged exposure to sunlight Drug–Drug Interactions **Increased levels/effects of:** corticosteroids. **Decreased levels/effects of:** anticoagulants, hydantoins. **Decreased levels/effects of estrogens:** hydantoins, barbiturates, rifampin.	ADRs Breakthrough bleeding, spotting, dysmenorrhea, PMS-like syndrome, amenorrhea, vaginal candidiasis, hemolytic uremic syndrome; endometrial cystic hyperplasia, nausea, vomiting, abdominal cramps, bloating, photosensitivity; urticaria, dermatitis, headache, dizziness, depression, edema, changes in libido, breast tenderness or enlargement. Pharmacokinetics Oral or transdermal; 98% protein bound; hepatically metabolized.	Contraindications Hypersensitivity; breast cancer (some exceptions); active thrombophlebitis; thromboembolic disorders; estrogen-dependent neoplasia; undiagnosed abnormal genital bleeding; pregnancy. Precautions Use cautiously in those with hepatic or renal dysfunction; monitor serum calcium. Pregnancy Category: X Lactation Issues Excreted in breast milk. Use only if benefit clearly outweighs risk.
Esterified Estrogens Estratab, Menest Tablets 0.3 mg, 0.625 mg, 1.25 mg, 2.5 mg	**Use cyclical pattern of therapy (3 weeks on, 1 week off) unless otherwise specified.** **Vasomotor symptoms associated with menopause, atrophic vaginitis, kraurosis vulvae:** 0.3–1.25 mg/d. Titrate to patient response.	Administration Issues Avoid prolonged exposure to sunlight. Drug–Drug Interactions **Increased levels/effects of:** corticosteroids. **Decreased levels/effects of:** anticoagulants, hydantoins.	ADRs Breakthrough bleeding, spotting, dysmenorrhea, PMS-like syndrome, amenorrhea, vaginal candidiasis, hemolytic uremic syndrome; endometrial cystic hyperplasia, nausea, vomiting, abdominal cramps, bloating, photosensitivity; urticaria, dermatitis, headache, dizziness, depression, edema, changes in libido, breast tenderness or enlargement.	Contraindications Hypersensitivity; breast cancer (some exceptions); active thrombophlebitis; thromboembolic disorders; estrogen-dependent neoplasia; undiagnosed abnormal genital bleeding; pregnancy. Precautions Use cautiously in those with hepatic or renal dysfunction; monitor serum calcium.

	Hypogonadism: 2.5–7.5 mg/d in divided doses for 20 days, followed by rest period of 10 days. **Female castration or primary ovarian failure:** 1.25 mg/d. **Breast Cancer:** 10 mg tid for 3 months (do not use cyclical therapy). **Prostatic carcinoma:** 1.25–2.5 mg tid (do not use cyclical therapy).	**Decreased levels/effects of estrogens:** hydantoins, barbiturates, rifampin.	Pharmacokinetics Oral or transdermal; 98% protein bound; hepatically metabolized.	Pregnancy Category: X Lactation Issues Excreted in breast milk. Use only if benefit clearly outweighs risk.
Estradiol Estrace, generic Tablets: 0.5 mg, 1 mg, 1.5 mg, 2 mg **Estradiol Transdermal System** Vivelle, Climara, Estraderm, Alora, Fempatch Patch 0.025 mg/24 hr 0.0375 mg/24 hr 0.05 mg/24 hr 0.06 mg/24 hr 0.075 mg/24 hr 0.1 mg/24 hr	**Vasomotor symptoms associated with menopause, atrophic vaginitis, kraurosis vulvae, hypogonadism:** Oral: 1–2 mg/d. Titrate to patient response. **Breast cancer** Oral: 10 mg tid for at least 3 months. **Prostatic carcinoma:** 1–2 mg tid. **Osteoporosis:** 0.5 mg/d for 23 days, then 5 days off. Continue the cycle. Transdermal for all indications: 0.05 mg/d system initially. For the Estraderm and Vivelle systems, must apply twice weekly. The Climara patch is applied once weekly. Titrate dose based on patient response. For patients with an intact uterus, therapy is given on a cyclical basis (3 weeks of therapy, 1 week off); if not, therapy is continuous.	Administration Issues Avoid prolonged exposure to sunlight. Apply patch to clean, dry area on the trunk of the body (including buttocks and abdomen). Drug–Drug Interactions **Increased levels/effects of:** corticosteroids. **Decreased levels/effects of:** anticoagulants, hydantoins. **Decreased levels/effects of estrogens:** hydantoins, barbiturates, rifampin.	ADRs Breakthrough bleeding, spotting, dysmenorrhea, PMS-like syndrome, amenorrhea, vaginal candidiasis, hemolytic uremic syndrome; endometrial cystic hyperplasia, nausea, vomiting, abdominal cramps, bloating, photosensitivity; urticaria, dermatitis, headache, dizziness, depression, edema, changes in libido, breast tenderness or enlargement. Pharmacokinetics Oral or transdermal; 98% protein bound; hepatically metabolized.	Contraindications Hypersensitivity; breast cancer (some exceptions); active thrombophlebitis; thromboembolic disorders; estrogen-dependent neoplasia; undiagnosed abnormal genital bleeding; pregnancy. Precautions Use cautiously in those with hepatic or renal dysfunction; monitor serum calcium. Pregnancy Category: X Lactation Issues Excreted in breast milk. Use only if benefit clearly outweighs risk.
Estropipate Ortho-Est, Ogen, various generics	**Use cyclical pattern of therapy (3 weeks on, 1 week off) unless otherwise specified.**	Administration Issues Avoid prolonged exposure to sunlight.	ADRs Breakthrough bleeding, spotting, dysmenorrhea, PMS-like syndrome, amenorrhea, vaginal candidiasis, hemolytic uremic syndrome; endometrial cystic	Contraindications Hypersensitivity; breast cancer (some exceptions); active thrombophlebitis; thromboembolic disorders; estrogen-

(continues on next page)

605.1 Estrogens *continued from previous page*

Drug and Dosage Forms	Usual Dosage Range	Administration Issues and Drug–Drug Interactions	Common Adverse Drug Reactions (ADRs) and Pharmacokinetics	Contraindications, Pregnancy Category, and Lactation Issues
Estropipate *cont.* Tablets 0.625 mg (0.75 mg estropipate) 1.25 mg (1.5 mg estropipate) 2.5 mg (3 mg estropipate) 5 mg (6 mg estropipate)	**Vasomotor symptoms associated with menopause, atrophic vaginitis, kraurosis vulvae:** 0.625–5 mg/d given for 25 days of a 31 day cycle. **Hypogonadism, female castration, primary ovarian failure:** 1.25–7.5 mg/d given cyclically. **Osteoporosis:** 0.625 mg qd for 25 days of a 31 day cycle.	Drug–Drug Interactions **Increased levels/effects of:** corticosteroids. **Decreased levels/effects of:** anticoagulants, hydantoins. **Decreased levels/effects of estrogens:** hydantoins, barbiturates, rifampin.	hyperplasia, nausea, vomiting, abdominal cramps, bloating, photosensitivity; urticaria, dermatitis, headache, dizziness, depression, edema, changes in libido, breast tenderness or enlargement. Pharmacokinetics Oral or transdermal; 98% protein bound; hepatically metabolized.	dependent neoplasia; undiagnosed abnormal genital bleeding; pregnancy. Precautions Use cautiously in those with hepatic or renal dysfunction; monitor serum calcium. Pregnancy Category: X Lactation Issues Excreted in breast milk. Use only if benefit clearly outweighs risk.
Ethinyl Estradiol Estinyl Tablets 0.02 mg, 0.05 mg, 0.5 mg	**Use cyclical pattern of therapy (3 weeks on, 1 week off) unless otherwise specified.** Vasomotor symptoms associated with menopause, atrophic vaginitis, kraurosis vulvae: 0.02–0.05 mg/d. **Hypogonadism, female castration, primary ovarian failure:** 0.05 mg 1-tid during 1st 2 weeks of theoretical menstrual cycle followed by progestin during last half of arbitrary cycle. Continue for 3–6 months. **Breast cancer:** 1 mg tid given chronically. **Prostatic carcinoma:** 0.15–2 mg/d given chronically.	Administration Issues Avoid prolonged exposure to sunlight. Drug–Drug Interactions **Increased levels/effects of:** corticosteroids. **Decreased levels/effects of:** anticoagulants, hydantoins. **Decreased levels/effects of estrogens:** hydantoins, barbiturates, rifampin.	ADRs Breakthrough bleeding, spotting, dysmenorrhea, PMS-like syndrome, amenorrhea, vaginal candidiasis, hemolytic uremic syndrome; endometrial cystic hyperplasia, nausea, vomiting, abdominal cramps, bloating, photosensitivity; urticaria, dermatitis, headache, dizziness, depression, edema, changes in libido, breast tenderness or enlargement. Pharmacokinetics Oral or transdermal; 98% protein bound; hepatically metabolized.	Contraindications Hypersensitivity; breast cancer (some exceptions); active thrombophlebitis; thromboembolic disorders; estrogen-dependent neoplasia; undiagnosed abnormal genital bleeding; pregnancy. Precautions Use cautiously in those with hepatic or renal dysfunction; monitor serum calcium. Pregnancy Category: X Lactation Issues Excreted in breast milk. Use only if benefit clearly outweighs risk.
Vaginal Estrogens Vaginal Creams and Ring Ogen Cream 1.5 mg estropipate Premarin Cream 0.625 mg conj, estrogens/g	**Atrophic vaginitis, kraurosis vulvae associated with menopause:** **Estropipate and conjugated estrogen:** Administer cyclically: 3 wks on and 1 wk off. Give 0.5 to 2 g daily of conjugated and 2 to 4 g daily of estropipate intrav-	Administration Issues Avoid prolonged exposure to sunlight. Cream: insert high into the vagina (the length of the applicator). Ring: press the ring into an oval and insert into the upper third of the vaginal vault.	ADRs Breakthrough bleeding, spotting, dysmenorrhea, PMS-like syndrome, amenorrhea, vaginal candidiasis, hemolytic uremic syndrome; endometrial cystic hyperplasia, nausea, vomiting, abdominal cramps, bloating, photosensitivity; urticaria, dermatitis, headache, dizziness,	Contraindications Hypersensitivity; breast cancer (some exceptions); active thrombophlebitis; thromboembolic disorders; estrogen-dependent neoplasia; undiagnosed abnormal genital bleeding; pregnancy.

Ortho Dienestrol Cream 0.01% dienestrol Estrace Cream 0.1 mg estradiol/g Estring 2 mg estradiol/ring	aginally depending on severity of condition. **Dienestrol:** 1 applicatorful 1–2 times daily for 1 or 2 wks, then reduce to one-half the inital dose for a similar period. A maintenance dose of 1 applicatorful 1 to 3 times/wk may be used after restoration of vaginal mucosa. **Estradiol:** Cream: 2 to 4 g daily for 2 wk. Gradually reduce dose to one-half initial dosage for a similar period. A maintenance dose of 1 g 1 to 3 times/wk may be used after restoration of vaginal mucosa. Ring: Insert deeply as possible unto the upper one-third of the vaginal vault. The ring should remain in place continuously for 3 months, then removed and replace by a new ring, if indicated. Assess need for continuation at 3- or 6-month interval.	Drug–Drug Interactions **Increased levels/effects of:** corticosteroids. **Decreased levels/effects of:** anticoagulants, hydantoins. **Decreased levels/effects of estrogens:** hydantoins, barbiturates, rifampin.	depression, edema, changes in libido, breast tenderness or enlargement.	Precautions Use cautiously in those with hepatic or renal dysfunction; monitor serum calcium. Pregnancy Category: X Lactation Issues Excreted in breast milk. Use only if benefit clearly outweighs risk.

605.2 Progestins

Drug and Dosage Forms	Usual Dosage Range	Administration Issues, Drug–Drug & Drug–Lab Interactions	Common Adverse Drug Reactions (ADRs)	Contraindications, Pregnancy Category, and Lactation Issues
Medroxyprogesterone Cycrin, Provera, Amen, Curretab, various generics Tablets 2.5 mg, 5 mg, 10 mg	**Secondary amenorrhea:** 5–10 mg/d for 5–10 days. **Abnormal uterine bleeding:** 5–10 mg/d for 5–10 days beginning on the 16th or 21st day of the cycle. **Stress urinary incontinence:** 2.5 to 10 mg qd, continuous or cyclic (days 16–25 if uterus present).	Administration Issues Take with food if GI upset occurs. Drug–Drug Interactions **Decreased levels/effects of progestin:** aminoglutethimide, rifampin. Drug–Lab Interaction The following tests may be affected by progestins: hepatic function, coagulation, thyroid, metyrapone, and endocrine function.	ADRs Insomnia, somnolence, mental depression, rash, acne, melasma, changes in weight, breakthrough bleeding, spotting, change in menstrual flow, amenorrhea, changes in cervical secretions, breast changes, masculinization of the female fetus, edema, cholestatic jaundice, hirsutism.	Contraindications Hypersensitivity, thrombophlebitis, thromboembolic disorders, cerebral hemorrhage, impaired liver function, carcinoma of the breast or genital organs, undiagnosed vaginal bleeding, missed abortion, for use as a diagnostic test for pregnancy. Pregnancy Category: D Lactation Issues Small amounts excreted in breast milk—effects on infant not known.

(continues on next page)

605.2 Progestins *continued from previous page*

Drug and Dosage Forms	Usual Dosage Range	Administration Issues, Drug–Drug & Drug–Lab Interactions	Common Adverse Drug Reactions (ADRs)	Contraindications, Pregnancy Category, and Lactation Issues
Megestrol Megace, generic Suspension 40 mg/mL Tablets 20 mg, 40 mg	**Appetite enhancement in AIDS patients, palliative treatment of advanced breast or endometrium cancer:** 800 mg/d. Titrate based on patient response to range of 400–800 mg/d.	Administration Issues Store at room temperature, protect from heat. Safety/efficacy in children is not established. Drug–Drug Interactions **Decreased levels/effects of progestin:** aminoglutethimide, rifampin. Drug–Lab Interaction The following tests may be affected by progestins: hepatic function, coagulation, thyroid, metyrapone, and endocrine function.	ADRs Impotence, rash, diarrhea, insomnia, fever, headache, hypertension.	Contraindications Hypersensitivity, pregnancy, prophylactic use to avoid weight loss; for use as a diagnostic test for pregnancy. Pregnancy Category: D Lactation Issues Small amounts excreted in breast milk—effects on infant not known.
Norethindrone Aygestin, generic Tablets: 5 mg	**Amenorrhea, abnormal uterine bleeding:** 2.5–10 mg/d for 5–10 days during 2nd half of menstrual cycle. **Endometriosis:** 5 mg/d for 2 weeks. Titrate by 2.5 mg/d every 2 weeks until 15 mg/d is reached. Continue for 6–9 months.	Administration Issues Take with food if GI upset occurs. Drug–Drug Interactions **Decreased levels/effects of progestin:** aminoglutethimide, rifampin. Drug–Lab Interaction The following tests may be affected by progestins: hepatic function, coagulation, thyroid, metyrapone, and endocrine function.	ADRs Insomnia, somnolence, mental depression, rash, acne, melasma, changes in weight, breakthrough bleeding, spotting, change in menstrual flow, amenorrhea, changes in cervical secretions, breast changes, masculinization of the female fetus, edema, cholestatic jaundice, hirsutism.	Contraindications Hypersensitivity, thrombophlebitis, thromboembolic disorders, cerebral hemorrhage, impaired liver function, carcinoma of the breast or genital organs, undiagnosed vaginal bleeding, missed abortion, for use as a diagnostic test for pregnancy. Pregnancy Category: D Lactation Issues Small amounts excreted in breast milk—effects on infant not known.

605.3 Estrogen/Progestin Combinations

Drug and Dosage Forms	Usual Dosage Range	Administration Issues, Drug-Drug & Drug-Lab Interactions	Common Adverse Drug Reactions (ADRs) and Pharmacokinetics	Contraindications, Pregnancy Category, and Lactation Issues
Conjugated estrogens & medroxyprogesterone acetate	**Symptoms associated with menopause, vulvar/vaginal atrophy, prevention of osteoporosis:**	Administration Issues Avoid prolonged exposure to sunlight. Drug-Drug Interactions **Increased levels/effects of:** corticosteroids.	**ADRs** Estrogen: Breakthrough bleeding, spotting, dysmenorrhea, PMS-like syndrome, amenorrhea, vaginal candidiasis, hemolytic uremic syndrome; endometrial cystic hyperplasia, nausea, vomiting, abdominal	Contraindications Hypersensitivity; breast cancer (some exceptions); active thrombophlebitis; thromboembolic disorders; estrogen-dependent neoplasia; undiagnosed abnormal genital bleeding; pregnancy, for use as a diagnostic test for pregnancy.

Tablets 0.625 mg estrogen alone and the combination of 0.625 mg/5 mg Tablets (Prempro) 0.625 mg/2.5 mg (in combination) 0.625 mg/5 mg 0.3 mg/1.5 mg 0.45 mg/1.5 mg	Premphase: combination tablet qd **or** 0.625 mg estrogen qd days 1–14 & combination 0.625 mg/5 mg qd days 15–28. Prempro One 0.625 mg/0.2.5 mg tablet qd; can increase to 0.625/5 mg qd.	**Decreased levels/effects of:** anticoagulants, hydantoins. **Decreased levels/effects of estrogens:** hydantoins, barbiturates, rifampin. **Decreased levels/effects of progestin:** aminoglutethimide, rifampin. Drug-Lab Interaction The following tests may be affected by progestins: hepatic function, coagulation, thyroid, metyrapone, and endocrine function.	cramps, bloating, photosensitivity; urticaria, dermatitis, headache, dizziness, depression, edema, changes in libido, breast tenderness or enlargement. **Progestin:** Insomnia, somnolence, mental depression, rash, acne, melasma, photosensitivity, changes in weight, breakthrough bleeding, spotting, change in menstrual flow, amenorrhea, changes in cervical secretions, breast changes, masculinization of the female fetus, edema, cholestatic jaundice, hirsutism. Pharmacokinetics See individual drugs.	Precautions Use cautiously in those with hepatic or renal dysfunction; monitor serum calcium. Pregnancy Category: X Lactation Issues Excreted in breast milk. Use only if benefit clearly outweighs risk.
Other Combinations Femhrt tablets 5 mg ethinyl estradiol 1 mg norethindrone Activella tablets 1 mg estradiol 0.5 mg norethindrone Ortho-Prefest tablets 1 mg estradiol 1 mg estradiol/0.09 mg norqestimate (in combination) Combi Patch (Transdermal) 0.05 mg estradiol/0.14 mg norethindrone 0.05 mg estradiol/0.25 mg norethindrone acetato	Femhrt/Activella One tablet/day Ortho-Prefest: One pink tablet/day for 3 days, followed by 1 white tablet for 3 days Repeat regimen continuously without interruption. Combi Patch: Replace patch twice weekly. Advise women that monthly withdrawl bleeding often occurs.	Same as Premphase/Prempro above.	Same as Premphase/Prempro above.	Same as Premphase/Prempro above.

605.4 Estrogen/Androgen Combinations

Drug and Dosage Forms	Usual Dosage Range	Administration Issues and Drug-Drug Interactions	Common Adverse Drug Reactions (ADRs) and Pharmacokinetics	Contraindications, Pregnancy Category, and Lactation Issues
Estratest Tablets 1.25 mg esterified estrogens/2.5 mg methyltestosterone **Estratest H.S.** Tablets 0.625 mg esterified estrogens/1.25 mg methyltestosterone	**Moderate to severe vasomotor symptoms associated with menopause in those patients not improved by estrogen alone** 1 tablet Estratest *or* 1 to 2 tablets Estratest HS.	Administration Issues Administration should be cyclic (e.g. three wk on and one wk off). Attempts to discontinue or taper medication should be done at 3- to 6-month intervals. Drug-Drug Interactions **Increased levels/effects of:** corticosteroids, imipramine (increased paranoid symptoms). **Decreased levels/effects of:** hydantoins. **Decreased levels/effects of estrogens:** hydantoins, barbiturates, rifampin. **Variable effects:** may increase or decrease effects of anticoagulants.	ADRs Estrogen: Breakthrough bleeding, spotting, dysmenorrhea, PMS-like syndrome, amenorrhea, vaginal candidiasis, hemolytic uremic syndrome; endometrial cystic hyperplasia, nausea, vomiting, abdominal cramps, bloating, photosensitivity; urticaria, dermatitis, headache, dizziness, depression, edema, changes in libido, breast tenderness or enlargement. Methyltestosterone: Amenorrhea, other menstrual irregularities, virilization (deepening of voice, clitoral enlargement). Pharmacokinetics Hepatically metabolized.	Contraindications Hypersensitivity; breast cancer (some exceptions); active thrombophlebitis; thromboembolic disorders; estrogen-dependent neoplasia; undiagnosed abnormal genital bleeding; pregnancy; breast-feeding; presence of severe liver damage. Precautions Use cautiously in those with hepatic or renal dysfunction; monitor serum calcium. Pregnancy Category: X Lactation Issues Do not use.

605.5 Selective Estrogen Receptor Modulators

Drug and Dosage Forms	Usual Dosage Range	Administration Issues and Drug-Drug Interactions	Common Adverse Drug Reactions (ADRs) and Pharmacokinetics	Contraindications, Pregnancy Category, and Lactation Issues
Raloxifene Evista Tablets 60 mg	**Prevention and treatment of Osteoporosis in Postmenopausal Women:** 60 mg daily.	**Administration Issues** May be taken any time of day without regards to meals. Discontinue raloxifine at least 72 hr before periods of prolonged immobilization and avoid prolonged restrictions of movement during travel due to increased risk of venous thromboembolic events. Raloxifene is not effective in reducing hot flashed or flushes. Drug-Drug Interactions **Decreased levels/effects of:** warfarin (decreases seen in PT). **Decreased levels/effects of raloxifine:** ampicillin (though both can be given concurrently), cholestyramine (avoid coadministration).	ADRs Hot flashes, leg cramps, abdominal pain, nausea, weight gain, arthralgia. Pharmacokinetics $T_{1/2}$ = 32 h; undergoes extensive first-pass metabolism.	Contraindications Hypersensitivity; women who are or may become pregnant, women with an active history of thromboembolic events (DVT, PE). Pregnancy Category: X Lactation Issues Unknown if excreted in milk; however it is not recommended to give to nursing mothers.

606. Drugs for Osteoporosis

For Selective Estrogen Receptor Modulators see Section 605.5.

606.1 Biphosphonates

Drug and Dosage Forms	Usual Dosage Range	Administration Issues and Drug–Drug Interactions	Common Adverse Drug Reactions (ADRs) and Pharmacokinetics	Contraindications, Pregnancy Category, and Lactation Issues
Alendronate Fosamax Tablets 5 mg, 10 mg, 35 mg, 40 mg, 70 mg Oral solution 70 mg/bottle	**Treatment of Postmenopausal osteoporosis:** 10 mg qd or 70 mg once weekly. Mild renal impairment or elderly patients: No dosage adjustments necessary. **Prevention of osteoporosis** 35 mg once weekly or 5 mg qd. **Paget's disease:** 40 mg once daily for 6 months. May retreat the patient after 6 months of evaluation.	Administration Issues **Take on an empty stomach, at least 30 minutes before a meal. Drink a full glass of water only. Remain upright after taking medication for at least 30 minutes.** Drug–Drug Interactions **Increased levels/effects of:** aspirin (increased toxic effects to GI). **Decreased levels/effects of alendronate:** calcium supplements, antacids, vitamins (decrease absorption).	ADRs Flatulence, acid regurgitation, esophageal ulcer, dysphagia, abdominal distention, gastritis, musculoskeletal pain. Pharmacokinetics Plasma levels decrease by >95% after 6 hrs; bone $T_{1/2} > 10$ yr.	Contraindications Hypersensitivity; hypocalcemia; severe renal impairment. Precautions Use cautiously in those with active upper GI problems. Pregnancy Category: C Lactation Issues Unknown if excreted in milk; however it is not recommended to give to nursing mothers.
Etidronate Didronel Tablets 200 mg, 400 mg	**Paget's disease:** 5–10 mg/kg/d for not more than 6 months or 11–20 mg/kg/d for not more than 3 months. May retreat patients if needed after etidronate-free period of at least 90 days. **Heterotopic ossification:** Spinal cord injury: 20 mg/kg/d for 2 weeks followed by 10 mg/kg/d for 10 weeks. **Total hip replacement:** 20 mg/kg/d for 2 weeks for 1 month preoperatively then 20 mg/kg/d for 3 months postoperatively. **Unlabeled use: Postmenopausal Osteoporosis:** 400 mg/d for 1 week followed by several weeks of calcium therapy. This cyclical treatment is repeated every 3 months.	Administration Issues Take on an empty stomach, 2 hrs before a meal. Drink a full glass of water. Drug–Drug Interactions **Increased levels/effects of:** aspirin (increased toxic effects to GI). **Decreased levels/effects of etidronate:** calcium supplements, antacids (decrease absorption).	ADRs Diarrhea, nausea, flatulence, musculoskeletal pain, hypersensitivity reactions (rarely). Pharmacokinetics $T_{1/2} = 6$ h; bone $T_{1/2} > 90$ days.	Contraindications Hypersensitivity; hypocalcemia; severe renal impairment. Precautions Use cautiously in those with active upper GI problems. Pregnancy Category B Lactation Issues Unknown if excreted in milk; however, it is not recommended to give to nursing mothers. Pediatrics Safety/efficacy not established for children.

(*continues on next page*)

606.1 Biphosphonates *continued from previous page*

Drug and Dosage Forms	Usual Dosage Range	Administration Issues and Drug–Drug Interactions	Common Adverse Drug Reactions (ADRs) and Pharmacokinetics	Contraindications, Pregnancy Category, and Lactation Issues
Risedronate Actonel **Tablets** 5 mg, 30 mg, 35 mg	**Prevention and treatment of postmenopausal osteoporosis** 5 mg orally taken daily or one 35 mg tablet orally taken once weekly.	Administration Issues Take at least 30 minutes before the first food or drink of the day other than water. To facilitate delivery to the stomach, take while in an upright position with a full glass (6 to 8 oz; 180 to 240 mL) of plain water and avoid lying down for 30 minutes. Patients should receive supplemental calcium and vitamin D if dietary intake is inadequate. Take calcium supplements and calcium-, aluminum-, and magnesium-containing medications at a different time of the day to prevent interference with risedronate absorption. Drug-Drug Interactions Deceased effects of risedronate if given with calcium supplements or antacids.	ADRs Most Frequent: Upper GI irritations/disorders; angina, hypertension, diarrhea, nausea, anxiety, insomnia, neuralgia, abdominal pain, rash, flatulence, anemia, bruising, arthralgia, back pain, leg/muscle cramps, infections, influenza-like illness, pharyngitis, rhinitis, vasodilation. Pharmacokinetics Initial $T_{1/2} = 1.5$ h; Terminal exponential $T_{1/2} = 480$ h.	Contraindications/Warnings Hypersensitivity to bisphosphonates or any component of the products; hypocalcemia, inability to stand or sit upright for at least 30 minutes. Pregnancy Category: C Lactation Issues Exercise caution when administering risedronate to nursing mothers.
Tiludronate Sodium Skelid Tablets 240 mg (contains 200 mg tiludronic acid)	**Paget's disease** 400 mg single daily dose with 6 to 8 ounces plain water for 3 months. Do not remove tablets from foil strips until they are to be used.	Administration Issues Drink a full glass of water. Beverages other than plain water (including mineral water), food and some medications may reduce absorption of tiludronate. Do not take within 2 h of food. Take calcium or mineral supplements at least 2 h before or after tiludronate. Take antacids at least 2 h after taking tiludronate. Do not take within 2 h of indomethacin. Drug–Drug Interactions **Increased levels/effects of tiludronate:** indomethacin. **Decreased levels/effects of tiludronate:** calcium supplements, antacids (decrease absorption), aspirin (due to decreased bioavailability).	ADRs Vertigo, involuntary muscle contractions, anxiety, pruritus, increased sweating, dry mouth, gastritis, asthenia, flushing. Pharmacokinetics Bioavailability reduced by food.	Contraindications Hypersensitivity; hypocalcemia; severe renal impairment. Precautions Use cautiously in those with active upper GI problems. Pregnancy Category C Lactation Issues Unknown if excreted in milk; however it is not recommended to give to nursing mothers. Pediatrics Safety/efficacy not established for children.

606.2 Miscellaneous Agents for Osteoporosis

Drug and Dosage Forms	Usual Dosage Range	Administration Issues and Drug–Drug Interactions	Common Adverse Drug Reactions (ADRs) and Pharmacokinetics	Contraindications, Pregnancy Category, and Lactation Issues
Calcitonin Miacalcin Injection 200 IU/mL Nasal Spray 200 IU/activation	**Postmenopausal osteoporosis** Injection: 100 IU/d SC or IM Nasal: 200 IU/d Patients must also receive 1.5 g of calcium daily and 400 U/d of Vitamin D. **Paget's disease:** (Injection only) 100 IU/d SC or IM. May decrease to 50 IU/d or 100 IU every other day as a maintenance dose.	Administration Issues Test dose of 1 IU is given intracutaneously on inner aspect of the forearm. Site is observed for 15 minutes. Injection is given either subcutaneously or intramuscularly. Intranasal administration—alternate nostrils daily. Store both the injection and unopened bottle of nasal spray in the refrigerator. Once the nasal spray is opened, store at room temperature. Drug–Drug Interactions None known.	ADRs Nasal spray: rhinitis, nasal irritation, back pain. Injection: flu-like symptoms, polymyalgia, stiffness, dizziness, insomnia, anxiety, migraine, injection site reactions, flushing of face or hands, nausea with or without vomiting. Pharmacokinetics Injection or inhalation; metabolized to smaller inactive fragments primarily in the kidneys, blood, peripheral tissues; $T_{1/2} = 43$ min.	Contraindications Hypersensitivity. Precautions Monitor closely for acute hypersensitivity reactions. Antibody formation has occurred after 2–18 months of treatment in many patients—monitor for decreasing efficacy. Pregnancy Category: C Lactation Issues Safety for use is not established.
Teriparatide Forteo Injectable: 20 mcg	**Treatment of osteoporosis in men and women.** 20 mcg SQ daily for 24 months	Administration issues: For self-administration. Must be kept refrigerated. Clear, colorless liquid, available in pre-measured injection pens with a 28 day supply. Thigh or abdomen are desired injection sites. Should only take when the person is able to sit or lie down if transient hypotension is experienced. Do not use if solid particles or discoloration seen. Drug–Drug Interactions: No significant interactions. In co-administration of digoxin, caution must be used due to the rare possibility of hypercalcemia.	ADRs: Nausea, vomiting, constipation, muscle weakness, decreased energy, transient orthostatic hypotension. Pharmacokinetics: Peak serum concentrations in 30 minutes after SQ administration, declining to non-quantifiable levels within three hours. **Warning:** In both male and female rats given teriparatide there was an increase in the incidence of osteosarcoma that was dose and duration of use dependent.	Contraindications: Hypersensitivity; Not to be used in the presence of Paget's or other diseases of bone metabolism, or children or young adults with open epiphyses. Concurrent use of radiation affecting the bones. Pregnancy Category: C Lactation: No clinical studies conducted.

607. Thyroid Agents

607.1 Antithyroid Agents

Drug and Dosage Forms	Usual Dosage Range	Administration Issues and Drug–Drug Interactions	Common Adverse Drug Reactions (ADRs) and Pharmacokinetics	Contraindications, Pregnancy Category, and Lactation Issues
Methimazole Tapazole, generics Tablets 5 mg, 10 mg	**Hyperthyroidism:** 15 mg/d for mild disease; 30–40 mg/d for moderately severe disease; 60 mg/d for severe disease. Once Euthyroid: 5–15 mg/d Daily doses usually given in 3 divided doses every 8 h; single daily doses (i.e., 30 mg qd) produce similar therapeutic results and may be used in noncompliant patients. **Pediatrics:** 0.4 mg/kg/d given in 3 divided doses, initially. Reduce to 1/2 dose as a maintenance dose. Another regimen: 0.5–0.7 mg/kg/d in 3 divided doses initially. Reduce to 1/2–2/3 of initial dose when patient is euthyroid. Max dose is 30 mg/d.	Drug–Drug Interactions None known	ADRs (<1%) Agranulocytosis, paresthesias, neuritis, headache, drowsiness, nausea, vomiting, skin rash, urticaria, jaundice, hepatitis, nephritis, abnormal hair loss, arthralgia, myalgia, edema, drug fever. Pharmacokinetics 80–95% bioavailable; no protein binding; hepatically metabolized; $T_{1/2}$ = 6–13 h; renal elimination of metabolites.	Contraindications Hypersensitivity; nursing mothers. Precautions Monitor closely for signs of agranulocytosis Pregnancy Category: D Lactation Issues Excreted in breast milk. Nursing is contraindicated.
Propylthiouracil (PTU) various generics Tablets 50 mg	**Hyperthyroidism:** 300 mg/d in 3 divided doses given every 8 hrs, initially. For severe disease, may use 400–900 mg/d initially. Once euthyroid: 100–150 mg/d in 3 divided doses. **Pediatrics:** 6–10 yr.: 50–150 mg/d in 3 divided doses given q 8 h. ≥10 yr.: 150–300 mg/d in 3 divided doses q 8 h. Once euthyroid: based on patient response. Another regimen: 5–7 mg/kg/d in 3 divided doses q 8 h. Once euthyroid—1/3–2/3 of the initial dose.	Administration Issues Monitor closely for hepatotoxicity in children. Drug–Drug Interactions **Increased effect of:** anticoagulants.	ADRs (<1%) Agranulocytosis, paresthesias, neuritis, headache, drowsiness, nausea, vomiting, skin rash, urticaria, jaundice, hepatitis, nephritis, abnormal hair loss, arthralgia, myalgia, edema, drug fever. Pharmacokinetics 80–95% bioavailable; 75–80% protein bound; hepatically metabolized; $T_{1/2}$ = 1–2 hrs; 35% renal elimination of unchanged drug.	Contraindications Hypersensitivity; nursing mothers. Precautions Monitor closely for signs of agranulocytosis; monitor the prothrombin time and for bleeding. Pregnancy Category: D Lactation Issues Excreted in breast milk. Nursing is contraindicated.

607.2 Iodine Products

Drug and Dosage Forms	Usual Dosage Range	Administration Issues and Drug–Drug Interactions	Common Adverse Drug Reactions (ADRs) and Pharmacokinetics	Contraindications, Pregnancy Category, and Lactation Issues
Iodine Lugol's Solution, Thyro-Block Tablets 130 mg potassium iodide Solution 5% iodine and 10% potassium iodide	**As an adjunct to an antithyroid drug in hyperthyroid patients in preparation for thyroidectomy:** 2–6 drops of solution 3 times daily for 10 days prior to surgery. **For thyroid blocking in a radiation emergency:** 130 mg tablet daily. Pediatrics (<1 yr.): 65 mg (1/2 tablet) crushed daily.	Administration Issues Strong iodide solution should be diluted with water or fruit juice. Drug–Drug Interactions **Increased effects:** lithium (increased potential for hypothyroidism).	ADRs Skin rash, swelling of salivary glands, iodism (metallic taste, burning mouth and throat, sore teeth and gums, symptoms of a head cold and sometimes stomach upset and diarrhea), allergic reactions (fever, joint pain, swelling of face/body, severe shortness of breath requiring immediate medical attention). Pharmacokinetics Onset of action = 24 h; maximum effects attained after 10–15 days of continuous therapy; chronic administration leads to therapeutic effects that may persist for up to 6 weeks after the crisis has abated.	Contraindications Hypersensitivity Pregnancy Category: D Lactation Issues It is excreted in breast milk, but breastfeeding is not contraindicated.

607.3 Thyroid Hormones

Drug and Dosage Forms	Usual Dosage Range	Administration Issues and Drug–Drug Interactions	Common Adverse Drug Reactions (ADRs) and Pharmacokinetics	Contraindications, Pregnancy Category, and Lactation Issues
Levothyroxine (T4) Synthroid, various generics, Unithrid, Levoxyl Tablets 0.025 mg, 0.05 mg 0.075 mg, 0.088 mg 0.1 mg, 0.112 mg 0.125 mg, 0.137 mg 0.15 mg, 0.175 mg 0.2 mg, 0.3 mg	**Hypothyroidism: Must individualize dose:** 0.025–0.05 mg/d initially. May titrate by 0.025 mg/d every 2–3 weeks up to max of 0.3 mg/d (most do not need more than 0.2 mg/d). **Pediatrics:** 0–6 mos (8–10 mcg/kg): 25–50 mcg/d 6–12 mos (6–8 mcg/kg): 50–75 mcg/d 1–5 yr. (5–6 mcg/kg): 75–100 mcg/d 6–12 yr. (4–5 mcg/kg): 100–150 mcg/d >12 yr. (2–3 mcg/kg): >150 mcg/d **Thyroid suppression therapy:** 2.6 mcg/kg/d for 7-10 days.	Administration Issues Take on an empty stomach (enhances absorption of T4). Do not change from one brand to another. Drug–Drug Interactions **Increased levels/effects of:** anticoagulants, theophylline. **Decreased levels/effects of:** beta-blockers, digoxin. **Decreased levels/effects of thyroid hormone:** cholestyramine, colestipol, estrogens.	ADRs Very few adverse effects noted unless indicating hyperthyroidism or overdose. Pharmacokinetics T4 bioavailability = 48–79%; 99% protein bound; 35% peripheral conversion of T4 to T3; biological potency of T4 = 1; $T_{1/2}$ = 6–7 days.	Contraindications Hypersensitivity; acute myocardial infarction and thyrotoxicosis uncomplicated by hypothyroidism; when hypothyroidism and hypoadrenalism coexist unless hypoadrenalism is treated first. Precautions Use cautiously in those with cardiac disease, other endocrine disorders (unless the other disorders are appropriately treated first). Use smaller doses in those with myxedema. Monitor bone density following long term therapy. Pregnancy Category: A Lactation Issues Minimally excreted in breast milk. Use cautiously.

(continues on next page)

607.3 Thyroid Hormones *continued from previous page*

Drug and Dosage Forms	Usual Dosage Range	Administration Issues and Drug–Drug Interactions	Common Adverse Drug Reactions (ADRs) and Pharmacokinetics	Contraindications, Pregnancy Category, and Lactation Issues
Liothyronine (T3) Cytomel, various generics Tablets 5 mcg, 25 mcg, 50 mcg	**Hypothyroidism: Must individualize dose:** 25 mcg/d initially. May titrate by 12.5–25 mcg/d q 1–2 wk. up to 0.1 mg/d prn. **Congenital hypothyroidism:** 5 mcg/d initially. May titrate by 5 mcg/d q 3–4 days prn. **Simple goiter:** 5 mcg/d initially. May titrate by 5–10 mcg/d q 1–2 wk. up to 75 mcg/d. **Myxedema:** 5 mcg/d initially. May titrate by 5–10 mcg/d q 1–2 wk. up to 100 mg/d. When 25 mcg/d is reached, may titrate by 12.5–25 mcg/d q 1–2 wk. **Elderly or pediatrics:** 5 mcg/d initially. May titrate by 5 mcg/d q 1–2 wk. as needed/tolerated.	Administration Issues Do not change from one brand to another. Drug–Drug Interactions **Increased levels/effects of:** anticoagulants, theophylline. **Decreased levels/effects of:** beta-blockers, digoxin. **Decreased levels/effects of thyroid hormone:** cholestyramine, colestipol, estrogens.	ADRs Very few adverse effects noted unless indicating hyperthyroidism or overdose. Pharmacokinetics T3 bioavailability = 95%; 99% protein bound; peripheral metabolism; biologic potency of T3 = 4; $T_{1/2} \leq 2$ days.	Contraindications Hypersensitivity; acute myocardial infarction and thyrotoxicosis uncomplicated by hypothyroidism; when hypothyroidism and hypoadrenalism coexist unless hypoadrenalism is treated first. Precautions Use cautiously in those with cardiac disease, other endocrine disorders (unless the other disorders are appropriately treated first). Use smaller doses in those with myxedema. Monitor bone density following long term therapy. Pregnancy Category: A Lactation Issues Minimally excreted in breast milk. Use cautiously.
Liotrix (T4/T3 = 4/1) Euthyroid, Thyrolar Tablets Thyroid equivalent (T4/T3 content) 15 mg (12.5 mcg/3.1 mcg) 30 mg (25 mcg/6.25 mcg) 60 mg (50 mcg/12.5 mcg) 120 mg (100 mcg/25 mcg) 180 mg (150 mcg/37.5 mcg)	**Hypothyroidism: Must individualize dose:** 30 mg/d of thyroid equivalent initially. May titrate by 15 mg/d q 2–3 wk. Maintenance doses range from 60–120 mg/d, rarely exceed 180 mg/d. **Myxedema:** Initially, 15 mg/d. **Pediatrics** (dose based on T4): 0–6 mos (8–10 mcg/kg): 25–50 mcg/d 6–12 mos (6–8 mcg/kg): 50–75 mcg/d 1–5 yr. (5–6 mcg/kg): 75–100 mcg/d 6–12 yr. (4–5 mcg/kg): 100–150 mcg/d >12 yr. (2-3 mcg/kg): >150 mcg/d	Administration Issues Take on an empty stomach (enhances absorption of T4). Do not change from one brand to another. Drug–Drug Interactions **Increased levels/effects of:** anticoagulants, theophylline. **Decreased levels/effects of:** beta-blockers, digoxin. **Decreased levels/effects of thyroid hormone:** cholestyramine, colestipol, estrogens.	ADRs Very few adverse effects noted unless indicating hyperthyroidism or overdose. Pharmacokinetics **T4:** T4 bioavailability = 48–79%; 99% protein bound; 35% peripheral conversion of T4 to T3; biological potency of T4 = 1; $T_{1/2}$ = 6–7 days. **T3:** T3 bioavailability = 95%; 99% protein bound; peripheral metabolism; biologic potency of T3 = 4; $T_{1/2} \leq 2$ days.	Contraindications Hypersensitivity; acute myocardial infarction and thyrotoxicosis uncomplicated by hypothyroidism; when hypothyroidism and hypoadrenalism coexist unless hypoadrenalism is treated first. Precautions Use cautiously in those with cardiac disease, other endocrine disorders (unless the other disorders are appropriately treated first). Use smaller doses in those with myxedema. Monitor bone density following long term therapy.

				Pregnancy Category: A Lactation Issues Minimally excreted in breast milk. Use cautiously.
Thyroglobulin (T4/T3 = 2.5/1) Proloid Tablets 30 mg, 60 mg, 90 mg, 120 mg, 180 mg	**Hypothyroidism: Must individualize dose:** 30 mg/d initially. May titrate by 15 mg/d q 2–3 weeks as needed. Maintenance doses range from 60–120 mg/d, rarely exceed 180 mg/d. **Myxedema:** Initially, 15 mg/d. **Pediatrics:** 0–6 mos (4.8–6 mg/kg): 15–30 mg/d 6–12 mos (3.6–4.8 mg/kg): 30–45 mg/d 1–5 yr. (3–3.6 mg/kg): 45–60 mg/d 6–12 yr. (2.4–3 mg/kg): 60–90 mg/d >12 yr. (1.2–1.8 mg/kg): >90 mg/d	Administration Issues Take on an empty stomach (enhances absorption of T4). Do not change from one brand to another. Drug–Drug Interactions: **Increased levels/effects of:** anticoagulants, theophylline. **Decreased levels/effects of:** beta-blockers, digoxin. **Decreased levels/effects of thyroid hormone:** cholestyramine, colestipol, estrogens.	ADRs Very few adverse effects noted unless indicating hyperthyroidism or overdose. Pharmacokinetics **T4:** T4 bioavailability = 48–79%; 99% protein bound; 35% peripheral conversion of T4 to T3; biological potency of T4 = 1; $T_{1/2}$ = 6–7 days. **T3:** T3 bioavailability = 95%; 99% protein bound; peripheral metabolism; biologic potency of T3 = 4; $T_{1/2} \leq 2$ days.	Contraindications Hypersensitivity; acute myocardial infarction and thyrotoxicosis uncomplicated by hypothyroidism; when hypothyroidism and hypoadrenalism coexist unless hypoadrenalism is treated first. Precautions Use cautiously in those with cardiac disease, other endocrine disorders (unless the other disorders are appropriately treated first). Use smaller doses in those with myxedema. Monitor bone density following long term therapy. Pregnancy Category: A Lactation Issues Minimally excreted in breast milk. Use cautiously.
Thyroid Desiccated Thyroid USP (T4/T3 = 2–5/1) Armour Thyroid, various generics Tablets 15 mg, 30 mg, 60 mg, 90 mg, 120 mg, 180 mg, 240 mg, 300 mg **Thyroid Strong (T4/T3 = 3.1/1) (each 60 mg is equivalent to 90 mg)** Tablets 30 mg, 60 mg, 120 mg Tablets, sugar coated 30 mg, 60 mg, 120 mg, 180 mg	**Hypothyroidism: Must individualize dose:** 30 mg/d initially. May titrate by 15 mg/d q 2–3 wk as needed. Maintenance doses range from 60–120 mg/d, rarely exceed 180 mg/d. **Myxedema:** Initially, 15 mg/d. **Pediatrics:** 0–6 mos (4.8–6 mg/kg): 15–30 mg/d 6–12 mos (3.6–4.8 mg/kg): 30–45 mg/d 1–5 yr. (3–3.6 mg/kg): 45–60 mg/d	Administration Issues Take on an empty stomach (enhances absorption of T4). Do not change from one brand to another. Drug–Drug Interactions **Increased levels/effects of:** anticoagulants, theophylline. **Decreased levels/effects of:** beta-blockers, digoxin.	ADRs Very few adverse effects noted unless indicating hyperthyroidism or overdose. Pharmacokinetics T4 bioavailability = 48–79%; 99% protein bound; 35% peripheral conver	Contraindications Hypersensitivity; acute myocardial infarction and thyrotoxicosis uncomplicated by hypothyroidism; when hypothyroidism and hypoadrenalism coexist unless hypoadrenalism is treated first. Precautions Use cautiously in those with cardiac disease, other endocrine disorders (unless the other disorders are appropriately treated first). Use smaller doses in those with myxedema. Monitor bone density following long term therapy. Pregnancy Category: A

(continues on next page)

607.3 Thyroid Hormones *continued from previous page*

Drug and Dosage Forms	Usual Dosage Range	Administration Issues and Drug–Drug Interactions	Common Adverse Drug Reactions (ADRs) and Pharmacokinetics	Contraindications, Pregnancy Category, and Lactation Issues
Thyroid Desiccated Thyroid USP (**T4/T3 = 2–5/1**) ***cont.*** **Thyrar** (**T4/T3 = 2–5/1**) **(Bovine thyroid)** Tablets 30 mg, 60 mg, 120 mg **S-P-T** (**T4/T3 = 2–5/1**) **(pork thyroid)** Capsules 60 mg, 120 mg, 180 mg, 300 mg	6–12 yr. (2.4–3 mg/kg): 60–90 mg/d >12 yr. (1.2–1.8 mg/kg): >90 mg/d	**Decreased levels/effects of thyroid hormone:** cholestyramine, colestipol, estrogens.	sion of T4 to T3; biologic potency of T4 = 1; $T_{1/2}$ = 6–7 days.	Lactation Issues Minimally excreted in breast milk. Use cautiously.

608. Gonadotropin-Releasing Hormones

Drug and Dosage Forms	Usual Dosage Range	Administration Issues and Drug–Drug Interactions	Common Adverse Drug Reactions (ADRs) and Pharmacokinetics	Contraindications, Pregnancy Category, and Lactation Issues
Gonadorelin acetate Factrel Powder for injection 100 mcg/vial 500 mcg/vial	**Primary hypothalamic amenorrhea:** 100 mcg SC or IV. Perform the test in the early follicular phase (days 1–7) of the menstrual cycle	Administration Issues Reconstitute as directed Drug Interactions **Decreased levels/effects:** oral contraceptives, digoxin, phenothiazines, dopamine antagonists. **Increased levels/effect:** androgens, estrogens, progestins, glucocorticoids, spironolactone, levodopa.	ADRs Pain at site of injection, flushing, headache, nausea, abdominal discomfort.	Contraindications Hypersensitivity Pregnancy Category: B
Nafarelin acetate Synarel Nasal solution 2 mg/ml	**Treatment of endometriosis:** 1 spray (200 mcg) in 1 nostril each morning and the other nostril each evening starting on days 2–4 of menstrual cycle for 6 months.	Administration Issues Begin treatment between days 2–4 of menstrual cycle; usually menstruation will stop (as well as ovulation) but is not a reliable form of contraception and use of a nonhormonal contraceptive is recommended. Full compliance is very important; do not use a nasal decongestant for at least 30 minutes after using nafarelin.	ADRs Headache, emotional lability, acne, hot flashes, decreased libido, decreased breast size, vaginal dryness, myalgia, nasal irritation, insomnia, rash, shortness of breath. Pharmacokinetics Not absorbed from GI tract.	Contraindications Hypersensitivity to GnRH, GnRH-agonist analogs; undiagnosed abnormal vaginal bleeding, pregnancy, lactation. Pregnancy Category: X Lactation Issues Nursing is contraindicated.

700. RESPIRATORY AGENTS

701. Respiratory Inhalants

701.1 Anticholinergics

Drug and Dosage Forms	Usual Dosage Range	Administration Issues	Common Adverse Drug Reactions (ADRs) and Pharmacokinetics	Contraindications, Pregnancy Category, and Lactation Issues
Ipratropium Atrovent Aerosol 18 mcg/dose Solution for Inhalation 0.02% Nasal Spray 0.03%, 0.06%	**Bronchospasm associated with chronic obstructive pulmonary disease:** **adults:** initial dose: 2 inhalations qid maximum dose: 12 inhalations/day **children** <12y: 1-2 puffs INH tid-qid. Alternate 250 mcg NEB q6-8h. **perennial rhinitis (0.03% nasal spray):** 2 sprays bid to tid. **rhinorrhea associated with the common cold (0.06% nasal spray):** 2 sprays tid to qid.	Administration Issues Nasal spray pump requires initial priming with 7 actuations; safety and efficacy beyond 4 days with the common cold have not been established. For children, consider use of mask/spacer with MDI; may mix neb solution with albuterol or metaproterenol if used within 1h.	ADRs **Aerosol/inhalation solution:** cough; dry mouth; nervousness; agitation; dizziness; headache; GI upset; palpitations; urinary retention; constipation; worsening narrow angle glaucoma. **Nasal spray:** headache; epistaxis; pharyngitis; GI upset; nasal dryness/irritation; dry mouth; hoarseness; cough. Pharmacokinetics Poorly absorbed; protein binding < 9%; metabolized to inactive metabolites; $t_{1/2} = 1.6$ h.	Contraindications Hypersensitivity to ipratropium, atropine, soya lecithin or related products (soya bean or peanut). Pregnancy Category: B Lactation Issues It is not known if ipratropium is excreted in breast milk; use caution when administering to a nursing mother.

701.2 Corticosteroids

Drug and Dosage Forms	Usual Dosage Range	Administration Issues	Common Adverse Drug Reactions (ADRs) and Pharmacokinetics	Contraindications, Pregnancy Category, and Lactation Issues
Beclomethasone Aerosol Beclovent, Vanceril 42 mcg/dose Vanceril Double Strength (84 mcg/dose) Becloforte Inhaler 250 mcg/dose	**Bronchial asthma in patients requiring chronic treatment with corticosteroids** **adults:** 2 inhalations tid to qid or 4 inhalations bid. Maximum dose: 20 inhalations (840 mcg) daily. **children 6–12 y:** 1–2 inhalations tid to qid or 2–4 inhalations bid. Maximum dose: 10 inhalations (420 mcg) daily.	Administration Issues Use bronchodilator therapy several minutes before using inhaled steroid therapy to enhance penetration; use as preventative therapy only; not to be used to abort an acute attack. Use spacer with children <8y.	ADRs Throat irritation; hoarseness; coughing; dry mouth; oral thrush; adrenal suppression may occur with large doses over a prolonged period of time; rare cases of immediate and delayed hypersensitivity reactions reported. Pharmacokinetics Systemic absorption occurs rapidly; principal route of elimination is via feces.	Contraindications Hypersensitivity to steroids; systemic fungal infections. Pregnancy Category: C Lactation Issues It is not known whether inhaled steroids are excreted in breast milk; decide whether to discontinue nursing or the drug.

Budesonide Pulmicort Turbuhaler 200 mcg/dose Rhinocort Turbuhaler 100 mcg/dose **Pulmicort Respules** Inhalation suspension 0.25 mg/2mL 0.50 mg/2mL	**Bronchial asthma in patients requiring chronic treatment with corticosteroids** For adults and children, starting and maintenance doses depend upon patient's previous therapy (bronchodilators alone, inhaled corticosteroids, oral steroids). **adults:** 1-2 puffs INH qd-bid, max 4 puffs bid. **children:** 1 puff INH bid, max 2 puffs INH bid.	Administration Issues Use bronchodilator therapy several minutes before using inhaled steroid therapy to enhance penetration; use as preventative therapy only; not to be used to abort an acute attack; safety/efficacy have not been established in children <6 years. Rinse mouth with water after each dose.	ADRs Throat irritation; hoarseness; coughing; dry mouth; oral thrush; adrenal suppression may occur with large doses over a prolonged period of time; rare cases of immediate and delayed hypersensitivity reactions reported. Pharmacokinetics Systemic absorption occurs rapidly; principal route of elimination is via feces.	Contraindications Hypersensitivity to steroids; systemic fungal infections. Pregnancy Category: C Lactation Issues It is not known whether inhaled steroids are excreted in breast milk; decide whether to discontinue nursing or the drug.
Flunisolide AeroBid, AeroBid-M Aerosol 250 mcg/dose	**Bronchial asthma in patients requiring chronic treatment with corticosteroids** **adults:** 2 inhalations bid Maximum dose: 8 inhalations daily **children 6–15 years:** 2 inhalations bid Maximum dose: 4 inhalations daily	Administration Issues Use bronchodilator therapy several minutes before using inhaled steroid therapy to enhance penetration; use as preventative therapy only; not to be used to abort an acute attack; safety/efficacy have not been established in children <6 years.	ADRs Throat irritation; hoarseness; coughing; dry mouth; oral thrush. Pharmacokinetics Systemic absorption = 40%; rapidly undergoes first pass metabolism; $T_{1/2}$ = 1.8 h.	Contraindications Hypersensitivity to steroids; systemic fungal infections. Pregnancy Category: C Lactation Issues It is not known whether inhaled steroids are excreted in breast milk; decide whether to discontinue nursing or the drug.
Fluticasone Flovent Aerosol 44 mcg/dose, 110 mcg/dose, 220 mcg/dose **Flovent Rotadisk** Powder for inhalation 50 mcg/actuation, 100 mcg/actuation, 250 mcg/actuation **Flovent Diskus** Powder for Intialation 50 mcg/actuation, 100 mcg/actuation, 250 mcg/actuation (see Advair Diskus for combination product.)	**Bronchial asthma in patients requiring chronic treatment with corticosteroids** For the maintenance treatment of asthma as prophylactic therapy in patients 4 years of age or older (Flovent Rotadisk and Flovent Diskes) and ≥ 12 years (Flovent) **adults and adolescents > 12 yr.:** Previous therapy with bronchodilators alone: 88 mcg bid initially, increase prn to a max of 440 mcg bid Previous therapy with Inhaled corticosteroids: 88–220 mcg bid initially, increase prn to max of 440 mcg bid	Administration Issues Use bronchodilator therapy several minutes before using inhaled steroid therapy to enhance penetration; use as preventative therapy only; not to be used to abort an acute attack. Rinse mouth after use.	ADRs Throat irritation; hoarseness; coughing; dry mouth; oral thrush, nasal congestion, nasal discharge, headache, upper respiratory infection. Pharmacokinetics $T_{1/2}$ = 7.8 hours.	Contraindications Hypersensitivity to steroids; systemic fungal infections. Pregnancy Category: C Lactation Issues It is not known whether inhaled steroids are excreted in breast milk; decide whether to discontinue nursing or the drug.

(continues on next page)

701.2 Corticosteroids *continued from previous page*

Drug and Dosage Forms	Usual Dosage Range	Administration Issues	Common Adverse Drug Reactions (ADRs) and Pharmacokinetics	Contraindications, Pregnancy Category, and Lactation Issues
Fluticasone *cont.*	Previous therapy with oral corticosteroids: 880 mcg bid (initial and max dose) **Children:** <4 not recommended. 4-11y, use rotadisk. previously on bronchodilator alone or previously on INH corticosteroids 50 mcg bid, max 100 mcg bid.			
Triamcinolone Azmacort Aerosol 100 mcg/dose	**Bronchial asthma in patients requiring chronic treatment with corticosteroids** **adults:** 2 inhalations tid to qid Alternate: 4 puffs INH bid. Maximum dose: 16 inhalations daily **children 6–12 years:** 1–2 inhalations tid to qid. Maximum dose: 12 inhalations daily	Administration Issues Use bronchodilator therapy several minutes before using inhaled steroid therapy to enhance penetration; use as preventative therapy only; not to be used to abort an acute attack; safety/efficacy have not been established in children <6 years. Rinse mouth after use.	ADRs Throat irritation; hoarseness; coughing; dry mouth; oral thrush; adrenal suppression may occur with large doses over a prolonged period of time. Pharmacokinetics Rapidly absorbed from lung; rapidly metabolized; mainly eliminated via feces.	Contraindications Hypersensitivity to steroids; systemic fungal infections. Pregnancy Category: D Lactation Issues It is not known whether inhaled steroids are excreted in breast milk; decide whether to discontinue nursing or the drug.

701.3 Miscellaneous Inhalants

Drug and Dosage Forms	Usual Dosage Range	Administration Issues	Common Adverse Drug Reactions (ADRs) and Pharmacokinetics	Contraindications, Pregnancy Category, and Lactation Issues
Cromolyn Intal, Nasalcrom, generics Capsules for Inhalation 20 mg/2 mL Nebulizer Solution 20 mg/amp Aerosol 800 mcg/dose Nasal Solution 5.2 mg/dose	**Severe asthma (nebulizer solution, capsules, aerosol):** 20 mg inhaled capsule or nebulizer solution or 2 sprays of aerosol qid. **Prevention of exercise-induced asthma (nebulizer solution, capsules, aerosol):** 20 mg inhaled capsule or nebulizer solution or 2 sprays of aerosol no more than 1 hour before exercise.	Administration Issues Must be used regularly to achieve benefit; safety and efficacy have not been established in children < 5 years of age (inhalation capsules/aerosol), < 2 years of age (nebulizer solution) and < 6 years of age (nasal solution).	**ADRs** **inhalation capsules/aerosol:** lacrimation; swollen parotid gland; urinary frequency; dizziness; headache; rash. **nebulizer solution:** cough; wheezing; nasal congestion/ itching; sneezing; epistaxis. **nasal solution:** sneezing; headache; nasal stinging/ burning/irritation; bad taste in mouth; epistaxis.	Contraindications Hypersensitivity to cromolyn. Pregnancy Category:B Lactation Issues It not known if cromolyn is excreted in breast milk; use caution when administering to a nursing mother.

	Allergic rhinitis (nasal spray) 1 spray in each nostril 3–6 times daily > 2 years: 20 mg neb qid.		Pharmacokinetics 7–8% absorbed from the lung; poorly absorbed from the GI tract.	
Fluticasone/ salmeterol Advair Diskus Powder for Inhalation 100 mcg fluticasone/50 mcg salmeterol 250 mcg fluticasone/50 mcg salmeterol 500 mcg fluticasone/50 mcg salmeterol	**For the long-term, twice-daily maintenance treatment of asthma in patients ≥ 12 years of age. If symptoms arise in the period between doses, administer an inhaled, short-acting beta$_2$-agonist for immediate relief.** **adults and children ≥ 12 y:** Start with 100/50 mcg bid (morning and evening, ≈ 12 h apart), if not on inhaled steroid. Use 100/50 to 500/50 mcg 1 inhalation bid if on other inhaled steroids. More frequent administration or a higher number of inhalations of the prescribed strength is not recommended, as some patients are more likely to experience adverse effects with higher doses of salmeterol. **Patients who are receiving fluticasone propionate/salmeterol twice daily should not use salmeterol for prevention of exercise-induced bronchospasm, or for any other reason.**	Administration Issues Administer by the orally inhaled route only. The maximum recommended dose of fluticasone propionate/salmeterol is 500 mcg/50 mcg twice daily. Taper to lowest effective dose Advise patients to rinse mouth after inhalation. Not indicated for the relief of acute bronchospasm. Do not use fluticasone propionate/salmeterol for transferring patients from systemic corticosteroid therapy. Drug Interactions Avoid other sympathomimetics (except short-acting bronchodilators) during or within 2 weeks of MAOIs, tricyclic antidepressants (increased cardiac effects). Antagonized by beta blockers. Use with caution with K+ depleting diuretics. Potentiated by CYP 3A4 inhibitors.	ADRs Bronchospasm, laryngospasm, angioedema, adrenal suppression, ventricular arrhythmias, headache, sinusitis, GI upset.	Contraindications Hypersensitivity to any components, status asthmaticus, pulmonary TB, arrhythmias, caution if CV disease, DM, seizure disorder. Pregnancy:C Lactation Issues Safety in nursing infants is unknown. Use with caution in nursing mothers.
Ipratropium Bromide/ Albuterol Sulfate Combivent, DuoNeb Aerosol Each actuation delivers 18 mcg ipratropium bromide and 103 mcg albuterol sulfate (equivalent to 90 mcg albuterol base) Inhalation solution 0.5 mg ipratropium bromide and 3 mg albuterol sulfate (equivalent to 2.5 mg albuterol base)	**For use in patients with chronic obstructive pulmonary disease (COPD) dh a regular aerosol bronchodilator who continue to have evidence of bronchospasm and require a second bronchodilator** **Combivent:** The recommended dose is 2 inhalations 4 times a day. Patients may take additional inhalations as required; however, advise the patient not to exceed 12 in 24 hours.	Administration Issues Shake well before using. Administer in COPD when a second aerosol bronchodilator is needed.	ADRs (serious) Paradoxical bronchospasm, arrhythmias. Common ADRs Bronchitis, cough, bronchospasm, headache, dyspnea, pharyngitis, URI, dry mouth, nausea, dizziness. Pharmacokinetics Anticholinergic plus beta 2 agonist properties; antagonized by beta blockers.	Contraindications Hypersensitivity to drug; caution if CV disease, arrhythmias, hypertension, DM, seizure disorder, BPH or bladder neck disorders, angle closure glaucoma. Extreme caution within 2 weeks of MAOIs or tricyclic antidepressants (increased cardiovascular. effects) Caution with other anticholinergics sympathomimetics, drugs that lower serum potassium. Pregnancy:C Lactation Issues Safety in nursing infants is unknown. Use with caution in nursing mothers.

(continues on next page)

701.3 Miscellaneous Inhalants *continued from previous page*

Drug and Dosage Forms	Usual Dosage Range	Administration Issues	Common Adverse Drug Reactions (ADRs) and Pharmacokinetics	Contraindications, Pregnancy Category, and Lactation Issues
Ipratropium Bromide/ Albuterol Sulfate *cont.*	**DuoNeb:** The recommended dose is one 3 mL vial administered 4 times/day via nebulization with up to 2 additional 3 mL doses allowed per day, if needed. Administer via jet nebulizer connected to an air compressor with an adequate air flow, equipped with mouthpiece or suitable face mask.			
Nedocromil Tilade Aerosol 1.75 mg/dose	**Asthma:** **adults and children > 6 y:** 2 inhalations qid	Administration Issues Must be used regularly to achieve benefit; safety and efficacy have not been established in children < 6 of age.	ADRs Cough; pharyngitis; rhinitis; bronchospasm; dry mouth; unpleasant taste; GI upset; dizziness; headache. Pharmacokinetics Poorly absorbed; protein binding = 89%.	Contraindications Hypersensitivity to nedocromil. Pregnancy Category:B Lactation Issues It not known if nedocromil is excreted in breast milk; use caution when administering to a nursing mother.
Dornase Alfa Pulmozyme Solution for Inhalation 1 mg/mL (2.5 mL)	**Cystic fibrosis** **adults and children > 5 y:** 2.5 mg inhaled qd to bid	Administration Issues Clinical efficacy documented with the use of the following nebulizers: Hudson T Up-draft II, Marquest Acorn II in conjunction with Pulmo-Aide compressor, Pari LC Jet in conjunction with the PARI PRONEB compressor; safety and efficacy < 5 y have not been established.	ADRs Voice alteration; pharyngitis; laryngitis; rash; cough. Pharmacokinetics Poorly absorbed.	Contraindications Hypersensitivity to domase or Chinese Hamster Ovary cell products. Pregnancy Category:B Lactation Issues It not known if domase is excreted in breast milk; use caution when administering to a nursing mother.

702. Bronchodilators

702.1 Sympathomimetics

Drug and Dosage Forms	Usual Dosage Range	Administration Issues and Drug–Drug Interactions	Common Adverse Drug Reactions (ADRs) and Pharmacokinetics	Contraindications, Pregnancy Category, and Lactation Issues
Albuterol Proventil, Ventolin, generics Tablets 2 mg, 4 mg Extended Release Tablets 4 mg, 8 mg Aerosol 90 mcg/dose Solution for Inhalation 0.083%, 0.5%, 0.63 mg/3 mL, 1.25 mg/3 mL Capsules for Inhalation 200 mcg (Ventolin Rotacaps) Syrup 2 mg/5 mL	**Asthma/bronchospasm:** aerosol **adults and children > 12 y:** 1–2 inhalations q 4–6 hours **2–12 y:** 10–15 kg: 1.25 mg > 15 kg: 2.5 mg solution for inhalation **adults and children > 12 y:** 2.5 mg tid to qid 10–15 kg: 1.25 mg bid-tid by NEB > 15 kg: 2.5 mg bid-tid by NEB capsules for inhalation **adults and children > 14yr:** 200–400 mcg q 4–6 hours tablets and syrup **adults and children > 14 y:** 2–4 mg tid to qid; max dose: 32 mg daily **children 6–14 y:** 2 mg tid to qid; max dose: 24 mg daily **children 2–6 y:** 0.1 mg/kg tid; max dose: 12 mg daily extended release tablets **adults and children > 12 y:** 4–8 mg q 12 hours; maximum dose: 32 mg daily **Prevention of exercise-induced asthma:** **adults and children > 12 y:** 2 inhalations 15 minutes prior to exercise	Administration Issues Shake well before using; allow one full minute between inhalations; safety and efficacy have not been established in children < 12 years (inhalation, extended release tablets), < 6 years (tablets), < 2 years (syrup). Drug–Drug Interactions Albuterol may decrease serum **digoxin** concentrations; increased risk of cardiac toxicity when given with theophylline.	ADRs Palpitations; tachycardia; anxiety; irritability; tremor; GI upset; cough; dry mouth; hoarseness; flushing; headache. Pharmacokinetics (Aerosol) onset = 5 minutes; duration = 3–8 hours; (tablets) onset = 30 minutes; duration = 4–8 h.	Contraindications Hypersensitivity to beta adrenergic agents; cardiac arrhythmias; narrow angle glaucoma. Pregnancy Category: C Lactation Issues It is not known if albuterol is excreted in breast milk; either the drug or the nursing should be discontinued.

(continues on next page)

702.1 Sympathomimetics *continued from previous page*

Drug and Dosage Forms	Usual Dosage Range	Administration Issues and Drug–Drug Interactions	Common Adverse Drug Reactions (ADRs) and Pharmacokinetics	Contraindications, Pregnancy Category, and Lactation Issues
Ephedrine Capsules 25 mg, 50 mg	**Asthma:** **adults:** 25–50 mg bid to tid **children:** 3 mg/kg/day in 4–6 divided doses	Administration Issues Do not exceed prescribed dosage. If GI upset occurs, take with food. Drug–Drug Interactions Increased risk of cardiac toxicity when given with **theophylline.**	ADRs Palpitations; tachycardia; anxiety; irritability; tremor; GI upset; cough; dry mouth; hoarseness; flushing; headache. Pharmacokinetics Onset = 60 minutes; duration = 3–5 h.	Contraindications Hypersensitivity to beta adrenergic agents; cardiac arrhythmias; narrow angle glaucoma. Pregnancy Category: C Lactation Issues It is not known if ephedrine is excreted in breast milk; either the drug or nursing should be discontinued.
Epinephrine Adrenalin, Primatene Mist, Bronkaid Mist Solution for Inhalation 1:100, 1:1,000, 1.125%, 1% Aerosol 0.35 mg, 0.5%, 0.2 mg	**Asthma/bronchospasm:** aerosol 1–2 inhalations q 4–6 h solution for inhalation 1 treatment q 4–6 h with 8–15 gtts in nebulizer reservoir	Administration Issues Shake well before using; allow one full minute between inhalations. Drug–Drug Interactions Increased risk of cardiac toxicity when given with **theophylline.**	ADRs Palpitations; tachycardia; anxiety; irritability; tremor; GI upset; cough; dry mouth; hoarseness; flushing; headache. Pharmacokinetics Onset = 1–5 minutes; duration = 1–3 h.	Contraindications Hypersensitivity to beta adrenergic agents; cardiac arrhythmias; narrow angle glaucoma. Pregnancy Category: C Lactation Issues Epinephrine is excreted in breast milk; either the drug or nursing should be discontinued.
Metaproterenol Alupent, generics Tablets 10 mg, 20 mg Syrup 10 mg/5 mL Aerosol 0.65 mg/dose Solution for Inhalation 0.4%, 0.6%, 5%	**Asthma/bronchospasm:** **adults and children > 12 yr:** inhaler: 2–3 inhalation q 3–4 h; maximum dose: 12 inhalations daily solution for inhalation: adults: 0.2–0.3 mL diluted in 2.5 mL saline tid-qid children: < 6y not recommended 6–12y: 0.1–0.2 mL diluted to 3 mL in saline tid-qid tablets **adults and children > 9 y.:** 20 mg tid to qid **children 6–9 y:** 10 mg tid to qid	Administration Issues Shake well before using; allow one full minute between inhalations; safety and efficacy have not been established in children < 6 years. Drug–Drug Interactions Increased risk of cardiac toxicity when given with **theophylline.**	ADRs Palpitations; tachycardia; anxiety; irritability; tremor; GI upset; cough; dry mouth; hoarseness; flushing; headache. Pharmacokinetics Onset = 5–30 minutes; duration = 2–6 h.	Contraindications Hypersensitivity to beta adrenergic agents; cardiac arrhythmias; narrow angle glaucoma. Pregnancy Category: C Lactation Issues It is not known if metaproterenol is excreted in breast milk; either the drug or the nursing should be discontinued.

	<u>syrup</u> **children < 6 y:** 1.3–2.6 mg/kg/day in divided doses			
Pirbuterol Maxair <u>Aerosol</u> 0.2 mg/dose	**<u>Asthma/bronchospasm</u>** **adults and children > 12 y:** 1–2 inhalations q 4–6 h maximum dose: 12 inhalations daily	<u>Administration Issues</u> Shake well before using; allow one full minute between inhalations; safety and efficacy have not been established in children < 12 years. <u>Drug–Drug Interactions</u> Increased risk of cardiac toxicity when given with **theophylline.**	<u>ADRs</u> Palpitations; tachycardia; anxiety; irritability; tremor; GI upset; cough; dry mouth; hoarseness; flushing; headache. <u>Pharmacokinetics</u> Onset within 5 minutes; duration =5 h.	<u>Contraindications</u> Hypersensitivity to beta adrenergic agents; cardiac arrhythmias; narrow angle glaucoma. <u>Pregnancy Category: C</u> <u>Lactation Issues</u> It is not known if metaproterenol is excreted in breast milk; either the drug or the nursing should be discontinued.
Salmeterol Serevent <u>Aerosol</u> 25 mcg/dose <u>Diskus</u> 50 mcg/dose (see Advair Disks for combination product)	**<u>Asthma/bronchospasm:</u>** <u>Aerosol:</u> 1–2 inhalations bid <u>Diskus:</u> 1 inhalation bid **<u>exercise-induced bronchospasm:</u>** <u>Aerosol:</u> 2 inhalations 30–60 minutes before exercise **<u>COPD:</u>** <u>Aerosol:</u> 1–2 inhalations bid	<u>Administration Issues</u> Shake well before using; allow one full minute between inhalations; should not be used for relief of acute asthmatic symptoms; safety and efficacy have not been established in children < 4 years. Do not exceed 4 inhalations per day of the aerosol product. <u>Drug–Drug Interactions</u> Increased risk of cardiac toxicity when given with **theophylline.**	<u>ADRs</u> Palpitations; tachycardia; anxiety; irritability; tremor; GI upset; cough; dry mouth; hoarseness; flushing; headache. <u>Pharmacokinetics</u> Onset = 20 minutes; duration = 12 hours.	<u>Contraindications</u> Hypersensitivity to beta adrenergic agents; cardiac arrhythmias; narrow angle glaucoma. <u>Pregnancy Category: C</u> <u>Lactation Issues</u> It is not known if salmeterol is excreted in breast milk; either the drug or nursing should be discontinued.
Terbutaline Brethine, Bricanyl <u>Tablets</u> 2.5 mg, 5 mg <u>Aerosol</u> 0.2 mg/dose	**<u>Asthma/bronchospasm:</u>** <u>aerosol</u> **adults and children > 12 y:** 1–2 inhalations q 4–6 h <u>tablets</u> **adults and children > 15 y:** 2.5–5 mg tid; maximum dose: 15 mg daily **children 12–15 y:** 2.5 mg tid maximum dose: 7.5 mg daily	<u>Administration Issues</u> Shake well before using; allow one full minute between inhalations; safety and efficacy have not been established in children < 12 years. <u>Drug–Drug Interactions</u> Increased risk of cardiac toxicity when given with **theophylline.**	<u>ADRs</u> Palpitations; tachycardia; anxiety; irritability; tremor; GI upset; cough; dry mouth; hoarseness; flushing; headache. <u>Pharmacokinetics (aerosol)</u> onset = 5–30 minutes; duration = 3–6 hours; (tablets) onset = 30 minutes; duration = 4–8 hours.	<u>Contraindications</u> Hypersensitivity to beta adrenergic agents; cardiac arrhythmias; narrow angle glaucoma. <u>Pregnancy Category: B</u> <u>Lactation Issues</u> Terbutaline is excreted in breast milk; either the drug or the nursing should be discontinued.

702.2 Xanthine Derivatives

Drug and Dosage Forms	Usual Dosage Range	Administration Issues and Drug–Drug Interactions	Common Adverse Drug Reactions (ADRs) and Pharmacokinetics	Contraindications, Pregnancy Category, and Lactation Issues
Aminophylline Tablets 100 mg, 200 mg Controlled Release Tablets 225 mg Liquid 105 mg/5 mL Suppositories 250 mg, 500 mg	**Asthma/bronchospasm:** regular release tablets: initial dose: 16 mg/kg (up to 400 mg) in 3–4 divided doses controlled release tablets: initial dose: 12 mg/kg (up to 450 mg) in 2–3 divided doses maximum dose: **adults:** 13 mg/kg/day **children 12–16 y:** 18 mg/kg/day **children 9–12 y:** 20 mg/kg/day **children 1–9 y:** 24 mg/kg/day	Administration Issues Do not chew or crush enteric-coated or sustained-release capsules or tablets; take at the same time, with or without food each day; do not change from one brand to another without consulting a physician. Drug–Drug Interactions Agent that may decrease aminophylline concentrations include **phenobarbital, phenytoin, ketoconazole, rifampin,** and **smoking,** agents that may increase aminophylline concentrations include **allopurinol, cimetidine, corticosteroids, erythromycin, ciprofloxacin.**	ADRs GI irritation; diarrhea; increased gastroesophageal reflux; palpitations, tachycardia; potentiation of diuresis; toxic levels may result in cardiac arrhythmias, convulsions, and death. **Aminophylline therapeutic range: 5–15 mcg/mL** Pharmacokinetics Liquids and regular release tablets are well absorbed; absorption of sustained release preparation may vary; $T_{\_}$ averages 3–15 h depending on age, smoking status; $T_{\_}$ prolonged in patients with CHF, liver disease, alcoholism, and respiratory infections.	Contraindications Hypersensitivity to xanthines or ethylenediamine; peptic ulcer disease; underlying seizure disorder unless well controlled. Pregnancy Category: C Lactation Issues Aminophylline is excreted in breast milk and may cause signs of irritability in the nursing infants; decide whether nursing or the drug should be discontinued.
Dyphylline Dilor, Lufyllin Tablets 200 mg, 400 mg Elixir 100 mg/15 mL, 160 mg/15 mL Combination Products w/guaifenesin	**Asthma/bronchospasm:** 200 mg–400 mg q 6 h maximum dose: 15 mg/kg every 6 hours	Administration Issues Take at the same time, with or without food each day; do not change from one brand to another without consulting a physician. Drug–Drug Interactions Agents that may decrease theophylline concentrations include **phenobarbital, phenytoin, ketoconazole, rifampin,** and **smoking,** agents that may increase theophylline concentrations include **allopurinol, cimetidine, corticosteroids, erythromycin, ciprofloxacin.**	ADRs GI irritation; diarrhea; increased gastroesophageal reflux; palpitations, tachycardia; potentiation of diuresis; toxic levels may result in cardiac arrhythmias, convulsions, and death. **Serum theophylline levels do not measure dyphylline.** Pharmacokinetics Absorption = 68–82%; 83% excreted unchanged in urine; $T_{1/2}$ = 2 hours; dyphylline is 70% theophylline by molecular weight ratio.	Contraindications Hypersensitivity to xanthines; peptic ulcer disease; underlying seizure disorder unless well controlled. Pregnancy Category: C Lactation Issues Theophylline is excreted in breast milk and may cause signs of irritability in the nursing infants; decide whether nursing or the drug should be discontinued.
Oxtriphylline Choledyl Tablets 100 mg, 200 mg Sustained-Release Tablets 400 mg, 600 mg	**Asthma/bronchospasm:** tablets, elixir, syrup **adults:** 4.7 mg/kg q 8 h **children 9–16 y and adult smokers:** 4.7 mg/kg q 6 h	Administration Issues Do not chew or crush enteric-coated or sustained-release capsules or tablets; take at the same time, with or without food each day; do not change from one brand to another without consulting a physician.	ADRs GI irritation; diarrhea; increased gastroesophageal reflux; palpitations, tachycardia; potentiation of diuresis; toxic levels may result in cardiac arrhythmias, convulsions, and death. Oxtriphylline therapeutic range: 5–15 mcg/mL	Contraindications Hypersensitivity to xanthines; peptic ulcer disease; underlying seizure disorder unless well controlled. Pregnancy Category: C

Elixir 100 mg/5 mL Pediatric Syrup 50 mg/5 mL	**children 1–9 y.:** 6.2 mg/kg q 6 h sustained release tablets 400–600 mg q 12 h	Drug–Drug Interactions Agents that may decrease oxtriphylline concentrations include **phenobarbital, phenytoin, ketoconazole, rifampin,** and **smoking,** agents that may increase oxtriphylline concentrations include **allopurinol, cimetidine, corticosteroids, erythromycin, ciprofloxacin.**	Pharmacokinetics Liquids and regular release tablets are well absorbed; absorption of sustained release preparation may vary; hepatically metabolized; $T_{1/2}$ averages 3–15 h depending on age and smoking status; $T_{1/2}$ may be prolonged in patients with CHF, liver disease, alcoholism, and respiratory infections.	Lactation Issues Oxtriphylline is excreted in breast milk and may cause signs of irritability in the nursing infant; decide whether nursing or the drug should be discontinued.
Theophylline Elixophyllin, Quibron-T, Slo-Phyllin, Theo-Dur, Theolair, Uniphyl, plus Regular Release Tablets 100 mg, 125 mg, 200 mg, 250 mg, 300 mg Regular Release Capsules 100 mg, 200 mg Syrup 80 mg/15 mL, 150 mg/15 mL Elixir 80 mg/15 mL Solution 80 mg/15 mL, 150 mg/15 mL Timed Release Capsules 50 mg, 60 mg, 75 mg, 100 mg, 125 mg, 130 mg, 200 mg, 250 mg, 260 mg, 300 mg Timed Release Tablets 100 mg, 200 mg, 250 mg, 300 mg, 400 mg, 450 mg, 500 mg Combination Products w/various combinations of guaifenesin, ephedrine, hydroxyzine, potassium iodide, phenobarbital	**Asthma/bronchospasm:** **regular release preparations** initial dose: 16 mg/kg (up to 400 mg) in 3–4 divided doses time release preparations Initial dose: 12 mg/kg (up to 400 mg) in 2–3 divided doses **maximum dose:** **adults:** 13 mg/kg/day **children 12–16 y:** 18 mg/kg/day **children 9–12 y:** 20 mg/kg/day **children 1–9 y:** 24 mg/kg/day	Administration Issues Do not chew or crush enteric-coated or sustained-release capsules or tablets; take at the same time, with or without food each day; do not change from one brand to another without consulting a physician. Drug–Drug Interactions Agents that may decrease theophylline concentrations include **phenobarbital, phenytoin, ketoconazole, rifampin,** and **smoking,** agents that may increase theophylline concentrations include **allopurinol, cimetidine, corticosteroids, erythromycin, ciprofloxacin.**	ADRs GI irritation; diarrhea; increased gastroesophageal reflux; palpitations, tachycardia; potentiation of diuresis; toxic levels may result in cardiac arrhythmias, convulsions, and death. **Theophylline therapeutic range: 5–15 mcg/mL** Pharmacokinetics Liquids and regular release tablets are well absorbed; absorption of sustained release preparation may vary; hepatically metabolized; $T_{1/2}$ averages 3–15 h depending on age and smoking status; $T_{1/2}$ may be prolonged in patients with CHF, liver disease, alcoholism, and respiratory infections.	Contraindications Hypersensitivity to xanthines; peptic ulcer disease; underlying seizure disorder unless well controlled. Pregnancy Category: C Lactation Issues Theophylline is excreted in breast milk and may cause signs of irritability in the nursing infant; decide whether nursing or the drug should be discontinued.

703. Nasal Decongestants

Drug and Dosage Forms	Usual Dosage Range	Administration Issues and Drug–Drug Interactions	Common Adverse Drug Reactions (ADRs) and Pharmacokinetics	Contraindications, Pregnancy Category, and Lactation Issues
Oxymetazoline Afrin, generics Solution (spray) 0.05%	**Relief of nasal and nasopharyngeal mucosal congestion due to common cold, hay fever, sinusitis or allergies** 0.05% solution: **adults and children > 6 years:** 2–3 sprays or drops in each nostril bid	Administration Issues Nasal sprays are preferred to drops because of the lesser risk of swallowing the drug and resultant systemic absorption; dropper and dispensers should not be used by more than one person; tips of the dispensers or droppers should be rinsed with hot water following use; do not use topical nasal sprays longer than 3–5 d.	ADRs Burning; stinging; sneezing; dryness; local irritation; rebound congestion. Pharmacokinetics Onset = 5–10 minutes; duration = 5–6 h; systemic absorption is minimal.	Contraindications Hypersensitivity to decongestants; monoamine oxidase (MAO) inhibitor therapy; severe hypertension or coronary artery disease. Pregnancy Category: C Lactation Issues It is not known whether topical decongestants are excreted in breast milk; use with caution.
Phenylephrine Neo-Synephrine Solution (oral drops) 0.125%, 0.25%, 0.5%, 1% Solution (spray) 0.25%, 0.5%, 1% Tablets, chewable 10 mg	**Relief of nasal and nasopharyngeal mucosal congestion due to common cold, hay fever, sinusitis or allergies** **adults and children > 12 y:** 2–3 sprays or drops in each nostril q 3–4 hours (1% solution should not be given more frequently than every 4 hours) 1 or 2 tablets every 4 hours **children:** 6 mo–2 y: Consult physician 2–6y: 0.125% 2–3 drops per nostril q3–4h, do not use > 3d or 0.25% oral drops: 1 dropperful (1 mL) by mouth every 4 hours not to exceed 6 doses in a 24-hour period 6–12y: 0.125% 2–3 drops per nostril q4h or 0.25% 2–3 drops or 1–2 sprays/nostril q4h, do not use >3d children (6 to < 12 yrs) 1 tablet every 4 hours	Administration Issues Nasal sprays are preferred to drops because of the lesser risk of swallowing the drug and resultant systemic absorption; dropper and dispensers should not be used by more than one person; tips of the dispensers or droppers should be rinsed with hot water following use; do not use topical nasal sprays longer than 3–5 d.	ADRs Burning; stinging; sneezing; dryness; local irritation; rebound congestion. Pharmacokinetics Onset = 30 minutes; systemic absorption is minimal.	Contraindications Hypersensitivity to decongestants; monoamine oxidase (MAO) inhibitor therapy; severe hypertension or coronary artery disease. Pregnancy Category: C Lactation Issues It is not known whether topical decongestants are excreted in breast milk; use with caution.
Pseudoephedrine Afrin, Sudafed	**Temporary relief of nasal congestion due to common cold, hay fever, allergies, and sinusitis; promote nasal and sinus drainage; relief of eustachian tube congestion**	Administration Issues Safety and efficacy have not been established in children < 12 years of age; do not crush or chew sustained release preparations.	ADRs Increased blood pressure; anxiousness; restlessness; GI upset.	Contraindications Hypersensitivity to decongestants; monoamine oxidase (MAO) inhibitor therapy; severe hypertension or coronary artery disease.

Tablets 30 mg, 60 mg Tablets, chewable 15 mg Sustained-Release Tablets 120 mg, 240 mg Capsules 60 mg Capsules, softgels 30 mg Sustained-Release Capsules 120 mg Liquid 15 mg/5 mL, 30 mg/5 mL Drops 7.5 mg/0.8 mL Combination Products w/ various combinations of antihistamines, non-narcotic analgesics, narcotic analgesics, expectorants, antitussives	**adults and children > 12 y:** Tablets: 30–60 mg q 4–6 h sustained release preparations: 120 mg q 12 h 240 mg q 24 h maximum dose: 240 mg daily **children 6–12 y:** 30 mg q 4–6 h. Maximum dose: 120 mg daily **children 2 to 5 y:** 15 mg q 4–6 h. Maximum dose: 60 mg daily Drops: **children 1–2 y:** 7 drops/kg q 4–6 h up to 4 doses **children 3–12 mo:** 3 drops/kg q 4–6 h up to 4 doses Stress Urinary Incontinence: 15 to 30 mg tid	Drug–Drug Interactions Concurrent use with **monoamine oxidase inhibitors** may result in severe headache, hypertension, hyperpyrexia, and possibly hypertensive crisis; concomitant administration with **reserpine, tricyclic antidepressants, guanethidine,** or **methyldopa** may result in hypertension; additive effects may occur when given with other **sympathomimetic agents.**	Pharmacokinetics Onset within 30 minutes; duration = 4–8 h (12 h for sustained release formulations).	Pregnancy Category: C Lactation Issues Oral pseudoephedrine is contraindicated because of the higher than usual risks to infants from sympathomimetic agents.

704. Antitussives

Drug and Dosage Forms	Usual Dosage Range	Administration Issues and Drug–Drug Interactions	Common Adverse Drug Reactions (ADRs) and Pharmacokinetics	Contraindications, Pregnancy Category, and Lactation Issues
Benzonatate Benzonatate softgels, Tessalon Perles, various generics Capsules 100 mg, 200 mg	**Symptomatic relief of cough** **adults and children > 10 years:** 100–200 mg po tid maximum dose = 600 mg/day	Administration Issues Do not chew or break capsules, swallow whole.	ADRs Sedation; headache; dizziness; constipation; GI upset; rash. Pharmacokinetics Onset = 15–20 minutes; duration = 3–8 h.	Contraindications Hypersensitivity to benzonatate or related compounds (tetracaine). Pregnancy Category: C Lactation Issues: It is not known whether benzo-natate is excreted in breast milk.
Codeine (CII) Tablets 15 mg, 30 mg, 60 mg Combination Products w/ various combinations of antihistamines, decongestants, expectorants Solution, Oral 15 mg/5 mL	**Cough suppression** **adults:** 10–20 mg q 4–6 hours; maximum dose = 120 mg/day **children (6–12 y):** 5–10 mg q 4–6 h; maximum dose = 60 mg/day **Children (2–6 y):** 2.5–5 mg q 4–6 h; maximum dose = 30 mg/day	Administration Issues Safety and efficacy in newborns have not been established; take with food to minimize GI upset; should not be used for the persistent cough associated with smoking, asthma or emphysema or for a cough accompanied by excessive secretions. Drug–Drug Interactions Additive effects occur with concomitant administration with other CNS depressants **(alcohol, sedatives, hypnotics, phenothiazines, antihistamines, tricyclic antidepressants, tranquilizers).**	ADRs Nausea; vomiting; sedation; dizziness; constipation; orthostatic hypotension; dry mouth. Pharmacokinetics Absorption = 100%; metabolized in the liver and excreted in the urine; $T_{1/2}$ = 3 h.	Contraindications Hypersensitivity to codeine; premature infants. Pregnancy Category: C Lactation Issues Codeine is excreted in breast, use with caution.
Dextromethorphan Robitussin, Benylin, Hold, Vicks 44, Benylin DM, Delsym, Silphen DM Lozenges 2.5 mg, 5 mg, 7.5 mg Gelcaps 15 mg, 30 mg Liquid 3.5 mg/5 mL, 7.5 mg/5 mL, 10 mg/5 mL, 15 mg/5 mL Syrup 10 mg/5 mL, 15 mg/15 mL Sustained Action Liquid: 30 mg/5 mL Combination Products w/ various combinations of antitussive, methylxanthines, decongestants	**Control of nonproductive cough** Lozenges, Liquid, Syrup: **adults:** 10–30 mg q 4–8 h; maximum dose = 120 mg/day **children (6–12 y):** 5–10 mg q 4 h or 15 mg q 6–8 h; maximum dose = 60 mg/day **children (2–6 y) syrup:** 2.5–7.5 mg q 4–8 h; maximum dose = 30 mg/day Sustained Action Liquid: **adults:** 60 mg q 12 h **children (6–12 y):** 30 mg q 12 h **children (2–6 y):** 15 mg q 12 h	Administration Issues Should not be used for the persistent cough associated with smoking, asthma or emphysema or for a cough accompanied by excessive secretions. Drug–Drug Interactions **MAO inhibitors** in combination with dextromethorphan may lead to hypotension, hyperpyrexia, nausea, myoclonic leg jerks, and coma.	ADRs GI upset; drowsiness; dizziness. Pharmacokinetics Rapidly absorbed from GI tract; onset = 15–30 minutes; duration = 3–6 h.	Contraindications Hypersensitivity to dextromethorphan; patients receiving MAO inhibitors.

705. Antihistamines

705.1 Antihistamines—First Generation

Drug and Dosage Forms	Usual Dosage Range	Administration Issues and Drug-Drug Interactions	Common Adverse Drug Reactions (ADRs) and Pharmacokinetics	Contraindications, Pregnancy Category, and Lactation Issues
Azatadine Optimine, Trinalin Repetabs Tablets 1 mg Trinalin Repetabs 1 mg/120 mg pseudoephedrine	**Allergic rhinitis and conjunctivitis; relief of runny nose and sneezing due to the common cold; pruritus and urticaria** **adults and children > 12 y:** Tablets 1–2 mg bid Trinalin Repetabs 1 tablet bid	Administration Issues Safety and efficacy in children < 12 have not been established. Drug-Drug Interactions **MAO inhibitors** may potentiate the anticholinergic effects of antihistamines; additive CNS depressant effects may occur with concurrent use of **alcohol** or **other CNS depressants.**	ADRs Drowsiness; GI upset; dry mouth; thickening of bronchial secretions; urinary retention; constipation. Pharmacokinetics Well absorbed; onset = 15–30 minutes; duration up to 12 h.	Contraindications Hypersensitivity to antihistamines; narrow-angle glaucoma; stenosing peptic ulcer, symptomatic prostatic hypertrophy; bladder neck obstruction; asthmatic attack; concurrent monoamine oxidase inhibitor (MAOI) therapy; newborns and premature infants; third trimester of pregnancy. Pregnancy Category: B Lactation Issues Antihistamine therapy is contraindicated in nursing mothers.
Azelastine HCL Astelin Nasal spray 137 mcg/spray	**Allergic rhinitis/seasonal rhinitis:** **adults:** 2 sprays/nostril bid **children (5–12 y):** 1 spray/nostril bid Not recommended in children < 5 years	Drug Interactions No significant interactions.	ADRs Bitter taste, headache, somnolence, nasal burning, pharyngitis, dry mouth.	Contraindications Hypersensitivity to antihistamines. Pregnancy Category: C Lactation Issues Antihistamine therapy is contraindicated in nursing mothers.
Brompheniramine Brovex, Brovex CT Tablets 4 mg, 8 mg, 12 mg Sustained Release Tablets 8 mg, 12 mg Elixir 2 mg/5 mL Combination Products w/ various combinations of decongestants, analgesics, antitussives	**Allergic rhinitis and conjunctivitis; relief of runny nose and sneezing due to the common cold; pruritus and urticaria** Tablets and elixir: **adults and children > 12 y:** 4 mg q 4–6 h; maximum dose: 24 mg daily **children 6–12 y:** 2 mg q 4–6 h; maximum dose: 12 mg daily **children < 6 y:** 0.125 mg/kg po q6h	Drug–Drug Interactions **MAO inhibitors** may potentiate the anticholinergic effects of antihistamines; additive CNS depressant effects may occur with concurrent use of **alcohol** or **other CNS depressants.**	ADRs Drowsiness; GI upset; dry mouth; thickening of bronchial secretions; urinary retention; constipation. Pharmacokinetics Well absorbed; onset = 15–30 minutes; duration = 4–6 h.	Contraindications Hypersensitivity to antihistamines; narrow-angle glaucoma; stenosing peptic ulcer, symptomatic prostatic hypertrophy; bladder neck obstruction; asthmatic attack; concurrent monoamine oxidase inhibitor (MAOI) therapy; newborns and premature infants; third trimester of pregnancy. Pregnancy Category: C Lactation Issues Antihistamine therapy is contraindicated in nursing mothers.

(*continues on next page*)

705.1 Antihistamines—First Generation *continued from previous page*

Drug and Dosage Forms	Usual Dosage Range	Administration Issues and Drug-Drug Interactions	Common Adverse Drug Reactions (ADRs) and Pharmacokinetics	Contraindications, Pregnancy Category, and Lactation Issues
Brompheniramine *cont.*	Sustained release tablets: **adults and children > 12 years:** 8–12 mg q 8–12 h			
Chlorpheniramine Chlor-Trimeton, generics Chewable Tablets 2 mg Tablets 4 mg, 8 mg, 12 mg Capsules 12 mg Extended-Release Tablets 8 mg, 12 mg, 16 mg Sustained-Release Capsules 8 mg, 12 mg Tablets, Chewable 2 mg Syrup 2 mg/5 mL Combination Products w/ various combinations of decongestants, analgesics, antitussives	**Allergic rhinitis and conjunctivitis; relief of runny nose and sneezing due to the common cold; pruritus and urticaria** Tablets and syrup: **adults and children > 12 y:** 4 mg q 4–6 h; maximum dose: 24 mg daily **children 6–12 y:** 2 mg q 4–6 h; maximum dose: 12 mg daily **children 2–6 y:** 1 mg q 4–6 h; maximum dose: 4 mg daily Sustained release forms: **adults and children > 12 y:** 8–12 mg q 8–12 h **children 6–12 y:** 8 mg q 8–12 h	Drug–Drug Interactions **MAO inhibitors** may potentiate the anticholinergic effects of antihistamines; additive CNS depressant effects may occur with concurrent use of **alcohol** or **other CNS depressants.**	ADRs Drowsiness; GI upset; dry mouth; thickening of bronchial secretions; urinary retention; constipation. Pharmacokinetics Well absorbed; onset = 15–30 minutes; duration = 4–6 h.	Contraindications Hypersensitivity to antihistamines; narrow-angle glaucoma; stenosing peptic ulcer, symptomatic prostatic hypertrophy; bladder neck obstruction; asthmatic attack; concurrent monoamine oxidase inhibitor (MAOI) therapy; newborns and premature infants; third trimester of pregnancy. Pregnancy Category: B Lactation Issues: antihistamine therapy is contraindicated in nursing mothers
Clemastine Tavist Tablets 1.34 mg, 2.68 mg Syrup 0.67 mg/5 mL	**Allergic rhinitis and conjunctivitis; relief of runny nose and sneezing due to the common cold; pruritus and urticaria** **adults and children > 12 y:** 1.34 mg 2.68 mg bid/tid prn Maximum dose: 8.04 mg daily	Drug–Drug Interactions **MAO inhibitors** may potentiate the anticholinergic effects of antihistamines; additive CNS depressant effects may occur with concurrent use of **alcohol** or **other CNS depressants.**	ADRs Drowsiness; GI upset; dry mouth; thickening of bronchial secretions; urinary retention; constipation. Pharmacokinetics Well absorbed; onset = 15–30 minutes; duration up to 12 h.	Contraindications Hypersensitivity to antihistamines; narrow-angle glaucoma; stenosing peptic ulcer, symptomatic prostatic hypertrophy; bladder neck obstruction; asthmatic attack; concurrent monoamine oxidase inhibitor (MAOI) therapy; newborns and premature infants; third trimester of pregnancy.

				Pregnancy Category: B Lactation Issues Antihistamine therapy is contraindicated in nursing mothers.
Cyproheptadine Periactin Tablets 4 mg Syrup 2 mg/5 mL	**Allergic rhinitis and conjunctivitis; relief of runny nose and sneezing due to the common cold; pruritus and urticaria** **adults:** Initial dose: 4 mg tid. Maintenance dose: 12–32 mg daily in divided doses **children 7–14 y:** 4 mg bid to tid; Maximum dose: 16 mg daily **children 2–6 y:** 2 mg bid to tid; Maximum dose: 12 mg daily	Administration Issues Safety and efficacy in children < 2 have not been established. Drug–Drug Interactions **MAO inhibitors** may potentiate the anticholinergic effects of antihistamines; additive CNS depressant effects may occur with concurrent use of **alcohol** or **other CNS depressants.**	ADRs Drowsiness; GI upset; dry mouth; thickening of bronchial secretions; urinary retention; constipation. Pharmacokinetics Well absorbed; onset = 15–30 minutes; duration up to 8 h.	Contraindications Hypersensitivity to antihistamines; narrow-angle glaucoma; stenosing peptic ulcer, symptomatic prostatic hypertrophy; bladder neck obstruction; asthmatic attack; concurrent monoamine oxidase inhibitor (MAOI) therapy; newborns and premature infants; third trimester of pregnancy. Pregnancy Category: B Lactation Issues Antihistamine therapy is contraindicated in nursing mothers.
Diphenhydramine Benadryl, generics Capsules 25 mg, 50 mg Tablets 25 mg, 50 mg Tablets, chewable 12.5 mg Elixir 12.5 mg/ 5 mL Syrup 12.5 mg/ 5 mL Combination Products w/ various combinations of decongestants, analgesics, antitussives	**Allergic rhinitis and conjunctivitis; relief of runny nose and sneezing due to the common cold; pruritus and urticaria** **adults:** 25–50 mg q 4–6 h **children > 10 kg:** 12.5–25 mg q 6–8 h **Motion sickness:** 25–50 mg given 30 minutes before exposure to motion **Nighttime sleep aid for adults:** 50 mg hs **Cough suppression (syrup):** **adults:** 25–50 mg q 6–8 h **children > 10 kg:** 12.5–25 mg q 6–8 h	Drug–Drug Interactions **MAO inhibitors** may potentiate the anticholinergic effects of antihistamines; additive CNS depressant effects may occur with concurrent use of **alcohol** or **other CNS depressants.**	ADRs Drowsiness; GI upset; dry mouth; thickening of bronchial secretions; urinary retention; constipation. Pharmacokinetics Well absorbed; onset = 15–30 minutes; duration = 6–8 h.	Contraindications Hypersensitivity to antihistamines; narrow-angle glaucoma; stenosing peptic ulcer, symptomatic prostatic hypertrophy; bladder neck obstruction; asthmatic attack; concurrent monoamine oxidase inhibitor (MAOI) therapy; newborns and premature infants; third trimester of pregnancy. Pregnancy Category: B Lactation Issues Antihistamine therapy is contraindicated in nursing mothers.

(continues on next page)

705.1 Antihistamines-First Generation *continued from previous page*

Drug and Dosage Forms	Usual Dosage Range	Administration Issues and Drug-Drug Interactions	Common Adverse Drug Reactions (ADRs) and Pharmacokinetics	Contraindications, Pregnancy Category, and Lactation Issues
Hydroxyzine Atarax, Vistaril, generics Tablets 10 mg, 25 mg, 50 mg, 100 mg Capsules 25 mg, 50 mg, 100 mg Syrup 10 mg/5 mL Oral Suspension 25 mg/5 mL	**Management of pruritus due to allergic conditions such as chronic urticaria and atopic or chronic dermatitis** **Adults:** 25 mg 3–4 times/d **children:** **> 6 y:** 50 to 100 mg daily in divided doses **< 6 y:** 50 mg daily in divided doses	Administration Issues Avoid alcohol use. Drug-Drug Interactions **MAO inhibitors** may potentiate the anticholinergic effects of antihistamines; additive CNS depressant effects may occur with concurrent use of **alcohol** or **other CNS depressants.**	ADRs Drowsiness; GI upset; dry mouth; thickening of bronchial secretions; urinary retention; constipation; photosensitivity; involuntary muscle movements. Pharmacokinetics Well absorbed; onset = 15–30 minutes; duration = 4–6 h.	Contraindications Hypersensitivity to antihistamines; narrow-angle glaucoma; prostatic hypertrophy. Pregnancy Category: C Lactation Issues Antihistamine therapy is contraindicated in nursing mothers.

705.2 Antihistamines—Second Generation

Drug and Dosage Forms	Usual Dosage Range	Administration Issues and Drug–Drug Interactions	Common Adverse Drug Reactions (ADRs) and Pharmacokinetics	Contraindications, Pregnancy Category, and Lactation Issues
Cetirizine (considered "low-sedating") Zyrtec Tablets 5 mg, 10 mg Tablets, chewable 5 mg, 10 mg Syrup 5 mg/5 mL	**Allergic rhinitis and conjunctivitis; relief of runny nose and sneezing due to the common cold; pruritus and urticaria** **adults and children > 6 y:** 5–10 mg qd **children <2y:** not recommended **2–5y;** initially 2.5 mg qd, max 5 mg/d **Patients with renal or hepatic dysfunction:** 5 mg qd	Administration Issues: Safety and efficacy in children < 2 have not been established; somewhat more sedating than others, but less than first generation. Not as effective as first generation; use in patients who cannot tolerate sedation. Drug–Drug Interactions: **MAO inhibitors** may potentiate the anticholinergic effects of antihistamines; additive CNS depressant effects may occur with concurrent use of **alcohol** or **other CNS depressants.**	ADRs Headache; dry mouth; GI upset; dizziness; insomnia; nervousness; thickening of bronchial secretions; drowsiness (less frequent). Pharmacokinetics Well absorbed; onset = 1 h; duration = 24 h.	Contraindications Hypersensitivity to antihistamines; narrow-angle glaucoma; stenosing peptic ulcer, symptomatic prostatic hypertrophy; bladder neck obstruction; asthmatic attack; concurrent monoamine oxidase inhibitor (MAOI) therapy; newborns and premature infants; third trimester of pregnancy. Pregnancy Category: C Lactation Issues Antihistamine therapy is contraindicated in nursing mothers.
Desloratadine Clarinex, Clarinex RediTabs Tablets 5 mg	**Seasonal allergic rhinitis/chronic urticaria:** **adults and children > 12 y:** 5 mg qd	Administration Issues Safety and efficacy in children < 12 have not been established. Does not readily cross blood-brain barrier so it is less likely to cause drowsiness.	ADRs GI upset, dry mouth, thickening of bronchial secretions, urinary retention, constipation.	Contraindications Hypersensitivity to antihistamines, narrow angle glaucoma, symptomatic prostatic hypertrophy, bladder neck obstruction. Pregnancy Category: C

Tablets, rapidly disintegrating 5 mg	**patients with renal dysfunction:** 5 mg qod	RediTabs Administration: Place rapidly disintegrating tablets on the tongue immediately after opening the blister; tablet disintegration occurs rapidly. Administer with or without water.	Pharmacokinetics $T_{1/2} = 27$ h.	Lactation Issues Antihistamine therapy is contraindicated in nursing mothers.
Fexofenadine Allegra Capsules 60 mg Tablets 30 mg, 60 mg 180 mg	**Allergic rhinitis and conjunctivitis; relief of runny nose and sneezing due to the common cold; pruritus and urticaria** allergic rhinitis: **adults > 12 y:** 60 mg BID or 180 mg QD **children 6–11y:** 30mg po bid chronic urticaria: **adults >12 y:** 60 mg po bid **children 6–11y:** 30 mg po bid Renal Function Impairment **adults and children > 12** 60 mg qd as a starting dose **children 6 to 11 yrs** 30 mg qd as a starting dose **Patients with hepatic dysfunction:** 60 mg qd as (starting dose)	Administration Issues Safety and efficacy in children < 6 have not been established. Drug–Drug Interactions **MAO inhibitors** may potentiate the anticholinergic effects of antihistamines; additive CNS depressant effects may occur with concurrent use of **alcohol** or **other CNS depressants.**	ADRs GI upset; headache; appetite increase with weight gain; nervousness; dizziness; diarrhea; dry mouth; thickening of bronchial secretions; drowsiness (less frequent). Pharmacokinetics Rapid onset of action.	Contraindications Hypersensitivity to antihistamines; narrow-angle glaucoma; stenosing peptic ulcer, symptomatic prostatic hypertrophy; bladder neck obstruction; asthmatic attack; concurrent monoamine oxidase inhibitor (MAOI) therapy; newborns and premature infants; third trimester of pregnancy. Pregnancy Category: C Lactation Issues Antihistamine therapy is contra-indicated in nursing mothers.
Loratadine (OTC) Claritin, generics Tablets 10 mg Reditabs (rapidly disintegrating tablets) 10 mg Syrup 1 mg/mL Combination 5 mg/120 mg pseudoephedrine 10 mg/240 mg pseudoephedrine	**Allergic rhinitis and conjunctivitis; relief of runny nose and sneezing due to the common cold; pruritus and urticaria** **adults and children > 12 y:** 10 mg qd **children 6–11 y:** 10 mg (10 mL) qd **children 2–5 y:** 5 mg po qd **Patients with hepatic or renal dysfunction:** 10 mg qod	Administration Issues Take on an empty stomach; safety and efficacy in children < 6 have not been established. If taking rapidly disintegrating tablets: place tablet on tongue and it should disintegrate rapidly (seconds). Dissolved tablet may then be swallowed with or without water. Drug–Drug Interactions **Fluconazole, itraconazole, ketoconazole, miconazole, erythromycin, azithromycin, clarithromycin, and troleandomycin** may increase loratadine levels. **MAO inhibitors** may potentiate the anticholinergic effects of antihistamines; additive CNS depressant effects may occur with concurrent use of **alcohol** or **other CNS depressants.**	ADRs GI upset; dry mouth; thickening of bronchial secretions; urinary retention; constipation; drowsiness (less frequent). Pharmacokinetics Well absorbed; onset = 1–3 h; duration = 24 h.	Contraindications Hypersensitivity to antihistamines; narrow-angle glaucoma; stenosing peptic ulcer, symptomatic prostatic hypertrophy; bladder neck obstruction; asthmatic attack; concurrent monoamine oxidase inhibitor (MAOI) therapy; newborns and premature infants; third trimester of pregnancy. Pregnancy Category: B Lactation Issues Antihistamine therapy is contraindicated in nursing mothers.

706. Intranasal Steroids

Drug and Dosage Forms	Usual Dosage Range	Administration Issues and Drug-Drug Interactions	Common Adverse Drug Reactions (ADRs)	Contraindications, Pregnancy Category, and Lactation Issues
Beclomethasone Beconase, Beconase AQ, Vancenase, Vancenase AQ Aerosol 42 mcg/dose Spray (AQ) 0.042% (Beconase AQ) 0.084% (Vancenase AQ)	**Symptomatic relief of seasonal or perennial rhinitis; prevention of recurrence of nasal polyps following surgical removal; nonallergic rhinitis (spray)** **adults and children > 12 y:** 1 inhalation in each nostril bid to qid AQ: 1–2 INH bid **children 6–12 y:** 1 inhalation in each nostril tid AQ: 1–2 INH bid Vancenase AQ **Adults and children ≥ 6 y:** 1–2 INH qid.	Administration Issues Safety and efficacy have not been established in children < 6 years of age; use smallest maintenance dose possible to control symptoms; discontinue therapy if no improvement is noted within three weeks.	ADRs Nasal irritation, burning, stinging and dryness; headache; delayed wound healing.	Contraindications Hypersensitivity to steroids; untreated nasal infection. Pregnancy Category: C Lactation Issues It is not known whether beclomethasone is excreted in breast milk; use caution if nursing.
Budesonide Rhinocort, Rhinocort Aqua Aerosol 32 mcg/dose Spray 32 mcg/spray	**Symptomatic relief of seasonal or perennial rhinitis in adults and children; nonallergic perennial rhinitis in adults** Rhinocort **adults and children > 6 y:** 2 sprays in each nostril bid or 4 sprays in each nostril qd Rhinocort Aqua Adults and children > 6 y: 1 spray/nostril qd. Titrate to minimum effective dose.	Administration Issues Not recommended for children < 6 years of age with nonallergic perennial rhinitis; use smallest maintenance dose possible to control symptoms; discontinue therapy if no improvement is noted within three weeks.	ADRs Nasal irritation, burning, stinging and dryness; headache; delayed wound healing.	Contraindications Hypersensitivity to steroids; untreated nasal infection. Pregnancy Category: C Lactation Issues It is not known whether budesonide is excreted in breast milk; use caution if nursing.
Flunisolide Nasalide, Nasarel Spray 25 mcg/dose Solution 25 mcg/dose	**Symptomatic relief of seasonal or perennial rhinitis:** **adults and children > 14 y:** Initial dose: 2 sprays in each nostril bid to tid. Maintenance dose: 1 spray in each nostril qd. Maximum dose: 8 sprays daily **Children 6–14 y:** 1 spray in each nostril tid or 2 sprays in each nostril bid. Maximum dose: 4 sprays daily	Administration Issues Use smallest maintenance dose possible to control symptoms; discontinue therapy if no improvement is noted within three weeks.	ADRs Nasal irritation, burning, stinging and dryness; headache; delayed wound healing.	Contraindications Hypersensitivity to steroids; untreated nasal infection. Pregnancy Category: C Lactation Issues It is not known whether llunisolide is excreted in breast milk; use caution if nursing.

Fluticasone Flonase Spray 50 mcg/dose	**Symptomatic relief of seasonal or perennial rhinitis** **adults:** 2 sprays in each nostril qd. Maximum dose: 4 sprays daily **children >4y:** 1–2 sprays in each nostril qd. Maximum dose: 4 sprays daily	Administration Issues Not recommended for nonallergic rhinitis in children < 12 y; use smallest maintenance dose possible to control symptoms.	ADRs Nasal irritation, burning, stinging and dryness; headache; delayed wound healing.	Contraindications Hypersensitivity to steroids; untreated nasal infection. Pregnancy Category: C Lactation Issues It is not known whether fluticasone is excreted in breast milk; use caution if nursing.
Triamcinolone Nasacort, Nasacort AQ Spray Inhaler 55 mcg/dose	**Symptomatic relief of seasonal or perennial rhinitis** **adults and children > 12 y:** Nasacort: Starting dose of 2 sprays in each nostril qd. May increase to 440 mcg/day either qd or divided up to qid. Patients may be maintained on as little as 1 spray each nostril qd. Nasacort AQ: Starting and maximum dose is 2 sprays each nostril qd. Patients may be maintained on as little as 1 spray each nostril qd.	Administration Issues Use smallest maintenance dose possible to control symptoms; discontinue therapy if no improvement is noted within three weeks.	ADRs Nasal irritation, burning, stinging and dryness; headache; delayed wound healing.	Contraindications Hypersensitivity to steroids; untreated nasal infection. Pregnancy Category: C Lactation Issues It is not known whether triamcinolone is excreted in breast milk; use caution if nursing.

707. Expectorants

Drug and Dosage Forms	Usual Dosage Range	Administration Issues and Drug–Drug Interactions	Common Adverse Drug Reactions (ADRs)	Contraindications, Pregnancy Category, and Lactation Issues
Guaifenesin Robitussin, Guiatuss, Humibid, Syrup Duratuss 100 mg/5 mL Capsules 200 mg Sustained-Release Capsules 300 mg Tablets 100 mg, 200 mg 400 mg Sustained Release Tablets 575 mg, 600 mg, 800 mg, 1000 mg, 1200 mg Capsules, sustained release 300 mg Combination Products w/ varying combinations of methylxanthines, antihistamines, decongestants, analgesics	**Symptomatic relief of dry, nonproductive cough** Immediate Release **adults:** 200–400 mg q 4 hours. Maximum dose: 2400 mg/day **children (6–12 y):** 100–200 mg q 4 hours; Maximum dose: 1200 mg/day **children (2–6 y):** 50–100 mg q 4 hours. Maximum dose: 600 mg/day Sustained-Release **adults** 575 to 1200 mg q 12h. Max dose: 2400 mg/day **children (6–12 y):** 575 to 600 mg every 12h. Max dose: 1200 mg/day **children (2–6 y):** 275 to 300 mg every 12h. Max dose: 600 mg/day	Administration Issues: should not be used for the persistent cough associated with smoking, asthma or emphysema or for a cough accompanied by excessive secretions	ADRs: nausea, vomiting, dizziness, headache, rash	Contraindications: hypersensitivity to guaifenesin Pregnancy Category: C Lactation Issues: No data available

708. Leukotriene Receptor Antagonists

Drug and Dosage Forms	Usual Dosage Range	Administration Issues and Drug–Drug Interactions	Common Adverse Drug Reactions (ADRs) and Pharmacokinetics	Contraindications, Pregnancy Category, and Lactation Issues
Montelukast Singulair Chewable Tablets 4 mg, 5 mg Film-coated Tablets 10 mg Granules 4 mg/pk	**Prophylaxis and chronic treatment of asthma in adults and children >6 years:** **adults and children >15 y:** 10 mg in the evening **children 6–14 y:** 5 mg po in the evening **children 2–5 y:** 4mg po q hs	Administration Issues Take regularly as prescribed, even during symptom-free periods. Do not use to treat acute episode of asthma. Drug Interactions None reported.	ADRs Headache, dizziness, nausea, diarrhea, abdominal pain. Pharmacokinetics Food does not effect bioavailability; $T_{1/2} = 3–6$ h.	Contraindications Hypersensitivity to montelukast. Pregnancy Category: B Lactation Issues It is not known if montelukast is excreted in breast milk.
Zafirlukast Accolate Tablets 10 mg, 20 mg	**Prophylaxis and chronic treatment of asthma in adults and children >12 y:** **adults and children >12 y:** 20 mg bid **children 7–11 y:** 10 mg po bid	Administration Issues Take zafirlukast at least 1 h before or 2 h after meals. Take regularly as prescribed, even during symptom-free periods. Do not use to treat acute episode of asthma. Drug Interactions Aspirin may increase Zafirlukast levels. **Erythromycin, terfenadine, theophylline** may decrease zafirlukast levels. Zafirlukast may increase the anticoagulant effects of **warfarin.**	ADRs Headache, dizziness, nausea, diarrhea, abdominal pain. Pharmacokinetics Food reduces bioavailability by 40%; $T_{1/2} = 10$ h.	Contraindications Hypersensitivity to zafirlukast. Pregnancy Category: B Lactation Issues Nursing women should not take this drug.

709. Leukotriene Receptor Inhibitors

Drug and Dosage Forms	Usual Dosage Range	Administration Issues and Drug–Drug Interactions	Common Adverse Drug Reactions (ADRs) and Pharmacokinetics	Contraindications, Pregnancy Category, and Lactation Issues
Zileutin Zyflo Tablets 600 mg	**Prophylaxis and chronic treatment of asthma in adults and children >12 y:** **adults and children >12 y:** 600 mg qid with meals and hs.	Administration Issues Take regularly as prescribed, even during symptom-free periods. Do not use to treat acute episode of asthma. Zileutin may be taken with food. If patients experience signs or symptoms of liver dysfunction (nausea, fatigue, right upper quadrant pain, lethargy, jaundice, "flu-like" symptoms), contact healthcare professional immediately. Drug Interactions Zileutin may increase levels of **propranolol, terfenadine, and theophylline.** Ziluetin may increase the anticoagulant effects of **warfarin.**	ADRs Headache, ALT elevations, chest pain, dizziness, fever, insomnia, malaise, dyspepsia, abdominal pain, constipation, flatulence, weakness, myalgia. Pharmacokinetics Rapidly absorbed; $T_{1/2} = 1.7$ h.	Contraindications Hypersensitivity to zileutin, active liver disease, transaminase elevations ≥ 3 times upper limits of normal. Pregnancy Category: C Lactation Issues Nursing women should not take this drug.

710. Monoclonal Antibodies

Drug and Dosage Forms	Usual Dosage Range	Administration Issues and Drug-Drug & Drug-Food Interactions	Common Adverse Drug Reactions (ADRs)	Contraindications, Pregnancy Category and Lactation Issues
Omalizumab Xolair Powder for injection 202.5 mg (150 mg/1.2 mL after reconstitution)	**Moderate to severe persistent asthma:** For adults and adolescents 12 years of age and older with moderate to severe persistent asthma who have a positive skin test or in vitro reactivity to a perennial aeroallergen and those symptoms are inadequately controlled with inhaled corticosteroids. Omalizumab 150 to 375 mg is administered SC every 2 or 4 weeks. Doses (mg) and dosing frequency are determined by serum total immunoglobulin E (IgE) level (units/mL), measured before the start of treatment, and body weight (kg). Use tables in product labeling to determine appropriate dose.	**Administration Issues** **Observe patients after injection of omalizumab; medications for the treatment of severe hypersensitivity reactions including anaphylaxis should be available. If a severe hypersensitivity reaction to omalizumab occurs, discontinue therapy.** Refrigerate during storage. Use within 4 hours of reconstitution if stored at room temperature or within 8 hours if refrigerated. Because the solution is slightly viscous, the injection may take 5 to 10 seconds to administer. Inject only 150 mg per site; divide larger doses and administer multiple injections at multiple sites. Inform patients receiving omalizumab to not decrease the dose of, or stop taking any other asthma medications unless otherwise instructed by their physicians. Inform patients that they may not see immediate improvement in their asthma after beginning omalizumab therapy.	ADRs **The most serious adverse reactions occurring in clinical studies with omalizumab are malignancies and anaphylaxis. Anaphylactic reactions were rare but temporally associated with omalizumab administration.** The most common ADRs were injection site reaction (45%), viral infections (23%), upper respiratory tract infection (20%), sinusitis (16%), headache (15%), and pharyngitis (11%). Pharmacokinetics: Peak serum concentrations after an average of 7 to 8 days; omalizumab serum elimination half-life averaged 26 days	Contraindications Severe hypersensitivity reaction to omalizumab. Pregnancy Category: B Lactation Issues: Exercise caution when administering omalizumab to a nursing woman.

800. TOPICAL PREPARATIONS
801. Acne Products (Topical and Oral)

Drug and Dosage Forms	Usual Dosage Range	Administration Issues and Drug–Drug Interactions	Common Adverse Drug Reactions (ADRs)	Contraindications, Pregnancy Category, and Lactation Issues
Benzoyl Peroxide many products on the market with the following strengths and dosage forms: Liquid 2.5%, 3%, 4%, 5%, 6%, 8%, 9%, 10% Bar 5%, 10% Mask 5% Lotion: 4%, 5%, 5.5%, 8%, 10% Cleanser 9%, 10% Cream: 5%, 10% Gel: 2.5%, 4%, 5%, 6%, 7%, 8%, 9%, 10%, 20% Combination Products Gel 1% clindamycin 5% benzoyl peroxide	**Treatment of mild to moderate acne vulgaris and oily skin** Wash with cleansers once or twice daily. Apply other dose forms qd, gradually increasing to 2 to 3 times daily as needed.	Administration Issues For external use only; keep preparation away from the eyes, mouth, angles of nose, and mucous membranes; wash hands thoroughly after application; avoid excessive exposure to the sunlight or sunlamps; shake lotion well prior to administration; normal use of water-based cosmetics is permissible; avoid contact with hair or colored fabric, bleaching may occur. Safety and efficacy in children < 12 years of age have not been established. Drug–Drug Interactions Concomitant use of **tretinoin** and benzoyl peroxide may cause significant skin irritation.	ADRs Excessive drying, erythema, hypersensitivity.	Contraindications Hypersensitivity to benzoyl peroxide, cross-sensitivity may occur with benzoic acid derivatives. Pregnancy Category: C Lactation Issues Excretion in breast milk is unknown, use with caution in nursing mothers.
Clindamycin Phosphate Cleocin T, generics: Gel 1% Lotion: 1%	**Treatment of acne vulgaris** Apply a thin film to affected area twice daily.	Administration Issues For external use only; keep preparation away from the eyes, mouth, angles of nose, and mucous membranes; wash hands thoroughly after application; shake lotion well prior to administration; remove pledget from foil wrapper just prior to administration; use pledget only once, then discard. Safety and efficacy in children <	ADRs Dryness, erythema, burning, peeling, itching, oily skin, diarrhea, abdominal pain, and colitis.	Contraindications Hypersensitivity to clindamycin or lincomycin; history of antibiotic-associated colitis. Pregnancy Category: B Lactation Issues Due to potential for serious adverse events in infants, discontinue nursing or

Topical Suspension 1% Combination Products Gel 1% clindamycin 5% benzoyl peroxide		12 years of age have not been established. Drug–Drug Interactions **Erythromycin** may antagonize the effects of clindamycin.		the drug, taking into account the importance of the drug to the mother.
Erythromycin generics Solution 1.5%, 2% Gel 2% Benzamycin generics 30 mg erythromycin 50 mg benzoyl peroxide per gm Ointment 2% Pledgets 2%	**Treatment of acne vulgaris** Apply twice daily to affected area in the morning and evening.	Administration Issues For external use only; keep preparation away from the eyes, mouth, angles of nose, and mucous membranes; wash hands thoroughly after application; cleanse areas to be treated before applying medication; store benzamycin gel in the refrigerator and discard unused portion after 3 months. Safety and efficacy in children < 12 years of age have not been established. Drug–Drug Interactions Concomitant use of other acne products (**benzoyl peroxide, tretinoin**) with erythromycin may cause increased irritant effects. Erythromycin may antagonize the effects of **clindamycin.**	ADRs Erythema, burning, dryness.	Contraindications Hypersensitivity to erythromycin. Pregnancy Category: B (Eryderm 2%, Erygel); C (A/T/S, T-Stat, Staticin) Lactation Issues Erythromycin is excreted in breast milk; use with caution in nursing mothers.
Isotretinoin Accutane, generics Capsules 10 mg, 20 mg, 40 mg Capsules, softgels 10 mg 20 mg 30 mg 40 mg	**Treatment of severe recalcitrant cystic acne** Initially, 0.5–1 mg/kg/d divided into 2 doses for 15 to 20 weeks; patients with severe disease or disease primarily manifest on the body may require up to 2 mg/kg/d. A second course of therapy may be initiated after ≥ 2 months off therapy if severe cystic acne persists or recurs.	Administration Issues Patient information leaflet should be discussed with the patient; do not crush capsule; take with meals; women of childbearing potential should practice contraception during therapy and for 1 month before and after therapy; a pregnancy test 2 weeks prior to starting therapy is advised. Safety and efficacy in children have not been established. Drug–Drug Interactions Concomitant use of **vitamin A** and isotretinoin may result in additive toxic effects.	ADRs Dry mouth, nausea, vomiting, abdominal pain, conjunctivitis, decreased night vision, hypertriglyceridemia, arthralgia, hepatotoxicity, photosensitivity. **Warning** **Isotretinoin must not be used by females who are pregnant due to the risk of birth deformities. Contact dispensing pharmacy for details.**	Contraindications Pregnancy; hypersensitivity to parabens. Pregnancy Category: X Lactation Issues Excretion in breast milk is unknown; unknown; due to potential for adverse effects, do not use in nursing mothers.
Metronidazole MetroGel, generics	**Treatment of inflammatory papules, pustules, and erythema of rosacea** Apply and rub into a thin film twice daily in the morning and evening; therapeutic	Administration Issues For external use only; keep preparation away from the eyes, mouth, angles of nose, and mucous membranes; wash	ADRs Transient redness, dryness, burning, skin irritation.	Contraindications Hypersensitivity to metronidazole and parabens.

(continues on next page)

801. Acne Products (Topical and Oral) *continued from previous page*

Drug and Dosage Forms	Usual Dosage Range	Administration Issues and Drug–Drug Interactions	Common Adverse Drug Reactions (ADRs)	Contraindications, Pregnancy Category, and Lactation Issues
Metronidazole *cont.* Gel 0.75% Lotion 0.75% Cream 0.75%, 1%	results should be noticed within 3 weeks; studies have shown continuing improvement through 9 weeks of therapy.	hands thoroughly after application; cleanse areas to be treated before applying medication. Safety and efficacy in children have not been established.		Pregnancy Category: B Lactation Issues Metronidazole is excreted in breast milk; discontinue nursing or the drug, taking into account the importance of the drug to the mother.
Tretinoin Retin-A, generics Cream: 0.02%, 0.025%, 0.05%, 0.1% Gel 0.025%, 0.01% 0.04%, 0.1% Liquid 0.05%	**Treatment of acne vulgaris** Apply lightly to affected area once daily, before bedtime Therapeutic results should be seen after 2 to 3 weeks, but may not be optimal until after 6 weeks.	Administration Issues For external use only; keep preparation away from the eyes, mouth, angles of nose, and mucous membranes; wash hands thoroughly after application; avoid excessive exposure to the sunlight or sunlamps; apply liquid with the fingertip, gauze pad, or cotton swab, do not oversaturate gauze or cotton; normal use of cosmetics is permissible. Drug–Drug Interactions Concomitant use of **sulfur, resorcinol, benzoyl peroxide, medicated soaps,** or **salicylic acid** with tretinoin may cause significant skin irritation.	ADRs Photosensitivity, skin irritation, hyperpigmentation, hypopigmentation.	Contraindications Hypersensitivity to tretinoin or any component of the product. Pregnancy Category: C Lactation Issues Excretion in breast milk is unknown; use with caution in nursing mothers.

802. Antipsoriatic Products

Drug and Dosage Forms	Usual Dosage Range	Administration Issues and Drug–Drug Interactions	Common Adverse Drug Reactions (ADRs)	Contraindications, Pregnancy Category, and Lactation Issues
Acitretin Soriatane Capsules 10 mg, 25 mg	**Treatment of severe psoriasis, including erythrodermic and generalized pustular types** Initiate therapy at 25 or 50 mg/d as a single dose with main meal. Maintenance doses of 25 to 50 mg/d may be given.	Administration Issues **Women should NOT become pregnant while taking acitretin and should use contraception during treatment and for 3 years after discontinuing therapy;** do not consume alcohol during therapy and for 2 months following discontinuation of acitretin since alcohol may interfere with the excretion of acitretin. Drug Interactions Acitretin may interfere with the contraceptive effect of **microdose progestin** preparations.	ADRs Fatigue, asthenia, headache, dysesthesia, dizziness, dry nose, dry eyes, conjunctivitis, chelitis, alopecia, nail fragility, pruritus, dermatitis, arthralgias, mylagias, chills, diaphoresis, hypertriglyceridemia (monitor lipids monthly × 4 months then q 2–3 months), LFT elevations (monitor monthly × 6 months then q 3 months). Pharmacokinetics $T_{1/2}$ (parent); 50 h; food increases bioavailability.	Contraindications Hypersensitivity to acitretin or etretinate, pregnancy, intention to become pregnant during therapy or within 3 yr after discontinuation. Pregnancy Category: X Lactation Issues Excretion in breast milk is unknown.
Anthralin Ointment Anthra-Derm, generics 0.1%, 0.25%, 0.5%, 1% Cream generics 0.25%, 1% Drithocreme 0.1%, 0.25%, 0.5% Drithocreme HP 1% Dritho-Scalp 0.25%, 0.5%	**Treatment of quiescent or chronic psoriasis** Rub gently into skin until absorbed once daily beginning with the lowest strength available; increase strength as needed; the optimal period of contact will vary according to the strength used and the patient's response to treatment; initial contact time is 0.1% to 2% for 15 to 20 minutes, followed by thorough removal of the anthralin with soap or petrolatum; continue treatment until the patient's skin is entirely clear.	Administration Issues For external use only; keep preparation away from the eyes, mouth, angles of nose, and mucous membranes; wash hands thoroughly after application; anthralin may stain fabrics, skin, fingernails, or hair. Safety and efficacy in children have not been established. Drug–Drug Interactions **Topical corticosteroids** may destabilize psoriasis, allow at least one week between the discontinuation of topical steroids and the commencement of anthralin therapy.	ADRs Skin irritation.	Contraindications Hypersensitivity to anthralin; use on the face; acutely or actively inflamed psoriatic eruptions. Pregnancy Category: C Lactation Issues Excretion in breast milk is unknown; due to the potential for tumorigenicity in animals, discontinue nursing or the drug, taking into account the importance of the drug to the mother.
Calcipotriene Dovonex Ointment 0.005% Cream 0.005% Solution 0.005%	**Treatment of moderate plaque psoriasis** Apply a thin layer to the affected area twice daily and rub in gently; improvement in clinical trials was shown after 2 weeks of therapy with 70% of patients showing at least marked improvement after 8 weeks	Administration Issues For external use only; keep preparation away from the eyes, mouth, angles of nose, and mucous membranes; wash hands thoroughly after application. Safety and efficacy in children have not been established.	ADRs Burning, itching, erythema, dry skin. Absorption Issues approximately 6% of the applied dose is absorbed systemically; most of the absorbed dose is converted to inactive metabolites within 24 h of application.	Contraindications Hypersensitivity to any component of the preparation; patients with demonstrated hypercalcemia or evidence of vitamin D toxicity; use on the face. Pregnancy Category: C Lactation Issues Excretion in breast milk is unknown; use with caution in nursing mothers.

(continues on next page)

802. Antipsoriatic Products *continued from previous page*

Drug and Dosage Forms	Usual Dosage Range	Administration Issues and Drug–Drug Interactions	Common Adverse Drug Reactions (ADRs)	Contraindications, Pregnancy Category, and Lactation Issues
Nitrofurazone Furacin, generics Solution 0.2% Ointment, soluble 0.2% Cream 0.2%	**Adjunctive therapy for patients with second and third degree burns when bacterial resistance to other agents is a potential problem and in skin grafting to prevent bacterial contamination** Apply once daily directly to lesion or place on gauze; may reapply every few days, depending on dressing technique.	Administration Issues For external use only; keep preparation away from the eyes, mouth, angles of nose, and mucous membranes; wash hands thoroughly after application; flush dressing with sterile saline to facilitate removal.	ADRs Rash, pruritis, superinfection. Antibacterial spectrum *Staphylococcus aureus,* Streptococcal sp., *E. coli, Clostridium perfringens, Aerobacter aerogenes,* and *Proteus* sp.	Contraindications Hypersensitivity to nitrofurazone. Pregnancy Category: C Lactation Issues Excretion in breast milk is unknown; discontinue nursing or the drug, taking into account the importance of the drug to the mother.
Tar-Containing Products The following types of products are available in varying strengths of coal tar: **creams, lotions, liquids, gels, soaps, oil**	**Adjunct treatment of psoriasis, seborrheic dermatitis, atopic dermatitis, and eczema** Add to bath water; soak 10 to 20 minutes; pat dry. **Do not use in children < 2 years**	Administration Issues For external use only; keep preparation away from the eyes, mouth, and mucous membranes; avoid prolonged exposure to the sun for 72 h after use; staining of hair, clothes, and plastic or fiberglass tubs may occur.	ADRs Irritation, photosensitivity, dermatitis.	Contraindications Open or infected lesions; acute inflammation. Pregnancy Category: C Lactation Issues Excretion in breast milk is unknown; decide whether to discontinue breastfeeding or discontinue the drug, taking into account the importance of coal tar to the mother.
Tar Derivative Shampoos (with varying concentrations of coal tar) Shampoo Neutrogena T/Gel, Tegrin Medicated, plus Conditioner Neutrogena T/Gel	**Treatment of scalp psoriasis, eczema, seborrheic dermatitis, dandruff, cradle-cap, and other oily, itchy conditions of the body and scalp** Rub shampoo liberally into wet hair and scalp; rinse thoroughly; repeat and leave on for 5 minutes; rinse thoroughly. Depending on product, use from once daily to at least twice a week; use daily for severe scalp problems.	Administration Issues For external use only; keep preparation away from the eyes, mouth, angles of nose, and mucous membranes; wash hands thoroughly after application; do not use on acutely inflamed skin; avoid prolonged exposure to sunlight for 24 h after application.	ADRs Rash, burning, photosensitivity, skin discoloration.	Contraindications Acute inflammation; open or infected lesions.

803. Antiseborrheic Products

Drug and Dosage Forms	Usual Dosage Range	Administration Issues	Common Adverse Drug Reactions (ADRs)	Contraindications, Pregnancy Category, and Lactation Issues
Chloroxine Capitrol Shampoo 2%	**Treatment of dandruff and mild to moderate seborrheic dermatitis of the scalp** Massage into wet hair, lather for 3 minutes, rinse, repeat, rinse thoroughly. Apply twice weekly.	Administration Issues For external use only; keep preparation away from the eyes, mouth, angles of nose, and mucous membranes; wash hands thoroughly after application.	ADRs Irritation, burning, discoloration of light-colored hair.	Contraindications Hypersensitivity to any of the ingredients. Pregnancy Category: C Lactation Issues Excretion in breast milk is unknown; use with caution in nursing mothers.
Povidone-Iodine Betadine Shampoo 7.5%	**Temporary relief of scaling and itching due to dandruff** Apply 2 teaspoonsful to hair and scalp, lather with warm water, rinse, repeat application, massage gently into scalp, allow to remain on scalp for 5 minutes, rinse scalp thoroughly; repeat twice weekly until improvement is noticed, thereafter use once weekly.	Administration Issues For external use only; keep preparation away from the eyes, mouth, angles of nose, and mucous membranes; wash hands thoroughly after application; do not use on acutely inflamed skin.	ADRs Rash, burning, irritation.	
Pyrithione Zinc Shampoo Zincon, Head & Shoulders, Head & Shoulders Dry Scalp 1%, 2% Soap ZNP Bar 2%	**Control dandruff and seborrheic dermatitis of the body (ZNP Bar) and scalp** Apply shampoo, lather, rinse, and repeat; use once or twice weekly.	Administration Issues For external use only; keep preparation away from the eyes, mouth, angles of nose, and mucous membranes; wash hands thoroughly after application; do not use on acutely inflamed skin.	ADRs Rash, burning.	
Selenium Sulfide Lotion-Shampoo Selsun Blue, Head & Shoulders Intensive Treatment Dandruff Shampoo, various 1% Selsun, Exsel, various generics 2.5%	**Treatment of dandruff and seborrheic dermatitis of the scalp** Massage 5 to 10 ml into wet scalp; allow to remain on the scalp for 2 to 3 minutes; rinse thoroughly. Usually 2 applications per week for 2 weeks will afford control; for maintenance therapy, it may be used once weekly, once every 2 weeks, or once every 3 to 4 weeks in some cases. **Treatment of tinea versicolor** Apply to affected areas and lather with a small amount of water; allow to remain	Administration Issues For external use only; keep preparation away from the eyes, mouth, angles of nose, and mucous membranes; wash hands thoroughly after application; do not use on acutely inflamed skin; may damage jewelry. Safety and efficacy in children have not been established.	ADRs Skin irritation, dryness of hair and scalp.	Contraindications Hypersensitivity to components of the product. Pregnancy Category: C (tinea versicolor)

(*continues on next page*)

803. Antiseborrheic Products *continued from previous page*

Drug and Dosage Forms	Usual Dosage Range	Administration Issues	Common Adverse Drug Reactions (ADRs)	Contraindications, Pregnancy Category, and Lactation Issues
Selenium Sulfide *cont.*	on skin for 10 minutes, rinse body thoroughly; repeat once daily for 7 days.			
Sulfacetamide Sodium Sebizon Lotion 10%	**Treatment of dandruff and seborrheic dermatitis** Apply at bedtime and allow to remain overnight, precede application by a shampoo if the hair and scalp are oily or greasy or if there is considerable debris; in severe cases with crusting, heavy scaling, and inflammation of the scalp, apply twice daily. The following morning wash the hair and scalp if desired, wash hair at least once weekly, continue treatment for 8 to 10 nights; increase the interval between applications as improvement occurs, once or twice weekly or every other week applications may prevent recurrence. **Treatment of secondary bacterial infection of the skin:** Apply 2 to 4 times daily until infection clears.	Administration Issues For external use only; keep preparation away from the eyes, mouth, angles of nose, and mucous membranes; wash hands thoroughly after application; completely moisten scalp and gently rub in with fingertips, brush hair thoroughly for 2 to 3 minutes after application. Safety and efficacy in children < 12 years have not been established.	ADRs Rash, burning, irritation, superinfection. Antibacterial spectrum Bacteriostatic effect against gram-positive and gram-negative organisms.	Contraindications Hypersensitivity to sulfonamides. Pregnancy Category: C Lactation Issues Excretion in breast milk is unknown; use with caution in nursing mothers.
Sulfur Preparations Adne lotion 10, others Cream 5% Lotion 4%, 10% Soap 5% Mask 6.4%	**Treatment of seborrheic dermatitis. May also be useful in the treatment of acne vulgaris, oily skin, rosacea, and tinea versicolor** Apply a thin layer. Use qd to tid.	Administration Issues For external use only. For best results, wash skin thoroughly with a mild cleanser prior to application. Keep away from eyes. If undue irritation develops discontinue use. Preferred treatment for infants, small children, patients with seizures or other neurologic disorders and pregnant or lactating women.	ADRs Skin irritation.	Contraindications Hypersensitivity to sulfur or any component of the product.
Antiseborrheic Combinations Shampoo Fostex Medicated Cleansing, plus	**Treatment of dandruff and mild to moderate seborrheic dermatitis of the scalp** Massage into wet hair, lather for 3 minutes, rinse, repeat, rinse thoroughly	Administration Issues For external use only; keep preparation away from the eyes, mouth, angles of nose, and mucous membranes; wash hands thoroughly after application.	ADRs Irritation, burning.	

804. Antihistamine-Containing Products

Drug and Dosage Forms	Usual Dosage Range	Administration Issues and Drug–Drug Interactions	Common Adverse Drug Reactions (ADRs)
Diphenhydramine Cream Benadryl (1% diphenhydramine) Maximum Strength Benadryl (2% diphenhydramine) Caladryl (1% diphenhydramine, 8% calamine) Lotion Caladryl (1% diphenhydramine) Ziradryl (1% diphenhydramine, 2% zinc oxide) Spray Benadryl (1% diphenhydramine, 85% alcohol) Caladryl (1% diphenhydramine, 8% calamine)	**Temporary relief of itching due to minor skin disorders, sunburn, insect bites and stings, and poison ivy, sumac, and oak** Apply to affected area 3 to 4 times daily as needed.	Administration Issues For external use only; keep preparation away from the eyes, mouth, angles of nose, and mucous membranes; wash hands thoroughly after application; do not apply to blistered, raw, or oozing areas of the skin; avoid prolonged use (> 7 days).	ADRs Irritation, burning.
Doxepin Zonalon Cream 5%	**Short-term management of moderate pruritis in adults** Apply to affected area 4 times daily with at least a 3 to 4 hour interval between applications. No safety or efficacy data for use > 8 days.	Administration Issues For external use only; keep preparation away from the eyes, mouth, angles of nose, and mucous membranes; wash hands thoroughly after application; do not use occlusive dressings that may increase the absorption of doxepin; apply a thin coat. Drug–Drug Interactions **Alcohol** ingestion may increase the potential for sedative effects of doxepin; **Cimetidine** may inhibit the metabolism of doxepin leading to increased toxic effects; Concurrent use of doxepin and **monoamine oxidase inhibitors** may lead to serious toxic adverse effects.	ADRs Drowsiness, dry mouth, headache, burning, stinging. Absorption Issues Topical; plasma concentrations ranged from 0–47 ng/ml, target therapeutic level following oral dosing is 30–150 ng/ml.

805. Anti-Infective Products (Topical and Vaginal)

Drug and Dosage Forms	Usual Dosage Range	Administration Issues	Adverse Drug Reaction (ADRs) Spectrum (If listed) and Absorption issues	Contraindications, Pregnancy Category, and Lactation Issues
Acyclovir Zovirax Ointment 5% Cream 5%	**Treatment of initial episodes of herpes genitalis and in limited mucocutaneous herpes simplex virus infections** Apply to affected areas q 3 to 6 hours for 7 days.	Administration Issues For external use only; keep preparation away from the eyes, mouth, angles of nose, and mucous membranes; initiate therapy as early as possible following onset of symptoms; apply using a finger cot or rubber glove to avoid autoinoculation of other body sites; acyclovir is not a cure for HSV infections.	ADRs Mild pain, burning, stinging. Antiviral spectrum *Herpes simplex* virus types 1 (HSV-1) and type 2 (HSV-2)	Contraindications Hypersensitivity or intolerance to components of the preparation. Pregnancy Category: C Lactation Issues Excretion in breast milk is unknown; use with caution in nursing mothers.
Amphotericin B Fungizone, generics Cream 3% Lotion 3% Ointment 3%	**Treatment of cutaneous and mucocutaneous infections caused by *Candida* sp.** Apply liberally to affected area 2 to 4 times daily for 1 to 3 weeks.	Administration Issues For external use only; keep preparation away from the eyes, mouth, and mucous membranes; cleanse the affected area with soap and water and dry thoroughly prior to application; wash hands thoroughly after application.	ADRs Skin discoloration, burning, itching.	Contraindications Hypersensitivity to any component of the product.
Bacitracin generics Ointment 500 units per gm	**Aid to healing and prophylaxis of infection in minor cuts, wounds, burns, and skin abrasions** Apply to affected area 1 to 4 times daily.	Administration Issues For external use only; keep preparation away from the eyes, mouth, and mucous membranes; wash hands thoroughly after application; area to be treated may be covered with a gauze dressing if desired.	ADRs Skin irritation, superinfection.	Contraindications Hypersensitivity to any ingredients in the preparation.
Butoconazole Gynazole-1, Mycelex-3 Vaginal Cream 2%	**Treatment of vulvovaginal candidiasis** 1 applicator of cream intravaginally once (Gynazole-1) or insert one applicatorful a day, preferably at bedtime 3 consecutive days.	Administration Issues For external use only. Follow patient information sheet.	ADRs Irritation, burning, discharge, swelling, itchy fingers (0.2%).	Contraindications Hypersensitivity to buconazole. Pregnancy Category: C Lactation Issues use with caution
Ciclopirox Olamine Loprox	**Treatment of athlete's foot, jock itch, ringworm, cutaneous candidiasis, and tinea versicolor**	Administration Issues For external use only; keep preparation away from the eyes, mouth, and mucous membranes; cleanse the affected area	ADRs Irritation, pruritis, burning.	Contraindications Hypersensitivity to ciclopirox olamine. Pregnancy Category: B

Cream 0.77% Lotion 0.77% Shampoo 1% Topical Solution 0.77% Pentac Nail Lacquer 8%	Apply to affected area twice daily, morning and evening; improvement should occur within 7 days (Loprox) **Treatment of onychomycosis of fingernails /toenails by *T. rubrum* (*Pentac*)** Apply daily to all infected nails.	with soap and water and dry thoroughly prior to application; wash hands thoroughly after application; for athlete's foot, wear well-fitting, ventilated shoes and change shoes and socks at least once daily; reevaluate therapy if no improvement occurs in 4 weeks.		Lactation Issues Excretion in breast milk is unknown; use with caution in nursing mothers.
Clioquinol Cream 3% Ointment 3%	**Treatment of inflamed conditions of the skin such as eczema, athlete's foot, and other fungal infections** Apply to affected area 2 times daily or as directed.	Administration Issues For external use only; keep preparation away from the eyes, mouth, and mucous membranes; cleanse the affected area with soap and water and dry thoroughly prior to application; wash hands thoroughly after application; for athlete's foot, wear well-fitting, ventilated shoes and change shoes and socks at least once daily; reevaluate therapy if no improvement occurs in 4 weeks.	ADRs Irritation, stinging; may have systemic reactions (if applied on large area of skin): iodism, hair loss, agranulocytosis.	Contraindications Hypersensitivity to chloroxine, iodine or iodine-containing preparations; severe renal or hepatic disease; thyroid disorder. Pregnancy Category: C Lactation Issues Safety not established.
Clotrimazole Topical Cream 1% Lotrimin, Lotrimin AF Mycelex, Mycelex OTC Topical Solution, 1% Lotrimin, Lotrimin AF Mycelex, Mycelex OTC Topical Lotion Lotrimin 1% Vaginal Suppositories Mycelex, Gyne-Lotrimin 100 mg, 200 mg Vaginal Cream 1%, 2%	**Treatment of athlete's foot, jock itch, ringworm, cutaneous candidiasis, and tinea versicolor** Topical: Apply to affected area twice daily, morning and evening; improvement should occur within 7 days **Treatment of vulvovaginal candidiasis** Vaginal Suppository Insert 1 suppository intravaginally at bedtime × 3 days (200 mg) Vaginal Cream: 1 applicatorful intravaginally × 3–7 d	Administration Issues Topical: For external use only; keep preparation away from the eyes, mouth, and mucous membranes; cleanse the affected area with soap and water and dry thoroughly prior to application; wash hands thoroughly after application; for athlete's foot, wear well-fitting, ventilated shoes and change shoes and socks at least once daily; reevaluate therapy if no improvement occurs in 4 weeks. Vaginal: For vaginal use only. Follow instructions carefully. Refrain from sexual intercourse during therapy.	ADRs Topical: Irritation, pruritis, burning Vaginal: Skin rash, lower abdominal cramps, vulval irritation, vaginal irritation, itching, burning.	Contraindications Hypersensitivity to clotrimazole. Pregnancy Category: B Lactation Issues Excretion in breast milk is unknown; use with caution in nursing mothers.

(continues on next page)

805. Anti-Infective Products (Topical and Vaginal) *continued from previous page*

Drug and Dosage Forms	Usual Dosage Range	Administration Issues	Adverse Drug Reaction (ADRs) Spectrum (If listed) and Absorption issues	Contraindications, Pregnancy Category, and Lactation Issues
Combination Anti-infectives Ointment Polysporin (10,000 units/gm polymyxin, 500 units/gm bacitracin) Maximum Strength Neosporin (10,000 units/gm polymyxin, 3.5 mg/gm neomycin, 500 units/gm bacitracin) Neosporin, Triple Antibiotic (5,000 units/gm polymyxin, 3.5 mg/gm neomycin, 400 units/gm bacitracin) Maximum Strength Mycitracin Triple Antibiotic (5,000 units/gm polymyxin, 3.5 mg/gm neomycin, 500 units/gm bacitracin) Mycitracin Plus (5,000 units/gm polymyxin, 3.5 mg/gm neomycin, 500 units/gm bacitracin, 40 mg/gm lidocaine) Cream Neosporin (10,000 units/gm polymyxin B sulfate, 3.5 mg/gm neomycin) Powder Polysporin (10,000 units/gm polymyxin, 500 units/gm bacitracin) Spray Polysporin (2222 units/ml polymyxin, 111 units/ml bacitracin)	**Aid to healing and prophylaxis of infection in minor cuts, wounds, burns, and skin abrasions** Apply to affected area 1 to 4 times daily.	Administration Issues For external use only; keep preparation away from the eyes, mouth, and mucous membranes; wash hands thoroughly after application; area to be treated may be covered with a gauze dressing if desired.	ADRs Skin irritation, superinfection.	Contraindications Hypersensitivity to any ingredients in the preparation.
Econazole Nitrate Spectazole, generics Cream 1%	**Treatment of athlete's foot, jock itch, ringworm, and tinea versicolor** Apply to affected area once daily; treat for 2 weeks, except athlete's foot treat for 4 weeks.	Administration Issues For external use only; keep preparation away from the eyes, mouth, and mucous membranes; cleanse the affected area with soap and water and dry thoroughly prior to application; wash hands thoroughly after application; for athlete's foot, wear well-fitting, ventilated shoes and change shoes and socks at least once daily; reevaluate therapy if no improvement occurs in 4 weeks.	ADRs Irritation, burning, itching, erythema.	Contraindications Hypersensitivity to econazole nitrate. Pregnancy Category: C Lactation Issues Excretion in breast milk is unknown; use with caution in nursing mothers.

	<u>Treatment of cutaneous candidiasis</u> Apply to affected area twice daily for 2 weeks.			
Erythromycin generics <u>Ointment</u> Akne-mycin 2% <u>Solution</u> 1.5%, 2% <u>Gel</u> 2% <u>Pledgets</u> 2%	**<u>Aid to healing and prophylaxis of infection in minor cuts, wounds, burns, and skin abrasions</u>** Apply to affected area bid.	<u>Administration Issues</u> For external use only; keep preparation away from the eyes, mouth, and mucous membranes; wash hands thoroughly after application; area to be treated may be covered with a gauze dressing if desired.	<u>ADRs</u> Skin irritation, superinfection.	<u>Contraindications</u> Hypersensitivity to any ingredients in the preparation.
Gentamicin Garamycin, generics <u>Ointment</u> 0.1% <u>Cream</u> 0.1%	**<u>Aid to healing and prophylaxis of infection in minor cuts, wounds, burns, and skin abrasions</u>** Apply to affected area 3 to 4 times daily.	<u>Administration Issues</u> For external use only; keep preparation away from the eyes, mouth, and mucous membranes; wash hands thoroughly after application; area to be treated may be covered with a gauze dressing if desired.	<u>ADRs</u> Skin irritation, superinfection.	<u>Contraindications</u> Hypersensitivity to any ingredients in the preparation.
Imiquimod Aldara <u>Cream</u> 5%	**<u>Treatment of genital and perianal warts</u>** Apply 3 times/wk, prior to normal sleeping hours and leave on skin for 6 to 10 h. Wash with soap and water after treatment period.	<u>Administration Issues</u> For external use only; keep preparation away from the eyes, mouth, and mucous membranes. Do not occlude area with bandages, covers or wraps. Imiquimod may weaken condoms and vaginal diaphragms.	<u>ADRs</u> Erythema, itching, erosion, burning, pain, excoriation, flaking, edema, induration, ulceration.	<u>Contraindications</u> Hypersensitivity to any component of the product. <u>Pregnancy Category:</u> Do not use in pregnant women. <u>Lactation Issues</u> Excretion in breast milk is unknown.
Ketoconazole Nizoral, generics <u>Cream</u> 2% <u>Shampoo</u> 1%, 2%	**<u>Treatment of athlete's foot, jock itch, ringworm, cutaneous candidiasis, and tinea versicolor</u>** Apply to affected area once daily for 2 weeks; treat athlete's foot for 6 weeks. **<u>Treatment of seborrheic dermatitis</u>** Apply to affected area twice daily for 4 weeks.	<u>Administration Issues</u> For external use only; keep preparation away from the eyes, mouth, and mucous membranes; cleanse the affected area with soap and water and dry thoroughly prior to application; moisten hair and scalp thoroughly prior to application; wash hands thoroughly after application.	<u>ADRs</u> Irritation, pruritis, stinging, mild dryness of skin.	<u>Contraindications</u> Hypersensitivity to any component of the product. <u>Pregnancy Category: C</u> <u>Lactation Issues</u> Safety for use in nursing mothers has not been established; use with caution.

(*continues on next page*)

805. Anti-Infective Products (Topical and Vaginal) *continued from previous page*

Drug and Dosage Forms	Usual Dosage Range	Administration Issues	Adverse Drug Reaction (ADRs) Spectrum (If listed) and Absorption issues	Contraindications, Pregnancy Category, and Lactation Issues
Ketoconazole *cont.*	**Treatment of dandruff and scaling** Apply to hair and scalp; lather and wash for 1 minute; rinse thoroughly; repeat, leaving shampoo on scalp for 3 minutes; rinse thoroughly; dry hair. Shampoo twice weekly for 4 weeks with at least 3 days between each shampooing; may shampoo intermittently as needed to maintain control.			
Miconazole Nitrate generics Powder 2% Spray 2% Spray liquid 2% Powder 2% Vaginal Suppositories 100 mg, 200 mg, 1200 mg Vaginal Cream 2% Ointment 2% Cream 2%	**Treatment of athlete's foot, jock itch, ringworm, and cutaneous candidiasis** Apply to affected area twice daily, morning and evening; treat for 2 weeks, except athlete's foot treat for 4 weeks. **Treatment of tinea versicolor** Apply to affected area once daily; clinical improvement should be seen in 2 weeks. **Treatment of vulvovaginal candidiasis** Vaginal suppository: 200 mg, 1 dose × 3 d or 100 mg, 1 dose × 7 d or 1200 mg, 1 dose × 1 day Vaginal cream: 1 applicatorful q hs × 3–7 d Cream: Apply to affected areas bid × 7 d	Administration Issues For external use only; keep preparation away from the eyes, mouth, and mucous membranes; cleanse the affected area with soap and water and dry thoroughly prior to application; wash hands thoroughly after application; for athlete's foot, wear well-fitting, ventilated shoes and change shoes and socks at least once daily; reevaluate therapy if no improvement occurs in 4 weeks.	ADRs Topical: Irritation, burning. Vaginal: Vulvovaginal burning, itching, irritation, headache, pelvic cramps, contact dermatitis.	Contraindications Hypersensitivity to any component of the product. Pregnancy Category: Topical safe in pregnancy. Lactation Issues Safety for use in nursing mothers has not been established; use with caution.

Mupirocin Bactroban, Bactroban Nasal generics **Ointment** 2% **Cream** 2%	**Treatment of impetigo** Apply a small amount to affected area 3 times daily; reevaluate patients not showing clinical response in 3 to 5 days. Nasal Divide ≈ ½ of the ointment from the single-use tube between the nostrils and apply bid × 5 days.	Administration Issues For external use only; keep preparation away from the eyes, mouth, and mucous membranes; wash hands thoroughly after application; area to be treated may be covered with a gauze dressing if desired Nasal: After application, close nostrils by pressing together and releasing sides of the nose repeatedly for ≈ 1 minute.	ADRs Burning, stinging, local pain. Antibacterial spectrum *Staphylococcus aureus* (methicillin-resistant and beta lactamase-producing strains), *S. saprophyticus, S. epidermidis* and *pyogenes.*	Contraindications Hypersensitivity to any components of the product. Pregnancy Category: B Lactation Issues Excretion in breast milk is unknown; temporarily discontinue nursing while using mupirocin.
Naftifine Naftin Cream 1% Gel 1%	**Treatment of athlete's foot, jock itch, and ringworm** Apply to affected area once daily with cream or twice daily with gel.	Administration Issues For external use only; keep preparation away from the eyes, mouth, and mucous membranes; cleanse the affected area with soap and water and dry thoroughly prior to application; wash hands thoroughly after application; reevaluate therapy if no improvement occurs in 4 weeks.	ADRs Burning, stinging, dryness, irritation. Absorption Issues Systemic absorption was approximately 6% of administered dose following topical administration.	Contraindications Hypersensitivity to naftifine. Pregnancy Category: B Lactation Issues Excretion in breast milk is unknown; use with caution in nursing mothers.
Neomycin Sulfate Generics Ointment 3.5 mg/gm Cream 3.5 mg/gm	**Aid to healing and prophylaxis of infection in minor cuts, wounds, burns, and skin abrasions** Apply to affected area 1 to 3 times daily	Administration Issues For external use only; keep preparation away from the eyes, mouth, and mucous membranes; wash hands thoroughly after application; area to be treated may be covered with a gauze dressing if desired.	ADRs Skin irritation, superinfection.	Contraindications Hypersensitivity to any ingredients in the preparation.
Nystatin Mycostatin, Nilstat, various generics Cream 100,000 units/gm Ointment 100,000 units/gm Powder 100,000 units/gm Vaginal Tablets 100,000 units	**Treatment of cutaneous and mucocutaneous infections caused by *Candida* sp.** Apply to affected area 2 to 3 times daily until healing is complete. For fungal infections of the feet, dust powder freely on the feet as well as the shoes and socks. **Treatment of vulvovaginal candidiasis** 1 tablet intravaginally qd × 2 wk	Administration Issues Topical: For external use only; keep preparation away from the eyes, mouth, and mucous membranes; cleanse the affected area with soap and water and dry thoroughly prior to application; massage a small amount into affected area; wash hands thoroughly after application; use the cream for infections involving the intertriginous areas; reevaluate therapy if no improvement occurs in 4 weeks. Vaginal: Symptomatic relief may occur in a few days; continue for full course of therapy.		Contraindications Hypersensitivity to any components of the product. Pregnancy Category: A Lactation Issues Excretion in breast milk is unknown; use with caution in nursing mothers.

(continues on next page)

805. Anti-Infective Products (Topical and Vaginal) *continued from previous page*

Drug and Dosage Forms	Usual Dosage Range	Administration Issues	Adverse Drug Reaction (ADRs) Spectrum (If listed) and Absorption issues	Contraindications, Pregnancy Category, and Lactation Issues
Oxiconazole Nitrate Oxistat Cream 1% Lotion 1%	**Treatment of athlete's foot, jock itch, and ringworm** Apply to affected area twice daily for 2 weeks; treat athlete's foot for 4 weeks to decrease possibility of recurrence.	Administration Issues For external use only; keep preparation away from the eyes, mouth, and mucous membranes; cleanse the affected area with soap and water and dry thoroughly prior to application; wash hands thoroughly after application; for athlete's foot, wear well-fitting, ventilated shoes and change shoes and socks at least once daily; reevaluate therapy if no improvement occurs in 4 weeks.	ADRs Pruritis, burning, stinging, irritation. Absorption Issues Systemic absorption is very low; < 0.3% of applied dose is recovered in urine 5 days after application	Contraindications Hypersensitivity to oxiconazole nitrate. Pregnancy Category: B Lactation Issues Excretion in breast milk is unknown; use with caution in nursing mothers.
Podofilox Condylox Topical Gel 0.5% Topical Solution 0.5%	**Topical treatment of anogenital warts (gel) and topical treatment of external warts (solution) due to HPV** Apply solution or gel bid × 3 days, then off for 4 days. May repeat cycle total of 4 times. Minimize application on surrounding normal tissue. Allow to dry before allowing the return of the opposing skin surfaces to normal positions.	Administration Issues Instruct patient to wash hands thoroughly before using and after each application. For external use only. Avoid contact with eyes. If no improvement after 4 weeks of treatment have patient consult health-care provider.	ADRs Burning, pain, inflammation, erosion, itching, bleeding Side effects more common in patients treated with the solution than with the gel.	Contraindications Hypersensitivity to product. Pregnancy Category: Do not use on pregnant patients. Lactation Issues Weigh risk to infant versus benefit to nursing mother.
Podophyllum Resin Podcon-25, Podofin Liquid 25% podophyllum resin in tincture of benzoin	**Treatment of soft genital (venereal) warts (condylomata acuminata) and other papillomas; CDC recommends podophyllum as an alternative treatment of HPV** Apply no more than 0.5 mL to the lesion per visit. Wash in 1–4 h. Retreat in 7 to 10 days. If no improvement after 3–4 treatments, refer to specialist.	Administration Issues To be applied only by a trained health-care professional. For external use only. Avoid contact with eyes.	ADRs Paresthesia, polyneuritis, pyrexia, leukopenia, diarrhea, abdominal pain, confusion, dizziness.	Contraindications Hypersensitivity to product; diabetics, patients using steroids or with poor blood circulation, bleeding warts. Pregnancy Category: Do not use on pregnant patients. Lactation Issues Do not use in nursing mothers.
Sulconazole Nitrate Exelderm Cream 1% Solution 1%	**Treatment of athlete's foot, jock itch, ringworm, and tinea versicolor** Apply to affected area 1 to 2 times daily for 3 to 4 weeks; athlete's foot should be treated twice daily for 4 weeks.	Administration Issues For external use only; keep preparation away from the eyes, mouth, and mucous membranes; cleanse the affected area with soap and water and dry thoroughly prior to application; massage a small amount into affected area; wash hands thoroughly after application; for athlete's foot, wear well-fitting, ventilated shoes	ADRs Itching, burning, stinging.	Contraindications Hypersensitivity to sulconazole nitrate. Pregnancy Category: C Lactation Issues Excretion in breast milk is unknown; use with caution in nursing mothers.

		and change shoes and socks at least once daily; reevaluate therapy if no improvement occurs in 4 to 6 weeks.		
Terbinafine Lamisi AT, Desenex Max Cream 1% Spray 1%	**Treatment of athlete's foot, jock itch, ringworm, cutaneous candidiasis, and tinea versicolor** Cream: Apply to affected area once or twice daily for 1 to 4 weeks. Spray: bid for 1 week or as directed.	Administration Issues For external use only; keep preparation away from the eyes, mouth, and mucous membranes; cleanse the affected area with soap and water and dry thoroughly prior to application; wash hands thoroughly after application; avoid the use of occlusive dressings; reevaluate therapy if no improvement occurs in 4 weeks.	ADRs Irritation, itching, dryness. Absorption Issues: Approximately 3.5% of a topical dose is recovered in the urine.	Contraindications Hypersensitivity to terbinafine. Pregnancy Category: B Lactation Issues Excreted in breast milk in small concentrations; due to potential for adverse events in nursing infants, discontinue nursing or the drug, taking into account the importance of the drug to the mother.
Terconazole Terazol 7, Terazol 3 Vaginal Cream 0.4%, 0.8% Vaginal Suppositories 80 mg	**Treatment of vulvovaginal candidiasis** Suppositories: Insert 1 dose (80 mg) × 3 d Cream: 0.4%: 1 applicatorful q hs × 7 d or 0.8%: 1 applicatorful q hs × 3 d	Administration Issues Before prescribing another course of therapy, reconfirm diagnosis by smears or culture to rule out other pathogens. The therapeutic effect of terconazole is not affected by menstruation.	ADRs Headache, body pain, dysmenorrhea, itching, pruritus.	Contraindications Hypersensitivity to terconazole. Pregnancy Category: C Lactation Issues Use with caution.
Tetracycline Achromycin Ointment 3%	**Aid to healing and prophylaxis of infection in minor cuts, wounds, burns, and skin abrasions** Apply to affected area 1 to 4 times daily.	Administration Issues For external use only; keep preparation away from the eyes, mouth, and mucous membranes; wash hands thoroughly after application; area to be treated may be covered with a gauze dressing if desired	ADRs Skin irritation, superinfection.	Contraindications Hypersensitivity to any ingredients in the preparation.
Tioconazole Vagistat-1, Mouistal-1 Vaginal Ointment 6.5%	**Treatment of vulvovaginal candidiasis** 1 applicatorful intravaginally × 1 dose	Administration Issues For external use only. Follow patient instruction information sheet.	ADRs Irritation, burning, discharge, vulvar edema.	Contraindications Hypersensitivity to tioconazole. Pregnancy Category: C Lactation Issues Use with caution.
Tolnaftate Tinactin, generics Cream 1%	**Treatment of athlete's foot, jock itch, ringworm, and tinea versicolor** Apply to affected area twice daily for 2 to 3 weeks.	Administration Issues For external use only; keep preparation away from the eyes, mouth, and mucous membranes; cleanse the affected area with soap and water and dry thoroughly	ADRs Irritation.	

(continues on next page)

805. Anti-Infective Products (Topical and Vaginal) *continued from previous page*

Drug and Dosage Forms	Usual Dosage Range	Administration Issues	Adverse Drug Reaction (ADRs) Spectrum (If listed) and Absorption issues	Contraindications, Pregnancy Category, and Lactation Issues
Tolnaftate *cont.* Solution 1% Gel 1% Powder 1% Spray Powder 1% Spray Liquid 1%		prior to application; powders are used mainly as adjunctive therapy; use a small quantity; wash hands thoroughly after application; for athlete's foot, wear well-fitting, ventilated shoes and change shoes and socks at least once daily; reevaluate therapy if no improvement occurs after 10 days.		
Triacetin Solution Fungoid Tincture 30 ml Fungoid 15 ml Cream Fungoid Creme 30 gm	**Treatment of athlete's foot, jock itch, ringworm, and monilial impetigo** Apply cream or solution to affected area 3 times daily; improvement should occur within 7 days; reevaluate therapy if no improvement occurs in 4 weeks. **Treatment of nail fungus** Apply tincture to nail surface, beds, edges, and under surface of nail 3 times daily; continued treatment for several months may be necessary to see results.	Administration Issues For external use only; keep preparation away from the eyes, mouth, and mucous membranes; cleanse the affected area with soap and water and dry thoroughly prior to application; wash hands thoroughly after application; for athlete's foot, wear well-fitting, ventilated shoes and change shoes and socks at least once daily.	ADRs Irritation; use with caution in diabetic or patients with impaired blood circulation.	Contraindications Sensitivity to any components of the product.
Trichloroacetic Acid Tri-Chlor Liquid 80%	**Treatment of genital and perianal warts** Apply once or twice weekly depending on patient's tolerance. Apply baking soda and water paste after treatment to the area to neutralize acid. If no improvement after 3 treatments, refer to specialist.	Administration Issues For external use only; keep preparation away from the eyes, mouth, and mucous membranes. Can pretreat with topical anesthetic to lessen burning.	ADRs Burning, irritation, pain.	Contraindications Sensitivity to any components of the product; severely irritated tissue. Pregnancy: Safe to use in pregnancy.

806. Scabicides and Pediculicides

Drug and Dosage Forms	Usual Dosage Range	Administration Issues	Adverse Drug Reactions (ADRs)	Contraindications, Pregnancy Category, and Lactation Issues
Crotamiton Eurax Cream 10% Lotion 10%	**Treatment of scabies** Apply a thin layer to dry skin from neck down and rub in thoroughly over entire body; a second application is advisable 24 h later; remove medication with a cleansing bath 48 h after the second application.	Administration Issues For external use only; keep preparation away from the eyes, mouth, and mucous membranes; avoid use on the face; apply with rubber gloves; flush eyes well with water several minutes if contact occurs; avoid use on cuts; shake lotion and cream well prior to administration; change clothing and bed linen the next day, contaminated clothing and linen may be dry cleaned or washed in the hot cycle and machine dried in the hot cycle for 20 minutes; consider treatment in other family members and close personal contacts.	ADRs Irritation.	Contraindications Hypersensitivity to crotamiton. Pregnancy Category: C
Lindane Generics Cream 1% Lotion 1% Shampoo 1%	**Treatment of head lice and pubic lice** Apply lotion thinly to cover the dry hair and skin of affected area and rub in thoroughly; leave on for 12 hours; remove thoroughly with washing; one application is usually curative. Apply shampoo to dry hair; lather with a small quantity of water; work thoroughly into hair for 4 minutes; rinse thoroughly and towel dry; one application is usually curative. **Treatment of scabies** Apply a thin layer of cream or lotion to dry skin from neck down and rub in thoroughly over entire body (generally 2 oz. of medication is adequate for adults); leave on for 8 to 12 h; remove thoroughly with washing; one application is usually curative.	Administration Issues For external use only; keep preparation away from the eyes, mouth, and mucous membranes; avoid use on the face; apply with rubber gloves; flush eyes well with water several minutes if contact occurs; avoid use on cuts; treat sexual contacts simultaneously; shake lotion and cream well prior to administration; a fine-toothed comb may be used to comb hair to remove any remaining nit shells; reapply if there are demonstrable nits after 7 days; change clothing and bed linen the next day; contaminated clothing and linen may be dry cleaned or washed in the hot cycle and machine dried in the hot cycle for 20 minutes; consider treatment in other family members and close personal contacts. **Use with caution in children, potential toxic effects are greater in the young due to enhanced topical absorption.**	ADRs Dizziness, irritation.	Contraindications Hypersensitivity to lindane; use in premature neonates; patients with known seizure disorders. Pregnancy Category: B Lactation Issues Excreted in breast milk; due to potential for serious adverse events in infants, use an alternate method of feeding while using lindane.
Permethrin Generics Cream 5%	**Treatment of scabies** Apply a thin layer to dry skin from neck down and rub in thoroughly over entire body (usually 30 gm is sufficient for adults); leave on for 8 to 14 h; remove	Administration Issues For external use only; keep preparation away from the eyes, mouth, and mucous membranes; avoid use on the face; apply with rubber gloves; flush eyes well with	ADRs Pruritis. burning, stinging.	Contraindications Hypersensitivity to synthetic pyrethroid or pyrethrin, chrysanthemums, or any component of the product.

(*continues on next page*)

806. Scabicides and Pediculicides *continued from previous page*

Drug and Dosage Forms	Usual Dosage Range	Administration Issues	Adverse Drug Reactions (ADRs)	Contraindications, Pregnancy Category, and Lactation Issues
Liquid (cream rinse) Nix 1% Lotion 1%	thoroughly with washing; one application is usually curative. **Treatment of head lice** Apply shampoo to dry hair; lather; leave on hair for 10 minutes; rinse thoroughly and towel dry; one application is usually curative.	water several minutes if contact occurs; avoid use on cuts; shake lotion and cream well prior to administration; wash hair with shampoo, rinse with water, and towel dry prior to apply medication; a fine-toothed comb may be used to comb hair to remove any remaining nit shells; reapply if there are demonstrable nits after 7 days; change clothing and bed linen the next day, contaminated clothing and linen may be dry cleaned or washed in the hot cycle and machine dried in the hot cycle for 20 minutes; consider treatment in other family members and close personal contacts.		Pregnancy Category: B Lactation Issues Excretion in breast milk is unknown; use an alternate method of feeding while using permethrin.
Malathion Ovide Lotion 0.5%	**Treatment of head lice and their ova** Sprinkle lotion on dry hair and rub gently until the scalp is thoroughly moistened. Allow to dry naturally; use no heat and leave uncovered. After 8–12 h, wash the hair with a nonmedicated shampoo. Rinse and use a fine-toothed comb to remove dead lice and eggs. If required, repeat with second application in 7 to 9 days.	Administration Issues For external use only; keep preparation away from the eyes, mouth, and mucous membranes; avoid use on the face; apply with rubber gloves; flush eyes well with water several minutes if contact occurs; avoid use on cuts.	ADRs Irritation.	Contraindications Hypersensitivity to product. Pregnancy Category: B Lactation Issues Excretion in breast milk is unknown; use caution in nursing mothers.
Miscellaneous Pediculicides Liquid Control-L, End Lice (0.3% pyrethrin, 3% piperonyl, butoxide) Shampoo A-200, R&C, RID (0.3% pyrethrin, 3% piperonyl butoxide)	**Treatment of head lice, body lice, and pubic lice** Apply to affected hairy and surrounding area, lather hair; allow to remain for 10 minutes; wash hair and surrounding area thoroughly and dry with a clean towel. A second treatment after 7–10 days is recommended to kill any newly hatched lice.	Administration Issues For external use only; keep preparation away from the eyes, mouth, and mucous membranes; avoid use on the face; apply with rubber gloves; flush eyes well with water several minutes if contact occurs; avoid use on cuts; treat sexual contacts simultaneously; a fine-toothed comb may be used to comb hair to remove any remaining nit shells; change clothing and bed linen the next day, contaminated clothing and linen may be dry cleaned or washed in the hot cycle and machine dried in the hot cycle for 20 minutes; consider treatment in other family members and close personal contacts.	ADRs Irritation.	Contraindications Hypersensitivity to pyrethrins, permethrins, or any component of the product.

807. Corticosteroid Products

Warnings about topical steroid products: Topical corticosteroids have a repository effect; with continuous use, 1 to 2 applications per day may be as effective as 3 or more applications. Short-term or intermittent therapy with high-potency agents (i.e., every other day, 3 to 4 consecutive days per week) may be more effective and cause fewer adverse effects than continuous regimens using lower potency products. After long-term use or after using a potent agent, in order to prevent a rebound effect, switch to a less potent agent or alternative use of topical corticosteroids and emollient products. Treatment with very high potency topical corticosteroids should not exceed 2 consecutive weeks

Drug and Dosage Forms	Usual Dosage Range	Administration Issues	Adverse Drug Reactions (ADRs) and Pharmacokinetics	Contraindications, Pregnancy Category, and Lactation Issues
Alclometasone Dipropionate Aclovate Ointment 0.05% Cream 0.05%	**Relief of inflammation associated with contact dermatitis, poison ivy, poison sumac, poison oak, eczema, insect bites, sunburn, and second-degree localized burns; adjunctive therapy in the treatment of psoriasis, seborrheic dermatitis, severe diaper rash, and chronic discoid lupus erythematosus** Apply to affected area 2 to 4 times daily. Topical corticosteroids have a repository effect; with continuous use, 1 to 2 applications per day may be as effective as 3 or more applications. Short-term or intermittent therapy with high potency agents (i.e. every other day, 3 to 4 consecutive days per week) may be more effective and cause fewer adverse effects than continuous regimens using lower potency products After long-term use or after using a potent agent, in order to prevent a rebound effect, switch to a less potent agent or alternative use of topical corticosteroids and emollient products. Treatment with very high potency topical corticosteroids should not exceed 2 consecutive weeks.	Administration Issues For external use only; keep preparation away from the eyes, mouth, and mucous membranes; apply sparingly in a light film and rub in gently; do not use tight-fitting diapers or plastic pants on children treated with corticosteroids in the diaper area; do not use occlusive dressings with very potent agents such as augmented betamethasone dipropionate, clobetasol, halobetasol propionate, and mometasone.	ADRs Burning, itching, irritation, erythema, dryness, skin atrophy (especially with potent preparations), HPA axis suppression (especially with potent preparations). Pharmacokinetics Systemic absorption through the skin depends on intrinsic properties of the drug itself, the vehicle used, the duration of exposure, and the surface area and condition of the skin involved; occlusive dressings greatly enhance skin penetration and drug absorption.	Contraindications Hypersensitivity to any component of the product; monotherapy in primary bacterial infections (i.e., impetigo). Pregnancy Category: C Lactation Issues Excretion in breast milk is unknown; use with caution in nursing mothers.
Amcinonide Cyclocort, generic	Apply to affected area 2 to 4 times daily.	Administration Issues For external use only; keep preparation away from the eyes, mouth, and mucous membranes; apply sparingly in a light film and rub in gently; shake lotion and	ADRs Burning, itching, irritation, erythema, dryness, skin atrophy (especially with potent preparations), HPA axis suppression (especially with potent preparations).	Contraindications Hypersensitivity to any component of the product; monotherapy in primary bacterial infections (i.e., impetigo).

(continues on next page)

807. Corticosteroid Products *continued from previous page*

Drug and Dosage Forms	Usual Dosage Range	Administration Issues	Adverse Drug Reactions (ADRs) and Pharmacokinetics	Contraindications, Pregnancy Category, and Lactation Issues
Amcinonide *cont.* Ointment 0.1% Cream 0.1% Lotion 0.1%	Apply to affected area 2 to 4 times daily.	spray preparations prior to administration; do not use tight-fitting diapers or plastic pants on children treated with corticosteroids in the diaper area.	Pharmacokinetics Systemic absorption through the skin depends on intrinsic properties of the drug itself, the vehicle used, the duration of exposure, and the surface area and condition of the skin involved; occlusive dressings greatly enhance skin penetration and drug absorption.	Pregnancy Category: C Lactation Issues Excretion in breast milk is unknown; use with caution in nursing mothers.
Augmented Betamethasone Dipropionate Ointment 0.05% Cream 0.05% Gel 0.05% Lotion 0.05%	Apply to affected area 2 to 4 times daily.	Administration Issues For external use only; keep preparation away from the eyes, mouth, and mucous membranes; apply sparingly in a light film and rub in gently; shake lotion and spray preparations prior to administration; do not use tight-fitting diapers or plastic pants on children treated with corticosteroids in the diaper area; do not use occlusive dressings with very potent agents such as augmented betamethasone dipropionate, clobetasol, halobetasol propionate, and mometasone.	ADRs Burning, itching, irritation, erythema, dryness, skin atrophy (especially with potent preparations), HPA axis suppression (especially with potent preparations). Pharmacokinetics Systemic absorption through the skin depends on intrinsic properties of the drug itself, the vehicle used, the duration of exposure, and the surface area and condition of the skin involved; occlusive dressings greatly enhance skin penetration and drug absorption.	Contraindications Hypersensitivity to any component of the product; monotherapy in primary bacterial infections (i.e., impetigo). Pregnancy Category: C Lactation Issues Excretion in breast milk is unknown; use with caution in nursing mothers.
Betamethasone Dipropionate Diprosone, Maxivate, various generics Ointment 0.05% Cream 0.05% Lotion 0.05% Aerosol Diprosone 0.1%	Apply to affected area 2 to 4 times daily.	Administration Issues For external use only; keep preparation away from the eyes, mouth, and mucous membranes; apply sparingly in a light film and rub in gently; shake lotion and spray preparations prior to administration; hold spray 3 to 6 inches away from affected area while in use, spray for about 2 seconds to cover an area the size of your hand; do not use tight-fitting diapers or plastic pants on children treated with corticosteroids in the diaper area.	ADRs Burning, itching, irritation, erythema, dryness, skin atrophy (especially with potent preparations), HPA axis suppression (especially with potent preparations). Pharmacokinetics Systemic absorption through the skin depends on intrinsic properties of the drug itself, the vehicle used, the duration of exposure, and the surface area and condition of the skin involved; occlusive dressings greatly enhance skin penetration and drug absorption. In some cases, generic ÅgequivalentsÅh have less vasoconstrictive activity compared to the name brand medication.	Contraindications Hypersensitivity to any component of the product; monotherapy in primary bacterial infections (i.e., impetigo). Pregnancy Category: C Lactation Issues Excretion in breast milk is unknown; use with caution in nursing mothers.

Betamethasone Valerate various generics Ointment 0.1% Cream 0.05%, 0.01%, 0.1% Lotion 0.1% Foam 1.2 mg/g	Apply to affected area 2 to 4 times daily.	Administration Issues For external use only; keep preparation away from the eyes, mouth, and mucous membranes; apply sparingly in a light film and rub in gently; shake lotion and spray preparations prior to administration; do not use tight-fitting diapers or plastic pants on children treated with corticosteroids in the diaper area; do not use occlusive dressings with very potent agents such as augmented betamethasone dipropionate, clobetasol, halobetasol propionate, and mometasone.	ADRs Burning, itching, irritation, erythema, dryness, skin atrophy (especially with potent preparations), HPA axis suppression (especially with potent preparations). Pharmacokinetics Systemic absorption through the skin depends on intrinsic properties of the drug itself, the vehicle used, the duration of exposure, and the surface area and condition of the skin involved; occlusive dressings greatly enhance skin penetration and drug absorption. In some cases, generic "equivalents" have less vasoconstrictive activity compared to the name brand medication.	Contraindications Hypersensitivity to any component of the product; monotherapy in primary bacterial infections (i.e., impetigo). Pregnancy Category: C Lactation Issues Excretion in breast milk is unknown; use with caution in nursing mothers.
Clobetasol Propionate Temovate, generics Ointment 0.05% Cream 0.05% Scalp application 0.05% Gel 0.05% Foam 0.05%	Apply to affected area 2 to 4 times daily.	Administration Issues For external use only; keep preparation away from the eyes, mouth, and mucous membranes; apply sparingly in a light film and rub in gently; do not use tight-fitting diapers or plastic pants on children treated with corticosteroids in the diaper area; do not use occlusive dressings with very potent agents such as augmented betamethasone dipropionate, clobetasol, halobetasol propionate, and mometasone.	ADRs Burning, itching, irritation, erythema, dryness, skin atrophy (especially with potent preparations), HPA axis suppression (especially with potent preparations). Pharmacokinetics Systemic absorption through the skin depends on intrinsic properties of the drug itself, the vehicle used, the duration of exposure, and the surface area and condition of the skin involved; occlusive dressings greatly enhance skin penetration and drug absorption.	Contraindications Hypersensitivity to any component of the product; monotherapy in primary bacterial infections (i.e., impetigo). Pregnancy Category: C Lactation Issues Excretion in breast milk is unknown; use with caution in nursing mothers.
Clocortolone Pivalate Cloderm Cream 0.1%	Apply to affected area 2 to 4 times daily.	Administration Issues For external use only; keep preparation away from the eyes, mouth, and mucous membranes; apply sparingly in a light film and rub in gently; do not use tight-fitting diapers or plastic pants on children treated with corticosteroids in the diaper area.	ADRs Burning, itching, irritation, erythema, dryness, skin atrophy (especially with potent preparations), HPA axis suppression (especially with potent preparations). Pharmacokinetics Systemic absorption through the skin depends on intrinsic properties of the drug itself, the vehicle used, the duration of exposure, and the surface area and condition	Contraindications Hypersensitivity to any component of the product; monotherapy in primary bacterial infections (i.e., impetigo). Pregnancy Category: C Lactation Issues Excretion in breast milk is unknown; use with caution in nursing mothers.

(*continues on next page*)

807. Corticosteroid Products *continued from previous page*

Drug and Dosage Forms	Usual Dosage Range	Administration Issues	Adverse Drug Reactions (ADRs) and Pharmacokinetics	Contraindications, Pregnancy Category, and Lactation Issues
Clocortolone Pivalate *cont.*	Apply to affected area 2 to 4 times daily.		of the skin involved; occlusive dressings greatly enhance skin penetration and drug absorption. In some cases, generic "equivalents" have less vasoconstrictive activity compared to the name brand medication.	
Desonide generics Ointment 0.05% Cream 0.05% Lotion 0.05%	Apply to affected area 2 to 4 times daily.	Administration Issues For external use only; keep preparation away from the eyes, mouth, and mucous membranes; apply sparingly in a light film and rub in gently; shake lotion and spray preparations prior to administration; do not use tight-fitting diapers or plastic pants on children treated with corticosteroids in the diaper area.	ADRs Burning, itching, irritation, erythema, dryness, skin atrophy (especially with potent preparations), HPA axis suppression (especially with potent preparations). Pharmacokinetics Systemic absorption through the skin depends on intrinsic properties of the drug itself, the vehicle used, the duration of exposure, and the surface area and condition of the skin involved; occlusive dressings greatly enhance skin penetration and drug absorption. In some cases, generic "equivalents" have less vasoconstrictive activity compared to the name brand medication.	Contraindications Hypersensitivity to any component of the product; monotherapy in primary bacterial infections (i.e., impetigo). Pregnancy Category: C Lactation Issues Excretion in breast milk is unknown; use with caution in nursing mothers.
Desoximetasone generics Ointment 0.25% Cream 0.05%, 0.25% Gel 0.05%	Apply to affected area 2 to 4 times daily.	Administration Issues For external use only; keep preparation away from the eyes, mouth, and mucous membranes; apply sparingly in a light film and rub in gently; do not use tight-fitting diapers or plastic pants on children treated with corticosteroids in the diaper area.	ADRs Burning, itching, irritation, erythema, dryness, skin atrophy (especially with potent preparations), HPA axis suppression (especially with potent preparations). Pharmacokinetics Systemic absorption through the skin depends on intrinsic properties of the drug itself, the vehicle used, the duration of exposure, and the surface area and condition of the skin involved; occlusive dressings greatly enhance skin penetration and drug absorption. In some cases, generic "equivalents" have less vasoconstrictive activity compared to the name brand medication.	Contraindications Hypersensitivity to any component of the product; monotherapy in primary bacterial infections (i.e., impetigo). Pregnancy Category: C Lactation Issues Excretion in breast milk is unknown; use with caution in nursing mothers.

Dexamethasone Aerosol Decaspray 0.04%	Apply to affected area 2 to 4 times daily.	Administration Issues For external use only; keep preparation away from the eyes, mouth, and mucous membranes; apply sparingly in a light film and rub in gently; shake lotion and spray preparations prior to administration; hold spray 3 to 6 inches away from affected area while in use, spray for about 2 seconds to cover an area the size of your hand; do not use tight-fitting diapers or plastic pants on children treated with corticosteroids in the diaper area.	ADRs Burning, itching, irritation, erythema, dryness, skin atrophy (especially with potent preparations), HPA axis suppression (especially with potent preparations). Pharmacokinetics Systemic absorption through the skin depends on intrinsic properties of the drug itself, the vehicle used, the duration of exposure, and the surface area and condition of the skin involved; occlusive dressings greatly enhance skin penetration and drug absorption. In some cases, generic "equivalents" have less vasoconstrictive activity compared to the name brand medication.	Contraindications Hypersensitivity to any component of the product; monotherapy in primary bacterial infections (i.e., impetigo). Pregnancy Category: C Lactation Issues Excretion in breast milk is unknown; use with caution in nursing mothers.
Dexamethasone Sodium Phosphate Decadron Phosphate Cream 0.1%	Apply to affected area 2 to 4 times daily.	Administration Issues For external use only; keep preparation away from the eyes, mouth, and mucous membranes; apply sparingly in a light film and rub in gently; do not use tight-fitting diapers or plastic pants on children treated with corticosteroids in the diaper area.	ADRs Burning, itching, irritation, erythema, dryness, skin atrophy (especially with potent preparations), HPA axis suppression (especially with potent preparations). Pharmacokinetics Systemic absorption through the skin depends on intrinsic properties of the drug itself, the vehicle used, the duration of exposure, and the surface area and condition of the skin involved; occlusive dressings greatly enhance skin penetration and drug absorption.	Contraindications Hypersensitivity to any component of the product; monotherapy in primary bacterial infections (i.e., impetigo). Pregnancy Category: C Lactation Issues Excretion in breast milk is unknown; use with caution in nursing mothers.
Diflorasone Diacetate generics Ointment 0.05% Cream 0.05%	Apply to affected area 2 to 4 times daily.	Administration Issues For external use only; keep preparation away from the eyes, mouth, and mucous membranes; apply sparingly in a light film and rub in gently; do not use tight-fitting diapers or plastic pants on children treated with corticosteroids in the diaper area.	ADRs Burning, itching, irritation, erythema, dryness, skin atrophy (especially with potent preparations), HPA axis suppression (especially with potent preparations). Pharmacokinetics Systemic absorption through the skin depends on intrinsic properties of the drug itself, the vehicle used, the duration of exposure, and the surface area and condition of the skin involved; occlusive dressings greatly enhance skin penetration and drug absorption.	Contraindications Hypersensitivity to any component of the product; monotherapy in primary bacterial infections (i.e., impetigo). Pregnancy Category: C Lactation Issues Excretion in breast milk is unknown; use with caution in nursing mothers.

(*continues on next page*)

807. Corticosteroid Products *continued from previous page*

Drug and Dosage Forms	Usual Dosage Range	Administration Issues	Adverse Drug Reactions (ADRs) and Pharmacokinetics	Contraindications, Pregnancy Category, and Lactation Issues
Fluocinolone Acetonide generics Ointment 0.025% Cream 0.01%, 0.025%, 0.2% Solution 0.01% Shampoo 0.01% Oil 0.01%	Apply to affected area 2 to 4 times daily.	Administration Issues For external use only; keep preparation away from the eyes, mouth, and mucous membranes; apply sparingly in a light film and rub in gently; do not use tight-fitting diapers or plastic pants on children treated with corticosteroids in the diaper area.	ADRs Burning, itching, irritation, erythema, dryness, skin atrophy (especially with potent preparations), HPA axis suppression (especially with potent preparations). Pharmacokinetics Systemic absorption through the skin depends on intrinsic properties of the drug itself, the vehicle used, the duration of exposure, and the surface area and condition of the skin involved; occlusive dressings greatly enhance skin penetration and drug absorption. In some cases, generic "equivalents" have less vasoconstrictive activity compared to the name brand medication.	Contraindications Hypersensitivity to any component of the product; monotherapy in primary bacterial infections (i.e., impetigo). Pregnancy Category: C Lactation Issues Excretion in breast milk is unknown; use with caution in nursing mothers.
Fluocinonide generics Ointment 0.05% Cream 0.05% Solution 0.05% Gel 0.05%	Apply to affected area 2 to 4 times daily.	Administration Issues For external use only; keep preparation away from the eyes, mouth, and mucous membranes; apply sparingly in a light film and rub in gently; do not use tight-fitting diapers or plastic pants on children treated with corticosteroids in the diaper area.	ADRs Burning, itching, irritation, erythema, dryness, skin atrophy (especially with potent preparations), HPA axis suppression (especially with potent preparations). Pharmacokinetics Systemic absorption through the skin depends on intrinsic properties of the drug itself, the vehicle used, the duration of exposure, and the surface area and condition of the skin involved; occlusive dressings greatly enhance skin penetration and drug absorption. In some cases, generic "equivalents" have less vasoconstrictive activity compared to the name brand medication).	Contraindications Hypersensitivity to any component of the product; monotherapy in primary bacterial infections (i.e., impetigo). Pregnancy Category: C Lactation Issues Excretion in breast milk is unknown; use with caution in nursing mothers.
Flurandrenolide Ointment 0.025%, 0.05% Cream 0.025%, 0.05%	Apply to affected area 2 to 4 times daily.	Administration Issues For external use only; keep preparation away from the eyes, mouth, and mucous membranes; apply sparingly in a light film and rub in gently; shake lotion and spray preparations prior to administra-	ADRs Burning, itching, irritation, erythema, dryness, skin atrophy (especially with potent preparations), HPA axis suppression (especially with potent preparations).	Contraindications Hypersensitivity to any component of the product; monotherapy in primary bacterial infections (i.e., impetigo). Pregnancy Category: C

Lotion 0.05% Tape 4 mcg/cm^2	Apply to affected area 2 to 4 times daily.	tion; do not use tight-fitting diapers or plastic pants on children treated with corticosteroids in the diaper area.	Pharmacokinetics Systemic absorption through the skin depends on intrinsic properties of the drug itself, the vehicle used, the duration of exposure, and the surface area and condition of the skin involved; occlusive dressings greatly enhance skin penetration and drug absorption.	Lactation Issues Excretion in breast milk is unknown; use with caution in nursing mothers.
Fluticasone Propionate Cutivate Ointment 0.005% Cream 0.05%	Apply to affected area 2 to 4 times daily.	Administration Issues For external use only; keep preparation away from the eyes, mouth, and mucous membranes; apply sparingly in a light film and rub in gently; do not use tight-fitting diapers or plastic pants on children treated with corticosteroids in the diaper area.	ADRs Burning, itching, irritation, erythema, dryness, skin atrophy (especially with potent preparations), HPA axis suppression (especially with potent preparations). Pharmacokinetics Systemic absorption through the skin depends on intrinsic properties of the drug itself, the vehicle used, the duration of exposure, and the surface area and condition of the skin involved; occlusive dressings greatly enhance skin penetration and drug absorption.	Contraindications Hypersensitivity to any component of the product; monotherapy in primary bacterial infections (i.e., impetigo). Pregnancy Category: C Lactation Issues Excretion in breast milk is unknown; use with caution in nursing mothers.
Halcinonide Halog Ointment 0.1% Cream 0.025%, 0.1% Solution 0.1%	Apply to affected area 2 to 4 times daily.	Administration Issues For external use only; keep preparation away from the eyes, mouth, and mucous membranes; apply sparingly in a light film and rub in gently; do not use tight-fitting diapers or plastic pants on children treated with corticosteroids in the diaper area.	ADRs Burning, itching, irritation, erythema, dryness, skin atrophy (especially with potent preparations), HPA axis suppression (especially with potent preparations). Pharmacokinetics Systemic absorption through the skin depends on intrinsic properties of the drug itself, the vehicle used, the duration of exposure, and the surface area and condition of the skin involved; occlusive dressings greatly enhance skin penetration and drug absorption.	Contraindications Hypersensitivity to any component of the product; monotherapy in primary bacterial infections (i.e., impetigo). Pregnancy Category: C Lactation Issues Excretion in breast milk is unknown; use with caution in nursing mothers.
Halobetasol Propionate Ultravate Ointment 0.05% Cream 0.05%	Apply to affected area 2 to 4 times daily.	Administration Issues For external use only; keep preparation away from the eyes, mouth, and mucous membranes; apply sparingly in a light film and rub in gently; do not use tight-fitting diapers or plastic pants on children treated with corticosteroids in the diaper area; do not use occlusive dressings with	ADRs Burning, itching, irritation, erythema, dryness, skin atrophy (especially with potent preparations), HPA axis suppression (especially with potent preparations).	Contraindications Hypersensitivity to any component of the product; monotherapy in primary bacterial infections (i.e., impetigo). Pregnancy Category: C

(*continues on next page*)

807. Corticosteroid Products *continued from previous page*

Drug and Dosage Forms	Usual Dosage Range	Administration Issues	Adverse Drug Reactions (ADRs) and Pharmacokinetics	Contraindications, Pregnancy Category, and Lactation Issues
Halobetasol Propionate *cont.*	Apply to affected area 2 to 4 times daily.	very potent agents such as augmented betamethasone dipropionate, clobetasol, halobetasol propionate, and mometasone.	Pharmacokinetics Systemic absorption through the skin depends on intrinsic properties of the drug itself, the vehicle used, the duration of exposure, and the surface area and condition of the skin involved; occlusive dressings greatly enhance skin penetration and drug absorption.	Lactation Issues Excretion in breast milk is unknown; use with caution in nursing mothers.
Hydrocortisone generics Ointment 0.5%, 1%, 2.5% Cream 0.5%, 1%, 2.5% Lotion 0.25%, 0.5%, 1%, 2.5% Gel 0.5%, 1% Liquid 1% Solution 1% Aerosol/Pump Spray 0.5% Stick, roll-on 1% Pump Spray 1%	Apply to affected area 2 to 4 times daily.	Administration Issues For external use only; keep preparation away from the eyes, mouth, and mucous membranes; apply sparingly in a light film and rub in gently; shake lotion and spray preparations prior to administration; hold spray 3 to 6 inches away from affected area while in use, spray for about 2 seconds to cover an area the size of your hand; do not use tight-fitting diapers or plastic pants on children treated with corticosteroids in the diaper area.	ADRs Burning, itching, irritation, erythema, dryness, skin atrophy (especially with potent preparations), HPA axis suppression (especially with potent preparations). Pharmacokinetics Systemic absorption through the skin depends on intrinsic properties of the drug itself, the vehicle used, the duration of exposure, and the surface area and condition of the skin involved; occlusive dressings greatly enhance skin penetration and drug absorption. In some cases, generic "equivalents" have less vasoconstrictive activity compared to the name brand medication.	Contraindications Hypersensitivity to any component of the product; monotherapy in primary bacterial infections (i.e., impetigo). Pregnancy Category: C Lactation Issues Excretion in breast milk is unknown; use with caution in nursing mothers.
Hydrocortisone Acetate Ointment Cortaid with Aloe, Lanacort-5, Maximum	Apply to affected area 2 to 4 times daily.	Administration Issues For external use only; keep preparation away from the eyes, mouth, and mucous membranes; apply sparingly in a light	ADRs Burning, itching, irritation, erythema, dryness, skin atrophy (especially with potent	Contraindications Hypersensitivity to any component of the product; monotherapy in primary bacterial infections (i.e., impetigo).

Strength Cortaid, Maximum, Anusol HC 0.5%, 1% Cream Corticaine, CaldeCort, Cortaid with Aloe, Lanacort 0.5%, 1%	Apply to affected area 2 to 4 times daily.	film and rub in gently; do not use tight-fitting diapers or plastic pants on children treated with corticosteroids in the diaper area.	preparations), HPA axis suppression (especially with potent preparations). Pharmacokinetics Systemic absorption through the skin depends on intrinsic properties of the drug itself, the vehicle used, the duration of exposure, and the surface area and condition of the skin involved; occlusive dressings greatly enhance skin penetration and drug absorption.	Pregnancy Category: C Lactation Issues Excretion in breast milk is unknown; use with caution in nursing mothers.
Hydrocortisone Valerate Westcort, generics Ointment 0.2% Cream 0.2%	Apply to affected area 2 to 4 times daily.	Administration Issues For external use only; keep preparation away from the eyes, mouth, and mucous membranes; apply sparingly in a light film and rub in gently; do not use tight-fitting diapers or plastic pants on children treated with corticosteroids in the diaper area.Apply to affected area 2 to 4 times daily.	ADRs Burning, itching, irritation, erythema, dryness, skin atrophy (especially with potent preparations), HPA axis suppression (especially with potent preparations). Pharmacokinetics Systemic absorption through the skin depends on intrinsic properties of the drug itself, the vehicle used, the duration of exposure, and the surface area and condition of the skin involved; occlusive dressings greatly enhance skin penetration and drug absorption.	Contraindications Hypersensitivity to any component of the product; monotherapy in primary bacterial infections (i.e., impetigo). Pregnancy Category: C Lactation Issues Excretion in breast milk is unknown; use with caution in nursing mothers.Apply to affected area 2 to 4 times daily.
Mometasone Furoate Elocon Ointment 0.1% Cream 0.1% Lotion 0.1%	Apply to affected area 2 to 4 times daily.	Administration Issues For external use only; keep preparation away from the eyes, mouth, and mucous membranes; apply sparingly in a light film and rub in gently; shake lotion and spray preparations prior to administration; do not use tight-fitting diapers or plastic pants on children treated with corticosteroids in the diaper area; do not use occlusive dressings with very potent agents such as augmented betamethasone dipropionate, clobetasol, halobetasol propionate, and mometasone.	ADRs Burning, itching, irritation, erythema, dryness, skin atrophy (especially with potent preparations), HPA axis suppression (especially with potent preparations). Pharmacokinetics Systemic absorption through the skin depends on intrinsic properties of the drug itself, the vehicle used, the duration of exposure, and the surface area and condition of the skin involved; occlusive dressings greatly enhance skin penetration and drug absorption.	Contraindications Hypersensitivity to any component of the product; monotherapy in primary bacterial infections (i.e., impetigo). Pregnancy Category: C Lactation Issues Excretion in breast milk is unknown; use with caution in nursing mothers.
Prednicarbate Dermatop Cream 0.1%	Apply to affected area 2 to 4 times daily.	Administration Issues For external use only; keep preparation away from the eyes, mouth, and mucous membranes; apply sparingly in a light film and rub in gently; do not use tight-	ADRs Burning, itching, irritation, erythema, dryness, skin atrophy (especially with potent preparations), HPA axis suppression (especially with potent preparations).	Contraindications Hypersensitivity to any component of the product; monotherapy in primary bacterial infections (i.e., impetigo).

(*continues on next page*)

807. Corticosteroid Products *continued from previous page*

Drug and Dosage Forms	Usual Dosage Range	Administration Issues	Adverse Drug Reactions (ADRs) and Pharmacokinetics	Contraindications, Pregnancy Category, and Lactation Issues
Prednicarbate *cont.* Ointment 0.1%	Apply to affected area 2 to 4 times daily	fitting diapers or plastic pants on children treated with corticosteroids in the diaper area.	Pharmacokinetics Systemic absorption through the skin depends on intrinsic properties of the drug itself, the vehicle used, the duration of exposure, and the surface area and condition of the skin involved; occlusive dressings greatly enhance skin penetration and drug absorption.	Pregnancy Category: C Lactation Issues Excretion in breast milk is unknown; use with caution in nursing mothers.
Triamcinolone Acetonide generics Ointment 0.025%, 0.1%, 0.5% Cream 0.025%, 0.1%, 0.5% Lotion 0.025%, 0.1% Aerosol 2 second spray	Apply to affected area 2 to 4 times daily. .	Administration Issues For external use only; keep preparation away from the eyes, mouth, and mucous membranes; apply sparingly in a light film and rub in gently; shake lotion and spray preparations prior to administration; hold spray 3 to 6 inches away from affected area while in use, spray for about 2 seconds to cover an area the size of your hand; do not use tight-fitting diapers or plastic pants on children treated with corticosteroids in the diaper area.	ADRs Burning, itching, irritation, erythema, dryness, skin atrophy (especially with potent preparations), HPA axis suppression (especially with potent preparations). Pharmacokinetics Systemic absorption through the skin depends on intrinsic properties of the drug itself, the vehicle used, the duration of exposure, and the surface area and condition of the skin involved; occlusive dressings greatly enhance skin penetration and drug absorption. In some cases, generic "equivalents" have less vasoconstrictive activity compared to the name brand medication.	Contraindications Hypersensitivity to any component of the product; monotherapy in primary bacterial infections (i.e., impetigo). Pregnancy Category: C Lactation Issues Excretion in breast milk is unknown; use with caution in nursing mothers.

808. Corticosteroid Combinations

Warnings about topical steroid products: Topical corticosteroids have a repository effect; with continuous use, 1 to 2 applications per day may be as effective as 3 or more applications. Short-term or intermittent therapy with high-potency agents (i.e., every other day, 3 to 4 consecutive days per week) may be more effective and cause fewer adverse effects than continuous regimens using lower potency products. After long-term use or after using a potent agent, in order to prevent a rebound effect, switch to a less potent agent or alternative use of topical corticosteroids and emollient products. Treatment with very high potency topical corticosteroids should not exceed 2 consecutive weeks.

Drug and Dosage Forms	Usual Dosage Range	Administration Issues	Adverse Drug Reactions (ADRs) and Pharmacokinetics	Contraindications, Pregnancy Category, and Lactation Issues
Betamethasone-Clotrimazole Lotrisone, generics Cream 0.05% betamethasone 1% clotrimazole	**Relief of inflammation associated with contact dermatitis, poison ivy, poison sumac, poison oak, eczema, insect bites, sunburn, and second-degree localized burns; adjunctive therapy in the treatment of psoriasis, seborrheic dermatitis, severe diaper rash, and chronic discoid lupus erythematosus** Apply to affected area 2 to 4 times daily.	Administration Issues For external use only; keep preparation away from the eyes, mouth, and mucous membranes; apply sparingly and rub in gently; do not use tight-fitting diapers or plastic pants on children treated with corticosteroids in the diaper area.	ADRs Burning, itching, irritation, erythema, dryness. Pharmacokinetics Systemic absorption through the skin depends on intrinsic properties of the drug itself, the vehicle used, the duration of exposure, and the surface area and condition of the skin involved; occlusive dressings greatly enhance skin penetration and drug absorption. In some cases, generic ÅgequivalentsÅh have less vasoconstrictive activity compared to the name brand medication.	Contraindications Hypersensitivity to any component of the product; monotherapy in primary bacterial infections (i.e., impetigo). Pregnancy Category: C Lactation Issues Excretion in breast milk is unknown; use with caution in nursing mothers.
Hydrocortisone-Clioquinol Ointment Various concentrations Cream Various concentrations	Apply to affected area 2 to 4 times daily.	Administration Issues For external use only; keep preparation away from the eyes, mouth, and mucous membranes; apply sparingly and rub in gently; shake lotion and spray preparations prior to administration; do not use tight-fitting diapers or plastic pants on children treated with corticosteroids in the diaper area.	ADRs Burning, itching, irritation, erythema, dryness. Pharmacokinetics Systemic absorption through the skin depends on intrinsic properties of the drug itself, the vehicle used, the duration of exposure, and the surface area and condition of the skin involved; occlusive dressings greatly enhance skin penetration and drug absorption.	Contraindications Hypersensitivity to any component of the product; monotherapy in primary bacterial infections (i.e., impetigo). Pregnancy Category: C Lactation Issues Excretion in breast milk is unknown; use with caution in nursing mothers.
Hydrocortisone-Pramoxine Ointment Various concentrations Cream Various combinations	Apply to affected area 2 to 4 times daily.	Administration Issues For external use only; keep preparation away from the eyes, mouth, and mucous membranes; apply sparingly and rub in gently; do not use tight-fitting diapers or plastic pants on children treated with corticosteroids in the diaper area.	ADRs Burning, itching, irritation, erythema, dryness. Pharmacokinetics Systemic absorption through the skin depends on intrinsic properties of the drug	Contraindications Hypersensitivity to any component of the product; monotherapy in primary bacterial infections (i.e., impetigo). Pregnancy Category: C

(continues on next page)

808. Corticosteroid Combinations *continued from previous page*

Drug and Dosage Forms	Usual Dosage Range	Administration Issues	Adverse Drug Reactions (ADRs) and Pharmacokinetics	Contraindications, Pregnancy Category, and Lactation Issues
Hydrocortisone-Pramoxine *cont.* Lotion Various combinations Foam 1% hydrocortisone/1% pramoxine	Apply to affected area 2 to 4 times daily.		itself, the vehicle used, the duration of exposure, and the surface area and condition of the skin involved; occlusive dressings greatly enhance skin penetration and drug absorption. In some cases, generic ÅgequivalentsÅh have less vasoconstrictive activity compared to the name brand medication.	Lactation Issues Excretion in breast milk is unknown; use with caution in nursing mothers.
Hydrocortisone-Iodoquinol Vytone Cream 1% hydrocortisone/1% iodoquinol	Apply to affected area 2 to 4 times daily.	Administration Issues For external use only; keep preparation away from the eyes, mouth, and mucous membranes; apply sparingly and rub in gently; do not use tight-fitting diapers or plastic pants on children treated with corticosteroids in the diaper area.	ADRs Burning, itching, irritation, erythema, dryness. Pharmacokinetics Systemic absorption through the skin depends on intrinsic properties of the drug itself, the vehicle used, the duration of exposure, and the surface area and condition of the skin involved; occlusive dressings greatly enhance skin penetration and drug absorption.	Contraindications Hypersensitivity to any component of the product; monotherapy in primary bacterial infections (i.e., impetigo). Pregnancy Category: C Lactation Issues Excretion in breast milk is unknown; use with caution.
Corticosteroid-Neomycin Combinations Ointment 0.5% hydrocortisone/0.5% neomycin 1% hydrocortisone/0.5% neomycin 1% hydrocortisone/0.5% neomycin/400 units bacitracin zinc/gm 5000 units polymyxin B sulfate/gm Cream 1% hydrocortisone/0.5% neomycin 0.025% fluocinolone/0.5% neomycin 0.1% dexamethasone/0.5% neomycin 0.5% hydrocortisone/0.5% neomycin/10,000 units polymyxin B sulfate/gm	Apply to affected area 2 to 4 times daily.	Administration Issues For external use only; keep preparation away from the eyes, mouth, and mucous membranes; apply sparingly and rub in gently; do not use tight-fitting diapers or plastic pants on children treated with corticosteroids in the diaper area.	ADRs Burning, itching, irritation, erythema, dryness. Pharmacokinetics Systemic absorption through the skin depends on intrinsic properties of the drug itself, the vehicle used, the duration of exposure, and the surface area and condition of the skin involved; occlusive dressings greatly enhance skin penetration and drug absorption. In some cases, generic ÅgequivalentsÅh have less vasoconstrictive activity compared to the name brand medication.	Contraindications Hypersensitivity to any component of the product; monotherapy in primary bacterial infections (i.e., impetigo). Pregnancy Category: C Lactation Issues Excretion in breast milk is unknown; use with caution in nursing mothers.

Corticosteroid-Antifungal Combinations Ointment Mycolog-II, various generics 0.1% triamcinolone acetonide 100,000 units nystatin/gm Cream Mycolog-II, various generics 0.1% triamcinolone acetonide 100,000 units nystatin/gm Lotrisone 0.05% betamethasone dipropionate 1% clotrimazole Fungoid-HC 0.5% hydrocortisone/triacetin	Apply to affected area 2 to 4 times daily.	Administration Issues For external use only; keep preparation away from the eyes, mouth, and mucous membranes; apply sparingly and rub in gently; do not use tight-fitting diapers or plastic pants on children treated with corticosteroids in the diaper area.	ADRs Burning, itching, irritation, erythema, dryness. Pharmacokinetics Systemic absorption through the skin depends on intrinsic properties of the drug itself, the vehicle used, the duration of exposure, and the surface area and condition of the skin involved; occlusive dressings greatly enhance skin penetration and drug absorption. In some cases, generic ÅgequivalentsÅh have less vasoconstrictive activity compared to the name brand medication.	Contraindications Hypersensitivity to any component of the product; monotherapy in primary bacterial infections (i.e., impetigo). Pregnancy Category: C Lactation Issues Excretion in breast milk is unknown; use with caution in nursing mothers.

809. Miscellaneous Topical Products

Drug and Dosage Forms	Usual Dosage Range	Administration Issues	Common Adverse Drug Reactions (ADRs)	Contraindications, Pregnancy Category, and Lactation Issues
Aluminum Acetate Solution Solution Burow's Solution 480 ml Tablet Domeboro Tablets 1 tablet in 1 pint of water = 1:40 Burow's solution Powder Domeboro Powder, Boropak Powder, Bluboro Powder 1 packet in 1 pint of water = 1:40 Burow's solution	**Astringent used for the relief of inflammation of the skin associated with insect bites, poison ivy, allergic reactions, and athlete's foot** Apply to affected area every 15 to 30 minutes for 4 to 8 h. Do not use for > 7 days, if symptoms persists, seek medical attention.	Administration Issues For external use only; keep preparation away from the eyes, mouth, and mucous membranes; apply as a wet dressing with a gauze pad saturated with solution. Drug Interactions Aluminum acetate solution may inhibit the effect of **collagenase;** remove aluminum acetate solution with repeated washings or normal saline before applying the enzyme ointment.	ADRs Irritation.	
Silver Sulfadiazine Silvadene, Thermazene, SSD Cream Cream 10 mg/g in a water miscible base	**Adjunct for prevention and treatment of sepsis in second- and third-degree burns** Apply under sterile conditions once or twice daily to a thickness of approximately 1/16 inch to the clean and debrided wound.	Administration Issues For external use only. Reapply immediately after hydrotherapy. Drug Interactions Silver sulfadiazine may inactivate topical proteolytic enzymes.	ADRs Leukopenia, skin necrosis, erythema multiforme, skin discoloration, rashes. **Up to 10% of sulfadiazine may be absorbed. Use in patients with G-6-PD deficiency may be hazardous.**	Contraindications Hypersensitivity, pregnant women at or near term, premature infants, infants < 2 months. Pregnancy Category: B Lactation Issues Sulfonamide derivatives can cause kernicterus; take into account risk to infant versus benefit to nursing mother.
Sunscreens Many products on market as lotions, creams, and gels with the following SPFs: 2, 4, 6, 8, 10, 15, 16, 17, 18, 25, 29, 30, 40, 45, 46 Waterproof formulas Maintain sunburn protection after being in the water up to 80 minutes. Water-resistant formulas Maintain sunburn protection after being in the water up to 40 minutes. Sweat-resistant formulas Maintain protection after < 30 minutes of continuous heavy perspiration.	**Sunburn prevention** Apply liberally to all exposed areas. **Do not use on infants < 6 months. Do not use SPFs as low as 2 or 3 on children < 2 years of age.**	Administration Issues Apply at least 30 minutes prior to sun exposure to allow penetration and binding to the skin; reapply after swimming or excessive sweating; for external use only; keep preparation away from the eyes, mouth, angles of nose, and mucous membranes; wash hands thoroughly after application; PABA containing sunscreens may cause permanent staining of clothes; wear protective eye coverings or sunglasses.	ADRs Contact dermatitis in PABA allergic patients.	Precautions Patients hypersensitive to PABA or its derivatives should avoid sunscreens containing PABA.

Lip balm SPFs 10, 15, 30, 45+	**Any benefits that might be derived from using sunscreen with SPFs > 30 are negligible; an SPF of at least 15 for most individuals is recommended by the Skin Cancer Foundation.**			

900. URINARY TRACT PRODUCTS

901. Antispasmodics

Drug and Dosage Forms	Usual Dosage Range	Administration Issues and Drug-Drug Interactions	Common Adverse Drug Reactions (ADRs)	Contraindications, Pregnancy Category, and Lactation Issues
Flavoxate Urispas, generics Tablet 100 mg	**Symptomatic relief of dysuria, urgency, frequency, and incontinence** 100 mg–200 mg 3 to 4 times daily; reduce dose when symptoms improve.	Administration Issues Flavoxate may be given without regard to meals. Safety and efficacy in children < 12 years has not been established.	ADRs Nausea, vomiting, dry mouth, headache, drowsiness, blurred vision, vertigo.	Contraindications Obstructive uropathies of the lower urinary tract. Pregnancy Category: C Lactation Issues Excretion in breast milk is unknown; use with caution in nursing mothers.
Oxybutynin Ditropan, Ditropan XL, various generics Tablet 5 mg Tablets, extended release 5 mg, 10 mg, 15 mg Syrup 5 mg/5 ml Transdermal system 36 mg of oxybutynin delivering 3.9 mg oxybutynin/day	**The relief of bladder instability symptoms (urgency, frequency, urinary leakage, urge incontinence, and dysuria) associated with voiding in patients with uninhibited and reflex neurogenic bladder, treatment of primary nocturnal enuresis in children** **adults:** 5 mg 2 to 3 times daily; maximum dose is 20 mg daily **children > 5 years:** 5 mg bid; maximum dose is 15 mg daily **stress urinary incontinence** 2.5 to 5 mg tid Ditropan XL 5 mg qd. Dosage may be adjusted in 5 gm increments to balance efficacy & tolerability. Adjustment can be made at weekly intervals. Maximum dose 30 mg/day. Transdermal System Apply twice weekly. Every 3 to 4 days	Administration Issues Periodic interruptions in therapy are recommended to assess continued need for drug. Tolerance has occurred in some patients. ER tablets must be swallowed whole. Apply transdermal system to dry, intact skin on the abdomen, hip or buttock. Select a new application site with each new system to avoid reapplication to the same site within 7 days. Drug-Drug Interactions Increased anticholinergic side effects may occur with concurrent **phenothiazine, amantadine, tricyclic antidepressant** administration.	ADRs Dry mouth, drowsiness, blurred vision, urinary hesitancy and retention, decreased GI motility.	Contraindications Angle-closure glaucoma, myasthenia gravis, partial or complete gastric obstruction, severe colitis. Pregnancy Category: C Lactation Issues Excretion in breast milk is unknown; use with caution in nursing mothers.

Tolterodine Tartrate Detrol, Detrol LA Tablets 1 mg, 2mg Tablets, extended-release 2 mg, 4 mg	**Treatment of patients with an overactive bladder with symptoms of urinary frequency, urgency, or urge incontinence.** **Immediate-release:** Initially, 2 mg bid. The dose may be lowered to 1 mg twice daily based on individual response and tolerability. For patients with significantly reduced hepatic function or who are currently taking drugs that are inhibitors of cytochrome P450 3A4, the recommended dose is 1 mg twice daily. **Extended-release (ER):** 4 mg qd. The dose may be lowered to 2 mg daily based on individual response and tolerability; however, limited efficacy data is available for the 2 mg capsules. For patients with significantly reduced hepatic or renal function or who are currently taking drugs that are potent inhibitors of CYP3A4, the recommended dose of the ER capsules is 2 mg daily.	Administration Issues Inform patients that antimuscarinic agents such as tolterodine may produce blurred vision, dizziness, or drowsiness. Drug-Drug Interactions **Cytochrome P450:** ***3A4 inhibitors:*** Patients receiving cytochrome P450 3A4 inhibitors, such as macrolide antibiotics (erythromycin and clarithromycin), antifungal agents (ketoconazole, itraconazole, and miconazole), or cyclosporine or vinblastine should not receive doses of tolterodine > 1 mg twice daily (> 2 mg daily for ER capsules).	ADRs Dry mouth, headache, constipation, vertigo/dizziness, and abdominal pain. Pharmacokinetics Tolterodine undergoes extensive and variable first-pass hepatic metabolism following oral dosing. Renal impairment can significantly alter the disposition of immediate-release tolterodine and its metabolites. Liver impairment can significantly alter the disposition of tolterodine.	Contraindications Urinary retention; gastric retention; uncontrolled narrow-angle glaucoma; hypersensitivity to the drug or its ingredients. Pregnancy Category: C Lactation Issues: Discontinue administration during nursing.

902. Cholinergic Stimulants

Drug and Dosage Forms	Usual Dosage Range	Administration Issues and Drug-Drug Interactions	Common Adverse Drug Reactions (ADRs) and Pharmacokinetics	Contraindications, Pregnancy Category, and Lactation Issues
Bethanechol Chloride Urecholine, various generics Tablet 5 mg, 10 mg, 25 mg, 50 mg	**Acute postoperative and postpartum treatment of nonobstructive urinary retention and neurogenic atony of the urinary bladder** 10 mg–50 mg 3 to 4 times daily; begin with 5 mg–10 mg initially and repeat dose every hour to a maximum of 50 mg or until satisfactory response.	Administration Issues Take on an empty stomach (1 h before or 2 h after meals). Drug-Drug Interactions **Quinidine and procainamide** may antagonize the cholinergic effects of bethanechol chloride. Additive cholinergic effects may occur with concurrent **cholinesterase inhibitor** use. A decrease in the cholinergic effects of bethanechol chloride may occur with concurrent **atropine, phenothiazine, or tricyclic antidepressant** administration.	ADRs Abdominal cramping, nausea, hypotension, urinary urgency. Pharmacokinetics Onset of action usually in 30–90 minutes; duration of action usually 1 h.	Contraindications Patients with hyperthyroidism, peptic ulcer disease, latent or active bronchial asthma, coronary heart disease, mechanical obstruction of the GI or urinary tract, vagotonia, epilepsy, parkinsonism, obstructive pulmonary disease, bradycardia, and atrioventricular conduction defects. Pregnancy Category: C Lactation Issues Excretion in breast milk is unknown; evaluate risk to infant versus importance of the drug to the mother.

903. Urinary Analgesics

For combination anti-infective/phenazopyridine products see Table 108.

Drug and Dosage Forms	Usual Dosage Range	Administration Issues, Drug-Drug and Drug-Lab Interactions	Common Adverse Drug Reactions (ADRs)	Contraindications, Pregnancy Category, and Lactation Issues
Phenazopyridine Azo-Standard, Pyridium, various generics Tablet 95 mg, 97.2 mg, 100 mg, 150 mg, 200 mg	**Symptomatic relief of pain, burning, urgency, frequency, and other discomforts of the lower urinary tract usually associated with a UTI** **adults:** 200 mg tid after meals **children:** 6–12 years, 12 mg/kg/d divided tid	Administration Issues Take after meals; may cause reddish-orange discoloration of the urine and may stain fabric. Staining of contact lenses has also occurred. **Administration should not exceed two days when given with an antibiotic for the treatment of UTI. Do not use chronically to treat undiagnosed urinary tract pain.** Drug-Lab Interactions Phenazopyridine may interfere with urinalysis based on spectrometry or color reactions.	ADRs Headache, rash, itching.	Contraindications Hypersensitivity to phenazopyridine. Pregnancy Category: B Lactation Issues No information is available on phenazopyridine and lactation.
Pyridium Plus Tablet 150 mg phenazopyridine 0.3 mg hyoscyamine 15 mg butabarbital	**Symptomatic relief of pain, burning, urgency, frequency, and other discomforts of the lower urinary tract usually associated with a UTI** 1 tablet qid after meals and at bedtime	Administration Issues Take after meals; may cause reddish-orange discoloration of the urine and may stain fabric. Staining of contact lenses has also occurred. Drug-Lab Interactions Phenazopyridine may interfere with urinalysis based on spectrometry or color reactions	ADRs Headache, rash, itching.	Contraindications Hypersensitivity to phenazopyridine. Pregnancy Category: B Lactation Issues: No information is available on phenazopyridine and lactation.

1000. MISCELLANEOUS AGENTS
1001. Agents for Impotence

Drug and Dosage Forms	Usual Dosage Range	Administration Issues and Drug—Drug Interactions	Common Adverse Drug Reactions (ADRs) and Pharmacokinetics	Contraindications, Pregnancy Category, and Lactation Issues
Alprostadil (PGE_1) Pellet *Muse* 125 mcg, 250 mcg, 500 mcg, 1000 mcg Injection, aqueous *Caverject, Edex* 10 mcg/ml, 20 mcg/ml, 40 mcg/2ml Powder for injection, lypholized *Caverject* 5 mcg/ml, 10 mcg/ml, 20 mcg/ml, 40 mcg/ml *Caverject Impulse* 10 mcg/0.5 mL, 20 mcg/0.5 mL	**Erectile dysfunction due to vasculogenic, psychogenic, or mixed etiology** **Caverject** Treatment initiation: Under medical care, administer 2.5 mcg. Partial response: titrate by 2.5 mcg, then by 5 to 10 mcg until produce erection suitable for intercourse but not exceeding 1 hour. No response to 2.5 mcg: titrate by 5 mcg, then by 5–10 mcg as above. Pt must stay in office until complete detumescence occurs. **Erectile dysfunction due to neurogenic etiology (spinal cord injury):** Treatment initiation: Under medical care, administer 1.25 mcg. Titrate by 1.25 mcg, then by 2.5–5 mcg as above. **Muse** Treatment initiation: Titrate dose under supervision of physician to lowest dose sufficient for sexual intercourse. Onset of effect is 30–60 minutes. Do not use more than two systems/24 h period.	Administration Issues **Caverject** Reconstitute using 1 mL of diluent (bacteriostatic or sterile water for injection preserved with benzyl alcohol). 1 mL of solution = 10 or 20 mcg depending on vial strength. Use immediately. Do not change dose of alprostadil established in physician's office Patient Instructions: – do not reuse needles/syringes – choose site of injection along side of the proximal third of the penis – alternate injection sites – avoid visible veins – cleanse injection site with alcohol **Muse** Do not change dose of alprostadil established in physician's office. Drug–Drug Interactions **Increased risk of bleeding:** anticoagulants (warfarin or heparin). Alprostadil may decrease **cyclosporine** concentrations. **Unknown effect:** Other vasoactive agents (do not use in combination).	ADRs **Caverject:** Local: Penile pain, prolonged erection (4–6 hrs), penile fibrosis, injection site hematoma or ecchymosis. Other penile disorders (local): numbness, yeast infection, irritation, sensitivity, etc. Priapism (>6 hrs): occurs rarely (0.4% incidence) Systemic effects: Upper respiratory infection, headache. **Muse:** Local: Penile pain, urethral pain, urethral bleeding. Systemic effects: Upper respiratory infection, headache, dizziness, hypotension. Pharmacokinetics: Injection into corpora cavernosa/Intraurethral: Systemic levels not significant.	Contraindications Hypersensitivity; conditions predisposing patients to priapism (e.g., sickle cell anemia, multiple myeloma, leukemia); anatomical deformation of the penis; penile implants; females; pediatrics; use in men in whom sexual activity is contraindicated. Other Considerations: Treat underlying causes of sexual dysfunction before using this agent. **Do not use alprostadil if female partner is pregnant unless the couple uses a condom barrier.** **Erection > 4 hours requires urgent physician intervention.**
Sildenafil Citrate Viagra Tablets 25 mg, 50 mg, 100 mg	**Erectile dysfunction in males** Usual: 50 mg 1 hour before sexual activity once daily. Dosage may be increased to 100 mg or decreased to 25 mg based on efficacy, tolerance. The maximum recommended dosing frequency is once per day.	Administration Issues: Take only once daily. Take 1 hour before anticipated sexual activity. Effective range is 0.5 to 4 hours.	ADRs: Headache (16%) Flushing (10%) Dyspepsia (7%) Nasal congestion (4%) Visual color changes (3%)	Contraindications: Current use of nitrates. Current use of alpha-blockers if sildenafil dose is > 25 mg and not within 4 hours if dose = 25 mg.

	For: Renal impairment (CrCl<30); Hepatic impairment; concomitant CYP3A4 inhibitor; age > 65 Start with 25 mg dose	Drug-Drug Interactions: CYP3A4 inhibitors will reduce sildenafil clearance (cimetidine, erythromycin, ketoconazole, saquinovir, ritonavir). Additive hypotensive effects with nitrates and alpha-blockers.	Pharmacokinetics: $T_{1/2}$ = 4 hours Hepatic elimination	**Erection > 4 hours requires immediate medical attention.** Pregnancy Category: B Not indicated for women or children.
Tadalafil Cialis Tablets 5 mg, 10 mg, 20 mg	**Erectile dysfunction in males** Usual: 10 mg once daily before anticipated sexual activity. Range is 5 to 20 mg daily based on efficacy and tolerance. Moderate renal failure (CrCL 31–50 mL/min): Use 5mg starting dose (max of 10mg not more than once every 48 hours) Mild or moderate hepatic impairment: Do not exceed 10mg once daily.	Administration Issues: Take only once daily. Take before anticipated sexual activity. Effective range is up to 36 hours. Drug-Drug Interactions: CYP3A4 inhibitors will reduce tadalafil clearance (cimetidine, erythromycin, ketoconazole, saquinovir, ritonavir). Additive hypotensive effects with nitrates and alpha-blockers.	ADRs: Headache (11%) Flushing (3%) Dyspepsia (8%) Nasal congestion (3%) Visual color changes (<0.1%) Back, lower limb pain (5%) Pharmacokinetics: $T_{1/2}$ = 36 hours Renal and hepatic elimination.	Contraindications: Current use of nitrates. Current use of alpha-blockers except for tamulosin 0.4 mg daily. **Erections > 4 hours require immediate medical attention.** Pregnancy Category: B Not indicated for women or children.
Vardenafil HCl Levitra Tablets 2.5 mg, 5 mg, 10 mg, 20 mg	**Erectile dysfunction in males** Usual: 10 mg once daily 1 hour before anticipated sexual activity. Range is 5 to 20 mg daily based on efficacy and tolerance. Mild to moderate hepatic failure: Start with 5 mg dose (10 mg max) Age > 65 years: Start with 5 mg dose With potent CYP3A4 inhibitors: Start with low dose	Administration Issues: Take only once daily. Take approximately 60 minutes before anticipated sexual activity. Effective range is up to 4 hours. Drug-Drug Interactions: CYP3A4 inhibitors will reduce vardenafil clearance (cimetidine, erythromycin, ketoconazole, saquinovir, ritonavir). Additive hypotensive effects with nitrates and alpha-blockers.	ADRs: Headache (15%) Flushing (11%) Dyspepsia (4%) Nasal congestion (9%) Visual color changes (<2%) Back, lower limb pain (2%) Pharmacokinetics: $T_{1/2}$ = 3.5–5 hours Hepatic elimination.	Contraindications: Current use of nitrates. Current use of alpha-blockers. **Erections > 4 hours require immediate medical attention.** Pregnancy Category: B Not indicated for women or children.
Yohimbine Aphrodyne, Dayto Himbin, Yocon, Yohimex, various generics Tablets 5.4 mg	**No FDA Approved Indications** **Unlabeled Uses: Impotence (vascular or diabetic origins)** 5.4 mg tid	Drug-Drug Interactions **Increased adverse effects:** antidepressants (do not use together).	ADRs CNS: Antidiuresis, nervousness, irritability, tremor, increased motor activity, dizziness, headache. Cardiovascular: Elevated blood pressure, increased heart rate. Overdose: Tachycardia, hypertension, paresthesias, incoordination, piloerection, rhinorrhea, tremulousness.	Contraindications Hypersensitivity; renal disease, pregnancy, pediatrics. High-risk patients to avoid: Geriatric, psychiatric, cardiorenal patients with history of gastric or duodenal ulcer.

1002. Agents for Obesity
For OTC agents used for obesity see Table 703 (Decongestants)

Drug and Dosage Forms	Usual Dosage Range	Administration Issues and Drug-Drug Interactions	Common Adverse Drug Reactions (ADRs) and Pharmacokinetics	Contraindications, Pregnancy Category, and Lactation Issues
Benzphetamine (CIII) Didrex Tablets 25 mg, 50 mg	**Short-term (8–12 weeks) adjunct in a regimen of weight reduction based on caloric restriction** Initiate dosage with 25 to 50 mg qd; increase according to response; dosage range = 25 to 50 mg qd to tid	Administration Issues Anorexiant effects are temporary, seldom lasting more than a few weeks; tolerance may occur; therefore, long-term use is not recommended. To avoid insomnia, daily dose should be taken no later than 6 h before bedtime. Abrupt termination of therapy following prolonged high doses may result in GI distress, stomach cramps, trembling, weakness, mental depression. Physical and/or psychological dependence may occur with long-term use or abuse. Drug Interactions Amphetamine elimination may be decreased by **acetazolamide, sodium bicarbonate.** Amphetamine elimination may be increased by **ammonium chloride** and **ascorbic acid.** Blood pressure effects may be increased by **furazolidone.** Amphetamines may decrease hypotensive effects of **guanethidine, guanadrel.** Hypertensive crisis and intracranial hemorrhage may occur when combined with **MAOIs** or **selegiline. Tricyclic antidepressants** may decrease effectiveness of amphetamines.	ADRs Restlessness, insomnia, palpitations. Pharmacokinetics Readily absorbed; duration = 4 h.	Contraindications Known hypersensitivity to sympathomimetic amines, angle-closure glaucoma, advanced arteriosclerosis, angina pectoris, severe cardiovascular disease, moderate to severe hypertension, hyperthyroidism, history of drug abuse, children < 12. Cautious Use In: Diabetes mellitus, elderly, psychosis. Pregnancy Category: X Lactation Issues Safety has not been established.
Diethylpropion (CIV) Tenuate, generics Tablets 25 mg Tablets, sustained release 75 mg	**Short-term (8–12 weeks) adjunct in a regimen of weight reduction based on caloric restriction** Tablets: 25 mg tid, 1 h before meals, and in midevening if needed to overcome nighttime hunger Sustained-release tablets: 75 mg qd, in midmorning	Administration Issues Sustained-release tablets should be swallowed whole and not chewed. Anorexiant effects are temporary, seldom lasting more than a few weeks; tolerance may occur; therefore, long-term use is not recommended. Abrupt termination of therapy following prolonged high doses may result in GI distress, stomach cramps, trembling, weakness, mental depression. Physical and/or psychological dependence may occur with long-term use or abuse.	ADRs Restlessness, insomnia, palpitations, ECG changes, decrease in seizure threshold in epileptics. Pharmacokinetics Readily absorbed; duration = 4 h, regular release; 10–14 h sustained release.	Contraindications Known hypersensitivity to sympathomimetic amines, angle-closure glaucoma, advanced arteriosclerosis, angina pectoris, severe cardiovascular disease, moderate to severe hypertension, hyperthyroidism, history of drug abuse, children < 12. Cautious Use In: Diabetes mellitus, elderly, psychosis, epilepsy

		Drug Interactions Amphetamine elimination may be decreased by **acetazolamide, sodium bicarbonate.** Amphetamine elimination may be increased by **ammonium chloride** and **ascorbic acid.** Blood pressure effects may be increased by **furazolidone.** Amphetamines may decrease hypotensive effects of **guanethidine, guanadrel.** Hypertensive crisis and intracranial hemorrhage may occur when combined with **MAOIs** or **selegiline. Tricyclic antidepressants** may decrease effectiveness of amphetamines.		Pregnancy Category: B Lactation Issues Safety has not been established.
Orlistat (CIV) Xenical Capsule 120 mg.	**Adjunct to reduced-calorie diet in obesity management, including weight loss and weight maintenance.** Take 120 mg 3 times a day with main meals or up to 1 hr after meals.	Administration Issues Diet should have ≤ 30% of calories from fat. If a meal is missed or contains no fat, dose may be skipped. Drug Interactions Decreases absorption of fat-soluble vitamins, Increases effect of Pravastatin.	ADRs Increased urgency, oily stools, fecal incontinence, flatus. Pharmacokinetics Blocks absorption of fat.	Contraindications Chronic malabsorption syndrome, cholestasis. Cautious use in: Hyperoxaluria, calcium oxalate nephrolithiasis, diabetes, patients on warfarin or cyclosporin. Pregnancy Category: B Lactation Issues Not recommended.
Phentermine (CIV) Pro-Fast, Adipet-P, Ionamin, generics Tablets 8 mg, 30 mg, 37.5 mg Capsules 15 mg, 18.75 mg, 30 mg, 37.5 mg Capsules, resin complex 15 mg, 30 mg	**Short-term (8–12 weeks) adjunct in a regimen of weight reduction based on caloric restriction** Take 8 mg tid, 30 minutes before meals, or 15 to 37.5 mg as a single daily dose before breakfast or 10 to 14 hours before bedtime. Take Pro-Fast HS and Pro-Fast SR capsules approx. 2 h after breakfast. Take Adipex-P capsules/tablets before breakfast or 1–2 h after breakfast.	Administration Issues Anorexiant effects are temporary, seldom lasting more than a few weeks; tolerance may occur; therefore, long-term use is not recommended. Abrupt termination of therapy following prolonged high doses may result in GI distress, stomach cramps, trembling, weakness, mental depression. Physical and/or psychological dependence may occur with long-term use or abuse. Drug Interactions Amphetamine elimination may be decreased by **acetazolamide, sodium bicarbonate.** Amphetamine elimination may be increased by **ammonium chloride**	ADRs Restlessness, insomnia, palpitations, hypertension, confusion, constipation. Pharmacokinetics Readily absorbed.	Contraindications Known hypersensitivity to sympathomimetic amines, angle-closure glaucoma, advanced arteriosclerosis, angina pectoris, severe cardiovascular disease, moderate to severe hypertension, hyperthyroidism, history of drug abuse, children < 12. Cautious Use In Diabetes mellitus, elderly, psychosis. Pregnancy Category: C Lactation Issues Safety has not been established.

(continues on next page)

1002. Agents for Obesity *continued from previous page*

Drug and Dosage Forms	Usual Dosage Range	Administration Issues and Drug-Drug Interactions	Common Adverse Drug Reactions (ADRs) and Pharmacokinetics	Contraindications, Pregnancy Category, and Lactation Issues
Phentermine (CIV) ***cont.***		and **ascorbic acid.** Blood pressure effects may be increased by **furazolidone.** Amphetamines may decrease hypotensive effects of **guanethidine, guanadrel.** Hypertensive crisis and intracranial hemorrhage may occur when combined with **MAOIs** or **selegiline. Tricyclic antidepressants** may decrease effectiveness of amphetamines.		
Sibutramine (CIV) Meridia Capsule 5 mg, 10 mg, 15 mg	**Approved for long-term management of obesity, including weight loss and the management of weight loss in conjunction with a reduced calorie diet** Initial dose is 10 mg qd. If there is inadequate weight loss, dose may be titrated after 4 weeks to a dose of 15 mg qd.	Administration Issues May be taken with or without food. It is recommended to take sibutramine in the morning. Routine monitoring of blood pressure should be done while taking this drug. Drug Interactions Sibutramine should not be taken concomitantly with **MAOIs**. Drugs that raise blood **pressure,** such as **pseudoephedrine** or **ephedrine** should be avoided while taking sibutramine. **Ketoconazole** may decrease the clearance of sibutramine.	ADRs Headache, back pain, flu syndrome, asthenia, abdominal pain, anorexia, constipation, increased appetite, nausea, dyspepsia, arthralgia, insomnia, dizziness, rhinitis, pharyngitis, rash, dysmenorrhea, increases in blood pressure. Pharmacokinetics Extensively metabolized, readily absorbed.	Contraindications Hypersensitivity to product, patients receiving MAOIs or other appetite suppressants, patients with anorexia nervosa, CAD, CHF, arrhythmias or stroke. Cautious Use In: Narrow angle glaucoma Pregnancy Category: C Lactation Issues Safety has not been established.

1003. Agents for Nicotine Withdrawal

Drug and Dosage Forms	Usual Dosage Range	Administration Issues and Drug-Drug Interactions	Common Adverse Drug Reactions (ADRs) and Pharmacokinetics	Contraindications, Pregnancy Category, and Lactation Issues
Bupropion Zyban Tablets, sustained release 100 mg, 150 mg	**An aid to smoking cessation:** Begin dosing at 150 mg/d qd × 3 d, followed by a dose increase for most patients to the recommended dose of 300 mg/d. Do not give doses > 300 mg/d. Combination treatment: Bupropion can be given in combination with nicotine transdermal system.	Administration Issues Initiate treatment while patient is still smoking since 1 wk is required to reach steady-state levels. Patients should set a "target quit date" within first 2 weeks of therapy, generally in the second week. Continue treatment for 7–12 wks. Drug Interactions **Carbamazepine** may decrease bupropion levels; **levodopa, MAO inhibitors and ritonavir** may increase bupropion levels; **do not coadminister with MAOIs**.	ADRs Abdominal pain, insomnia, anxiety, dizziness, myalgia, nervousness, nausea, dry mouth, arthralgia, constipation, diarrhea, rhinitis. Pharmacokinetics Extensively metabolized; $T_{1/2} = 21$ h.	Contraindications Hypersensitivity to bupropion; coadministration with a MAOI; prior diagnosis of bulimia or anorexia nervosa, seizure disorder. Pregnancy Category: B Lactation Issues Bupropion is secreted in breast milk; due to potential serious adverse effects on the infant, decide whether to discontinue breastfeeding or discontinue drug, taking into account the importance of the drug to the mother.
Nicotine Transdermal System Patches generics (Steps 1, 2, 3) 21 mg/d, 14 mg/d, 7 mg/d Nicoderm CQ (Steps 1, 2, 3) 21 mg/d, 14 mg/d, 7 mg/d Nicotrol (Steps 1, 2, 3) 15 mg/d, 10 mg/d, 5 mg/d	**As an aid for smoking cessation for the relief of nicotine withdrawal symptoms. Use as part of a comprehensive behavioral smoking-cessation program** Apply 1 patch q 24 h by the following schedule: **Habitrol, Nicoderm:** 21 mg/d × 6 wk, 14 mg/d × 2 wk, 7 mg/d × 2 wk. If weight <45 kg (100 lb.), smoke < 1/2 pack/d or have cardiovascular disease: 14 mg/d × 6 wk Apply 1 patch q 16 h by the following schedule **Nicotrol:** 15 mg/d × 4–12 wk, 10 mg/d × 2–4 wk	Administration Issues Immediately after removing patch from protective container, apply to a nonhairy, clean, dry skin site. Always remove old patch before apply next patch. Dispose of old patches in a way that makes them inaccessible to children and pets. Follow written instructions in package. Drug-Drug Interactions A decrease in theophylline dose may be required at cessation of smoking.	ADRs Erthythema, pruritus, local edema, rash. Pharmacokinetics 75–90% absorbed through the skin; duration of action = 24 h; $T_{1/2} = 1-2$ h.	Contraindications Hypersensitivity to nicotine, nonsmokers, immediate post-MI patients, serious arrhythmias, severe angina, pregnancy, nursing mothers. Cautious Use: Hypertensive patients, hyperthyroidism, IDDM, hepatic or renal impairment, history of esophagitis, peptic ulcer disease. Pregnancy Category: D Lactation Issues Nicotine passes freely into breast milk; weight risk of exposure of the infant to nicotine against risks associated with the mother's continued smoking.
Nicotine Polacrilex (Nicotine Resin Complex) Nicotine Gum, Nicorette Chewing Gum 2 mg/square 4 mg/square	**As an aid for smoking cessation for the relief of nicotine withdrawal symptoms. Use as part of a comprehensive behavioral smoking-cessation program**	Administration Issues Patients using the 2 mg strength of gum should not exceed 30 pieces/day; those taking 4 mg strength should not exceed 20 pieces/day.	ADRs Headache, dizziness, lightheadedness, jawache, nausea, indigestion, sore mouth or throat, hiccups, irritation/tingling of tongue.	Contraindications Hypersensitivity to nicotine, nonsmokers, immediate post-MI patients, serious arrhythmias, severe angina, women with childbearing potential (unless effective contraception used).

(continues on next page)

1003. Agents for Nicotine Withdrawal *continued from previous page*

Drug and Dosage Forms	Usual Dosage Range	Administration Issues and Drug-Drug Interactions	Common Adverse Drug Reactions (ADRs) and Pharmacokinetics	Contraindications, Pregnancy Category, and Lactation Issues
Nicotine Polacrilex (Nicotine Resin Complex) ***cont.*** Lozenge (Commit) 2 mg/lozenge, 4 mg/lozenge	Chew 1 piece of gum when patient has urge to smoke; may be repeated as needed; max for 2 mg = 30 pieces/d; max for 4 mg = 20 pieces/d If patient smokes first cigarette more than 30 minutes after waking up, start with the 2 mg lozenge. If patient smokes first cigarette within 30 minutes of waking up, start with 4 mg lozenge. Follow instructions in package insert.	Lozenge Place lozenge in mouth and allow it to dissolve slowly over 20 to 30 minutes. Minimize swallowing. Advise patient not to chew or swallow lozenge and to occassionally move lozenge from one side of the mouth to the other until completely dissolved Do not eat or drink 15 minutes before or while using lozenge. Use at least 9 lozenges/day for first 6 weeks. Follow written instructions in package. Drug-Drug Interactions May increase the metabolism of caffeine and theophylline.	Pharmacokinetics Approximately 90% of nicotine is absorbed over a 15–30 min period; rate of release is controlled by vigor and duration of chewing.	Cautious Use: Hypertensive patients, hyperthyroidism, IDDM, hepatic or renal impairment, history of esophagitis, peptic ulcer disease, patients with dentures. Pregnancy Category: X Lactation Issues Nicotine passes freely into breast milk; weight risk of exposure of the infant to nicotine against risks associated with the mother's continued smoking.
Nicotine Inhalation System Nicotrol Inhaler Inhaler 4 mg delivered (10 mg/cartridge)	**As an aid to smoking cessation for the relief of nicotine withdrawal symptoms. The nasal spray should be used as a part of a comprehensive behavioral smoking cessation program.** Dosage The initial dosage of the nicotine inhaler is individualized. Patients may self-titrate to the level of nicotine they require. Most successful patients in the clinical trials used between 6 and 16 cartridges a day. Best effect was achieved by frequent continuous puffing (20 minutes). The recommended duration of treatment is 3 months, after which patients may be weaned from the inhaler by gradual reduction of the daily dose over the following 6 to 12 weeks. The safety and efficacy of the continued use of the nicotine inhaler for periods > 6 months have not been studied and such use is not recommended.	Administration Issues See patient information sheet for instructions on handling and disposal. After using the inhaler, carefully separate the mouthpiece, remove the used cartridge and throw it away, out of the reach of children and pets. Store the mouthpiece in the plastic storage case for further use. The mouthpiece is reusable and should be cleaned regularly with soap and water. Patients should be encouraged to use at least 6 cartridges/day at least for the first 3 to 6 weeks of treatment. Additional doses may be needed to control the urge to smoke with a maximum of 16 cartridges daily for up to 12 weeks. Regular use of the inhaler during the first week of treatment may help patients adapt to the irritant effects of the product. Some patients may exhibit signs or symptoms of nicotine withdrawal or excess, which will require an adjustment of the dosage.	ADRs Local irritation (mouth, throat), coughing, rhinitis, dyspepsia, headache, taste complaints, pain in neck and jaw, influenza-like symptoms, pain, back pain, allergy, paresthesias, flatulence, fever, nausea, diarrhea, hiccough, chest discomfort, bronchitis, hypertension. **Withdrawal:** Dizziness, anxiety, sleep disorder, depression, withdrawal syndrome, drug dependence, fatigue, myalgia (≥ 3%). Pharmacokinetics Most of the nicotine released from the inhaler is deposited in the mouth with only a fraction of the dose released (< 5%) reaching the lower respiratory tract. Eight deep inhalations over 20 minutes releases on average 4 mg of nicotine content from each cartridge, of which 2 mg is systemically absorbed. Peak plasma concentrations are typically reached within 15 minutes after inhalation ends.	Contraindications Hypersensitivity to nicotine or any components of the products, including menthol. Pregnancy Category: D Lactation Issues Decide whether to discontinue nursing or to discontinue the drug, weighing the risk of exposure of the infant to nicotine from replacement therapy against the risks associated with the infant's exposure to nicotine from continued smoking by the mother and from nicotine therapy alone or in combination with continued smoking.

	Gradual reduction of dose (up to 12 weeks): Most patients will need to gradually discontinue the use of the inhaler after the initial treatment period. Gradual reduction of dose may begin after 12 weeks of initial treatment and may last for up to 12 weeks.	Drug-Drug Interactions Smoking cessation, with or without nicotine substitutes, may alter response to concomitant medication in ex-smokers. Cigarette smoking is an inducer of CYP1A2 enzymes, the primary mechanism for drug interactions. For drugs whose metabolism is stimulated by enzyme inducers, the dose may need to be increased upon initiation of inducer (smoking) therapy and decreased when the inducer (smoking) is discontinued.		
Nicotine Nasal Spray Nicotrol NS Spray Pump 0.5 mg nicotine/actuation (10mg/mL) Each actuation of the nasal spray delivers a metered 50 mcL spray containing 0.5 mg nicotine. One dose is 1 mg of nicotine (2 sprays, 1 in each nostril). **Safety and handling:** Take care in handling the nasal spray during periods of opening and closing the container. Should even a small amount of the nasal spray come in contact with the skin, lips, mouth, eyes, or ears, immediately rinse the affected areas with water. Dispose of used bottles with the child-resistant cap in place. Used bottles should be disposed of in way as to prevent access by children and pets.	**As an aid to smoking cessation for the relief of nicotine withdrawal symptoms. The nasal spray should be used as a part of a comprehensive behavioral smoking cessation program.** Safety and efficacy of continued use of nicotine nasal spray for periods longer than 6 months have not been adequately studied and such use is not recommended. **Dosage:** Start patients with 1 or 2 doses per hour, which may be increased up to a maximum recommended dose of 40 mg (80 sprays, somewhat less than 1/2 of the bottle) per day. For best results, encourage patients to use at least the recommended minimum of 8 doses/day, as less is unlikely to be effective. **Drug abuse and dependence:** Nicotine nasal spray has a dependence potential intermediate between other nicotine-based therapies and cigarettes. The nasal spray is distinct from other nicotine-based smoking cessation therapies in its greater speed of onset, greater capacity of self-titration of dose, and frequent, rapid fluctuations of plasma nicotine concentration.	Administration Issues Instruct patients to stop smoking completely when they begin using the product. Instruct them not to sniff, swallow, or inhale through the nose as the spray is being administered. They should also be advised to administer the spray with the head tilted back slightly. If a patient is unable to stop smoking by the fourth week of therapy, discontinue treatment. Drug-Drug Interactions Smoking cessation, with or without nicotine substitutes, may alter response to concomitant medication in ex-smokers. Cigarette smoking is an inducer of CYP1A2 enzymes, the primary mechanism for drug interactions. For drugs whose metabolism is stimulated by enzyme inducers, the dose may need to be increased upon initiation of inducer (smoking) therapy and decreased when the inducer (smoking) is discontinued.	ADRs **Common complaints:** Chest tightness, dyspepsia, paresthesias in limbs, constipation, and stomatitis. **Withdrawal symptoms:** Anxiety, irritability, restlessness, cravings, dizziness, impaired concentration, weight increase, emotional lability, somnolence, fatigue, increased sweating, insomnia, confusion, depression, apathy, tremor, increased appetite, incoordination, increased dreaming. **Local irritation:** Moderate-to-severe during the first 2 days of treatment, runny nose; throat irritation; watering eyes; sneezing; cough; nasal congestion; transient epistaxis; eye irritation; transient changes in sense of smell; pharyngitis; paresthesias of the nose, mouth, or head; numbness of the nose or mouth; burning of the nose or eyes; earache; facial flushing; transient changes in sense of taste; hoarseness; nasal ulcer or blister. Pharmacokinetics Following administration ≈ 53% enters the systemic circulation. The absorption $T_{1/2} \approx$ 3 minutes.	Contraindications Hypersensitivity to nicotine or any components of the products, including menthol. Pregnancy Category: D Lactation Issues Decide whether to discontinue nursing or to discontinue the drug, weighing the risk of exposure of the infant to nicotine from replacement therapy against the risks associated with the infant's exposure to nicotine from continued smoking by the mother and from nicotine therapy alone or in combination with continued smoking.

1100. VITAMINS, MINERALS, AND TRACE ELEMENTS
1101. Fat-Soluble Vitamins

Source: Reproduced, by permission, from Williams, S.R. Nutrition and Diet Therapy, *8th ed. (1997, p. 177). St. Louis: Mosby.*

Vitamin	Physiologic Functions	Results of Deficiency	Requirement	Food Sources
Vitamin A Provitamin: beta-carotene Vitamin: retinol	Production of rhodopsin and other light-receptor pigments Formation and maintenance of epithelial tissue Growth Reproduction Toxic in large amounts	Poor dark adaptation, night blindness, xerosis, xerophthalmia Keratinization of epithelium Growth failure Reproductive failure	Adult male: 1000 μg or RE (5000 IU) Adult female: 800 μg or RE (4000 IU) Pregnancy: 1000 μg or RE (5000 IU) Lactation: 1200 μg or RE (6000 IU) Children: 400 μg or RE (2000 IU) to 800 μg or RE (4000 IU)	Liver, cream, butter, whole milk, egg yolk Green and yellow vegetables, yellow fruits Fortified margarine
Vitamin D Provitamins: ergosterol (plants); 7-dehydrocholesterol (skin) Vitamins D_2 (ergocholecalciferol) and D_3 (cholecaliciferol)	Calcitriol a major hormone regulator of bone mineral (calcium and phosphorus) metabolism Calcium and phosphorus absorption Toxic in large amounts	Faulty bone growth; rickets, osteomalacia	Adult: 5–10 μg cholecalciferol (200–400 IU) Pregnancy and lactation: 10–12.5 μg (400–500 IU) depending on age Children: 10 μg (400 IU)	Fortified milk Fortified margarine Fish oils Sunlight on skin
Vitamin E Tocopherols	Antioxidant Hemopoiesis Related to action of selenium	Anemia in premature infants	Adult: 8–10 mg α-TE Pregnancy and lactation: 10–11 mg α-TE Children: 3–10 mg α-TE	Vegetable oils
Vitamin K K_1 (phylloquinone) K_2 (menaquinone) Analog: K_3 (menadione)	Activates blood-clotting factors (e.g., prothrombin) by alpha-carboxylating glutamic acid residues Toxicity can be induced by water-soluble analogs	Hemorrhagic disease of the newborn Defective blood clotting Deficiency symptoms are produced by coumarin anticoagulants and by antibiotic therapy	Adult: 70–140 μg Children: 15–100 μg Infants: 12–20 μg	Cheese, egg yolk, liver Green leafy vegetables Synthesized by intestinal bacteria

1102. Water-Soluble Vitamins

Source: Reproduced, by permission, from Williams, S.R. Nutrition and Diet Therapy, *8th ed. (1997, p. 196). St. Louis: Mosby.*

Vitamin	Coenzymes: Physiologic Function	Clinical Applications	Requirement	Food Sources
Thiamin	Carbohydrate metabolism Thiamin pyrophosphate (TPP): oxidative decarboxylation	Beriberi (deficiency) Neuropathy Wernicke-Korsakoff syndome (alcoholism) Depressed muscular and secretory symptoms	0.5 mg/1000 kcal	Pork, beef, liver, whole or enriched grains, legumes
Riboflavin	General metabolism Flavin adenine dinucleotide (FAD) Flavin mononucleotide (FMN)	Cheilosis, glossitis, seborrheic dermatitis	0.6 mg/1000 kcal	Milk, liver, enriched cereals
Niacin (nicotinic acid, nicotinamide)	General metabolism Nicotinamine-adenine dinucleotide (NAD) Nicotinamide-adenine dinucelotide phosphate (NADP)	Pellagra (deficiency) Weakness, anorexia Scaly dermatitis Neuritis	6.6 NE/1000 kcal*	Meat, peanuts, enriched grains (protein foods containing tryptophan)
Vitamin B_6 (pyridoxine, pyridoxal, pyridoxamine)	General metabolism Pyridoxal phosphate (PLP): transamination and decarboxylation	Reduced serum levels associated with pregnancy and use of oral contraceptives Antagonized by isoniazid, penicillamine, and other drugs	2 mg (men) 1.6 mg (women)	Wheat, corn, meats, liver
Pantothenic acid	General metabolism CoA (coenzyme A): acetylation	Many roles through acyltransfer reactions (e.g., lipogenesis, amino acid activation, and formation of cholesterol, steroid hormones, heme)	4 to 7 mg	Liver, egg, milk
Biotin	General metabolism *N*-Carboxybiotinyl lysine: CO_2 transfer reactions	Deficiency induced by avidin (a protein in raw egg white) and by antibiotics Synthesis of some fatty acids and amino acids	30 to 100 µg	Egg yolk, liver Synthesized by intestinal microorganisms

* NE = niacin equivalents.

(*continues on next page*)

1102. Water-Soluble Vitamins *continued from previous page*

Vitamin	Coenzymes: Physiologic Function	Clinical Applications	Requirement	Food Sources
Folate (folic acid, folacin)	General metabolism Single-carbon transfer reactions (for example, purine nucleotide, thymine, heme synthesis)	Megaloblastic anemia	200 μg (men) 180 μg (women)	Liver, green leafy vegetables
Cobalamin	General metabolism Methylcobalamin: methylation reactions (e.g., synthesis of amino acids, heme)	Pernicious anemia induced by lack of intrinsic factor Megaloblastic anemia Methylmalonic aciduria Homocystinuria Peripheral neuropathy (strict vegetarian diet)	2 μg	Liver, meat, milk, egg, cheese
Vitamin C (ascorbic acid)	Antioxidant Collagen biosynthesis General metabolism Makes iron available for hemoglobin synthesis Influences conversion of folic acid to folinic acid Oxidation-reduction of the amino acids phenylalanine and tyrosine	Scurvy (deficiency) Wound healing, tissue formation Fevers and infections Stress reactions Growth	60 mg	Fresh fruits, especially citrus Vegetables such as tomatoes, cabbage, potatoes, chili peppers, and broccoli

1103. Major Minerals

Source: Reproduced, by permission, from Williams, S.R. Nutrition and Diet Therapy, *8th ed. (1997, p. 223). St. Louis: Mosby.*

Mineral	Metabolism	Physiologic Functions	Clinical Applications	Requirements	Food Sources
Calcium (Ca)	Absorption according to body need; requires Ca-binding protein and regulated by vitamin D, parathyroid hormone, and calcitonin; absorption favored by protein, lactose, acidity Excretion chiefly in feces; 70%–90% of amount ingested Deposition-mobilization in bone tissue constant, regulated by vitamin D and parathyroid hormone	Constituent of bones and teeth Participates in blood clotting, nerve transmission, muscle action, cell membrane permeability, enzyme activation	Tetany (decrease in serum Ca) Rickets, osteomalacia Osteoporosis Resorptive hypercalciuria, renal calculuses Hyperthyroidism and hypothyroidism	Adults: 800 mg (Premenopause: 1000 mg; Menopause: 1500 mg) Pregnancy and lactation: 1200 mg Infants: 400–600 mg Children: 800–1200 mg	Milk, cheese Green, leafy vegetables Whole grains Egg yolk Legumes, nuts
Phosphorus (P)	Absorption with Ca aided by vitamin D and parathyroid hormone as for calcium; hindered by binding agents Excretion chiefly by kidney according to serum level, regulated by parathyroid hormone Deposition-mobilization in bone compartment constant	Constituent of bones and teeth, ATP, phosphorylated intermediary metabolites Participates in absorption of glucose and glycerol, transport of fatty acids, energy metabolism, and buffer system	Growth Recovery from diabetic acidosis Hypophosphatemia: bone disease, malabsorption syndromes, primary hyperparathyroidism Hyperphosphatemia: renal insufficiency, hypothyroidism, tetany	Adults: 800 mg Pregnancy and lactation: 1200 mg Infants: 300–500 mg Children: 800–1200 mg	Milk, cheese Meat, egg yolk Whole grains Legumes, nuts
Magnesium (Mg)	Absorption according to intake load; hindered by excess fat, phosphate, calcium, protein Excretion (regulated by kidney)	Constituent of bones and teeth Coenzyme in general metabolism, smooth muscle action, neuromuscular irritability Cation in intracellular fluid	Low serum level following gastrointestinal losses Tremor, spasm in deficiency induced by malnutrition, alcoholism	Adults: 280–350 mg Pregnancy and lactation: 290–355 mg Infants: 40–60 mg Children: 80–170 mg	Milk, cheese Meat, seafood Whole grains Legumes, nuts
Sodium (Na)	Readily absorbed Excretion chiefly by kidney, controlled by aldosterone	Major cation in extracellular fluid, water balance, acid-base balance Cell membrane permeability, absorption of glucose Normal muscle irritability	Losses in gastrointestinal disorders, diarrhea Fluid-electrolyte and acid-base balance problems Muscle action	Adults 500 mg Infants: 120–200 mg Children: 225–500 mg	Salt (NaCl) Sodium compounds in baking and processing Milk, cheese Meat, eggs Carrots, beets, spinach, celery

(continues on next page)

1103. Major Minerals *continued from previous page*

Mineral	Metabolism	Physiologic Functions	Clinical Applications	Requirements	Food Sources
Potassium (K)	Readily absorbed Secreted and resorbed in gastrointestinal circulation Excretion chiefly by kidney, regulated by aldosterone	Major cation in intracellular fluid, water balance, acid-base balance Normal muscle irritability Glycogen formation Protein synthesis	Losses in gastrointestinal disorders, diarrhea Fluid-electrolyte, acid-base balance problems Muscle action, especially heart action Losses in tissue catabolism Treatment of diabetic acidosis; rapid glycogen production reduces serum potassium level Losses with diuretic therapy	Adults: 2000 mg Infants: 500–700 mg Children: 1000–2000 mg	Fruits Vegetables Legumes, nuts Whole grains Meat
Chlorine (Cl)	Readily absorbed Excretion controlled by kidney	Major anion in extracellular fluid, water balance, acid-base balance, chloride-bicarbonate shift Gastric hydrochloride—digestion	Losses in gastrointestinal disorders, vomiting, diarrhea, tube drainage Hypochloremic alkalosis	Adults: 750 mg Infants: 180–300 mg Children: 350–750 mg	Salt (NaCl)
Sulfur (S)	Elemental form absorbed as such; split from amino acid sources (methionine and cystine) in digestion and absorbed into portal circulation Excreted by kidney in relation to protein intake and tissue catabolism	Essential constituent of protein structure Enzyme activity and energy metabolism through free sulfhydryl group (–SH) Detoxification reactions	Cystine renal calculuses Cystinuria	Diet adequate in protein contains adequate sulfur	Meat, eggs Milk, cheese Legumes, nuts

1104. Trace Elements

Source: Reproduced, by permission, from Williams, S.R. Nutrition and Diet Therapy, *8th ed. (1997, p. 226). St. Louis: Mosby.*

Mineral	Metabolism	Physiologic Functions	Clinical Applications	Requirements	Food Sources
Iron (Fe)	Absorption controls bioavailability; favored by body need, acidity, and reduction agents such as vitamins; hindered by binding agents, reduced gastric HCl, infection, gastrointestinal losses Transported as transferrin, stored as ferritin or hemosiderin Excreted in sloughed cells, bleeding	Hemoglobin synthesis, oxygen transport Cell oxidation, heme enzymes	Anemia (hypochromic, microcytic) Excess: hemosiderosis, hemochromatosis Growth and pregnancy needs	Adults: men—10 mg, women—15 mg Pregnancy and lactation: 30 and 15 mg, respectively Infants: 6–10 mg Children: 10–12 mg	Liver, meat, eggs Whole grains Enriched breads and cereals Dark green vegetables Legumes, nuts (Iron cookware)
Iodine (I)	Absorbed as iodides, taken up by thyroid gland under control of thyroid-stimulating hormone Excretion by kidney	Synthesis of thyroxin, which regulates cell metabolism, basal metabolic rate	Endemic colloid goiter, cretinism Hypothyroidism and hyperthyroidism	Adults: 150 μg Infants: 40–50 μg Children: 70–150 μg	Iodized salt Seafood
Zinc (Zn)	Absorbed with zinc-binding ligand from pancreas Transported in blood by albumin; stored in many sites Excretion largely intestinal	Essential coenzyme constituent: carbonic anhydrase, carboxypeptidase, lactic dehydrogenase	Growth: hypogonadism Sensory impairment: taste and smell Wound healing Malabsorption disease	Adults: 12–15 mg Infants: 5 mg Children: 10–15 mg	Widely distributed Seafood, oysters Liver, meat Milk, cheese, eggs Whole grains
Copper (Cu)	Absorbed with copper-binding protein metallothionein Transported in blood by histidine and albumin Stored in many tissues	Associated with iron in enzyme systems, hemoglobin synthesis Metalloprotein enzyme constituent	Hypocupremia: nephrosis and malabsorption Wilson's disease, excess copper storage Menke's syndrome, kinky hair, disordered copper metabolism	Adults: 1.5–3 mg Infants: 0.4–0.7 mg Children: 0.7–2.5 mg	Widely distributed Liver, meat Seafood Whole grains Legumes, nuts (Copper cookware)

(*continues on next page*)

1104. Trace Elements *continued from previous page*

Mineral	Metabolism	Physiologic Functions	Clinical Applications	Requirements	Food Sources
Manganese (Mn)	Absorbed poorly Excretion mainly by intestine	Enzyme component in general metabolism	Low serum levels in diabetes, protein-energy malnutrition Inhalation toxicity	Adults: 2–5 mg Infants: 0.3–1.0 mg Children: 1–5 mg	Cereals, whole grains Legumes, soybeans
Chromium (Cr)	Absorbed in association with zinc Excretion mainly by kidney	Associated with glucose metabolism; improves faulty glucose uptake by tissues; glucose tolerance factor	Potentiates action of insulin in persons with diabetes Lowers serum cholesterol, LDL-cholesterol* Increases HDL*	Adults: 50–200 µg Infants: 10–60 µg Children: 20–200 µg	Leafy vegetables Cereals Whole grains Brewer's yeast Animal protein
Cobalt (Co)	Absorbed as component of food source, vitamin B_{12} Elemental form shares transport with iron Stored in liver	Constituent of vitamin B_{12}, functions with vitamin	Deficiency assocciated only with deficiency of vitamin B_{12}	Unknown; evidently minute	Vitamin B_{12} source
Selenium (Se)	Absorption depends on solubility of compound form Excreted mainly by kidney	Constituent of enzyme glutathione peroxidase Synergistic antioxidant with vitamin E Structural component of teeth	Marginal deficiency when soil content is low Deficiency secondary to parenteral nutrition; malnutrition Toxicity observed in livestock	Adults: 55–70 µg Infants: 10–15 µg Children: 20–50 µg	Varies with soil content Seafood Legumes Whole grains Low-fat meats and dairy products Vegetables
Molybdenum (Mo)	Readily absorbed Excreted rapidly by kidney Small amount excreted in bile	Constituent of oxidase enzymes, xanthine oxidase	Deficiency unknown in humans	Adults: 75–250 µg Infants: 15–30 µg Children: 25–250 µg	Legumes Whole grains Milk Organ meats Leafy vegetables

* LDL = low-density lipoprotein; HDL = high-density lipoprotein.

Fluoride (F)	Absorption in small intestine; little known of bioavailability Excreted by kidney—80%	Accumulates in bones and teeth, increasing hardness	Dental caries inhibited Osteoporosis: may help control Excess: dental fluorosis	Adults: 1.5–4 mg Infants: 0.1–0.5 mg Children: 0.5–2.5 mg	Fish Fish products Tea Foods cooked in fluoridated water Drinking water

INDEX

References in boldface denote drug table entries. Page numbers followed by *f* or *t* indicate figures or tables, respectively.

A

Augmentin, 61
dose-response relationships, 31
for pneumonia, 422
Auranofin, 1107
Aurothioglucose, 1108
Autohaler, 371
Automatic implantable cardiac defibrillator (AICD), 325
Autonomic dysreflexia, in disabled individuals, 201, 202t
Azapirones
for anxiety disorders, 728, 729, 730
monitoring for toxicity, 732
Azathioprine, 474, 1108
for hyperuricemia, 513
for rheumatoid arthritis, 498–499
Azatadine, 1239
Azelastine HCl, 1125, 1239
Azithromycin, 880–881
for chlamydia, 814, 815
for cystic fibrosis, 404
drug-food interactions, 98t
for folliculitis, 780
for gonorrhea, 810, 812
for granuloma inguinale, 819
for influenza, 360
for lymphogranuloma vernereum, 818
for otitis media, 456
for pelvic inflammatory disease, 823
for pharyngitis, 363
for pneumonia, 410, 416
for pneumonia, in pregnancy, 420, 422
for urethritis, 766

B

Babinski's sign, 201
Baccillus anthracis, 161
Bacille Calmette-Guerin (BCG), 211
Bacitracin, 442, 1120, 1258
Baciofen, 1082
Back pain, low
assessment, 515
etiology, 513–514
followup, 517
monitoring, 517
nonpharmacologic therapy, 514–515
patient/caregiver information, 515–516
pharmacotherapy
goals, 514
initiation, time frame for, 515
selecting appropriate agents for, 516–517
Baclofen, 602, 604
for low back pain, 517
Bacterial infections
medications for, 237t
Bacterial skin infections, 525–528
Bacterial vaginosis (BV), 237, 829–831
Bacteroides, 829
Bactroban, 780
Balsalazide disodium, 1165
Barrier methods. *See* Contraception, barrier methods
Basal body temperature (BBT), 253
Basal cell carcinoma, 555
Bearberry
common/scientific names, 119t
dosage, 134
for urinary infection/inflammation, 134
Beclomethasone, 1226, 1244
for allergic rhinitis, 352
Belladonna, 1142–1143
Benazepril, 960
Bendroflumethiazide, 984–985
Benemid. *See* Probenecid
Benign paroxysmal positional vertigo (BPPV), 607, 608, 609, 610
Benign prostatic hyperplasia
assessment/history taking, 772t, 773t
defined, 771
monitoring, 773
patient/caregiver information, 772, 773t
pharmacotherapy
goals, 772
initiation, time frame for, 772

for flatulence, 124
for mouth ulcers, 130
Charcoal, 1168
Chaste tree berry
for breast tenderness, 121
common/scientific names, 119t
dosage, 132
for menopausal symptoms, 130
for premenstrual symptoms, 131–132
Chemical antagonism, 36
Chemotherapy, nausea/vomiting associated with, 463–464
Chest x-rays, 418
for heart failure, 314
for pneumonia, 412
Chicken pox. *See* Varicella-zoster virus
Childhood Immunization Program, 166
Children
common antibiotics for, 180t–181t
distribution, 177
doses of over-the-counter drugs, 182t
drug absorption, 177
drug use in, 173–174
pain in, 184
Chlamydia, 249, 797
assessment/history taking, 813t, 813–814
CDC treatment recommendations, 814t
etiology, 812
monitoring, 815
pharmacotherapy, 812–813, 814–815
during pregnancy, 238
in pregnancy, 812–813
Chlamydia pneumoniae, 360, 361
Chlamydia trachomatis, 445, 446, 455, 762, 770, 812, 813, 814, 817, 822, 823
Chlamydophilia pneumonia, 410, 411
Chloral hydrate, 1050
Chlordiazepoxide, 1039, 1078
Chloroquine, 159, 904
Chloroxine, 1255
Chlorphenesin carbamate, 1082
Chlorpheniramine, 352, 1240
Chlorpromazine, 1068
Chlorpropamide, 686, 687, 1196
Chlorzoxazone, 1083, 1087
Cholera, 159, 468
Cholestatic jaundice, 687
Cholestyramine
drug interactions, 18
Choline salicylate, 1022
Cholinesterase inhibitors, 614
Chronic bacterial prostatitis (CBP), 767, 768, 770
Chronicity, 513
Chronic obstructive pulmonary disease (COPD)
assessment for, 395, 395t
definition of, 392
diagnosis of, 393, 393t
drugs to avoid, 399, 400t
monitoring for, 399–400
nonpharmacologic therapy, 394–395
outcomes management, 396–399
patient/caregiver information, 395–396
pharmacotherapy
goals, 394
initiation, time frame for, 395
selecting appropriate agents for, 396t, 396–399
risk factors for, 393t
severity
classification of, 394t
Chronopharmacology, defined, 7
Ciclopirox olamine, 1258–1259
Ciliary neurotrophic factor (CNTF), 705
Cilostazol, 328, 978
Cimetidine, 852, 1147
creatine clearance and, 46
drug interactions, 23, 44
receptors and, 32
Cinoxacin, 936
Ciprofloxacin, 156, 467, 874–875, 1120, 1131
absorption and, 18
drug interactions, avoiding, 100
for pharyngeal infection, 811, 812

D

E

F

G

Goldenrod
  common/scientific names, 119t
  dosage, 134
  for urinary infection/inflammation, 134
Gold sodium thiomalate, 1109
Gold therapy
  for rheumatoid arthritis, 499
Gonadorelin acetate, 1225
Gonadotropin measurements, in menopause diagnosis, 283
Gonorrhea, 249, 797
  assessment/history taking, 810
  CDC treatment recommendations, 811t
  contraceptives and, 245
  etiology, 809
  monitoring, 812
  pharmacotherapy, 810–812
  during pregnancy, 238
  symptoms, 809, 810
Gout
  assessment, 510
  epidemiology, 508–509
  monitoring, 513
  nonpharmacologic therapy, 509
  pathogenesis, 509
  patient/caregiver information, 510
  pharmacotherapy
    commonly prescribed durgs, 508t
    goals, 509
    initiation, time frame for, 509
    selecting appropriate agents for, 510–513
  prophylactic treatment for, 511–512
Gram's stain, 410, 757, 810
Gransitron, 1173
Granuloma inguinale, 818–819
Graves' disease, 652, 656
"Gray-baby" syndrome, 173
Griseofulvin, 531, 900–901
  drug-nutrient interactions, 98t
Guaifenesin, 1246
  COPD and, 398
Guanabenz, 966
Guanadrel, 966–967
Guanethidine, 329, 967
Guanfacine, 966

H

Haemophilus influenzae
  dose-response relationships, 31
Haemophilus influenzae, 358, 360, 363, 407, 410, 411, 416, 420, 421, 422, 445, 451, 454, 455, 456, 526
Haemophilus influenzae Type B, 148–149
Halcinonide, 1275
Haldol, 11, 583, 584
  for vertigo, 609
Half-life, 28–29
Halobetasol proprionate, 1275–1276
Haloperidol, 616, 1072–1073
  for traumatic brain injury, 583
Handbook of Pediatric Drug Therapy, 174
Hawthorn
  common/scientific names, 119t
Hay fever
  herbal remedies, 125
Headache
  diagnosis, 617, 618t
  herbal remedies, 125–126
  migraine, nausea/vomiting associated with, 463
  monitoring, 621
  nonpharmacologic therapy, 620
  from oral contraceptive usage, 266
  patient/caregiver information, 621
  pharmacotherapy
    assessment, 620–621
    drug classes, 620
    goals, 619
    initiation, time frame for, 620
    selecting appropriate agents for, 621
  during pregnancy, 233–234
Health belief model (HBM), 66, 69

Herpes genitalis
assessment/history taking, 815–816
CDC treatment guidelines, 816t
etiology, 815
pharmacotherapy, 815, 816–817
Herpes simplex virus (HSV), 536–537
HIV and, 845
nonpharmacologic therapy, 539
pharmacotherapy, 539, 542
signs/symptoms, 536–537
Herpes whitlow, 536
Herpes zoster, 538
Heterotopic ossification, in disabled individuals, 200–201
Hevea brasiliensis, 203
High-flux membranes, 51
Hirsutism, 662, 663
causes of, 662t
Hismanal. *See* Astemizole
Hispanic Americans, medication-taking behavior of, 64–65
Histamine
receptors and, 32
HIV/AIDS, 158
in adult/adolescents, 839–844
assessment/history taking, 841, 842t, 843t, 844t
in children, 846–850
assessment, 848–849
initiation of treatment, 849
monitoring, 849–850
nonpharmacologic therapy, 848
opportunistic diseases, treating, 849
pharmacotherapy, 846–847, 848
prevention, 847–848
chlamydia and, 814
cutaneous reactions, 90
fusion inhibitors, 844–845
nonpharmacologic therapy, 840–841
opportunistic diseases and, 845
pathogenesis of, 840t
patient/caregiver information, 841, 844
pharmacotherapy
goals, 840
selecting appropriate agents for, 840t, 841t, 843–844
postexposure prophylaxis, 845–846
in pregnancy, 848
prevention, 840
scabies and, 542
self-efficacy and, 67
spectrum of infection, 840t
symptoms, 845t
tuberculosis with, 426
Homatropine, 440
Homeless population
health problems in, 209
medication/treatment considerations for, 209–211, 210t
Homeostastis, 563
Homeostatic mechanisms, age-related changes, 190–191
Hordeolum (stye), 441
Horehound
for colds/flu, 122
common/scientific names, 119t
for cough, 123
dosage, 123
Hormone replacement therapy (HRT), 276, 277, 278, 279, 280, 284, 286, 287–289, 508, 786
duration of, 290
risks, 284–285
side effects of, 285
stroke and, 591
Hot flashes (flushes), 276, 280, 286, 287, 289, 290
Human diploid cell vaccine (HDCV), 157, 158
Human papillomavirus (HPV)
nonpharmacologic therapy, 820
pharmacotherapy, 820–821
types, 819
Human rabies immune globulin (HRIG), 157, 158
Human tetanus immune globulin (TIG), 146
Humulin, 681
Hydralazine, 976
allergic responses to, 851

J

K

Lidocaine, 198, 539, 820
for cirrhosis, 47
patch, 223
Ligands, 30–32
Ligase chain reaction (LCR), 813
Lindane, 545, 546, 824, 825, 1267
Linezolid, 898
Lioresal (Baclofen), 203
Liothyronine, 1222
Liotrix, 1222–1123
Lipids
management, 677
metabolism, oral contraceptive usage and, 258, 260
Lipophilic drugs, 13, 20
Liquid supplements, for cystic fibrosis, 405
Lisinopril, 316, 961–962
Lispro, 1205
Lithium, 1080
for anxiety disorders, 730
for bacterial vaginosis, 831
for bipolar disorder, 722, 723
breastfeeding and, 723
drug-drug interactions, 97t
for eating disorders, 735
for PMS, 793
Liver
blood flow, 22
disease, absorption and, 18
Lodoxemide, 1126
Lomefloxacin, 877
Long-acting progestin contraceptives, 266–268
Loperamide, 159, 1155
Lopinavir/ritonavir, 927–928
Loracarbef, 869
Loratadine, 352, 1243
Lorazepam, 583, 1041
for anxiety disorders, 730
for dementia, 616
metabolism, 44
for seizures, 636
Losartan, 964–965
Lovastatin, 343, 957–958
drug-nutrient interactions, 98t
Loxapine, 1073–1074
Loxosceles reclusa, 543
Lunelle, 265
Lupron, 798
Lyme disease, 544, 607
Lymphogranuloma venereum (LGV), 817–818

M

Macolides
for lymphogranuloma vernereum, 818
Macrobid, 9
Macrocytosis, 571
Macrodantin. *See* Nitrofurantoin
Magaldrate, 1139, 1141
Magnesium carbonate, 1141
Magnesium citrate, 1159
Magnesium deficiency
hormonal therapy and, 289
Magnesium hydroxide, 1139–1140, 1141, 1159
Magnesium oxide, 1140
Magnesium salicylate, 1022–1023
Magnesium trisilicate, 1141
Magnetic resonance imaging (MRI), 527
Maintenance, in transtheoretical model of behavior change, 68
Malabsorptive disorders, oral drug absorption and, 18
Malaria, 159
Malathion, 1268
Male condoms, 245t, 245–246, 264, 827
syphilis and, 806
Malignant melanoma, 555
Mammography, in menopause diagnosis, 283–284
Manufacturer's sales representatives (MSRs), 86
Maprotiline, 1060
Marfan's syndrome, 335, 337
Marijuana
ADHD and, 589
interaction with drugs, 99
Maximal efficacy, 30
Mazindol, 702

osteoporosis. *See* Osteoporosis
rheumatoid arthritis. *See* Rheumatoid arthritis
sprains, 517–519
strains, 517–519
tendinitis, 517–519
Mycobacterium tuberculosis, 158
Mycoplasma pneumoniae, 361, 410, 411, 412, 829
Myocardial infarction, 334
oral contraceptive usage and, 257, 260
Myocardial ischemia, 330–331, 333

N

Nabumetone, 1016
Nadolol, 971
Nafarelin, 798, 1225
Nafitifine, 1263
Nalidixic acid, 937
Naloxone
opioid receptor blockade, 35
Naltrexone, 744, 745
Naprosyn. *See* Naproxen
Naproxen, 1012–1013
for dysfunctional uterine bleeding and, 787
for dysmenorrhea, 795
for epididymitis, 764
formulation, 9
for gout, 511
for osteoarthritis, 502
for PMS, 792
for rheumatoid arthritis, 494
Naratriptan HCl, 1096
Narcan. *See* Naloxone
Narcotic combination drugs, 994–1004
Nasal cromolyn
for allergic rhinitis, 350
Nasolacrimal obstruction (NLO), 174
Natamycin, 1124
Nateglinide, 1202–1203
National Center for Complementary and Alternative Medicine (NCCAM), 115, 117
National Infant Immunization Week, 166
National Institutes of Health (NIH), 115
Native Americans, medication-taking behavior of, 65
Nausea
assessment, 462–463
herbal remedies, 131
monitoring, 464–465
nonpharmacologic therapy, 462
patient/caregiver information, 463
pharmacotherapy
goals, 462
initiation, time frame for, 462
selecting appropriate agents for, 463–464
during pregnancy, 235
in pregnancy, 462
symptoms of, 461
treatment of, 462t
Nedocromil, 1126, 1230
Nefazodone, 1061
for depression, 713, 716, 717
for sexual dysfunction, 801
Neisseria gonorrhoeae, 445, 447, 751, 762, 809, 810, 811, 812, 813, 822, 823
Neisseria meningitidis, 156
Nelfinavir, 928
Neomycin, 780, 946, 1263, 1280
Neonates
acne, 532–533
administration of drugs and, 177
conjunctivitis, 447
distribution, 175–176
drug absorption, 174–175
excretion, 176
metabolism, 176
over-the-counter drugs, 174
Neosporin, 527
Nettle
common/scientific names, 119t
dosage, 125, 132
for hay fever, 125
for prostate enlargement (benign), 132
Neurogenic bladder, 198–200

P

Q

R

Risedronate, 1218
for osteoporosis, 285, 286
Risperidone, 615, 1077
Ritalin. *See* Methylphenidate
Ritonavir, 844, 929
Rivastigmine, 614, 615, 1090
Rizatriptan benzoate, 1096–1097
Robitussin, 112, 112t
Rocky Mountain spotted fever, 544
Rofecoxib, 796, 1020
Ropinirole, 623, 625, 1105
Rosiglitazone, 688, 689, 1203–1204
Rotarix, 166
RotaTeg, 166
RU 486, 269
Rubella (German measles), 539
childhood immunizations, 147–148
immunization, 232–233
Rubeola (measles), 538–539
Rubivirus, 147

S

Safety issues
medications, 185t
Salicylates
for chronic pain, 217–218
Salicylic acid
for warts, 540
Saline laxatives, 470
Salmeterol, 404, 1229, 1233
Salmonella, 159
Salsalate, 1023–1024
Santmyer swallow reflex, 177
Saquinavir, 844, 929–930
SARS, 408
Saw palmetto
common/scientific names, 119t
dosage, 132
for prostate enlargement (benign), 132–133
Scabies, 824, 825
etiology, 542
nonpharmalogic therapy, 544
pharmacotherapy, 545
School-agers
administration of drugs, 178–179
Scopolamine, 1171
Seborrhea
HIV and, 845
Seborrheic dermatitis, 547, 549
Secobarbital, 1046
Second messengers, 35
Seizures
anticonvulsant regimen, planning, 630t
antidepressants and, 221
classification of, 629
defined, 628
febrile, 628
management, 597
monitoring, 631–632
nonpharmacologic treatment, 630
patient/caregiver information, 631
pharmacotherapy
assessment, 630–631
goals, 629–630
selecting appropriate agents for, 631
posttraumatic, 584–585
Selective estrogen receptor modulators (SERMs), 286
Selective serotonin reuptake inhibitors (SSRI), 4
for ADHD, 588
for anxiety disorders, 731
for bipolar disorder, 723
dementia and, 616
for depression, 238, 239, 627, 711, 712, 715–716, 717, 718
drug-herb interactions, 99t
drug interactions, avoiding, 100
for eating disorders, 734
for obesity, 706
for OCD, 726
for Parkinson's disease, 625
for PMS, 789, 792, 793
for sexual dysfunction, 801
for stroke, 598, 599
Selegiline, 624, 625, 1105

T

U

V

W

X

Y

Z